ANDREOLI AND CARPENTER'S
CECIL ESSENTIALS OF MEDICINE

9TH EDITION

ANDREOLI AND CARPENTER'S CECIL ESSENTIALS OF MEDICINE

9TH EDITION

Editor-in-Chief

Ivor J. Benjamin, MD, FACC, FAHA
Professor of Medicine, Physiology, Pharmacology and Toxicology, Cell Biology, and
    Surgery
Director, Cardiovascular Center
Chief, Division of Cardiovascular Medicine
Vice Chair, Translational Research, Department of Medicine
Medical College of Wisconsin
Milwaukee, Wisconsin

Editors

Robert C. Griggs, MD, FACP, FAAN
Professor of Neurology, Pediatrics, Pathology, and Laboratory Medicine
Center for Human Experimental Therapeutics
University of Rochester School of Medicine and Dentistry
Rochester, New York

Edward J. Wing, MD, FACP, FIDSA
Professor of Medicine
The Warren Alpert Medical School
Brown University
Providence, Rhode Island

J. Gregory Fitz, MD
Executive Vice President for Academic Affairs and Provost
Dean, University of Texas Southwestern Medical School
University of Texas Southwestern Medical Center
Dallas, Texas

ELSEVIER
SAUNDERS

SAUNDERS

1600 John F. Kennedy Blvd.
Ste 1800
Philadelphia, PA 19103-2899

ANDREOLI & CARPENTER'S CECIL ESSENTIALS OF MEDICINE   ISBN: 978-1-4377-1899-7
INTERNATIONAL EDITION   ISBN: 978-0-323-29617-5

Notices

Knowledge and best practice in this field are constantly changing. As new research and experience broaden our understanding, changes in research methods, professional practices, or medical treatment may become necessary.

Practitioners and researchers must always rely on their own experience and knowledge in evaluating and using any information, methods, compounds, or experiments described herein. In using such information or methods they should be mindful of their own safety and the safety of others, including parties for whom they have a professional responsibility.

With respect to any drug or pharmaceutical products identified, readers are advised to check the most current information provided (i) on procedures featured or (ii) by the manufacturer of each product to be administered, to verify the recommended dose or formula, the method and duration of administration, and contraindications. It is the responsibility of practitioners, relying on their own experience and knowledge of their patients, to make diagnoses, to determine dosages and the best treatment for each individual patient, and to take all appropriate safety precautions.

To the fullest extent of the law, neither the Publisher nor the authors, contributors, or editors, assume any liability for any injury and/or damage to persons or property as a matter of products liability, negligence or otherwise, or from any use or operation of any methods, products, instructions, or ideas contained in the material herein.

Previous editions copyrighted 2010, 2007, 2004, 2001, 1997, 1993, 1990, 1986 by Saunders, an imprint of Elsevier Inc.

Library of Congress Cataloging-in-Publication Data

Andreoli and Carpenter's Cecil essentials of medicine / editor-in-chief,
Ivor J. Benjamin, editors, Robert C. Griggs, Edward J. Wing,
J. Gregory Fitz.—9th edition.
    p. ; cm.
  Cecil essentials of medicine
  Essentials of medicine
  Includes bibliographical references and index.
  ISBN 978-1-4377-1899-7 (pbk. : alk. paper)
  I. Title Benjamin, Ivor J., editor.   II. Griggs, Robert C., 1939- , editor.   III. Wing, Edward J., editor.
IV. Fitz, J. Gregory, editor.   V. Title: Cecil essentials of medicine.   VI. Title: Essentials of medicine.
  [DNLM: 1. Internal Medicine.   WB 115]
  RC46
  616–dc23
                                                                    2014049765

Senior Content Strategist: James Merritt
Content Development Manager: Taylor Ball
Publishing Services Manager: Patricia Tannian
Project Manager: Amanda Mincher
Design Specialist: Paula Catalano

Printed in China

Last digit is the print number: 9 8 7 6 5 4 3 2 1

Lloyd Hollingsworth (Holly) Smith, Jr., MD   Fred Plum, MD (Deceased)

This ninth edition of Andreoli and Carpenter's Cecil Essentials of Medicine *had as its progenitor* Cecil Essentials of Medicine. *The idea for* Essentials *was originally conceived in the mid-1980s by Holly Smith and by Fred Plum. At the time, Charles C.J. (Chuck) Carpenter and I were Consulting Editors for* The Cecil Textbook of Medicine *for Infectious Diseases and Nephrology, respectively. Holly and Fred entrained the two of us into participating in a new venture that, happily, has become a successful force in Internal Medicine. The entire idea was to make Internal Medicine accessible in a compact but critical format to medical students, residents, and other practitioners of medicine. It is a privilege to pay tribute to Holly and Fred by dedicating this ninth edition of* Essentials *to them.*

Lloyd H. Smith, Jr., MD

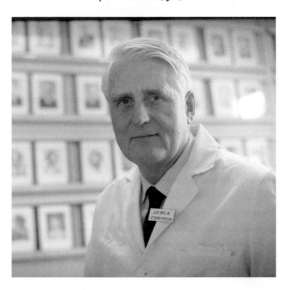

Dr. Smith, universally known as Holly Smith, is one of the true giants of academic medicine. A thoroughly engaging and courtly Southern gentleman, Holly was educated at Washington and Lee University, where he received a bachelor's degree, summa cum laude, *in 1944. He then went north to Harvard Medical School where, in 1948, he received his MD,* magna cum laude.

Following his residency in internal medicine at the Massachusetts General Hospital, Holly joined the Army Medical Corps where he provided, among other clinical activities, early dialysis in soldiers afflicted with epidemic hemorrhagic fever in the Korean Conflict. Investigatively, Holly's work was an exemplar for the early beginnings of molecular biology. In particular, he found that there was a double enzyme defect in a rare genetic disorder, orotic aciduria. Subsequently, working with Hibbard Williams, he discovered the enzyme defects of two distinct forms of primary hyperoxaluria.

One can see from the above narrative that Holly excelled in clinical medicine and in research. But perhaps his most powerful impact on internal medicine was his acceptance of the position as chair of internal medicine at the University of California, San Francisco, which he held from 1964 through 1985. He is now a professor of medicine and associate dean emeritus at UCSF. Holly's contribution as chair of internal medicine at UCSF was, in a word, dazzling. He developed a faculty that is peerless among departments of internal medicine in the United States. Following his tenure as chair of internal medicine at UCSF, Holly became associate dean, a position he held between 1985 and 2000, where his exceptional administrative talents provided a major impetus to the further expansion of UCSF.

For his contributions, Holly has been recognized as the president of virtually all the major societies in internal medicine, including the American Society for Clinical Investigation (1969), the Association of American Physicians (1975), and the Association of Professors of Medicine (1978). He has received the George M. Kober Medal from the Association of American Physicians, as well as membership in the American Academy of Arts and Sciences and the Institute of Medicine of the National Academy of Sciences.

Fred Plum, MD (Deceased)

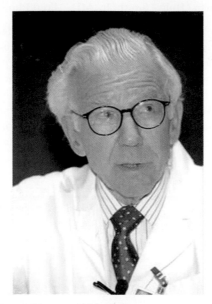

Fred Plum, attending neurologist at New York Presbyterian Hospital and university professor at Weill Medical College of Cornell University, was, together with Holly Smith, one of the two progenitors of Essentials. *Fred was a truly remarkable individual who had an exceptional mastery of the neurologic sciences, both basic and clinical. One could hardly imagine two more different personalities than Holly and Fred. As I mentioned above, Holly is a classic Southern gentleman. Fred was born and raised in Atlantic City, New Jersey, and carried with him the charming but demanding characteristics of a resident of that city.*

Fred trained in medicine and neurology at New York Hospital and at the neurologic division of Bellevue Hospital. Subsequently, he became an instructor in medicine at Cornell University Medical College, then an assistant professor, associate professor, and professor of medicine (neurology) at the University of Washington School of Medicine, all between 1953 and 1963. In 1963, Fred became the Anne Parrish Titzell Professor and Chair of the Department of Neurology at Cornell University Medical College, a position he held for 31 years. After stepping down as chairman of neurology, he was recognized for his remarkable accomplishments by having been made a university professor at Weill Medical College of Cornell University in 1998.

Fred was a member of virtually all distinguished societies in internal medicine and in neurology. He held honorary doctorates from at least two medical schools, including the Karolinska Institute in Stockholm.

Fred was not only a spectacular clinician but an extraordinary teacher. His textbook, Diagnosis of Stupor and Coma, *written together with J.B. Posner, is one of the classics of its field.*

Fred, like Holly, recognized in the mid-1980s the need for providing a textbook which was sufficiently concise yet comprehensive to be usable by students, house staff, young physicians, and physicians outside his own discipline of neurology. I remember particularly well the editorial meetings in the early years of Essentials, *involving Fred, Holly Smith, Chuck Carpenter, and myself. Fred's exceptional analytic reasoning, coupled with remarkable flexibility, was clearly a tutorial in how one deals with a pleomorphic group such as the four editors: flexibility on the one hand and an insistence on excellence on the other.*

Holly and Fred were the two prime movers in the development of what was originally Cecil Essentials of Medicine *and is now titled* Andreoli and Carpenter's Cecil Essentials of Medicine. *Medical students, residents in internal medicine, young physicians, and others interested in internal medicine owe a great deal to Holly and Fred for their vision in generating the notion of* Essentials. *And the other editors of* Essentials *owe Holly and Fred a great debt for tutoring us in how one assembles a textbook of internal medicine.*

Thomas E. Andreoli, MD (Deceased)

Ivor J. Benjamin, MD, FACC, FAHA

Editors-in-Chief

Contributors

I Introduction to Molecular Medicine

Ivor J. Benjamin, MD, FACC, FAHA
Professor of Medicine, Physiology, Pharmacology and Toxicology, Cell Biology, and Surgery, Director, Cardiovascular Center, Chief, Division of Cardiovascular Medicine, Vice Chair, Translational Research, Department of Medicine, Medical College of Wisconsin, Milwaukee, Wisconsin

II Cardiovascular Disease

Contributors
Mohamed F. Algahim, MD
Resident, Cardiothoracic Surgery, Medical College of Wisconsin, Milwaukee, Wisconsin

Ivor J. Benjamin, MD, FACC, FAHA
Professor of Medicine, Physiology, Pharmacology and Toxicology, Cell Biology, and Surgery, Director, Cardiovascular Center, Chief, Division of Cardiovascular Medicine, Vice Chair, Translational Research, Department of Medicine, Medical College of Wisconsin, Milwaukee, Wisconsin

Marcie G. Berger, MD
Associate Professor, Director of Electrophysiology, Department of Medicine, Medical College of Wisconsin, Milwaukee, Wisconsin

Michael P. Cinquegrani, MD
Director, Heart and Vascular Service Line, Cardiovascular Medicine, Froedtert and Medical College of Wisconsin, Milwaukee, Wisconsin

Scott Cohen, MD
Wisconsin Adult Congenital Heart Disease Program (WAtCH), Adult Cardiovascular Medicine and Pediatric Cardiology, Medical College of Wisconsin, Milwaukee, Wisconsin

Michael G. Earing, MD
Director, Wisconsin Adult Congenital Heart Disease Program (WAtCH), Adult Cardiovascular Medicine and Pediatric Cardiology, Medical College of Wisconsin, Milwaukee, Wisconsin

Panayotis Fasseas, MD, FACC
Cardiovascular Medicine, Medical College of Wisconsin, Milwaukee, Wisconsin

Nunzio A. Gaglianello, MD
Assistant Professor, Division of Cardiovascular Medicine, Medical Director, Advanced Heart Failure and Mechanical Circulatory Support, Medical College of Wisconsin, Milwauke, Wisconsin

James Kleczka, MD
Associate Professor, Department of Medicine, Medical College of Wisconsin, Milwaukee, Wisconsin

Nicole L. Lohr, MD, PhD
Assistant Professor of Medicine, Medical College of Wisconsin, Milwaukee, Wisconsin

Robert B. Love, MD, FACS, FRCS
Professor, Cardiothoracic Surgery, Medical College of Wisconsin, Milwaukee, Wisconsin

Claudius Mahr, DO
Advanced Heart Failure and Transplant Cardiology, Director, Clinical Integration, UW Regional Heart Center; Medical Director, Mechanical Circulatory Support Program, University of Washington Medical Center; Associate Professor of Clinical Medicine and Cardiac Surgery, University of Washington, Seattle, Washington

James A. Roth, MD
Associate Professor, Division of Cardiovascular Medicine, Medical College of Wisconsin, Milwaukee, Wisconsin

Jason C. Rubenstein, MD, FACC
Assistant Professor, Department of Medicine, Medical College of Wisconsin, Milwaukee, Wisconsin

Jennifer L. Strande, MD, PhD
Cardiovascular Medicine, Medical College of Wisconsin, Milwaukee, Wisconsin

Ronald G. Victor, MD
Burns and Allen Professor of Medicine, Director, Hypertension Center, Associate Director, The Heart Institute, Cedars-Sinai Medical Center, Los Angeles, California

Wanpen Vongpatanasin, MD
Norman and Audrey Kaplan Professor of Medicine, University of Texas Southwestern Medical Center, Dallas, Texas

Timothy D. Woods, MD
Internal Medicine–Cardiology, University of Tennessee Health Science Center, Memphis, Tennessee

III Pulmonary and Critical Care Medicine

Contributors
Jason M. Aliotta, MD
Assistant Professor of Medicine, Alpert Medical School of Brown University; Division of Pulmonary, Critical Care, and Sleep Medicine, Rhode Island Hospital, Providence, Rhode Island

Rizwan Aziz, MBBS, MRCP UK, MRCPE
Respiratory Registrar, University Hospital Limerick, Dooradoyle, Limerick, Ireland

Brian Casserly, MD
Assistant Professor of Medicine, Alpert Medical School of Brown University, Providence, Rhode Island

Lauren M. Catalano, MD
Fellow, Pulmonary Disease and Critical Care Medicine, Alpert Medical School of Brown University, Providence, Rhode Island

Eric J. Gartman, MD
Assistant Professor of Medicine, Alpert Medical School of Brown University, Providence, Rhode Island; Memorial Hospital of Rhode Island, Pawtucket, Rhode Island

Matthew D. Jankowich, MD
Assistant Professor of Medicine, Alpert Medical School of Brown University; Staff Physician, Pulmonary and Critical Care Medicine, Providence VA Medical Center, Providence, Rhode Island

F. Dennis McCool, MD
Professor of Medicine, Division of Pulmonary and Critical Care Medicine, Alpert Medical School of Brown University, Providence, Rhode Island; Memorial Hospital of Rhode Island, Pawtucket, Rhode Island

Sharon Rounds, MD
Professor of Medicine, Alpert Medical School of Brown University; Chief, Medical Service, Providence VA Medical Center, Providence, Rhode Island

Narendran Selvakumar, BSc, MBBCh
University of Limerick, Limerick City, Ireland

Jigme M. Sethi, MD, FCCP
Associate Professor of Medicine, Division of Pulmonary and Critical Care Medicine, Alpert Medical School of Brown University, Providence, Rhode Island; Memorial Hospital of Rhode Island, Pawtucket, Rhode Island

IV Preoperative and Postoperative Care

Contributors
Kim A. Eagle, MD
Albion Walter Hewlett Professor of Internal Medicine, Chief, Clinical Cardiovascular Medicine, Director, Cardiovascular Center, University of Michigan Medical School, Ann Arbor, Michigan

Prashant Vaishnava, MD
Clinical Lecturer in Medicine–Cardiology, University of Michigan Cardiovascular Center, Ann Arbor, Michigan

V Renal Disease

Lead Author
Biff F. Palmer, MD
Professor, Department of Internal Medicine, University of Texas Southwestern Medical Center, Dallas, Texas

Contributors
Rajiv Agarwal, MD
Indiana University School of Medicine, Richard L. Roudebush Veterans Administration Medical Center, Indianapolis, Indiana

Jeffrey S. Berns, MD
Professor of Medicine and Pediatrics, Renal, Electrolyte, and Hypertension Division, Perelman School of Medicine, University of Pennsylvania, Philadelphia, Pennsylvania

Kerri L. Cavanaugh, MD, MHS
Assistant Professor of Medicine, Division of Nephrology, Vanderbilt University Medical Center, Nashville, Tennessee

An De Vriese, MD, PhD
Division of Nephrology, AZ Sint-Jan Brugge Hospital, Bruges, Belgium

Fernando C. Fervenza, MD, PhD
Professor of Medicine, Division of Nephrology and Hypertension, Mayo Clinic, Rochester, Minnesota

T. Alp Ikizler, MD
Catherine McLaughlin-Hakim Professor of Medicine, Division of Nephrology, Vanderbilt University Medical Center, Nashville, Tennessee

Orson W. Moe, MD
Professor of Medicine, The Charles Pak Distinguished Chair in Mineral Metabolism, Donald W. Seldin Professorship in Clinical Investigation, Department of Internal Medicine, Division of Nephrology, University of Texas Southwestern Medical Center, Dallas, Texas

Javier A. Neyra, MD
Postdoctoral Fellow, Department of Internal Medicine, Division of Nephrology, University of Texas Southwestern Medical Center, Dallas, Texas

Mark A. Perazella
Professor of Medicine, Director, Nephrology Fellowship Program, Medical Director, Yale Physician Associate Program, Department of Medicine, Section of Nephrology, Yale University School of Medicine; Director, Acute Dialysis Services, Yale–New Haven Hospital, New Haven, Connecticut

Nilum Rajora, MD
Associate Professor, Department of Internal Medicine, Division of Nephrology, UT Southwestern Medical Center, Dallas, Texas

Ramesh Saxena, MD, PhD
Professor, Department of Internal Medicine, Division of Nephrology, UT Southwestern Medical Center, Dallas, Texas

Sanjeev Sethi, MD, PhD
Professor of Laboratory Medicine and Pathology, Division of Anatomic Pathology, Mayo Clinic, Rochester, Minnesota

Shani Shastri, MD, MPH, MS
Assistant Professor, Department of Internal Medicine, Division of Nephrology, UT Southwestern Medical Center, Dallas, Texas

Jeffrey M. Turner, MD
Assistant Professor of Medicine, Section of Nephrology, Yale University School of Medicine, New Haven, Connecticut

VI Gastrointestinal Disease

Lead Author
M. Michael Wolfe, MD
Charles H. Rammelkamp, Jr. Professor of Medicine, Case Western Reserve University; Chair, Department of Medicine, MetroHealth System, Cleveland, Ohio

Contributors
Charles M. Bliss, Jr., MD
Assistant Professor of Medicine, Boston University School of Medicine; Section of Gastroenterology, Boston Medical Center, Boston, Massachusetts

Francis A. Farraye, MD, MSc
Professor of Medicine, Boston University School of Medicine; Clinical Director, Section of Gastroenterology, Boston Medical Center, Boston, Massachusetts

Ronnie Fass, MD
Professor of Medicine, Case Western Reserve University; Director, Division of Gastroenterology and Hepatology, Head, Esophageal, and Swallowing Center, MetroHealth Medical Center, Cleveland, Ohio

D. Roy Ferguson, MD
Associate Professor of Medicine, Case Western Reserve University School of Medicine; Director of Endoscopy, Division of Gastroenterology and Hepatology, MetroHealth System, Cleveland, Ohio

Christopher S. Huang, MD
Assistant Professor, Internal Medicine, Boston University School of Medicine, Boston, Massachusetts

David R. Lichtenstein, MD, FACG, AGAF, FASGE
Director of Gastrointestinal Endoscopy, Associate Professor of Medicine, Boston University School of Medicine, Boston, Massachusetts

Robert C. Lowe, MD
Associate Professor, Department of Medicine, Boston University School of Medicine, Boston, Massachusetts

Carla Maradey-Romero, MD
Postdoctoral Fellow, Division of Gastroenterology and Hepatology, Department of Medicine, MetroHealth Medical Center, Cleveland, Ohio

John S. Maxwell, MD
Assistant Professor of Medicine, Case Western Reserve University School of Medicine; Division of Gastroenterology and Hepatology, MetroHealth System, Cleveland, Ohio

Hannah L. Miller, MD
Assistant Professor of Medicine, Department of Gastroenterology, Boston University School of Medicine, Boston, Massachusetts

Elihu M. Schimmel, MD
Professor of Medicine, Boston University School of Medicine; Section of Gastroenterology, VA Boston Healthcare System, Boston, Massachusetts

Sharmeel K. Wasan, MD
Assistant Professor of Medicine, Boston University School of Medicine; Section of Gastroenterology, Boston Medical Center, Boston, Massachusetts

VII   Diseases of the Liver and Biliary System

Lead Author
Michael B. Fallon, MD
Dan and Lillie Sterling Professor of Medicine, Division of Gastroenterology, Hepatology, and Nutrition, The University of Texas Health Science Center at Houston, Houston, Texas

Contributors
Brendan M. McGuire, MD
Professor of Medicine, Medical Director of Liver Transplantation, Department of Medicine, University of Alabama at Birmingham, Birmingham, Alabama

Klaus Mönkemüller, MD
Professor of Medicine, Director of the Basil I. Hirschowitz Endoscopic Center of Excellence, University of Alabama School of Medicine, Birmingham, Alabama

Helmut Neumann, MD
Faculty of Medicine, Division of Gastroenterology, Hepatology, and Infectious Diseases, Otto-von-Guericke University, Magdeburg, Germany

Jen-Jung Pan, MD, PhD
Assistant Professor of Medicine, Division of Gastroenterology, Hepatology, and Nutrition, Department of Internal Medicine, The University of Texas Health Science Center at Houston, Houston, Texas

Shaheryar A. Siddiqui, MD
Hepatology and Gastroenterology, University of Texas Houston, Houston, Texas

Matthew P. Spinn, MD
Assistant Professor, Department of Internal Medicine, The University of Texas Health Science Center at Houston, Houston, Texas

VIII   Hematologic Disease

Contributors
Nancy Berliner, MD
Chief, Division of Hematology, Department of Medicine, Brigham and Women's Hospital; Professor of Medicine, Harvard Medical School, Boston, Massachusetts

Jill Lacy, MD
Associate Professor of Medicine, Yale Cancer Center, Yale University, New Haven, Connecticut

Henry M. Rinder, MD
Professor, Laboratory and Internal Medicine, Hematology, Yale University School of Medicine, New Haven, Connecticut

Michal G. Rose, MD
Associate Professor of Medicine, Yale University School of Medicine, New Haven, Connecticut; Director, Cancer Center, VA Connecticut Healthcare System, West Haven, Connecticut

Stuart Seropian, MD
Associate Professor of Medicine, Yale Cancer Center, Yale University, New Haven, Connecticut

Alexa J. Siddon, MD
Assistant Professor, Pathology and Laboratory Medicine, Yale University School of Medicine, New Haven, Connecticut

Christopher A. Tormey, MD
Assistant Professor of Laboratory Medicine, Lecturer in Molecular Biophysics and Biochemistry, Director, Transfusion Medicine Fellowship, Yale University School of Medicine, New Haven, Connecticut

Richard Torres, MD
Attending Hematopathologist, Yale University School of Medicine, New Haven, Connecticut

Eunice S. Wang, MD
Associate Professor of Oncology, Department of Medicine, Roswell Park Cancer Institute, Buffalo, New York

IX   Oncologic Disease

Lead Author
Alok A. Khorana, MD, FACP
Professor of Medicine, Cleveland Clinic Lerner College of Medicine, Case Western Reserve University; Sondra and Stephen Hardis Chair in Oncology Research, Vice Chair (Clinical Services), Director GI Malignancies Program, Taussig Cancer Institute, Cleveland Clinic, Cleveland, Ohio

Contributors
Robert Dreicer, MD, MS, FACP, FASCO
Department of Hematology/Oncology, Taussig Cancer Institute, Cleveland Clinic, Cleveland, Ohio

Bassam Estfan, MD
Assistant Professor, Cleveland Clinic Lerner College of
 Medicine, Department of Hematology and Medical
 Oncology, Taussig Cancer Institute, Cleveland Clinic,
 Cleveland, Ohio

Jorge Garcia, MD, FACP
Department of Hematology/Oncology, Taussig Cancer
 Institute, Cleveland Clinic, Cleveland, Ohio

Timothy Gilligan, MD
Department of Hematology/Oncology, Taussig Cancer
 Institute, Cleveland Clinic, Cleveland, Ohio

Aram F. Hezel, MD
Associate Professor of Medicine, Division of Hematology/
 Oncology, University of Rochester Medical Center,
 Rochester, New York

Nicole M. Kuderer, MD
Instructor in Medicine, Division of Hematology, University of
 Washington School of Medicine, Seattle, Washington

Gary H. Lyman, MD, MPH, FASCO
Co-Director, Hutchinson Institute for Cancer Outcomes
 Research, Fred Hutchinson Cancer Research Center;
 Professor of Medicine, University of Washington School of
 Medicine, Seattle, Washington

Patrick C. Ma, MD, MSc
Director, Aerodigestive Oncology Translational Research,
 Translational Hematology and Oncology Research, Staff
 Physician, Solid Tumor Oncology, Taussig Cancer Institute,
 Cleveland Clinic, Cleveland, Ohio

Michael J. McNamara, MD
Department of Solid Tumor Oncology, Taussig Cancer
 Institute, Cleveland Clinic, Cleveland, Ohio

Brian Rini, MD
Department of Hematology/Oncology, Taussig Cancer
 Institute, Cleveland Clinic, Cleveland, Ohio

Davendra P.S. Sohal, MD, MPH
Assistant Professor of Medicine, Lerner College of Medicine;
 Director, Clinical Genomics Program, Taussig Cancer
 Institute, Cleveland Clinic, Cleveland, Ohio

X   Endocrine Disease and Metabolic Disease

Contributors
Glenn D. Braunstein, MD
The James R. Klinenberg, MD Professor of Medicine, Vice
 President for Clinical Innovation, Cedars-Sinai Medical
 Center, Los Angeles, California

Theodore C. Friedman, MD, PhD
Charles R. Drew University of Medicine and Science, Los
 Angeles, California

Geetha Gopalakrishnan, MD
Associate Professor of Medicine, The Warren Alpert Medical
 School at Brown University, Division of Diabetes and
 Endocrinology, Providence, Rhode Island

Osama Hamdy, MD, PhD
Medical Director, Obesity Clinical Program, Director of
 Inpatient Diabetes Program, Joslin Diabetes Center;
 Assistant Professor of Medicine, Harvard Medical School,
 Boston, Massachusetts

Kawaljeet Kaur, MD
Assistant Professor of Medicine, Division of Endocrinology,
 Metabolism, and Clinical Nutrition, Medical College of
 Wisconsin, Milwaukee, Wisconsin

Diana Maas, MD
Associate Professor of Medicine, Division of Endocrinology,
 Metabolism, and Clinical Nutrition, Medical College of
 Wisconsin, Milwaukee, Wisconsin

Robert J. Smith, MD
Professor of Medicine, The Warren Alpert School of Medicine,
 Brown University; Research Staff, Ocean State Research
 Institute, Providence Veterans Administration Medical
 Center, Providence, Rhode Island

Thomas R. Ziegler, MD
Professor of Medicine, Division of Endocrinology, Metabolism,
 and Lipids, Emory University School of Medicine; Atlanta
 Clinical and Translational Science Institute, Emory
 University Hospital, Atlanta, Georgia

XI   Women's Health

Contributors
Michelle Anvar, MD
Clinical Assistant Professor of Medicine, Department of
 Internal Medicine, Alpert Medical School at Brown
 University, Providence, Rhode Island

Kimberly Babb, MD
Clinical Instructor of Medicine and Pediatrics, Department of
 Internal Medicine, Alpert Medical School at Brown
 University, Providence, Rhode Island

Christine Duffy, MD, MPH
Assistant Professor of Medicine, Department of Internal
 Medicine, Alpert Medical School at Brown University,
 Providence, Rhode Island

Laura Edmonds, MD
Clinical Assistant Professor of Medicine, Department of Internal Medicine, Alpert Medical School at Brown University, Providence, Rhode Island

Jennifer Jeremiah, MD, FACP
Clinical Associate Professor of Medicine, Department of Internal Medicine, Alpert Medical School at Brown University, Providence, Rhode Island

Kelly McGarry, MD, FACP
Associate Professor of Medicine, Department of Internal Medicine, Alpert Medical School at Brown University, Providence, Rhode Island

XII   Men's Health

Douglas F. Milam, MD
Associate Professor, Urologic Surgery, Vanderbilt University Medical Center, Nashville, Tennessee

David James Osborn, MD
Walter Reed National Military Medical Center, Bethesda, Maryland

Joseph A. Smith, Jr., MD
Professor and Chairman, Urologic Surgery, Vanderbilt University, Nashville, Tennessee

XIII   Diseases of Bone and Bone Mineral Metabolism

Lead Author
Andrew F. Stewart, MD
Director, Diabetes, Obesity, and Metabolism Institute; Irene and Dr. Arthur M. Fishberg Professor of Medicine, Icahn School of Medicine at Mount Sinai, New York, New York

Contributors
Susan L. Greenspan, MD, FACP
Professor of Medicine, Director, Osteoporosis Prevention and Treatment Center; Director, Bone Health Program, Magee-Women's Hospital, University of Pittsburgh School of Medicine, Pittsburgh, Pennsylvania

Steven P. Hodak, MD
Professor of Medicine, Associate Director of Clinical Affairs, Division of Endocrinology, Diabetes, and Metabolism, New York University School of Medicine, New York, New York

Mara J. Horwitz, MD
Division of Endocrinology, University of Pittsburgh School of Medicine, Pittsburgh, Pennsylvania

XIV   Musculoskeletal and Connective Tissue Disease

Robyn T. Domsic, MD, MPH
Assistant Professor, Department of Medicine, University of Pittsburgh School of Medicine, Pittsburgh, Pennsylvania

Yong Gil Hwang, MD
Assistant Professor, Department of Rheumatology, University of Pittsburgh, Pittsburgh, Pennsylvania

Rayford R. June, MD
Assistant Professor of Medicine, Division of Rheumatology, Penn State College of Medicine, Hershey, Pennsylvania

Amy H. Kao, MD, MPH, MS
Associate Medical Director, Immunology Clinical Development, Cambridge, Massachusetts

C. Kent Kwoh, MD
Professor of Medicine and Medical Imaging, The Charles A.L. and Suzanne M. Stephens Chair of Rheumatology, Chief, Division of Rheumatology, University of Arizona, Tucson, Arizona

Kimberly P. Liang, MD
Assistant Professor of Medicine, Division of Rheumatology and Clinical Immunology, University of Pittsburgh, Pittsburgh, Pennsylvania

Douglas W. Lienesch, MD
Assistant Professor of Medicine, Division of Rheumatology and Clinical Immunology, University of Pittsburgh, Pittsburgh, Pennsylvania

Susan Manzi, MD, MPH
Professor of Medicine, Temple University School of Medicine; Chair, Department of Medicine, Lupus Center of Excellence, Allegheny Health Network, Pittsburgh, Pennsylvania

Niveditha Mohan, MBBS
Assistant Professor, Department of Medicine, Division of Rheumatology and Clinical Immunology, University of Pittsburgh, Pittsburgh, Pennsylvania

Larry W. Moreland, MD
Chief, Division of Rheumatology and Clinical Immunology, Margaret J. Miller Endowed Professor of Arthritis Research, Professor of Medicine, Immunology, Clinical, and Translational Science, University of Pittsburgh, Pittsburgh, Pennsylvania

Ghaith Noaiseh, MD
Assistant Professor of Medicine, Division of Rheumatology and Clinical Immunology, University of Pittsburgh, Pittsburgh, Pennsylvania

XV Infectious Disease

Contributors

Philip A. Chan, MD, MS
Assistant Professor of Medicine, Division of Infectious Diseases, Brown University, The Miriam Hospital, Providence, Rhode Island

Kimberle Chapin, MD
Director, Department of Pathology, Rhode Island Hospital, Providence, Rhode Island

Cheston B. Cunha, MD
Assistant Professor of Medicine, Infectious Disease Division, Warren Alpert Medical School at Brown University, Providence, Rhode Island

Susan Cu-uvin, MD
Professor of Obstetrics and Gynecology, Professor of Medicine and Professor of Health Services, Policy and Practice, Division of Infectious Diseases, Brown University, Providence, Rhode Island

Staci A. Fischer, MD, FACP, FIDSA
Director, Transplant Infectious Diseases, Rhode Island Hospital; Associate Professor of Medicine, Warren Alpert Medical School at Brown University, Providence, Rhode Island

Timothy P. Flanigan, MD
Professor of Medicine, Brown University, Providence, Rhode Island

Ekta Gupta, MD
Fellow, Infectious Diseases, Warren Alpert Medical School at Brown University, Providence, Rhode Island

Sajeev Handa, MD, SFHM
Director, Division of Hospital Medicine, Rhode Island Hospital; Clinical Assistant Professor of Medicine, Alpert Medical School of Brown University, Providence, Rhode Island

Marjorie A. Janvier, MD
Warren Alpert Medical School at Brown University, Providence, Rhode Island

Erna Milunka Kojic, MD
Associate Professor of Medicine, Division of Infectious Disease, Warren Alpert Medical School at Brown University, Providence, Rhode Island

Awewura Kwara, MD, MPH&TM
Associate Professor, Department of Medicine, Warren Alpert Medical School at Brown University, Providence, Rhode Island

Jerome Larkin, MD
Assistant Professor of Medicine, Division of Infectious Diseases, Warren Alpert Medical School at Brown University, Providence, Rhode Island

John R. Lonks, MD
Associate Professor, Department of Medicine, Warren Alpert Medical School at Brown University, Providence, Rhode Island

Russell J. McCulloh, MD
Assistant Professor, Pediatric and Adult, Infectious Diseases, Children's Mercy Hospital, Kansas City, Missouri

Maria D. Mileno, MD
Associate Professor of Medicine, Infectious Diseases, Warren Alpert Medical School at Brown University; Co-Director, Travel Medicine, Infectious Diseases, The Miriam Hospital, Providence, Rhode Island

Brian T. Montague, DO, MS, MPH
Assistant Professor of Medicine, Warren Alpert Medical School at Brown University, Providence, Rhode Island

Eleftherios Mylonakis, MD, PhD, FIDSA
Professor of Medicine, Infectious Disease Division, Alpert School of Medicine, Brown University, Providence, Rhode Island

Avindra Nath, MD
Chief, Section of Infections of the Nervous System, National Institute of Neurological Diseases and Stroke, National Institutes of Health, Bethesda, Maryland

Steven M. Opal, MD
Professor of Medicine, Infectious Disease Division, Warren Alpert Medical School at Brown University, Providence, Rhode Island; Chief, Infectious Disease Division, Memorial Hospital of Rhode Island, Pawtucket, Rhode Island

Bharat Ramratnam, AB, MD
Associate Professor of Medicine, Laboratory of Retrovirology, Division of Infectious Diseases, The Warren Alpert Medical School at Brown University; Attending Physician, Miriam and Rhode Island Hospitals, Providence, Rhode Island

Aadia I. Rana, MD
Assistant Professor of Medicine, Warren Alpert Medical School at Brown University, Providence, Rhode Island

Rebecca Reece, MD
Division of Infectious Diseases, Warren Alpert Medical School of Brown University, Providence, Rhode Island

Steven "Shaefer" Spires, MD
Assistant Professor of Medicine, Division of Infectious Diseases, Vanderbilt University School of Medicine; Hospital Epidemiologist, Williamson Medical Center; Medical Director of Infection Control, Antimicrobial Stewardship, VA Tennessee Valley Healthcare System, Nashville, Tennessee

Thomas R. Talbot, MD, MPH
Associate Professor of Medicine and Health Policy, Vanderbilt University School of Medicine; Chief, Hospital Epidemiologist, Vanderbilt University Medical Center, Nashville, Tennessee

Joao Tavares, MD
Infectious Disease Specialist, Cape Cod Hospital, Hyannis, Massachusetts

Allan R. Tunkel, MD, PhD
Professor of Medicine, Associate Dean for Medical Education, Warren Alpert Medical School of Brown University, Providence, Rhode Island

Edward J. Wing, MD, FACP, FIDSA
Professor of Medicine, Warren Alpert Medical School at Brown University, Providence, Rhode Island

XVI   Neurologic Disease

Contributors

Selim R. Benbadis, MD
Professor of Neurology, University of South Florida, Tampa, Florida

Michel J. Berg, MD
Associate Professor of Neurology, University of Rochester Medical Center, Rochester, New York

Kevin M. Biglan, MD, MPH
Associate Chair of Clinical Research, Associate Professor of Neurology, Director, National Parkinson Foundation Center of Excellence; Director, Huntington Disease Society of America Center of Excellence, University of Rochester School of Medicine and Dentistry, Strong Memorial Hospital, Rochester, New York

Bryan J. Bonder, MD
Department of Neurology, University Hospitals Case Medical Center, Cleveland, Ohio

William P. Cheshire, Jr., MD
Professor of Neurology, Mayo Clinic, Jacksonville, Florida

Mohamad Chmayssani, MD
Clinical Instructor, Department of Neurosurgery, David Geffen School of Medicine at UCLA, Los Angeles, California

Emma Ciafaloni, MD
Professor of Neurology and Pediatrics, Department of Neurology, University of Rochester, Rochester, New York

Timothy J. Counihan, MD, FRCPI
Honorary Senior Clinical Lecturer in Medicine, School of Medicine, National University of Ireland Galway, Galway, Ireland

Anne Haney Cross, MD
Professor of Neurology, Washington University School of Medicine, Saint Louis, Missouri

Mitchell S.V. Elkind, MD, MS
Professor of Neurology and Epidemiology, Fellowships Director, Head, Division of Neurology Clinical Outcomes Research and Population Sciences, Department of Neurology and Sergievsky Center, Columbia University, New York, New York

Robert C. Griggs, MD, FACP, FAAN
Professor of Neurology, Medicine, Pathology and Laboratory Medicine, Pediatrics, Center for Human Experimental Therapeutics, University of Rochester School of Medicine and Dentistry, Rochester, New York

Carlayne E. Jackson, MD
Professor of Neurology, University of Texas Health Science Center, San Antonio, Texas

Kevin A. Kerber, MD, MS
Associate Professor, Department of Neurology, University of Michigan Health System, Ann Arbor, Michigan

Jennifer M. Kwon, MD
Associate Professor, Departments of Neurology and Pediatrics, University of Rochester Medical Center, Rochester, New York

Geoffrey S.F. Ling, MD, PhD
Professor of Neurology, Uniformed Services University of the Health Sciences, Bethesda, Maryland; Attending Physician in Neuro Critical Care Medicine, Johns Hopkins Medical Institutions, Baltimore, Maryland

Jeffrey M. Lyness, MD
Senior Associate Dean for Academic Affairs, Professor of
Psychiatry and Neurology, University of Rochester School of
Medicine and Dentistry, Rochester, New York

Frederick J. Marshall, MD
Associate Professor, Department of Neurology, University of
Rochester, Rochester, New York

Eavan McGovern, MD
Department of Neurology, St. Vincent's University Hospital,
Dublin, Ireland

Sinéad M. Murphy, MB, MD, FRCPI
Consultant Neurologist, The Adelaide and Meath Hospitals
incorporating the National Children's Hospital, Tallaght,
Dublin; Senior Lecturer, Department Medicine, Trinity
College Dublin, Dublin, Ireland

Lisa R. Rogers, DO
Medical Director, Neuro-oncology Program, Brain Tumor and
Neuro-oncology Center, The Neurological Institute,
Cleveland, Ohio

Maxwell H. Sims
Halterman Research Lab, Center for Neural Development and
Disease, University of Rochester, Rochester, New York

Jeffrey M. Statland, MD
Assistant Professor of Neurology, University of Kansas Medical
Center, Kansas City, Kansas

Paul M. Vespa, MD, FCCM, FAAN, FNCS
Professor, Departments of Neurology and Neurosurgery, David
Geffen School of Medicine at UCLA, Los Angeles,
California

XVII Geriatrics

Contributors
Harvey Jay Cohen, MD
Walter Kempner Professor of Medicine and Director, Center
for the Study of Aging and Human Development, Duke
University School of Medicine, Durham, North Carolina

Mitchell T. Heflin, MD, MHS
Associate Professor, Department of Medicine, Duke University
School of Medicine, Durham, North Carolina

XVIII Palliative Care

Contributors
Robert G. Holloway, MD, MPH
Professor of Neurology, Chairman, Department of Neurology,
Palliative Care Program, University of Rochester Medical
Center, Rochester, New York

Timothy E. Quill, MD
Professor of Medicine, Psychiatry and Medical Humanities,
Palliative Care Program, University of Rochester Medical
Center, Rochester, New York

XIX Alcohol and Substance Abuse

Contributors
L. David Hillis, MD
Professor and Chair, Department of Internal Medicine,
University of Texas Health Science Center, San Antonio,
Texas

Richard A. Lange, MD, MBA
President, Dean, Paul L. Foster School of Medicine, Texas Tech
University Health Sciences Center, El Paso, Texas

Preface

This is the ninth edition of *Andreoli and Carpenter's Cecil Essentials of Medicine*. *Essentials IX*, like its predecessors, is intended to be comprehensive but concise. *Essentials IX*, therefore, provides an exacting and thoroughly updated treatise on internal medicine, without excessive length, for students of medicine at all levels of their careers.

We welcome with enthusiasm a new editor, J. Gregory Fitz, MD, provost and dean of medicine at the University of Texas Southwestern Medical Center at Dallas.

Essentials IX has maintained its three cardinal components and added a fourth. First, at the beginning of each section—kidney, for example—we provide a brief but rigorous summary of the fundamental biology of the kidney and/or the cardinal signs and symptoms of diseases of the kidney. The same format has been used in all the sections of the book. Second, the main body of each section contains a detailed but, again, concise description of the diseases of the various organ systems together with their pathophysiology and their treatment.

Essentials IX relies heavily on the internet. Along with the print publication, *Essentials IX* is published in its entirety online. In the online version of *Essentials IX*, we provide a substantial amount of supplemental material, indicated in the hard copy text by various icons in the margins of the pages. These icons are present throughout the hard copy of the book as well as in the Internet version and direct the reader to a series of illustrations, tables, or videos in the online version of *Essentials*. This material is clearly crucial to understanding modern medicine, but we hope that, in this manner, the supplemental material will enrich *Essentials IX* without having enlarged the book significantly.

Finally, *Essentials IX* is being published simultaneously with *Goldman-Cecil Medicine*, 25th Edition, which is edited by Lee Goldman, MD, and Andrew I. Schafer, MD. Accordingly, the student has both the depth and breadth of two complementary textbooks, which were written and edited by contributors who number among the most recognized and respected authorities in the field. We feel that such integration and partnership expose students at all levels to the latest developments in biology with current evidence-based diagnosis, therapy, and practices.

As in prior editions, we make abundant use of four-color illustrations and each section has been reviewed first by one or another of the editors and finally by the editor-in-chief.

We thank James T. Merritt, senior acquisitions editor, medical education, of Elsevier, Inc., and especially Taylor Ball, content development manager, Elsevier, Inc. Both Jim Merritt and Taylor Ball contributed heartily to the preparation of this ninth edition of *Essentials*. Lastly, we thank our very able secretarial staff, Ms. Deborah Lamontange and Rachel Trower (Milwaukee), Ms. Patricia Hopkins (Rochester), Ms. Diane DiLolle (Dallas), and Ms. Carrie Gridelli and Ms. Lola Wright (Providence).

The Editors

Contents

Video Table of Contents

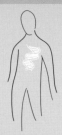

Introduction to Molecular Medicine

1 Molecular Basis of Human Disease
Ivor J. Benjamin

1

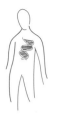

Molecular Basis of Human Disease

Ivor J. Benjamin

INTRODUCTION

Medicine has evolved dramatically during the past century—from a healing art in which standards of practice were established on the basis of personal experience passed on from one practitioner to the next to a rigorous intellectual discipline reliably steeped in the scientific method. This process tests the validity of a hypothesis or prediction through experimentation, the foundation of current advances in the fields of physiology, microbiology, biochemistry, and pharmacology.

These advances have served as the basis for new diagnostic and therapeutic approaches to illness and disease while challenging providers and practitioners to adopt their use at an accelerated pace in 21st century. Since the 1980s, for example, understanding of the molecular basis of genetics has expanded dramatically, and advances in this field have identified new and exciting dimensions for defining the basis of conventional genetic diseases (e.g., sickle cell disease) and complex genetic traits (e.g., hypertension). Insights into the interactions between genes and environment that independently influence the noncoding genome laid the foundation for the field of epigenetics.

Armed with a variety of sensitive and specific molecular techniques, contemporary medicinal practice seeks to provide the molecular underpinning of complex pathobiologic processes and identify individuals at risk for common diseases. To fully exploit modern medicine, clinical teams are increasingly relying on a detailed understanding of cellular mechanisms and on precision drugs that disrupt the fine-structural targets underlying the molecular basis of disease. The outcomes of large clinical trials that yield mean responses to therapy will likely evolve into personalized medicine, defining more effective treatments for specific patient subpopulations. This introductory chapter offers an overview of these complex and rapidly evolving topics and summarizes the principles of molecular medicine that are highlighted in specific sections throughout this text.

DEOXYRIBONUCLEIC ACID AND THE GENOME

All organisms possess a scheme to transmit the essential information containing the genetic makeup of the species through successive generations. Human cells have 23 pairs of chromosomes, and each pair contains a unique sequence of genetic information. In the human genome, about 6×10^9 nucleotides, or 3×10^9 pairs of nucleotides, associate in the double helix. The specificity of DNA is determined by the base sequence that is stored in complementary form in the double-helical structure. It facilitates correction of sequence errors and provides a mechanistic basis for replication of information during cell division. Each DNA strand provides a template for replication, which is accomplished by the action of DNA-dependent polymerases that unwind the double-helical DNA and copy each single strand with remarkable fidelity.

Except for gametocytes, all cells contain the duplicate, diploid number of genetic units, one half of which is referred to as the *haploid number*. The genetic information contained in chromosomes is separated into discrete functional elements known as *genes*. A gene is a unit of base sequences that (with rare exception) encodes a specific polypeptide sequence. New evidence suggests that small, noncoding RNAs play critical roles in the expression of this essential information. An estimated 30,000 genes constitute the human haploid genome, and they are interspersed among sequence regions that do not code for protein and whose function is as yet unknown. For example, noncoding RNAs (e.g., transfer RNAs [tRNAs], ribosomal RNAs [rRNAs], other small RNAs) are components of enzyme complexes such as the ribosome and spliceosome. The average chromosome contains 3000 to 5000 genes, which range in size from about 1 kilobase (kb) to 2 megabases (Mb).

RIBONUCLEIC ACID SYNTHESIS

Transcription, or RNA synthesis, is the process of transferring information contained in nuclear DNA to an intermediate molecular species known as messenger RNA (mRNA). Two biochemical differences distinguish RNA from DNA. The polymeric backbone is made up of ribose rather than deoxyribose sugars linked by phosphodiester bonds, and the base composition is different in that uracil is substituted for thymine.

RNA synthesis from a DNA template is performed by three types of DNA-dependent RNA polymerases, each a multisubunit complex with distinct nuclear location and substrate specificity. RNA polymerase I, located in the nucleolus, directs the transcription of genes encoding the 18S, 5.8S, and 28S ribosomal RNAs, forming a molecular scaffold with catalytic and structural functions within the ribosome. RNA polymerase II, which is located in the nucleoplasm instead of the nucleoli, primarily transcribes precursor mRNA transcripts and small RNA molecules. The carboxyl terminus of RNA polymerase II is uniquely modified with a 220-kD protein domain, which is the site of enzymatic regulation by protein phosphorylation of critical serine and threonine

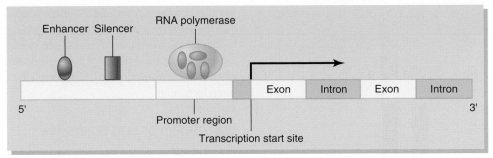

FIGURE 1-1   Transcription. Genomic DNA is shown with enhancer and silencer sites located 5' upstream of the promoter region, to which RNA polymerase is bound. The transcription start site is shown downstream of the promoter region, and this site is followed by exonic sequences interrupted by intronic sequences. The former sequences are transcribed one after another (ad seriatim) by the RNA polymerase.

residues. All tRNA precursors and other rRNA molecules are synthesized by RNA polymerase III in the nucleoplasm.

RNA polymerases are synthesized from precursor transcripts that must be cleaved into subunits before further processing and assembling with ribosomal proteins into macromolecular complexes. Ribosomal architectural and structural integrity are derived from the secondary and tertiary structures of rRNA, which assume a series of folding patterns containing short duplex regions. Precursors of tRNA in the nucleus undergo the removal of the 5' leader region, splicing of an internal intron sequences, and modification of terminal residues.

Precursors of mRNA are produced in the nucleus by the action of DNA-dependent RNA polymerase II, which copies the *antisense* strand of the DNA double helix to synthesize a single strand of mRNA that is identical to the *sense* strand of the DNA double helix in a process called *transcription* (Fig. 1-1). The initial, immature mRNA first undergoes modification at the 5' and 3' ends. A special nucleotide structure called the *cap* is added to the 5' end, which increases binding to the ribosome and enhances translational efficiency. The 3' end undergoes modification by nuclease cleavage of about 20 nucleotides, followed by the addition of a length of polynucleotide sequence containing a uniform stretch of adenine bases, the so-called poly-A tail that stabilizes the mRNA.

In addition to these changes that occur uniformly in all mRNAs, more selective modifications can occur. Because each gene contains exonic and intronic sequences and the precursor mRNA is transcribed without regard for exon-intron boundaries, this immature message must be edited so that all exons are spliced together in an appropriate sequence. The process of splicing, or removing intronic sequences to produce the mature mRNA, is an exquisitely choreographed event that involves the intermediate formation of a spliceosome, which is a large complex consisting of small nuclear RNAs and specific proteins that contains a loop or lariat-like structure that includes the intron targeted for removal. Only after splicing, a catalytic process requiring adenosine triphosphate hydrolysis, has concluded is the mature mRNA able to transit from the nucleus into the cytoplasm, where the encoded information is translated into protein.

Alternative splicing is a process for efficiently generating multiple gene products that often are dictated by tissue specificity, developmental expression, and pathologic state. Gene splicing allows the expression of multiple isoforms by expanding the repertoire for molecular diversity. An estimated 30% of genetic

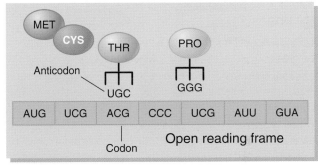

FIGURE 1-2   Translation. The open reading frame of a mature messenger RNA is shown with its series of codons. Transfer RNA molecules are shown with their corresponding anticodons, charged with their specific amino acid. A short, growing polypeptide chain is depicted. A, Adenine; C, cytosine; CYS, cysteine; G, guanine; MET, methionine; PRO, proline; THR, threonine; U, uracil.

diseases in humans arise from defects in splicing. The resulting mature mRNA then exits the nucleus to begin the process of *translation* or conversion of the base code to polypeptide (Fig. 1-2). Alternative splicing pathways (i.e., alternative exonic assembly pathways) for specific genes also serve at the level of transcriptional regulation. The discovery of catalytic RNA, which enables self-directed internal excision and repair, has advanced the view that RNA serves as a template for translation of the genetic code and simultaneously as an enzyme (see Transcriptional Regulation).

Protein synthesis, or translation of the mRNA code, occurs on ribosomes, which are macromolecular complexes of proteins and rRNA located in the cytoplasm. Translation involves the conversion of the linear code of a triplet of bases (i.e., codon) into the corresponding amino acid. A four-base code generates 64 possible triplet combinations ($4 \times 4 \times 4$), and they correspond to 20 different amino acids, many of which are encoded by more than one base triplet. To decode mRNA, an adapter molecule (tRNA) recognizes the codon in mRNA through complementary base pairing with a three-base anticodon that it bears; each tRNA is charged with a unique amino acid that corresponds to the anticodon (Fig. 1-3).

Translation on the mRNA template proceeds without punctuation of the non-overlapping code with the aid of rRNA on an assembly machine called a *ribosome*—essentially a polypeptide polymerase. At least one tRNA molecule exists for each of the 20 amino acids, although degeneracy in the code expands the

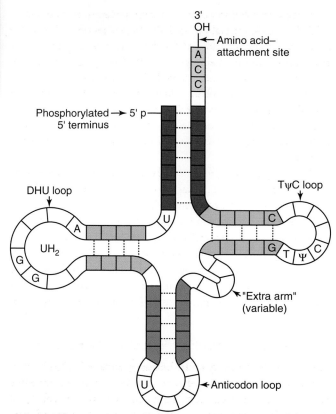

FIGURE 1-3 Secondary structure of transfer RNA (tRNA). The structure of each tRNA serves as an adapter molecule that recognizes a specific codon for the amino acid to be added to the polypeptide chain. About one half the hydrogen-bonded bases of the single chain of ribonucleotides are shown paired in double helices like a cloverleaf. The 5′ terminus is phosphorylated, and the 3′ terminus contains the hydroxyl group on an attached amino acid. The anticodon loop is typically located in the middle of the tRNA molecule. C, Cytocide; DHU, dihydroxyuridine; G, guanine; UH_2, dihydrouridine; ψ, pseudouridine; T, ribothymidine; U, uracil. (Data from Berg JM, Tymoczko JL, Strayer JL: Berg, Tymoczko, and Strayer's biochemistry, ed 5, New York, 2006, WH Freeman.)

number of available tRNA molecules, mitigates the chances of premature chain termination, and ameliorates the potential deleterious consequences of single-base mutations. The enzymatic activity of the ribosome then links amino acids through the synthesis of a peptide bond, releasing the tRNA in the process.

Consecutive linkage of amino acids in the growing polypeptide chain represents the terminal event in the conversion of information contained within the nuclear DNA sequence into mature protein (DNA → RNA → protein). Proteins are directly responsible for the form and function of an organism. Abnormalities in protein structure or function brought about by changes in primary amino acid sequence are the immediate precedent cause of changes in phenotype, adverse forms of which define a disease state.

Inhibition of RNA synthesis is a well-recognized mechanism of specific toxins and antibiotics. Toxicity from the ingestion of the poisonous mushroom (*Amanita phalloides*), for example, leads to the release of the toxin α-amanitin, a cyclic octapeptide that inhibits the RNA polymerase II and blocks elongation of RNA synthesis. The antibiotic actinomycin D binds with high affinity to double-helical DNA and intercalates between base pairs, precluding access of DNA-dependent RNA polymerases and the selective inhibition of transcription. Several major antibiotics inhibit translation. For example, the aminoglycoside antibiotics disrupt the mRNA-tRNA codon-anticodon interaction, whereas erythromycin and chloramphenicol inhibit peptide bond formation.

CONTROL OF GENE EXPRESSION

Overview

The timing, duration, localization, and magnitude of gene expression are all important elements in the complex tapestry of cell form and function governed by the genome. Gene expression represents the flow of information from the DNA template into mRNA transcripts and the process of translation into mature protein.

Four levels of organization involving transcription factors, RNAs, chromatin structure, and epigenetic factors orchestrate gene expression in the mammalian genome. Transcriptional regulators bind to specific DNA motifs that positively or negatively control the expression of neighboring genes. The information contained in the genome must be transformed into functional units of RNA or protein products. How DNA is packed and modified represents additional modes of gene regulation by disrupting the access of transcription factors from DNA-binding motifs.

In the postgenomic era, the challenge is to understand the architecture by which the genome is organized, controlled, and modulated. Transcription factors, chromatin architecture, and modifications of nucleosomal organization make up the major mechanisms of gene regulation in the genome.

Transcriptional Regulation

The principal regulatory step in gene expression occurs at the level of gene transcription. A specific DNA-dependent RNA polymerase performs the transcription of information contained in genomic DNA into mRNA transcripts. Transcription begins at a proximal (i.e., toward the 5′ end of the gene) transcription start site containing nucleotide sequences that influence the rate and extent of the process (see Fig. 1-1). This *promoter region* of the gene often includes a sequence rich in adenine and thymine (i.e., TATA box) along with other sequence motifs within about 100 bases of the start site. These regions of DNA that regulate transcription are known as *cis*-acting regulatory elements. Some of these regulatory regions of promoter sequence bind proteins known as *trans*-acting factors (i.e., transcription factors), which are themselves encoded by other genes. The *cis*-acting regulatory sequences to which transcription factors bind are often referred to as *response elements*. Families of transcription factors have been identified and are often described by unique aspects of their predicted secondary protein structure, including helix-turn-helix motifs, zinc finger motifs, and leucine zipper motifs. Transcription factors make up an estimated 3% to 5% of the protein-coding products of the genome.

In addition to gene-promoter regions, enhancer sites are distinct from promoter sites in that they can exist at distances quite remote from the start site, either upstream or downstream (i.e., beyond the 3′ end of the gene), and without clear orientation requirements. *Trans*-acting factors bind to these enhancer sites and are thought to alter the tertiary structure or conformation of the DNA in a manner that facilitates the binding and assembly of the transcription-initiation complex at the promoter region, perhaps in some cases by forming a broad loop of DNA in the process. Biochemical modification of select promoter or enhancer sequences, such as methylation of cytosine-phosphate-guanine (CpG)–rich sequences, can also modulate transcription; methylation typically suppresses transcription. The terms *silencer* and *suppressor* elements refer to *cis*-acting nucleotide sequences that reduce or shut off gene transcription and do so through association with *trans*-acting factors that recognize these specific sequences.

Regulation of transcription is a complex process that occurs at several levels. The expression of many genes is regulated to maintain high basal levels; they are known as *housekeeping* or *constitutively expressed* genes. They typically yield protein products that are essential for normal cell function or survival and must be maintained at a specific steady-state concentration in all circumstances. Many other genes are not expressed or are only modestly expressed under basal conditions; however, with the imposition of some stress or exposure of the cell to an agonist that elicits a cellular response distinct from that of the basal state, expression of these genes is induced or enhanced. For example, the heat shock protein genes encoding *stress proteins* are rapidly induced in response to diverse pathophysiologic stimuli (e.g., oxidative stress, heavy metals, inflammation) in most cells and organisms. Increased heat shock protein expression is complementary to the basal level of heat shock proteins, which are molecular chaperones that play key roles during protein synthesis to prevent protein misfolding, increase protein translocation, and accelerate protein degradation. These adaptive responses often mediate changes in phenotype that are homeostatically protective to the cell or organism.

Micro-RNAs and Gene Regulation

Less is known about the determinants of translational regulation than is known about transcriptional regulation. The recent discovery and identification of small RNAs (21-mer to 24-mer clusters), called *micro-RNAs* (miRNAs), adds further complexity to the regulation of gene expression in the eukaryotic genome. First discovered in worms more than 15 years ago, miRNAs are conserved noncoding strands of RNA that bind by Watson-Crick base pairing to the 3′-untranslated regions of target mRNAs, enabling gene silencing of protein expression at the translational level. Gene-encoding miRNAs exhibit tissue-specific expression and are interspersed in regions of the genome unrelated to known genes.

Transcription of miRNAs proceeds in multiple steps from sites under the control of an mRNA promoter. RNA polymerase II transcribes the precursor miRNA, called *primary miRNA* (primiRNA), containing 5′ caps and 3′ poly-A tails. In the nucleus, the larger pri-miRNAs of 70 nucleotides form an internal hairpin loop, embedding the miRNA portion that undergoes recognition and subsequent excision by a double-stranded RNA–specific ribonuclease called *Drosha*. Gene expression is silenced by the effect of miRNA on nascent RNA molecules targeted for degradation.

Because translation occurs at a fairly invariant rate among all mRNA species, the stability or half-life of a specific mRNA also serves as another checkpoint for the regulation of gene expression. The 3′-untranslated region of mRNAs contains regions of sequence that dictate the susceptibility of the message to nuclease cleavage and degradation. Stability appears to be sequence specific, and in some cases, it depends on *trans*-acting factors that bind to the mRNA. The mature mRNA contains elements of untranslated sequence at the 5′ and 3′ ends that can regulate translation.

Beginning in the organism's early development, miRNAs may facilitate much more intricate ways for the regulation of gene expression, as have been shown for germline production, cell differentiation, proliferation, and organogenesis. Because studies have implicated the expression of miRNAs in brain development, cardiac organogenesis, skeletal muscle regeneration, colonic adenocarcinoma, and viral replication, this novel mechanism for gene silencing has potential therapeutic roles for congenital heart defects, viral disease, neurodegeneration, regenerative medicine, and cancer.

Chromatin Remodeling and Gene Regulation

The size and complexity of the human genome with 23 chromosomes ranging in size between 50 and 250 Mb pose formidable challenges for transcription factors to exert the specificity of DNA-binding properties in gene regulation. Control of gene expression takes place in diverse types of cells, often with exquisite temporal and spatial specificity throughout the lifespan of the organism. In eukaryotic cells, the genome is highly organized into densely packed nucleic acid DNA- and RNA-protein structures, called *chromatin*. The building blocks of chromatin are called *histones*, a family of small basic proteins that occupy one half of the mass of the chromosome. Histones derive their basic properties from the high content of basic amino acids, arginine, and lysine. Five major types of histones—H1, H2A, H2B, H3, and H4—have evolved to form complexes with genomic DNA. Two pairs each of the four types of histones form a protein core, the histone octomer, which is wrapped by 200 base pairs of DNA to form the nucleosome (Fig. 1-4). The core proteins within the nucleosomes have protruding amino-terminal ends, exposing critical lysine and arginine residues for covalent modification. Further DNA condensation is achieved as higher-order structure is imposed on the chromosomes. The nucleosomes are further compacted in layered stacks with a left-handed superhelix resulting in negative supercoils that provide the energy for DNA strand separation during replication.

Condensation of DNA in chromatin precludes the access of regulatory molecules such as transcription factors. Reversal of chromatin condensation typically occurs in response to environmental and other developmental signals in a tissue-dependent manner. Promoter sites undergoing active transcription and relaxation of chromatin structure that become susceptible to enzymatic cleavage by nonspecific DNAase I are called *hypersensitive sites*. Transcription factors on promoter sites may gain access by protein-protein interactions to enhancer elements containing tissue-specific proteins at remote sites (several thousand bases away), resulting in transcription activation or repression.

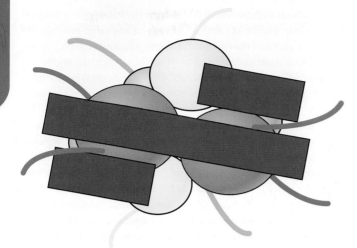

FIGURE 1-4 Schematic representation of a nucleosome. Rectangular blocks represent the DNA strand wrapped around the core that consists of eight histone proteins. Each histone has a protruding tail that can be modified to repress or activate transcription.

Epigenetic Control of Gene Expression

Complex regulatory networks revolve around transcription factors, nucleosomes, chromatin structure, and epigenetic markings. *Epigenetics* refers to heritable changes in gene expression without changes in the DNA sequence. Examples include DNA methylation, gene silencing, chromatin remodeling, and X-chromosome inactivation. This form of inheritance involves alterations in gene function without changes in DNA sequence. The chemical marking of DNA methylation is cell specific and developmentally regulated. Methylation of the 5'-CpG dinucleotide by specific methyl transferases, which occurs in 70% of the mammalian genome, is another mechanism of gene regulation. Steric hindrance from the bulky methyl group of 5'-methylcytosine precludes occupancy by transcription factors that stimulate or attenuate gene expression. Most genes are found in CpG islands, reflecting sites of gene activity across the genome.

In an analogous manner, modifications of histone by phosphorylation, methylation, ubiquitination, and acetylation are transmitted and reestablished in an inheritable manner. It is conceivable that other epigenetic mechanisms do not involve genomic modifications of DNA. For example, modification of the gene encoding the estrogen receptor-α has been implicated in gene silencing at 5-methylcytosine (^{5m}C) sites of multiple downstream targets in breast cancer cells. Powerful approaches are being developed to examine feedback and feed-forward loops in the transmission of epigenetic markings.

The concept that dynamic modifications (i.e., DNA methylation and acetylation) of histones or epigenesis contribute in part to tumorigenic potential for progression has already been translated into therapies. Histone acetyltransferases (HATs) and histone deacetyltransferases (HDACs) play antagonistic roles in the addition and removal of acetylation in the genome. Genome-wide analysis of HATs and HDACs is beginning to provide important insights into complex modes of gene regulation. Several inhibitors of histone deacetylases with a range of biochemical and biologic activities are being developed and tested as anticancer agents in clinical trial. Results of phase I clinical trials have suggested that these drugs are well tolerated. Inhibition of deacetylase remodels chromatin assembly and reactivates transcription of the genome. Because the mechanisms of actions of HDACs extend to apoptosis, cell cycle control, and cellular differentiation, current clinical trials are seeking to determine the efficacy of these novel reagents in the drug compendium for human cancers.

GENETIC SEQUENCE VARIATION, POPULATION DIVERSITY, AND GENETIC POLYMORPHISMS

A stable, heritable change in DNA is defined as a *mutation*. This strict contemporary definition does not depend on the functional relevance of the sequence alteration and implicates a change in the primary DNA sequence. Considered in a historical context, mutations were first defined on the basis of identifiable changes in the heritable phenotype of an organism. As biochemical phenotyping became more precise in the mid-20th century, investigators demonstrated that many proteins exist in more than one form in a population, and these forms were viewed as a consequence of variations in the gene coding for that protein (i.e., allelic variation). With advances in DNA-sequencing methods, the concept of mutation evolved from one that could be appreciated only by identifying differences in phenotype to one that could precisely be defined at the level of changes in the structure of DNA. Although most mutations are stably transmitted from parents to offspring, some are genetically lethal and cannot be passed on. The discovery of regions of the genome that contain sequences that repeat in tandem a highly variable number of times (i.e., tandem repeats) suggests that some mutations are less stable than others. These tandem repeats are further described later.

The molecular nature of mutations is varied (Table 1-1). A mutation can involve the deletion, insertion, or substitution of a single base, all of which are referred to as *point mutations*. Substitutions can be further classified as *silent* when the amino acid encoded by the mutated triplet does not change, as *missense* when the amino acid encoded by the mutated triplet changes, and as *nonsense* when the mutation leads to premature termination of translation (i.e., stop codon). Occasionally, point mutations can alter the processing of precursor mRNA by producing alternate splice sites or eliminating a splice site. When a single- or double-base deletion or insertion occurs in an exon, a frameshift mutation results, usually leading to premature termination of translation at a now in-frame stop codon. The other end of the spectrum of mutations includes large deletions of an entire gene or a set of contiguous genes; deletion, duplication, and translocation of a segment of one chromosome to another; or duplication or deletion of an entire chromosome. These chromosomal mutations play a large role in the development of many cancers.

Each individual possesses two alleles, one from each parent, for any given gene locus. Identical alleles define homozygosity and nonidentical alleles define heterozygosity for any gene locus. The heritability of these alleles follows typical mendelian rules. With a clearer understanding of the molecular basis of mutations and of allelic variation, their distribution in populations can be analyzed precisely by following specific DNA sequences.

TABLE 1-1	MOLECULAR BASIS OF MUTATIONS
TYPE	**EXAMPLES**
POINT MUTATIONS	
Deletion	α-Thalassemia, polycystic kidney disease
SUBSTITUTIONS	
Silent	Cystic fibrosis
Missense	Sickle cell anemia, polycystic kidney disease, congenital long QT syndrome
Nonsense	Cystic fibrosis, polycystic kidney disease
LARGE MUTATIONS (GENE OR GENE CLUSTER)	
Deletion	Duchenne's muscular dystrophy
Insertion	Factor VIII deficiency (hemophilia A)
Duplication	Duchenne's muscular dystrophy
Inversion	Factor VIII deficiency
Expanding triplet	Huntington's disease
VERY LARGE MUTATIONS (CHROMOSOMAL SEGMENT OR CHROMOSOME)	
Deletion	Turner's syndrome (45,X)
Duplication	Trisomy 21
Translocation	XX male [46,X; t(X;Y)]*

*Translocation onto an X chromosome of a segment of a Y chromosome that bears the locus for testicular differentiation.

Differences in DNA sequences studied within the context of a population are referred to as *genetic polymorphisms*, and these polymorphisms underlie the diversity observed within a given species and among species.

Despite the high prevalence of benign polymorphisms in a population, the occurrence of harmful mutations is rare because of selective pressures that eliminate the most harmful mutations from the population (i.e., lethality) and the variability within the genomic sequence in response to polymorphic change. Some portions of the genome are remarkably stable and free of polymorphic variation, whereas other portions are highly polymorphic, the persistence of variation within which is a consequence of the functional benignity of the sequence change. In other words, polymorphic differences in DNA sequence between individuals can be categorized as those producing no effect on phenotype, those causing benign differences in phenotype (i.e., normal genetic variation), and those producing adverse consequences in phenotype (i.e., mutations). The latter group can be further subdivided into the polymorphic mutations that alone are able to produce a functionally abnormal phenotype such as monogenic disease (e.g., sickle cell anemia) and those that alone are unable to do so but in conjunction with other mutations can produce a functionally abnormal phenotype (i.e., complex disease traits such as essential hypertension).

Polymorphisms are more common in noncoding regions of the genome than they are in coding regions, and one common type involves the tandem repetition of short DNA sequences a variable number of times. If these tandem repeats are long, they are called *variable number tandem repeats* (VNTRs); if the repeats are short, they are called *short tandem repeats* (STRs). During mitosis, the number of tandem repeats can change, and the frequency of this kind of replication error is high enough to make alternative lengths of the tandem repeats common in a population. However, the rate of change in length of the tandem repeats is low enough to make the size of the polymorphism useful as a stable genotypic trait in families, and polymorphic tandem repeats are useful in determining the familial heritability of specific genomic loci.

Polymorphic tandem repeats are sufficiently prevalent along the entire genomic sequence, enabling them to serve as genetic markers for specific genes of interest by analysis of their linkage to those genes during crossover and recombination events. Analyses of multiple genetic polymorphisms in the human genome (i.e., genotyping) reveal that a remarkable variation exists among individuals at the level of the sequence of genomic DNA. A single-nucleotide polymorphism (SNP), the most common variant, differs by a single base between chromosomes on a given stretch of DNA sequence (Fig. 1-5). From genotyping of the world's representative population, 10 million variants (i.e., one site per 300 bases) are estimated to make up 90% of the common SNP variants in the population, with the rare variants making up the remaining 10%. With each generation of a species, the frequency of polymorphic changes in a gene is 10^{-4} to 10^{-7}. In view of the number of genes in the human genome, between 0.5% and 1.0% of the base sequence of the human genome is polymorphic. In this context, the new variant can be traced historically to the surrounding alleles on the chromosomal background present at the time of the mutational event.

A haplotype is a specific set or combination of alleles on a chromosome or part of a chromosome (see Fig. 1-5). When parental chromosomes undergo crossover, new *mosaic* haplotypes that contain additional mutations are created from the recombination. SNP alleles within haplotypes can be co-inherited with other alleles in the population, a mechanism called *linkage disequilibrium* (LD). The association between two SNPs declines with increasing distance, enabling patterns of LD to be identified from the proximity of nearby SNPs. Conversely, a few well-selected SNPs are often sufficient to predict the location of other common variants in the region.

Haplotypes associated with a mutation are expected to become common by recombination in the general population over thousands of generations. In contrast, genetic mapping with LD departs from traditional mendelian genetics by using the entire human population as a large family tree without an established pedigree. Of the possible 10 million variants, the International HapMap Project and the Perlegen private venture have deposited more than 8 million variants comprising the public human SNP map from more than 341 people representing different population samples. The SNPs distributed across the genome of unrelated individuals provide a sufficiently robust sample set for statistical associations to be drawn between genotypes and modest phenotypes. A mutation is now defined as a specific type of allelic polymorphism that causes a functional defect in a cell or organism.

The causal relationship between monogenic diseases with well-defined phenotypes that co-segregate with the disease requires only a small number of affected individuals compared with unaffected control individuals. In contrast, complex disorders (e.g., diabetes, hypertension, cancer) necessitate the combinatorial effects of environmental factors and genes with subtle effects. Only by searching for variations in genetic frequency between patients and the general population can the causation of

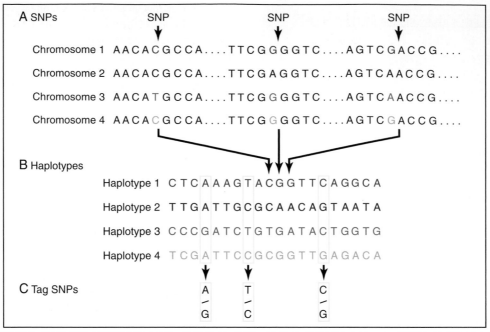

FIGURE 1-5 Single nucleotide polymorphisms (SNPs), haplotypes, and tag SNPs. Stretches of mostly identical DNA on the same chromosome are shown for four individuals. SNP refers to the variation of the three bases shown in a DNA region. The combination of nearby SNPs (**A**) defines a haplotype. Tag SNPs (**C**) are useful tools for genotyping four unique haplotypes from the 20 haplotypes (**B**). (Modified from International HapMap Consortium: The International HapMap Project, Nature 426:789–796, 2003.)

disease be discerned. In the postgenomic era, gene mapping entails the statistical association with the use of LD and high-density genetic maps that span thousands to 100,000 base pairs. To enable comprehensive association studies to become routine in clinical practice, inexpensive genotyping assays and denser maps with all common polymorphisms must be linked to all possible manifestations of the disease. Longitudinal studies of the HapMap and Perlegen cohorts can determine the effects of diet, exercise, environmental factors, and family history on future clinical events. Without similar approaches to securing adequate sample sizes and datasets, the promise of genetic population theory will not overcome the inherent limitations of linking human sequence variation with complex disease traits.

● GENE MAPPING AND THE HUMAN GENOME PROJECT

The process of gene mapping involves identifying the relative order and distance of specific loci along the genome. Maps can be of two types: genetic and physical. Genetic maps identify the genomic location of specific genetic loci by a statistical analysis based on the frequency of recombination events of the locus of interest with other known loci. Physical maps identify the genomic location of specific genetic loci by direct measurement of the distance along the genome at which the locus of interest is located in relation to one or more defined markers. The precise location of genes on a chromosome is important for defining the likelihood that a portion of one chromosome will interchange, or cross over, with the corresponding portion of its complementary chromosome when genetic recombination occurs during meiosis (Fig. 1-6).

During meiotic recombination, genetic loci or alleles that have been acquired from one parent interchange with those acquired from the other parent to produce new combinations of alleles, and the likelihood that alleles will recombine during meiosis varies as a function of their linear distance from one another in the chromosomal sequence. This recombination probability (i.e., distance) is commonly quantitated in centimorgan (cM) units; 1 cM is the chromosomal distance over which there is a 1% chance that two alleles will undergo a crossover event during meiosis. Crossover events serve as the basis for mixing parental base sequences during development, promoting genetic diversity among offspring. Analysis of the tendency for specific alleles to be inherited together indicates that the recombination distance in the human genome is about 3000 cM.

Identifying the gene or genes responsible for a specific polygenic disease phenotype requires an understanding of the topographic anatomy of the human genome, which is inextricably linked to interactions with the environment. The Human Genome Project, first proposed in 1985, represented an international effort to determine the complete nucleotide sequence of the human genome, including the construction of its detailed genetic, physical, and transcript maps, with identification and characterization of all genes. This foray into large-scale biology was championed by Nobel Laureate James Watson as the defining moment in his lifetime for witnessing the path from the double helix to the sequencing of 3 billion bases of the human genome, paving the way for understanding human evolution and harnessing the benefits for human health.

Among the earliest achievements of the Human Genome Project was the development of 1-cM resolution maps, each containing 3000 markers, and the identification of 52,000 sequenced tagged sites. For functional analysis on a genome-wide scale, major technologic advances were made, including as high-throughput oligonucleotide synthesis, normalized and subtracted complementary DNA (cDNA) libraries, and DNA microarrays.

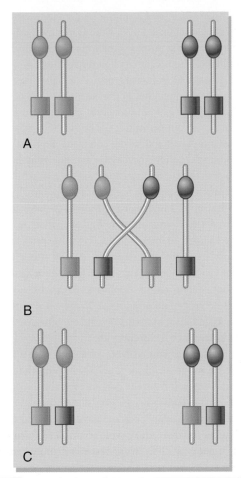

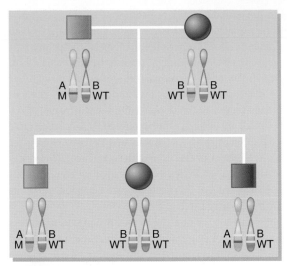

FIGURE 1-7 Linkage analysis. Analysis of the association (i.e., genomic contiguity) of a mutation *(M)* and a polymorphic allelic marker *(A)* shows close linkage in that the mutation segregates with the *A* allele, whereas the wild-type gene locus *(WT)* associates with the *B* allele.

In 1998, the Celera private venture proposed a goal similar to that of the Human Genome Project using a revolutionary approach, called *shotgun sequencing*, to determine the sequence of the human genome (http://www.dnai.org/c/index.html). The shotgun sequencing method was designed for random, large-scale sequencing and subsequent alignment of sequenced segments using computational and mathematic modeling. In the end, the Human Genome Project in collaboration with the Celera private venture produced a refined map of the entire human genome in 2001.

Because of the differences in genomic sequence that arise as a consequence of normal biologic variations or sequence polymorphisms, the resulting restriction fragment length polymorphisms (RFLPs) differ among individuals and are inherited according to mendelian principles. These polymorphisms can serve as genetic markers for specific loci in the genome. One of the most useful types of RFLP for localization of genetic loci in the genome is that produced by tandem repeats of sequence. Tandem repeats arise through *slippage* or stuttering of the DNA polymerase during replication in the case of STRs; longer variations arise through unequal crossover events. STRs are distributed throughout the genome and are highly polymorphic. These markers have

two different alleles at each locus that are derived from each parent; the origins of the two chromosomes can be discerned through this analysis.

The use of highly polymorphic tandem repeats that occur throughout the genome as genomic markers has provided a basis for mapping specific gene loci by establishing the association or linkage with select markers. Linkage analysis is predicated on a simple principle: the likelihood that a crossover event will occur during meiosis decreases the closer the locus of interest is to a given marker. The extent of genetic linkage can be ascertained for any group of loci, one of which may contain a disease-producing mutation (Fig. 1-7).

IDENTIFYING MUTANT GENES

Deducing the identity of a specific gene sequence thought to cause a specific human disease requires identification of mutations in the gene of interest. If the gene suspected to be responsible for the disease phenotype is known, its sequence can be determined by conventional cloning and sequencing strategies, and the mutation can be identified. A variety of techniques are available for detecting mutations. Mutations that involve insertion or deletion of large segments of DNA can be detected by Southern blot, in which the isolated DNA is annealed to a radioactively labeled fragment of a cDNA sequence. Prior incubation of the DNA with a specific restriction endonuclease cleaves the DNA sequence of interest at specific sites to produce smaller fragments that can be monitored by agarose gel electrophoresis. Shifts in mobility on the gel in comparison with wild-type sequence become apparent as a function of changes in the molecular size of the fragment. Alternatively, the polymerase chain reaction (PCR) can be used to identify mutations.

In the PCR approach, small oligonucleotides (20 to 40 bases long), which are complementary to regions of DNA that bracket the sequence of interest and are complementary to each strand of the double-stranded DNA, are synthesized and used as primers for the amplification of the DNA sequence of interest. These primers are added to the DNA solution. The temperature of the solution is increased to dissociate the individual DNA strands and is then reduced to permit annealing of the primers to their complementary template target sites. A thermostable DNA polymerase is included in the reaction to synthesize new DNA in the 5′ to 3′ direction from the primer annealing sites. The temperature is then increased to dissociate duplex structures, after which it is reduced, enabling another cycle of DNA synthesis to occur. Several temperature cycles (usually up to 40) are used to amplify progressively the concentration of the sequence of interest, which can be identified as a PCR product by agarose gel electrophoresis with a fluorescent dye. The product can be isolated and sequenced to identify the suggested mutation.

If the gene is large and the site of the mutation is unknown (especially if it is a point mutation), other methods can be used to identify the likely mutated site in the exonic sequence. A common approach involves scanning the gene sequence for mutations that alter the structural conformation of short complexes between parent DNA and PCR products, leading to a shift in mobility on a nondenaturing agarose gel (i.e., single-strand conformational polymorphism). A single-base substitution or deletion can change the conformation of the complex compared with wild-type complexes and yield a shift in mobility. Sequencing this comparatively small region of the gene facilitates precise identification of the mutation.

When the gene thought to cause the disease phenotype is unknown, when its likely position on the genome has not been identified, or when only limited mapping information is available, a candidate gene approach can be used to identify the mutated gene. In this strategy, potential candidate genes are identified on the basis of analogy to animal models or by analysis of known genes that map to the region of the genome for which limited information is available. The candidate gene is then analyzed for potential mutations. Regardless of the approach used, mutations identified in candidate genes should always be correlated with functional changes in the gene product because some mutations may be functionally silent, representing a polymorphism without phenotypic consequences. Functional changes in the gene product can be evaluated through the use of cell culture systems to assess protein function by expressing the mutant protein through transiently transfecting the cells with a vector that carries the cDNA coding for the gene of interest and incorporating the mutation of interest. Alternatively, unique animal models can be developed in which the mutant gene is incorporated in the male pronucleus of oocytes taken from a superovulating, impregnated female. This union produces an animal that overexpresses the mutant gene; it produces a transgenic animal, an animal with more than the usual number of copies of a given gene, or an animal in which the gene of interest is disrupted and the gene product is not synthesized (i.e., a gene *knockout* animal or an animal with one half [heterozygote] or none [homozygote] of the usual number of a given gene).

Molecular Diagnostics

The power of molecular techniques extends beyond their use in defining the precise molecular basis of an inherited disease. By exploiting the exquisite sensitivity of PCR to amplify rare nucleic acid sequences, it is possible to diagnose rapidly a range of infectious diseases for which unique sequences are available. In particular, infections caused by fastidious or slow-growing organisms can be rapidly diagnosed, similar to the case for *Mycobacterium tuberculosis*. The presence of genes conferring resistance to specific antibiotics in microorganisms can also be verified by PCR techniques. Sequencing of the entire genome of organisms such as *Escherichia coli*, *M. tuberculosis*, and *Treponema pallidum* offers unparalleled opportunities to monitor the epidemiologic structures of infections, follow the course of acquired mutations, tailor antibiotic therapies, and develop unique gene-based therapies (discussed later) for infectious agents for which conventional antibiotic therapies are ineffective or marginally effective.

The application of molecular methods to human genetics has revolutionized the field. Through the use of approaches that incorporate linkage analysis and PCR, point mutations can be precisely localized and characterized. At the other end of the spectrum of genetic changes that underlie disease, chromosomal translocations, deletions, or duplications can be identified by conventional cytogenetic methods. Large deletions that can incorporate many kilobase pairs and many genes can be visualized with fluorescence in situ hybridization (FISH), a technique in which a segment of cloned DNA is labeled with a fluorescent tag and hybridized to chromosomal DNA. With the deletion of the segment of interest from the genome, the chromosomal DNA fails to fluoresce in the corresponding chromosomal location.

Advances in molecular medicine have elucidated the mechanisms of carcinogenesis and revolutionized the diagnosis and treatment of neoplastic diseases. According to current views, a neoplasm arises from the clonal proliferation of a single cell that is transformed from a regulated, quiescent state into an unregulated growth phase. DNA damage accumulates in the parental tumor cell as a result of exogenous factors (e.g., radiation exposure) or heritable determinants. In early phases of carcinogenesis, certain genomic changes may impart intrinsic genetic instability that increases the likelihood of additional damage. One class of genes that becomes activated during carcinogenesis is oncogenes, which are primordial genes that normally exist in the mammalian genome in an inactive (proto-oncogene) state but, when activated, promote unregulated cell proliferation through specific intracellular signaling pathways.

Molecular methods based on the acquisition of specific tumor markers and unique DNA sequences that result from oncogenetic markers of larger chromosomal abnormalities (i.e., translocations or deletions that promote oncogenesis) are broadly applied to the diagnosis of malignancies. These methods can be used to establish the presence of specific tumor markers and oncogenes in biopsy specimens, to monitor the presence or persistence of circulating malignant cells after completion of a course of chemotherapy, and to identify the development of genetic resistance to specific chemotherapeutic agents. Through the use of conventional linkage analysis and candidate gene approaches, future studies will be able to identify individuals with a heritable predisposition to malignant transformation. Many of these topics are discussed in later chapters.

The advent of *gene chip* technologies or expression arrays has revolutionized molecular diagnostics and has begun to clarify the pathobiologic structures of complex diseases. These methods involve labeling the cDNA generated from the entire pool of mRNA isolated from a cell or tissue specimen with a radioactive or fluorescent marker and annealing this heterogeneous population of polynucleotides to a solid-phase substrate to which many different polynucleotides of known sequence are attached. The signals from the labeled cDNA strands bound to specific locations on the array are monitored, and the relative abundance of particular sequences is compared with that from a reference specimen. Using this approach, microarray patterns can be used as molecular fingerprints to diagnose a particular disease (i.e., type of malignancy and its susceptibility to treatment and prognosis) and to identify the genes whose expression increases or decreases in a specific disease state (i.e., identification of disease-modifying genes).

Many other applications of molecular medicine techniques are available in addition to those in infectious diseases and oncology. Molecular methods can be used to sort out genetic differences in metabolism that may modulate pharmacologic responses in a population of individuals (i.e., pharmacogenomics), address specific forensic issues such as paternity or criminal culpability, and approach epidemiologic analysis on a precise genetic basis.

Genes and Human Disease

Human genetic diseases can be divided into three broad categories: those caused by a mutation in a single gene (e.g., monogenic disorders, mendelian traits), those caused by mutations in more than one gene (e.g., polygenic disorders, complex disease traits), and those caused by chromosomal abnormalities (Table 1-2). In all three groups of disorders, environmental factors can contribute to the phenotypic expression of the disease by modulating gene expression or unmasking a biochemical abnormality that has no functional consequence in the absence of a stimulus or stress.

Classic monogenic disorders include sickle cell anemia, familial hypercholesterolemia, and cystic fibrosis. These genetic diseases can be exclusively produced by a single specific mutation (e.g., sickle cell anemia) or by any one of several mutations (e.g., familial hypercholesterolemia, cystic fibrosis) in a given family (i.e., Pauling paradigm). Some of these disorders evolved to protect the host. For example, sickle cell anemia evolved as

protection against *Plasmodium falciparum* malaria, and cystic fibrosis developed as protection against cholera. Examples of polygenic disorders or complex disease traits include type 1 (insulin-dependent) diabetes mellitus, atherosclerotic cardiovascular disease, and essential hypertension. A common example of a chromosomal disorder is the presence of an extra chromosome 21 (i.e., trisomy 21).

The overall frequency of monogenic disorders is about 1%. About 60% of these include polygenic disorders, which includes those with a genetic substrate that develops later in life. About 0.5% of monogenic disorders include chromosomal abnormalities. Chromosomal abnormalities are frequent causes of spontaneous abortion and malformations.

Contrary to the view held by early geneticists, few phenotypes are entirely defined by a single genetic locus. Monogenic disorders are comparatively uncommon; however, they are still useful as a means to understanding some basic principles of heredity. Three types of monogenic disorders occur: autosomal dominant, autosomal recessive, and X-linked. *Dominance* and *recessiveness* refer to the nature of the heritability of a genetic trait and correlate with the number of alleles affected at a given locus. If a mutation in a single allele determines the phenotype, the mutation is said to be dominant; that is, the heterozygous state conveys the clinical phenotype to the individual. If a mutation is necessary at both alleles to determine the phenotype, the mutation is said to be recessive; that is, only the homozygous state conveys the clinical phenotype to the individual. Dominant or recessive mutations can lead to a loss or a gain of function of the gene product. If the mutation is present on the X chromosome, it is defined as X-linked (which in males can, by definition, be viewed only as dominant); otherwise, it is autosomal.

The importance of identifying a potential genetic disease as inherited by one of these three mechanisms is that the disease must involve a single genomic abnormality that leads to an abnormality in a single protein. Classically identified genetic diseases are produced by mutations that affect coding (exonic) sequences. However, mutations in intronic and other untranslated regions of the genome occur that may disturb the function or expression of specific genes. Examples of diseases with these types of mutations include myotonic dystrophy and Friedreich ataxia.

An individual with a dominant monogenic disorder typically has one affected parent and a 50% chance of transmitting the mutation to his or her offspring. Men and women are equally likely to be affected and equally likely to transmit the trait to their offspring. The trait cannot be transmitted to offspring by two unaffected parents. In contrast, an individual with a recessive monogenic disorder typically has parents who are clinically normal. Affected parents, each heterozygous for the mutation, have a 25% chance of transmitting the clinical phenotype to their offspring but a 50% chance of transmitting the mutation to their offspring (i.e., producing an unaffected carrier).

Notwithstanding the clear heritability of common monogenic disorders (e.g., sickle cell anemia), the clinical expression of the disease in an individual with a phenotype expected to produce the disease may vary. *Variability in clinical expression* is defined as the range of phenotypic effects observed in individuals carrying a given mutation. *Penetrance* refers to a smaller subset of individuals with variable clinical expression of a mutation and is defined

TABLE 1-2 MOLECULAR BASIS OF MUTATIONS

TYPE	EXAMPLES
MONOGENIC DISORDERS	
Autosomal dominant	Polycystic kidney disease 1, neurofibromatosis 1
Autosomal recessive	β-Thalassemia, Gaucher's disease
X-linked	Hemophilia A, Emery-Dreifuss muscular dystrophy
One of multiple mutations	Familial hypercholesterolemia, cystic fibrosis
POLYGENIC DISORDERS	
Complex disease traits	Type 1 (insulin-dependent) diabetes, essential hypertension, atherosclerotic disease, cancer
CHROMOSOMAL ABNORMALITIES	
Deletions, duplications	Turner Syndrome (monosomy), Down Syndrome (Trisomy)

as the proportion of individuals with a given genotype who exhibit any clinical phenotypic features of the disorder.

Three principal determinants of variability in clinical expression or incomplete penetrance of a given genetic disorder can occur: environmental factors, the effects of other genetic loci, and random chance. Environmental factors can modulate disease phenotype by altering gene expression in several ways, including acting on transcription factors (e.g., transcription factors that are sensitive to cell redox state, such as nuclear factor-κB) or on *cis*-elements in gene promoters (e.g., folate-dependent methylation of CpG-rich regions) and post-translationally modifying proteins (e.g., lysine oxidation). That other genes can modify the effects of disease-causing mutations is a reflection of the overlay of genetic diversity on primary disease phenotype. Numerous examples exist of the effects of these *disease-modifying genes* producing phenotypic variations among individuals with the identical primary disease-causing mutations (i.e., gene-gene interactions) and the effects of disease-modifying genes interacting with environmental determinants to alter phenotype further (i.e., gene-environment interactions). These interactions are important in polygenic diseases; gene-gene and gene-environment interactions can modify the phenotypic expression of the disease. Among patients with sickle cell disease, for example, some experience painful crises, others exhibit acute chest syndrome, and still other presentations include hemolytic crises.

Genetic disorders affecting a unique pool of DNA, mitochondrial DNA, have been identified. Mitochondrial DNA is is inherited only from the mother. Mutations in mitochondrial DNA can vary among mitochondria within a given cell and within a given individual (i.e., heteroplasmy). Examples of disorders of the mitochondrial genome are Kearns-Sayre syndrome and Leber hereditary optic neuropathy. The list of known mitochondrial genomic disorders is growing rapidly, and mitochondrial contributions to a large number of common polygenic disorders may also exist.

Molecular Medicine

A principal goal of molecular strategies is to restore normal gene function to individuals with genetic mutations. Methods to do so are currently primitive, and a number of obstacles must be surmounted for this approach to be successful.

Delivering a complete gene into a cell is not easy, and persistent expression of the new gene cannot be ensured because of the variability in its incorporation in the genome and the consequent variability in its regulated expression. Many approaches have been used, but none has been completely successful. They include the following: (1) packaging the cDNA in a viral vector, such as an attenuated adenovirus, and using the cell's ability to take up the virus as a means for the cDNA to gain access to the cell; (2) delivering the cDNA by means of a calcium phosphate–induced perturbation of the cell membrane; and (3) encapsulating the cDNA in a liposome that can fuse with the cell membrane and thereby deliver the cDNA.

After the cDNA has been successfully delivered to the cell of interest, the magnitude and durability of expression of the gene product are important variables. The magnitude of expression is determined by the number of copies of cDNA taken up by a cell and the extent of their incorporation in the genome of the cell. The durability of expression appears to depend partly on the antigenicity of the sequence and protein product.

Notwithstanding these technical limitations, gene therapy has been used to treat adenosine deaminase deficiency successfully, which suggests that the principle on which the treatment is based is reasonable. Clinical trials of gene therapy slowed considerably after unexpected deaths were widely reported in the scientific and lay media. Efforts in other genetic disorders and as a means to induce expression of a therapeutic protein (e.g., vascular endothelial cell growth factor to promote angiogenesis in ischemic tissue) are ongoing.

Understanding the molecular basis of disease leads naturally to the identification of unique disease targets. Examples of this principle have led to the development of novel therapies for diseases that have been difficult to treat. Imatinib, a tyrosine kinase inhibitor that is particularly effective at blocking the action of the BCR-ABL kinase, is effective for the treatment of chronic-phase chronic myelogenous leukemia. Monoclonal antibody to tumor necrosis factor-α (infliximab) and soluble tumor necrosis factor-α receptor (etanercept) are prime examples of *biologic modifiers* that are effective in the therapy of chronic inflammatory disorders, including inflammatory bowel disease and rheumatoid arthritis. This approach to molecular therapeutics is rapidly expanding and holds great promise for improving the therapeutic armamentarium for a variety of diseases.

Beyond cancer-related categories (e.g., DNA, RNA repair), gene expression arrays have identified additional interactions of regulatory pathways of clinical interest. The limitation of gene expression profiling using microarrays, which does not account for post-transcriptional and other post-translational modifications of protein-coding products, will likely be overcome by advances in proteomics. Such processes by signaling networks tend to amplify or attenuate gene expression on time scales lasting seconds to weeks. Much work remains to improve current knowledge about the pathways that initiate and promote tumors. The basic pathways and nodal points of regulation will be identified for rational drug design and targets from mechanistic insights gleaned from expression profiling of cultured cell lines, from small animal models of human disease, and from human samples. Although accounting for tissue heterogeneity and variation among different cell types, the new systems' approach for incorporating genomic and computational research appears particularly promising for deciphering the pathways that promote tumorigenesis. Biologists and clinicians will use information derived from these tools to understand the events that promote survival, proangiogenesis, and immune escape, all of which may confer metastatic potential and progression.

What potential diagnostic tools are available to establish genetic determinants of drug response? Genome-wide approaches from the Human Genome Project in combination with microarrays, proteomic analysis, and bioinformatics will identify multiple genes encoding drug targets (e.g., receptors). Similar high-throughput screening should provide insights into the predisposition to adverse effects or outcomes from treatments that are linked to genetic polymorphisms.

Genome Editing

Improvements of genome editing tools are revolutionizing the ability of researchers to make precision changes in the genomes of stem cells from humans, facilitating the fast and cost-effective production of genetically engineered animals (e.g., mouse and rat) and human cells. The clustered regularly interspaced short palindromic repeats (CRISPR) pathway was first discovered in bacteria, in which it provides an immunologic memory of previous viral infection.

Along with CRISPR-associated protein 9 (Cas9) and guide RNA (gRNA), this relatively simple prokaryotic system has been shown to function as an efficient site-specific nuclease with low off-targeting effects at recognition sequences in mammalian cells. From dermal fibroblasts of an affected organism or patient, for example, we can generate induced pluripotent stem cells (iPSCs) used for the differentiation of iPSC-derived cardiomyocytes or skeletal muscle, or both. Correction of the mutation involves a co-targeting strategy in which a selection cassette capable of the zinc finger–stimulated homologous recombination is targeted to the affected locus at the same time as the mutation is corrected. The CRISPR system is increasingly being used to target a variety of mammalian loci of stem cells and functionality of this targeting vector containing an excisable piggyback construct, allowing the stem cells to be gene corrected "without a trace."

Pharmacogenetics

The future of pharmacogenetics is to know all the factors that influence adverse drug effects. In this way, the premature abandonment of special drug classes can be avoided in favor of rational drug design and therapy.

Many hurdles must be overcome for pharmacogenetics to become more widespread and to be integrated into medical practice. Current approaches of trial and error in medical practice are well engrained, but the allure of blockbuster drugs produced by the pharmaceutical industry warrants a new model for approaching individualized doses. Training for physicians in molecular biology and genetics should complement clinical pharmacogenomic studies that determine efficacy in an era of evidence-based medicine. Pharmacogenetic polymorphisms, unlike other clinical variables such as renal function, need only a single test, ideally performed for newborns.

Polygenic models of therapeutic optimization still face hurdles that reduce the chances for abuse of genetic information and additional costs. However, SNP haplotyping has the potential to identify genetically similar subgroups of the population and to randomize therapies based on more robust genetic markers. On a population level, genomic variability is much greater within than among distinct racial and ethnic groups.

Therapeutic efficacy and host toxicity are influenced by the patient's specific disease, age, renal function, nutritional status, and other comorbid factors. New challenges will be posed for the selection of drug therapy for patients with cancer, hypertension, and diabetes. Treatment of multisystem disorders (e.g., metabolic syndrome) may be derived from novel therapeutics based on individual, interacting, and complementary molecular pathways.

Regenerative Medicine

Regenerative medicine entails the uses of novel applications and approaches to repair damaged cells or tissues with the anticipated full restoration of normal function. By harnessing the compendium of biologics, drugs, medical devices, and cell-based therapies, this emerging field represents the convergence of multiple disciplines that integrate tissue engineering, stem cell biology, biomaterials, and gene therapy. Over 50 years, the transplantation of solid organs such as corneas, hearts, lungs, kidneys, and living-donor livers has become a well-established medical-surgical intervention, but the limited availability of organs restricts widespread applications. Tissue-engineered grafts for skin replacement of wounds after burns and diabetic foot ulcers are the antecedent strategies for the use of a patient's own cells, grown outside the body, to ultimately replace a bladder or vascular grafts used for bypass surgery.

A new era of regenerative biology has emerged with the discoveries by James Thompson that human embryonic stem cells can be cultured in a Petri dish and by Shinya Yamanaka that adult mammalian cells can be reprogrammed to become iPSCs. The iPSCs share the common features of somatic cell reprogramming but with the aid of one to four transcription factors. Embryonic stem (ES) cells share common features of clonagenicity, self-renewal, and multipotentiality, a prerequisite for differentiation into diverse cell lineages of multicellular adult organism. Technical and ethical concerns propelled the search for new sources, including the isolation of ES cells from a single blastomere, which circumvents destruction of the embryo, and the use of postimplantation embryos as ES cell donors. Somatic cell nuclear transplantation (SCNT) or nuclear transfer is a technique for successful cloning and reprogramming of adult animal cell nuclei from healthy oocyte host cells. SCNT provides a source of stem cells tailored to the donor organism and promises to accelerate the pace for human use. Because stem and precursor cells can be obtained from a variety of sources (e.g., embryos, adult tissues), their manipulation and transplantation in animal models and pilot human studies are increasingly providing alternative and complementary strategies to solid organ transplantation, thereby expanding the platform for regenerative medicine.

Previous dogmas that postmitotic, terminally differentiated organs are devoid of regenerative capacity have been overturned by evidence for cellular plasticity and low-level regeneration of adult solid organs throughout adult life. Age, gender, disease status, and other risk factors influence cellular regenerative plasticity, proliferation, and cellular functions.

Can progenitor cells derived from bone marrow or circulating blood be administered safely and efficaciously? Clinical and translational scientists are actively pursuing clinical trials to address whether stem cell therapy has efficacy for the victims of stroke, heart attack, and spinal cord injury. Given the large investments from federal, state, and private agencies, there have been concerns raised about the claims of stem cell therapy to engender false hopes. Notwithstanding, stem cell transplantation of bone marrow has become the standard of care for several blood dyscrasias, and new combinatorial strategies are in clinical trials. Beyond the questions of feasibility related to benefits from transplantation originating from embryonic, fetal, or adult stem cell lineages, the era of large-scale clinical trials will be increasingly challenged as precision medicine that tailors therapy to the individual's genome and disease profile enters the clinic.

SUGGESTED READINGS

Cheng H, Force T: Why do kinase inhibitors cause cardiotoxicity and what can be done about it? Prog Cardiovasc Dis 53:114–120, 2010.

Collins FS, Green ED, Guttmacher AE: A vision for the future of genomics research, Nature 422:835–847, 2003.

Evans WE, McLeod HL: Pharmacogenomics: drug disposition, drug targets, and side effects, N Engl J Med 348:538–549, 2003.

Kim H, Kim JS: A guide to genome engineering with programmable nucleases, Nat Rev Genet 15:321–334, 2014.

Orlando G, Wood KJ, Stratta RJ, et al: Regenerative medicine and organ transplantation: past, present, and future, Transplantation 91:1310–1317, 2011.

Willard HF, Ginsburg GS, editors: Genomic and personalized medicine, New York, 2009, Elsevier.

Zamore PD, Haley B: Ribo-gnome: the big world of small RNAs, Science 309:1519–1524, 2005.

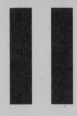

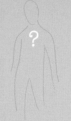
ESSENTIALS

Cardiovascular Disease

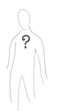

Structure and Function of the Normal Heart and Blood Vessels

Nicole L. Lohr and Ivor J. Benjamin

DEFINITION

The circulatory system comprises the heart, which is connected in series to the arterial and venous vascular networks, which are arranged in parallel and connect at the level of the capillaries (Fig. 2-1). The heart is composed of two atria, which are low-pressure capacitance chambers that function to store blood during ventricular contraction (systole) and then fill the ventricles with blood during ventricular relaxation (diastole). The two ventricles are high-pressure chambers responsible for pumping blood through the lungs (right ventricle) and to the peripheral tissues (left ventricle). The left ventricle is thicker than the right, in order to generate the higher systemic pressures required for perfusion.

There are four cardiac valves that facilitate unidirectional blood flow through the heart. Each of the four valves is surrounded by a fibrous ring, or annulus, that forms part of the structural support of the heart. Atrioventricular (AV) valves separate the atria and ventricles. The mitral valve is a bileaflet valve that separates the left atrium and left ventricle. The tricuspid valve is a trileaflet valve that separates the right atrium and right ventricle. Strong chords (chordae tendineae) attach the ventricular aspects of these valves to the papillary muscles of their respective ventricles. Semilunar valves separate the ventricles from the arterial chambers: the aortic valve separates the left ventricle from the aorta, and the pulmonic valve separates the right ventricle from the pulmonary artery.

A thin, double-layered membrane called the pericardium surrounds the heart. The inner, or visceral, layer adheres to the outer surface of the heart, also known as the epicardium. The outer layer is the parietal pericardium, which attaches to the sternum, vertebral column, and diaphragm to stabilize the heart in the chest. Between these two membranes is a pericardial space filled with a small amount of fluid (<50 mL). This fluid serves to lubricate contact surfaces and limit direct tissue-surface contact during myocardial contraction. A normal pericardium exerts minimal external pressure on the heart, thereby facilitating normal movement of the interventricular septum during the cardiac cycle. Too much fluid in this space (i.e., pericardial effusion), can cause impaired ventricular filling and abnormal septal movement. Please refer to Chapter 77, "Pericardial Diseases," in *Goldman-Cecil Medicine*, 25th Edition.

CIRCULATORY PATHWAY

The purpose of the circulatory system is to bring deoxygenated blood, carbon dioxide, and other waste products from the tissues to the lungs for disposal and reoxygenation (see Fig. 2-1A). Deoxygenated blood drains from peripheral tissues through venules and veins, eventually entering the right atrium through the superior and inferior venae cavae during ventricular systole. Venous drainage from the heart enters the right atrium through the coronary sinus. During ventricular diastole, the blood in the right atrium flows across the tricuspid valve and into the right ventricle. Blood in the right ventricle is ejected across the pulmonic valve and into the main pulmonary artery, which bifurcates into the left and right pulmonary arteries and perfuses the lungs. After multiple bifurcations, blood reaches the pulmonary capillaries, where carbon dioxide is exchanged for oxygen across the alveolar-capillary membrane. Oxygenated blood then enters the left atrium from the lungs via the four pulmonary veins. Blood flows across the open mitral valve and into the left ventricle during diastole and is ejected across the aortic valve and into the aorta during systole. The blood reaches various organs, where oxygen and nutrients are exchanged for carbon dioxide and metabolic wastes, and the cycle begins again.

The heart receives its blood supply through the left and right coronary arteries, which originate in outpouchings of the aortic root called the *sinuses of Valsalva*. The left main coronary artery is a short vessel that bifurcates into the left anterior descending (LAD) and the left circumflex (LCx) coronary arteries. The LAD supplies blood to the anterior and anterolateral left ventricle through diagonal branches and to the anterior interventricular septum through septal perforator branches. The LAD travels anteriorly in the anterior interventricular groove and terminates at the cardiac apex. The LCx traverses posteriorly in the left AV groove (between left atrium and left ventricle) to perfuse the lateral aspect of the left ventricle (through obtuse marginal branches) and the left atrium. The right coronary artery (RCA) courses down the right AV groove to the *crux* of the heart, the point at which the left and right AV grooves and the inferior interventricular groove meet. The RCA gives off branches to the right atrium and acute marginal branches to the right ventricle.

The blood supply to the diaphragmatic and posterior aspects of the left ventricle varies. In 85% of individuals, the RCA bifurcates at the crux to form the posterior descending coronary artery (PDA), which travels in the inferior interventricular groove to supply the inferior left ventricule and the inferior third of the interventricular septum, and the posterior left ventricular (PLV) branches. This course is termed a *right-dominant circulation*. In 10% of individuals, the RCA terminates before reaching the crux, and the LCx supplies the PLV and PDA. This course is termed a *left-dominant circulation*. In the remaining individuals, the RCA

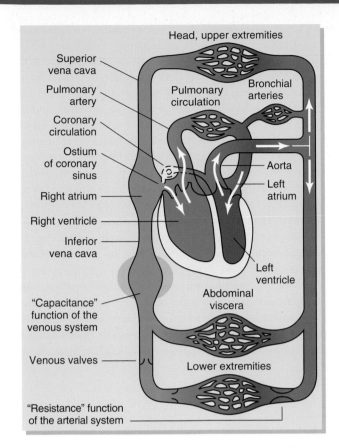

A

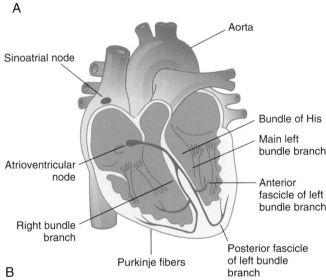

B

FIGURE 2-1 **A,** Schematic representation of the systemic and pulmonary circulatory systems. The venous system contains the greatest amount of blood at any one time and is highly distensible, accommodating a wide range of blood volumes (high capacitance). The arterial system is composed of the aorta, arteries, and arterioles. Arterioles are small muscular arteries that regulate blood pressure by changing tone (resistance). **B,** A schematic representation of the cardiac conduction system.

gives rise to the PDA and the LCx gives rise to the PLV in a *co-dominant circulation.*

CONDUCTION SYSTEM

The sinoatrial (SA) node is a collection of specialized pacemaker cells, 1 to 2 cm long, that is located in the right atrium between

the superior vena cava and the right atrial appendage (see Fig. 2-1B). The SA node is supplied by the SA nodal artery, which is a branch of the RCA in about 60% of the population and a branch of the LCx in about 40%. An electrical impulse originates in the SA and is conducted to the AV node by internodal tracts within the atria.

The AV node is a critical electrical interface between the atria and ventricles, because it facilitates electromechanical coupling. The AV node is a located at the inferior aspect of the right atrium, between the coronary sinus and the septal leaflet of the tricuspid valve. The AV node is supplied by the AV nodal artery, which is a branch of the RCA in about 90% of the population and a branch of the LCx in 10%. Electrical impulse conduction slows through the AV node and continues to the ventricles by means of the His-Purkinje system. The increased impulse time through the AV node allows for adequate ventricular filling.

The bundle of His extends from the AV node down the membranous interventricular septum to the muscular septum, where it divides into the left and right bundle branches, finally terminating in Purkinje cells, which are specialized cells that facilitate the rapid propagation of electrical impulses. The Purkinje cells directly stimulate myocytes to contract. The right bundle and the left bundle are supplied by septal perforator branches from the LAD. The distal and posterior portion of the left bundle has an additional blood supply from the AV nodal artery (PDA origin); for that reason, it is more resistant to ischemia. Conduction can be impaired at any point, from ischemia, medications (e.g., β-blockers, calcium channel blockers), infection, or congenital abnormalities. Please refer to Chapter 61, "Principles of Electrophysiology," in *Goldman-Cecil Medicine*, 25th Edition.

NEURAL INNERVATION

The autonomic nervous system is an integral component in the regulation of cardiac function. In general, sympathetic stimulation increases the heart rate (HR) (chronotropy) and the force of myocardial contraction (inotropy). Sympathetic stimulation commences in preganglionic neurons located within the superior five or six thoracic segments of the spinal cord. They synapse with second-order neurons in the cervical sympathetic ganglia and then propagate the signal through cardiac nerves that innervate the SA node, AV node, epicardial vessels, and myocardium. The parasympathetic system produces an opposite physiologic effect by decreasing HR and contractility. Its neural supply originates in preganglionic neurons within the dorsal motor nucleus of the medulla oblongata, which reach the heart through the vagus nerve. These efferent neural fibers synapse with second-order neurons located in ganglia within the heart which terminate in the SA node, AV node, epicardial vessels, and myocardium to decrease HR and contractility. Conversely, afferent vagal fibers from the inferior and posterior aspects of the ventricles, the aortic arch, and the carotid sinus conduct sensory information back to the medulla, which mediates important cardiac reflexes.

MYOCARDIUM

The proper cellular organization of cardiac tissue (myocardium) is critical for the generation of efficient myocardial contraction. Disruptions in this structure and organization lead to cardiac dyssynchrony and arrhythmias, which cause significant morbidity and mortality. Atrial and ventricular myocytes are specialized, branching muscle cells that are connected end to end by intercalated disks. These disks aid in the transmission of mechanical tension between cells. The myocyte plasma membrane, or sarcolemma, facilitates excitation and contraction through small transverse tubules (T tubules). Subcellular features specific for myocytes include increased mitochondria number for production of adenosine triphosphate (ATP); an extensive network of intracellular tubules, called the *sarcoplasmic reticulum*, for calcium storage; and *sarcomeres*, which are myofibrils comprised of repeating units of overlapping thin actin filaments and thick myosin filaments and their regulatory proteins troponin and tropomyosin. Specialized myocardial cells form the cardiac conduction system (described earlier) and are responsible for the generation of an electrical impulse and organized propagation of that impulse to cardiac myocytes, which, in turn, respond by mechanical contraction.

MUSCLE PHYSIOLOGY AND CONTRACTION

Calcium-induced calcium release is the primary mechanism for myocyte contraction. When a depolarizing stimulus reaches the myocyte, it enters special invaginations within the sarcolemma called T tubules. Specialized channels open in response to depolarization, permitting calcium flux into the cell (Fig. 2-2). The sarcoplasmic reticulum is in close proximity to the T tubules, and the initial calcium current triggers the release of large amounts of calcium from the sarcoplasmic reticulum into the cell cytosol. Calcium then binds to the calcium-binding regulatory subunit, troponin C, on the actin filaments of the sarcomere, resulting in a conformational change in the troponin-tropomyosin complex. The myosin binding site on actin is now exposed, to facilitate binding of actin-myosin cross-bridges, which are necessary for cellular contraction. The energy for myocyte contraction is derived from ATP. During contraction, ATP promotes dissociation of myosin from actin, thereby permitting the sliding of thick filaments past thin filaments as the sarcomere shortens.

The force of myocyte contraction is regulated by the amount of free calcium released into the cell by the sarcoplasmic reticulum. More calcium allows for more frequent actin-myosin interactions, producing a stronger contraction. On repolarization of the sarcolemmal membrane, intracellular calcium is rapidly and

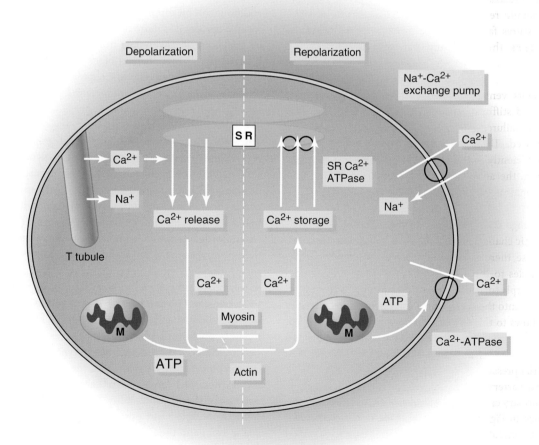

FIGURE 2-2 Calcium dependence of myocardial contraction. (1) Electrical depolarization of the myocyte results in an influx of Ca^{2+} ions into the cell through channels in the T tubules. (2) This initial phase of calcium entry stimulates the release of large amounts of Ca^{2+} from the sarcoplasmic reticulum (SR). (3) The Ca^{2+} then binds to the troponin-tropomyosin complex on the actin filaments, resulting in a conformational change that facilitates the binding interaction between actin and myosin. In the presence of adenosine triphosphate (ATP), the actin-myosin association is cyclically dissociated as the thick and thin filaments slide past each other, resulting in contraction. (4) During repolarization, the Ca^{2+} is actively pumped out of the cytosol and sequestered in the SR. ATPase, Adenosine triphosphatase; M, mitochondrion.

actively resequestered into the sarcoplasmic reticulum, where it is stored by various proteins, including calsequestrin, until the next wave of depolarization occurs. Calcium is also extruded from the cytosol by various calcium pumps in the sarcolemma. The active removal of intracellular calcium by ATP ion pumps facilitates ventricular relaxation, which is necessary for proper ventricular filling during diastole.

Circulatory Physiology and the Cardiac Cycle

The term *cardiac cycle* describes the pressure changes within each cardiac chamber over time (Fig. 2-3). This cycle is divided into *systole*, the period of ventricular contraction, and *diastole*, the period of ventricular relaxation. Each cardiac valve opens and closes in response to pressure gradients generated during these periods. At the onset of systole, ventricular pressures exceeds atrial pressures, so the AV valves passively close. As myocytes contract, the intraventricular pressures rise initially, without a change in ventricular volume (isovolumic contraction), until they exceed the pressures in the aorta and pulmonary artery. At this point, the semilunar valves open, and ventricular ejection of blood occurs. When intracellular calcium levels fall, ventricular relaxation begins; arterial pressures exceed intraventricular pressures, so the semilunar valves close. Ventricular relaxation initially does not change ventricular volume (isovolumic relaxation). At the point at which intraventricular pressures fall below atrial pressures, the AV valves open. This begins the rapid and passive ventricular filling phase of diastole, during which blood in the atria empties into the ventricles. At the end of diastole, active atrial contraction augments ventricular filling. When the myocardium exhibits increased stiffness due to age, hypertension, diabetes, or systolic heart failure, the early passive phase of ventricular filling is decreased. The end result is reliance on atrial contraction to sufficiently fill the ventricle during diastole. In atrial fibrillation, the atrium does not contract; patients often have worse symptoms because this additional ventricular filling is lost.

Pressure tracings obtained from the periphery complement the hemodynamic changes exhibited in the heart. In the absence of valvular disease, there is no impediment to blood flow moving from the ventricles to the arterial beds, so the systolic arterial pressure rises sharply to a peak. During diastole, no further blood volume is ejected into the aorta, so the arterial pressure gradually falls as blood flows to the distal tissue beds and elastic recoil of the arteries occurs.

Atrial pressure can be directly measured in the right atrium, but the left atrial pressure is indirectly measured by occluding a small pulmonary artery branch and measuring the pressure distally (the pulmonary capillary *wedge* pressure). An atrial pressure tracing is shown in Figure 2-3. It is composed of several waves. The *a wave* represents atrial contraction. As the atria subsequently relax, the atrial pressure falls, and the *x descent* is seen on the pressure tracing. The x descent is interrupted by a small *c wave*, which is generated as the AV valve bulges toward the atrium during ventricular systole. As the atria fill from venous return, the *v wave* is seen, after which the *y descent* appears as the AV valves open and blood from the atria empties into the ventricles. The normal ranges of pressures in the various cardiac chambers are shown in Table 2-1.

Cardiac Performance

The amount of blood ejected by the heart each minute is referred to as the cardiac output (CO). It is the product of the stroke volume (SV), which is the amount of blood ejected with each ventricular contraction, and the HR:

$$CO = SV \times HR$$

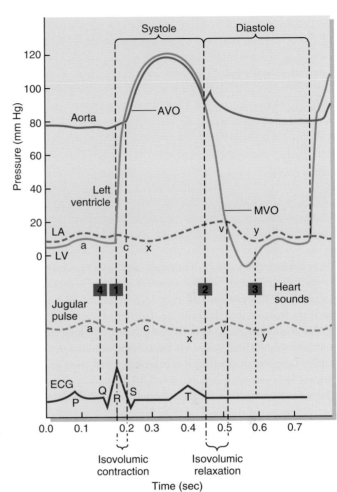

FIGURE 2-3 Simultaneous electrocardiogram (ECG) and pressure tracings obtained from the left atrium (LA), left ventricle (LV), and aorta and the jugular venous pressure during the cardiac cycle. (For simplification, pressures on the right side of the heart have been omitted. Normal right atrial (RA) pressure closely parallels that of the LA, and right ventricular and pulmonary artery pressures are timed closely with their corresponding left-sided counterparts; they are reduced only in magnitude. Normally, closure of the mitral and aortic valves precedes closure of the tricuspid and pulmonic valves; whereas valve opening reverses this order. The jugular venous pulse lags behind the RA pulse.) During the course of one cardiac cycle, the electrical (ECG) events initiate and therefore precede the mechanical (pressure) events, and the latter precede the auscultatory events (heart sounds) that they themselves produce *(red boxes)*. Shortly after the P wave, the atria contract to produce the a wave. The QRS complex initiates ventricular systole, followed shortly by LV contraction and the rapid buildup of LV pressure. Almost immediately, LV pressure exceeds LA pressure, closing the mitral valve and producing the first heart sound. After a brief period of isovolumic contraction, LV pressure exceeds aortic pressure and the aortic valve opens (AVO). When the ventricular pressure once again falls to less than the aortic pressure, the aortic valve closes to produce the second heart sound and terminate ventricular ejection. The LV pressure decreases during the period of isovolumic relaxation until it drops below LA pressure and the mitral valve opens (MVO). See text for further details.

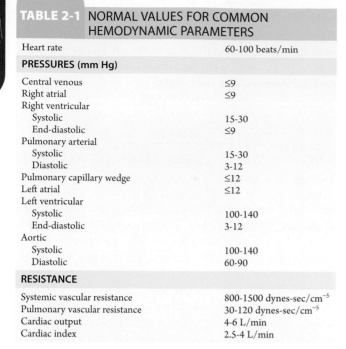

TABLE 2-1	NORMAL VALUES FOR COMMON HEMODYNAMIC PARAMETERS
Heart rate	60-100 beats/min
PRESSURES (mm Hg)	
Central venous	≤9
Right atrial	≤9
Right ventricular	
Systolic	15-30
End-diastolic	≤9
Pulmonary arterial	
Systolic	15-30
Diastolic	3-12
Pulmonary capillary wedge	≤12
Left atrial	≤12
Left ventricular	
Systolic	100-140
End-diastolic	3-12
Aortic	
Systolic	100-140
Diastolic	60-90
RESISTANCE	
Systemic vascular resistance	800-1500 dynes-sec/cm^{-5}
Pulmonary vascular resistance	30-120 dynes-sec/cm^{-5}
Cardiac output	4-6 L/min
Cardiac index	2.5-4 L/min

The cardiac index is a way of normalizing the CO to body size. It is the CO divided by the body surface area and is measured in L/min/m^2. The normal CO is 4 to 6 L/min at rest and can increase fourfold to sixfold during strenuous exercise.

The main determinants of SV are preload, afterload, and contractility (Table 2-2). *Preload* is the volume of blood in the ventricle at the end of diastole; it is primarily a reflection of venous return. Venous return is determined by the plasma volume and the venous compliance. Clinically, intravenous fluids increase preload, whereas diuretics or venodilators such as nitroglycerin decrease preload. When the preload is increased, the ventricle stretches, and the ensuing ventricular contraction becomes more rapid and forceful, because the increased sarcomere length facilitates actin and myosin cross-bridge kinetics by means of an increased sensitivity of troponin C to calcium. This phenomenon is known as the Frank-Starling relationship. Ventricular filling pressure (ventricular end-diastolic pressure, atrial pressure, or pulmonary capillary wedge pressure) is frequently used as a surrogate measure of preload.

Afterload is the force against which the ventricles must contract to eject blood. The main determinants of afterload are the arterial pressure and the dimensions of the left ventricle. As the arterial blood pressure increases, the amount of blood that can be ejected into the aorta decreases. Wall stress, an often overlooked determinant of afterload, is directly proportional to the size of the ventricular cavity and inversely proportional to the ventricular wall thickness (Laplace's law). Therefore, ventricular wall hypertrophy is a compensatory mechanism to reduce afterload. Drugs such as angiotensin-converting enzyme (ACE) inhibitors and hydralazine reduce blood pressure (BP) by reducing afterload. Diuretics decrease left ventricular volume and size, which can reduce wall stress–mediated afterload.

Contractility, or inotropy, represents the force of ventricular contraction in the presence of constant preload and afterload. Inotropy is regulated at a cellular level through stimulation of

TABLE 2-2	FACTORS AFFECTING CARDIAC PERFORMANCE
PRELOAD (LEFT VENTRICULAR DIASTOLIC VOLUME)	

Total blood volume
Venous (sympathetic) tone
Body position
Intrathoracic and intrapericardial pressures
Atrial contraction
Pumping action of skeletal muscle

AFTERLOAD (IMPEDANCE AGAINST WHICH THE LEFT VENTRICLE MUST EJECT BLOOD)

Peripheral vascular resistance
Left ventricular volume (preload, wall tension)
Physical characteristics of the arterial tree (elasticity of vessels or presence of outflow obstruction)

CONTRACTILITY (CARDIAC PERFORMANCE INDEPENDENT OF PRELOAD OR AFTERLOAD)

Sympathetic nerve impulses
Increased contractility
Circulating catecholamines
Digitalis, calcium, other inotropic agents
Increased heart rate or post-extrasystolic augmentation
Anoxia, acidosis
Decreased contractility
Pharmacologic depression
Loss of myocardium
Intrinsic depression

HEART RATE

Autonomic nervous system
Temperature, metabolic rate
Medications, drugs

cathecholminergic (epinephrine, norepinephrine, and dopamine) receptors, intracellular signaling cascades (phosphodiesterase inhibitors), and intracellular calcium levels (affected by levosimendan and, indirectly, by digoxin). Many antihypertensive medications (e.g., β-blockers, calcium channel antagonists) interfere with adrenergic receptor activation or intracellular calcium levels, which can decrease the strength of ventricular contractions. Please refer to Chapter 53, "Cardiac Function and Circulatory Control," in *Goldman-Cecil Medicine*, 25th Edition.

Physiology of the Coronary Circulation

The normally functioning heart maintains equilibrium between the amount of oxygen delivered to myocytes and the amount of oxygen consumed by them (myocardial oxygen consumption, or Mvo_2). If a myocyte works harder because it is contracting with increased frequency (HR), with increased intensity (contractility), or against an increased load (wall stress), then it will use more oxygen and its Mvo_2 will increase. In order to meet this increase in demand for more oxygen, the heart will have to either increase blood flow or increase its efficiency in extracting oxygen. The heart is unique in that its oxygen extraction is almost maximal at resting conditions. Therefore, increasing blood flow is the only reasonable means of increasing oxygen supply.

Microvascular blood flow in the coronary circulation is impaired during systole because the intramyocardial blood vessels are compressed by contracting myocardium. Therefore, most coronary flow occurs during diastole. Accordingly, the diastolic pressure is the major pressure driving flow within the coronary circulation. Systolic pressure impedes intramyocardial arterial blood flow but augments venous flow. On a clinical note, tachycardia is particularly detrimental because coronary flow is reduced when the diastolic filling time is abbreviated, and the Mvo_2 increases with increasing HR. In order to sustain constant perfusion to the myocardium, coronary blood flow is maintained constant over a wide range of pressures in a process called autoregulation.

In response to a change in Mvo_2, the coronary arteries dilate or constrict, which changes the vascular resistance and thereby appropriately changes flow. This regulation of arterial resistance occurs at the arterioles and is mediated by several factors. Adenosine, a metabolite of ATP, is released during contraction and acts as a potent vasodilator. Other consequences of myocardial metabolism, such as decreased oxygen tension, increased carbon dioxide, acidosis, and hyperkalemia, also mediate coronary vasodilation. The endothelium produces several potent vasodilators, including nitric oxide and prostacyclin. Nitric oxide is released by the endothelium in response to acetylcholine, thrombin, adenosine diphosphate (ADP), serotonin, bradykinin, platelet aggregation, and an increase in shear stress (called *flow-dependent vasodilation*). Finally, the coronary arteries are innervated by the autonomic nervous system, and activation of sympathetic neurons mediates vasoconstriction or vasodilation through α- or β-receptors, respectively. Parasympathetic neurons from the vagus nerve secrete acetylcholine, which mediates vasodilation. Vasoconstricting factors, notably endothelin, are produced by the endothelium and may be important in conditions such as coronary vasospasm. Please refer to Chapter 53, "Cardiac Function and Circulatory Control," in *Goldman-Cecil Medicine*, 25th Edition.

Physiology of the Systemic Circulation

The normal cardiovascular system delivers appropriate blood flow to each organ of the body under a wide range of conditions. This regulation is achieved by maintaining BP through adjustments in cardiac output and tissue blood flow resistance by neural and humoral factors.

Poiseuille's law generally describes the relationship between pressure and flow in a vessel. Fluid flow (F) through a tube is proportional (proportionality constant = K) to the pressure (P) difference between the ends of the tube:

$$F = K \times \Delta P$$

K is equivalent to the inverse of resistance to flow (R); that is, $K = 1/R$. Resistance to flow is determined by the properties of both the fluid and the tube. In the case of a steady, streamlined flow of fluid through a rigid tube, Poiseuille found that these factors determine resistance:

$$R = 8\eta L / \pi r^4$$

Where r is the radius of the tube, L is its length, and η is the viscosity of the fluid. Notice that changes in radius have greater influence than changes in length, because resistance is inversely proportional to the fourth power of the radius. Poiseuille's law incorporates the factors influencing flow, so that:

$$F = \Delta P / R = \Delta P \pi r^4 / 8\eta L$$

Therefore, the most important determinants of blood flow in the cardiovascular system are ΔP and r^4. Small changes in arterial radius can cause large changes in flow to a tissue or organ. Practically, systemic vascular resistance (SVR) is the total resistance to flow caused by changes in the radius of resistance vessels (small arteries and arterioles) of the systemic circulation. The SVR can be calculated as the pressure drop across the peripheral capillary beds (mean arterial pressure − right atrial pressure) divided by the blood flow across the beds (i.e., SVR = BP/CO). It is normally in the range of 800 to 1500 dynes-sec/$^{cm-5}$.

The autonomic nervous system alters systemic vascular tone through sympathetic and parasympathetic innervation as well as metabolic factors (local oxygen tension, carbon dioxide levels, reactive oxygen species, pH) and endothelium-derived signaling molecules (NO, endothelin). Neural regulation of BP occurs by means of constitutive and reflex changes in autonomic efferent outflow to modulate cardiac chronotropy, inotropy, and vascular resistance.

The baroreflex loop is the primary mechanism by which BP is neurally modulated. Baroreceptors are stretch-sensitive nerve endings that are distributed throughout various regions of the cardiovascular system. Those located in the carotid artery (e.g., carotid sinus) and aorta are sometimes referred to as *high-pressure baroreceptors* and those in the cardiopulmonary areas as *low-pressure baroreceptors*. After afferent impulses are transmitted to the central nervous system, the signals are integrated, and the efferent arm of the reflex projects neural signals systemically through the sympathetic and parasympathetic branches of the autonomic nervous system. In general, an increase in systemic BP increases the firing rate of the baroreceptors. Efferent sympathetic outflow is inhibited (reducing vascular tone, chronotropy, and inotropy), and parasympathetic outflow is increased (reducing cardiac chronotropy). The opposite occurs when BP decreases. Please refer to Chapter 53, "Cardiac function and Circulatory Control," in *Goldman-Cecil Medicine*, 25th Edition.

Physiology of the Pulmonary Circulation

Like the systemic circulation, the pulmonary circulation consists of a branching network of progressively smaller arteries, arterioles, capillaries, and veins. The pulmonary capillaries are separated from the alveoli by a thin alveolar-capillary membrane through which gas exchange occurs. The partial pressure of oxygen (Po_2) is the main regulator of pulmonary blood to optimize blood flow toward well-ventilated lung segments and away from poorly ventilated segments.

SUGGESTED READINGS

Berne RM, Levy MN: Physiology: part IV. The cardiovascular system, ed 6 with Student Consult Access, St. Louis, 2010, Elsevier.
Guyton AC, Hall JE: Textbook of medical physiology, ed 12, St. Louis, 2011, Elsevier.

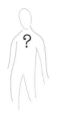

Evaluation of the Patient with Cardiovascular Disease

James Kleczka and Ivor J. Benjamin

DEFINITION AND EPIDEMIOLOGY

Cardiovascular disease is a major cause of morbidity and mortality around the world, and its spectrum is wide-reaching. Included in this population of patients are people with coronary artery disease (CAD), congestive heart failure, stroke, hypertension, peripheral arterial disease, atrial fibrillation and other arrhythmias, valvular disease, and congenital heart disease. In the United States alone, these diseases affect more than 82 million individuals at any given time. The impact of cardiovascular disease is unmistakable: It accounted for more inpatient hospital days in the years of 1990-2009 than other disorders such as chronic lung disease and cancer. The high number of inpatient days associated with cardiovascular disease led to a total economic cost of more than $297 billion in the year 2008 alone. Cardiovascular disease was also the number one cause of death in the United States in 2008; more than half of these deaths were from CAD, which was the top cause of mortality among individuals older than 65 years of age.

Given these facts, the proper evaluation of a patient with cardiovascular disease can have a major impact on multiple fronts, from an economic standpoint as well as an individual's morbidity and mortality. Therefore, one must obtain a very thorough history and detailed physical examination to accurately assess and manage patients with cardiovascular disease.

PATHOLOGY

A patient with cardiovascular disease may have one or more of a number of problems. *Coronary artery disease*, discussed in depth in Chapter 8, is a leading cause of morbidity and mortality. At presentation, patients with CAD may have stable angina or an acute coronary syndrome such as unstable angina, non–ST segment elevation myocardial infarction (NSTEMI), or ST segment elevation myocardial infarction (STEMI). For some patients, their first presentation with CAD is sudden cardiac death, the result of arrhythmia often caused by atherosclerosis of the coronary vasculature.

Congestive heart failure is the end result of many cardiac disorders and is generally classified as systolic or diastolic in etiology. Various forms of cardiomyopathy, such as dilated cardiomyopathy or hypertrophic cardiomyopathy, may lead to systolic dysfunction and a decline in ejection fraction. Without proper management, this will inevitably lead to alterations in hemodynamics that result in development of pulmonary vascular congestion, edema, and a decline in functional capacity. Diastolic dysfunction can be present with systolic dysfunction and is often the result of uncontrolled hypertension or infiltrative disorders such as hemochromatosis or amyloidosis. Heart failure with a preserved ejection fraction is often caused by diastolic dysfunction. Various forms of heart failure are further discussed in Chapter 5.

Stroke is caused by cerebral hypoperfusion, which can result from such problems as carotid disease, thromboembolism, or emboli of infectious origin. A more detailed discussion can be found in Chapter 116.

Peripheral arterial disease (PAD), addressed in Chapter 12, includes such entities as aneurysms of the ascending, descending, and abdominal aorta; aortic dissection; carotid disease; and atherosclerosis of branch vessels of the aorta and vessels in the limbs. PAD is often present in patients with CAD.

Atrial fibrillation and *hypertension* (see Chapters 9 and 12) are not uncommon and increase in prevalence with age. Although they are not typically the primary cause of mortality, these problems often predispose to other causes of cardiovascular disease mortality, such as stroke and heart failure. Arrhythmias other than atrial fibrillation are also common and can lead to significant morbidity and mortality.

Valvular heart disease may lead to cardiomyopathy and is found in all age groups.

Congenital heart disease includes a wide variety of disorders, ranging from valve abnormalities and coronary anomalies to cardiomyopathy and other structural abnormalities including shunts and malformations of the cardiac chambers. With advances in surgical techniques and medical therapy, these patients are often living beyond previous expectations, increasing the likelihood that they will live into adulthood. For more detailed information on congenital heart diseases, see Chapter 6.

CLINICAL PRESENTATION

There have been major advances in technology over the years that allow for specialized testing to assist in the diagnosis of cardiovascular diseases. We now rely on such tests as angiography, ultrasound scanning, and advanced imaging modalities such as high-resolution computed tomography and magnetic resonance imaging to determine how to manage an individual case. However, these techniques should be used not as a primary method of assessment but rather to supplement the findings from a thorough history and physical examination. Despite the availability of rather costly imaging techniques and laboratory tests, a relatively inexpensive but detailed history and physical examination is often all that is required to establish a diagnosis.

When evaluating patients with cardiovascular disease, it is important to allow them to express their symptoms in their own words. For example, many patients who deny chest pain when asked specifically about this symptom, will, in their very next breath, describe the chest pressure they feel, which they do not consider to be "pain." It is very important to delve into details regarding the setting in which the symptom occurs (e.g., at rest, with activity, with extreme emotional stress). The location, quality, intensity, and radiation of the symptom should be elicited. One should ask whether there are aggravating or alleviating factors and whether there are other symptoms that accompany the primary symptom. It is also important to note the pattern of the symptom in terms of stability or progression in intensity or frequency over time. An assessment of functional status should always be a part of the history in a patient with cardiovascular disease, because a recent decline in exercise tolerance can be very telling in regard to severity of disease.

A detailed past medical history and review of systems are necessary because cardiovascular conditions can be associated with other medical conditions; for example, patient may have arrhythmias in the setting of hyperthyroidism. A comprehensive list of medications must be reviewed, and a social history must be taken detailing alcohol use, smoking, and occupational history. Patients should also be questioned regarding major risk factors such as hypertension, hyperlipidemia, and diabetes mellitus. A thorough family history is needed, not only to identify such entities as early-onset CAD but also to assess for other potentially inherited disorders, such as familial cardiomyopathy or arrhythmic disorders (e.g., long-QT syndrome).

Chest Pain

Chest pain is one of the cardinal symptoms of cardiovascular disease, but it may also be present in many noncardiovascular diseases (Tables 3-1 and 3-2). Chest pain may be caused by cardiac ischemia but also may be related to aortic pathology such as dissection, pulmonary disease such as pneumonia, gastrointestinal pathology such as gastroesophageal reflux, or musculoskeletal pain related to chest wall trauma. Issues with organs in the abdominal cavity such as the gallbladder or pancreas can also cause chest pain. It is therefore very important to characterize the pain in terms of location, quality, quantity, location, duration, radiation, aggravating and alleviating factors, and associated symptoms. These details will help determine the origin of the pain.

Myocardial ischemia due to obstructive CAD often leads to typical angina pectoris. Angina is often described as tightness, pressure, burning, or squeezing discomfort that patients may not identify as true pain. Patients frequently describe angina as a sensation of "bricks on the center of the chest" or an "elephant standing on the chest." Angina is more common in the morning, and the intensity may be affected by heat or cold, emotional stress, or eating. This discomfort is typically located in the substernal region or left side of the chest. If it is reproduced by palpation, it is unlikely to be angina. Anginal pain often radiates to the left shoulder and arm, particularly the ulnar aspect. It may also radiate to the neck, jaw, or epigastrium. Pain that radiates to the back, the right or left lower anterior chest, or below the epigastric region is less likely to be anginal in etiology. Anginal chest pain is usually brought on with exertion, in particular with more intense activity or walking up inclines, in extremes of weather, or after large meals. It is typically brief in duration, lasting 2 to 10 minutes, and resolves with rest or administration of nitroglycerine within 1 to 5 minutes. Associated symptoms often include nausea, diaphoresis, dyspnea, palpitations, and dizziness. Patients typically report a stable pattern of angina that is relatively predictable and reproducible with a given amount of exertion. When this pain begins to increase in frequency and severity or occurs with lesser amounts of exertion or at rest, one must then consider unstable angina. Anginal pain that occurs at rest with increased

TABLE 3-1   CARDIOVASCULAR CAUSES OF CHEST PAIN

CONDITION	LOCATION	QUALITY	DURATION	AGGRAVATING OR ALLEVIATING FACTORS	ASSOCIATED SYMPTOMS OR SIGNS
Angina	Retrosternal region; radiates to or occasionally isolated to neck, jaw, shoulders, arms (usually left), or epigastrium	Pressure, squeezing, tightness, heaviness, burning, indigestion	<2-10 min	Precipitated by exertion, cold weather, or emotional stress; relieved by rest or nitroglycerin; variant (Prinzmetal) angina may be unrelated to exertion, often early in the morning	Dyspnea; S_3, S_4, or murmur of papillary dysfunction during pain
Myocardial infarction	Same as angina	Same as angina, although more severe	Variable; usually >30 min	Unrelieved by rest or nitroglycerin	Dyspnea, nausea, vomiting, weakness, diaphoresis
Pericarditis	Left of the sternum; may radiate to neck or left shoulder, often more localized than pain of myocardial ischemia	Sharp, stabbing, knifelike	Lasts many hours to days; may wax and wane	Aggravated by deep breathing, rotating chest, or supine position; relieved by sitting up and leaning forward	Pericardial friction rub
Aortic dissection	Anterior chest; may radiate to back, interscapular region	Excruciating, tearing, knifelike	Sudden onset, unrelenting	Usually occurs in setting of hypertension or predisposition, such as Marfan's syndrome	Murmur of aortic insufficiency; pulse or blood pressure asymmetry; neurologic deficit

TABLE 3-2 NONCARDIAC CAUSES OF CHEST PAIN

CONDITION	LOCATION	QUALITY	DURATION	AGGRAVATING OR ALLEVIATING FACTORS	ASSOCIATED SYMPTOMS OR SIGNS
Pulmonary embolism (chest pain often not present)	Substernal or over region of pulmonary infarction	Pleuritic (with pulmonary infarction) or angina-like	Sudden onset (minutes to hours)	Aggravated by deep breathing	Dyspnea, tachypnea, tachycardia; hypotension, signs of acute right ventricular heart failure, and pulmonary hypertension with large emboli; pleural rub; hemoptysis with pulmonary infarction
Pulmonary hypertension	Substernal	Pressure; oppressive	—	Aggravated by effort	Pain usually associated with dyspnea; signs of pulmonary hypertension
Pneumonia with pleurisy	Located over involved area	Pleuritic	—	Aggravated by breathing	Dyspnea, cough, fever, bronchial breath sounds, rhonchi, egophony, dullness to percussion, occasional pleural rub
Spontaneous pneumothorax	Unilateral	Sharp, well localized	Sudden onset; lasts many hours	Aggravated by breathing	Dyspnea; hyperresonance and decreased breath and voice sounds over involved lung
Musculoskeletal disorders	Variable	Aching, well localized	Variable	Aggravated by movement; history of exertion or injury	Tender to palpation or with light pressure
Herpes zoster	Dermatomal distribution	Sharp, burning	Prolonged	None	Vesicular rash appears in area of discomfort
Esophageal reflux	Substernal or epigastric; may radiate to neck	Burning, visceral discomfort	10-60 min	Aggravated by large meal, postprandial recumbency; relief with antacid	Water brash
Peptic ulcer	Epigastric, substernal	Visceral burning, aching	Prolonged	Relief with food, antacid	—
Gallbladder disease	Right upper quadrant; epigastric	Visceral	Prolonged	Spontaneous or after meals	Right upper quadrant tenderness may be present
Anxiety states	Often localized over precordium	Variable; location often moves from place to place	Varies; often fleeting	Situational	Sighing respirations; often chest wall tenderness

intensity and lasts longer than 30 minutes may represent acute myocardial infarction. Angina-like pain at rest may also occur with coronary vasospasm and noncardiac chest pain.

There are several other potential causes of chest pain that may be confused with angina pectoris (see Table 3-2). Pain associated with acute pericarditis is typically sharp, is located to the left of the sternum, and radiates to the neck, shoulders, and back. This may be rather severe pain that is present at rest and can last for hours. It typically improves with sitting up and forward and worsens with inspiration. Acute aortic dissection usually causes sudden onset of severe tearing chest pain which radiates to the back between the scapulae or to the lumbar region. Typically, there is a history of hypertension, and pulses may be asymmetric between the extremities. A murmur of aortic regurgitation may also be heard. Pain associated with pulmonary embolism is also acute in onset and is usually accompanied by shortness of breath. This pain is typically pleuritic, worsening with inspiration.

Dyspnea

Dyspnea is another hallmark symptom of cardiovascular disease, but it is also a primary symptom of pulmonary disease. It is defined as an uncomfortable heightened awareness of breathing.

This can be an entirely normal sensation in individuals performing moderate to extreme exertion, depending on their level of conditioning. When it occurs at rest or with minimal exertion, dyspnea is considered abnormal. Dyspnea may accompany a large number of noncardiac conditions such as anemia due to a lack of oxygen-carrying capacity, pulmonary disorders such as obstructive or restrictive lung disease and asthma, obesity due to an increased work of breathing and restricted filling of the lungs, and deconditioning. In the cardiovascular patient, dyspnea is typically caused by left ventricular dysfunction, either systolic or diastolic; CAD and resultant ischemia; or valvular heart disease which, when severe, can lead to a drop in cardiac output. In cases of left ventricular dysfunction and valvular disease, the mechanism of dyspnea often involves increased intracardiac pressures that lead to pulmonary vascular congestion. Fluid then leaks into the alveolar space, impairing gas exchange and causing dyspnea.

Breathing difficulties can also be secondary to a low-output state without pulmonary vascular congestion. Patients often notice dyspnea with exertion, but it can also occur at rest in patients with severe cardiac disease. Shortness of breath at rest is also a symptom in patients with pulmonary edema, large pleural effusions, anxiety, or pulmonary embolism. A patient with left ventricular systolic or diastolic failure may describe the acute onset of breathing difficulty when sleeping. This problem, called paroxysmal nocturnal dyspnea (PND), is caused by pulmonary edema that is redistributed in a prone position; it is usually secondary to left ventricular failure. These patients often notice the acute onset of dyspnea followed by coughing roughly 2 to 4 hours after going to sleep. This can be a very uncomfortable feeling, and it leads the patient to sit up immediately or get out of bed. Symptoms typically resolve over 15 to 30 minutes. Patients with left ventricular failure also often complain of orthopnea, which is dyspnea that occurs when one assumes a prone position. This is relieved by sleeping on multiple pillows or remaining seated to sleep.

Patients with sudden onset of dyspnea may be experiencing flash pulmonary edema, which is very rapid and acute accumulation of fluid in the lungs. This can be associated with severe CAD and may also be a cause of dyspnea in patients with coarctation of the aorta and renal artery stenosis. Sudden dyspnea is associated with pulmonary embolism, and this symptom is typically accompanied by pleuritic chest pain and possibly hemoptysis in such patients. Pneumothorax can cause dyspnea accompanied by acute chest pain. Dyspnea due to lung disease is present with exertion, although in severe cases it may be present at rest. This is often accompanied by hypoxia and is relieved by pulmonary bronchodilators or steroids or both. Dyspnea may also be an "angina equivalent." Not all patients with CAD develop typical anginal chest pain. Dyspnea that comes on with exertion or emotional stress, is relieved with rest, and is relatively brief in duration might be a manifestation of significant CAD. This type of dyspnea is also usually improved with the administration of nitroglycerine.

Palpitation

Palpitation is another symptom commonly seen in the cardiovascular patient. This is the subjective sensation of rapid or forceful beating of the heart. Patients often are able to describe in detail the sensation they feel, such as jumping, skipping, racing, fluttering, or an irregularity in the heartbeat. It is important to ask the patient about the onset of the palpitations because they may begin abruptly at rest, only with exertion, with emotional stress, or with ingestion of certain foods such as chocolate. One should also inquire about associated symptoms such as chest pain, dyspnea, dizziness, and syncope. It is important to note other medical issues, such as thyroid disease, and bleeding, which can lead to anemia, because these conditions may be associated with arrhythmias. A social history focusing on drug use and intake of alcohol is important because use of these substances can lead to certain rhythm disturbances. The family history is also important, because there are many inherited disorders (e.g., long-QT syndromes) that might lead to significant arrhythmias.

Potential etiologies of palpitation include premature atrial or ventricular beats, which are typically described as isolated skips and can be uncomfortable. Supraventricular tachycardias such as atrial flutter, AV nodal reentrant tachycardia, and paroxysmal atrial tachycardia often start and stop abruptly and can be rapid. Atrial fibrillation is usually rapid and very irregular. Ventricular arrhythmias are more often associated with severe dizziness or

syncope. Gradual onset of tachycardia with a gradual decline in HR is more indicative of sinus tachycardia or anxiety.

Syncope

Syncope may be caused by a variety of cardiovascular diseases. It is the transient loss of consciousness due to inadequate cerebral blood flow. In the patient presenting with syncope as a primary complaint, one must try to differentiate true cardiac causes from neurologic issues such as seizure and metabolic causes such as hypoglycemia. Determination of the timing of the syncopal event and associated symptoms is very helpful in determining the etiology. True cardiac syncope is typically very sudden, with no prodromal symptoms. It is typically caused by an abrupt drop in cardiac output which may be due to tachyarrhythmias such as ventricular tachycardia or fibrillation, bradyarrhythmias such as complete heart block, severe valvular heart disease such as aortic or mitral stenosis, or obstruction of flow due to left ventricular outflow tract (LVOT) obstruction. True cardiac syncope often has no accompanying aura. In situations such as aortic stenosis or LVOT obstruction, syncope typically occurs with exertion. Patients usually regain consciousness rather quickly with true cardiac syncope.

Neurocardiogenic syncope involves an abnormal reflexive response to a change in position. When one rises from a prone or seated position to a standing position, the peripheral vasculature usually constricts and the HR increases to maintain cerebral perfusion. With neurocardiogenic syncope, the peripheral vasculature abnormally dilates or the HR slows or both. This leads to a reduction in cerebral perfusion and syncope. A similar mechanism is responsible for carotid sinus syncope and syncope associated with micturition and cough. The patient usually describes a gradual onset of symptoms such as flushing, dizziness, diaphoresis, and nausea before losing consciousness, which lasts seconds. When these patients wake, they are often pale and have a lower HR. In the patient with syncope due to seizures, a prodromal aura is typically present before loss of consciousness occurs. Patients regain consciousness much more slowly and at times are incontinent, complain of headache and fatigue, and have a post-ictal confusional state. Syncope due to stroke is rare, because there must be significant bilateral carotid disease or disease of the vertebrobasilar system causing brainstem ischemia. Neurologic deficits accompany the physical examination findings in these patients.

The history is very important in determining the cause of a syncopal episode. This was previously studied by Calkins and colleagues, who found that men older than 54 years of age who had no prodromal symptoms were more likely to have an arrhythmic cause of their episodes. However, those with prodromal symptoms such as nausea, diaphoresis, dizziness, and visual disturbances before passing out were more likely to have neurocardiogenic syncope. Many inherited disorders such as long-QT syndrome and other arrhythmias, hypertrophic cardiomyopathy with LVOT obstruction, and familial dilated cardiomyopathy lead to states conducive to syncope. For this reason, a very detailed family history is necessary.

Edema

Edema often accompanies cardiovascular disease but may be a manifestation of liver disease (cirrhosis), renal disease (nephrotic syndrome), or local issues such as chronic venous insufficiency or thrombophlebitis. Edema related to cardiac disease is caused by increased venous pressures that alter the balance between hydrostatic and oncotic forces. This leads to extravasation of fluid into the extravascular space. Peripheral edema is common with right-sided heart failure, whereas the same process in left-sided heart failure leads to pulmonary edema.

Edema due to a cardiac etiology is typically bilateral and begins distally with progression in a proximal fashion. The feet and ankles are affected first, followed by the lower legs, thighs, and, ultimately, the abdomen, sometimes accompanied by ascites. If edema is visible, it is usually preceded by a weight gain of at least 5 to 10 pounds. Edema with heart disease is typically pitting, leaving an indentation in the skin after pressure is applied to the area. The edema is usually worse in the evening, and patients often describe an inability to fit into their shoes. While these patients are lying prone, the edema can shift to the sacral region after several hours, only to accumulate again the next day when they are on their feet again (dependent edema).

Total body edema, or anasarca, may be caused by heart failure but is also seen in nephrotic syndrome and cirrhosis. Unilateral edema is more likely associated with a localized issue such as deep venous thrombosis or thrombophlebitis. Other parts of the history may shed light on the etiology of edema. Patients who report PND and orthopnea are likely have a cardiac etiology. If there is a history of alcohol abuse and jaundice is present, liver disease is a probable cause. Edema of the eyes and face in addition to lower-extremity edema is more likely related to nephrotic syndrome. Edema associated with discoloration or ulcers of the lower extremities is often seen with chronic venous insufficiency. In a patient with insidious onset of edema progressing to anasarca and ascites, one must consider constrictive pericarditis.

Cyanosis

Cyanosis is defined as an abnormal bluish discoloration of the skin resulting from an increase in the level of reduced hemoglobin or abnormal hemoglobin in the blood. When present, it typically represents an oxygen saturation of less than 85% (normal, >90%). There are several types of cyanosis. Central cyanosis often manifests in discoloration of the lips or trunk and usually represents low oxygen saturations due to right-to-left shunting of blood. This can occur with structural cardiac abnormalities such as large atrial or ventricular septal defects, but it also happens with impaired pulmonary function, as in with severe chronic obstructive lung disease. Peripheral cyanosis is typically secondary to vasoconstriction in the setting of low cardiac output. This can also occur with exposure to cold and can represent local arterial or venous thrombosis. When localized to the hands, peripheral cyanosis suggests Raynaud's phenomenon. Cyanosis in childhood often indicates congenital heart disease with resultant right-to-left shunting of blood.

Other

There are other, nonspecific symptoms that may indicate cardiovascular disease. Although fatigue is present with a myriad of medical conditions, it is very common in patients with cardiac disease when low cardiac output is present. It can be seen with hypotension due to aggressive medical treatment of hypertension or with overdiuresis in patients with heart failure. Fatigue may also be a direct result of medical therapy for cardiac disease itself, such as with β-blocking agents. Although cough is commonly associated with pulmonary disease, it may also indicate high intracardiac pressures which can lead to pulmonary edema. Cough may be present in patients with heart failure or significant left-sided valve disease. A patient with congestive heart failure may describe a cough productive of frothy pink sputum, as opposed to frank bloody or blood-tinged sputum, which is seen more typically with primary lung pathology. Nausea and emesis can accompany acute myocardial infarction and may also be a reflection of heart failure leading to hepatic or intestinal congestion due to high right heart pressures. Anorexia, abdominal fullness, and cachexia may occur with end-stage heart failure. Nocturia is also a symptom described with heart failure; renal perfusion improves when the patient lies in a prone position, leading to an increase in urine output. Hoarseness of voice can occur due to compression of the recurrent laryngeal nerve. This may happen with enlarged pulmonary arteries, enlarged left atrium, or aortic aneurysm.

Despite the myriad symptoms of cardiovascular disease described here, many patients with significant cardiac disease are asymptomatic. Patients with CAD may have periods of asymptomatic ischemia that can be documented on ambulatory electrocardiographic monitoring. Up to one third of patients who have suffered a myocardial infarction are unaware that they had an event. This is more common in diabetics and in older patients. A patient may have severely depressed ventricular function for some time before presenting with symptoms. In addition, patients with atrial fibrillation can be entirely asymptomatic, with this rhythm discovered only after a physical examination is performed.

At times, patients do not report having symptoms related to usual activities of daily living, yet symptoms are present when functional testing is performed. Therefore, assessing functional capacity is a very important part of the history in a patient with known or suspected cardiovascular disease. The ability or inability to perform various activities plays a substantial role in determining the extent of disability and in assessing response to therapy and overall prognosis, and it can influence decisions regarding the timing and type of therapy or intervention. The New York Heart Association Functional Classification is a commonly used method to assess functional status based on "ordinary activity" (Table 3-3). Patients are classified in one of four functional classes. Functional class I includes patients with known cardiac disease who have no limitations with ordinary activity. Functional classes II and III describe patients who have symptoms with less and less activity, whereas patients in functional class IV have symptoms at rest. The Canadian Cardiovascular Society has provided a similar classification of functional status specifically for patients with angina pectoris. These tools are very useful in classifying a patient's symptoms at a given time, allowing comparison at a future point and determination as to whether the symptoms are stable or progressive.

● DIAGNOSIS AND PHYSICAL EXAMINATION
General

Like the detailed history, the physical examination is also vital when assessing a patient with cardiovascular disease. This consists of more than simply auscultating the heart. Many diseases of the cardiovascular system can affect and be affected by other organ systems. Therefore, a detailed general physical examination is essential. The general appearance of a patient is helpful: Such observations as skin color, breathing pattern, whether pain is present, and overall nutritional status can provide clues regarding the diagnosis. Examination of the head may reveal evidence of hypothyroidism, such as hair loss and periorbital edema, and examination of the eyes may reveal exophthalmos associated with hyperthyroidism. Both conditions can affect the heart. Retinal examination may reveal macular edema or flame hemorrhages which can be associated with uncontrolled hypertension. Findings such as clubbing or edema when examining the extremities, and jaundice or cyanosis when evaluating the skin, may provide clues to undiagnosed cardiovascular disease.

Examination of the Jugular Venous Pulsations

Examination of the neck veins can provide a great deal of insight into right heart hemodynamics. The right internal jugular vein should be used, because the relatively straight course of the right innominate and jugular veins allows for a more accurate reflection of the true right atrial pressure. The longer and more winding course of the left-sided veins does not allow for as accurate a transmission of hemodynamics. For examination of the right internal jugular vein, the patient should be placed at a 45-degree angle—higher in patients with suspected elevated venous pressures and lower in those with lower venous pressures. The head should be turned to the left and light shined at an angle over the neck. Although the internal jugular vein itself is not visible, the pulsations from that vessel are transmitted to the skin and can be seen in most cases. The carotid artery lies in close proximity to the jugular vein, and its pulsations can sometimes be seen as well. Therefore, one must be certain one is observing the correct vessel. This can be accomplished by applying gentle compression at the site of pulsations. An arterial pulse will not be obliterated by this maneuver, whereas a venous pulse likely will become diminished or absent with compression. In addition, an arterial pulse is usually much more forceful and vigorous.

Both the level of venous pressure and the morphology of the venous waveforms should be noted. Once the pulsations have been located, the vertical distance from the sternal angle (angle of Louis) to the top of the pulsations is determined. Because the right atrium lies about 5 cm vertically below the sternal angle,

this number is added to the previous measurement to arrive at an estimated right atrial pressure in centimeters of water. The right atrial pressure is normally 5 to 9 cm H_2O. It can be higher in patients with decompensated heart failure, disorders of the tricuspid valve (regurgitation or stenosis), restrictive cardiomyopathy, or constrictive pericarditis.

With inspiration, negative intrathoracic pressure develops, venous blood drains into the thorax, and venous pressure in the normal patient falls; the opposite occurs during expiration. In a patient with conditions such as decompensated heart failure, constrictive pericarditis, or restrictive cardiomyopathy, this pattern is reversed (Kussmaul sign), and the venous pressure increases with inspiration. When the neck veins are examined, firm pressure should be applied for 10 to 30 seconds to the right upper quadrant over the liver. In a normal patient, this will cause the venous pressure to increase briefly and then return to normal. In the patient with conditions such as heart failure, constrictive pericarditis, or substantial tricuspid regurgitation, the neck veins will reveal a sustained increase in pressure due to passive congestion of the liver. This finding is called hepatojugular reflux.

The normal waveforms of the jugular venous pulse are depicted in Figure 3-1A. The *a* wave results from atrial contraction. The *x* descent results from atrial relaxation after contraction and the pulling of the floor of the right atrium downward with right ventricular contraction. The *c* wave interrupts the *x* descent and is generated by bulging of the cusps of the tricuspid valve into the right atrium during ventricular systole. This occurs at the same time as the carotid pulse. Atrial pressure then increases as a result of venous return with the tricuspid valve closed during ventricular systole; this generates the *v* wave, which is typically smaller than the *a* wave. The *y* descent follows as the tricuspid valve opens and blood flows from the right atrium to the right ventricle during diastole.

Understanding of the normal jugular venous waveforms is paramount, because these waveforms can be altered in different disease states. Abnormalities of these waveforms reflect underlying structural, functional, and electrical abnormalities of the heart (see Fig. 3-1B to G). Elevation of the right atrial pressure leading to jugular venous distention can be found in heart failure (both systolic and diastolic), hypervolemia, superior vena cava syndrome, and valvular disease. The *a* wave is exaggerated in any condition in which a greater resistance to right atrial emptying occurs. Such conditions include pulmonary hypertension, tricuspid stenosis, and right ventricular hypertrophy or failure. *Cannon a waves* occur when the atrium contracts against a closed tricuspid valve, which can occur with complete heart block or any other situation involving AV dissociation. The *a* wave is absent during atrial fibrillation. With significant tricuspid regurgitation, the *v* wave becomes very prominent and may merge with the *c* wave, diminishing or eliminating the *x* descent. With tricuspid stenosis, there is impaired emptying of the right atrium, which leads to an attenuated *y* descent. In pericardial constriction and restrictive cardiomyopathy, the *y* descent occurs rapidly and deeply, and the *x* descent may also become more prominent, leading to a waveform with a w-shaped appearance. With pericardial tamponade, the *x* descent becomes very prominent while the *y* descent is diminished or absent.

TABLE 3-3	CLASSIFICATION OF FUNCTIONAL STATUS*	
Class I	Uncompromised	Ordinary activity does not cause symptoms; symptoms occur only with strenuous or prolonged activity.
Class II	Slightly compromised	Ordinary physical activity results in symptoms; no symptoms at rest.
Class III	Moderately compromised	Less than ordinary activity results in symptoms; no symptoms at rest.
Class IV	Severely compromised	Any activity results in symptoms; symptoms may be present at rest.

*Symptoms refers to undue fatigue, dyspnea, palpitations, or angina in the New York Heart Association classification and refers specifically to angina in the Canadian Cardiovascular Society classification.

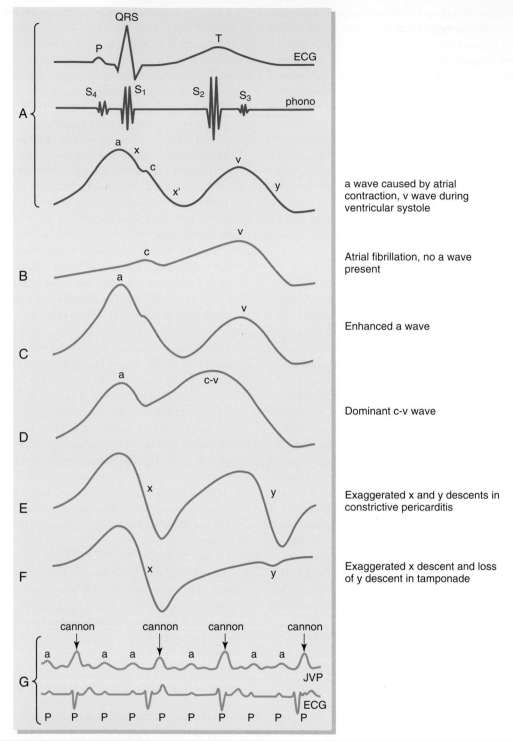

FIGURE 3-1 Normal and abnormal jugular venous pulse (JVP) tracings. **A,** Normal jugular pulse tracing with simultaneous electrocardiogram (ECG) and phonocardiogram. **B,** Loss of the *a* wave in atrial fibrillation. **C,** Large *a* wave in tricuspid stenosis. **D,** Large *c-v* wave in tricuspid regurgitation. **E,** Prominent *x* and *y* descents in constrictive pericarditis. **F,** Prominent *x* descent and diminutive *y* descent in pericardial tamponade. **G,** JVP tracing and simultaneous ECG during complete heart block demonstrates cannon *a* waves occurring when the atrium contracts against a closed tricuspid valve during ventricular systole. P, P waves correlating with atrial contraction; S_1 to S_4, heart sounds.

Examination of Arterial Pressure and Pulse

Arterial blood pressure is measured noninvasively with the use of a sphygmomanometer. Before the blood pressure is taken, the patient ideally should be relaxed, allowed to rest for 5 to 10 minutes in a quiet room, and seated or lying comfortably. The cuff is typically applied to the upper arm, approximately 1 inch above the antecubital fossa. A stethoscope is then used to auscultate under the lower edge of the cuff. The cuff is rapidly inflated to approximately 30 mm Hg above the anticipated systolic pressure and then slowly deflated (at approximately 3 mm Hg/sec) while the examiner listens for the sounds produced by blood entering the previously occluded artery. These sounds are the Korotkoff sounds. The first sound is typically a very clear tapping sound which, when heard, represents the systolic pressure. As the cuff continues to deflate, the sounds will disappear; this point represents the diastolic pressure.

In normal situations, the pressure in both arms is relatively equal. If the pressure is measured in the lower extremities rather than the arms, the systolic pressure is typically 10 to 20 mm Hg higher. If the pressures in the arms are asymmetric, this may suggest atherosclerotic disease involving the aorta, aortic dissection, or obstruction of flow in the subclavian or innominate arteries. The pressure in the lower extremities can be lower than arm pressures in the setting of abdominal aortic, iliac, or femoral disease. Coarctation of the aorta can also lead to discrepant pressures between the upper and lower extremities. Leg pressure that is more than 20 mm Hg higher than the arm pressure can be found in the patient with significant aortic regurgitation, a finding called Hill's sign. A common mistake in taking the arterial blood pressure involves using a cuff of incorrect size. Use of a small cuff on a large extremity leads to overestimation of pressure. Similarly,

use of a large cuff on a smaller extremity underestimates the pressure.

Examination of the arterial pulse in a cardiovascular patient should include palpation of the carotid, radial, brachial, femoral, popliteal, posterior tibial, and dorsalis pedis pulses bilaterally. The carotid pulse most accurately reflects the central aortic pulse. One should note the rhythm, strength, contour, and symmetry of the pulses. A normal arterial pulse (Fig. 3-2A) rises rapidly to a peak in early systole, plateaus, and then falls. The descending limb of the pulse is interrupted by the incisura or dicrotic notch, which is a sharp deflection downward due to closure of the aortic valve. As the pulse moves toward the periphery, the systolic peak is higher and the dicrotic notch is later and less noticeable.

The normal pattern of the arterial pulse can be altered by a variety of cardiovascular diseases (see Fig. 3-2B to F). The amplitude of the pulse increases in conditions such as anemia, pregnancy, thyrotoxicosis, and other states with high cardiac output. Aortic insufficiency, with its resultant increase in pulse

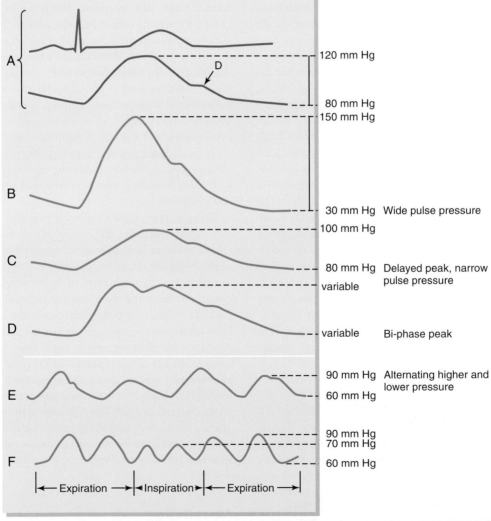

FIGURE 3-2 Normal and abnormal carotid arterial pulse contours. **A,** Normal arterial pulse with simultaneous electrocardiogram (ECG). The dicrotic wave (D) occurs just after aortic valve closure. **B,** Wide pulse pressure in aortic insufficiency. **C,** Pulsus parvus et tardus (small amplitude with a slow upstroke) associated with aortic stenosis. **D,** Bisferiens pulse with two systolic peaks, typical of hypertrophic obstructive cardiomyopathy or aortic insufficiency, especially if concomitant aortic stenosis is present. **E,** Pulsus alternans, characteristic of severe left ventricular failure. **F,** Paradoxic pulse (systolic pressure decrease >10 mm Hg with inspiration), most characteristic of cardiac tamponade.

pressure (difference between systolic and diastolic pressure), leads to a bounding carotid pulse often referred to as a Corrigan pulse or a water-hammer pulse. The amplitude of the pulse is diminished in low-output states such as heart failure, hypovolemia, and mitral stenosis. Tachycardia, with shorter diastolic filling times, also lowers the pulse amplitude. Aortic stenosis, when significant, leads to a delayed systolic peak and diminished carotid pulse, referred to as *pulsus parvus et tardus*. A bisferiens pulse is most perceptible on palpation of the carotid artery. It is characterized by two systolic peaks and can be found in patients with pure aortic regurgitation. The first peak is the percussion wave, which results from the rapid ejection of a large volume of blood early in systole. The second peak is the tidal wave, which is a reflected wave from the periphery. A bisferiens pulse may also be found in those with hypertrophic cardiomyopathy, in which the initial rapid upstroke of the pulse is interrupted by LVOT obstruction. The reflected wave produces the second impulse. Pulsus alternans is beat-to-beat variation in the pulse and can be found in patients with severe left ventricular systolic dysfunction.

Pulsus paradoxus is an exaggeration of the normal inspiratory fall in systolic pressure. With inspiration, negative intrathoracic pressure is transmitted to the aorta, and systolic pressure typically drops by as much as 10 mm Hg. In pulsus paradoxus, this drop is greater than 10 mm Hg and can be palpable when marked (>20 mm Hg). It is characteristic in cardiac tamponade but can also be seen in constrictive pericarditis, pulmonary embolism, hypovolemic shock, pregnancy, and severe chronic obstructive lung disease.

Because peripheral vascular disease often accompanies CAD, a detailed examination of the peripheral pulses is an absolute necessity in patients with known ischemic heart disease. In addition to the carotid, brachial, radial, femoral, popliteal, dorsalis pedis, and posterior tibial pulses, the abdominal aorta should be palpated. When the abdominal aorta is palpable below the umbilicus, the presence of an abdominal aortic aneurysm is suggested. Impaired blood flow to the lower extremities can cause claudication, a cramping pain located in the buttocks, thigh, calf, or foot, depending on the location of disease. With significant stenosis in the peripheral vasculature, the distal pulses may be significantly reduced or absent. Blood flow in a stenotic artery may be turbulent, creating an audible bruit. With normal aging, the peripheral arteries become less compliant and this change may obscure abnormal findings.

Examination of the Precordium

A complete cardiovascular examination should always include careful inspection and palpation of the chest, because this may reveal valuable clues regarding the presence of cardiac disease. Abnormalities of the chest wall including skin findings should be observed. The presence of pectus excavatum is associated with Marfan's syndrome and mitral valve prolapse. Pectus carinatum can also be found in patients with Marfan's syndrome. Kyphoscoliosis can lead to right-sided heart failure and secondary pulmonary hypertension. One should also assess for visible pulsations, in particular in the regions of the aorta (second right intercostal space and suprasternal notch), pulmonary artery (third left intercostal space), right ventricle (left parasternal region), and left ventricle (fourth to fifth intercostal space at the left midclavicular line). Prominent pulsations in these areas suggest enlargement of these vessels or chambers. Retraction of the left parasternal area can be observed in patients with severe left ventricular hypertrophy, whereas systolic retraction at the apex or in the left axilla (Broadbent sign) is more characteristic of constrictive pericarditis.

Palpation of the precordium is best performed when the patient, with chest exposed, is positioned supine or in a left lateral position with the examiner located on the right side of the patient. The examiner should then place the right hand over the lower left chest wall with fingertips over the region of the cardiac apex and the palm over the region of the right ventricle. The right ventricle itself is typically best palpated in the subxiphoid region with the tip of the index finger. In those patients who have chronic obstructive lung disease, are obese, or are very muscular, the normal cardiac pulsations may not be palpable. In addition, chest wall deformities may make pulsations difficult or impossible to palpate. The normal apical cardiac impulse is a brief and discrete (1 cm in diameter) pulsation located in the fourth to fifth intercostal space along the left midclavicular line. In a patient with a normal heart, this represents the point of maximal impulse (PMI). If the heart cannot be palpated with the patient supine, a left lateral position should be tried. If the left ventricle is enlarged for any reason, the PMI will typically be displaced laterally. With volume overload states such as aortic insufficiency, the left ventricle dilates, resulting in a brisk apical impulse that is increased in amplitude. With pressure overload, as in long-standing hypertension and aortic stenosis, ventricular enlargement is a result of hypertrophy, and the apical impulse is sustained. Often, it is accompanied by a palpable S_4 gallop. Patients with hypertrophic cardiomyopathy can have double or triple apical impulses. Those with apical aneurysm may have an apical impulse that is larger and dyskinetic.

The right ventricle is usually not palpable. However, in those with right ventricular dilation or hypertrophy, which can be related to severe lung disease, pulmonary hypertension, or congenital heart disease, an impulse may be palpated in the left parasternal region. In some cases of severe emphysema, when the distance between the chest wall and right ventricle is increased, the right ventricle is better palpated in the subxiphoid region. With severe pulmonary hypertension, the pulmonary artery may produce a palpable impulse in the second to third intercostal space to the left of the sternum. This may be accompanied by a palpable right ventricle or a palpable pulmonic component of the second heart sound (S_2). An aneurysm of the ascending aorta or arch may result in a palpable pulsation in the suprasternal notch. Thrills are vibratory sensations best palpated with the fingertips; they are manifestations of harsh murmurs caused by such problems as aortic stenosis, hypertrophic cardiomyopathy, and septal defects.

Auscultation
Techniques

Auscultation of the heart is accomplished by the use of a stethoscope with dual chest pieces. The diaphragm is ideal for high-frequency sounds, whereas the bell is better for low-frequency sounds. When one is listening for low-frequency tones, the bell should be placed gently on the skin with minimal pressure applied. If the bell is applied more firmly, the skin will stretch and higher-frequency sounds will be heard (as when using the diaphragm). Auscultation should ideally be performed in a quiet setting with the patient's chest exposed and the examiner best positioned to the right of the patient. Four major areas of auscultation are evaluated, starting at the apex and moving toward the base of the heart. The mitral valve is best heard at the apex or location of the PMI. Tricuspid valve events are appreciated in or around the left fourth intercostal space adjacent to the sternum. The pulmonary valve is best evaluated in the second left intercostal space. The aortic valve is assessed in the second right intercostal space. These areas should be evaluated from apex to base using the diaphragm and then evaluated again with the bell. Auscultation of the back, the axillae, the right side of the chest, and the supraclavicular areas should also be done. Having the patient perform maneuvers such as leaning forward, exhaling, standing, squatting, and performing a Valsalva maneuver may help to accentuate certain heart sounds (Table 3-4).

Normal Heart Sounds

All heart sounds should be described according to their quality, intensity, and frequency. There are two primary heart sounds heard during auscultation: S_1 and S_2. These are high-frequency

sounds caused by closure of the valves. S_1 occurs with the onset of ventricular systole and is caused by closure of the mitral and tricuspid valves. S_2 is caused by closure of the aortic and pulmonic valves and marks the beginning of ventricular diastole. All other heart sounds are timed based on these two sounds.

S_1 has two components, the first of which (M_1) is usually louder, heard best at the apex, and caused by closure of the mitral valve. The second component (T_1), which is softer and thought to be related to closure of the tricuspid valve, is heard best at the lower left sternal border. Although there can be two components, S_1 is typically heard as a single sound. S_2 also has two components, which typically can be easily distinguished. A_2, the component caused by closure of the aortic valve, is usually louder and is best heard at the right upper sternal border. P_2, caused by closure of the pulmonic valve, is recognized best over the left second intercostal space. With expiration, a normal S_2 is perceived as a single sound. With inspiration, however, venous return to the right heart is augmented, and the increased capacitance of the pulmonary vascular bed results in a delay in pulmonic valve closure. A slight decline in pulmonary venous return to the left ventricle leads to earlier aortic valve closure. Therefore, physiologic splitting of S_2, with A_2 preceding P_2 during inspiration, is a normal finding.

Additional heart sounds can at times be heard in normal individuals. A third heart sound can sometimes be heard in healthy children and young adults. This is referred to as a physiologic S_3, which is rarely heard after the age of 40 years in a normal individual. A fourth heart sound is caused by forceful atrial contraction into a noncompliant ventricle; it is rarely audible in normal young patients but is relatively common in older individuals.

Murmurs are auditory vibrations generated by high flow across a normal valve or normal flow across an abnormal valve or structure. Murmurs that occur early in systole and are soft and brief in duration are not typically pathologic and are termed *innocent murmurs*. These usually are caused by flow across normal left ventricular or right ventricular outflow tracts and are found in children and young adults. Some systolic murmurs may be associated with high-flow states such as fever, anemia, thyroid disease, and pregnancy and are not innocent, although they are not typically associated with structural heart disease. They are called *physiologic murmurs* because of their association with altered physiologic states. All diastolic murmurs are pathologic.

Abnormal Heart Sounds

Abnormalities in S_1 and S_2 are related to either intensity (Table 3-5) or respiratory splitting (Table 3-6). S_1 is accentuated with tachycardia and with short PR intervals, whereas it is softer in the setting of a long PR interval. S_1 varies in intensity if the relationship between atrial and ventricular systole varies. In those patients with atrial fibrillation, atrial filling and emptying is not consistent because the variable HR leading to beat-to-beat changes in the intensity of S_1. This also can occur with heart block or AV dissociation. In early mitral stenosis, S_1 is often accentuated, but with severe stenosis, there is decreased leaflet excursion and S_1 is diminished in intensity or altogether absent (Figs. 3-3 and 3-4). As previously mentioned, splitting of S_1 is not frequently heard.

TABLE 3-4	EFFECTS OF PHYSIOLOGIC MANEUVERS ON AUSCULTATORY EVENTS	
MANEUVER	**MAJOR PHYSIOLOGIC EFFECTS**	**USEFUL AUSCULTATORY CHANGES**
Respiration	↑ Venous return with inspiration	↑ Right heart murmurs and gallops with inspiration; splitting of S_2 (see Fig. 3-3)
Valsalva (initial ↑ BP, phase I; followed by ↓ BP, phase II)	↓ BP, ↓ venous return, ↓ LV size (phase II)	↓ HCM ↓ AS, MR MVP click earlier in systole; murmur prolongs
Standing	↑ Venous return ↑ LV size	↑ HCM ↓ AS, MR MVP click earlier in systole; murmur prolongs
Squatting	↑ Venous return ↑ Systemic vascular resistance ↑ LV size	↑ AS, MR, AI ↓ HCM MVP click delayed; murmur shortens
Isometric exercise (e.g., handgrip)	↑ Arterial pressure ↑ Cardiac output	↑ Gallops ↑ MR, AI, MS ↓ AS, HCM
Post PVC or prolonged R-R interval	↑ Ventricular filling ↑ Contractility	↑ AS Little change in MR
Amyl nitrate	↓ Arterial pressure ↑ Cardiac output ↓ LV size	↑ HCM, AS, MS ↓ AI, MR, Austin Flint murmur MVP click earlier in systole; murmur prolongs
Phenylephrine	↑ Arterial pressure ↑ Cardiac output ↓ LV size	↑ MR, AI ↓ AS, HCM MVP click delayed; murmur shortens

↑, Increased intensity; ↓, decreased intensity; AI, aortic insufficiency; AS, aortic stenosis; BP, blood pressure; HCM, hypertrophic cardiomyopathy; LV, left ventricle; MR, mitral regurgitation; MS, mitral stenosis; MVP, mitral valve prolapse; PVC, premature ventricular contraction; R-R, interval between the R waves on an electrocardiogram.

ventricular septal defect is typically associated with a loud murmur.

The frequency of a murmur can be high or low; higher-frequency murmurs are more correlated with high velocity of flow at the site of turbulence. It is also important to notice the configuration or shape of a murmur, such as crescendo, crescendo-decrescendo, decrescendo, or plateau (Fig. 3-5). The quality of a murmur (e.g., harsh, blowing, rumbling) and the pattern of radiation are also helpful in diagnosis. Physical maneuvers can sometimes help clarify the nature of a particular murmur (see Table 3-4).

Murmurs can be divided into three different categories (Table 3-8). Systolic murmurs begin with or after S_1 and end with or before S_2. Diastolic murmurs begin with or after S_2 and end with or before S_1. Continuous murmurs begin in systole and continue through diastole. Murmurs can result from abnormalities on the left or right side of the heart or in the great vessels. Right-sided murmurs become louder with inspiration because of increased venous return. This can help differentiate them from left-sided murmurs, which are unaffected by respiration.

Systolic murmurs should be further differentiated based on timing (i.e., early systolic, midsystolic, late systolic, and holosystolic murmurs). Early systolic murmurs begin with S_1, are decrescendo, and end typically before mid systole. Ventricular septal defects and acute mitral regurgitation may lead to early systolic murmurs. Midsystolic murmurs begin after S_1 and end before S_2, often in a crescendo-decrescendo shape. They are typically caused by obstruction to left ventricular outflow, accelerated flow through the aortic or pulmonic valve, or enlargement of the aortic root or pulmonary trunk. Aortic stenosis, when

less than severe in degree, causes a midsystolic murmur that may be harsh and may radiate to the carotids. Pulmonic stenosis leads to a similar murmur that does not radiate to the carotid arteries but may change with inspiration. The murmur of hypertrophic cardiomyopathy may be mistaken for aortic stenosis; however, it does not radiate to the carotids and becomes exaggerated with diminished venous return. Innocent or benign murmurs may also occur as a result of aortic valve sclerosis, vibrations of a left ventricular false tendon, or vibration of normal pulmonary leaflets. They are generally less harsh and shorter in duration. High-flow states such as those found in patients with fever, during pregnancy, or with anemia may also lead to midsystolic murmurs.

Holosystolic murmurs begin with S_1 and end with S_2; the classic examples are the murmurs associated with mitral regurgitation and tricuspid regurgitation. They may also occur with ventricular septal defects and patent ductus arteriosus. Late systolic murmurs begin in mid to late systole and end with S_2. They can be characteristic of more severe aortic stenosis and are also typical of murmurs associated with mitral valve prolapse.

Diastolic murmurs are also classified by timing (i.e., early diastolic, mid diastolic, and late diastolic). Early diastolic murmurs begin with S_2 and can result from aortic or pulmonic regurgitation; they are usually decrescendo in shape. Shorter and quieter murmurs typically represent an acute process or mild regurgitation, whereas longer-lasting and louder murmurs are likely due to more severe regurgitation. Mid-diastolic murmurs begin after S_2 and are usually caused by mitral or tricuspid stenosis. They are low pitched and are often referred to as *diastolic rumbles*. Because

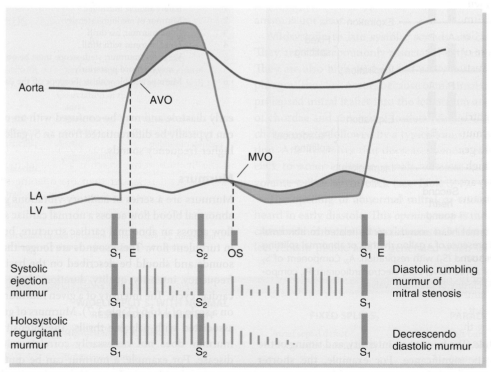

FIGURE 3-5 Abnormal sounds and murmurs associated with valvular dysfunction displayed simultaneously with left atrial (LA), left ventricular (LV), and aortic pressure tracings. The *shaded areas* represent pressure gradients across the aortic valve during systole or across mitral valve during diastole; they are characteristic of aortic stenosis and mitral stenosis, respectively. AVO, Aortic valve opening; E, ejection click of the aortic valve; MVO, mitral valve opening; OS, opening snap of the mitral valve; S_1, first heart sound; S_2, second heart sound.

TABLE 3-8 CLASSIFICATION OF HEART MURMURS

CLASS	DESCRIPTION	CHARACTERISTIC LESIONS
SYSTOLIC		
Ejection	Begins in early systole; may extend to mid or late systole Crescendo-decrescendo pattern Often harsh in quality Begins after S_1 and ends before S_2	Valvular, supravalvular, and subvalvular aortic stenoses Hypertrophic cardiomyopathy Pulmonic stenosis Aortic or pulmonary artery dilation Malformed but nonobstructive aortic valve ↑ Transvalvular flow (e.g., aortic regurgitation, hyperkinetic states, atrial septal defect, physiologic flow murmur)
Holosystolic	Extends throughout systole* Relatively uniform in intensity	Mitral regurgitation Tricuspid regurgitation Ventricular septal defect
Late	Variable onset and duration, often preceded by a nonejection click	Mitral valve prolapse
DIASTOLIC		
Early	Begins with A_2 or P_2 Decrescendo pattern with variable duration Often high pitched, blowing	Aortic regurgitation Pulmonic regurgitation
Mid	Begins after S_2, often after an opening snap Low-pitched *rumble* heard best with bell of stethoscope Louder with exercise and left lateral position Loudest in early diastole	Mitral stenosis Tricuspid stenosis ↑ Flow across atrioventricular valves (e.g., mitral regurgitation, tricuspid regurgitation, atrial septal defect)
Late	Presystolic accentuation of mid-diastolic murmur	Mitral stenosis Tricuspid stenosis
CONTINUOUS		
	Systolic and diastolic components "Machinery murmurs"	Patent ductus arteriosus Coronary atrioventricular fistula Ruptured sinus of Valsalva aneurysm into right atrium or ventricle Mammary soufflé Venous hum

A_2, Component of S_2 caused by closure of aortic valve; P_2, component of S_2 caused by closure of pulmonic valve; S_1, first heart sound; S_2, second heart sound.
*Encompasses both S_1 and S_2.

they are of low frequency, they are better auscultated with the bell of the stethoscope. Similar murmurs can be heard with obstructing atrial myxomas. Severe chronic aortic insufficiency can lead to premature closure of the mitral valve, causing a mid-diastolic rumble called an Austin-Flint murmur. Late diastolic murmurs occur immediately before S_1 and reflect presystolic accentuation of the mid-diastolic murmurs resulting from augmented mitral or tricuspid flow after atrial contraction.

Continuous murmurs begin with S_1 and last though part or all of diastole. They are generated by continuous flow from a vessel or chamber with high pressure into a vessel or chamber with lower pressure. They are referred to as *machinery murmurs* and are caused by aortopulmonary connections such as a patent ductus arteriosus, AV malformations, or disturbances of flow in arteries or veins.

Other Cardiac Sounds

Pericardial rubs occur in the setting of pericarditis and are coarse, scratching sounds similar to rubbing leather. They are typically heard best at the left sternal border with the patient leaning forward and holding the breath at end-expiration. A classic pericardial rub has three components: atrial systole, ventricular systole, and ventricular diastole. One might also hear a pleural rub caused by localized irritation of surrounding pleura. Continuous venous murmurs, or *venous hums*, are almost always present in children. They can be heard in adults during pregnancy, in the setting of anemia, or with thyrotoxicosis. They are heard best at the base of the neck with the patient's head turned to the opposite direction.

Prosthetic Heart Sounds

Prosthetic heart valves produce characteristic findings on auscultation. Bioprosthetic valves produce sounds that are similar to those of native heart valves, but they are typically smaller than the valves that they replace and therefore have an associated murmur. Mechanical valves have crisp, high-pitched sounds related to valve opening and closure. In most modern valves such as the St. Jude valve, which is a bileaflet mechanical valve, the closure sound is louder than the opening sound. An ejection murmur is common. If there is a change in murmur or in the intensity of the mechanical valve closure sound, dysfunction of the valve should be suspected.

For a deeper discussion of this topic, please see Chapter 51, "Approach to the Patient with Possible Cardiovascular Disease," in Goldman-Cecil Medicine, 25th Edition.

SUGGESTED READINGS

Agency for Healthcare Research and Quality, U.S. Department of Health and Human Services: Total expenses and percent distribution for selected conditions by type of service: United States, 2008. Medical Expenditure Panel Survey: Household Component Summary Tables. Available at: http://www.meps.ahrq.gov/mepsweb/data_stats/quick_tables_search.jsp?component=1&subcomponent=0. Accessed August 5, 2014.

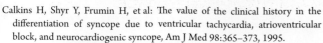
Calkins H, Shyr Y, Frumin H, et al: The value of the clinical history in the differentiation of syncope due to ventricular tachycardia, atrioventricular block, and neurocardiogenic syncope, Am J Med 98:365–373, 1995.

Go AS: The epidemiology of atrial fibrillation in elderly persons: the tip of the iceberg, Am J Geriatr Cardiol 14:56–61, 2005.

Goldman L, Ausiello D: Cecil Medicine: part VIII. Cardiovascular disease, Philadelphia, 2012, Saunders.

Hirsch AT, Criqui MH, Treat-Jacobson D, et al: Peripheral arterial disease: detection, awareness, and treatment in primary care, JAMA 286:1317–1324, 2001.

Hoffman JI, Kaplan S, Liberthson RR: Prevalence of congenital heart disease, Am Heart J 147:425–439, 2004.

National Vital Statistics System, Centers for Disease Control and Prevention: Mortality tables. Available at http://www.cdc.gov/nchs/nvss/mortality _tables.htm. Accessed August 5, 2014.

National Heart, Lung and Blood Institute, National Institutes of Health. Unpublished tabulations of National Vital Statistics System mortality data. 2008. Available at: http://www.cdc.gov/nchs/nvss/mortality_public_use _data.htm. Accessed August 5, 2014.

National Heart, Lung and Blood Institute, National Institutes of Health, Unpublished tabulations of National Hospital discharge survey, 2009. Available at http://www.cdc.gov/nchs/nhds/nhds_questionnaires.htm. Accessed August 5, 2014.

National Heart, Lung and Blood Institute. Unpublished tabulations of National Health interview survey, 1965-2010. Available at: http://www.cdc.gov/nchs/ nhis/nhis_questionnaires.htm. Accessed August 5, 2014.

National Heart, Lung and Blood Institute, National Institutes of Health. Morbidity and mortality: 2012 chart book on cardiovascular, lung, and blood diseases. Available at https://www.nhlbi.nih.gov/research/reports/2012-mortality -chart-book.htm. Accessed September 26, 2014.

Pickering TG, Hall JE, Appel LJ, et al: Recommendations for blood pressure measurement in humans and experimental animals: part 1. Blood pressure measurement in humans: a statement for professionals from the Subcommittee of Professional and Public Education of the American Heart Association Council on High Blood Pressure Research, Circulation 111:697–716, 2005.

Diagnostic Tests and Procedures in the Patient with Cardiovascular Disease

Ivor J. Benjamin

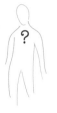

CHEST RADIOGRAPHY

The chest radiograph is an integral part of the cardiac evaluation, and it gives valuable information regarding the structure and function of the heart, lungs, and great vessels. A routine examination includes posteroanterior and lateral projections (Fig. 4-1).

In the posteroanterior view, cardiac enlargement may be identified when the transverse diameter of the cardiac silhouette is greater than one half of the transverse diameter of the thorax. The heart may appear falsely enlarged when it is displaced horizontally, such as with poor inflation of the lungs, and when the film is an anteroposterior projection, which magnifies the heart shadow. Left atrial enlargement is suggested when the left-sided heart border is straightened or bulges toward the left. The main bronchi may be widely splayed, and a circular opacity or *double density* may be seen in the cardiac silhouette. Right atrial enlargement may be confirmed when the right-sided heart border bulges toward the right. Left ventricular enlargement results in

downward and lateral displacement of the apex. A rounding of the displaced apex suggests ventricular hypertrophy. Right ventricular enlargement is best assessed on the lateral view and may be diagnosed when the right ventricular border occupies more than one third of the retrosternal space between the diaphragm and thoracic apex.

The aortic arch and thoracic aorta may become dilated and tortuous in patients with severe atherosclerosis, long-standing hypertension, and aortic dissection. Dilation of the proximal pulmonary arteries may occur when pulmonary pressures are elevated and pulmonary vascular resistance is increased. Disease states associated with increased pulmonary artery flow and normal vascular resistance, such as atrial or ventricular septal defects, may result in dilation of the proximal and distal pulmonary arteries.

Pulmonary venous congestion due to elevated left ventricular heart pressure results in redistribution of blood flow in the lungs and prominence of the apical vessels. Transudation of fluid into the interstitial space may result in fluid in the fissures and along

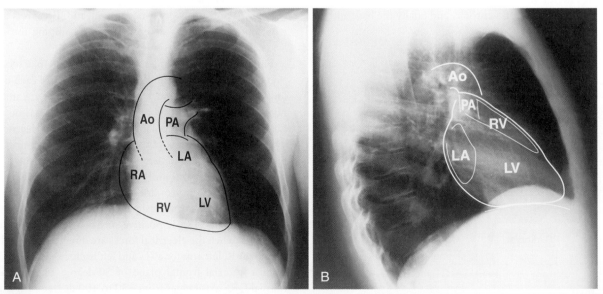

FIGURE 4-1 Schematic illustration of the parts of the heart, whose outlines can be identified on a routine chest radiograph. **A,** Posteroanterior chest radiograph. **B,** Lateral chest radiograph. Ao, Aorta; LA, left atrium; LV, left ventricle; PA, pulmonary artery; RA, right atrium; RV, right ventricle.

the horizontal periphery of the lower lung fields (i.e., Kerley B lines). As venous pressures further increase, fluid collects in the alveolar space, which early on collects preferentially in the inner two thirds of the lung fields, resulting in a characteristic butterfly appearance.

Fluoroscopy or plain films may identify abnormal calcification involving the pericardium, coronary arteries, aorta, and valves. Fluoroscopy can be instrumental in evaluating the function of mechanical prosthetic valves. Specific radiographic signs of congenital and valvular diseases are discussed in later sections.

Electrocardiography

The electrocardiogram (ECG) represents the electrical activity of the heart recorded by skin electrodes. This wave of electrical activity is represented as a sequence of deflections on the ECG (Fig. 4-2). The horizontal axis of the graph paper represents time, and at a standard paper speed of 25 mm/second, each small box (1 mm) represents 0.04 second, and each large box (5 mm) represents 0.20 second. The vertical axis represents voltage or amplitude (10 mm = 1 mV). The heart rate can be estimated by dividing the number of large boxes between complexes (i.e., R-R interval) into 300.

In the normal heart, the electrical impulse originates in the sinoatrial (SA) node and is conducted through the atria. Given that depolarization of the SA node is too weak to be detected on the surface ECG, the first, low-amplitude deflection on the surface ECG represents atrial activation and is called the *P wave.* The interval between the onset of the P wave and the next rapid deflection (QRS complex) is known as the *PR interval.* It primarily represents the time taken for the impulse to travel through the atrioventricular (AV) node. The normal PR segment ranges from 0.12 to 0.20 second. A PR interval greater than 0.20 second defines AV nodal block.

After the wave of depolarization has moved through the AV node, the ventricular myocardium is depolarized in a sequence of four phases. The interventricular septum depolarizes from left to right. This phase is followed by depolarization of the right ventricle and inferior wall of the left ventricle, then the apex and central portions of the left ventricle, and finally the base and the

posterior wall of the left ventricle. Ventricular depolarization results in a high-amplitude complex on the surface ECG known as the *QRS complex.* The first downward deflection of this complex is the Q wave, the first upward deflection is the R wave, and the subsequent downward deflection is the S wave. In some individuals, a second upward deflection may occur after the S wave, and it is called *R prime* (R′). Normal duration of the QRS complex is less than 0.10 second. Complexes greater than 0.12 second are usually secondary to some form of interventricular conduction delay.

The isoelectric segment after the QRS complex is the ST segment, which represents a brief period during which relatively little electrical activity occurs in the heart. The junction between the end of the QRS complex and the beginning of the ST segment is the J point. The upward deflection after the ST segment is the T wave, which represents ventricular repolarization. The QT interval, which reflects the duration and transmural gradient of ventricular depolarization and repolarization, is measured from the onset of the QRS complex to the end of the T wave. The QT interval varies with heart rate, but for rates between 60 and 100 beats/minute, the normal QT interval ranges from 0.35 to 0.44 second. For heart rates outside this range, the QT interval can be corrected (QT$_c$) using the following formula (all measurements in seconds):

$$QT_c = QT / R\text{-}R \text{ interval}^{1/2}$$

In some individuals, the T wave may be closely followed by a U wave (0.5 mm deflection, not shown in Figure 4-2), the cause of which is unknown.

The standard ECG consists of 12 leads: six limb leads (I, II, III, aVR, aVL, and aVF) and six chest or precordial leads (V$_1$ to V$_6$) (Fig. 4-3). The electrical activity recorded in each lead represents the direction and magnitude (i.e., vector) of the electrical force as seen from that lead position. Electrical activity directed toward a particular lead is represented as an upward deflection, and an electrical impulse directed away from a particular lead is represented as a downward deflection. Although the overall direction of electrical activity can be determined for any of the waveforms previously described, the mean QRS axis is the most clinically useful and is determined by examining the six limb leads.

Figure 4-4 illustrates the axial reference system, a reconstruction of the Einthoven triangle, and the polarity of each of the six limb leads of the standard ECG. Skin electrodes are attached to both arms and legs, with the right leg serving as the ground. Leads I, II, and III are bipolar leads and represent electrical activity between two leads. Lead I represents electrical activity between the right and left arms (left arm positive), lead II between the right arm and left leg (left leg positive), and lead III between the left arm and left leg (left leg positive). Leads aVR, aVL, and aVF are designated the *augmented leads.* Using these leads, the QRS is positive or has a predominant upward deflection when the electrical forces are directed toward the right arm for aVR, left arm for aVL, and left leg for aVF. These six leads form a hexaxial frontal plane of 30-degree arc intervals. The normal QRS axis ranges from −30 to +90 degrees. An axis more negative than −30 defines left axis deviation, and an axis greater than +90 defines right axis deviation. A positive QRS complex

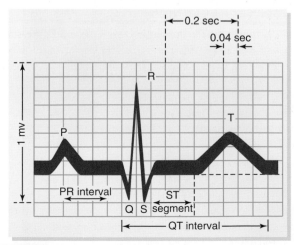

FIGURE 4-2 Normal electrocardiographic complex with labeling of waves and intervals.

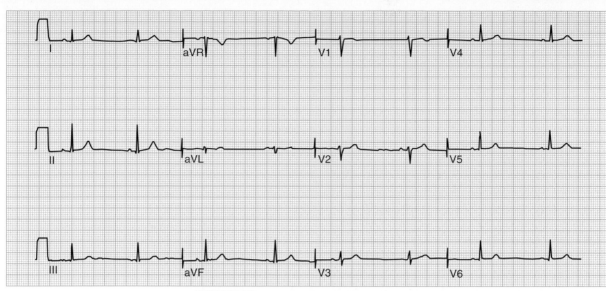

FIGURE 4-3 Normal 12-lead electrocardiogram.

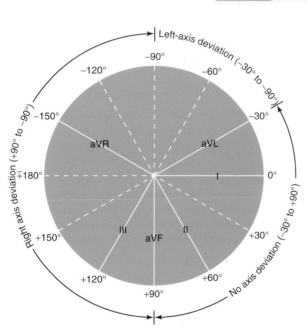

FIGURE 4-4 Hexaxial reference figure for frontal plane axis determination, indicating values for abnormal left and right QRS axis deviations.

in leads I and aVF suggests a normal QRS axis between 0 and 90 degrees.

The six standard precordial leads (V_1 to V_6) are attached to the anterior chest wall (Fig. 4-5). Lead placement should be as follows: V_1: fourth intercostal space, right sternal border; V_2: fourth intercostal space, left sternal border; V_3: midway between V_2 and V_4; V_4: fifth intercostal space, left midclavicular line; V_5: level with V_4, left anterior axillary line; V_6: level with V_4, left midaxillary line. The chest leads should be placed under the breast.

Electrical activity directed toward these leads results in a positive deflection on the ECG. Leads V_1 and V_2 are closest to the right ventricle and interventricular septum, and leads V_5 and V_6 are closest to the anterior and anterolateral walls of the left ventricle. Normally, a small R wave occurs in lead V_1, reflecting septal depolarization, along with a deep S wave, reflecting predominantly left ventricular activation. From V_1 to V_6, the R wave becomes larger (and the S wave smaller) because the predominant forces directed at these leads originate from the left ventricle. The transition from a predominant S wave to a predominant R wave usually occurs between leads V_3 and V_4.

Right-sided chest leads are used to look for evidence of right ventricular infarction. ST-segment elevation in V_{4R} has the best sensitivity and specificity for making this diagnosis. For right-sided leads, standard V_1 and V_2 are switched, and V_{3R} to V_{6R} are placed in a mirror image of the standard left-sided chest leads. Some groups have advocated the use of posterior leads to increase the sensitivity for diagnosing lateral and posterior wall infarction or ischemia—areas that are often deemed to be *electrically silent* on traditional 12-lead ECGs. To do this, six additional leads are placed in the fifth intercostal space continuing posteriorly from the position of V_6.

ABNORMAL ELECTROCARDIOGRAPHIC PATTERNS

Chamber Abnormalities and Ventricular Hypertrophy

The P wave is normally upright in leads I, II, and F; inverted in aVR; and biphasic in V_1. Left atrial abnormality (i.e., enlargement, hypertrophy, or increased wall stress) is characterized by a wide P wave in lead II (0.12 second) and a deeply inverted terminal component in lead V_1 (1 mm). Right atrial abnormality is identified when the P waves in the limb leads are peaked and at least 2.5 mm high.

Left ventricular hypertrophy may result in increased QRS voltage, slight widening of the QRS complex, late intrinsicoid deflection, left axis deviation, and abnormalities of the ST-T segments (see Fig. 4-5A). Multiple criteria with various degrees of sensitivity and specificity for detecting left ventricular hypertrophy are available. The most frequently used criteria are given in Table 4-1.

Right ventricular hypertrophy is characterized by tall R waves in leads V_1 through V_3; deep S waves in leads I, aVL, V_5, and V_6;

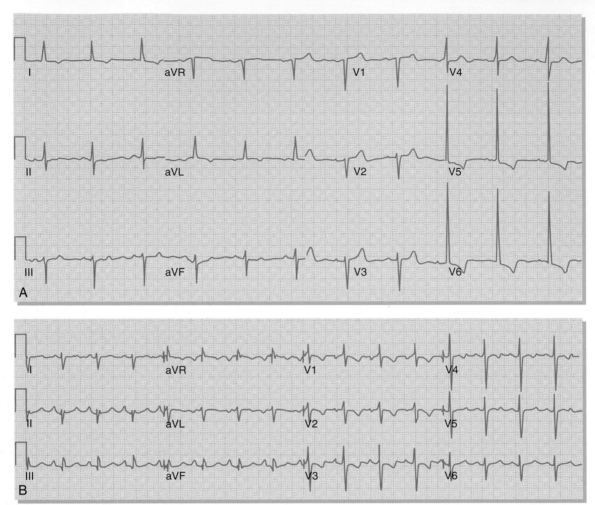

FIGURE 4-5   **A,** Left ventricular hypertrophy as seen on an electrocardiographic recording. Characteristic findings include increased QRS voltage in precordial leads (i.e., deep S in lead V_2 and tall R in lead V_5) and downsloping ST depression and T-wave inversion in lateral precordial leads (i.e., strain pattern) and leftward axis. **B,** Right ventricular hypertrophy with tall R wave in right precordial leads, downsloping ST depression in precordial leads (i.e., RV strain), right axis deviation, and evidence of right atrial enlargement.

and right axis deviation (see Fig. 4-5B). In patients with chronically elevated pulmonary pressures, such as with chronic lung disease, a combination of ECG abnormalities reflecting a right-sided pathologic condition may be identified and include right atrial abnormality, right ventricular hypertrophy, and right axis deviation. In patients with acute pulmonary embolus, ECG changes may suggest right ventricular strain and include right axis deviation; incomplete or complete right bundle branch block (RBBB); S waves in leads I, II, and III; and T-wave inversions in leads V_1 through V_3.

Interventricular Conduction Delays

The ventricular conduction system consists of two main branches, the right and left bundles. The left bundle further divides into the anterior and posterior fascicles. Conduction block can occur in either of the major branches or in the fascicles (Table 4-2).

Fascicular block results in a change in the sequence of ventricular activation but does not prolong overall conduction time (i.e., QRS duration remains <0.10 second). Left anterior fascicular block is a relatively common ECG abnormality and is sometimes associated with RBBB. This conduction abnormality is identified when extreme left axis deviation occurs (i.e., more

negative than −45 degrees), when the R wave is greater than the Q wave in leads I and aVL, and when the S wave is greater than the R wave in leads II, III, and aVF. Left posterior fascicular block is uncommon but is associated with right axis deviation (>90 degrees); small Q waves in leads II, III, and aVF; and small R waves in leads I and aVL. The ECG findings associated with fascicular blocks can be confused with myocardial infarction (MI). For example, with left anterior fascicular block, the prominent QS deflection in leads V_1 and V_2 can mimic an anteroseptal MI, and the rS deflection in leads II, III, and aVF can be confused with an inferior MI. Similarly, the rS deflection in leads I and aVL in left posterior fascicular block may be confused with a high lateral infarct. Abnormal ST- and T-wave segments and pathologic Q waves (see Myocardial Ischemia and Infarction) are helpful findings for differentiating MI from a fascicular block.

Bundle branch blocks are associated with a QRS duration longer than 120 milliseconds. In left bundle branch block (LBBB), depolarization proceeds down the right bundle, across the interventricular septum from right to left, and then to the left ventricle. Characteristic electrocardiographic findings include a wide QRS complex; a broad R wave in leads I, aVL, V_5, and V_6; a deep QS wave in leads V_1 and V_2; and ST depression and

TABLE 4-1	ELECTROCARDIOGRAPHIC MANIFESTATIONS OF ATRIAL ABNORMALITIES AND VENTRICULAR HYPERTROPHY

LEFT ATRIAL ABNORMALITY

P-wave duration ≥0.12 second
Notched, slurred P wave in leads I and II
Biphasic P wave in lead V_1 with a wide, deep, negative terminal component

RIGHT ATRIAL ABNORMALITY

P-wave duration ≤0.11 second
Tall, peaked P waves of ≥2.5 mm in leads II, III, and aVF

LEFT VENTRICULAR HYPERTROPHY

Voltage criteria
R wave in lead aVL ≥12 mm
R wave in lead I ≥15 mm
S wave in lead V_1 or V_2 + R wave in lead V_5 or V_6 ≥35 mm
Depressed ST segments with inverted T waves in the lateral leads
Left axis deviation
QRS duration ≥0.09 second
Left atrial enlargement

RIGHT VENTRICULAR HYPERTROPHY

Tall R waves over right precordium (R-to-S ratio in lead V_1 >1.0)
Right axis deviation
Depressed ST segments with inverted T waves in leads V_1 to V_3
Normal QRS duration (if no right bundle branch block)
Right atrial enlargement

TABLE 4-2	ELECTROCARDIOGRAPHIC MANIFESTATIONS OF FASCICULAR AND BUNDLE BRANCH BLOCKS

LEFT ANTERIOR FASCICULAR BLOCK

QRS duration ≤0.1 second
Left axis deviation (more negative than −45 degrees)
rS pattern in leads II, III, and aVF
qR pattern in leads I and aVL

RIGHT POSTERIOR FASCICULAR BLOCK

QRS duration ≤0.1 second
Right axis deviation (+90 degrees or greater)
qR pattern in leads II, III, and aVF
rS pattern in leads I and aVL
Exclusion of other causes of right axis deviation (e.g., chronic obstructive pulmonary disease, right ventricular hypertrophy)

LEFT BUNDLE BRANCH BLOCK

QRS duration ≥0.12 second
Broad, slurred, or notched R waves in lateral leads (I, aVL, V_5, and V_6)
QS or rS pattern in anterior precordium leads (V_1 and V_2)
ST-T-wave vectors opposite to terminal QRS vectors

RIGHT BUNDLE BRANCH BLOCK

QRS duration ≥0.12 second
Large R′ wave in lead V_1 (rsR′)
Deep terminal S wave in lead V_6
Normal septal Q waves
Inverted T waves in leads V_1 and V_2

T-wave inversion opposite the QRS deflection (Fig. 4-6A). Given the abnormal sequence of ventricular activation with LBBB, many ECG abnormalities, such as Q-wave MI and left ventricular hypertrophy, are difficult to evaluate. In some cases, acute MI is apparent even with LBBB. An LBBB typically indicates underlying myocardial disease—most commonly fibrosis due to ischemic injury or hypertrophy. With RBBB, the interventricular septum depolarizes normally from left to right, the initial QRS deflection remains unchanged, and ECG abnormalities such as Q-wave MI can still be interpreted. After septal activation, the left ventricle depolarizes, followed by the right ventricle. The ECG is characterized by a wide QRS complex; a large R′ wave in lead V_1 (R-S-R′); and deep S waves in leads I, aVL, and V_6, representing delayed right ventricular activation (see Fig. 4-6B). Although RBBB may be associated with underlying cardiac disease, it may also appear as a normal variant or be seen intermittently when heart rate is elevated. In the latter case, it is referred to as *rate-related bundle branch block*.

Myocardial Ischemia and Infarction

Myocardial ischemia and MI may be associated with abnormalities of the ST segment, T wave, and QRS complex. Myocardial ischemia primarily affects repolarization of the myocardium and is often associated with horizontal or down-sloping ST-segment depression and T-wave inversion. These changes may be transient, such as during an anginal episode or an exercise stress test, or they may be long-lasting in the setting of unstable angina or MI. T-wave inversion without ST-segment depression is a nonspecific finding and must be correlated with the clinical findings. Localized ST-segment elevation suggests more extensive myocardial injury and is often associated with acute MI (Fig. 4-7). Vasospastic or Prinzmetal angina may be associated with reversible ST-segment elevation without MI. ST-segment elevation may occur in other settings not related to acute ischemia or infarction. Persistent, localized ST-segment elevation in the same leads as pathologic Q waves is consistent with a ventricular aneurysm. Acute pericarditis is associated with diffuse ST-segment elevation and PR depression. Diffuse J-point elevation in association with upward-coving ST segments is a normal variant common among young men and is often referred to as *early repolarization.*

A Q wave is one of the criteria used to diagnose MI. Infarcted myocardium is unable to conduct electrical activity, and electrical forces are directed away from the surface electrode overlying the infarcted region, producing a Q wave on the surface ECG. Knowing which region of the myocardium each lead represents enables the examiner to localize the area of infarction (Table 4-3). A pathologic Q wave has a duration greater than or equal to 0.04 second or a depth one fourth or more of the height of the corresponding R wave.

Not all MIs result in the formation of Q waves. Small R waves can return many weeks to months after an MI.

Abnormal Q waves, or *pseudoinfarction,* may be associated with nonischemic cardiac disease, such as ventricular preexcitation, cardiac amyloidosis, sarcoidosis, idiopathic or hypertrophic cardiomyopathy, myocarditis, and chronic lung disease.

Abnormalities of the ST Segment and T Wave

A number of drugs and metabolic abnormalities may affect the ST segment and T wave (Fig. 4-8). Hypokalemia may result in prominent U waves in the precordial leads and prolongation of the QT interval. Hyperkalemia may result in tall, peaked T waves. Hypocalcemia typically lengthens the QT interval, whereas hypercalcemia shortens it. A commonly used cardiac medication, digoxin, often results in diffuse, scooped ST-segment depression. Minor or *nonspecific* ST-segment and T-wave abnormalities may occur in many patients and have no definable cause. In these

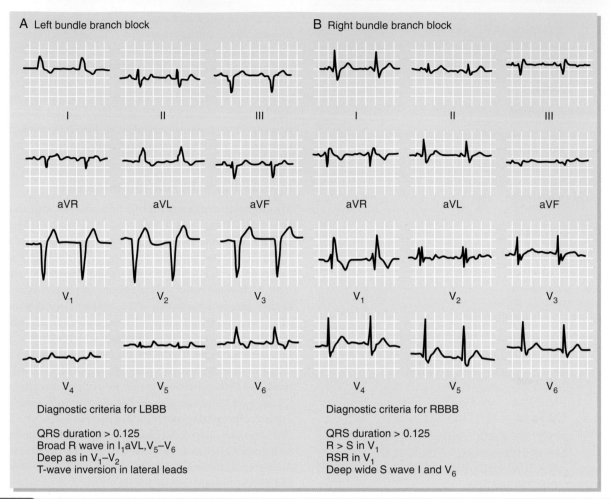

A Left bundle branch block

B Right bundle branch block

Diagnostic criteria for LBBB

QRS duration > 0.125
Broad R wave in I_1aVL, V_5-V_6
Deep as in V_1-V_2
T-wave inversion in lateral leads

Diagnostic criteria for RBBB

QRS duration > 0.125
$R > S$ in V_1
RSR in V_1
Deep wide S wave I and V_6

FIGURE 4-6 **A,** Left bundle branch block (LBBB). **B,** Right bundle branch block (RBBB). Criteria for bundle branch blocks are summarized in Table 4-2.

instances, the physician must determine the significance of the abnormalities based on clinical findings. Several excellent websites containing examples of normal and abnormal ECGs are available.

⬤ LONG-TERM AMBULATORY ELECTROCARDIOGRAPHIC RECORDING

An ambulatory ECG (i.e., Holter monitoring) is a widely used, noninvasive method to evaluate cardiac arrhythmias and conduction disturbances over an extended period and to detect electrical abnormalities that may be brief or transient. With this approach, ECG data from two to three surface leads are stored on a tape recorder that the patient wears for at least 24 to 48 hours. The recorders have patient-activated event markers and time markers so that any abnormalities can be correlated with the patient's symptoms or time of day. These data can then be printed in a standard, real-time ECG format for review.

For patients with intermittent or rare symptoms, an event recorder, which can be worn for several weeks, may be helpful in identifying the arrhythmia. The simplest device is a small, hand-held monitor that is applied to the chest wall when symptoms occur. The ECG data are recorded and can be transmitted later by telephone to a monitoring center for analysis. A more sophisticated system uses a wrist recorder that allows continuous-loop

storage of 4 to 5 minutes of ECG data from one lead. When the patient activates the system, ECG data preceding the event and for 1 to 2 minutes after the event are recorded and stored for further analysis. With both devices, the patient must be physically able to activate the recorder during the episode to store the ECG data. Implantable (subcutaneous) recording devices are sometimes used to diagnose infrequent events over extended periods (i.e., months).

Stress Testing

Stress testing is an important noninvasive tool for evaluating patients with known or suggested coronary artery disease (CAD). During exercise, the increased demand for oxygen by the working skeletal muscles is met by increases in heart rate and cardiac output. In patients with significant CAD, the increase in myocardial oxygen demand cannot be met by an increase in coronary blood flow, and myocardial ischemia may produce chest pain and characteristic ECG abnormalities. Combined with the hemodynamic response to exercise, these changes can give useful diagnostic and prognostic information for the patient with cardiac abnormalities. The most common indications for stress testing include establishing a diagnosis of CAD in patients with chest pain, assessing prognosis and functional capacity of patients with chronic stable angina or after an MI, evaluating exercise-induced

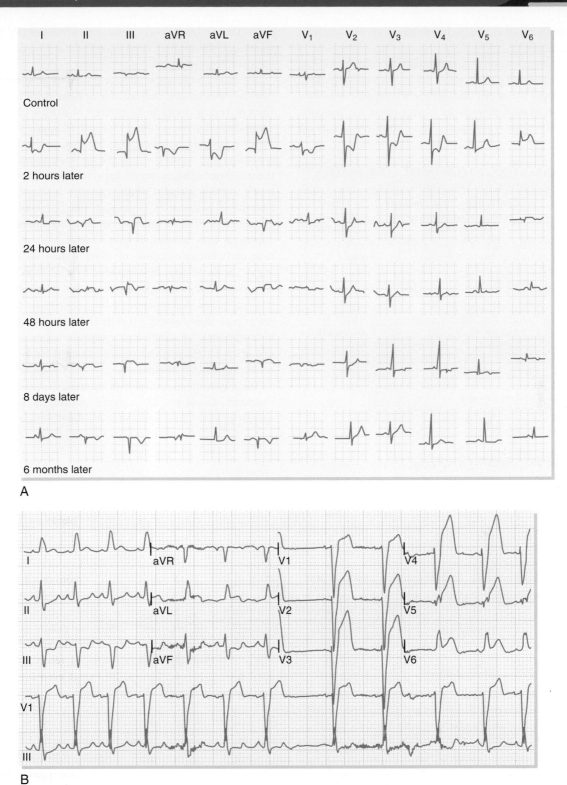

FIGURE 4-7 **A,** Evolutionary changes in a posteroinferior myocardial infarction (MI). Control tracing is normal. The tracing recorded 2 hours after onset of chest pain demonstrated development of early Q waves, marked ST-segment elevation, and hyperacute T waves in leads II, III, and aVF. A larger R wave, ST-segment depression, and negative T waves have developed in leads V_1 and V_2. These early changes indicate acute posteroinferior MI. The 24-hour tracing demonstrates further evolutionary changes. In leads II, III, and aVF, the Q wave is larger, the ST segments have almost returned to baseline, and the T wave has begun to invert. In leads V_1 to V_2, the duration of the R wave exceeds 0.04 seconds, the ST segment is depressed, and the T wave is upright. (In this example, electrocardiographic changes of true posterior involvement extend past lead V_2; ordinarily, only leads V_1 and V_2 may be involved.) Only minor further changes occur through the 8-day tracing. Six months later, the electrocardiographic pattern shows large Q waves, isoelectric ST segments, and inverted T waves in leads II, III, and aVF and shows large R waves, isoelectric ST segment, and upright T waves in leads V_1 and V_2, indicative of an old posteroinferior MI. **B,** Electrocardiogram from a patient with an underlying left bundle branch block (LBBB) who experienced an acute anterior MI. Characteristic ST segment elevation and hyperacute T waves are seen in leads V_1 through V_6 and leads I and aVL despite the presence of the LBBB. This is not always the case, and a patient with typical symptoms, an LBBB, and no definite ischemic ST-segment elevations should be treated as if the individual is having a myocardial infarction or acute coronary syndrome.

arrhythmias, and assessing for ischemia after a revascularization procedure.

The most common form of stress testing uses continuous ECG monitoring while the patient walks on a treadmill. With each advancing stage, the speed and incline of the belt increases, increasing the amount of work the patient performs. The commonly used Bruce protocol employs 3 minutes of exercise at each stage. The modified Bruce protocol incorporates two beginning stages with slower speeds and lesser inclines than are used in the standard Bruce protocol.

The modified Bruce or similar protocols are used for older, markedly overweight, and unstable or more debilitated patients. Exercise testing may also be performed using a bicycle or arm ergometer. The stress test is deemed adequate if the patient achieves 90% of his or her predicted maximal heart rate, which is equal to 220 minus the patient's age. Indications for stopping the test include fatigue, severe hypertension (>220 mm Hg systolic), worsening angina during exercise, developing marked or widespread ischemic ECG changes, significant arrhythmias, or hypotension. The diagnostic accuracy of stress testing is improved with adjunctive echocardiography or radionuclide imaging. Contraindications to stress testing include unstable angina, acute MI, poorly controlled hypertension (blood pressure >220/110 mm Hg), severe aortic stenosis (valve area <1.0 cm^2), and decompensated congestive heart failure. In the era of reperfusion therapy (i.e. thrombolytic and percutaneous interventions), for acute coronary syndromes or acute MI, little role exists for the predischarge submaximal stress test that was commonly used in the past.

The diagnostic accuracy of the exercise test depends on the pretest likelihood of CAD in a given patient, the sensitivity and specificity of the test results in that patient population, and the

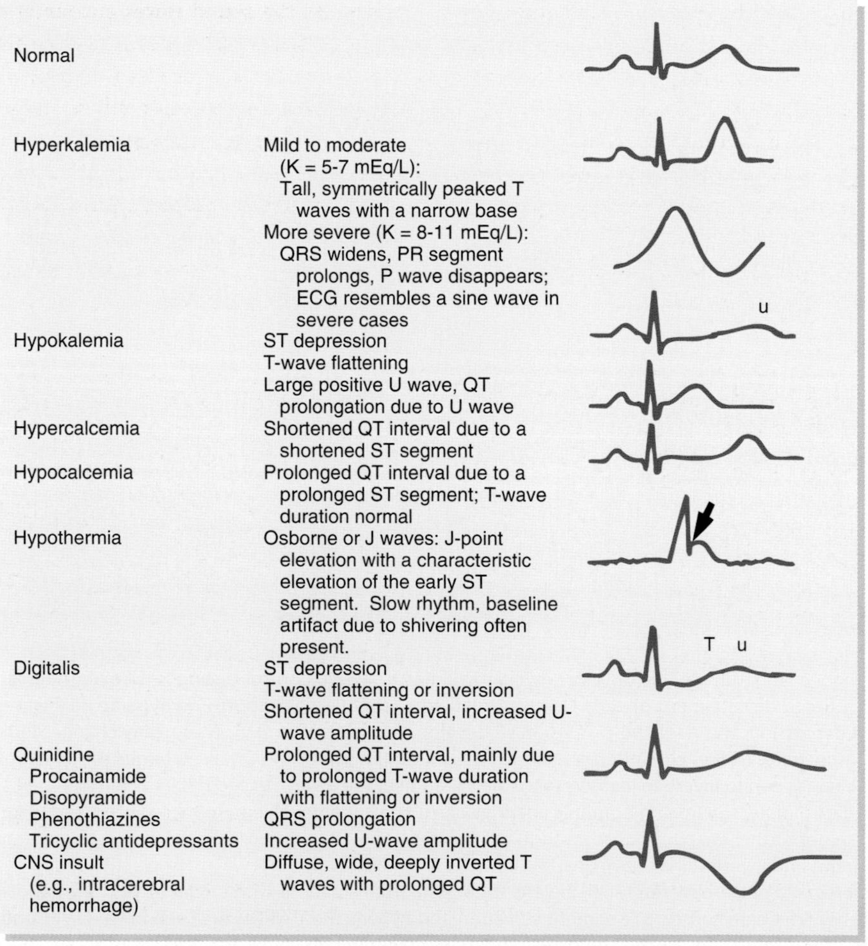

TABLE 4-3 ELECTROCARDIOGRAPHIC LOCALIZATION OF MYOCARDIAL INFARCTION

INFARCT LOCATION	LEADS DEPICTING PRIMARY ELECTROCARDIOGRAPHIC CHANGES	LIKELY VESSEL INVOLVED*
Inferior	II, III, aVF	RCA
Septal	V_1, V_2	LAD
Anterior	V_3, V_4	LAD
Anteroseptal	V_1 to V_4	LAD
Extensive anterior	I, aVL, V_1 to V_6	LAD
Lateral	I, aVL, V_5 to V_6	CIRC
High lateral	I, aVL	CIRC
Posterior[†]	Prominent R in V_1	RCA or CIRC
Right ventricular[‡]	ST elevation in V_1; more specifically, V_4R in setting of inferior infarction	RCA

CIRC, Circumflex artery; LAD, left anterior descending coronary artery; RCA, right coronary artery.

*This is a generalization; variations occur.

[†]Usually in association with inferior or lateral infarction.

[‡]Usually in association with inferior infarction.

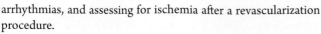

Normal		
Hyperkalemia	Mild to moderate (K = 5-7 mEq/L): Tall, symmetrically peaked T waves with a narrow base	
	More severe (K = 8-11 mEq/L): QRS widens, PR segment prolongs, P wave disappears; ECG resembles a sine wave in severe cases	
Hypokalemia	ST depression T-wave flattening	
	Large positive U wave, QT prolongation due to U wave	
Hypercalcemia	Shortened QT interval due to a shortened ST segment	
Hypocalcemia	Prolonged QT interval due to a prolonged ST segment; T-wave duration normal	
Hypothermia	Osborne or J waves: J-point elevation with a characteristic elevation of the early ST segment. Slow rhythm, baseline artifact due to shivering often present.	
Digitalis	ST depression T-wave flattening or inversion Shortened QT interval, increased U-wave amplitude	
Quinidine Procainamide Disopyramide Phenothiazines Tricyclic antidepressants	Prolonged QT interval, mainly due to prolonged T-wave duration with flattening or inversion QRS prolongation Increased U-wave amplitude	
CNS insult (e.g., intracerebral hemorrhage)	Diffuse, wide, deeply inverted T waves with prolonged QT	

FIGURE 4-8 Metabolic and drug influences on the electrocardiographic recording. CNS, Central nervous system; ECG, electrocardiogram.

ECG criteria used to define a positive test. Clinical features that are most useful for predicting important angiographic coronary disease before exercise testing include advanced age, male sex, and typical (versus atypical) anginal chest pain.

The diagnostic accuracy and cost-effectiveness of exercise testing is best for patients at intermediate risk for CAD (30% to 70%) and when ischemic ECG changes are accompanied by chest pain during exercise. Exercise testing is less cost-effective in diagnosing CAD in a patient with classic symptoms of angina because a positive test result does not significantly increase the post-test probability of CAD, and a negative test result likely represents a false-negative result. Nonetheless, prognostic information and objective information about the efficacy of pharmacologic therapy may still be obtained. Similarly, exercise testing in young patients with atypical chest pain may not be diagnostically useful because an abnormal test result is likely a false-positive result and does not significantly increase the post-test probability of CAD.

The normal physiologic response to exercise is an increase in heart rate and systolic and diastolic blood pressures. The ECG maintains normal T-wave polarity, and the ST segment remains unchanged or, if depressed, has a rapid upstroke back to baseline. An ischemic ECG response to exercise is defined as 1.5 mm of up-sloping ST-segment depression measured 0.08 second past the J point, at least 1 mm of horizontal ST depression, or 1 mm of down-sloping ST-segment depression measured at the J point. Given the large amount of artifact on the ECG that may occur with exercise, these changes must be seen in at least three consecutive depolarizations. Other findings that suggest more extensive CAD include early onset of ST depression (6 minutes); marked, down-sloping ST depression (>2 mm), especially if present in more than five leads; ST changes persisting into recovery for more than 5 minutes; and failure to increase systolic blood pressure to 120 mm Hg or more or a sustained decrease of 10 mm Hg or more below baseline.

The ECG is not diagnostically useful for left ventricular hypertrophy, LBBB, Wolff-Parkinson-White syndrome, or chronic digoxin therapy. In these instances, nuclear or echocardiographic imaging is needed to diagnose ischemia. For patients who are unable to exercise, pharmacologic stress testing with myocardial imaging has the sensitivity and specificity for detecting CAD equal to those of exercise stress imaging. Intravenous dipyridamole and adenosine and newer selective adenosine A2A receptor agonists are coronary vasodilators that increase blood flow in normal arteries without significantly changing the flow in diseased vessels. The resulting heterogeneity in blood flow can be detected by nuclear imaging techniques, and the regions of myocardium supplied by diseased vessels can be identified.

Another commonly used technique to evaluate ischemia is dobutamine-stress echocardiography. Dobutamine is an inotropic agent that increases myocardial oxygen demand by increasing heart rate and contractility. The echocardiogram is used to monitor for ischemia, which is defined as new or worsening wall motion abnormalities during the infusion. Demonstrating improvement in wall thickening with low-dose dobutamine suggests that there is myocardial viability of abnormal segments (i.e., segments that are hypokinetic or akinetic at baseline).

Echocardiography

Echocardiography is a widely used, noninvasive technique in which sound waves are used to image cardiac structures and evaluate blood flow. A piezoelectric crystal housed in a transducer placed on the patient's chest wall produces ultrasound waves. As the sound waves encounter structures with different acoustic properties, some of the ultrasound waves are reflected to the transducer and recorded. Ultrasound waves emitted from a single, stationary crystal produce an image of a thin slice of the heart (M mode), which can be followed through time. Steering the ultrasound beam across a 90-degree arc multiple times per second creates two-dimensional imaging (Fig. 4-9). Transthoracic echocardiography is safe, simple, fast, and relatively inexpensive. It is the most commonly used test to assess cardiac size, structure, and function.

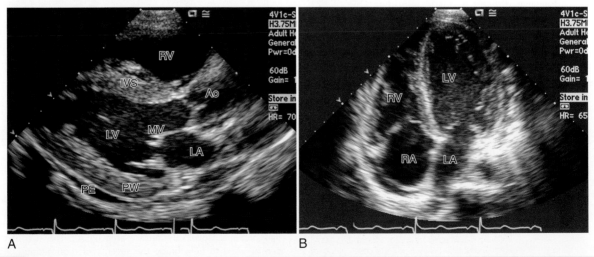

A   B

FIGURE 4-9 Portions of standard two-dimensional echocardiograms show the major cardiac structures in a parasternal long-axis view (**A**) and apical four-chamber view (**B**). Video 4-3 shows a moving image of a two-dimensional echocardiogram. Ao, Aorta; IVS, interventricular septum; LA, left atrium; LV, left ventricle; MV, mitral valve; PE, pericardial effusion; PW, posterior left ventricular wall; RV, right ventricle. (Image courtesy Sheldon E. Litwin, MD, Division of Cardiology, University of Utah, Salt Lake City, Utah.)

The development of three-dimensional echocardiographic imaging techniques offers great promise for more accurate measurements of chamber volumes and mass, as well as the assessment of geometrically complex anatomy and valvular lesions. Video 4-1 shows a three-dimensional image.

Doppler echocardiography allows assessment of the direction and velocity of blood flow in the heart and great vessels. When ultrasound waves encounter moving red blood cells, the energy reflected to the transducer is altered. The magnitude of this change (i.e., Doppler shift) is represented as velocity on the echocardiographic display and can be used to determine whether the blood flow is normal or abnormal (Fig. 4-10). The velocity of a particular jet of blood can be converted to pressure using the modified Bernoulli equation ($\Delta P \cong 4v^2$). This process allows assessment of pressure gradients across valves or between chambers. Color Doppler imaging allows visualization of blood flow through the heart by assigning a color to the red blood cells based on their velocity and direction (Fig. 4-11, Video 4-2). By convention, blood moving away from the transducer is represented in shades of blue, and blood moving toward the transducer is represented in red. Color Doppler imaging is particularly useful in identifying valvular insufficiency and abnormal shunt flow between chambers. The use of Doppler techniques to record myocardial velocities or strain rates has provided insights into myocardial function and hemodynamics.

Two-dimensional echocardiography and Doppler echocardiography are often used in conjunction with exercise or pharmacologic stress testing. Although sensitivity and specificity values vary among studies, the sensitivity of stress echocardiography is apparently slightly lower and the specificity slightly higher compared with myocardial perfusion imaging using nuclear tracers. The estimated cost-effectiveness of stress echocardiography is significantly better than nuclear perfusion imaging because of the lower cost.

The development of ultrasound contrast agents composed of microbubbles that are small enough to transit through the pulmonary circulation has greatly improved the ability to use ultrasound to image obese patients, patients with lung disease, and those with otherwise difficult acoustic windows (Fig. 4-12). Video 4-3 shows a dynamic contrast echocardiographic image.

These agents are being developed for molecular imaging by complexing the bubbles to compounds that can selectively bind to the target site of interest (i.e., clots, neovessels).

Transesophageal echocardiography (TEE) allows two-dimensional and Doppler imaging of the heart through the esophagus by having the patient swallow a gastroscope mounted with an ultrasound crystal in its tip. Given the proximity of the esophagus to the heart, high-resolution images can be obtained, especially of the left atrium, mitral valve apparatus, and aorta. TEE is particularly useful in diagnosing aortic dissection, endocarditis, prosthetic valve dysfunction, and left atrial masses (Fig. 4-13, Video 4-4).

Nuclear Cardiology

Radionuclide imaging of the heart allows quantification of left ventricular size, systolic function, and myocardial perfusion. For radionuclide ventriculography, the patient's red blood cells are labeled with a small amount of a radioactive tracer (usually technetium-99m).

Left ventricular function can then be assessed by one of two methods. With the first-pass technique, radiation emitted by the tagged red blood cells as they initially flow though the heart is detected by a gamma camera positioned over the patient's chest. With the gated equilibrium method, or multigated acquisition (MUGA) method, the tracer is allowed to achieve an equilibrium distribution throughout the blood pool before count acquisition begins. This second method improves the resolution of the ventriculogram. For both techniques, the gamma camera can be gated to the ECG, allowing determination of the total emitted end-diastole counts (EDCs) and end-systole counts (ESCs). Left

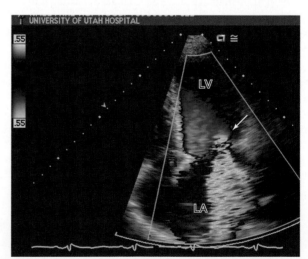

FIGURE 4-11 Color Doppler recording demonstrates severe mitral regurgitation. The regurgitant jet seen in the left atrium is represented in *blue* because blood flow is directed away from the transducer. The *yellow* components are the mosaic pattern traditionally assigned to turbulent or high-velocity flow. The *arrow* points to the hemisphere of blood accelerating proximal to the regurgitant orifice (i.e., proximal isovelocity surface area [PISA]). The size of the PISA can be used to help grade the severity of regurgitation. Video 4-2 shows a dynamic echocardiographic image in a patient with mitral regurgitation. LA, Left atrium; LV, left ventricle. (Image courtesy Sheldon E. Litwin, MD, Division of Cardiology, University of Utah, Salt Lake City, Utah.)

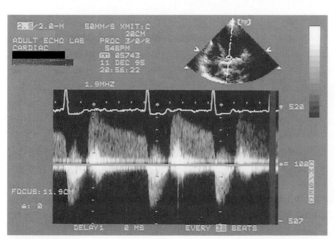

FIGURE 4-10 Doppler tracing in a patient with aortic stenosis and regurgitation. The velocity of systolic flow is related to the severity of obstruction.

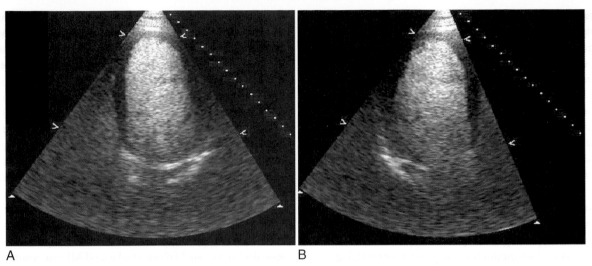

A   B

FIGURE 4-12 Echocardiogram enhanced with intravenous ultrasound contrast agent: apical four-chamber view (**A**) and apical long-axis view (**B**). Highly echo-reflectant microbubbles make the left ventricular cavity appear white, whereas the myocardium appears dark. Video 4-3 shows a dynamic image of echocardiographic contrast. (Image courtesy Sheldon E. Litwin, MD, Division of Cardiology, University of Utah, Salt Lake City, Utah.)

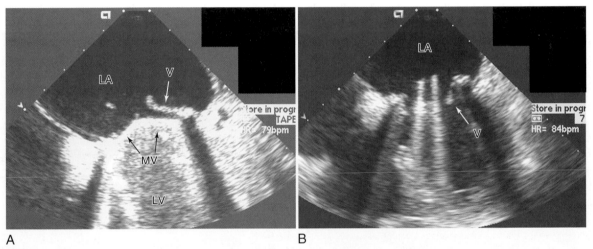

A   B

FIGURE 4-13 Transesophageal echocardiogram demonstrates a vegetation *(arrow)* adherent to the ring of a bileaflet, tilting-disk mitral valve prostheses. **A,** In systole, the leaflets are closed with the vegetation seen in the left atrium. **B,** In diastole, the leaflets are open, with the vegetation prolapsing into the left ventricle. Transesophageal echocardiography is the diagnostic test of choice for assessing prosthetic mitral valves because the esophageal window allows unimpeded views of the atrial surface of the valve. Video 4-4 shows a dynamic transesophageal echocardiographic image. *LA,* Left atrium; *LV,* left ventricle; *MV,* prosthetic mitral valve disks; *V,* vegetation. (Courtesy Sheldon E. Litwin, MD, Division of Cardiology, University of Utah, Salt Lake City, Utah.)

ventricular ejection fraction (LVEF) can then be calculated as follows:

$$LVEF = (EDC - ESC)/EDC$$

If scintigraphic information is collected throughout the cardiac cycle, a computer-generated image of the heart can be displayed in a cinematic fashion. This allows assessment of wall motion.

Myocardial perfusion imaging is usually performed in conjunction with exercise or pharmacologic (vasodilator) stress testing. Dipyridamole (Persantine), or more commonly adenosine, is used as the coronary vasodilator. Each agent can increase myocardial blood flow by fourfold to fivefold. Adenosine is more expensive, but it has the advantage over dipyridamole of a very short half-life. Newer adenosine-like agents with reduced side effect profiles are starting to be used clinically.

Technetium-99m sestamibi is the most frequently used radionuclide, and it is usually injected just before completion of the stress test. Single-photon emission computed tomography (SPECT) images of the heart are obtained for qualitative and quantitative analyses at rest and after stress. In the normal heart, the radioisotope is relatively equally distributed throughout the myocardium. In patients with ischemia, a localized area of decreased uptake occurs after exercise but partially or completely fills in at rest (i.e., redistribution). A persistent defect at peak exercise and rest (i.e., fixed defect) is consistent with MI or scarring. However, in some patients with apparently fixed defects, repeat rest imaging at 24 hours or after reinjection of a smaller quantity of isotope demonstrates improved uptake, indicating viable, but severely ischemic myocardium.

The use of new approaches such as combined low-level exercise and vasodilators, prone imaging, attenuation correction, and

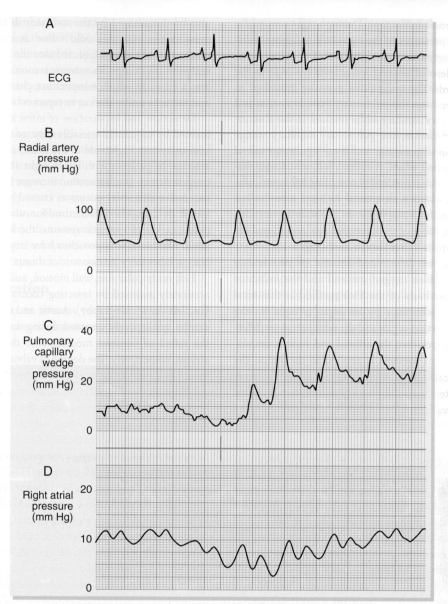

A
ECG

B
Radial artery
pressure
(mm Hg)

100

0

C
Pulmonary
capillary
wedge
pressure
(mm Hg)

40

20

0

D
Right atrial
pressure
(mm Hg)

20

10

0

FIGURE 4-16 Electrocardiographic (ECG) (**A**) and Swan-Ganz flotation catheter (**C**) recordings are shown. The recordings of a catheter in the radial artery and Swan-Ganz floating catheter in the right atrium are shown in **B** and **D**, respectively. The left portion of tracing **C** was obtained with the balloon inflated, yielding the pulmonary arterial wedge pressure. The right portion of tracing **C** was recorded with the balloon deflated, depicting the pulmonary arterial pressure. In this patient, the pulmonary arterial wedge pressure (i.e., left ventricular filling pressure) is normal, and the pulmonary artery pressure is elevated because of lung disease.

TABLE 4-4   DIFFERENTIAL DIAGNOSIS USING A BEDSIDE BALLOON FLOW-DIRECTED (SWAN-GANZ) CATHETER

DISEASE STATE	THERMODILUTION CARDIAC OUTPUT	PCW PRESSURE	RA PRESSURE	COMMENTS
Cardiogenic shock	↓	↑	nl or ↓	↑ Systemic vascular resistance
Septic shock (early)	↑	↓	↓	↑ Systemic vascular resistance; myocardial dysfunction can occur late
Volume overload	nl or ↑	↑	↑	
Volume depletion	↓	↓	↓	
Noncardiac pulmonary edema	nl	nl	nl	
Pulmonary heart disease	nl or ↑	nl	↑	↑ PA pressure
RV infarction	↓	↓ or nl	↑	
Pericardial tamponade	↓	nl or ↑	↑	Equalization of diastolic RA, RV, PA, and PCW pressure
Papillary muscle rupture	↓	↑	nl or ↑	Large *v* waves in PCW tracing
Ventricular septal rupture	↑	↑	nl or ↑	Artifact caused by RA → PA sampling higher in PA than RA; may have large *v* waves in PCW tracing

nl, Normal; PA, pulmonary artery; PCW, pulmonary capillary wedge; RA, right atrium; RV, right ventricle; ↑, increased; ↓, decreased.

improvements in outcomes of critically ill patients in whom pulmonary artery catheterization was performed. Improvements in noninvasive imaging techniques have made the pulmonary artery catheter much less important in diagnosing cardiac conditions, such as pericardial tamponade, constrictive pericarditis, right ventricular infarction, and ventricular septal defect.

Magnetic Resonance Imaging

Magnetic resonance angiography or imaging (MRI) is a noninvasive method that is increasingly used for studying the heart and vasculature, especially in patients who have contraindications to standard contrast angiography. MRI offers high-resolution dynamic and static images of the heart that can be obtained in any plane. Good-quality images can be obtained in a higher number of subjects than is typically possible with echocardiography. Obesity, claustrophobia, inability to perform multiple breath-holds of 10 to 20 seconds, and arrhythmias are causes of reduced image quality. The presence of cardiac pacemakers or implantable defibrillators is considered a contraindication for MRI. Magnetic resonance angiography is useful in the evaluation of cerebral, renovascular, and lower extremity arterial disease.

MRI offers significant advantages over other imaging techniques for the characterization of tissues (e.g., muscle, fat, scar). MRI is useful in the evaluation of ischemic heart disease because

stress-rest myocardial perfusion (Fig. 4-17A) and areas of prior infarction (see Fig. 4-17B to D) can be visualized with excellent special resolution. Delayed gadolinium contrast enhancement in the myocardium is characteristic of scar or permanently damaged tissue (Video 4-6). The greater the transmural extent of delayed enhancement in a given segment, the lower is the likelihood of improved function in that segment after revascularization. Because of the better spatial resolution, delayed enhancement imaging can depict localized or subendocardial scars that are not detectable with nuclear imaging techniques. The combined use of stress-rest perfusion and delayed enhancement imaging has performance characteristics for diagnosing CAD that are as good as and probably superior to those of conventional stress tests using nuclear scintigraphy or echocardiography.

MRI is excellent for evaluating a variety of cardiomyopathies (Fig. 4-18). In addition to morphology and function, characteristic patterns of delayed enhancement have been reported in myocarditis, hypertrophic cardiomyopathy, and cardiac amyloidosis. MRI has also been used to help assess right ventricular morphology and function in patients with suspected arrhythmogenic right ventricular cardiomyopathy.

Computed Tomography of the Heart

Newer applications of computed tomography (CT) have greatly advanced our ability to diagnose cardiovascular disease

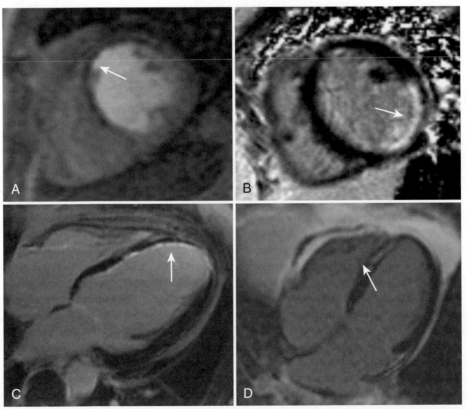

FIGURE 4-17 Use of cardiac magnetic resonance imaging in the evaluation of chest pain or ischemic heart disease. **A,** First-pass perfusion study during vasodilator stress shows a large septal perfusion defect *(arrow)*. The hypoperfused area appears dark compared with the myocardium with normal perfusion. **B,** Example of delayed enhancement imaging of an almost transmural infarction of the mid-inferolateral wall, including the posterior papillary muscle. Infarcted myocardium appears *white*, whereas normal myocardium is *black (arrow)*. **C,** Nontransmural (subendocardial) infarction of the septum and apex *(arrow)*. **D,** Patient with acute myocarditis mimicking an acute coronary syndrome. Mid-myocardial, rather than subendocardial, delayed enhancement is characteristic of myocarditis *(arrow)*.

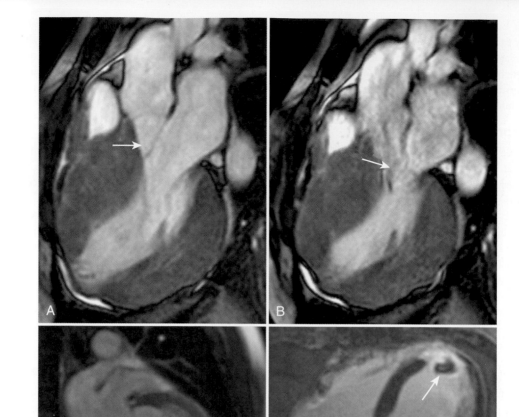

FIGURE 4-18 Cardiac magnetic resonance imaging (MRI) is used in the evaluation of cardiomyopathies. **A,** Severe left ventricular hypertrophy in a patient with hypertrophic cardiomyopathy. Diastolic frame shows open mitral valve *(arrow).* **B,** Systolic frame shows systolic anterior motion of the mitral valve with flow disturbance in the left ventricular outflow tract *(arrow).* **C,** Patient has left ventricular noncompaction as evidenced by deep trabeculations in the left ventricular apex *(arrow).* **D,** Patient with ischemic cardiomyopathy has transmural apical infarction and adjacent mural thrombus *(arrow).* Video 4-6 shows a dynamic cardiac MRI image. (Images courtesy Sheldon E. Litwin, MD, Division of Cardiology, University of Utah, Salt Lake City, Utah.)

noninvasively. The development of fast gantry rotation speeds and the addition of multiple rows of detectors (i.e., multidetector CT) have allowed unprecedented visualization of the great vessels, heart, and coronary arteries with images acquired during a single breath-hold lasting 10 to 15 seconds. CT is used to diagnose aortic aneurysm, acute aortic dissection, pulmonary embolism, and it is useful for defining congenital abnormalities and detecting pericardial thickening or calcification associated with constrictive pericarditis. ECG-gated dynamic CT images have been used to quantify ventricular size, function, and regional wall motion (Video 4-7), and in contrast to echocardiography, CT is not limited by lung disease or chest wall deformity. However, obesity and implanted prosthetic materials (i.e., mechanical valves or pacing wires) may affect image quality.

The greatest excitement and controversy about cardiac CT relates to the evaluation of coronary atherosclerosis. Electron beam and multidetector CT scans can be used to quickly and reliably visualize and quantitate the extent of coronary artery calcification (Fig. 4-19). The presence of coronary calcium is pathognomonic of atherosclerosis, and the extent of coronary calcium (usually reported as an Agatston score) is a powerful marker of future cardiac events. The coronary calcium score adds substantial, independent improvement in risk prediction to the commonly employed clinical risk scores (e.g., Framingham risk score). Although the extent of coronary artery calcification does not reliably predict the severity of stenoses, the calcium score is a good marker of the overall atherosclerotic burden.

Contrast-enhanced coronary computed tomography angiography (CTA) has improved dramatically in recent years. Coronary CTA has a sensitivity of more than 95% in diagnosing significant coronary artery obstruction. This is superior to the sensitivity of stress echo or nuclear myocardial perfusion scanning. Given the speed and accuracy of this test, it is likely to assume a major role in the evaluation of patients with acute chest pain syndromes.

Some advocates of cardiac CT have proposed the use of CTA for the *triple rule-out* in patients with acute chest pain—the ability to diagnose pulmonary embolism, aortic dissection, and CAD

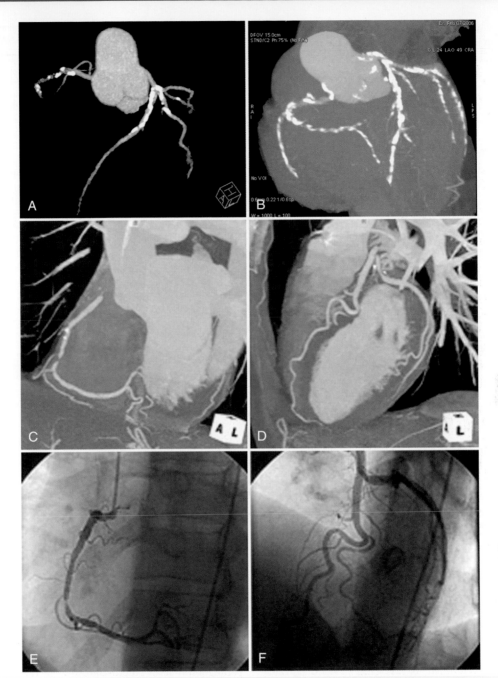

FIGURE 4-19 Computed tomography coronary angiography compared with conventional radiographic contrast angiography. **A** and **B,** Volume-rendering technique demonstrates stenosis of the right coronary artery and normal left coronary artery. **C** and **D,** Maximal intensity projection of the same arteries demonstrates severe noncalcified plaque in the right coronary artery with superficial calcified plaque. **E** and **F,** Invasive angiography of the same arteries. (From Raff GL, Gallagher MJ, O'Neill WW, et al: Diagnostic accuracy of noninvasive coronary angiography using 64-slice spiral computed tomography, J Am Coll Cardiol 46:552–557, 2005.)

with one imaging study. Formal evaluation of this hypothesis needs to be undertaken. Detractors of cardiac CT most frequently cite the risks of radiation and contrast exposure and the lack of prospective studies showing improvement in outcome with this testing modality. The calculated radiation exposure of cardiac CTA is about double that of a diagnostic invasive coronary angiogram, but it is similar to that of a typical nuclear myocardial perfusion scan. The future role of cardiac CTA in routine clinical practice remains uncertain.

Noninvasive Vascular Testing

Assessment for the presence and severity of peripheral vascular disease is an important component of the cardiovascular evaluation. Comparison of the systolic blood pressure in the upper and lower extremities is one of the simplest tests to detect hemodynamically important arterial disease. Normally, the systolic pressure in the thigh is similar to that in the brachial artery. An ankle-to-brachial pressure ratio (i.e., ankle-brachial index) of less than or equal to 0.9 is abnormal. Patients with claudication usually have an index ranging from 0.5 to 0.8, and patients with rest pain have an index less than 0.5. In some patients, measuring the ankle-brachial index after treadmill exercise may help to determine the importance of borderline lesions. During normal exercise, blood flow increases to the upper and lower extremities and decreases in peripheral vascular resistance, whereas the ankle-brachial index remains unchanged. In the presence of a hemodynamically significant lesion, the increase in systolic blood pressure in the arm is not matched by an increase in blood pressure in the leg. As a result, the ankle-brachial index decreases, the magnitude of which is proportional to the severity of the stenosis.

After significant vascular disease in the extremities has been identified, plethysmography can be used to determine the location and severity of the disease. With this method, a pneumatic cuff is positioned on the leg or thigh, and when inflated, it temporarily obstructs venous return. Volume changes in the limb segment below the cuff are converted to a pressure waveform, which can be analyzed. The degree of amplitude reduction in the pressure waveform corresponds to the severity of arterial disease at that level.

Doppler ultrasound uses reflected sound waves to identify and localize stenotic lesions in the peripheral arteries. This test is particularly useful for patients with severely calcified arteries, for whom pneumatic compression is not possible and ankle-brachial indices are inaccurate. In combination with real-time imaging (i.e., duplex imaging), this technique is useful in assessing specific arterial segments and bypass grafts for stenotic or occlusive lesions.

Magnetic resonance angiography and CTA allow high-quality and comprehensive imaging of the entire peripheral arterial circulation in a single study. The three-dimensional nature of these studies and the ability to perform extensive postprocessing views, including cross-sectional views, of all vessels, even those that are very tortuous, are attractive features of these modalities.

SUGGESTED READINGS

Cheitlin MD, Armstrong WF, Aurigemma GP, et al: ACC/AHA/ASE 2003 guideline update for the clinical application of echocardiography: summary article. A report of the American College of Cardiology/American Heart Association Task Force on Practice Guidelines (ACC/AHA/ASE Committee to Update the 1997 Guidelines for the Clinical Application of Echocardiography), J Am Soc Echocardiogr 16:1091–1110, 2003.

Fleisher LA, Beckman JA, Brown KA, et al: ACC/AHA 2006 guideline update on perioperative cardiovascular evaluation for noncardiac surgery: focused update on perioperative beta-blocker therapy executive summary: a report of the American College of Cardiology/American Heart Association Task Force on Practice Guidelines (Writing Committee to Update the 2002 Guidelines on Perioperative Cardiovascular Evaluation of Noncardiac Surgery), Circulation 113:2662–2674, 2006.

Fraker TD Jr, Fihn SD, Gibbons RJ, et al: 2007 Chronic angina focused update of the ACC/AHA 2002 Guidelines for the management of patients with chronic stable angina: a report of the American College of Cardiology/American Heart Association Task Force on Practice Guidelines Writing Group to develop the focused update of the 2002 Guidelines for the management of patients with chronic stable angina, Circulation 116:2762–2772, 2007.

Gibbons RJ, Balady GJ, Bricker JT, et al: ACC/AHA 2002 guideline update for exercise testing: summary article. A report of the American College of Cardiology/American Heart Association Task Force on Practice Guidelines (Committee to Update the 1997 Exercise Testing Guidelines), J Am Coll Cardiol 40:1531–1540, 2002.

Klein C: Nekolla SG: Assessment of myocardial viability with contrast-enhanced magnetic resonance imaging: comparison with positron emission tomography, Circulation 105:162–167, 2002.

Morey SS: ACC and AHA update guidelines for coronary angiography. American College of Cardiology. American Heart Association, Am Fam Physician 60:1017–1020, 1999.

Raff GL, Goldstein JA: Coronary angiography by computed tomography, J Am Coll Cardiol 49:1830–1833, 2007.

Sandham JD, Hull RD, Brant RF, et al: A randomized, controlled trial of the use of pulmonary artery catheters in high-risk surgical patients, N Engl J Med 348:5–14, 2003.

Heart Failure and Cardiomyopathy

Nunzio A. Gaglianello, Claudius Mahr, and Ivor J. Benjamin

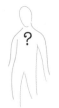

⬤ HEART FAILURE

Definition

Heart failure (HF) is a clinical syndrome characterized by structural or functional impairment of ventricular filling or ejection of blood that results in inadequate blood flow to meet the metabolic needs of the body's tissues and organs. HF can be caused by numerous disease processes (Table 5-1).

HF can be classified as HF with reduced ejection fraction (HFrEF) or HF with preserved ejection fraction (HFpEF). HFrEF (i.e., systolic HF) is defined as a left ventricular ejection fraction (LVEF) of less than 40%. Efficacious therapies have been demonstrated for this patient population. HFpEF (i.e., diastolic dysfunction) is defined as an LVEF greater than 50%, and it is more common in women than in men. No efficacious therapies have been discovered for this patient population.

The New York Heart Association (NYHA) functional classification (Table 5-2) defines four functional classes. Class I HF requires no limitations of physical activity; ordinary physical activity does not cause symptoms. Class II requires slight limitations of physical activity; patients are comfortable at rest, but ordinary physical activity results in HF symptoms. Class III requires marked limitations of physical activity; patients are comfortable at rest, but less than ordinary activity causes symptoms of HF. Patients with class IV HF are unable to carry on any physical activity without HF symptoms or have symptoms when at rest.

The American College of Cardiology Foundation and American Heart Association (ACCF/AHA) staging system (Fig. 5-1) classifies patients either as being at risk for HF or as having the clinical syndrome of HF. Stage A HF includes patients with risk factors for the development of HF, such as hypertension, obesity, atherosclerotic disease, and the metabolic syndrome. Stage B HF includes patients with structural heart disease (i.e., previous myocardial infarction [MI], asymptomatic valvular disease, and LV hypertrophy) but without symptoms of HF. Stage C HF is structural heart disease with prior or current symptoms of HF. Stage D HF is refractory or end-stage HF.

HF should further be characterized by cause (e.g., ischemic, nonischemic, valvular). It can be classified as predominantly left, right, or biventricular; high output or low output; and acute or chronic.

Idiopathic cardiomyopathy is a primary abnormality of the myocardium in the absence of structural or systemic disease. Secondary cardiomyopathies may be related to a significant number of disorders, but in the United States, it is most often the result

TABLE 5-1 CAUSES OF CONGESTIVE HEART FAILURE AND CARDIOMYOPATHY

CORONARY ARTERY DISEASE	Doxorubicin (Adriamycin)
Acute ischemia	Methamphetamine
Myocardial infarction	**METABOLIC-ENDOCRINE CONDITIONS**
Ischemic cardiomyopathy with hibernating myocardium	Thiamine deficiency
IDIOPATHIC CONDITIONS	Diabetes
	Hemochromatosis
Idiopathic dilated cardiomyopathy*	Thyrotoxicosis
Idiopathic restrictive cardiomyopathy	Obesity
Peripartum cardiomyopathy	Hemochromatosis
PRESSURE OVERLOAD	**INFILTRATIVE CONDITIONS**
Hypertension	Amyloidosis
Aortic stenosis	**INFLAMMATORY CONDITIONS**
VOLUME OVERLOAD	Viral myocarditis
Mitral regurgitation	**HEREDITARY CONDITIONS**
Aortic insufficiency	Hypertrophic cardiomyopathy
Anemia	Dilated cardiomyopathy
Atrioventricular fistula	
TOXINS	
Ethanol	
Cocaine	

*Genetic bases for these cardiomyopathies have been identified in many individual patients and families. Most of the mutations have been found in cardiac contractile or structural proteins.

TABLE 5-2 NEW YORK HEART ASSOCIATION FUNCTIONAL CLASSIFICATION OF HEART FAILURE

CLASS	SYMPTOMS
I (Mild)	No limitation of physical activity. Ordinary physical activity does not cause undue fatigue, palpitation, or dyspnea (shortness of breath).
II (Mild)	Slight limitation of physical activity. Comfortable at rest, but ordinary physical activity results in fatigue, palpitation, or dyspnea.
III (Moderate)	Marked limitation of physical activity. Comfortable at rest, but less than ordinary activity causes fatigue, palpitation, or dyspnea.
IV (Severe)	Unable to carry out any physical activity without discomfort. Symptoms of include cardiac insufficiency at rest. If physical activity is undertaken, discomfort is increased.

From the Heart Failure Society of America: Questions about heart failure. Available at http://www.abouthf.org/questions_stages.htm. Accessed August 2, 2014.

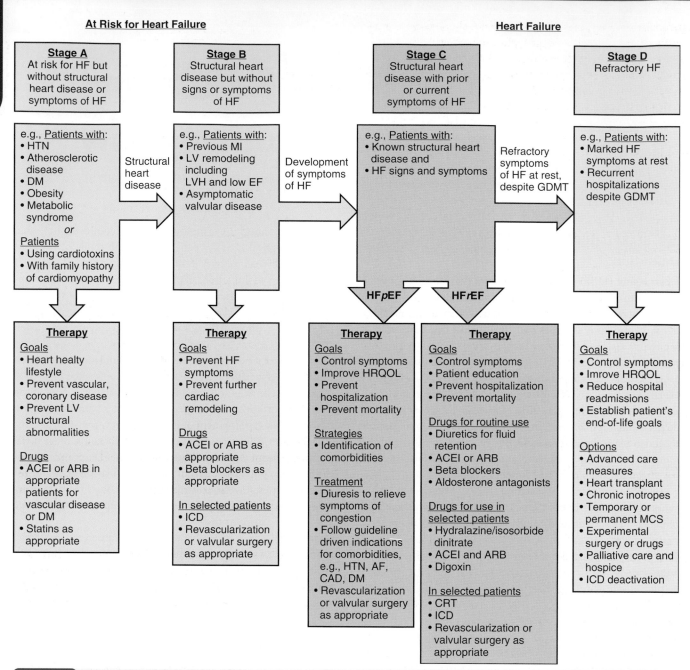

At Risk for Heart Failure   **Heart Failure**

Stage A At risk for HF but without structural heart disease or symptoms of HF	**Stage B** Structural heart disease but without signs or symptoms of HF	**Stage C** Structural heart disease with prior or current symptoms of HF	**Stage D** Refractory HF

e.g., Patients with:
• HTN
• Atherosclerotic disease
• DM
• Obesity
• Metabolic syndrome
  or
Patients
• Using cardiotoxins
• With family history of cardiomyopathy

→ Structural heart disease →

e.g., Patients with:
• Previous MI
• LV remodeling including LVH and low EF
• Asymptomatic valvular disease

→ Development of symptoms of HF →

e.g., Patients with:
• Known structural heart disease and
• HF signs and symptoms

Refractory symptoms of HF at rest, despite GDMT →

e.g., Patients with:
• Marked HF symptoms at rest
• Recurrent hospitalizations despite GDMT

HF*p*EF   **HF*r*EF**

Therapy

Goals
• Heart healty lifestyle
• Prevent vascular, coronary disease
• Prevent LV structural abnormalities

Drugs
• ACEI or ARB in appropriate patients for vascular disease or DM
• Statins as appropriate

Therapy

Goals
• Prevent HF symptoms
• Prevent further cardiac remodeling

Drugs
• ACEI or ARB as appropriate
• Beta blockers as appropriate

In selected patients
• ICD
• Revascularization or valvular surgery as appropriate

Therapy

Goals
• Control symptoms
• Improve HRQOL
• Prevent hospitalization
• Prevent mortality

Strategies
• Identification of comorbidities

Treatment
• Diuresis to relieve symptoms of congestion
• Follow guideline driven indications for comorbidities, e.g., HTN, AF, CAD, DM
• Revascularization or valvular surgery as appropriate

Therapy

Goals
• Control symptoms
• Patient education
• Prevent hospitalization
• Prevent mortality

Drugs for routine use
• Diuretics for fluid retention
• ACEI or ARB
• Beta blockers
• Aldosterone antagonists

Drugs for use in selected patients
• Hydralazine/isosorbide dinitrate
• ACEI and ARB
• Digoxin

In selected patients
• CRT
• ICD
• Revascularization or valvular surgery as appropriate

Therapy

Goals
• Control symptoms
• Imrove HRQOL
• Reduce hospital readmissions
• Establish patient's end-of-life goals

Options
• Advanced care measures
• Heart transplant
• Chronic inotropes
• Temporary or permanent MCS
• Experimental surgery or drugs
• Palliative care and hospice
• ICD deactivation

FIGURE 5-1 The American College of Cardiology Foundation and American Heart Association staging system. ACEI, Angiotensin-converting enzyme inhibitor; AF, atrial fibrillation; ARB, angiotensin receptor blocker; CAD, coronary artery disease; CRT, cardiac resynchronization therapy; DM, diabetes mellitus; EF, ejection fraction; GDMT, guideline-directed medical therapy; HF, heart failure; HRQOL, health-related quality of life; HTN, hypertension; ICD, implantable cardiac defibrillator; LV, left ventricular; LVH, left ventricular hypertrophy; MCS, mechanical circulatory support.

of ischemic heart disease. Ventricular dysfunction can result from excessive pressure overload, as in long-standing hypertension or aortic stenosis, or from volume overload, as in aortic insufficiency or mitral regurgitation. Diseases that result in infiltration and replacement of normal myocardial tissue, such as amyloidosis, are rare causes of HF. Hemochromatosis can cause a dilated cardiomyopathy that is thought to result from iron-mediated mitochondrial damage. Diseases of the pericardium, such as chronic pericarditis or pericardial tamponade, can impair cardiac function without directly affecting the myocardial tissue. Long-standing tachyarrhythmias have been associated with myocardial dysfunction that is often reversible.

High-output failure is an uncommon disorder characterized by an elevated resting cardiac index of greater than 2.5 to 4.0 L/min/m² and low systemic vascular resistance. Causes of high-output failure are severe anemia, vascular shunting, hyperthyroidism, and vitamin B_1 deficiency. It results from ineffective blood volume and pressure, which stimulate the sympathetic nervous system and renin-angiotensin-aldosterone system (RAAS), causing release of antidiuretic hormone (ADH), which results in ventricular enlargement, negative remodeling, and HF. Treatment targets the specific cause.

Low-output failure is much more common than high-output failure. It is characterized by insufficient forward cardiac output, particularly during times of increased metabolic demand. Cardiac dysfunction may predominantly affect the left ventricle, as with a large MI, or the right ventricle, as with an acute pulmonary embolus. However, in many disease states, both ventricles are impaired (i.e., biventricular HF).

Acute HF usually refers to the situation in which an individual who was previously asymptomatic develops HF signs or symptoms after an acute injury to the heart, such as MI, myocarditis, or acute valvular regurgitation. Chronic HF refers to situations in which symptoms have developed over a long period, most often in the setting of preexisting cardiac disease. However, a patient with myocardial dysfunction from any cause may remain compensated for extended periods and then develop acute HF symptoms in the setting of arrhythmia, anemia, hypertension, ischemia, systemic illness, dietary or medication noncompliance, and progression of chronic HF.

The severity of HF symptoms does not correlate closely with the usual clinical measures of cardiac function, although the LVEF is a reasonable prognostic marker. This situation likely reflects the fact that ventricular filling pressures are a more important determinant of symptoms than myocardial function. The predisposing conditions for HF (e.g., hypertension, advanced age, coronary artery disease, renal dysfunction) are similar, and the prognosis is similar whether the LVEF is preserved or reduced. Despite many similarities, medical treatments that have proved beneficial in HF with reduced EF have not shown similar efficacy in HF with preserved ejection fraction.

HEART FAILURE WITH PRESERVED EJECTION FRACTION

Slowed relaxation of the left ventricle and increased chamber stiffness impairs ventricular filling and may contribute to elevated left ventricular (LV), left atrial, and pulmonary venous pressures. Some patients with a diagnosis of HF have normal or almost normal EFs. These patients are diagnosed with HFpEF, which is the preferred terminology for describing this condition. Relaxation abnormalities occur in most people older than 65 years and are almost universal after age 75 years; however, most of these individuals do not have HF. Isolated abnormalities of LV relaxation are insufficient to directly cause HF in the absence of other predisposing conditions. In patients with a variety of cardiovascular diseases, relaxation abnormalities appear at earlier ages than otherwise expected. No therapeutic agents that specifically target impaired relaxation have been developed. The use of diuretics to manage volume overload and the vigorous treatment of hypertension with evidence-based therapy, including angiotensin-converting enzyme (ACE) inhibitors, are the mainstay of pharmacotherapy for this condition.

Epidemiology

Prevalence

The lifetime risk of developing HF is 20%, or 1 in 5 Americans 40 years of age or older. HF affects almost 7 million Americans, and the incidence of HF has largely remained stable in the United States, with approximately 670,000 new HF cases diagnosed annually (Fig. 5-2). As patients continue to live longer, it is expected that the incidence of HF will continue to rise.

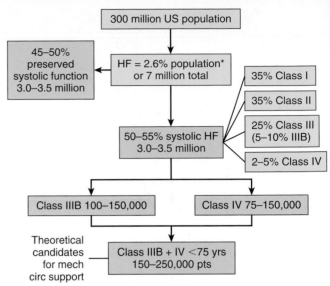

FIGURE 5-2 The lifetime risk of developing heart failure (HF) is 20%, or 1 in 5 for Americans 40 years of age or older. As patients continue to live longer, it is expected that the incidence of HF will continue to rise. HF affects almost 7 million Americans, and the incidence of HF has largely remained stable in the United States, with approximately 670,000 new HF cases diagnosed annually.

Incidence

The rate of HF increases with age, rising from 20 per 1000 people 65 to 69 years of age to more than 80 per 1000 people older than 85 years. African Americans have higher incidence and 5-year mortality rates compared with non-Hispanic whites. Despite advances in medical therapy, the mortality rate for HF remains 50% at 5 years after diagnosis.

Risk Factors

Risk factors for the development of HF include increasing age, gender (males > females), race (black > white), coronary artery disease (the cause of 60% to 75% of symptomatic HF in developed countries), hypertension, LV hypertrophy, diabetes mellitus, and obesity.

Pathogenesis

Numerous cardiac diseases can lead to HFrEF (see Table 5-1). Adaptive mechanisms maintain cardiac output and blood flow to vital organs. They include compensatory increases in ventricular volume and pressure achieved through the Frank-Starling mechanism and neurohormonal activation. Left untreated, these adaptive responses ultimately are detrimental and result in sodium and fluid retention, which worsen ventricular remodeling and further deteriorate systolic function (Fig. 5-3).

Normally, increasing either the stroke volume or the heart rate can augment cardiac output. Stroke volume depends on the contractility of the myocardium, LV filling (i.e., preload), and resistance to LV emptying (i.e., afterload). According to the Frank-Starling law, stroke volume can be increased with minimal elevation in LV pressure as long as contractility is normal.

When there is depressed contractility (Fig. 5-4A), the end-diastolic volume is increased in an attempt to maintain stroke volume. However, when the LV end-diastolic pressure approaches 20 to 25 mm Hg, pulmonary edema may develop due to

Pathophysiology of Heart Failure

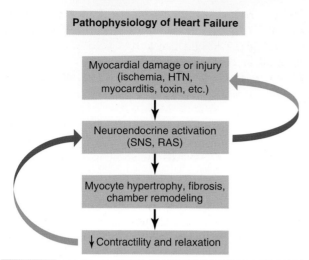

FIGURE 5-3 The diagram illustrates the progressive nature of left ventricular dysfunction that can follow an initial cardiac insult. Attenuation of the neurohumoral activation (or blockade of the downstream effects) may interrupt the positive feedback and slow or reverse the progression of heart failure. HTN, Hypertension; RAS, renin-angiotensin system; SNS, sympathetic nervous system.

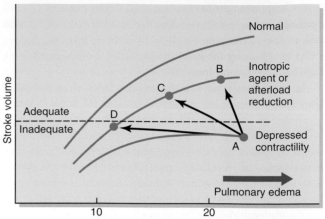

FIGURE 5-4 Normal and abnormal ventricular function curves. When the left ventricular end-diastolic pressure acutely rises above 20 mm Hg (point A), pulmonary edema often occurs. The effect of diuresis or venodilation is to move leftward along the same curve, with a resultant improvement in pulmonary congestion and with minimal decrease in cardiac output. The stroke volume is poor at any point along this depressed contractility curve; therapeutic maneuvers to raise it more toward the normal curve are necessary to improve cardiac output significantly. Unlike the effect of diuretics, the effect of vasodilator therapy in a patient with heart failure is to move the patient into another ventricular function curve intermediately between the normal and depressed curves. When the patient's ventricular function moves from point A to B by the administration of one of these agents, the LVEDP may also decrease because of improved cardiac function. Further administration of diuretics or venodilators may shift the patient further to the left along the same curve from point B to C and eliminate the risk for pulmonary edema. A vasodilating agent that has arteriolar and venous dilating properties (e.g., nitroprusside) would shift this patient directly from point A to C. If this agent shifts the patient from point A to D because of excessive venodilation or administration of diuretics, the cardiac output may fall too low, even though the LVEDP would be normal (10 mm Hg) for a normal heart. LVEDPs between 15 and 18 mm Hg are usually optimal in the failing heart to maximize cardiac output but avoid pulmonary edema. (Modified from the Heart Failure Society of America: Questions about heart failure. Available at http://www.abouthf.org/questions_stages.htm. Accessed August 2, 2014.)

differences between the hydrostatic pressure in the pulmonary capillaries and the oncotic pressure of the lungs. Depressed myocardial contractility (in HFrEF) and increased chamber stiffness (in HFpEF) can lead to pulmonary congestion through this same mechanism.

After the initial compensatory mechanism, the failing heart undergoes ventricular remodeling, characterized by myocardial structural and functional abnormalities resulting in a dilated, spherical ventricle with reduced contractility. Ventricular remodeling occurs in response to pressure and volume overload, myocyte loss, or a combination of these factors, resulting in progressive decline in contractility. Ventricular remodeling begins with ventricular hypertrophy in response to increased wall stress to decrease myocardial oxygen consumption. If the extent of hypertrophy is inadequate to normalize wall stress, a vicious cycle is established.

The remodeling changes occur to make the failing ventricle more efficient and can be understood in the context of LaPlace's law ($T = P \times r/w_t$), where T = tension, P = pressure, r = the radius of the chamber or vessel, and W_t = the thickness of the wall. As tension (force) increases, pressure increases proportionally. Untreated, this mechanism leads to progressive ventricular dilation and chamber enlargement, causing increased wall stress, increased myocardial oxygen consumption, and progressively worsening contractility.

Neurohormonal Activation

Activation of the sympathetic nervous system is the first response to decreased cardiac output. It results in the release of epinephrine and norepinephrine, which bind all adrenergic receptors. This results in stimulation or inhibition of G proteins (i.e., G_s and G_i subtypes). G protein activation upregulates adenylate cyclase, which converts adenosine triphosphate (ATP) to cyclic adenosine monophosphate (cAMP). cAMP signals protein kinase A, which phosphorylates ryanodine receptors, leading to increased intracellular calcium levels, which increase contractility by phosphorylating and inhibiting phospholamban. Stimulation of the

sympathetic nervous system also increases ventricular relaxation (i.e., lusitropy) and increases the basal heart rate. These effects, although beneficial initially, are ultimately detrimental to the myocardium.

The RAAS is stimulated by the sympathetic nervous system and by decreased blood flow to the afferent arteriole of the nephron, resulting in the release of renin. This ultimately leads to activation of angiotensin II, which is a potent vasoconstrictor, with the initial response to supply adequate blood to vital organs. However, angiotensin II increases afterload, wall stress, and myocardial oxygen consumption and leads to a decrease in stroke volume. Angiotensin II also leads to sympathetic nervous system activation, aldosterone release, and myocardial fibrosis, perpetuating the cycle.

The release of aldosterone prompts sodium reabsorption, promoting water retention to effectively maintain cardiac output. Aldosterone also has fibrotic properties. The release of vasopressin promotes free water absorption by the kidney. These changes are responsible for many of the clinical signs and symptoms associated with HF.

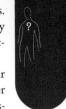

The body attempts to counter these effects by secreting atrial natriuretic peptide and brain natriuretic peptide (BNP) from the myocardium. Endogenous natriuretic peptides promote salt and water excretion by the kidneys and cause arterial vasodilation, but they are relatively ineffective at reversing the changes associated with stimulating the sympathetic nervous system and the RAAS.

Clinical Presentation and Diagnosis

The approach to the patient with suspected HF starts with the history, physical examination, and testing to help establish the diagnosis. The history should assess for NYHA functional class, including symptoms of fatigue, weakness, dyspnea, orthopnea, edema, abdominal distention, and chest discomfort. The examiner should also assess for comorbidities, including hypertension, diabetes mellitus, dyslipidemia, obesity, and sleep-disordered breathing.

The medical history should inquire about exposure to cardiotoxic agents, including anthracycline-based chemotherapy. The social history evaluates past and current use of tobacco products, alcohol, and illicit drugs. The family history assesses for sudden cardiac death, coronary artery disease, and cardiomyopathy. For patients with an idiopathic dilated cardiomyopathy, a three-generation history should be obtained to establish a familial component.

The physical examination starts by assessing vital signs. Worrisome vital signs for significant cardiac dysfunction include faint pulses, a narrow pulse pressure due to peripheral vasoconstriction and low stroke volume, and resting tachycardia. Assessment of the peripheral pulse includes evaluating the patient for pulsus alternans, which is defined as beat-to-beat variation in the amplitude of the peripheral pulse, and it is pathognomonic for severe LV dysfunction.

Most symptoms of HF are related to elevated filling pressures. Dyspnea (in men) and fatigue (in women) are some of the most common symptoms of HF. They may have an acute onset resulting in pulmonary edema, or they may be chronic and progressive and occur at rest. Dyspnea on exertion has a sensitivity of 84% to 100% but a specificity of 17% to 34%. Dyspnea from HF is often exacerbated in the supine position (i.e., orthopnea), and it is caused by increased distribution of blood to the pulmonary circulation when lying flat. Patients with HF tend to use increased numbers of pillows to overcome orthopnea. Orthopnea has a sensitivity of 22% to 50% and a specificity of 74% to 77% for HF. Episodes of paroxysmal nocturnal dyspnea (PND) awaken patients from sleep and are likely caused by central redistribution of edema, leading to a sudden rise in intracardiac pressures. The sensitivity of PND for the diagnosis of HF is 39% to 41%, and the specificity ranges from 80% to 84%. Patients with stage D HF may exhibit Cheyne-Stokes respirations, which is associated with a poor prognosis.

Evaluation of volume status includes assessment of serial weights, jugular venous pressure, pulmonary congestion, and peripheral edema. The jugular venous pressure is best assessed using the right internal jugular vein with the patient lying at a 30- to 45-degree angle. Patients with markedly elevated venous pressures may need to be positioned at a higher angle. The jugular venous pressure is an estimate of the central venous pressure

(CVP) (i.e., right atrial pressure) and therefore of volume status. A normal CVP is in the range of 5 to 9 cm H_2O. An abnormally elevated CVP may be seen in hypervolemia, pericardial constriction, or pulmonary hypertension.

Evaluating the abdominal jugular reflux (i.e., hepatojugular reflux) involves gently compressing the abdomen or right upper quadrant for 15 to 30 seconds and assessing jugular venous distention. This method assesses volume status and right ventricular dysfunction and compliance. An abnormal abdominal jugular reflux is defined as a sustained increase in jugular venous pressure of more than 4 cm H_2O.

On lung auscultation, crackles may be heard. Crackles are a specific finding for HF, but they are not detected in approximately 60% of patients with chronic HF. Before auscultation, the precordium should be examined and the point of maximal impulse (PMI) evaluated. An abnormal PMI is defined as displacement below the fifth intercostal space and lateral to the midclavicular line. It offers the clinician an assessment of heart size and function if it is sustained for more than one third of systole or is palpable over two intercostal spaces.

On auscultation of the heart, abnormal findings include an early diastolic third heart sound (S_3). A third heart sound is compatible with elevated atrial pressures and increased ventricular chamber stiffness. The sound results from rapid deceleration of the passive component of blood flow from the atrium into the noncompliant ventricle. An S_3 sound can be generated from the left or right ventricle; the latter changes in intensity with respiration. A fourth heart sound (S_4) results from an exaggerated atrial contribution to LV filling, but it is not specific for HF. Patients may also have an accentuated P_2 pulmonic valve component of S_2 if pulmonary hypertension also exists. Poor prognostic signs on physical examination include elevated jugular venous pressures and an S_3 sound.

Peripheral edema usually involves the lower extremities, but edema can involve the thighs and abdomen. Abdominal ascites may develop, particularly in the setting of worsening right ventricular failure and severe tricuspid regurgitation. Lower extremity edema can occur in many other disease states, including nephrotic syndrome, cirrhosis, venous stasis, and lymphedema, and it is not specific for HF.

The murmurs of mitral and tricuspid regurgitation are common in patients with HF. They may become worse during an acute decompensation.

Diagnostic Testing

The electrocardiogram in patients with congestive HF usually is nonspecific, but it may reveal changes suggesting a prior MI, conduction system disease, and chamber enlargement. The chest radiograph may show cardiomegaly and signs of pulmonary congestion (Fig. 5-5). Treatment of HF improves the vascular congestion seen on the chest radiograph, but radiographic changes may lag 24 to 48 hours behind clinical improvement.

Transthoracic echocardiography (TTE) is recommended for all patients with suspected HF. A noninvasive echocardiogram can assess ventricular chamber sizes, ventricular wall thickness, systolic function, diastolic function, and valvular stenosis or regurgitation. It can provide an estimation of left and right atrial pressures and quantification of stroke volume and cardiac output (Fig. 5-6). These measurements, including chamber size,

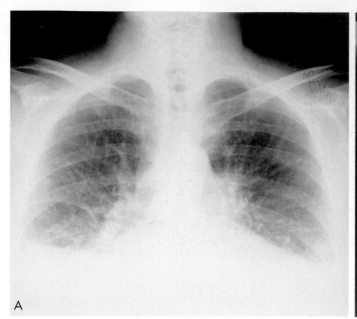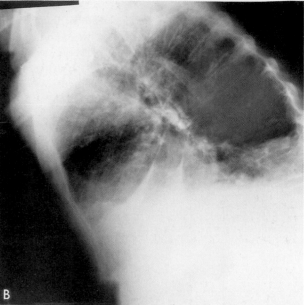

FIGURE 5-5 **A,** Posteroanterior chest radiograph showing cardiomegaly. **B,** Lateral chest radiograph showing pulmonary vascular congestion that is typical of pulmonary edema.

ventricular hypertrophy, and ventricular function, have been used in clinical trials to assess the efficacy of therapies.

Laboratory Evaluation

Initial laboratory evaluation includes a complete blood count (CBC) to assess for anemia and a basic chemistry panel for electrolyte abnormalities. The serum sodium level may be impaired, and there may be evidence of renal dysfunction due to decreased cardiac output and renal artery vasoconstriction or elevated venous pressures reflected in the renal veins (i.e., cardiorenal syndrome). Patients should be evaluated for hyperthyroidism or hypothyroidism and for hemochromatosis (i.e., with a serum ferritin level) because it is a reversible cause of HF. Patients should be tested for human immunodeficiency virus (HIV) infection. Laboratory tests for other modifiable risk factors include a fasting lipid panel and a blood glucose level. Liver function enzymes may be elevated in patients with HF and hepatic congestion, which can result from volume overload and significant LV dysfunction and may be seen in cases of right ventricular HF or severe tricuspid regurgitation.

Tests for plasma natriuretic peptide levels (BNP or NT-pro-BNP) were initially developed to evaluate patients with acute dyspnea when the diagnosis of HF was in doubt. When results are normal, this test has strong discriminatory power to eliminate HF as the cause of dyspnea. The Valsartan Heart Failure Trial (Val-HeFT) established that serial measurements of natriuretic peptide levels correlate with prognosis.

Acute Treatment

After the clinical diagnosis of HF is established, a model proposed by Stevenson and colleagues (Fig. 5-7) focuses on assessing volume status and perfusion and then further characterizes the patient according to volume overload/congestion-related and perfusion/output-related presentations. Using the history and physical examination findings, a physician can make astute clinical decisions based on one of four profiles for patients with HF.

In patients with acute onset of pulmonary edema, initial management should be directed at improving oxygenation and providing hemodynamic stability. Patients commonly have marked elevation of blood pressure, myocardial ischemia, and worsening mitral regurgitation. Standard therapy includes supplemental oxygen and an intravenous loop diuretic.

Nitroglycerin helps to reduce preload through venodilation and may provide symptomatic relief for patients with ischemic and nonischemic ventricular dysfunction. For patients with hypertensive urgency, severe hypertension, or decompensated HF related to aortic or mitral regurgitation, an arterial vasodilator such as nitroprusside may be helpful in reducing afterload. Evaluation of the patient's response to treatment requires serial assessment of blood pressure, heart rate, end-organ perfusion, and oxygen saturation. For severely decompensated patients with refractory hypoxia or respiratory acidosis, mechanical ventilation or continuous positive airway pressure (CPAP) therapy may be necessary.

Pulmonary artery catheterization may be helpful in documenting filling pressures and the cardiac index and in hemodynamically guiding the response to therapy. Although invasive monitoring has not been associated with improved outcomes, it is impossible to adjust these studies for disease severity. In patients with refractory pulmonary edema or a markedly impaired cardiac index, inotropic agents or short-term mechanical circulatory support (e.g., intra-aortic balloon pump) may become necessary.

Treatment of Heart Failure

Treatment of HF is directed at relieving the patient's symptoms, mitigating the underlying or precipitating causes (Table 5-3), and slowing disease progression. Patients should be educated about the importance of adherence to medical therapy and restriction of dietary sodium and fluid. Rhythm disturbances such as atrial

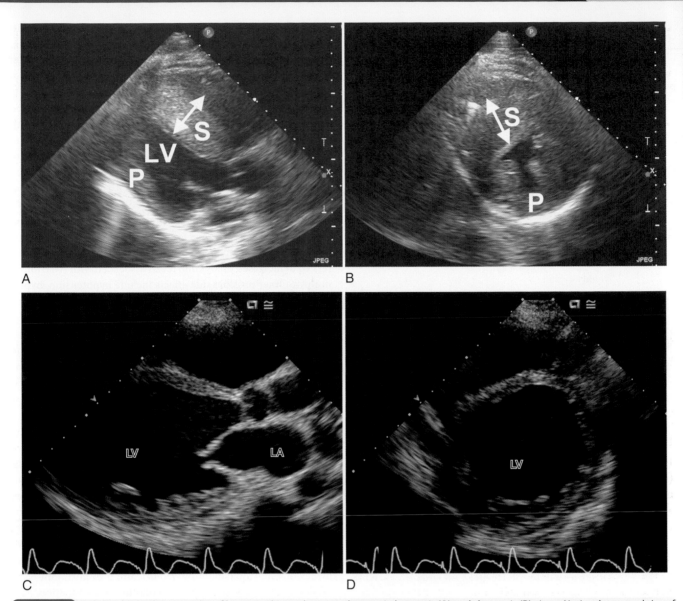

FIGURE 5-6 Echocardiographic examples of hypertrophic cardiomyopathy seen in long-axis (**A**) and short-axis (**B**) views. Notice the normal size of the left ventricular (LV) cavity and marked thickening of the interventricular septum (S) compared with posterior wall (P). In contrast, similar views of a patient with dilated cardiomyopathy (**C** and **D**) reveal a markedly enlarged LV cavity with diffuse wall thinning.

fibrillation may precipitate decompensated HF and may require specific therapy. Treatment of coronary artery disease with active ischemia, hypertension, or valvular disease may improve HF symptoms. Correction of concomitant medical problems (e.g., sleep-disordered breathing, pulmonary hypertension) may improve heart function.

Nonpharmacologic Treatment

All patients with HF should be encouraged to restrict sodium intake to about 2 g/day. Fluid intake should also be limited to avoid hyponatremia. Weight reduction by the obese patient helps to reduce the workload of the failing heart. A structured cardiovascular exercise program can reduce HF symptoms and improve functional capacity in most patients.

Pharmacologic Treatment

Table 5-4 lists all medications approved for HF and their dosing requirements.

Diuretics

Symptoms of volume overload are commonly seen in HF due to activation of the RAAS, and diuretics help to promote renal excretion of sodium and water and provide rapid relief of pulmonary congestion and peripheral edema. Loop diuretics, such as furosemide, torsemide or bumetanide, are the preferred agents in the treatment of hypervolemic HF due to their quick onset and rapid relief of symptoms by decreasing preload and lowering ventricular filling pressures. Unfortunately, there are no randomized, controlled trial data that support a mortality benefit for diuretics. Diuretics actually activate the RAAS and sympathetic nervous system, both of which can potentiate the progression of HF. The Diuretic Optimization Strategies Evaluation (DOSE) trial attempted to discern whether continuous intravenous administration of loop diuretics compared with intermittent bolus infusion would produce better outcomes for patients with acute decompensated HF. Results were equivocal according to

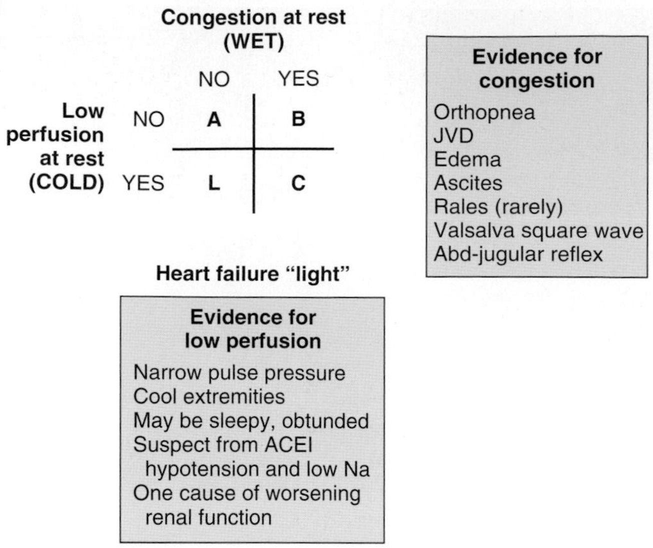

Congestion at rest
(WET)

		NO	YES
Low perfusion at rest (COLD)	NO	A	B
	YES	L	C

Heart failure "light"

Evidence for congestion

Orthopnea
JVD
Edema
Ascites
Rales (rarely)
Valsalva square wave
Abd-jugular reflex

Evidence for low perfusion

Narrow pulse pressure
Cool extremities
May be sleepy, obtunded
Suspect from ACEI
  hypotension and low Na
One cause of worsening
  renal function

FIGURE 5-7 Diagram of a 2×2 table of hemodynamic profiles for patients with heart failure. Most patients can be classified in a 2-minute bedside assessment according to the signs and symptoms shown, although in practice, some patients may be on the border between the warm-and-wet and cold-and-wet profiles. The classification helps guide initial therapy and prognosis for patients with advanced heart failure. Most patients with hypoperfusion also have elevated filling pressures (i.e., cold and wet profile). Patients with symptoms of heart failure at rest or minimal exertion without clinical evidence of elevated filling pressures or hypoperfusion (i.e., warm and dry profile) should be carefully evaluated to determine whether their symptoms result from heart failure. A, Warm and dry profile; Abd, abdominal; ACEI, angiotensin-converting enzyme inhibitor; B, warm and wet profile; C, cold and wet profile; JVD, jugular venous distention; L, cold and dry profile; Na, serum sodium. (Modified from Nohria A, Lewis E, Stevenson LW: Medical management of advanced heart failure, JAMA 287:628–640, 2002.)

TABLE 5-3   PRECIPITANTS OF HEART FAILURE

Dietary (sodium and fluid) indiscretion
Noncompliance with medications
Development of cardiac arrhythmia
Anemia
Uncontrolled hypertension
Superimposed medical illness (pneumonia, renal dysfunction)
New cardiac abnormality (acute ischemia, acute valvular insufficiency)

patient symptom reports, and there was no significant change in renal function.

If a patient remains volume overloaded and does not adequately respond to loop diuretic monotherapy, adding additional agents (i.e., metolazone, thiazide diuretics, carbonic anhydrase inhibitors, aldosterone receptor blocker, and arginine vasopressin blockers) that block reabsorption at other locations in the nephron may provide adequate diuresis, an approach called *sequential nephron blockade.* This strategy is particularly useful for patients with intrinsic renal dysfunction or significant hyponatremia due to volume overload.

Angiotensin-Converting Enzyme Inhibitors and Angiotensin Receptor Blockers

ACE inhibitors and angiotensin receptor blockers (ARBs) inhibit the RAAS and reduce afterload primarily by vasodilation. Both drug classes have an excellent safety profile and significant morbidity and mortality benefits for symptomatic and asymptomatic LV dysfunction with or without coronary artery disease. On a cellular level, ACE inhibitors slow the progression of cardiovascular disease by multiple pleiotropic effects, including improved endothelial function; antiproliferative effects on smooth muscle cells, neutrophils, and monocytes; and antithrombotic effects. Meta-analyses suggest a 23% reduction in mortality and a 35% reduction in the combination end point of mortality and hospitalizations for HF among patients treated with ACEI inhibitors.

ACE inhibitors should be avoided in pregnant patients, patients considering pregnancy, and patients with a history of angioedema. The major side effect of ACE inhibitors is a persistent dry cough, which occurs in up to 20% of patients and is related to increased bradykinin levels associated with ACE inhibitor use. Other possible side effects include hypotension, hyperkalemia, and azotemia. Renal function and potassium levels should be checked 1 week after initiation and after dose titration.

ARBs prevent the binding of angiotensin II to its receptor, which decreases the release of bradykinin. ARBs should be reserved for patients who proved to be ACE inhibitor intolerant, primarily because of cough. Angioedema occurs in less than 1%.

β-Blockers

Historically, β-blockers were considered contraindicated in HF for many years due to the reliance on sympathetic tone to maintain adequate cardiac output and end-organ perfusion. Because unopposed adrenergic stimulation was ultimately found to be deleterious to the myocardium, β-blockers were introduced into clinical practice. The beneficial effects were thought to result from decreasing heart rate, β-receptor upregulation, altered myocardial metabolism, improved calcium transport, inhibition of the RAAS, improvement in endothelial dysfunction, and decreased levels of circulating cytokines.

The three approved β-blockers used in HF are metoprolol succinate, carvedilol, and bisoprolol. The estimated reduction in all-cause mortality in the Metoprolol CR/XL Randomised Intervention Trial in Congestive Heart Failure (MERIT-HF), Carvedilol Post-Infarct Survival Control in Left Ventricular Dysfunction Study (CAPRICORN), Carvedilol Prospective Randomized Cumulative Survival (COPERNICUS), and Cardiac Insufficiency Bisoprolol Study II (CIBIS-II) trials was approximately 35%. These effects largely result from prevention of sudden cardiac death through mechanisms inhibiting the adrenergic pathway and its deleterious effects.

Long-term treatment with β-blockers can lessen the symptoms of HF, improve the patient's clinical status, and improve the overall sense of well-being. β-Blockers should be withheld from patients with markedly decompensated acute HF until they are clinically stable, because the drugs are negatively chronotropic and acutely result in diminished cardiac output. β-Blockers should be titrated to the maximum doses achieved in clinical trials because they have been proved to improve LVEF and reduce or reverse the degree of negative LV remodeling.

TABLE 5-4 MEDICATIONS USED AND APPROVED FOR HEART FAILURE

DRUG	INITIAL DOSES	MAXIMUM DOSES	MEAN DOSES ACHIEVED IN CLINICAL TRIALS*
ANGIOTENSIN-CONVERTING ENZYME INHIBITORS			
Captopril	6.25 mg tid	50 mg tid	122.7 mg/day (421)
Enalapril	2.5 mg bid	10 to 20 mg bid	16.6 mg/day (412)
Fosinopril	5 to 10 mg qd	40 mg qd	—
Lisinopril	2.5 to 5 mg qd	20 to 40 mg qd	32.5 to 35.0 mg/day (444)
Perindopril	2 mg qd	8 to 16 mg qd	—
Quinapril	5 mg bid	20 mg bid	—
Ramipril	1.25 to 2.5 mg qd	10 mg qd	—
Trandolapril	1 mg qd	4 mg qd	—
ANGIOTENSIN-RECEPTOR BLOCKERS			
Candesartan	4 to 8 mg qd	32 mg qd	24 mg/day (419)
Losartan	25 to 50 mg qd	50 to 150 mg qd	129 mg/day (420)
Valsartan	20 to 40 mg bid	160 mg bid	254 mg/day (109)
ALDOSTERONE ANTAGONISTS			
Spironolactone	12.5 to 25 mg qd	25 mg qd or bid	26 mg/day (424)
Eplerenone	25 mg qd	50 mg qd	42.6 mg/day (445)
β-BLOCKERS			
Bisoprolol	1.25 mg qd	10 mg qd	8.6 mg/day (118)
Carvedilol	3.125 mg bid	50 mg bid	37 mg/day (446)
Carvedilol CR	10 mg qd	80 mg qd	—
Metoprolol succinate extended release (metoprolol CR/XL)	12.5 to 25 mg qd	200 mg qd	159 mg/day (447)
HYDRALAZINE AND ISOSORBIDE DINITRATE			
Fixed dose combination (423)	37.5 mg hydralazine and 20 mg isosorbide dinitrate tid	75 mg hydralazine and 40 mg isosorbide dinitrate tid	≈175 mg hydralazine/90 mg isosorbide dinitrate qd
Hydralazine and isosorbide dinitrate (448)	Hydralazine, 25 to 50 mg tid or qid, and isosorbide dinitrate, 20 to 30 mg tid or qid	Hydralazine, 300 mg qd in divided doses, and isosorbide dinitrate, 120 mg qd in divided doses	—

Modified from Yancy CW, Jessup M, Bozkurt B, et al: 2013 ACCF/AHA guidelines for the management of heart failure: a report of the American College of Cardiology Foundation/American Heart Association Task Force on Practice Guidelines, J Am Coll Cardiol 62:e147–e239, 2013.
*Number of patients enrolled is given in parentheses.

Carvedilol is the least β-selective of the three drugs, and bisoprolol and metoprolol succinate are much more β_1-selective. Carvedilol is also an antioxidant and an α-blocker, which may result in lowered blood pressure and improved endothelial function and may be beneficial in patients with HF. Compared with bisoprolol or metoprolol, carvedilol can cause hypotension and may cause more bronchospasm in patients with underlying lung disease. According to the American College of Cardiology and American Heart Association (ACC/AHA) 2013 HF guidelines, use of one of the three β-blockers proven to reduce mortality (i.e., bisoprolol, carvedilol, and sustained-release metoprolol succinate) is recommended for all patients with current or prior symptoms of HFrEF (LVEF <40%), unless contraindicated, to reduce morbidity and mortality.

Aldosterone Receptor Antagonists

After initiating first-line therapy with ACE inhibitors and β-blockers, the next class of beneficial agents is aldosterone receptor antagonists. Two agents studied are spironolactone and eplerenone. Aldosterone receptor antagonists are weak diuretics and have important antifibrotic properties. Use of aldosterone receptor antagonists is a class I indication according to the ACC/AHA 2013 HF guidelines, and they are recommended for patients with NYHA class II through IV HF and who have an LVEF of 35% or less, unless otherwise contraindicated, to reduce morbidity and mortality. The landmark Randomized Aldactone Evaluation Study (RALES), which evaluated spironolactone in patients with NYHA class III or IV HF with an EF less than 35% demonstrated a 30% relative risk reduction for death from progressive HF and sudden death from cardiac causes. Eplerenone was studied in the Eplerenone in Mild Patients Hospitalization and Survival Study in Heart Failure (EMPHASIS-HF) trial, which evaluated patients with NYHA class II symptoms and found a relative risk reduction of 37% for the primary end point of death and hospital readmissions.

Hydralazine and Nitrates

Hydralazine in combination with oral nitrates has reduced mortality rates for African American patients with ongoing symptomatic HF after institution of the three regimens previously described (i.e., ACE inhibitors or ARBs, β-blockers, and aldosterone receptor antagonists). This combination provides an alternative for patients who are ACE inhibitor intolerant or may require additional therapy for blood pressure control. Although this drug combination has not proved to be efficacious in non–African Americans, all patients who cannot tolerate ACE inhibitors or ARBs may use this regimen.

The ACC/AHA HF guidelines class I recommendation states that the combination of hydralazine and isosorbide dinitrate can be used to reduce morbidity and mortality for patients self-described as African Americans with NYHA class III through IV HFrEF receiving optimal therapy with ACE inhibitors and β-blockers, unless contraindicated. The class IIa recommendation states that a combination of hydralazine and

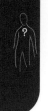

isosorbide dinitrate can be used to reduce morbidity or mortality rates among patients with current or prior symptomatic HFrEF who cannot be given an ACE inhibitor or ARB because of drug intolerance, hypotension, or renal insufficiency, unless contraindicated.

Digoxin

Perhaps the oldest treatment of HF, digoxin works through the inhibition of the sodium-potassium pump to increase intracellular calcium and increase contractility. Unlike the medications previously described, there is no proven mortality benefit from treatment with digoxin, but there may be a reduction in the number of rehospitalizations. Digoxin has been proved to improve symptoms, exercise tolerance, and health-related quality of life in men, but not women. Digoxin has many potential side effects, including nausea, vomiting, induction of ventricular or atrial arrhythmias, and heart block, and it may cause hyperkalemia. It is most famously known for causing visual color disturbances. Caution should be used to avoid toxicity for patients with intrinsic renal disease because digoxin is renally cleared.1

Drugs to Avoid

Nonsteroidal Anti-inflammatory Drugs

Nonsteroidal anti-inflammatory drugs (NSAIDs) cause sodium retention, vasoconstriction, renal impairment, and increased blood pressure. They enhance the toxicity of diuretics, ACE inhibitors, and ARBs.

Calcium-Channel Blockers

Calcium-channel blockers should be avoided in patients with HFrEF. Diltiazem and the nondihydropyridines are contraindicated in patients with an LVEF less than 40% due to their negative inotropic effects and reflex adrenergic system activation.

Antiarrhythmics

Two antiarrhythmic medications are approved for patients with a reduced LVEF. They are amiodarone and dofetilide, and both appear to be mortality neutral in properly selected patients.

Thiazolidinediones

Thiazolidinediones are used in the treatment of diabetes mellitus. They lead to increased sodium reabsorption and ultimately to fluid retention. They are contraindicated for patients with HF.

Hormonal Therapy and Nutritional Supplements

There are no proven benefits for hormonal therapies, unless there is needed replacement due to a specific hormonal deficiency. There are no data to support using nutritional supplements to improve HF symptoms or outcomes. However, some data support the use of omega-3 fatty acids by HF patients

Implantable Cardiac Defibrillators and Cardiac Resynchronization Therapy

Patients with cardiomyopathies of ischemic and nonischemic origins and reduced LVEFs are prone to ventricular arrhythmias. Many studies have demonstrated the survival benefits of implanting a defibrillator for primary prevention of sudden cardiac death.

The guidelines recommend implantable cardiac defibrillator (ICD) therapy for patients with nonischemic dilated cardiomyopathy or ischemic heart disease at least 40 days after an MI with an LVEF of 35% or less and NYHA class II or III HF and who have been treated with optimal medical therapy for a minimum of 3 to 6 months and have a life expectancy of more than 1 year. An ICD is also recommended for patients with NYHA class I symptoms and an LVEF less of than 30% 40 days after an MI and who have been treated with optimal medical therapy for 3 to 6 months.

Resynchronization Therapy

Intraventricular conduction delays, demonstrated as a prolonged QRS duration of more than 120 milliseconds by surface ECG, are a common complication in patients with HF. The delay leads to dyssynchronous contraction of the left ventricle and can result in reduced systolic function, decreased cardiac output, and reduced exercise capacity.

Cardiac resynchronization therapy (i.e., biventricular pacing) aims to improve intraventricular synchrony and has been associated with improved cardiac output and LVEF. Biventricular pacing may have a beneficial effect on LV remodeling by reducing LV volume, LV mass, and severity of mitral regurgitation. These hemodynamic and structural changes have translated into a clinical improvement of functional capacity, exercise tolerance, and quality of life.

Biventricular pacing has reduced mortality rates and hospitalization for HF in multiple randomized, controlled trials. A systematic review of 14 randomized trials was published in 2007 by McAlister and colleagues. It evaluated 4420 patients with LVEF values less than 35%, QRS duration longer than 120 msec, NYHA class III and IV HF, and optimal medical therapy. They reported that cardiac resynchronization therapy (CRT) improved LVEF by 3% and improved LV remodeling, quality of life, and exercise capacity; 59% of patients had improvement by at least one NYHA class. Hospitalizations were decreased by 37%, and all-cause mortality was decreased by 22%. CRT was beneficial for patients with NYHA class III and IV symptoms, and there was a mortality benefit for patients with NYHA class I and II symptoms.

One third of patients undergoing biventricular pacemaker placements are found to be nonresponders. Patients with the best response to CRT have a wide QRS in a left bundle branch block pattern. The class I recommendation from the ACC guidelines proposes CRT for patients who have an LVEF of 35% or less, sinus rhythm, left bundle branch block with a QRS duration of 150 milliseconds or greater, and NYHA class II, III, or ambulatory IV symptoms who are receiving optimal medical therapy (Fig. 5-8).

Anticoagulation

Patients with HF; persistent, paroxysmal, or permanent atrial fibrillation; and one other risk factor in the CHADS2 index (i.e., congestive heart failure, hypertension, age 75 years or greater, diabetes mellitus, and stroke) should receive chronic anticoagulant therapy. According to the guidelines, it is reasonable to anticoagulate patients with HF and atrial fibrillation without additional risk factors.

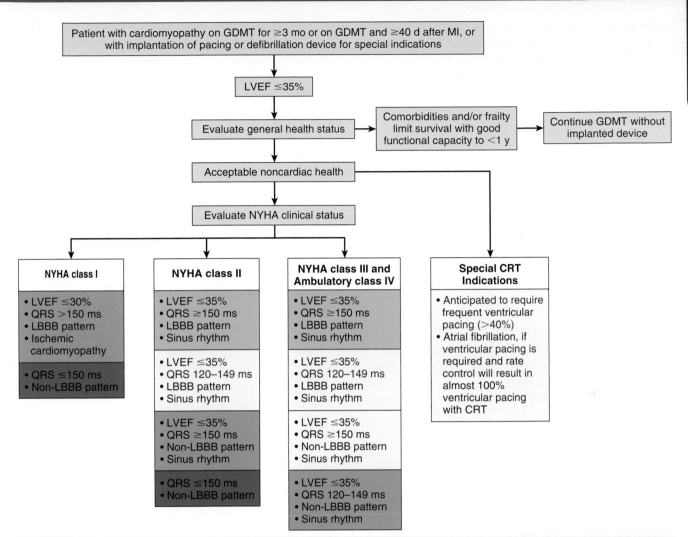

FIGURE 5-8 Left ventricular ejection fraction (LVEF) and New York Heart Association (NYHA) functional class that correlates with the American College of Cardiology and American Heart Association (ACC/AHA) guidelines for recommendations for defibrillators and cardiac resynchronization therapy (CRT). Class I recommendations are shown in *green*, class IIa recommendations are shown in *yellow*, class IIb recommendations are shown in *orange*, and class III recommendations are shown in *red*. GDMT, Guideline-directed medical therapy; LBBB, left bundle branch block; MI, myocardial infarction.

Stage D Heart Failure

Despite optimal medical therapy, many patients with HF fail to have significant improvement in symptoms. In these instances, a trial of hemodynamically guided (i.e., using a Swan-Ganz catheter) HF therapy may be necessary to optimize volume status and perfusion and to assess the degree of impairment of the cardiac index.

This approach allows assessment of candidacy for advanced HF therapies, such as cardiac transplantation and mechanical circulatory support with ventricular assist devices. One commonly used agent is milrinone, an intravenous phosphodiesterase inhibitor that has similar effects on contractility and afterload. Administration increases the cardiac index and promotes spontaneous diuresis. In patients with markedly elevated systemic vascular resistance, the use of intravenous vasodilators (e.g., nitroglycerin, sodium nitroprusside) can significantly reduce afterload and may improve cardiac output.

If the previously described measures fail to produce a satisfactory diuretic response, dopamine given in doses ranging from 2 to 5 μg/kg/min may facilitate sodium and water excretion by stimulating renal dopaminergic receptors. Table 5-5 shows the clinical signs and laboratory values that a clinician should recognize in patients with stage D or advanced HF. The Interagency Registry for Mechanically Assisted Circulatory Support (INTERMACS) scale is used to appropriately risk-stratify these patients for potential mechanical circulatory support.

Mechanical Circulatory Support

Two permanent ventricular assist devices (VADs) are approved by the U.S. Food and Drug Administration. The first device is the HeartMate II, which is an axial flow device that is approved for bridge-to-transplantation use and for destination therapy in transplantation-ineligible patients. The second device is a third-generation VAD called Heartware (HVAD), which is a centrifugal pump. Both pumps require chronic anticoagulation and antiplatelet therapy. The current estimated aggregate survival rate is approximately 80% at 1 year and approximately 70% at 2 years.

TABLE 5-5 IDENTIFYING ADVANCED HEART FAILURE

Repeated (≥2) hospitalizations or ED visits for HF in the past year

Progressive deterioration in renal function (e.g., rise in BUN and creatinine)

Weight loss without other cause (e.g., cardiac cachexia)

Intolerance to ACE inhibitors due to hypotension and/or worsening renal function

Intolerance to β-blockers due to worsening HF or hypotension

Frequent systolic blood pressure <90 mm Hg

Persistent dyspnea with dressing or bathing requiring rest

Inability to walk 1 block on the level ground due to dyspnea or fatigue

Recent need to escalate diuretics to maintain volume status, often reaching daily furosemide equivalent dose >160 mg/day and/or use of supplemental metolazone therapy

Progressive decline in serum sodium, usually to <133 mEq/L

Frequent ICD shocks

Modified from Yancy CW, Jessup M, Bozkurt B, et al: 2013 ACCF/AHA guidelines for the management of heart failure: a report of the American College of Cardiology Foundation/American Heart Association Task Force on Practice Guidelines, J Am Coll Cardiol 62:e147–e239, 2013.

ACE, Angiotensin-converting enzyme; BUN, blood urea nitrogen; ED, emergency department; HF, heart failure; ICD, implantable cardiac defibrillator.

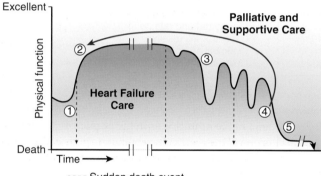

FIGURE 5-9 Conceptualizing comprehensive heart failure (HF) care. Early in therapy (1), supportive efforts focus on education for the patient and family about HF and self-management. Diuresis and evidence-based therapies achieve a plateau of improved function (2). Even when a plateau of improved function is achieved, the patient and family can benefit from efforts that improve symptoms and assist them in coping with HF and its impact on their lives. Functional status declines with intermittent exacerbations of HF that respond to rescue efforts (3). Heart transplantation or destination therapy ventricular assist devices (4) improve function for patients for a period and carry a different burden of chronic illness. At the end of life or when significant physical frailty or comorbidities predominate (5), the major focus of care is palliation, but some HF therapies remain important. HF is different from cancer, for which potentially curative treatments are discontinued as the patient reaches the end stage. (Modified from Goodlin S: Palliative care in congestive heart failure, J Am Coll Cardiol 54:386–396, 2009.)

Prognosis

The disease trajectory of HF is complex and characterized by variable intervals of clinical stability (Fig. 5-9). Although many randomized, controlled trials have demonstrated a symptom and mortality benefit with ACE inhibitors, ARBs, β-blockers, mineralocorticoid receptor blockers, and ICD and CRT therapy, the sobering 5-year mortality rate for HF remains at 50%, and the 10-year survival rate for patients with symptomatic HF is only 20%.

For a deeper discussion on this topic, please see Chapter 58, "Heart Failure: Pathophysiology and Diagnosis," in Goldman-Cecil Medicine, 25th Edition.

SUGGESTED READINGS

Bardy GH, Lee KL, Mark DB, et al: Amiodarone or an implantable cardioverter-defibrillator for congestive heart failure, N Engl J Med 352:225–237, 2005.

Cook D, Simel DL: The rational clinical examination: does this patient have abnormal central venous pressure? JAMA 275:630–634, 1996.

Digitalis Investigation Group: The effect of digoxin on mortality and morbidity in patients with heart failure, N Engl J Med 336:525–533, 1997.

Drazner MH, Rame JE, Stevenson LW, et al: Prognostic importance of elevated jugular venous pressure and a third heart sound in patients with heart failure, N Engl J Med 345:574–581, 2001.

Felker M, O'Connor CM, Braunwald E, et al: Loop diuretics in acute decompensated heart failure: necessary? Evil? A necessary evil? Circ Heart Fail 2:56–62, 2009.

Felker M, Lee KL, Bull DA, et al: Diuretic strategies in patients with acute decompensated heart failure, N Engl J Med 364:797–805, 2011.

McAlister FA, Ezekowitz J, Hooton N, et al: Cardiac resynchronization therapy for patients with left ventricular systolic dysfunction: a systematic review, JAMA 297:2502–2514, 2007.

Nohria A, Lewis E, Stevenson LW: Medical management of advanced heart failure, JAMA 287:628–640, 2002.

Packer M: Effect of carvedilol on survival in severe chronic heart failure, N Engl J Med 344:1651–1658, 2001.

Pitt B, Zannad F, Remme WJ, et al: The effect of spironolactone on morbidity and mortality in patients with severe heart failure. Randomized Aldactone Evaluation Study Investigators, N Engl J Med 341:709–717, 1999.

Roger VL, Go AS, Lloyd-Jones DM, et al: Heart disease and stroke statistics—2011 update: a report from the American Heart Association, Circulation 123:e18–e209, 2011.

SOLVD Investigators: Effect of enalapril on survival in patients with reduced left ventricular ejection fractions and congestive heart failure. The SOLVD Investigators, N Engl J Med 325:293–302, 1991.

Taylor AL, Ziesche S, Yancy C, et al: African-American Heart Failure Trial Investigators: Combination of isosorbide dinitrate and hydralazine in blacks with heart failure, N Engl J Med 351:2049–2057, 2004.

Yancy CW, Jessup M, Bozkurt B, et al: 2013 ACCF/AHA guidelines for the management of heart failure: a report of the American College of Cardiology Foundation/American Heart Association Task Force on Practice Guidelines, J Am Coll Cardiol 62:e147–e239, 2013.

Congenital Heart Disease

Scott Cohen and Michael G. Earing

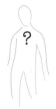

INTRODUCTION

Congenital heart defects are the most common group of birth defects, occurring in approximately 9 of 1000 live births. Without treatment, most patients die in infancy or childhood, with only 5% to 15% surviving into adulthood. Advancements in surgical and medical practices have resulted in survival of approximately 90% of these children to adulthood. For the first time in history, estimates suggest that more adults than children are living with congenital heart disease in the United States and that there is a 5% increase every year.

Most adults living with congenital heart disease have had interventions performed (Table 6-1). Although most children who undergo surgical intervention survive to adulthood, total correction usually is not the rule. Adult patients with congenital heart disease are surviving longer than ever before, and it is becoming apparent that even the simplest lesions can be associated with long-term cardiac complications (i.e., arrhythmias and conduction abnormalities, ventricular dysfunction, residual shunts, valvular lesions, hypertension, and aneurysms) and noncardiac complications (i.e., renal dysfunction, restrictive lung disease, anxiety, depression, and liver dysfunction). Most adults with congenital heart disease need lifelong follow-up.

ACYANOTIC HEART DISEASE

Atrial Septal Defects

Definition and Epidemiology

Atrial septal defects (ASDs) are communications between the atria that allow shunting of blood from one atrium to the other. They are among the most common congenital anomalies seen in adolescents and young adults, occurring in 1 of 1500 live births and constituting 6% to 10% of all congenital heart defects.

There are four main types of ASDs. Ostium secundum defects are the most common, accounting for 75% of all ASDs. This defect occurs in the region of the fossa ovalis and results from excessive absorption of the septum primum or insufficient development of the septum secundum, or both.

Ostium primum defects represent about 20% of all ASDs and represent a form of atrioventricular septal defect (i.e., partial or incomplete atrioventricular canal). These defects are located in the inferior aspect of the atrial septum adjacent to the mitral and tricuspid valves. The defects result from lack of closure of the ostium primum by the endocardial cushions, which are embryologic swellings in the heart that form the primum atrial septum, the inlet portion of the ventricular septum, and parts of the mitral and tricuspid valve. The lesions often are associated with clefts in the mitral and tricuspid valves.

Sinus venosus ASDs represent 5% of all ASDs and are located at the entry of the superior vena cava into the right atrium. Frequently, there is associated partial anomalous drainage of the right upper pulmonary vein. This defect results from resorption of the wall between the vena cava and pulmonary veins.

An unroofed coronary sinus is a rare form of ASD, representing less than 1% of all ASDs. The coronary sinus is in apposition to the posterior aspect of the left atrium, but the orifice is in the right atrium. When a defect exists in the roof of the coronary sinus, a communication between the left atrium and right atrium exists, allowing shunting.

Pathology

All four types of ASDs allow oxygenated blood to pass from the left atrium into the right atrium, resulting in volume overload of the right atrium and right ventricle (Fig. 6-1). The degree of shunting is determined by the size of the ASD and the compliance of the left and right cardiac chambers. Comorbidities that increase left-sided filling pressures (i.e., left ventricular [LV] diastolic dysfunction, myocardial infarction, and mitral stenosis) may result in an increased left-to-right shunt. Over time, significant left-to-right shunting can cause enlargement of the right atrium and right ventricle, eventually leading to right ventricular (RV) systolic dysfunction and failure. Pulmonary hypertension may occur in approximately 26% of patients with a secundum ASD. However, significant elevation in pulmonary vascular resistance is rare.

TABLE 6-1	MOST COMMON CONGENITAL HEART DEFECTS SURVIVING TO ADULTHOOD WITHOUT SURGERY OR INTERVENTIONAL CATHETERIZATION

Mild pulmonary valve stenosis
Bicuspid aortic valve
Small to moderate size atrial septal defect
Small ventricular septal defect
Small patent ductus arteriosus
Mitral valve prolapse
Partial atrioventricular canal (ostium primum atrial septal defect and cleft mitral valve)
Marfan syndrome
Ebstein's anomaly
Congenitally corrected transposition (atrioventricular and ventriculoarterial discordance)

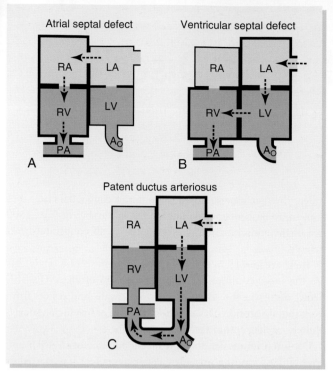

Atrial septal defect

Ventricular septal defect

Patent ductus arteriosus

FIGURE 6-1 The diagram shows three types of shunt lesions that commonly survive until adulthood and their effects on chamber size. **A,** Uncomplicated atrial septal defect with left-to-right shunt flow across the interatrial septum, resulting in dilation of the right atrium (RA), right ventricle (RV), and pulmonary artery (PA). **B,** Uncomplicated ventricular septal defect, resulting in dilation of the RV, left atrium (LA), and left ventricle (LV). **C,** Uncomplicated patent ductus arteriosus, resulting in dilation of the LA, LV, and PA. Ao, Aorta. (From Liberthson RR, Walkman H: Congenital heart disease in the adult. In Kloner RA, editor: Guide to cardiology, ed 3, Greenwich, Conn., 1991, Le Jacq Communications, pp 24–27.)

Clinical Presentation

Although most individuals with an ASD are diagnosed during childhood after a murmur is noticed, a few patients have symptoms for the first time as adults. Most patients are asymptomatic during the first and second decades of life. In the third decade, an increasing numbers of patients develop exercise intolerance, palpitations due to atrial arrhythmias, and cardiac enlargement on the chest radiograph. In patients with ASDs, the RV impulse at the left lower sternal border often has increased force compared with normal. On auscultation, the second heart sound typically is widely split and fixed (i.e., does not vary with inspiration).

All patients have a systolic ejection murmur, which is best heard at the left upper sternal border and is related to increased flow across a usually normal pulmonary valve. When there is a large left-to-right shunt, a mid-diastolic murmur can be heard at the left lower sternal border; it is related to increased flow across a normal tricuspid valve. When a mid-diastolic murmur is identified, the degree of left-to-right shunt is considered to be 1.5 times normal. In the setting of a primum ASD, an additional holosystolic murmur at the apex may be caused by a cleft in the anterior leaflet of the mitral valve, resulting in mitral regurgitation.

Diagnosis

On the electrocardiogram (ECG), the features of ASD depend on the size and type of defect. In the setting of a large ostium secundum, sinus venosus, or unroofed coronary sinus defect, the ECG typically demonstrates evidence of right atrial (RA) enlargement, RV hypertrophy, and right axis deviation. In the setting of an ostium primum ASD, like other forms of atrioventricular defects, there is a superior axis. The chest radiograph is helpful for evaluating the degree of left-to-right shunting. With a small shunt, the radiograph will be normal. As the shunt increases in size, the heart size and pulmonary vascular markings also increase.

The diagnosis of an ASD and its location is confirmed by transthoracic echocardiography in most cases. A sinus venosus ASD is the exception. In this setting, transesophageal echocardiography may be necessary. Cardiac catheterization is rarely performed to diagnose an ASD. However, transcatheter closure has become the preferred treatment option for most ostium secundum defects.

Treatment

The treatment of ASDs involves surgical or transcatheter device closure. For secundum ASD, surgical closure and transcatheter device closure are accepted treatment options. Device closure is the most commonly used technique for closure of secundum defects. This technique, however, requires an adequate rim of septal tissue around the entire defect to allow for device stabilization. For ostium primum, sinus venosus, and unroofed coronary sinus forms of ASDs, surgical closure remains the only option.

Prognosis

Most patients who have undergone early closure of a defect have excellent long-term survival rates with low morbidity rates if repair is undertaken before 25 years of age. Older age at repair is associated with decreased late survival rates and an associated increased risk of atrial arrhythmias, thromboembolic events, and pulmonary hypertension. After the age of 40 years for patients with unrepaired ASDs, the mortality rate increases by 6% per year, and more than 20% of patients develop atrial fibrillation. By 60 years of age, the number of patients with atrial fibrillation increases to more than 60%. Long-term rates of late complications and survival after transcatheter device closure remain unknown.

Ventricular Septal Defects
Definition and Epidemiology

Ventricular septal defects (VSDs) occur in 1.5 to 3.5 of 1000 live births. They constitute 20% of congenital heart defects.

There are four types of VSD: perimembranous, muscular, supracristal, and inlet. Perimembranous VSDs are the most common, comprising 70% of all VSDs. The membranous septum is relatively small and sits directly under the aortic valve. Perimembranous VSDs involve the membranous septum and typically extend into the muscular tissue adjacent to the membranous septum. If not large, these defects may close spontaneously by tissue from the septal leaflet of the tricuspid valve.

Muscular VSDs are the second most common VSD and account for 5% to 20% of all VSDs. Multiple muscular VSDs commonly are found at the time of diagnosis. Muscular VSDs have the highest rate of spontaneous closure.

Supracristal VSDs represent 5% to 8% of all VSDs. These defects are located superior to the crista supraventricularis (i.e., within the RV outflow tract directly below the right cusp of the aortic valve). These defects are associated with prolapse of the right aortic cusp, which can lead to progressive aortic regurgitation. In some cases, the prolapsed right aortic cusp may restrict the defect, but rarely do they spontaneously close.

Inlet VSDs are located in the posterior ventricular septum, just inferior to the tricuspid and mitral valve. They account for 5% to 8% of all VSDs and never close spontaneously.

Pathology

Shunting through a VSD is typically left to right and can cause overcirculation of the pulmonary vasculature and increased pulmonary venous return, resulting in left-sided chamber enlargement (see Fig. 6-1). The degree of shunting depends on the size of the defect and the pulmonary vascular resistance. Small defects (i.e., restrictive defects) typically have a small degree of shunting and normal pulmonary artery pressure. Moderate-sized defects have enough left-to-right shunting to cause mildly elevated pulmonary artery pressures and some left-sided chamber enlargement. Large defects (i.e., nonrestrictive defects) allow LV systolic pressures to be transmitted to the pulmonary circulation. This can cause irreversible obstructive pulmonary vascular disease early in childhood. Eventually, if the pulmonary vascular resistance exceeds the systemic vascular resistance, the shunt may reverse to right to left (i.e. Eisenmenger's physiology).

Clinical Presentation

The physical findings for a patient with a VSD depend on the size of the VSD, magnitude of the shunt, and the level of pulmonary artery hypertension. For patients with a small VSD, the apical impulses of the right ventricle and left ventricle typically have normal intensity on palpation, but there may be a palpable thrill. The first and second heart sounds typically are normal, and in most cases, there is a holosystolic murmur of moderate intensity at the left lower sternal border.

Patients with Eisenmenger's syndrome have cyanosis and secondary erythrocytosis. The RV impulse usually is increased at the left lower sternal border, and the pulmonary component of the second heart sound may be palpable. Typically, no systolic murmur is detected, but a diastolic murmur is often heard at the left upper sternal border due to a severely dilated main pulmonary artery and resultant pulmonary regurgitation.

Diagnosis

The ECG should be normal for patients with small VSDs. For those with Eisenmenger's syndrome, the ECG usually demonstrates RV hypertrophy with right axis deviation. Patients with a small VSD have a normal chest radiograph. Patients with Eisenmenger's syndrome may have mild cardiac enlargement with enlarged proximal pulmonary arteries and peripheral pruning

with oligemic lung fields. Echocardiography allows confirmation of the diagnosis, localization of defect, identification of long-term complications, and estimation of pulmonary artery pressure. Cardiac catheterization allows direct measurement of the degree of left-to-right shunting, pulmonary artery pressure, and pulmonary vascular reactivity.

Treatment

Because patients with small VSDs are asymptomatic, they should be treated conservatively. Because of the long-term risks, they need intermittent follow-up for life to monitor for the development of late complications. The exceptions to this rule are those with small supracristal or perimembranous VSDs with associated prolapse of the aortic cusp into the defect that results in progressive aortic regurgitation. These patients should be considered for surgical repair at the time of diagnosis to prevent progressive aortic valve damage.

Prognosis

Although isolated VSDs are common forms of congenital heart disease, the diagnosis of a VSD in an adult is rare. Most patients with a hemodynamically significant VSD have undergone repair in childhood or died earlier in life. As result, the spectrum of isolated VSDs in adults is limited to those with small restrictive defects, those with Eisenmenger's syndrome, and those who had their defects closed in childhood.

For patients with small restrictive VSDs, long-term survival is excellent, with an estimated 25-year survival rate of 96%. The rate of long-term morbidity for patients with a restrictive VSD also appears to be low. However, the clinical course is not completely benign. Reported long-term complications include endocarditis, progressive aortic regurgitation due to prolapse of aortic valve into the defect (i.e., highest risk for the supracristal type but can occur with a perimembranous defect), and the development of right and left outflow tract obstruction from a double-chamber right ventricle or a subaortic membrane.

For patients who develop Eisenmenger's syndrome, survival into the third decade is common. However, with increasing age, the long-term complications of right heart failure, paradoxical emboli, and erythrocytosis usually result in a progressive drop in survival, with an average age of death of 37 years. Adults with previous VSD closure and without pulmonary hypertension or residual defects have a normal life expectancy.

Complete Atrioventricular Septal Defects
Definition and Epidemiology

Complete atrioventricular septal defects (AVSDs) consist of several cardiac malformations that result from abnormal development of the endocardial cushions. AVSDs account for 4% to 5% of congenital heart defects. Down syndrome is a common association; 40% of Down syndrome patients have congenital heart disease, and 40% of these have some form of AVSD.

AVSDs are categorized as partial (or incomplete) or complete. Both forms share common structural abnormalities—ostium primum ASD, inlet VSD, and cleft anterior mitral and septal tricuspid valve—in various combinations.

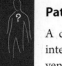

Pathology

A combination of the previously described defects results in interatrial and interventricular shunts, LV-to-RA shunt, and atrioventricular regurgitation. Because these defects include deficiency of the inlet portion of the ventricular septum, the LV outflow tract is lengthened and may be narrowed, producing the characteristic goose-neck deformity.

The natural history for patients with complete AVSD is characterized by the early development of pulmonary vascular disease, leading to irreversible damage that often occurs by 1 year of age, particularly for patients with Down syndrome. Surgery needs to be undertaken early if it is to be successful. Patients who are diagnosed in adulthood can be categorized in two groups: those with Eisenmenger's syndrome and those who had their defects closed in childhood.

Clinical Presentation

On physical examination, most previously repaired patients are cardiovascularly normal. However, patients with significant left atrioventricular (AV) valve regurgitation have a grade 3 or 4 (of 6) holosystolic regurgitant murmur at the apex. For the rare patient with subaortic stenosis, a grade 2 or 3 systolic murmur can be detected at the left midsternal border and radiating to the neck. The physical examination findings for patients with Eisenmenger's syndrome are similar to those for patients with unoperated VSDs.

Diagnosis

On the ECG, first-degree heart block is a common finding for patients with AVSD. All patients have a superior, leftward QRS axis. For those with Eisenmenger's syndrome, the chest radiograph demonstrates cardiomegaly, large proximal pulmonary arteries, and small peripheral pulmonary arteries (i.e., peripheral pruning). Patients who underwent previous repair and have significant systemic left AV valve regurgitation have cardiomegaly with increased vascular markings.

Treatment

Patients who underwent previous repair with significant left AV valve regurgitation causing symptoms, atrial arrhythmias, or deterioration in ventricular function should undergo elective repair or replacement. Previously repaired patients who develop significant subaortic stenosis (i.e., peak cardiac catheterization or echo gradient of ≥50 mm Hg) should undergo surgical repair.

Prognosis

Overall, for patients who underwent early repair before the development of pulmonary vascular disease, the long-term prognosis is good. The most common long-term complication is left AV valve regurgitation, with approximately 5% to 10% of patients requiring surgical revision for left AV valve repair or replacement during follow-up. The second most common long-term complication for this group is subaortic stenosis, occurring in up to 5% of patients after repair. Other long-term complications include residual atrial- or ventricular-level shunts, complete heart block, atrial and ventricular arrhythmias, and endocarditis.

Patients with Eisenmenger's syndrome are symptomatic with exertional dyspnea, fatigue, palpitations, edema, and syncope. Survival is similar to that for other forms of Eisenmenger's syndrome, with a mean age at death of 37 years. In retrospective studies, strong predictors for death included syncope, age at presentation of symptoms, poor functional class, low oxygen saturation (≤85%), increased serum creatinine and serum uric acid concentrations, and Down syndrome.

Coarctation of the Aorta

Definition

Coarctation of the aorta is an abnormal narrowing of the aortic lumen. It constitutes 5% of congenital heart defects. Coarctation of the aorta may occur anywhere along the descending aorta, even below the diaphragm, but in more than 95% of cases, the narrowing is just below the takeoff of the left subclavian artery. In 50% to 85% of cases, there is an associated bicuspid aortic valve. Other associated lesions include VSDs, subaortic stenosis, and mitral valve stenosis.

Pathology

Coarctation of the aorta is an aortopathy of the entire aorta rather than a localized abnormality. In the young, significant coarctation can decrease blood flow to the kidneys, gut, and lower extremities, resulting in severe acidosis and shock requiring immediate treatment. Unrepaired coarctation of the aorta can be seen in adults, but it is rare. Affected individuals develop extensive arterial collateralization to maintain distal perfusion. Most patients seen in adulthood are patients who have had previous coarctation of the aorta repair using a variety of different techniques.

Even after successful repair to relieve the obstruction, multiple studies have demonstrated that patients have persistent abnormalities in the media of the aorta proximal and distal to the coarctation repair site. The stiff aortic wall is characterized by decreased distensibility and endothelial and vascular dysfunction. Examples include resting and exercise-induced hypertension, increased carotid intimal thickness, and abnormal peripheral arterial responses to augmented blood flow and nitroglycerin. Patients with coarctation of the aorta are at increased risk for other left-sided obstructive lesions, particularly a bicuspid aortic valve, which occurs in 50% of cases.

Clinical Presentation

The clinical presentation of coarctation of the aorta depends on the severity of obstruction and the associated anomalies. Unrepaired coarctation of the aorta typically manifests with symptoms before adulthood. Symptoms include headaches related to hypertension, leg fatigue or cramps, exercise intolerance, and systemic hypertension. Untreated patients surviving to adulthood typically have only mild coarctation of the aorta.

Cardinal clinical features in the setting of a significant coarctation of the aorta include upper body hypertension, weak and delayed femoral pulses, and a blood pressure gradient between the right arm and right leg determined by blood pressure cuff. On auscultation, the aortic valve closure sound is usually loud; in the setting of a bicuspid aortic valve, an ejection click, often with a

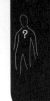

crescendo-decrescendo systolic murmur, is heard at the right upper sternal border. Often, a continuous systolic murmur is heard over the left scapula. It is related to continuous flow across the coarctation of the aorta.

Diagnosis

Patients with significant coarctation of the aorta typically show various degrees of left atrial (LA) and LV enlargement on an ECG. The chest radiograph typically demonstrates normal heart size with dilation of the ascending aorta and kinking or double contouring in the region of the descending aorta in the area of the coarctation, producing the characteristic figure-3 sign.

Most adult patients have rib notching. It is caused by the dilated intercostal collateral arteries eroding the undersurface of the ribs. Echocardiography is used to identify site, structure, and degree of stenosis or restenosis. Echocardiography is valuable for identifying other lesions, LV systolic function, and degree of LV hypertrophy.

Cardiac catheterization remains the gold standard for determining the anatomy and absolute degree of stenosis. In adult patients, cardiac catheterization with balloon dilation and stent placement has become the procedure of choice for the treatment of recoarctation. Newer magnetic resonance imaging (MRI) methods are quite good for imaging coarctation, defining the arch vessel anatomy, and identifying collaterals.

Treatment

Patients with significant native or residual coarctation of the aorta (i.e., symptomatic with a peak gradient across the coarctation of ≥30 mm Hg) should be considered for surgical repair or catheter intervention with balloon angioplasty with or without stent placement. Surgical repair in the adult patient is technically difficult and is associated with high rates of morbidity. As result, catheter based intervention has become the preferred method in most experienced congenital heart disease centers.

Prognosis

After surgical repair, long-term survival is good but directly correlates with the age at repair. Those repaired after 14 years of age have a lower 20-year survival rate than those repaired earlier (79% vs. 91%). Long-term outcome data for catheter-based treatment is limited, but studies suggest that stented patients have lower acute and long-term complications at 60 months (25% for surgery vs. 12.5% for stents). Irrespective of the type of repair, the most common long-term complication is persistent or new systemic hypertension at rest or during exercise. Other long-term complications include aneurysms of the ascending or descending aorta (especially after Dacron patch repair), recoarctation at the site of previous repair, coronary artery disease, aortic stenosis or regurgitation (in the setting of a bicuspid aortic valve), rupture of an intracranial aneurysm, and endocarditis.

Patent Ductus Arteriosus

Definition and Epidemiology

Patent ductus arteriosus (PDA) represents 9% to 12% of congenital heart defects. It is patent in the fetus but normally closes within several days of birth. However, it remains open in about 1

of 2500 to 5000 births. In infants born prematurely, the incidence is even higher, occurring in 8 of 1000 live births. The incidence of PDA is 30 times greater for babies born at high altitudes than for those born at sea level.

Pathology

A PDA allows transit of blood from the aorta into the pulmonary artery and recirculation through the pulmonary vasculature and the left side of the heart. This can result in left-sided chamber enlargement (see Fig. 6-1). As with VSDs, the size of the defect is the primary determinant of the clinical course in the adult patient. PDAs can be clinically categorized as silent PDAs; small, hemodynamically insignificant PDAs; moderate-size PDAs; large PDAs; and previously repaired PDAs.

Clinical Presentation

A silent PDA is a tiny defect that cannot be heard by auscultation and is detected only by other nonclinical means such as echocardiography. Life expectancy is always normal for this population, and the risk of endocarditis is extremely low.

Patients with a small PDA have an audible, long-ejection or continuous murmur that is heard best at the left upper sternal border and radiating to the back. They have normal peripheral pulses. Because there is negligible left-to-right shunting, these patients have normal LA and LV sizes and normal pulmonary artery pressure. Like those with silent PDAs, these patients are asymptomatic and have a normal life expectancy. However, they do have a higher risk of endocarditis.

Patients with moderate-size PDAs may be diagnosed during adulthood. These patients often have wide, bouncy peripheral pulses and an audible, continuous murmur. They have significant volume overload and develop some degree of LA and LV enlargement and some degree of pulmonary hypertension. These patients are symptomatic with dyspnea, palpitations, and heart failure. Patients with large PDAs typically have signs of severe pulmonary hypertension and Eisenmenger's syndrome. By adulthood, the continuous murmur is typically absent, and there is differential cyanosis (i.e., lower extremity saturations are lower than the right arm saturation).

Diagnosis

Patients with silent and small PDAs appear normal by echocardiography and chest radiography. Calcifications may be seen on the posteroanterior and lateral films of an older patient with a PDA. In patients with significant left-to-right shunting, there typically is dilation of the central pulmonary arteries with increased pulmonary vascular markings. On an ECG, broad P waves and tall QRS complexes suggest LA and LV volume overload. A tall R wave in lead V_1 with a right axis deviation suggests significant pulmonary hypertension. Echocardiography is important to estimate the size of the defect, degree of LA or LV enlargement, and degree of pulmonary artery hypertension.

Treatment

All patients with clinical evidence of a PDA are at increased risk for endocarditis. Except for patients with small or silent PDAs and those with severe, irreversible pulmonary hypertension, PDA closure should be considered. Catheter device closure is the preferred method in most centers. Surgical closure is reserved for

patients with PDAs too large for device closure and for distorted anatomy such as a large ductal aneurysm.

Prognosis

Patients with a large PDA who have developed Eisenmenger's syndrome have a prognosis similar to that of other patients with Eisenmenger's syndrome. Patients who underwent PDA repair before the development of pulmonary hypertension have a normal life expectancy without restrictions.

Pulmonary Valve Stenosis

Definition and Epidemiology

Pulmonary valve stenosis occurs in approximately 4 of 1000 live births and constitutes 5% to 8% of congenital cardiac defects. It is one of the most common adult forms of unoperated congenital heart disease. It can occur in isolation or with other congenital heart defects, such as an ASD.

Pathology

In congenital pulmonary valve stenosis, the pulmonary valve leaflets are often fused or thickened, which obstructs blood flow out of the right ventricle. The obstruction elevates RV pressure, and compensatory RV hypertrophy develops. Pulmonary stenosis is often tolerated better than aortic stenosis. Over time, RV dilation and dysfunction may occur.

Clinical Presentation

Most patients with pulmonary valve stenosis are asymptomatic and have a cardiac murmur at presentation. Most unoperated adults with severe stenosis have jugular venous distention, and on palpation, a RV lift at the left lower sternal border and a thrill at the left upper sternal border can be identified. On auscultation, the second heart sound is widely split, and a systolic ejection click may or may not be heard, depending on the mobility of the pulmonary valve leaflets. In most cases, there is a harsh, crescendo-decrescendo systolic ejection murmur, which is heard best at the left upper sternal border; it radiates to the back and varies with inspiration.

Diagnosis

With moderate to severe pulmonary valve stenosis, the ECG demonstrates right axis deviation, RV hypertrophy, and RA enlargement. The ECG is usually normal for patients with mild pulmonary valve stenosis. On the chest radiograph, a prominent main pulmonary artery caused by poststenotic dilatation is a common finding regardless of the degree of stenosis. In patients with severe pulmonary valve stenosis, cardiomegaly due to RA and RV enlargement is often seen.

Echocardiography is the diagnostic method of choice. It allows visualization of the valve anatomy and degree of stenosis and enables estimation of the valve gradient.

Treatment

Survival into adult life and the need for intervention directly correlate with the degree of obstruction. In the Second Natural History Study of Congenital Heart Disease, patients with trivial stenosis (i.e., peak gradient ≤25 mm Hg) who were followed for 25 years remained asymptomatic and had no significant progression of obstruction over time. For those with moderate pulmonary valve stenosis (i.e., peak gradient between 25 and 49 mm Hg), there was an approximately 20% chance of requiring intervention by 25 years of age. Most patients with severe stenosis (i.e., peak gradient of ≥50 mm Hg) require intervention (i.e., surgery or balloon valvuloplasty) by age 25 years. Patients with moderate to severe pulmonary stenosis should be considered for intervention even in the absence of symptoms.

Since 1985, percutaneous balloon valvuloplasty has been the accepted treatment for patients of all ages. Before 1985, surgical valvotomy had been the gold standard. Today, surgical valvotomy is reserved for patients who are unlikely to have successful results from balloon valvuloplasty, such as those with an extremely dysplastic or calcified valve.

Prognosis

After surgical valvotomy for isolated pulmonary stenosis, long-term survival is excellent. However, with longer follow-up the incidence of late complications and the need for reintervention do increase. The most common indication for reintervention is pulmonary valve replacement for severe pulmonary regurgitation. Other long-term complications include recurrent atrial arrhythmias, endocarditis, and residual subpulmonary obstruction.

Aortic Valve Stenosis

Definition and Epidemiology

Aortic valve stenosis is a common abnormality in adults with congenital heart disease. It is usually caused by a bicuspid aortic valve, which occurs in 1% to 2% of adults and is three times more common in males. It typically is an isolated lesion but can be associated with other defects such as coarctation of the aorta or VSD.

Pathology

Aortic valve stenosis results in pressure overload of the left ventricle, which increases wall stress and causes compensatory LV hypertrophy. Diastolic dysfunction and oxygen delivery-demand mismatch ensues. The patient may remain well compensated and asymptomatic for many years, but compensatory mechanisms eventually begin to fail, and LV dysfunction can develop. Patients with a bicuspid aortic valve have abnormal structure of the aortic wall that often leads to ascending aortic dilation.

Clinical Presentation

Most patients with aortic valve stenosis are asymptomatic and are diagnosed after a murmur is detected. The severity of obstruction at the time of diagnosis correlates with the pattern of progression. Symptoms are rare until patients have severe aortic valve stenosis (i.e., mean gradient by echocardiography of ≥40 mm Hg). Symptoms include chest pain, exertional dyspnea, near-syncope, and syncope. With any of these symptoms, the risk of sudden cardiac death is very high, and surgical intervention is mandated.

Patients with moderate to severe stenosis typically have decreased peripheral pulses, an increased apical impulse, and a

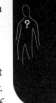

palpable thrill at the base of the heart. On auscultation, these patients have an ejection click followed by a crescendo-decrescendo systolic murmur, which is heard best at the left mid-sternal border and radiating to the right upper sternal border and the neck. Correlation between the degree of stenosis and the intensity of the murmur is not good. However, it is rare for a murmur of 2/6 or less to be associated with severe stenosis. Some patients with aortic stenosis also have aortic regurgitation, in which case a decrescendo diastolic murmur at the left midsternal border that radiates to the apex is detected at presentation.

Diagnosis

Many patients with significant aortic stenosis have LV hypertrophy identified on the ECG. However, the correlation between the severity of stenosis and the finding of LV hypertrophy on the ECG is unreliable. On chest radiography, most patients with severe aortic stenosis have a normal heart size unless there is concurrent aortic regurgitation. Post-stenotic dilation of the ascending aorta is common irrespective of degree of stenosis, and ascending aorta dilation is a common finding. It appears on the chest radiograph as a widened mediastinum.

Echocardiography is the gold standard for evaluation of the severity of aortic valve stenosis and the anatomic morphology of the aortic valve. Cardiac catheterization is primarily indicated to evaluate coronary artery disease before surgical intervention, because approximately one half of adults with symptomatic aortic valve stenosis have concurrent coronary artery disease.

Treatment

Patients with severe aortic stenosis and symptoms or asymptomatic patients with severe aortic valve stenosis and reduced LV systolic function (<50%) should be considered for intervention. Treatment involves manipulating the valve to reduce stenosis. This can be accomplished by transvenous balloon dilation of the valve, open surgical valvotomy, or surgical or catheter-based valve replacement. In absence of significant aortic regurgitation, most centers favor balloon dilation or surgical valvotomy for children and young adults who have pliable valves with fusion of the commissures. In older adults, aortic valve replacement is the treatment of choice.

Prognosis

The natural history of aortic valve stenosis in adults varies but is characterized by progressive stenosis over time. By 45 years of age, approximately 50% of bicuspid aortic valves have some degree of stenosis. Most patients requiring surgical valvotomy to relieve the stenosis before adulthood do well. However, by the 25-year follow-up, up to 40% of patients required a second operation for residual stenosis or regurgitation.

⬤ CYANOTIC HEART DISEASE
Tetralogy of Fallot
Definition and Epidemiology

Tetralogy of Fallot (TOF) is the most common cyanotic heart disease seen in adulthood, and it represents 10% of congenital heart defects. It consists of a large VSD, pulmonary stenosis (which may be valvular, subvalvular, and or supravalvular), an aorta that overrides the VSD, and RV hypertrophy.

Pathology

Newborns with TOF are cyanotic because of the right-to-left shunt through the VSD and decreased pulmonary blood flow. The amount of pulmonary blood flow depends on the severity of the obstruction through the RV outflow tract. By the time TOF patients reach adulthood, most have had complete repair or palliative surgery.

Many adults with repaired TOF have had a transannular patch (i.e., synthetic patch across the pulmonary annulus) placed to relieve the RV outflow tract obstruction. This patch causes obligatory free pulmonary regurgitation. Free pulmonary regurgitation can be well tolerated by the right ventricle for many years, but usually in the third or fourth decades, the right ventricle begins to dilate, and it may become dysfunctional. Significant RV dilation and dysfunction can lead to LV dysfunction, significant tricuspid regurgitation, and atrial or ventricular arrhythmias. Almost 29% of adults with repaired TOF also have a dilated ascending aorta due to increased blood flow through the aorta before repair.

Clinical Presentation

Patients with repaired TOF typically have normal oxygen saturation levels. On palpation, there often is an RV lift at the left lower sternal border. On auscultation, there typically is a widely split second heart sound with a to-and-fro murmur in the pulmonary area due to significant pulmonary regurgitation or, less commonly, aortic regurgitation. A holosystolic murmur due to tricuspid regurgitation may be heard at the left lower sternal border. Symptoms in the adult with repaired TOF may include exertional dyspnea, palpitations, syncope, and sudden cardiac death.

Diagnosis

The ECG almost universally reveals a right bundle branch block pattern in patients who underwent repair of TOF. The QRS duration from the standard surface ECG correlates with the degree of RV dilation and dysfunction. A maximum QRS duration of 180 milliseconds or more is a highly sensitive and relatively specific marker for sustained ventricular tachycardia and sudden cardiac death. Patients with significant pulmonary regurgitation often have cardiomegaly with dilated central pulmonary arteries identified on the chest radiograph. A right aortic arch occurs in 25% of cases, and it can be detected by close observation of the chest radiograph. An echocardiogram is useful for evaluating the RV outflow tract (e.g., pulmonary regurgitation, residual stenosis), biventricular size and function, tricuspid valve function, and ascending aortic size. MRI is the gold standard for assessing RV size and function (Fig. 6-2). It can also give an accurate assessment of the degree of pulmonary insufficiency and branch pulmonary artery anatomy.

Treatment

Treatment for TOF is surgical repair. Repair is typically performed between 3 to 12 months of age and consists of patch closure of the VSD and relief of the pulmonary outflow tract obstruction by patch augmentation of the RV outflow tract or

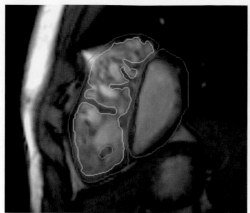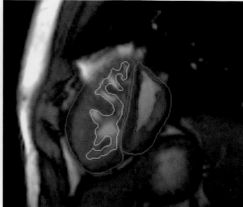

FIGURE 6-2 Short axis magnetic resonance images of the right and left ventricles with epicardial and endocardial tracings of both ventricular cavities. There are a predefined number of slices through the heart with a constant thickness. The volumes of the left and right ventricles in each slice are calculated and summed together in end diastole and end systole to determine the total right and left ventricular volumes (i.e., Simpon's method).

pulmonary valve annulus, or both. Reintervention is necessary in approximately 10% of adults with repaired TOF after 20 years of follow-up. With longer follow-up, the incidence of reintervention continues to increase. The most common indication for reintervention is pulmonary valve replacement for severe pulmonary valve regurgitation.

Prognosis

In the developed world, the unoperated adult with TOF has become a rarity because most patients undergo palliation (i.e., stenting) or repair in childhood. Survival of the unoperated patient to the seventh decade has been described but is rare. Only 11% of unrepaired patients are alive at 20 years of age and only 3% at 40 years.

Late survival after repair of TOF is excellent. Survival rates at 32 and 35 years are 86% and 85%, respectively, compared with 95% for age- and sex-matched controls. Importantly, most patients live an unrestricted life. However, many patients over time develop late symptoms related to numerous, long-term complications after TOF repair. Late complications include endocarditis, aortic regurgitation with or without aortic root dilation (typically due to damage of the aortic valve during VSD closure or to an intrinsic aortic root abnormality), LV dysfunction (from inadequate myocardial protection during previous repair or chronic LV volume overload due to long-standing palliative arterial shunts), residual pulmonary obstruction, residual pulmonary valve regurgitation, RV dysfunction (due to pulmonary regurgitation or pulmonary stenosis), atrial arrhythmias (typically atrial flutter), ventricular arrhythmias, and heart block.

Transposition of the Great Arteries
Definition and Epidemiology

Transposition of the great arteries (TGA) represents 3.8% of all congenital heart disease. In complete TGA, the aorta arises from the right ventricle and the pulmonary artery from the left ventricle. As a result, the systemic venous flow (i.e., blood with low oxygen content) is returned to the right ventricle and is then pumped to the body through the aorta without passing through the lungs for gas exchange. The pulmonary venous flow (i.e., oxygenated blood) returning to the left ventricle is then pumped back to the lungs. As a result, the systemic and pulmonary circulations run in parallel. Oxygenation and survival depend on mixing between the systemic and pulmonary circulations at the atrial, ventricular, or PDA level. In 50% of cases, there are other anomalies: VSD (30%), pulmonary stenosis (5% to 10%), aortic stenosis, and coarctation of the aorta (≤5%).

The first definitive operations for TGA (i.e., atrial switch procedures) were described by Senning in 1959 and Mustard in 1964. In these procedures, the systemic and pulmonary venous returns are rerouted in the atrium by constructing baffles. The systemic venous return from the superior and inferior vena cavae is directed through the mitral valve and into the left ventricle, which is connected to the pulmonary artery. The pulmonary venous return is then directed through the tricuspid valve into the right ventricle, which is connected to the aorta. These procedures leave the left ventricle as the pulmonary ventricle and the right ventricle as the systemic ventricle.

Over the past 10 to 20 years, the arterial switch procedure has gained popularity. During the procedure, the great arteries are transected and reanastomosed to the correct ventricle (i.e., left ventricle to the aorta and right ventricle to the pulmonary artery) along with coronary artery transfer. Operative survival after the arterial switch procedure is very good, with a surgical mortality rate of 2% to 5%.

Pathology

Most infants who do not have surgical intervention die in the first few months of life. For adults born with complete TGA who have had an atrial switch procedure, the right ventricle continues to be the systemic ventricle, and the left ventricle is the subpulmonic ventricle. Long-term follow-up series have demonstrated that the right ventricle can function as the systemic ventricle for 30 to 40 years, but with longer follow-up, systemic ventricular dysfunction continues to increase. At the 35-year follow-up, approximately 61% of patients have developed moderate or severe RV dysfunction.

Another common postoperative problem is the tricuspid valve. After the atrial switch procedure, the tricuspid valve remains the systemic atrioventricular valve and must tolerate systemic pressures. Due to changes in RV morphology and abnormal chordal attachments, the tricuspid valve is prone to become dysfunctional and develop significant regurgitation.

Significant coronary lesions, such as occlusions or stenoses, occur in 6.8% of patients who have had the arterial switch procedure. These lesions are likely related to suture lines or kinking at the time of reimplantation of the coronary arteries into the neo-aorta. Systemic LV function is usually normal. LV dysfunction is associated with coronary anomalies.

Clinical Presentation

In the repaired adult with an atrial switch procedure, the physical examination may reveal a murmur consistent with tricuspid valve insufficiency and a prominent second heart sound due to the anterior position of the aorta. Patients who have had an atrial switch procedure tend to have worsening functional status as the length of follow-up increases. They often have resting sinus bradycardia or a junctional rhythm. Palpitations due to atrial arrhythmias are common, occurring in up to 48% of patients 23 years after the atrial switch procedure.

In those who undergo the arterial switch procedure, the physical examination may reveal a murmur of neo-aortic or neo-pulmonic regurgitation. These patients usually have normal function status, but because of denervation of the heart, myocardial ischemia may manifest as atypical chest discomfort.

Diagnosis

After the atrial switch procedure, the ECG may show a loss of sinus rhythm with evidence of RV hypertrophy. Chest radiographs may show an enlarged cardiac silhouette in those with a dilated systemic right ventricle. An echocardiogram can demonstrate qualitative systemic RV size and function and the degree of tricuspid regurgitation. MRI is often used to accurately quantify systemic RV size and function, tricuspid valve function, and atrial baffle anatomy.

Echocardiography is used to assess pulmonary artery and branch pulmonary artery stenosis, neo-aortic and neo-pulmonic valve regurgitation, and ventricular function. MRI or computed tomography may be used to assess the anatomy of the branch pulmonary arteries. An exercise stress test is often used to evaluate myocardial ischemia.

Treatment

Treatment options are limited for adults with complete TGA repaired by atrial switch who have failing systemic right ventricles or significant tricuspid regurgitation, and evidence of significant benefit is lacking. However, potential treatments include medical therapy, revision of atrial baffles, pulmonary artery banding, resynchronization therapy, ventricular assist devices, and possible transplantation.

After the arterial switch procedure, catheter-based or surgical reintervention for pulmonary artery stenosis may be required in 5% to 25% of patients, Coronary artery revascularization is rarely required (0.46% of patients), as is neo-aortic valve repair or replacement (1.1% of patients).

Prognosis

Long-term follow-up studies after the atrial switch procedure show a small but ongoing attrition rate, with numerous intermediate- and long-term complications. Long-term complications include systemic RV dysfunction and tricuspid valve regurgitation, loss of sinus rhythm with the development of atrial arrhythmias (50% incidence by age 25), endocarditis, baffle leaks, baffle obstruction, and sinus node dysfunction requiring pacemaker placement. Intermediate-term complications include coronary artery compromise, pulmonary outflow tract obstruction (at the supravalvular level or takeoff of the peripheral pulmonary arteries), neo-aortic valve regurgitation, endocarditis, and neo-aorta dilation.

As a result of the long-term complications associated with the atrial switch procedure, the arterial switch operation has been the procedure of choice since 1985. Long-term data on the survival after the arterial switch operation do not exist, but intermediate-term results are promising: 88% at 10 and 15 years.

For a deeper discussion on this topic, please see Chapter 69, "Congenital Heart Disease in Adults," in Goldman-Cecil Medicine, *25th Edition.*

SUGGESTED READINGS

Campbell M: Natural history of atrial septal defect, Br Heart J 32:820–826, 1970.

Cohen M, Fuster V, Steele PM, et al: Coarctation of the aorta. Long-term follow-up and prediction of outcome after surgical correction, Circulation 80:840–845, 1989.

Cohen SB, Ginde S, Bartz PJ, et al: Extracardiac complications in adults with congenital heart disease, Congenit Heart Dis 8:370–380, 2013.

Co-Vu JG, Ginde S, Bartz PJ, et al: Long-term outcomes of the neoaorta after arterial switch operation for transposition of the great arteries, Ann Thorac Surg 95:1654–1659, 2013.

Cramer JW, Ginde S, Bartz PJ, et al: Aortic aneurysms remain a significant source of morbidity and mortality after use of Dacron patch aortoplasty to repair coarctation of the aorta: results from a single center, Pediatr Cardiol 34:296–301, 2013.

Earing MG, Connolly HM, Dearani JA, et al: Long-term follow-up of patients after surgical treatment for isolated pulmonary valve stenosis, Mayo Clin Proc 80:871–876, 2005.

Earing MG, Webb GD: Congenital heart disease and pregnancy: maternal and fetal risks, Clin Perinatol 32:913–919, 2005.

Gatzoulis MA, Freeman MA, Siu SC, et al: Atrial arrhythmia after surgical closure of atrial septal defects in adults, N Engl J Med 340:839–846, 1999.

Gunther T, Mazzitelli D, Haehnel CJ, et al: Long-term results after repair of complete atrioventricular septal defects: analysis of risk factors, Ann Thorac Surg 65:754–759, discussion 759–760, 1998.

Hickey EJ, Gruschen V, Bradely TJ, et al: Late risk of outcomes for adults with repaired tetralogy of Fallot from an inception cohort spanning four decades, Eur J Cardiothorac Surg 35:156–164, 2009.

Losai J, Touchot A, Serraf A, et al: Late outcome after arterial switch operation for transposition of the great arteries, Circulation 104(Suppl 1):I1121–I1126, 2001.

Perloff JK, Warnes CA: Challenges posed by adults with repaired congenital heart disease, Circulation 103:2637–2643, 2001.

Soto B, Becker AE, Moulaert AJ, et al: Classification of ventricular septal defects, Br Heart J 43:332–343, 1980.

Warnes CA: Transposition of the great arteries, Circulation 114:2699–2709, 2006.

Warnes CA, Williams RG, Bashore TM, et al: ACC/AHA 2008 guidelines for the management of adults with congenital heart disease: a report of the American College of Cardiology/American Heart Association Task Force on Practice Guidelines (writing committee to develop guidelines on the management of adults with congenital heart disease), Circulation 118:e714–e833, 2008.

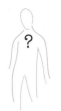

Valvular Heart Disease

Timothy D. Woods

● INTRODUCTION

Although rheumatic fever remains a major cause of valvular heart disease in undeveloped countries, degenerative disease is the most common etiology in industrialized countries. As expected, the prevalence increases with age, to as high as 13.2% in those 75 years of age and older. The aortic and mitral valves are by far the most commonly affected valves.

There have been few randomized studies in valvular heart disease to guide management, and most of the joint guideline recommendations from the American College of Cardiology (ACC) and American Heart Association (AHA) are based on single-center studies or expert consensus (level C evidence).

● AORTIC STENOSIS

Definition

When three normal aortic valve leaflets open fully in systole, they permit the left ventricular (LV) stroke volume to pass through the valve with little resistance to ejection. In aortic stenosis, leaflet excursion becomes progressively restricted over time. In advanced disease, the high resistance to ejection in systole invokes a cascade of physiologic sequelae that lead to the symptoms and physical examination findings of severe aortic stenosis.

Pathology

Aortic leaflet motion can become restricted for a variety of reasons. In westernized societies, the most common cause is senile degeneration. This term is a misnomer, in that this is not a degenerative disease but an active process involving the leaflet tissue that shares many characteristics with atherosclerosis. As plaques progress over time, calcified deposits accumulate on leaflets and increasingly restrict their motion.

A less common but important cause of aortic stenosis is congenitally abnormal leaflets. A two-leaflet, or bicuspid, aortic valve occurs in approximately 2% of the general population. Many patients with this condition develop premature thickening, fusion of the commissures, and calcification, resulting in abnormal flow characteristics and aortic stenosis at a relatively young age. Bicuspid aortic valves also put patients at increased risk for aortic enlargement and dissection and are associated with coarctation of the aorta.

Rheumatic fever is an uncommon cause of aortic stenosis in developed countries but is still seen in economically depressed regions. Rheumatic aortic stenosis is almost always associated with concomitant involvement of the mitral valve. See Table 7-1 for differential diagnosis of the valve lesions most commonly encountered clinically.

Clinical Presentation

Patients typically remain asymptomatic from aortic stenosis until the lesion reaches the severe range. Even after that point, most patients still experience an asymptomatic period of variable length. The onset of symptoms heralds an increase in mortality risk, as first described in 1968 by Ross and Braunwald, and guides management of this disorder. In order of increasing severity and decreasing survival, these symptoms are angina, syncope, and congestive heart failure (Fig. 7-1). Evaluation of patients with severe aortic stenosis must include careful screening for the development of these symptoms, and their detection can be especially challenging in sedentary individuals.

Diagnosis

The physical examination can be both sensitive and specific for the detection of aortic valve stenosis. The findings in severe stenosis either result from the outflow obstruction itself or are based on the direct physiologic sequelae of the obstruction.

The resistance to flow causes a pressure overload state of the left ventricle, resulting in concentric LV hypertrophy. This is

TABLE 7-1	MAJOR CAUSES OF VALVULAR HEART DISEASE IN ADULTS	
AORTIC STENOSIS	**MITRAL REGURGITATION**
Bicuspid aortic valve	**Chronic**
Rheumatic fever	Mitral valve prolapse
Degenerative stenosis	Left ventricular dilation
AORTIC REGURGITATION	Posterior wall myocardial infarction
	Rheumatic fever
Bicuspid aortic valve	Endocarditis
Aortic dissection	**Acute**
Endocarditis	Posterior wall or papillary muscle ischemia
Rheumatic fever	Papillary muscle or chordal rupture
Aortic root dilation	Endocarditis
MITRAL STENOSIS	Prosthetic valve dysfunction
	Systolic anterior motion of mitral valve
Rheumatic fever	
	TRICUSPID REGURGITATION
	Functional (annular) dilation
	Tricuspid valve prolapse
	Endocarditis
	Carcinoid heart disease

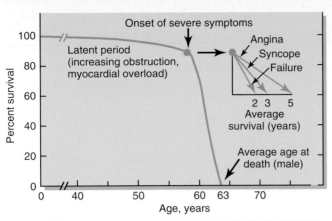

FIGURE 7-1 Natural history of severe aortic stenosis without surgery once symptoms develop. (From Ross J Jr, Braunwald E: Aortic stenosis, Circulation 38:61, 1968)

identified as increased voltages on the electrocardiogram (ECG) and a sustained but nondisplaced point of maximal impulse on palpation. The resistance to blood flow in systole results in the classic harsh crescendo-decrescendo systolic murmur. Although it is typically heard best in the aortic position, the murmur may radiate to the apical region (known as Gallivardin's phenomenon). Because the stiff, calcified, and restricted aortic valve leaflets make little excursion in systole, their closing no longer produces a sound; this results in an inaudible aortic component of S_2. The ventricle cannot quickly eject blood through the small aortic orifice, and the carotid pulses may have a resulting low amplitude (described in Latin as *pulsus parvus*) and delay in reaching their peak (*et tardus*). See Table 7-2 for a summary of physical examination, ECG, and chest radiography findings for chronic valvular heart lesions.

Transthoracic echocardiography (TTE) has become the "gold standard" for confirming the presence of severe aortic valve stenosis. It offers the ability to visualize the valve as well as the use of Doppler imaging to estimate the peak instantaneous and mean valve gradients. Importantly, an estimated valve area can be derived for a more reliable measure of stenosis severity. Criteria for differentiating mild, moderate, and severe stenosis have been published (Table 7-3). In most cases, echocardiography is sufficiently accurate for clinical decision making regarding the valve, but patients may still require invasive coronary or computed tomographic (CT) angiography to exclude obstructive coronary disease before valve replacement. If doubt remains regarding stenosis severity, hemodynamic measurements at the time of cardiac catheterization can confirm the degree of stenosis.

Treatment

For decades, surgical replacement of the aortic valve was the only treatment proven to prolong life in symptomatic severe aortic valve stenosis. Aortic valve replacement (AVR) is a class I indication (level B evidence) for symptomatic patients with severe aortic stenosis. AVR is also a class I indication in patients with asymptomatic aortic stenosis who have LV systolic dysfunction that is believed to be the result of the stenosis (level C evidence). AVR can restore survival rates in these patients almost to normal.

For patients who are deemed to be at acceptable surgical risk, there are two prosthetic options that may be considered for AVR. Mechanical prosthetic valves (see example in Fig. 7-2) have the advantage of excellent flow characteristics; they typically last for the patient's lifetime but require anticoagulation. Bioprosthetic valves (Fig. 7-3), which are made from either porcine or bovine material, have the advantage of not requiring long-term anticoagulation. Because the leaflets are made of biologic tissue, the lifespan and durability of bioprosthetic valves are finite, and valve re-replacement is invariably required 10 to 20 years after implantation.

In those for whom open surgical replacement of their aortic valve would pose an inappropriately high risk, a third option became available in the United States in November of 2012 when the U.S. Food and Drug Administration (FDA) approved the use of a percutaneously placed bioprosthetic valve (Fig. 7-4). In appropriately selected patients, this valve may be delivered via a catheter through the femoral artery to the aortic valve, and then expanded into position by a balloon, effectively squeezing the native valve against the aortic wall. It can also be placed through a small apical incision in the chest wall, entering the heart through the LV apex. Complications may include regurgitation around the prosthesis, stroke, and damage to the peripheral vessels during catheter insertion. Currently, these techniques are approved in the United States only for patients with symptomatic severe stenosis who have been declared ineligible for open surgical valve replacement due to excessive risk.

Prognosis

The mortality risk of asymptomatic severe aortic valve stenosis appears to be very low based on available studies, probably less than 1% per year. However, in sedentary individuals, absence of symptoms can be deceiving. On occasion, it is reasonable to perform carefully monitored exercise stress testing in patients professing to be asymptomatic. Once symptoms have appeared, the survival rate with severe stenosis, as demonstrated by Ross and Braunwald, is abysmal, with about half of those patients who develop heart failure dying within 2 years after symptom onset.

● AORTIC REGURGITATION

Definition

When aortic valve leaflets fail to adequately coapt in diastole, blood regurgitates into the left ventricle. As with other compensatory mechanisms of the body, the left ventricle can tolerate large volumes if the progression to severe regurgitation occurs slowly enough. When severe regurgitation develops rapidly, hemodynamic collapse and death can occur. Therefore, the causes, clinical presentation, and management of acute versus chronic severe aortic regurgitation should be considered separately.

Pathology

Aortic regurgitation may occur as a result of leaflet abnormalities, aortic root disease, or a combination of these factors. Infectious endocarditis and aortic dissection are the two most

TABLE 7-2 CHARACTERISTIC PHYSICAL, ELECTROCARDIOGRAPHIC, AND CHEST RADIOGRAPHIC FINDINGS IN CHRONIC ACQUIRED VALVULAR HEART DISEASE

CAUSE	PHYSICAL FINDINGS*	ELECTROCARDIOGRAM	RADIOGRAPH
Aortic stenosis	Pulsus parvus et tardus (may be absent in older patients or in patients with associated aortic regurgitation); carotid *shudder* (coarse thrill) Ejection murmur radiates to base of neck; peaks late in systole if stenosis is severe Sustained but not significantly displaced LV impulse A_2 decreased, S_2 single or paradoxically split S_4 gallop, often palpable	LV hypertrophy Left bundle branch block is also common Rare heart block from calcific involvement of conduction system	LV prominence without dilation Post-stenotic aortic root dilation Aortic valve calcification
Aortic regurgitation	Increased pulse pressure Bifid carotid pulses Rapid pulse upstroke and collapse LV impulse hyperdynamic and displaced laterally Diastolic decrescendo murmur; duration related to severity Systolic flow murmur S_{3G} common	LV hypertrophy, often with narrow deep Q waves	LV and aortic dilation
Mitral stenosis	Loud S_1 OS S_2-OS interval inversely related to stenosis severity S_1 not loud and OS absent if valve heavily calcified Signs of pulmonary arterial hypertension	LA abnormality Atrial fibrillation common RV hypertrophy pattern may develop if associated pulmonary arterial hypertension is present	Large LA: double-density sign, posterior displacement of esophagus, elevation of left mainstem bronchus Straightening of left heart border as a result of enlarged left appendage Small or normal-sized LV Large pulmonary artery Pulmonary venous congestion
Mitral regurgitation	Hyperdynamic LV impulse S_3 Widely split S_2 may occur Holosystolic apical murmur radiating to axilla (murmur may be atypical with acute mitral regurgitation, papillary muscle dysfunction, or mitral valve prolapse)	LA abnormality LV hypertrophy Atrial fibrillation	Enlarged LA and LV Pulmonary venous congestion
Mitral valve prolapse	One or more systolic clicks, often midsystolic, followed by late systolic murmur Auscultatory findings dynamic Symptoms may include tall thin habitus, pectus excavatum, straight back syndrome	Often normal Occasionally ST-segment depression or T wave changes or both in inferior leads	Depends on degree of valve regurgitation and presence or absence of those abnormalities
Tricuspid stenosis	Jugular venous distention with prominent *a* wave if sinus rhythm Tricuspid OS and diastolic rumble at left sternal border; may be overshadowed by concomitant mitral stenosis Tricuspid OS and rumble increased during inspiration	Right atrial abnormality Atrial fibrillation common	Large RA
Tricuspid regurgitation	Jugular venous distention with large regurgitant (systolic) wave Systolic murmur at left sternal border, increased with inspiration Diastolic flow rumble RV S_3 increased with inspiration Hepatomegaly with systolic pulsation	RA abnormality; findings are often related to the cause of the tricuspid regurgitation	RA and RV enlarged; findings are often related to the cause of the tricuspid regurgitation

LA, Left atrium; LV, left ventricle; OS, opening snap; RA, right atrium; RV, right ventricle; S_{3G}, S_3 gallop.
*Findings are influenced by the severity and chronicity of the valve disorder.

common causes of acute severe aortic valve regurgitation. Congenitally abnormal (most commonly bicuspid) aortic valve leaflets often lead to chronic severe aortic regurgitation (see Table 7-1).

Clinical Presentation

Acute Severe Regurgitation

Patients may have symptoms related to their underlying pathology, such as fever and malaise from endocarditis or severe chest pain due to aortic dissection. In addition, they are likely to suffer progressive signs and symptoms of cardiogenic shock, including tachycardia and hypotension caused by severely impaired cardiac

output and fulminant pulmonary edema due to markedly elevated filling pressures. In general, the more rapidly the severity of regurgitation evolves, the less well it is hemodynamically tolerated.

Chronic Severe Aortic Regurgitation

When severe regurgitation develops slowly over months to years, compensatory mechanisms such as LV remodeling lead to chamber dilatation and increased compliance, permitting even large regurgitant volumes to be well tolerated. At onset, the symptoms are typically exertional, including dyspnea and fatigue. Orthopnea and occasionally chest pain can develop in the absence of epicardial coronary disease.

TABLE 7-3	MEASURES OF AORTIC STENOSIS SEVERITY			
INDICATOR	**NORMAL**	**MILD**	**MODERATE**	**SEVERE**
Aortic valve area (cm^2)	>2.0	1.5-2.0	1.0-1.5	<1.0
Mean gradient (mm Hg)		<25	25-40	>40
Peak jet velocity (m/sec)	<2.0	2-3	3-4	>4

Data from Baumgartner H, Hung J, Bermego J, et al: Echocardiographic assessment of valve stenosis: EAE/ASE recommendations for clinical practice, J Am Soc Echocardiogr 22:1–22, 2009.

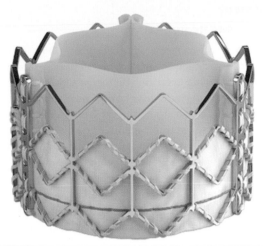

FIGURE 7-4   Edwards SAPIEN transcatheter heart valve. (Courtesy of Edwards Lifesciences LLC, Irvine, Calif.)

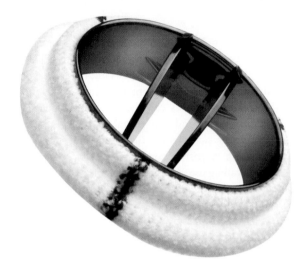

FIGURE 7-2   Medtronic bileaflet mechanical prosthetic valve. (Courtesy of Medtronic, Inc.)

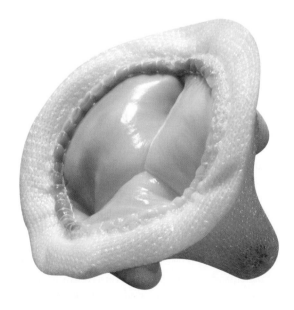

FIGURE 7-3   Medtronic Hancock II bioprosthetic valve. (Courtesy of Medtronic, Inc.)

Diagnosis

Acute Severe Regurgitation

The sudden development of severe regurgitation is poorly tolerated by the normal left ventricle. Left heart filling pressures rise rapidly, and respiratory failure from pulmonary edema develops.

The decreased effective cardiac output results in a resting tachycardia and hypotension. The patient's tachypnea and rapid heart rate impede recognition of the typical diastolic decrescendo murmur because of marked shortening of diastole and early termination of the murmur. The diagnosis can be easily missed, particularly with hasty and errant performance of a cursory examination of an unstable patient in a noisy emergency room. A chest radiograph showing a normal-size heart with pulmonary edema should raise suspicions. Timely TTE or transesophageal echocardiography (TEE) is key to establishing the diagnosis early in the disease course.

Chronic Severe Regurgitation

When time permits compensatory mechanisms such as LV dilation to gradually evolve, even a very large regurgitant volume can be tolerated well for many years. The resulting large stroke volume, along with the regurgitation, is responsible for many of the findings on physical examination.

The enlarged heart caused by ventricular volume overload results in a laterally displaced and diffuse point of maximal impulse (PMI), as well as cardiomegaly by chest radiography. A low diastolic blood pressure is present and results in a large pulse pressure. The increased diastolic filling results in a soft S$_1$ heart sound, and an S$_3$ gallop may be present even in the absence of clinical heart failure. Auscultation of the typical diastolic decrescendo murmur, heard at either the left or the right sternal border, can be improved by examining the patient as he or she is leaning forward at end-expiration. A diastolic flow rumble at the left sternal border may be confused with mitral stenosis; this is known as an Austin-Flint murmur. A soft systolic murmur may be present because of the large stroke volume ejected in systole (see Table 7-2). The large stroke volume also results in a number of peripheral physical examination findings such as Quincke's pulse (systolic plethora and diastolic nail bed blanching with pressure), Musset's sign (head bobbing) and Corrigan's pulse (a bounding full carotid pulse with rapid downstroke). These findings, including the increased pulse pressure, are present only after compensatory cardiac changes have evolved and are not present with acute severe regurgitation.

Treatment

Acute Severe Regurgitation

The mainstay of management in the patient with cardiogenic shock consists of attempts at medical stabilization through afterload reduction while preparing for urgent surgery. Death due to pulmonary edema, ventricular arrhythmias, or hemodynamic collapse is well described, and surgery is the established standard of care for these severely ill patients.

Drugs such as intravenous nitroprusside can be useful to rapidly achieve afterload reduction and improve cardiac output while the patient is prepared for urgent surgery. Diuretics may be used simultaneously to improve pulmonary edema. β-Blockers, although useful with aortic dissection, can cause further hemodynamic deterioration when acute severe regurgitation accompanies the dissection.

Chronic Severe Regurgitation

Patients may tolerate this lesion well due to compensatory mechanisms, remaining asymptomatic for many years. Although one study suggested that antihypertensive therapy with a dihydropyridine calcium blocker delays the need for surgery, a more recent study called into question the efficacy of either calcium blocker or angiotensin-converting enzyme (ACE) inhibitor therapy. These antihypertensives are considered a class IIb indication (level B evidence) for use in cases of asymptomatic severe aortic regurgitation with LV enlargement and normal systolic function. No studies of level A evidence have been completed to evaluate indications for AVR. Level B and C evidence indicates that AVR should be recommended based on the development of symptoms or asymptomatic structural changes in the heart. Specifically, a decrease in LV ejection fraction to 50% or less, even in an asymptomatic patient, is considered a class I indication for surgery. Similarly, marked diastolic (>75 mm) or systolic (>55 mm) LV enlargement, despite an absence of symptoms, is a class IIa indication for AVR. Finally, AVR has a class I indication in symptomatic patients, regardless of the status of their LV systolic function.

Options for prosthetic valve selection are similar to those for aortic stenosis, with the exception that a percutaneous method of valve replacement has not been approved by the FDA for this indication.

Prognosis

Acute Severe Regurgitation

Any cardiac surgery that has to be performed urgently entails greater surgical risk. When the cause of aortic regurgitation is infectious endocarditis, the long-term mortality rate, even with surgery, can be as high as 50%.

Chronic Severe Regurgitation

Close monitoring of patients for the evolution of surgical indications, as described earlier, leads to an excellent prognosis with acceptably low surgical mortality rates and survival curves that approach those of an otherwise normal population.

⬤ MITRAL STENOSIS

Definition

When the mitral leaflets open in diastole, they permit the entire stroke volume to pass from the atria to the left ventricle at relatively low pressure gradients. If mitral leaflet motion becomes restricted in opening, resistance to flow develops. The resulting severity of stenosis can be described by the pressure gradient that develops between the left atrium and left ventricle during diastole or by the size of the mitral valve opening.

Pathology

Both leaflet- and non–leaflet-related causes of stenosis can occur. Although restricted mitral leaflet motion due to rheumatic heart disease is by far the most common cause, immune disease affecting the valve and congenital abnormalities can also result in stenosis. Mitral inflow stenosis can also occasionally occur from severe calcification around the mitral annulus. A left atrial myxoma may lodge persistently or intermittently in the mitral annulus, resulting in obstruction to ventricular inflow. Finally, mitral stenosis can be the inadvertent outcome of surgical mitral valve repair or replacement.

Regardless of the etiology, the symptoms of mitral stenosis develop as left atrial pressure increases in response to forward flow limitation. As this increased pressure is reflected back to the lungs, pulmonary congestion evolves and, if severe enough, ultimately leads to pulmonary edema. The resulting pulmonary hypertension eventually results in right ventricular (RV) failure.

The mean gradient between the left atrium and left ventricle, measured at the valve orifice during diastole, is the most common way of describing the stenosis severity. The normal mitral valve area is 4 to 5 cm^2, and a normal gradient is less than 2 mm Hg. Although symptoms typically do not develop until the valve area is reduced to less than 2.5 cm^2, both cardiac output and heart rate can significantly affect the onset of symptoms for any particular degree of stenosis. Increased cardiac output, with a resulting increase in gradient, can lead to symptoms in a previously asymptomatic patient without change in mitral valve area (Fig. 7-5). Pregnancy is an example of a physiologic state of increased cardiac output that may produce symptoms in someone who was previously asymptomatic without any change in valve area. Shortening of the diastolic filling period after onset of a tachyarrhythmia is another reason that symptoms may suddenly develop without any anatomic change in valve size.

Rheumatic Valve Disease

In some patients who develop group A streptococcal pharyngitis, an abnormal immune response results in rheumatic fever, which can occur anywhere from 10 days to 3 weeks after the initial infection if left untreated. It typically occurs in children 6 to 15 years of age, with clinical manifestations leading to a diagnosis as summarized in the revised Jones Criteria (Table 7-4). The diagnosis is made based on the presence of two major or one major and two minor Jones criteria occurring after a recent documented group A streptococcal infection.

The pancarditis that occurs affects the pericardium and the myocardium as well as the valve tissue. The inflammation eventually leads to chordal thickening, shortening, and together with

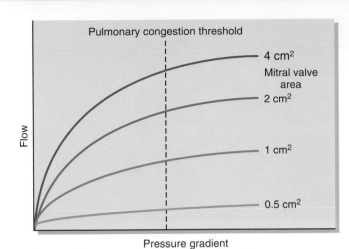

FIGURE 7-5 Graphic illustration of the relationship between the diastolic gradient across the mitral valve and the flow through the mitral valve. As the mitral valve becomes more stenotic, the pressure gradient across the valve must increase to maintain flow into the left ventricle. If the mitral opening is 1 cm² or smaller, the flow rate into the left ventricle cannot be significantly increased, despite a significantly elevated pressure gradient across the mitral valve. (Modified from Wallace AG: Pathophysiology of cardiovascular disease. In Smith LH Jr, Thier SO, editors: The international textbook of medicine (vol 1), Philadelphia, 1981, Saunders, p. 1192.)

TABLE 7-4 REVISED JONES CRITERIA FOR DIAGNOSIS OF RHEUMATIC FEVER*	
MAJOR CRITERIA	**MINOR CRITERIA**
Carditis (pleuritic chest pain, friction rub, heart failure)	Fever
Polyarthritis	Arthralgia
Chorea	Previous rheumatic fever or known rheumatic heart disease
Erythema marginatum	
Subcutaneous nodules	

*Rheumatic fever is diagnosed based on the presence of two major criteria or one major and two minor criteria after a recent documented group A streptococcal infection.

leaflet commissural fusion, a funnel-shaped, flow-limiting orifice forms. Although the aortic valve can be affected as well, it is almost never involved without concomitant mitral valve involvement. In less developed countries, the incidence is much higher than in westernized societies, and the time from acute rheumatic fever to symptomatic stenosis is often years instead of decades.

Clinical Presentation

Patients typically remain asymptomatic until the valve area is reduced to approximately 1.5 cm² or less. Initial symptoms are usually exertional in nature, with noticeable dyspnea or fatigue that resolves with rest. As the stenosis progresses, symptoms develop earlier with exercise, until ultimately they are markedly limiting. If the cause remains undetected, the markedly elevated left atrial and pulmonary pressures will lead to significant left atrial enlargement. Even in the absence of atrial fibrillation, there is increased risk of thromboembolism. When atrial fibrillation occurs, it carries an approximate 18-fold increased risk of cerebrovascular accident. Secondary changes in the pulmonary vasculature may occur over time, rarely resulting in fixed pulmonary hypertension that is not relieved by valve surgery performed at this late stage. Finally, the right ventricle responds adversely to the chronic severe pulmonary hypertension, and clinical right-sided heart failure ensues.

Diagnosis

Only about 60% of patients with rheumatic heart disease recall having rheumatic fever as a child, and the history cannot be relied on to suspect the diagnosis. Elicitation of the symptoms, followed by confirming physical examination findings, is the cornerstone of diagnosis.

Early in the disease course, there is typically a prominent S_1 sound. As motion of the leaflets becomes increasingly restricted, S_1 may become soft. The opening in diastole begins with a snap and is followed by a low-pitched diastolic rumble, heard best with the bell of a stethoscope at the apex in the left lateral decubitus position. The length of time from S_2 to the mitral opening snap can help in estimating stenosis severity, with shorter intervals indicating proportionally increased severity.

The ECG may show left atrial enlargement and, ultimately, right atrial enlargement; right axis deviation and right bundle branch block are possible in later stages. Left atrial enlargement and dilation of the main pulmonary artery are often identified by chest radiography. In advanced cases, RV enlargement may be evident (see Table 7-2).

Confirmation is typically by echocardiography, and the valve can be evaluated by several methods. The restricted motion of the mitral leaflets in diastole is highly characteristic of rheumatic disease. The valve leaflets appear to dome or form the shape of a hockey stick. The motion of the valve leaflets forms an overall funnel-shaped mitral orifice (Fig. 7-6). Finally, a Doppler examination can be used to estimate the mitral valve area and to measure the mean diastolic gradient across the valve. If doubt remains regarding mitral stenosis severity despite these techniques, invasive pressure measurements taken directly from the left ventricle and atrium will permit calculation of a valve area and mean mitral gradient.

Treatment

In general, symptoms guide the treatment of mitral stenosis. It is believed that asymptomatic cases do not require treatment unless significant pulmonary hypertension has developed (class I indication, level C evidence) or new-onset atrial fibrillation has occurred (class IIb, level C).

In most patients, exertional symptoms drive the need for therapy. As with all other valve lesions, a mechanical (percutaneous or surgical) intervention is required to alter the natural history. In the case of mitral stenosis, an invasive procedure that can be performed in a catheterization laboratory, known as percutaneous balloon mitral valvuloplasty (PBMV), has gained favor over the past 2 decades. A balloon is delivered through the femoral vein across the mitral orifice and inflated (Fig. 7-7); this procedure is repeated with successively larger balloons until the valve area is significantly improved. PBMV has a class I indication for symptomatic patients with moderate or severe mitral stenosis, providing their leaflet morphology is acceptable for this technique.

If the patient is deemed a poor candidate for PBMV, surgical commissurotomy or valve replacement is considered to be a class IIa indication in the symptomatic patient. Because mitral stenosis

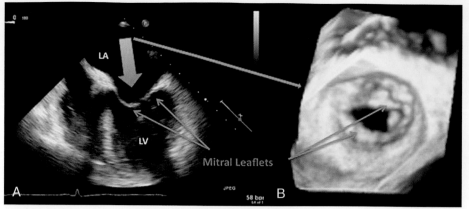

FIGURE 7-6 Abnormal motion of the mitral valve in rheumatic mitral stenosis. **A**, Transesophageal echocardiographic (TEE) image demonstrates the abnormal doming motion of the mitral leaflets in diastole. The *blue arrow* denotes the orientation of image **B. B,** Three-dimensional TEE image demonstrates the appearance of the mitral opening if viewed looking down at the valve from inside the left atrium (LA), a surgeon's orientation to the valve. The area of the mitral opening between anterior and posterior leaflets is well visualized, and the area measured from this view is used to estimate stenosis severity. LV, Left ventricle.

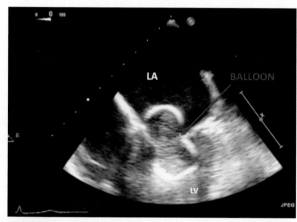

FIGURE 7-7 Balloon inflation during percutaneous balloon mitral valvuloplasty for treatment of mitral stenosis. Orientation is the same as in Figure 7-6A, and the inflated balloon is visible between the leaflets. LA, Left atrium; LV, left ventricle.

is primarily an anatomic problem, there is a limited role for medical therapy in improving survival. However, diuretics and heart rate slowing can be very helpful in controlling symptoms while a definitive mechanical solution to the problem is sought. Anticoagulation is key to prevent thromboembolism in any patient with a previous event or with onset of atrial fibrillation.

Prognosis

Although survival in asymptomatic patients is good, onset of symptoms heralds a rise in risk. Given the physiology of the disease, these risks understandably include heart failure, thromboembolism, and death. One study suggested a 5-year survival rate of only 44% in symptomatic patients who declined treatment.

⬤ MITRAL REGURGITATION
Definition

Mitral leaflet coaptation in systole should produce a tight seal to prevent regurgitation. This mechanism can fail for a variety of reasons, resulting in a problem for the left ventricle similar to that caused by aortic regurgitation—both being states of volume overload. Severe mitral regurgitation is also similar to aortic regurgitation in that its hemodynamic and clinical significance depend on the rapidity of onset.

Pathology

In considering the causes of mitral regurgitation, it is important to understand the anatomic components, which act collectively to provide valvular competence. Correct function of this system starts at the LV wall where the papillary muscles attach. A system of primary, secondary, and tertiary chordae provides the anatomic and structural attachments between the papillary muscles and the mitral leaflets. The leaflets, in turn, are attached at their circumference to the annulus. When one or more of these components are defective, regurgitation occurs. Given the complexity of this system, it is useful to divide major causes into valve leaflet abnormalities (i.e., primary or organic etiology) and causes related to structures other than the leaflets (i.e., secondary or functional etiology) (see Table 7-1).

Valvular etiologies include mitral valve prolapse (Fig. 7-8) and rheumatic valvular disease. When the LV wall fails to contract (after myocardial infarction) or the mitral annulus is enlarged, the normal valve leaflets are prevented from coapting properly, resulting in functional regurgitation.

Some causes, such as endocarditis of the valve leaflet or rupture of valve chordae, can occur suddenly and result in acute severe mitral regurgitation. Like aortic regurgitation, this condition is poorly tolerated medically and can be life-threatening without surgical intervention. In contrast, mitral valve prolapse can result in slow progression to chronic severe mitral regurgitation.

Acute severe mitral regurgitation results in a sudden increase in left atrial pressure. Given that a significant portion of the LV stroke volume then passes into the low-impedance left atrium during systole, cardiac output drops. The resulting pulmonary edema and hypotension often become life-threatening if the progression is not interrupted.

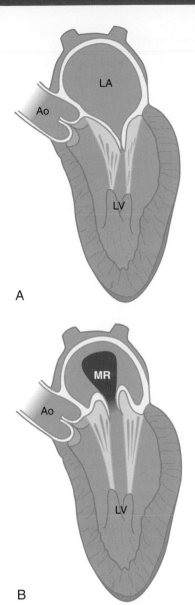

A

B

FIGURE 7-8 Degenerative mitral valve disease is an inheritable leaflet abnormality that often results in mitral valve prolapse, the most common cause of mitral regurgitation. **A,** Diagram shows normal leaflet position during closure in systole. **B,** Prolapsing motion of the mitral leaflets above the mitral annulus during systole results in mitral regurgitation (MR). Ao, Aorta; LA, left atrium; LV, left ventricle.

When the regurgitation develops slowly over months to years, the heart typically compensates with ventricular remodeling, enlargement, and increased compliance. This permits the stroke volume to be maintained at normal filling pressures for prolonged periods, preventing symptoms. Eventually, the systolic function declines or the patient develops symptoms, heralding the need for surgery.

Clinical Presentation

Patients with acute severe mitral regurgitation are acutely ill at presentation and often are in cardiogenic shock. In addition to dyspnea, hypotension, and tachycardia, they may have signs and symptoms of the primary etiology. For example, a patient who has a ruptured papillary muscle due to a myocardial infarction may also have chest pain and ECG changes at presentation.

When the heart has time to develop compensatory mechanisms with chronic severe regurgitation, patients may remain asymptomatic and not even realize the condition is present until it is identified by physical examination. Over time, exertional fatigue and shortness of breath develop. If the condition is not identified in these early stages, the patient will ultimately develop typical signs and symptoms of chronic congestive heart failure and arrhythmia.

Diagnosis

In patients with acute severe regurgitation, the examination findings typically observed with mitral regurgitation may be absent or difficult to detect. Rapid rise in left atrial pressure during systole results in an abbreviated systolic murmur. When tachypnea and tachycardia are present as additional confounders to the physical examination, the diagnosis can be easily missed at the bedside (see Table 7-2). If clinical suspicion is present, echocardiography is an essential tool in rapidly confirming the diagnosis.

A patient with chronic severe mitral regurgitation is more likely to have a classic holosystolic murmur present at the LV apex. If the cause of the regurgitation is mitral valve prolapse, there is often a mid-systolic click followed by a late-peaking systolic murmur. The cardiac enlargement that has evolved may be appreciated by a diffuse, laterally displaced PMI. An S_3 gallop may be present, even in the absence of congestive heart failure.

Diagnosis is best confirmed by TTE. This technique is important, not only for quantitatively estimating the regurgitation severity but for defining the anatomic mechanism, which has significant implications for management. If the valvular abnormality cannot be confirmed by transthoracic imaging, both two- and three-dimensional TEEs are very sensitive for identifying the anatomic mechanism of regurgitation.

Techniques in the cardiac catheterization laboratory can be useful in evaluating the severity of regurgitation, but these are less commonly used and have been largely supplanted by echocardiography.

Treatment

As in patients with acute severe aortic regurgitation, the primary objective is to stabilize the patient while urgently arranging for definitive mechanical correction—namely, repair or replacement of the mitral valve. In contrast to acute severe aortic regurgitation, an intraortic balloon pump is an option for reducing afterload and improving cardiac output in patients with mitral regurgitation. Otherwise, intravenous sodium nitroprusside or hydralazine can be attempted to lower afterload, or a diuretic can be used to reduce pulmonary edema if hypotension is not prohibitive.

In patients with chronic severe mitral regurgitation, the clinical status may remain stable, and many experts advocate a strategy of "watchful waiting." In general, the active patient may be monitored for development of exertional symptoms. However, even in the absence of symptoms, patients can develop occult LV systolic dysfunction. Therefore, periodic echocardiographic surveillance in asymptomatic patients is critical to prevent irreversible systolic dysfunction.

When a patient develops exertional symptoms or congestive heart failure, providing there has not already been a large decline in LV systolic function, mitral repair or replacement surgery is considered a class I indication (level B evidence). When an asymptomatic patient develops an LV ejection fraction of 60% or less, surgery is again a class I level B recommendation. When patients with chronic severe mitral regurgitation develop new-onset atrial fibrillation or confirmed significant pulmonary hypertension, surgery is advised with a class IIa recommendation (level C evidence). There are no medications that have been confirmed as able to alter the natural history of chronic severe mitral regurgitation, and no specific medical therapy in the absence of hypertension is recommended.

Prognosis

Rarely, patients with acute severe mitral regurgitation rapidly improve and enter a prolonged compensated phase in which watchful waiting is appropriate. However, most patients require urgent surgical intervention for survival. In chronic severe mitral regurgitation, it has been demonstrated that a program of watchful waiting, if diligently followed for appearance of a surgical indication as described, leads to excellent patient outcomes. However, failure to act when surgical criteria are met clearly leads to increased risk of morbidity and mortality.

⬤ TRICUSPID VALVE DISEASE

Definition

Anatomic requirements for tricuspid competence are similar to those described for the mitral valve: A complex of valve tissue and supportive structures must work in concert to maintain competence. With the tricuspid valve, however, three leaflets must come together appropriately to prevent regurgitation.

Tricuspid valve stenosis is similar to mitral stenosis in that the restriction of leaflet motion results in obstruction of right atrial emptying in diastole. The degree of stenosis determines the onset and severity of symptoms.

Pathology

Tricuspid stenosis in adults most often occurs as a result of rheumatic heart disease, which is uncommon in developed countries. Tricuspid valve involvement is less common than mitral and aortic valve involvement in rheumatic disease, and it almost never occurs without the mitral valve also being affected. Congenital abnormalities resulting in stenosis occur but are typically identified in childhood. Large leaflet vegetations and carcinoid disease may rarely cause stenosis, as may orifice obstruction from a large myxoma.

Tricuspid regurgitation can result from leaflet abnormalities (primary) or from another pathology affecting the right ventricle (functional). Functional tricuspid regurgitation is more common clinically; it occurs in patients with significant pulmonary hypertension, often caused by left-sided heart disease or lung disease. RV enlargement resulting from an atrial septal defect or anomalous pulmonary venous return can lead to severe functional tricuspid regurgitation. Primary leaflet abnormalities can occur from infectious endocarditis, carcinoid, or blunt chest trauma or iatrogenically from pacemaker or defibrillator leads (see Table 7-1).

Clinical Presentation

Because patients with tricuspid stenosis most often have mitral or aortic valve disease, or both, it is difficult to differentiate those symptoms that are solely caused by tricuspid disease. Symptoms of isolated tricuspid stenosis are similar to those of right-sided heart failure, although RV function is typically normal. These symptoms include edema and ascites as well as fatigue and dyspnea from low cardiac output.

Tricuspid regurgitation similarly results in heart failure symptoms of peripheral edema and low cardiac output that can include fatigue and exertional dyspnea. As RV systolic function deteriorates over time, symptoms progress and become more challenging to treat. Eventually, bowel edema results in decreased appetite and decreased absorption of oral diuretics, leading to malnutrition and a downward clinical spiral. As in tricuspid stenosis, the enlarging right atrium can precipitate atrial arrhythmias that further confound therapy.

Diagnosis

Physical examination for tricuspid stenosis is confounded by findings from left-sided valve disease in most cases. In normal sinus rhythm, an atrium contracting against a restricted tricuspid orifice can result in a prominent *a* wave on inspection of jugular venous pulsations. An opening snap may be audible. A soft diastolic-flow rumble may be identified by placing the bell of a stethoscope at the right parasternal border but may be inaudible. The key to distinguishing murmurs of right-sided origin is the respiratory variation in intensity, which augments with inspiration. Chest radiography may demonstrate right atrial enlargement, but there is no RV or pulmonary artery enlargement or prominence (see Table 7-2). A normal tricuspid valve has an area of 4 to 5 cm². Severe stenosis is thought to be present when the area is reduced to less than 1 cm² or the mean tricuspid valve gradient is 7 mm Hg or greater. Right heart catheterization is possible but is rarely needed to confirm the diagnosis of tricuspid stenosis.

The holosystolic murmur of tricuspid regurgitation can be soft or absent, and the diagnosis may go unsuspected. When present, the murmur is typically loudest at the left sternal border and increases with inspiration. Inspection of the jugular veins may demonstrate a characteristic *v* wave. Hepatic enlargement, with a pulsatile liver in systole, may be felt. Right atrial and ventricular enlargement may be seen on a chest radiograph.

TTE is the gold standard imaging modality for identifying the presence, cause, and severity of both tricuspid stenosis and tricuspid regurgitation. If the right heart cannot be adequately visualized by this technique, TEE or magnetic resonance imaging (MRI) can be helpful.

Treatment

There is no effective medical treatment for symptomatic isolated severe tricuspid valve stenosis. Diuretics typically reduce the cardiac output further, improving fluid status at the cost of worsening fatigue and dyspnea. Although percutaneous valvuloplasty of the tricuspid valve has been described, patients do poorly if there is resulting significant regurgitation. Although there are no studies to confirm optimal treatment of isolated symptomatic severe tricuspid stenosis, the European Society of Cardiology rates valvuloplasty or valve replacement in symptomatic patients, or in those undergoing left-sided valve intervention, as a class I indication (level C evidence).

Severe tricuspid regurgitation is associated with increased risks of morbidity and mortality. Diuretics are useful initially to improve edema. As the disease progresses, increasing doses are required, until eventually patients become unresponsive. The improvement in their edema also comes at the expense of more fatigue and dyspnea due to limited cardiac output. Tricuspid valve repair or replacement is the only proven method of interrupting this clinical progression. Severe symptomatic tricuspid regurgitation therefore carries a class I recommendation for surgery (level C evidence).

Prognosis

There are few data on the natural history of isolated unoperated tricuspid valve stenosis. Guideline recommendations for therapy are based on expert consensus, and individual patient management is largely based on clinical judgment given the infrequency of isolated stenosis.

A study performed at the Mayo Clinic examined 60 patients with severe tricuspid regurgitation treated over a 20-year period. Patients with unoperated tricuspid regurgitation had a 4.5% per year mortality rate, significantly higher than that for a matched U.S. population, supporting the class I recommendation for surgery.

● PULMONARY VALVE DISEASE

Definition

Pulmonary valve stenosis, similar to stenosis of the aortic valve, results from incomplete opening of the three valve leaflets in systole and leads to a pressure gradient between right ventricle and the pulmonary artery. The severity of the resulting obstruction to flow determines the clinical sequelae. Isolated significant pulmonary valve regurgitation is uncommon and is well tolerated unless severe.

Pathology

Pulmonary valve stenosis is rare. It is caused predominantly by congenital heart disease and typically is identified in childhood. It is very common in certain congenital disorders, such as Noonan's syndrome. Rare acquired causes of the disease include carcinoid tumor and rheumatic heart disease, but other valves are typically involved as well in these conditions.

Moderate or severe pulmonary valve regurgitation can similarly result from congenital heart disease or, even more likely, from previous mechanical treatment of congenital pulmonary valve stenosis. Valvular causes include trauma, carcinoid, and endocarditis. RV outflow tract and pulmonary artery enlargement may also result in failed central leaflet coaptation with resulting regurgitation.

Clinical Presentation

Although the diagnosis of pulmonary valve stenosis is most often made in childhood, it is occasionally first identified in an adult.

The RV pressure overload of severe stenosis results most commonly in symptoms of fatigue and dyspnea. Angina, exertional lightheadedness, or syncope can occur in more advanced stages of the disease.

Pulmonary regurgitation typically has a benign course unless it becomes severe. Even after that point, the volume overload of the right ventricle may be tolerated well for many years, similar to the overload of the left ventricle in aortic regurgitation. The right ventricle eventually enlarges, with some increased risk of arrhythmia. Ultimately, there is loss of RV systolic function, and patients develop signs and symptoms of right-sided heart failure, as previously described.

Diagnosis

On physical examination, the patient with severe pulmonary stenosis may have an RV lift as a result of the RV hypertrophy that develops. A prominent *a* wave may be identifiable on inspection of jugular venous pulsations. A crescendo-decrescendo systolic murmur is best heard at the left upper sternal border and may vary with respiration. S_2 may have relative fixed slitting, with the P_2 pulmonic component becoming soft or absent as the stenosis progresses. Chest radiography may demonstrate right heart and pulmonary artery enlargement with decreased vascular markings.

Similarly, the RV enlargement of pulmonary valve regurgitation may result in an RV lift. A diastolic decrescendo murmur may be present at the left sternal border and varies with respiration, but it may be inaudible if pulmonary pressures are normal. Chest radiography demonstrates right-sided heart enlargement.

TTE is sensitive and specific for diagnosis of both stenosis and regurgitation of the pulmonary valve if actively sought on the examination. Severe pulmonary valve stenosis is considered to be present when the peak gradient is greater than 64 mm Hg. Cardiac MRI may be useful in quantitating regurgitation severity or in estimating the gradient in stenosis if echocardiography is inconclusive.

Treatment

Percutaneous balloon valvuloplasty is an effective treatment for symptomatic severe pulmonary valve stenosis (class I indication, level C evidence). Surgical valvotomy or valve replacement is used only when anatomic features prevent balloon valvuloplasty or if there has been a poor result from previous attempts.

Valve replacement for severe pulmonary valve regurgitation is thought by most to be indicated when patients become symptomatic or RV systolic dysfunction develops, although there is no consensus on recommendations for the approach to this problem.

Prognosis

Studies have suggested that survival in pulmonary stenosis is related to the pressure gradient, with decreased survival in those with gradients greater than 50 mm Hg. Therefore, balloon valvuloplasty is a class I (level C evidence) recommendation for asymptomatic patients with peak pulmonary valve gradients at catheterization of at least 40 mm Hg and a class IIb recommendation for asymptomatic patients with a gradient of 30 to 39 mm Hg (level C evidence).

SUGGESTED READINGS

Bonow RO, Carabello BA, Chatterjee K, et al: Focused update incorporated into the ACC/AHA 2006 guidelines for the management of patients with valvular heart disease: a report of the American College of Cardiology/American Heart Association Task Force on Practice Guidelines (Writing Committee to Revise the 1998 Guidelines for the Management of Patients With Valvular Heart Disease); endorsed by the Society of Cardiovascular Anesthesiologists, Society for Cardiovascular Angiography and Interventions, and Society of Thoracic Surgeons, Circulation 118:e523–e661, 2008.

Makkar RR, Fontana GP, Jilaihawi H, et al: Transcatheter aortic-valve replacement for inoperable severe aortic stenosis, N Engl J Med 366:1696–1704, 2012.

Messika-Zeitoun D, Thomson H, Bellamy M, et al: Medical and surgical outcome of tricuspid regurgitation caused by flail leaflets, J Thorac Cardiovasc Surg 128:296–302, 2004.

Nkomo VT, Gardin JM, Skelton TN, et al: Burden of valvular heart diseases: a population-based study, Lancet 368:1005–1011, 2006.

Vahanian A, Baumgartner H, Bax J, et al: Guidelines on the management of valvular heart disease: The Task Force on the Management of Valvular Heart Disease of the European Society of Cardiology, Eur Heart J 28:230–268, 2007.

Coronary Heart Disease

Michael P. Cinquegrani

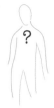

DEFINITION AND EPIDEMIOLOGY

The term *coronary heart disease* (CHD) describes a number of cardiac conditions that result from the presence of atherosclerotic lesions in the coronary arteries. The development of atherosclerotic plaque within the coronary arteries can result in obstruction to blood flow, producing ischemia, which can be acute or chronic in nature. Atherosclerosis is a disease process that starts at a young age and can be present for years in an asymptomatic form until the degree of vessel obstruction leads to ischemic symptoms. Obstructive atherosclerotic lesions can cause chronic symptoms of exercise- or stress-related angina; or, in the case of plaque rupture and acute thrombosis, sudden death, unstable angina, or myocardial infarction (MI) may ensue.

In the United States, more than 17 million people experience some form of CHD. Approximately 10 million suffer from symptoms of angina, and at least 380,000 deaths occur each year from acute MI or CHD-related sudden death. Despite progress in therapy and overall reductions in CHD-related mortality, CHD remains the number one cause of death in both men and women, accounting for 27% of deaths in women (more than deaths due to cancer). The incidence of CHD increases with age for both men and women. There are at least 1.2 million MIs per year in the United States, and many more cases of unstable angina. CHD frequently results in lifestyle-limiting symptoms due to angina or impairment of left ventricular (LV) function. The cost of care related directly to CHD and indirectly to lost productivity from CHD is in the range of $156 billion per year. CHD remains a major life-threatening disease process associated with significant economic impact.

RISK FACTORS FOR ATHEROSCLEROSIS

Before delving into discussion of the pathology of atherosclerosis, a description of risk factors is warranted. There are a number of well-known risk factors for coronary artery disease (CAD), some of which are modifiable (Table 8-1). Although women ultimately also carry a significant atherosclerotic burden, men develop CAD at younger ages, and the prevalence of the disease also increases as men age. Another potent risk factor for the development of CAD is a family history of premature CAD. This speaks to a nonmodifiable, genetically based risk. Commonly, multiple family members develop symptomatic CAD before the age of 55 years (65 years for women). Risks are additive, making it very important to appreciate the modifiable risk factors such as hyperlipidemia, hypertension, diabetes mellitus, metabolic syndrome, cigarette smoking, obesity, sedentary lifestyle, and heavy alcohol intake.

Metabolic syndrome deserves particular attention given that up to 25% of the adult U.S. population may satisfy the definition of the disorder as laid out by the National Cholesterol Education Program Adult Treatment Panel. The definition of metabolic syndrome requires the presence of at least three of the following five criteria: waist circumference greater than 201 cm in men or 88 cm in women, triglyceride level 150 mg/dL or higher, high-density lipoprotein (HDL) cholesterol level lower than 40 mg/dL in men or 50 mg/dL in women, blood pressure 130/85 mm Hg or higher, and fasting serum glucose level 110 mg/dL or higher. The features of metabolic syndrome are largely modifiable risk factors for CAD.

Hyperlipidemia, in particular elevated levels of low-density lipoprotein (LDL) cholesterol, plays a pivotal role in the development and evolution of atherosclerosis. HDL-cholesterol is believed to be protective, likely due to its role in transporting cholesterol from the vessel wall to the liver for degradation. Increased levels of HDL are inversely proportional to the risk of CAD-related problems. The interplay among circulating lipids is complex. Elevated levels of triglycerides are a risk factor for CAD and are frequently associated with reduced levels of protective HDL. Hyperlipidemia is highly modifiable, and clinical trials have shown that drug treatment directed at lowering LDL-cholesterol significantly reduces the risk of CAD-related complications or death.

TABLE 8-1	RISK FACTORS AND MARKERS FOR CORONARY ARTERY DISEASE
NONMODIFIABLE RISK FACTORS	
Age	
Male sex	
Family history of premature coronary artery disease	
MODIFIABLE INDEPENDENT RISK FACTORS	
Hyperlipidemia	
Hypertension	
Diabetes mellitus	
Metabolic syndrome	
Cigarette smoking	
Obesity	
Sedentary lifestyle	
Heavy alcohol intake	
MARKERS	
Elevated lipoprotein(a)	
Hyperhomocysteinemia	
Elevated high-sensitivity C-reactive protein (hsCRP)	
Coronary arterial calcification detected by EBCT or MDCT	

EBCT, Electron beam computed tomography; MDCT, multidetector computed tomography.

As with hyperlipidemia, hypertension (systolic pressure >140 mm Hg or diastolic pressure >90 mm Hg) contributes to the risk of CAD-related complications. Hypertension, probably through sheer stress, causes vessel injury that supports the development of atherosclerotic plaque. Increasing severity of hypertension is associated with greater risk of CAD. Control of hypertension is associated with a reduced risk of CAD.

Diabetes mellitus is a prominent risk factor for CAD, and the disease is becoming epidemic. Diabetes mellitus typically is associated with other risk factors, such as elevated triglycerides, reduced HDL, and hypertension, which accounts for the enhanced risk of CAD-related problems in diabetic patients. It is not clear that control of hyperglycemia in diabetic patients translates into a reduced risk of CAD, but the presence of diabetes mellitus drives the need to ensure good treatment of other modifiable risk factors.

Cigarette smoking has long been known as a significant risk factor for both CAD and lung cancer. Cigarette smoking is associated with increased platelet reactivity and increased risk of thrombosis, as well as lipid abnormalities. This addictive habit is modifiable, and smoking cessation can lead to a decrease in CAD event rates by 50% in the first 2 years of cessation.

Similar to diabetes mellitus, obesity (body mass index >30 kg/m^2) is associated with risk factors such as hypertension, hyperlipidemia, and glucose intolerance. Although multiple risk factors are frequently present in obese people, obesity itself carries some independent risk for CAD. The location and type of adipose tissue appear to influence CAD risk, with abdominal obesity posing a greater risk for CAD in men and women.

Numerous clinical studies have shown the benefit of regular aerobic exercise in decreasing the risk for CAD-related problems, both in the people without known CAD and in those with the disease. Sedentary lifestyles carry an increased risk that is modifiable through exercise.

Another common attribute of life, alcohol consumption, can influence the risk of CAD in both directions. One to two ounces of alcohol per day may reduce the risk for CAD-related events, but more than 2 ounces of alcohol per day is associated with an increased risk of events. Lower levels of alcohol consumption can increase HDL levels, although it is not clear that this is the mechanism of benefit. In contrast, excessive alcohol consumption is associated with hypertension, a definite risk for CAD, although other effects of high-dose alcohol may also be at play.

Additional factors that may have some role in adding CAD risk include lipoprotein(a) and homocysteine. Lipoprotein(a) is structurally similar to plasminogen and may interfere with the activity of plasmin, thus contributing to a prothrombotic state. Hyperhomocysteinemia has been associated with increased vascular risks, including coronary, cerebral, and peripheral vascular disease. It is not clear that a causal link exists, and the use of folic acid supplementation to lower homocysteine levels has not been shown to reduce the risk of MI or stroke.

C-reactive protein (CRP) is a marker of systemic inflammation, and it indicates an increased risk for coronary plaque rupture. High-sensitivity assays for CRP (hsCRP) have measured elevated levels that correlate with risk for MI, stroke, peripheral vascular disease, and sudden cardiac death. Another marker for the presence of CAD is coronary calcification. The process of atherosclerosis is often associated with deposition of calcium within the plaque. Coronary artery calcification can be detected by fluoroscopy during cardiac catheterization as well by computed tomography (CT) scanning using either multidetector computed tomography (MDCT) or electron beam computed tomography (EBCT). CT technology allows for a quantitative measure of coronary calcium deposits that correlates with the probability of having significant obstructive lesions. The value of routine use of either hsCRP or CT for coronary calcification remains unclear, but patients in whom coronary calcification is identified should be approached with aggressive risk-factor modification.

PATHOLOGY

The process of atherosclerosis is known to begin at a young age. Autopsies of teenagers frequently demonstrate the presence of atherosclerotic changes in coronary arteries. Atherosclerosis is a process linked to the subintimal accumulation of small lipoprotein particles that are rich in LDL. Subintimal deposits of LDL are oxidized, setting off a cascade of events that culminate in not only the development of atherosclerotic plaque but also vascular inflammation. Vascular inflammation drives progression of atherosclerosis as well as the potential rupture of plaque leading to vessel occlusion. The process of lipoprotein uptake by the vessel wall is enhanced by vascular endothelial injury, which may be triggered by hypercholesterolemia, the toxic effects of cigarette smoking, sheer stresses associated with hypertension, or vascular effects of diabetes mellitus.

Oxidized LDL aggregates trigger the expression of endothelial cell surface adhesion molecules, including vascular adhesion molecule-1, intracellular adhesion molecule-1, and selectins, which results in the binding of circulating macrophages to the endothelium. In response to cytokines and chemokines released by endothelial and smooth muscle cells, macrophages migrate into the subintimal region, where they ingest oxidized LDL aggregates. These LDL-laden macrophages are also called foam cells (based on the microscopic appearance), and the accumulation of foam cells represents the development of atherosclerosis.

Foam cells break down, releasing pro-inflammatory substances that promote ongoing accumulation of both macrophages and T lymphocytes. This process potentiates the development of atherosclerotic plaque. Growth factors are also released that promote smooth muscle cell and fibroblast proliferation. The net result is the development of a fibrous cap, which covers a lipid-rich core.

Important contributors to the pathologic evolution of atherosclerotic plaque include impaired endothelial synthesis of nitric oxide and prostacyclin, both of which play major roles in vascular homeostasis. The loss of these vasodilators leads to abnormal regulation of vascular tone and also plays a role in evolving a local prothrombotic state. Platelets adhere to areas of vascular injury and are not only prothrombotic but also release growth factors that help drive the aforementioned proliferation of smooth muscle cells and fibroblasts. A key structural constituent of the fibrous cap is collagen, and its synthesis by fibroblasts is inhibited by cytokines elaborated by accumulating T lymphocytes. Foam cell degradation also releases matrix metalloproteinases that break down collagen, leading to weakening of the fibrous core and making it prone to rupture. T lymphocytes tends to accumulate at the border of plaque, which is the frequent site of plaque rupture.

As the fibrous cap thins through collagen degradation and eventually ruptures, blood is exposed to the thrombogenic triggers of collagen and lipid. In this setting, platelets are activated and begin to aggregate at the site of rupture. Platelets release vasoconstrictor substances thromboxane and serotonin, but more importantly, they serve as the trigger for thrombin formation, which leads to local thrombosis. Thrombin accumulation along with ongoing platelet activation can lead to rapid accumulation of thrombus in the vessel lumen. The combination of platelet-mediated thrombus accumulation and vasoconstriction can significantly limit blood flow, leading to myocardial ischemia. The degree of ischemia and its duration can culminate in MI. Complete vessel occlusion by thrombus leads to the greatest degree of myocardial ischemia and infarction, typically resulting in an ST elevation myocardial infarction (STEMI). Incomplete vessel occlusion limits blood flow enough to cause symptomatic myocardial ischemia and lesser degrees of MI, resulting in the syndromes of unstable angina or non–ST elevation myocardial infarction (NSTEMI).

MI is the most profound consequence of atherosclerotic plaque pathology, but significant disability can also develop when atherosclerotic plaques expand in size, leading to obstruction of blood flow and resultant myocardial ischemia. Plaque growth, driven by smooth muscle cell proliferation, initially causes the vessel to expand toward the adventitia (Glagov remodeling). Once a limit of lateral expansion is reached, the enlarging plaque encroaches on the vessel lumen. Typically, when the diameter of the lumen is decreased by at least 70%, myocardial ischemia and symptoms of angina can develop under conditions of increasing demand for blood flow. In the case of exercise, increases in heart rate and blood pressure lead to increasing myocardial oxygen demand; when flow-limiting atherosclerotic lesions are present,

oxygen demand may not be met by supply and myocardial ischemia ensues. The greater the degree of vessel obstruction, the more likely it is that myocardial ischemia and angina will occur at low workloads, even to the point of angina at rest (Fig. 8-1). Other forms of stress, such as emotional stress or cold exposure, can also cause symptoms of angina in patients with significant obstructive plaque through mechanisms such has hypertension (increased myocardial oxygen demand) or sympathetically mediated vasoconstriction.

● CLINICAL PRESENTATIONS OF CORONARY ARTERY DISEASE

The clinical syndromes that patients experience due to the presence of CAD principally relate to the occurrence of myocardial ischemia. Myocardial ischemia develops when there is a mismatch of oxygen delivery and oxygen demand. Given that extraction of oxygen by the myocardium is very high, any increase in oxygen demand must be met with an increase in coronary blood flow. Oxygen demand is directly related to increases in heart rate, myocardial contractility, and wall stress (which are related to blood pressure and cardiac dimensions). There is a reflex increase in myocardial oxygen demand driven by these factors as the heart is required to deliver more systemic blood flow in the face of various stresses, the most common of which is increased exertion. Coronary blood flow also depends on the vascular tone of arterioles that are under the control of vasodilators derived from normal functioning endothelium and autonomic tone.

Coronary blood flow increases to meet an increase in myocardial oxygen demand through endothelium-mediated vasodilation. In the face of atherosclerosis, endothelial dysfunction may develop, resulting in reduced endothelium-mediated vasodilation. Endothelial dysfunction coupled with a flow-limiting stenosis sets the stage for the development of myocardial ischemia. The coronary vessel distal to a flow-limiting stenosis tends to be maximally dilated. As myocardial oxygen demand increases, the

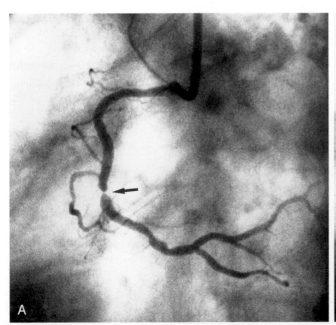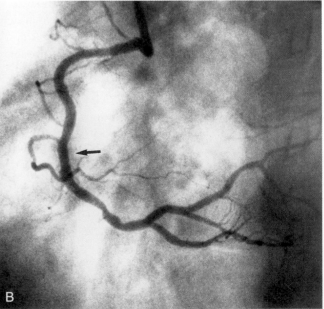

FIGURE 8-1 Angiograms of the right coronary artery. **A,** Discrete stenosis is observed in the middle segment of the artery *(arrow)*. **B,** The same artery is shown after successful balloon angioplasty of the stenosis and placement of an intracoronary stent *(arrow)*.

myocardium distal to a flow-limiting stenosis is no longer able to augment flow by additional dilation. An overall limitation in the ability to increase coronary blood flow due to flow-limiting stenosis and endothelial dysfunction results in supply/demand mismatch and myocardial ischemia.

The major clinical manifestation of myocardial ischemia is chest discomfort (angina pectoris), which is usually described as a pressure or sensation of midsternal tightness. It may be quite pronounced in intensity or relatively subtle. Myocardial ischemia produces not only the sensation of angina pectoris but also a number of derangements in myocyte function. As in any tissue, inadequate oxygen delivery leads to a transition to anaerobic glycolysis, increased lactate production causing cellular acidosis, and abnormal calcium homeostasis. The net consequences of these cellular abnormalities include reductions in myocardial contractility and relaxation. Decreased myocardial contractility results in systolic wall motion abnormalities in the area of ischemia, and the abnormality of relaxation causes reduced ventricular compliance. These changes cause an increase in LV filling pressures above the normal range. The cellular abnormalities related to myocardial ischemia also translate into changes in cellular electrical activity that appear as abnormalities in the electrocardiogram (ECG). Myocardial ischemia may result in either ST depression or ST elevation, depending on the duration, severity, and location of the ischemia. The cellular, mechanical, and electrical abnormalities caused by ischemia typically precede the patient's perception of angina.

Myocardial dysfunction due to ischemia may recover quickly to normal if the duration of ischemia is brief. Prolonged myocardial ischemia can lead to conditions of myocardial stunning or myocardial hibernation. In the case of stunning, the mechanical dysfunction induced by prolonged ischemia persists for hours or days until function returns to normal. In the face of chronic ischemia, myocyte viability may be maintained, but because of ischemia, mechanical dysfunction persists; in this condition, known as hibernation, restoration of blood flow can result in recovery of myocardial function.

The heart's conduction system is less prone to ischemic injury, but ischemia can lead to impaired conduction. Ischemic disruption of myocyte electrical homeostasis also sets the stage for potentially life-threatening arrhythmias.

Angina Pectoris and Stable Ischemic Heart Disease

Definition

Angina pectoris is a clinical manifestation of obstructive CAD, which in turn is usually the result of atherosclerotic plaque formation over a number of years. The term *angina pectoris* refers to the symptom of chest discomfort that may be described by the patient as a sensation of chest tightness or burning. Of the 17,600,000 adults in the United States with heart disease, as many as 10,200,00 have angina pectoris. It is estimated that 785,000 people experience a new ischemic episode annually, and recurrent events occur in at least 470,000 Americans each year.

Pathology

As a symptom, angina pectoris is experienced when myocardial ischemia develops. Myocardial ischemia and angina pectoris may occur in the face of obstructive atherosclerotic plaque that limits blood flow in the face of increased demand such as exertion or emotional excitement. Myocardial oxygen demand is directly related to increases in heart rate and blood pressure; these variables, in turn, can be manipulated with medical therapy to reduce the demand. Restricted oxygen supply, in the form of reduced blood flow, can also induce myocardial ischemia. Blood flow reduction is a prominent feature of acute presentations of CAD such as NSTEMI and STEMI, but atherosclerosis-mediated coronary vasoconstriction, or coronary vasospasm, is also a potential cause of flow limitation leading to myocardial ischemia. Another example of supply limitation is anemia, whereby reduced oxygen-carrying capacity coupled with obstructive lesions leads to myocardial ischemia and symptoms of angina pectoris. The term *stable* angina pectoris refers to myocardial ischemia caused by either plaque-mediated flow limitation in the face of excess demand or supply limitation due to coronary vasospasm.

Clinical Presentation

Angina pectoris may manifest in either stable or unstable patterns (Table 8-2), but the symptom expression is similar. Typically, patients complain of retrosternal discomfort that they may describe as pressure, tightness, or heaviness. The symptom can be subtle in its presentation, and inquiry as to the presence of

TABLE 8-2	ANGINA PECTORIS			
TYPE	**PATTERN**	**ECG**	**ABNORMALITY**	**MEDICAL THERAPY**
Stable	Stable pattern, induced by physical exertion, exposure to cold, eating, emotional stress	Baseline often normal or nonspecific ST-T changes	≥70% Luminal narrowing of one or more coronary arteries from atherosclerosis	Aspirin Sublingual nitroglycerin
	Lasts 5-10 min Relieved by rest or nitroglycerin	Signs of previous MI ST-segment depression during angina		Anti-ischemic medications Statin
Unstable	Increase in anginal frequency, severity, or duration Angina of new onset or now occurring at low level of activity or at rest May be less responsive to sublingual nitroglycerin	Same as stable angina, although changes during discomfort may be more pronounced Occasional ST-segment elevation during discomfort	Plaque rupture with platelet and fibrin thrombus, causing worsening coronary obstruction	Aspirin and clopidogrel Anti-ischemic medications Heparin or LMWH Glycoprotein IIb/IIIa inhibitors
Prinzmetal or variant angina	Angina without provocation, typically occurring at rest	Transient ST-segment elevation during pain Often with associated AV block or ventricular arrhythmias	Coronary artery spasm	Calcium channel blockers Nitrates

AV, Atrioventricular; ECG, electrocardiography; LMWH, low-molecular-weight heparin; MI, myocardial infarction.

"chest pain" may lead to a negative response in a patient experiencing angina pectoris. When taking a history aimed at discerning angina pectoris, one needs to seek answers to these more nuanced descriptions of symptoms. In addition to chest discomfort, patients may have associated discomfort in the arm, throat, back, or jaw. They also may experience dyspnea, diaphoresis, or nausea associated with angina pectoris.

There is a good deal of variability in the expression of symptoms related to myocardial ischemia, although each person tends to have a unique signature of symptoms. Some have no chest discomfort but only radiated arm, throat, or back symptoms; dyspnea; or abdominal discomfort. Myocardial ischemia can also manifest in a "silent" form, particularly in the elderly and in patients with long-standing diabetes mellitus. The duration of angina pectoris varies, probably depending on the magnitude of the underlying myocardial ischemia. Exertion-related angina pectoris, the hallmark of stable obstructive CAD, typically resolves with rest or with decreased intensity of exercise. In stable angina pectoris, the duration of events is usually in the range of 1 to 3 minutes. Prolonged symptoms in the 20- to 30-minute range are indicative of a more serious problem such as NSTEMI or STEMI.

The physical examination of patients with CAD is typically normal. However, if the patient is physically examined during an episode of myocardial ischemia, either at rest or after exertion, significant changes may be present. As with any form of discomfort, there may be a reflex increase in heart rate and blood pressure. Elevated heart rate and blood pressure may act to sustain the duration of angina by increasing myocardial oxygen demand in the face of supply-limiting coronary stenosis. Acute mitral regurgitation can develop if the distribution of myocardial ischemia includes a papillary muscle, the supporting structure of the mitral valve. The physical examination in such cases would demonstrate a new systolic murmur consistent with mitral regurgitation. If severe enough in degree, this mitral regurgitation will cause decreased LV compliance and, consequently, an acute elevation in left atrial and pulmonary vein pressure leading to pulmonary congestion. In this setting, the patient will have not only the symptom of angina pectoris but also the symptom of dyspnea and the physical finding of rales. Ischemia-induced increases in LV filling pressure due to diminished compliance also can occur independently of ischemia-induced mitral regurgitation. Decreased LV compliance can produce the abnormal heart sound S_4; in the case of severe diffuse myocardial ischemia causing LV systolic dysfunction, an S_3 may also be perceived. Resolution of myocardial ischemia results in not only a cessation of angina pectoris but also a return to the patient's baseline physical examination status.

Diagnosis and Differential Diagnosis

Three basic forms of testing have played major roles in assessing patients with chest discomfort possibly due to CAD. All of these tests capitalize on the effect of myocardial ischemia on various aspects of cardiac physiology. First, myocardial ischemia induced by exercise or by spontaneous coronary occlusion results in subendocardial ischemia, which appears on an ECG as diffuse ST depression (Fig. 8-2). Once ischemia resolves, the ECG returns to normal. Second, myocardial ischemia typically affects a segment of heart muscle, and that territory develops a wall

motion abnormality that can be detected by either echocardiography or nuclear scintigraphy. Third, the basis for myocardial ischemia is a decrease in coronary and myocardial blood flow. This abnormality can be detected by assessing the distribution of radioactive tracers such as thallium 201 or technetium sestamibi using specialized detectors for imaging myocardial perfusion. All stress test techniques used in diagnosing patients with possible CAD rely on these means of detecting the impact of myocardial ischemia on cardiac electrical activity, mechanical function, or myocardial perfusion.

Stress testing in its various forms frequently plays a pivotal role in the assessment of patients with possible CAD. In using stress testing, it is important to understand the significance of pretest probability of CAD in interpreting the results of any stress test method. For a patient with a high pretest probability of CAD, a positive test is highly predictive of underlying CAD, and a negative test carries the weight of being falsely negative. The opposite is true in a patient with a low pretest probability of CAD: A negative test is associated with a high negative predicative value for the presence of CAD, but a positive test is likely to be falsely positive. These factors play into a clinician's interpretation of test results and must always factor into decision making regarding the need for additional testing.

Stress testing is useful not only as a diagnostic tool but also in the long-term management of established CAD. Exercise stress testing, through its ability to quantify exercise capacity, can monitor the effectiveness of medical therapy directed at reducing myocardial ischemia. The findings of an exercise stress test also have predictive value in that patients with ischemia induced at low workloads are more likely to have extensive multivessel disease, whereas those who achieve high workloads are less prone to ischemic complications of CAD. A higher risk for poor outcomes related to CAD is implied by (1) ECG changes of ST depression early during exercise and persisting late into recovery; (2) exercise-induced reduction in systolic blood pressure; and (3) poor exercise tolerance (<6 minutes on the Bruce stress test protocol).

Patients with a normal resting ECG can reliably be assessed by standard exercise stress testing with ECG monitoring (Fig. 8-3). The specificity of ST changes with exertion is significantly reduced in the face of baseline ECG abnormalities related to LV hypertrophy, left bundle branch block (LBBB), pre-excitation, or use of digoxin. Various imaging techniques (echocardiography, nuclear scintigraphy, magnetic resonance imaging) have been developed to overcome the impact of baseline ECG abnormalities on the validity of stress testing. Because women also have lower specificity for ECG changes during exercise testing than men, an imaging technique is frequently used in the assessment of women. Overall, the addition of an imaging technique to stress testing significantly improves the sensitivity, specificity, and predictive value of the stress test but also greatly increases its cost.

Radionuclide stress testing is a common form of imaging-based stress test. Near peak exertion, a radionuclide tracer (thallium 201, technetium 99, or tetrofosmin) is administered intravenously. The tracer is distributed to the myocardium in a quantity directly proportional to blood flow. This type of image testing relies on a disparity of tracer uptake to detect an area of ischemia. Thallium 201 redistributes over 4 hours to viable

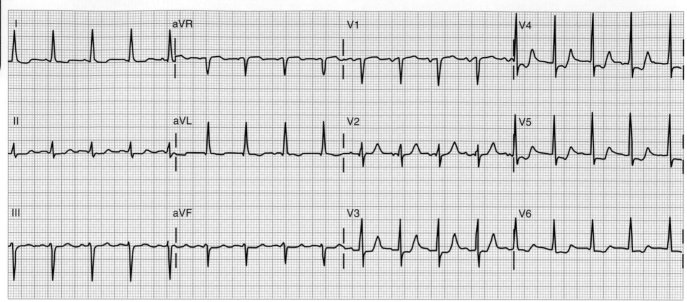

A

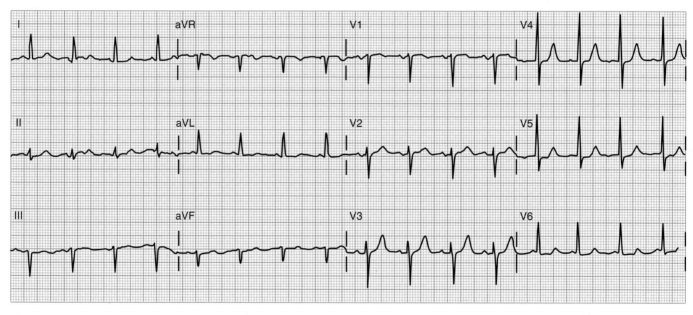

B

FIGURE 8-2 Electrocardiogram obtained during angina **(A)** and after the administration of sublingual nitroglycerin and subsequent resolution of angina **(B)**. During angina, transient ST-segment depression and T-wave abnormalities are present.

myocardium, allowing for comparison of stress-induced ischemia to a baseline state. The other tracers do not share this redistribution feature, and tests using technetium 99 or tetrofosmin require both "rest" and "stress" injections of tracer to differentiate ischemic myocardium. Patients with normal perfusion studies have a low risk of coronary events (<1%/year). The presence of a positive perfusion study confers a risk of about 7%/year for coronary events, with the risk increasing relative to the extent of perfusion abnormality.

An alternative means of imaging for exercise testing is the use of echocardiography to detect ischemia-induced wall motion abnormalities. This form of testing is increasingly favored because there is no radiation associated with its use, whereas radionuclide tracers expose the patient to a significant dose of radiation. Stress echocardiography carries with it the same enhancement in sensitivity, specificity, and predictive value as radionuclide imaging. An additional benefit of echocardiography imaging is more discrete anatomic data on valve function. If it is coupled with Doppler flow imaging, information regarding exercise-induced mitral regurgitation can be obtained.

Another means of assessing for exercise-induced wall motion abnormalities is the use of radionuclide ventriculography or multigated acquisition scanning (MUGA). This technique is usually included as part of the interpretation of an exercise stress

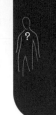

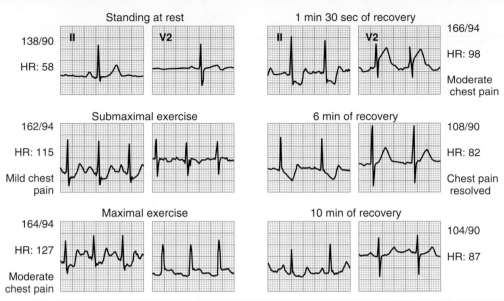

FIGURE 8-3 Treadmill exercise test demonstrates a markedly ischemic electrocardiogram (ECG) response. The resting ECG is normal. The test was stopped when the patient developed angina at a relatively low workload, accompanied by ST-segment depression in lead II and ST-segment elevation in lead V₂. These changes worsened early in recovery and resolved after administration of sublingual nitroglycerin. Only leads II and V₂ are shown; however, ischemic changes were seen in 10 of the 12 recorded leads. Severe atherosclerotic disease of all three coronary arteries was documented at subsequent cardiac catheterization.

radionuclide study. This imaging technique does not provide the anatomic detail associated with echocardiography, and it has the negative feature of significant radiation exposure.

An emerging imaging technique for stress testing is the use of magnetic resonance imaging. Radiation is not a concern, and cardiac structural imaging can match echocardiography (or exceed it in patients with poor images on echocardiography). The technique is not as easy to execute as echocardiography, but magnetic resonance imaging is likely to gain favor in exercise testing.

Not all patients who require noninvasive testing for CAD are able to exercise to a degree sufficient to induce ischemia, and for some patients exercise testing is not an option at all. For these patients, pharmacologic stress testing has evolved as a viable alternative to exercise testing. The prognostic benefit of exercise workload is not available from this form of testing, but information regarding the presence of ischemia-inducing atherosclerosis is obtainable. One common form of pharmacologic testing relies on inducing coronary vasodilation (as with dipyridamole, adenosine, or regadenosine), which produces a disparity of myocardial blood flow based on the presence of coronary stenosis. Radionuclide administered during the infusion of the coronary vasodilator allows for detection of myocardial ischemia similar to that observed with exercise testing. An alternative pharmacologic approach uses the inotropic and chronotropic effects of dobutamine to increase myocardial oxygen demand and induce segmental ischemia. Echocardiography is commonly used to detect dobutamine-induced wall motion abnormalities with this approach, although radionuclide or magnetic resonance imaging could also be used.

All of the stress testing techniques discussed here are able to assess for the presence of inducible myocardial ischemia associated with CAD. The presence of CAD can also be determined by assessment of coronary calcification using either EBCT or the now more common MDCT. Coronary calcification is present only because of underlying CAD. Although detecting its presence does not directly indicate the presence of obstructive CAD as would an abnormal imaging stress test, studies have shown a direct correlation between the amount of coronary calcification and the probability that a 70% stenosis is present. At the least, this type of information informs the physician that CAD is present and directs aggressive attention toward risk factor modification. MDCT scanners can reliably perform coronary angiography with the use of intravenous contrast agents and specifically timed imaging protocols. This technique is becoming increasingly used to detect the presence of obstructive CAD, although it cannot precisely define the severity of stenosis. MDCT is also valuable in defining coronary anomalies, and a negative study carries a high negative predictive value for the occurrence of coronary events.

Invasive coronary angiography has been considered the "gold standard" for detecting the extent and severity of underlying CAD. This approach carries a small risk of MI, stroke, or death, so it must not be taken lightly. In the case of patients with positive stress tests, particularly those with high-risk features, coronary angiography adds more discrete information regarding the underlying disease and guides the potential use of revascularization techniques (i.e., percutaneous coronary intervention or coronary artery bypass surgery) versus medical therapy to treat CAD (Table 8-3). Additional tools, such as pressure wires used to perform fractional flow reserve studies (FFR), add to the diagnostic power of invasive catheterization by allowing one to discriminate between physiologically significant lesions and those not likely to cause ischemia. Revascularization is not indicated for lesions that do not cause ischemia.

The physician must also be cognizant of the fact that not all chest discomfort is related to CAD. Although CAD as a cause of chest discomfort poses the biggest risk for poor outcomes, other

TABLE 8-3	INDICATIONS FOR CORONARY ANGIOGRAPHY IN PATIENTS WITH STABLE ANGINA PECTORIS

Unacceptable angina despite medical therapy (for consideration of revascularization)
Noninvasive testing results with high-risk features
Angina or risk factors for coronary artery disease in the setting of depressed left ventricular systolic function
For diagnostic purposes, in the individual in whom the results of noninvasive testing are unclear

TABLE 8-4   GOALS OF RISK FACTOR MODIFICATION

RISK FACTOR	GOAL
Dyslipidemia	
Elevated LDL-cholesterol level	
Patients with CAD or CAD equivalent*	LDL <70 mg/dL
Without CAD, ≥2 risk factors†	LDL <130 mg/dL (or <100 mg/dL‡)
Without CAD, 0-1 risk factors†	LDL <160 mg/dL
Elevated TG	TG <200 mg/dL
Reduced HDL-cholesterol level	HDL >40 mg/dL
Hypertension	Systolic blood pressure <140 mm Hg Diastolic blood pressure <90 mm Hg
Smoking	Complete cessation
Obesity	<120% of ideal body weight for height
Sedentary lifestyle	30-60 min moderately intense activity (e.g., walking, jogging, cycling, rowing) five times per week

CAD, Coronary artery disease; CRP, C-reactive protein; HDL, high-density lipoprotein; hsCRP, high-sensitivity C-reactive protein; LDL, low-density lipoprotein; TG, triglycerides.

*CAD equivalents include diabetes mellitus, noncoronary atherosclerotic vascular disease, or >20% 10-year risk for a cardiovascular event as predicted by the Framingham risk score.

†Risk factors include cigarette smoking, blood pressure ≥140/90 mm Hg or taking antihypertensive medication, HDL-cholesterol level <40 mg/dL, family history of premature coronary atherosclerosis (male, <45 yr; female, <55 yr).

‡Target of 100 mg/dL should be strongly considered for men ≥60 yr and for individuals with a high burden of subclinical atherosclerosis (coronary calcification >75th percentile for age and sex), hsCRP >3 mg/dL, or metabolic syndrome.

considerations of chest discomfort include esophageal disease (esophageal reflux may mimic typical angina pectoris), chest wall–related pain, pulmonary embolism, pneumonia, and trauma. The clinical presentation of the patient usually points in one direction or another, but patients with chest discomfort commonly undergo an evaluation for CAD, typically with the use of stress testing. Once CAD is reliably ruled out, the physician needs to consider alternative causes of the symptom. In the acute setting of severe chest discomfort, particularly in a hemodynamically unstable patient, the differential diagnosis includes acute MI, pulmonary embolism, and aortic dissection. Prompt and accurate diagnostic evaluation, commonly with the use of invasive angiography, can be lifesaving in this situation.

Treatment

Medical Management of Stable Angina

The treatment of CAD and angina pectoris is multifaceted. The presence of CAD with or without angina requires the physician to recommend risk factor modification, frequently associated with lifestyle changes. For angina pectoris, pharmacologic therapy is typically used to control symptoms, allowing for maintenance of reasonable exercise tolerance. Revascularization is commonly used to control symptoms to a degree better than what can be achieved with medications alone, but only a small group of patients with CAD benefit from revascularization in terms of increased longevity.

It is also incumbent on the physician to recognize other medical conditions that can lower the threshold for angina, thus worsening symptoms and affecting quality of life. Anemia is a common medical problem that, when addressed, can significantly reduce the frequency of angina pectoris. Hyperthyroidism, with its increased metabolic demand and tachycardia, can increase the frequency of angina pectoris. Uncompensated congestive heart failure lowers the anginal threshold through the effects of LV dilation and filling pressure elevation on myocardial oxygen demand. Chronic obstructive pulmonary disease (COPD) and obstructive sleep apnea leading to hypoxemia can trigger angina pectoris.

Attention to the major modifiable risk factors for CAD is a cornerstone of therapy. Poorly controlled diabetes mellitus, hypertension, hyperlipidemia, and ongoing smoking all drive the progression of CAD and increase the risk for catastrophic events such as MI or sudden death. The wealth of clinical research on preventing death and disability from CAD has led to the development of evidence-based guidelines that form the basis of contemporary therapy for CAD (Table 8-4). Complete smoking cessation is a must for patients with CAD regardless

of the presence of symptoms. The use of statin medications to reduce LDL cholesterol (to <100 mg/dL, with possible additional benefit if ≤70 mg/dL) has revolutionized the therapy for CAD. Statins have been shown to reduce the risk of MI in patients with proven CAD and in those at significant risk. There is also interest low HDL levels, which appear to confer increased risk for coronary events. It is unclear whether niacin, which raises HDL, actually reduces the risk of MI or death. Exercise increases HDL levels and may confer protective effects through other mechanisms. Pharmacologic strategies to elevate HDL and hopefully reduce risk are under development.

Antiplatelet therapy is known to reduce the risk of MI in those who have known CAD or are at risk. Patients should be instructed to take aspirin, 81 to 325 mg/day (clopidogrel 75 mg/day may be used in those who are aspirin intolerant or allergic). Angiotensin-converting enzyme (ACE) inhibitors reduce the risk of recurrent MI and are also beneficial for patients with diabetes mellitus or reduced LV function. Angiotensin receptor blockers (ARBs) can be substituted in those who experience significant side effects from ACE inhibitors.

Regular aerobic exercise can benefit patients with CAD by reducing their risk for complications related to the disease. Aerobic exercise also increases exercise tolerance and may reduce the frequency of exercise-related angina pectoris. Positive benefits also accrue from weight loss related to exercise and improved blood pressure control. In sedentary individuals, isometric activities such as snow shoveling can trigger MI and should be avoided. There may be some benefits to judicious weight training in patients with CAD.

In addition to antiplatelet therapy, the commonly employed medications to control angina pectoris include β-blockers, nitrates, and calcium channel blockers. These agents work by correcting supply/demand blood flow mismatch that is the cause of myocardial ischemia and angina pectoris (Table 8-5). Interestingly, these drugs principally control symptoms in chronic stable angina pectoris, but they do not reduce mortality risk as therapy with aspirin or statins does.

Nitrates in various forms have a long history of use in patients with symptomatic CAD and can be very effective in controlling exertion-related angina. Nitrates work by venodilating large-capacitance veins and thus shifting blood out of the heart, reducing preload and myocardial oxygen demand. Nitrates are also potent coronary vasodilators and can reverse coronary spasm, allowing for improved perfusion. Short-duration but quick-acting sublingual nitroglycerin has been a mainstay both for treatment of an anginal episode and for prophylaxis against angina in situations where it is likely to occur. Patients who respond well to nitrates are frequently treated with long-acting oral or topical preparations. Both methods can effectively prevent angina pectoris, but continued use can induce tolerance. There is a recognized need for patients to have a nitrate-free period of about 8 hours every day to prevent tolerance. This usually involves cessation of use during sleep. Intravenous nitroglycerin administered by continuous drip is reserved for patients with unstable angina or acute MI.

β-Blocker therapy is very effective at reducing the likelihood of exertion-related angina. β-Blockers bind to cell surface β-receptors and by so doing reduce heart rate, contractility, and blood pressure, all of which tip the balance in favor of reduced oxygen demand and less angina. The use of β-blockers can be limited by the degree of bradycardia they induce or by baseline atrioventricular (AV) conduction abnormalities. Patients with higher degrees of AV block, β-blockers can induce complete heart block. These drugs also vary in their β-receptor selectivity. Blockade of β2-adrenergic receptors can lead to bronchospasm and vasoconstriction. Even selective β1-adrenergic antagonists such as atenolol and metoprolol have some β2 activity at higher doses. Intolerance of β-blockers can limit their use in patients with significant COPD or peripheral vascular disease. β-Blockers may also add to glucose intolerance and may affect lipids by increasing triglycerides or reducing HDL. In general, these effects do not preclude their use if they prove effective in controlling angina pectoris.

Calcium channel blocking drugs can decrease myocardial oxygen demand by causing arterial vasodilation, bradycardia, and decreased contractility. The magnitude of these effects varies according to the class of agent used. Dihydropyridines such as nifedipine and amlodipine cause arterial vasodilation leading to a blood pressure–lowering effect. In the dose ranges administered, they have no significant effect on contractility or heart rate. In contrast, verapamil, a phenylalkylamine, has significant effects on heart rate, AV conduction, and contractility. Benzothiazepine agents such as diltiazem manifest less vasodilation than dihydropyridines and less effect on contractility than phenylalkyamine drugs. The net effect of calcium channel blocking drugs is reduced myocardial oxygen demand and less angina pectoris. Diltiazem should be used with caution in patients who are also taking a β-blocker, because severe bradycardia or heart block can occur. Verapamil should not be co-administered with a β-blocker.

A newer class of antianginal drug is represented by ranolazine. This drug is a selective inhibitor of late sodium current and reduces sodium-induced calcium overload in myocytes. Although it has no effect on heart rate or blood pressure, ranolazine demonstrates antianginal properties. It is typically used when other medical therapy is insufficient in controlling angina.

Revascularization Therapy for Chronic Stable Angina Pectoris

Revascularization therapy is an option to be considered when medical therapy is not sufficiently controlling symptoms leading to impaired lifestyle. It is also frequently pursued in the face of high-risk situations such as unstable angina, STEMI, heart failure complicated by angina, arrhythmias associated with angina, or

TABLE 8-5 MEDICATIONS FOR ANGINA PECTORIS

DRUG CLASS	EXAMPLES	ANTIANGINAL EFFECT	PHYSIOLOGIC SIDE EFFECTS	COMMENTS
Nitroglycerin	Sublingual Topical Intravenous Oral	Decreased preload and afterload Coronary vasodilation Increased collateral blood flow	Headache Flushing Orthostasis	Tolerance develops with continuous use
β-Adrenergic blocking agents	Metoprolol Atenolol Propranolol Nadolol	Decreased heart rate Decreased blood pressure Decreased contractility	Bradycardia Hypotension Bronchospasm Depression	May worsen heart failure and AV conduction block; avoid in vasospastic angina
Calcium channel blocking agents (non-dihydropyridine)	Phenylalkylamine (verapamil) Benzothiazepine (diltiazem)	Decreased heart rate Decreased blood pressure Decreased contractility Coronary vasodilation	Bradycardia Hypotension Constipation with verapamil	May worsen heart failure and AV conduction
Calcium channel blocking agents	Dihydropyridine (nifedipine, amlodipine)	Decreased blood pressure Coronary vasodilation	Hypotension, reflex tachycardia Peripheral edema	Short-acting nifedipine is associated with increased risk for cardiovascular events.
Late sodium current blocking agents	Ranolazine	Inhibits cardiac late I_{Na} Prevents calcium overload	Dizziness Headache Constipation Nausea	No effects on blood pressure or heart rate Modest QTc prolongation

AV, Atrioventricular; I_{Na}, sodium current.

the presence of large areas of myocardial ischemia documented by noninvasive imaging. The two types of revascularization procedures are coronary bypass grafting (CABG) and percutaneous coronary intervention (PCI).

Percutaneous transluminal coronary angioplasty was the initial mode of catheter-based revascularization introduced in the late 1970s (see Video, Angioplasty, http://www.heartsite.com/html/ptca.html). In this technique, a guidewire is placed through a stenotic segment of artery, after which a balloon-tipped catheter is threaded over the wire to the area of stenosis and then inflated. Angioplasty of this form enlarges the vessel lumen in an irregular geometry through disruption of the plaque and injury to the vessel intima. Plain old balloon angioplasty (POBA), as the procedure later became to be known, was effective at improving myocardial perfusion and reducing exercise-related angina. However, because of plaque disruption, there was a 2% to 5% risk of abrupt vessel closure frequently leading to MI. In addition, there was a high incidence of injury-mediated restenosis (up to 50%) during the first 3 to 6 months after the procedure. The process of restenosis involved intimal hyperplasia and remodeling, yielding a recurrent stenosis sometimes more severe in nature than the original lesion.

The innovation of coronary stents pioneered through the 1980s and clinically available in the early 1990s represented a significant advance in PCI (see Video, Intracoronary Stenting, http://www.heartsite.com/html/stent.html). Coronary stents are expandable metallic mesh tubes that are mounted on an angioplasty balloon, allowing delivery to an area of stenosis, where balloon inflation expands the stent into the vessel wall. The stent becomes permanently embedded in the vessel wall and scaffolds the artery to keep it open. This procedure not only reduces the risk of abrupt vessel occlusion to 1% or less, but it is also associated with a significant reduction in restenosis risk (20% to 25%, compared with 50% for POBA). The benefit of stenting for a patient is clear in terms of less risk of procedure-related acute MI and less need for repeat procedures. Vessels smaller than 2 mm in diameter are not good targets for stenting, because the smallest-diameter stent is 2 mm. Stents do have a risk of thrombosis, necessitating lifelong aspirin therapy and the use of clopidogrel for 4 weeks to 1 year after the procedure (there may be some advantage to longer-duration clopidogrel for 1 year).

Despite the reduction achieved with coronary stents, there was still a significant risk of restenosis, leading investigators to search for a means to lower that risk. Drug-eluting stents (DES) were found to significantly reduce the risk of restenosis compared to bare metal stents. The first DES, released for use in 2003, was coated with either sirolimus or paclitaxel, both of which inhibited the hyperplastic response in the vessel wall triggered by PCI. The current generations of DES are coated with either zotarolimus or everolimus, both very effective at reducing restenosis. The predicted restenosis rate for current-generation DES is in the range of 5% to 10%. Vessel diameter affects restenosis risk, with larger-diameter vessels demonstrating less restenosis. The benefit of inhibiting tissue overgrowth within the stent is also associated with delayed endothelialization of the stent, which increases the risk of stent thrombosis for a longer time than with bare metal stents. Therefore, dual antiplatelet therapy with aspirin and clopidogrel should be maintained for at least 1 year.

Aspirin should never be discontinued after 1 year, to minimize the risk of late stent thrombosis. Decision making regarding the use of DES needs to take into account the patient's ability to tolerate long-term dual antiplatelet therapy, the potential for noncompliance with medications, and any need for major surgery in the near future after stent placement. The benefits of DES also confer the need for additional planning and caution.

A host of other devices to treat stenotic coronary arteries have come and gone over time. In this era, rotational atherectomy plays a role in treating calcified lesions in about 5% of patients. Catheter-based aspiration of thrombus has gained a role in patients with STEMI. Intravascular ultrasound is an important imaging adjunct than can be helpful in interrogating lesions or defining the end result of stent placement.

CABG emerged in the 1970s as an effective means of coronary revascularization for the control of angina. Bypass grafts take the form of saphenous vein from the leg, free radial artery segments, or intact left or right internal mammary artery grafts. The vein or radial artery grafts are placed on the ascending aorta and then anastomosed to the coronary vessels distal to the site of obstruction. In contrast, left or right internal mammary arteries are left intact at their origins and anastomosed distal to the obstruction. The left internal mammary artery is typically placed onto the left anterior descending coronary artery. This is the most important vessel to graft because of its size and distribution, and the left internal mammary artery is ideal given an expected patency rate of 90% at 10 years. Saphenous vein grafts degenerate over time, leading to episodes of symptomatic abrupt occlusion and a 50% patency rate at 10 years. Free radial artery grafts perform better than vein grafts but less well than intact mammary artery grafts. CABG is a major cardiac surgical procedure, but in skilled hands the mortality rate is expected to be 1% to 2%, with a similar risk of stroke. Periprocedural MI rates are in the range of 5% to 10%. There has been controversy over whether the use of the heart-lung machine to support CABG causes more problems for patients than "beating heart" surgery does. Recent studies suggest there is no long term difference in outcomes, such as death, MI, or stroke, for patients undergoing CABG, either on- or off-pump.

Most CABG procedures are performed for symptom control and are not likely to enhance longevity. The categories of patients likely to have life prolonged by CABG include those with a left main coronary artery more than 50% narrowed, those with severe three-vessel obstructive disease associated with a decrease in ejection fraction (EF, 35% to 50%), and those with two- or three-artery disease whose proximal left anterior descending artery is severely stenosed.

Clinical trials comparing CABG and PCI have consistently shown that patients undergoing CABG require fewer repeat procedures during the first 2 years after surgery. In the first 2 years, it is more likely that patients with PCI will experience symptomatic restenosis than that patients with CABG will have graft failure. Over time, this advantage is lost as vein grafts begin to fail 5 to 10 years after surgery. However, there is evidence that a survival advantage exists for diabetic patients with multivessel CAD who undergo CABG as opposed to PCI. A recent study also demonstrated long-term survival benefit for CABG over PCI in the face of multivessel CAD. Some of the survival advantage in favor of CABG may be linked to the use of the left internal mammary artery as a graft.

Despite the use of either revascularization technique, patients remain prone to progressive atherosclerotic disease with the potential to form plaque at previously unaffected sites. This necessitates aggressive long-term medical therapy and risk factor modification to achieve the lowest possible risk of symptomatic progression or MI. Retreatment with CABG is possible but is fraught with higher risk, and the outcome of repeat stenting for in-stent restenosis is never as good as for de novo lesions.

In a small group of patients, PCI and/or CABG fails and the patient has refractory angina. Once medical therapy has been maximized, few truly effective options remain. Transmyocardial laser revascularization in areas of ischemia has been used to reduce symptoms, but this technique is now of uncertain value. External counterpulsation is a technique whereby blood pressure cuffs are placed on each leg, inflated during diastole and deflated during systole. Patients typically have a 1-hour session that may be repeated 35 times. Angina relief has been reported with this procedure and may reflect some beneficial effect on endothelial function. Spinal cord stimulation using electrodes placed in the C7-T1 dorsal epidural space can reduce anginal symptoms in the short term, although the long-term role needs definition.

Other Anginal Syndromes

Variant Angina

Whereas typical angina pectoris is usually triggered by physical or emotional stress, some patients experience a syndrome termed *variant angina*. Variant angina was first described in 1959 by Prinzmetal and colleagues, who observed patients with chest discomfort at rest, not triggered by physical or emotional stress, and associated with ST segment elevation (Fig. 8-4). Episodes of AV block and ventricular ectopy were observed, but MI was not a common feature. These patients typically did not have the common CAD risk factors other than smoking. Coronary angiography demonstrated these patients to be experiencing transient coronary vasospasm. The vasospasm tended to occur in an area of atherosclerotic plaque, but some patients had spasm in angiographically normal segments of coronary artery.

In the course of investigating the pathophysiology of variant angina, a number of provocative tests were developed to induce coronary spasm in susceptible individuals. Intracoronary ergonovine or acetylcholine can induce spasm in patients with variant angina, probably as a result of underlying endothelial dysfunction. Other spasm-inducing provocations include the cold pressor test (placing a hand in an ice bath), the induction of alkalosis (hyperventilation or intravenous bicarbonate), and histamine infusion. Provocative testing to induce coronary vasospasm has fallen out of favor in the routine assessment of patients with angina.

Coronary vasospasm usually resolves promptly with the administration of nitroglycerin (sublingual, intravenous, or intra-arterial). The combination of oral nitrates and calcium channel blockers is often used to prevent spasm. β-Blockers may aggravate coronary spasm by inhibiting the action of vasodilating β_2-receptors, allowing for unopposed α-receptor induced vasoconstriction. Rare patients do not respond to vasodilator medical therapy and may benefit from coronary stent placement in spasm-prone atherosclerotic lesions.

Microvascular Angina with Normal Coronary Arteries

Angina can occur in some patients in the face of normal-appearing coronary arteries and no provocable spasm. Decreased endothelium-dependent vasodilation may be the underlying pathophysiology of microvascular angina. Patients with this condition may demonstrate an increase in coronary resistance and an inability to increase coronary blood flow sufficiently when challenged by increases in myocardial oxygen demand. Women are more likely to be affected with microvascular angina, and the symptoms not uncommonly occur at rest or with emotional stress. Exercise can also trigger angina.

A host of diagnostic tests can detect the presence of ischemia in patients with microvascular angina. In the case of stress testing, ST changes of ischemia can be detected as well as nuclear

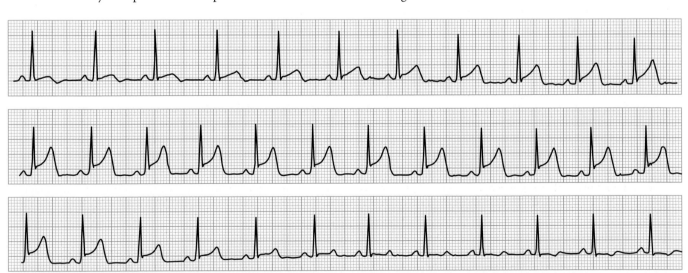

FIGURE 8-4 Continuous electrocardiogram recording in a patient with Prinzmetal (variant) angina. The spontaneous onset of chest discomfort began during the *top strip,* accompanied by transient ST-segment elevation. By the *bottom strip,* several minutes later, both discomfort and ST-segment elevation had resolved.

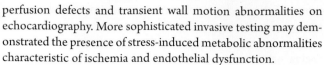

perfusion defects and transient wall motion abnormalities on echocardiography. More sophisticated invasive testing may demonstrated the presence of stress-induced metabolic abnormalities characteristic of ischemia and endothelial dysfunction.

Exercise-related ischemic symptoms may respond to β-blocker therapy. Microvascular angina also tends to respond well to nitrates, both short-acting sublingual nitroglycerin and long-acting oral nitrates. Calcium channel antagonists are sometimes used together with nitrates to control angina related to microvascular ischemia.

Silent Myocardial Ischemia

Not all episodes of myocardial ischemia are associated with angina. Some patients may only experience episodes of silent myocardial ischemia as evidenced by transient ST depression with ECG monitoring. Such patients can also have silent MI. It is also possible, and probably not uncommon, for patients to have both silent myocardial ischemia episodes and typical angina; this is termed *mixed angina*. Episodes of silent myocardial ischemia can be observed in all settings of CAD: chronic stable angina, unstable angina, and coronary vasospasm. Silent ischemia is more common in diabetic patients. Medical therapy directed at controlling symptomatic angina also reduces the number of episodes of silent ischemia.

Prognosis

Contemporary therapies for stable ischemic heart disease have significantly reduced the risks of cardiac events and mortality. The annual rate of major ischemic events such as MI is in the range of 1% to 2%, and the yearly mortality rate is 1% to 3%. CAD is frequently associated with systemic vascular disease, making these patients prone to a host of other events. Patients with stable ischemic heart disease have a yearly combined outcome risk for cardiovascular death, MI, or stroke in the range of 4.5%.

Despite advances in medical and revascularization therapies, up to 30% of patients face some limiting symptoms of recurrent angina. Revascularization does not abolish the need for ongoing antianginal medical therapy in 80% of patients.

Patients with stable ischemic heart disease should first be treated with medical therapy appropriate to reduce the risk of ischemic events (aspirin, statins) and to control symptoms of angina (nitrates, β-blockers, calcium channel antagonists). Revascularization therapy with either PCI or CABG is an option for patients who continue to have lifestyle-limiting symptoms despite the use of medical therapy and risk factor modification. The goal of all therapies for patients with stable ischemic heart disease should be individualized, taking advantage of information from controlled trials and directed at improving overall lifestyle and reducing the risk of death and disability due to progressive CAD or systemic vascular disease.

Acute Coronary Syndrome: Unstable Angina and NSTEMI

Definition

Asymptomatic CAD or chronic stable angina may undergo transition to a more aggressive stage of disease called acute coronary syndrome (ACS). ACS comprises a spectrum of clinical presentations, ranging from unstable angina to NSTEMI or STEMI. Unstable angina represents the new onset of angina at rest or on exertion, or an increase in frequency of previously stable anginal symptoms, particularly at rest. ACS manifesting as MI, either NSTEMI or STEMI, is differentiated from unstable angina on the basis of prolonged symptoms, characteristic ECG changes, and the presence of biomarkers in blood. Unstable angina may be a harbinger of either NSTEMI or STEMI, and the diagnosis of unstable angina identifies a patient who requires careful assessment and treatment.

Epidemiology

The occurrence of ACS represents a significant clinical event in up to 1.4 million Americans annually. One third of those categorized as having ACS are diagnosed with NSTEMI. More than half of patients with NSTEMI are 65 years of age or older, and approximately one-half are women. NSTEMI is more common in patients with diabetes, peripheral vascular disease, or chronic inflammatory disease (e.g., rheumatoid arthritis).

Primary ACS is the most common form of the disease and reflects underlying plaque rupture leading to intracoronary thrombus formation and limitation of blood flow. Secondary ACS reflects imbalances in myocardial oxygen supply and demand leading to myocardial ischemia. Examples of decreased oxygen supply include profound anemia, systemic hypotension, and hypoxemia. Increased demand occurs in the face of severe systemic hypertension, fever, tachycardia, and thyrotoxicosis. Secondary ACS not uncommonly unmasks previously asymptomatic obstructive CAD, but it may also occur in the absence of CAD. Treatment of secondary ACS is directed at correcting the underlying medical condition.

Pathology

Most patients who experience NSTEMI do so as a result of plaque rupture with subsequent thrombosis causing subtotal occlusion of the coronary artery. The limitation of coronary blood flow in this situation leads to subendocardial ischemia in the distribution of the affected coronary artery. The same pathology underlies STEMI, although in that case complete vessel occlusion occurs, leading to more extensive MI. It is possible for patients with obstructive CAD to develop collateral support of the affected artery, and in that case plaque rupture with complete vessel occlusion may lead to NSTEMI as opposed to STEMI.

A smaller percentage of patients have ACS due to coronary vasospasm, which, if severe and prolonged, can lead to myocardial necrosis. Vasospasm may occur in regions of endothelial dysfunction induced by atherosclerotic plaque, or it may be triggered by exogenous vasoconstrictors such as cocaine ingestion, the use of serotonin agonists (for migraine therapy), or chemotherapeutic agents (e.g., 5-fluorouracil). Less common causes of ACS include coronary vasculitis and spontaneous coronary dissection (peripartum coronary dissection).

Atherosclerotic plaques rich in LDL are prone to develop inflammation, which in turn degrades the collagen-rich fibrous cap, leading to rupture and thrombosis. Oxidized LDL within the plaque leads to accumulation of macrophages and T lymphocytes, causing inflammation within the plaque. Cytokines elaborated in the inflammatory process inhibit collage synthesis. The fibrous structure of the plaque is further compromised by matrix metalloproteinases released by macrophages. Degradation of the plaques' fibrous structure makes them prone to rupture. Systemic inflammatory conditions may also play a role in plaque rupture in some patients. It is possible to have multiple sites of plaque ulceration or rupture.

Plaque rupture leads to platelet adherence and subsequent activation at the site of rupture. As platelets aggregate, the thrombosis cascade is triggered, leading to progressive accumulation of intravascular thrombus. The severity of myocardial ischemia and MI depends on the degree to which thrombus occludes the vessel. It is also possible for ACS to occur as a result of embolization of platelet aggregates or thrombus.

Clinical Presentation

ACS may manifest as a first symptom of angina pectoris in a previously asymptomatic patient. Alternatively, patients with pre-existing angina pectoris experience more frequent angina, angina at lower levels of exertion, or angina at rest. Patients who have developed ACS commonly experience their typical symptom of angina in terms of location and radiation but with increased intensity and duration. Patients with subtotal or total occlusion of a coronary artery may be much less responsive or completely unresponsive to the effects of nitroglycerin.

Physical examination during myocardial ischemia may reveal a patient is who is clearly anxious and uncomfortable and who may also be experiencing dyspnea, nausea, or vomiting. Sinus tachycardia and hypertension is a common response to the discomfort of ACS, but in some instances sinus bradycardia and varying degrees of heart block may be observed. Bradyarrhythmias may also be associated with hypotension. Auscultation may reveal the presence of an S_4, reflecting diminished LV compliance, or an S_3 if there is extensive LV dysfunction. In the case of ischemia-induced papillary muscle dysfunction, the systolic murmur of mitral regurgitation can be heard. Patients with large areas of ischemic myocardium develop elevated LV filling pressures leading to pulmonary congestion, dyspnea, and the physical finding of rales on lung auscultation.

Diagnosis

Patients presenting with ACS require urgent care directed at rapid diagnosis and treatment. The ECG is critically important in early diagnosis of presumed ACS. The finding of ST elevation in multiple leads (Fig. 8-5) is diagnostic of STEMI and portends a more extensive MI and the need for prompt revascularization. The distribution of ST elevation reflects the region of myocardium affected by thrombotic coronary occlusion. For example, ST elevation in leads II, III, and aVF reflects an inferior MI due to occlusion of the right coronary artery (or circumflex coronary artery in some cases). ST elevation in leads V_2 through V_6 (see Fig. 8-5) reflects an anterior MI caused by obstruction of the left anterior descending coronary artery.

Unstable angina or NSTEMI is caused by subtotal vessel occlusion by thrombus leading to reduced coronary blood flow. This results in subendocardial ischemia and the characteristic ECG changes of ST depression (Fig. 8-6). It is important to recognize that up to half of patients with acute MI do not have significant ECG abnormalities on the initial study. Sequential ECGs are frequently required to establish a diagnosis. If there is a high index of suspicion for MI and ECGs are persistently nondiagnostic, the use of leads extending to the patient's back (V_7 to V_9) may demonstrate ST changes related to posterior LV ischemia (usually a circumflex coronary artery occlusion). Echocardiography showing regional wall motion abnormalities can also help to establish the diagnosis of acute MI.

Serum biomarkers also play an important role in the diagnosis of acute MI. Myocardial necrosis leads to the release of biomarkers that can be measured in serial fashion to document the occurrence of MI. The presence of specific biomarkers is

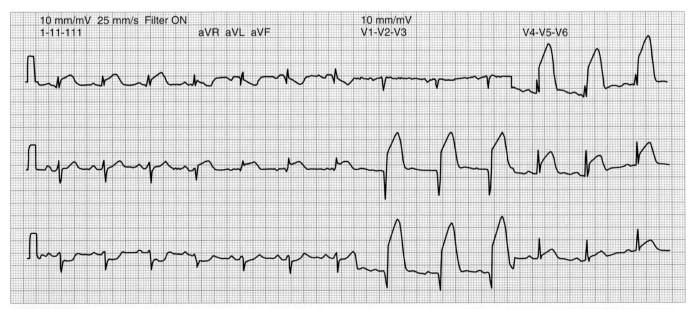

FIGURE 8-5 Acute anterolateral myocardial infarction. Leads I, aVL, and V_2 to V_6 demonstrate ST-segment elevation. Reciprocal ST-segment depression is seen in leads II, III, and aVF. Deep Q waves have developed in leads V_2 and V_3.

Boston University Hospital

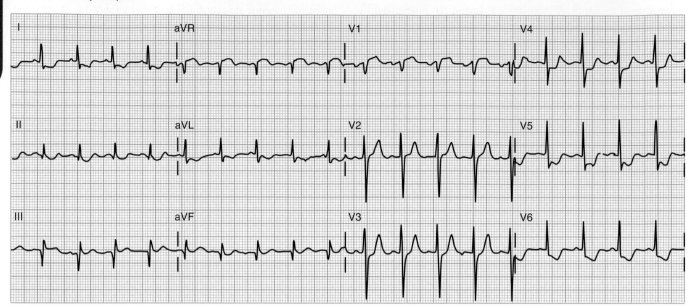

FIGURE 8-6 Marked ST-segment depression in a patient with prolonged chest pain resulting from an acute non–ST-segment elevation myocardial infarction. Between 1 and 3 mm of ST-segment depression is seen in leads I, aVL, and V_4 to V_6. The patient was known to have had a previous inferior myocardial infarction.

definitive evidence of MI, and they are particularly helpful to provide prognostic significance when symptoms are mild and ECG changes are minimal. Common biomarkers include creatine kinase (CK), troponin I, troponin T, lactate dehydrogenase (LDH), and aspartate aminotransferase (AST). Sequential measurement of biomarkers demonstrates their various time courses for abnormal elevation after an acute MI (Fig. 8-7). This information can be helpful in retrospectively timing the occurrence of an event. In contemporary practice, troponin has become the most frequently measured biomarker, although CK is still used. LDH and AST are no longer routinely measured for the diagnosis of MI.

Troponins I and T are the most sensitive and most specific markers of myocardial necrosis, and as a consequence, they have become the standard in the biochemical diagnosis of acute MI. The myocardial-specific isozyme CK-MB may be in the normal range while concomitant measurement of troponin I or T reveals the presence of myocardial necrosis. Troponins I and T begin to rise within 4 hours of myocardial necrosis and remain elevated for 7 to 10 days after the MI event. Confounding elevations of troponin T occur in patients with renal failure and congestive heart failure not related to ACS. Troponin release also occurs in the case of demand ischemia not related to coronary thrombosis. This requires careful attention to the entire clinical presentation in discerning the likelihood of underlying ACS due to coronary thrombosis.

In the absence of clear evidence of NSTEMI (i.e., normal examination, ECG findings, and biomarkers), patients who present with the diagnosis of unstable angina should undergo stress testing. A negative exercise stress test is very helpful for distinguishing those patients who require more aggressive diagnostic testing (e.g., catheterization) from those who can be monitored as outpatients. Some centers have embraced the use of CT coronary angiography in the assessment of low-risk patients. This

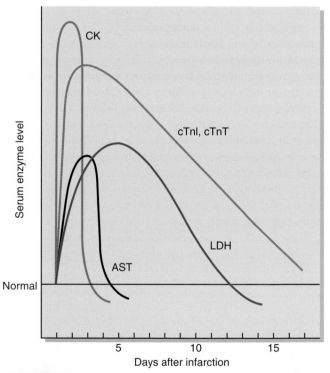

FIGURE 8-7 Typical time course for the detection of enzymes released after myocardial infarction. AST, Serum aspartate aminotransferase; CK, creatine kinase; cTnI, cardiac troponin I; cTnT, cardiac troponin T; LDH, lactate dehydrogenase.

technique has a high negative predictive value in establishing a diagnosis of CAD.

Echocardiography can be helpful in patients with equivocal ECG findings for ischemia and normal biomarkers. The presence of regional wall motion abnormalities, particularly if they correlate with the distribution of ECG abnormalities, raises the risk for underlying CAD as a cause of symptoms. The echocardiogram may also show evidence of other abnormalities as causes of chest discomfort, such as pericarditis, pulmonary embolism, or aortic dissection.

Patients with a high risk for future coronary events should be directed toward coronary angiography. In the absence of contraindications, coronary angiography is indicated for patients with clear evidence of NSTEMI based on clinical presentation of symptoms, ECG changes, and positive biomarkers. Patients undergoing evaluation for unstable angina who have significant stress test abnormalities are also candidates for coronary angiography. Some patients who have ambiguous stress test findings or ongoing symptoms in the absence of other findings of NSTEMI require coronary angiography to resolve the issue as to whether underlying CAD is present.

Up to 15% of patients undergoing coronary angiography for NSTEMI have no significant obstructive CAD. In a number of patients, there will be a clear "culprit" lesion showing the earmarks of plaque rupture with ulceration, associated thrombus, or reduced coronary flow. Lesions that may have played a role in symptoms, ECG findings, or biomarker release that are not clearly stenotic may be assessed for physiologic significance with the use of a fractional flow reserve (FFR) study using a pressure wire device.

Patients who have new-onset chest pain require careful monitoring in an appropriate care setting that allows for rhythm monitoring as well as repeat evaluations of ECG findings and biomarker measurements. Risk assessment is aided by the use of risk scores calculated with either the Thrombolysis in Myocardial Infarction (TIMI) or the Global Registry of Acute Coronary Events (GRACE) algorithms (see Chapter 72, "Acute Coronary Syndrome: Unstable Angina and Non-ST Elevation Myocardial Infarction," in *Goldman-Cecil Medicine,* 25th Edition). The overall assessment in cases of new symptoms of chest discomfort aims to triage patients based on risk for coronary events. Low-risk patients can be spared aggressive anticoagulation protocols and coronary angiography, whereas high-risk patients are likely to benefit from these approaches. The use of appropriate therapies in high-risk patients (medical therapy or revascularization or both) leads to a 20% to 40% decrease in recurrent ischemic events and a 10% reduction in mortality.

Differential Diagnosis

The initial assessment of patients with possible ACS should include consideration of other potentially life-threatening conditions such as pulmonary embolism and aortic dissection. These considerations are particularly important if the patient's presentation does not entirely fit that of ACS. Pulmonary embolism can be associated with ECG changes and troponin elevation, and such findings lead to early use of coronary angiography. If there is no CAD-related explanation of the patient's presentation, prompt investigation for pulmonary embolism is warranted. If the patient has findings suggestive of aortic dissection, that diagnosis should be aggressively pursued with appropriate imaging techniques, given the high risk of mortality associated with that disease. Valvular heart diseases such as aortic stenosis or regurgitation and hypertrophic cardiomyopathy can manifest with symptoms and ECG findings suggestive of ACS. Physical examination should aid in consideration of these conditions. Pericarditis and myopericarditis can also present diagnostic dilemmas related to chest pain, ECG abnormalities (ST and T-wave changes mimicking ischemia), and positive biomarkers. Stress cardiomyopathy (Takotsubo's syndrome) also manifests with chest pain, T-wave inversion, and positive biomarkers. Patients with this diagnosis frequently undergo urgent catheterization to assess for CAD. The absence of a culprit lesion and findings of characteristic wall motion abnormalities establish the diagnosis.

Treatment

Patients with chest pain suggestive of ACS need urgent evaluation for evidence of ischemia (serial ECGs) and myocardial necrosis (serial biomarkers). Serial biomarker measurements, in the current era usually troponin, establish the diagnosis of MI. Continuous ECG monitoring is important given the risk of ischemia-mediated arrhythmias, and serial ECGs establish a pattern of ST changes consistent with ischemia. Patients are also prescribed bedrest and supplemental oxygen. Those with a high index of suspicion for ACS require hospital admission for observation and appropriate diagnostic testing. Chest pain lends itself well to diagnosis and treatment algorithms that guide the clinician through decision trees based on expert opinion and evidence-based medicine (see Chapter 72, "Acute Coronary Syndrome: Unstable Angina and Non-ST Elevation Myocardial Infarction," in *Goldman-Cecil Medicine,* 25th Edition). STEMI is typically diagnosed at the time of initial presentation. Those without evidence of ST elevation can be risk stratified, as discussed earlier, using the guidance of recurrent symptoms, ECG changes, or abnormal biomarker levels. Treatment of patients who are categorized as having unstable angina or NSTEMI is directed by their allocation to either low- or high-risk status.

Once recognized as having ACS, patients require antiplatelet therapy with aspirin (75 to 162 mg per day) and clopidogrel, because plaque rupture and thrombosis is a frequent underlying pathology. Prasugrel, another thienopyridine, is an option in place of clopidogrel for those going to coronary angiography. Antiplatelet therapy significantly reduces mortality risk in patients with NSTEMI. The aspirin/clopidogrel combination is indicated as ongoing therapy in the year following diagnosis of NSTEMI. Symptoms of chest discomfort can be treated with nitrates (sublingual, topical, or intravenous drip) and β-blockers. The latter therapy slows heart rate and reduces blood pressure, effects that translate into reduced myocardial oxygen demand in the face of limited supply. It is important not to give nitrates to patients who have taken phosphodiesterase-5 inhibitors (sildenafil, tadalafil, or vardenafil) within the previous 24 to 48 hours. Attention to this detail minimizes the risk for nitrate-induced hypotension. Calcium channel antagonists may be used in lieu of β-blockers, particularly if there is a need for blood pressure control, but they should be avoided in patients with reduced EF or overt heart failure. The dihydropyridine calcium channel blocker nifedipine can be effective in controlling blood pressure and promoting coronary vasodilation, but it should be given in conjunction with a β-blocker because of the potential for the drug to induce reflex tachycardia and thereby increase myocardial oxygen demand.

Glycoprotein IIb/IIIa inhibitors block platelet aggregation and can reduce ischemic events in patients undergoing PCI as treatment for NSTEMI. These drugs are usually reserved for high-risk patients at the time of PCI. They require intravenous administration and are given for 12 to 24 hours after PCI. The use of this class of drugs for PCI has decreased in light of data suggesting advantages of bivalirudin, a direct thrombin inhibitor, over the glycoprotein IIb/IIIa inhibitors.

Heparin, given in its unfractionated form or as a low-molecular-weight (LMW) preparation, has been shown to reduce the risk of ischemic complications in patients with NSTEMI. Heparin acts by activating antithrombin and thereby inhibiting the formation and activity of thrombin. The anti-ischemic effect of heparin is additive to that of aspirin. Unfractionated heparin is given by continuous intravenous drip for up to 48 hours. It is usually not continued after revascularization. Heparin may be associated with mild thrombocytopenia, and 1% to 5% of patients experience profound antibody-mediated thrombocytopenia. These patients usually have been exposed to heparin in the past, and a known diagnosis of heparin-induced thrombocytopenia necessitates the use of alternative antithrombin therapy.

LMW heparins are fragments of unfractionated heparin that are more predictable in their antithrombin activity and are associated with reduced risks for thrombocytopenia and bleeding complications. The drug should be avoided in patients who have a history of heparin-induced thrombocytopenia. Clinical studies of patients with NSTEMI have shown superiority of LMW heparin over unfractionated heparin in reducing the end point of death or MI during hospitalization. LMW heparin, either enoxaparin or dalteparin, is administered subcutaneously for up to 8 days after hospitalization. As with unfractionated heparin, LMW heparin is not continued after revascularization. Dosing of LMW heparin in based on renal function status, age, and weight. LMW heparin has a long duration of action and cannot be reversed with protamine. Unfractionated heparin has a shorter duration of action and is reversible with protamine, making unfractionated heparin the preferred anticoagulant for patients who may require CABG.

Fondaparinux is a selective factor Xa inhibitor that does not induce thrombocytopenia. It can reduce ischemic events in patients with NSTEMI and is associated with a lower risk of bleeding than is seen with enoxaparin. There is an increased risk of catheter-related thrombosis in patients treated with fondaparinux who are undergoing coronary angiography. This drug is reserved for cases that will be managed noninvasively and where there is a higher risk for heparin-related bleeding.

Bivalirudin, a direct thrombin inhibitor, is an alternative to heparin for patients who are undergoing PCI. It is as effective as the combination of heparin and glycoprotein IIb/IIIa inhibitor in reducing the risk of ischemic complications related to PCI, and it is associated with a reduced risk of postprocedure bleeding. Bivalirudin is used preferentially in patients with a history of heparin-induced thrombocytopenia.

Statin therapy is also indicated in patients with NSTEMI at presentation. Statins act to stabilize plaque and improve endothelial function. These drugs should be initiated at the time of admission to the hospital and continued after discharge. There is

evidence that high-dose atorvastatin (80 mg/day) given to patients with NSTEMI reduces the risk of subsequent ischemic events.

Risk stratification is important in appropriately evaluating patients with ACS. Low-risk patients (age <75 years, normal troponin levels, 0 to 2 TIMI risk factors) should be evaluated with noninvasive testing, either exercise or pharmacologic stress testing. before hospital discharge. Those with tests are positive for ischemia should be considered for predischarge coronary angiography. This approach leads to selective use of invasive testing and subsequent revascularization. Patients with high-risk ACS profiles (age >75 years, elevated troponin levels, ≥3 TIMI risk factors) are candidates for coronary angiography and, when appropriate, revascularization. The high-risk ACS patient group will have fewer subsequent ischemic events when approached in this way. Risk stratification occurs early after admission for possible ACS. An early invasive strategy (coronary angiography within 24 hours of admission) for high-risk patients has been shown to reduce the combined end point of death, MI, or stroke compared with a delayed invasive approach. The occurrence of acute heart failure, hypotension, or ventricular arrhythmias in the face of ACS prompts urgent coronary angiography to identify patients with high-risk coronary anatomy that requires urgent revascularization (see Video, Cardiac Cath, http://www.heartsite.com/html/cardiac_cath.html).

Invasive coronary angiography always carries with it a risk of bleeding complications that is no doubt enhanced by the concomitant use of potent antiplatelet and antithrombin therapies. Those at increased risk for bleeding complications include patients with female gender, low body weight, diabetes mellitus, renal insufficiency, low hematocrit, and hypertension. Some cardiologists recommend the preferential use of a radial artery approach to catheterization in order to minimize bleeding complications that are associated with the femoral artery approach.

Prognosis

The extent and magnitude of ST depression noted on ECG in patients with NSTEMI predicts mortality risk. Patients who exhibit 2 mm or more of ST depression in multiple leads have a 10-fold increased mortality rate at 1 year. The degree of elevation in troponin also identifies patients with an increased risk of mortality during the following year. It has also been observed that the combined measurement of troponin, hsCRP, and brain natriuretic peptide (BNP) predicts an increased mortality risk better than any individual biomarker.

Contemporary practice significantly reduced the risk of mortality for patients with ACS at presentation. Risk stratification with appropriate revascularization and use of antiplatelet therapy, statins, and overall coronary risk factor reduction also contribute to this decrease in mortality risk. Whereas the immediate mortality risk for patients with NSTEMI is lower than for patients with STEMI (5% vs. 7%), those with NSTEMI are more prone to subsequent recurrent coronary events. The cumulative mortality rate for STEMI and NSTEMI is similar at 6 months after presentation (12% vs.13%). NSTEMI identifies a patient group with significant long-term mortality risk who require aggressive attention to modifiable coronary risk factors.

Acute STEMI and Complications of Myocardial Infarction

Definition and Epidemiology

Sustained myocardial ischemia, regardless of its cause, can result in myocardial necrosis, which underlies the clinical syndrome of MI. MI represents a spectrum of myocardial necrosis, from relatively small amounts of muscle in the case of demand ischemia, to more extensive subendocardial MI that characterizes NSTEMI, to typically large transmural MIs commonly manifesting as STEMI. The current accepted definition of acute MI accounts for clinical setting and mechanism. STEMI represents the range of large MIs that are almost always caused by total occlusion of an epicardial coronary artery resulting in extensive transmural myonecrosis (Fig. 8-8). In contrast, NSTEMI reflects subtotal coronary occlusion leading to subendocardial myonecrosis. Whereas both NSTEMI and STEMI are life-threatening, their different underlying mechanisms mandate different therapeutic strategies and affect the urgency with which they are applied.

One half of all deaths in the United States and developed countries are related to cardiovascular disease. In the United States, there are approximately 1.2 million nonfatal or fatal MIs each year. CAD plays a role in 650,000 deaths each year, and 250,000 deaths are caused by acute MI. One half of patients with acute MI at presentation die within 1 hour of onset, before therapy can be instituted. Of the 5 million patients who come to emergency rooms with chest pain, 1.5 million are admitted to hospital with ACS. In this group of patients, the presence of ST elevation on ECG or an LBBB indicates the diagnosis of STEMI and the need for prompt intervention to open an occluded coronary artery. STEMI accounts for 30% of all MIs, but this mechanism of MI is associated with the highest immediate mortality risk, prompting the need for urgent therapeutic intervention.

Pathology

Lipid-rich coronary plaques are subject to inflammation incited by the response to oxidation of LDL-cholesterol within the plaque. A sequence of inflammatory events leads to macrophage accumulation and the elaboration of metalloproteinases that degrade collagen in the fibrous cap of the plaque. Thinning of the fibrous cap makes the plaque vulnerable to rupture and exposure of blood to thrombogenic stimuli, resulting in platelet aggregation and activation, thrombin generation, and the evolution of fibrin-based thrombus. If the occlusion is total, transmural myocardial ischemia and necrosis ensue and the ECG demonstrates ST elevation. In contrast, partially occlusive thrombus can result in unstable angina or NSTEMI (subendocardial MI). The presence of coronary collaterals can limit the extent of ischemia and necrosis in either scenario. Both STEMI and NSTEMI can set the stage for arrhythmias and LV dysfunction. Whereas coronary thrombosis is the cause of most MIs, there are patients who develop MI related to coronary embolization, coronary vasospasm, vasculitis, coronary anomalies, dissection of the aorta or a coronary artery, or trauma.

One key feature of the pathology of MI is its time-dependent nature. Experimental and clinical studies have documented that coronary occlusion leads to ischemia and myonecrosis in a wave-front manner, from endocardium to epicardium. Restoration of flow to the vessel within 6 hours after occlusion is associated with limitation of infarct size and a favorable effect on mortality risk. The principle of time dependency of MI drives the need to aggressively reperfuse occluded coronary arteries, and this is the cornerstone of contemporary therapy for STEMI.

Clinical Presentation

Patients with acute MI usually have a combination of chest discomfort, ECG changes (ST elevation in contiguous leads or LBBB), and elevation in biomarkers such as CK-MB and troponin. The high sensitivity and high specificity of troponin have made it the preferred biomarker in the diagnosis of MI. The chest discomfort associated with MI is similar to angina pectoris but more severe in nature. It is usually described as substernal pressure, tightness, or fullness. Patients may have symptoms of discomfort that radiate to the neck, jaw, one or both arms, or the back. Not uncommonly, patients with symptoms of acute MI also experience nausea, vomiting, diaphoresis, apprehension, dyspnea, or weakness. In contrast to angina pectoris associated with stable CAD, acute MI symptoms last longer than 20 to 30 minutes (up to hours).

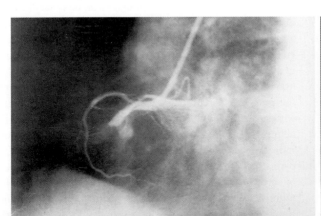
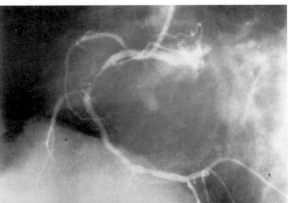

FIGURE 8-8 Right coronary artery angiogram in a patient with acute inferior myocardial infarction. The *left panel* demonstrates total occlusion of the right coronary artery. The *right panel* depicts restoration of flow 90 minutes after the intravenous administration of tissue-type plasminogen activator.

Occasionally, patients only have symptoms in the non-chest areas usually associated with radiation. Up to 20% of patients, particularly the elderly and diabetics, do not have typical chest discomfort at presentation. The index of suspicion for acute MI should be high in these groups if the patient exhibits profound weakness, acute dyspnea or pulmonary edema, nausea, vomiting, ventricular arrhythmias, or hypotension. The differential diagnosis for patients with chest discomfort suspicious for acute MI includes aortic dissection, pulmonary embolism, chest wall pain, esophageal reflux, acute pericarditis, pleuritis, and panic attacks. Given the life-threatening nature of aortic dissection and pulmonary embolism, these diagnoses should always be paramount, along with acute MI, in patients presenting with chest discomfort.

Physical Examination

A comprehensive examination should be undertaken if acute MI is suspected. Attention must be paid to vital signs, because patients may be either hypertensive or hypotensive during the course of an MI. In some cases, such as inferior MI, profound bradycardia may be present. Auscultation of the heart may reveal an S_4. In the case of a large MI, the patient may have symptoms and signs of heart failure such as dyspnea, rales, elevated central venous pressure, and an S_3. Severe heart failure may lead to cardiogenic shock with hypotension and vasoconstriction causing the extremities to be cool to touch. Patients with acute MI are also subject to mechanical problems such as mitral regurgitation due to papillary muscle dysfunction.

Electrocardiogram

The ECG is an important tool in the diagnosis of acute MI. ST elevation of 1 mm or greater in contiguous leads is seen in most patients with acute MI. The initial ECG may be nondiagnostic, so it is important to obtain serial tracings no more than 20 minutes apart to detect the evolutionary changes characteristic of STEMI. The first stage of ECG presentation is ST elevation that subtends the region of the heart affected by transmural ischemia. ST depression may be present in opposing leads, and these are termed *reciprocal changes* (see Chapter 73, "ST Elevation Acute Myocardial Infarction and Complications of Myocardial Infarction," in *Goldman-Cecil Medicine*, 25th Edition). The presence of reciprocal changes may indicate a larger and more threatening MI. As the MI progresses, ST elevation gives way to T wave inversion. Varying degrees of resolution of ST and T wave changes occur over time, but patients with transmural MI develop pathologic Q waves in the leads subtending the infarcted muscle. Other causes of ST elevation include pericarditis and a chronic repolarization finding of "early repolarization." The presence of either cause of ST elevation can confound the early ECG diagnosis of acute MI.

Approximately 30% of acute MIs originate from the circumflex coronary artery on the posterior wall of the heart. This type of MI appears on the ECG as precordial ST depression. The presence of precordial ST depression should raise suspicion of the presence of "true posterior MI," and additional leads placed through the axilla to the back may reveal the presence of posterior ST elevation. Echocardiography demonstrating posterior hypokinesis is also useful in discriminating true posterior MI. Acute inferior MI due to occlusion of the right coronary artery can also be associated with right ventricular infarction if the right coronary artery's acute marginal branch is compromised. Right ventricular infarction can lead to some challenging management issues, and its diagnosis is aided by the use of right precordial leads to detect ST elevation.

LBBB can mask ST elevation due to acute MI. Patients with clinical features of acute MI who have an LBBB (particularly a new LBBB) should be presumed to have STEMI and treated appropriately. Right bundle branch block (RBBB) does not mask the ST elevation of STEMI.

Differential Diagnosis

The diagnosis of STEMI is usually straightforward based on symptoms and ECG findings, but a number of conditions can mimic the ST elevation of STEMI and confound the diagnosis. The ECG changes of early repolarization, Takotsubo's syndrome, acute myocarditis, or pericarditis can be difficult or impossible to distinguish from those of STEMI. In the face of ST elevation and chest discomfort, it may be necessary to perform coronary angiography in patients who ultimately are diagnosed with a condition other than STEMI so as to not miss this critical diagnosis.

Diagnostic Testing

Cardiac troponins (cTnI and cTnT) are sarcomere proteins that, when measured in blood, are specific for myocardial injury. The troponin level becomes elevated 2 to 4 hours after the onset of injury, and the abnormal elevation can persist for up to 2 weeks after the event. The CK-MB isomere is not as specific for heart injury as troponin, but it can still be useful in documenting the presence of MI. CK-MB is found elevated within 4 hours after an acute MI, but it clears more rapidly than troponin. In the case of persistently elevated troponin, a measurable increase in CK-MB may herald another episode of myocardial necrosis. Chronic renal insufficiency is associated with false-positive elevations of troponin T, more so than troponin I. In addition to biomarkers of myocardial injury, other laboratory studies obtained in patients with acute MI include a complete blood count, blood chemistries, lipid panel, prothrombin time (PT), and partial thromboplastin time (PTT). Leukocytosis is a common finding in acute MI, reflecting the inflammatory nature of myocardial necrosis.

At the time of admission, chest radiographs are obtained to assess for the presence of pulmonary edema or mediastinal widening suspicious for dissection. Echocardiography is important in delineating the extent of MI and assessing EF. In cases of diagnostic ambiguity, early use of echocardiography can demonstrate the presence of regional wall motion abnormalities consistent with acute MI. Echocardiography with color Doppler is also helpful in diagnosing complications of acute MI such as infarct-related mitral regurgitation or ventricular septal defect (VSD), pericardial effusion, or evidence of pseudoaneurysm as a result of myocardial rupture. Follow-up echocardiography in the months after acute MI can also reveal recovery of LV function. Radionuclide tracer studies are not useful in diagnosing acute MI. CT, cardiac MRI, and transesophageal echocardiography are all useful in diagnosing aortic dissection when there is an increased index of suspicion. Cardiac MRI can also distinguish myopericarditis.

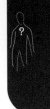

Treatment

Acute STEMI is caused by occlusion of the epicardial coronary artery by thrombus after rupture of a vulnerable plaque. The process of myocardial necrosis is time dependent, so diagnosis and treatment of STEMI to preserve myocardium must occur as quickly as possible. More than half of deaths occur within 1 hour after onset of symptoms, before the patient can be reached for emergency care. Patients often delay seeking care for symptoms of acute MI despite efforts to alert the public to the risk of ignoring symptoms of chest discomfort. Emergency medical personnel who respond to patients with possible MI begin to institute initial therapy in the field. Patients are monitored with ECG for rhythm disturbances such as ventricular tachycardia (VT) or ventricular fibrillation (VF) that require prompt cardioversion or defibrillation. Oxygen is administered via nasal cannula, and intravenous access is established. Aspirin (162 to 325 mg) is administered to the patient, and sublingual nitroglycerin may also be given in attempt to relieve chest discomfort. Some emergency response systems perform 12-lead ECGs and telemeter the results to the emergency department, allowing for early diagnosis of STEMI and early decision making regarding revascularization strategies.

Once the patient arrives in the emergency department, an ECG, if not already available, will be preformed within 5 minutes. If the ECG is nondiagnostic, a second study is obtained no more than 20 minutes after presentation. A diagnosis of STEMI triggers decision making regarding reperfusion strategies that are used by the particular institution (see Chapter 73, "ST Elevation Acute Myocardial Infarction and Complications of Myocardial Infarction," in *Goldman-Cecil Medicine*, 25th Edition). Hospitals that are capable of performing emergency cardiac catheterization for the purpose of reperfusion therapy have an established rapid response system to activate the catheterization laboratory for this urgent therapy. There is evidence that primary PCI therapy for STEMI is superior to fibrinolytic therapy, but its use depends on the timely availability of a well-trained catheterization team. The quality of primary PCI is signified by a so-called door-to-balloon time of less than 90 minutes. Likewise, the standard for fibrinolytic therapy is a door-to-needle time of less than 30 minutes. Regardless of the means of reperfusion, it is important for the hospital treating patients with STEMI to have a structured protocol for timely diagnosis, decision making, and initiation of therapy.

In addition to aspirin, the patient should be given a loading dose of thienopyridine (clopidogrel 600 mg or prasugrel 60 mg), assuming he or she will be treated with primary PCI. Unfractionated heparin in a dose of 60 IU/kg should be administered (no more than 4000 IU bolus) with a drip rate of 12 IU/kg/hour (maximum dose, 1000 IU/hour). LMW heparin may also be used (enoxaparin 30 mg IV bolus with 1 mg/kg subcutaneously every 12 hours for patients younger than 75 years of age who have normal renal function). Other agents such as glycoprotein IIb/IIIa inhibitors or bivalirudin are administered depending on the protocols of the catheterization laboratory.

Intravenous morphine (2 to 4 mg, repeated every 5 to 15 minutes as needed) is frequently used for pain control. Patients also are commonly given sublingual nitroglycerin 0.4 mg (repeat every 5 minutes for no more than three total doses), which may help to diminish chest discomfort. Intravenous nitroglycerin may be helpful for control of both pain and hypertension if present. Intravenous β-blockers such as metoprolol (5-mg bolus every 10 minutes for a total dose of 15 mg) is indicated in the treatment of STEMI, but it should be avoided in the face of heart failure, severe COPD, hypotension, or bradycardia. β-Blockers (metoprolol, propranolol, atenolol, timolol, and carvedilol) have been shown to significantly reduce the risk of future MI and cardiovascular mortality. Statin therapy, as mentioned for NSTEMI, is recommended for all patients with STEMI as a presenting symptom regardless of their history of hypercholesterolemia. Other adjunctive measures include bedrest for the first 12 hours, ongoing oxygen by nasal cannula with pulse oximeter monitoring, continuous rhythm monitoring, anxiolytic agents as needed, and stool softeners. Atropine is kept in reserve for the treatment of hemodynamically significant bradycardia, which may occur with inferior MI.

ACE-inhibitor therapy also plays an important role in the long-term survival of patients after STEMI. ACE-inhibitor therapy has been shown to reduce the incidence of heart failure, recurrent MI, and long-term mortality after STEMI. ACE inhibitors commonly used for this purpose include lisinopril, captopril, enalapril, and ramipril. The decision to initiate ACE-inhibitor therapy is directed by the patient's tolerance. Care is warranted early after STEMI, because the patient may be prone to hypotension related to ACE-inhibitor therapy. A low dose should be administered first, with gradual upward titration.

Aldosterone receptor blockade with eplerenone (25 to 50 mg/day) reduces cardiovascular mortality after MI in patients with heart failure and a reduced EF of less than 40% or diabetes. Spironolactone also reduces mortality in patients with heart failure and a history of remote MI.

Reperfusion Therapy

Timely reperfusion therapy, either thrombolytic therapy or primary PCI, is critical to limiting the extent of MI and reducing the risks of future morbidity and mortality. Primary PCI has been shown to have advantages over thrombolytic therapy, with higher immediate and long-term vessel patency. Primary PCI depends on the availability of cardiac catheterization facilities and staff to conduct the reperfusion procedure quickly (see earlier discussion). If the patient has not had access to a catheterization facility for longer than 2 hours after presentation, thrombolytic therapy is a reasonable alternative.

In the randomized, placebo-controlled Gruppo Italiano per lo Studio della Streptochinasi nell'Infarto (GISSI) study, thrombolytic therapy with intravenous streptokinase was shown to reduce the risk of mortality in patients with STEMI if it was administered early after presentation. The time-dependent nature of therapy was also demonstrated, in that patients treated more than 12 hours after the onset of symptoms had no measurable benefit from thrombolysis. The next generation of thrombolytic agents, recombinant tissue-type plasminogen activators (rt-PA), improved on mortality reduction when compared with streptokinase (30-day mortality rate, 7.3% with streptokinase vs. 6.3% with rt-PA). The advantage of rt-PA appeared to be related to enhanced vessel patency at 90 minutes after administration (80% with rt-PA vs. 53% to 60% with streptokinase). Subsequent forms of rt-PA, although easier to administer, did not further reduce mortality. The major attribute of thrombolytic therapy is its ease of administration, but there is a significant risk (0.5% to 1%) of catastrophic bleeding complications in the form of intracerebral hemorrhage. Age older than 75 years, female gender, hypertension, and concomitant use of heparin increase the risk of this complication. In the case of failed thrombolytic therapy, rescue PCI may be pursued.

Primary PCI has been shown to be superior to thrombolytic therapy based on lower overall mortality rates and reduced risk of recurrent nonfatal MI. It is also associated with higher vessel patency rates and a low risk of intracranial hemorrhage. Primary PCI is frequently performed by mechanical aspiration of thrombus and placement of a coronary stent. Balloon angioplasty may or may not be needed during this procedure. Patients should receive preprocedure thienopyridine (clopidogrel 600 mg or prasugrel 60 mg). Bivalirudin was shown in a clinical trial of primary PCI to be superior to both heparin- and glycoprotein IIb/IIIa–based anticoagulation with lower post-MI mortality and fewer bleeding complications. Centers that are dedicated to primary PCI as the preferred therapy are likely to have the best outcomes when operators are sufficiently skilled and the institution cares for this patient population on a regular basis. Primary PCI is the best option for patients in cardiogenic shock (within 18 hours after onset of shock), for patients with prior CABG (graft occlusion is not amenable to thrombolysis), and for patients older than 70 years of age (conferring a reduced risk of intracerebral hemorrhage compared with thrombolysis).

Complications of Myocardial Infarction

Recurrent Chest Pain

MI is associated with a number of possible problems related to the extent of injury (Table 8-6). Patients can experience post-infarction angina which may reflect re-occlusion of the infarct related vessel. This can occur either in patients who underwent primary PCI with stent placement (stent thrombosis) or thrombolysis. Post-infarction angina usually requires cardiac catheterization for appropriate diagnosis and treatment. Patients with transmural MI are also subject to pericarditis 2 to 4 days after the event. This diagnosis is usually established by the symptom nature and pattern (worse with inspiration or supine position,

improved with sitting), which is different from their initial presentation with acute MI. A less common event is the development of pericarditis due to Dressler's syndrome up to 10 weeks after acute MI. This is likely an immune-mediated phenomenon. Pericarditis is treated with aspirin or nonsteroidal anti-inflammatory drugs.

Arrhythmias

The highest risk of life-threatening arrhythmias is during the first 24 to 48 hours after the onset of acute MI. Ischemic myocardium is susceptible to arrhythmia generation, probably based on micro-re-entry associated with ischemic myocardium. The significant mortality risk in the early hours of acute MI is largely attributed to arrhythmias such as VF or VT. The risk of VF is about 3% to 5% in the early hours of MI and diminishes over 24 to 48 hours. One of the benefits of rhythm monitoring during the first 48 hours after presentation is prompt recognition and treatment of life-threatening ventricular arrhythmias.

Accelerated idioventricular rhythm occurs early in the course of MI and may be associated with reperfusion. This arrhythmia is well tolerated and does not require specific therapy.

Ventricular arrhythmias occurring late (>48 hours) after acute MI usually are associated with large underlying MIs and heart failure. Late episodes of VF or VT portend a poor prognosis. Immediate therapy for VF is electrical defibrillation. VT that causes hemodynamic embarrassment is treated with synchronized electrical cardioversion. β-Blocker therapy may help to suppress arrhythmias in patients who are prone to them, as may the use of amiodarone. Correction of residual ischemia may also play a role in controlling VF or VT events. Patients with late VF or hemodynamically significant VT are candidates for an implantable cardioverter defibrillator device (ICD). An ICD can also improve survival in asymptomatic patients with a persistently reduced EF less than 30% at 40 days after their acute MI. ICD therapy is also indicated if the EF is less than 35% at 40 days after MI in a patient with symptomatic heart failure.

Atrial fibrillation (AF) occurs in 10% to 15% of patients after MI. Those more prone to AF include patients with older age, large MI, hypokalemia, hypomagnesemia, hypoxia, or increased sympathetic activity. Rate control with β-blockers (e.g., metoprolol), digoxin, calcium channel blockers (e.g., diltiazem) or some combination of these agents is warranted, as is the use of intravenous heparin to reduce the risk of systemic embolization. Cardioversion is warranted in the face of rapid rates that cause ischemia, heart failure, or hypotension. Amiodarone is sometimes used to help maintain sinus rhythm for the first few months after MI-related AF.

Sinus bradycardia or AV block due to increased vagal tone is common in cases of inferior MI (30% to 40%). Reperfusion of the right coronary artery may be associated with significant bradycardia (Bezold-Jarisch reflex). Atropine (0.5 to 1.5 mg IV) can resolve severe inferior MI–related bradycardia. In contrast, heart block and wide-complex escape rhythms associated with anterior MI suggest an infra–AV node block. This may be worsened by the use of atropine.

Advanced degrees of heart block may require the placement of a permanent pacemaker. Intermittent second-degree or third-degree AV block associated with bundle branch block or

TABLE 8-6   COMPLICATIONS OF ACUTE MYOCARDIAL INFARCTION

FUNCTIONAL

Left ventricular failure
Right ventricular failure
Cardiogenic shock

MECHANICAL

Free-wall rupture
Ventricular septal defect
Papillary muscle rupture with acute mitral regurgitation

ELECTRICAL

Bradyarrhythmias (first-, second-, and third-degree atrioventricular blocks)
Tachyarrhythmias (supraventricular, ventricular)
Conduction abnormalities (bundle branch and fascicular blocks)

symptomatic AV block are indications for a permanent pace-maker. Type I AV block (Wenckebach) is usually not persistent and rarely causes symptoms that warrant a permanent pacemaker.

Heart Failure and Low-Output States

MI involving 20% to 25% of the left ventricle can result in significant heart failure manifesting with dyspnea due to pulmonary congestion and findings of LV dysfunction such as an S_3 or S_4. Cardiogenic shock is associated with loss of 40% of the myocardium. This condition carries a very high risk of mortality. In the era of widespread use of reperfusion therapy, the incidence of post-MI heart failure or cardiogenic shock has declined. Early use of reperfusion therapies limits infarct size and the risk of complications related to heart failure. When acute heart failure occurs with MI, therapeutic interventions including oxygen, intravenous morphine, and diuretics can help stabilize the patient. Nitroglycerin can also help by reducing the elevated preload. Long-term therapy for heart failure related to reduced EF after acute MI includes the use of ACE inhibitors (or ARBs), appropriate β-blockers, aldosterone receptor antagonists such as eplerenone or spironolactone, and diuretics as needed.

The acutely infarcted ventricle requires an increased filling pressure and volume to optimize its performance. Patients with acute MI may become relatively fluid depleted due to nausea, vomiting, or decreased fluid intake, leading to reduced LV volume and a fall in cardiac output. This can translate into hypotension that is best treated by judicious administration of fluids.

Acute inferior MI is usually associated with a low mortality risk once the early arrhythmia-prone hours have passed. Occlusion of the right coronary artery and a significant acute marginal branch can lead to right ventricular infarction. Approximately 10% to 15% of patients with inferior MI have associated right ventricular infarction. This condition produces a significant increase in mortality risk (in-hospital mortality, 25% to 30% vs. <6%). Hallmarks of right ventricular infarction include elevated jugular venous pressure with Kussmaul sign and hypotension. Right ventricular function frequently recovers, but it may be necessary to administer sufficient volume to maintain right heart output. Short-term inotropic support with dobutamine in sometimes needed, and venodilators and diuretics should be avoided. High-degree AV block, usually transient with inferior MI, may worsen hemodynamics and necessitate temporary AV sequential pacing. AF may not be tolerated and may require cardioversion.

Cardiogenic Shock

Cardiogenic shock is a clinical syndrome associated with extensive loss of myocardium, which leads to a reduced cardiac index (<1.8 L/min/m^2) in the face of elevated LV filling pressures (pulmonary capillary wedge pressure >18 mm Hg), resulting in systemic hypotension and reduced organ perfusion. This shock state is associated with mortality rates in the range of 70% to 80%. Aggressive diagnosis with hemodynamic monitoring and appropriate support with an intra-aortic balloon pump (IABP) and inotropic agents as indicated can help to stabilize the patient. IABP therapy is at best temporizing, and the patient's survival depends on the presence of reversible factors such as ischemia

that respond to revascularization or correction of a mechanical complication of MI (e.g., mitral regurgitation or VSD. IABP therapy cannot be used in the face of significant aortic insufficiency and may not be feasible in the presence of significant peripheral vascular disease. Some centers now resort to ventricular assist devices to stabilize the patient with cardiogenic shock, but recovery of LV function is not guaranteed with this approach.

Mechanical Complications

Mechanical complications of acute MI include mitral regurgitation (due to ischemic papillary muscle dysfunction or rupture), VSD, free wall rupture, and LV aneurysm formation. These problems usually occur during the first week after MI, and they account for as much as 15% of MI-related mortality. A new murmur, sudden onset of heart failure, or hemodynamic collapse should also raise suspicion of a mechanical complication of MI. Patients who either were not reperfused or were reperfused late after onset of MI are most at risk for these problems. Echocardiography usually identifies the mechanical problem, and hemodynamic assessment with right heart catheterization can aid the diagnosis. Surgical correction of the defect is usually required.

Papillary muscle rupture or dysfunction leading to acute severe mitral regurgitation results in severe heart failure and up to 75% mortality within 24 hours after onset. Afterload reduction with intravenous nitroprusside and the use of IABP can help to stabilize the patient, but surgical valve repair or replacement will be needed to provide some chance of survival. Surgery is associated with a 25% to 50% mortality risk, but that still is better than the risk with medical or IABP therapy only.

Elderly patients, particularly those with hypertension, are more prone to MI-related VSD. Thrombolytic therapy may also place patients at risk for this complication. Acute VSD with resultant left-to-right shunting can produce severe hemodynamic instability. As with acute mitral regurgitation, afterload reduction and IABP may help to stabilize the patient, but ultimately surgical repair will be required. Moderate to large VSDs are not well tolerated and are associated with significant mortality risk. VSDs related to anterior MI may offer a better opportunity for surgical repair than those resulting from inferior MI. Some patients have been helped by the use of percutaneous closure devices, which can afford an opportunity to delay surgery until there is better tissue healing in the infarct area.

LV free wall rupture is similar to VSD in terms of risk for occurrence and underlying myocardial pathology. Free wall rupture is usually associated with sudden death due to cardiac tamponade. On occasion, a pseudoaneurysm forms and the patient can be treated surgically.

Thromboembolic Complications

In earlier years, thromboembolism in the form of either cardioembolic stroke or pulmonary embolism contributed to 25% of post-MI in-hospital mortality, and clinical events were diagnosed in 10% of patients. The risk of thromboembolism is linked to the presence of LV mural clot, which is more likely to be found in anterior MI with associated apical akinesis and deep venous thrombosis due to prolonged bed-rest. Contemporary methods of care for acute MI have greatly reduced the risk of post-MI thromboembolism.

Reperfusion therapy, when applied in a timely fashion, results in less extensive MI and less impairment of LV function. Patients with anterior MI treated with reperfusion therapy are less likely to have extensive apical akinesis, which is the breeding ground for mural thrombus. It is advised that patients treated for acute MI have an echocardiogram to assess for overall LV function; in the case of anterior MI, the presence of apical mural thrombus can be detected by echocardiography. If LV mural thrombus is present, the patient should receive therapeutic anticoagulation with unfractionated or LMW heparin while oral anticoagulation with warfarin is initiated. Warfarin therapy should be continued for 6 months after MI when LV apical mural thrombus is detected. Early ambulation after MI, along with the use of compression stockings and subcutaneous heparin prophylaxis (unfractionated or LMW) for deep venous thrombosis, has greatly diminished the threat of pulmonary embolism.

⬤ PROGNOSIS

Risk Stratification after Myocardial Infarction

Key to understanding an individual patient's risk for future coronary events or mortality related to MI is a thorough assessment of drivers for those risks: status of LV function and its impact on clinical functional status, residual myocardial ischemia, and spontaneous or exercise-induced arrhythmias. Appropriate predischarge assessments provide a comprehensive picture of the patient's risk status and prognosis.

Electrocardiographic Monitoring

Patients are routinely monitored by telemetry systems that capture arrhythmic events in the first 48 hours after MI. Late ventricular arrhythmias such as VF or sustained VT identify patients who are likely to benefit from ICD therapy. This is particularly true if EF is reduced to less than 40%. ICD implantation is also indicated for patients with persistently reduced EF (<30%).

Cardiac Catheterization and Noninvasive Testing

Predischarge risk stratification may involve cardiac catheterization, submaximal predischarge exercise stress testing (on days 4 to 6), or maximal exercise stress testing after discharge (at 2 to 6 weeks). The presence or absence of high-risk coronary anatomy is demonstrated for patients who have undergone primary PCI at the time presentation. Many patients who have been treated with thrombolytic therapy undergo coronary angiography before discharge to determine the extent and severity of underlying CAD as well as the status of the culprit lesion. If coronary angiography is not performed, predischarge submaximal exercise testing (up to 70% of maximal predicted heart rate) is done to identify those who are at increased risk for postdischarge coronary ischemic events. Patients who undergo submaximal exercise stress testing in lieu of coronary angiography frequently have a follow-up maximal exercise stress test within 2 to 6 weeks after discharge. During stress testing, positive results that suggest the need for coronary angiography include exercise-induced angina, ST changes of ischemia (ST depression), exercise-induced hypotension, exercise-induced ventricular arrhythmias, and low functional capacity. The sensitivity and specificity of stress testing after MI is enhanced by the use of imaging modalities such as stress echocardiography or nuclear perfusion imaging. All patients should have their EF assessed, typically by echocardiography, before discharge.

Secondary Prevention, Patient Education, and Rehabilitation

The goal of secondary prevention is to reduce the risk of recurrent MI and cardiovascular mortality. Risk factor modification is key to the secondary prevention strategy. All patients should have their lipid status assessed at the time of admission, but statin therapy is warranted in patients with acute MI at presentation. The target LDL level is less than 100 mg/dL, preferably closer to 70 mg/dL. Smoking cessation is of critical importance because it can reduce the risk of reinfarction, and ongoing smoking can double the risk of recurrent MI or mortality in the first year after MI. Structured smoking cessation programs and the use of pharmacologic aids (e.g., nicotine patches or gum, bupropion, varenicline) can increase the success of smoking cessation efforts.

Antiplatelet therapy with aspirin (75 to 162 mg/day) is given indefinitely to all patients after MI. Regardless of whether primary PCI has been performed, patients will benefit from the use of clopidogrel 75 mg/day for the first year after MI. Those patients who have received a stent during primary PCI should continue either clopidogrel 75 mg/day or prasugrel 10 mg/day for a duration appropriate for the type of stent employed. At the least, patients should receive dual antiplatelet therapy (aspirin + thienopyridine) for 1 month for a bare metal stent, 3 months for a sirolimus-based stent, and 6 months for a paclitaxel-eluting stent. Most patients who have been treated with any type of stent receive dual antiplatelet therapy for the first year after their MI. The use of antiplatelet therapy in any form should be tempered by an individual patient's risk of hemorrhagic complications.

The use of warfarin anticoagulation (target international normalized ratio [INR], 2.0 to 3.0) is indicated for patients with persistent or paroxysmal AF, guided by their CHADS-2 score (congestive heart failure, hypertension, age ≥75 years, diabetes mellitus, and stroke). Patients who have experienced pulmonary or systemic thromboembolism also warrant warfarin therapy. Patients who are at high risk for thromboembolism after acute MI, such as those with low EF related to anterior MI, should also be considered for warfarin. The concomitant use of dual antiplatelet therapy along with warfarin requires careful monitoring for bleeding complications.

Acute anterior MI that has resulted in significant injury to the ventricle with an EF of less than 40% places the patient at risk for future negative remodeling of the left ventricle and potential heart failure. ACE-inhibitor therapy has been shown to reduce the risk of negative remodeling and the occurrence of heart failure in such patients. This group of patients also experiences a reduction in future recurrent MI risk with the use of ACE-inhibitor therapy. This observation does not appear to carry over to patients with stable CAD. ACE-inhibitor therapy (captopril, ramipril, lisinopril) is indicated for all patients after MI. The use

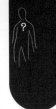

of ARBs (e.g., valsartan, losartan) is reasonable for patients who are intolerant of ACE-inhibitor therapy. The aldosterone receptor antagonist eplerenone (25 mg/day, titrated to 50 mg/day) is indicated as additive therapy to ACE or ARB in MI patients who have reduced EF (<40%) or diabetes. Careful monitoring of serum potassium is required after initiation of eplerenone together with ACE or ARB.

Beta blocker therapy reduces mortality risk in patients who have reduced EF post-MI. This therapy should be avoided in patients with uncompensated heart failure early after MI or the presence of other contraindications. Metoprolol succinate (25 mg/day titrated up to 200 mg/day) or carvedilol (3.125-6.25 mg titrated to 25 mg twice each day) should be initiated at low doses and titrated upward as tolerated. The role of beta blockers in patients with no residual myocardial ischemia, arrhythmias, or normal EF is not clear.

Nitrates, either short-acting sublingual nitroglycerin or long-acting versions, may be useful in the treatment of stable angina. Calcium channel blocking drugs should be avoided in patients with reduced EF (<40%). In patients with normal EF, either diltiazem or verapamil may useful as a substitute in patients who are intolerant of β-blockers when either antianginal therapy or rate control for AF is needed. The dihydropyridine, amlodipine, may be a useful adjunct for control of hypertension or treatment of angina. It should be used with caution in the face of reduced EF.

After acute MI, women should refrain from initiating hormone therapy with estrogen or estrogen/progesterone preparations; these agents do not decrease the risk of recurrent MI but do increase the risk of thromboembolic events. The ongoing use of hormone therapy in women already receiving treatment should be individualized, with a bias toward discontinuing therapy. Diabetic patients need attention to their degree of glycemic control, with a target of hemoglobin A_{1c} less than 7%. Vitamin supplements have no clear role in therapy for MI patients. Fish oil supplements do not appear to benefit patients who have experienced acute MI.

Patient Education and Cardiac Rehabilitation

It is important to begin the education of patients early after acute MI so that they understand the value of their various prescribed medical therapies and the need for risk factor modification. Cardiac rehabilitation programs are very useful in the ongoing education of patients; they reinforce positive lifestyle changes and provide exercise training in the post-MI period. Such programs not only educate patients but also help them to regain confidence in their ability to perform the tasks of daily living and other activities they enjoy. Early follow-up with the physician after discharge is also important to ensure clinical stability and tolerance of medical therapy and to monitor the progress of lifestyle changes.

SUGGESTED READINGS

Anderson JL, Adams CD, Antman EM, et al: 2012 ACCF/AHA focused update incorporated into the ACCF/AHA 2007 guidelines for the management of patients with unstable angina/non–ST-elevation myocardial infarction: a report of the American College of Cardiology Foundation/American Heart Association Task Force on Practice Guidelines, J Am Coll Cardiol 61:e179–e347, 2013.

Fihn SD, Gardin JM, Abrams J, et al: ACCF/AHA/ACP/AATS/PCNA/SCAI/STS guideline for the diagnosis and management of patients with stable ischemic heart disease: a report of the American College of Cardiology Foundation/American Heart Association Task Force on Practice Guidelines, and the American College of Physicians, American Association for Thoracic Surgery, Preventive Cardiovascular Nurses Association, Society for Cardiovascular Angiography and Interventions, and Society of Thoracic Surgeons, J Am Coll Cardiol 60:e44–e164, 2012.

Hillis LD, Smith PK, Anderson JL, et al: 2011 ACCF/AHA guideline for coronary artery bypass graft surgery: a report of the American College of Cardiology Foundation/American Heart Association Task Force on Practice Guidelines. Developed in collaboration with the American Association for Thoracic Surgery, Society of Cardiovascular Anesthesiologists, and Society of Thoracic Surgeons, J Am Coll Cardiol 58:e123–e210, 2011.

Levine GN, Bates ER, Blankenship JC, et al: 2011 ACCF/AHA/SCAI guideline for percutaneous coronary intervention: a report of the American College of Cardiology Foundation/American Heart Association Task Force on Practice Guidelines and the Society for Cardiovascular Angiography and Interventions, J Am Coll Cardiol 58:e44–e122, 2011.

O'Gara PT, Kushner FG, Ascheim DD, et al: 2013 ACCF/AHA guideline for the management of ST-elevation myocardial infarction: a report of the American College of Cardiology Foundation/American Heart Association Task Force on Practice Guidelines, J Am Coll Cardiol 61:e78–e140, 2013.

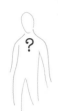

Cardiac Arrhythmias

Marcie G. Berger, Jason C. Rubenstein, and James A. Roth

● BASIC CELLULAR ELECTROPHYSIOLOGY

Cardiac myocytes actively maintain a negative resting membrane potential (E_m) through the differential distribution of ions between intracellular and extracellular compartments, which is an energy-dependent process that relies on ion channels, pumps, and exchangers. Transmembrane differences in voltage and ionic concentration create electrical and chemical forces that drive charged ions in and out of cells.

The resting E_m of cardiac myocytes is controlled by potassium ions (K^+). Active K^+ transport by the sodium-potassium adenosine triphosphatase pump (Na^+, K^+-ATPase) produces a transmembrane ionic gradient, with the intracellular concentration of K^+ exceeding the extracellular concentration. This favors the net efflux of K^+ from cells, yielding a resting negative charge within the cardiac myocytes. K^+ continues to flow from the intracellular to the extracellular compartment until the negative intracellular charge counterbalances the transmembrane K^+ concentration gradient at a potential called the *equilibrium potential* for K^+. This potential, at which the net K^+ current is zero, is close to the resting E_m of nonpacemaker cardiac myocytes. Pacemaker cells (i.e., sinoatrial and atrioventricular [AV] nodal cells) are characterized by a resting E_m of −50 to −60 mV. The resting E_m of atrial and ventricular myocytes is typically −80 to −90 mV.

The depolarization of a cardiac myocyte to threshold potential triggers a sequence of ionic movements resulting in a cardiac action potential (Fig. 9-1). The action potential is divided into five phases. Phase 0 is the rapid depolarization of nonpacemaker myocytes resulting from rapid sodium ion (Na^+) entry through fast Na^+ channels. These channels have three conformational states: closed (resting state), open (conducting Na^+ current), and inactivated, from which recovery is voltage dependent. Phase 1 is early, rapid, partial repolarization of the cell mediated by K^+ efflux. During phase 2, the plateau phase, there is a small net current flow, with inward calcium ion (Ca^{2+}) flow balanced by outward K^+ flow.

During phase 3, repolarization is mediated by an increase in K^+ efflux and a decline in Ca^{2+} influx. The dominant repolarizing current is I_{Kr}, the rapidly activating delayed rectifier K^+ current, a channel encoded by the *KCNE2* gene (also called *HERG*). The I_{Ks} current, or slowly activating delayed rectifier K^+ current, also contributes to repolarization. Phase 3 determines to a large degree the cellular refractory period. Importantly, I_{Kr} is inhibited by a large number of drugs that prolong the action potential duration.

Phase 4 is particularly significant in cardiac pacemaker cells because slow depolarization occurs from the resting membrane potential to the threshold potential. The resting E_m, rate of spontaneous phase 4 depolarization, and rate of phase 0 depolarization differentiate slow-response from fast-response cardiac myocytes. Slow-response cells, located in the sinoatrial node and AV node, normally display automaticity or spontaneous depolarization during phase 4. Resting E_m in slow-response cells is less negative, and Ca^{2+} current mediates phase 0 depolarization. Conduction in these pacemaker cells is slow, and recovery from

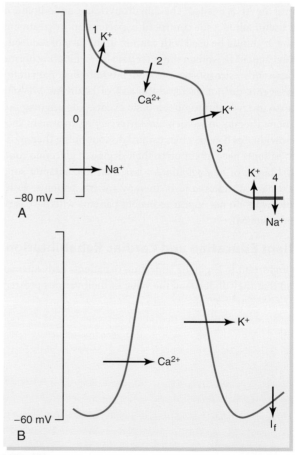

FIGURE 9-1 Electrophysiologic basis of the cardiac cellular action potential. **A,** Fast-response cells found in working myocardium and the specialized infranodal conduction system maintain a strongly negative resting membrane potential and a brisk phase 0 upstroke mediated by rapid sodium influx at the start of the action potential. **B,** In contrast, slow-response cells found in the sinus node and atrioventricular nodal tissue exhibit less-negative resting membrane potentials, slower calcium-channel–dependent action potential upstrokes, and phase 4 depolarization.

inactivation is time dependent. The fast-response cells found in atrial myocytes, ventricular myocytes, and the His-Purkinje system display slow phase 4 depolarization and do not typically display automaticity. The resting E_m is more negative, and the fast Na^+ current drives rapid phase 0 depolarization and rapid conduction. Recovery from inactivation in these cells is voltage dependent.

The sinus node typically displays the fastest phase 4 depolarization. Other cardiac tissues have the capacity to depolarize spontaneously, and subsidiary pacemakers may take over when sinus rates slow and under conditions of increased automaticity. Typically, the AV node, located above the AV ring, serves as the heart's secondary pacemaker, with a spontaneous rate of depolarization of 40 to 50 beats per minute. Automaticity of cardiac myocytes is increased when the slope of phase 4 depolarization increases, with a shift of threshold potentials to more negative values, or in the presence of more positive maximal diastolic potentials.

The sinus node is the primary intrinsic pacemaker, and spontaneous depolarization leads to action potential generation, with normal resting rates of 60 to 100 beats per minute. Depolarization then spreads through the atria to the AV node, where conduction slows, introducing a delay between atrial and ventricular activation, and then to the His-Purkinje system fibers, which originate at the AV node with the bundle of His and split to form the left bundle branch and the right bundle branch, rapidly conducting depolarization to the ventricular myocardium. Cardiac myocytes are joined by electrical synapses called *gap junctions*, which permit the flow of intracellular current from cell to cell.

Classification of Arrhythmias

Mechanistically, cardiac arrhythmias can be broadly divided into disorders of action potential formation and disorders of impulse conduction. Clinically, arrhythmias are classified as bradycardias and tachycardias, with further categorization according to arrhythmia origin. This information is used to guide evaluation and management strategies.

Electrophysiologic Mechanisms of Arrhythmias

Automaticity is a normal function of pacemaker cells, occurring during phase 4 depolarization. *Enhanced automaticity* occurs when pacemaker cells depolarize at a faster rate due to an increased slope of phase 4 depolarization, a shift of threshold potential to a more negative value, or a shift of the maximal diastolic potential to a more positive value. These changes may occur with sympathetic stimulation. Enhanced automaticity may be normal (e.g., appropriate sinus tachycardia) or abnormal (e.g., inappropriate sinus tachycardia). Spontaneous depolarization occurring in nonpacemaker cardiac myocytes is called *abnormal automaticity*. Conditions as ischemia, electrolyte abnormalities, and sympathetic stimulation may produce abnormal automaticity. Premature atrial and ventricular depolarizations, atrial tachycardia, and ventricular tachycardia (VT) may result.

Triggered activity occurs when secondary cardiac depolarizations are initiated by prior depolarizations. If these secondary

depolarizations reach threshold potential, they may generate action potentials during or immediately after phase 3 of the action potential. *Early afterdepolarizations* (EADs) are observed when triggered depolarization occurs during phase 3 of the action potential. Inciters of EADs include QT-prolonging drugs, hypokalemia, and bradycardia. Patients with congenital long QT syndrome (LQTS) are prone to develop EADS, resulting in *torsades de pointes* (TdP).

When triggered activity occurs during phase 4, *delayed afterdepolarizations* (DADs) result. DADs are exaggerated at rapid heart rates and observed with digoxin toxicity and high-level catecholamine states, conditions that are associated with intracellular calcium overload. DADs are thought to be the chief arrhythmic mechanism underlying catecholaminergic polymorphic VT (CPVT).

Reentry is the dominant mechanism underlying clinical tachyarrhythmias. Reentry describes the reexcitation of a localized region of cardiac tissue by the same impulse, requiring bifurcating conduction pathways with different velocities and refractory periods. To permit reentry, unidirectional block in one pathway and slowed conduction in the other are required. Reentry is further categorized as anatomic, circling around a fixed anatomic obstacle, or functional, in which the inexcitable center of a reentrant circuit is not fixed but functionally refractory. Figure 9-2 illustrates reentry as an arrhythmic mechanism. The two pathways join proximally and distally. Pathway *A* conducts rapidly but has a long refractory period. Pathway *B* is slowly conducting but has a shorter refractory period. A normally timed impulse enters the two pathways through the proximal common pathway, conducting rapidly down *A* and slowly down *B*. As the impulse from pathway *A* reaches the distal common pathway, while continuing distally, it may also turn around to activate *B* retrogradely. This impulse collides with the slowly conducting antegrade impulse in pathway *B*, extinguishing the impulse. However, a sufficiently premature stimulus may enter the proximal common pathway, finding pathway *A* with its long refractory period inexcitable, traveling slowly down pathway *B*, and finally reaching the distal common pathway. Due to the slow conduction velocity in pathway *B*, pathway *A* may no longer be refractory, and the impulse may successfully travel retrograde up pathway *A*, potentially repeatedly activating the circuit. Reentry is the most common mechanism producing supraventricular tachycardia (SVT) and VT.

For a deeper discussion on this topic, please see Chapter 61, "Principles of Electrophysiology," in Goldman-Cecil Medicine, *25th Edition.*

GENERAL APPROACH TO MANAGEMENT
Diagnostic Procedures
Electrocardiography

The baseline 12-lead electrocardiogram (ECG) is essential for the initial evaluation of patients with arrhythmic symptoms. The baseline ECG may indicate an underlying structural heart disease, with Q waves or fractionated QRS complexes suggesting prior myocardial infarction (MI). Slow sinus rates or AV conduction

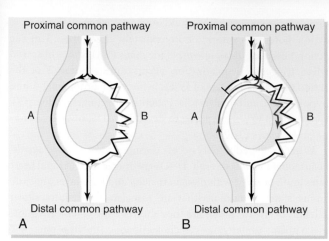

Proximal common pathway — Proximal common pathway

A   B   A   B

Distal common pathway — Distal common pathway

A   B

FIGURE 9-2 Mechanism of reentry. Reentry requires two distinct pathways with different refractoriness and a region of slowed conduction. One pathway (A) has normal rapid conduction but a long refractory period. The second pathway (B) has slowed conduction but a relatively shorter refractory period. To initiate reentry, conduction must fail down one pathway in the antegrade direction but then permit later retrograde reactivation of this pathway. This is referred to as a *unidirectional block*. A fixed or functional obstacle must maintain separation of the two pathways. Although drawn schematically as a circular loop, the anatomy of circuits is often complex and circuitous and is different in different arrhythmia mechanisms. **A,** In normal rhythm, the circuit is activated in an antegrade direction down both pathways. However, because of slowed conduction in the B limb, distal activation is mediated by the faster A pathway, which arrives first and may activate the slowly conducting pathway in a retrograde direction. This retrograde conduction is electrocardiographically concealed (invisible), collides with the antegrade wave front, and is extinguished, and no tachycardia results. **B,** Reentry is usually initiated by a premature beat originating independently of the circuit. The premature beat fails to propagate down the rapidly conducting A limb due to differential refractoriness of the two limbs, but it is able to propagate down the slowly conducting B pathway, where it may encounter substantial delay due to increased conduction time with prematurity (i.e., decremental conduction), allowing recovery of the previously blocked rapidly conducting A limb. This permits the rapidly conducting A limb to act as a return path and for ultimate reentrant reactivation of the slowly conducting B pathway, initiating sustained reentrant tachycardia in the circuit.

abnormalities may point to susceptibility to symptomatic bradycardia. Delta waves confirm an accessory pathway and direct the evaluation of arrhythmic symptoms toward the diagnosis of Wolff-Parkinson-White (WPW) syndrome while localizing the accessory pathway.

Evidence for hereditary cardiomyopathies and cardiac ion channel disorders that predispose to sudden death may be detected on a baseline ECG. Patients with arrhythmogenic right ventricular (RV) dysplasia may have epsilon waves and inverted T waves in the right precordial leads. QT interval prolongation or shortening may indicate congenital or acquired long QT or short QT syndrome, respectively. Brugada syndrome can be diagnosed based on coved ST-segment elevation in leads V_1 and V_2.

A 12-lead ECG obtained during arrhythmic symptoms can establish the cause of a patient's symptoms. A symptom ECG is most useful in discriminating between SVT and VT. The specific mechanism underlying narrow complex tachycardia can often be inferred from the ECG. Documentation of QRS morphology

during VT on a 12-lead ECG aids in localizing the site of origin, identifying the VT mechanism, and guiding catheter ablation.

Ambulatory Monitoring

Although a 12-lead ECG obtained during arrhythmic symptoms is ideal, it is difficult to obtain in practice because of the transient and intermittent nature of these symptoms. Ambulatory recording devices permit electrocardiographic monitoring over longer periods to establish symptom-rhythm correlations.

Three types of monitoring devices are available. *Holter monitors* provide continuous electrogram storage for 24 to 48 hours. Holter monitoring is helpful for patients with frequent symptoms. The prolonged sampling period provides useful information about heart rate variability, rate control with atrial fibrillation (AF), AF burden, asymptomatic arrhythmias, and the frequency of ventricular ectopy.

External event monitors or loop recorders, which can be worn for 30 days, store electrograms when triggered by patients for symptoms or are autoactivated based on heart rate detection above or below a programmed threshold value. Some external loop monitors have algorithms to detect AF. Episode storage varies from seconds to minutes. After events are recorded, patients transmit the data by telephone. External loop recorders are intended to identify cardiac rhythm disturbances underlying infrequent symptoms.

For patients with arrhythmia symptoms occurring less than once per month, *implantable loop recorders* may be useful. These small devices implanted in a subcutaneous pocket in the left chest record patient-triggered and autotriggered ECGs based on programmed heart rate parameters. With a 3-year anticipated battery longevity, implantable loop recorders are valuable in establishing the cause of recurrent infrequent syncope.

Electrophysiologic Testing

To perform electrophysiologic studies, temporary transvenous pacing catheters are positioned in multiple locations in the heart, permitting pacing and recording of intracardiac electrograms. Catheters are typically placed in the right atrium, the right ventricle, close to the bundle of His, and in the coronary sinus for left atrial recording and pacing. Electrophysiologic studies can define the mechanism of tachyarrhythmias and guide therapy. In patients with prior MI, induction of VT may assist in determining patient susceptibility to life-threatening arrhythmias and inform decisions regarding defibrillator implantation. Electrophysiologic testing also can evaluate sinus node function and AV conduction.

Pharmacologic Therapy

Antiarrhythmic drugs are traditionally divided according to the Singh–Vaughan Williams classification, which categorizes agents based on their primary physiologic effect (Table 9-1). When this classification system was first proposed, knowledge of electrophysiologic mechanisms was limited. Although the simplicity of categorizing antiarrhythmic drugs according to Singh–Vaughan Williams classes I through IV is appealing, the system has many limitations. As hybrid classifications, class I and III agents block ion channels, and class II and IV drugs block receptors. Some drugs cross classes and have several mechanisms of action. There

TABLE 9-1	SINGH–VAUGHAN WILLIAMS CLASSIFICATION OF ANTIARRHYTHMIC DRUGS	
CLASS	**PHYSIOLOGIC EFFECT***	**EXAMPLES**
I	Blocks sodium channels; predominantly reduces the maximum velocity of the upstroke of the action potential (phase 0)	
IA	Intermediate-potency blockade	Quinidine, procainamide, disopyramide
IB	Least-potent blockade	Lidocaine, tocainide, mexiletine, phenytoin
IC	Most-potent blockade	Flecainide, propafenone, moricizine
II	β-Adrenergic receptor blockade	Propranolol, metoprolol, atenolol
III	Potassium channel blockade: predominantly prolongs action potential duration	Amiodarone, sotalol, bretylium, ibutilide, dofetilide, dronedarone
IV	Calcium-channel blockade	Verapamil, diltiazem

*Several agents have physiologic effects characteristic of more than one class.

are drugs with antiarrhythmic action that are excluded from the classification, such as digitalis and adenosine. The system categorizes drugs based on their in vitro electrophysiologic effects in normal cardiac tissues.

Available antiarrhythmic drugs have limited efficacy and carry the risk of adverse events, including proarrhythmic potential. Knowledge of drug metabolism, interactions, electrophysiologic effects, and side effects is essential. Certain antiarrhythmics may suppress left ventricular systolic function and may affect pacing and defibrillation thresholds. Excepting β-blockers, none of the antiarrhythmics has been demonstrated to reduce mortality rates. The use of antiarrhythmic agents may confer an increased risk of cardiovascular mortality, particularly in heart failure patients. Tables 9-2 and 9-3 summarize major characteristics and side effects of commonly used antiarrhythmic drugs.

Class I Antiarrhythmic Agents

Class I antiarrhythmic drugs include sodium-channel blockers that bind fast sodium channels in their open and inactivated states and dissociate from sodium channels during their resting state. Blocking voltage-gated fast sodium channels slows phase 0 depolarization and conduction velocity. Class I agents demonstrate use-dependent blockade, and their effect is potentiated at faster heart rates. The drug dissociation rate from sodium channels during phase 4 of the action potential determines the degree to which these agents depress cardiac conduction velocity.

Class IA agents have a slow rate of drug dissociation from sodium channels, conferring moderate potency. In addition to blocking voltage-gated fast sodium channels, class IA drugs block delayed rectifier potassium channels. Slowing of conduction velocity and action potential prolongation are observed. All are antimuscarinic, especially disopyramide. Clinical applications include SVT, AF, atrial flutter, and VT. In the setting of atrial flutter and AF, class IA drugs are vagolytic. They may improve AV nodal conduction and should be used in conjunction with a β-blocker or calcium-channel blocker to avoid uncontrolled ventricular response rates. Quinidine is infrequently used due to its

side effect profile, including diarrhea, thrombocytopenia, and QT prolongation, triggering polymorphic VT. Clinical studies highlight the proarrhythmic risk and increased mortality associated with quinidine therapy. Procainamide, available as an intravenous formulation, has an active metabolite N-acetylprocainamide (NAPA) and may induce a reversible lupus-like syndrome. Disopyramide, with its potent negative inotropic and antimuscarinic activity, has been used to treat vagally mediated AF.

Class IB agents rapidly dissociate from sodium channels during phase 4, providing weak sodium-channel blockade. Their therapeutic role is restricted to ventricular arrhythmias due to a lack of effect on the sinoatrial node, AV node, and atrial tissue. Lidocaine, which is available parentally, undergoes extensive first-pass hepatic inactivation. Lidocaine is more effective in relatively depolarized ventricular tissue due to preferential affinity for inactivated sodium channels; the drug is more potent in ischemic tissue. Mexiletine, which is available orally, has slower hepatic metabolism and a longer half-life than lidocaine.

Class IC drugs are potent fast sodium-channel blockers with little effect on K^+ current. These agents have a role in the therapy of SVTs and VTs. Their use is relegated to patients without coronary disease or significant structural heart disease. The Cardiac Arrhythmia Suppression Trial proved that the use of flecainide and moricizine to suppress ventricular arrhythmias after MI increased mortality rates. These agents may convert AF to atrial flutter and slow atrial conduction sufficiently to permit 1 : 1 AV conduction during atrial flutter, necessitating the simultaneous use of AV nodal–blocking therapies in patients with atrial arrhythmias. Flecainide is associated with bronchospasm, leukopenia, thrombocytopenia, and neurologic side effects. Flecainide, which inhibits Ca^{2+} release from the sarcoplasmic reticulum cardiac ryanodine receptor, may be useful in the therapy for CPVT. Propafenone has β-blocking effects and can cause agranulocytosis, anemia, and thrombocytopenia.

Class II and IV Antiarrhythmic Agents

β-Adrenoceptor antagonists, the class II agents, inhibit sympathetic activation of cardiac automaticity and conduction, resulting in slowing of the heart rate, decreased AV node conduction velocity, and prolongation of the AV node refractory period. Side effects include bradycardia, hypotension, exacerbation of reactive airway disease, fatigue, worsening symptoms of peripheral vascular disease, and depression. β-Blockers have different half-lives, lipid solubilities, elimination routes, and specificities for $β_1$ and $β_2$ receptors.

Class IV agents include the nondihydropyridine calcium-channel blockers. Blockade of voltage-gated L-type calcium channels decreases AV nodal conduction velocity, increases AV nodal refractory period, slows sinus node automaticity, and decreases myocardial contractility. Calcium-channel blockers may cause hypotension, bradycardia, and heart failure. Clinical applications for these agents include rate control for atrial tachyarrhythmias, termination and suppression of SVT, and normal heart VT. In the setting of atrial arrhythmias with underlying WPW, they can potentiate accessory pathway conduction and should be avoided.

TABLE 9-2 SELECTED CHARACTERISTICS OF ANTIARRHYTHMIC DRUGS

DRUG	EFFECT ON SURFACE ECG	EFFECT ON LV FUNCTION	IMPORTANT DRUG INTERACTIONS	EFFECT ON PACING AND DEFIBRILLATION THRESHOLDS	MAJOR ROUTE OF ELIMINATION
Quinidine	Prolongs QRS and QT	Negative inotrope	Increases digoxin level and warfarin effect Cimetidine increases quinidine level Phenobarbital, phenytoin, and rifampin decrease quinidine level	Increases PT and DT at high doses	Liver and kidney
Procainamide	Prolongs PR, QRS, and QT	Negative inotrope	Cimetidine, alcohol, and amiodarone increase procainamide level	Increases PT at high doses	Liver and kidney
Disopyramide	Prolongs QRS and QT	Negative inotrope	Phenobarbital, phenytoin, and rifampin decrease disopyramide level	Increases PT at high doses	Liver and kidney
Lidocaine	Shortens QT	None	Propranolol, metoprolol, and cimetidine increase lidocaine level	Increases DT	Liver
Mexiletine	Shortens QT	None	Increases theophylline level Phenobarbital, phenytoin, and rifampin decrease mexiletine level	Various effects	Liver
Flecainide	Prolongs PR and QRS	Negative inotrope	Increases digoxin level	Increases PT; variable effect on DT	Liver and kidney
Propafenone	Prolongs PR and QRS	Negative inotrope	Increases digoxin, theophylline, and cyclosporine levels; increases warfarin effect Phenobarbital, phenytoin, and rifampin decrease propafenone level Cimetidine and quinidine increase propafenone level	Increases PT; variable effect on DT	Liver
Dronedarone	Prolongs PR and QT; slows sinus rate	Negative inotrope	CYP3A inhibitors (ketoconazole, clarithromycin, calcium-channel blockers) increase dronedarone levels; additive effect with drugs that prolong QT (macrolides, class I and III antiarrhythmics) increasing risk of TdP; increases dabigatran levels	Little effect	Liver
Amiodarone	Prolongs PR and QT; slows sinus rate	None	Increases digoxin and cyclosporine levels; increases warfarin effect	Increases DT	Liver
Sotalol	Prolongs PR and QT; slows sinus rate	Negative inotrope	Additive effects with other β-blockers	Decreases DT	Kidney
Ibutilide	Prolongs PR and QT	None	Additive effect on QT prolongation with class IA and other class III anti-arrhythmic agents	Decreases DT	Liver
Dofetilide	Prolongs QT	None	Verapamil, diltiazem, Cimetidine, and ketoconazole increase dofetilide level	Decreases DT	Liver and kidney

DT, Defibrillation threshold; ECG, electrocardiogram; LV, left ventricle; PT, pacing threshold; TdP, torsades de pointes.

Class III Antiarrhythmic Agents

Class III antiarrhythmic agents are a heterogeneous group of drugs that block the potassium rectifier currents responsible for phase 3 cardiac repolarization, prolonging the cardiac action potential duration and refractory period. These agents demonstrate reverse-use dependence, with more potent potassium-channel blockade at slower heart rates. Prolonging the action potential duration can be therapeutic or proarrhythmic (e.g., TdP). This class represents the dominant category of antiarrhythmic agents in use.

Amiodarone is an iodinated compound available orally and parentally. With oral administration, it is slowly absorbed.

Deposition of amiodarone in body fat stores prolongs the time to reach steady-state levels. The elimination half-life of the drug is 35 to 100 days. Amiodarone's pharmacology is complex, with class I through IV activity, although its primary therapeutic mechanism is prolongation of the action potential duration. It is effective in treating SVTs and VTs. It is hepatically metabolized and proven safe to use in the setting of congestive heart failure. Amiodarone is commonly used to treat atrial and ventricular arrhythmias in patients with structural heart disease and renal failure. Amiodarone is superior to other parental antiarrhythmic agents used to treat cardiac arrest and recurrent VT or ventricular fibrillation (VF). Widespread use of amiodarone has been limited by significant side effects necessitating drug discontinuation in

TABLE 9-3 COMMON SIDE EFFECTS OF SELECT ANTIARRHYTHMIC DRUGS

DRUG	MAJOR SIDE EFFECTS
Quinidine	Nausea, diarrhea, abdominal cramping Cinchonism: decreased hearing, tinnitus, blurred vision, delirium Rash, thrombocytopenia, hemolytic anemia Hypotension, torsades de pointes (quinidine syncope)
Procainamide	Drug-induced lupus syndrome Nausea, vomiting Rash, fever, hypotension, psychosis, agranulocytosis Torsades de pointes
Disopyramide	Anticholinergic: dry mouth, blurred vision, constipation, urinary retention, closed angle glaucoma Hypotension, worsening heart failure
Lidocaine	CNS: dizziness, perioral numbness, paresthesias, altered consciousness, coma, seizures
Mexiletine	Nausea, vomiting CNS: dizziness, tremor, paresthesias, ataxia, confusion
Flecainide	CNS: blurred vision, headache, ataxia Congestive heart failure, ventricular proarrhythmia
Propafenone	Nausea, vomiting, constipation, metallic taste to food Dizziness, headache, exacerbation of asthma, ventricular proarrhythmia
β-Blockers	Bronchospasm, bradycardia, fatigue, depression, impotence Congestive heart failure
Calcium-channel blockers	Congestive heart failure, bradycardia, heart block, constipation
Amiodarone	Agranulocytosis, pulmonary fibrosis, hepatopathy, hyperthyroidism or hypothyroidism, corneal microdeposits, bluish discoloration of the skin, nausea, constipation, bradycardia
Sotalol	Same as β-blockers, torsades de pointes
Dronedarone	Diarrhea, QT prolongation and torsades de pointes, death, bradycardia, congestive heart failure, hepatocellular injury, interstitial lung disease
Ibutilide	Torsades de pointes
Dofetilide	Torsades de pointes, headache, dizziness, diarrhea

CNS, Central nervous system.

up to 20% of patients. Serious adverse effects include potentially irreversible pulmonary fibrosis, optic neuropathy producing visual impairment, hyperthyroidism, and severe hepatic toxicity. Less serious adverse effects include hypothyroidism, neurologic toxicity, sun sensitivity, QT prolongation, and bradycardia.

Sotalol blocks β-adrenoreceptors and delayed rectifier K^+ channels, decreasing sinoatrial node automaticity, slowing AV conduction velocity, and prolonging repolarization. It effectively treats a large number of ventricular and supraventricular arrhythmias.

Dofetilide, a selective class III agent used primarily to treat atrial arrhythmias, blocks delayed rectifier K^+ channels to prolong action potential duration and QT intervals. The risk of TdP is about 1% among patients without structural heart disease but as high as 4.8% among patients with congestive heart failure.

Ibutilide, an intravenous class III agent, is used for the acute termination of recent-onset AF and atrial flutter. The risk of polymorphic VT with administration of ibutilide is 8.3%.

Dronedarone is an orally available class III drug demonstrated to reduce the risk of first hospitalization due to cardiovascular events or death from any cause for patients in sinus rhythm

with a history of paroxysmal or persistent AF. Dronedarone may not be used in the setting of permanent AF or in patients with New York Heart Association (NYHA) class IV heart failure or symptomatic heart failure with recent decompensation because the drug increases the risk of cardiovascular death in these populations. Other major side effects of dronedarone are severe hepatotoxicity, interstitial lung disease, bradycardia, and QT prolongation.

Other Antiarrhythmic Agents

The Singh–Vaughn Williams classification scheme does not describe several agents commonly used in cardiac arrhythmia management. *Adenosine* is a parental agent with an elimination half-life of 1 to 6 seconds. The drug binds to A1 receptors to activate K^+ channels, decreasing the action potential duration and hyperpolarizing membrane potentials in the atria, sinoatrial node, and AV node. Indirectly, adenosine blocks catecholamine-stimulated adenylate cyclase activation, decreasing cAMP and consequently decreasing Ca^{2+} influx. Used clinically for its ability to produce transient AV block, adenosine can terminate SVT when the AV node contributes to the reentrant circuit.

Digoxin inhibits Na^+, K^+-ATPase, increasing intracellular Na^+ concentrations and stimulating the Na^+-Ca^{2+} exchanger to increase intracellular Ca^{2+}, accounting for its positive inotropic effect. Digoxin also acts through the autonomic nervous system to enhance vagal tone, slowing sinus rates, shortening the atrial refractory period, and prolonging AV conduction. Digoxin is therefore used for rate control in patients with atrial arrhythmias.

Cardioversion and Defibrillation

Direct current cardioversion and defibrillation represent the cornerstone of acute therapy for unstable tachyarrhythmias and play an important role in the termination of medication-refractory stable tachyarrhythmias. Organized VTs and SVTs may be terminated by synchronized cardioversion—shock delivery synchronized to the QRS complex—to restore normal rhythm. Synchronization is critical to avoid induction of VF by delivering energy during the relative refractory period of the cardiac cycle. Defibrillation entails the asynchronous delivery of electrical current to depolarize a critical mass of myocardium and terminate VF. Successful defibrillation is time dependent, with the likelihood of success declining by approximately 10% per minute from the onset of VF.

Defibrillation may be delivered internally through an implantable cardioverter-defibrillator (ICD) or externally through an automatic external defibrillator (AED). Current-generation AEDs use biphasic waveforms, achieving greater first-shock efficacy compared with older devices delivering monophasic waveforms. ICDs, implanted in patients for primary and secondary prevention of sudden cardiac death (SCD), deliver defibrillation shocks directly to the endocardium through an RV lead. With direct delivery of energy, relatively lower energy levels (<40 J) are typically effective.

Ablation

Catheter ablation plays an important role in the therapy of a broad range of arrhythmias, such as SVT, atrial arrhythmias, and VT. The ascendance of catheter ablation derives in part from the poor efficacy and side effect profiles of available antiarrhythmic drugs. Radiofrequency ablation (i.e., applying radiofrequency-range energy) and cryoablation (i.e., administering freezing temperatures, to produce localized cellular and tissue injury) are commonly used.

Focal and reentrant arrhythmias are defined and localized, permitting targeted delivery of ablation energy to eliminate the tachyarrhythmia. Ablation is associated with varied success and complication rates, depending on the mechanism and location of the arrhythmogenic focus. Cure rates for tricuspid and caval isthmus–dependent atrial flutter, AV nodal reentry tachycardia (AVNRT), and accessory pathway–mediated tachycardias exceed 95%, with low complication rates of about 2%. Although an important therapeutic option in the treatment of AF and VT, success rates are lower and procedural risks are higher.

 For a deeper discussion on this topic, please see Chapter 62, "Approach to the Patient with Suspected Arrhythmia," in Goldman-Cecil Medicine, *25th Edition.*

 BRADYCARDIA

Bradycardia, defined as a heart rate of less than 60 beats per minute, may occur as a consequence of physiologic adaptations or pathology. Bradycardia always results from failure of sinus node function or AV conduction disturbances, or both processes. Clinically significant bradycardia or pauses may result from autonomic disturbances, drugs, chronic intrinsic conduction system disease, or acute cardiac damage as occurs with endocarditis or infarction.

Normal Conduction System: Anatomy and Physiology

Because of the normal gradient of intrinsic automaticity, heart rate usually is determined by intrinsic automaticity of the sinus node. The sinus node is a complex of cells that extends from the superior vena cava and along the upper right atrial free wall in the sulcus terminalis. Blood supply is derived from the sinus node artery, which arises from the right coronary in 66% or left coronary in 34% of patients.

Activation proceeds through the right atrium to the AV node, which is located in the low interatrial septum adjacent to the tricuspid annulus. The AV node is a complex structure with at least three preferential atrial insertions. The anterior atrial insertion has a short conduction time and usually determines the normal AV conduction time in sinus rhythm. The posterior right and left atrial insertions have long conduction times. Because they do not normally mediate AV conduction in humans, they are functionally vestigial. However, the posterior slowly conducting insertions become important in mediating paroxysmal supraventricular tachycardia (PSVT). The AV node derives its blood supply from the AV nodal artery, which is supplied by the right coronary artery in 73% or the left coronary artery in 27% of patients.

After entry into the AV node, conduction proceeds to the His bundle through the fibrous annulus and along the membranous septum before splitting into a leftward Purkinje branch, which ramifies over the left ventricular endocardium, and a rightward branch, which similarly ramifies over the RV endocardium. The leftward branch may be damaged proximally, resulting in full left bundle branch block, or damaged more distally in its anterior or posterior divisions, resulting in fascicular hemiblock patterns.

Normal Autonomic Regulation of Heart Rate

Normal heart rate is a consequence of tonic and phasic autonomic modulation of intrinsic sinus node automaticity. The intrinsic heart rate in the absence of autonomic modulation ranges from 85 to 110 beats per minute and is somewhat faster than normal resting heart rates. That the normal heart rate is slower than the intrinsic rate is a consequence of the dominance of parasympathetic tone over adrenergic tone in the resting state.

Based on a review of Holter recordings in a normal population, the normal resting heart rate is 46 to 93 beats per minute in men and 51 to 95 beats per minute in women. It has been proposed that 50 to 90 is a clinically more accurate working definition of normal heart rate for adults than the traditional 60 to 100 beats per minute commonly used by consensus. However, heart rates well below these estimates may be seen in normal people, especially during hours of sleep. For these reasons, defining a cutoff value for pathologic bradycardia in the absence of symptoms is problematic for an otherwise healthy patient.

The maximal stress-induced heart rate (HR_{max}) is related to maximal sympathetic stimulation, accompanied by withdrawal of parasympathetic tone. This is commonly estimated as $HR_{max} = (220 - age)$.

Sinus Node Dysfunction

Sick sinus syndrome, also called *sinus node dysfunction,* is a common clinical syndrome that increases in prevalence with age. The estimated prevalence is 1 case per 600 patients older than 65 years of age, and it accounts for about one half of all pacemaker implantations. Sinus node dysfunction is a consequence of two distinct processes: failure of intrinsic automaticity and failure of propagation of sinus node impulses to the surrounding atrial tissue, also referred to a *sinus node exit block.*

Sinus node dysfunction manifests clinically as one of several patterns: persistent or episodic sinus bradycardia, inability to appropriately augment rate with exercise (i.e., chronotropic incompetence), sinus pauses, or commonly a combination of these patterns. The sinus node is at the top of a cascade of automaticity and is normally backed up by a competent AV junctional escape mechanism. Severe bradycardia and associated symptoms due to sinus node dysfunction always imply sinus node dysfunction and simultaneous failure of normal subsidiary escape mechanisms. In the setting of a competent escape mechanism, even severe sinus node dysfunction may be completely asymptomatic, clinically well tolerated, and require no specific therapy.

Resting Sinus Bradycardia

Sinus bradycardia is frequently observed during routine clinical practice. Modest sinus bradycardia in the high 40s in men and 50s in women is normal and called *bradycardia* only because of the conventional choice of 60 beats per minute as the lower limit of normal rates. Because there is no set rate at which sinus bradycardia can be labeled as pathologic, pathologic sinus node dysfunction is best defined as significant bradycardia associated with symptoms plausibly attributable to bradycardia.

Modest persistent bradycardia is often asymptomatic. When symptoms occur, they are commonly nonspecific, such as fatigue, listlessness, or dyspnea, making the attribution of symptoms to resting bradycardia difficult. Sinus bradycardia may also exacerbate congestive heart failure and limit effective use of β-blocker therapy, a cornerstone of therapy for heart failure, coronary disease, and tachyarrhythmias. When inappropriate sinus bradycardia is persistent, especially when severe, plausible symptoms are present, and alternate causes of symptoms have been excluded, pacemaker implantation is reasonable. Asymptomatic sinus bradycardia should rarely be treated with pacing unless a need for medical therapy is expected to further exacerbate bradycardia.

Chronotropic Incompetence

Cardiac output during exercise is increased by augmentation in stroke volume and an increase in heart rate. If heart rate rise with exercise is inadequate, exertional symptoms such as fatigue or dyspnea may ensue. As in the case of resting sinus bradycardia, unless severe, attribution of symptoms to chronotropic incompetence is difficult. Various criteria for this condition have been proposed that rely on the inability to achieve a set fraction of age-predicted heart rate or heart rate reserve. As for resting sinus bradycardia, the decision to implant a pacemaker for chronotropic incompetence is a matter of judgment more than criteria.

Sinus Pauses or Arrest

An abrupt failure of sinus node automaticity or failure of propagation from the sinus node to the atrium can result in a pause in atrial activity. P waves are absent, and if of adequate duration and not accompanied by a competent subsidiary escape mechanism, it can result in abrupt symptoms of lightheadedness, presyncope or true syncope. Sinus pauses of less than 3 seconds are commonly seen for normal subjects, who are rarely symptomatic. Sinus pauses exceeding 3 seconds and not occurring during sleep are often pathologic and may result in symptoms. Sinus pauses associated with simultaneous symptoms and documentation of pauses lasting 3 seconds or longer in patients with a history of symptoms plausibly related to bradycardia are indications for pacemaker therapy.

Sinoatrial Exit Block

Sinus node dysfunction is often accompanied by significant atrial fibrosis, which may lead to a block in the tissues surrounding the sinus node complex and impede propagation to the atrial tissue. Bradycardia due to sinus node dysfunction may result, not from a failure of automaticity, but from failure of propagation from the sinus node complex to the atrium. Because sinus node activity is not directly apparent from the surface ECG, the diagnosis is made indirectly by the observation of abrupt halving in the sinus P-wave rate, followed by an abrupt return to the baseline sinus rate (Fig. 9-3C and D). Although other patterns may be observed, 2 : 1 exit block is the most common. Therapy for sinoatrial exit block is identical to that for intermittent sinus bradycardia (discussed earlier).

Bradycardia-Tachycardia Syndrome as a Consequence of Sinus Node Dysfunction

Bradycardia-tachycardia ("brady-tachy") syndrome refers to a clinically significant tachyarrhythmia sometimes accompanied by clinically significant bradycardia. The term may be confusing because the mechanism of tachycardia is often unrelated to the mechanism of bradycardia.

This syndrome most commonly manifests as intermittent pathologic atrial arrhythmias, often intermittent AF with concomitant sinus node dysfunction resulting in long pauses or symptomatic sinus bradycardia when the patient is in sinus rhythm. A typical manifestation of this syndrome is a prolonged period of asystole after termination of AF (see Fig. 9-3E) due to slow recovery of sinus node automaticity with resultant presyncope or syncope.

The combination of two seemingly independent processes is in part a consequence of the high prevalence of AF and sinus node dysfunction in the elderly and the need to use potent drugs to decrease ventricular response during AF with resultant unintended secondary sinus node dysfunction between periods of atrial arrhythmias. This type of bradycardia-tachycardia syndrome represents an important form of clinical sinus node dysfunction and is a common indication for pacemaker implantation.

Sinus node dysfunction causing bradycardia-tachycardia should be distinguished from a common, unrelated form of bradycardia-tachycardia syndrome, which is characterized by chronic rather than intermittent AF with periods of rapid and slow ventricular responses. This condition is often incorrectly referred to as *sick sinus syndrome*. However, in this syndrome, the atrium is chronically fibrillating, and the sinus node therefore has no influence on heart rate. Bradycardia or protracted pauses in the setting of chronic AF is a consequence of impaired AV conduction and is unrelated to sinus node dysfunction.

Atrioventricular Conduction Disturbances

AV conduction disturbances include disorders in which the normal physiologic AV relationship is not maintained due to pathologic delay in AV conduction or to intermittent or complete loss of AV conduction. The PR interval includes three distinct phases of AV conduction. Although the individual components of AV conduction can be readily recorded by a His bundle catheter in an electrophysiology laboratory, the salient features of AV conduction disturbances can usually be elucidated by careful interpretation of the surface ECG without resorting to invasive recording techniques.

The right atrial conduction time from the area of the sinus node where the P wave begins to the region of the AV node occupies a short first portion of the PR interval and usually lasts no more than 30 milliseconds. Because the atrial conduction time is short and does not change much over time in a given patient, it can conveniently be ignored when assessing AV conduction. The second portion of the PR interval is the propagation time through the AV node, which is normally 50 to 120 milliseconds. The last component of the PR interval is the time for propagation through the His bundle and bundle branches, which is typically 30 to 55 milliseconds. Although this last portion,

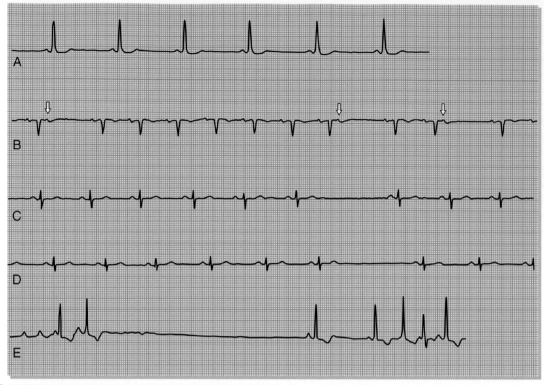

FIGURE 9-3 Sinus node dysfunction. **A,** Sinus bradycardia in a patient receiving metoprolol. This bradycardia results from diminished normal automaticity of the sinus node. **B,** Pauses related to blocked premature atrial contractions (PACs). Blocked PACs are a common cause for apparent sinus pauses because the PAC may be early enough to be concealed by the T wave of the preceding beat *(arrows)*. The pauses are not a sign of sinus node dysfunction but rather a physiologic response to an early coupled PAC. **C,** The sinus pause is an abnormal finding that suggests sinus node disease. The pause is exactly two sinus cycles and may represent sinoatrial exit block. **D,** Sinoatrial Wenckebach type exit block. As is the case with the RR interval preceding atrioventricular nodal Wenckebach, progressive shortening of the PP interval preceding a doubling in sinus cycle length likely represents Wenckebach exit block from the sinus node tissue to the atrium. **E,** Bradycardia tachycardia syndrome due to sinus node dysfunction. An episode of rapidly conducted atrial fibrillation or flutter terminates and is followed for a protracted period of sinus arrest before recovery of sinus rhythm and ultimate relapse of rapidly conducted atrial fibrillation. These pauses may result in syncope or near-syncope.

constituting His-Purkinje conduction, is short, it is the major prognostic component of AV conduction and therefore clinically important. Because the last portion of the PR interval is the time from the onset of His bundle to the time of ventricular activation, it is commonly referred to as the HV interval. Although the HV interval cannot be measured directly from the surface ECG, a block in the His-Purkinje system can be inferred from the characteristic features that can be gleaned from review of the surface ECG.

First-Degree Atrioventricular Block

First-degree AV block is defined as a PR interval exceeding 0.2 seconds (200 milliseconds) in the setting of otherwise preserved AV conduction (Fig. 9-4A). First-degree block implies a conduction delay in one of the components of AV conduction, usually at the level of the AV node or His-Purkinje system (i.e., infranodal conduction system). First-degree AV block is usually asymptomatic, but it is a sign of AV conduction system disease and may be a diagnostic clue to the mechanism of intermittent electrocardiographically undocumented symptoms in a patient with unexplained syncope.

Second-Degree Atrioventricular Bock

Second-degree AV block is defined as intermittent failure of AV conduction with interspersed periods of intact AV conduction.

Second-degree AV block, like sinus bradycardia and pauses, may be seen normally during hours of sleep as well as in athletes with high parasympathetic tone. Alone, it is not an indication of AV conduction system disease.

Second-degree block may be asymptomatic, may be associated with mild symptoms such as palpitations, or if resulting in protracted pauses or persistent bradycardia, may result in hemodynamic symptoms, including lightheadedness, syncope, and fatigue. Second-degree AV block at the level of the AV node is usually indolent and gradually progressive. Because of stable junctional escape mechanisms associated with progression to complete heart block at the level of the AV node, second-degree AV block at this level tends to have a benign prognosis and, in the absence of symptoms, can be followed safely without intervention.

Second-degree block in the infranodal conduction system, which is composed of the His bundle and bundle branches, can be malignant with a tendency to progress abruptly and unpredictably to higher degrees of AV block accompanied by unstable or absent subsidiary escape mechanisms. After a patient becomes symptomatic, the infranodal block may progress to complete heart block and, in some cases, to sudden death. Despite its malignant nature, SCD is rarely attributable to complete heart block, suggesting that most patients have symptoms permitting intervention before progression to sudden death.

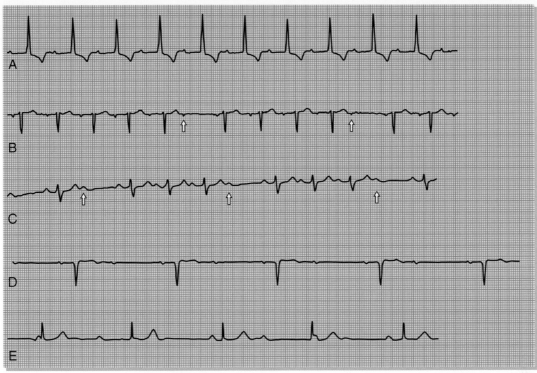

FIGURE 9-4　Heart block. **A,** First-degree atrioventricular (AV) block is associated with 1:1 conduction but a prolonged PR interval more than 200 milliseconds. **B,** Mobitz type I (Wenckebach) second-degree AV block. Notice the progressive PR prolongation preceding the blocked P wave (arrows) followed by recovery of conduction with a shorter PR interval before repetition of the same pattern. **C,** Mobitz type II second-degree AV block. Notice that the PR interval does not prolong in the beat preceding the blocked P wave (arrows). **D,** A 2:1 second-degree AV block. Notice that every other P wave fails to conduct. Because there are never two consecutively conducted P waves to assess for the presence or absence of progressive prolongation, this type of block is neither Mobitz I nor Mobitz II. **E,** Complete heart bock with a junctional escape rhythm. Notice that the atrial rate is faster than the ventricular rate and that there is AV dissociation. The narrow QRS escape rhythm implies a level of block high in the conduction system near the AV node.

Because of the profound difference in natural history of second-degree AV block at the AV node and that at an infranodal level, the major clinical task in evaluating patients with second-degree AV block is to establish the probable level of the block. The surface ECG and pattern of block are quite useful.

Mobitz Type I Second-Degree Atrioventricular Block

Also referred to a Wenckebach block, *Mobitz type I second-degree AV block* is a progressive prolongation in the PR interval before development of AV block, usually for one cycle followed by recovery of conduction with a return to the baseline PR interval (see Fig. 9-4B). Because the degree of prolongation of the PR interval is less with each successive beat before the block, the RR intervals can paradoxically shorten in the final beats before the block.

Mobitz I AV block typically is associated with block at the level of the AV node. However, this pattern is rarely seen with advanced infranodal disease in the His bundle and bundle branches. Because Mobitz type I AV block usually occurs at the level of the AV node, infranodal conduction is commonly normal and associated with a narrow conducted QRS complex. In ambiguous cases, other clues may be helpful. Because AV node function is improved with exercise, Mobitz I block tends to normalizes with activity and return at rest. Second-degree block at the level of the AV node is improved with atropine and exacerbated by carotid sinus massage. If associated with periods of complete heart block,

a block at the level of the AV node is associated with a junctional escape with a QRS morphology similar to that in conducted sinus rhythm. In contrast, the observation of a wide complex escape that is different from the conducted QRS points to infranodal causes of block in the His-Purkinje system. The block may be malignant (discussed later) and require expeditious use of ventricular pacing to prevent catastrophic bradycardia.

Mobitz Type II Second-Degree Atrioventricular Block

Mobitz type II second-degree AV block is intermittent failure of AV conduction during stable atrial rates without antecedent PR prolongation and followed by recovery of AV conduction (see Fig. 9-4C). Mobitz II AV block is believed to always be a sign of block in the infranodal tissues, including the His bundle and bundle branches. Whereas infranodal block may rarely display Mobitz I (Wenckebach) periodicity, AV block at the level of the AV node does not result in true Mobitz II AV block periodicity.

The finding of Mobitz II AV block is always reason for concern. Although it may result from block in the His bundle or subsidiary bundle branches. Block within the His bundle accompanied by a narrow QRS complex is uncommon. In practice, Mobitz II AV block is usually preceded by the development of fixed bundle branch block. It has been believed that such bundle branch block patterns implied disease of the bundle branches themselves as they ramify within the ventricles. However in many cases of left bundle branch block, the disease process may actually be within

the His bundle affecting fibers which will ultimately extend to the left bundle branch. Regardless of the exact anatomical level of clinical bundle branch block, it remains a good clinical rule that most patients exhibiting Mobitz II AV Block will also exhibit a full bundle branch block pattern during periods of conduction between episodes of second degree AV block.

In ambiguous cases, other clues may be helpful. Because infranodal function improves relatively little with exercise, infranodal block tends to worsen with the increasing heart rates associated with exercise or stress. Atropine is not helpful for infranodal block, and because it may accelerate sinus rates, it may cause a patient to progress to higher degrees of AV block with a consequent decrease in the conducted ventricular rate. Exogenous catecholamines such as isoproterenol infusion may be helpful acutely but should not be relied on. Because of its malignant potential, hemodynamically significant Mobitz II AV block should be addressed with early temporary or permanent pacing.

2 : 1 and High-Degree Atrioventricular Blocks

2 : 1 AV block is a failure of conduction of every other P wave (see Fig. 9-4D). This pattern is most commonly seen with an infranodal block in the His bundle or bundle branches. However, 2 : 1 AV block may also be observed in advanced AV nodal disease. It can be distinguished from the more common infranodal form of 2 : 1 block by the typical Mobitz I periodicity accompanied by a usually narrow QRS complex at other times in the same patient. Because two consecutive conducted P waves are not available to assess the Mobitz pattern, a 2 : 1 AV block is neither Mobitz I nor Mobitz II.

High-degree AV block is second-degree AV block with conduction failure of two or more consecutive P waves. High-degree AV block is neither Mobitz I nor Mobitz II. Although Mobitz periodicity cannot be assigned, like other forms of second-degree AV blocks, the level of block must be established to assess prognosis and guide therapy. In this case, the ancillary clues described for Mobitz blocks remain useful.

Third-Degree Atrioventricular Block

Third-degree AV block or equivalently complete heart block is a complete failure of AV conduction. In the setting of underlying sinus rhythm, this is an atrial rate faster than the ventricular rate associated with AV dissociation (see Fig. 9-4E). However, when the underlying rhythm is AF, the definition of complete heart block cannot rely on the demonstration of AV dissociation. Because conducted AF always results in an *irregular* ventricular response, the finding of a *regular and slow* ventricular response during AF implies an associated complete heart block.

As is the case for second-degree AV block, the level of the third-degree block determines the clinical behavior and prognosis of complete heart block. Complete heart block at the level of the AV node is associated with a generally stable junctional escape with rates between 40 and 50 beats per minute and usually with a narrow QRS complex. If the patient had a bundle branch block before the development of complete heart block, a block at the level of the AV node is associated with a wide QRS escape, identical to the conducted QRS before the development of a block.

Complete heart block at an infranodal level is associated with a wide and slow ventricular escape rhythm, which often is slower than 40 beats per minute with a QRS different from the antecedent conducted morphology. Unfortunately, infranodal escape rhythms may be absent entirely, leading to asystole and loss of consciousness. When infranodal complete heart block is suspected, regardless of tolerance of the ventricular escape rhythm, prompt institution of temporary or permanent ventricular pacing is appropriate.

⬤ TACHYCARDIAS
Overview and Classification

Tachyarrhythmias are categorized as supraventricular and ventricular arrhythmias. SVT relies mechanistically on the atrium or the AV node, or both. During SVT, normal depolarization of the ventricles by the His-Purkinje system produces a narrow complex tachycardia. SVT can manifest as a wide complex tachycardia in the setting of aberrancy or antegrade conduction down an accessory pathway, producing an abnormal sequence of ventricular activation. Ventricular tachyarrhythmias do not depend on the atrium or AV node; they originate in the ventricles, generating a wide complex tachycardia.

Supraventricular Tachycardias

SVTs can be categorized as PSVT, focal atrial tachycardia, atrial flutter and related organized reentrant atrial tachycardias, and AF. This classification scheme, which addresses the underlying arrhythmic mechanism, clinical presentation, and prognosis, guides evaluation and therapy.

PSVT typically manifests in young patients without structural heart disease. The PSVT syndrome is characterized by recurrent tachypalpitations with abrupt onset and offset. Focal atrial tachycardia is more often observed in patients with underlying atrial enlargement and valvular heart disease. AF and atrial flutter are associated with advancing age, hypertension, structural heart disease, diabetes, obstructive sleep apnea, and pulmonary disease. Unlike PSVT, AF carries an increased risk of stroke, heart failure, and death.

Paroxysmal Supraventricular Tachycardia

The incidence of PSVT is 35 cases per 100,000 person-years, with a prevalence of 2.25 per 1000 person-years. Patients report recurrent tachypalpitations. Associated symptoms may include shortness of breath, lightheadedness, chest pain, and syncope. Anginal chest pain and ischemic ST-segment depression are common and related to increased myocardial oxygen demand coupled with the loss of normal diastolic coronary perfusion time. These findings do not necessarily indicate underlying coronary artery disease and typically resolve with tachycardia termination.

PSVT typically occurs independent of structural heart disease and may manifest at any point from infancy to advanced age. PSVT relies on reentry, which is localized in the AV node in approximately 60% of cases and uses a concealed or manifest accessory pathway in 40%. Unless a delta wave indicative of WPW is identified, the underlying mechanism of PSVT is not usually apparent on initial clinical presentation.

An ECG obtained during PSVT can provide useful clues to establish the diagnosis and guide management. The AV relationship should be assessed during tachycardia. By ascertaining the relationship of the P wave to the preceding QRS complex, it is possible to classify PSVT as a *short RP tachycardia* or a *long RP tachycardia*. Short RP tachycardias demonstrate a short RP pattern with P waves embedded within or occurring closely after the preceding QRS complex. Short RP tachycardias occur with reentrant SVT when the retrograde VA conduction time is shorter than the antegrade AV conduction time. This pattern is observed in the two most common forms of PSVT: typical AV nodal reentry tachycardia and reciprocating AV tachycardia related to an accessory pathway.

Long RP tachycardias are characterized by an RP interval that is longer than the next PR interval during tachycardia. This pattern occurs when the retrograde VA conduction time in reentrant arrhythmias is long due to a slowly conducting retrograde pathway during tachycardia. Atypical AV node reentry, in which retrograde conduction occurs over the slow AV nodal pathway, is the most common example of a long RP reentrant tachycardia.

Atrioventricular Nodal Reentry Tachycardia

AVNRT is the most common form of PSVT. The arrhythmic mechanism depends on two distinct pathways in the AV node: a slowly conducting pathway with a short effective refractory period (i.e., slow pathway) and a rapidly conducting pathway with a longer refractory period (i.e., fast pathway). The atrial insertion sites of the two pathways are different. The fast pathway inserts anteriorly near the bundle of His, and the slow pathway inserts posteriorly near the coronary sinus ostium. Although the dual pathways are a normal feature of the AV node, patients with clinical tachycardia have more robust slow pathway conduction.

Tachycardia is most commonly triggered by a premature atrial contraction that blocks the fast pathway due to its prolonged refractory period and conducts slowly antegrade down the slow pathway, producing a long PR interval on the ECG. On reaching the distal common pathway where the fast and slow AV nodal inputs meet, if the fast pathway is no longer refractory, the impulse may penetrate the fast pathway in a retrograde direction and rapidly activate the atrium, producing a short RP interval and reinitiating reentry down the slow pathway and up the fast pathway. In typical slow-fast AVNRT, the RP interval is so short that the P wave is often buried in the preceding QRS complex (Fig. 9-5A).

Atypical fast-slow AVNRT may occur with antegrade conduction over the fast pathway and retrograde conduction over the slow pathway. This form of AVNRT is uncommon and produces a long RP pattern on the ECG with characteristically deeply inverted retrograde P waves in leads II, III, and aVF.

Vagal maneuvers cause temporary AV nodal blockade and may terminate sustained AVNRT. Alternatively, intravenous adenosine is a highly effective acute therapy. The need for chronic or definitive therapy is determined by symptoms, arrhythmia frequency, and patient preference. Catheter ablation of the slow pathway at the posterior AV node is highly successful, eliminating AVNRT with a greater than 90% success rate and a low risk of complications. Drug therapy with β-blockers and calcium-channel blockers directed at the AV node may be helpful for chronic suppression. Occasionally, class IC and III antiarrhythmics may be required. AVNRT should be easily distinguished

from automatic junctional tachycardia, with a narrow complex and rapid, irregular rhythm typically demonstrating AV dissociation (see Fig. 9-5B).

Reciprocating Atrioventricular Tachycardia and Preexcitation Syndromes

Congenital anomalous extranodal AV muscle fibers or accessory pathways may arise as a consequence of incomplete development of the AV annulus. These pathways are usually observed in patients with otherwise anatomically normal hearts, although right-sided accessory pathways are associated with Ebstein's anomaly and left-sided accessory pathways with hypertrophic cardiomyopathy.

Accessory pathways, or bypass tracts, may conduct antegradely, retrogradely, or bidirectionally. They typically fail to demonstrate decremental conduction or the slowed conduction with increasingly frequent stimulation that characterizes the AV node. Accessory pathways capable of antegrade conduction produce early activation of the ventricle in sinus rhythm because conduction over the accessory pathway surpasses conduction over the AV node. The relatively rapid AV conduction produces a shortened PR interval, and eccentric ventricular activation over the pathway slurs the QRS onset, resulting in a delta wave (see Fig. 9-5C). If the accessory pathway is capable only of retrograde conduction, the baseline ECG in sinus rhythm does not show evidence of an accessory pathway, and the extranodal AV connection is called *concealed*.

Short PR intervals are also observed in patients with Lown-Ganong-Levine syndrome. These patients have a normal-appearing QRS complex without a delta wave because ventricular activation occurs through the His-Purkinje system (see Fig. 9-5D).

Whether accessory pathways are concealed or manifest, the most common associated arrhythmia is *orthodromic AV reentrant tachycardia* (AVRT). Tachycardia is mediated by antegrade conduction down the AV node to the ventricle and subsequent retrograde conduction up the accessory pathway to activate the atrium and then move back down the AV node. Because the ventricles are activated during tachycardia exclusively over the AV node, the resulting tachycardia is typically a narrow complex unless aberrancy occurs (see Fig. 9-5E). A short RP pattern is observed on the ECG, although the RP is slightly longer than commonly observed in a typical AVNRT. Because the atria and ventricles constitute portions of the reentrant circuit, tachycardia depends on 1 : 1 AV conduction.

Less frequently, *antidromic AV reentrant tachycardia* is seen in patients with accessory pathways capable of antegrade conduction. The accessory pathway provides the antegrade limb of the reentrant circuit, and the AV node serves as the retrograde pathway, resulting in a wide QRS tachycardia due to complete preexcitation of the ventricles.

Special Considerations for Patients with Supraventricular Tachycardia and Delta Waves in Sinus Rhythm

Asymptomatic patients may have delta waves on the ECG, which is called a *WPW pattern*. Prevalence of the WPW pattern in the general population is approximately 1 case per 1000 people. Accessory pathways may be poorly conducting and less likely to

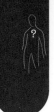

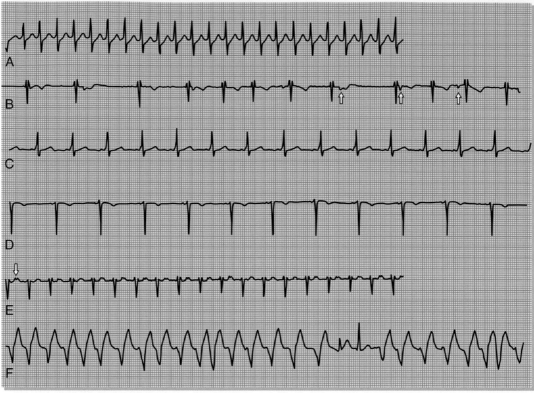

FIGURE 9-5 Atrioventricular (AV) nodal (junctional) rhythm disturbances. **A,** Supraventricular tachycardia. The lack of visible P waves during tachycardia suggests that they are concealed within the QRS complex, a pattern indicative of underlying AV nodal reentrant tachycardia. **B,** Automatic junctional tachycardia. Notice the AV dissociation during tachycardia. The P waves *(arrows)* are dissociated from the QRS complexes. **C,** Sinus rhythm with a short PR interval due to the presence of delta waves in a patient with Wolff-Parkinson-White (WPW) syndrome. The slurred QRS upstroke of the delta wave results from early activation of the ventricle by the extranodal bypass tract, followed by fusion with rapid conduction down the normal conduction system and resulting in narrowing of the terminal QRS. **D,** Sinus rhythm with a short PR interval but no delta waves. Despite the short PR, the P wave is normally vectored, excluding a junctional rhythm that appears similar but with an inverted P wave. A short PR interval in sinus rhythm without delta waves is caused by an abnormally rapid AV nodal conduction and is described as a Lown-Ganong-Levine pattern. **E,** Supraventricular tachycardia. Unlike tracing **A,** there is a clear P wave *(arrow)* inscribed immediately after each QRS in the ST segment. This pattern is seen most commonly with orthodromic AV reciprocating tachycardia in a patient with WPW syndrome. The early P wave in WPW is caused by retrograde conduction up the accessory pathway after ventricular activation during tachycardia. **F,** Preexcited atrial fibrillation (AF) in a patient with WPW syndrome. Notice the rapid and irregular ventricular response with widening of the QRS due to preexcitation. This pattern results from rapid conduction of the AF down the accessory pathway, bypassing the normal conduction system. As in this arrhythmia, occasional conduction down the AV node may occur during ongoing tachycardia, resulting in periods with a narrow QRS complex.

promote tachycardia, accounting for the absence of symptoms. These patients have a favorable prognosis, particularly if spontaneous and abrupt cessation of preexcitation occurs with exercise or during ambulatory monitoring. In most cases, no specific therapy is required.

Occasionally, patients participating in high-risk activities with WPW pattern may be subjected to invasive electrophysiologic testing for risk stratification. Patients with delta waves demonstrating SVT or suggestive arrhythmic symptoms are said to have WPW syndrome, and invasive electrophysiologic testing is ordinarily recommended in these patients. Testing helps to stratify the risk of SCD.

Curative ablation is highly effective, with a success rate of 95%, and poses a low risk of procedural complications. Chronic therapy with antiarrhythmic drugs that prolong the accessory pathway refractory period (i.e., class IA, IC, or III agents) may be effective, but the potential for adverse drug effects has made accessory pathway ablation the treatment of choice for symptomatic patients.

The use of agents that slow AV nodal conduction in patients with WPW syndrome warrants special mention. Digoxin, β-blockers, and calcium-channel blockers should not be used in patients with WPW because they slow conduction through the AV node, resulting in preferential excitation of the ventricles over the accessory pathway. In the setting of AF or atrial flutter, this may cause rapid ventricular rates and hemodynamic instability.

Wolff-Parkinson-White Syndrome and Atrial Fibrillation

WPW syndrome is associated with a 0.25% per year risk of SCD, which is related to the development of AF with rapid antegrade conduction over the accessory pathway and to VF. This risk is greatest for patients demonstrating very short preexcited RR intervals during AF. For some WPW patients, SCD may be the initial presentation. Successful catheter ablation of the accessory pathway eliminates this possibility.

Patients with WPW and rapidly conducted AF have the characteristic electrocardiographic findings of a rapid, irregularly irregular, wide QRS rhythm with various degrees of QRS widening or preexcitation from beat to beat (see Fig. 9-5F). During AF in the setting of underlying WPW, activation of the ventricle over the AV node produces concealed retrograde activation of the accessory pathway, prolonging the refractory period of the pathway and moderating the rate of antegrade accessory pathway conduction.

Treating patients with AV nodal–blocking therapy decreases concealed retrograde activation of the pathway, facilitating antegrade accessory pathway conduction and potentiating hemodynamic instability. Appropriate acute therapy includes drugs that prolong the accessory pathway refractory period, such as intravenous procainamide, ibutilide, or amiodarone. In the event of hemodynamic instability, electrical cardioversion is preferred.

Role of Catheter Ablation in Wolff-Parkinson-White Syndrome

Catheter ablation is highly effective for treating WPW, with success rates of approximately 95% and recurrence rates of only 5%. Procedural complications are uncommon, with major complications occurring in 2% to 4% of cases and deaths related to ablation occurring in 0.1%.

Although antiarrhythmic drug therapy may control symptoms, the expense and risks of pharmacologic therapy along with the safety and efficacy of ablation have made radiofrequency ablation the first-line therapy for symptomatic WPW. Because most patients with asymptomatic WPW patterns have a favorable prognosis, they should not be subjected to ablation.

Atrial Arrhythmias
Overview and Classification

Atrial arrhythmias depend entirely on the atria but are mechanistically independent of AV conduction. As a consequence, intra-atrial arrhythmias persist despite the development of spontaneous or pharmacologically induced AV block. Tachycardias originating in the atria may be organized and repetitive, resulting from automaticity or intra-atrial reentry, or may be chaotic and disorganized, as is the case in AF. Therapy is directed at moderating the ventricular response during episodes of tachycardia or suppressing the underlying atrial arrhythmia.

Focal arrhythmias originate from a point source in one of the atria, and circumferential spread encompasses the remainder of the atrium. These arrhythmias display distinct P waves separated by a clear isoelectric segment. Focal arrhythmias commonly have an automatic mechanism, but in some cases, they may result from micro-reentry involving a geographically small portion of the atrium (e.g., around a single pulmonary vein), followed by radial spread to the rest of the atrium. Although most commonly a single abnormal focus may be active, in the setting of severe physiologic stress, multiple foci may be active simultaneously, leading to a chaotic electrocardiographic appearance with multiple distinct P waves, referred to as *multifocal atrial tachycardia* (MAT) (Fig. 9-6B). Automatic arrhythmias tend to be episodic and nonsustained, sometimes recurring incessantly. Cycle length often varies within a run, between runs, and with changes in autonomic tone.

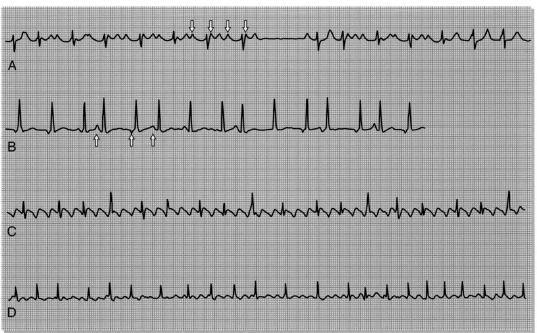

FIGURE 9-6   Atrial arrhythmias. **A,** Runs of focal atrial tachycardia with variable atrioventricular (AV) block. The tachycardia occurs in salvos with interspersed periods of sinus rhythm. The P waves *(arrows)* during tachycardia appear uniform although their cycle length varies, resulting in variable patterns of AV conduction and an irregular ventricular rate. **B,** Multifocal atrial tachycardia. Notice the incessant atrial premature beats *(arrows)* with at least three distinct morphologies. Because of the irregularly irregular response, this arrhythmia can be easily misdiagnosed as atrial fibrillation (which lacks discrete P waves) if the tracing is not carefully reviewed. **C,** Atrial flutter with rapid, variable conduction. Notice the continuous sawtooth atrial activity. Although commonly manifesting with stable 2:1 block and a regular response, the block varies in this patient, progressing through periods of 2:1 and 3:1 ratios and resulting in an irregular ventricular response. **D,** Atrial fibrillation with a rapid ventricular response. Notice the wavering baseline without distinct P waves and an irregularly irregular response.

Macro-reentrant atrial arrhythmias are a consequence of stable reentrant circuits, which encompass large portions of the atria. All such circuits require a central obstacle and a region of slowed atrial conduction related to atrial dilation or fibrosis. The most common of these arrhythmias is *typical atrial flutter,* which is mediated by right atrial reentry around normal anatomic obstacles. In addition to typical flutter, reentry may occur around acquired obstacles, most commonly scars resulting from prior cardiac surgery or ablation involving the atria. Reentrant arrhythmias tend to manifest clinically as paroxysmal sustained or persistent arrhythmias. Although they may be self-terminating and episodic, individual episodes tend to be protracted.

The final mechanism of atrial arrhythmia is AF. This arrhythmia involves components of focal automatic mechanisms and reentry. The major advances made in the understanding and management of this common arrhythmia are reviewed in the following sections.

Focal Atrial Tachycardia

Focal atrial tachycardia also is referred to as ectopic atrial tachycardia and automatic atrial tachycardia. These terms describe a characteristic clinical pattern that usually manifests as runs of unifocal PACs lasting for seconds or minutes, usually followed by spontaneous termination and subsequent spontaneous reinitiation of additional salvos of tachycardia (see Fig. 9-6A). This arrhythmia less commonly manifests as a paroxysmal sustained tachycardia. When mapped in the electrophysiologic laboratory, these arrhythmias have a focal origin, and although they are sometimes triggered by rapid pacing, suggesting triggered activity, they appear to be automatic rather than a reentrant mechanism.

The electrocardiographic features are characteristic and usually permit accurate diagnosis. Because the arrhythmia is focal and automatic, the morphology of the first PAC of the run is identical to the subsequent PACs. Cycle length tends to vary between and within runs, and tachycardia is unaffected by intermittent AV block, which may occur during the runs. The same focus often fires erratically between runs, resulting in frequent atrial ectopy that is morphologically similar to the P wave observed during the runs.

The arrhythmia appears to be caused by intracellular calcium overload and resultant triggered activity related to delayed afterdepolarizations, making it responsive to calcium-channel blockers and β-blockers. The paroxysmal sustained form of this arrhythmia is also adenosine responsive, giving the false impression of dependence on AV conduction. The use of digoxin may exacerbate triggered causes of atrial tachycardia. Class IC agents, such as flecainide and propafenone, may be useful in patients without structural heart disease or coronary artery disease. Amiodarone can also be used in these patients for rhythm control. The arrhythmia is readily amenable to catheter ablation if ectopy occurs frequently enough to permit mapping.

Typical Atrial Flutter

Atrial flutter is a persistent atrial arrhythmia with an atrial rate of at least 250 beats per minute (see Fig. 9-6C). Because the normal AV node cannot conduct 1 : 1 at these rates, this arrhythmia characteristically manifests with 2 : 1 conduction and a ventricular response of about 140 to −150 beats per minute. During 2 : 1 conduction, the difficulty in perceiving flutter waves may lead to diagnostic confusion. Typical atrial flutter is the most common form of this arrhythmia, and it is mediated by macro-reentry restricted to the right atrium. The central obstacles in this circuit consist of normal anatomic structures, accounting for its stereotyped pattern.

Typical atrial flutter is mediated by counterclockwise reentry around the tricuspid valve as viewed from the ventricle. The valve prevents anterior collapse of the circuit, and posteriorly a long ridge in the atrial wall (i.e., crista terminalis) forms a functional line of block, preventing the circuit from collapsing posteriorly. Because the normal obstacles already exist, flutter development results from the abnormally slowed conduction related to atrial enlargement, fibrosis, or edema, which sometimes is combined with shortened atrial refractory periods due to catecholamine stress. Typical counterclockwise atrial flutter demonstrates a deeply negative F wave in leads II, III, and aVF; a sharply positive F wave in V_1; and a negative F wave in V_6.

A less common reversed form of this arrhythmia is caused by clockwise reentry around the tricuspid valve. It demonstrates an ECG exactly opposite to the counterclockwise form, with a strongly positive F wave in leads II, III, and aVF; a sharply negative F wave in V_1; and a positive F wave in V_6. In both cases, the F waves are often difficult to perceive because of 2 : 1 conduction. If the unusual F-wave vector is not recognized, the ECG may be misinterpreted as sinus tachycardia. Clues to identification of atrial flutter are persistent, unexplained heart rates of about 150 beats per minute with a variation of only a few beats per minute over time and the finding of a negative P wave in the inferior leads, which is expected to be positive in sinus rhythm.

The most fruitful method of diagnosis is the provocation of transient AV block with carotid sinus massage or adenosine infusion. This transiently exposes the underlying flutter waves but does not terminate the arrhythmia.

Although acute therapy involves rate control or cardioversion if drugs are poorly tolerated, long-term rate control for this arrhythmia is difficult. Drug doses that result in acceptable block at rest often fail to control exercise rates, and doses that result in exercise rate control often provoke bradycardia at rest. Early restoration of sinus rhythm is preferred for this arrhythmia.

Atrial flutter is a common transient arrhythmia in acute care hospital settings. The right atrial wall is thin, and pericarditis resulting from cardiac or thoracic surgery results in atrial edema and inflammation that may permit adequate slowing and promote transient atrial flutter. Acute pulmonary decompensation may result in right heart failure and may promote transient atrial flutter. In all of these settings, endogenous or pharmacologic catecholamine stimulation exacerbates the arrhythmia. Transient therapy for up to a month is appropriate in these settings.

When atrial flutter occurs in the absence of an acute precipitant, long-term therapy is required. Given the difficulty of achieving rate control in atrial flutter and the need for antiarrhythmic agents with associated potential morbidity to maintain sinus rhythm, catheter ablation has become the primary means of treating this arrhythmia. Antiarrhythmic therapy for atrial flutter is similar to that for AF (discussed later). Antiarrhythmic drug

therapy should be reserved for temporary treatment of likely transient flutter or for patients who are not suitable candidates for invasive management. Catheter ablation of typical atrial flutter is a low-risk procedure with a long-term success rate exceeding 90% in experienced centers.

Atypical Atrial Flutter and Macro-reentrant Atrial Tachycardia

In addition to the typical atrial flutter circulating around normal anatomic obstacles, atrial disease with associated fibrosis or, more commonly, atrial scars created at the time of cardiac surgery for valvular or congenital heart disease may create alternative substrates for intra-atrial reentry. Common to these arrhythmias is a significant region of scar with a channel of surviving myocardium bridging the scar or between the scar and a normal anatomic obstacle. Within the channel, conduction is slow and electrocardiographically silent, resulting in an isoelectric PP interval. Because the circuit is different from that of typical atrial flutter, the P-wave morphology is atypical.

When the rate is 250 beats per minute or greater, the arrhythmia is arbitrarily classified as atypical atrial flutter, and when the rate is less than 250 beats per minute, it is arbitrarily classified as atrial tachycardia. Like typical atrial flutter, these arrhythmias are paroxysmal sustained or persistent arrhythmias, and when manifesting with 2 : 1 conduction, they may be misdiagnosed as sinus tachycardia if the abnormal P-wave vector and fixed heart rate over time are not recognized. Therapy and prognosis are otherwise similar to those for typical atrial flutter.

Atrial Fibrillation

Overview and Classification

AF is a chaotic atrial rhythm related to continuous and variable activation of the atria. There are no distinct P waves or periods of atrial quiescence. It is characterized electrocardiographically by a wavering baseline associated with an irregular ventricular response (see Fig. 9-6D).

AF is the most common clinically significant arrhythmia. It affects 2.2 million people in the United States. Its prevalence is between 0.4% and 1% in the general population, and it increases with age, reaching 8% in those older than 80 years. Patients with AF have a higher risk of stroke, heart failure, and mortality. However, the role of AF as an independent determinant of mortality is uncertain because it commonly coexists with other important conditions. Patients with lone AF do not have an increased mortality rate, and carefully designed trials exploring the benefit of maintenance of sinus rhythm over rate control show no survival benefit for sinus rhythm. Whether AF is merely a marker for increased mortality or a mechanism remains uncertain.

AF is often classified by its clinical presentation and pattern. When AF is first detected, it is called *new onset*, and its ultimate pattern is initially undetermined. When AF relapses during follow-up, it is called *recurrent* and classified by its clinical pattern. If AF terminates spontaneously, it is called *paroxysmal* AF. Although episodes lasting up to 7 days are defined as paroxysmal, most episodes of paroxysmal AF terminate within the first 24 hours and many terminate within minutes or hours of onset.

When AF lasts longer than 7 days, it is designated as *persistent*. AF that persists for a long interval, typically more than a year, without return of an interim period of sinus rhythm (spontaneously or as a result of medical intervention such as cardioversion) is often called *permanent* AF.

Mechanisms of Atrial Fibrillation

Because of its chaotic nature, it has been difficult to study AF, and its mechanisms remain incompletely understood. The initiation of spontaneous AF is a consequence of rapid electrical firing from preferential focal sites of origin. The most common site of focal origin is from left atrial muscle sleeves extending along the outer surface of the pulmonary veins. When firing does not originate from a pulmonary vein, it is commonly from the left atrial tissue immediately adjacent to one of the veins or occasionally from one of the other thoracic veins such as the ostium of the superior vena cava or the ostium of the coronary sinus. Atrial rates recorded in and around the pulmonary veins are significantly higher than at other atrial sites, suggesting that activity in the region of the veins is important in perpetuating AF after initiation.

These insights have produced highly effective techniques for the cure of AF. Ablation techniques designed to isolate these trigger sites from the atrium have success rates of 70% to 80% for the cure of paroxysmal AF and somewhat lower rates for the cure of persistent AF. Ablation restricted to the region of the pulmonary veins and adjacent left atrium is curative in most patients with AF, implying that most cases of AF are arrhythmias entirely contained within and maintained by the left atrium and connecting veins. In the same way that typical atrial flutter is the characteristic arrhythmia of the right atrium, AF is the characteristic arrhythmia of the left atrium.

Anticoagulation and Atrial Fibrillation

During AF (and to some extent, atrial flutter), the atria have incomplete and ineffective contractions. Blood stasis occurs and may result in the formation of intracardiac thrombus, which may lead to thromboembolism and stroke. The overall risk of stroke in patients with AF is 5% per year. Certain risk factors may adjust this risk, including age, gender, rheumatic heart disease, prior stroke, left ventricular dysfunction, left atrial enlargement, hypertension, and diabetes.

Scoring systems have been developed to estimate a patient's AF-related stroke risk based on his or her constellation of risk factors. The most used system is the $CHADS_2$ score (*c*ardiac failure, *h*ypertension, *a*ge ≥75 years, *d*iabetes mellitus, and prior *s*troke). This system has been well validated in assessing the stroke risk of patients with AF. It assigns a single point for age of 75 years or older, diabetes, history of heart failure, and hypertension. It assigns two points for a history of stroke or transient ischemic attack. A score of 0 correlates with a relatively low risk of stroke at 1.9% per year, a score of 1 has a stroke risk of 2.8% per year, a score of 2 has a risk of 4.0% per year, and a score of 3 or higher has a stroke risk of more than 5.9% per year.

The $CHADS_2$ underwent further refinement to increase the granularity of stroke risk stratification with the creation of the CHA_2DS_2-VASc (*v*ascular disease, *a*ge, and *s*ex) scoring system. In this system, congestive heart failure, hypertension, diabetes mellitus, vascular disease, age between 65 and 74 years, and female gender are assigned 1 point, and age of 75 years or older and prior stroke are assigned 2 points. A CHA$_2$DS$_2$-VASc score of 0 was associated with a 0% stroke rate, a score of 1 with a 0.6% per year risk, a score of 2 with a 1.6% risk, and a score of 3 with a risk of 3.9%. This system may be most useful for patients with an intermediate risk based on a CHADS$_2$ score of 1 or 2.

After a patient's individualized stroke risk is determined, it can be balanced against the risk of anticoagulation to determine what would be appropriate for stroke prevention. A useful tool for estimating bleeding risk due to oral anticoagulation is the HAS-BLED (*h*ypertension, *a*bnormal renal/liver function, *s*troke, *b*leeding history or predisposition, *l*abile international normalized ratio, *e*lderly, *d*rugs/alcohol) score. Patients with a HAS-BLED score of 0 had a risk of 0.59 severe bleeds per 100 patient-years, those with a score of 1 had a risk of 1.51, those with a score of 2 had a risk of 3.20, and those with a score of 3 had a risk of 19.51.

Aspirin and warfarin are the longest-studied antithrombotics used for reducing the rate of AF-related stroke. Aspirin reduces the risk of AF-related stroke by 25%, and warfarin reduces the risk by 50%. Warfarin can be difficult to administer; the level of blood-thinning effect must be constantly monitored with international normalized ratio (INR) blood testing. An INR less than 2.0 is associated with higher rates of ischemic stroke; a level greater than 3.0 is associated with increased intracranial bleeding. On average, a therapeutic INR (between 2.0 and 3.0) is maintained in only two thirds of cases, and there are many drug and dietary interactions with warfarin.

The combination of aspirin plus clopidogrel is somewhat more effective than aspirin alone in preventing stroke (2.4% versus 3.3% per year), but it comes at the cost of almost twice the major bleeding rate. Coumadin is superior to the combination of aspirin and clopidogrel, especially if the INR can be kept within the therapeutic range at least 65% of the time.

Several newer oral anticoagulants have effectiveness and bleeding risk rates similar to warfarin, but they do not require drug level monitoring. They include dabigatran, rivaroxaban, and apixaban, which have been studied in large patient groups and found to be noninferior to warfarin, and some may be superior in certain aspects.

The highest risk of stroke related to AF occurs at time of conversion to sinus rhythm achieved spontaneously or by chemical or electrical cardioversion. If thrombus has formed within the left atrium or left atrial appendage, it may not leave the atria during AF due to ineffective atrial mechanics. However, after sinus rhythm is restored, the improved atrial function may eject the thrombus and cause embolic stroke or other systemic embolic sequelae. Even with restoration of electrical atrial systole, the recovery of normal atrial mechanics may be delayed several days to weeks (i.e., atrial stunning). To reduce the risk of pericardioversion stroke, it is important to reduce the risk of preexisting thrombus and to prevent formation in the time period immediately after cardioversion.

The risk of preexisting thrombus can be reduced by 3 weeks of oral anticoagulation or Doppler transesophageal echocardiography (TEE) before cardioversion. These steps are recommended for any patient who has been in AF for an unknown period or has been documented to be in AF more than 48 hours. Although thrombi have been identified in patients with AF for shorter periods, current clinical practice presumes that most thrombus formation requires at least 48 hours. Thrombus related to AF occurs most commonly in the left atrial appendage, which cannot be well visualized by transthoracic echocardiography; TEE is often recommended before cardioversion for optimal imaging of the left atrial appendage. After cardioversion, at least 4 weeks of oral anticoagulation is recommended (regardless of CHADS$_2$ score).

Acute Management of Atrial Fibrillation: Rate Control

The acute management of AF centers on the control of the ventricular response, timely restoration of sinus rhythm, and identification of potentially reversible factors that might have precipitated the arrhythmia. AF with rapid ventricular response results in acute deterioration in stroke volume and cardiac output and an increase in myocardial oxygen demand with the potential for coronary ischemia. Patients who are symptomatic must be controlled promptly. When pursuing rate control for acute AF of recent onset, the fastest way to achieve rate control is the restoration of sinus rhythm. If rate control proves difficult or is not well tolerated, cardioversion should be undertaken early.

For the acute control of rapidly conducted AF, intravenous administration of a β-blocker (i.e., esmolol, metoprolol, or propranolol) or a nondihydropyridine calcium-channel blocker (i.e., diltiazem or verapamil) is preferred. In the setting of decompensated heart failure, the use of a calcium-channel blocker may exacerbate heart failure and should be avoided. In this setting, digoxin is a useful agent for resting rate control. Digoxin is also a useful second-line drug in addition to a calcium-channel or β-blocker for resting rate control. If this therapy is ineffective or not tolerated, intravenous amiodarone is a useful rate control agent, especially in the setting of congestive heart failure, and it may facilitate restoration of sinus rhythm.

Long-term targets for rate control of permanent AF have been a matter of debate. The recently completed Rate Control Efficacy in Permanent Atrial Fibrillation II (RACE II) study showed no advantage to strict rate control. Targeting a resting rate of less than 80 beats per minute showed no advantage over a target of less than 110 and was much harder to achieve. For long-term management, the results suggest that achieving a resting heart rate of less than 110 beats per minute may be sufficient and safe.

Acute Management of Atrial Fibrillation: Restoration of Sinus Rhythm

When sinus rhythm is restored in the first 48 hours of acute AF, the thromboembolic risk is low, and anticoagulation is not required. New-onset AF should be managed with a plan to restore sinus rhythm during this period if possible. At least one half of new-onset AF episodes terminate spontaneously in the first 24 to 48 hours.

Pharmacologic Conversion of Atrial Fibrillation

Pharmacologic conversion of AF can be undertaken when restoration of sinus rhythm is not urgent. Several antiarrhythmic drugs have been effective in increasing the rate of early conversion of AF. Pharmacologic conversion usually is more successful with AF of recent onset than with chronic AF.

Oral agents with efficacy in the early conversion of AF include flecainide, propafenone, and dofetilide. Oral amiodarone and sotalol have been associated with a 27% and 24% conversion rate, respectively, occurring after 28 days of therapy. However, due to low early conversion rates, these oral drugs are not recommended for conversion. Intravenous agents with efficacy for early conversion include ibutilide and amiodarone. Ibutilide is limited by a relatively high 4% rate of drug-induced QT prolongation and TdP VT. This risk is even higher in the setting of LV dysfunction, electrolyte disturbances, or heart failure. Ibutilide should be reserved for the pharmacologic conversion of stable patients with a baseline normal QT interval. In contrast, intravenous amiodarone is well tolerated by unstable patients and is the preferred pharmacologic agent for conversion in the critically ill.

Electrical Cardioversion of Atrial Fibrillation

Electrical cardioversion should be performed urgently in the case of severe compromise related to acute AF, including angina, heart failure, hypotension, and shock. Cardioversion should also be attempted at least once electively in most cases of new-onset AF regardless of tolerance. When performing electrical cardioversion, an anterior-posterior patch or paddle position is more effective than the conventional anterior-to-lateral patch or paddle position used for ventricular defibrillation. Although low-output discharges may be effective in some patients, a strategy of starting at higher outputs decreases the number of shocks required and the average cumulative energy delivered. An initial shock energy of 200 J is recommended. After a failed initial shock, full output should be used for the next attempt.

Long-Term Maintenance of Sinus Rhythm

Antiarrhythmic Therapy

Despite the association of AF with an increase in stroke-related and all-cause mortality, no study has established a benefit for pharmacologic maintenance of sinus rhythm in terms of stroke risk or survival. This may be because AF is merely a marker and not a mechanism of mortality. It may also be a consequence of the relative inefficacy of pharmacologic therapy in the maintenance of sinus rhythm and the difficulty establishing whether patients thought to be in sinus rhythm are consistently in sinus rhythm at follow-up.

The largest and best designed trial addressing this issue was the Atrial Fibrillation Follow-up Investigation of Rhythm Management (AFFIRM) trial. The study included 4060 patients randomly assigned to rhythm control with antiarrhythmic drugs, most commonly amiodarone, or to rate control without attempts to maintain sinus rhythm. AFFIRM demonstrated no advantage in stroke or mortality rates using a strategy of sinus rhythm maintenance compared with rate control. Either strategy can be offered to patients with an expectation of similar outcomes with regard to hard end points. The decision to pursue sinus rhythm usually is determined by the management of symptoms that may be better addressed by maintaining sinus rhythm in selected patients.

In the absence of antiarrhythmic drugs, more than 80% of patients relapse during the first year after cardioversion of AF. Antiarrhythmic drugs remain the primary strategy for maintaining sinus rhythm after cardioversion and for preventing symptomatic episodes in patients with paroxysmal AF. However, antiarrhythmic therapy has many limitations, and alternative ablative therapies may over time overtake antiarrhythmic therapy in the management of AF.

All antiarrhythmic drugs have the potential for proarrhythmia, the unintended precipitation of a new arrhythmic problem caused by the drug. Adverse rhythm effects of drugs may include sinus node dysfunction, heart block, promotion of drug-slowed atrial flutter permitting rapid 1 : 1 conduction, and promotion of potentially lethal ventricular arrhythmias. Class I drugs such as flecainide, propafenone, and disopyramide may result in significant direct myocardial depression and consequent exacerbation of heart failure. The array of potential adverse effects of antiarrhythmic drugs is beyond the scope of this chapter, but certain essential concepts are important to recognize.

Class I drugs such as flecainide and propafenone, which work by slowing conduction, have a high risk of ventricular proarrhythmia and potential for sudden death in the setting of heart failure, LV dysfunction, and coronary artery disease. Use of these drugs is restricted to patients with preserved cardiac function and no evidence of obstructive coronary artery disease. However, in this selected group of patients with normal hearts, these drugs are exceedingly safe, well tolerated, and often effective.

Class III drugs, which prolong repolarization and refractoriness, include sotalol, dofetilide, dronedarone, and amiodarone. They are safe for patients with coronary artery disease, and in the case of dofetilide and amiodarone, they are safe for those with congestive heart failure. However, sotalol and dofetilide may provoke TdP, even in patients with normal cardiac function, and they must be used with caution. Amiodarone has greater long-term efficacy than other drugs and a lower risk of proarrhythmia, but long-term somatic toxicity consisting of thyroid dysfunction, pulmonary, and occasional hepatotoxicity limits the use of this drug in older patients or those with limited expected longevity or an inability to safely tolerate alternative agents due to advanced cardiac disease or proarrhythmia. Amiodarone is highly effective for the short-term, acute management of arrhythmias in critically ill patients when the potential risk of long-term toxicity is not an issue.

Dronedarone, which was approved in 2009, was derived by modification of the amiodarone molecule. Like amiodarone, the drug has a low risk of proarrhythmia and TdP VT. Unlike amiodarone, the drug does not cause thyroid toxicity. In common use, hepatotoxicity is also uncommon with dronedarone. However, rare cases of hepatic failure have been associated with dronedarone use. Dronedarone has increased mortality rates for patients with recently decompensated heart failure and when used as a simple rate control agent in patients with permanent AF. It is contraindicated in these settings.

In addition to being useful agents for the prevention of AF, sotalol, dronedarone, and amiodarone provide substantial rate control during relapses of AF. However, rate control with other antiarrhythmic agents may not be adequate to prevent rapid conduction with relapse, and class I drugs such as flecainide may accelerate response at the time of relapse. Antiarrhythmic drugs other than sotalol, dronedarone, or amiodarone should therefore be combined with a rate control agent such as a β-blocker or nondihydropyridine calcium-channel blocker during long-term therapy. Figure 9-7 is a proposed strategy for antiarrhythmic drug selection for the long-term maintenance of sinus rhythm in patients with AF.

Surgical Ablation of Atrial Fibrillation

The surgical treatment of AF was pioneered by Cox with the development of the atrial maze procedure. The procedure was predicated on the concept that AF was maintained by multiple interacting wave fronts of activity. By surgically dividing the atria into narrow channels, most with connection back to the sinus node, it was thought that AF could be abolished while preserving physiologic activation and contraction of the atrium. The circuitous path left for atrial activation and the multiple barriers created in the atrium intended to prevent AF gave rise to the term *maze procedure* to describe the technique. The initial procedure was thought to be highly successful but was associated with significant surgical risks and problems with sinus node dysfunction. Because of the surgical complexity of making and then closing multiple incisions in the atria and the complications associated with the procedure, the initial cut-and-sew maze procedure has fallen out of clinical use.

Although the original maze procedure is no longer used, many techniques have been developed to simplify the operation by

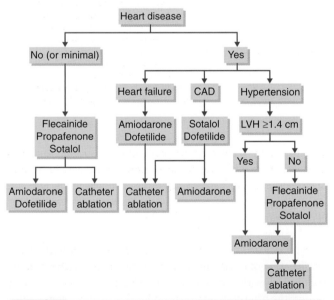

FIGURE 9-7 A strategy for the selection of therapy to maintain sinus rhythm in patients with recurrent atrial fibrillation. Patients are stratified by the presence of absence of structural heart disease, and drugs expected to have the greatest efficacy and lowest therapeutic risk in each group are selected. Catheter ablation becomes a therapeutic option after failure of at least one antiarrhythmic drug. The class 1C drugs flecainide and propafenone are not advised for patients with heart failure or coronary artery disease (CAD). Amiodarone is an acceptable first-line drug for those with heart failure and severe left ventricular hypertrophy. Because of its potential for somatic toxicity, amiodarone is otherwise reserved as a second-line agent that is used as an alternative to catheter ablation.

substituting linear thermal ablation (by heating or cooling tissue) to create lines of conduction block in the atria without the need for extensive atrial dissection and reconstruction. Surgical ablation is commonly applied in patients with a history of AF who are undergoing concomitant heart operations for other indications such as valvular or coronary disease. Less frequently, surgical ablation has been applied as a stand-alone procedure for the sole management of AF. In that setting, various minimally invasive techniques have been developed. However, the techniques used vary widely from one center to another and long-term reporting of outcomes is inconsistent. In a large series that included 282 patients undergoing an open bi-atrial ablation procedure, 78% were in sinus rhythm without antiarrhythmic therapy at the 1 year follow-up evaluation.

Another important potential benefit of surgical ablation for AF is that it provides an opportunity to eliminate the left atrial appendage as a potential site of thrombus formation and source of thromboembolism. This can be accomplished by complete amputation of the appendage with oversewing of the appendage or clamping off the opening to the appendage with special devices designed for this purpose. This may be especially important in patients with absolute or relative contraindications to anticoagulation.

Catheter Ablation of Atrial Fibrillation

Catheter ablation has become a common procedure for the management of AF after failure of initial attempts at medical therapy of AF. Initial attempts to cure AF using catheter techniques were based on attempts in the early 1990s to emulate the linear lesion set of the Cox maze procedure with multiple endocardial lesions. High complication rates and limited efficacy led to abandonment of this approach.

In 1998, Haissaguerre reported the important role of rapid activity originating in the musculature of the pulmonary veins in initiation of paroxysmal AF. This led to the development of procedures designed to target the pulmonary veins and eventuated in the technique of electrical pulmonary vein isolation (PVI), which is currently the primary ablative approach to treatment of paroxysmal AF by catheter techniques. This technique has had acceptably high success rates (≈70%) at multiple centers for the treatment of paroxysmal AF without antiarrhythmic therapy.

Despite the high success rate of catheter PVI ablation for the treatment of paroxysmal AF, this technique has not proved reliably effective in the management of more persistent forms of AF, especially long-standing persistent AF. This likely reflects the importance of factors other than pulmonary vein activity in the initiation and maintenance of persistent AF that are not addressed by PVI ablation. Multiple ablative techniques are currently used in an attempt to increase the success rates for patients with persistent AF. They have included addition of linear lesions to block reentrant wave fronts, ablation of regions of unusually rapid atrial activity during ongoing AF, and interruption of stable rotors of atrial activity identified during multisite mapping of AF. Although these techniques have improved success rates in limited series, it is uncertain which, if any, of these methods represents the optimal approach to the ablation of long-standing persistent AF.

In summary, catheter ablation is the preferred secondary strategy for treatment of symptomatic AF after initial attempts at medical therapy have failed. Simple pulmonary vein isolation has a high success rate for the management of patients with paroxysmal AF. Success rates for all ablative techniques are lower for persistent AF, especially for long-term AF. As in the case of surgical ablation, multiple techniques are used at various centers, and the different strategies for follow-up and definitions of response have made it difficult to ascertain the relative efficacy of the various approaches in common use.

Catheter Ablation of the Atrioventricular Node

Although less commonly used today than in the past, the older technique of catheter ablation of the AV node resulting in complete heart block followed by placement of a ventricular pacemaker to maintain physiologic heart rates remains an option for patients when rate control cannot be achieved medically. This technique continues to have an important role in the management of patients who are too infirm to safely undergo AF ablation or in patients for whom ablative techniques have failed to control the arrhythmia.

For a deeper discussion on this topic, please see Chapter 64, "Cardiac Arrhythmias with Supraventricular Origin," in Goldman-Cecil Medicine, *25th Edition.*

SYNCOPE

Syncope is a sudden loss of consciousness that is transient. Syncope has cardiac causes (e.g., low cerebral blood pressure) and noncardiac causes. Common causes and categories of syncope are outlined in Table 9-4. Cerebrovascular disease or stroke uncommonly manifests as syncope unless a large cerebral territory is involved. Syncope is a common reason for emergency room or hospital admission.

The diagnostic approach to a patient with syncope is given in Figure 9-8. Most causes can be identified by the medical history and physical examination alone. Conditions surrounding the syncopal episode often suggest a cause. For example, vasovagal episodes often occur during stress, pain, straining, coughing, or urination. Exercise-induced syncope may indicate obstructive coronary disease, channelopathies such as long QT or CPVT, obstructive cardiomyopathy, aortic stenosis, or arrhythmia. A history of palpitations or syncope with no warning may be related to cardiac arrhythmias. Very long episodes of syncope (>5 minutes) suggest noncardiac causes. A recent change in medications or dizziness with position changes suggests orthostatic hypotension. Witnessed limb movements or posturing is not specific for neurologic causes and can result from any type of cerebral hypoperfusion, even from cardiac causes.

Beyond the history, physical examination, and routine ECG, further testing has little diagnostic utility. Holter or loop recorders may be useful. Implantable loop recorders may have utility in cases of recurrent, infrequent syncope. Electrophysiologic testing may be useful in some patients with other abnormalities suggesting an arrhythmic cause.

Despite thorough evaluations, more than 30% of patients with syncope have no identifiable cause. Cardiac causes of syncope have the highest morbidity and mortality rates. Because patients

TABLE 9-4 CAUSES OF SYNCOPE	
CAUSE	**FEATURES**
PERIPHERAL VASCULAR OR CIRCULATORY	
Vasovagal syncope (neurally mediated)	Prodrome of pallor, yawning, nausea, diaphoresis; precipitated by stress or pain; occurs when patient is upright, aborted by recumbency; fall in blood pressure with or without a decrease in heart rate
Micturition syncope	Syncope with urination (probably vagal)
Post-tussive syncope	Syncope after paroxysm of coughing
Hypersensitive carotid sinus syndrome	Vasodepressor and/or cardioinhibitory responses with light carotid sinus massage
Drugs	Orthostasis; occurs with antihypertensive drugs, tricyclic antidepressants, phenothiazines
Volume depletion	Orthostasis; occurs with hemorrhage, excessive vomiting or diarrhea, Addison's disease
Autonomic dysfunction	Orthostasis; occurs in diabetes, alcoholism, Parkinson's disease, deconditioning after a prolonged illness
CENTRAL NERVOUS SYSTEM	
Cerebrovascular	Transient ischemic attacks and strokes are unusual causes of syncope; associated neurologic abnormalities are usually identified
Seizures	Warning aura sometimes present, jerking of extremities, tongue biting, urinary incontinence, postictal confusion
METABOLIC	
Hypoglycemia	Confusion, tachycardia, jitteriness before syncope; patient may be taking insulin
CARDIAC	
Obstructive	Syncope is often exertional; physical findings consistent with aortic stenosis, hypertrophic obstructive cardiomyopathy, cardiac tamponade, atrial myxoma, prosthetic valve malfunction, Eisenmenger's syndrome, tetralogy of Fallot, primary pulmonary hypertension, pulmonic stenosis, massive pulmonary embolism
Arrhythmias	Syncope may be sudden and occurs in any position; episodes of dizziness or palpitations; may be history of heart disease; bradyarrhythmias or tachyarrhythmias may be responsible—check for hypersensitive carotid sinus

with unknown causes of syncope have long-term outcomes similar to those with noncardiac syncope, and the major goal of an evaluation is to identify cardiac causes of syncope.

VENTRICULAR ARRHYTHMIAS AND SUDDEN CARDIAC DEATH

Ventricular ectopy is defined as cardiac beats that originate from within the right or left ventricular muscle or conduction system. Premature ventricular contractions (PVCs) can occur singly or as ventricular couplets or triplets. VT is four or more consecutive beats that originate from the ventricle at a rate of at least 100 beats per minute. VT is classified as *sustained* if it lasts longer than 30 seconds or requires termination due to hemodynamic instability; otherwise, it is classified as *nonsustained* VT (NSVT).

Ventricular ectopy also may be classified based on maintenance of a similar electrocardiographic morphology. The beats of monomorphic VT (MMVT) appear to be identical and usually originate from the same area of the heart. *Ventricular flutter* is a term that may be used to describe MMVT with rates of more than 300 beats per minute. Polymorphic VT (PMVT) has a more

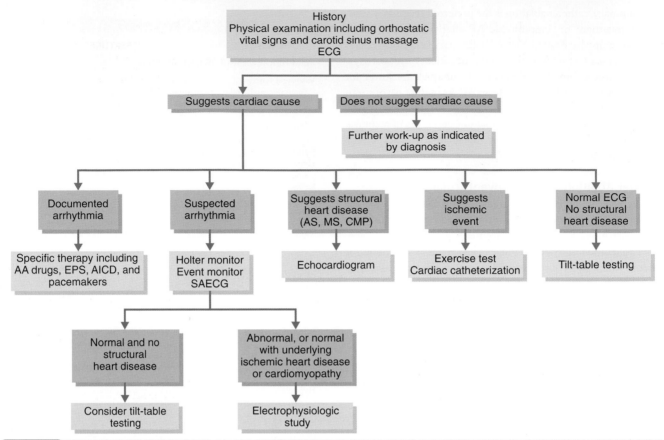

```
                    History
        Physical examination including orthostatic
         vital signs and carotid sinus massage
                      ECG
```

```
        Suggests cardiac cause          Does not suggest cardiac cause

                                          Further work-up as indicated
                                                by diagnosis
```

```
  Documented      Suspected     Suggests structural     Suggests        Normal ECG
  arrhythmia      arrhythmia     heart disease           ischemic        No structural
                                 (AS, MS, CMP)           event           heart disease
```

```
  Specific therapy including    Holter monitor
  AA drugs, EPS, AICD, and      Event monitor        Echocardiogram     Exercise test       Tilt-table testing
  pacemakers                    SAECG                                   Cardiac catheterization
```

```
  Normal and no            Abnormal, or normal
  structural               with underlying
  heart disease            ischemic heart disease
                           or cardiomyopathy
```

```
  Consider tilt-table      Electrophysiologic
  testing                  study
```

FIGURE 9-8 Approach to the evaluation of syncope. AA, Antiarrhythmic; AICD, automatic implantable cardioverter-defibrillator; AS, aortic stenosis; CMP, cardiomyopathy; ECG, electrocardiogram; EPS, electrophysiologic study; MS, mitral stenosis; SAECG, signal-averaged ECG.

variable appearance on the ECG than MMVT. TdP is a special form of PMVT that has a repetitive, undulating periodicity and usually implies a long-QT triggered mechanism. VF is the most chaotic form of ventricular ectopy. It is associated with no meaningful cardiac output and usually leads to death unless rapidly treated. The other forms of VT may eventually degrade into VF.

Determining whether a patient has a rhythm of ventricular origin usually is done by 12-lead surface ECG. Ventricular ectopy typically has a wide QRS morphology (Fig. 9-9). Not all wide QRS morphologies are ventricular in origin, and there are criteria for determining whether a wide complex tachycardia is supraventricular or ventricular. SVT may appear as a wide complex tachycardia if it conducts to the ventricle with aberrancy (e,g., bundle branch block) or through an accessory pathway (e.g., WPW syndrome). Features that may help distinguish between SVT and VT include AV dissociation with capture beats and fusion beats and the QRS morphology and duration (Table 9-5). The Brugada algorithm is commonly used for determining the site of origin of wide complex tachycardia. The tachycardia has a ventricular origin in more than 90% of patients with a history of ischemic heart disease.

VT may occur by the same mechanisms as other tachycardias, such as reentry, enhanced automaticity, or triggered activity. VT often occurs as a reentrant tachycardia around an area of prior MI scar in the left ventricle. VT in the chronic phase of ischemic heart disease is mediated by reentry through channels or sheets of surviving myocardium, especially in the partially spared border zone of a region of scar resulting from a prior MI. In these

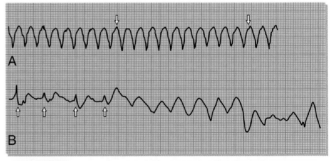

FIGURE 9-9 Ventricular arrhythmias. **A,** Monomorphic ventricular tachycardia (VT). Notice the wide QRS with a stable appearance with each beat. Detecting P waves during VT is difficult due to the overlying ventricular activity, but it is visible at several points on this tracing, some of which are marked by *arrows*. The AV dissociation is diagnostic of VT and excludes supraventricular tachycardia. **B,** An initially organized agonal (preterminal) rhythm *(arrows)* degenerates into coarse ventricular fibrillation. Notice the irregular baseline and the absence of organized QRS complexes. During ventricular fibrillation, there is no forward cardiac output, and cardiac arrest immediately ensues.

channels, conduction is abnormally slow due to poor coupling between sparse surviving myocytes. Susceptibility to sustained VT increases with worsening left ventricular dysfunction, likely due to the greater extent of ventricular scar.

VT can occur in the absence of ischemic heart disease in the form of idiopathic VT, nonischemic cardiomyopathies, hypertrophic cardiomyopathies, arrhythmogenic RV dysplasia, bundle branch reentry, cardiac ion channel disorders, or electrolyte

TABLE 9-5 DIFFERENTIATION OF VENTRICULAR TACHYCARDIA FROM SUPRAVENTRICULAR TACHYCARDIA WITH ABERRANCY

HELPFUL FEATURES	IMPLICATIONS
Positive QRS concordance	Diagnostic of VT
AV dissociation, capture beats, or fusion beats	Diagnostic of VT
Atypical RBBB (monophasic R, QR, RS, or triphasic QRS in V_1; R:S ratio <1, QS or QR, monophasic R in V_6)	Suggests VT
Atypical LBBB (R >30 min or R to S [nadir or notch] >60 min in V_1 or V_2; R:S ratio <1, QS or QR in V_6)	Suggests VT
Shift of axis from baseline	Suggests VT
History of CAD	Suggests VT
QRS during tachycardia identical to QRS during sinus rhythm	Suggests SVT
Termination with adenosine	Suggests SVT

AV, Atrioventricular; CAD, coronary artery disease; LBBB, left bundle branch block; RBBB, right bundle branch block; SVT, supraventricular tachycardia; VT, ventricular tachycardia.

TABLE 9-6 CAUSES OF SUDDEN CARDIAC DEATH

NONCARDIAC CAUSES

Central nervous system hemorrhage
Massive pulmonary embolus
Drug overdose
Hypoxia secondary to lung disease
Aortic dissection or rupture

CARDIAC CAUSES

Ventricular fibrillation
Myocardial ischemia or injury
Long QT syndrome
Short QT syndrome
Brugada syndrome
Arrhythmogenic right ventricular dysplasia
Ventricular tachycardia

Bradyarrhythmias, sick sinus syndrome
Aortic stenosis
Tetralogy of Fallot
Pericardial tamponade
Cardiac tumors
Complications of infective endocarditis
Hypertrophic cardiomyopathy (arrhythmia or obstruction)
Myocardial ischemia
Atherosclerosis
Prinzmetal angina
Kawasaki arteritis

disturbances. The right ventricular outflow tract (RVOT) is the most common origin of idiopathic VT, which is likely caused by triggered activity. This form of VT (or PVCs) is usually sensitive to catecholamines and may terminate with adenosine (i.e., adenosine-sensitive VT). Another common form of idiopathic VT originates from the left ventricular conduction system (i.e., fascicular VT) and may be verapamil sensitive. Idiopathic VTs are common targets for successful catheter ablation.

Nonsustained VT usually does not require specific therapy unless the patient is symptomatic. The Cardiac Arrhythmia Suppression Trial treated PVCs and NSVT after the acute phase of MI with class I antiarrhythmic drugs, and the trial demonstrated increased mortality rates when the arrhythmias were treated. If VT is attributed to reversible causes such as electrolyte disturbances or acute ischemia, the underlying mechanism should be treated. VT not due to reversible causes may be treated with β-blockers, antiarrhythmic drug therapy (e.g., amiodarone), or catheter ablation. If urgent treatment is required due to hemodynamic instability, direct current cardioversion is performed. It should be synchronized to the QRS complex if a regular morphology exists; otherwise, it should be nonsynchronized. Performing direct current cardioversion during the refractory period (T wave) of MMVT may degrade the rhythm to VF. An ICD often is used in patients who survive VT or VF to quickly treat recurrent episodes. Endocardial and epicardial catheter ablation has become an effective treatment for VT.

Prevention of Sudden Cardiac Death

SCD is defined as death within 1 hour of the onset of symptoms. It may result from a variety of cardiac or noncardiac conditions (Table 9-6). SCD is one of the most common causes of death, with 400,000 events occurring annually in the United States. The most common cause of SCD is VT or VF. Cardiac conditions that increase the risk of SCD include LQTS, hypertrophic cardiomyopathy, Brugada syndrome, arrhythmogenic RV dysplasia, and nonischemic or ischemic cardiomyopathy. The most common cardiac condition that may lead to SCD is acute or distant MI.

The successful treatment of SCD due to VF usually requires rapid access to cardioversion; if treatment is delayed by more than 5 to 10 minutes, permanent brain injury is common. AEDs can reduce the time to defibrillation and improve survival when placed in public areas, although they have been less effective when installed in private residences, even for patients at risk for SCD.

ICDs used in the treatment of SCD have improved mortality rates. Patients who are at high risk for SCD are often offered an ICD to enable rapid defibrillation before the onset of anoxic brain injury. If a patient survives the first episode of SCD due to documented or presumed VT or VF from nonreversible or unknown causes, he or she is offered an ICD. ICDs are extremely successful in the detection and treatment of VT or VF. They do not always prevent loss of consciousness because it takes 15 to 20 seconds to treat the arrhythmia, and low cardiac output may cause syncope before restoration of normal rhythm, especially if several cardioversions are required.

The earliest ICD trials examined their use in the secondary prevention of SCD (i.e., treating patients who had already survived an episode of cardiac arrest). The largest study was the Antiarrhythmics Versus Implantable Defibrillators (AVID) trial, which randomized patients with a history of poorly tolerated sustained VT or cardiac arrest to empirical amiodarone or ICD implantation. In this trial and several others, ICD therapy was associated with a lower risk of arrhythmic and all-cause death compared with antiarrhythmic therapy.

Several trials have examined the use of ICDs for the primary prevention of SCDs (i.e., treating patients who are at risk for SCD). The first was the Multicenter Automatic Defibrillator Implantation Trial (MADIT), which enrolled patients with a prior MI and an ejection fraction of 35% or less who had frequent ventricular ectopy and inducible VT at electrophysiologic testing. The study demonstrated a substantial mortality reduction with ICD therapy. MADIT-II enrolled patients with a prior MI and an ejection fraction of 30% or less in the chronic phase, without requiring invasive testing. A significant mortality benefit was associated with ICD therapy.

The Sudden Cardiac Death in Heart Failure trial enrolled a broader population consisting of patients with ischemic and nonischemic cardiomyopathy, symptomatic heart failure, and an ejection fraction of 35% or less. A survival benefit was found for patients treated with an ICD compared with conventional therapy or empirical amiodarone therapy. The degree of benefit was similar for patients with ischemic or nonischemic cardiomyopathy, suggesting that primary prevention with ICDs for patients with prior MI or nonischemic cardiomyopathy and heart failure was appropriate.

The risk of SCD after MI is highest in the few months after the index event. However, ICDs have not been effective when implanted immediately after MI or revascularization procedures. The reason for this is unclear; it may reflect the large percentage of patients who have improved cardiac function early on, which decreases the risk of SCD and therefore the benefit of an ICD. Alternatively, the mechanism for SCD in the early period after an MI or revascularization procedure may be recurrent ischemia rather than reentrant tachycardia and therefore less amenable to ICD therapy. The Defibrillator in Acute Myocardial Infarction Trial (DINAMIT) randomized 675 patients with low ejection fractions immediately after MI to ICD or medical therapy; no difference in mortality rates was seen. The current recommendations are to avoid primary prevention with ICDs within 40 days of an MI or 3 months of revascularization.

A significant challenge in modern medicine is identifying patients who are have an elevated risk of SCD to allow effective use of primary prevention interventions such as ICDs. Some known predictors of SCD after MI are shown in Table 9-7, but many are not specific or sensitive enough for practical use. Reduced ejection fraction has been the most successful noninvasive measure that can predict increased risk of SCD. An electrophysiologic study is a minimally invasive catheter procedure that with electrical stimulation can help to identify patients who are prone to VT. Electrophysiologic studies are most sensitive in patients with prior MI, but they may be less useful in other cardiac conditions. Cardiac magnetic resonance imaging (MRI), which can directly image cardiac function and cardiac scar or fibrosis, is showing great promise as a more sensitive and specific, noninvasive risk predictor of SCD.

Ventricular Tachycardia and Ventricular Fibrillation without Evident Heart Disease

Ventricular arrhythmias occurring in the absence of structural heart disease usually carry a benign prognosis but can be associated with SCD in patients with genetic arrhythmic syndromes predisposing to life-threatening polymorphic VT. Genetic screening for these syndromes is important to identify at-risk family members.

Idiopathic Ventricular Tachycardia

Idiopathic VT most commonly originates from the outflow tracts, with approximately 80% localized to the RVOT and the remainder originating in the left ventricular outflow tract (LVOT), the aortic sinuses of Valsalva, and the region of the aortomitral continuity. Idiopathic RVOT VT manifests with the characteristic electrocardiographic findings of left bundle branch block and inferior axis VT QRS morphology. Triggered activity is the mechanism underlying outflow tract tachycardias. This calcium-dependent mechanism explains why an outflow tract VT often terminates with adenosine, β-blockers, and calcium-channel blockers.

Patients in their third or fourth decade typically have palpitations, shortness of breath, and lightheadedness at presentation. Reports of cardiac arrest are rare, and treatment is directed at controlling symptoms. β-Blockers and calcium-channel blockers are often used initially, although some patients require catheter ablation or antiarrhythmic drug therapy. A subset of asymptomatic patients may develop tachycardia-mediated cardiomyopathy due to frequent ventricular ectopy. The PVC burden posing the greatest risk for producing left ventricular dysfunction is likely more than 10,000 PVCs daily. Fortunately, PVC suppression with catheter ablation usually improves ventricular function.

Arrhythmogenic Right Ventricular Cardiomyopathy or Dysplasia

Arrhythmogenic right ventricular cardiomyopathy (ARVC) is an inherited cardiomyopathy with typically autosomal dominant transmission. It is associated with mutations affecting desmosomes, which are molecular complexes of cell adhesion proteins that bind cardiac myocytes. Although morphologic changes in the RV free wall predominate, biventricular or primary left ventricular variants occur. Due to myocyte death, large portions of the right ventricle are replaced with adipose tissue, leading to wall motion abnormalities, cardiac dysfunction, and aneurysm formation. Structural changes spread from the epicardium to the endocardium. RV imaging classically demonstrates RV enlargement with focal wall motion abnormalities and RV hypokinesis. The RV free wall is not well imaged by routine cardiac echocardiography, and MRI has become the gold standard for the diagnosis of ARVC.

ARVC patients develop ventricular arrhythmias with associated symptoms, including palpitations, lightheadedness, syncope, and SCD. Given the typical RV origin of arrhythmias in ARVC, the ventricular arrhythmias have a left bundle branch morphology. The surface ECG during sinus rhythm may demonstrate inverted T waves in the V_1 to V_3 leads or epsilon waves, which are low-amplitude deflections at the end of the QRS complex in the right precordial leads resulting from slowed RV conduction.

Distinguishing ARVC from idiopathic RVOT VT is essential because of the different prognostic and therapeutic implications of the two diagnoses. The diagnosis of ARVC is established by the ARVC Task Force Criteria. Risk factors for SCD of ARVC patients include prior aborted episodes of SCD, syncope, young age, LV dysfunction, and markedly diminished RV function.

Patients with documented ARVC typically receive ICDs. Adjunctive therapy with antiarrhythmic drugs or ablation, particularly strategies incorporating combined epicardial and endocardial ablation, may be useful in treating symptomatic VT.

TABLE 9-7	PREDICTORS OF SUDDEN CARDIAC DEATH AFTER MYOCARDIAL INFARCTION

Decreased left ventricular ejection fraction
Residual ischemia
Delayed enhancement on cardiac MRI
Late potentials on signal-averaged electrocardiography
Decreased heart rate variability
Prolonged QT on ECG
Induction of sustained MMVT with programmed electrical stimulation
Complex ventricular ectopy (e.g., NSVT) on ambulatory monitoring

ECG, Electrocardiogram; MMVT, monomorphic ventricular tachycardia; MRI, magnetic resonance imaging; NSVT, nonsustained ventricular tachycardia.

Congenital Long QT Syndrome

Congenital LQTS is a genetic disorder characterized by abnormal cardiac repolarization producing QT prolongation on the ECG (corrected QT [QTc] >440 milliseconds in men and >460 milliseconds in women). It is a leading cause of SCD in the young.

Mutations in 16 genes that participate in cardiac repolarization have been identified in patients with LQTS. Mutations of *KCNQ1* (encodes the α-subunit of the I_{Ks} potassium channel) produce LQT1; mutations of *KCNH2* (encodes the α-subunit of the I_{Kr} potassium channel) produce LQT2; and mutations of *SCN5A* (encodes the α-subunit of the cardiac sodium channel) cause LQT3. Together, they account for 75% of cases of congenital LQTS.

Decreased outward potassium currents or increased inward sodium currents prolong action potential duration, predisposing to early afterdepolarizations and TdP, a specific type of polymorphic VT. Symptoms typically begin during adolescence and include syncope, seizures, and SCD. The arrhythmia triggers in LQTS are gene specific. Patients with LQT1 are at risk during high adrenergic states, such as exercise; arrhythmias in LQT2 are triggered by sudden noises such as alarms; and LQT3 patients are more likely to experience arrhythmias during sleep. The autosomal dominant Romano-Ward variant has a prevalence of 1 case in 2000 live births.

Chronic treatment is directed at prevention of SCD. Initial therapy includes avoidance of QT-prolonging agents and initiation of β-blockers in symptomatic patients and asymptomatic patients with significant QT prolongation. ICDs are recommended after resuscitation from a cardiac arrest and for recurrent syncope despite β-blockade. The acute treatment of TdP is different from that of other forms of VT because many antiarrhythmic agents prolong the QT interval and should therefore be avoided.

Brugada Syndrome

The Brugada syndrome is a genetic disorder predisposing to polymorphic VT and SCD. The ECG characteristically displays coving ST elevation in the right precordial leads, V_1 to V_3, and a right bundle branch block pattern. These electrocardiographic abnormalities may be dynamic, and they are characteristically exacerbated by fever and therapy that blocks sodium channels.

In most cases, the syndrome is linked to mutations in *SCN5A*, which encodes the cardiac sodium channel. Mutations result in a reduction in the sodium current. The mode of transmission is autosomal dominant. Patients typically have syncope or cardiac arrest, often occurring during sleep.

Although quinidine, by virtue of its ability to block transient outward potassium current (I_{to}), may have a therapeutic role, there are no established medical therapies to prevent VT in Brugada syndrome. Intravenous β-adrenergic stimulation with isoproterenol or a similar agent, by virtue of its ability to augment the sodium current, is potentially useful in the acute management of recurrent VT or VF in Brugada syndrome. Paradoxically, because of a protective effect of catecholamine stimulation, β-blockers are potentially harmful in patients with Brugada syndrome and should be avoided.

ICDs represent the only proven therapy for prevention of cardiac arrest. ICD therapy is recommended for secondary prevention of SCD. For high-risk patients with a spontaneous Brugada electrocardiographic pattern and syncope, primary prevention with an ICD is indicated.

Catecholaminergic Polymorphic Ventricular Tachycardia

CPVT is a genetic disorder that alters myocardial calcium handling, resulting in exercise-induced polymorphic or bidirectional VT. Exercise-triggered syncope or SCD during childhood is the common presenting symptom. About 50% to 60% of patients have an inherited or sporadic autosomal dominant mutation affecting the cardiac ryanodine receptor gene *(RYR2)*, producing abnormal calcium-induced calcium release from the sarcoplasmic reticulum and intracellular calcium overload.

β-Blockers along with exercise restriction represent the primary therapy, although arrhythmia breakthrough is common. ICD therapy may be used for secondary prevention, although ICD shocks can produce catecholamine surges that may exacerbate the underlying arrhythmia. Left cardiac sympathetic denervation is useful in selected cases.

Acquired Long QT Syndrome

Environmental factors may prolong cardiac repolarization and produce QTc prolongation, leading to the development of early afterdepolarizations and TdP. Patients with acquired LQTS may have background genetics predisposing them to develop excessive QTc prolongation and polymorphic VT in response to electrolyte abnormalities (i.e., hypokalemia, hypomagnesemia, and hypocalcemia), bradycardia, and the use of QT-prolonging medications. Most QTc-prolonging drugs block the rapid component of the delayed rectifier potassium channel (I_{Kr}) encoded by the *KCNE2* gene. Drugs known to prolong the QTc interval are updated on an Internet registry. Therapy for acquired LQTS requires reversal of inciting physiologic factors and discontinuation of offending medications.

Genetic Testing for Channelopathies

Commercial laboratories offer genetic testing for congenital LQTS, Brugada syndrome, and CPVT. The yields of genetic testing vary from 25% for Brugada syndrome up to 80% for congenital LQTS. The limited sensitivity of current assays and the common finding of genetic variants of unknown significance represent ongoing challenges. Despite these considerations, cascade screening or screening of family members for a disease-causing mutation once characterized in a proband has been effectively used to identify mutation carriers.

Mutation-positive family members may benefit from prophylactic therapy. Reassurance for mutation-negative individuals is also valuable. Before ordering genetic testing, patients should be thoroughly informed of the risks, benefits, and limitations of testing. Genetic counselors ideally play an important advisory role.

For a deeper discussion on this topic, please see Chapter 65, "Ventricular Arrhythmias," in Goldman-Cecil Medicine, *25th Edition.*

SUMMARY

Cardiac arrhythmias are caused by disorders of action potential formation or propagation and are broadly categorized as abnormally slow rhythms (i.e., bradycardias) or abnormally rapid rhythms (i.e., tachycardias). The cardiac cellular action potential is composed of five phases determined by the activity of multiple ion channels, including the rapid sodium channel, several potassium channels, and a calcium current. Disruptions of these currents may lead to abnormal automaticity and triggered activity, which may mediate pathologic tachyarrhythmias. Reentry is the dominant mechanism of clinically significant tachyarrhythmias and requires a functional or fixed obstacle to propagation, an area of slowed conduction, and differential refractoriness for initiation and perpetuation of the arrhythmia.

Antiarrhythmic drugs are commonly divided into four broad groups using the Singh–Vaughn Williams classification. Despite its clinical utility, many antiarrhythmic drugs have multiple effects and do not fit neatly into this framework. Some, such as adenosine and digoxin, fall completely outside of it. Class I drugs slow membrane conduction by blockade of the sodium channel. Class II drugs, or β-blockers, function by blockade of the cardiac β-receptor. Class III drugs prolong repolarization and the QT interval. Class IV drugs block the slow calcium channel and are primarily active in slow-response myocytes such as the sinus and AV node.

All bradycardia is a consequence of impairment of sinus node function or AV conduction, or both. Sinus and AV nodal function is strongly influenced by autonomic tone. Parasympathetic tone dominates at rest, and significant bradycardia and second-degree AV block may be observed in normal patients due to increased parasympathetic tone, especially during sleep or athletic training. Clinical sinus node dysfunction manifests as one of several syndromes, including sinus bradycardia, chronotropic incompetence, exit block, and bradycardia-tachycardia syndrome due to sinus pauses and bradycardia when concomitant atrial arrhythmias terminate to sinus rhythm.

AV conduction disturbances may occur at the AV nodal level or infranodal level. A block at the level of the AV node tends to be indolent, characterized by gradual progression and competent subsidiary escapes that usually protect the patient from catastrophic bradycardia. This permits asymptomatic patients to be followed clinically for the development of symptoms before intervention. In contrast, second- or third-degree infranodal block at the His bundle, or more commonly at the level of the bundle branches, is potentially malignant and is often not accompanied by stable escape mechanisms. If not managed appropriately, it can cause sudden death. Clues to an infranodal level of block are Mobitz II periodicity, associated bundle branch block, worsening heart block with tachycardia or exercise, and a wide QRS escape rhythm different from the conducted QRS in the setting of a high-degree or third-degree AV block.

Tachycardias are broadly categorized as SVTs, which depend on the atrium and AV conduction system, and ventricular arrhythmias, which depend on the ventricular myocardium. Supraventricular arrhythmias are further categorized as PSVTs, which depend on AV nodal conduction, and intra-atrial arrhythmias, which depend only on atrial tissue and not on AV conduction. The PSVTs include AVNRT and AV reciprocating tachycardia related to WPW syndrome. Intra-atrial arrhythmias include organized atrial arrhythmias, such as focal atrial tachycardia, atrial flutter, macro-reentrant atrial tachycardia, and AF, a common disorganized atrial arrhythmia. Recurrent atrial flutter and AF carry a risk of thromboembolism and, based on risk stratification, should be treated with antithrombotic therapy when appropriate. Catheter ablation has an important role in the management of all supraventricular arrhythmias but remains a second-line strategy for AF, for which success rates are lower and complication rates are higher than for other supraventricular arrhythmias.

Ventricular arrhythmias include isolated ventricular premature beats; short, nonsustained runs of tachycardia; and sustained ventricular arrhythmias. Sustained VT lasts more than 30 seconds or requires intervention before then. It is classified as monomorphic if beats all share a single electrocardiographic morphology, polymorphic if the electrocardiographic morphology is variable, TdP when the morphology is variable and the arrhythmia is associated with pathologic QT prolongation, and VF when the surface ECG continuously varies without distinct QRS complexes. VT is poorly tolerated and is the major cause of cardiac arrest. Although commonly seen in the setting of ischemic heart disease, idiopathic VT may be seen in the absence of structural heart disease.

Antiarrhythmic drugs have not been effective in reducing the risk of SCD after MI. In contrast, ICDs have been shown to improve mortality rates for patients with impaired LV function after an MI and patients with heart failure and impaired LV function with or without coronary disease.

In addition to advanced structural heart disease as a cause for VT, several syndromes may result in VT in the absence of evident structural heart disease. They include the syndrome of idiopathic VT, ARVC, arrhythmogenic RV dysplasia, congenital LQTS, Brugada syndrome, and CPVT. Several of these conditions are familial, and genetic testing and family screening have important roles in their management.

SUGGESTED READINGS

Calkins H, Kuck KH, Cappato R, et al: 2012 HRS/EHRA/ECAS expert consensus statement on catheter and surgical ablation of atrial fibrillation: recommendations for patient selection, procedural techniques, patient management and follow-up, definitions, endpoints, and research trial design: a report of the Heart Rhythm Society (HRS) Task Force on Catheter and Surgical Ablation of Atrial Fibrillation. Developed in partnership with the European Heart Rhythm Association (EHRA), a registered branch of the European Society of Cardiology (ESC) and the European Cardiac Arrhythmia Society (ECAS); and in collaboration with the American College of Cardiology (ACC), American Heart Association (AHA), the Asia Pacific Heart Rhythm Society (APHRS), and the Society of Thoracic Surgeons (STS). Endorsed by the governing bodies of the American College of Cardiology Foundation, the American Heart Association, the European Cardiac Arrhythmia Society, the European Heart Rhythm Association, the Society of Thoracic Surgeons, the Asia Pacific Heart Rhythm Society, and the Heart Rhythm Society, Heart Rhythm 9:632.e21–696.e21, 2012.

Fuster V, Rydén LE, Cannom DS, et al: 2011 ACCF/AHA/HRS focused updates incorporated into the ACC/AHA/ESC 2006 Guidelines for the management of patients with atrial fibrillation; a Report of the American College of Cardiology Foundation/American Heart Association Task Force on Practice Guidelines developed in partnership with the European Society of Cardiology

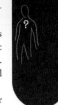

and in collaboration with the European Heart Rhythm Association and the Heart Rhythm Society, J Am Coll Cardiol 57:e101–e198, 2011.

Hohnloser SH, Kuck KH, Dorian P, et al: Prophylactic use of an implantable cardioverter-defibrillator after acute myocardial infarction, N Engl J Med 351:2481–2488, 2004.

Køber L, Torp-Pedersen C, McMurray JJ, et al: Increased mortality after dronedarone therapy for severe heart failure, N Engl J Med 358:2678–2687, 2008.

Pisters R, Lane DA, Nieuwlaat R, et al: A novel user-friendly score (HAS-BLED) to assess 1-year risk of major bleeding in patients with atrial fibrillation: the euro heart survey, Chest 138:1093–1100, 2010.

Roth JA: American College of Chest Physicians (AACP) Critical Care Board Review Course, presented August 24-26, 2007. Phoenix, Ariz.

Tracy CM, Epstein AE, Darbar D, et al: 2012 ACCF/AHA/HRS focused update of the 2008 guidelines for device-based therapy of cardiac rhythm abnormalities: a report of the American College of Cardiology Foundation/American Heart Association Task Force on Practice Guidelines, J Am Coll Cardiol 60:1297–1313, 2012.

Van Der Werf C, Kannankeril PJ, Sacher F, et al: Flecainide therapy reduces exercise-induced ventricular arrhythmias in patients with catecholaminergic polymorphic ventricular tachycardia, J Am Coll Cardiol 57:2244–2254, 2011.

Van Gelder IC, Groenveld HF, Crijns HJ, et al: Lenient versus strict rate control in patients with atrial fibrillation, N Engl J Med 362:1363–1373, 2010.

Zipes DP, Camm AJ, Borggrefe M, et al: ACC/AHA/ESC 2006 guidelines for management of patients with ventricular arrhythmias and the prevention of sudden cardiac death: a report of the American College of Cardiology/American Heart Association Task Force and the European Society of Cardiology Committee for Practice Guidelines (Writing Committee to Develop Guidelines for Management of Patients with Ventricular Arrhythmias and the Prevention of Sudden Cardiac Death), J Am Coll Cardiol 48:e247–e346, 2006.

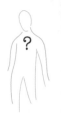

Pericardial and Myocardial Disease

Jennifer L. Strande, Panayotis Fasseas, and Ivor J. Benjamin

⬤ PERICARDIAL DISEASE

The pericardium is a thin, fibrous sac that envelops the heart and consists of two layers: visceral and parietal. The space between these two layers contains a small amount of fluid (15 to 50 mL), which is a plasma ultrafiltrate. The pericardium has mechanical, immunologic, and anatomic barrier functions.

Due to a paucity of randomized trial data and absence of practice guideline statements, the recommendations for assessment and treatment of pericardial disorders in this chapter are largely based on expert opinion and professional consensus.

Acute Pericarditis

Definition and Epidemiology

Acute pericarditis is an inflammatory disorder of the pericardium that has several causes. It is difficult to determine the exact incidence of acute pericarditis because a subclinical course is common.

Pathology

About 85% of cases are idiopathic or viral. Less common causes include infection (other than viral), uremia, trauma, metabolic disorders, autoimmune disorders, and neoplastic involvement. Causes of acute pericarditis are listed in Table 10-1.

Clinical Presentation

Patients may have symptoms of low-grade fever, malaise, dyspnea, and less frequently, hiccups (i.e., phrenic nerve irritation). The classic manifestation of acute pericarditis is chest pain, which is often severe, sharp, and positional. It is aggravated by a supine position, inspiration, and cough, and it is relieved by sitting up and leaning forward. The pain is usually substernal and left precordial, and it may radiate to the neck, shoulder, and scapular ridge, mimicking that of myocardial ischemia. Chest discomfort may be mild or absent in patients with connective tissue disorders, uremia, or neoplastic involvement.

In the absence of significant pericardial effusion, results of the inspection and palpation of the precordium are normal. A high-pitched, rasping pericardial friction rub is heard on cardiac auscultation in most patients with acute pericarditis. It may have three components corresponding to atrial contraction, ventricular systole, and early diastole, and it is best appreciated at end expiration with the patient leaning forward. It can be intermittent, and serial auscultation is recommended.

Diagnosis

The electrocardiographic (ECG) changes of acute pericarditis typically evolve over days to weeks. In the early stages, there is diffuse ST segment elevation (i.e., concave upward) with upright T waves and PR depression, which occasionally precedes the ST segment elevation. Resolution of the ST elevations is followed by diffuse T wave inversion. These ECG changes are not always seen, and serial tracings should be obtained.

The laboratory findings of acute idiopathic pericarditis are not specific and consist of mild elevation of the white blood cell count, sedimentation rate, and C-reactive protein level. If indicated, specific testing for tuberculosis, human immunodeficiency virus (HIV), thyroid disease, or autoimmune disorders is recommended. However, routine performance of viral serologic testing has limited utility. Elevation of serum cardiac biomarkers (e.g., creatine kinase, troponin) reflects involvement of the adjacent

TABLE 10-1 CAUSES OF PERICARDITIS

Idiopathic
Infectious
    Viral (echovirus, coxsackievirus, adenovirus, cytomegalovirus, hepatitis B virus, Ebstein-Barr virus, human immunodeficiency virus)
    Bacterial (*Staphylococcus, Streptococcus,* and *Mycoplasma* species; *Borrelia burgdorferi, Haemophilus influenzae, Neisseria meningitidis*)
    Mycobacterial (*Mycobacterium tuberculosis, Mycobacterium avium-intracellulare*)
    Fungal (*Histoplasma* and *Coccidioides* species)
    Protozoal
Immune or inflammatory
    Connective tissue disease (systemic lupus erythematosus, rheumatoid arthritis, scleroderma)
    Arteritis (polyarteritis nodosa, temporal arteritis)
    Late after myocardial infarction (Dressler's syndrome), late postcardiotomy or thoracotomy
Drug induced
    Procainamide, hydralazine, isoniazid, cyclosporine
Trauma or damage to adjacent structures
    Penetrating trauma
    Acute myocardial infarction, cardiac surgery, coronary angioplasty, implantable defibrillators, pacemakers
    Pneumonia
Neoplastic disease
    Primary: mesothelioma, fibrosarcoma, lipoma
    Secondary (metastatic or direct extension): breast, lung, thyroid carcinoma, lymphoma, leukemia, melanoma
Radiation induced
Miscellaneous
    Uremia
    Hypothyroidism
    Gout

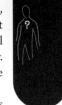

myocardium. In uncomplicated acute pericarditis, the chest radiograph and echocardiographic findings are normal. Although not essential for the diagnosis of pericarditis, echocardiography is the diagnostic imaging modality of choice for the detection and determination of the hemodynamic significance of a pericardial effusion.

Treatment

Patients with uncomplicated idiopathic or viral pericarditis can be managed as outpatients. For patients with fever, large pericardial effusions, or elevated levels of cardiac biomarkers and for those with possible secondary causes or immunocompromised status, hospitalization for further investigation and treatment should be considered. Treatment consisting of high-dose nonsteroidal anti-inflammatory drugs (NSAIDs) is usually effective. Colchicine with NSAIDs or as monotherapy provides prompt resolution of symptoms and decreases the recurrence rate. The use of glucocorticoids results in rapid symptomatic improvement. However, it is associated with higher rates of symptomatic recurrence.

Prognosis

Most patients with idiopathic or viral pericarditis have an uneventful clinical course with complete recovery. Possible complications include recurrent pericarditis, cardiac tamponade, and constrictive pericarditis.

Pericardial Effusion and Cardiac Tamponade

Definition and Epidemiology

Pericardial effusion, an abnormal collection of fluid in the pericardial space, is a relatively common and incidental echocardiographic finding that is encountered in approximately 10% of studies. Cardiac tamponade occurs when fluid accumulation results in increased intrapericardial pressure, leading to cardiac compression, impaired ventricular filling, and reduced cardiac output. Accumulation of pericardial fluid can be caused by virtually any type of acute pericarditis. Pericardial effusions due to bacterial pericarditis (including tuberculosis), neoplastic involvement, uremic pericarditis, and trauma have a high incidence of progression to tamponade.

Pathology

The hemodynamic consequences of a pericardial effusion depend on the rate of accumulation. The normal pericardium has relatively limited reserve volume. The mechanical properties of the parietal pericardium are such that when stretched, it becomes rapidly inelastic and resistant to further expansion. As a result of these physical characteristics, rapidly accumulating effusions may result in significant hemodynamic compromise with only 100 to 200 mL of fluid. Conversely, when the accumulation of fluid is slow, the pericardium undergoes adaptive changes and can accommodate large (>1500 mL) effusions without the development of tamponade.

Clinical Presentation

The clinical manifestations of a pericardial effusion depend on the size and rate of fluid accumulation and may range from dyspnea, chest discomfort, and orthopnea to circulatory collapse, pulseless electrical activity, and death. Compression of adjacent structures such as the phrenic nerve and the recurrent laryngeal nerve can result in cough or hiccups and hoarseness, respectively. A complaint of dysphasia may indicate compression of the esophagus.

A normal cardiac examination is not uncommon in patients with small effusions. With larger effusions, the apical impulse can be decreased or absent, and the cardiac sound may be muffled. In patients with acute pericarditis, disappearance of the pericardial friction rub may indicate development of an effusion. Compression of the base of the left lung can result in dullness to percussion, egophony, and bronchial breath sounds under the left scapula (i.e., Ewart's sign).

Patients with tamponade usually appear to be in distress with tachypnea and tachycardia. The classic physical findings are hypotension, jugular venous distention with absent y descent, and muffled or absent heart sounds. Pulsus paradoxus, defined as a greater than 10 mm Hg of inspiratory decline of the systolic blood pressure, is a characteristic physical finding. It is the result of the inspiratory decrease of the left ventricular stroke volume and systemic blood pressure. Under normal conditions, the intrathoracic pressure decreases during inspiration, resulting in enhanced right ventricular filling and enlargement. In cases of cardiac tamponade, the total heart volume is fixed, and the right ventricular expansion displaces the interventricular septum toward the left ventricle, with consequent reduction of the left ventricular stroke volume and systemic hypotension. Pulsus paradoxus is not pathognomonic of cardiac tamponade and can be detected in severe chronic obstructive airway disease, pulmonary embolism, bronchial asthma, constrictive pericarditis, and hypovolemic shock.

Diagnosis

The ECG findings of moderate to large pericardial effusions include low-voltage QRS complexes and occasionally include electrical (QRS) alternans caused by the heart's swinging motion within the fluid-filled pericardium. The chest radiograph demonstrates an enlarged cardiac silhouette. Transthoracic echocardiography, the imaging modality of choice, provides information regarding the size, location (circumferential vs. loculated), and most importantly, the hemodynamic consequences of the pericardial effusion suggesting tamponade.

The two-dimensional findings of tamponade include right atrial and right ventricular collapse, distention of the inferior vena cava, and evidence of increased ventricular interdependence (Fig. 10-1). Doppler quantification of the mitral and tricuspid inflow velocity respiratory variation is more sensitive than two-dimensional echocardiography for determining the hemodynamic significance of pericardial effusions. Right heart catheterization demonstrates decreased cardiac output, elevated right atrial pressure with diminished or absent y descent, and equalization of the cardiac filling pressures (i.e., right atrial, pulmonary wedge, and diastolic pulmonary artery pressures).

Computed tomography (CT) and magnetic resonance imaging (MRI) can accurately identify pericardial effusions and may be used with echocardiography in the assessment of loculated effusions, pericardial thickening, and extracardiac

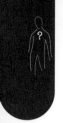

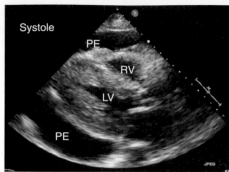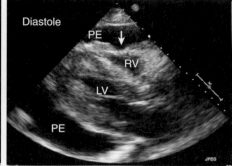

FIGURE 10-1 Parasternal long axis echocardiographic views of the right ventricle in systole and diastole show right ventricular diastolic collapse *(arrow)* in a patient with a large, circumferential pericardial effusion. LV, Left ventricle; PE, pericardial effusion; RV, right ventricle.

surrounding structures. A diagnostic pericardiocentesis is the procedure of choice for evaluating for bacterial, tuberculous, or malignant causes.

Treatment

Routine drainage of pericardial effusions is unnecessary in the absence of hemodynamic compromise. Cardiac tamponade is a life-threatening emergency requiring urgent drainage of the pericardial effusion. Fluid resuscitation should be initiated to increase preload and filling of the cardiac chambers. Inotropic and vasopressor support has limited utility. Surgical drainage is appropriate and therapeutic for loculated, purulent, and tuberculous effusions and for tissue biopsy.

Fluid should be analyzed for pH, cell count, glucose, protein, cholesterol, triglycerides, and acid-fast bacilli by Gram stain, culture, cytology, and laboratory tests. For patients with chronic, recurring effusions, the surgical creation of a pleuropericardial window provides a long-term solution.

Prognosis

The underlying cause of the pericardial effusion and the availability of effective treatment determine the prognosis.

Constrictive Pericarditis

Definition and Epidemiology

Pericardial constriction is a condition characterized by a rigid, scarred pericardium that limits diastolic filling of the ventricles, resulting in increased intracardiac pressures. It can be caused by any type of pericardial inflammation. The most common causes are infection, prior cardiac surgery, trauma, and irradiation. Less common causes include connective tissue disorders, uremia, and neoplastic involvement of the pericardium. In developing countries, tuberculous pericarditis is a common cause of pericardial constriction. Often a specific cause cannot be determined.

Pathology

Constriction is the end result of pericardial inflammation with scarring, fibrosis, calcification, and adhesion of the parietal and visceral layers of the pericardium. Although pericardial thickening is a usual pathologic finding, its absence does not exclude constriction.

Clinical Presentation

In the early stages, symptoms consist of dyspnea, fatigue, decreased exercise tolerance, and lower extremity edema. As the disease progresses, early signs and symptoms may be accompanied by ascites, anasarca, cachexia, and muscle wasting.

Physical examination reveals jugular venous distention with prominent x and y descents and an increase (or failure to decrease) of central venous pressure with inspiration (i.e., Kussmaul sign). The arterial blood pressure is usually normal, and pulsus paradoxus is absent in most patients. Ascites and hepatomegaly can be prominent with advanced disease. On cardiovascular examination, the apical impulse may be decreased and the cardiac sounds muffled. An early diastolic sound (i.e., pericardial knock) corresponding to the abrupt cessation of early ventricular diastolic filling is pathognomonic of pericardial constriction, but it is not always detected.

Diagnosis

The diagnosis of pericardial constriction may be challenging and frequently requires the use of multiple imaging modalities. The electrocardiogram may display low QRS voltage, left atrial enlargement, and nonspecific T-wave changes. Atrial fibrillation occurs in one third of cases. The chest radiograph may reveal pleural effusions and pericardial calcification, which are best appreciated in the lateral projection.

Transthoracic echocardiography shows dilation of the inferior vena cava, abnormal interventricular septal motion, and pericardial thickening. Doppler echocardiography demonstrates abnormal respirophasic variations of the pulmonary and hepatic venous flow and mitral valve inflow. CT and MRI can accurately measure pericardial thickness.

Cardiac catheterization is essential in the diagnosis of pericardial constriction and differentiation from restrictive cardiomyopathy (RCM). The right atrial pressure tracing shows prominent x and y descents with equalization of the end-diastolic atrial and ventricular pressures. The ventricular pressure tracings show a rapid early diastolic filling of the ventricles, with abrupt cessation in middle and end diastole due to the finite volume of the rigid pericardium (i.e., dip-and-plateau morphology or the square root sign) (Fig. 10-2). Enhanced ventricular interdependence demonstrated by simultaneous measurement of right and left ventricular pressures during respiration is a more specific finding of pericardial constriction.

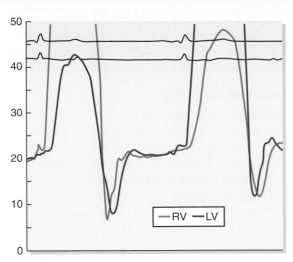

FIGURE 10-2 Pressure recordings from a patient with constrictive pericarditis. Simultaneous right ventricular and left ventricular pressure tracings show equalization of diastolic pressure and dip-and-plateau morphology. LV, Left ventricle; RV, right ventricle.

Treatment

Medical therapy with sodium restriction and diuretics is of limited efficacy and is only appropriate in patients who are not surgical candidates in view of comorbidities. Pericardiectomy is the only definitive treatment for constrictive pericarditis.

Prognosis

Pericardiectomy is associated with substantial operative risk that depends on the extent of cardiac involvement and existence of comorbid conditions. Successful pericardial resection leads to resolution of the symptoms of constriction over a period of weeks to months. For patients who are not surgical candidates, the prognosis is poor.

Effusive Constrictive Pericarditis

Effusive constrictive pericarditis is characterized by a pericardial effusion and a noncompliant or fibrotic parietal and visceral pericardium. Although it may result from any type of pericardial inflammation, it is usually seen after cardiac surgery or radiation injury. It likely represents a transition stage between acute pericarditis with effusion and pericardial constriction. It shares the clinical and hemodynamic features of both conditions.

Typically, drainage of the effusion does not result in resolution of symptoms, and the central venous and right atrial pressures remain elevated. In the early stage of the disease, patients may respond to prolonged treatment with NSAIDs. However, visceral and parietal pericardiectomy is often required. For a deeper discussion of this topic, please see Chapter 77, "Pericardial Diseases," in *Goldman-Cecil Medicine*, 25th Edition.

● DISEASES OF THE MYOCARDIUM

Myocarditis

Definition and Epidemiology

Myocarditis is an inflammation of the myocardium caused by a variety of toxins, medications, and viruses. Viral myocarditis, which accounts for about 20% of cases of dilated cardiomyopathy

(DCM), is commonly caused by the enteroviruses, specifically Coxsackie group B serotypes and, less commonly, adenoviruses, parvovirus B19, hepatitis C virus, cytomegalovirus, and HIV.

Other causes include bacterial infections such as diphtheria, brucellosis, clostridial infections, legionnaires disease, and meningococcal, streptococcal, and *Mycoplasma pneumoniae* infections. Rickettsial infections (e.g., Q fever, Rocky Mountain spotted fever), spirochetal infections (e.g., leptospirosis, Lyme disease), fungal infections, and parasitic infections (e.g., *Trypanosoma cruzi* [Chagas' disease]) are also known causes of myocarditis.

Pathology

The pathogenesis of viral myocarditis is thought to begin with direct viral invasion of the myocardium and subsequent immunologic activation. Normal cellular and antibody-mediated immune responses lead to viral clearing and myocardial healing. However, a few patients go on to develop DCM and heart failure due to an abnormal immune response, furthering myocardial damage. The exact mechanisms are unknown, but they involve cytokines, autoantibodies, and possibly other processes associated with persistent, low-level viral replication in myocytes, leading to myocyte atrophy, myocyte apoptosis, and adverse remodeling of the ventricles. In nonviral infections, the damage is attributed to the bacterial toxins or abnormal immune responses, and in parasitic infections, it is largely immune mediated.

Multiple chemicals and drugs can lead to myocardial inflammation by direct effect or as part of a hypersensitivity reaction. Some of the common causes include cocaine, chemotherapeutics (e.g., daunorubicin, doxorubicin), and antibiotics.

Giant cell myocarditis is a rare disorder of uncertain origin, but it can be rapidly fatal. It is usually associated with ventricular arrhythmias and progressive, severe heart failure. Multinucleated giant cells seen on myocardial biopsy are pathognomonic.

Clinical Presentation

The clinical manifestations range from asymptomatic ECG abnormalities to cardiogenic shock. Patients report heart failure symptoms, including exercise intolerance, shortness of breath, fluid retention, and persistent fatigue, and in the case of viral myocarditis, they often report a viral prodrome, including fever, myalgia, fatigue, respiratory symptoms, and gastroenteritis that precedes the heart failure symptoms. Patients are often tachycardic and hypotensive, and they may have an elevated jugular venous pressure, S_3 gallop, crackles, and peripheral edema. Myocarditis can masquerade as an acute coronary syndrome.

Diagnosis

Testing is performed to determine a possible infectious cause. Rising viral titers are often seen in cases of viral myocarditis. Serum cardiac enzymes (e.g., troponin, creatine kinase) are measured when myocarditis is suspected. Sinus tachycardia and nonspecific ST- and T-wave abnormalities are common ECG findings. When pericardium is also involved by the inflammatory process, diffuse ST-segment elevations typical for acute pericarditis are also seen. Ventricular ectopy is common, and atrioventricular

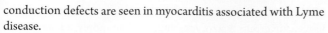

conduction defects are seen in myocarditis associated with Lyme disease.

Echocardiography is recommended in the initial diagnostic evaluation to identify ventricular remodeling, including increasing chamber size and ventricular systolic dysfunction. Cardiac MRI is a promising technique to detect myocardial inflammation and injury based on small, observational clinical studies.

Transvenous endomyocardial biopsy should be performed only when there is rapid deterioration of the clinical condition (level of evidence B). Histopathologic abnormalities such as infiltrating white cells (i.e., macrophages, lymphocytes, and eosinophils), evidence of myocardial damage, and a finding of interstitial fibrosis are used to establish acute myocarditis, but the determination is subject to significant intraobserver and interobserver variability, and the biopsy often does not provide a conclusive diagnosis. The endomyocardial biopsy is helpful in diagnosing giant cell myocarditis (i.e., multinucleated giant cells are seen) or hypersensitivity myocarditis (i.e., eosinophilic infiltrate is seen). The polymerase chain reaction can detect specific viral genomes in the myocardium.

Treatment

Supportive care is the mainstay of treatment. A few patients with fulminant or acute myocarditis require an intensive level of hemodynamic support and aggressive pharmacologic intervention similar to that for patients with advanced heart failure.

After initial hemodynamic stabilization, treatment should follow current American College of Cardiology and American Heart Association (ACC/AHA) recommendations for the management of left ventricular systolic dysfunction. Treatment includes β-adrenergic blockers, angiotensin-converting enzyme inhibitors, aldosterone receptor blockers, and diuretics.

No evidence-based guided therapy for viral myocarditis has been established. Clinical trials of various forms of antiviral or immunosuppressive therapy (e.g., prednisone, cyclosporine, azathioprine, intravenous immunoglobulin, interferon immunoadsorption) have not resulted in conclusive evidence of benefit. Treatment of nonviral myocarditis is aimed at eradication of the specific infectious agent. For Chagas disease, treatment with antiprotozoal therapy, if initiated early in the course of infection, may be beneficial.

Hypersensitivity myocarditis and myocarditis associated with toxins respond to withdrawal of the offending agent. Immunosuppressive therapy has been effective in giant cell myocarditis.

Prognosis

Understanding the natural history of myocarditis has been limited by its diverse clinical presentations and causes. It is thought that one third of the patients fully recover, one third of the patients have some sequelae in the form of left ventricular systolic dysfunction but are stable on medical therapy, and one third of patients progress to advanced heart failure. Patients who progress to chronic DCM have 5-year survival rates of less than 50%.

Cardiomyopathies

Cardiomyopathies are a heterogeneous group of diseases in which the major structural abnormality is limited to the myocardium. The four main cardiomyopathic groups are dilated, hypertrophic, restrictive, and arrhythmogenic right ventricular cardiomyopathy. Familial (genetic) and nonfamilial (acquired) forms of the diseases have been described.

Dilated Cardiomyopathy

Definition and Epidemiology

Cardiac enlargement and systolic dysfunction in DCM result from a wide spectrum of genetic, inflammatory, toxic, and metabolic causes (Table 10-2), although most cases are idiopathic. Abnormal loading conditions such as hypertension, valvular disease, or coronary artery disease can lead to similar structural and functional changes; these conditions are not considered to be part of the DCM group and are discussed elsewhere.

Most cases are thought to result from acute viral myocarditis, a process described earlier. Exposures to cardiac toxins such as chemotherapeutic agents, alcohol, cocaine, and radiation, along with deficiency of nutrients such as thiamine (causes beriberi), vitamin C (causes scurvy), carnitine, selenium, phosphate, and calcium, can cause DCM. Peripartum cardiomyopathy is a rare cause of DCM that can develop during the last month of pregnancy and up to 6 months after delivery.

The pathogenesis of this often life-threatening disease is not completely understood, and it is a diagnosis of exclusion. Risk factors include older maternal age, being African American, and having multiple pregnancies. Prolonged periods of supraventricular or ventricular tachycardia can lead to idiopathic DCM (i.e., tachycardia-induced cardiomyopathy). The structural and functional changes usually reverse after the rapid heart rhythm is controlled.

Familial forms of DCM may be responsible for 20% to 30% of cases. Specific mutations described involve genes that encode proteins of the sarcomere, cytoskeleton, nuclear membrane, and mitochondria; many mutations remain unknown. The mode of inheritance is typically autosomal dominant, but it can be an X-linked or mitochondrial pattern.

Pathology

Marked enlargement of all four cardiac chambers is typical of DCM, although the disease sometimes is limited to the left or right chambers. The dilation is out of proportion to the ventricular thickness. Histology reveals evidence of myocyte degeneration with irregular hypertrophy and atrophy of myofibers with often extensive interstitial and perivascular fibrosis.

Clinical Presentation

DCM usually manifests with symptoms of heart failure, including fatigue, weakness, dyspnea, and edema. In some patients, the presenting episode is related to arrhythmia or an embolic event. On physical examination, signs of decreased cardiac output are often found, including cool extremities, narrow pulse pressure, and tachycardia. The cardiac examination reveals a laterally displaced apex. An S_3 gallop is common, along with murmurs of mitral and tricuspid regurgitation. Pulmonary edema manifests as auscultatory crackles over the lung fields, and breath sounds may be diminished if there are pleural effusions. In some patients, the clinical features of right ventricular heart failure may

TABLE 10-2 CARDIOMYOPATHIES

DISORDER	DESCRIPTION AND CAUSE
Dilated cardiomyopathy	Dilation and impaired systolic function of the left or both ventricles
Familial (genetic)	Known or unknown genetic mutations
Nonfamilial	Viral myocarditis, nonviral infective myocarditis, idiopathic (immune) myocarditis
	Toxins (drugs, alcohol)
	Pregnancy (peripartum cardiomyopathy)
	Nutritional (thiamine deficiency [beriberi], vitamin C deficiency [scurvy], selenium deficiency)
	Endocrine (diabetes mellitus, hyperthyroidism, hypothyroidism, hyperparathyroidism, pheochromocytoma, acromegaly)
	Autoimmune (rheumatoid arthritis, systemic lupus erythematosus, dermatomyositis)
	Tachycardia induced
Hypertrophic cardiomyopathy	Left and/or right ventricular hypertrophy, often asymmetrical (usually more prominent hypertrophy of the interventricular septum)
Familial (genetic)	Mutations of sarcoplasmic proteins (several hundred described)
	Metabolic storage diseases of the myocyte
Restrictive cardiomyopathy	Restrictive filling of the ventricles; ventricles are usually small, atria are markedly enlarged
Familial (genetic)	Mutations of sarcomeric proteins
	Familial amyloidosis (transthyretin, apolipoprotein)
	Hemochromatosis
	Desminopathy, pseudoxanthoma elasticum, glycogen storage diseases
	Unknown genetic mutations
Nonfamilial	Amyloidosis, sarcoidosis, carcinoid, scleroderma
	Endomyocardial fibrosis (hypereosinophilic syndrome, idiopathic, chromosomal defect, drugs)
	Radiation, metastatic cancer, anthracycline toxicity
Arrhythmogenic right ventricular	Progressive fibrofatty replacement of the right and, to a lesser degree, left ventricular cardiomyopathy
Familial	Unknown gene mutation
	Mutations of intercalated disk protein, cardiac ryanodine receptor, transforming growth factor-β3

UNCLASSIFIED CARDIOMYOPATHIES

Takotsubo (stress-induced) cardiomyopathy	Transient dilation and dysfunction of the distal parts of the left ventricle (apical ballooning) in the setting of a stressful situation; usually resolves within weeks
Left ventricular noncompaction	Characterized by prominent left ventricular trabeculae and deep intertrabecular recesses; familial in most cases, caused by arrest in the normal embryogenesis of the heart; apex and periapical regions of the left ventricle most affected; some patients remain asymptomatic, but others develop left ventricular dilation and systolic dysfunction
Cardiomyopathies associated with muscular dystrophies and neuromuscular disorders	Duchenne-Becker muscular dystrophy, Emery-Dreifuss muscular dystrophy, myotonic dystrophy, Friedreich's ataxia, neurofibromatosis, tuberous sclerosis
Ion channelopathies	Disorders caused by mutations in genes encoding ionic channel proteins; not considered cardiomyopathies because they are not associated with typical structural changes of the heart but rather manifest with electrical dysfunction; some classifications include these disorders as cardiomyopathies: long QT syndrome, short QT syndrome, Brugada syndrome, catecholaminergic polymorphic ventricular tachycardia

predominate, with jugular venous distention hepatomegaly, ascites, and peripheral edema.

Diagnosis

Standard diagnostic procedures include a chest radiograph, an electrocardiogram, serum markers, and echocardiography. The radiograph shows cardiomegaly, pulmonary venous congestion, and pleural effusions. The electrocardiogram may reveal enlargement of the heart chambers along with other nonspecific ST- and T-wave abnormalities. Serum B-type natriuretic peptide (BNP) levels are elevated.

Echocardiography provides a comprehensive evaluation of ventricular size and function and valvular function, and it can show a ventricular thrombus. Similar information can be obtained with MRI.

A complete work-up should rule out ischemic, valvular, and hypertensive heart disease as the cause of myocardial dysfunction, and it should include evaluation for potentially reversible causes of DCM (e.g., alcohol, nutritional deficiencies). Myocardial biopsy may be considered if the cause of DCM is in question. In patients with a strong family history, a referral for genetic testing should be considered.

Treatment

Potential reversible causes of DCM should be addressed (e.g., alcohol cessation, correction of nutritional deficiencies, removal of cardiotoxic agents). Treatment should follow current ACC/AHA recommendations for the management of left ventricular systolic dysfunction and include β-adrenergic blockers, angiotensin-converting enzyme inhibitors, aldosterone receptor blockers, and diuretics.

Patients with idiopathic DCM who have persistent, moderate to severe symptoms of heart failure and a QRS duration longer than 120 milliseconds may benefit from cardiac resynchronization therapy with a biventricular pacemaker. Survival of patients with a left ventricular ejection fraction less than 35% despite maximal medical management is improved with the use of implantable cardioverter-defibrillators (ICDs). Patients with limiting heart failure symptoms despite use of the previously described therapies may be considered for heart transplantation or support with a left ventricular assist device.

Prognosis

The prognosis of patients with DCM depends on the response to medical therapy. Some patients have a significant improvement in symptoms and cardiac function, but in others, the disease is progressive and associated with a high mortality rate.

Hypertrophic Cardiomyopathy

Definition and Epidemiology

Hypertrophic cardiomyopathy (HCM) is a disease state characterized by unexplained left ventricular hypertrophy with nondilated ventricular chambers in the absence of an apparent cause for hypertrophy (e.g., hypertensive disease, aortic stenosis). This is a relatively common genetic disease (1 case in 500 people in the general population) with autosomal dominant inheritance, although spontaneous mutations have been described. More than 1400 mutations identified among at least eight genes encoding proteins of the cardiac sarcomere have been described, with mutations of the β-myosin heavy chain being the most common.

Pathology

The main pathophysiologic abnormalities seen in HCM are left ventricular outflow obstruction, diastolic dysfunction, mitral regurgitation, and arrhythmias. Obstruction of left ventricular outflow occurs in roughly one half of the patients. During systole, the hypertrophied septum bulges into the left ventricular outflow tract, creating a gradient between the lower part of the left ventricular cavity and the left ventricular outflow. This causes high-velocity turbulent flow through the narrowed path, which results in a suction force (i.e., Venturi effect) that pulls the anterior leaflet of the mitral valve into the outflow tract. This worsens the obstruction and causes mitral regurgitation. Diastolic dysfunction from impaired relaxation properties of the abnormal myocardium causes marked elevation of left ventricular filling and pulmonary venous pressures, pulmonary congestion, and limitation in cardiac output. Patients with HCM are also predisposed to supraventricular and ventricular arrhythmias.

Clinical Presentation

HCM is a heterogeneous cardiac disease with a diverse course and clinical manifestations. Most patients probably do not suffer sequelae from this disease during their lifetimes. When the disease does result in complications, there are three relatively discrete but not mutually exclusive clinical manifestations: sudden cardiac death due to unpredictable ventricular tachyarrhythmia, most commonly in young asymptomatic patients (<35 years of age); heart failure characterized by exertional dyspnea (with or without chest pain) that may progress despite preserved systolic function and sinus rhythm; and atrial fibrillation that associates with various degrees of heart failure.

Heart failure symptoms result from the dynamic obstruction to left ventricular outflow and diastolic dysfunction. The most frequent symptom is dyspnea on exertion, followed by ischemic chest pain due to the increased oxygen demand by the hypertrophied ventricle and elevated wall tension that reduces blood flow to the subendocardium. Abnormalities of the structure of small myocardial arteries in HCM can contribute to myocardial ischemia. Presyncope or syncope can result from outflow tract obstruction and an inability to increase cardiac output during exertion or from arrhythmias that can be triggered by exertion. In some, sudden death caused by ventricular arrhythmia is the initial manifestation of the disease.

Physical examination findings include pulsus bisferiens, a brisk initial upstroke in pulse followed by a mid-systolic dip corresponding to the development of left ventricular outflow tract obstruction, followed by another rise in late systole. Cardiac examination may shows a forceful and sustained apical impulse, an audible S_4 gallop, and a harsh crescendo-decrescendo systolic murmur best heard along the left sternal border with radiation to the base of the heart.

Patients may also have an apical holosystolic murmur of mitral regurgitation. The intensity of the murmur of HCM varies with changing degrees of obstruction. This can be observed with physiologic or pharmacologic maneuvers that change preload (i.e., left ventricular filling) or contractility. The intensity of the murmur increases with a Valsalva maneuver, with assuming a standing position, and after administration of nitroglycerin or inotropic drugs. The intensity of the murmur decreases with squatting, volume loading, and administration of β-blockers.

Diagnosis

Clinical diagnosis is made most commonly with echocardiography and increasingly with cardiac MRI. The diagnosis is based on a maximal left ventricular wall thickness of 15 mm or more; a wall thickness of 13 to 14 mm is considered borderline. The diagnosis can be made in the setting of other compelling information (e.g., family history of HCM). Genetic testing is available to confirm the diagnosis and to screen family members.

Treatment

The ACC/AHA hypertrophic cardiomyopathy guideline recommends tailored therapy based on the individual patient. For asymptomatic patients, the usefulness of β-blockade and verapamil is a class IIb recommendation. For patients symptomatic with dyspnea or angina, β-blockers and verapamil are recommended (level of evidence B). If patients remain symptomatic, it is reasonable to add disopyramide to a β-blocker or verapamil (level of evidence B).

Nonpharmacologic therapies should be considered in patients with considerable symptoms despite medical management. Septal reduction therapy is recommended only for patients with severe drug-refractory symptoms and left ventricular outflow tract obstruction (level of evidence C) (Fig. 10-3). Use of ICD therapy is guided by the perceived risk for ventricular arrhythmias in individual patients; it can prevent sudden death in these patients (level of evidence C). Some of the characteristics that have been associated with this risk are prior cardiac arrest or sustained ventricular tachycardia; great (>30 mm) ventricular wall thickness; syncope, especially if exertional or recurrent; and a first-degree relative with sudden cardiac death. Certain genotypes appear to convey an increased risk of sudden cardiac death. Patients with HCM should be excluded from most competitive sports and should avoid strenuous exercise.

Prognosis

The clinical course of HCM varies. Sudden cardiac death is the leading cause of mortality. Heart failure symptoms may gradually progress, and some patients who are unresponsive to conventional therapy may require heart transplantation.

Restrictive Cardiomyopathies

Definition and Epidemiology

RCM is an uncommon form of cardiomyopathy characterized by impaired ventricular filling of nondilated ventricles. RCM can be genetic or acquired. Causes include infiltrative disorders (e.g., amyloidosis, sarcoidosis, Gaucher's disease, Hurler's syndrome, fatty infiltration), storage diseases (e.g., hemochromatosis, Fabry's disease, glycogen storage disease), other disorders (e.g., hypereosinophilic syndrome, carcinoid heart disease), drugs (e.g., serotonin, methysergide, ergotamine), and cancer treatment (e.g., irradiation, chemotherapy).

Pathology

In the purest form of the disease, the atria are disproportionately dilated compared with the normal ventricular size, and the left ventricle has normal or near-normal systolic function in the absence of hypertrophy. Histology is normally nondistinctive and can reveal normal findings or nonspecific degenerative changes, including myocyte hypertrophy, disarray, and degrees of interstitial fibrosis.

Clinical Presentation

Patients often have symptoms and signs of pulmonary and systemic congestion. The most common symptoms include dyspnea, palpitations, fatigue, weakness, and exercise intolerance due to poor cardiac output. As central venous pressure continues to increase in advanced cases, there may be hepatosplenomegaly, ascites, and anasarca. The chest radiograph shows atrial enlargement, pulmonary venous congestion, and pleural effusions.

Diagnosis

The diagnosis of RCM should be considered for patients with predominantly right ventricular heart failure without evidence of cardiomegaly or systolic dysfunction. The correct diagnosis often is not made until months or years after symptom onset. Constrictive pericarditis can mimic RCM, and establishing the correct diagnosis can be challenging. Distinctive features of the two disorders are described in Table 10-3.

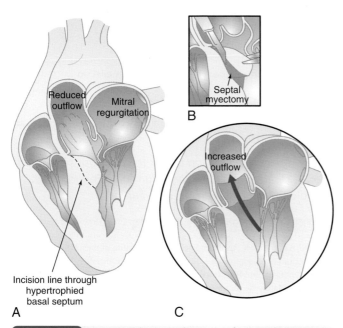

FIGURE 10-3 **A** to **C,** Schematic diagrams of a septal myectomy. (From Nishimura RA, Holmes DR Jr: Clinical practice: hypertrophic obstructive cardiomyopathy, N Engl J Med 350:1320–1327, 2004.)

TABLE 10-3   DIFFERENTIATION OF RESTRICTIVE CARDIOMYOPATHY FROM CONSTRICTIVE PERICARDITIS

TYPE OF EVALUATION	RESTRICTIVE CARDIOMYOPATHY	CONSTRICTIVE PERICARDITIS
Physical examination	Kussmaul sign present Apical impulse may be prominent Regurgitant murmurs are common	Kussmaul sign may be present Apical impulse usually not palpable Pericardial knock may be present
Electrocardiography	Low QRS voltage (especially in amyloidosis) Pseudoinfarction pattern Bundle branch blocks AV conduction disturbances Atrial fibrillation	Low QRS voltage Repolarization abnormalities
Chest radiography		Calcification of the pericardium may be present
Echocardiography	Marked enlargement of the atria Increased wall thickness (especially in amyloidosis)	Atria usually of normal size Normal wall thickness Pericardial thickening may be seen
Doppler echocardiography	Restrictive mitral inflow (dominant E wave with short deceleration time) No significant variation (<10%) of transvalvular velocities with respiration Reversal of forward flow in hepatic veins during inspiration	Restrictive mitral inflow (dominant E wave with short deceleration time) Increased velocity of RV filling and decreased velocity of LV filling with inspiration; opposite with expiration; variation in velocity exceeds 15% Reversal of forward flow in hepatic veins during expiration
Cardiac catheterization	Prominent atrial *x* and *y* descents (w sign) Dip-and-plateau appearance of ventricular diastolic pressure Diastolic pressures increased but not equalized; LV diastolic pressure higher than RV diastolic pressure	Prominent atrial *x* and *y* descents (w sign) Dip-and-plateau appearance of ventricular diastolic pressure Increase and equalization of diastolic pressures Discordance of RV and LV peak systolic pressures (with inspiration, RV systolic pressure increases and LV systolic pressure decreases)
Endomyocardial biopsy	May reveal specific cause of restrictive cardiomyopathy	No specific findings on endomyocardial biopsy Pericardial biopsy may reveal abnormality
Computed tomography, magnetic resonance imaging		Pericardial thickening

AV, Atrioventricular; *LV,* left ventricular; *RV,* right ventricular.

Treatment

Treatment of RCM focuses on alleviating the symptoms of heart failure. Diuretics are used for decongestion, but intravascular depletion may compromise ventricular filling and lead to reduced cardiac output and hypotension. Supraventricular tachyarrhythmias are poorly tolerated. In patients with conduction system disease such as advanced atrioventricular block, a permanent pacemaker may be indicated. Specific therapies for underlying disorders include chemotherapy in amyloidosis, phlebotomy and iron chelation therapy in hemochromatosis, and steroids in sarcoidosis and endomyocardial fibrosis.

Prognosis

The course of RCM depends on the pathology, and treatment is often unsatisfactory. In the adult population, the prognosis usually is poor, with progressive deterioration and death due to low-output heart failure.

Arrhythmogenic Right Ventricular Cardiomyopathy

Definition and Epidemiology

Arrhythmogenic right ventricular cardiomyopathy (ARVC) is an autosomal dominant disease characterized by specific myocardial pathology. The estimated prevalence of ARVC is about 1 case in 2000 to 5000 people, and it has a male predominance.

Pathology

The myocardium of the right ventricular free wall is progressively replaced by fibrous and adipose tissue. Right ventricular function is abnormal, with regional akinesis or dyskinesis or global right ventricular dilation and dysfunction.

Clinical Presentation

The disease typically manifests in young adults as palpitations, dizziness or syncope, or sudden cardiac death. Symptoms of right ventricular failure are rare, despite evidence of right ventricular dysfunction on imaging studies.

Diagnosis

The clinical diagnosis of ARVC is suggested by integration of the information from the clinical presentation (e.g., arrhythmias), electrocardiogram, family history, and imaging studies. When available, histologic examination of the right ventricle confirms the diagnosis. The resting electrocardiogram may be normal, but common abnormalities include incomplete or complete right bundle branch block, the so-called epsilon waves that follow the QRS complex, and inverted T waves in the precordial leads. Right ventricular dilation and systolic dysfunction can be seen with echocardiography and MRI. The latter modality can also show myocardial fat.

Treatment

Treatment consists of ICD therapy to prevent sudden cardiac death, but the indications for implantation are not well defined. Antiarrhythmics and radiofrequency ablation of ventricular tachycardia are used in patients with frequent arrhythmias, but they have not been shown to reduce the risk of sudden cardiac death. Patients with a probable or definite diagnosis of ARVC should be excluded from competitive sports.

Prognosis

The prognosis for these patients remains uncertain.

Unclassified Cardiomyopathies

Some cardiomyopathies that do not fit the current categories are described in Table 10-2.

For a deeper discussion of this topic, please see Chapter 60, "Diseases of the Myocardium and Endocardium," in Goldman-Cecil Medicine, 25th Edition.

SUGGESTED READINGS

Elliott P, Andersson B, Arbustini E, et al: Classification of the cardiomyopathies: a position statement from the European Society of Cardiology Working Group on Myocardial and Pericardial Diseases, Eur Heart J 29:270–276, 2008.

Gersh BJ, Maron BJ, Bonow RO, et al: 2011 ACCF/AHA guideline for the diagnosis and treatment of hypertrophic cardiomyopathy: a report of the American College of Cardiology Foundation/American Heart Association Task Force on Practice Guidelines. Developed in collaboration with the American Association for Thoracic Surgery, American Society of Echocardiography, American Society of Nuclear Cardiology, Heart Failure Society of America, Heart Rhythm Society, Society for Cardiovascular Angiography and Interventions, and Society of Thoracic Surgeons, J Am Coll Cardiol 58:e212–e260, 2011.

Kindermann I, Barth C, Mahfoud F, et al: Update on myocarditis, J Am Coll Cardiol 59:779–792, 2012.

Maron BJ, Ackerman MJ, Nishimura RA, et al: Task Force 4: HCM and other cardiomyopathies, mitral valve prolapse, myocarditis, and Marfan syndrome, J Am Coll Cardiol 45:1340–1345, 2005.

Maron BJ, Towbin JA, Thiene G, et al: Contemporary definitions and classification of the cardiomyopathies: an American Heart Association scientific statement from the Council on Clinical Cardiology, Heart Failure and Transplantation Committee; Quality of Care and Outcomes Research and Functional Genomics and Translational Biology Interdisciplinary Working Groups; and Council on Epidemiology and Prevention, Circulation 113:1807–1816, 2006.

Yancy CW, Jessup M, Bozkurt B, et al: 2013 ACCF/AHA guideline for the management of heart failure: a report of the American College of Cardiology Foundation/American Heart Association Task Force on Practice Guidelines, Circulation 128:1810–1852, 2013.

Other Cardiac Topics

Mohamed F. Algahim, Robert B. Love, and Ivor J. Benjamin

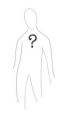

● CARDIAC TUMORS

Primary cardiac tumors are extremely rare, with a prevalence of less than 0.3% in most pathologic series (Table 11-1). Myxoma, the most common primary tumor of the heart, is usually benign. Myxomas are frequently isolated lesions, arising most often in the left atrium in the region of the fossa ovalis. Less commonly, they may be detected in the right atrium, in the right or left ventricle, or in multiple sites within the heart. A familial pattern of myxomas can occur and is transmitted in an autosomal dominant manner. In these patients, multiple cardiac myxomas may be present in association with a constellation of extracardiac abnormalities including pigmented nevi, cutaneous myxomas, breast fibroadenomas, and pituitary and adrenal gland disease. In addition, patients with familial myxoma may have recurrence of the tumors after surgical excision. Whether sporadic or familial, fewer than 10% of myxomas are malignant.

Symptoms associated with myxoma are usually related to embolization of tumor fragments and obstruction of the mitral valve. Tumor involvement of the conduction system may manifest as sick sinus syndrome and dysrhythmias. In addition, patients may exhibit a constellation of nonspecific symptoms and laboratory abnormalities including fever, malaise, weight loss, anemia, and elevated erythrocyte sedimentation rate. The diagnosis is usually made with echocardiography; the transesophageal approach is the most sensitive method for detecting small left atrial tumors. Considering the propensity for embolization, most myxomas are surgically removed when diagnosed. Tumors may recur, so follow-up echocardiograms should be performed. Because of the low incidence right-sided tumors and subsequent low index of suspicion by physicians, these tumors are often misdiagnosed as thrombus on echocardiography. This leads to delayed diagnosis or inappropriate long-term commitment to anticoagulation therapy. Cardiac magnetic resonance imaging is often warranted to differentiate cardiac thrombus from a mass when the initial findings are not consistent with the clinical signs and symptoms (Fig. 11-1).

Other, less common benign tumors include papillary fibroelastomas, fibromas, and rhabdomyomas. Fibroelastomas are pedunculated tumors with frondlike attachments that usually arise from the surface of the mitral and aortic valve leaflets. These tumors do not result in valve dysfunction but may be a source of systemic embolization. Fibromas most often arise within the interventricular septum and may be associated with arrhythmias or conduction disturbances. Rhabdomyomas are the most common cardiac tumors found in children and are often associated with tuberous sclerosis.

Cardiac lipomas may occur throughout the heart and pericardium. Pericardial lipomas can be large, whereas intramyocardial lipomas are small and often encapsulated. Surgical excision is the treatment of choice. Lipomatous hypertrophy of the interatrial septum should be considered in the differential diagnosis of atrial masses. This lesion is a consequence of nonencapsulated adipose tissue hyperplasia. Although it is occasionally found incidentally at autopsy, it may be associated with supraventricular arrhythmias, conduction disturbances, and, in rare cases, sudden cardiac death.

About one fourth of all primary cardiac tumors are malignant, and most of these are sarcomas. These tumors grow rapidly and often result in chamber obliteration and obstruction of blood flow. If there is involvement of the pericardium, a hemorrhagic effusion with pericardial tamponade may develop. The prognosis in affected individuals is poor; surgical excision is possible in rare cases. Irradiation and chemotherapy may provide palliative relief.

In contrast to primary cardiac tumors, metastatic disease involving the heart is common, occurring in up to one in five patients dying with malignancy. The most common tumors to metastasize to the heart are carcinomas of the lung, breast, and kidney; melanoma and lymphoma may also have cardiac involvement. Metastasis to the pericardium is common and is often complicated by a hemorrhagic effusion and pericardial tamponade. Infiltration of the myocardium may result in conduction disturbances and arrhythmias. Intracavitary masses are unusual but may result from local tumor invasion or direct extension of the malignancy through the venous system (e.g., renal cell carcinoma may metastasize to the heart through the inferior vena cava). Treatment is directed at the underlying malignancy. If pericardial tamponade is present, immediate drainage will help stabilize the patient. A pericardotomy is often necessary to prevent reaccumulation of fluid within the pericardial sac. Surgical excision of an obstructing tumor mass is usually palliative.

TABLE 11-1	EXAMPLES OF TUMORS OF THE HEART AND PERICARDIUM
PRIMARY	Mesothelioma
Benign	Fibrosarcoma
Myxoma lipoma	**METASTATIC**
Papillary fibroelastoma	
Rhabdomyoma	Melanoma
Fibroma	Lung
Malignant	Breast
	Lymphoma
Angiosarcoma	Renal cell
Rhabdomyosarcoma	

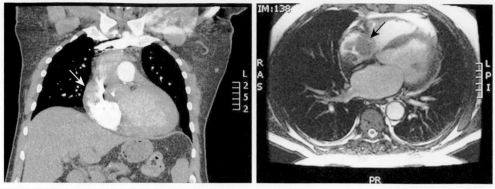

FIGURE 11-1 Cardiac magnetic resonance images of right atrial mass found to be primary cardiac lymphoma. The image on the *left* is a coronal cut, and the image on the *right* is an axial cut of the chest. *Arrows* point to the lobulated mass within the right atrium. (Courtesy Mohamed F. Algahim, MD, Division of Cardiothoracic Surgery, The Medical College of Wisconsin, Milwaukee, Wis.)

TABLE 11-2	CARDIAC LESIONS FROM NONPENETRATING TRAUMA	
PERICARDIUM	**VALVES**
Hematoma	Rupture (e.g., leaflets, chordae,
Hemopericardium	papillary muscle)
Rupture	**CORONARY ARTERIES**
Pericarditis	
Constriction (late complication)	Laceration
MYOCARDIUM	**GREAT VESSELS**
Contusion	Aortic rupture
Intracavitary thrombus	
Aneurysms and pseudoaneurysms	
Rupture (e.g., free wall, septum)	
Acute rupture (e.g., atrium, ventricle, septa)	

Data from Schick EC: Nonpenetrating cardiac trauma, Cardiol Clin 13:241–247, 1995.

⬤ TRAUMATIC HEART DISEASE

Nonpenetrating Cardiac Injuries

Blunt cardiac trauma accounts for about 10% of all traumatic heart disease (Table 11-2). Motion-related injuries secondary to abrupt body deceleration (e.g., motor vehicle accidents) and chest wall compression (e.g., steering wheel impact, athletic blow, cardiac resuscitative maneuvers) are the most common causes of blunt injury to the heart. Changes in the myocardium range from small ecchymotic areas in the subepicardium to transmural injury with myocardial hemorrhage and necrosis. Pericarditis is present in most patients and may be complicated by a tear or rupture of the pericardium or cardiac tamponade. Less common complications include rupture of a papillary muscle or chordae tendineae and coronary artery laceration.

Patients most often experience precordial pain that is similar to that associated with myocardial infarction (MI). However, musculoskeletal pain secondary to chest wall injury may confuse the clinical presentation. Congestive heart failure is unusual unless myocardial injury has been extensive or valve dysfunction has occurred. Life-threatening ventricular arrhythmias may occur with severe trauma and are a frequent cause of death in such patients. The electrocardiogram (ECG) most often demonstrates nonspecific repolarization abnormalities or ST-segment and T-wave changes consistent with acute pericarditis. If myocardial injury is extensive, localized ST-segment elevation and pathologic Q waves may be present.

Elevation of the myocardial component of the creatine kinase muscle band (CK-MB) is supportive of a diagnosis of cardiac contusion but is of limited diagnostic use in patients with massive chest wall trauma because the CK-MB fraction may be elevated as a result of severe skeletal muscle injury. Newer markers of myocardial injury, such as troponins T and I, may be more specific for establishing a diagnosis of myocardial contusion. Echocardiography is a useful, noninvasive tool to assess for wall motion abnormalities, valve dysfunction, and the presence of hemodynamically significant pericardial effusion.

Treatment of cardiac contusion is similar to that of MI, with initial observation and monitoring, followed by a gradual increase in physical activity. Anticoagulants and thrombolytic agents are contraindicated given the risk for hemorrhage into the myocardium and pericardial sac. Most patients who survive the initial injury will have partial or complete recovery of myocardial function. However, patients should be monitored for late complications that include aneurysm formation, free-wall or papillary muscle rupture, and significant arrhythmias.

Great Vessel Injury

Rupture of the aorta is one of the most common cardiovascular injuries resulting from blunt chest wall trauma. In more than 90% of cases, rupture occurs in the descending thoracic aorta just distal to the origin of the subclavian artery. Most individuals die immediately of exsanguination. However, up to 20% of patients may survive the initial injury if the blood is confined within the aortic adventitia and surrounding mediastinal tissues (pseudoaneurysm). Characteristic symptoms and findings on presentation include chest and interscapular back pain, increased arterial pressure and pulse amplitude in the upper extremities, decreased pressure and pulse amplitude in the lower extremities, and mediastinal widening on the chest radiograph.

Previously, aortography was the standard for diagnosis of blunt aortic injury. However, aortography is a relatively invasive, time-consuming procedure with the potential for additional morbidity in this critically ill group of patients. Although conventional chest computed tomography (CT) cannot match the diagnostic accuracy of aortography, helical thin-cut CT angiography has emerged as a superior alternative to aortography for diagnosing blunt

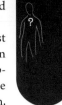

aortic injury. Helical CT scanning is an ideal diagnostic method for aortic injury because of its relatively low cost compared with aortography, its almost universal availability in emergency departments, and its lack of operator dependence. In addition, at most trauma centers, CT scanning is already an integral part of the diagnosis and management of serious blunt injury, with patients typically undergoing simultaneous CT scanning of other areas of the body to evaluate potential injuries. The overall diagnostic accuracy for helical CT scanning in the setting of blunt aortic injury exceeds 99%, and the positive and negative predictive values meet or exceed those of aortography. Patients without direct helical CT evidence of blunt aortic injury require no further evaluation. Aortography should be reserved for indeterminate helical CT scans. Such a strategy helps to substantially reduce the morbidity and cost of unnecessary aortograms for blunt aortic injury.

The force from rapid deceleration that is sufficient to tear the aorta often leads to injuries of other organs as well. Associated injuries are present in more than 90% of patients with aortic transection, and 24% of these patients require a major surgical procedure before aortic repair. The extremely high death rate of acute blunt rupture of the thoracic aorta has led surgeons in the past to repair the tear as quickly as possible. However, this form of management results in high rates of death and complications, often because of associated injuries in other organs.

Patients with traumatic rupture of the aorta fall into two broad categories. About 5% are hemodynamically unstable or deteriorate within 6 hours of admission. These patients require emergent surgical correction because without intervention mortality exceeds 90%. The second group, 95% of patients, are hemodynamically stable at the time of presentation, allowing time for a work-up and staging of any intervention. Mortality in this group is as low as 25% and is rarely the result of free rupture if the blood pressure is controlled. In the past decade, the philosophy of managing traumatic rupture of the aorta in this subgroup of patients has changed to emphasizing blood pressure control and assessing the need for emergent repair against the risks of operation. Prospective studies have demonstrated the value of initial antihypertensive therapy to allow delayed repair of blunt aortic injury in patients with severe coexistent injuries to other organ systems. In a substantial number of cases, associated injuries or comorbidities make the risks of immediate surgical repair prohibitive.

The current indications for considering delayed aortic repair include trauma to the central nervous system, contaminated wounds, respiratory insufficiency from lung contusion or other causes, body surface burns, blunt cardiac injury, tears of solid organs that will undergo nonoperative management, and retroperitoneal hematoma, as well as age older than 50 years and the presence of medical comorbidities. Patients with significant neurologic, pulmonary, or cardiac injuries have better outcomes if their confounding pathologic condition can be ameliorated before thoracotomy.

Penetrating Cardiac Injuries

Penetrating cardiac injuries are frequently the result of physical violence leading to bullet and knife wounds. Similar wounds may result from the inward displacement of bone fragments or fractured ribs due to blunt chest wall injury. Iatrogenic injuries may occur during placement of central venous catheters and wires.

With traumatic perforations, the right ventricle is the most frequently involved chamber, considering its anterior location in the chest. It is often associated with pericardial laceration. Symptoms are related to the size of the wound and the nature of the concomitant pericardial injury. If the pericardium remains open, extravasated blood drains freely into the mediastinum and pleural cavity, and symptoms are related to the resulting hemothorax. If the pericardial sac limits blood loss, pericardial tamponade results. In this situation, treatment includes emergent pericardiocentesis followed by emergent surgical closure of the wound. Small penetrating wounds to the ventricles that are not associated with extensive cardiac damage have the highest rate of survival. Late complications include chronic pericarditis, arrhythmias, aneurysm formation, and ventricular septal defects.

CARDIAC SURGERY
Coronary Artery Bypass Grafting

Despite the effectiveness of current medical therapy for the treatment of coronary artery disease, many patients require revascularization. Coronary artery bypass grafting (CABG) is an effective means of reducing or eliminating symptoms of angina pectoris. CABG may improve survival in certain subgroups of patients, including patients with angina refractory to medical therapy, patients with greater than 50% stenosis of the left main coronary artery, and patients with severe three-vessel coronary artery disease associated with left ventricular dysfunction. In addition, patients with two-vessel coronary artery disease in which a severe stenosis (>75%) is present in the proximal left anterior descending artery appear to benefit from CABG even if left ventricular function is normal.

Standard CABG is performed through a median sternotomy incision with cardiopulmonary bypass (CPB) and cardioplegic arrest. Operative mortality is 1% or less in stable patients with normal left ventricular function; the incidences of perioperative MI and stroke range from 1% to 4%. An increase in adverse events is associated with advancing age, female gender, short stature, diabetes, unstable angina or recent MI, and severely reduced left ventricular function. Overall survival at 10 years is about 80%, with recurrent or progressive angina occurring in about 50% of patients.

Long-term success of surgery is dependent on the type of conduit used during the surgery (saphenous vein versus internal mammary artery grafts) and the progression of atherosclerotic disease in the native and graft vessels. The internal mammary artery is particularly resistant to atherosclerotic disease and has a patency rate of about 90% at 10 years. In comparison, venous grafts are subject to closure both during the immediate postoperative period (usually secondary to technical factors) and months to years after surgery (secondary to intimal hyperplasia and progression of atherosclerosis). As a result, only 50% of venous grafts are patent 7 to 10 years after CABG.

The major predictor of development of atherosclerotic disease in the surgically placed bypass grafts is the ability of patients to control their risk factors for the development of atherosclerotic disease generally after surgery, particularly cigarette smoking,

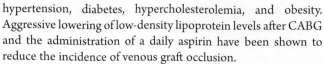

hypertension, diabetes, hypercholesterolemia, and obesity. Aggressive lowering of low-density lipoprotein levels after CABG and the administration of a daily aspirin have been shown to reduce the incidence of venous graft occlusion.

Most cases of recurrent angina can be managed successfully with medication (see Chapter 9). In many cases, percutaneous revascularization of a native vessel or graft can provide symptomatic relief and is the initial procedure of choice in this setting. In patients with refractory symptoms not amenable to percutaneous revascularization, repeat CABG is an option; however, in this setting, repeat CABG is associated with increased perioperative mortality and less satisfactory long-term control of angina.

Minimally Invasive Cardiac Surgery

Minimally invasive approaches for cardiac surgery can be broadly grouped into two categories: those that avoid the performance of a sternotomy and those that avoid the use of CPB. During the last 15 years, progressive experience incorporating these approaches has led to the application of minimally invasive techniques to selected patients undergoing cardiac surgery. However, many of the approaches have significant limitations, and the field continues to evolve.

In highly selected patients, minimally invasive direct coronary artery bypass (MIDCAB) can be performed through a limited thoracotomy, sparing the patient the perioperative morbidity associated with a median sternotomy. This technique also avoids the use of CPB. The most common approach is through a small left anterior thoracotomy incision. This allows for harvesting of the left internal mammary artery under direct visualization. This technique is most suitable for patients with proximal disease in the distribution of the left anterior descending coronary artery, although other coronary arteries can be bypassed with the use of different thoracotomy approaches. The major limitation of this approach has been the lower patency rates in the left internal mammary grafts placed using this technique and a higher incidence of recurrent ischemia compared with conventional CABG. The MIDCAB procedure therefore is applicable only to highly selected patients with disease in the distribution of the left anterior descending coronary artery and significant comorbidities that preclude the performance of a median sternotomy and use of CPB.

The initial experience with the MIDCAB approach and the subsequent demonstration of its limitations prompted the development of port-access cardiac surgery. This technique incorporates the MIDCAB approach of a limited lateral thoracotomy, thereby avoiding a median sternotomy, but uses CPB to facilitate performance of intracardiac procedures and potential access to other coronary artery distributions beyond the left anterior descending coronary artery for CABG. The port-access approach uses an endoaortic balloon inserted through cannulas placed in the femoral vessels for CPB. A few centers have successfully used the port-access platform for performance of selected cardiac surgical procedures, particularly mitral valve repair or replacement. The widespread adoption of this platform has been limited by persistent difficulties with access to all areas of the heart for coronary revascularization and the potentially catastrophic complication of aortic dissection in a small number of patients.

The limitations encountered with both the MIDCAB and port-access platforms have spurred interest in coronary bypass surgery performed through a median sternotomy but without CPB (e.g., off-pump coronary artery bypass [OPCAB]), allowing for surgery on the beating heart. The advantages of OPCAB over other platforms for minimally invasive coronary surgery are that complete revascularization can be performed and both internal mammary arteries can be harvested. Compared with conventional CABG, OPCAB is associated with decreased blood loss, decreased need for transfusion, decreased myocardial enzyme release up to 24 hours after surgery, decreased renal dysfunction, and, typically, decreased number of grafts placed per patient. OPCAB is not associated with a decreased length of hospital stay, a decreased mortality rate, or improved long-term neurologic function compared with conventional CABG. Although the OPCAB platform has become the most widely adopted approach for minimally invasive cardiac surgery, major questions remain regarding the intermediate and long-term patencies of the bypass grafts placed with this technique and whether the decreased number of grafts placed per patient compromises the long-term cardiac outcomes, compared with conventional CABG. Large-scale prospective clinical trials need to be conducted to answer these questions definitively.

Advances in minimally invasive cardiac surgery have led to the development of robotically assisted cardiac surgery. In this approach, the surgeon sits behind a computer console and uses telemanipulation to guide robotic arms that are placed through ports in the chest wall. On- or off-pump surgeries can be performed, and CPB is achieved through the peripheral cannulation. Although a variety of cardiac surgeries are possible in selected patients, the most commonly performed robotically assisted cardiac procedure is repair or replacement of the mitral valve. CABG can be performed on a beating or arrested heart. The internal mammary artery is typically taken down with the use of the robot, and the distal anastomosis is performed freehand through a mini-thoracotomy or mini-sternotomy incision. Alternatively, totally endoscopic robotic coronary bypass (TECAB) can be performed with good results. Similar procedures using this approach include ablation of atrial fibrillation, resection of intracardiac tumors, closure of atrial septal defects, and implantation or revision of the left ventricular lead of a device.

Other benefits of minimally invasive techniques include a smaller incision, less pain, and shorter length of hospital stay. Advocates of robotically assisted cardiac surgery highlight the improved visualization, panoramic 360-degree views, wrist-like articulation of instruments, improved dexterity, and elimination of hand tremor. These procedures are continually evolving, but their widespread adoption is limited to specialized centers due to significant costs for purchase and maintenance. As the experience with the technology improves, use of robotic approaches is likely to increase and to play a substantial role in the field of minimally invasive cardiac surgery.

Valvular Surgery

Surgical repair or replacement of a diseased valve is dependent on multiple factors, including the type and severity of the valve lesion, the presence of symptoms, and the functional status of the left and, in some cases, the right ventricle (see Chapter 8). In most adults, the diseased valve is replaced with a prosthesis, although some forms of valve disease, such as mitral valve regurgitation or mitral stenosis without significant valvular or chordal calcification, may be amenable to repair. Because prosthetic heart valves are associated with a number of complications (e.g., thrombosis, endocarditis, hemolysis), the decision to proceed with valve surgery should made only after the risks of valve replacement have been weighed against the potential benefits of symptom relief and improved survival.

Valve surgery is performed in a manner similar to CABG, with most cases requiring a median sternotomy, CPB, and cardioplegic arrest. Minimally invasive surgery through a modified sternotomy or thoracotomy incision may be possible in selected patients with isolated aortic or mitral valve disease. Operative mortality for all techniques ranges from 1% to 8% for most patients with preserved left ventricular function and good exercise capacity. The risk of surgery increases with advancing age, depressed left ventricular ejection fraction, presence of severe coronary artery disease, and replacement of multiple valves. Symptomatic patients usually have significant clinical improvement after valve surgery; however, long-term survival is strongly dependent on the patient's preoperative functional status and ventricular function.

Mechanical Circulatory Support and Cardiac Transplantation

The term *mechanical circulatory support* refers to total or partial mechanical support of the heart to allow for continued circulation of blood and adequate tissue perfusion. John H. Gibbon performed the first clinical application of mechanical circulatory support in 1953 when he used a CPB machine for closure of an atrial septal defect. The ability to operate on a motionless and bloodless field led to the birth of cardiac surgery as a discipline and spawned the current era by providing a surgical alternative approach for the treatment of coronary artery disease, valvular heart disease, and diseases of the great vessels.

Since the advent of the CPB machine, several mechanical support systems have become available, including intra-aortic balloon pumps (IABP), extracorporeal membrane oxygenators (ECMO), ventricular assist devices (VADs), and total artificial hearts (TAHs). Because the surgical management of heart failure continues to evolve, this section focuses on the indications and associated complications of left VADs (LVADs), especially in relation to heart transplantation. Further details on the disease process and medical management of heart failure are covered in Chapter 6.

Cardiopulmonary Bypass

A CPB procedure not only circumvents the normal functions of the heart and lungs during an operation but enables surgery to be carried out in a bloodless and motionless field while simultaneously providing adequate oxygenation of blood and perfusion of end organs. The heart is arrested with the use of a cardioplegic solution of blood or normal saline that is highly concentrated with potassium. Aside from creating a motionless surgical field, cardiac arrest and cooling of the heart provide cardiac protection against ischemia by decreasing metabolic demand during bypass. Other important functions of the CPB

are intraoperative regulation of blood volume and pressure, cooling and rewarming of the patient, administration of medications, filtering the blood, and providing rapid laboratory analysis of blood samples to achieve successful CPB surgery

In a schematic diagram of standard CPB circuit shown in Figure 11-2, deoxygenated blood is first drained from the right side of the heart by cannulas placed in the inferior and superior venae cavae. The blood is transported into a reservoir and then pumped through a heat exchanger, oxygenator, and filtration unit before it is returned through a cannula into the ascending aorta for whole-body circulation. Peripheral cannulation is achieved through the femoral vessels or the axillary artery or both, the latter approach being reserved for complex aortic arch surgery or in instances when standard cannulation of the great vessels is not possible.

The CPB operation is well tolerated by most patients. Similar to MCS devices discussed later, the secondary complications from contact of circulating blood with the synthetic surface of the circuit promote the activation of inflammatory pathways, systemic responses, and hypercoagulability. All patients undergoing CPB require heparin anticoagulation to a goal activated clotting time of at least 480 seconds. Corticosteroids may be administered to suppress the inflammatory response, and protamine is routinely used for reversal of heparin before decannulation. Postoperatively, patients should be monitored for heparin-induced thrombocytopenia (see also Chapter 54).

Extracorporeal Membrane Oxygenation

ECMO is the use of a simplified CPB circuit for temporary life support in patients with reversible cardiac or respiratory failure in the intensive care unit. The mechanical oxygenation and organ perfusion allows for cardiopulmonary recovery. Improved survival has been demonstrated in neonates and adults with isolated pulmonary or cardiac failure for whom maximal medical therapy has failed. As with CPB, cannulas are placed in the right side of the heart to drain blood into the ECMO circuit for oxygenation, but blood can be returned to either the right heart or the arterial system (the proximal or distal aorta). Return of blood to the right heart (i.e., veno-venous ECMO) is indicated for patients with isolated pulmonary failure. In patients with pulmonary and concomitant cardiac failure with hemodynamic instability, veno-arterial ECMO is used to return oxygenated blood to the proximal aorta to augment cardiac output and recovery. Patients on veno-arterial ECMO require anticoagulation. As with CPB, complications associated with ECMO include bleeding, thromboembolism, and heparin-induced thrombocytopenia.

Intraaortic Balloon Pump

The physiologic basis of an IABP is to provide counterpulsation and to improve the peripheral oxygen demands in the patient with a failing heart. Common indications for IABP are hemodynamic support during or after heart catheterization, cardiogenic shock, weaning from CBP, preoperative stabilization in high-risk patients, refractory unstable angina, refractory ventricular failure, and mechanical complications due to acute MI.

A helium-filled balloon is placed percutaneously or under direct vision through the femoral artery into the thoracic aorta, just distal to the left subclavian artery. The balloon is

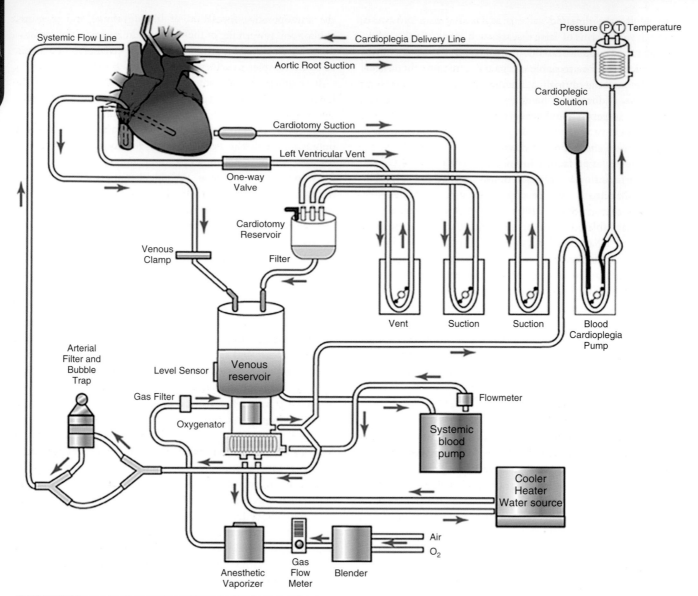

FIGURE 11-2 Diagram of a standard cardiopulmonary bypass circuit. See text for details. (Cohn LH: Cardiac surgery in the adult, ed 4, New York, 2011, McGraw-Hill.)

synchronized with the ECG or arterial waveform of the patient to fill during diastole and deflate during systole. Balloon inflation during diastole increases aortic pressure, referred to as diastolic augmentation, allowing for maximal delivery of oxygenated blood to the coronary arteries. Deflation during systole decreases the afterload and oxygen consumption of the heart while improving cardiac output. Potential major complications include balloon leak, severe bleeding (e.g., retroperitoneal), major limb ischemia, and death.

Ventricular Assist Devices

VAD was first successfully applied in 1966 by Michael E. DeBakey for cardiogenic shock after cardiac surgery in a 37 year-old female patient. She was maintained on the device for 10 days before being discharged home. The early cardiac assist devices were developed to improve weaning off the CPB machine in cardiac surgery patients. Today, distinct VADs have been designed for short-term and long-term management of failure of the right, left, or both ventricles.

Although cardiac transplantation remains the standard of care for refractory heart failure, the number of available donor hearts has plateaued, limiting the number of heart transplantations performed in the United States to just 2000 per year. Between 15% to 25% of patients with end-stage heart failure die while awaiting transplantation. As a result, the use of VADs, in particular LVADs, has significantly increased over the last 2 decades. As discussed later, LVADs have demonstrated a viable alternative for patients awaiting transplantation and for those who do not meet heart transplant criteria. This technology of surgical intervention has changed the dynamic and expanded management capabilities for patients with advanced heart failure. For the medical management of heart failure, refer to Chapter 60.

Compared with optimal medical therapy, LVADs have demonstrated improved 1- and 2-year survival rates in patients with end-stage heart failure, when compared to optimal medical therapy. The use of LVADs continues to evolve as clinical insights of the consequences of current devices are recognized and newer devices become available. Few randomized clinical trials exist, and current recommendations for LVADs are primarily based on level C evidence (i.e., consensus based). The goal of LVAD therapy is to support cardiac function and maintain adequate end-organ perfusion to provide meaningful recovery and quality of life. In the acute setting (e.g., cardiogenic shock), a LVAD may be placed temporarily, either as a bridge to decision for a longer-term VAD and assessment of alternative management options or as a bridge to recovery if the heart failure is deemed reversible (e.g., viral myocarditis, nonischemic cardiomyopathy). Patients with chronic heart failure who have failed maximal medical therapy and are candidates for transplantation may receive a LVAD as a bridge to transplantation while awaiting the availability of a donor heart. Survival from the time of implantation of the cardiac assist device to the time of cardiac transplantation varies from 51% to 71% worldwide.

In patients with lifestyle-limiting heart failure despite maximal medical therapy who are not candidates for transplantation, a LVAD may be indicated for destination therapy. In this setting, the LVAD is placed indefinitely to maintain tissue perfusion and improve quality of life or, in some cases, until recovery is achieved or the patient becomes a candidate for heart transplantation. Destination therapy is the most common indication for LVAD placement; approximately 40% of all VADs placed in 2012 were for that purpose.

Before implantation of any MCS device, medical and psychosocial factors as well as operative risk factors should be taken into consideration and assessed by a multidisciplinary team devoted to such longitudinal care. VADs are not recommended for patients with irreversible end-organ damage and without anticipation of meaningful improvement in quality of life.

Table 11-3 lists the VADs currently approved by the U.S. Food and Drug Administration (FDA). Several types of VADs that can be placed percutaneously or surgically in the acute setting exist for longer support. In general, LVADs decompress the left ventricle by draining blood into the aorta using a mechanical pump; they also contain a power source, such as a portable battery pack, and a cardiac and device monitoring system (Fig. 11-3). First-generation LVADs were pneumatically driven pulsatile pumps that drew blood from the apex of the heart and ejected it into the proximal aorta. The Heartmate XVE (Thoratec Corp., Pleasanton, Calif.), a first-generation LVAD, was approved by the FDA in 1994 as a bridge to transplantation. Although these pulsatile pumps are considered more physiologic, they are bulky and technically difficult to implant because they require a large body surface area, and they have a high incidence of infection and pump thrombosis. These flaws led to the development of the smaller, second-generation LVADs that were driven by axial or centrifugal pumps to provide continuous flow of blood from the left ventricle apex into the aorta (Fig. 11-4; see Fig. 11-3).

In the United States, two continuous-flow pumps are currently approved by the FDA: the HeartMate II (Thoratec), an axial pump LVAD, for destination therapy and as a bridge to transplantation, and the HeartWare (HeartWare CT, HeartWare, Inc., Miami Lakes, Fla.), a centrifugal pump LVAD, as a bridge to transplantation. Improved survival and technical ease of implantation have become the hallmarks of these pumps, rendering the use of the first-generation pumps almost obsolete. Nevertheless, the risks of infection, thrombosis, and stroke are considerable.

Increased use and improved survival rates have brought to light new complications associated with the second-generation pumps. The diminished left ventricular excursion and low pulsatility of continuous-flow pumps are associated with the development of gastrointestinal arteriovenous malformations and acquired von Willibrand's disease. Such complications can lead to potentially catastrophic gastrointestinal bleeding because these patients require chronic anticoagulation. Risk factors for increased mortality in patients with continuous-flow pumps include older age and associated fragility, renal dysfunction, respiratory dysfunction, right-sided heart failure, and history of previous or concomitant cardiac surgery at the time of device implantation. Third-generation LVADs, which use hydrodynamic or electromagnetic pump technology with few moving parts, are currently under investigation.

Surgical management of heart failure is a continually evolving field, and further technological advances are needed to address issues of size, infection, thrombosis, and diminished pulsatility. A multidisciplinary approach involving cardiac surgeons, cardiologists, intensivists, anesthesiologists, perfusionists, and specialized nurses and social workers is essential to ensure successful management of the LVAD patient and the family. Continuous emphasis on the education and training of the patient, family, local paramedics, among others, requires meticulous coordination among all team members to ensure successful outpatient management, avoid potentially lethal complications, and provide improved patient safety and health outcomes.

Total Artificial Heart

The first successful application of a TAH in humans was by Denton Cooley, in 1969, to wean a 47-year-old male patient off CPB. The TAH functioned for 64 hours until successful cardiac

TABLE 11-3	MECHANICAL CIRCULATORY SUPPORT DEVICES APPROVED FOR USE IN THE UNITED STATES	
TYPE	**DEVICE**	
DURABLE DEVICES		
Continuous flow	Thoratec HeartMate II	
	HeartWare HVAD	
	MicroMed DeBakey Child VAD	
Pulsatile extracorporeal	Thoratec PVAD	
	Heart Excor	
Pulsatile intracorporeal	HeartMate IP	
	HeartMate VE	
	HeartMate XVE	
	Thoratec IVAD	
	NovaCor PC	
	NovaCor PCq	
Total artificial heart	SynCardia CardioWest	
	AbioCor TAH	
TEMPORARY DEVICES		
Short-term devices	Abiomed AB5000	
	Abiomed BVS 5000	
	Levitronix Centrimag	
	Biomedicus	
	Tandem Heart	

Data from Kirklin JK, Naftel DC, Kormos RL, et al: Fifth INTERMACS annual report: risk factor analysis from more than 6,000 mechanical circulatory support patients, J Heart Lung Transplant 32:141–156, 2013.

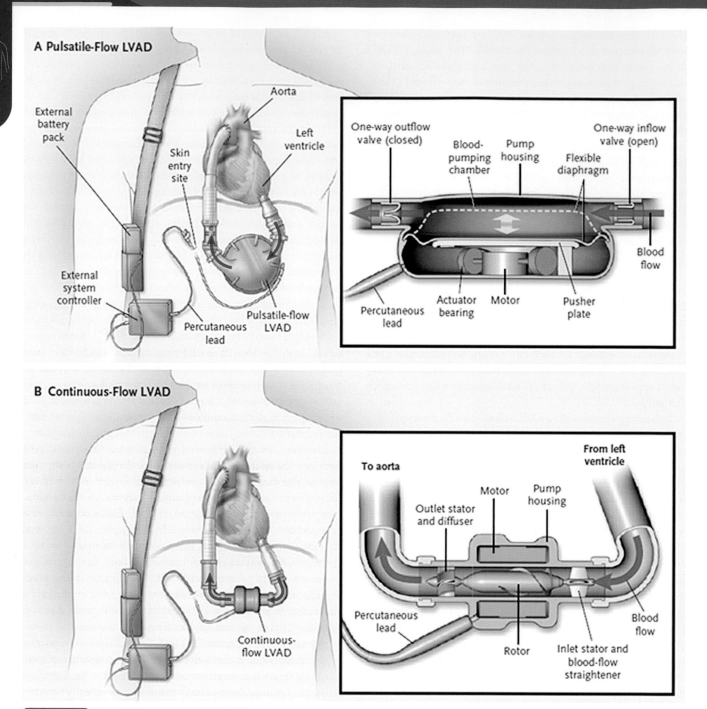

A Pulsatile-Flow LVAD

External battery pack

Skin entry site

Aorta

Left ventricle

External system controller

Pulsatile-flow LVAD

Percutaneous lead

One-way outflow valve (closed)

Blood-pumping chamber

Pump housing

One-way inflow valve (open)

Flexible diaphragm

Blood flow

Percutaneous lead

Actuator bearing

Motor

Pusher plate

B Continuous-Flow LVAD

Continuous-flow LVAD

To aorta

From left ventricle

Motor

Pump housing

Outlet stator and diffuser

Percutaneous lead

Blood flow

Rotor

Inlet stator and blood-flow straightener

FIGURE 11-3 **A,** HeartMate XVE left ventricular assist device (LVAD) with pneumatically driven pulsatitle pump system. **B,** HeartMate II LVAD with axial flow pump system. See text for details. (Slaughter MS, Rogers JG, Milano CA, et al: Advanced heart failure treated with continuous-flow left ventricular assist device, N Engl J Med 361:2241–2251, 2009.)

transplantation was achieved. The TAH seeks to entirely restore cardiac function, and it is indicated in patients who are at risk of death from irreversible biventricular failure not amenable to medical or surgical therapy.

In the United States, the pneumatically driven SynCardia CardioWest TAH-t (temporary) (SynCardia, Inc., Tucson, Ariz.) and the hydraulically driven AbioCor TAH (Abiomed, Danvers, Mass.) are presently approved by the FDA. These pulsatile pumps are placed in the orthotropic position by excising the right and left ventricles for total replacement of bilateral valvular and ventricular function (Fig. 11-5). The CardioWest TAH-t is approved as a bridge to transplantation and has a survival rate

similar to LVAD implantation for that indication. To date, the longest survival time with the CardioWest is 1374 days. The AbioCor is currently approved for humanitarian device use. Such instances involve the compassionate use of the device, without prior evidence of effectiveness, to potentially benefit patients with a rare disease. The AbioCor TAH is entirely implantable and is intended for permanent cardiac replacement in patients younger than 75 years of age who have severe heart failure and are not candidates for transplantation but meet the criteria for humanitarian device use. Initial clinical trials in 14 patients demonstrated adequate support; the longest survival time with the AbioCor was 512 days.

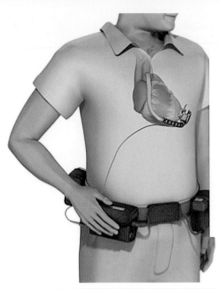
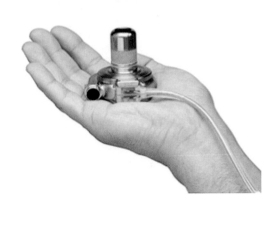

FIGURE 11-4 *Left image* shows placement of the HeartWare ventricular assist device; *right image* demonstrates its relatively small size. See text for details. (Courtesy HeartWare Inc., Framingham, Mass.)

In both the CardioWest and the AbioCor TAH, morbidity and mortality are associated with significant risks of bleeding, infection, thromboembolism, and stroke. These complications are the target of current research for device improvement. Further studies are underway to assess the utility of the CardioWest TAH for destination therapy, and the AbioCor II is in development as a smaller and more durable device than the original.

Cardiac Transplantation

During the last 2 decades, cardiac transplantation has become a life-saving treatment choice for patients with end-stage congestive heart failure. With advances in surgical techniques and immunosuppressive therapy, 1- and 5-year survival rates are about 90% and 75%, respectively. These rates are far superior to the 1-year survival rate for patients with advanced heart failure, which approaches 50%. Many patients who are eligible for cardiac transplantation die before surgery because of the limited number of donor hearts available each year. The development and widespread application of LVADs has allowed many of these patients who would otherwise die awaiting transplantation to survive until a donor heart becomes available. In many centers today, more than half of patients undergoing cardiac transplantation have previously undergone placement of a LVAD.

The major indications for cardiac transplantation are to prolong survival and improve quality of life. Determining which patients are suitable for cardiac transplantation can be difficult because many patients have clinical and hemodynamic improvement with intensification of medical therapy. In general, functional capacity, as assessed by exercise stress testing with measurement of maximal oxygen consumption at peak exercise, is the best predictor of whether a patient should be selected for cardiac transplantation. Individuals with severely impaired exercise capacity (e.g., peak oxygen consumption <10 to 12 mL/kg/min, with the lower limit of normal being 20 mL/kg/min) are most likely to experience a survival benefit from transplantation. Exclusion criteria include irreversible pulmonary vascular hypertension, malignancy, active infection, diabetes mellitus with end-organ damage, and advanced liver or kidney disease. Although advanced age is associated with higher surgical and 1-year mortality rates, an age limit for cardiac transplantation is no longer strictly enforced at most centers, with patients instead being listed for transplantation based on an overall assessment of their physiologic status and potential for long-term survival after transplantation.

The procedure is performed through a median sternotomy incision. The posterior walls of the left and right atria with their venous connections are left in place and used to suture to the donor heart. The aorta and pulmonary artery are directly anastomosed to the recipient's great vessels. Immunosuppressive therapy is begun immediately after surgery and continued throughout the patient's life. Although new immunosuppressive agents are available, most regimens still include combinations of cyclosporine, azathioprine, and prednisone. Common complications during the first year include infection and rejection of the donor heart. In addition, hyperlipidemia and hypertension are common medical problems that may require treatment.

The major long-term complication is the development of coronary vasculopathy in the transplanted heart. In contrast to coronary artery atherosclerosis, which tends to be a focal process affecting primarily the proximal vessels, this disease is characterized by diffuse myointimal proliferation involving primarily the medial and distal segments of the coronary arteries. Although the cause of this disease is not entirely known, coronary vasculopathy is thought to be related to an immune-mediated response directed against the donor vessels. Monitoring for this complication can be difficult because angina is not provoked in the denervated heart and standard exercise stress testing has a low sensitivity for detecting this disease.

Coronary angiography is performed after transplantation and yearly thereafter to monitor for significant narrowing of the coronary arteries. However, the diffuse nature of the vasculopathy reduces the accuracy of coronary angiography for detection of this disease. Intracoronary ultrasound, with measurements of the intimal layer and coronary artery lumen size, is a new technique that appears to be more sensitive than coronary angiography for detection of this complication. Treatment options are limited,

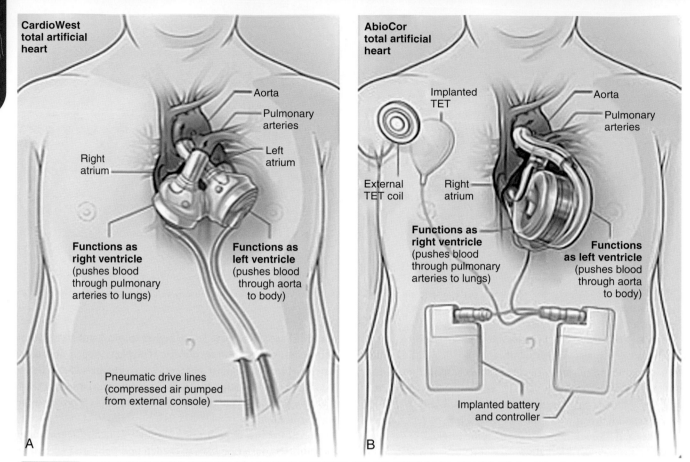

FIGURE 11-5 Total artificial hearts approved by the U.S. Food and Drug Administration: **A,** CardioWest total artificial heart. **B,** AbioCor total artificial heart. See text for details. TET, Transcutaneous energy transfer device. (Modified from National Heart, Lung, and Blood Institute, U.S. Department of Health and Human Services: What is a total artificial heart? Available at http://www.nhlbi.nih.gov/health/health-topics/topics/tah/. Accessed August 15, 2014.)

but aggressive management of hypercholesterolemia and the use of calcium-channel blockers, specifically diltiazem, have been associated with a slowing of disease progression and a higher survival rate. Retransplantation is reserved for patients who have severe, three-vessel coronary artery disease with reduced left ventricular function and symptoms of congestive heart failure.

Noncardiac Surgery in the Patient with Cardiovascular Disease

Noncardiac surgery in patients with known cardiovascular disease may be associated with an increased risk for death or cardiac complications such as MI, congestive heart failure, and arrhythmias. To determine an individual patient's risk for a procedure, the consulting physician must have knowledge of the type and severity of the patient's cardiac disease, the comorbid risk factors, and the type and urgency of surgery. In general, the preoperative evaluation and management are the same as in the nonoperative setting; for patients who are at risk, additional noninvasive and invasive testing may be performed if the results would affect treatment or outcome.

Usually, estimation of a patient's perioperative risk can be determined by a careful clinical evaluation, including a history, physical examination, and review of the ECG. Patients at highest risk for a perioperative cardiac event are those with a recent MI (defined as occurring >7 days but <1 month earlier), unstable or

severe angina, decompensated congestive heart failure, significant arrhythmias, or severe valvular disease (Table 11-4). Predictors of moderate or intermediate cardiac risk include a history of stable angina, compensated heart failure, prior MI, or diabetes mellitus. Advanced age, an abnormal ECG, low functional capacity, and poorly controlled hypertension are associated with cardiovascular disease but are not independent predictors of a perioperative cardiac event.

In regard to the type of surgery, risks are highest in patients who are undergoing major emergency procedures, especially older adults (Table 11-5). Cardiac complications are also common after vascular surgery, considering that the prevalence of underlying coronary artery disease is high in this patient population. In addition, any surgery associated with large volume shifts or blood loss may place increased demands on an already diseased heart. Procedures associated with the lowest risk in patients with cardiac disease are cataract extraction and endoscopy. Several risk stratification calculators have been developed and validated for patients undergoing going cardiac surgery. The Society for Thoracic Surgeons risk calculator (available at http://riskcalc.sts.org/STSWebRiskCalc273/) and the recently updated EuroSCORE II risk calculator (available at http://www.euroscore.org/calc.html) are used in the United States and Europe to assess risk of in-hospital mortality and morbidity and risk of 30-day in-hospital mortality, respectively.

TABLE 11-4	CLINICAL PREDICTORS OF INCREASED PERIOPERATIVE CARDIOVASCULAR RISK (MYOCARDIAL INFARCTION, CONGESTIVE HEART FAILURE, DEATH)

MAJOR

Unstable coronary syndromes
Recent myocardial infarction (e.g., >1 wk and <1 mo)
Unstable or severe angina (Canadian Cardiovascular Society angina class III or IV)
Decompensated heart failure
Significant arrhythmias
High-grade atrioventricular block
Symptomatic ventricular arrhythmias
Supraventricular arrhythmias with uncontrolled ventricular response
Severe valvular disease

INTERMEDIATE

Mild angina (Canadian Cardiovascular Society angina class I or II)
Prior myocardial infarction
Compensated or prior congestive heart failure
Diabetes mellitus

MINOR

Advanced age
Abnormal electrocardiogram (e.g., left ventricular hypertrophy, left bundle branch block)
Rhythm other than sinus
Low functional capacity (i.e., unable to climb one flight of stairs with a bag of groceries)
History of a stroke
Uncontrolled systemic hypertension

TABLE 11-5	CARDIAC RISK STRATIFICATION FOR NONCARDIAC SURGICAL PROCEDURES

HIGH (REPORTED CARDIAC RISK >5%)

Emergent major operations, particularly in the older adult population
Major vascular surgery, aortic aneurysm repair
Peripheral vascular surgery
Prolonged procedures associated with large fluid shifts or blood loss or both

INTERMEDIATE (REPORTED CARDIAC RISK <5%)

Carotid endarterectomy
Head and neck
Intraperitoneal and intrathoracic
Orthopedic
Prostate

LOW (REPORTED CARDIAC RISK <1%)

Endoscopic procedures
Cataract extraction
Breast biopsy

Data from Eagle KA, Brundage BH, Chaitman BR, et al: Guidelines for perioperative cardiovascular evaluation for noncardiac surgery: report of the ACC/AHA Task Force on Practice Guidelines, J Am Coll Cardiol 27:910–948, 1996.

Once the clinical evaluation is complete and the type of surgery is known, the need for additional testing and treatment can be determined. If emergency surgery is contemplated, little in the way of cardiac assessment can be performed, and recommendations may be directed at perioperative medical management and surveillance. If surgery is not urgent, additional evaluation is based on the clinical assessments of the risk and type of surgery. Patients with major risk factors for cardiac complications should have surgery delayed until the cardiac condition has been treated and stabilized. Patients with intermediate predictors of cardiac risk who are scheduled for high-risk surgery should undergo noninvasive testing such as exercise or pharmacologic stress testing or echocardiography. The results of these tests will help determine future management, such as cardiac catheterization or intensification of medical therapy. Patients scheduled for low- or intermediate-risk surgery, especially those who have good exercise capacity, should proceed to surgery with appropriate medical management and postoperative surveillance. Noncardiac surgery is generally safe for patients with minor or no clinical risk factors for cardiac complications, although some patients with poor functional capacity who are scheduled for high-risk operations may benefit from additional cardiac evaluation.

DISEASE-SPECIFIC APPROACHES

Coronary Artery Disease and Myocardial Infarction

About 70% of MIs occur within the first 6 days after an operation, with the peak incidence between 24 and 72 hours. Mortality associated with noncardiac surgery has been reported to be as high as 30% to 40%, especially if associated with congestive heart failure or significant arrhythmias. Multiple stresses associated with surgery can provoke ischemia. Physiologic tachycardia and hypertension secondary to volume shifts, anemia, infection, and the stress of wound healing increase myocardial oxygen demand and may provoke ischemia. In addition, increased platelet reactivity during the postoperative period may increase the risk for coronary thrombosis and subsequent infarction.

Despite the high mortality rate associated with perioperative MI, few studies have examined the effects of anti-ischemic therapy to prevent this complication. Several small, uncontrolled trials have suggested that β-blockers reduce intraoperative ischemia. More recently, the use of atenolol before and after surgery was associated with a reduction in MI and cardiac death, especially during the first 6 to 12 months after surgery. Although the data are limited, the use of a perioperative β-blocker therapy should be considered for all patients with suggested or known coronary artery disease unless a specific contraindication to its use is present. The data available on the usefulness of calcium-channel blockers and nitrates are even more limited, but this approach may be appropriate for the treatment of symptomatic coronary disease in individuals who are not candidates for revascularization. Coronary angiography and revascularization should be reserved for individuals in whom this treatment would otherwise result in significant improvement in symptoms or long-term survival. In rare cases, revascularization may be indicated for high-risk patients undergoing major noncardiac surgery.

All patients with suggested or known cardiac disease should have routine ECGs the first 3 days after surgery to monitor for ischemia. If the ECG is inconclusive, measurement of troponin levels may be helpful to document an ischemic event. Treatment of an MI in this setting is similar to that for the nonsurgical patient (see Chapter 9), although the use of anticoagulants and thrombolytic agents may be contraindicated in the immediate postoperative period. Special attention should be paid to correcting abnormalities that may provoke additional ischemia (e.g., hypoxia, anemia).

Congestive Heart Failure

Several studies have shown that decompensated heart failure is associated with increased perioperative cardiac complications. In these patients, surgery should be postponed until appropriate treatment is instituted and symptoms have been stabilized. If planned surgery is associated with large blood loss or fluid shifts, a pulmonary artery catheter may be helpful.

During the postoperative period, congestive heart failure most commonly occurs in the first 24 to 48 hours, when fluid administered during surgery is mobilized from the extravascular space. However, heart failure may also result from myocardial ischemia and new arrhythmias. Initial management includes identification and treatment of the underlying cause. In addition, intravenous diuretics usually provide rapid relief of pulmonary congestion. If heart failure is complicated by hypotension or poor urine output, insertion of a pulmonary artery catheter may be helpful to guide additional therapy (see Chapter 6).

Valvular Heart Disease

In regard to valvular heart disease the greatest risk for complications after noncardiac surgery is in those with aortic or mitral stenosis. Patients with symptomatic, severe aortic stenosis should have valve replacement before noncardiac surgery. In patients with mild to moderate mitral stenosis, careful attention to volume status and heart rate control are necessary to optimize left ventricular filling and avoid pulmonary congestion. Patients with severe mitral stenosis should be considered for percutaneous valvuloplasty or mitral valve replacement before high-risk surgery. In patients with valve disease or prosthetic heart valves, prophylactic antibiotics are recommended if appropriate.

Arrhythmias and Conduction Defects

Patients with symptomatic, high-grade conduction disturbances, such as third-degree atrioventricular (AV) block, have an increased perioperative risk for cardiac complications and should have a temporary pacemaker inserted before surgery. Patients with first-degree AV block, Mobitz type I AV block, or bifascicular block (right bundle branch block and left anterior fascicular block) do not require prophylactic pacemaker insertion.

Atrial arrhythmias such as atrial fibrillation are common after surgery and usually are not associated with significant complications if the ventricular rate is well controlled. Ventricular premature beats and nonsustained ventricular tachycardia are also common after noncardiac surgery and do not require specific therapy unless they are associated with myocardial ischemia or heart failure. In most instances, treatment of the underlying cause (e.g., hypoxia, metabolic abnormalities, ischemia, volume overload) results in significant improvement or resolution of the rhythm disturbance without specific antiarrhythmic therapy.

Cardiac Disease in Pregnancy

Pregnancy is associated with dramatic changes in the cardiovascular system that may result in significant hemodynamic stress to the patient with underlying heart disease. During a normal pregnancy, plasma volume increases an average of 50%, beginning in the first trimester and peaking between the 20th and 24th weeks of gestation. This change is accompanied by increases in stroke volume, heart rate, and, accordingly, cardiac output. In addition, a concomitant fall in systemic vascular resistance and mean arterial pressure occurs because of the effects of gestational hormones on the vasculature and the creation of a low-resistance circulation in the pregnant uterus and placenta. During labor, uterine contractions result in a transient increase of up to 500 mL of blood in the central circulation, resulting in further increases in stroke volume and cardiac output. After delivery, intravascular volume and cardiac output increase further as compression of the inferior vena cava by the gravid uterus is relieved and extravascular fluid is mobilized. Symptoms and signs that may mimic cardiac disease often accompany these hemodynamic changes; they include fatigue, reduced exercise tolerance, lower-extremity edema, distention of the neck veins, S_3 gallop, and new systolic murmurs. Differentiating symptoms produced by cardiac disease from those attributable to a normal pregnancy can be difficult. Under such circumstances, echocardiography can be a safe and helpful noninvasive test to assess cardiac structure and function in the pregnant patient.

Many pregnant women with known cardiac disease can complete a normal pregnancy and delivery without significant harm to the mother or fetus. However, certain cardiac conditions, including irreversible pulmonary hypertension, cardiomyopathy associated with severe heart failure, and Marfan syndrome with a dilated aortic root, are associated with a high risk for cardiovascular complications and death. Under these circumstances, patients should be advised against having children. If pregnancy occurs, a first-trimester therapeutic abortion should be strongly recommended.

⬤ SPECIFIC CARDIAC CONDITIONS
Mitral Stenosis

Mitral stenosis secondary to rheumatic heart disease frequently occurs in young women of childbearing age. The physiologic increases in heart rate and cardiac output during pregnancy result in a significant increase in the gradient across the mitral valve and a rise in left atrial and pulmonary venous pressures. Congestive heart failure may develop as the pregnancy progresses through the second and third trimesters, or it may occur more acutely with the onset of atrial fibrillation.

The management of mitral stenosis depends on the patient's prepregnant functional capacity and the severity of the valve obstruction. In general, patients with severely symptomatic mitral valve stenosis should have percutaneous or surgical correction of the valve before conception. Women with minimal symptoms (New York Heart Association functional classes I to II) usually tolerate pregnancy and vaginal delivery well, even if moderate to severe stenosis is present. Management includes salt restriction, diuretic therapy, and aggressive treatment of pulmonary infections. Patients who develop atrial fibrillation with a rapid ventricular response should be treated with AV nodal blocking agents and cardioversion if possible. Patients who develop refractory heart failure during pregnancy should be considered for mitral balloon valvuloplasty because surgical commissurotomy or valve replacement may be associated with fetal demise.

Aortic Stenosis

Aortic stenosis in a pregnant woman is usually congenital in origin. Patients with significant outflow obstruction may develop angina or heart failure during the later portion of the pregnancy as cardiac output increases. Supportive therapy includes bedrest and prevention of hypovolemia. If these measures fail to control symptoms and the fetus is not near term, balloon valvuloplasty, transaortic valve replacement, or aortic valve surgery should be considered to reduce the risk for maternal death.

Marfan Syndrome

Pregnant women with Marfan syndrome are at an increased risk for aortic dissection and rupture, especially during the third trimester and the first postpartum month. Patients with an aortic root diameter greater than 40 mm are at greatest risk for this complication and should strongly consider therapeutic abortion during the first trimester. Women with an aortic root diameter less than 40 mm should have serial echocardiograms to monitor the size of the aortic root during pregnancy. In addition, restriction in physical activity and treatment with a β-blocker may help prevent further dilation of the aorta.

Congenital Heart Disease

Survival to reproductive age is common in patients with corrected congenital defects. The risk for pregnancy in these patients is related to the completeness of the repair and the mother's functional capacity. Uncomplicated atrial or ventricular septal defects not associated with symptoms or pulmonary hypertension are usually well tolerated during pregnancy. Intracardiac shunts associated with pulmonary vascular hypertension are associated with a high maternal mortality rate during pregnancy as a result of increased right-to-left shunting and worsening oxygen desaturation of the blood. In these women, pregnancy is contraindicated. If pregnancy occurs, a therapeutic abortion during the first trimester should be recommended. Women with uncorrected tetralogy of Fallot should undergo palliative or definitive repair before conception to improve maternal and fetal outcomes. Women with residual obstruction of the right ventricular outflow tract remain at high risk for right ventricular heart failure during pregnancy.

Prosthetic Heart Valves

Most patients with a normal-functioning prosthetic valve tolerate pregnancy without complications. However, in patients with mechanical valves, special attention to the choice and dose of anticoagulant therapy is necessary to avoid thromboembolic complications in the mother and teratogenic effects in the fetus. Women should start subcutaneous heparin before conception to avoid the potential teratogenic effects of warfarin during the first several months of critical fetal organ development. This therapy can be continued throughout pregnancy, or, alternatively, warfarin can be reinstituted late in the second trimester or during the third trimester. Although heparin therapy confers less risk of teratogenicity than warfarin use, it is associated with a high risk for maternal bleeding complications. Low-molecular-weight heparin may be an acceptable alternative, but no firm data are available to support this recommendation. At the time of delivery, anticoagulation therapy is interrupted to avoid bleeding complications. Antibiotic prophylaxis is usually not recommended at the time of delivery.

Heart Disease Arising During Pregnancy

Cardiovascular disease can develop during pregnancy and may pose a significant risk to the mother and fetus. Hypertension is not an uncommon problem during pregnancy and is defined as a consistent increase in blood pressure of 30/15 mm Hg or an absolute blood pressure greater than 140/90 mm Hg. The three major forms of hypertension that may develop during pregnancy are chronic hypertension, gestational hypertension, and toxemia. Toxemia is a form of hypertension that develops during the second half of pregnancy and is associated with proteinuria, edema, and, in severe forms, seizures. This problem is primarily managed by the obstetrician and is not discussed in this text. Gestational hypertension is an elevation in blood pressure that occurs late in the pregnancy, during delivery, or during the first postpartum days. This disease entity is not associated with proteinuria or edema and resolves within 2 weeks after delivery.

Chronic hypertension is presumed to be present if an elevation in blood pressure is detected before the 20th week of pregnancy. No matter what the cause, fetal mortality correlates with the severity of the hypertension and begins to rise when the diastolic pressure exceeds 75 mm Hg during the second trimester or 85 mm Hg during the third trimester. Initial treatments include a reduction in physical activity and salt restriction. If the blood pressure remains greater than 150/90 mm Hg, then antihypertensive treatment should be instituted. Agents that have been safely used in pregnancy include hydralazine, α-methyldopa, clonidine, β-blockers, and labetalol. Diuretics should be used with caution because of the increased risk for placental hypoperfusion.

Peripartum cardiomyopathy (PCM) is a form of dilated cardiomyopathy that may begin during the last trimester of pregnancy or within the first 6 months after delivery in a woman without prior heart disease or other definable causes for cardiac dysfunction. The true incidence of the disease is unknown, but estimates conclude that 1 in every 3000 to 4000 pregnancies is affected. Although the cause of PCM is unknown, myocardial injury is thought to be immunologically mediated. Women usually exhibit symptoms and signs of congestive heart failure. Echocardiography is useful to assess chamber size and degree of ventricular dysfunction. The outcome with PCM is variable, with death or progressive heart failure occurring in about one third of affected women. The prognosis is particularly poor if symptoms develop before delivery. Despite this risk, many patients have complete recovery of ventricular function, although recurrence is possible, especially with subsequent pregnancies. Treatment is similar to that for congestive heart failure (see Chapter 6) and usually includes the use of vasodilators such as hydralazine, digoxin, and diuretics. Angiotensin-converting enzyme inhibitors have been associated with increased fetal wastage in pregnant animals and should be avoided. A thorough evaluation of cardiac function should be performed before subsequent pregnancies. If a woman decides to proceed with another pregnancy, she should be monitored regularly for signs of cardiac decompensation.

About 50% of aortic dissections that occur in women younger than 40 years of age are associated with pregnancy. Although the cause of aortic dissection during pregnancy is unknown, it has been postulated that hemodynamic and hormonal changes associated with pregnancy may weaken the aortic wall. The highest incidence of dissection is during the third trimester, although it can occur at any time during the pregnancy or in the early postpartum period. The presenting symptoms and diagnostic work-up are similar to those for the nonpregnant patient (see Chapter 13). Transesophageal echocardiography is highly sensitive and specific for the detection of aortic dissection and offers the advantage of not exposing the fetus to ionizing radiation. Management includes aggressive blood pressure control and β-blocker therapy to reduce shear forces of the ejected blood. Recommendations for corrective surgery are similar to those for the nonpregnant patient and are discussed in Chapter 13.

● PROSPECTUS FOR THE FUTURE

CABG remains an important but now less commonly used mode for revascularization in symptomatic coronary artery disease. Technical advances in percutaneous coronary angioplasty (PTCA) have emboldened such attempts for revascularization of unprotected left main disease, the established domain for CABG, even in octogenarians. Prospective studies are needed to evaluate the efficacy, health outcomes, and costs and benefits for combined approaches of CABG and PTCA with drug-eluting stents. Percutaneous and minimally invasive surgical options are gaining more widespread application in the management of heart disease. With the limited donor pool for cardiac transplantation, advanced heart failure will be managed with resynchronization therapy, LVADs, and stem- and cell-based therapies.

SUGGESTED READINGS

Butany J, Nair V, Naseemuddin A, et al: Cardiac tumours: diagnosis and management, Lancet Oncol 6:219–228, 2005.

Elkayam U, Bitar F: Valvular heart disease and pregnancy. Part I: native valves, J Am Coll Cardiol 46:223–230, 2005.

Elkayam U, Bitar F: Valvular heart disease and pregnancy. Part II: prosthetic valves, J Am Coll Cardiol 46:403–410, 2005.

Feldman D, Pamboukian SV, Teuteberg JJ, et al: The 2013 International Society for Heart and Lung Transplantation guidelines for mechanical circulatory support: executive summary, J Heart Lung Transplant 32:157–187, 2013.

Froehlich JB, Karavite D, Russman PL, et al: ACC/AHA preoperative assessment guidelines reduce resource utilization before aortic surgery, J Vasc Surg 36:758–763, 2002.

Gray DT, Veenstra DL: Comparative economic analyses of minimally invasive direct coronary artery bypass surgery, J Thorac Cardiovasc Surg 125:618–624, 2003.

Kirklin JK, Naftel DC, Kormos RL, et al: Fifth INTERMACS annual report: risk factor analysis from more than 6,000 mechanical circulatory support patients, J Heart Lung Transplant 32:141–156, 2013.

Pal B, Hossain MA: Stress fracture of the tibia mimicking deep venous thrombosis or rupture of the popliteal cyst, Br J Rheumatol 25:319–320, 1986.

Rodés-Cabau J, DeBlois J, Bertrand OF, et al: Nonrandomized comparison of coronary artery bypass surgery and percutaneous coronary intervention for the treatment of unprotected left main coronary artery disease in octogenarians, Circulation 118:2374–2381, 2008.

Rose EA, Gelijns AC, Moskowitz AJ, et al: Long-term use of a left ventricular assist device for end-stage heart failure, N Engl J Med 345:1435–1443, 2001.

Stoney WS: Evolution of cardiopulmonary bypass, Circulation 119:2844–2853, 2009.

Vascular Diseases and Hypertension

Wanpen Vongpatanasin and Ronald G. Victor

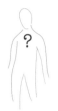

INTRODUCTION

Diseases of the systemic and pulmonary vasculature are among the most common clinical problems encountered in internal medicine. Yet these important diseases are not often given the emphasis they deserve; they fall between the cracks of traditional medical subspecialties. Early clinical recognition is important because effective therapy often can prevent or at least delay needless suffering and death. This chapter reviews the causes, clinical manifestations, diagnostic evaluations, and therapeutic approaches to the major forms of systemic and pulmonary vascular diseases as well as arterial hypertension.

SYSTEMIC VASCULAR DISEASE

Peripheral Arterial Disease

The term *peripheral arterial disease* (PAD) refers to atherosclerotic vascular disease of mainly the lower extremities. Similar to other atherosclerotic vascular diseases, PAD is more prevalent in men than it is in women, particularly before the age of menopause. The prevalence increases with age, ranging from 2% to 6% for adults younger than 60 years to 20% to 30% for those older than 70 years. As with coronary atherosclerosis, the major reversible risk factors are cigarette smoking, diabetes mellitus, hyperlipidemia, and hypertension. Only 30% to 50% of patients with PAD become symptomatic. The classic syndrome of intermittent claudication refers to ischemic muscle pain or weakness brought on by exertion and promptly relieved by rest. Claudication is associated with a significant 10-year risk of morbidity and mortality. Approximately 25% of patients will develop worsening claudication, 5% will require amputation, 10% to 20% will require revascularization, and 30% will die of a cardiovascular event (e.g., heart attack, stroke) as a result of concomitant coronary artery and/or cerebrovascular atherosclerosis. To minimize progression of PAD and avoid complications, risk factor modification is absolutely essential. This includes tight control of blood pressure (BP), plasma lipids, and blood glucose. Complete cessation of tobacco use is a must.

The diagnosis of PAD begins with a careful history and physical examination and is confirmed by noninvasive laboratory testing. Ischemic pain occurs in the leg muscles supplied by arterial segments that are distal to the site of stenosis. Calf claudication is the hallmark of femoral-popliteal disease, whereas discomfort in the thigh, hip, or buttock associated with impotence indicates aortoiliac disease (Leriche's syndrome).

Depending on the severity of the stenosis, the pain is experienced at a predictable walking distance and is promptly relieved by rest. Claudication must be differentiated from the pseudoclaudication of lumbar degenerative spinal canal stenosis. In the latter condition, walking can also aggravate leg pain, but it is not relieved simply by the cessation of exercise. Rather, assuming positions that minimize lumbar extension, such as stooping forward or sitting, alleviates the pain. The characteristic physical findings of PAD are absent or diminished pulses distal to the stenosis, bruits over the diseased artery, hair loss, thin shiny skin, and muscle atrophy. Severe ischemia causes pallor, cyanosis, decreased skin temperature, ulceration, and gangrene.

Noninvasive techniques are quite good. The *ankle-brachial index* (ABI) is the ratio of the highest systolic BP measured from either the dorsalis pedis or the posterior tibialis artery to the highest systolic BP obtained from the brachial artery using a Doppler stethoscope. The normal ABI range is 1.0 to 1.4. An ABI of 0.9 or less indicates PAD. This simple noninvasive test has a sensitivity and specificity of 95% and 99%, respectively. In some patients with diabetes mellitus or renal failure, the media of the affected leg vessels become so heavily calcified that they resist compression except during very high levels of cuff inflation. The result is a falsely elevated ankle BP and an artificially normal or supernormal ABI (Table 12-1).

Duplex ultrasonography is an important adjunct to the ABI and has a similar sensitivity and specificity. This test is particularly useful to diagnose PAD in patients with noncompressible vessels due to medial wall calcification. The Doppler velocity waveform remains abnormal despite a spuriously normal or elevated ABI. Magnetic resonance (MR) angiography and computed tomographic (CT) angiography permit excellent visualization of vascular stenosis and identification of runoff vessels. With these noninvasive imaging modalities, spatial resolution is comparable to that of traditional invasive

TABLE 12-1	INTERPRETATION OF ANKLE-BRACHIAL INDEX	
ANKLE-BRACHIAL INDEX	**INTERPRETATION**
1.00-1.40	Normal
0.90-0.99	Borderline
0.70-0.89	Mild PAD
0.40-069	Moderate PAD
<0.40	Severe PAD
>1.40	Noncompressible vessels

PAD, Peripheral arterial disease.

angiography, which now is reserved for patients undergoing revascularization.

The medical management of PAD includes lifestyle and risk factor modification as well as antiplatelet therapy. Smoking cessation reduces the risks of limb loss, myocardial infarction, and death. Lipid-lowering therapy with a statin (hydroxymethylglutaryl–coenzyme A [HMG-CoA] reductase inhibitor) should be initiated and intensified if the serum low-density lipoprotein (LDL) cholesterol level is greater than 100 mg/dL. Antihypertensive medication should be initiated and intensified until the BP is lower than 140/90 mm Hg. β-Adrenergic receptor blockers do not reduce walking capacity or worsen intermittent claudication in patients with PAD. Aspirin reduces the risks of myocardial infarction, death, and stroke. However, clopidogrel is an effective alternative treatment and is more effective than aspirin in reducing cardiovascular events (level B of evidence). Each patient needs an exercise prescription because exercise training improves walking capacity and quality of life. Pentoxifylline is a methylxanthine derivative that may improve maximal walking distance, but the data are inconclusive. Better data are available with cilostazol, a phosphodiesterase-3 (PDE3) inhibitor (whereas sildenafil is a PDE5 inhibitor). In several studies of patients with symptomatic PAD, cilostazol consistently improved walking capacity and quality of life. It is one of the most effective agents for intermittent claudication. However, cilostazol must be avoided in patients with congestive heart failure because its use may increase mortality in those patients.

Revascularization (percutaneous or surgical) is indicated for patients with severe claudication that is resistant to medical therapy, limb-threatening ischemia, or ischemia-induced impotence. Percutaneous revascularization offers a comparable patency rate with less morbidity and mortality than surgery in patients with short, focal stenoses of large arteries such as the distal aorta or iliac arteries (Fig. 12-1). Surgical revascularization is more suitable for longer areas of stenosis or obstructive lesions

distal to the origin of the iliac arteries. The selection of surgery versus percutaneous intervention as the initial mode of revascularization in patients with limb-threatening ischemia also depends on the patients' life expectancy. In general, bypass surgery is preferable to balloon angioplasty in patients with an expected life expectancy of more than 2 years because of greater overall long-term survival and amputation-free survival times (level B evidence). In contrast, percutaneous intervention is preferable for those with limited life expectancy because of less short-term morbidity (level B evidence).

Acute limb ischemia is a vascular emergency. Sudden occlusion of a peripheral artery is caused by either arterial embolism or thrombosis in situ. Arterial emboli usually originate in the cardiac chambers in the setting of preexisting cardiac disease such as myocardial infarction (e.g., left ventricular mural thrombus), congestive heart failure, or atrial arrhythmias (e.g., left atrial thrombus in a patient with atrial fibrillation). Thrombosis in situ usually occurs in arteries with a preexisting severe stenosis in the setting of long-standing PAD with or without previous vascular surgery. Patients with arterial embolism usually experience sudden onset of symptoms without a history of claudication, whereas those with thrombosis in situ typically have a history of claudication that has previously been stable and then suddenly assumes a crescendo pattern over a period of days. In either case, the physical examination reveals a cold, cyanotic (bluish) extremity with absent pulses distal to the site of arterial occlusion and diminished motor and/or sensory function. A handheld Doppler device is used to assess signals at various arterial segments and confirms the diagnosis of acute vascular occlusion. Anticoagulation should be initiated immediately with intravenous heparin titrated to maintain the activated partial thromboplastin time equal to 2.0 to 2.5 times control. Patients with acute limb ischemia who have symptoms for more than 14 days or occlusion in suprainguinal sites usually require surgical thromboembolectomy or bypass surgery. In contrast, patients with more recent onset of symptoms or infrainguinal occlusion should undergo

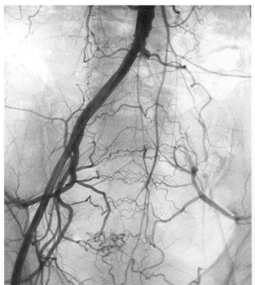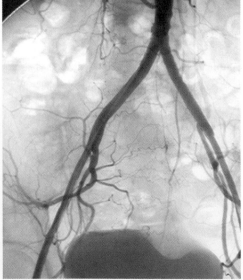

FIGURE 12-1   Angiogram of the distal abdominal aorta and iliac arteries demonstrates an occluded left common iliac artery with extensive collateral circulation from the contralateral internal iliac artery *(left)*, which resolved after successful stent implantation *(right)*. (Courtesy Bart Domatch, MD, Radiology Department, University of Texas Southwestern Medical Center, Dallas, Tex.)

catheter-directed infusion of thrombolytic therapy or percutaneous thrombus extraction. Irreversible tissue necrosis, regardless of the cause, should be treated with emergent amputation rather than revascularization to reduce the risk of kidney failure (myoglobinuria), sepsis, and multiorgan failure.

Aortic Aneurysm

Abdominal aortic aneurysm (AAA) is a common vascular disease in older adults, affecting 4% to 8% of men and 0.5% to 1.5% of women older than 65 years of age. Thoracic aortic aneurysm is much less prevalent (0.4% to 0.5%). Besides age, the major risk factors for AAAs are cigarette smoking, hypertension, and a family history of aortic aneurysms. Atherosclerosis is responsible for most cases of AAA, but other causes include cystic medial necrosis (Marfan syndrome, Ehlers-Danlos syndrome), vasculitis with connective tissue disease (Takayasu's arteritis, giant-cell arteritis), chronic infection (syphilitic aortitis), and trauma. AAAs grow gradually, at an average rate of 1 to 4 mm/year. The risk of rupture is low until the diameter reaches 5 cm, and then it increases exponentially. The risk of aortic rupture is 1% per year for aneurysms between 3.5 and 4.9 cm in diameter and 5% per year for aneurysms larger than 5 cm.

Most patients with AAA are asymptomatic, but some develop vascular complications such as aneurysm expansion with compression of adjacent structures. Occasionally, mural thrombi form within the aneurysm and embolize, causing acute occlusion of distal arterial segments. Patients with iliac aneurysm may develop hydronephrosis or recurrent urinary tract infections from ureteral compression. Others develop neurologic symptoms from compression of sciatic or femoral nerves. The classic physical finding is a pulsatile, nontender mass below the umbilicus (distal to the origin of the renal arteries). In thin patients, normal aortic pulsations are often palpable but above the umbilicus. Hypotension and acute abdominal pain should prompt consideration of aneurysm rupture, which requires emergent operative repair. Duplex ultrasonography is an accurate and reliable diagnostic tool for abdominal aortic and iliac aneurysms. Routine screening for AAA with ultrasonography is recommended for all men between the ages of 65 and 75 years and for men older than 60 years of age with a family history of AAA among first-degree relatives. Such screening is of proven benefit in reducing mortality. CT and MR angiography allow visualization of the thoracic and abdominal aorta as well as the iliac arteries and its branches (Fig. 12-2).

Medical treatment for aortic aneurysm includes smoking cessation, tight BP control, and cholesterol reduction. β-Blockade reduces the rate of aortic root enlargement in patients with Marfan syndrome but has not proved beneficial in patients with AAA from other causes. Patients with large aneurysms or rapid aneurysm expansion regardless of size should undergo aneurysm repair (Table 12-2). Elective AAA repair carries a perioperative mortality rate of 2% to 6%. Furthermore, a large randomized study failed to demonstrate any benefit of surgery in patients with aneurysms 4.0 to 5.5 cm in diameter (level A evidence). For these reasons, patients with small aortic aneurysms should be treated medically with close monitoring of aneurysm size by periodic imaging studies every 6 to 12 months (see Table 12-2).

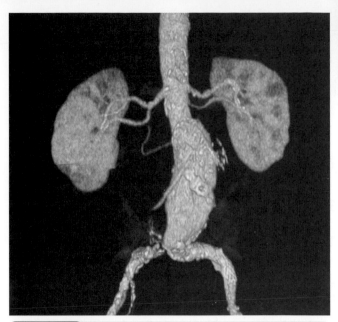

FIGURE 12-2 Computed tomographic angiogram of the distal abdominal aorta shows abdominal aortic aneurysm, 6.2 cm in largest diameter, with severe stenosis at the origin of the right common iliac artery. (Courtesy Bart Domatch, MD, Radiology Department, University of Texas Southwestern Medical Center, Dallas, Tex.)

TABLE 12-2   INDICATIONS FOR SURGICAL TREATMENT OF ARTERIAL ANEURYSMS

Symptoms from expansion of aneurysm or compression of adjacent structure
Rupture of aneurysm
Rapid aortic aneurysm expansion of ≥1 cm/yr
Large aneurysm
  Ascending aorta >4.5 cm for patients with Marfan syndrome and >5.0 cm for all others
  Aortic arch >5.5 cm
  Descending thoracic aorta >5.0 cm
  Abdominal aorta >5.5 cm
  Iliac aneurysm >3 cm

Percutaneous endovascular aneurysm repair (EVAR) is an alternative to open surgical repair for treatment of AAA. EVAR offers a lower rate of perioperative death than surgical repair with equivalent long-term survival (level A evidence). However, EVAR should be reserved for patients who are able to return for follow-up visits and repeated imaging studies of the aneurysm site to ensure that the stent graft is free from endovascular leaks or displacement (level A evidence). EVAR has not been shown to improve mortality in patients with multiple comorbidities, who are considered to be unfit for surgery, when compared to conservative management. Therefore, it should be offered only to selected patients with symptoms from compression of adjacent organs or vascular complications.

Aortic Dissection

In aortic dissection, the intimal layer is torn from the aortic wall, resulting in the formation of a false lumen in parallel with the true lumen. Risk factors include hypertension, cocaine use, trauma, hereditary connective tissue disease (e.g., Marfan syndrome, Ehlers-Danlos syndrome), vasculitis (e.g., Takayasu's arteritis, giant-cell arteritis), Behçet's disease, bicuspid aortic valve, and aortic coarctation. Aortic dissection can be divided into types A and B (Stanford system). Type A dissection involves the ascending aorta, whereas type B involves the distal aorta. The DeBakey system subdivides aortic dissection into three subtypes: I, II, and III. Type I dissection involves the entire aorta, whereas type II involves only the ascending aorta and type III involves only the descending aorta. Aortic dissection involving the ascending aorta carries a high mortality rate of 1% to 2% per hour during the first 24 to 48 hours. Patients usually develop acute onset of severe chest or back pain. Abdominal pain, syncope, and stroke are common. Retrograde propagation of the dissection can cause pericardial tamponade or coronary artery dissection with acute myocardial infarction. Dissection involving the aortic valve causes acute severe aortic insufficiency with acute pulmonary edema. The dissection plane may propagate in an antegrade direction to compromise flow in the carotid and subclavian arteries, producing a stroke or acute upper limb ischemia.

Patients with distal (type B) aortic dissection exhibit acute onset of back pain or chest pain, often accompanied by lower-extremity ischemia and ischemic neuropathy. The physical findings include pulse deficits, neurologic deficits, or a diastolic murmur of aortic regurgitation. However, acute aortic regurgitation into an unprepared ventricle produces only a short, soft diastolic murmur that is often missed. Widened pulse pressure and associated physical findings of chronic aortic regurgitation are absent, and the clinical picture is that of an acutely ill patient with tachypnea, tachycardia, and a narrow pulse pressure. Hypotension, jugular venous distention, and pulsus paradoxus should prompt the diagnosis of pericardial tamponade. Transesophageal echocardiography, MR angiography, or CT angiography confirm the diagnosis by demonstrating an intimal flap that separates the true lumen from the false lumen (Fig. 12-3).

Type A aortic dissection is uniformly fatal without emergent surgical repair. With surgery, mortality is reduced to 10% at 24

hours and 20% at 30 days. Patients with type B aortic dissection should be treated medically because the 1-year survival rate is higher with medical therapy than with surgery (75% vs. 50%). However, surgery is indicated if type B dissection compromises blood flow to the legs, kidneys, or other viscera. Tight control of BP is essential because aortic aneurysm develops in 30% to 50% of patients with type B aortic dissection studied for 4 years.

Penetrating Aortic Ulcers and Intramural Hematoma

Penetrating aortic ulcers and intramural hematomas exhibit chest pain that is indistinguishable from that of aortic dissection. In contrast to aortic dissection, however, the pathologic condition is localized. No identifiable intimal flap, and therefore no branch vessel occlusion, is produced. Disruption of the internal elastic lamina produces aortic ulcers that erode into the medial wall and protrude into the surrounding structures. Rupture of the vasa vasorum causes formation of localized hematoma underneath the adventitia with resultant asymmetric thickening of the aortic wall. Patients with either condition typically are older than those with aortic dissection, have a larger aortic size, and have a higher prevalence of AAA. Aortic rupture is the major complication of both penetrating ulcers and intramural hematomas, particularly if the aneurysm is located in the ascending aorta. The diagnosis is made with invasive angiography, CT angiography, or MR angiography (Fig. 12-4). Surgical intervention should be considered for ulcers and hematomas of the ascending aorta, for deeply penetrating ulcers, and for severely bulging hematomas, irrespective of their location. Ulcers and hematomas of the descending aorta may be managed successfully with β-blockade and tight control of BP.

Other Arterial Diseases

Buerger's Disease

Buerger's disease is a nonatherosclerotic disease of the arteries, veins, and nerves of the arms and legs that affects mostly men

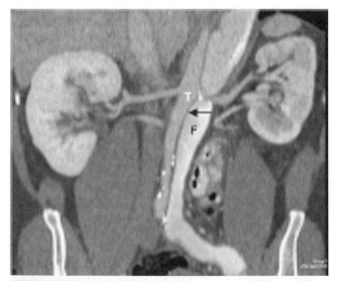

FIGURE 12-3   Computed tomographic angiogram of the aorta shows type B aortic dissection. The intimal flap *(arrow)* separates the true lumen *(T)* from the false lumen *(F)* and compromises blood flow to the right kidney, causing renal atrophy and cortical thinning. (Courtesy Bart Domatch, MD, Radiology Department, University of Texas Southwestern Medical Center, Dallas, Tex.)

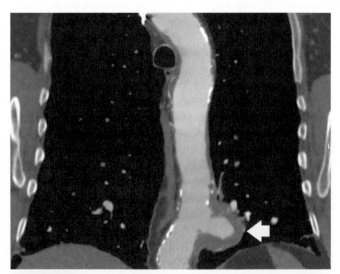

FIGURE 12-4   Computed tomographic angiogram of the descending thoracic aorta shows a large penetrating aortic ulcer above the diaphragm *(arrow)*. (Courtesy Bart Domatch, MD, Radiology Department, University of Texas Southwestern Medical Center, Dallas, Tex.)

younger than 45 years of age. The mechanism is unknown, but all patients have a history of heavy tobacco addiction. The presenting symptom is claudication of the feet, legs, hands, or arms. Multiple-limb involvement and superficial thrombophlebitis are common. The C-reactive protein level and erythrocyte sedimentation rate (Westergren method) typically are normal, and a search for serologic markers for connective tissue disease (e.g., antinuclear antibody, rheumatoid factor, antiphospholipid antibody) is negative. The diagnosis is based on the typical clinical presentation. If the presentation is atypical, then biopsy is needed to make the diagnosis. The histologic hallmark is inflammatory intramural thrombi within the arteries and veins with sparing of internal elastic lamina and other arterial wall structures. The most effective treatment for Buerger's disease is complete tobacco abstinence. The prostacyclin analogue iloprost constitutes adjunctive therapy to reduce limb ischemia and improve wound healing.

Raynaud's Phenomenon

Raynaud's phenomenon is a vasospastic disease of the small arteries of mainly the fingers and toes. Primary (idiopathic) Raynaud's phenomenon occurs in the absence of underlying disorders. Secondary Raynaud's phenomenon occurs in association with connective tissue diseases (e.g., scleroderma, polymyositis, rheumatoid arthritis, systemic lupus erythematosus) repeated mild physical trauma (e.g., use of jack hammers), use of certain drugs (e.g., antineoplastic chemotherapeutic agents, interferon, monamine-reuptake inhibitors such as tricyclic antidepressants, serotonin agonists), and Buerger's disease. Patients usually complain of recurrent episodes of ischemia of the digits, which exhibit a characteristic white-blue-red color sequence: Pallor is followed by cyanosis if ischemia is prolonged and then by erythema (reactive hyperemia) when the episode resolves. Episodes are precipitated by cold temperature or emotional stress. The physical examination can be entirely normal between attacks with normal radial, ulnar, and pedal pulses. Some patients have digital ulcers or thickening of the fat pad (sclerodactyly). Patients should be instructed to avoid cold temperatures and dress warmly. Calcium-channel blockers (CCBs) reduce the frequency and severity of vasospastic episodes.

Giant-Cell Arteritis

Giant-cell arteritis is an immune-mediated vasculitis that predominantly involves medium-sized and large arteries such as the subclavian artery, axillary artery, and aorta of older adults, with a strong male predominance. Approximately 40% of patients with giant-cell arteritis also have polymyalgia rheumatica, a syndrome characterized by severe stiffness and pain originating in the muscles of the shoulders and pelvic girdle. Patients may exhibit headache from temporal arteritis, jaw claudication from ischemia of the masseter muscles, or visual loss from involvement of the ophthalmic artery. Chest pain suggests the coexistence of aortic aneurysm or dissection. Physical findings include low-grade fever, scalp tenderness in the temporal area, pale and edematous fundi, or a diastolic murmur of aortic regurgitation. A BP difference of more than 15 mm Hg between the arms suggests subclavian artery stenosis. Laboratory findings include a significantly elevated C-reactive protein level and Westergren sedimentation

rate plus anemia. The diagnosis is confirmed by histologic examination of the arterial tissue (frequently obtained by temporal artery biopsy) showing infiltration of lymphocytes and macrophages (i.e., giant cells) in all layers of the vascular wall. High-dose corticosteroids are highly effective. To minimize complications from long-term corticosteroid administration, the steroid dose should be tapered to find the lowest dose needed to suppress symptoms, which often wane. Every attempt should be made to discontinue corticosteroids over time.

Takayasu's Arteritis

Takayasu's arteritis is an idiopathic granulomatous vasculitis of the aorta, its main branches, and the pulmonary artery. This condition is particularly common in young women of Asian descent, but it also occurs in non-Asian women and in men. The inflammatory process in the vascular wall can lead to stenosis or aneurysm formation or both. Hypertension, as a result of renal artery stenosis or aortic coarctation, is the most common manifestation and is present in as many as 80% of affected individuals. Because the vascular involvement is so widespread, patients may have symptoms and signs of coronary ischemia, congestive heart failure, stroke, vertebrobasilar insufficiency, or intermittent claudication. Physical findings include bruits over the subclavian arteries or aorta with diminished brachial pulses and therefore a low brachial artery BP. The diagnosis is based primarily on this clinical presentation. First-line treatment is with corticosteroids. Other immunosuppressive agents such as methotrexate or cyclophosphamide are often added to prevent disease progression and relapse. Immunosuppressive therapy does not cause regression of preexisting vascular stenoses or aneurysms. For this reason, percutaneous or surgical revascularization is usually required.

Arteriovenous Fistula

Arteriovenous (AV) fistulas are abnormal vascular communications that shunt blood flow from the arterial system directly into the venous system, bypassing the capillary beds that normally ensure optimal tissue perfusion and nutrient exchange. AV fistulas may be congenital, as in AV malformation, or acquired. The main causes of acquired AV fistula are penetrating trauma (e.g., gunshot, knife wound) and shunts created surgically for hemodialysis access. Patients may exhibit a pulsatile mass, symptoms related to compression of an adjacent organ, or bleeding from spontaneous rupture of an AV malformation. Systolic and diastolic bruits or thrills may be detectable over the fistula or malformation. An AV malformation in skeletal muscle may lead to bone malformation or a pathologic fracture, whereas an AV malformation in the brain may result in neurologic deficits or seizures. High-output heart failure is another complication from a large AV malformation or fistula. MR angiography, CT angiography, or conventional angiography confirms the diagnosis. Depending on the size and location of the lesion, treatment options include surgical resection, transcatheter embolization, or pulse laser irradiation. Patients with acquired AV fistulas from trauma usually need surgical closure.

⬤ PULMONARY VASCULAR DISEASE

Pulmonary hypertension is characterized by elevated mean pulmonary artery pressure of greater than 25 mm Hg at rest or greater than 30 mm Hg during exercise. The many causes of pulmonary hypertension are summarized in Table 12-3.

Patients with pulmonary hypertension not only have an elevated pulmonary arterial pressure but also a low cardiac output, causing symptoms of exertional dyspnea, fatigue, and syncope. Pulmonary capillary wedge pressure is usually normal ($\leq$15 mm Hg) except in patients with pulmonary hypertension due to impaired left ventricular systolic or diastolic function or left-sided valvular heart disease.

Pulmonary Arterial Hypertension

Pulmonary arterial hypertension (PAH) is caused by a combination of pulmonary vasoconstriction, endothelial cell and/or smooth muscle proliferation, intimal fibrosis, and thrombosis in the pulmonary capillaries and arterioles. PAH is either idiopathic (primary pulmonary hypertension) or secondary to connective tissue disease, congenital heart disease, portal hypertension, human immunodeficiency virus (HIV) infection, or anorexigenic drugs or toxins. Connective tissue diseases, particularly scleroderma, are the most common secondary causes of PAH.

Patients with mild PAH can be asymptomatic, but patients with more advanced disease complain of dyspnea, chest pain, syncope, or presyncope. Physical findings include a left parasternal lift, loud pulmonary component of the second heart sound, murmur of tricuspid or pulmonic regurgitation, hepatomegaly, peripheral edema, or ascites. Associated electrocardiogram (ECG) abnormalities indicate right ventricular hypertrophy, right atrial enlargement, or right axis deviation. Echocardiography provides important information about the severity of the pulmonary hypertension (e.g., estimated pulmonary artery pressure, right ventricular dimensions and function) and its potential causes (e.g., left ventricular failure, valvular lesions, congenital heart disease with left-to-right shunt). Pulmonary function tests, ventilation-perfusion ($\dot{V}/\dot{Q}$) lung scans, polysomnography or overnight oximetry, autoantibody tests, HIV serology, and liver function tests also should be performed to determine other potential causes. Right ventricular catheterization should be performed in all patients with suspected PAH. Under basal conditions in the catheterization laboratory, an elevated mean pulmonary artery pressure exceeding 25 mm Hg, a pulmonary capillary wedge pressure of less than 15 mm Hg, and a pulmonary vascular resistance exceeding 3 units confirm the diagnosis. Acute vasodilator drug challenge should be performed during right ventricular catheterization to guide appropriate treatment.

Without treatment, the prognosis of PAH is poor, with a median survival time of less than 3 years. Patients with severe symptoms should be treated with prostacyclin or epoprostenol (an intravenous prostacyclin analogue) because of their proven efficacy in improving exercise capacity, quality of life, and survival. Other prostacyclin analogues, such as treprostinil and iloprost, are also effective in reducing pulmonary artery pressure and improving exercise capacity. Other classes of drugs approved for treatment of PAH include endothelin-receptor blockers (bosentan or ambrisentan) and PDE5 inhibitors (sildenafil, tadalafil). Much higher daily doses of PDE5 inhibitors are needed to treat PAH than to treat erectile dysfunction or prostatism. Oral CCBs are indicated for the small subset of patients with mild to moderate symptoms who demonstrate significant reduction in pulmonary pressure with acute CCB challenge (decrease in mean pulmonary artery pressure of at least 10 mm Hg to an absolute level of less than 40 mm Hg without a decrease in cardiac output). Supplemental home oxygen is indicated for all patients with hypoxemia. Travel to high elevations exacerbates hypoxia, and relocation to sea level improves symptoms. Oral anticoagulation is recommended for all patients with PAH. Diuretics should be prescribed for patients with peripheral edema or hepatic congestion. Lung transplantation is recommended only for patients in whom severe symptoms occur despite intensive medical therapy.

⬤ VENOUS THROMBOEMBOLIC DISEASE

The term *venous thromboembolism* (VTE) encompasses both deep vein thrombosis (DVT) and pulmonary embolism (PE). Among the adult population in the United States, the overall combined annual incidence is as high as 1 new case per 1000 persons. The incidence of VTE is higher in men than in women and higher in African Americans and whites than in Asians and Hispanics. More than 150 years ago, Rudolf Virchow recognized three predisposing factors: endothelial damage, venous stasis, and hypercoagulation (now known as Virchow's triad). Endothelial damage is common with surgery or trauma; venous stasis is common with prolonged bedrest or immobilization (e.g., leg cast); and hypercoagulation is common with cancer. Trousseau's syndrome consists of migratory thrombophlebitis with noninfectious vegetations on the heart valves (nonbacterial thrombotic endocarditis, formerly known as marantic endocarditis), typically in the setting of mucin-secreting adenocarcinoma. Trousseau, a pathologist, diagnosed his own pancreatic carcinoma on the basis of the association that now bears his name. Hypercoagulable states include hereditary diseases such as deficiencies in antithrombin III, protein C, or protein S; mutation in the factor V gene (factor V Leiden) or the factor II gene (prothrombin G20210A); and hyperhomocysteinemia. However, a thorough search for identifiable risk factors will remain negative in 25% to 50% of patients with VTE.

TABLE 12-3	CLASSIFICATION OF PULMONARY HYPERTENSION	
CATEGORY	**EXAMPLES**
1. Pulmonary arterial hypertension (PAH)	
A. Primary or idiopathic PAH	Sporadic Familial
B. Secondary PAH	Connective tissue disease Congenital heart disease Portal hypertension Human immunodeficiency virus infection Drugs and toxins: anorexigens, cocaine
2. Pulmonary venous hypertension	Left ventricular heart failure Left ventricular valvular heart disease
3. Pulmonary hypertension associated with chronic respiratory disease or hypoxemia	Chronic obstructive pulmonary disease Obstructive sleep apnea
4. Pulmonary hypertension associated with chronic venous thromboembolism	Deep vein thrombosis
5. Pulmonary hypertension due to miscellaneous disorders directly affecting the pulmonary vasculature	Sarcoidosis, histiocytosis X, compression of pulmonary vessels (adenopathy, tumor, fibrosing mediastinitis)

Deep Vein Thrombosis

Most DVT starts in the calf veins. Without treatment, 15% to 30% of these clots propagate to the proximal calf veins. The risk of a subsequent PE is much higher with proximal DVT than with clots confined to the distal calf vessels (40% to 50% vs. 5% to 10%, respectively). Involvement of the upper extremities is much less common, but subclavian or axillary vein thrombosis also can lead to PE in as many as 30% of affected individuals. The same risk factors that cause lower-extremity DVT also cause upper-extremity DVT. In addition, other specific causes of upper-extremity DVT include traumatic damage of the vessel intima due to heavy exertion such as rowing, wrestling, or weight lifting (Paget-Schroetter syndrome), extrinsic compression at the level of thoracic inlet (thoracic outlet obstruction), or insertion of central venous catheters or pacemakers.

Pain and swelling are the major complaints from patients with DVT; however, a large number of patients are asymptomatic, particularly if the DVT is restricted to the calf. Patients with upper-extremity DVT can develop the superior vena cava syndrome of facial swelling, blurred vision, and dyspnea. Thoracic outlet obstruction can compress the brachial plexus, leading to unilateral arm pain associated with hand weakness. Physical examination frequently reveals tenderness, erythema, warmth, and swelling below the site of thrombosis. Pain with dorsiflexion of the foot (Homan's sign) may be present, but the low sensitivity and the low specificity limit the usefulness of this sign in the diagnosis of lower-extremity DVT. A palpable tender cord, dilated superficial veins, and low-grade fever occur in some patients. Upper-extremity DVT can cause brachial plexus tenderness in the supraclavicular fossa and atrophic hand muscles. For patients with probable thoracic outlet obstruction, several provocative tests should be performed. Adson's test is positive if the radial pulses weaken during inspiration and during extension of the arm of the affected side while rotating the head to the same side. Wright's test is positive if the radial pulses become weaker and painful symptoms are reproduced while the shoulder of the affected side is abducted with the humerus externally rotated.

The laboratory diagnosis of DVT includes measurement of D-dimers, which are fibrin degradation products. D-dimer elevation is a highly sensitive indicator of DVT that can be performed rapidly in the emergency department. In a patient in whom the index of probability is low, a negative D-dimer test effectively excludes the diagnosis of DVT. However, the test is not specific and can be elevated in many other conditions frequently encountered in hospitalized patients (e.g., inflammation, recent surgery, malignancy). Duplex ultrasonography can be used to demonstrate the presence of a blood clot or noncompressibility of the affected veins proximal to the site of occlusion. Duplex ultrasonography has greater sensitivity in detecting proximal DVT (90% to 100%) than distal DVT (40% to 90%) of the lower extremities. With upper-extremity DVT, acoustic shadowing of the clavicle may obscure detection of thrombosis in subclavian vein segments. MR angiography is particularly helpful in making the diagnosis of upper-extremity DVT and pelvic vein thrombosis. Contrast venography is the conventional "gold standard" test, but it is invasive and technically difficult in patients with edematous extremities. Therefore, invasive venography should be reserved for patients in whom the clinical suggestion is high despite negative or inconclusive results from noninvasive imaging.

Patients with proximal lower-extremity DVT and those with upper-extremity DVT should be treated initially with subcutaneous low-molecular-weight heparin (LMWH), intravenous or subcutaneous unfractionated heparin (UFH) or the subcutaneous selective factor Xa inhibitor fondaparinux to prevent thrombus propagation and to maintain the patency of venous collaterals (level A evidence). Intravenous UFH should be given as a bolus, followed by continuous infusion to maintain an activated partial thromboplastin time of at least 1.5 times the control value. Both LMWH and fondaprinux have a longer half-life than UFH and can be given once or twice daily with similar efficacy. Oral warfarin should be initiated together with LMWH, UFH, or fondaprinux without delay and titrated until the international normalized ratio (INR) reaches a value between 2 and 3. Alternatively, rivaroxaban, an oral factor Xa inhibitor, may be used without initial parenteral anticoagulation and continued for at least 3 months. Direct thrombin inhibitors such as dabigatran have been shown to be efficacious in this clinical setting and were recently approved for treatment of DVT and pulmonary embolism in the United States. When DVT is confined to the calf, the risk of PE is low, and the risk-to-benefit ratio of anticoagulation remains controversial.

When upper-extremity DVT occurs in young patients who are otherwise healthy, two invasive approaches to thrombus removal should be considered: infusion of a fibrinolytic drug through a catheter inserted directly into the affected vein and mechanical fragmentation of the thrombus via catheter-based technology. The purpose of these invasive procedures is to prevent or minimize the post-thrombotic syndrome, which includes chronic arm pain, swelling, hyperpigmentation, and ulceration from residual venous obstruction.

Catheter-based placement of a filter in the inferior vena cava should be considered for patients with proximal DVT who either have an absolute contraindication to anticoagulation or develop recurrent PE despite an adequate trial of anticoagulation. Vena cava filters are effective in reducing the incidence of PE, but they increase the risk of recurrent DVT. Some proximal or distal migration of the filter occurs in up to 50% of cases; however, clinically evident filter embolization is limited to case reports.

Pulmonary Embolism

PE occurs when a thrombus dislodges from the deep veins of the upper or lower extremities and travels to the lungs. Pulmonary vascular resistance and pulmonary arterial pressure increase from two mechanisms: anatomic reduction in cross-sectional area of the pulmonary vascular bed and functional hypoxia-induced pulmonary vasoconstriction. The pressure overload on the right ventricle can lead to dilation, hypokinesis, and tricuspid regurgitation. Elevated right ventricular end-diastolic pressure, if severe, can compress the right coronary artery, causing subendocardial ischemia. In acute PE, areas of lung tissue are ventilated but underperfused. This $\dot{V}/\dot{Q}$ mismatch and the resultant redistribution of pulmonary blood flow from the obstructed pulmonary artery to other lung regions with lower $\dot{V}/\dot{Q}$ ratios cause arterial hypoxemia. In patients with a patent foramen ovale, hypoxemia worsens when the sudden elevation in right atrial pressure causes right-to-left shunting across the foramen.

The classic symptoms of acute PE are sudden onset of dyspnea and pleuritic chest pain. Additional symptoms include anginal chest pain from right ventricular ischemia, hemoptysis from pulmonary infarction, and syncope or presyncope from massive PE with acute right ventricular failure (cor pulmonale). The most common physical findings are tachypnea and tachycardia. Additional physical findings include a right ventricular lift, inspiratory crackles, a loud pulmonary component of the second heart sound, expiratory wheezing, and a pleural rub. Symptoms and signs of proximal DVT are present in 10% to 20% of patients. Arterial blood gas analysis often reveals hypoxemia, respiratory alkalosis, and a high alveolar-to-arterial oxygen tension gradient. However, normal arterial blood gas values do not exclude the diagnosis.

The most common finding with ECG analysis is sinus tachycardia. Atrial fibrillation, premature atrial contraction, and supraventricular tachycardia are less common. Other ECG changes suggest acute right ventricular strain. These include the S1-Q3-T3 pattern, a new right bundle branch block or right axis deviation, and P-wave pulmonale. However, these findings are present in only 30% of patients even with massive PE. Common but nonspecific abnormalities on chest radiographic studies include atelectasis, pleural effusion, and pulmonary infiltrates. Less common but more specific radiographic findings include Hampton's hump (i.e., wedge-shaped infiltrate in the peripheral lung field), which is indicative of pulmonary infarction, and Westermark's sign (decreased vascularity).

The plasma D-dimer level is elevated in most patients with PE as a result of activation of the endogenous fibrinolytic system, which is not sufficient to dissolve the clot. Commercially available D-dimer assays have a high sensitivity and negative predictive value but low specificity. Therefore, a normal D-dimer test effectively excludes the diagnosis of PE in patients in whom the clinical suggestion is low or intermediate, but the should not be used to screen patients with high index of suspicion because of the low negative predictive value. Elevated levels of cardiac troponin I and troponin T and other markers of myocardial injury can be found in patients with PE and are indicative of right ventricular dysfunction and a poor prognosis. Similarly, elevated natriuretic peptides, including brain natriuretic peptide (BNP) and N-terminal pro-BNP, have been shown to be predictive of adverse outcomes. In patients with suspected PE, a completely normal $\dot{V}/\dot{Q}$ scan effectively excludes the diagnosis without further testing. However, fewer than 10% of $\dot{V}/\dot{Q}$ scans are interpreted as definitively normal. In patients in whom a moderate or high level of clinical probability of PE exists, a high-probability $\dot{V}/\dot{Q}$ scan has a diagnostic accuracy of 90% to 100%; however, a low or intermediate probability scan is no more helpful than a coin flip.

More recently, multidetector CT angiography has become the imaging modality of choice in patients with acute PE because of its excellent visualization of the pulmonary artery (Fig. 12-5). The resolution of 1 mm or less rivals that of conventional invasive angiography. The speed of newer-generation scanners allows acquisition of all images within a single breath-hold, avoiding respiratory motion artifacts. The overall negative predictive value

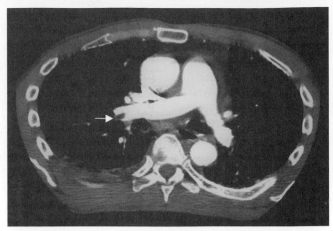

FIGURE 12-5 Spiral chest computed tomographic angiogram shows a large thrombus in the right main pulmonary artery *(arrow)*. (Courtesy Michael Landay, MD, Department of Radiology, University of Texas Southwestern Medical Center, Dallas, Tex.)

of multidetector CT angiography exceeds 99%. A negative CT scan excludes the diagnosis of PE and eliminates the need for further diagnostic testing. The CT scan also permits detection of other pathologic conditions involving the lung parenchyma, pleura, and mediastinal structures. Such pathologic findings may mimic PE and constitute alternative causes of chest pain and dyspnea. Multidetector CT angiography is not yet available at all centers. The requirement for intravenous injection of iodinated contrast material restricts its applicability to those without a history of kidney disease or an allergic reaction to contrast dye.

Figure 12-6 presents an algorithm for the work-up of PE based on current evidence. Echocardiography may directly detect thrombi in the right atrium, right ventricle, or pulmonary artery or may indirectly demonstrate right ventricular dysfunction, signifying the presence of hemodynamically significant emboli. Therefore, it is helpful in diagnosis of PE in patients with hypotension or shock, particularly if multidetector CT is not immediately available. Invasive pulmonary angiography should be reserved for patients for whom noninvasive testing is inconclusive.

Treatment of acute PE includes immediate anticoagulation with UFH, LMWH, or fondaparinux (level A evidence). LMWH and fondaparinux are preferred agents in patients with normal renal function because of the ease of subcutaneous administration and their lower rates of thrombocytopenia. These drugs are excreted by the kidney, so they should be avoided in patients with renal failure, and intravenous UFH should be used instead. Thrombolytic therapy with recombinant tissue-type plasminogen activator (rt-PA) is indicated for patients with either (1) hypotension or shock or (2) right ventricular enlargement or dysfunction from massive PE (level B evidence). Surgical or percutaneous removal of emboli should be considered in patients with massive PE who have contraindications for thrombolytic therapy. After initiation of heparin or fondaparinux, warfarin should be administered. Infusion of heparin or fondaparinux needs to be continued for at least the first 5 days of warfarin therapy until a therapeutic INR of 2 to 3 is reached. Oral rivaroxaban without initial treatment with heparin or fondaparinux is an alternative strategy and is considered to be another option for

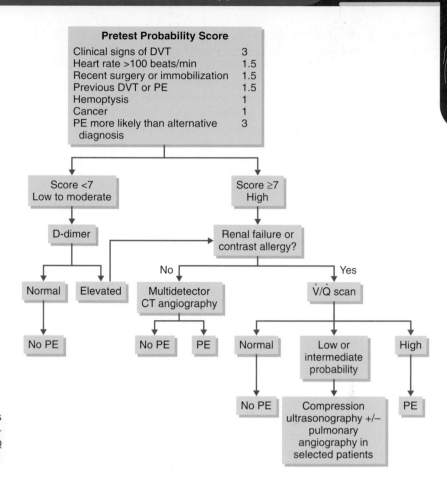

FIGURE 12-6 Diagnostic algorithm for patients with suggested pulmonary embolism (PE). CT, Computed tomographic; DVT, deep vein thrombosis; V̇/Q̇ scan, ventilation-perfusion scan.

patients with advanced chronic kidney disease, in whom LMWH use is generally prohibited.

The time for which anticoagulation should be continued after an acute PE or DVT episode depends on the presence of reversible risk factors for recurrent VTE. Patients with a history of trauma or surgery typically have a low rate of recurrent VTE; therefore, warfarin can be discontinued after 3 months of administration. Patients with cancer and VTE should be treated initially with subcutaneous fixed-dose LMWH for 3 to 6 months because of the greater efficacy of LMWH compared with warfarin in preventing recurrent thromboembolism in this setting. After this initial period, treatment with LMWH or warfarin should be continued indefinitely unless the cancer is cured. Patients with idiopathic VTE and a low risk of bleeding should be treated with warfarin for longer than 3 months, whereas those with high bleeding risk should remain on treatment for at least 3 months. Beyond the 3- to 6-month period, aspirin is an alternative to long-term warfarin and should be considered for patients who have contraindications for anticoagulation or high bleeding risk.

Venous Thromboembolism Prophylaxis

Patients who are at high risk for VTE should receive prophylaxis with subcutaneous UFH or LMWH. Patients at high risk include those who are hospitalized with acute medical illness (particularly congestive heart failure, acute respiratory illness, or acute inflammatory disease), those who are expected to be immobilized for 3 days or longer, and patients with previous VTE. Major surgery, either elective or emergent, is an important indication for VTE prophylaxis.

Subcutaneous UFH is as effective as LMWH and fondaparinux in preventing symptomatic DVT in patients undergoing general surgery, gynecologic surgery, or neurosurgery. However, LMWH, fondaparinux, and warfarin (dose-adjusted to an INR between 2 and 3) are preferred to UFH for prevention of DVT in cases of orthopedic surgery such as hip surgery or total knee replacement because their superior efficacy in this setting (level A evidence). More recently, rivaroxaban has been approved by the U.S. Food and Drug Administration for prevention of VTE after knee or hip surgery; it has a higher efficacy than LMWH in reducing risks without increasing perioperative bleeding. DVT prophylaxis should be continued for 10 to 14 days after knee surgery and for 35 days after hip surgery. Patients undergoing major cancer surgery should receive continued prophylaxis after discharge up to 28 days. Mechanical prophylaxis with intermittent pneumatic compression provides additional protection from VTE and should be administered to all surgical patients whenever possible.

● ARTERIAL HYPERTENSION

Arterial hypertension affects almost one third of the adult population—75 million people in the United States and 1 billion worldwide. It is the leading cause of death in the world, the most common cause for an outpatient visit to a physician, and the most easily recognized treatable risk factor for stroke, myocardial infarction, heart failure, peripheral vascular disease, aortic dissection, atrial fibrillation, and end-stage kidney disease. Despite this knowledge and unequivocal scientific proof that treating hypertension with medication dramatically reduces its attendant morbidity and mortality, hypertension remains untreated or undertreated in the majority of affected individuals in all countries, including those with the most advanced systems of medical care. Currently, fewer than one in two Americans with hypertension have their BP treated and controlled to below 140/90 mm Hg. For this reason, hypertension remains one of the world's great public health problems. The asymptomatic nature of the condition impedes early detection, which requires regular BP measurement. Because most cases of hypertension cannot be cured, BP control requires lifelong treatment with prescription medications, which can be costly and may cause more symptoms than the underlying disease process. Effective hypertension management requires continuity of care by a regular and knowledgeable medical provider as well as sustained active participation by an educated patient. This section reviews the most important principles in the early detection and effective treatment of hypertension.

Initial Evaluation for Hypertension

The initial evaluation for hypertension needs to accomplish three goals: staging of BP, assessing the patient's overall cardiovascular risk, and detecting clues of secondary hypertension. The initial clinical data needed to accomplish these goals are obtained through a thorough history and physical examination, routine blood tests, a spot (preferably first morning) urine specimen, and a resting 12-lead ECG. Home BP monitoring is indicated in most patients to confirm the diagnosis of hypertension and to exclude the so-called white coat syndrome. In some cases, 24-hour ambulatory BP monitoring and an echocardiogram provide helpful additional data about the time-integral burden of BP on the cardiovascular system.

Goal 1: Accurate Assessment of Blood Pressure

Across populations, the risks of heart disease and stroke increase continuously and logarithmically with increasing systolic and

diastolic BP levels of 115/75 mm Hg or higher (Fig. 12-7). Therefore, the dichotomous separation of *normal* from *high* BP is artificial. BP is currently staged as normal, prehypertension, or hypertension based on the average of two or more readings taken at two or more office visits. When a patient's average systolic and diastolic pressures fall into different stages, the higher stage applies (Table 12-4).

Prehypertension is defined as BP levelss in the range of 120 to 139 mm Hg systolic and 80 to 89 mm Hg diastolic. Prehypertensive individuals are twice as likely to progress to hypertension as are those with lower values.

BP normally varies dramatically throughout a 24-hour period. To minimize variability in readings, BP should be measured at least twice after 5 minutes of rest with the patient seated, the back supported, and the arm bare and at heart level. The most common mistake in measuring BP is using a standard-issue cuff that is too small for a large arm, producing spuriously elevated readings. Most overweight adults require a large adult cuff. Tobacco and caffeine should be avoided for at least 30 minutes. To avoid underestimation of systolic pressure in older adults who may have an *auscultatory gap* as a result of arteriosclerosis, radial artery palpation should be performed first to estimate systolic pressure. The cuff should be inflated to a value 20 mm Hg higher than the

TABLE 12-4 STAGING OF OFFICE BLOOD PRESSURE*

BLOOD PRESSURE STAGE	SYSTOLIC BLOOD PRESSURE (MM HG)	DIASTOLIC BLOOD PRESSURE (MM HG)
Normal	<120	<80
Prehypertension	120-139	80-89
Stage 1 hypertension	140-159	90-99
Stage 2 hypertension	≥160	≥100

From Chobanian AV, Bakris GL, Black HR, et al: The seventh report of the Joint National Committee on the Prevention, Evaluation, and Treatment of High Blood Pressure: the JNC 7 report, JAMA 289:2560–2572, 2003.
*Calculation of seated blood pressure is based on the mean of two or more readings on two separate office visits.

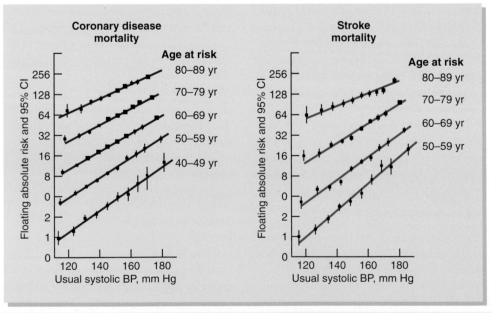

FIGURE 12-7 Floating absolute risk of coronary artery disease and stroke mortality by usual systolic blood pressure (BP) levels. CI, Confidence interval. (From Lewington S, Clarke R, Qizilbash N, et al: Age-specific relevance of usual blood pressure to vascular mortality: a meta-analysis of individual data for one million adults in 61 prospective studies, Lancet 360:1903–1913, 2002.)

level that obliterates the radial pulse and then deflated at a rate of 3 to 5 mm Hg per second. BP should be measured in both arms and after 5 minutes of standing, the latter to exclude a significant postural fall in BP, particularly in older persons and in those with diabetes or other conditions (e.g., Parkinson's disease) that predispose the patient to autonomic insufficiency.

However, out-of-office readings either obtained by home or ambulatory BP monitoring are required to accurately assess a person's typical BP. Because of the anxiety of going to the physician, BPs often are higher in the physician's office than when measured at home or during normal daily life outside the home. Self-monitoring of BP outside the physician's office actively engages a patient in his or her own health care and provides a better estimate of the usual BP for medical decision making. BP should be measured in the early morning and in the evening. Three BP readings should be obtained during each measurement, separated by at least 1 minute. Because the first BP measurement tends to be the highest, average BP should be used to assess home BP levels. Many electronic home monitors are available, but only a handful of models have been rigorously validated against mercury sphygmomanometry and can be recommended.

Ambulatory monitoring provides automated measurements of BP over a 24- or 48-hour period while patients are engaged in their usual activities, including sleep (Fig. 12-8). With ambulatory monitoring, current recommendations for *upper limits of normal* are a mean daytime BP of less than 135/85 mm Hg, a mean nighttime BP of 120/70 mm Hg, and a mean 24-hour BP of less than 130/80 mm Hg. However, an *optimal* mean daytime ambulatory BP is lower, less than 130/80 mm Hg. To avoid undertreating hypertension, these lower treatment thresholds must be used when incorporating ambulatory monitoring in medical decision making. With self-monitoring of BP at home, an average value of less than 135/85 mm Hg should be considered the upper limit of normal.

Up to one third of patients with elevated office BP levels have normal home or ambulatory BPs. If the 24-hour BP profile is completely normal and no target organ damage has occurred despite consistently elevated office readings, then the patient has *office-only*, or *white-coat*, hypertension, presumably the result of a transient adrenergic response to the measurement of BP in the physician's office (see Fig. 12-8).

In other patients, office readings underestimate ambulatory BPs, presumably because of sympathetic overactivity in daily life owing to job or home stress, tobacco abuse, or other adrenergic stimulation that dissipates when coming to the office (Fig. 12-9). Such documentation prevents underdiagnosis and undertreatment of this *masked hypertension*, which is also associated with high cardiovascular risks. Masked hypertension is identified in 10% of all hypertensive patients, in up to 40% of those with diabetes, and in 70% of African American patients with hypertensive kidney disease.

Goal 2: Cardiovascular Risk Stratification

The great majority of patients with BPs in the prehypertensive or hypertensive range have one or more additional modifiable risk factors for atherosclerosis (e.g., hypercholesterolemia, cigarette smoking, diabetes). The patient's global cardiovascular risk should be calculated from the 2013 ACC/AHA pooled atherosclerotic cardiovascular disease (ASCVD) risk calculator (http://www.cardiosource.org/Science-And-Quality/Practice-Guidelines-and-Quality-Standards/2013-Prevention-Guideline-Tools.aspx).

Goal 3: Identification of Secondary (Identifiable) Causes of Hypertension

A thorough search for secondary causes is not cost-effective in most patients with hypertension, but it becomes critically important in two circumstances: (1) when a compelling cause is found on the initial evaluation, or (2) when the hypertensive process is so severe that it either is refractory to intensive multiple-drug therapy or necessitates hospitalization. Table 12-5 summarizes the major causes of secondary hypertension that should be

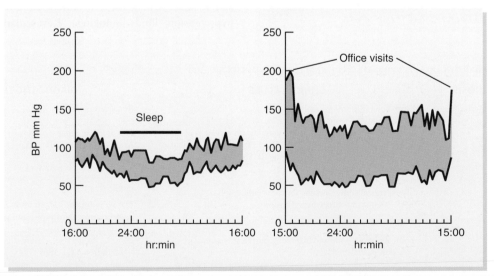

FIGURE 12-8 Twenty-four hour ambulatory blood pressure (BP) monitor tracings in two different patients. **A,** Optimal BP in a healthy 37-year-old woman. The normal variability in BP, the nocturnal dip in BP during sleep, and the sharp increase in BP on awakening are shown. **B,** Pronounced white-coat syndrome in an 80-year-old woman referred for evaluation of medically refractory hypertension. Documentation of the white-coat effect prevented overtreatment of the patient's isolated systolic hypertension.

suggested on the basis of a good history, physical examination, and routine laboratory tests.

Renal Parenchymal Hypertension

Chronic kidney disease is the most common cause of secondary hypertension. Hypertension is present in more than 85% of patients with chronic kidney disease and is a major factor causing their increased cardiovascular morbidity and mortality. The mechanisms causing the hypertension include an expanded

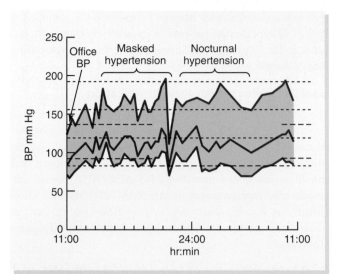

FIGURE 12-9 Twenty-four hour ambulatory blood pressure (BP) monitor tracing shows both masked hypertension and nocturnal hypertension in a 55-year-old man with stage 3 chronic kidney disease. Treatment with three different antihypertensive medications produced an office BP of 125/75 mm Hg, which seemed to be at goal. However, progressive hypertensive heart disease and deterioration of renal function suggested masked hypertension. Ambulatory monitoring revealed that the patient's treated BP was much higher out of the office, documenting both masked hypertension (ambulatory BP of 175/95 mm Hg) and sustained nocturnal hypertension (BP of 175/90 mm Hg). Additional medication was added. (Courtesy Ronald G. Victor, MD, Hypertension Division, Department of Internal Medicine, University of Texas Southwestern Medical Center, Dallas, Tex.)

plasma volume and peripheral vasoconstriction, with the latter caused by both activation of vasoconstrictor pathways (renin-angiotensin and sympathetic nervous systems) and inhibition of vasodilator pathways (nitric oxide). Renal insufficiency should be considered when proteinuria is found by dipstick or when the serum creatinine level is greater than 1.2 mg/dL in women with hypertension or greater than 1.4 mg/dL in men with hypertension.

Renovascular Hypertension

Unilateral or bilateral renal artery stenosis is present in fewer than 2% of patients with hypertension in a general medical practice but in up to 30% of patients with medically refractory hypertension. The main causes of renal artery stenosis are atherosclerosis (85% of patients), typically in older adults with other clinical manifestations of systemic atherosclerosis, and fibromuscular dysplasia (15% of patients), typically in women between the ages of 15 and 50 years. Unilateral renal artery stenosis leads to underperfusion of the juxtaglomerular cells, resulting in renin-dependent hypertension even though the contralateral kidney is able to maintain normal blood volume. In contrast, bilateral renal artery stenosis (or unilateral stenosis with a solitary kidney) constitutes a potentially reversible cause of progressive renal failure and volume-dependent hypertension.

The following clinical clues increase the suggestion of renovascular hypertension: any hospitalization for urgent or emergent hypertension; recurrent *flash* pulmonary edema; recent worsening of long-standing, previously well-controlled hypertension; severe hypertension in a young adult or after 50 years of age; precipitous and progressive worsening of renal function in response to angiotensin-converting enzyme (ACE) inhibition or angiotensin-receptor blockade (ARB); unilateral small kidney by any radiographic study; extensive peripheral arteriosclerosis; or a flank bruit. The diagnosis is confirmed by noninvasive testing with MR or spiral CT angiography (Fig. 12-10).

Renal artery angioplasty often cures fibromuscular dysplasia. Atherosclerotic renal artery stenosis should be treated with intensive medical management of atherosclerotic risk factors (e.g., hypertension, lipids, smoking). Revascularization should be

TABLE 12-5 GUIDE TO EVALUATION OF SECONDARY HYPERTENSION

PROBABLE DIAGNOSIS	CLINICAL CLUES	DIAGNOSTIC TESTING
Renal parenchymal hypertension	Estimated GFR <60 mL/min/1.73m² Urine albumin : creatinine >30 mg/g	Renal ultrasound
Renovascular disease	New elevation in serum creatinine, significant elevation in serum creatinine with initiation of ACEIs or ARBs, refractory hypertension, flash pulmonary edema, abdominal bruit Coarctation of the aorta Arm BP > leg BP BP, chest bruits, rib notching on chest radiograph	MR or CT angiography, invasive angiogram Arm pulses > leg pulses, chest MR or CT, aortogram
Primary aldosteronism	Hypokalemia, refractory hypertension	Plasma renin and aldosterone, 24-hr urine potassium, 24-hr urine aldosterone and potassium after salt loading, adrenal CT scan, adrenal vein sampling
Cushing's syndrome	Truncal obesity, wide and blanching purple striae, muscle weakness, diabetes	24-hr Urine cortisol, dexamethasone suppression test, adrenal CT scan
Pheochromocytoma	Spells of paroxysmal hypertension, palpitations, perspiration, pallor, pain in the head	Plasma and 24-hr urine metanephrines and catecholamines, adrenal CT scan
Obstructive sleep apnea	Loud snoring, daytime somnolence, obesity, large neck	Sleep study

Modified from Kaplan NM: Clinical hypertension, ed 8, Philadelphia, 2002, Williams & Wilkins.
ACEIs, Angiotensin-converting enzyme inhibitors; ARBs, angiotensin-receptor blockers; BP, blood pressure; CT, computed tomography; GFR, glomerular filtration rate; MR, magnetic resonance.

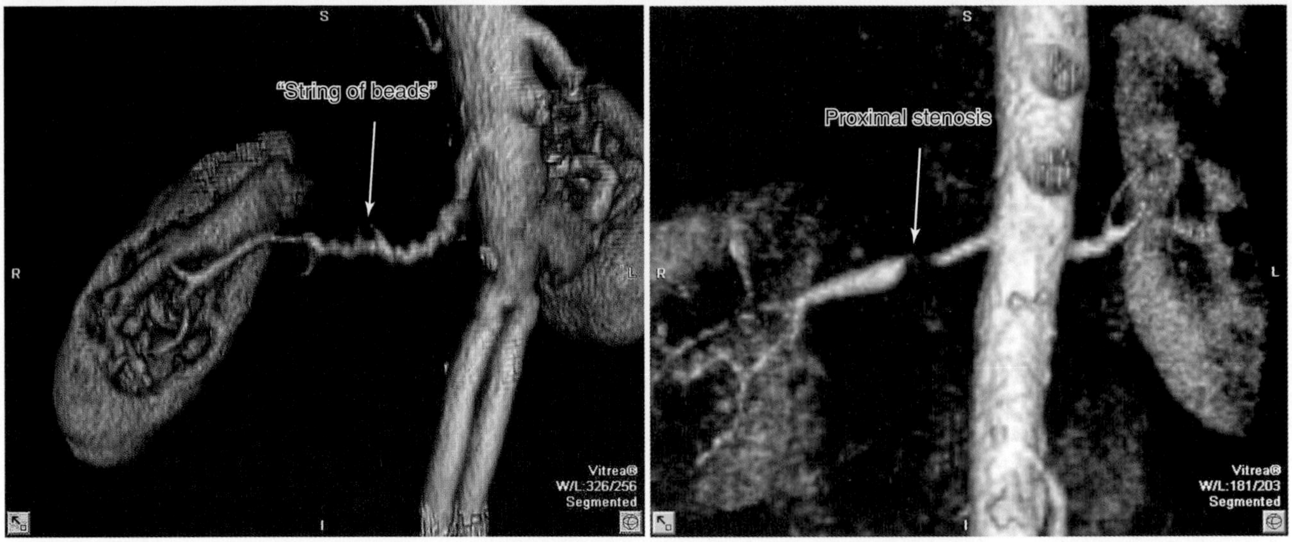

FIGURE 12-10 Computed tomography angiogram with three-dimensional reconstruction. **A,** Classic string-of-beads lesion of fibromuscular dysplasia. **B,** Severe proximal atherosclerotic stenosis of the right renal artery. (Courtesy Bart Domatch, MD, Radiology Department, University of Texas Southwestern Medical Center, Dallas, Tex.)

considered for medically refractory hypertension, progressive renal failure while on medical therapy, and bilateral renal artery stenosis or stenosis of a solitary functioning kidney.

Primary Aldosteronism

The most common causes of primary aldosteronism are a unilateral aldosterone-producing adenoma and bilateral adrenal hyperplasia. Because aldosterone is the principal ligand for the mineralocorticoid receptor in the distal nephron, excessive aldosterone production causes excessive renal Na^+-K^+ exchange, often resulting in hypokalemia. The diagnosis should always be suggested when hypertension is accompanied by either unprovoked hypokalemia (serum K^+ <3.5 mmol/L in the absence of diuretic therapy) or a tendency to develop excessive hypokalemia during diuretic therapy (serum K^+ <3.0 mmol/L). However, more than one third of patients do not have hypokalemia on initial presentation, and the diagnosis should be considered in any patient with refractory hypertension.

The diagnosis is confirmed by the demonstration of nonsuppressible hyperaldosteronism during salt loading, followed by adrenal vein sampling to distinguish between a unilateral adenoma and bilateral hyperplasia. Laparoscopic adrenalectomy is the treatment of choice for unilateral aldosterone-producing adenoma, whereas pharmacologic mineralocorticoid-receptor blockade with eplerenone is the treatment for bilateral adrenal hyperplasia.

Mendelian Forms of Hypertension

Nine very rare forms of severe early-onset hypertension are inherited as mendelian traits. In each case, the hypertension is mineralocorticoid induced and involves excessive activation of the epithelial sodium channel ($E_{Na}C$), the final common pathway for reabsorption of sodium from the distal nephron. The resultant salt-dependent hypertension can be caused by gain-of-function mutations of $E_{Na}C$ (Liddle's syndrome) or the mineralocorticoid receptor (a rare form of pregnancy-induced hypertension) or by increased production or decreased clearance of mineralocorticoids including aldosterone (glucocorticoid-remediable aldosteronism), deoxycorticosterone (17-hydroxylase deficiency), and cortisol (syndrome of apparent mineralocorticoid excess). Mutations in the potassium-channel subunit KCNJ5 and in TWIK-related acid-sensitive K^+ channel (TASK) have been linked to familial aldosteronism because they increase aldosterone release or increase proliferation of zona glomerulosa cells.

Pheochromocytoma and Paraganglioma

Pheochromocytomas are rare catecholamine-producing tumors of the adrenal chromaffin cells. Paragangliomas are even rarer extra-adrenal catecholamine-producing or nonfunctional tumors of sympathetic and parasympathetic ganglia. The diagnosis should be suggested when hypertension is accompanied by paroxysms of headaches, palpitations, pallor, or diaphoresis. However, the most common presentation of pheochromocytoma is that of an adrenal incidentaloma—an incidental adrenal mass discovered unexpectedly on abdominal imaging for another indication. In some patients, pheochromocytoma is misdiagnosed as panic disorder. A family history of early-onset hypertension may suggest pheochromocytoma as part of the multiple endocrine neoplasia (MEN) syndromes or familial paraganglioma. If the diagnosis is missed, then outpouring of catecholamines from the tumor can cause an unsuspected hypertensive crisis during unrelated radiologic or surgical procedures; the perioperative mortality rate exceeds 80% in such circumstances.

Laboratory confirmation of pheochromocytoma is made by demonstration of elevated levels of plasma or urinary metanephrines; these are methylated derivatives of norepinephrine and epinephrine that are made in the adrenal medulla and continually leak out into the plasma even between BP spikes. Pheochromocytomas are typically large adrenal tumors that can usually be localized by CT or MR imaging, although nuclear scanning with

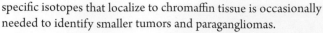

specific isotopes that localize to chromaffin tissue is occasionally needed to identify smaller tumors and paragangliomas.

Treatment of these tumors is by surgical resection. Patients must receive adequate preoperative management with α-blockade followed by β-blockade and volume expansion to prevent the hemodynamic swings that can occur during surgical manipulation of the tumor. For unresectable tumors, chronic therapy with the α-adrenergic blocker phenoxybenzamine is usually effective.

Pheochromocytoma is a great masquerader, and the large differential diagnosis includes causes of neurogenic hypertension such as sympathomimetic agents (e.g., cocaine, methamphetamine), baroreflex failure, and obstructive sleep apnea. A history of surgery and radiation therapy for head and neck tumors suggests the possibility of baroreceptor damage. Loud snoring, obesity, and somnolence suggest obstructive sleep apnea. Weight loss, continuous positive airway pressure, and corrective surgery improve BP control in some patients with sleep apnea.

Other causes of secondary hypertension include nonsteroidal anti-inflammatory drugs (NSAIDs), hypothyroidism, hyperthyroidism, coarctation of the aorta, and immunosuppressive drugs, especially cyclosporine and tacrolimus.

TREATMENT OF HYPERTENSION

Prescription medication is the cornerstone for treatment of hypertension. Lifestyle modification should be used as an essential adjunct but not as an alternative to life-saving BP pharmacotherapy. Most dietary sodium comes from processed foods, and daily salt consumption can be reduced from 10 to 6 g by teaching patients to read food labels (6 g of NaCl = 2.4 g of Na$^+$ = 100 mmol of Na$^+$). The Dietary Approach to Stop Hypertension (DASH) diet, which is rich in fresh fruits and vegetables (for high potassium content) and low-fat dairy products, has been shown to lower BP in feeding trials. Other lifestyle modifications that can lower BP include weight loss in overweight patients with hypertension, regular aerobic exercise, smoking cessation, and moderation in alcohol intake.

The list of drugs marketed for the treatment of hypertension in the United States is shown in Table 12-6. Major contraindications and side effects of these drugs are summarized in Table 12-7. The following sections describe which drugs should be used for which groups of patients.

Patients with Uncomplicated Hypertension

Current guidelines (Figure 12-11) recommend blood pressure goals of less than 150/90 mm Hg for elderly patients and less than 140/90 mm Hg for most other patients. Some experts recommend the goal of less than 140/90 mm Hg in patients older than 60 years if they are not frail and are able to tolerate such treatment without side effects. Multiple guidelines recommend initiating drug treatment with one or more of three classes of first-line drugs, which have additive or synergistic effects when used in combination: (1) CCBs, (2) renin-angiotensin system blockers—either ACE inhibitors or ARBs, and (3) thiazide diuretics.

The European Society of Hypertension makes no specific drug class recommendation, arguing that the most effective drugs are those that the patient can tolerate and will take. Long-term patient adherence is best with an ARB, intermediate with an ACEI or CCB, and worst with a thiazide. The British Hypertension Society advocates a treatment strategy that is based on the patient's age and ethnicity. It recommends initiating therapy with an ACEI or ARB for younger white patients (<55 years of age), who often have high-renin hypertension, but a CCB or diuretic for older and black patients, who often have low-renin hypertension.

A growing body of evidence from clinical trials emphasizes the overriding importance of lowering BP with combinations of drugs rather than belaboring the choice of a single, best agent to begin therapy. Primary hypertension is multifactorial, and typically several medications with different mechanisms of action (see Table 12-4) are required simultaneously to reach the BP goal. In most patients with hypertension, low-dose combination drug therapy is the only way to control BP adequately while minimizing side effects. With many classes of antihypertensive medications, the dose-response relationship for BP is rather flat. Most of the BP lowering occurs at the lower end of the dose range. However, many of the side effects are steeply dose dependent, becoming problematic mainly at the high end of the clinical dose range. Therefore, low-dose combinations achieve therapeutic synergy and minimize side effects. Fixed-dose combinations reduce pill burden and cost.

One highly effective, well-tolerated combination is a CCB plus an ACEI or ARB. A recent clinical trial demonstrated a large benefit of combination therapy with an ACEI plus a dihydropyridine CCB, compared with the combination of an ACEI plus a thiazide diuretic, in reducing cardiovascular events in high-risk patients (level A evidence). In contrast, the combination of an ARB plus an ACEI ("dual renin-angiotensin system blockade") should be avoided because it results in deterioration of renal function and increases the risk of hypotension without added cardiovascular benefit (level A evidence).

Kaiser-Permanente of Northern California, a large managed care organization, has increased the control of hypertension among its membership over the last decade from 44% to an astounding 80% by increasing access through walk-in BP checks by medical assistants, establishing registry rounds to identify and contact patients with elevated office BP, and instituting a system-wide simple medication treatment protocol that features once-daily combination therapy.

Along with antihypertensive medication, lipid-lowering medication should be strongly considered as an integral part of most antihypertensive regimens. A sizeable cardiovascular benefit of adding 10 mg of the HMG-CoA reductase inhibitor atorvastatin to antihypertensive therapy was demonstrated in patients older than 60 years of age who had moderate hypertension and an average LDL-cholesterol level of only 130 mg/dL (level A evidence).

Hypertension in African Americans

Hypertension disproportionately affects African Americans. The explanation is unknown, but the dominant importance of environmental factors is indicated by geographic variation in hypertension prevalence among African-origin and European-origin populations. Hypertension is rare among Africans living in Africa and is more prevalent in several European countries than it is in

TABLE 12-6 ORAL ANTIHYPERTENSIVE AGENTS

DRUG	DOSE RANGE, TOTAL (MG/DAY)	DOSES PER DAY	DRUG	DOSE RANGE, TOTAL (MG/DAY)	DOSES PER DAY
DIURETICS			**ANGIOTENSIN-RECEPTOR BLOCKERS**		
Thiazide Diuretics			Azilsartan	40-80	1
			Candesartan	8-32	1
Hydrochlorothiazide (HCTZ)	6.25-50	1	Eprosartan	400-800	1-2
Chlorthalidone	6.25-25	1	Irbesartan	150-300	1
Indapamide	1.25-5	1	Losartan	25-100	2
Metolazone	2.5-5	1	Olmesartin	5-40	1
			Telmisartan	20-80	1
Loop Diuretics			Valsartan	80-320	1-2
Furosemide	20-160	2	**DIRECT RENIN INHIBITOR**		
Torsemide	2.5-20	1-2	Aliskiren	75-300	1
Bumetanide	0.5-2	2	**α-BLOCKERS**		
Ethacrynic acid	25-100	2	Doxazosin	1-16	1
Potassium-Sparing Diuretics			Prazosin	1-40	2-3
Amiloride	5-20	1	Terazosin	1-20	1
Triamterene	25-100	1	Phenoxybenzamine	20-120	2 for pheochromocytoma
Spironolactone	12.5-400	1-2	**CENTRAL SYMPATHOLYTICS**		
Eplerenone	25-100	1-2	Clonidine	0.2-1.2	2-3
β-BLOCKERS			Clonidine patch	0.1-0.6	Weekly
Acebutolol	200-800	2	Guanabenz	2-32	2
Atenolol	25-100	1	Guanfacine	1-3	1 (at bedtime)
Betaxolol	5-20	1	Methyldopa	250-1000	2
Bisoprolol	2.5-20	1	Reserpine	0.05-0.25	1
Carteolol	2.5-10	1	**DIRECT VASODILATORS**		
Metoprolol	50-450	2	Hydralazine	10-200	2
Metoprolol XL	50-200	1-2	Minoxidil	2.5-100	1
Nadolol	20-320	1	**FIXED-DOSE COMBINATIONS**		
Nebivolol	5-40	1	Azilsartan/chlorthalidone	40-80/12.5-25	1
Penbutolol	10-80	1	Aliskiren/HCTZ	75-300/12.5-25	1
Pindolol	10-60	2	Amiloride/HCTZ	5/50	1
Propranolol	40-180	2	Amlodipine/benazepril	2.5-5/10-20	1
Propranolol LA	60-180	1-2	Amlodipine/valsartan	5-10/160-320	1
Timolol	20-60	2	Amlodipine/olmesartan	5-10/20-40	1
β/α-BLOCKERS			Atenolol/chlorthalidone	50-100/25	1
Labetalol	200-2400	2	Benazepril/HCTZ	5-20/6.25-25	1
Carvedilol	6.25-50	2	Bisoprolol/HCTZ	2.5-10/6.25	1
CALCIUM-CHANNEL BLOCKERS			Candesartan/HCTZ	16-32/12.5-25	1
Dihydropyridines			Enalapril/HCTZ	5-10/25	1-2
Amlodipine	2.5-10	1	Eprosartan/HCTZ	600/12.5-25	1
Felodipine	2.5-20	1-2	Fosinopril/HCTZ	10-20/12.5	1
Isradipine CR	2.5-20	2	Irbesartan/HCTZ	15-30/12.5-25	1
Nicardipine SR	30-120	2	Losartan/HCTZ	50-100/12.5-25	1
Nifedipine XL	30-120	1	Olmesartan/amlodipine	20-40/5-10	1
Nisoldipine	10-40	1-2	Olmesartan/HCTZ	20-40/12.5-25	1
Nondihydropyridines			Olmesartan/amlodipine/HCTZ	20-40/5-10/12.5-25	1
Diltiazem CD	120-540	1	Spironolactone/HCTZ	25/25	0.5-1
Verapamil HS	120-480	1	Telmisartan/HCTZ	40-80/12.5-25	1
ANGIOTENSIN-CONVERTING ENZYME INHIBITORS			Trandolapril/verapamil	2-4/180-240	1
			Triamterene/HCTZ	37.5/25	0.5-1
Benazepril	10-80	1-2	Valsartan/HCTZ	80-160/12.5-25	1
Captopril	25-150	2	Valsartan/amlodipine/HCTZ	80-160/5-10/12.5-25	1
Enalapril	2.5-40	2			
Fosinopril	10-80	1-2			
Lisinopril	5-80	1-2			
Moexipril	7.5-30	1			
Perindopril	4-16	1			
Quinapril	5-80	1-2			
Ramipril	2.5-20	1			
Trandolapril	1-8	1			

TABLE 12-7 MAJOR CONTRAINDICATIONS AND SIDE EFFECTS OF ANTIHYPERTENSIVE DRUGS

DRUG CLASS	MAJOR CONTRAINDICATIONS	SIDE EFFECTS
DIURETICS		
Thiazides	Gout	Insulin resistance, new-onset type 2 diabetes (especially in combination with β-blockers)
		Hypokalemia, hyponatremia
		Hypertriglyceridemia
		Hyperuricemia, precipitation of gout
		Erectile dysfunction (more than other drug classes)
		Potentiate nondepolarizing muscle relaxants
		Photosensitive dermatitis
Loop diuretics	Hepatic coma	Interstitial nephritis
		Hypokalemia
		Potentiate succinylcholine
		Potentiate aminoglycoside ototoxicity
Potassium-sparing diuretics	Serum K >5.5 mEq/L	Fatal hyperkalemia if used with salt substitutes, ACEIs, ARBs, high-potassium foods, NSAIDs
	GFR <30 mg/mL/1.73 m^2	
β-Blockers	Heart block	Insulin resistance, new-onset type 2 diabetes (especially in combination with thiazides)
	Asthma	
	Depression	Heart block, acute decompensated CHF
	Cocaine and/or methamphetamine abuse	Bronchospasm
		Depression, nightmares, fatigue
		Cold extremities, claudication (β$_2$ effect)
		Stevens-Johnson syndrome
		Agranulocytosis
ACEIs	Pregnancy	Cough
	Bilateral renal artery stenosis	Hyperkalemia
	Hyperkalemia	Angioedema
		Leukopenia
		Fetal toxicity
		Cholestatic jaundice (rare fulminant hepatic necrosis if the drug is not discontinued)
ARBs	Pregnancy	Hyperkalemia
	Bilateral renal artery stenosis	Angioedema (very rare)
	Hyperkalemia	Fetal toxicity
Direct renin inhibitors	Pregnancy	Hyperkalemia
	Bilateral renal artery stenosis	Diarrhea
	Hyperkalemia	Fetal toxicity
Dihydropyridine CCBs	As monotherapy in chronic kidney disease with proteinuria	Headaches
		Flushing
		Ankle edema
		CHF
		Gingival hyperplasia
		Esophageal reflux
Nondihydropyridine CCBs	Heart block	Bradycardia, atrioventricular block (especially with verapamil)
	Systolic heart failure	Constipation (often severe with verapamil)
		Worsening of systolic function, CHF
		Gingival edema and/or hypertrophy
		Increase cyclosporine blood levels
		Esophageal reflux
α-Blockers	Monotherapy for hypertension	Orthostatic hypotension
	Orthostatic hypotension	Drug tolerance (in the absence of diuretic therapy)
	Systolic heart failure	Ankle edema
	Left ventricular dysfunction	CHF
		First-dose effect (acute hypotension)
		Potentiate hypotension with PDE5 inhibitors (e.g., sildenafil)
Central sympatholytics	Orthostatic hypotension	Depression, dry mouth, lethargy
		Erectile dysfunction (dose dependent)
		Rebound hypertension with clonidine withdrawal
		Coombs-positive hemolytic anemia and elevated LFTs with α-methyldopa
Direct vasodilators	Orthostatic hypotension	Reflex tachycardia
		Fluid retention
		Hirsutism, pericardial effusion with minoxidil
		Lupus with hydralazine

ACEIs, Angiotensin-converting enzyme inhibitors; ARBs, angiotensin-receptor blockers; CCBs, calcium-channel blockers; CHF, congestive heart failure; GFR, glomerular filtration rate; LFTs, liver function tests; MI, myocardial infarction; NSAIDs, nonsteroidal anti-inflammatory drugs; PDE5, phosphodiesterase type 5.

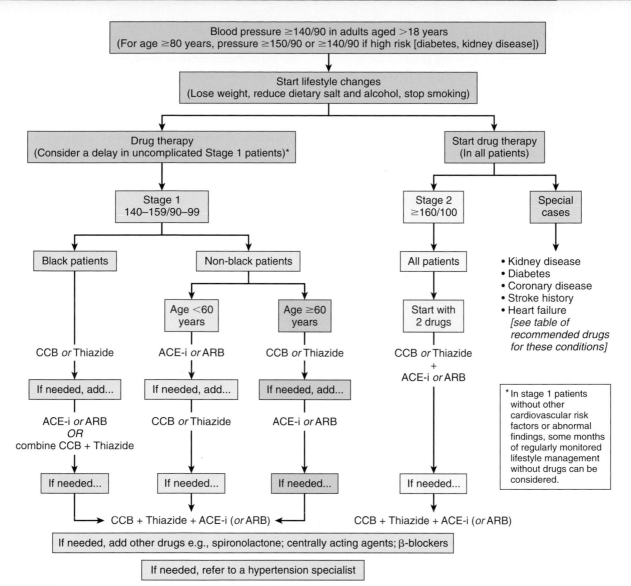

FIGURE 12-11 2014 Hypertension Management Algorithm Recommended by the American Society of Hypertension and the International Society of Hypertension. At any stage it is entirely appropriate to seek help from a hypertension expert if treatment is proving difficult. In patients with stage 1 hypertension in whom there is no history of cardiovascular, stroke, or renal events or evidence of abnormal findings and who do not have diabetes or other major risk factors, drug therapy can be delayed for a short trial of lifestyle modification; however, most patients will require medication to achieve recommended blood pressure targets. In all other patients (including those with stage 2 hypertension), it is recommended that drug therapy be started as soon as the diagnosis of hypertension is made. Blood pressure values are in mm Hg. ACE-i, Angiotensin-convertingenzyme inhibitors; ARB, angiotensin receptor blocker; CCB, calcium channel blocker; thiazide, thiazide or thiazide-like diuretics. (From Weber MA, Schiffrin EL, White WB et al: Clinical practice guidelines for the management of hypertension in the community. A statement by the American Society of Hypertension and the International Society of Hypertension, J Clin Hypertens 16:14–26, 2014.)

the United States. As monotherapy for hypertension, an ACEI (or ARB) typically yields a smaller decrease in BP in an African American patient than it does in a non–African American patient and therefore affords less protection against stroke. However, when an ACEI or ARB is used in combination with a CCB or a diuretic, antihypertensive efficacy is amplified and ethnic differences disappear. When used as part of an appropriate multidrug regimen, an ACEI-based treatment can achieve excellent control of hypertension in African American patients with hypertensive nephrosclerosis, and it slows the deterioration in renal function.

Hypertensive Nephrosclerosis

Hypertension is the second most common cause of chronic kidney disease, accounting for more than 25% of cases.

Hypertensive nephrosclerosis is the result of persistently uncontrolled hypertension causing chronic glomerular ischemia. Typically, proteinuria is mild (<0.5 g/24 hours). Nondiabetic chronic kidney disease is a compelling indication for ACEI-based or ARB-based antihypertensive therapy. ACEIs cause greater dilation of the efferent renal arterioles, thereby minimizing intraglomerular hypertension. In contrast, arterial vasodilators such as dihydropyridine CCBs, when used without an ACEI or ARB, preferentially dilate the afferent arteriole and impair renal autoregulation. Glomerular hypertension can result if the systemic BP is not sufficiently lowered. The ACEI should be withdrawn only if the rise in serum creatinine exceeds 30% of the baseline value or the serum potassium level increases to greater than 5.6 mmol/L.

Hypertensive Patients with Diabetes

Compared with its 25% prevalence in the general adult population, hypertension is present in 75% of patients with diabetes and is a major factor contributing to excessive risk of myocardial infarction, stroke, heart failure, microvascular complications, and diabetic nephropathy progressing to end-stage renal disease. The Action to Control Cardiovascular Risk in Diabetes blood pressure trial (ACCORD BP) failed to show reduced overall mortality or cardiovascular mortality from lowering the systolic BP to less than 120 mm Hg in patients with type 2 diabetes mellitus. However, the risk of stroke was reduced by 60% in these patients. The findings from the ACCORD trial have led to revised European and British hypertension guidelines increasing the target BP goal from 130/80 mm Hg to 140/90 mm Hg in most diabetic patients. However, the benefits of lowering systolic BP to less than 130 mm Hg in reducing the risk of stroke in diabetics and nondiabetic patients with high cardiovascular risks remains to be further determined. An ACEI or ARB plus a CCB is an excellent combination to treat hypertension in patients with diabetes. Thiazide diuretics and standard β-blockers exacerbate glucose intolerance, whereas the vasodilating β-blockers such as carvedilol and nebivolol have neutral or possibly beneficial effects.

Hypertensive Patients with Coronary Artery Disease

To lower myocardial oxygen demands in patients with coronary artery disease, the antihypertensive regimen should reduce BP without causing reflex tachycardia. For this reason, a β-blocker is often prescribed in conjunction with a dihydropyridine CCB such as amlodipine. β-Blockers are indicated for patients with hypertension who have sustained a myocardial infarction and for most patients with chronic heart failure. ACEIs are indicated for almost all patients with left ventricular systolic dysfunction and may be considered after myocardial infarction even in the absence of ventricular dysfunction. Among patients with stable coronary artery disease, a cardioprotective effect of ACE inhibition has also been demonstrated in those with moderate cardiovascular risk profiles but not in those with lower risk profiles.

Isolated Systolic Hypertension in Older Adults

In developed countries, systolic pressure rises progressively with age; if individuals live long enough, then almost all (>90%) develop hypertension. Diastolic pressure rises until the age of 50 years and decreases thereafter, producing a progressive rise in pulse pressure (i.e., systolic pressure minus diastolic pressure) (Fig. 12-12).

Different hemodynamic faults underlie hypertension in younger and older persons. Patients who develop hypertension before 50 years of age typically have *combined systolic and diastolic hypertension*: systolic pressure greater than 140 mm Hg *and* diastolic pressure greater than 90 mm Hg. The main hemodynamic fault is vasoconstriction at the level of the resistance arterioles. In contrast, most patients who develop hypertension after 50 years of age have *isolated systolic hypertension*: systolic pressure greater than 140 mm Hg but diastolic pressure lower than 90 mm Hg (often <80 mm Hg). In isolated systolic hypertension, the primary hemodynamic fault is decreased distensibility of the aorta and other large conduit arteries (see Fig. 12-12). Collagen replaces elastin in the elastic lamina of the aorta, an age-dependent process that is accelerated by atherosclerosis and hypertension. The cardiovascular risk associated with isolated systolic hypertension is related to pulsatility, the repetitive pounding of the blood vessels with each cardiac cycle and a more rapid return of the arterial pulse wave from the periphery, both begetting more systolic hypertension. In the United States and Europe, the majority of uncontrolled hypertension occurs in older patients with isolated systolic hypertension. A BP of 160/60 mm Hg (pulse pressure, 100 mm Hg) carries twice the

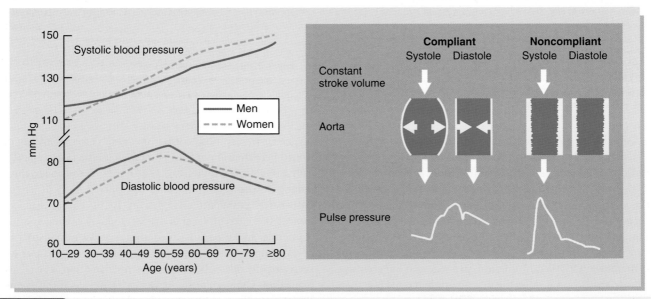

FIGURE 12-12 Age-dependent changes in systolic and diastolic blood pressure in the United States *(left).* Schematic diagram explains the relation between aortic compliance and pulse pressure *(right).* (*Left,* From Burt V, Whelton P, Rocella EJ, et al: Prevalence of hypertension in the U.S. adult population: results from the Third National Health and Nutrition Examination Survey, 1988–1991, Hypertension 25:305–313, 1995; *Right,* Courtesy Dr. Stanley Franklin, University of California, Irvine, Calif.)

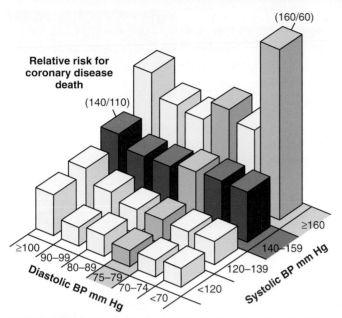

FIGURE 12-13 Joint influences of systolic blood pressure (BP) and diastolic BP on the risk of fatal coronary heart disease in the Multiple Risk Factor Intervention Trial. (Neaton JD, Wentworth D: Serum cholesterol, blood pressure, cigarette smoking, and death from coronary heart disease: overall findings and differences by age for 316,099 white men, Arch Intern Med 152:56–64, 1992.)

risk of fatal coronary heart disease as a BP of 140/110 mm Hg (pulse pressure, 30 mm Hg) (Fig. 12-13).

In older persons with isolated systolic hypertension, lowering the systolic pressure from more than 160 to less than 150 mm Hg reduces the risks of stroke, myocardial infarction, and overall cardiovascular mortality; it also reduces heart failure admissions and slows the progression of dementia (level A evidence). Trial data do not yet exist in older persons to determine whether treatment of isolated elevations in systolic pressure below 140 mm Hg is beneficial. However, in the absence of such data, treatment may be warranted to prevent progression of systolic hypertension, if the patient can tolerate the treatment without side effects such as orthostatic hypotension.

The combination of a low-dose thiazide diuretic with a dihydropyridine CCB or an ACEI reduces the risk of cardiovascular events in older patients with isolated systolic hypertension (level A evidence). To prevent orthostatic hypotension, medication should be titrated to standing BP, and one low-dose medication should be started at a time.

Blood Pressure Lowering for Secondary Prevention of Stroke

Most neurologists do not recommend BP reduction during an acute stroke. After the acute phase, BP should be lowered with a thiazide diuretic, and an ACEI or additional drugs should be added as needed to achieve BP levels lower than 140/90 mm Hg; whether BP should be lowered further is unclear.

Hypertensive Disorders of Women

Oral contraceptives cause a small increase in BP in most women but rarely cause a large increase into the hypertensive range. If hypertension develops, oral contraceptive therapy should be

discontinued in favor of other methods of contraception. Oral estrogen replacement therapy seems to cause a small increase in BP. In contrast, transdermal estrogen (which bypasses first-pass hepatic metabolism) seems to cause a small but consistent decrease in BP.

Hypertension, the most common nonobstetric complication of pregnancy, is present in 10% of all pregnant women. One third of these cases are caused by chronic hypertension, and two thirds are caused by preeclampsia, which is defined as an increase in BP to 160/110 mm Hg or greater after the 20th week of gestation accompanied by proteinuria (>300 mg/24 hours) and pathologic edema, sometimes accompanied by seizures (eclampsia) and the multisystem HELLP syndrome of hemolysis (H), elevated liver enzymes (EL), and low platelets (LP). Oral drug therapy should be initiated with any one of three preferred drugs: labetalol (400 to 2400 mg daily). Intravenous labetalol (0.5 to 2 mg/minute up to a cumulative dose of 300 mg) has replaced hydralazine as the drug of choice to treat severe preeclampsia/eclampsia.

Resistant Hypertension

Resistant hypertension, defined as persistence of usual BP above 140/90 mm Hg despite treatment with full doses of three or more different classes of medications in rational combination and including a diuretic, is the most common reason for referral to a hypertension specialist. In practice, most of these patients have pseudoresistant hypertension due to (1) *white-coat aggravation*, a white-coat reaction superimposed on chronic hypertension that is well controlled with medication outside the physician's office; (2) an inadequate medical regimen; (3) nonadherence; or (4) ingestion of pressor substances. Common shortcomings of the medical regimen include undertreatment of hypertension with monotherapy and use of clonidine, a potent central sympatholytic that causes rebound hypertension between doses particularly, with PRN dosing. Several common causes of pseudoresistant hypertension are related to the patient's behavior, including medication nonadherence, recidivism with lifestyle modification (e.g., obesity, high-salt diet, excessive alcohol intake), and habitual use of pressor substances such as sympathomimetics (e.g., tobacco, cocaine, methamphetamine, phenylephrine-containing cold or herbal remedies) or NSAIDs, with the latter causing renal sodium retention. Once these behavioral factors have been excluded, the search should begin for causes of secondary hypertension.

The most common forms of secondary hypertension are chronic kidney disease and primary aldosteronism. Significant impairment in renal function can be present with serum creatinine in the range of 1.2 to 1.4 mg/dL or even lower, particularly in older patients with little muscle mass. To avoid this pitfall, calculation of the glomerular filtration rate (GFR) by equations based on serum creatinine, age, weight, and measurement of the urinary albumin-to-creatinine ratio from a spot-urine specimen should be an essential part of the routine evaluation of every patient with hypertension. Either a loop diuretic (e.g., a furosemide) or a potent thiazide-type diuretic (e.g, chlorthalidone) may be required to control hypertension in patients with chronic kidney disease. The treatment of primary aldosteronism was discussed earlier.

After exclusion of pseudoresistant hypertension and secondary hypertension, some patients have severe drug-resistant primary hypertension. Fourth- and fifth-line therapies include a vasodilating β-blocker and spironolactone (even in the absence of primary aldosteronism). Percutaneous catheter-based renal denervation is being investigated as a novel interventional approach to treat drug-resistant hypertension.

Acute Severe Hypertension

Of all the patients in the emergency department, 25% have an elevated BP. *Hypertensive emergencies* are acute, often severe, elevations in BP that are accompanied by acute or rapidly progressive target-organ dysfunction such as myocardial or cerebral ischemia or infarction, pulmonary edema, or renal failure. *Hypertensive urgencies* are severe elevations in BP without severe symptoms and without evidence of acute or progressive target-organ dysfunction. The key distinction and approach to the patient depends on the state of the patient and the assessment of target-organ damage, not simply the absolute level of BP. The full-blown clinical picture of a hypertensive emergency is a critically ill patient with a BP greater than 220/140 mm Hg, headaches, confusion, blurred vision, nausea and vomiting, seizures, heart failure, oliguria, and grade III or IV hypertensive retinopathy (Fig. 12-14).

Hypertensive emergencies require immediate admission in an intensive care unit for intravenous therapy and continuous BP monitoring, whereas hypertensive urgencies can often be managed with oral medications and appropriate outpatient follow-up in 24 to 72 hours. The most common hypertensive cardiac emergencies are acute aortic dissection, hypertension after coronary artery bypass grafting, acute myocardial infarction, and unstable angina. Other hypertensive emergencies include eclampsia, head trauma, severe body burns, postoperative bleeding from vascular suture lines, and epistaxis that cannot be controlled with anterior and posterior nasal packing. Neurologic emergencies, which include acute ischemic stroke, hemorrhagic stroke, subarachnoid hemorrhage, and hypertensive encephalopathy, can be difficult to distinguish from one another. Hypertensive encephalopathy is characterized by severe hypertensive retinopathy (i.e., retinal hemorrhages and exudates with or without papilledema) and a posterior leukoencephalopathy affecting mainly the white matter of the parieto-occipital regions as seen on cerebral MR imaging or CT scanning. A new focal neurologic deficit suggests a stroke-in-evolution, which demands a much more conservative approach to correcting the elevated BP.

In most other hypertensive emergencies, the goal of parenteral therapy is to achieve a controlled and gradual lowering of BP. A good rule of thumb is to lower the initially elevated arterial pressure by 10% in the first hour and by an additional 15% over the next 3 to 12 hours to a BP of no less than 160/110 mm Hg. BP can be reduced further over the next 48 hours. Unnecessarily rapid correction of the elevated BP to completely normal values places the patient at high risk for worsening cerebral, cardiac, and renal ischemia. In chronic hypertension, cerebral autoregulation is reset to higher-than-normal BPs. This compensatory adjustment prevents tissue overperfusion (i.e., increased intracranial pressure) at very high BPs, but it also predisposes the patient to

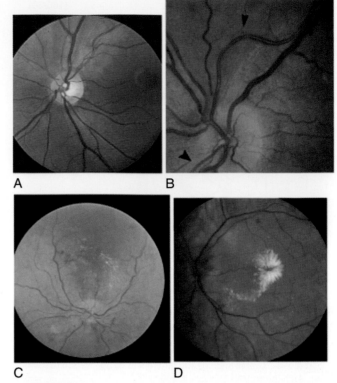

A   B

C   D

FIGURE 12-14 Hypertensive retinopathy is traditionally divided into four grades. **A,** Grade 1 shows very early and minor changes in a young patient; increased tortuosity of a retinal vessel and increased reflectiveness (silver wiring) of a retinal artery are seen at the one o'clock position in this view. Otherwise, the fundus is completely normal. **B,** Grade 2 also shows increased tortuosity and silver wiring *(arrowheads)*. In addition, nipping of the venules at arteriovenous crossings is visible *(arrow)*. **C,** Grade 3 shows the same changes as grade 2 plus flame-shaped retinal hemorrhages and soft cotton-wool exudates. **D,** In grade 4, swelling of the optic disc (papilledema) is observed, retinal edema is present, and hard exudates may collect around the fovea, producing a typical macular star. (From Forbes CD, Jackson WF: Color atlas and text of clinical medicine, ed 3, London, 2003, Mosby.)

tissue underperfusion (i.e., cerebral ischemia) when an elevated BP is lowered too quickly. In certain clinical settings, such as aortic dissection or acute pulmonary edema, more rapid reduction in BP may be required to avoid further propagation of dissection or to minimize myocardial oxygen demand and increase oxygenation. Secondary causes of hypertension should be considered in every patient who is admitted to the intensive care unit with hypertensive crisis.

Parenteral agents for the treatment of hypertensive emergency are summarized in Table 12-8. Intravenous labetalol (a combined α- and β-blocker) is an effective first-line drug for many hypertensive crises, particularly myocardial ischemia with preserved ventricular function. Sodium nitroprusside, a nitric oxide donor, is popular because it can be titrated rapidly to control BP. Intravenous nitroglycerin, another nitric oxide donor, is indicated mainly for hypertension in the setting of acute coronary syndrome or decompensated heart failure. Nicardipine is a parenteral dihydropyridine CCB that is particularly useful in the postoperative cardiac patient and in patients with renal failure to avoid the thiocyanate toxicity with nitroprusside. Urapidil is a new central sympatholytic agent.

TABLE 12-8 INTRAVENOUS DRUGS FOR HYPERTENSIVE EMERGENCIES

DRUG	ONSET OF ACTION	HALF-LIFE	DOSE	CONTRAINDICATIONS AND SIDE-EFFECTS
Labetalol	5-10 min	3-6 hours	0.25-0.5 mg/kg; 2-4 mg/min until goal BP is reached, thereafter 5-20 mg/hr	2nd or 3rd degree AV block; systolic heart failure, COPD (relative); bradycardia
Nicardipine	5-15 min	30-40 min	5-15 mg/hr as continuous infusion, starting dose 5 mg/hr, increase Q 15-30 min with 2.5 mg until goal BP, thereafter decrease to 3 mg/hr	Liver failure
Nitroprusside	Immediate	1-2 min	0.3-10 μg/kg/min, increase by 0.5 μg/kg/min Q 5 min until goal BP	Liver/kidney failure (relative), cyanide toxicity
Nitroglycerine	1-5 min	3-5 min	5-200 μg/min, 5 μg/min increase Q 5 min	
Urapadil	3-5 min	4-6 hrs	12.5-25 mg as bolus injections; 5-40 mg/hr as continuous infusion	
Esmolol	1-2 min	10-30 min	0.5-1.0 mg/kg as bolus; 50-300 μg/kg/min as continuous infusion	2nd or 3rd degree AV block, systolic heart failure, COPD (relative); bradycardia
Phentolamine	1-2 min	3-5 min	1-5 mg, repeat after 5-15 min until goal BP is reached; 0.5-1 mg/hr as continuous infusion	Tachyarrhythmia, angina pectoris

Modified from van den Born BJ, Beutler JJ, Gaillard CA, et al: Dutch guideline for the management of hypertensive crisis–2010 revision, Neth J Med 69:248–255, 2011.

Most patients in the emergency department with hypertensive urgencies are nonadherent to their medical regimen or are being treated with an inadequate regimen. To expedite the necessary changes in medications, outpatient follow-up should be arranged within 72 hours. To manage BP during the short interim period, effective oral medication includes labetalol, clonidine, or captopril, which is a short-acting ACEI.

BPs greater than 160/110 mm Hg are a common incidental finding among patients in emergency departments and other acute care settings for urgent medical or surgical care of symptoms that are unrelated to BP (e.g., musculoskeletal pain, orthopedic injury). In these settings, the elevated BP is more often the first indication of chronic hypertension than a simple physiologic stress reaction, providing an important opportunity to initiate primary care referral for formal evaluation and treatment of chronic hypertension. Home and ambulatory BP monitoring are indicated to determine whether the patient's BP normalizes completely once the acute illness has resolved.

PROGNOSIS

One of the most important prognostic factors in hypertension is ECG or echocardiographic left ventricular hypertrophy, the latter of which is already present in as many as 25% of patients with newly diagnosed hypertension. Left ventricular hypertrophy predisposes the patient to heart failure, atrial fibrillation, and sudden cardiac death.

Because of their relatively short duration (typically <5 years), randomized controlled trials underestimate the lifetime protection against premature disability and death afforded by several decades of antihypertensive therapy in clinical practice. In the Framingham Heart Study, treatment of hypertension for 20 years in middle-aged adults reduced total cardiovascular mortality by 60%, which is considerably greater than the results achieved in most randomized trials, despite the less intense treatment guidelines when therapy was initiated in the 1950s through the 1970s.

PROSPECTUS FOR THE FUTURE

1. Further delineation of genetic causes of hypertension and application of this research to the treatment and prevention of hypertension, including development of pharmacologic and nonpharmacologic therapies that target the various signaling pathways in hypertension and prehypertension.
2. Further work to define the efficacy of catheter-based renal denervation to treat resistant hypertension.
3. Evaluation of drug-eluting stents for the prevention of restenosis after percutaneous revascularization of infrainguinal vascular disease.
4. Further assessment of safety and efficacy of emerging antithrombotic therapies in patients with atrial fibrillation, venous thromboembolism, and vascular disease.
5. Improvements in techniques for noninvasive imaging of the vasculature, including three-dimensional reconstruction using CT angiography, MR angiography, and duplex ultrasonography.

For a deeper discussion on this topic, please see Chapters 67, "Arterial Hypertension," and 68, "Pulmonary Hypertension," in Goldman-Cecil Medicine, *25th Edition.*

SUGGESTED READINGS

ACCORD Study Group: Effects of intensive blood-pressure control in type 2 diabetes mellitus, N Engl J Med 362:1575–1585, 2010.
Bhatt DL, Kandzari DE, O'Neill WW, et al: A controlled trial of renal denervation for resistant hypertension, N Engl J Med 370:1393–1401, 2014.
Eckel RH, Jakicic JM, ARd JD, et al: 2013 AHA/ACC guideline on lifestyle management to reduce cardiovascular risk: a report of the American College of Cardiology/American Heart Association Task Force on Practice Guidelines, J Am Coll Cardiol 63(25 Pt B):2960–2984, 2014.
EINSTEIN–PE Investigators: Oral rivaroxaban for the treatment of symptomatic pulmonary embolism, N Engl J Med 366:1287–1297, 2012, 2012.
Kearon C, Akl E, Comerota A, et al: Antithrombotic therapy for VTE disease: antithrombotic therapy and prevention of thrombosis, 9th ed: American College of Chest Physicians evidence-based clinical practice guidelines, Chest 141(Suppl):e419S–e494S, 2012.
Jaff M, McMurtry S, Archer S, et al: Management of massive and submassive pulmonary embolism, iliofemoral deep vein thrombosis, and chronic thromboembolic pulmonary hypertension: a scientific statement from the American Heart Association, Circulation 123:1788–1830, 2011.
Jamerson K, Weber MA, Bakris GL, et al: for the ACCOMPLISH Trial Investigators: Benazepril plus amlodipine or hydrochlorothiazide for hypertension in high-risk patients, N Engl J Med 359:2417–2428, 2008.
James PA, Oparil S, Carter BL, et al: 2014 evidence-based guideline for the management of high blood pressure in adults: report from the panel members

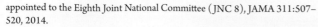
appointed to the Eighth Joint National Committee (JNC 8), JAMA 311:507–520, 2014.

National Institute for Health and Care Excellence: Hypertension: clinical management of primary hypertension in adults, August 2011. NICE guidelines GC127. Available at http://www.nice.org.uk/guidance/CG127. Accessed August 20, 2014.

Mancia G, Fagard R, Narkiewica K, et al: 2013 ESH/ESC guidelines for the management of arterial hypertension: the Task Force for the Management of Arterial Hypertension of the European Society of Hypertension (ESH) and of the European Society of Cardiology (ESC), Eur Heart J 34:2159–2219, 2013.

McLaughlin VV, Archer SL, Badesch DB, et al: ACCF/AHA 2009 expert consensus document on pulmonary hypertension: a report of the American College of Cardiology Foundation Task Force on Expert Consensus Documents and the American Heart Association developed in collaboration with the American College of Chest Physicians; American Thoracic Society, Inc.; and the Pulmonary Hypertension Association, J Am Coll Cardiol 53:1573–1619, 2009.

Rooke T, Hirsch AT, Misra S, et al: 2011 ACCF/AHA focused update of the guideline for the management of patients with peripheral artery disease (updating the 2005 guideline): a report of the American College of Cardiology Foundation/American Heart Association Task Force on Practice Guidelines, J Am Coll Cardiol 58:2020–2045, 2011.

van den Born BJ, Beutler JJ, Gaillard CA, et al: Dutch guideline for the management of hypertensive crisis–2010 revision, Neth J Med 69:248–255, 2011.

Weber MA, Schiffrin EL, White WB, et al: Clinical practice guidelines for the management of hypertension in the community. A statement by the American Society of Hypertension and the International Society of Hypertension, J Clin Hypertens 16:14–26, 2014.

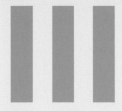

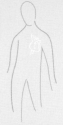

III

Pulmonary and Critical Care Medicine

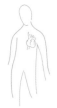

13

Lung in Health and Disease

Sharon Rounds and Matthew D. Jankowich

INTRODUCTION

The lung is part of the respiratory system (Fig. 13-1). The respiratory system includes the centers for respiratory control in the brain cortex and medulla, the spinal cord, and peripheral nerves that innervate the skeletal muscles of respiration and the airways and vessels. The upper airway, including the nose, pharynx, and larynx, is where inspired air is humidified and particulate matter is filtered. The bony structure of the chest wall protects the heart, lungs, and liver, and the lungs are maintained in an inflated state by mechanical coupling of the chest wall with the lungs. The skeletal muscles of respiration include the diaphragm and the accessory muscles; the latter are important when disease causes diaphragm fatigue.

The lung consists of conducting airways, blood vessels, and gas exchange units with alveolar gas spaces and capillaries. The lung is a complex organ with an extensive array of airways and vessels arranged to efficiently transfer the gases necessary for sustaining life. The organ has an immense capacity for gas exchange. It is not a limiting factor in exercise tolerance in healthy individuals, but

The Respiratory System

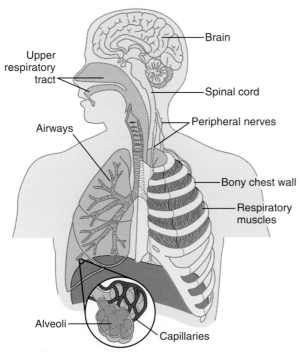

FIGURE 13-1 The respiratory system includes neural structures that control breathing, the chest wall and skeletal muscles of breathing, the upper airway, and lung parenchyma.

gas exchange becomes compromised in lung disease, rendering the host unable to function properly. The most dramatic consequence of acute and chronic abnormalities in lung function is systemic hypoxemia, which causes tissue hypoxia. The sequelae of lung dysfunction include detrimental effects to other organs.

In addition to gas exchange, the lungs have other functions, such as defense against inhaled infectious agents and environmental toxins. The entire cardiac output passes through the pulmonary circulation, which serves as a filter for blood-borne clots and infections. The massive surface area of endothelial cells lining the pulmonary circulation has metabolic functions, such as conversion of angiotensin I to angiotensin II.

Lung disorders are common and range from well-known conditions such as asthma and chronic obstructive pulmonary disease (COPD) to rarely encountered disorders such as lymphangioleiomyomatosis. The chapters in Section III discuss the diagnosis, evaluation, and management of pulmonary disorders that develop in direct response to lung injury and those that develop indirectly through injuries to other organs. Section III also addresses illnesses requiring critical care, such as acute lung injury and sepsis, which are often triggered by injuries to the lung and are frequently managed by pulmonary or critical care specialists.

This chapter reviews the structural-functional relationships of the lung during development, the epidemiology of pulmonary disease, and the classification of pulmonary disorders.

LUNG DEVELOPMENT

The lung begins to develop during the first trimester of pregnancy through complex and overlapping processes that transform the embryonic lung bud into a functioning organ with an extensive airway network, two complete circulatory systems, and millions of alveoli responsible for the transfer of gases to and from the body. Lung development occurs in five consecutive stages: embryonic, pseudoglandular, canalicular or vascular, saccular, and alveolar postnatal (Table 13-1).

During the embryonic stage (between 21 days and 7 weeks' gestation), the rudimentary lung emerges from the foregut as a single epithelial bud surrounded by mesenchymal tissue. This stage is followed by the pseudoglandular stage (between 5 and 17 weeks' gestation), during which repeated monochotomous and dichotomous branching forms rudimentary airways, a process called *branching morphogenesis* (Fig. 13-2). Coinciding with airway formation, new bronchial arteries arise from the aorta.

The canalicular stage (between 17 and 24 weeks' gestation) is characterized by the formation of the acinus, differentiation of the acinar epithelium, and development of the distal pulmonary circulation. Through the processes of angiogenesis and vasculogenesis, capillary networks derived from endothelial cell precursors are formed, extend from and around the distal air spaces, and connect with the developing pulmonary arteries and veins. By the end of this stage, the thickness of the alveolar capillary membrane is similar to that in the adult.

During the saccular or prenatal alveolar stage (between 24 and 38 weeks' gestation), vascularized crests emerging from the parenchyma divide the terminal airway structures called *saccules.* Thinning of the interstitium continues, bringing capillaries from adjacent alveolar structures into close apposition and producing a double capillary network. Near birth, capillaries from opposing networks fuse to form a single network, and capillary volume increases with continuing lung growth and expansion.

During the alveolar postnatal stage (between 36 weeks' gestation and 2 years of age), alveolar development continues, and maturation occurs. The lung continues to grow through the first few years of childhood with the creation of more alveoli through septation of the air sacs. By age 2 years, the lung contains double arterial supplies and venous drainage systems, a complex airway system designed to generate progressive decreases in resistance to airflow as the air travels distally, and a vast alveolar network that efficiently transfers gases to and from the blood.

The processes that drive lung development are tightly controlled, but mishaps occur. Congenital lung disorders include cystic adenomatoid malformation of the lung, lung hypoplasia or agenesis, bullous changes in the lung parenchyma, and abnormalities in the vasculature, including aberrant connections between systemic vessels and lung compartments (e.g., lung sequestration) and congenital absence of one or both pulmonary arteries. In children without congenital abnormalities, lung disorders are uncommon, except for those caused by infection and accidents.

Congenital lung disorders are rare compared with the number of infants born annually with abnormal lung function as a result of prematurity. In premature infants, the type II pneumocytes of the lung are underdeveloped and produce insufficient quantities of surfactant, a surface-active substance produced by specific alveolar epithelial cells that helps to decrease surface tension and prevent alveolar collapse. This disorder is called *infant respiratory distress syndrome* (IRDS). The treatment of IRDS is administration of exogenous surfactant and corticosteroids to enhance lung maturation. To sustain life while allowing maturation, mechanical ventilation and oxygen supplementation are required but may promote the development of bronchopulmonary dysplasia.

● PULMONARY DISEASE
Epidemiology

Diseases of the adult respiratory system are some of the most common clinical entities confronted by physicians. According to the Centers for Disease Control and Prevention data for 2010, three of the top 10 causes of death due to medical illnesses in the United States are lung diseases: lung cancer, chronic lower respiratory diseases, and influenza or pneumonia.

Chronic obstructive pulmonary disease (COPD) is the third leading cause of death and the second leading cause of disability in the United States. At a time when the age-adjusted death rate for other common disorders such as coronary artery disease and stroke is a decreasing, the death rate for COPD continues to increase. More than 16 million Americans are estimated to have COPD, but the number is expected to rise because COPD takes years to develop and the incidence of cigarette smoking (the most common etiologic factor for COPD) is staggering. In 2010, more than 46.6 million Americans were daily smokers, and 40% of

TABLE 13-1	STAGES OF LUNG DEVELOPMENT	
STAGE	**PERIOD**	**COMMENTS**
Embryonic	3-7 wk	Embryonic lung bud emerges from the foregut.
Pseudoglandular	5-17 wk	Airway tree is formed through a process of monochotomous and dichotomous branching accompanied by growth.
Canalicular	17-24 wk	Angiogenesis and vasculogenesis form the developing vascular network.
Saccular	24-38 wk	Alveoli begin to form through thinning of the mesenchyme, apposition of vascular structures with the air spaces, and maturation.
Alveolar (postnatal)	36 wk-2 yr	Further alveoli development and maturation occurs.

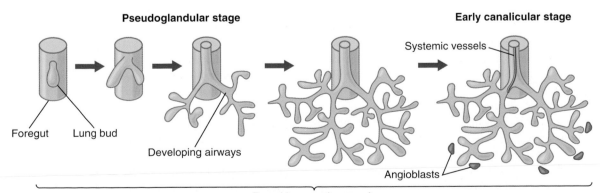

FIGURE 13-2 Lung branching morphogenesis occurs during the pseudoglandular stage of lung development. It is the process by which the embryonic lung develops the primitive airway system through monochotomous and dichotomous branching.

nonsmokers were exposed to secondhand smoke. The true disease burden of COPD is much greater than these numbers indicate.

Other pulmonary conditions are common. Asthma affects 8% of adults and 9.5% of children in the United States. The prevalence, hospitalization rate, and mortality rate related to asthma continue to increase. In 2010, there were 1.1 million hospital discharges for pneumonia and almost 50,000 deaths. Sleep-disordered breathing affects an estimated 7 to 18 million people in the United States, and 1.8 to 4 million of them have severe sleep apnea. Interstitial lung diseases are increasingly recognized, and their true incidence appears to have been underestimated. For example, idiopathic pulmonary fibrosis, the most common of the idiopathic interstitial pneumonias, affects 85,000 to 100,000 Americans annually.

These conditions affect males and females of all ages and races. However, a disproportionate increase in the incidence, morbidity, and mortality related to lung diseases exists for minority populations. This finding is true for COPD, asthma, certain interstitial lung disorders, and other diseases. Although these differences point to genetic differences among these populations, they also indicate differences in culture, socioeconomic status, exposure to pollutants (e.g., inner-city living), and access to health care.

Classification

Lung diseases are often classified on the basis of the affected anatomic areas of the lung (e.g., interstitial lung diseases, pleural diseases, airways diseases) and the physiologic abnormalities detected by pulmonary function testing (e.g., obstructive lung diseases, restrictive lung diseases). Classification schemes based exclusively on physiologic factors are inaccurate because distinctly different disorders with different causes, consequences, and responses to therapy have similar physiologic abnormalities (Fig. 13-3).

The obstructive lung diseases have in common a limitation of airflow, called an *obstructive pattern,* as determined by pulmonary function testing. Obstructive lung diseases include COPD, asthma, and bronchiectasis.

The interstitial lung diseases are less common disorders but are more difficult to categorize because they include more than 120 distinct entities, some of which are inherited, but most do not have an obvious cause. These disorders are characterized by a restrictive physiologic condition due to decreased lung compliance and small lung volumes, which is the reason they are often referred to as *restrictive lung disorders* (e.g., idiopathic pulmonary fibrosis). However, not all interstitial lung diseases exhibit a purely restrictive pattern on pulmonary function testing. They may have airflow limitation as a result of small airway involvement (e.g., sarcoidosis, cryptogenic organizing pneumonia).

In the pulmonary vascular diseases, involvement of the pulmonary vasculature causes increased pulmonary vascular resistance. These diseases range from disorders caused by obstruction to blood flow as a result of blood clots (e.g., pulmonary embolus) to disorders characterized by tissue remodeling and obliteration of blood vessels by vascular remodeling (e.g., pulmonary arterial hypertension, formerly known as primary pulmonary hypertension).

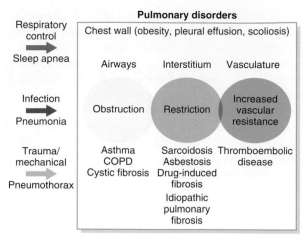

FIGURE 13-3 Lung diseases are caused by abnormalities in the lung structure (e.g., airways, interstitium, vasculature) or in the chest wall or by external forces (e.g., infection). Disorders affecting the lung structure cause physiologic derangements (e.g., obstruction to airflow, restricted lung volumes, pulmonary hypertension, hypoxia). These derangements are not necessarily specific to any particular Lung diseases, but there is extensive overlap among them, so that different disorders can have similar physiologic abnormalities. COPD, Chronic obstructive pulmonary disease.

Disorders of respiratory control include conditions in which extrapulmonary abnormalities cause respiratory system dysfunction and abnormal ventilation. Included are sleep disorders such as obstructive sleep apnea and neuromuscular system disorders such as myasthenia gravis and polymyositis, in which ventilatory abnormalities result from poor excursion of the respiratory muscles.

Disorders of the pleura, chest wall, and mediastinum are classified as such because they affect these structures. Infectious agents, commonly viruses and bacteria, cause infectious diseases of the lung. Neoplastic disorders of the lung include benign (e.g., hamartomas) and malignant (e.g., lung carcinoma) tumors, which can affect the lung parenchyma or its surrounding pleura (e.g., mesothelioma).

● PROSPECTUS FOR THE FUTURE

Important questions about lung development remain. What are the primary stimuli for branching morphogenesis? How does gene regulation alter lung development? How is lung airway and blood vessel development coordinated? What are the environment-gene interactions that cause abnormal lung development and subsequent lung diseases?

There are important fundamental questions about the epidemiology of lung diseases. For example, it is not clear whether or how childhood asthma and adult COPD are related. The role of fine particulate matter air pollution in the pathogenesis of lung diseases is unknown, and the causes and pathogenesis of many lung diseases, such as sarcoidosis, are unclear.

SUGGESTED READINGS

Schraufnagel DE, editor: Breathing in America: diseases, progress, and hope, New York, 2010, American Thoracic Society.

Whitsett JA, Haitchi HM, Maeda Y: Intersections between pulmonary development and disease, Am J Respir Crit Care Med 184:401–406, 2011.

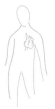

14

General Approach to Patients with Respiratory Disorders

Rizwan Aziz and Brian Casserly

INTRODUCTION

Effective assessment of a patient who may have pulmonary disease requires a detailed history and review of symptoms. Patients with lung disorders often complain of one or more of the following symptoms: dyspnea, fatigue, exercise intolerance, chest tightness, cough, sputum production, and chest pain. Although individually these symptoms are not diagnostic, a combination of symptoms in an individual may point to a specific diagnosis.

Common symptoms of respiratory disease, such as dyspnea and cough, frequently occur with diseases of other organ systems (Table 14-1). For example, dyspnea is a cardinal symptom of heart disease, and cough may be caused by gastroesophageal reflux or chronic sinusitis. An organized approach to the patient, starting with a careful history and a detailed physical examination, further focuses the investigation to determine the cause of the symptom.

For a deeper discussion on this topic, please see Chapter 83, "Approach to the Patient with Respiratory Disease," in Goldman-Cecil Medicine, 25th Edition.

CLINICAL PRESENTATION

Dyspnea (i.e., shortness of breath) is a common complaint of patients with pulmonary disease (Table 14-2). Timing and acuity of onset, exacerbating and alleviating factors, and degree of functional impairment are key elements of the history. Associated symptoms such as cough, hemoptysis, chest pain, wheezing, orthopnea, and paroxysmal nocturnal dyspnea and the environmental triggers are helpful in developing a differential diagnosis. If dyspnea is recent, of sudden onset, and accompanied by chest pain, pneumothorax, pulmonary embolism, and pulmonary edema should be considered. If the dyspnea is slowly progressive, chronic conditions such as chronic obstructive pulmonary disease (COPD), pulmonary fibrosis, pulmonary arterial hypertension, and neuromuscular disorders are in the differential diagnosis.

The progression of chronic dyspnea may be insidious. Asking specific questions to quantify changes in functional status over time is important. Dyspnea may occur during exertion or at rest and may be episodic or continuous. Episodic dyspnea associated with exertion suggests parenchymal lung disease or cardiac dysfunction. Dyspnea that is seasonal or triggered by

TABLE 14-1 MAJOR SYMPTOMS OF RESPIRATORY DISEASE

Cough	Chest pain
Sputum	Fever
Hemoptysis	Hoarseness
Dyspnea (acute, progressive, or paroxysmal)	Night sweats
Wheezing	

TABLE 14-2 CAUSES OF DYSPNEA

CAUSE	EXAMPLES
Airways disease	Chronic obstructive lung diseases
	Laryngeal disorders
	Epiglottitis, bronchiolitis, and croup in children
	Tracheal obstruction or stenosis
	Tracheomalacia
Parenchymal lung disease	Pneumonia
	Interstitial lung diseases
	Obliterative bronchiolitis
	Pulmonary edema due to increased vascular permeability (acute respiratory distress syndrome)
	Infiltrative and metastatic malignancies
Pulmonary circulation disorders	Pulmonary thromboembolism
	Pulmonary arterial hypertension
	Pulmonary arteriovenous malformation
Chest wall and pleural disorders	Pneumothorax
	Pleural effusion or massive ascites
	Pleural tumor
	Fractured ribs, flail chest
	Chest wall deformities
	Neuromuscular diseases
	Bilateral diaphragmatic paresis
Cardiac disorders	Pulmonary edema due to left heart failure
	Myocardial infarction
	Pericardial effusion or constrictive pericarditis
	Intracardiac shunt
Hematologic disorders	Anemia, hemolysis, methemoglobinemia, carbon monoxide poisoning
Noncardiorespiratory disorders	Psychogenic diseases
	Midbrain lesion
Metabolic or endocrine disorders	Metabolic acidosis (diabetic ketoacidosis, sepsis, severe dehydration, inborn errors of metabolism)
	Hyperthyroidism
	Hypothyroidism
	Hyperammonemia
	Hypocalcemia (laryngospasm)
	Anaphylaxis
	Smoke inhalation
	Chemical agent exposures (phosgene, chlorine, cyanide)
Other causes	Biologic and chemical weapons (anthrax, tularemia, phosgene, nitrogen mustard, nerve agents, ricin)
	Submersion injury (near-drowning)
	Acute chest syndrome (sickle cell disease)

environmental exposure suggests diseases such as asthma and hypersensitivity pneumonitis. Positional dyspnea can occur in patients with severe obstructive lung disease, diaphragmatic paralysis, or neuromuscular weakness.

Orthopnea is dyspnea that occurs in the supine position. This condition may result from a decrease in vital capacity caused by abdominal contents exerting force against the diaphragm. Paroxysmal nocturnal dyspnea is dyspnea that occurs 1 to several hours after lying down and is associated with congestive heart failure. Increased venous return to the heart causes this condition, resulting in mild interstitial pulmonary edema. Asthma can also be associated with nocturnal dyspnea and is thought to result from decreased vital capacity in the supine position, decreased production of endogenous agents with bronchodilator functions, and increased exposure to allergens in bedding. Exercise-induced asthma causes dyspnea out of proportion to the degree of exertion, with dyspnea often being most severe in the 15 to 30 minutes after the cessation of exercise.

Wheezing has many causes, including asthma. However, the absence of wheezing does not rule out asthma in any setting, and the presence of wheezing does not establish the diagnosis. Other conditions that cause wheezing are congestive heart failure; endobronchial obstruction by tumor, foreign body, or mucus; vocal cord abnormalities; and acute bronchitis.

Cough is a frustrating symptom for the patient and the physician. The three most common causes of chronic cough are postnasal drip, asthma, and gastroesophageal reflux disease. Cough may be mild and infrequent, or it may be severe enough to induce emesis or syncope. Cough may be dry or may produce sputum or blood (i.e., hemoptysis). The symptom may begin months after initiation of a drug (e.g., angiotensin-converting enzyme [ACE] inhibitors), leading to a dry, hacking cough. *Bordetella pertussis* infection (i.e., whooping cough) and viral lower respiratory tract infections can produce a cough that may last for 3 months or longer. Patients with asthma often have a cough. Occasionally, cough is their only symptom, a condition referred to as *cough-variant asthma*. Nocturnal cough suggests asthma, heart failure, or gastroesophageal reflux disease.

More than occasional production of sputum is abnormal and should be characterized with regard to quantity, color, timing, and presence or absence of blood. The physician should ask the patient to estimate the frequency and volume of sputum produced in 24 hours and describe diurnal variations. Chronic bronchitis is defined as a persistent cough resulting in sputum production for more than 3 months in each of the past 3 years. Patients with asthma often have a productive cough resulting from excess mucus production. Colored sputum does not always signify a bacterial infection because the concentration of cellular debris—predominantly white cells in inflammatory processes—influences sputum color. Patients with difficult to control asthma who report brown plugs or casts of the small bronchi in their sputum may have allergic bronchopulmonary aspergillosis.

Hemoptysis is a frightening symptom. The volume of blood may be scant or large enough to cause asphyxiation or exsanguination. The most common cause of hemoptysis in the United States is bronchitis, whereas the most common cause worldwide is pulmonary tuberculosis. Most cases of hemoptysis are small in volume and self-limited, and they resolve with the treatment of the underlying process. Massive hemoptysis, defined as more than 500 mL of blood in 24 hours, is rare and considered a medical emergency when it occurs. Causes of massive hemoptysis include lung cancer, lung cavities containing mycetomas, cavitary tuberculosis, pulmonary hemorrhage syndromes, pulmonary arteriovenous malformations, and bronchiectasis. The physician should distinguish among hemoptysis, epistaxis, and hematemesis. Because many patients have trouble identifying the source of the bleeding, a careful upper airway physical examination is essential.

Chest pain attributable to the lungs usually results from pleural disease, pulmonary vascular disease, or musculoskeletal pain precipitated by coughing because no pain receptors exist in the lung parenchyma. Lung cancer, for example, does not cause pain until it invades the pleura, chest wall, vertebral bodies, or mediastinal structures. Disease or inflammation of the pleura causes pleuritic chest pain characterized as a sharp or stabbing pain with deep inspiration. Pain caused by pulmonary emboli, infection, pneumothorax, and collagen vascular disease is usually pleuritic. Pulmonary hypertension may produce dull anterior chest pain unrelated to respiration caused by right ventricular strain and demand ischemia. Other examples of noncardiac causes of chest pain are esophageal disease, herpetic neuralgia, musculoskeletal pain, and trauma. Older patients or those with a history of chronic systemic steroid use may have thoracic pain resulting from vertebral compression or rib fractures.

Adequate analgesia, including narcotics, is essential in the treatment of chest pain in patients with underlying lung disease to prevent the reduction in vital capacity caused by splinting of the chest in reaction to the pain. The diagnosis of musculoskeletal chest pain should be considered after other causes have been ruled out. This pain is usually reproducible with movement or palpation over the affected area.

⬤ HISTORY

The examiner should always ask about previous respiratory illness, including pneumonia, tuberculosis, or chronic bronchitis, and abnormalities seen on the chest radiograph that have been previously reported to the patient. Patients with the acquired immunodeficiency syndrome (AIDS) are at high risk for *Pneumocystis jiroveci* pneumonia and other chest infections, including tuberculosis. Immunosuppression from long-standing steroid use may predispose to tuberculosis and other lung infections.

Most classes of drug can be associated with lung toxicity. Examples include pulmonary embolism from use of the oral contraceptive pill, interstitial lung disease from cytotoxic agents (e.g., methotrexate, cyclophosphamide, bleomycin), bronchospasm from β-adrenergic receptor blockers or nonsteroidal anti-inflammatory drugs, and cough from ACE inhibitors. Some drugs known to cause lung disease may not be mentioned by the patient because they are illegal (e.g., cocaine, heroin).

An accurate history of tobacco use and other toxic and environmental exposures is essential for patients with respiratory complaints. Tobacco smoke is the most prevalent environmental toxin causing lung disease. Asking about tobacco use and attempting to motivate patients to quit smoking are the physician's duty. The risk for lung disease from smoking is directly related to individual genetic susceptibility and the total pack-years of exposure, and it is inversely related to the age at onset of smoking and, in the case of lung cancer, the interval since smoking cessation.

A history of exposure to other inhaled toxins, irritants, or allergens should be elicited. A careful occupational history often uncovers exposure to inorganic dust or fibers such as asbestos, silica, or coal dust. Organic dusts may cause hypersensitivity pneumonitis and other interstitial lung diseases. Solvents and corrosive gases also cause pulmonary disease. The presence of pets in the home should be documented. Cats are the most allergenic for asthma, and birds may cause hypersensitivity or fungal lung disease.

A travel history is important in evaluating infectious causes of pulmonary disease. For example, histoplasmosis is common in the Ohio and Mississippi River valleys, and coccidioidomycosis is found in the desert Southwest. Travel to developing countries increases the risk of exposure to tuberculosis. A family history is important in assessing the risk for genetic lung diseases such as cystic fibrosis and α_1-antitrypsin deficiency and susceptibility to asthma, emphysema, or lung cancer.

PHYSICAL EXAMINATION

The physical examination should be complete, with emphasis on areas highlighted by the history. The first steps in the physical examination of the patient with pulmonary disease are observation and inspection, which must be done when the patient's chest is bare. The physician should start by evaluating the general appearance of the patient. Particular attention should be given to the presence or absence of respiratory distress. This observation helps in making the diagnosis and suggests the urgency of the case.

Body habitus is important because morbid obesity in a patient with exercise intolerance and sleepiness may point to a diagnosis of sleep-disordered breathing, whereas dyspnea in a thin, middle-aged man with pursed lips may suggest emphysema. Race and sex should be considered because certain conditions are more frequently encountered in specific populations. For example, sarcoidosis is most common in African Americans in the Southeast, whereas lymphangioleiomyomatosis is a rare disorder that essentially affects young women of childbearing age. Tachycardia and pulsus paradoxus are important signs of severe asthma.

The physician should watch the patient breathe and notice the effort required for breathing. Increased respiratory rate, use of accessory muscles of respiration, pursed-lip breathing, and paradoxical abdominal movement indicate increased work of breathing. Paradoxical abdominal movement indicates diaphragm weakness and impending respiratory failure. The patient's inability to speak in full sentences indicates severe airway obstruction or neuromuscular weakness. The physician should listen for cough during the history and physical examination and should observe the strength of the cough because it may signal respiratory muscle weakness or severe obstructive lung disease. The patient's rib cage should expand symmetrically with inspiration. The shape of the thoracic cage should be considered. Increased anteroposterior diameter is observed in those with lung hyperinflation due to obstructive lung disease. Severe kyphoscoliosis, pectus excavatum, ankylosing spondylitis, and morbid obesity

can produce restrictive ventilatory disease as a consequence of distortion and restriction of the volume of the thoracic cavity.

The patient's hands may reveal important signs of lung diseases. Clubbing is commonly associated with respiratory disease. An uncommon association with clubbing is hypertrophic pulmonary osteoarthropathy (HPO). HPO is characterized by periosteal inflammation at the distal ends of long bones, the wrists, the ankles, and the metacarpal and metatarsal bones. There is swelling and tenderness over the wrists and other involved areas. Rarely, HPO may occur without clubbing. The causes of HPO include pleural mesothelioma, pulmonary fibrosis, and chronic lung infections, such as lung abscess.

Staining of the fingers (caused by tar because nicotine is colorless) is a sign of cigarette smoking. The patient should be asked to dorsiflex the wrists with the arms outstretched and to spread out the fingers. A flapping tremor (i.e., asterixis) may be seen with severe carbon dioxide retention. Wasting and weakness are signs of cachexia due to malignancy or end-stage emphysema. Compression and infiltration by a peripheral lung tumor of a lower trunk of the brachial plexus results in wasting of the small muscles of the hand and weakness of finger abduction.

Examination of the head and neck is important. The eyes are inspected for evidence of Horner's syndrome (i.e., constricted pupil, partial ptosis, and loss of sweating), which can be caused by an apical lung tumor compressing the sympathetic nerves in the neck. The voice is assessed for hoarseness, which may indicate recurrent laryngeal nerve palsy associated with carcinoma of the lung (usually left sided) or laryngeal carcinoma. However, the most common cause is laryngitis.

The patient is examined for nasal polyps (associated with asthma), engorged turbinates (various allergic conditions), and a deviated septum (nasal obstruction). Sinusitis is indicated by tenderness over the sinuses on palpation.

The tongue is assessed for central cyanosis. The mouth may hold evidence of an upper respiratory tract infection (i.e., reddened pharynx and tonsillar enlargement with or without a coating of pus). A broken tooth or gingivitis may predispose to lung abscess or pneumonia. There may be facial plethora or cyanosis if the superior vena cava is obstructed. Some patients with obstructive sleep apnea are obese and have a receding chin, a small pharynx, and a short, thick neck.

Palpation of the chest is performed by first palpating the accessory muscles (i.e., scalene and sternocleidomastoid) of respiration in the patient's neck. Hypertrophy and contraction indicate increased respiratory effort. The trachea should be palpated and should lie in the midline of the neck. Deviation of the trachea may suggest lung collapse or a mass. Neck masses should be documented.

The physician should place both hands on the lower half of the patient's posterior thorax with thumbs touching and fingers spread; the hands should be kept in place while the patient takes several deep inspirations. The physician's thumbs should separate slightly and the hands should move symmetrically apart during the patient's inspiration.

Fremitus is a faint vibration felt best with the edge of the hand against the patient's chest wall while the patient speaks. Fremitus is increased in areas with underlying lung consolidation, and it is decreased over a pleural effusion. Next, the patient's chest should be percussed. The level of the diaphragms on each side should be observed. The percussion note should be compared on the two sides starting at the apex and moving down, including the posterior, anterior, and lateral aspects. A pleural effusion, consolidation, mass, or elevated diaphragm can cause dullness to percussion; a pneumothorax or hyperinflation can cause hyperresonance.

Auscultation of the lungs is performed to evaluate the quality of the breath sounds and to detect extra sounds not heard in normal lungs. Normal breath sounds have two qualities, vesicular and bronchial. Bronchial breath sounds are heard over the central airways and are louder and coarser than vesicular breath sounds, which are heard at the periphery and base of the lungs. Bronchovesicular sounds are a combination of the two and are heard over medium-sized airways. Bronchial sounds have a longer inhaled component, whereas vesicular sounds have a much longer expiratory component and are much softer. Bronchial breath sounds and bronchovesicular breath sounds at the periphery of the lungs are abnormal and may be caused by underlying consolidation. In the setting of consolidation, increased transmission of vocal sounds, called *whispered pectoriloquy,* occurs; *egophony,* in which the spoken letter *e* sounds like an *a* over the area of consolidation, is heard and sometimes compared with the bleating of a goat.

Abnormal or extrapulmonary sounds are crackles, wheezes, and rubs. Crackles can be coarse rattles or fine, Velcro-like sounds. Mucus in the airways or the opening of large- and medium-sized airways often causes coarse crackles. In bronchiectasis, the crackles are altered with coughing. Fine crackles, heard during inspiration and caused by the opening of collapsed alveoli, are most common at the bases. Crackles are heard in pulmonary edema and interstitial fibrosis.

Wheezing is a higher-pitched sound, and when heard locally, it suggests large airway obstruction. The wheezing of patients with asthma or congestive heart failure is lower in pitch and heard diffusely over all lung fields. Localized wheezing can be heard in conditions such as pulmonary embolism, obstruction of a bronchus by a tumor, and foreign-body aspiration.

A rub is a pleural sound caused by inflamed pleural surfaces rubbing together. A rub has been described as the sound of pieces of leather rubbing against each other. Rubs are often evanescent and depend on the amount of fluid in the pleural space. Often, pleuritic chest pain and a rub develop after large-volume thoracentesis.

A crunching sound timed with the cardiac cycle, called *Hamman's crunch* or *Hamman's sign,* is heard in patients with a pneumomediastinum. The complete absence of breath sounds on one side should cause the examiner to think of pneumothorax, hydrothorax, or hemothorax; obstruction of a main stem bronchus; or surgical or congenital absence of the lung.

● EVALUATION

The clinician should be able to develop a differential diagnosis based on a detailed history and a thorough physical examination. The preliminary differential diagnosis is the basis for ordering a battery of tests, recognizing that these tests may reveal disorders not considered in the initial assessment. The objective of this extended evaluation is twofold: to confirm a diagnosis

or discard other disorders and to assess the severity of the lung derangement.

Patients with a suggested lung disorder should undergo pulmonary function testing (see Chapter 15). Spirometry evaluates airflow and helps to distinguish between the obstructive pattern characteristic of COPD, asthma, and related disorders and the restrictive pattern observed in fibrosing lung disease. Spirometry also provides information regarding the severity of the physiologic derangement.

Lung volume measurements are helpful in assessing hyperinflation or confirming a restrictive process. Measuring the diffusing capacity of the lung for carbon monoxide (D_{LCO}) provides information about alterations in gas-exchanging capability. Further assessment of gas exchange can be obtained by the determination of oxygen saturation using pulse oximetry.

Information regarding oxygenation and acid-base status is obtained from arterial blood gas determination. A 6-minute walk test can evaluate oxygenation during exertion; through this test, patients are often found to require supplemental oxygen for the first time. Other, more specialized tests (e.g., bronchoprovocation, cardiopulmonary stress testing, polysomnography) may be required, depending on the circumstances.

Imaging studies of the chest are extremely useful in evaluating lung structure. The chest radiograph provides information about the lung parenchyma and pleura, the cardiac silhouette, mediastinal structures, and body habitus. Examining old chest radiographic images is essential for assessing progression of disease.

Computed tomography (CT) provides more accurate information about the pulmonary and mediastinal structures, and it is essential in the assessment of interstitial lung disease, lung masses, and other disorders. Together with ventilation-perfusion scanning and pulmonary angiography, CT is one of the many tools available to evaluate the lung vasculature. Positron emission tomography is used to assess metabolic activity of lung masses and can suggest a diagnosis of malignancy.

Standard blood tests such as the blood counts and blood chemistry point to specific disorders or may provide information about the severity of a lung disorder (e.g., polycythemia in chronic hypoxemia, leukocytosis in lung infection). Some specialized tests should be reserved for specific diagnoses such as connective tissue disorders (e.g., rheumatoid factor, antinuclear antibodies) or hypersensitivity pneumonitis (hypersensitivity profile).

Together with the history and physical examination, these tests are useful for narrowing a diagnosis to establish a specific plan of treatment. The plan can often be created in a single visit. However, patients frequently require several visits to a clinician. During these follow-up visits, the physician assesses progression of disease, patient compliance with therapy, and response to management.

If noninvasive tests do not allow a diagnosis of the problem, more invasive tests may be necessary. Fiberoptic or rigid bronchoscopy allows direct visualization of the airways and acquisition of valuable clinical samples for study. Transthoracic percutaneous needle aspiration or navigational bronchoscopy is useful in evaluating peripheral lung lesions. Ultimately, surgery may be required to obtain tissue through open or video-assisted thoracoscopically guided lung biopsy.

For a deeper discussion on this topic, please see Chapter 84, "Imaging in Pulmonary Disease," and Chapter 101, "Interventional and Surgical Approaches to Lung Disease," in Goldman-Cecil Medicine, 25th Edition.

PROSPECTUS FOR THE FUTURE

The predictive values of various aspects of the history and physical examination need to be clarified. The role of quantitative CT analysis in the diagnosis and assessment of disability from lung diseases should be refined. The role of interventional pulmonary procedures must be ascertained for the diagnosis and treatment of lung diseases.

SUGGESTED READINGS

Fitzgerald FT, Murray JF: History and physical examinations. In Mason RJ, Murray JF, Broaddus VC, et al, editors: Murray and Nadel's textbook of respiratory medicine, ed 4, Philadelphia, 2005, Elsevier.

Ryder REJ, Mir MA, Freeman EA: An aid to the MRCP PACES, vol 1, ed 3, Oxford, 2007, Blackwell Publishing.

Weiner DL: Causes of acute respiratory compromise in children. Available at: http://www.uptodate.com/contents/causes-of-acute-respiratory-compromise-in-children?source=search_result&search=Causes+of+acute+respiratory+compromise+in+children&selectedTitle=1%7E150. Accessed August 25, 2014.

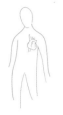

15

Evaluating Lung Structure and Function

Jigme M. Sethi and F. Dennis McCool

INTRODUCTION

The satisfactory functioning of all organ systems depends on their capacity to consume oxygen and eliminate carbon dioxide. The primary function of the lung is to deliver oxygen to the pulmonary capillary blood and to excrete carbon dioxide. To accomplish this, the lung must generate a flux of air into and out of the alveoli (ventilation) while absorbing oxygen into the pulmonary blood and eliminating carbon dioxide from alveolar air (gas exchange). This is accomplished in a manner that attempts to optimize gas exchange (ventilation-perfusion matching). This remarkably efficient process allows the human to maintain optimal oxygenation and acid-base balance over a range of activities, from resting breathing to moderately strenuous activity. This chapter provides an overview of the anatomy and physiology that enable the respiratory system to perform its life-sustaining functions as well as a discussion of tests available to evaluate lung structure and function.

ANATOMY

Airway

Inspired air travels through the nose and nasopharynx, where it is warmed to body temperature, humidified, and filtered of airborne particles greater than 10 μm in diameter. Air then enters a complex system of dichotomously branching airways that form a tree occupying the thorax. The first 15 divisions, beginning with the trachea, the mainstem bronchi, segmental and subsegmental bronchi down to the terminal bronchioles, are simply a set of conducting tubes that do not participate in gas exchange. Together, they constitute the *conducting zone* of the lung, also known as the *anatomic dead space* (about 1 mL per pound of ideal body weight, or approximately 150 mL) (Fig. 15-1). Cartilaginous rings help to maintain the patency of these large airways. In the mainstem bronchi, the rings are circumferential, whereas in the trachea, the cartilaginous rings are U-shaped, with the posterior membrane of the trachea sharing a wall with the esophagus.

Airway subdivision	Order No.	Cross-sectional area (cm^2)	Resistance (cm H$_2$O $\cdot$ L^{-1} $\cdot$ sec)
Larynx	0		0.5
Trachea	0	2.5	0.5
Bronchi	1	2.0	
	2		
Bronchioles		5.0	0.2
	16	1.8 x 10^2	
Respiratory bronchioles	17		
	19	9.4 x 10^2	
Alveolar ducts			
	22	5.8 x 10^3	
Alveoli	23	5.6 x 10^7	

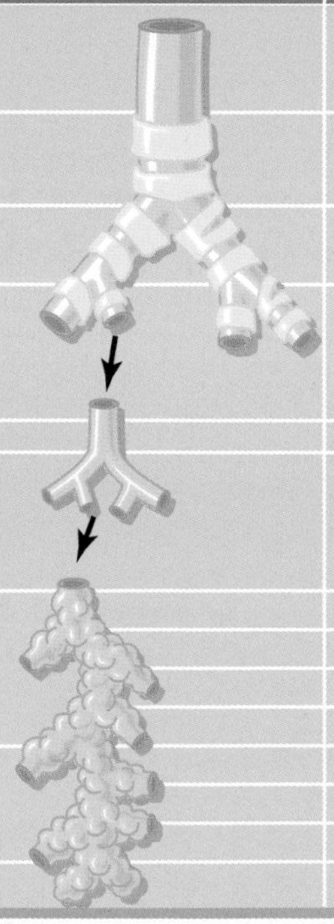

FIGURE 15-1 The subdivisions of the airways and their nomenclature. (Modified from Weibel ER: Morphometry of the human lung, Berlin, 1963, Springer.)

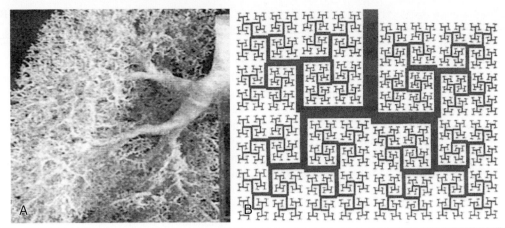

FIGURE 15-2   **A**, Cast of the right lung demonstrates branching of airways. **B**, The branching airways can be modeled by use of the principles of fractal geometry, which allow for efficient filling of the thoracic space.

The branching pattern of these first 15 divisions of the airways follows the principles of fractal geometry: The reduction of airway diameter and length between each generation is similar, by a factor of 0.79, serving to densely compact the airways into the available space of the thorax (Fig. 15-2A and B). This geometry reduces bronchial path length from the trachea to the periphery and minimizes both dead space volume and resistance to convective airflow.

The remaining eight generations of airways comprise the respiratory bronchioles and alveolar ducts lined with alveolar sacs. This area of the lung is referred to as the *respiratory zone*, and the terminal respiratory unit is called the acinus. Gas exchange commences in the respiratory zone but primarily occurs in the alveoli. Inspired air moves down the conducting zone primarily by bulk convective flow, whereas the movement of oxygen in the respiratory zone is by diffusion.

In total, there are an average of 23 subdivisions of the airway from the trachea to the alveolar ducts. Although it might be suspected that resistance to convective flow would be highest in the small airways because of their small diameter, the opposite is the case. The enormous number of small airways together provide a huge net cross-sectional area for airflow. For example, the cross-sectional area of the trachea is 2.5 cm^2, compared with a total cross-sectional area of 300 cm^2 for all of the alveolar ducts combined. As a result, 80% of the resistance to airflow occurs in the first seven generations of bronchi, and the remaining "small" airways (diameters <2 mm) contribute only 20% of the resistance to airflow (Fig. 15-3). As the lung expands during inspiration, the net cross-sectional area of the alveolar ducts doubles, further reducing resistance to airflow.

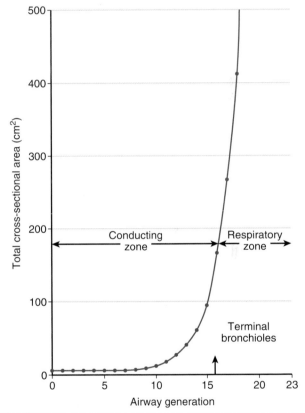

FIGURE 15-3   Total cross-sectional area of the airways is depicted for several generations of airways. The total cross-sectional area increases dramatically in the respiratory zone. Consequently, the velocity of gas entering the respiratory zone decreases and resistance is low.

Alveoli

The alveoli are the grapelike clusters of air sacs that interface with the pulmonary capillaries. There are about 300 million individual alveolar sacs, or 10,000 in each of the 30,000 acini. The alveoli are thin-walled structures with a total surface area of about 130 m^2. This is roughly half the size of a doubles tennis court. The surface of the alveoli is lined by two types of cells. The flat type I pneumocytes constitute 95% of the cells. Type II pneumocytes, which account for about 5% of the alveolar lining cells, secrete surfactant, a complex lipoprotein whose role in lowering surface tension in the alveolar space is critical to reducing the forces needed to expand the lung. Surfactant is also important in preventing alveolar collapse at low lung volumes and thereby promoting normal gas exchange. The capillaries run in the exceedingly thin septa that separate the alveoli and are therefore exposed to the air from surrounding alveoli. The epithelial lining of the alveoli, the endothelial lining of the capillaries, and the intervening fused basement membrane form the alveolar-capillary interface. Normally, this interface is less than 1 μm thick and does not significantly interfere with gas exchange.

Blood Vessels

The pulmonary artery arises from the right ventricle and branches until it terminates in a meshwork of capillaries that surround the alveoli. This creates a large surface area that facilitates gas exchange. Blood returns to the heart through pulmonary veins that course through the lungs, coalesce into four main pulmonary veins, and empty into the left atrium. The pulmonary circulation is a low-resistance circuit; pulmonary vascular resistance is about one tenth of the resistance in the systemic circulation. Pulmonary vessels can be easily recruited to accommodate increases in blood flow while maintaining low pressure and resistance. Accordingly, during exercise, any increase in cardiac output can be distributed through the lung without significantly increasing pulmonary arterial pressures.

A separate vascular system, the bronchial system, also supplies the lung. The bronchial arteries originate from the aorta and, in contrast to the pulmonary arteries, are under systemic pressure. These vessels provide nutrients to lung structures proximal to the alveoli. Two thirds of the bronchial circulation drains into the pulmonary veins and then empties into the left atrium. This blood, which has low oxygen content, mixes with the freshly oxygenated blood from the pulmonary veins to lower the oxygen content of the blood that enters the systemic circulation.

● PHYSIOLOGY

Ventilation

Ventilation refers to the bulk transport of air from the atmosphere to the alveolus. The product of tidal volume (V_T) and breathing frequency (f) represents the total volume of air delivered to the lung per minute (minute ventilation). However, not all air entering the lung is in contact with gas-exchanging units. The portion of V_T that fills the respiratory zone and alveoli and is available for gas exchange constitutes the alveolar volume (V_A), whereas the portion remaining in the conducting airways is the anatomic dead space volume (V_D) (Fig. 15-4). The ratio of V_D to V_T is called the *dead space ratio* (V_D/V_T). Normally, one third of a breath is dead space ($V_D/V_T = \frac{1}{3}$). The amount of fresh air reaching the alveoli is $V_A - V_D$. With large breaths, the dead space becomes a smaller fraction of the total tidal volume. Therefore, for a given V_T, slow, deep breathing results in greater V_A and improved gas exchange compared with rapid, shallow breathing.

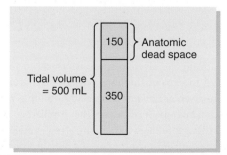

FIGURE 15-4   Schematic diagram of the inspired volume of air that participates in gas exchange (V_A, 350 mL) and the volume of anatomic dead space (V_D, 150 mL), which together provide a tidal breath (V_T) of 500 mL.

The V_D/V_T ratio can be calculated by the Bohr method, as follows:

$$V_D/V_T = (Pa_{CO_2} - PE_{CO_2})/Pa_{CO_2}$$

where Pa_{CO_2} is the arterial partial pressure of carbon dioxide and PE_{CO_2} is the partial pressure of carbon dioxide in mixed expired gas (i.e., the mixture of CO_2-rich gas that enters the alveoli from the pulmonary capillaries and dead space gas, which is devoid of CO_2). PE_{CO_2} increases during expiration, reaching a plateau at end-expiration. At end-expiration, the PE_{CO_2} represents exhaled alveolar gas that has been in equilibrium with pulmonary capillary blood. In healthy individuals, the PE_{CO_2} at end-expiration is equivalent to the Pa_{CO_2}.

Ventilation of the dead space is wasted ventilation, because only V_A participates in gas exchange. Therefore, as the metabolic rate and carbon dioxide production increase, V_A must increase to maintain an arterial P_{CO_2} of 40 mm Hg. The relationship among these variables is described by the alveolar carbon dioxide equation:

$$Pa_{CO_2} = CO_2 \text{ production}/\dot{V}_A$$

where Pa_{CO_2} is the partial pressure of carbon dioxide in the alveolus and $\dot{V}_A$ is alveolar ventilation. From this equation, one appreciates that the partial pressure of carbon dioxide in the alveolus is inversely proportional to alveolar ventilation.

The relationship described by the alveolar oxygen equation is similar:

$$Pa_{O_2} = O_2 \text{ consumption}/\dot{V}_A$$

However, this relationship is more complicated because Pa_{O_2} also is proportional to the fraction of inspired oxygen, the water vapor pressure, and the partial pressure of carbon dioxide in the alveolus (discussed later). The implications of the alveolar carbon dioxide and oxygen relationships are that (1) maintenance of a constant alveolar gas composition depends on a constant ratio of ventilation to metabolic rate; (2) if ventilation is too high (hyperventilation), alveolar P_{CO_2} will be low and alveolar P_{O_2} will be high; and (3) if ventilation is too low (hypoventilation), alveolar P_{CO_2} will be high and alveolar P_{O_2} will be low.

Mechanics of Breathing

Respiratory mechanics is the study of forces needed to deliver air to the lung and how these forces govern the volume and flow of gases. Mechanically, the respiratory system consists of two structures: the lungs and the chest wall. The lungs are elastic (spring-like) structures that are situated within another elastic structure, the chest wall. At end-expiration, with absent respiratory muscle activity, the inward recoil of the lung is exactly balanced by the outward recoil of the chest wall, representing the equilibrium position of the lung–chest wall unit. Normally, the recoil of the lung is always inward (favoring lung deflation), and the recoil of the chest wall is outward (favoring inflation); at high lung volumes, however, the chest wall also recoils inward (Fig. 15-5). The energy required to stretch the respiratory system beyond its equilibrium state (end-expiration during quiet breathing) is provided by the inspiratory muscles. With normal quiet breathing, gas flow out of the lung is usually accomplished by passive recoil of the respiratory system.

Normal

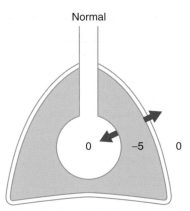

FIGURE 15-5 Schematic diagram of the lung and chest wall at functional residual capacity (FRC). The *arrows* show that the expanding elastic force of the chest wall equals the collapsing elastic force of the lung. The intrapleural pressure is −5 at FRC because both forces are tugging on the pleural space in opposite directions.

During a typical breath, inspiratory muscle contraction lowers the intrapleural pressure, which in turn lowers the intra-alveolar pressure. Once alveolar pressure becomes subatmospheric, air can flow from the mouth through the airways to the alveoli. At the end of inspiration, the inspiratory muscles are turned off, and the lungs and chest wall recoil passively back to their equilibrium states. This passive recoil of the respiratory system causes alveolar pressure to become positive throughout expiration until the resting position of the lung and chest wall are reestablished and alveolar pressure once again equals atmospheric pressure. During quiet breathing, pleural pressure is always subatmospheric, whereas alveolar pressure oscillates below and above zero (atmospheric) pressure (Fig. 15-6).

The major inspiratory muscle is the diaphragm. Others include the sternocleidomastoid muscles, the scalenus muscles, the parasternals, and the external intercostals. Diaphragm contraction results in expansion of the lower rib cage and compression of the intra-abdominal contents. The latter action results in expansion of the abdominal wall. The expiratory muscles consist of the internal intercostal muscles and the abdominal muscles. Expiratory flows can be enhanced by recruiting the expiratory muscles; this occurs during exercise or with cough.

To inflate the respiratory system, the inspiratory muscles must overcome two types of forces: the elastic forces imposed by the lung and the chest wall (elastic loads) and the resistive forces related to airflow (resistive loads). The elastic loads on the inspiratory muscles result from the respiratory system's tendency to resist stretch. The elastic forces are volume dependent; that is, the respiratory system becomes more difficult to stretch at volumes greater than the functional residual capacity (FRC) and more difficult to compress at volumes lower than the FRC. The elastic forces can be characterized by examining the relationship between lung volume and recoil pressure (Fig. 15-7). When either deflated or inflated, the lung and chest wall have characteristic recoil pressures. The slope of the relationship between lung volume and elastic recoil pressure of the chest wall or lung represents the *compliance* of each structure. The sum of the chest wall and lung recoil pressures represents the recoil pressure of the total respiratory system.

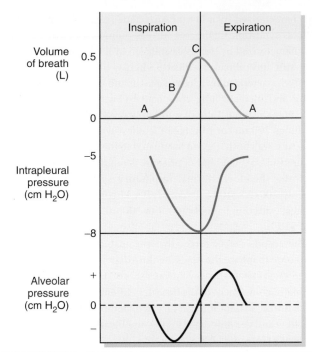

FIGURE 15-6 Volume, intrapleural pressure, and alveolar pressure during a normal breathing cycle. The letters correspond to the various phases of the cycle: A, end-expiration; B, inspiration; C, end-inspiration; and D, expiration. Alveolar pressure is biphasic, with zero crossings at times of no flow (i.e., end-expiration and end-inspiration). Intrapleural pressure remains subatmospheric throughout.

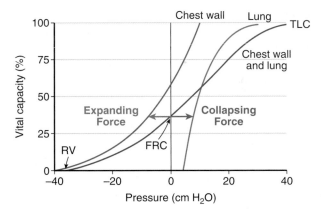

FIGURE 15-7 Volume-pressure relationship of the respiratory system and its components, the lung and chest wall. Respiratory system recoil pressure at any volume is the sum of the lung and chest wall recoil pressures. Forces creating negative pressures expand the respiratory system, whereas forces creating positive pressures collapse the respiratory system. The slope of the volume-pressure curve represents the compliance of each structure. FRC, Functional residual capacity; RV, residual volume; TLC, total lung capacity.

The elastic properties of the lung are related to two factors: the elastic behavior of collagen and elastin in the lung parenchyma and the surface tension in the alveolus at the air-liquid interface. Both factors contribute equally to lung elastic recoil. A surface-active substance called *surfactant* is produced by type II alveolar cells and lines the alveoli. This substance consists primarily of phospholipids. It lowers the surface tension of the air-liquid interface, making it easier to inflate the lung. The lungs are stiff (less compliant) and difficult to inflate in diseases that are characterized by a loss of surfactant (e.g., infant respiratory distress syndrome). Diseases such as pulmonary fibrosis, which are characterized by excessive collagen in the lung, can make the lung stiff and difficult to inflate, whereas those such as emphysema, characterized by a loss of elastin and collagen, reduce lung recoil and increase lung compliance (Fig. 15-8). Normally, at FRC, it takes about 1 cm of water pressure (1 cm H_2O) to inflate the lungs 200 mL or to inflate the chest wall 200 mL. The lung and chest wall both need to be inflated to the same volume during inspiration, so 2 cm H_2O of pressure is required to inflate both to 200 mL. Therefore, normal respiratory system compliance is roughly 200/2 or100 mL/cm H_2O and compliance of the lung or chest wall compliance is 200/1 or 200 mL/cm H_2O at volumes near FRC.

The second set of forces that the inspiratory muscles must overcome to inflate the lungs are flow-dependent forces; namely, tissue viscosity and airway flow resistance, the latter constituting the major component of the flow-dependent forces. Airway resistance during inspiration can be calculated by measuring inspiratory flow and the difference in pressure between the alveolus and the airway opening (ΔP_{A-ao}).

$$Resistance = \Delta P_{A-ao}/\dot{V}$$

The airflow velocity, the type of airflow (laminar or turbulent), and the physical attributes of the airway (radius and length) are the key determinants of airway resistance. Of the physical properties, the radius of the airways is the major factor. Resistance increases to the fourth power as the diameter decreases under conditions of laminar flow (streamline flow profile) and to the fifth power under conditions of turbulent flow (chaotic flow profile). Because airway diameter increases

as lung volume increases, airway resistance decreases as lung volume increases (Fig. 15-9). Airway diameter also contributes to regional differences in airway resistance. Although the peripheral airways are narrower than the central airways, their total cross-sectional area is much greater than that of the central airways, as described earlier. Consequently, resistance to airflow of the peripheral airways is low relative to the central airways (see Fig. 15-3).

The type of airflow is another key determinant of airway resistance. Resistance is directly proportional to flow rate when flow is laminar. Resistance is much greater with turbulent flow because it is proportional to the square of the flow rate. The velocity of airflow determines, in part, whether the flow pattern is laminar or turbulent. Clinically, increased airway resistance can be seen in diseases associated with airway obstruction caused by an intrinsic mass, mucus within the airway, airway smooth muscle contraction, or extrinsic compression of the airways.

Lung elastic recoil also influences airway resistance and airflow. Decreased lung recoil increases resistance by promoting collapse of the small airways (E-Fig. 15-1). Normal resistance when breathing at FRC at low flow rates is in the range of 1 to 2 cm H_2O/L per second.

Distribution of Ventilation

The distribution of inhaled volume throughout the lung is unequal. In general, more of the inhaled volume goes to the bases of the lung than to the apex when the individual is inhaling while in an the upright body position. This pattern of volume distribution leads to greater ventilation of the bases than at the apices. This inhomogeneity of ventilation results largely from regional differences in lung compliance. The alveoli at the lung apex are relatively more inflated at FRC than the alveoli at the lung base. The difference in alveolar distention from apex to base is related to pleural pressure differences from apex to base. The weight of the lung causes pleural pressure to be more negative at the apex

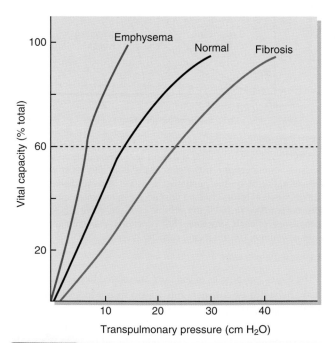

FIGURE 15-8 Compliance curves for normal individuals and for patients with emphysema or pulmonary fibrosis. The transpulmonary pressure required to achieve a given lung volume is greatest for the patient with pulmonary fibrosis (notice the horizontal dashed line at 60% of the vital capacity). This increases the work of breathing.

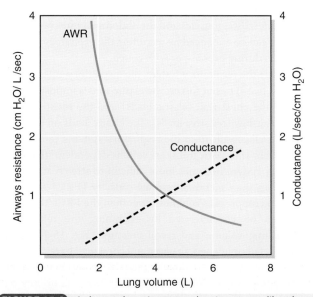

FIGURE 15-9 As lung volume increases, the airways are dilated, and airways resistance (AWR) decreases. The reciprocal of resistance (conductance) increases as lung volume increases.

and less negative at the base. The normal difference in pleural pressure from apex to base in an adult is about 8 cm H_2O (Fig. 15-10). Because the apical alveoli are more stretched at FRC, they are operating on a stiffer, less compliant region of their volume-pressure curve than the alveoli at the bases, making them more difficult to inflate than the basilar alveoli. Therefore, at the beginning of inspiration, more volume is directed toward the base than to the apex of the lung.

Control of Ventilation

Maintenance of adequate oxygenation and acid-base balance is accomplished through the respiratory control system. This system consists of the neurologic respiratory control centers, the respiratory effectors (muscles that provide the power to inflate the lungs), and the respiratory sensors. The respiratory center that automatically controls inspiration and expiration is located in the medulla of the brain stem. The respiratory center in the brain stem has an intrinsic rhythm generator (pacemaker) that drives breathing. The output of this center is modulated by inputs from peripheral and central chemoreceptors, from mechanoreceptors in the lungs, and from higher centers in the brain, including conscious control from the cerebral cortex. The respiratory center in the medulla is primarily responsible for determining the level of ventilation.

Carbon dioxide is the primary factor controlling ventilation. Carbon dioxide in the arterial blood diffuses across the blood-brain barrier, thereby reducing the pH of the cerebral spinal fluid and stimulating the central chemoreceptors. A change in $Paco_2$ above or below normal will increase or decrease ventilation, respectively. During quiet, resting breathing, the level of $Paco_2$ is thought to be the major factor controlling breathing. Only when the Pao_2 (i.e., the partial pressure of oxygen dissolved in the blood that is not bound to hemoglobin) falls substantially does ventilation respond significantly. Typically, Pao_2 needs to fall to

less than 50 mm Hg before ventilation dramatically increases (Fig. 15-11). Low oxygen levels in the blood are not sensed by the respiratory center in the brain but are sensed by receptors in the carotid body. These vascular receptors are located between the internal and external branches of the carotid artery. Changes in Pao_2 are sensed by the carotid sinus nerve. Neural traffic projects to the respiratory center through the glossopharyngeal nerve, which serves to modulate ventilation. The carotid body also senses changes in $Paco_2$ and pH. Nonvolatile acids (e.g., ketoacids) stimulate ventilation through their effects on the carotid body.

The outcome of this complex respiratory control system is that variables such as Pao_2, $Paco_2$, and pH are held within narrow limits under most circumstances. The respiratory control center also can adjust tidal volume and frequency of breathing to minimize the energetic cost of breathing and can adapt to special circumstances such as speaking, swimming, eating, and exercise. Breathing can be stimulated by artificial manipulation of the Pco_2, Po_2, and pH. For example, ventilation is increased by rebreathing of carbon dioxide, inhalation of a concentration of low oxygen, or infusion of acid into the bloodstream.

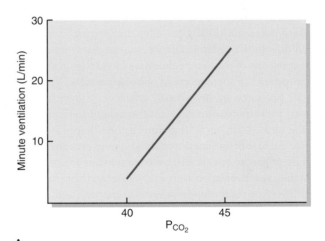

A

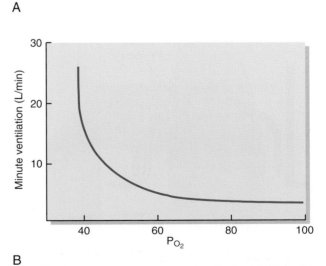

B

FIGURE 15-11 **A,** A rising partial pressure of carbon dioxide (Pco_2) leads to a linear increase in minute ventilation. **B,** The ventilatory response to hypoxemia is less sensitive and is clinically relevant only when the partial pressure of oxygen (Po_2) has dropped significantly.

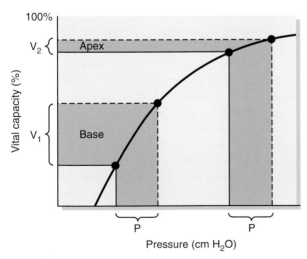

FIGURE 15-10 Transpulmonary pressure and volume for lung units at the base and apex of the lung. Because pleural pressure is more negative at the apex of the lung. Therefore, the alveoli in that region are stretched, placing them on a less compliant part of the volume-pressure curve. For a given change (*P*) in transpulmonary pressure during inspiration, the more compliant base inflates to a greater degree than the apex (V_1 and V_2, respectively).

Perfusion

The pulmonary vascular bed differs from the systemic circulation in several respects. The pulmonary vascular bed receives the entire cardiac output of the right ventricle, whereas the cardiac output from the left ventricle is dispersed among several organ systems. Despite receiving the entire cardiac output, the pulmonary system is a low-resistance, low-pressure circuit. The normal mean systemic arterial pressure is about 100 mm Hg, whereas the normal mean pulmonary artery pressure is in the range of 15 mm Hg. The vascular bed can passively accommodate an increase in blood flow without raising arterial pressure by recruiting more vessels in the lung. During exercise, for example, there is little increase in pulmonary artery resistance despite a large increase in pulmonary blood flow. Hypoxic vasoconstriction, another feature unique to the pulmonary vascular system, regulates regional blood flow. This regulation aids in matching blood flow to ventilation by reducing flow to poorly ventilated regions of the lung.

Perfusion ($\dot{Q}$) refers to the blood flow through an organ (i.e., the lung). In the upright individual, there is greater perfusion of the lung bases than of the apices (Fig. 15-12). In a low-pressure system such as the pulmonary circulation, the effects of gravity on blood flow need to betaken into account. The arterial-venous pressure difference usually provides the "driving" pressure for blood flow in the systemic circulation, but this is true only for certain regions of the lung. Pulmonary blood flow also needs to be considered in the context of alveolar pressure. Venous and arterial pressures are importantly affected by gravity, whereas alveolar pressure remains constant throughout the lung, assuming the airways are open. Therefore, as one descends from the apex to the base of the lung, arterial and venous pressures increase because of gravity but alveolar pressure remains constant.

At the apex, alveolar pressure may be greater than arterial pressure. This region of the lung is referred to as *zone 1,* and, in theory,

it receives no blood flow. The alveolar pressure may be greater than arterial pressure, for example, in special circumstances such as hypovolemic shock, which lowers the arterial pressure, or with very high levels of positive end-expiratory pressure (PEEP), which increases alveolar pressure.

As one descends from the apex toward the midzone of the lung, arterial and venous pressures increase, whereas alveolar pressure remains constant. At some point, arterial pressure becomes greater than alveolar pressure. In this region, the driving pressure for blood flow is the arterial-alveolar pressure difference. This region is referred to as *zone 2* of the lung. Normally, zone 2 is very small because alveolar pressure is less than venous pressure in most of the lung. However, with high levels of PEEP, alveolar pressure becomes greater than venous pressure in more lung regions.

Further toward the base of the lung, the effects of gravity on arterial and venous pressures are more pronounced, venous pressure becomes greater than alveolar pressure, and the arterial-venous pressure difference provides the driving pressure for blood flow, as in the systemic circulation. This region is referred to as *zone 3* of the lung.

Normally, most of the lung is in zone 3, and most of the perfusion is to the lung base. This inequality in perfusion from apex to base is *qualitatively* similar to the inequality of ventilation from apex to base. However, blood flow increases from apex to base *more* than ventilation does, and this accounts for the small amount of ventilation-perfusion inequality that exists in the normal lung.

Gas Transfer

Oxygen and carbon dioxide are easily dissolved in plasma. Nitrogen is much less soluble and is not significantly exchanged across the alveolar-capillary interface. The driving force for the diffusion of a gas across a tissue barrier is the difference in partial pressure of the gas across the barrier. The partial pressure of oxygen in inspired room air entering the trachea is 150 mm Hg; this is derived from the equation, $\text{Po}_2 = (\text{P}_{atm} - \text{PH}_2\text{O}) \times \text{Fio}_2$, assuming that P_{atm} (atmospheric pressure) is 760 mm Hg, PH_2O (the partial pressure of water vapor) is 47 mm Hg, and Fio_2 (the fraction of oxygen in inspired air) is 20.9%. In the alveolus, however, the partial pressure of oxygen is reduced to 100 mm Hg because the inspired VT mixes with about 3 L of "oxygen-poor" air already in the lungs and is diluted by carbon dioxide moving into the alveolus from the pulmonary capillaries. The partial pressure of oxygen in the alveolus (Pao_2) is set by the balance of these processes. Increasing minute ventilation increases the amount of oxygen added to the alveolus while lowering the Paco_2—the opposite result from hypoventilation. This reciprocal relationship between alveolar carbon dioxide and alveolar oxygen is described by the *alveolar gas equation*:

$$\text{PAO}_2 = [(\text{P}_{atm} - \text{PH}_2\text{O}) \times \text{Fio}_2] - (\text{Paco}_2 / \text{RER})$$

where RER is the respiratory exchange ratio, usually about 0.8.

The pressure gradient that drives diffusion of oxygen from the alveolus to the capillary is the difference between the alveolar Po_2 (100 mm Hg) and the arterial Po_2 (40 mm Hg) in the capillary blood entering the alveolus. By the time the blood leaves the alveolus, the Po_2 in the capillary blood has risen to 100 mm Hg.

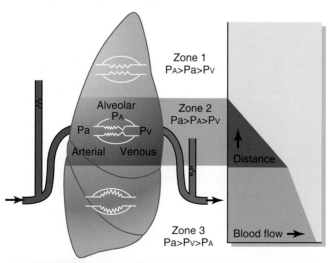

FIGURE 15-12 Zonal model of blood flow in the lung. Because of the inter-relationship of arterial (Pa) and venous (Pv) vascular pressures and alveolar (PA) pressures, the lung base receives the most flow (see text for explanation). (From West JB, Dollery CT, Naimark A: Distribution of blood flow in isolated lung: relation to vascular and alveolar pressures, J Appl Physiol 19:713–724, 1964.)

However, because small regions of ventilation-perfusion inequality and shunt exist in the normal lung, the P_{O_2} in the pulmonary veins from the lungs as a whole is usually about 90 mm Hg. Therefore, the difference between the alveolar and arterial partial pressures of oxygen, known as the *A-a gradient*, is typically about 10 mm Hg in health.

The pressure gradient that drives carbon dioxide from the mixed venous blood into the alveolus is the difference in partial pressure of carbon dioxide (45 mm Hg in mixed venous blood and 40 mm Hg in the alveolus). Despite the lower driving pressure for carbon dioxide compared with oxygen, the greater solubility of carbon dioxide allows complete equilibration between the alveolus and plasma during each respiratory cycle (Fig. 15-13).

Most of the oxygen contained in the blood is bound to hemoglobin; a small fraction is dissolved and measured as the Pa_{O_2}. The amount of oxygen dissolved is about 3 mL/L in arterial blood, whereas the amount of oxygen bound to hemoglobin is about 197 mL/L, assuming a normal hematocrit. Each molecule of hemoglobin is capable of carrying four molecules of oxygen. The shape of the oxyhemoglobin association curve reflects the cooperative binding of oxygen to hemoglobin (Fig. 15-14). In general, the hemoglobin saturation is between 80% and 100% with Pa_{O_2} values greater than 60 mm Hg and drops dramatically when the Pa_{O_2} is less than 60 mm Hg. Factors that decrease the affinity of hemoglobin for oxygen include a reduction in blood pH, an increase in temperature, an increase in Pa_{CO_2}, and an increase in the concentration of 2,3-diphosphoglyceric acid (2,3-DPG) (Fig. 15-15). These factors facilitate unloading of oxygen into tissues, which is seen as a shift of the oxyhemoglobin dissociation curve to the right. The oxygen-carrying capacity of hemoglobin is also affected by competitive inhibitors for binding sites, such as carbon monoxide. Carbon monoxide has an affinity for hemoglobin that is 240 times greater than that of oxygen and preferentially binds to the hemoglobin molecule. However, this does not affect the amount of oxygen dissolved in the blood. Someone with carbon monoxide poisoning may have a normal Pa_{O_2} but a very low blood oxygen content because of the high amount of desaturated hemoglobin.

About 5% of carbon dioxide in the blood is dissolved in plasma, and about 10% is bound to hemoglobin. However, carbon dioxide does not exhibit cooperative binding; therefore, the shape of the carbon dioxide–hemoglobin dissociation curve is linear. Carbon dioxide binds to the protein component of the hemoglobin molecule and to the amino groups of the polypeptide chains of plasma proteins to form carbamino compounds. About 10% of carbon dioxide is transported in this fashion. Most of the carbon dioxide is transported as bicarbonate ion: As carbon dioxide diffuses from metabolically active tissue into the blood, it reacts with water to form carbonic acid. This reaction primarily occurs in the red blood cells because it is catalyzed by the enzyme carbonic anhydrase, which resides in those cells. Carbonic acid then dissociates to bicarbonate and hydrogen ion. Although there is more carbon dioxide dissolved in blood than oxygen, it is still a small fraction of the total carbon dioxide transported by blood.

Abnormalities of Pulmonary Gas Exchange

The arterial P_{O_2} and P_{CO_2} are determined by the degree of equilibration between the alveolar gas and capillary blood, which depends on four major factors: ventilation, matching of ventilation with perfusion, shunt, and diffusion. *Hypoxemia* refers to a reduction in the oxygen content of the blood and is determined by measuring the P_{O_2} of arterial blood. In contrast, *hypoxia* refers to a decrease in oxygen content of an organ, for example, myocardial hypoxia. Aberrations in the four factors listed can result in hypoxemia. A fifth cause of hypoxemia is a low inspired P_{O_2}, which may occur at altitude.

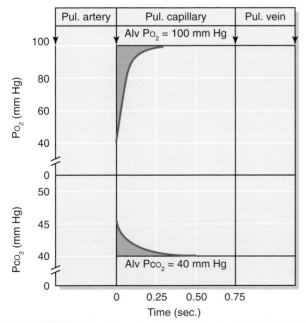

FIGURE 15-13 Changes in the partial pressures of oxygen (P_{O_2}) and carbon dioxide (P_{CO_2}) as blood courses from the pulmonary artery through the capillaries and into the pulmonary veins. The diffusion gradient is greater for O_2 than for CO_2. However, equilibration of capillary and alveolar gas occurs for both molecules within the 0.75 second it takes for blood to traverse the capillaries. Alv, Alveolar; Pul., pulmonary.

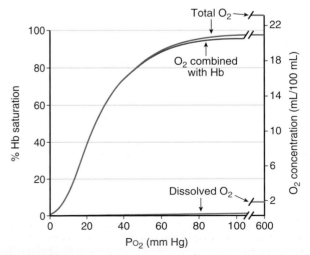

FIGURE 15-14 The oxyhemoglobin dissociation curve. The bulk of the oxygen (O_2) is combined with hemoglobin (Hb). Little is dissolved in plasma. P_{O_2}, Partial pressure of oxygen.

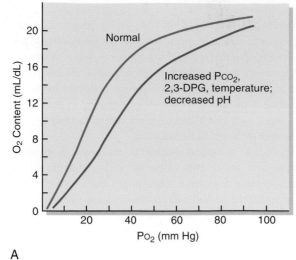

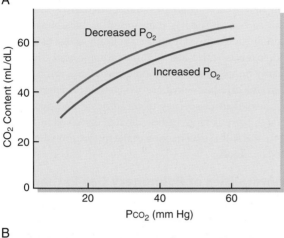

FIGURE 15-15 **A,** The various factors that decrease the oxygen affinity of hemoglobin are shown shifting the curve to the right. **B,** The carbon dioxide dissociation curve is more linear than the oxyhemoglobin curve throughout the physiologic range. Increased partial pressure of oxygen in the arteries (Pao_2) shifts the curve to the right, decreasing the carbon dioxide content for any given arterial partial pressure of carbon dioxide ($Paco_2$) and thereby facilitating carbon dioxide off-loading in the lungs. The shift to the left at a lower Pao_2 facilitates carbon dioxide on-loading at the tissues. 2,3-DPG, 2,3-Diphosphoglycerate.

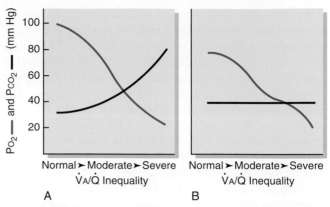

FIGURE 15-16 **A,** The effects of increasing inequality of alveolar ventilation and perfusion (decreasing $\dot{V}A/\dot{Q}$) on the arterial partial pressures of oxygen (Po_2) and carbon dioxide (Pco_2) when cardiac output and minute ventilation are held constant. **B,** The gas tensions change when minute ventilation is allowed to increase. Increased ventilation can maintain a normal arterial Pco_2 but can only partially correct the hypoxemia. (Modified from Dantzker DR: Gas exchange abnormalities. In Montenegro H, editor: Chronic obstructive pulmonary disease, New York, 1984, Churchill Livingstone, pp 141–160.)

Hypoventilation is defined as ventilation that is inadequate to keep Pco_2 from increasing above normal. Hypoxemia may occur when increased carbon dioxide in the alveoli displaces alveolar oxygen. As alveolar ventilation falls and $Paco_2$ rises, Pao_2 will have to fall. Administration of supplemental oxygen (i.e., increasing the Fio_2) can reverse hypoventilation-induced hypoxemia. When one is breathing room air, the difference between alveolar oxygen and arterial oxygen (A-a gradient) is normally about 10 mm Hg. Typically, this difference increases when hypoxemia is present. However, if the hypoxemia is caused by hypoventilation, the A-a gradient will be within normal limits. Causes of hypoventilation are varied and range from diseases or drugs that depress the respiratory control center to disorders of the chest wall or respiratory muscles that impair respiratory pump function. Disorders associated with hypoventilation include inflammation, trauma, or hemorrhage in the brain stem; spinal cord pathology; anterior horn cell disease; peripheral neuropathies; myopathies; abnormalities of the chest wall such as kyphoscoliosis; and upper airway obstruction. Administration of a higher Fio_2 alleviates the hypoxemia but does little to improve the elevated $Paco_2$.

The most common cause of hypoxemia in disease states is ventilation-perfusion mismatch. In regions where the ratio of ventilation $\dot{V}$ to perfusion $\dot{Q}$ is low, the blood receives little oxygen from the poorly ventilated alveoli. By contrast, in regions where $\dot{V}/\dot{Q}$ is high, the blood is well oxygenated but receives little additional oxygen despite the higher ventilation because the shape of the oxyhemoglobin dissociation curve plateaus at levels of high Pao_2. As a result, lung units with high $\dot{V}/\dot{Q}$ cannot completely correct for the low oxygen content of blood flowing past units with low $\dot{V}/\dot{Q}$. Thus, the oxygen uptake of the whole lung is lowered, causing hypoxemia. In the ideal lung, ventilation and perfusion would be perfectly matched (i.e., $\dot{V}/\dot{Q} = 1$). However, the $\dot{V}/\dot{Q}$ normally ranges from 0.5 at the base to 3 at the apex, with an overall value of 0.8. If lung disease develops, ventilation-perfusion inequality may be amplified. If the $\dot{V}/\dot{Q}$ is less than 0.8, the A-a gradient is increased and hypoxia ensues. The $Paco_2$ is usually within the normal range but increases slightly at extremely low $\dot{V}/\dot{Q}$ ratios (Fig. 15-16). Typically, hypoxemia in diseases that affect the airways, such as chronic obstructive pulmonary disease (COPD), is caused by ventilation-perfusion mismatch. As with hypoxemia due to hypoventilation, administration of a higher Fio_2 improves hypoxemia by improving the Pao_2 in areas of *low* $\dot{V}/\dot{Q}$.

The third cause of hypoxemia is shunt. A right-to-left shunt occurs when a portion of blood travels from the right side to the left side of the heart without the opportunity to exchange oxygen and carbon dioxide in the lung. Right-to-left shunts can be classified as anatomic or physiologic. With an anatomic shunt, a portion of the blood bypasses the lung by traversing through an anatomic canal. In all healthy individuals, there is a small fraction of blood in the bronchial circulation that passes to the pulmonary veins and empties into the left atrium, thereby reducing the Pao_2

of the systemic circulation. A smaller portion of the normal shunt is related to the coronary circulation draining through the thebesian veins into the left ventricle. Anatomic shunts found in disease states can be classified as intracardiac or intrapulmonary shunts. Intracardiac shunts occur when right atrial pressures are elevated and deoxygenated blood travels from the right atrium to the left atrium through an atrial septal defect or patent foramen ovale. Intrapulmonary anatomic shunts consist primarily of arteriovenous malformations or telangiectasias. With a physiologic right-to-left shunt, a portion of the pulmonary arterial blood passes through the normal vasculature but does not come into contact with alveolar air. This is an extreme example of ventilation-perfusion mismatch ($\dot{V}/\dot{Q}=0$). Physiologic shunt can be caused by diffuse flooding of the alveoli with fluid, as seen in congestive heart failure or acute respiratory distress syndrome. Alveolar flooding with inflammatory exudates, as seen in lobar pneumonia, also causes a shunt. The fraction of blood shunted (Qs/Qt) can be calculated when the FIO_2 is 100% by the following equation:

$$Qs/Qt = (Cco_2 - Cao_2)/(Cco_2 - Cvo_2)$$

where Qs is the shunted blood flow, Qt is the total blood flow, Cco_2 is the end-pulmonary capillary oxygen content; Cao_2 is the arterial oxygen content; and Cvo_2 is the mixed venous oxygen content.

If the shunt is severe enough, mechanical ventilation and PEEP are required to improve arterial oxygenation. At values less than 50% of the cardiac output, a shunt has very little effect on $Paco_2$ (Fig. 15-17). With shunting, the A-a gradient is elevated while the $Paco_2$ is within normal range or may be low. In contrast to hypoxemia due to hypoventilation or low $\dot{V}/\dot{Q}$, oxygen administration does not correct hypoxemia due to shunt because the shunted blood has no exposure to oxygen in the alveoli. However, the Pao_2 may increase somewhat because the higher

FIO_2 improves oxygenation of blood traveling to low $\dot{V}/\dot{Q}$ areas that commonly coexist with shunt.

The fourth cause of hypoxemia is diffusion impairment. With normal cardiopulmonary function, the blood spends, on average, 0.75 second in the pulmonary capillaries. Typically, it takes only 0.25 second for the alveolar oxygen to diffuse across the thin alveolar capillary membrane and equilibrate with pulmonary arterial blood (see Fig. 15-13). However, if there is impairment to diffusion across this membrane, such as thickening of the alveolar capillary membrane by fluid, fibrous tissue, cellular debris, or inflammatory cells, it will take longer for the oxygen in the alveoli to equilibrate with pulmonary arterial blood. If the impediment to diffusion is such that it takes longer than 0.75 second for oxygen to diffuse, hypoxemia ensues, and the A-a gradient widens. Alternatively, if the time a red blood cell spends traversing the pulmonary capillary decreases to 0.25 second or less, hypoxemia may develop. Hypoxemia may be evident only during exercise in individuals with diffusion impairment because of the shortened red cell transit time. In these cases, the A-a gradient may be normal at rest but increases with exercise. With diffusion impairment, the $Paco_2$ usually is within the normal range. As with hypoxemia due to hypoventilation or ventilation-perfusion mismatch, administration of a higher FIO_2 improves hypoxemia due to impaired diffusion by raising the alveolar Po_2.

An additional cause of hypoxemia is low inspired oxygen. This may occur at high altitude: The FIO_2 is normal, but the Po_2 is low because the barometric pressure (P_{atm}) is low. Rarely, circumstances occur in which the FIO_2 is low (e.g., rebreathing air). Hypoxemia due to low inspired oxygen is associated with a normal A-a gradient and is usually accompanied by a low $Paco_2$. Supplemental oxygen corrects this form of hypoxemia. Finally, a low mixed venous Po_2 predisposes individuals to hypoxia (Fig. 15-18).

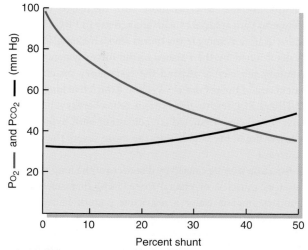

FIGURE 15-17 The effects of increasing shunt on the arterial partial pressures of oxygen (Po_2) and carbon dioxide (Pco_2). The minute ventilation has been held constant in this example. Under usual circumstances, the hypoxemia would lead to increased minute ventilation and a fall in the Pco_2 as the shunt increased. (From Dantzker DR: Gas exchange abnormalities. In Montenegro H, editor: Chronic obstructive pulmonary disease, New York, 1984, Churchill Livingstone, pp 141–160.)

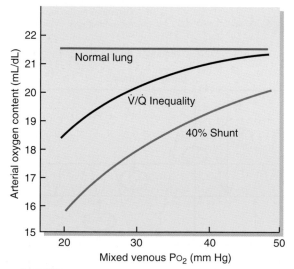

FIGURE 15-18 The effects of increasing mixed venous partial pressure of oxygen (Po_2) on the arterial oxygen content under three assumed conditions: a normal lung, severe ventilation-perfusion inequality ($\dot{V}/\dot{Q}$), and the presence of a 40% shunt. For each situation, the patient is breathing 50% oxygen and the mixed venous Po_2 is altered, keeping all other variables constant. (From Dantzker DR: Gas exchange in the adult respiratory distress syndrome, Clin Chest Med 3:57–67, 1982.)

EVALUATION OF LUNG FUNCTION

Pulmonary function tests evaluate one or more major aspects of the respiratory system. Accurate measurements of lung volumes, airway function, and gas exchange require a pulmonary function testing laboratory. Pulmonary function tests are commonly used to aid in the diagnosis of disease and assess disease severity. In addition, they are helpful in monitoring the course of disease, assessing the risk for surgical procedures, and measuring the effects of varied environmental exposures. The response to bronchodilators or other forms of treatment also can be assessed with serial pulmonary function tests (Table 15-1). Accurate interpretation of pulmonary function tests requires the appropriate reference standards. Variables that affect the predicted standards include age, height, gender, race, and hemoglobin concentration.

Spirometry, the simplest means of measuring lung function, can be performed in an office practice. A spirometer is an apparatus that measures inspiratory and expiratory volumes. Flow rates can be calculated from tracings of volume versus time. Typically, vital capacity (VC) is measured as the difference between a full inspiration to total lung capacity (TLC) and a full exhalation to residual volume (RV) (Fig. 15-19). Flow rates are measured after the patient is instructed to forcefully exhale from TLC to RV. Such a forced expiratory maneuver allows one to calculate the forced expiratory volume in 1 second (FEV_1) and the forced vital capacity (FVC) (Fig. 15-20). A value that is 80% to 120% of the predicted value is considered normal for FVC. Normally, people can exhale more than 75% to 80% of their FVC in the first second, and the majority of the FVC can be exhaled in 3 seconds. The ratio of FEV_1/FVC is normally greater than 0.80.

Spirometry can reveal abnormalities that are classified into two patterns: obstructive and restrictive. Obstructive impairments are defined by a low FEV_1/FVC ratio. Diseases that are characterized by an obstructive pattern include asthma, chronic bronchitis, emphysema, bronchiectasis, cystic fibrosis, and some central airway lesions. The reduction in FEV_1 (expressed as % predicted FEV_1) is used to determine the severity of airflow obstruction (E-Fig. 15-2). Peak expiratory flow rate (PEFR) can be measured as the maximal expiratory flow rate obtained during spirometry or when using a handheld peak flowmeter. The lower the PEFR, the more significant the obstruction. The peak flowmeter can be used at home or in the emergency department to evaluate the presence of obstruction. Severe attacks of asthma, for example, are usually associated with PEFRs of less than 200 L/minute (normal, 500 to 600 L/minute). A restrictive pattern is characterized by loss of lung volume. With spirometry, both the FVC and the FEV_1 are reduced, so the FEV_1/FVC ratio remains normal. The restrictive pattern must be confirmed by measurements of lung volumes.

Lung volumes are measured by body plethysmography or by dilution of an inert gas such as helium. Lung volumes that can be measured with these techniques include FRC, TLC, and RV (see Fig. 15-19). As described earlier, FRC is the lung volume at which the inward elastic recoil of the lung equals the outward elastic recoil of the chest wall. Changes in FRC reflect abnormalities in lung elastic recoil. Diseases associated with increased elastic recoil (e.g., pulmonary fibrosis) are associated with a reduction in FRC, whereas those with decreased recoil (e.g., emphysema) are associated with an increase in FRC. TLC is the amount of air remaining in the thorax after a maximal inspiration. It is determined by the balance of the forces generated by the respiratory muscles to expand the respiratory system and the elastic recoil of the respiratory system. Restrictive lung disease is defined as a TLC less than 80% predicted, whereas values of TLC greater than 120% predicted are consistent with hyperinflation. The lower the % predicted TLC, the more severe the restrictive impairment.

Restriction may be caused by disorders of the lung, chest wall, respiratory muscles, or pleural space. Lung diseases that cause pulmonary fibrosis cause a restrictive pattern because of the increased elastic recoil of the respiratory system. Diseases of the chest wall, such as kyphoscoliosis, obesity, or ankylosing spondylitis, can also cause restriction by reducing the elasticity of the chest wall. Weakness of the respiratory muscles causes restriction by reducing the force available to inflate the respiratory system. Myasthenia gravis, amyotrophic lateral sclerosis, diaphragm paralysis, and Guillain-Barré syndrome can be associated with weakness sufficient to cause restrictive lung disease. Finally, space-occupying lesions involving the pleural space, such as

TABLE 15-1	INDICATIONS FOR PULMONARY FUNCTION TESTING

Evaluation of signs and symptoms:
  Shortness of breath
  Exertional dyspnea
  Chronic cough
Screening of at-risk populations
Monitoring of pulmonary drug
  toxicity
	Follow-up after abnormal study
	  results:
	    Chest radiograph
	    Electrocardiogram
	    Arterial blood gases
	    Hemoglobin
	Preoperative assessment:
	    Assess severity
	    Follow response to therapy
	    Determine further treatment goals
	    Assess disability

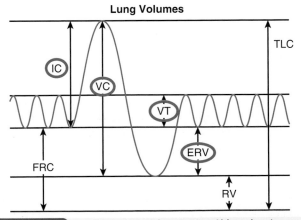

FIGURE 15-19 Lung volumes and capacities. Although spirometry can measure vital capacity and its subdivisions *(red circles)*, calculation of residual volume (RV) requires measurement of functional residual capacity (FRC) by one of the following techniques: body plethysmography, helium dilution, or nitrogen washout. IC, Inspiratory capacity; ERV, expiratory reserve volume; TLC, total lung capacity; VC, vital capacity; VT, tidal volume.

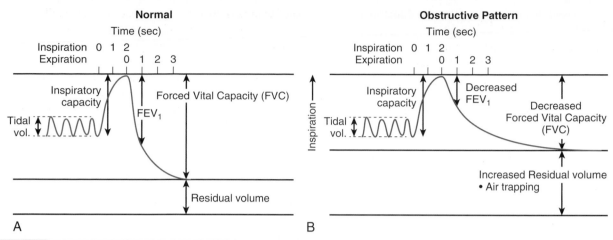

FIGURE 15-20 Spirometry in a normal individual (**A**) and in a patient with obstructive lung disease (**B**). FEV₁ represents the forced expiratory volume in 1 second, and FVC represents the forced vital capacity. The FEV₁/FVC ratio is normally greater than 0.80. With obstruction, the FEV₁/FVC ratio is less than 0.70.

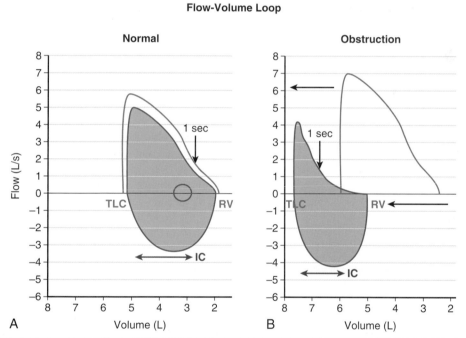

FIGURE 15-21 The maximum expiratory flow and volume curve in a normal individual (**A**) and in an individual with obstructive lung disease (in this case, COPD) (**B**). Hyperinflation and air trapping *(arrows)* push the total lung capacity (TLC) and residual volume (RV) to the left (i.e., toward higher lung volumes). In addition, characteristic scalloping of the expiratory limb of the flow-volume curve develops. IC, Inspiratory capacity.

pleural effusions, pneumothorax, or pleural tumors, can cause restriction. Occasionally, RV and FRC may be elevated with no increase in TLC. This pattern, referred to as *air trapping,* and can be seen with COPD or asthma.

The forced expiratory maneuver can be analyzed in terms of flow and volume by construction of a flow-volume loop (Fig. 15-21). Flow-volume loops are useful to identify obstructive and restrictive patterns. The characteristic appearance of obstructive impairment is concavity ("scooping") of the expiratory loop, whereas with restrictive impairments, the loops have a normal shape but are reduced in size. In addition, flow-volume loops are the primary means of identifying upper airway obstruction. Upper airway obstruction is characterized by a truncated (clipped) inspiratory or expiratory loop. A fixed obstruction

produces clipping of both inspiratory and expiratory loops. Variable intrathoracic upper airway obstruction exhibits clipping of the expiratory loop, whereas variable extrathoracic obstruction exhibits clipping of the inspiratory loop (Fig. 15-22).

Bronchoprovocation Testing

Bronchoprovocation testing is typically used to determine the presence or absence of hyperreactive airways disease. Some individuals with a clinical suspicion of asthma have normal expiratory flow rates and lung volumes. Bronchoprovocation testing in these individuals can be important to identify hyperreactive airways disease and support the diagnosis of asthma. Methacholine is a cholinergic agonist that causes bronchoconstriction. During the bronchoprovocation test, the subject inhales

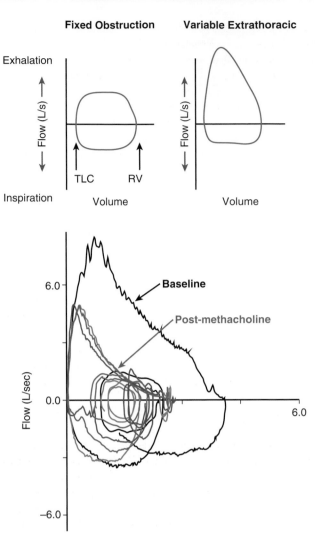

Fixed Obstruction

Variable Extrathoracic

Variable Intrathoracic

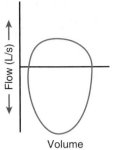

FIGURE 15-22 The flow-volume loops display different patterns of upper airway obstruction. With fixed obstruction, both inspiratory and expiratory flows are reduced (clipped). With variable extrathoracic obstruction, only the inspiratory flows are clipped. With variable intrathoracic obstruction, only the expiratory flows are clipped. RV, Residual volume; TLC, total lung capacity.

FIGURE 15-23 In bronchoprovocation challenge, patients are exposed to increasing concentrations of an inhaled challenge (e.g., methacholine, histamine), followed by evaluation of the forced expiratory volume in 1 second (percentage of baseline value) or airways conductance. The FEV$_1$ falls by more than 20% (compared to baseline), and airways conductance by more than 40%, at lower concentrations of the challenge drug in individuals with asthma.

TABLE 15-2 NORMAL VALUES FOR ARTERIAL BLOOD GASES

Partial pressure of oxygen (Pao$_2$): $104 - (0.27 \times \text{age})$
Partial pressure of carbon dioxide (Paco$_2$): 36-44
pH: 7.35-7.45
Alveolar-arterial O$_2$ difference $= 2.5 + (0.21 \times \text{age})$

capillary blood, carbon monoxide is used rather than oxygen to assess diffusion capacity. Carbon monoxide diffuses across the alveolar capillary membranes much as oxygen does. However, carbon monoxide has the advantage of binding completely to hemoglobin. Therefore, the partial pressure of carbon monoxide in the pulmonary venous blood is negligible. The D$_{LCO}$ is then measured as the rate of disappearance of carbon monoxide from the alveolus and is used as a surrogate for oxygen diffusion capacity.

The D$_{LCO}$ measurement provides an overall assessment of gas exchange and depends on factors such as the surface area of the lung, the physical properties of the gas, perfusion of ventilated areas, hemoglobin concentration, and the thickness of the alveolar-capillary membrane. Therefore, an abnormal value may not only signify disruption of the alveolar-capillary membrane but may also be related to a reduction in surface area of the lung (pneumonectomy), poor perfusion (pulmonary embolus), or poor ventilation of alveolar units (COPD). A low D$_{LCO}$ may be seen in interstitial lung diseases that alter the alveolar-capillary membrane or in diseases such as emphysema that destroy both alveolar septa and capillaries (E-Fig. 15-3). Anemia lowers the D$_{LCO}$. Most laboratories provide a hemoglobin correction for diffusion capacity. An increased D$_{LCO}$ may be associated with engorgement of the pulmonary circulation by red blood cells or polycythemia.

Arterial Blood Gases

The measurement of Pao$_2$ and Paco$_2$ provides information about the adequacy of oxygenation and ventilation. This requires arterial blood sampling through arterial puncture or indwelling cannula (Table 15-2). Oxygenation also can be measured through noninvasive devices such as the pulse oximeter, which measures hemoglobin oxygen saturation, and through transcutaneous devices that measure Pao$_2$ and Paco$_2$. These devices are particularly useful for measuring oxygenation during exertion or sleep. Often, alterations in oxygenation are not detected at rest but are unveiled during exertion. The 6-minute walk

increasing concentrations of methacholine. Measurements of FEV$_1$, FVC, and specific airways conductance are obtained after the inhalation of each concentration until the maximal dose of methacholine has been administered. If the FEV$_1$ is reduced by 20% or more or the specific airways conductance is reduced by 40% or more, a diagnosis of hyperreactive airways disease is established. Patients with asthma demonstrate a fall in FEV$_1$ at considerably smaller doses than in normal individuals (Fig. 15-23).

Lung Diffusion Capacity

The diffusion of oxygen from the alveolus into the capillary can be assessed by measuring the diffusion capacity for carbon monoxide (D$_{LCO}$). To calculate the diffusion capacity for oxygen, one would need to know the alveolar volume and the partial pressures of oxygen in the alveolus and in the pulmonary capillary. Because it is not practical to measure the oxygen tension of pulmonary test is a standardized test in which the patient walks for 6 minutes while the oxygen hemoglobin saturation is measured. A decrease in saturation is abnormal and suggests impaired gas exchange capabilities, and a reduction in distance walked is a means of detecting deterioration of overall function due to lung disease.

In summary, pulmonary function tests, in conjunction with the history and physical examination, can be used to diagnose pulmonary disorders and assess severity and response to therapy, as illustrated in the flow diagram (E-Fig. 15-4).

Analysis of Exhaled Breath

Exhaled breath includes monoxides (nitric oxide and carbon monoxide) and volatile organic compounds (VOCs) that are produced endogenously by normal metabolism or in pathologic states such as cancer and inflammation. These compounds can be measured by gas chromatography, spectroscopy or other chemical means and serve as biomarkers of pulmonary inflammation or cancer. Exhaled nitric oxide is elevated in asthma, and clinical use of this biomarker has been approved by the U.S. Food and Drug Administration for diagnosis and evaluation of asthma exacerbation or quiescence. Similarly, unique patterns of exhaled VOCs provide a "fingerprint" that may identify lung cancer. Cytokines and other similar compounds in the condensate phase of exhaled breath are being investigated for possible applications in inflammatory lung diseases (e.g., cystic fibrosis, bronchiectasis). Other nonpulmonary diseases such as malabsorption syndromes and *Helicobacter pylori* infection are also detected by analysis of exhaled breath.

⬤ EVALUATION OF LUNG STRUCTURE
Chest Radiography

Generally, the evaluation of a patient with lung disease begins with routine chest radiography and then proceeds to more specialized techniques such as computed tomography (CT) or magnetic resonance imaging (MRI). Ideally, the chest radiograph consists of two different films, a posteroanterior (PA) radiograph and a lateral radiograph (E-Fig. 15-5). Many pathologic processes can be identified on a PA chest radiograph, and the lateral view adds valuable information about areas that are not well seen on the PA projection. In particular, the retrocardiac region, the posterior bases of the lung, and the bony structure of the thorax (e.g., the vertebral column) are better visualized on the lateral radiograph. The PA chest radiograph is obtained with the patient standing with his or her back to the x-ray beam and the anterior chest wall placed against the film cassette. The chest radiograph should be obtained while the patient takes the deepest breath possible. If the patient is too weak to stand or too sick to travel to the radiology department, the cassette is placed behind the patient's back, and the x-ray beam travels from anterior to posterior (AP film). The quality of a portable film is not that of a standard PA film, but it still provides valuable information.

The examination of a chest radiograph should be systematic so that subtle abnormalities are not missed. It should include evaluation of the lungs and pulmonary vasculature, the bony thorax, the heart and great vessels, the diaphragm and pleura, the mediastinum, the soft tissues, and the subdiaphragmatic areas. Abnormalities that are visible on a chest radiograph include pulmonary infiltrates, nodules, interstitial disease, vascular disease, masses, pleural effusions and thickening, cavitary lung disease, cardiac enlargement, some airway diseases, and vertebral or rib fractures. In addition to the PA and lateral chest radiographs, the lateral decubitus projection is often used to identify the presence or absence of pleural effusion. The decubitus view is particularly useful in determining whether blunting of the costal phrenic sulcus is caused by freely flowing pleural fluid or related to pleural thickening. Chest radiography, in concert with a good history and physical examination, allows the clinician to diagnose chest disease in many circumstances.

Fluoroscopy

Fluoroscopic examination of the chest is useful for evaluating motion of the diaphragm. This technique is particularly helpful in diagnosing unilateral diaphragm paralysis. A paralyzed hemidiaphragm moves paradoxically when the patient is instructed to inhale or to forcefully sniff. However, fluoroscopy is limited when evaluating for bilateral diaphragm paralysis. Apparently normal descent of the diaphragm during inspiration, caused by compensatory respiratory strategies employed by the patient with bilateral diaphragm paralysis, leads to false-negative results. False-positive results are caused by paradoxical hemidiaphragm motion, which can be seen in as many as 6% of normal subjects during the sniff maneuver. Alternatively, two-dimensional B-mode ultrasound imaging of the diaphragm can be used to visualize diaphragm contraction during inspiration. With this technique, the diaphragm muscle is visualized in the zone of apposition of the diaphragm to the rib cage. Absence of contraction correlates with absence of active transdiaphragmatic pressure and indicates diaphragm paralysis. This technique can be used to diagnose both bilateral and unilateral diaphragm paralysis.

Ultrasonography

In ultrasonographic studies, sound waves in the frequency range of 3 to 10 MHz are reflected off internal tissues to produce images of viscera such as the liver, kidney, and heart. The air-filled lung cannot be imaged directly, but over the last decade, an understanding of various *artifacts* generated by ultrasound beams traversing normal and abnormal lung have led to increased application of ultrasound for imaging of the lung, particularly in the intensive care unit. Ultrasonography can rapidly and reliably detect a pneumothorax, pleural effusion, consolidation, and even pulmonary edema with sensitivity and specificity similar to those of a chest radiograph (Fig 15-24). It is routinely used in real time to direct invasive procedures such as thoracentesis, pericardiocentesis, and placement of a pleural, central venous, or arterial catheter. Other applications of pulmonary ultrasound include assessment of volume status by imaging inferior vena cava collapsibility with respiration and assessment of right ventricular function. Ultrasound can be used to evaluate diaphragm function, as described earlier. Ultrasonic imaging is noninvasive, rapidly and easily applied, relatively low-cost, readily portable to the bedside, and, because it does not use radiation, safe for repeated use on a patient.

neoplasia. Finally, new insights into the function of the respiratory control centers in the cortex and brain stem may be attained from the use of functional MRI studies of the brain.

SUGGESTED READINGS

McCool FD, Hoppin FG Jr: Respiratory mechanics. In Baum GL, editor: Textbook of pulmonary diseases, Philadelphia, 1998, Lippincott-Raven, pp 117–130.

McCool FD, Tzelepis GE: Current clinical aspects of diaphragm dysfunction, N Engl J Med 366:932–942, 2012.

Miller WT: Radiographic evaluation of the chest. In Fishman AP, editor: Fishman's pulmonary diseases and disorders, New York, 2008, McGraw-Hill, pp 455–510.

Pellegrino R, Viegi G, Brusasco V, et al: Interpretative strategies for lung function tests, Eur Respir J 26:948–968, 2005.

Wagner PD: Ventilation, pulmonary blood flow, and ventilation-perfusion relationships. In Fishman AP, editor: Fishman's pulmonary diseases and disorders, New York, 2008, McGraw-Hill, pp 173–189.

Weibel ER: It takes more than cells to make a good lung, Am J Respir Crit Care Med 187:342–346, 2013.

West JB: Respiratory physiology: the essentials, ed 5, Baltimore, 1995, Williams & Wilkins.

West JB, Wagner PD: Pulmonary gas exchange, Am J Respir Crit Care Med 157:S82–S87, 1988.

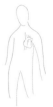

16

Obstructive Lung Diseases

Matthew D. Jankowich

INTRODUCTION

The obstructive lung diseases are a group of pulmonary disorders that result in dyspnea characterized by an obstructive pattern of expiratory airflow limitation on spirometry. These disorders include chronic obstructive pulmonary disease (COPD), asthma, cystic fibrosis (CF), bronchiectasis, and the bronchiolar disorders. In some cases, these disorders overlap clinically (Fig. 16-1), sharing several features aside from the presence of expiratory airflow limitation. These features may include symptoms of wheezing and sputum production, chronic airway-centered inflammation, presence of airway structural changes resulting in remodeling of the airways, and episodic periods of temporarily worsened clinic status, known as exacerbations. However, the causes, locations, and patterns of airway inflammatory changes and remodeling, as well as the treatments, prognoses, and natural histories, are often significantly different, making clinical distinction among these disorders important.

COPD is characterized in general by abnormal airway inflammation and abnormal lung structure in response to an inhaled irritant (typically cigarette smoke); this results in irreversible or incompletely reversible airflow limitation and is typically progressive over time. *Asthma* is distinguished from COPD by characteristic smooth muscle hyperreactivity and reversible airflow

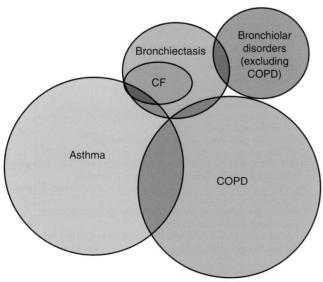

FIGURE 16-1 Classification of obstructive lung diseases. Although most patients with chronic obstructive pulmonary disease (COPD) have small airways disease, the bronchiolar disorders do not overlap with COPD. CF, Cystic fibrosis.

limitation, by its variable clinical course, and by its frequent association with atopy. These disorders are epidemic in the general population worldwide and account for a significant proportion of the morbidity and mortality associated with the obstructive lung diseases. *Bronchiectasis* is a permanent abnormal dilation of the bronchi that results in chronic cough, purulent sputum production, and hemoptysis; it is caused by diverse conditions, including CF, a genetic disorder resulting from mutations in the *CFTR* gene. The *bronchiolar disorders*, also called *small airways disorders*, result from inflammation and/or fibrosis of the small airways of the lung that leads to dyspnea. They may be difficult to diagnose because loss or obstruction of a majority of the small airways must occur before the appearance of expiratory airflow limitation on spirometry.

The basis for expiratory airflow obstruction varies among these disorders. The flow of air through the bronchial tree is directly proportional to the driving pressure and inversely proportional to the resistance. In obstructive lung disease, alterations in one or both of these processes may be present. Loss of lung elastic tissue, frequently present in COPD, results in decreased lung elastic recoil on expiration and therefore decreased driving pressure for expiratory airflow. By contrast, airflow limitation in asthma is primarily caused by smooth muscle contraction resulting in bronchoconstriction that increases airway resistance. Increases in airway resistance are also present in COPD and are related to small airway inflammation and fibrosis as well as small airway collapse due to decreased "tethering" of the airways in the setting of loss of surrounding lung elastic tissue. Mucus obstruction of airway lumens contributes to increased airway resistance in all the obstructive lung diseases.

Obstruction to airflow causes characteristic changes in lung volumes. The residual volume (RV) and functional residual capacity (FRC) are increased, whereas the total lung capacity (TLC) remains normal or is increased. Vital capacity, and particularly inspiratory capacity, is eventually reduced by the increase in RV. Several factors may contribute to the increase in FRC and RV in obstructive lung disease. Decreased lung elastic recoil in COPD increases the FRC because of reduced opposition to the outward force exerted by the chest wall. Loss of airway tone and decreased tethering by the surrounding lung in COPD, as well as bronchoconstriction and mucus plugging in acute asthma, allow airways to collapse at higher lung volumes and trap excessive air. Finally, under demands for increased minute ventilation (e.g., during exercise), the increased resistance to airflow may not allow the lungs to empty completely in the time available for expiration; this leads to so-called dynamic hyperinflation of the lungs as the volume of trapped air progressively increases while pro-inflammatory response in this condition. Pro-inflammatory gene expression promotes cytokine production and release, contributing to further inflammatory cell recruitment and activation. Systemic inflammation, triggered by ongoing pulmonary inflammation, may lead to nonpulmonary abnormalities associated with emphysema, including cachexia and skeletal muscle alterations. Finally, increased apoptosis of pneumocytes and endothelial cells has been observed in lungs with emphysema and could contribute to the loss of alveoli.

Understanding of emphysema pathogenesis has improved with the recognition that inflammation, oxidative stress, protease-antiprotease balance, and apoptosis are linked in a complex interaction induced by cigarette smoke. This improved understanding has broadened the range of potential therapies that may be effective in ameliorating the destructive process. To date, however, therapies targeted at molecular pathways involved in emphysema pathogenesis have not been successful in altering disease progression, with the possible exception of α_1-antitrypsin replacement therapy in individuals with α_1-antitrypsin deficiency.

α_1-Antitrypsin, an acute phase reactant, is produced primarily in the liver, from which it travels to the lung. By its effect on elastases in the lung, α_1-antitrypsin prevents the uncontrolled degradation of elastin in the lung parenchyma and protects against the development of emphysema. Individuals with the ZZ genotype of α_1-antitrypsin deficiency produce mutant forms of α_1-antitrypsin that have a tendency to inappropriately polymerize within the hepatocyte, leading to a deficiency in secreted α_1-antitrypsin and, in some cases, collateral damage to the liver caused by accumulation of intracellular misfolded, mutant α_1-antitrypsin. Patients who develop emphysema at a young age (<40 years) should be evaluated for this condition whether or not they smoke, as should patients with bronchiectasis and unexplained liver disease or cirrhosis. Testing shows reduced α_1-antitrypsin levels. Genotyping can reveal specific mutations (most commonly ZZ in severe deficiency). Polymorphisms in various other genes (e.g., *MMP12*) that appear to be relevant to susceptibility to COPD have been uncovered, and other factors contributing to COPD heritability and susceptibility are under active investigation. α_1-Antitrypsin supplementation has been used for patients with α_1-antitrypsin deficiency and appears to result in a decreased loss of lung density (surrogate for emphysema) by computed tomographic measurement (level 1 evidence).

Large and Small Airways Disease in COPD

Chronic bronchitis often coincides with emphysema in patients with COPD, but it may occur independently from either emphysema or COPD and is defined in clinical terms (described earlier). Cigarette smoking is the major cause, although exposure to pollutants such as dusts and smokes may pay a role. Pathologic findings are goblet cell hyperplasia, mucus hypersecretion and plugging, and airway inflammation and fibrosis (Fig. 16-3).

The disease mechanisms involved in the development of emphysema are also important in the pathogenesis of chronic bronchitis. However, in contrast to emphysema, chronic bronchitis is a disease of the large airways and not of the lung parenchyma. Therefore, the relationship of chronic bronchitis to airflow obstruction is less robust than for emphysema, and

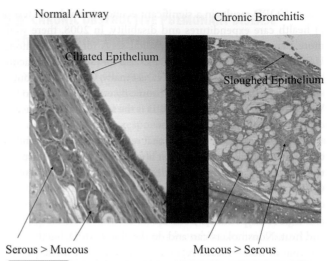

Normal Airway — Chronic Bronchitis

FIGURE 16-3 Pathology of chronic bronchitis: Normally, airway submucosal serous glands outnumber mucous glands and the epithelium includes ciliated cells. In chronic bronchitis, mucous glands are more prevalent than serous glands and the epithelium is abnormal. (Courtesy Dr. Charles Kuhn.)

airflow limitation consistent with COPD in a patient with symptoms of chronic bronchitis may be more reflective of concomitant emphysema and small airways disease. Inflammation in chronic bronchitis leads to effects on the airway epithelium, including excess mucus production and impairment in mucociliary clearance.

Neurogenic stimuli are also important in the pathogenesis of airway obstruction in chronic bronchitis. The conducting airways are surrounded by smooth muscle, which contains adrenergic and cholinergic receptors. Stimulation of β_2-adrenergic receptors by circulating catecholamines dilates airways, whereas stimulation of airway irritant receptors constricts airways through a cholinergic mechanism by means of the vagus nerve. The irritant bronchoconstrictive pathways are normally present to protect against inhalation of noxious agents, but in pathologic states, these pathways may contribute to airway hyperreactivity. A host of endogenous chemical mediators such as proteases, growth factors, and cytokines can also affect airway tone.

By definition, the predominant symptom in chronic bronchitis is sputum production. Bronchospasm may also be prominent. Recurrent bacterial airway infections are typical. As with patients with COPD, the evaluation of patients with chronic bronchitis should include pulmonary function tests and a chest radiograph in addition to standard laboratory testing.

Damage to the small airways (those less than about 2 mm in diameter) is integral to the pathogenesis of COPD. The small airways are the major site of resistance to airflow in COPD. Respiratory bronchiolitis, in which there is an accumulation of pigmented macrophages in and around the bronchioles (E-Fig. 16-5), may be an incidental finding in asymptomatic smokers without COPD. However, as COPD develops, other inflammatory cells are recruited to the small conducting airways, presumably in reaction to ongoing irritation from cigarette smoke or inhaled particles. With inflammation, the small airways in COPD can be affected by remodeling, leading to airway wall thickening and fibrosis, smooth muscle hypertrophy, and airway luminal narrowing, all of which contribute to airflow obstruction. Mucus plugs and inflammatory exudates can occlude the small airways, leading to increased resistance to airflow.

Recently, demonstration of profound decreases in small airway numbers and cross-sectional area in lungs of individuals with COPD has provided important evidence that loss of the small airways occurs with sufficient severity to result in the spirometrically detectable expiratory airflow limitation that characterizes COPD. Indeed, there is evidence that small airway loss may precede emphysema development in COPD.

Immune-mediated abnormalities are also seen at the level of the small airways in COPD. Lymphoid follicles may form around these airways in response to ongoing antigenic stimulation and bacterial infection, with a prominence of B cells and CD8+ T cells in more advanced COPD. Emphysema is associated with airflow obstruction of the small airways caused by destruction of the alveoli tethered to the airways, which normally provide a force opposing airway closure. These myriad changes at the small airway level contribute significantly to the physiologic abnormalities and altered local immune response in COPD.

Clinical Presentation

COPD related to chronic tobacco exposure is characterized by slowly progressive dyspnea that is first noticed during exertion but progresses over years until it is evident with minimal exertion (e.g., when dressing) or even at rest. Affected individuals complain of exercise intolerance and fatigue, and the disease eventually may lead to weight loss, depression, and anxiety as a result of increased work of breathing. Chronic cough can be present and is productive or dry, depending on the degree of mucus metaplasia (e.g., chronic bronchitis). In general, emphysema caused by chronic cigarette smoking is almost never observed in patients before 40 years of age. If it is, consideration should be given to genetic disorders such as α_1-antitrypsin deficiency.

During the early stages of COPD, the physical examination may be normal. Normal examination results and the absence of symptoms often delay diagnosis. Inspection of the thorax and palpation may fail to reveal findings. As the disease progresses, the lungs may become hyperresonant to percussion, and auscultation may show diminished breath sounds with rhonchi or wheezes. The chest wall may begin to remodel, giving the patient the appearance of a "barrel chest." During the late stages of COPD, patients show evidence of increased work of breathing with use of accessory muscles, pursed-lip breathing, and weight loss. Skeletal muscle wasting may also become evident. Despite their respiratory insufficiency, some patients are able to sustain relatively normal oxygen levels in blood until very late in the disease, leading to the classic clinical presentation of the "pink puffer." Other patients tend to retain carbon dioxide and diminish their work of breathing, resulting in chronic respiratory acidosis and, in extreme cases, polycythemia and cyanosis; this is the prototypical "blue bloater" phenotype. There is also an overlap of COPD with other respiratory disorders, such as obstructive sleep apnea, that may contribute to carbon dioxide retention.

Although COPD results in chronic, progressive dyspnea, periodic acute exacerbations are also characteristic. A rapidly worsening of pulmonary function and an increased burden of respiratory symptoms such as dyspnea, cough, and sputum production characterize COPD exacerbations. Acute exacerbations are associated with various triggers, most importantly viral or bacterial respiratory infections, air pollution or other environmental factors, pulmonary embolism, and cardiac failure. Exacerbations are more common with increasing severity of COPD, with increasing age, and during the winter months. Exacerbations vary widely in severity. Severe exacerbations may lead to hospitalization, acute respiratory failure, and death. After an exacerbation, it may take weeks for the patient to return to a baseline level of function. Patients with frequent exacerbations of COPD experience an accelerated rate of decline in FEV_1. Patients who have experienced a COPD exacerbation are more likely to experience future exacerbations, suggesting that exacerbation is an important event in the natural history of COPD. On occasion, an exacerbation of COPD leading to acute respiratory failure is the first event leading to the diagnosis of COPD in an individual patient.

COPD is associated with a number of comorbid conditions, such as atherosclerotic heart disease, lung cancer, osteoporosis, and depression. These comorbidities may be related to smoking, to the chronic systemic inflammation present in patients with COPD, to the impaired quality of life resulting from COPD, or to treatments (e.g., corticosteroids) administered during the course of COPD. Monitoring for and appropriate management of these coexisting disorders is an important part of the ongoing assessment of patients with COPD.

As COPD progresses, the lung volumes increase (hyperinflation) and the diaphragms flatten, rendering inspiratory excursions inefficient. Tidal volume decreases and respiratory rate increases in an effort to decrease the work of breathing. In advanced disease, the cardiovascular system becomes affected as a result of the loss of vasculature in destroyed alveolar walls and vasoconstriction and vascular remodeling due to chronic hypoxia. With a limited area for blood flow, pulmonary vascular resistance is increased, leading to increased right ventricular afterload and development of pulmonary hypertension. This accelerates the development of right ventricular failure, which is referred to as cor pulmonale in the setting of lung disease. Right heart gallop, distended neck veins, hepatojugular reflux, and leg edema characterize cor pulmonale.

Diagnosis and Differential Diagnosis
Diagnosis

Pulmonary function tests, especially spirometry, are essential for the diagnosis of COPD. A reduced FEV_1/FVC ratio (<0.70) on spirometry performed after administration of a bronchodilator is diagnostic of COPD. Although some degree of reversibility of the obstruction may be detected with bronchodilators, and airway hyperreactivity can be unveiled by bronchoprovocation challenges if performed, the obstructive defect is not entirely reversible in COPD. This characteristic and the consistent and progressive nature of the expiratory flow limitation represent key features that help distinguish COPD from asthma, a major differential diagnostic consideration. The severity of disease and prognosis can be estimated by the FEV_1:

GOLD 1/mild COPD	$FEV_1 \geq 80\%$ predicted
GOLD 2/moderate COPD	$FEV_1 \geq 50\%$ but less than 80% predicted
GOLD 3/severe COPD	$FEV_1 \geq 30\%$ but less than 50% predicted
GOLD 4/very severe COPD	$FEV_1 < 30\%$ predicted

An FEV_1 of about 1 L (usually 50% predicted) suggests severe obstruction and, in the case of COPD, predicts a mean survival rate of 50% at 5 years. For a better predictor of mortality than FEV_1 alone, the BODE index can be used: *b*ody mass index, degree of *o*bstruction as measured by FEV_1, modified Medical Research Council *d*yspnea score, and *e*xercise capacity as denoted by 6-minute walk distance.

Lung volumes should be measured along with pulmonary function testing because the limitation to expired airflow and decreased elastic recoil lead to lung hyperinflation, as evidenced by increased RV, FRC, and, ultimately, TLC.

Destruction of alveoli decreases the surface area for gas exchange in emphysema. This loss of surface area, coupled with bronchial obstruction and altered distribution of ventilated air, results in ventilation-perfusion inequality or mismatch, a cause of hypoxemia. Hyperinflation of the lungs increases zone 1 conditions, in which alveolar pressure exceeds pulmonary arterial pressure, and this process decreases perfusion and increases physiologic dead space. Hypercarbia can be avoided by increasing the minute ventilation, even with substantial ventilation-perfusion mismatching. However, eventually, the metabolic costs of breathing become excessive, and respiratory muscles fatigue. Over time, chemoreceptors reset, allowing the level of partial pressure of carbon dioxide in arterial blood ($Paco_2$) to rise, which increases the efficiency of ventilation by eliminating a higher concentration of carbon dioxide per breath, thereby lowering the metabolic cost of breathing. Significant individual variation is observed in the degree of mechanical impairment and in the magnitude of increase in $Paco_2$. Derangements in gas exchange can be detected by measuring arterial blood gases, by showing a decrease in D_{LCO}, or by evaluating hemoglobin oxygen desaturation during exertion. The degree of decrease in D_{LCO} correlates well with the radiologic extent of emphysema in COPD.

Chest radiography may fail to reveal abnormalities during the early stages of COPD, but in later stages, radiographic studies show hyperinflation, hyperlucency, flattening of the diaphragms, and bullous changes in lung parenchyma (E-Fig. 16-6). Pleural abnormalities, lymphadenopathy, and mediastinal widening are not characteristic of emphysema and should point to other diagnoses, such as lung cancer. Computed tomography is more sensitive than plain radiography because it allows for a more detailed evaluation of the lung parenchyma and surrounding structures. Computed tomography is useful in assessing the distribution of emphysema (E-Fig. 16-7) in patients for whom operative interventions such as lung volume reduction surgery are being contemplated (see later discussion). HRCT is highly sensitive for the detection of occult emphysema and can reveal the pattern of emphysematous changes. Electrocardiography might show evidence of right ventricular strain. Echocardiography can reveal evidence of right ventricular hypertrophy or dilation and can often provide an estimate of pulmonary arterial pressures in patients with advanced COPD. A high blood hemoglobin level might reveal erythrocytosis in the setting of chronic hypoxemia, whereas increased white blood cell counts might suggest infection. The arterial blood gas analysis may show hypoxemia, hypercarbia, or both, whereas acidemia due to acute hypercarbia may be present during an exacerbation.

Differential Diagnosis

The differential diagnosis of COPD includes the other major obstructive lung disorders: asthma, bronchiectasis, and the bronchiolar disorders. Asthma can occur at any age and sometimes overlaps with COPD, such as in patients with childhood asthma who smoke as adults. However, patients with COPD are typically older than 40 years of age and have a lengthy smoking history, whereas patients with asthma often have a history of atopy, have more variable symptoms that are often worse at night, and typically have marked improvements in lung function after bronchodilator administration. Patients with asthma may have normal pulmonary function during periods in which their asthma is well controlled, whereas those with COPD demonstrate ongoing airway obstruction even during periods of relative clinical stability.

It can be difficult to distinguish COPD with chronic bronchitis from bronchiectasis, and HRCT is necessary to assess for the abnormal bronchial dilation that is diagnostic of bronchiectasis.

Bronchiolar disorders can also be difficult to distinguish from COPD but should be considered in patients with risk factors, such as connective tissue disease or occupational exposures. Again, more sophisticated testing, such as HRCT with inspiratory and expiratory views to demonstrate peripheral areas of gas trapping and centrilobular nodules consistent with mucus impaction of the small airways, or even lung biopsy, may be needed to diagnose bronchiolitis.

Nonpulmonary causes of dyspnea on exertion, such as congestive heart failure or coronary artery disease, should also be considered in the differential diagnosis of COPD.

Treatment

Prevention

Because a cure for COPD does not exist, the best approach to this condition is prevention. Most cases of COPD in the United States are caused by cigarette smoking. Therefore, an appropriate major emphasis has been placed on the development of community education programs that focus on smoking prevention and promote smoking cessation. Legislative measures banning smoking in various public settings and levying increased taxes on cigarettes have been used to diminish the effects of environmental or second-hand exposure to tobacco smoke and to discourage smoking. Although smoking cessation interventions are effective in only a minority of patients, smoking cessation decreases mortality in patients with COPD who do succeed in quitting (level 1 evidence).

Most patients who are successful at smoking cessation have had at least one prior failed attempt, so physicians should encourage smoking cessation with at least brief interventions at every opportunity, even in patients who have tried but failed to quit in the past. Long-term physician and group support increases the success of cessation attempts, and pharmacologic smoking cessation aides, including nicotine replacement with gum or transdermal patches, bupropion, and varenicline, may provide additional benefit.

Pharmacologic Therapies

After COPD is established, therapy is directed at avoiding complications such as exacerbations, relieving airflow obstruction through use of bronchodilators, and providing supplemental oxygen to patients with hypoxemia. Commonly used inhaled bronchodilators include sympathomimetic agents (β_2-adrenoreceptor agonists) and anticholinergic agents. Ipratropium bromide, a short-acting anticholinergic agent, is effective at decreasing dyspnea and improving FEV_1 in COPD (level 1 evidence). Albuterol is the most commonly used β_2-agonist; its bronchodilator effect is rapid in onset and relatively short lived. In practice, a combination of albuterol and ipratropium is frequently prescribed because these agents produce greater benefits when used in combination than individually.

Short-acting agents are typically prescribed for patients with mild disease or intermittent symptoms on an as-needed basis. Short-acting bronchodilators can be delivered by metered-dose inhaler (MDI) or by nebulizer. The MDI offers advantages of portability and ease of administration and convenience. When used correctly with a spacer, MDIs are as effective as nebulizers in delivering the drug. Nebulization has no advantage over the use of MDIs in the long-term management of obstructive lung disease except in patients who are unable to use an MDI properly.

Long-acting bronchodilators are effective for maintenance therapy in patients who have at least moderate COPD. Long-acting agents include the long-acting β_2-agonists (LABAs), which are available in once- or twice-daily formulations, and the long-acting anticholinergic/muscarinic antagonists (LAMAs), which are administered once daily. Both the LABAs and the LAMAs provide effective bronchodilation with resultant improvements in FEV_1 and symptoms (level 1 evidence). Tiotropium, a LAMA, as well as salmeterol, indacaterol, and formoterol, all LABAs, have been shown to reduce exacerbation rates in COPD (level 1). Initiation of either a LABA or a LAMA is reasonable for patients with COPD who require a long-acting bronchodilator. Tachycardia, hypokalemia, and tremor are potential adverse effects of LABAs, whereas dry mouth and urinary retention may occur with LAMA administration. In more advanced disease, there is some evidence (level 2) of additional benefits from the combination of a LABA and a LAMA.

Current data suggest that the chronic use of inhaled corticosteroids improves symptoms and decreases the frequency of exacerbations (level 1). Inhaled long-acting corticosteroids (e.g., beclamethasone, budesonide, fluticasone propionate) should be considered for individuals with COPD and a history of exacerbations but should not be used as monotherapy. Inhaled corticosteroids are less clearly effective in COPD than in asthma, and pneumonia occurs more frequently in patients with COPD treated with inhaled corticosteroids (level 1). Inhaled corticosteroids can be combined with LABAs; the combination salmeterol with fluticasone in patients with moderate to severe COPD was shown to improve health-related quality of life and to reduce exacerbations to a greater extent than either component alone (level 2).

Systemic use of corticosteroids is indicated during acute exacerbations, and intravenous corticosteroids are useful in the acute setting. Intravenous corticosteroids have also proved effective for the management of acute exacerbations of most obstructive lung diseases, including asthma (Fig. 16-4). Patients with acute exacerbations are usually transitioned from intravenous to oral steroids within 72 hours, with a subsequent tapering of the oral steroid dose over 2 weeks, although shorter courses may also be effective. Other agents with anti-inflammatory capabilities, such as leukotriene inhibitors, are not indicated for treatment of COPD.

Theophylline, a methylxanthine, is a weak systemic sympathomimetic agent with a narrow therapeutic window. It is not a first-line drug in the treatment of COPD, although long-acting derivatives with improved safety profiles have been developed. Theophylline preparations have some anti-inflammatory activity and may provide additional bronchodilation in patients with COPD who do not respond adequately to inhaled β-agonists. When these preparations are used, blood concentrations should be maintained in the lower end of the therapeutic range (between 8 and 12 μg/mL). Toxicity is common at concentrations higher than 20 μg/mL. The metabolism of theophylline is decreased by many commonly used drugs (e.g., erythromycin), and toxic serum concentrations of theophylline can be reached quickly when these other drugs are administered unless the theophylline dose is adjusted appropriately. Toxic effects of theophylline may be observed in the gastrointestinal, cardiac, and neurologic systems. Severe theophylline toxicity can be fatal, and treatment with charcoal hemoperfusion may be required.

Phosphodiesterase type 4 (PDE4) inhibitors have been investigated for the treatment of COPD, and an oral PDE4 inhibitor was recently approved as add-on therapy for treatment of severe COPD with chronic bronchitis and a history of exacerbations. PDE4 inhibitors act to inhibit breakdown of cyclic adenosine monophosphate (cAMP), resulting in a weak bronchodilator effect (approximately 50 mL improvement in FEV_1); they should not be used as acute bronchodilators. However, roflumilast was demonstrated to reduce exacerbation rates in patients who had severe COPD with chronic bronchitis and a history of exacerbation in the prior year and were not using inhaled corticosteroids (level 2 evidence). Adverse effects include weight loss, nausea and loss of appetite, and an increase in psychiatric adverse reactions including suicidality.

Oxygen Therapy and Mechanical Ventilation

Continuous oxygen therapy has been shown to improve survival in patients with COPD and hypoxemia (level 1 evidence). Oxygen supplementation is recommended once the partial pressure of oxygen in arterial blood (Pao_2) drops below 55 mm Hg or the hemoglobin oxygen saturation decreases to 88%. Oxygen supplementation is indicated at higher levels of Pao_2 if end-organ damage, such as pulmonary hypertension, is present.

Oxygen therapy is frequently necessary for treatment of acute exacerbations of obstructive lung disease. In patients who hypoventilate chronically and therefore have an elevated $Paco_2$, elevating the inspired oxygen content may acutely worsen hypercarbia by inhibiting the hypoxic ventilatory drive and by promoting the dissociation of carbon dioxide from oxygenated hemoglobin (the Haldane effect). High-flow oxygen has been

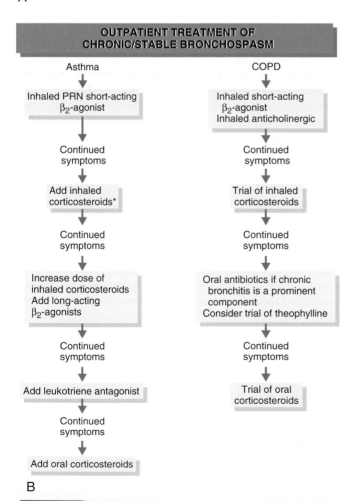

EMERGENCY DEPARTMENT TREATMENT OF ACUTE BRONCHOSPASM

Oxygen
Inhaled β₂-agonist
Consider inhaled anticholinergic
Oral or IV corticosteroids

Inadequate response → Inhaled anticholinergics if not given previously → Persistent bronchospasm → Admit to hospital → Respiratory failure → Consider aminophylline / Heliox (helium = oxygen) / IV magnesium / Endotracheal intubation and mechanical ventilation

Good response → Discharge on inhaled β₂-agonist ± inhaled anticholinergic / Corticosteroids × 5 days / Arrange outpatient follow-up within 5 days

A

OUTPATIENT TREATMENT OF CHRONIC/STABLE BRONCHOSPASM

Asthma → Inhaled PRN short-acting β₂-agonist → Continued symptoms → Add inhaled corticosteroids* → Continued symptoms → Increase dose of inhaled corticosteroids / Add long-acting β₂-agonists → Continued symptoms → Add leukotriene antagonist → Continued symptoms → Add oral corticosteroids

COPD → Inhaled short-acting β₂-agonist / Inhaled anticholinergic → Continued symptoms → Trial of inhaled corticosteroids → Continued symptoms → Oral antibiotics if chronic bronchitis is a prominent component / Consider trial of theophylline → Continued symptoms → Trial of oral corticosteroids

B

FIGURE 16-4 Algorithms for the treatment of bronchospasm in patients in the emergency department (**A**) and in outpatients with stable disease (**B**). IV, Intravenous; PRN, as needed. *Leukotriene antagonists could be considered.

shown to be harmful in the setting of prehospital emergency treatment for COPD (level 1 evidence). Therefore, oxygen should be closely titrated to maintain normoxia and to avoid either hypoxemia or excessively elevated PaO_2. An oxygen saturation of 90% to 92% is a reasonable target in the absence of further data (level 3). During exacerbations of COPD leading to hypercarbic respiratory failure, noninvasive positive airway pressure ventilation has proved useful in reducing the work of breathing, alleviating diaphragm fatigue, and reducing the need for endotracheal intubation and mechanical ventilation (level 1).

Antibiotics

Exacerbations of airway obstruction may result from viral or bacterial infection. The most common bacterial pathogens in COPD are *Streptococcus pneumoniae, Haemophilus influenzae,* and *Moraxella catarrhalis.* Management of acute exacerbations should include empiric administration of antibiotics, which have been shown to improve the success rate in exacerbation treatment (level 2 evidence). The role of chronic prophylactic antibiotic use in COPD is uncertain, and a trial of oral azithromycin resulted in a reduction in exacerbations but an increased risk of hearing loss (level 2). Immunization with influenza vaccines directed at specific epidemic strains reduces exacerbations of COPD (level 1). Pneumococcal vaccination is also recommended in patients with COPD.

Nonpharmacologic Therapies

Multiple airway clearance techniques aid in clearing of airway secretions, but their effectiveness in the management of emphysema and other obstructive lung diseases in adults is questionable. If needed, chest physiotherapy and postural drainage might be useful in patients with chronic bronchitis and increased sputum production. Few data support the use of specific mucolytics or expectorant agents for patients with COPD.

Patients with pulmonary disease of sufficient severity to compromise normal activities of daily living commonly demonstrate improved quality of life and less subjective dyspnea when enrolled in a comprehensive, high-quality pulmonary rehabilitation program (level 1 evidence). Pulmonary rehabilitation has not been shown to improve objective measures of pulmonary function, to affect the rate of decline in lung function, or to improve survival. However, it has been shown to improve the quality of life in motivated patients. An important part of pulmonary rehabilitation is nutritional assessment and careful attention to maintaining adequate nutrition. Malnutrition and cachexia are common in later stages of obstructive lung disease, and they result in decreased respiratory muscle strength and compromised immune function.

The role of surgery in COPD is generally limited. Bullectomy, lung volume reduction surgery (LVRS), and lung transplantation are all potentially effective surgical options for selected patients. Resection of nonfunctional areas of lung (e.g., bullectomy) may allow for compressed functional areas to expand and may improve symptoms, airflow, and oxygenation by improving ventilation-perfusion matching in a subgroup of patients. In addition, resection of bullae can decrease lung volumes, resulting in enhanced diaphragmatic function and decreased work of breathing. The best candidates for LVRS are those with predominantly upper lobe disease who have a low exercise tolerance despite rehabilitation and are without other major comorbidities. This subgroup may have reduced mortality after LVRS (level 2 evidence). In general, a high surgical mortality risk exists in patients referred for LVRS who have an FEV_1 or D_{LCO} of less than 20% predicted and in those who have more homogeneous distribution of emphysema. Endoscopic therapies to deflate regions of lung with emphysema are currently under investigation.

Single or bilateral lung transplantation is an option for patients with end-stage airflow obstruction. The average survival after lung transplantation is 4 to 5 years. Rejection, viral infections, transplant-associated lymphoproliferative disease, and late occurrence of bronchiolitis obliterans remain significant problems, but the procedure can improve the quality of life in properly selected patients.

Palliative Care

Although the disease course can be unpredictable, discussion of end-of-life issues with the patient is an important component of longitudinal care as COPD progresses to an advanced stage. Preparation of advance directives regarding use of intensive care measures at the end of life may be desirable. Opioid narcotics can be highly effective for relieving dyspnea in patients with terminal complications of COPD (level 1 evidence).

Prognosis

COPD is a chronic and progressive disease with a variable and typically prolonged clinical course. As discussed previously, measurement of lung function (FEV_1 % predicted) has prognostic significance, and use of the multifactorial BODE index can improve prognostication compared with use of FEV_1 alone. Patients who have frequent exacerbations of COPD appear to have more rapid loss of lung function than those without exacerbations, suggesting that frequent exacerbations result in a worse clinical course.

At present, aside from smoking cessation and the addition of long-term oxygen therapy for patients with hypoxemia, interventions to improve survival in COPD are limited. No pharmacologic therapy for COPD has been definitively demonstrated to improve survival. In mild COPD, mortality is frequently related to comorbidities such as ischemic heart disease and lung cancer; in more advanced stages, a greater proportion of patients die from respiratory causes.

⬤ BRONCHIOLAR DISORDERS
Definition and Epidemiology

The bronchioles are defined as the small noncartilaginous airways (<2 mm in diameter). The bronchiolar disorders, or bronchiolitides, encompass a spectrum of diseases of widely varying causes primarily affecting these small airways. Although small airways disease contributes significantly to the syndrome of COPD, and respiratory bronchiolitis may be found incidentally in smokers, bronchiolar disorders with different etiologies than cigarette smoking also exist. These disorders are associated with patchy inflammation and epithelial injury, fibrosis, mucoid impaction, or obliteration of the bronchioles (E-Fig. 16-8). These changes result in airflow limitation due to increased airway resistance.

Acute bronchiolitis related to respiratory syncytial virus infection is epidemic among infants and young children, but primary bronchiolar disorders, including infectious or postinfectious bronchiolitis, are rare in the adult general population and tend to affect certain specific patient populations.

Pathology

The pathology of the bronchiolar disorders is complex. A variety of terms are used to describe or classify the various histopathologic patterns of small airways disease, including *cellular bronchiolitis* (inflammatory cell infiltration of the small airway wall resulting in small airway narrowing), *follicular bronchiolitis* (formation of abundant lymphoid follicles in close apposition to the small airways, resulting in airway compression), *obliterative* or *constrictive bronchiolitis* (fibrosis surrounding the small airways resulting in narrowing of the affected airways), and *bronchiolitis obliterans* (formation of endoluminal fibrous lesions, sometimes called *Masson bodies*, obstructing the small airway lumen). The histopathologic pattern of small airways disease may suggest a likely underlying etiology; for example, follicular bronchiolitis is often, although not exclusively, seen in the context of Sjögren's syndrome.

Clinical Presentation

In general, the bronchiolar disorders manifest nonspecifically with dyspnea, which may be severe or progressive, in some cases accompanied by cough or sputum production. The physical examination may reveal inspiratory squeaks or wheezes but may be surprisingly normal. The possibility of a bronchiolar disorder should be considered in particular settings. For example, bronchiolitis may complicate the course of rheumatoid arthritis, Sjögren's syndrome, or inflammatory bowel disease.

Diffuse panbronchiolitis is a rare idiopathic disorder, most common in Japan, that is characterized by cough with purulent sputum, sinusitis, and dyspnea. Recurrent respiratory infections with bacterial organisms such as *Pseudomonas aeruginosa* complicate the course of diffuse panbronchiolitis. Bronchiolitis obliterans (in this context a clinical, not a histopathologic, term) is seen with the bronchiolitis obliterans syndrome of chronic allograft rejection after lung transplantation, in graft-versus-host disease after allogeneic hematopoietic stem cell transplantation, and after occupational toxin exposures. For example, occupational clusters of bronchiolitis obliterans have been described after exposure to diacetyl, a flavoring chemical used in the manufacture of microwave popcorn.

Diagnosis and Differential Diagnosis

In general, the bronchiolar disorders cause an obstructive pattern of expiratory airflow limitation on pulmonary function testing without evidence of reversibility. The bronchiolitis obliterans syndrome is diagnosed clinically by a decline in FEV_1 of 20% from a stable baseline value on serial testing after lung transplantation. HRCT is valuable in the diagnosis and assessment of the bronchiolar disorders. Characteristic findings on HRCT include centrilobular nodules or tree-in-bud opacities, reflecting impacted inflammatory exudates or sloughed epithelial cells in the bronchioles. A "mosaic attenuation" pattern, with decreased attenuation in geographic regions of lung reflecting areas of air trapping distal to obstructed bronchioles, is often seen on inspiration. CT scanning during the expiratory phase can confirm that this finding is caused by air trapping as opposed to decreased perfusion from pulmonary vascular disease. Lung biopsy may be of limited value because of the scattered, patchy nature of the abnormalities present in the bronchiolar disorders. The differential diagnosis includes COPD, which also causes poorly reversible obstruction on spirometry.

Treatment

Treatment of the bronchiolar disorders is challenging. Acute bronchiolitis typically resolves without treatment; bronchodilators and steroids are not clearly beneficial, although they are often prescribed. The bronchiolitis obliterans syndrome responds poorly to increased immunosuppression and is a frequent cause of death after lung transplantation. Azithromycin, a macrolide antibiotic, has been reported to increase FEV_1 in the bronchiolitis obliterans syndrome. Macrolide antibiotics have also been reported to positively affect the clinical course of diffuse panbronchiolitis, possibly reflecting immunomodulatory or antifibrotic effects of these medications (level 2 evidence). Lung transplantation may be necessary in progressive bronchiolitis obliterans, and retransplantation has sometimes been performed in patients affected by the bronchiolitis obliterans syndrome after transplant rejection.

Prognosis

These disorders may be self-limited, as in acute bronchiolitis caused by respiratory syncytial virus, or relentlessly progressive and fatal, as in the bronchiolitis obliterans syndrome occurring after lung transplantation.

⬤ BRONCHIECTASIS

Definition and Epidemiology

Bronchiectasis (E-Fig. 16-9) is defined as an abnormal dilation of the bronchi (the large airways containing cartilage within their walls) resulting from inflammation and permanent destructive changes of the bronchial walls. The incidence of bronchiectasis is unknown, but it may affect more than 100,000 individuals in the United States and is more frequent in older age groups. There is likely a higher incidence of bronchiectasis in developing countries where there are lower childhood vaccination rates and a higher prevalence of pulmonary tuberculosis.

Pathology

Bronchiectasis may be localized to a bronchial segment or lobe of the lung, or it may be diffuse. The involved bronchi are abnormally dilated and demonstrate chronic inflammation within the bronchial wall with neutrophilic inflammation and bacterial colonization and infection in the bronchial lumen. The inflammation in bronchiectasis is associated with structural changes in the walls of the bronchi, including destructive changes affecting the elastic fibers, smooth muscle, and cartilage. As with COPD, there is also involvement of the small airways. Small airway obstruction leads to increased resistance to airflow that results in airflow obstruction despite the presence of dilation of the larger airways. The classic pathologic classifications of bronchiectasis are *tubular*

(the most common form, in which there is smooth dilation of the bronchi), *varicose* (dilated bronchi with indentations reminiscent of varicose veins), and *cystic* (end-stage bronchiectasis with dilated bronchi ending in sac-like structures resembling clusters of grapes).

Bronchiectasis is hypothesized to result from an environmental insult leading to bronchial damage in a susceptible host. This in turn leads to impaired infection clearance, bacterial colonization and infection or reinfection, ongoing inflammation of the airways, and further bronchial damage, creating a classic vicious cycle. An inciting infection, sometimes occurring in childhood, is thought to initiate the development of bronchial damage leading to bronchiectasis in many cases (post-infectious bronchiectasis). This may be a viral infection (e.g., measles), a necrotizing pneumonia (e.g., *Staphylococcus aureus* pneumonia), tuberculosis, or infection with an atypical mycobacteria (e.g., *Mycobacterium avium-intracellulare*). Because infections such *M. avium-intracellulare* also complicate the course of bronchiectasis, determination of whether a mycobacterial infection was an initiator or a consequence of bronchiectasis may be difficult.

Localized bronchiectasis may also result from anatomic obstruction by an endobronchial foreign body, tumor, or broncholith or from extrinsic compression by lymphadenopathy. The right middle lobe syndrome results from narrowing of the right middle lobe bronchial orifice, often by lymph node enlargement in the setting of tuberculosis, which leads to localized bronchiectasis distal to the site of obstruction. Anatomic obstruction results in chronic or recurrent bacterial infections and inflammation leading to bronchial distortion and destruction over time.

Diffuse bronchiectasis can result from various impairments in host defenses that create a vulnerability to persistent or recurrent lung infection leading to bronchial damage. For example, bronchiectasis may occur with congenital defects that impair mucus clearance in the airways such as CF (discussed later) or primary ciliary dyskinesia, a rare inherited abnormality of the ciliary microtubules. The classic triad of sinusitis, situs inversus, and infertility is diagnostic of Kartagener's syndrome, a form of primary ciliary dyskinesia. Immunodeficiency states, such as hypogammaglobulinemia in combined variable immunodeficiency, may also result in bronchiectasis. α_1-Atitrypsin deficiency results in deficient antiprotease activity in the lung and is also associated with bronchiectasis. Bronchiectasis also complicates certain connective tissue disorders such as rheumatoid arthritis.

Finally, bronchiectasis overlaps with the more common obstructive lung disorders, COPD and asthma. Certain patients with COPD also have bronchiectasis, often in the lower lobes. Allergic bronchopulmonary aspergillosis is a condition that occurs in asthmatics with hypersensitivity to aspergillus fungi. It is associated with central bronchiectasis, high levels of immunoglobulin E (IgE), and precipitins for *Aspergillus* species.

Clinical Presentation

Patients with bronchiectasis exhibit chronic cough and copious, sometimes foul-smelling sputum. The sputum produced may be greater in volume and purulence than with COPD or asthma. Shortness of breath and fatigue may also be present. Blood-streaked sputum is common, and massive hemoptysis may occur during the course of bronchiectasis. Localized crackles and clubbing may be present. Periodic exacerbations due to infection with bacterial pathogens, including *H. influenzae* and *P. aeruginosa*, are common. Nontuberculous mycobacterial colonization or infection may also occur. Pulmonary function tests typically show mild to moderate obstruction. Evidence of bronchial hyperresponsiveness is not infrequent.

Diagnosis and Differential Diagnosis

Chest radiographs may be normal or may show increased interstitial markings. The classic finding is parallel lines in peripheral lung fields, described as "tram tracks," which represent thickened bronchial walls that do not taper from proximal to distal sites. However, HRCT is more sensitive for the detection of dilated airways and is the diagnostic test of choice in the evaluation of suspected bronchiectasis. Bronchiectasis on HRCT is diagnosed by demonstration of lack of airway tapering, airways that are larger in diameter than their accompanying blood vessel, and the presence of visible bronchi at the lung periphery (outer 1 to 2 cm of the lung). Bronchoscopy may be indicated in localized bronchiectasis to assess for endobronchial abnormalities or foreign body. Sputum can be cultured to assess for fungal or mycobacterial organisms that may be causative or for identification of specific bacterial pathogens during exacerbations. Once the diagnosis of bronchiectasis is established, investigation to determine the underlying cause, such as assessment of immunoglobulin levels to rule out combined variable immunodeficiency, is indicated.

The differential diagnosis includes chronic bronchitis and COPD, asthma, and, in the setting of hemoptysis and clubbing, lung cancer.

Treatment

Treatment of the underlying cause of the bronchiectasis should be undertaken if possible. An anatomic obstruction, such as from a foreign body or benign tumor, should be relieved. Atypical mycobacterial infection should be treated with an appropriate multidrug regimen in symptomatic patients after confirmation of the diagnosis with multiple smears and cultures. Allergic bronchopulmonary aspergillosis is typically treated with corticosteroids; addition of azole antifungals may also be beneficial (level 3 evidence). Bacterial exacerbations of bronchiectasis should be treated with a broad-spectrum antibiotic that is effective against the likely pathogens, such as amoxicillin or, in patients known to be colonized or infected by *Pseudomonas*, a fluoroquinolone (level 2). Aerosolized antibiotics are of benefit to suppress bacterial growth in bronchiectasis associated with CF and may be beneficial in non-CF bronchiectasis if *Pseudomonas* infection is present or if frequent exacerbations occur (level 3). Chronic administration of macrolide antibiotics has been shown to reduce inflammation and exacerbations in bronchiectasis but may also promote development of macrolide-resistant bacteria (level 2).

Immunoglobulin supplementation may aid in the host defense against bacterial infection in individuals with hypogammaglobulinemia. Airway clearance and postural drainage are frequently employed in bronchiectasis. Bronchodilators may provide symptomatic relief. Massive hemoptysis should be managed with airway protection and identification of the bleeding site; bronchial artery angiography with embolization of the causative bleeding vessels can be life-saving (level 3). The role of surgery

is mainly in resection of obstructing lesions that are causing distal bronchiectasis, in removal of a badly damaged isolated segment of bronchiectatic lung, and, on occasion, as a salvage therapy in resection of a site with uncontrolled hemorrhage (level 3).

Prognosis

The prognosis of patients with bronchiectasis is generally thought to be favorable, although deterioration of lung function over time has been shown to occur. Quality of life may be affected adversely, for example by chronic production of copious sputum or frequent exacerbations. Massive hemoptysis is an emergency situation that requires intensive management and may be fatal.

CYSTIC FIBROSIS
Definition and Epidemiology

CF is an autosomal recessive genetic disorder that results from mutations in the *CFTR* gene. CF affects about 30,000 children and adults in the United States. This disorder affects many organs, including the lungs, pancreas, and reproductive organs, although most mortality related to CF is due to lung disease. It is the most common lethal genetic disorder in the white population, with a carrier frequency of about 1 in 29, affecting 1 in 3300 live births. About 1000 new cases of CF are diagnosed each year. Although most patients are diagnosed in infancy and childhood, some are not diagnosed until adulthood. About 45% of the population with CF in the United States is older than 18 years of age, but before 1940, infants with CF rarely lived to their first birthday. Currently, the median predicted life span for a person with CF is about 37 years.

Pathology

CF results from pathogenic mutations in both alleles of a single gene, *CTFR*, which encodes the cystic fibrosis transmembrane conductance regulator (CFTR), a cAMP-regulated chloride channel that is present on the apical surface of epithelial cells (E-Fig. 16-10). The most common mutation is the ΔF508 mutation, a three-base-pair deletion that results in absence of the phenylalanine residue at the 508 position of the protein. However, more than 1600 mutations in CFTR have been identified to date.

The abnormal CFTR protein results in defective chloride transport and increased sodium reabsorption in airway and ductal epithelia; this leads to abnormally thick and viscous secretions in the respiratory, hepatobiliary, gastrointestinal, and reproductive tracts. The thick secretions do not easily clear from the airways, resulting in respiratory symptoms, and they cause luminal obstruction and destruction of exocrine ducts in other organs, leading to exocrine organ fibrosis and dysfunction, including pancreatic damage.

In patients with CF, the airways become colonized initially with *S. aureus* or *H. influenzae*, followed by *P. aeruginosa* in ensuing years. Persistent inflammation and infection cause bronchial wall destruction and bronchiectasis. Mucus plugging of small airways results in postobstructive cystic airway dilation and parenchymal destruction; progressive airflow obstruction and eventually hypoxemia ensue. The course of CF may additionally be complicated by the development of allergic bronchopulmonary aspergillosis or by nontuberculous mycobacterial infection.

Colonization and infection with multidrug-resistant organisms such as the *Burkholderia cepacia* complex may occur in advanced CF, creating challenging management issues. Most patients die of respiratory failure.

Clinical Presentation

Neonatal screening programs for CF exist nationwide in the United States to identify infants with possible CF who should undergo further testing (e.g., genotyping). Infants with CF may have meconium ileus or failure to thrive with steatorrhea. Salty-tasting skin may be noticed by caregivers. Patients with CF typically have chronic cough with thick sputum production, wheezing, and dyspnea. Pancreatic insufficiency and diabetes are common, and male patients have azoospermia. Nasal polyps are often present, and clubbing is typical.

CF should be considered in the differential diagnosis of patients with unexplained chronic sinus disease, bronchiectasis, male infertility associated with absence of the vas deferens, pancreatitis, or malabsorption. Pulmonary function tests demonstrate hyperinflation and obstruction; a bronchodilator response may be present. Chest imaging studies show hyperinflation, bronchial wall thickening, and bronchiectasis.

Diagnosis and Differential Diagnosis

Measurement of the concentration of chloride in sweat (sweat test) is used to diagnose CF. The diagnosis is considered definitive if the clinical picture is consistent with CF and if the chloride concentration measured in a certified laboratory is greater than 60 mEq/L on at least two occasions. Genotyping can also confirm the diagnosis if known mutations are identified in both gene alleles and may be used if sweat testing is equivocal.

Treatment

The treatment of CF currently relies on supportive measures such as aggressive airway hygiene, nutritional support including pancreatic enzyme replacement, antibiotics, and bronchodilators. Aerosolized recombinant human deoxyribonuclease I (Dornase alfa) decreases sputum viscosity, improves lung function, and reduces exacerbations in CF (level 1 evidence). Inhaled hypertonic saline helps to hydrate secretions, allowing them to be coughed out more easily, and also improves pulmonary function, although likely to a lesser extent than Dornase alfa (level 2). Inhaled tobramycin provided twice daily every other month is indicated for patients with moderate to severe CF who have pseudomonal infections (level 1). Inhaled aztreonam also appears to be beneficial in this patient group (level 2). Anti-inflammatory therapy with ibuprofen and azithromycin may be helpful in certain patients with CF (level 2 for both). However, chronic inhaled and oral corticosteroids are not beneficial and should not be used (level 1).

Specific treatments to improve the function of the defective CFTR chloride channel in CF are under investigation. Recent studies have shown ivcaftor to have positive benefits on CFTR function and FEV_1 in patients with a specific CF mutation (G551D) (level 1 evidence). As with other obstructive lung diseases, the ultimate therapy for patients with CF and end-stage lung disease is lung transplantation. Bilateral lung transplantation is preferred in this condition.

Prognosis

CF is ultimately a fatal disease, although supportive care measures have led to considerable improvement in median survival time. There clinical course of may be variable, in part related to the underlying mutations in the *CFTR* gene.

⬤ ASTHMA

Definition and Epidemiology

Asthma is described by the Global Initiative for Asthma as "a chronic inflammatory disorder of the airways in which many cells and cellular elements play a role. The chronic inflammation is associated with airway hyperresponsiveness that leads to recurrent episodes of wheezing, breathlessness, chest tightness, and coughing, particularly at night or in the early morning. These episodes are usually associated with widespread but variable airflow obstruction within the lung that is often reversible either spontaneously or with treatment."

The incidence of asthma is highest in children, but it affects all ages and occurs worldwide, with a preponderance of the disease in developed industrialized countries. Asthma affects millions of individuals worldwide. In the United States in 2008, 8.2% of the population (approximately 24,000,000 persons) were estimated to have asthma based on survey data, an increase from 7.3% in 2001. The prevalence of asthma has increased markedly over recent decades. Nevertheless, after rising in the late 20th century, the number of deaths from asthma has declined since 2000; in 2010, there were 3404 deaths from asthma in the United States, compared with 5637 deaths in 1995. Asthma death rates are higher in older age groups, females, and blacks.

Pathology

Underlying chronic airway inflammation is considered to be a major pathogenic feature of asthma. Patients with asthma have higher numbers of activated inflammatory cells within the airway wall, and the epithelium is typically infiltrated with eosinophils, mast cells, macrophages, and T lymphocytes, which produce multiple soluble mediators such as cytokines, leukotrienes, and bradykinins. Airway inflammation in asthma is typified by a type 2 helper T-cell (T_H2) response with predominantly eosinophilic inflammation, but some patients with severe asthma exhibit neutrophilic airway inflammation and cytokine production more characteristic of T_H1 inflammation.

The hallmark of asthma is airway hyperresponsiveness—a tendency of the airway smooth muscle to constrict in response to levels of inhaled allergens or irritants that would not typically elicit such a response in normal hosts. Inhaled allergens provoke airway mast cell degranulation by binding to and cross-linking IgE on the mast cell surface. Mast cell degranulation leads to the release of chemical mediators, which cause acute bronchoconstriction and thus increased airway resistance and wheezing as well as mucus hypersecretion (E-Fig. 16-11). Disruption of the continuity of the ciliated columnar epithelium and increased vascularity and edema of the airway wall also follow antigen exposure. In addition to allergens, factors such as stimulation of irritant receptors, respiratory tract infections, and airway cooling can provoke bronchoconstriction in asthmatic individuals.

Airway cooling appears to be responsible for exercise-induced bronchoconstriction as well as some wintertime asthma attacks.

Asthma is associated with airway wall remodeling, which is characterized by hyperplasia and hypertrophy of smooth muscle cells (E-Fig. 16-12), edema, inflammatory infiltration, angiogenesis, and increased deposition of connective tissue components such as type I and type III collagen. This last effect leads not only to a thickening of the subepithelial lamina reticularis (E-Fig. 16-13) but also to an expansion of the entire airway wall. Airway remodeling may begin fairly early in the course of the disease. Whether inflammation leads to remodeling or whether these processes represent two independent manifestations of the disease is unknown. Pulmonary function does seem to decline at an accelerated rate over time in patients with asthma, and airway wall remodeling may play a role in this functional loss. Over time, airway wall remodeling may lead to irreversible airflow limitation, which can worsen the disease by rendering bronchodilator drugs less effective. In this way, airway wall remodeling may make the clinical distinction between asthma and COPD difficult.

The cause of asthma is unknown, but it is likely to be a polygenic disease influenced by environmental factors. Atopy is strongly linked to asthma. Asthma is associated with an allergic-type activation of the immune system, typified by a T_H2-predominant T-cell response to inhaled antigens with consequent IgE production and allergic airway inflammation. Exposure to indoor allergens such as dust mites, cockroaches, furry pets, and fungi is a significant factor; outdoor pollution and other irritants, including cigarette smoke, are also important.

Current concepts of asthma pathogenesis include a focus on impairment of the shift from a T_H2-predominant immunity to a T_H1 immune response early in life. Paradoxically, in the developed world, the perpetuation of T_H2 immune responses and the development of inappropriate allergic responses may be related to a relative lack of exposure of the immune system to appropriate infectious antigenic stimuli in childhood, the so-called hygiene hypothesis. Farming, for example, appears to be protective against the development of asthma and allergic disease, possibly in part because of the increased exposure to microbial antigens eliciting a T_H1 response. Increased exposure to other children (as in daycare settings) and less frequent use of antibiotics may also decrease asthma risk, supporting this hypothesis. On the other hand, asthma is common in poor urban settings in which there is heavy exposure to allergic antigens from dust mites and cockroaches. The timing and roles of particular environmental exposures in utero and in early life in the pathogenesis of asthma and allergic diseases remain to be fully elucidated, and there is no current theory that completely explains asthma pathogenesis or the recent increased incidence of asthma. The interplay of other aspects of modern life, such as changes in the microbiome, with regard to asthma propensity continues to be explored.

Several genetic polymorphisms have been associated with asthma, including variations in the β-adrenergic receptor leading to diminished responsiveness to β-agonists. Identification of other genetic polymorphisms that are important in asthma is a subject of ongoing research. Although asthma is more common in male children than in female children, the prevalence of asthma changes after puberty, and it is more common in adult women than in men. These facts, along with evidence of variation in asthma symptoms during the menstrual cycle and during pregnancy, suggest possible hormonal influences on asthma pathogenesis.

Asthma can be induced by workplace exposures in persons having no previous history of asthma (occupational asthma). Certain substances, such as isocyanates (used in spray paints) and Western red cedar wood dust, are strongly provocative agents for the development of occupational asthma. Obesity has been linked to a higher incidence of asthma. The mechanisms by which obesity may influence asthma development are unclear. Certain infectious agents and other conditions can cause acute bronchospasm even in patients without the diagnosis of asthma. Examples include viral infections, gastroesophageal reflux disease (GERD), and exposure to gases or fumes. These disorders may play a role in the development or control of some cases of asthma.

Clinical Presentation

Major symptoms of asthma are wheezing, episodic dyspnea, chest tightness, and cough. The clinical manifestations vary widely, from mild intermittent symptoms to catastrophic attacks resulting in asphyxiation and death. Although wheezing is not a pathognomonic feature of asthma, in the setting of a compatible clinical picture, asthma is the most common diagnosis. Often symptoms worsen at night or during the early hours of the morning. Other associated symptoms are sputum production and chest pain or tightness. Patients may exhibit only one or a combination of symptoms, such as chronic cough only (cough-variant asthma). Wheezing may occur several minutes after exercise (exercise-induced bronchoconstriction). Physical examination typically shows evidence of wheezing, although findings may be normal in between symptomatic periods. Rhinitis or nasal polyps may be present. In the case of an acute episode of bronchospasm or an exacerbation, the clinician may find that the patient has difficulty talking, is using accessory muscles of inspiration, has pulsus paradoxus, is diaphoretic, and has mental status changes ranging from agitation to somnolence. In patients with these findings, treatment should be immediate and aggressive.

Diagnosis and Differential Diagnosis

A diagnosis of asthma requires documentation of bronchial hyperreactivity and reversible airway obstruction. The history may provide sufficient documentation because most patients complain of characteristic periodic episodes of wheezing and other symptoms that respond to use of a bronchodilator. However, spirometry is recommended to assess formally for expiratory flow limitation, and reversibility is demonstrated by repeat spirometry after bronchodilator administration. At least 12% and 200 mL improvement in FEV_1 after bronchodilator use indicates reversibility. Because asthma is episodic, airflow limitation is variable and patients may exhibit symptoms at a time when spirometry cannot be performed. Peak expiratory flow measurements can be performed at home and may be helpful in establishing evidence of variability in expiratory flow.

Depending on the circumstances, formal testing for airway hyperactivity by bronchoprovocation challenge may be necessary. A stimulant with bronchoconstrictor activity, most commonly methacholine, is applied to the patient's airway. Methacholine, a synthetic form of acetylcholine, is preferred to histamine because there are fewer systemic side effects. Exercise can also be used to trigger an attack. Although most patients with or without asthma develop some degree of airflow limitation during bronchoprovocation testing, those with asthma develop airflow limitation at much lower doses. For methacholine challenge, the concentration of methacholine required to produce a 20% decline in FEV_1 from baseline is reported. Although a positive bronchoprovocation challenge result is not by itself diagnostic of asthma, a negative result is helpful in ruling out asthma as a diagnosis.

Lung volume measurements may show hyperinflation during active disease, but the D_{LCO} is typically normal or even elevated. During acute exacerbations of asthma, analysis of arterial blood gases is useful to determine gas-exchange status. A chest radiograph should be obtained if a concern for pulmonary infection exists, but routine chest radiography is not necessary. Fleeting or migratory infiltrates on chest radiographs in a patient with difficult asthma should suggest the possibility of allergic bronchopulmonary aspergillosis. Blood tests in asthma might reveal eosinophilia and increased levels of IgE. Skin tests might be useful to identify household products or other antigens that could precipitate asthma attacks in a specific patient.

The differential diagnosis includes tracheal disorders, respiratory tract tumors and foreign bodies, COPD, and bronchiectasis. In patients whose primary presenting complaint is chronic cough, the differential diagnosis includes other causes of chronic cough, such as GERD and postnasal drip. A major differential consideration in patients not responding to typical asthma treatment is vocal cord dysfunction.

Treatment

The management of asthma requires education and cooperation on the part of the patient. Simple, inexpensive peak expiratory flow meters can be used at home to monitor airflow obstruction. A diary should be maintained, and a clear written plan should be in place for using symptoms and peak flow information to intervene early in exacerbations and to alter long-term therapy for optimal control of symptoms. Short-acting β-agonists are used for acute relief of symptoms such as wheezing (level 1 evidence). However, the cornerstone of maintenance therapy in all but mild intermittent asthma is administration of inhaled corticosteroids, which are highly effective in improving asthma control (level 1). Long-acting β-agonists may be added for additional symptomatic control as needed (level 1). LABAs should not be used as a monotherapy for asthma control because they do not control airway inflammation and increased mortality has been demonstrated with this therapeutic approach (level 1). However, these medications may be added to inhaled corticosteroids to provide additional symptom control.

Alternatively, leukotriene modifiers can be used in maintenance therapy (level 1 evidence), although they appear to be somewhat less effective than inhaled corticosteroids (see Fig. 16-4). Theophylline preparations may have additional beneficial effects in some patients, but the narrow therapeutic window and modest efficacy of these preparations limit their value. Recent evidence suggests that use of long-acting anticholinergics in patients with poor control on LABAs and inhaled corticosteroids may increase the time to exacerbation and provide additional bronchodilation (level 2). Oral or intravenous corticosteroids are used during acute asthma exacerbations. Long-term use of oral corticosteroids should be avoided, if possible, given the various side effects associated with chronic glucocorticoid administration.

Allergen avoidance is a reasonable measure in asthma, although the effects of specific interventions, such as mattress barrier protection to reduce dust mite exposure, appear limited. Treatment of associated conditions that may exacerbate asthma, such as allergic rhinitis and GERD, may be clinically beneficial and may aid in achieving asthma control. Use of recombinant human anti-IgE monoclonal antibody may be effective at reducing exacerbations in certain patients with allergic asthma (level 2 evidence). Therapies targeting other specific cytokines involved in asthma remain under active investigation. Bronchial thermoplasty is a new endoscopic technique in which radiofrequency energy delivered in a series of treatments is used to destroy airway smooth muscle. It has been shown to reduce exacerbations and improve quality of life in the months following treatment (level 2).

Acute severe asthma, or status asthmaticus, is an attack of severe bronchospasm that is unresponsive to routine therapy. Such attacks may be sudden (hyperacute asthma) and can be rapidly fatal, often before medical care can be obtained. In most cases, however, patients have a history of progressive dyspnea over hours to days, with increasing bronchodilator use. Treatment of status asthmaticus should be aggressive, including administration of nebulized bronchodilators and intravenous steroids and continuous monitoring of blood oxygen saturation by pulse oximetry, often supplemented by arterial blood gas analysis to evaluate for hypercarbia. A rising $PaCO_2$ in a patient with asthma is an ominous sign and may portend need for ventilatory support. Noninvasive ventilation has been used successfully to decrease the work of breathing and avoid the need for endotracheal intubation in patients with exacerbations of asthma, but intubation and mechanical ventilation are necessary for the management of respiratory failure in status asthmaticus. Mechanical ventilation of the patient with status asthmaticus can be extremely challenging and may require the use of paralytic agents to control the breathing pattern or even use of inhaled general anesthesia to relieve bronchospasm.

Prognosis

The prognosis in most patients with asthma is excellent. Although there is no cure, most patients can achieve appropriate control of their asthma.

For a deeper discussion on this topic, please see Chapter 88 ("Chronic Obstructive Pulmonary Disease"), Chapter 87 ("Asthma"), Chapter 89, ("Cystic Fibrosis"), and Chapter 90 ("Bronchiectasis, Atelectasis, Cysts, and Localized Lung Disorders") in Goldman-Cecil Medicine, *25th Edition.*

SUGGESTED READINGS

Buist AS, McBurnie MA, Vollmer WM, et al; on behalf of the BOLD Collaborative Research Group: International variation in the prevalence of

COPD (the BOLD Study): a population-based prevalence study, Lancet 370:741–750, 2007.

Burgel P-R, Bergeron A, de Blic J, et al: Small airways diseases, excluding asthma and COPD: an overview, Eur Respir Rev 22:131–147, 2013.

Decramer M, Janssens W, Miravitlles M: Chronic obstructive pulmonary disease, Lancet 379:1341–1351, 2012.

Global Initiative for Asthma: GINA report: global strategy for asthma management and prevention (updated 2012), Available at: www.ginasthma.org. Accessed August 29, 2014.

Global Initiative for Chronic Obstructive Lung Disease: Global strategy for the diagnosis, management, and prevention of chronic obstructive pulmonary disease (updated 2013), Available at: www.goldcopd.org. Accessed August 29, 2014.

Kim V, Criner GJ: Chronic bronchitis and chronic obstructive pulmonary disease, Am J Respir Crit Care Med 187:228–237, 2013.

King PT: The pathophysiology of bronchiectasis, Int J COPD 4:411–419, 2009.

McDonough JE, Yuan R, Suzuki M, et al: Small-airway obstruction and emphysema in chronic obstructive pulmonary disease, N Engl J Med 365:1567–1575, 2011.

Mogayzel PJ, Naureckas ET, Robinson KA, et al: and the Pulmonary Clinical Practice Guidelines Committee: Cystic fibrosis pulmonary guidelines: chronic medications for maintenance of lung health, Am J Respir Crit Care Med 187:680–689, 2013.

Pasteur MC, Bilton D, Hill AT; on behalf of the British Thoracic Society Bronchiectasis (Non-CF) Guideline Group: British Thoracic Society guideline for non-CF bronchiectasis, Thorax 65:i1–i58, 2010.

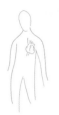

17

Interstitial Lung Diseases

Matthew D. Jankowich

INTRODUCTION

The interstitial lung diseases (ILDs) are a complex group of dozens of disorders with heterogeneous clinical courses and prognoses. ILDs are characterized by diffuse and typically chronic lung injury occurring in the setting of various degrees of inflammation, which often leads to lung fibrosis. These diseases are daunting for the clinician because the differential diagnosis may be broad, and the work-up required to make the appropriate diagnosis may be extensive.

Understanding of these disorders has been hampered in the past by use of confusing and nonspecific terminology, especially for the idiopathic interstitial pneumonias (IIPs). Current classifications use histopathology and clinical syndromes to categorize them in understandable groups: idiopathic interstitial pneumonitides, granulomatous disorders, connective tissue–related ILDs, drug-induced ILDs, pulmonary vasculitic disorders, and distinct entities of unknown origin that exhibit well-defined syndromes such as pulmonary Langerhans cell histiocytosis (LCH) and lymphangioleiomyomatosis.

ILD manifests with nonspecific, common clinical symptoms, including dyspnea on exertion, dry cough, and sometimes, constitutional symptoms. Pulmonary function tests usually show restriction and gas-exchange abnormalities. Imaging usually demonstrates diffuse lung disease. However, early radiographic changes may be subtle, and other clinical entities such as congestive heart failure or lymphangitic carcinomatosis may manifest with similar clinical, physiologic, and radiographic findings. The diagnosis may sometimes be delayed until other clinical entities are excluded and biopsy is undertaken. High-resolution computed tomography (HRCT) has contributed greatly to the diagnostic work-up of patients with suspected ILD because typical HRCT patterns in appropriate clinical settings may be sufficient for diagnosis.

Most ILDs, including more common entities such as idiopathic pulmonary fibrosis (IPF), manifest with chronic, progressive symptoms. However, some ILDs manifest in an acute fashion. They include acute pneumonitis due to systemic lupus erythematosus, acute hypersensitivity pneumonitis (HP), some drug reactions, and acute interstitial pneumonia. Infection often needs to be ruled out in these cases, and the diagnosis may be challenging for critically ill individuals.

When ILD is suspected in a patient with typical symptoms and diffuse lung disease on identified on imaging, the epidemiologic background, including the age, race, and sex of the patient, is helpful in formulating the diagnostic possibilities. For example, IPF typically occurs in middle-aged or elderly individuals, whereas sarcoidosis often occurs in young individuals and is most common among African Americans in the United States. Sex is also a consideration because lymphangioleiomyomatosis manifests almost exclusively in women of childbearing age, and pulmonary LCH most often occurs in young male smokers. These background data can help to focus the initial differential diagnosis.

The history can further narrow the differential diagnosis for suspected ILD. Important factors to elicit are rash, dysphagia, arthritis, and Raynaud's phenomenon, which may suggest an underlying connective tissue disorder. If the patient has a diagnosis of connective tissue disease, the work-up may be limited if imaging findings are typical of the pulmonary manifestations of that disease. A history of severe or poorly controlled asthma for a patient with radiographic infiltrates and constitutional symptoms should lead to consideration of Churg-Strauss syndrome, whereas a history of severe sinus disease should raise the possibility of granulomatosis with polyangiitis (formerly called *Wegener's granulomatosis*).

Drug-induced ILD should be considered for all patients with diffuse lung disease seen on imaging, and a careful evaluation of medication use is critical. The smoking history is important because several ILDs are associated with cigarette smoking, including respiratory bronchiolitis–associated interstitial lung disease, desquamative interstitial pneumonitis, and pulmonary LCH.

Environmental exposures should be elicited. For example, an exposure to pet birds or hot tubs may suggest HP. Home visits can be informative, and the occupational history is important. Although the pneumoconioses due to asbestos and silica exposure are becoming much less common with modern safeguards and restrictions, these diseases continue to manifest long after exposure. High-technology manufacturing has particular hazards, such as beryllium exposure leading to berylliosis in susceptible individuals. Nonindustrial professions also carry occupational risks. For example, outbreaks of granulomatous pneumonitis have been described in indoor lifeguards exposed to molds.

The physical examination may reveal only oxygen desaturation with exertion in early ILD. Patients may have evidence of decreased chest expansion during inspection. Auscultation of the lungs typically reveals Velcro-like crackles at the lung bases. The patient may have clubbing. Skin rashes, arthritis with joint deformities, Raynaud's phenomenon, and dysphagia may point to a connective tissue–related ILD such as dermatomyositis or polymyositis, progressive systemic sclerosis, or mixed connective tissue disorder. Evidence of right ventricular heart failure with jugular vein distention, a cardiac gallop, a loud P_2 sound, and leg edema suggests pulmonary hypertension. Right ventricular heart failure is usually the result of chronic hypoxemia and is often related to end-stage lung disease.

Laboratory studies may be of benefit. For example, eosinophilia suggests the particular group of disorders associated with pulmonary infiltrates and peripheral blood eosinophilia.

A chest radiograph can narrow the diagnosis based on the distribution of the typical reticulonodular changes found in ILD. For example, sarcoidosis, lymphangioleiomyomatosis, silicosis, HP, eosinophilic granuloma, and ankylosing spondylitis most often affect the upper- and mid-level lung fields, whereas IPF, asbestosis, and many connective tissue–related ILDs typically involve the lower-level lung fields.

Disease patterns are best analyzed with the use of HRCT of the chest, a test considered essential in the evaluation of patients thought to have ILD. HRCT can reveal patterns of disease that allow the diagnostic considerations to be significantly narrowed. For example, upper lobe–predominant cystic lung disease on HRCT suggests LCH, sarcoidosis, or lymphangioleiomyomatosis. Lower lobe and peripheral reticular opacities with associated traction bronchiectasis and honeycombing suggest IPF, asbestosis, or certain connective tissue disease–related ILDs. Visualization of abnormalities of the mediastinum or pleura associated with parenchymal lung disease is helpful. Sarcoidosis, for example, typically exhibits hilar and mediastinal lymphadenopathy associated with beadlike septal nodules, whereas pleural plaques associated with lower lobe fibrosis are consistent with asbestosis. Incorporation of HRCT imaging data with clinical history sometimes may be sufficient for diagnosis.

Pulmonary function tests for ILD typically reveal a restrictive pattern characterized by proportionately decreased airflow with a preserved ratio of forced expiratory volume in 1 second to forced vital capacity (FEV_1/FVC) (i.e., no obstruction to airflow) and decreased lung volumes as highlighted by decreased total lung capacity and functional residual capacity. The diffusion capacity of the lung for carbon dioxide (D_{LCO}) is often decreased and may be the earliest change seen in drug-induced ILD or connective tissue disease–related ILD. The restrictive abnormality found in most forms of ILD results from decreased compliance of the lung in the setting of fibrosis.

Histologically, ILD affects the interstitium of the lung, the space located between the basement membrane of the vascular structures in the distal air spaces and the basement membranes of the epithelial cells that line the alveoli (Fig. 17-1). This space extends proximally toward the alveolar ducts and respiratory bronchioles. Normally, the interstitium of the lung contains a few fibroblasts and connective tissue components within a very thin wall that allows efficient diffusion of gases. In ILD, however, this space expands with the accumulation of fibroblasts or other

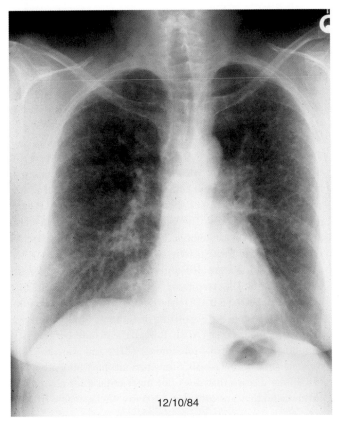

12/10/84

Preserved lung volumes

Sarcoidosis
Hypersensitivity pneumonitis

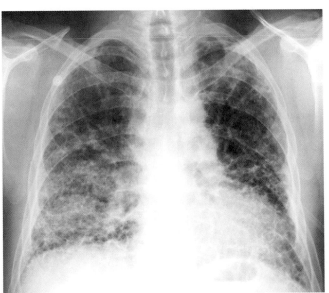

Small lung volumes

Idiopathic pulmonary fibrosis
Asbestosis

FIGURE 17-1 Radiographic manifestations of interstitial lung diseases. Well-preserved lung volumes with bilateral interstitial reticulonodular infiltrates *(left)* are seen in diseases similar to sarcoidosis and hypersensitivity pneumonitis. Reduced lung volumes with bilateral basilar infiltrates *(right)* are seen in idiopathic pulmonary fibrosis.

cells and the deposition of an aberrant matrix that increases the distance between the alveolar space and vascular structures, delaying and sometimes preventing gas exchange. This thickened interstitium accounts for poor oxygenation with exercise, increased lung stiffness exhibited as decreased compliance, small lung volumes, and increased work of breathing.

Because lung involvement by ILD may be sporadic, with areas of normal lung adjacent to areas of fibrosis, local differences in compliance may result in ventilation-perfusion mismatching, contributing to hypoxemia. The processes previously outlined account for the physiologic manifestations seen in disorders such as IPF and asbestosis.

In some ILDs, an obstructive rather than restrictive abnormality or mixed patterns are identified on pulmonary function testing, and lung volumes are relatively preserved on physiologic testing and imaging (Fig. 17-2). In diseases such as lymphangioleiomyomatosis, pulmonary LCH, and some cases of HP or sarcoidosis, obstructive or mixed patterns on pulmonary function testing occur with preservation of lung volumes. This pattern of disease is caused by proximal extension of the interstitial disease in the lung parenchyma with consequent involvement of the small airways. For example, in lymphangioleiomyomatosis, the small airways are narrowed by the proliferation of surrounding abnormal smooth muscle–like cells. This leads to increased airway resistance and airflow obstruction. Endobronchial disease with direct narrowing of the airways can occur in sarcoidosis, leading to similar effects. The finding of airflow obstruction does not rule out a diagnosis of ILD but may help to focus the differential diagnosis on particular diseases.

In ILD, a synthesis of clinical, functional, and imaging data, often in the context of a multidisciplinary approach, can determine the appropriate diagnosis. In many circumstances, however, clinical and imaging data are insufficiently specific, and lung biopsy must be undertaken. Surgical lung biopsy, typically using a thoracoscopic approach, is the preferred method of obtaining tissue for examination. Transbronchial lung biopsy through the bronchoscope yields small fragments of tissue, typically too small to allow appropriate examination of the lung architecture, and it is not recommended for the assessment of suspected IPF. However, transbronchial biopsies may be useful for certain ILDs, including sarcoidosis, cryptogenic organizing pneumonia, and HP.

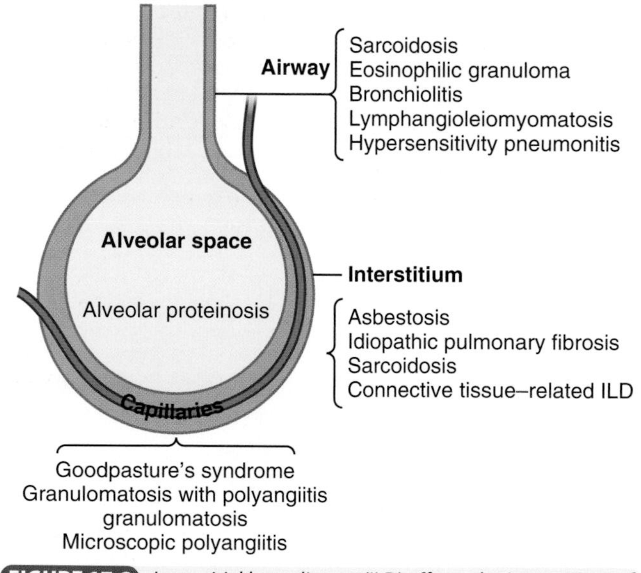

The lung's response to injury is relatively stereotyped, and particular biopsy patterns of injury, such as usual interstitial pneumonia or granulomatous inflammation, are seen in a variety of disorders. Interpretation of lung biopsy results must be done in the appropriate context and with incorporation of clinical and imaging data. For example, a biopsy result of usual interstitial pneumonitis may carry a different prognosis in the setting of rheumatoid arthritis–associated ILD than in the setting of IPF. The typical manifestations of several ILDs are summarized in Table 17-1.

Management of ILD depends on the underlying cause, and treatments appropriate to specific entities are discussed later. Exposure avoidance is critical for HP, smoking-related ILD, and drug-induced ILD. Immunosuppressants are employed in a variety of the ILDs, with results depending on the specific disease. Supplemental oxygen and pulmonary rehabilitation may be helpful in advanced disease. Lung transplantation is performed in patients with limited life expectancy, and early referral is suggested for patients with a poor prognosis, as in IPF.

For a deeper discussion on this topic, please see Chapter 92, "Interstitial Lung Disease," in Goldman-Cecil Medicine, *25th Edition.*

IDIOPATHIC INTERSTITIAL PNEUMONIAS

The IIPs are a group of ILDs of unknown origins. In the 1970s, these conditions were considered to be different variations of IPF. However, the distinct clinical presentations, natural courses, and responses to treatment observed in these patients led to their reclassification as IIPs. The classification scheme suggested in a 2002 consensus statement by the American Thoracic and European Respiratory Societies was updated in 2013.

The major IIPs are IPF, idiopathic nonspecific interstitial pneumonia (NSIP), respiratory bronchiolitis–associated interstitial lung disease (RB-ILD), desquamative interstitial pneumonia (DIP), cryptogenic organizing pneumonia (COP), and acute interstitial pneumonia (AIP). Rare IIPs include lymphoid (or lymphocytic) interstitial pneumonia (LIP) and idiopathic pleuroparechymal fibroelastosis. Some patients have idiopathic interstitial lung disease that does not meet criteria for any of these entities, and they are considered to have unclassifiable IIP.

FIGURE 17-2 Interstitial lung disease (ILD) affects the interstitium of the lung at different locations. Depending on the site of disease activity, its consequences may vary. Diseases that affect the interstitium that surrounds the distal part of the alveoli lead to physiologic restrictions with reduced lung volumes. Diseases that preferentially affect the interstitium located near the more proximal parts of the acinus near the distal bronchioles may exhibit predominantly well-preserved lung volumes and physiologic obstruction.

Idiopathic Pulmonary Fibrosis
Definition and Epidemiology

Of the IIPs, IPF, formerly called *cryptogenic fibrosing alveolitis*, is the most common, affecting 85,000 to 100,000 individuals in the United States. IPF was defined in a consensus statement as a

TABLE 17-1 MANIFESTATIONS OF INTERSTITIAL LUNG DISEASE

DISEASE	PHYSICAL EXAMINATION	RADIOGRAPHS	LABORATORY FINDINGS	HISTOLOGIC FINDINGS
Pneumoconioses				
Silicosis	Various findings	Large nodules Eggshell calcification of hilar nodes PMF, upper lobes Emphysema, nodules	Restrictive PFTs	Silica: inflammation, birefringent crystals, alveolar proteinosis
Coal worker's pneumoconiosis	Normal	PMF	FEV1 and FVC may be decreased	Coal: pigmented macules, anthracotic pigment
Asbestosis	Crackles	Pleural plaques, lower lobe fibrosis	Restrictive PFTs	Asbestos: UIP pattern, asbestos bodies, mesothelioma
Beryllium exposure	Nonspecific findings	Lymphadenopathy, lung nodules	Nonspecific except beryllium: lymphocyte transformation test	Beryllium: noncaseating granulomas
Hypersensitivity pneumonitis	Fever, cough, crackles	Centrilobular nodules, air trapping, fibrosis	Serum precipitins to specific proteins CD8>CD4 cells Lymphocytic BAL fluid Obstructive and/or restrictive PFTs	Chronic airway centered inflammation, poorly formed granulomas
Idiopathic interstitial pneumonias				
DIP, RB-ILD	Various findings	Centrilobular nodules, ground-glass infiltrates	Nonspecific	DIP: Intra-alveolar accumulation of pigmented macrophages
IPF	Crackles, clubbing	Basilar predominant fibrosis, honeycombing	Restrictive PFTs	IPF: UIP pattern with heterogeneous areas of fibrosis, fibroblast foci
AIP	Tachypnea, respiratory distress	Bilateral alveolar infiltrates	Nonspecific	AIP: Diffuse alveolar damage
NSIP	Crackles, possible clubbing	Ground-glass, subpleural reticulations	Restrictive PFTs	NSIP: Uniform thickening of interstitium with inflammatory cells and fibrosis
Collagen vascular	Collagen vascular disease, crackles, pleural rub	Pleural effusions Diffuse interstitial infiltrates, nodular infiltrates Occasional cavities	Serologic findings for specific disease Occasionally obstructive, usually restrictive PFTs	Interstitial inflammation Vasculitis Bronchiolar obstruction Organizing pneumonia Fibrosis: UIP, NSIP, LIP
Drug-induced ILD	Fever, crackles, pleural rub	Fibrosis Migratory infiltrates, diffuse interstitial infiltrates Pulmonary edema	Restrictive PFTs	Alveolar macrophages with lamellar bodies in amiodarone Interstitial inflammation Fibrosis Eosinophilic infiltration
Sarcoidosis	Fever, malaise, weight loss Erythema nodosum, lupus pernio, and skin plaques Salivary and lacrimal gland enlargement Arthritis Iritis, uveitis, chorioretinitis; keratoconjunctivitis Cranial nerve palsies Occasional rales or wheezes	Reticulonodular infiltrates Nodules Hilar adenopathy Mediastinal adenopathy Fibrosis	Lymphocytic BAL, T4 > T8 cell subsets Obstructive and/or restrictive PFTs Elevated transaminases with liver involvement Occasional hypercalcemia	Noncaseating granuloma with giant cells and negative acid-fast bacilli and fungal staining Fibrosis
Radiation exposure	Crackles, fever	Focal interstitial infiltrates corresponding to radiation port Occasional diffuse infiltrates Fibrosis	Restrictive PFTs	Acute: endothelial and alveolar lining cell damage Chronic: fibrosis
Pulmonary Langerhans cell histiocytosis	None to cough, dyspnea, chest pain Fatigue, weight loss, occasional fever	Spontaneous pneumothorax Nodules Reticulonodular infiltrates Middle and upper lobe predominance Honeycombing Sparing of costophrenic angle Cysts and nodules on HRCT	Normal lung volumes with decreased D_{LCO}	OKT-6 (CD1) and S100-positive immunostaining Few eosinophils Peribronchiolar inflammation Macrophages filling lumen of bronchioles and intraluminal fibrosis

TABLE 17-1 MANIFESTATIONS OF INTERSTITIAL LUNG DISEASE—cont'd

DISEASE	PHYSICAL EXAMINATION	RADIOGRAPHS	LABORATORY FINDINGS	HISTOLOGIC FINDINGS
Lymphangioleiomyomatosis	Dyspnea, cough, chest pain Decreased breath sounds or rales Hemoptysis, ascites	Spontaneous pneumothorax Pleural effusions Reticulonodular infiltrate Miliary pattern Honeycombing Hyperinflation Diffuse, small, thin-walled cysts on HRCT	Obstructive and/or restrictive PFTs Chylous pleural effusions Chylous ascites	HMB-45–positive immunostaining Atypical smooth muscle cell proliferation around bronchovascular bundles
COP	Fever, chills, malaise, fatigue, cough, dyspnea on exertion, weight loss	Peripheral patchy infiltrates, occasionally migratory CT: patchy consolidation, ground-glass opacities, small nodules	Restrictive and occasionally obstructive PFTs for smokers	Patchy peribronchiolar distribution Foamy macrophages in alveolar spaces Intraluminal buds of granulation tissue

AIP, Acute interstitial pneumonia; BAL, bronchoalveolar lavage; BOOP, bronchiolitis obliterans and organizing pneumonia; COP, cryptogenic organizing pneumonia; CT, computed tomography; DIP, desquamative interstitial pneumonia; DLCO, diffusing capacity of the lung for carbon monoxide; HRCT, high-resolution computed tomography; ILD, interstitial lung disease; IPF, idiopathic pulmonary fibrosis; LIP, lymphoid interstitial pneumonia; NSIP, nonspecific interstitial pneumonia; PFT, pulmonary function test; PMF, progressive massive fibrosis; RB, respiratory bronchiolitis; RNP, anti-ribonucleoprotein antibodies; UIP, usual interstitial.

"specific form of chronic, progressive fibrosing interstitial pneumonia of unknown cause, occurring primarily in older adults, limited to the lungs, and associated with the histopathologic and/or radiologic pattern of usual interstitial pneumonitis."

Although initially thought to be a rare disease, IPF is now considered one of the most common ILDs, with a prevalence in some populations of up to 29 cases per 100,000 people; the prevalence is much higher among patients older than 70 years. Among most patients with IPF, the disease is sporadic. However, IPF has been found in members of certain families and is called *familial IPF,* indicating that genetic alterations predispose some patients to this illness. Genetic abnormalities associated with familial IPF include abnormalities of the telomerase complex and surfactant proteins.

The disease is idiopathic, but risk factors include cigarette smoking and possibly gastroesophageal reflux disease. Many environmental, occupational, and infectious agents can cause lung fibrosis, including asbestos, silica, and tuberculosis. Distinguishing IPF from other lung disorders is important because of the implications for prognosis and therapy.

Pathology

The underlying histopathologic pattern found in the lungs of patients with IPF is called *usual interstitial pneumonia* (UIP). This histologic pattern shows areas of scar tissue deposition and honeycombing interspersed with areas with relatively normal alveolar structures, resulting in a heterogeneous pattern on microscopy (Fig. 17-3). An interesting pathologic feature is the finding of fibroblastic foci, which are areas in which fibroblasts accumulate. They are thought to be sites of disease activity.

The UIP pattern can accompany other disorders (e.g., connective tissue–related ILD in rheumatoid arthritis, asbestosis). The diagnosis of IPF depends on a clinical, radiographic, and histologic picture that includes the syndrome of ILD in the absence of an obvious cause and a histologic manifestation consistent with UIP.

Clinical Presentation

IPF is characterized by progressive fibrosis of the lungs, resulting in nonproductive cough and shortness of breath that worsens

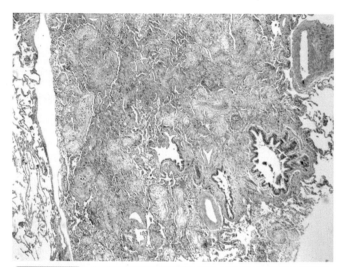

FIGURE 17-3 Pulmonary fibrosis in idiopathic pulmonary fibrosis with usual interstitial pneumonia pathology that is adjacent to normal lung parenchyma. (Courtesy Dr. Charles Kuhn.)

with exertion and ultimately causes hypoxemic respiratory failure. The typical patient with IPF is older than 50 years, and the symptoms frequently develop 1 to 2 years before a diagnosis is confirmed.

Physical examination often reveals inspiratory crackles in the bases of both lungs, indicating the predominant site of scarring. Clubbing may exist, but extrapulmonary findings such as rash or joint arthritis are absent. With increased connective tissue deposition, the lung becomes stiff as evidenced by decreased compliance. Pulmonary function tests show decreased lung volumes consistent with a restrictive process, and the DLCO is reduced. Impaired oxygenation in IPF, initially with exercise and later at rest, often requires long-term oxygen supplementation.

The chest radiograph shows reticular infiltrates that are most predominant at the bases and periphery of the lungs. HRCT allows better visualization of the lung and is useful in evaluating the extent of disease. It delineates the areas of fibrosis and provides information about other structures in the chest. The classic HRCT findings of IPF are bilateral reticulonodular infiltrates, which are more pronounced at the lung bases and have a peripheral, subpleural distribution, and detection of honey-combing and traction bronchiectasis in the absence of ground-glass opacification, lymphadenopathy, and pleural disease (Fig. 17-4; E-Fig. 17-1). In the setting of a typical clinical presentation and classic HRCT findings, a lung biopsy is unnecessary. A lung biopsy may be required for confirmation in some patients.

Diagnosis and Differential Diagnosis

IPF is diagnosed on the basis of typical clinical, radiographic (HRCT), and if available, pathologic features (e.g., biopsy showing a UIP pattern). Other potential causes of ILD, such as connective tissue disease, hypersensitivity pneumonitis, and asbestosis, must be ruled out by the history, examination, and selected laboratory testing.

HRCT of the chest should show a compatible UIP pattern, with subpleural reticulations, honeycombing, and traction bronchiectasis. If honeycombing is absent on HRCT or atypical features such as ground-glass infiltrates, lymphadenopathy, nodules, or air trapping are found, the radiographic diagnosis becomes less certain. In these cases, a lung biopsy may be needed, and it should show a UIP pattern to confirm a diagnosis of IPF. Multidisciplinary discussion during the diagnostic process, with input from experienced clinicians, radiologists, and pathologists, is ideal.

Treatment

There is insufficient clinical evidence to suggest that any pharmacologic treatment improves survival or the quality of life for patients with IPF. A commonly used immunosuppressive combination of corticosteroids, azathioprine, and N-acetylcysteine was shown in a multicenter clinical trial to be more harmful than a placebo or N-acetylcysteine alone (level 1 evidence). N-acetylcysteine treatment did not show any clear advantage over placebo.

The antifibrotic drug pirfenidone has been approved in some countries based on evidence from a study showing a reduced decline in lung function with this medication, although a parallel study did not show the same results (level 2 evidence). An ongoing clinical trial of this drug showing better preserved lung function with pirfenidone compared to placebo was recently completed in the United States.

Lung transplantation should be considered for patients with IPF. Because survival of patients with IPF on the lung transplantation waiting list is worse than for patients with other indications for lung transplantation, early referral for transplantation evaluation should be initiated (level 2 evidence). Unfortunately, the 5-year survival rate for lung transplant recipients with IPF is only 40% to 50%.

Some patients with IPF experience acute respiratory deterioration in the absence of any clinically apparent cause (e.g., heart failure, pulmonary embolism, pneumonia). These episodes of idiopathic acute deterioration have been called *acute exacerbations of IPF* and are associated with a poor prognosis. HRCT findings include new ground-glass opacities and consolidation superimposed on a background reticular or honeycomb pattern consistent with UIP. Histologically, evidence of acute lung injury (i.e., diffuse alveolar damage) can be found on the background of UIP. Acute exacerbations of IPF are typically treated with high doses of corticosteroids (level 3 evidence).

Prognosis

The prognosis for IPF is poor. The disease is progressive, ultimately leading to death from respiratory failure or other complications such as lung cancer. Median survival is often reported to be 2 to 3 years from the diagnosis, although this may be an underestimate.

Other Idiopathic Pneumonias

The second most common IIP is NSIP. This condition exhibits a histologic picture that is nonspecific and characterized by diffuse, uniform interstitial inflammation (i.e., cellular NSIP, which is less common) with or without fibrosis (i.e., fibrotic NSIP, which is more common), as distinguished by the heterogeneous pattern seen in UIP or IPF. Patients with NSIP exhibit progressive dyspnea, cough, and bilateral interstitial infiltrates. Affected patients are middle-aged and commonly women.

Although NSIP may be idiopathic, the NSIP pathologic pattern also may occur in conditions such as connective tissue disorders (e.g., systemic lupus erythematosus, rheumatoid arthritis, polymyositis). The association with these disorders is so strong that histologic confirmation of NSIP should prompt a search for these conditions, which occasionally manifest only after the development of NSIP. The differential diagnosis also includes IPF, COP, and HP. Pulmonary function tests most commonly show a restrictive pattern. Ground-glass infiltrates, subpleural reticulation, and traction bronchiectasis are often seen by HRCT, but honeycombing is minimal or absent.

NSIP may be more responsive to immunosuppressants than IPF, and a trial period with immunosuppressive agents should be considered (level 3 evidence). Lung transplantation should be considered in these patients if they exhibit progressive disease. However, the overall prognosis is much better than for IPF, with a 5-year survival rate of more than 82% in one series.

DIP is a rare idiopathic pneumonia usually seen in younger individuals. It is associated in most cases with a history of cigarette smoking. Patients exhibit a progressive shortness of breath

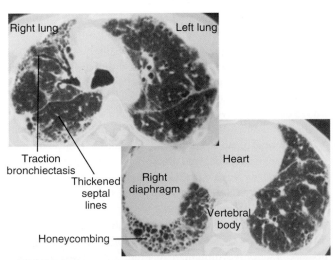

FIGURE 17-4 Computed tomography of the chest of a patient with idiopathic pulmonary fibrosis.

and bilateral infiltrates on chest radiographs. The HRCT pattern shows extensive ground-glass infiltrates, and a biopsy is often required for diagnosis. Tissue histologic findings show the accumulation of so-called smoker's macrophages, which contain yellow-brown pigment and fill the alveolar spaces, and some degree of interstitial inflammation and fibrosis.

Treatment of DIP relies on immunosuppressant therapy and the avoidance of tobacco exposure. Prognosis is fair, with some individuals developing progressive lung disease. DIP is considered by some experts to be part of a continuum with RB-ILD, which produces a similar clinical presentation; has a somewhat different pathology, with macrophages centered at the small airways as opposed to the alveolar level; and is associated with tobacco exposure. RB-ILD has a better prognosis. Respiratory bronchiolitis may be found incidentally in asymptomatic smokers, and it does not constitute an ILD if not extensive and associated with clinical symptoms.

AIP is an IIP that manifests acutely. There is no sex predominance in AIP and no association with smoking. Dyspnea and radiographic alveolar lung opacities develop and progress over days to a few weeks, invariably leading to respiratory failure. Patients often have a prior illness suggesting a viral upper respiratory infection with constitutional symptoms such as myalgias, arthralgias, fever, chills, and malaise. The histologic pattern shows diffuse alveolar damage with hyaline membrane formation or with organization. Although a trial of immunosuppressants is recommended (level 3 evidence), this condition is frequently fatal independent of treatment, and relapse may occur even after apparent improvement.

COP manifests over a subacute time course. Patients with COP exhibit dyspnea, cough, and systemic symptoms. Radiographically, patients with COP typically have areas of air space consolidation mimicking a bacterial pneumonia but that do not resolve with antibiotics. The radiographic infiltrates may be unilateral or bilateral and may be migratory. Pulmonary function tests may show restriction or obstruction. Histologically, COP is characterized by distal airway and interstitial inflammation and obliteration of distal small airways and air spaces with plugs of fibroblasts and fibrotic tissue called *Masson bodies*.

Similar to NSIP and DIP, COP is likely to respond to immunosuppressant therapy and is usually treated with prednisone (level 2 evidence). Relapses are typical and may occur when the steroid treatment is tapered. Connective tissue disorders, inhaled irritants, and drugs (e.g., methotrexate) can cause a type of inflammation known as *secondary organizing pneumonia*.

LIP is a rare disease that is seen predominantly in women. Patients have gradual-onset dyspnea and cough and occasionally have fever, weight loss, chest pain, and arthralgias. Cases of apparently idiopathic LIP must be investigated for known causes, such as collagen vascular diseases (especially Sjögren syndrome and rheumatoid arthritis) and immunodeficiency diseases (e.g., acquired immunodeficiency syndrome [AIDS]).

For LIP, HRCT shows interstitial reticulations, centrilobular nodules, ground-glass opacities, and thin-walled cysts. Histologically, infiltration of cells, including lymphocytes, plasma cells, and histiocytes, can be seen within alveolar septa. Type II pneumocyte hyperplasia and an increase in the number of alveolar macrophages can be seen in cases of LIP. Lymphoid follicles are often identified, usually in the distribution of pulmonary lymphatics.

Corticosteroids are used to treat LIP with various degrees of success (level 3 evidence); however, more than one third of patients progress to diffuse fibrosis. It is unclear whether treatment influences the course of the disease or has a significant effect on lung physiology.

● GRANULOMATOUS DISORDERS

Interstitial Lung Diseases with Granuloma Formation

Several noninfectious ILDs are characterized by granuloma formation in the lungs, including granulomatosis with polyangiitis, HP, and chronic beryllium disease. These disorders are discussed elsewhere in this chapter. Of the ILDs characterized by granulomatous lung inflammation, sarcoidosis is the most common.

Sarcoidosis

Definition and Epidemiology

Sarcoidosis is a multisystem granulomatous disorder of unknown cause. The lungs and thoracic lymph nodes are frequent sites of involvement. Sarcoidosis is relatively common, with a prevalence of 1 to 40 cases per 100,000 people worldwide. A higher incidence of sarcoidosis is reported among Scandinavian, German, and Irish individuals residing in northern Europe. In the United States, the prevalence rates of sarcoidosis are 10.9 cases per 100,000 whites and 35.5 cases per 100,000 African Americans, with women in both groups being more frequently affected. Because sarcoidosis may be asymptomatic, the true prevalence may be higher. Sarcoidosis typically occurs in individuals between 10 and 40 years old.

Pathology

Sarcoidosis is characterized by the formation in tissues of noncaseating granulomas that organize in an inner core of epithelioid histiocytes, $CD4^+$ T lymphocytes, and giant cells, which are surrounded by a rim of lymphocytes, fibroblasts, and connective tissue (Fig. 17-5). Granulomas are found in the airways or lung parenchyma in more than 90% of patients with sarcoidosis. Granulomatous angiitis may also be found in the lungs. The upper respiratory system, lymph nodes, skin, and eyes are commonly involved. Virtually any other organ may be affected, including the liver, bone marrow, spleen, musculoskeletal system, heart, salivary glands, and nervous system.

The granulomas may be clinically silent or, if extensive, may disrupt normal organ structure and function. The cause of these lesions is unknown, but given the frequency of lung involvement, inhaled antigens ranging from bacteria (especially mycobacteria and *Propionibacterium*) to environmental substances have been hypothesized to trigger the onset of granulomatous inflammation. This inflammation may be self-limited or may be propagated, possibly by repeated exposure to the unknown antigen or because of defective immune regulation.

Familial susceptibility to sarcoidosis exists, and alleles of human leukocyte antigen (HLA) genes involved in antigen

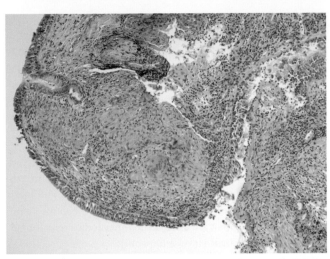

FIGURE 17-5 Subepithelial noncaseating granuloma, which is characteristic of sarcoidosis, from an endobronchial biopsy.

TABLE 17-2	RADIOGRAPHIC STAGING OF SARCOIDOSIS	
STAGE		**RADIOGRAPHIC FINDINGS**
0		Normal radiograph
I		Adenopathy without parenchymal abnormality
II		Adenopathy and parenchymal disease
III		Parenchymal disease without lymphadenopathy
IV		End-stage fibrosis

presentation and a mutation in the butyrophilin-like 2 gene (*BTNL2*), a possible immunoregulatory gene, have been associated with susceptibility to sarcoidosis. A single causative antigen initiating granuloma formation may not exist, and sarcoidosis instead may represent a stereotypical inflammatory reaction to various antigens in a genetically susceptible host.

Sarcoidosis is associated with abnormal immune function as evidenced by cutaneous anergy and as exhibited in lung by an increased ratio of $CD4^+$ to $CD8^+$ T lymphocytes and increased concentrations of pro-inflammatory cytokines such as interferon-γ, interleukin-12, and tumor necrosis factor-α (TNF-α). These derangements can be detected in the bronchoalveolar lavage (BAL) fluid and are consistent with an imbalance in the production of type 1 (T_H1) and type 2 (T_H2) helper T-cell cytokines, favoring the production of the former and promoting persistent inflammation. Sarcoidosis may occur in the setting of immunomodulatory therapy, especially with interferon alfa, or the immune reconstitution syndrome, occurring after initiation of antiretroviral therapy for human immunodeficiency virus (HIV) infection, highlighting the role of immune imbalances in the disorder.

Clinical Presentation

The clinical presentation of patients with sarcoidosis varies. The disease is frequently detected incidentally on routine chest radiographs of asymptomatic individuals. Others may have diverse acute or chronic symptoms. Patients may develop well-described acute syndromes such as Löfgren syndrome, which includes erythema nodosum, fever, arthritis, and hilar adenopathy, or uveoparotid fever (i.e., Heerfordt's syndrome), which exhibits the triad of uveitis, parotitis, and facial nerve palsy. Both syndromes are associated with better outcomes than for other clinical presentations of sarcoidosis.

In many cases, symptoms are vague and chronic, and they may include systemic symptoms such as low-grade fevers, fatigue, night sweats, or joint pains. Respiratory manifestations, including shortness of breath, wheezing, dry cough, and chest pain, occur in one third to one half of patients. Skin manifestations include erythema nodosum, plaques, nodules, and lupus pernio, a

violaceous, often disfiguring, nodular lesion of the nose and cheeks. Ocular symptoms are also common, and the onset of uveitis may eventually lead to the diagnosis of sarcoidosis when granulomatous extraocular organ involvement is uncovered. Neurosarcoidosis may manifest with cranial nerve palsies or with headache in the setting of lymphocytic meningitis. Sarcoidosis can involve the heart, resulting in a cardiomyopathy. Arrhythmias and sudden cardiac death can occur as a result of the disruption of the conducting system by granulomatous infiltration. Pulmonary hypertension may result from pulmonary fibrosis or directly from granulomatous vasculitis.

In 90% of patients, the chest radiograph shows abnormalities that include bilateral hilar adenopathy (E-Fig. 17-2), infiltrates (E-Fig. 17-3), and fibrosis. The radiographic changes characteristic of sarcoidosis have been classified as stages 0 through IV (Table 17-2), but this staging system does not imply a typical chronologic progression. However, stage I patients have a better prognosis for resolution than those with more advanced stages of disease.

As in other ILDs, computed tomography (CT) is more sensitive for the detection of parenchymal abnormalities, and it more clearly demonstrates the extent of mediastinal adenopathy. Parenchymal HRCT findings include nodularity along the bronchovascular bundles emanating from the hila (E-Fig. 17-4). Lung parenchyma involvement in sarcoidosis is more prominent in the upper lobes. Positron emission tomography (PET) or gallium-67 scans may reveal other sites of organ involvement.

Pulmonary function tests show restriction or obstruction. Liver involvement may cause mild elevation of transaminase levels, and cirrhosis and liver failure have been reported, although they are rare. Hypercalcemia and hypercalciuria may be detected and are caused by increased intestinal absorption of calcium as a result of increased conversion of vitamin D to its active form in sarcoid granulomas. Kidney stones may result from the abnormal calcium metabolism. Elevated levels of angiotensin-converting enzyme (ACE) are common but are not specific. The use of ACE levels in the diagnosis or management of sarcoidosis is controversial.

Diagnosis

The diagnosis of sarcoidosis depends on a typical clinical, radiographic, and histologic picture and is a diagnosis of exclusion. Patients with classic syndromes such as the Löfgren syndrome or uveoparotid fever may not require biopsy; however, most patients require tissue biopsy of an affected organ. Tissue samples show noncaseating granulomas, but because this finding is nonspecific, careful attention should be given to ruling out other causes of granulomatous inflammation (e.g., mycobacterial infection) through stains and cultures.

Necrotizing granulomas have rarely been reported in sarcoidosis, but this finding should prompt an intense search for infection. In contrast to most ILDs, in which tissue diagnosis requires open lung biopsy, the granulomas in sarcoidosis can be identified in skin nodules or in lymph nodes. Due to frequent lung and lymph node involvement, bronchoscopy is commonly used to diagnose sarcoidosis. Results of bronchoscopy with transbronchial lung biopsy are positive for 50% to 60% of patients, but the procedure poses the risks of hemorrhage and pneumothorax. Because airway involvement is common, endobronchial biopsies may also demonstrate granulomas. However, there is increasing evidence that transbronchial needle aspiration of mediastinal and hilar lymph nodes using endobronchial ultrasound guidance may have a higher diagnostic yield for granulomas than conventional bronchoscopic techniques (level 1 evidence).

After the diagnosis is made, all patients should have an ophthalmologic evaluation and a 24-hour collection of urine to assess for hypercalciuria. Electrocardiographic examination and sometimes Holter monitoring should be performed to assess for conduction system abnormalities or arrhythmias resulting from involvement of the heart by sarcoidosis. If cardiac sarcoidosis is suspected, magnetic resonance imaging (MRI) or PET scanning may be helpful.

Treatment

Corticosteroids are the standard therapy, but they should not be used indiscriminately in all patients with the diagnosis of sarcoidosis because sarcoidosis may not cause symptoms or complications and the disease may undergo spontaneous remission. Whether corticosteroids alter the disease course is uncertain. However, corticosteroid therapy should be considered in patients with extrapulmonary organ involvement or progressive pulmonary symptoms. In patients with pulmonary involvement, oral prednisone at a dosage of 20 to 40 mg per day may be initiated (level 2 evidence). Because the duration of treatment may be prolonged, steroid-sparing agents, particularly methotrexate, have been used (level 2). Infliximab, an anti-TNF agent, has resulted in a small improvement in vital capacity compared with placebo in patients with pulmonary sarcoidosis (level 1).

Patients with erythema nodosum in the setting of Löfgren syndrome may be treated with nonsteroidal anti-inflammatory medications alone. Other skin involvement may respond to hydroxychloroquine or topical corticosteroids. The treatment of lupus pernio is challenging, but it may respond to infliximab (level 3 evidence). Given the role of TNF in $T_H 1$-type immunity, anti-TNF agents may also have roles in treating other forms of extrapulmonary disease not responding to conventional therapy (level 3).

Anterior uveitis may be treated with topical steroids, but other eye involvement may require systemic corticosteroids. Systemic corticosteroids are also used for the treatment of cardiac sarcoidosis (level 3 evidence). Conduction system disease and arrhythmias may necessitate placement of pacemakers or automatic implantable cardioverter-defibrillators (level 3). Neurosarcoidosis and hypercalcemia are among the other indications for systemic steroid treatment (level 3 for both).

Prognosis

The course of sarcoidosis varies. Spontaneous remission is common, and death and disability occur rarely, making decisions regarding treatment initiation difficult. The acute sarcoidosis syndromes tend to remit and not recur. However, about one third of patients with sarcoidosis have chronic, progressive disease, and some patients develop pulmonary fibrosis or other end-organ damage.

For a deeper discussion on this topic, please see Chapter 95, "Sarcoidosis," in Goldman-Cecil Medicine, 25th Edition.

INTERSTITIAL LUNG DISEASES RELATED TO CONNECTIVE TISSUE DISORDERS

In patients with ILD, a thorough history and physical examination may reveal abnormalities such as arthritis and hand deformities, rashes, esophageal dysmotility, Raynaud's syndrome, and skin changes suggesting an underlying connective tissue disease. Connective tissue disorders, such as systemic lupus erythematosus, rheumatoid arthritis, mixed connective tissue disorder, systemic sclerosis (i.e., scleroderma), polymyositis or dermatomyositis, and Sjögren syndrome, can cause ILD and a wide variety of other pulmonary manifestations (Table 17-3). Lung disease is a major cause of morbidity and mortality in some of these conditions, especially systemic sclerosis. Although not typical, a connective tissue disorder–related ILD (CTD-ILD)

TABLE 17-3   PULMONARY INVOLVEMENT IN CONNECTIVE TISSUE DISORDERS

DISORDER	RA	LUPUS	SS	PM/DM	SJÖGREN SYNDROME
Pleural effusion	+ (5-40%)	+ (30-40%)			
Necrobiotic nodules	+				
Fibrosis	+ (20-60%)	+ (3%)	+ (15-90%)	+ (10-40%)	+ (33%)
Bronchiolitis	+	+			+
Pulmonary arteriopathy	+	+	+	+	
Atelectasis		+			
Pulmonary edema		+			
Pneumonitis, hemorrhage		+			
Diaphragm dysfunction		+			
Aspiration			+	+ (14%)	
Secondary carcinoma			+		

DM, Dermatomyositis; PM, polymyositis; RA, rheumatoid arthritis; SS, systemic sclerosis.

can develop before other symptoms such as arthritis manifest, making the diagnosis more difficult.

Clinical manifestations of CTD-ILD are nonspecific and include exertional dyspnea and dry cough. Exertional dyspnea may be obscured by disabilities caused by the underlying connective tissue disorder. CTD-ILD may be relatively asymptomatic, manifesting as an incidental finding on imaging. Lung examination in patients with CTD-ILD may reveal bibasilar crackles, and pulmonary function tests often show a restrictive pattern with decreased diffusion capacity. If obstruction is identified on pulmonary function testing, airway manifestations of the connective tissue disorder, such as obliterative bronchiolitis in the setting of rheumatoid arthritis, must be considered.

Chest imaging studies are useful because they may reveal typical patterns associated with the underlying connective tissue disorder, often obviating the need for biopsy. These patterns include apical fibrocavitary disease in ankylosing spondylitis and basilar fibrotic changes in rheumatoid arthritis, polymyositis, and systemic sclerosis. Imaging may also reveal pulmonary nodules in RA or pleural disease in the setting of rheumatoid arthritis or systemic lupus erythematosus.

Pulmonary hypertension in the absence of fibrosis can occur in these patients, especially those with limited scleroderma (e.g., CREST syndrome [calcinosis, Raynaud's phenomenon, esophageal dysmotility, sclerodactyly, and telangiectasia]) and systemic lupus erythematosus. Echocardiography may be helpful in patients with these disorders and otherwise unexplained dyspnea.

Drug-induced lung disorders related to immunosuppressant therapy should always be considered in patients with connective tissue disorders. Although CTD-ILD typically is chronic in nature, acute or fulminant pneumonitis that may be difficult to distinguish from opportunistic infection can be seen in systemic lupus erythematosus, Sjögren syndrome, polymyositis, and dermatomyositis.

Bronchoscopy with BAL is often used to rule out infection in acute presentations or when imaging reveals areas of consolidation, as may occur with organizing pneumonia in rheumatoid arthritis. Lung biopsy may be necessary if the clinical presentation or imaging findings are atypical. Biopsies of areas of typical basilar fibrosis in connective tissue disorders frequently reveal patterns consistent with NSIP or UIP. In Sjögren syndrome with ILD, LIP or lymphoma may be found on biopsy. Diffuse alveolar damage is found in the setting of acute lupus pneumonitis.

Immunosuppressants are the mainstay of treatment for CTD-ILD. These disorders are more responsive to this therapy than IPF.

DRUG-INDUCED LUNG DISORDERS

A large number and variety of drugs can induce adverse reactions in the lung, often in the form of an ILD (Table 17-4). These reactions vary in severity from self-limited hypersensitivity reactions (E-Fig. 17-5) to diffuse alveolar damage resulting in respiratory failure and death. A high index of suspicion is needed to make the association between a drug and a pulmonary reaction, and a careful review of medications and other pharmacologic substances used by a patient is necessary in the setting of diffuse lung disease. Illicit drugs such as heroin and cocaine commonly produce adverse pulmonary reactions. Substances

such as talc may be injected or inhaled inadvertently during the use of illicit drugs, resulting in pulmonary vascular or interstitial disease.

The clinical presentation of a drug-induced ILD is often nonspecific, with fever, cough, and dyspnea accompanied by radiographic infiltrates. Eosinophilia is sometimes found. Tests results for antinuclear antibodies are positive, but those for anti–double-stranded DNA antibodies are negative in the setting of drug-induced lupus. Pulmonary function tests, if performed, usually reveal decreases in DLCO and often show a restrictive pattern. ILD caused by medications usually does not produce a unique radiographic or histologic pattern of lung injury but may result in a variety of nonspecific reactions, including pulmonary infiltrates with peripheral eosinophilia, an HP pattern, and interstitial fibrosis. Alveolar filling may also occur in the setting of drug-induced organizing pneumonia and acute lung injury or diffuse alveolar damage. Pleural and pericardial effusions may occur in lupus-like drug reactions. Because the clinical presentation of patients with drug-induced ILDs lacks specificity, ILDs are typically diagnoses of exclusion.

There are settings in which drug-induced lung disease may be especially relevant and should be strongly considered in the differential diagnosis. They include the use of chemotherapeutic agents, the use of illicit drugs, patients with lupus-like illness, and patients using agents known to produce pulmonary toxicity, such as amiodarone or nitrofurantoin. Many chemotherapeutic agents, ranging from the newer tyrosine kinase inhibitors to older agents such as bleomycin and methotrexate, may produce lung injury and ILD. Diagnosis of a drug-induced ILD may be challenging in patients treated with chemotherapy because atypical infections and chemotherapy-induced heart failure may result in similar symptoms and radiographic findings.

Heroin use typically results in pulmonary edema or aspiration injury rather than ILD. Cocaine use can produce a variety of pulmonary effects, including organizing pneumonia, alveolar hemorrhage, and diffuse alveolar damage. "Crack lung" is a clinical diagnosis typified by dyspnea, hemoptysis, and pulmonary infiltrates occurring in the setting of crack cocaine use. Drug-induced lupus occurs with drugs such as procainamide or hydralazine. Amiodarone lung toxicity is a classic drug-induced lung disorder that results in alveolar or interstitial infiltrates accompanied by dyspnea on exertion. Although foamy macrophages can be detected by BAL, they indicate amiodarone use, not toxicity. Nitrofurantoin may cause an acute pulmonary syndrome with fever, dyspnea, and cough soon after initiation of the drug or cause a chronic pulmonary fibrosis with long-standing use. Amiodarone and nitrofurantoin reactions necessitate drug withdrawal and often require corticosteroids for resolution.

Pulmonary toxicity from drugs may be dose dependent, as with bleomycin, for which the risk of lung toxicity increases with cumulative doses exceeding 450 U. Amiodarone lung disease typically occurs with dosages greater than 400 mg per day. Synergistic lung toxicities may occur. For example, exposure to high levels of inspired oxygen may precipitate bleomycin lung injury and should be avoided if possible in exposed patients.

An online drug reference website (http://www.pneumotox.com) is available. It tabulates the reported pulmonary

TABLE 17-4 COMMON DRUG-INDUCED LUNG DISEASES

DRUG	DOSE RELATIONSHIP	MANIFESTATION
CHEMOTHERAPEUTIC		
Bevacizumab	Acute	Hemoptysis, pulmonary hemorrhage
Bleomycin	Acute or delayed, >450 U increases risk	Pneumonitis, fibrosis, OP, lung nodules
Busulfan	Chronic	Fibrosis, alveolar proteinosis
Cyclophosphamide	Chronic	Fibrosis, OP
Cytosine arabinoside	Acute	Pulmonary edema, ARDS
Gefitinib	Acute	Pulmonary fibrosis, interstitial pneumonitis, diffuse alveolar damage
Gemcitabine	Acute	Dyspnea, bronchospasm, capillary leak syndrome with pulmonary edema, ARDS, alveolar hemorrhage
Imatinib	Acute, chronic	Pulmonary edema, pneumonitis
Interferon alfa	Chronic	Sarcoidosis
Irinotecan	Acute	Pneumonitis
Methotrexate	Acute or chronic	Hypersensitivity pneumonitis, resolves with discontinuation, OP
Mitomycin C	Acute or delayed	Pneumonitis, ARDS, OP, hemolytic uremic syndrome
Paclitaxel and docetaxel	Acute	Interstitial and hypersensitivity pneumonitis
ANTIMICROBIAL		
Nitrofurantoin	Acute or chronic	Acute pneumonitis, chronic fibrosis
Sulfasalazine	Acute or chronic	Pulmonary infiltrates with eosinophilia, OP
CARDIOVASCULAR		
Amiodarone	Acute or chronic, >400 mg/day	Pneumonitis, fibrosis
Flecainide	Acute	ARDS, LIP
Tocainide	Weeks or months	Pneumonitis
Procainamide	Subacute or chronic	Drug-induced SLE, pleural effusions, pulmonary infiltrates
ANTI-INFLAMMATORY		
Aspirin	Acute	Pulmonary edema, bronchospasm
ILLICIT		
Opiates	Acute	Pulmonary edema
Cocaine	Acute	Pulmonary edema, diffuse alveolar damage, pulmonary hemorrhage, OP
Talc (in intravenous and inhaled illicit drugs)	Acute or chronic	Granulomatous interstitial fibrosis, granulomatous pulmonary artery occlusion, particulate embolization
TOCOLYTIC		
Terbutaline, albuterol, ritodrine	Acute	Pulmonary edema

ARDS, Acute respiratory distress syndrome; OP, organizing pneumonia; LIP, lymphoid interstitial pneumonia; SLE, systemic lupus erythematosus.

toxicities of various drugs, and it is searchable by drug name and by pattern of lung involvement.

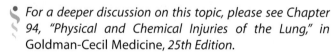 *For a deeper discussion on this topic, please see Chapter 94, "Physical and Chemical Injuries of the Lung," in Goldman-Cecil Medicine, 25th Edition.*

PULMONARY VASCULITIS AND DIFFUSE ALVEOLAR HEMORRHAGE

Diffuse Alveolar Hemorrhage

Definition and Epidemiology

Diffuse alveolar hemorrhage (DAH) syndromes encompass a diverse group of entities that are characterized by disruption of the alveolar-capillary membrane, resulting in bleeding into the alveolar spaces from the alveolar capillaries and intra-alveolar accumulation of red blood cells. DAH is a rare condition of uncertain incidence in the general population, but it occurs with increased frequency in specific patient populations, such as those after hematopoietic stem cell transplantation.

Pathology

The DAH syndromes are characterized by three distinct histologic patterns. Bland pulmonary hemorrhage is caused by alveolar hemorrhage without inflammation or destruction of the alveolar structures. This pattern is seen in conditions with elevated pulmonary capillary hydrostatic pressure, such as congestive heart failure or mitral stenosis, or with the use of anticoagulation medications.

DAH can be seen in diffuse alveolar damage (DAD), which is caused by a variety of pulmonary infections, connective tissue diseases, and medications. DAD is also seen in acute respiratory distress syndrome (ARDS) from any cause. Histologically, alveolar walls appear edematous and are lined with hyaline membranes.

The most common histologic pattern seen on lung biopsy obtained from patients with DAH is pulmonary capillaritis, which is characterized by neutrophilic infiltration of the alveolar septa. It sequentially leads to necrosis, loss of capillary structural integrity, and extravasation of red blood cells into the interstitium and alveolar spaces. This pattern is seen in a variety of connective tissue diseases and in some of the pulmonary vasculitides.

Clinical Presentation

All DAH syndromes are characterized by the abrupt onset of cough and dyspnea. Hemoptysis is common but not universal; it may be absent in up to one third of patients with DAH. Fever may occur in patients with underlying vasculitis. Physical findings are usually nonspecific, although ocular, nasopharyngeal, or cutaneous abnormalities may suggest systemic vasculitis or collagen vascular disease as a cause. The cardiopulmonary examination is often normal but may reveal inspiratory crackles, a systolic murmur suggesting mitral stenosis, or evidence of pulmonary hypertension.

Falling hemoglobin levels in the setting of new patchy alveolar infiltrates (E-Fig 17-6) seen on chest imaging favor the diagnosis of DAH, especially in the setting of a predisposing condition such as connective tissue disease. Pertinent laboratory abnormalities may include azotemia, suggesting a pulmonary-renal syndrome. In this setting, an abnormal urinalysis result with proteinuria, hematuria, and red blood cell casts is usually seen.

Some lung disorders characterized by DAH are associated with the production of antineutrophil cytoplasmic antibodies (ANCAs) directed against neutrophil cytoplasmic antigens or antibodies directed at the glomerular basement membrane. ANCA testing in particular can play an important role in the work-up of DAH because it is used in the diagnosis and classification of various pulmonary vasculitides that cause DAH. Two major immunofluorescent patterns can be seen in ANCA testing: diffuse staining throughout the cytoplasm (cANCA) or staining around the nucleus (pANCA). Specific antigens that ANCAs are directed against include proteinase 3 (PR3), typically causing the cANCA pattern, and myeloperoxidase (MPO), which typically causes the pANCA pattern. The Goodpasture or antiglomerular basement membrane syndrome is a cause of DAH and pulmonary-renal syndrome characterized by the finding of anti–basement membrane antibodies.

Diagnosis and Differential Diagnosis

Increasingly hemorrhagic fluid seen on sequential BAL studies confirms the diagnosis of DAH, but it does not give insight into the cause. The presence and quantity of hemosiderin-laden macrophages in BAL fluid should be determined. Biopsy of the lung shows accumulation of red blood cells in the alveolar spaces and may show evidence of associated capillaritis or diffuse alveolar damage.

After the diagnosis of DAH is established, the specific cause must be determined based on whether there is apparently bland pulmonary hemorrhage (e.g., mitral stenosis); pulmonary capillaritis with positive ANCA staining (e.g., granulomatosis with polyangiitis, which is typically positive for anti-PR3 ANCA and sometimes for anti-MPO ANCA); microscopic polyangiitis (typically anti-MPO positive); Goodpasture's syndrome with positive anti–basement membrane antibodies; pulmonary capillaritis due to connective tissue disease; or DAH due to diffuse alveolar damage (e.g., ARDS, bone marrow transplantation). Some cases of DAH are associated with idiopathic recurrent bland hemorrhage, resulting in accumulation of hemosiderin-laden macrophages in the lungs, a condition called *idiopathic pulmonary hemosiderosis*. This syndrome is most common in children, who have a worse prognosis than adults.

Treatment

Treatment of DAH is based on the underlying cause. Immunosuppressives are used for capillaritis due to vasculitis or connective tissue disease, such as a combination of cortico-steroids and cyclophosphamide for the treatment of granulomatosis with polyangiitis (level 1 evidence).

Prognosis

DAH is a serious condition. The underlying illnesses such as granulomatosis with polyangiitis are associated with significant morbidity and mortality rates.

Pulmonary Vasculitides

The pulmonary vasculitides represent a group of entities, many of which are associated with elevated serum ANCA levels. They include granulomatosis with polyangiitis, microscopic polyangiitis, Churg-Strauss syndrome, and certain drug-induced vasculitis syndromes. The conditions are rare.

Granulomatosis with polyangiitis is a systemic necrotizing granulomatous vasculitis that often involves the small and medium-sized vessels of the upper airway, the lower respiratory tract, and the kidney. Although this triad is not always seen at initial presentation because only 40% of those affected have renal disease at that time, 80% to 90% of patients eventually develop glomerulonephritis. The most frequent manifestations of this illness are pulmonary, as highlighted by cough, chest pain, hemoptysis, and dyspnea. Constitutional symptoms such as fever and weight loss and symptoms due to involvement of the skin, eye, heart, nervous system, and musculoskeletal system are also common.

Chest imaging may show bilateral disease and infiltrates that evolve over the course of the illness. Lung nodules are common and may cavitate. Effusions and adenopathy are uncommon. Sinus films or CT scans can diagnose upper airway involvement. The diagnosis of granulomatosis with polyangiitis is supported by clinical findings and by circulating ANCAs, which are seen in 90% of patients. The remaining 10% of patients are ANCA negative. In ANCA-positive patients, antibodies are usually directed against PR3; however, 10% to 20% may have anti-MPO antibodies.

Tissue biopsy at a site of active disease is usually needed to confirm granulomatosis with polyangiitis. Necrotizing granulomatous inflammation is common, but actual vasculitis is seen in only 35% of patients. A renal biopsy is preferred because it is easier to perform and more often diagnostic. In the absence of renal involvement, a lung biopsy should be considered. Pathologically, granulomatosis with polyangiitis is characterized by small and medium-sized vessel necrotizing vasculitis and granulomatous inflammation. Special stains and cultures should be performed to exclude infections that can produce similar findings.

Microscopic polyangiitis is a form of systemic necrotizing small vessel vasculitis that universally affects the kidneys, whereas pulmonary involvement occurs in only 10% to 30% of patients. This rare condition has a prevalence of 1 to 3 cases per 100,000 people, but it is the most common cause of pulmonary-renal syndrome.

Microscopic polyangiitis often is heralded by a long prodromal phase, characterized by constitutional symptoms followed by the development of rapidly progressive glomerulonephritis. In patients who develop lung involvement, DAH due to capillaritis is the most common manifestation. Joint, skin, peripheral nervous system, and gastrointestinal involvement also can be seen.

Seventy percent of patients with microscopic polyangiitis are ANCA positive, and most have anti-MPO antibodies. Because anti-MPO and anti-PR3 antibodies can occur in microscopic polyangiitis and granulomatosis with polyangiitis, these diseases cannot be distinguished based on their ANCA pattern. However, they can be distinguished pathologically because microscopic polyangiitis is characterized by a focal, segmental necrotizing vasculitis affecting venules, capillaries, arterioles, and small arteries without clinical or pathologic evidence of necrotizing granulomatous inflammation. The absence or paucity of immunoglobulin localization in vessel walls distinguishes microscopic polyangiitis from immune complex–mediated small vessel vasculitis such as Henoch-Schönlein purpura and cryoglobulinemic vasculitis.

Treatments for granulomatosis with polyangiitis and microscopic polyangiitis are similar. Combination therapy with corticosteroids and cyclophosphamide is the standard of care to induce remission (level 1 evidence). Rituximab is also an option in this setting (level 1). Plasma exchange is added in cases of severe disease and provides better renal outcomes (level 1). Azathioprine (level 1) or methotrexate (level 1) can be substituted for cyclophosphamide if remission is achieved. Rituximab may be used for induction of remission in place of cyclophosphamide (level 1 evidence) or for relapsing disease (level 1). Novel therapies, including co-trimoxazole (sulfamethoxazole/trimethoprim) for remission maintenance (level 1) and TNF inhibitors for persistent disease, have been tried with some success.

Allergic granulomatosis or Churg-Strauss syndrome is characterized by the triad of asthma, hypereosinophilia, and necrotizing vasculitis. Many other organ systems, including the nervous system, skin, heart, and gastrointestinal tract, may be involved. The vasculitis can be associated with skin nodules and purpura. Although DAH and glomerulonephritis may occur, they are much less common than in the other small vessel vasculitides. Morbidity and mortality often result from cardiac or gastrointestinal complications or status asthmaticus and respiratory failure.

ANCAs are less helpful in the diagnosis of Churg-Strauss syndrome because only 50% of patients are ANCA positive. Anti-MPO antibodies are more commonly seen in these patients. Pathologically, a necrotizing small vessel vasculitis and an eosinophil-rich inflammatory infiltrate with necrotizing granulomas are seen. Most patients respond well to corticosteroids, but other immunosuppressants such as cyclophosphamide may be required for patients with refractory disorders.

Other well-known causes of pulmonary capillaritis include the collagen vascular disorders, anti–glomerular membrane antibody syndrome (i.e., Goodpasture's syndrome), and Henoch-Schönlein purpura. Goodpasture's syndrome causes DAH associated with glomerulonephritis due to anti–glomerular basement membrane antibodies to the α_3 chain of type IV collagen that is also found in the lung basement membrane. More than 90% of patients with Goodpasture's syndrome have anti–glomerular basement membrane antibodies detectable in the serum. For those without circulating antibodies, the diagnosis may be confirmed by lung biopsy, although the kidney is the preferred site. Up to 40% may also be ANCA positive, primarily with anti-MPO antibodies. Pathologically, linear deposition of antibody along the alveolar or glomerular basement membrane is visible by direct immunofluorescence.

The treatment of Goodpasture's syndrome is plasmapheresis and immunosuppression. The disease is fatal if left untreated.

ENVIRONMENTAL AND OCCUPATIONAL INTERSTITIAL LUNG DISEASES

Several environmental and occupational exposures may cause ILDs. They include the pneumoconioses, drug-induced ILD (discussed earlier), and HP. Pneumoconioses are lung diseases resulting from the inhalation of mineral dusts, including silica, coal dust, or asbestos. HP is caused by the inhalation of organic dusts.

For a deeper discussion on this topic, please see Chapter 93, "Occupational Pulmonary Disorders," in Goldman-Cecil Medicine, 25th Edition.

Pneumoconiosis

The pneumoconioses result from the effects of accumulation of mineral dusts in the lungs; the typical reaction is fibrosis. The risk and extent of these diseases are related to the intensity and cumulative amount of exposure over time. Prevention of the pneumoconioses through occupational safeguards or, in the case of asbestos, legislative bans on use, is important because there are no effective treatments for these diseases.

Silicosis is a lung disease caused by exposure to crystalline-free silica, which results in an inflammatory and fibrotic reaction and the formation of the characteristic silicotic nodule. Occupations with a higher likelihood of exposure to silica include mining, stone cutting, carving, polishing, foundry work, and abrasive clearing (e.g., sandblasting). Although exposure is usually chronic (over years), accelerated and acute disease manifestations have been described in the setting of heavier short-term exposures.

Acute silicosis causes a pulmonary alveolar proteinosis and accumulation of surfactant in the alveolar spaces. Chronic silicosis results in simple nodular silicosis, which is usually asymptomatic unless the patient is also exposed to tobacco, and progressive massive fibrosis, which is characterized by extensive bilateral apical fibrosis resulting from the confluence of many silicotic nodules.

Patients with silicosis may have dyspnea or may be relatively asymptomatic but require further evaluation of an abnormal chest radiograph. Chest radiographs in uncomplicated silicosis show upper lobe nodular opacities, which may be subtle, whereas progressive massive fibrosis results in marked architectural distortion of the upper lobes (E-Fig 17-7). Hilar node enlargement may be accompanied by eggshell nodal calcification (E-Fig 17-8). Pulmonary function tests in simple nodular silicosis may be normal or show a mixed obstructive or restrictive pattern, whereas progressive massive fibrosis is typically associated with severe restriction and hypoxemia. Patients with silicosis are at elevated risk for tuberculosis and should be screened for latent tuberculosis infection; there is also an association between silicosis and rheumatoid arthritis.

Coal worker's pneumoconiosis is an uncommon cause of pulmonary fibrosis, occurring in workers exposed to coal dust and graphite. Usually, the patients are exposed while working in underground mines. Coal worker's pneumoconiosis results in the formation of pigmented lesions in the lung surrounded by emphysema, called *coal macules*. Progressive massive fibrosis may subsequently occur. Most patients have chronic cough, which is usually productive, resulting from bronchitis related to coal exposure or to tobacco. The chest radiograph shows diffuse, small, rounded opacities. As with silicosis, there is an association with rheumatoid arthritis. Caplan's syndrome is the occurrence of multiple, large, sometimes cavitary lung nodules in association with rheumatoid arthritis after coal dust exposure.

Asbestosis results from chronic exposure to asbestos, which is a fibrous silicate used for insulation, for friction-bearing surfaces, and to strengthen materials. The inhaled asbestos fibers are deposited in the lungs, where the small fibers may be phagocytosed and cleared through lymphatics to the pleural space, but the longer fibers are often retained. Asbestos exposure typically leads to pleural disease characterized by pleural plaques, effusion, and fibrosis, but it does not necessarily affect the lung parenchyma. If it does, it is called *asbestosis*, with interstitial lung fibrosis resulting from asbestos exposure.

Asbestosis is characterized by a gradual onset of dyspnea. As with other pneumoconioses, the risk and severity of disease are related to the extent and duration of exposure. Asbestosis is often diagnosed after exposure has ceased, and disease progression may continue in the absence of ongoing exposure because of the reaction to retained asbestos fibers in the lung.

The clinical presentation, pulmonary function tests, and imaging studies are similar to those for restrictive lung diseases such as IPF. However, the detection of significant pleural disease is useful in distinguishing this illness from other ILDs.

The diagnosis is made from the history of exposure and demonstration of concomitant pleural plaques and lower lobe–predominant fibrotic changes on the chest radiograph or CT scan. In uncertain cases, the demonstration of asbestos in tissue specimens may be necessary. Asbestos bodies are the characteristic finding and consist of asbestos fibers coated by iron-containing (ferruginous) material. Asbestos exposure increases the incidence of malignancy, including lung carcinoma and mesothelioma, especially among people who also smoke. It is uncertain whether asbestosis itself confers a heightened risk of malignancy independent of the effects of asbestos exposure alone. No specific treatment for asbestosis exists.

Berylliosis results from exposure to beryllium, a rare metal useful in modern, high-technology industries. Exposure to beryllium can lead to an acute chemical bronchitis and pneumonitis or chronic beryllium disease. Chronic beryllium disease is characterized by a multisystemic granulomatosis that is difficult to distinguish from sarcoidosis. The diagnosis is made by history of exposure, histologic examination, and laboratory confirmation using the beryllium lymphocyte proliferation test that is available at specialized centers. Corticosteroids may be useful in the treatment of berylliosis, but patients should avoid further exposure to beryllium.

Hypersensitivity Pneumonitis

Definition and Epidemiology

HP (formerly called *extrinsic allergic alveolitis*) is a relatively common ILD resulting from an exaggerated immune reaction in the alveoli and small airways to various small, inhaled organic antigens in sensitized individuals. Potential sensitizing antigens are diverse, ranging from bacterial, fungal, and animal proteins to low-molecular-weight chemicals (Table 17-5). Although evocative descriptions have been given to occupational forms of this disease (e.g., paprika splitter's lung resulting from sensitivity to inhaled paprika dust contaminated with *Mucor stolonifer)*, more prosaic exposures may occur in everyday life, such as to contaminated hot tub water or to antigens from pet birds. The incidence and prevalence of HP are not well known, and underdiagnosis occurs.

Pathology

HP occurs as the result of an abnormally exuberant immune response in the alveoli and small airways to inhaled antigens, typically organic molecules, but also small chemical compounds such as isocyanates, which bind to haptens. This response occurs in a susceptible host; the underlying reasons for susceptibility are unclear but probably include genetic and environmental factors (e.g., pesticide exposure). Smokers are less likely than nonsmokers to develop HP, but they may have a more severe disease course if HP does occur. After exposure to an antigen, a susceptible individual develops an alveolitis with influx of neutrophils and lymphocytes. A T_H1-type immune response then leads to granuloma formation.

Typical lung biopsy findings include granulomatous inflammation with poorly formed granulomas containing foreign body giant cells, interstitial chronic inflammation with a bronchiolocentric component, and bronchiolitis. In chronic or end-stage disease, fibrosis occurs, and biopsies may feature areas with a UIP or NSIP pattern in addition to areas of granulomatous and airway-centered inflammation.

Clinical Presentation

The disease may manifest in an acute fashion (i.e., acute HP) several hours after intense exposure to a provocative antigen, with

TABLE 17-5	HYPERSENSITIVITY PNEUMONITIS	
ANTIGEN	**SOURCE**	**DISEASES**
Thermophilic bacteria	Moldy hay, sugar cane, compost	Farmer's lung, bagassosis, mushroom worker's disease
Other bacteria, including atypical mycobacteria	Contaminated water, wood dust, fertilizer, paprika dust	Humidifier, detergent worker's disease, and familial hypersensitivity pneumonitis
Fungi	Moldy cork, contaminated wood dust, barley, maple logs	Suberosis, sequoiosis, and maple bark stripper's disease, malt worker's disease, and paprika splitter's lung
Animal protein	Bird droppings, animal urine, bovine and porcine pituitary powder	Pigeon breeder's lung, duck fever, turkey handler's disease, pituitary snuff-taker's disease, laboratory worker's hypersensitivity pneumonitis
Chemically altered human proteins (e.g., albumin)	Toluene diisocyanate, trimellitic anhydride, diphenylmethane diisocyanate	Hypersensitivity pneumonitis
Phthalic anhydride	Heated epoxy resin	Epoxy resin lung

a flulike illness featuring fever, chills, cough, dyspnea, and malaise that lasts for up to 24 hours (e.g., farmer's lung from exposure to thermophilic actinomycetes). Subacute and chronic HP may occur with repeated or prolonged lower-level antigen exposure, which results in chronic dyspnea and cough with eventual progression to pulmonary fibrosis (e.g., pigeon breeder's lung from exposure to avian droppings and other antigens).

The patient with acute HP may be febrile. Diffuse wheezes are common physical findings in acute HP, whereas crackles may be auscultated in chronic HP. Patients with chronic HP may have clubbing. Hypoxemia with exertion may occur in earlier stages of disease, progressing to hypoxemia at rest in chronic fibrotic HP. Pulmonary function tests usually show a restrictive pattern with abnormal gas exchange in subacute and chronic HP, although obstructive or mixed patterns are sometimes seen.

HP is characterized by nonspecific infiltrates in the middle and upper lung fields on chest radiographs, although chest radiographs may be normal in acute disease. CT scanning is more sensitive than chest radiography, revealing ground-glass opacities, centrilobular nodules, and mosaic attenuation and air trapping patterns resulting from airway obstruction. Chronic HP may have architectural distortion with traction bronchiectasis and honeycombing.

Emphysema occurs in some cases of advanced farmer's lung. BAL may demonstrate a lymphocytic alveolitis, with CD4$^+$ T-lymphocyte predominance. Patients with HP may have precipitating antibodies to the offending antigen, but serum precipitins are not sufficiently sensitive or specific for diagnosis, and the specific antigen may not be known or may not be tested for with standard test panels.

Diagnosis and Differential Diagnosis

An appropriate exposure, clinical history, BAL, and HRCT imaging findings can suggest the diagnosis, but a lung biopsy may be necessary for confirmation, especially in subacute and chronic HP. Transbronchial biopsy may be sufficient, but surgical lung biopsy can collect larger samples from different lung regions. The differential diagnosis includes acute viral infection in acute HP; in chronic HP, the differential includes other fibrosing lung diseases such as IPF, NSIP, and sarcoidosis.

Treatment

Clinical improvement often occurs in the hospital setting when patients are isolated from the offending antigen, and relapse may occur after discharge. This pattern of illness can point to the diagnosis of HP. Corticosteroids can relieve symptoms in the acute phase, but their long-term efficacy in chronic forms of the disease is less clear (level 3 evidence). Identification of the cause of HP is important because chronic disease management requires avoidance of exposure to the antigen, which can be financially or psychologically challenging for patients in the setting of occupational, pet, or residential exposures. For advanced HP with fibrosis, lung transplantation may be necessary.

Prognosis

The prognosis for HP varies. Acute HP usually has a good prognosis, but chronic HP can lead to end-stage pulmonary fibrosis and death.

⬤ SPECIFIC DISEASES

Pulmonary Langerhans Cell Histiocytosis

Definition and Epidemiology

Pulmonary LCH, formerly called *eosinophilic granuloma*, is a rare disease of young and middle-aged adults. It is characterized by an abnormal infiltration of Langerhans cells, which are dendritic cells, into the lung parenchyma. The disease almost always occurs in smokers.

Pathology

Pulmonary LCH results in the formation of cysts and nodules in the lungs. The accumulation of activated Langerhans cells results in stellate nodular infiltrates around the small airways, with eventual destruction and dilation of the airway walls, resulting in cystic changes in the lung parenchyma. Although a multisystem Langerhans cell disease related to clonal proliferation of Langerhans cells occurs in children, isolated pulmonary LCH in adult smokers does not appear to be a clonal neoplastic disorder.

Smoking may alter local immune signaling, attracting the Langerhans cells to the lungs, or it may cause local proliferation and increased survival of Langerhans cells in the lungs. Biopsy of the lung demonstrates multiple stellate lung nodules that may be cellular or fibrotic, containing Langerhans cells that stain for Cd1a and S100. Electron microscopy may reveal Birbeck granules, distinctive racquet-shaped structures in the Langerhans cells

Clinical Presentation

Patients may be asymptomatic or may exhibit constitutional symptoms, dyspnea on exertion, and cough, possibly with hemoptysis. Spontaneous pneumothorax may also occur. Chest imaging shows nodules that may be cavitary and cysts that predominate in the middle and upper lung zones. Pulmonary function tests show impaired diffusion capacity, and an obstructive or restrictive pattern may be seen.

Diagnosis and Differential Diagnosis

A specific diagnosis can be made with open lung biopsy. In the right clinical setting and with a typical HRCT, a biopsy may not be needed for a presumptive diagnosis. The differential diagnosis includes other cystic lung diseases, such as lymphangioleiomyomatosis, sarcoidosis, and smoking-related idiopathic pneumonias such as RB-ILD and DIP complicated by emphysema.

Treatment

The main treatment is tobacco cessation (level 3 evidence). Corticosteroids and cytotoxic agents are sometimes employed as adjunctive therapy (level 3). Lung transplantation may be considered in cases of advanced disease.

Prognosis

In contrast to systemic LCH, pulmonary LCH is not a neoplastic disorder, and spontaneous regression may occur with smoking cessation. Although some patients have a benign course, others develop progressive disease or complications such as pulmonary hypertension, which may be fatal.

Lymphangioleiomyomatosis

Definition and Epidemiology

Lymphangioleiomyomatosis is a rare, slowly progressive, neoplastic disorder resulting in cystic lung disease and kidney angiomyolipomas that occurs in association with the tuberous sclerosis complex or sporadically in women of childbearing age.

Pathology

The disease is characterized by extensive infiltration of the lungs and lymphatics with growths of smooth muscle–like lymphangioleiomyomatosis cells. Mutations in the *TSC1* or *TSC2* gene, which encodes tumor suppressor proteins that normally act as inhibitors of protein synthesis and cell growth, may result in tuberous sclerosis or lymphangioleiomyomatosis. Mutations in *TSC2* are associated with greater disease severity.

Clinical Presentation

Dyspnea and spontaneous pneumothorax are the most common presentations, with chylous pleural effusions and hemoptysis also occurring. These clinical presentations result from lung parenchymal destruction, airway narrowing, and lymphatic obstruction caused by the abnormal proliferation of the smooth muscle–like cells.

Imaging studies show an interstitial pattern with middle and upper lung predominance; multiple, thin-walled cystic lesions; and characteristically preserved lung volumes. Pleural effusion or pneumothorax may be seen on imaging. CT of the abdomen may reveal fat-containing kidney lesions consistent with angiomyolipomas. Pulmonary function tests typically show a progressive obstructive pattern, although mixed obstruction and restriction may also be seen.

Diagnosis

Although the clinical features coupled with characteristic imaging are often diagnostic, lung biopsy may be necessary in some cases. It demonstrates interstitial nodules composed centrally of spindle-shaped cells that stain for smooth muscle cell actin and for HMB-45, an antibody to the melanocytic glycoprotein 100, with staining involving the alveolar walls, lobular septa, venules, small airways, and pleura.

Treatment

Treatment involves management of pleural complications, including the use of pleurodesis to prevent recurrent pneumothorax or effusion, bronchodilator and oxygen therapy, and avoidance of pharmacologic estrogens, which may exacerbate the disease. Progesterones have been used in an attempt to modulate disease progression, but efficacy data are limited.

Because the products of the *TSC1* and *TSC2* genes normally act as inhibitors of the mammalian target of rapamycin (mTOR), pharmacologic mTOR inhibitors such as sirolimus and everolimus have been studied in lymphangioleiomyomatosis. Sirolimus stabilized lung function in lymphangioleiomyomatosis (level 1 evidence), and sirolimus and everolimus treatment resulted in angiomyolipoma shrinkage (level 1). Lung transplantation can be performed in patients with severe pulmonary dysfunction.

Prognosis

Lymphangioleiomyomatosis is a slowly progressive disease that can result in potentially fatal complications, especially respiratory failure.

Eosinophilic Lung Disease

Eosinophilic lung diseases are characterized by pulmonary infiltrates and eosinophilia of the peripheral blood or lung. Because eosinophilia is a feature of many diseases, distinguishing primary pulmonary eosinophilic lung disorders from lung disorders in which eosinophilia has a specific cause is important.

Eosinophilic lung diseases can be categorized as follows: primary pulmonary eosinophilic disorders (e.g., acute and chronic eosinophilic pneumonia, hypereosinophilic syndrome), pulmonary disorders of known cause associated with eosinophilia (e.g., asthma, allergic bronchopulmonary aspergillosis, drug reactions, parasitic infections), lung diseases associated with eosinophilia (e.g., HP, COP, IPF), malignancies associated with eosinophilia (e.g., lung cancer, leukemia, lymphoma), and systemic disease associated with eosinophilia (e.g., rheumatoid arthritis, sarcoidosis, Sjögren syndrome).

Acute eosinophilic pneumonia is characterized by fever, a nonproductive cough, and dyspnea of less than 7 days' duration, often leading to acute respiratory failure. This disease typically affects male smokers between the ages of 20 and 40 years who are otherwise healthy. Chest imaging reveals diffuse bilateral pulmonary infiltrates. Eosinophilia is not found in the peripheral blood initially but may occur 7 to 30 days after onset. Abundant eosinophils can be found in BAL fluid, and a level of greater than 25% of all nucleated cells is helpful in making the correct diagnosis. Although lung biopsy is typically not required to make the diagnosis, it can show eosinophilic infiltration with acute and organizing diffuse alveolar damage. Treatment with corticosteroids typically offers rapid and complete clinical and radiographic resolution without recurrence or residual sequelae (level 3 evidence).

Chronic eosinophilic pneumonia is an idiopathic disease predominantly of middle-aged women with a history of asthma. Also called *prolonged pulmonary eosinophilia*, this illness is characterized by a productive cough, dyspnea, malaise, weight loss, night sweats, and fever associated with progressive peripheral lung infiltrates that have been described as resembling the photographic negative of pulmonary edema on chest radiographs (E-Fig 17-9). On presentation, most patients with chronic eosinophilic pneumonia have a peripheral eosinophilia of greater than 30% and BAL fluid eosinophilia.

Histologic examination shows eosinophils and histiocytes in the lung parenchyma and interstitium, areas of COP, but minimal fibrosis. Spontaneous remissions have been reported, but respiratory failure can develop. Typically, treatment with corticosteroids is rapidly effective. Prolonged therapy is recommended because relapses are common (level 3 evidence), unlike treatment for acute eosinophilic pneumonia.

Simple pulmonary eosinophilia (i.e., Löffler syndrome) is characterized by transient migratory infiltrates that last less than 1 month. Some cases are asymptomatic, but dyspnea and dry cough may occur. Pathologic examination of tissues reveals interstitial and intra-alveolar accumulation of eosinophils, macrophages, and edema. The syndrome may be idiopathic or caused by parasitic infections (e.g., *Ascaris* species, *Strongyloides* species, hookworms) or drugs (e.g., nitrofurantoin, minocycline, sulfonamides, penicillin, nonsteroidal anti-inflammatory drugs). Treatment requires removal of the offending agent or treatment of the parasitic infection. In idiopathic cases, corticosteroids may be used.

Allergic bronchopulmonary aspergillosis is a hypersensitivity reaction that occurs when *Aspergillus* species colonizes the airways in patients with asthma or cystic fibrosis. Patients may have fever; malaise; a cough productive of thick, brown mucous plugs; and occasionally hemoptysis. On the chest radiograph, pulmonary infiltrates, which are often transient and migratory, and central bronchiectasis may be seen. Peripheral eosinophilia of greater than 10%, elevated immunoglobulin E (IgE) levels (and *Aspergillus*-specific IgE), and precipitating antibodies to *Aspergillus* are among the laboratory abnormalities seen in allergic bronchopulmonary aspergillosis. Response to corticosteroids is good. Itraconazole can be added to the treatment regimen.

Pulmonary Alveolar Proteinosis

Definition and Epidemiology

Pulmonary alveolar proteinosis (PAP) is a rare disorder in which surfactant accumulates within the alveoli. PAP occurs more frequently in middle-aged patients and in smokers.

Pathology

PAP results from impaired surfactant clearance by alveolar macrophages. PAP has a congenital form, characterized most commonly by mutations of the genes encoding surfactant proteins or for the receptor for granulocyte-macrophage colony-stimulating factor (GM-CSF). Secondary PAP occurs in conditions in which there is a functional impairment or decrease in the number of alveolar macrophages, as seen in various hematologic malignancies (e.g., leukemia), infections (e.g., pneumocystis pneumonia), and inhalation of toxic dusts (e.g., silica, aluminum) or after allogeneic bone marrow transplantation. The acquired or idiopathic form of PAP is an autoimmune disease, with neutralizing antibodies directly targeting GM-CSF, resulting in abnormal surfactant metabolism by alveolar macrophages. Lung biopsy in PAP shows intra-alveolar accumulation of eosinophilic, acellular material staining positive with the periodic acid–Schiff (PAS) stain, which is consistent with surfactant.

Clinical Presentation

Patients with PAP may be asymptomatic, or they may have progressive dyspnea on exertion, malaise, low-grade fever, and cough. Examination may reveal clubbing. The chest radiograph typically shows bilateral perihilar opacities. The CT scan may show thickening of the intralobular and interlobular septa, creating a pattern called *crazy paving*, which is a nonspecific finding because it is seen in many other diseases of the lung. The course of PAP may be complicated by opportunistic lung infection.

Diagnosis

BAL fluid can establish the diagnosis because it has a milky, opaque appearance. The fluid contains large, foamy alveolar macrophages and extracellular surfactant material that stains positive with PAS. Surgical or transbronchial lung biopsy may also be performed to establish the diagnosis if the BAL is nondiagnostic.

Treatment

Asymptomatic patients and those with mild symptoms require no immediate treatment. Sequential whole lung lavage with warmed saline (level 3 evidence) is indicated for patients with hypoxemia or severe dyspnea, and in up to 40% of patients, it may be required only one time. Limited lobar lavage may be performed in milder disease (level 3). GM-CSF administration in patients with acquired PAP may be beneficial (level 2). Rituximab has been used in refractory PAP (level 2).

Prognosis

The prognosis of autoimmune PAP is good, with excellent survival since the introduction of whole lung lavage.

🔴 PROSPECTUS FOR THE FUTURE

IPF, the most common of the IIPs, is usually fatal, and current treatment strategies are ineffective. The National Institutes of Health have established the Idiopathic Pulmonary Fibrosis Clinical Research Network to accelerate clinical research trials. These trials have demonstrated the ineffectiveness or even hazard of proposed or commonly used therapies, such as the triple-therapy regimen of prednisone, azathioprine, and N-acetylcysteine. A deeper understanding of the pathogenesis of IPF is needed to implement more effective therapies.

The advent of technology able to evaluate genetic abnormalities related to disease has unveiled mutations associated with IPF, sarcoidosis, and other ILDs, with the prospect for further insights into disease pathogenesis. The use of mTOR inhibitors in lymphangioleiomyomatosis, which affects women of childbearing age, is an example of the successful translation of the molecular pathobiology of a specific interstitial lung disease into effective therapy.

Further work linking basic science and clinical therapeutics is needed in other ILDs. Until new and effective treatment strategies are generated, lung transplantation represents the only hope for an increasing number of patients with fibrosing ILDs, and efforts to better allocate donors and decrease complications from lung transplantation remain priorities.

SUGGESTED READINGS

Allen TC: Pulmonary Langerhans cell histiocytosis and other pulmonary histiocytic diseases: a review, Arch Pathol Lab Med 132:1171–1181, 2008.

American Thoracic Society, European Respiratory Society: American Thoracic Society/European Respiratory Society international multidisciplinary consensus classification of the idiopathic interstitial pneumonias, Am J Respir Crit Care Med 165:277–304, 2002.

Borle R, Danel C, Debray MP, et al: Pulmonary alveolar proteinosis, Eur Respir Rev 20:98–107, 2011.

Culver DA: Sarcoidosis, Immunol Allergy Clin North Am 32:487–511, 2012.

Drakopanagiotakis F, Paschalaki K, Abu-Hijleh M, et al: Cryptogenic and secondary organizing pneumonia: clinical presentation, radiographic findings, treatment response, and prognosis, Chest 139:893–900, 2011.

Frankel SK, Cosgrove GP, Fischer A, et al: Update in the diagnosis and management of pulmonary vasculitis, Chest 129:452–465, 2006.

Judson MA: The treatment of pulmonary sarcoidosis, Respir Med 106:1351–1361, 2012.

Krymakaya VP: Smooth muscle-like cells in pulmonary lymphangioleiomyomatosis, Proc Am Thorac Soc 5:119–126, 2008.

Lara AR, Schwarz MI: Diffuse alveolar hemorrhage, Chest 137:1164–1171, 2010.

Noble PW, Albera C, Bradford WZ, et al: Pirfenidone in patients with idiopathic pulmonary fibrosis (CAPACITY): two randomized trials, Lancet 377:1760–1769, 2011.

Raghu G, Anstrom KJ, King TE Jr, et al: Idiopathic Pulmonary Fibrosis Clinical Research Network: Prednisone, azathioprine, and N-acetylcysteine for pulmonary fibrosis, N Engl J Med 366:1968–1977, 2012.

Raghu G, Collard HR, Egan JJ, et al: An official ATS/ERS/JRS/ALAT statement: idiopathic pulmonary fibrosis: evidence-based guidelines for diagnosis and management, Am J Respir Crit Care Med 183:788–824, 2011.

Rose DM, Hrncir DE: Primary eosinophilic lung diseases, Allergy Asthma Proc 34:19–25, 2013.

Selman M, Pardo A, King TE: Hypersensitivity pneumonitis: insights in diagnosis and pathobiology, Am J Respir Crit Care Med 186:314–324, 2012.

Suri HS, Yi ES, Nowakowski GS, et al: Pulmonary Langerhans cell histiocytosis, Orphanet J Rare Dis 7:16, 2012.

Tazelaar HD, Wright JL, Churg A: Desquamative interstitial pneumonia, Histopathology 58:509–516, 2011.

Trapnell BC, Whitsett JA, Nakata K: Pulmonary alveolar proteinosis, N Engl J Med 349:2527–2539, 2003.

Travis WD, Costabel U, Hansell DM, et al: An official American Thoracic Society/European Respiratory Society statement: update of the international multidisciplinary classification of the idiopathic interstitial pneumonias, Am J Respir Crit Care Med 188:733–748, 2013.

Travis WD, Hunninghake G, King TE, et al: Idiopathic nonspecific interstitial pneumonia: report of an American Thoracic Society project, Am J Respir Crit Care Med 177:1338–1347, 2008.

von Bartheld MB, Dekkers OM, Szlubowski A, et al: Endosonography vs conventional bronchoscopy for the diagnosis of sarcoidosis: the GRANULOMA randomized clinical trial, JAMA 309:2457–2464, 2013.

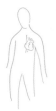

18

Pulmonary Vascular Diseases

Sharon Rounds and Matthew D. Jankowich

INTRODUCTION

Pulmonary vascular diseases are a heterogenous group of disorders with multiple causes that directly affect the pulmonary vessels, as in idiopathic pulmonary arterial hypertension (PAH), or are caused by other disorders, as in pulmonary hypertension associated with lung disease and hypoxemia. This chapter considers diseases of the pulmonary circulation characterized by vascular remodeling and pulmonary hypertension, followed by pulmonary thromboembolism.

The World Health Organization (WHO) classification of pulmonary hypertensive disorders is presented in Table 18-1. The hallmark of these disorders is pulmonary hypertension, defined by a mean pulmonary artery pressure greater than 25 mm Hg at rest. Factors that increase pulmonary arterial pressure include increases in cardiac output, left atrial pressure, or blood viscosity, and most importantly, loss of cross-sectional area of the vascular bed, which increases vascular resistance. Loss of cross-sectional area may result from mechanical occlusion, loss of vessels, vascular remodeling, or vasoconstriction.

Clinical manifestations of pulmonary hypertension may not be exhibited until late in the course of the disease because the normal pulmonary vasculature is a high-flow, low-resistance, highly compliant system with very high capacitance. The normal pulmonary circulation can accept the entire output of the right ventricle with only slight increases in pressure.

§ *For a deeper discussion on this topic, please see Chapter 68, "Pulmonary Hypertension," in* Goldman-Cecil Medicine, *25th Edition.*

IDIOPATHIC PULMONARY ARTERIAL HYPERTENSION

Definition and Epidemiology

Idiopathic PAH is an uncommon disorder that is progressive and usually fatal without treatment. The median survival time after diagnosis of the disease is about 3 years without treatment (level 1 evidence). Variables associated with poor survival include heart failure, Raynaud's phenomenon, elevated right atrial pressure, significantly elevated mean pulmonary arterial pressure, and decreased cardiac index.

The peak incidence of idiopathic PAH occurs between the ages of 20 and 45 years, and it affects women more frequently than men. The cause of idiopathic PAH is unknown. However, some cases occur in families, called *heritable pulmonary arterial*

hypertension. Heritable PAH is caused by mutations in the genes for bone morphogenetic protein receptor type 2 (*BMPR2*) and related receptors in the transforming growth factor-β family. PAH may also be associated with other disorders, such as human immunodeficiency virus (HIV) infection, scleroderma, hepatic cirrhosis, and anorectic drug use (see Table 18-1).

Pathology

The histologic characteristics of PAH include changes in the arterial and venous systems. The arteries are more commonly affected, with changes in the intima, media, and adventitia. There is medial vascular smooth muscle hypertrophy, adventitial thickening, and in situ thromboses of small pulmonary arteries. Plexogenic pulmonary arteriopathy is the classic pathologic finding in PAH, consisting of medial hypertrophy, intimal proliferation and fibroelastosis, and necrotizing arteritis. The plexiform lesion is an abnormal proliferation of pulmonary endothelial cells with slit-like channels seen only in PAH (E-Fig. 18-1).

Clinical Presentation

The clinical presentation of idopathic PAH can be subtle. The usual symptoms are dyspnea on exertion or chest pains that are not typical of angina pectoris. In more severe cases, patients may have syncope on exertion caused by the inability of the restricted pulmonary circulation to accommodate increased cardiac output with exercise. The WHO has classified the severity of symptoms in PAH (i.e., dyspnea, fatigue, chest pain, and syncope) in terms of functional ability: class I (symptoms with strenuous activity only), class II (symptoms with normal activity), class III (symptoms with activities of daily living), and class IV (symptoms with any physical activity; right heart failure, dyspnea, or fatigue may occur at rest).

Chest radiographs may reveal prominent pulmonary arteries or right ventricular enlargement (E-Fig. 18-2). Pulmonary function test results are usually normal, with the exception of diffusing capacity, which is usually decreased, reflecting the restricted circulation and decreased surface area available for gas exchange.

Diagnosis and Differential Diagnosis

The diagnosis of PAH depends on exclusion of other underlying heart or lung diseases that might cause pulmonary hypertension (see Table 18-1). In cases of PAH (group 1), the echocardiogram may reveal enlarged right atrial and right ventricular cavity size and encroachment of the interventricular septum on the left ventricle (E-Fig. 18-3). The echocardiogram also may be used to

TABLE 18-1 WORLD HEALTH ORGANIZATION CLASSIFICATION OF PULMONARY HYPERTENSION

Group 1: pulmonary arterial hypertension (PAH)
- Idiopathic PAH
- Heritable PAH
  - Bone morphogenic protein receptor type II
  - ALK-1, endoglin , SMAD9, caveolin-1, KCNK3
  - Unknown
- Drug- and Toxin-Induced
- Associated with PAH:
  - Connective tissue disease
  - Human immunodeficiency virus infection
  - Portal hypertension
  - Congenital heart diseases
  - Schistosomiasis

Pulmonary veno-occlusive disease and/or pulmonary capillary hemangiomatosis

Persistent pulmonary hypertension of the newborn

Group 2: pulmonary hypertension due to left heart disease
- Left ventricular systolic dysfunction
- Left ventricular diastolic dysfunction
- Valvular disease
- Congenital/acquired left heart inflow/outflow tract obstruction and congenital cardiomyopathies

Group 3: pulmonary hypertension due to lung diseases and/or hypoxia
- Chronic obstructive pulmonary disease
- Interstitial lung disease
- Other pulmonary diseases with mixed restrictive and obstructive pattern
- Sleep-disordered breathing
- Alveolar hypoventilation disorders
- Chronic exposure to high altitude
- Developmental lung diseases

Group 4: chronic thromboembolic pulmonary hypertension

Group 5: pulmonary hypertension with unclear multifactorial mechanisms
- Hematologic disorders: chronic hemolytic anemia, myeloproliferative disorders, splenectomy
- Systemic disorders: sarcoidosis, pulmonary histiocytosis, lymphangioleiomyomatosis
- Metabolic disorders: glycogen storage disease, Gaucher disease, thyroid disorders
- Others: tumoral obstruction, fibrosing mediastinitis, chronic renal failure, segmental PH

Modified from Simonneau G, Gatzoulis MA, Adatia L, et al: Updated clinical classification of pulmonary hypertension, J Am Coll Cardiol 62:D34–41, 2013.

estimate the level of pulmonary artery systolic pressure. Echocardiography also is useful for excluding group 2 pulmonary hypertension caused by heart diseases that increase pulmonary venous pressures (e.g., mitral valve stenosis).

Pulmonary function tests, lung imaging, and tests for conditions causing hypoxemia (e.g., obstructive sleep apnea) are important for excluding group 3 pulmonary hypertension. Acute pulmonary thromboembolism rarely causes pulmonary hypertension, but recurrent pulmonary emboli or nonresorbed clots that obstruct proximal pulmonary arteries can cause group 4 pulmonary hypertension. The diagnosis of group 4 disease requires a ventilation-perfusion $(\dot{V}/\dot{Q})$ scan, computed tomography (CT) angiography, or pulmonary arteriography.

Definitive diagnosis of PAH requires right heart catheterization and documentation of increased pulmonary arterial pressures and resistance with normal left-sided filling pressures as assessed by pulmonary capillary wedge pressure. Left-to-right intracardiac shunts can also cause pulmonary hypertension due to increased blood flow through the lungs. This can be diagnosed

at the time of right heart catheterization by measuring the difference in oxygen content between blood from the superior vena cava and the main pulmonary artery. At the time of right heart catheterization, short-acting vasodilators are usually administered, and hemodynamic responses are recorded. These vasodilator trials are useful in predicting whether patients are likely to respond to calcium-channel blockers (a minority of patients).

Treatment

Modern treatment of PAH includes drugs with vasodilator activity such as calcium-channel blockers, prostacyclin, endothelin receptor antagonists, and phosphodiesterase inhibitors that increase vascular cyclic guanosine monophosphate (cGMP) levels. Continuous intravenous prostacyclin is the only therapy that has been shown to prolong survival and is the recommended treatment for patients with WHO class IV symptoms (level 1 evidence). However, because of the cost and technical challenges of intravenous prostacyclin, oral endothelin receptor antagonists or phosphodiesterase inhibitors, or inhaled or subcutaneous prostacyclin derivatives are preferred for patients with WHO class II or III symptoms.

Most studies of the effects of vasodilator drugs have used the 6-minute walk test as a surrogate for hemodynamic improvement and have demonstrated benefits for exercise tolerance and symptoms (level 1 evidence). Combination therapy may improve symptoms when one agent is not sufficient (level 2-1). In addition to relaxing vascular smooth muscle constriction, vasodilator drugs may stabilize or reverse vascular remodeling in PAH (level 3).

Other interventions include supplemental oxygen, anticoagulation (level 2-1 evidence), and judicious use of diuretic medications. Pulmonary rehabilitation also can improve exercise tolerance (level 1). Heart-lung, double-lung, or single-lung transplantations have been performed in these patients with some success, but the overall 5-year survival rate for PAH patients undergoing lung transplantation is only 50%.

● SECONDARY PULMONARY HYPERTENSION

Pulmonary hypertension is associated with many disorders that increase pulmonary venous pressure (e.g., mitral valve stenosis, group 2 pulmonary hypertension) and diseases of the lungs associated with hypoxemia (e.g., sleep apnea, chronic obstructive pulmonary disease, group 3 pulmonary hypertension). These conditions have been called *secondary pulmonary hypertension.*

Vasoconstriction and vascular remodeling contribute to increased pulmonary vascular resistance in secondary pulmonary hypertension. For example, alveolar hypoxia causes intense pulmonary vasoconstriction. Long-standing hypoxia causes vascular remodeling that is similar to plexogenic pulmonary arteriopathy but does not include in situ thromboses or formation of plexiform lesions (E-Fig. 18-4).

Treatment of secondary pulmonary hypertension is directed at the underlying heart or lung disease. If the patient has hypoxia, home oxygen therapy should be used. It is not known whether vasodilator therapy is useful in group 2 or 3 diseases. Group 4 pulmonary hypertension caused by proximal, unresolved clot can be improved by pulmonary thromboembolectomy (level 1 evidence).

COR PULMONALE

The most frequent cause of death of patients with PAH is right ventricular failure, also called *cor pulmonale*. Prolonged increased afterload causes the right ventricle to hypertrophy and then dilate. The interventricular septum shifts to the left, and filling of the left ventricle is decreased, with subsequent decreased cardiac output. Dilation of the right atrium causes atrial tachyarrhythmias and further decreased cardiac output.

Treatment of cor pulmonale is directed at the underlying cause of pulmonary hypertension. The existence of cor pulmonale is a bad prognostic sign in group 1 pulmonary hypertension (level 1 evidence).

PULMONARY THROMBOEMBOLISM

Definition and Epidemiology

Pulmonary thromboembolism refers to the passage of a clot from the venous system or the right ventricle that lodges in a pulmonary artery. Other materials, such as tumor or injected foreign bodies (e.g., talc) can also lodge in the lung circulation, but pulmonary thromboembolism is a complication of venous thrombosis.

Pulmonary thromboembolic disease is a relatively common entity, with an incidence ranging from 400,000 to 650,000 cases per year in the United States. The deep veins of the femoral and popliteal systems of the lower extremities are most often involved, but right atrial, right ventricular, and upper extremity thromboses can also embolize to the lung. The predisposing factors for pulmonary embolism are the same as those for venous thrombosis and include venous stasis, hypercoagulability, and endothelial injury. Congenital or acquired procoagulant disorders (e.g., activated protein C deficiency, factor V Leiden) are also considered predisposing factors.

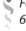 *For a deeper discussion on this topic, please see Chapter 68, "Pulmonary Hypertension," in* Goldman-Cecil Medicine, *25th Edition.*

Pathology

After a clot dislodges from the lower extremity circulation, it travels to the pulmonary circulation, where it can obstruct a branch of the pulmonary artery. The affected lung segment develops an increased $\dot{V}/\dot{Q}$ ratio. This increases overall dead space ventilation, which can lead to inefficient excretion of carbon dioxide, potentially raising the partial pressure of carbon dioxide in arterial blood ($Paco_2$). Blood flow is shifted from the obstructed site to other areas, which may include areas with a low $\dot{V}/\dot{Q}$ ratio, leading to shunting and hypoxemia.

Infarction of the lung distal to the occlusion is rare because of the redundancy of the pulmonary circulation and because of oxygenation of lung parenchyma by bronchial arteries and by alveolar oxygen. However, pulmonary thromboembolism causes deficiency or inactivation of surfactant and commonly causes collapse of alveolar units perfused by the obstructed vessel.

Clinical Presentation

The most common symptom of pulmonary thromboembolism is shortness of breath (level 1 evidence). Other, less common symptoms include chest pain, hemoptysis, and syncope. A careful history is paramount when evaluating patients for thromboembolic disease to determine risk factors, such as recent immobilization or surgery, malignancy, or a history of pulmonary embolus or deep vein thrombosis. Using a validated clinical scoring system to assess the pretest probability of pulmonary embolism, such as calculation of the Wells or Geneva score, is helpful in the integration of subsequent laboratory and radiologic testing results.

The most common physical examination findings are tachycardia and tachypnea (level 1 evidence). The physical examination may be normal or may reveal isolated crackles or even diffuse wheezing. Pleural effusions are identified by areas of dullness to percussion. Edema of the extremities, especially if the edema is asymmetrical, may point to venous thrombosis. In deep vein thrombosis, dorsiflexion of the foot may cause calf pain as a result of stretching the calf muscles and deep veins (Homan's sign). Signs of pulmonary hypertension and right ventricular strain, such as increased pulmonary component of the second heart sound or right ventricular heave, are not usually appreciated unless there is a massive pulmonary embolus or preexisting heart or lung disease.

Arterial blood gas determinations usually reveal respiratory alkalosis with a normal Pao_2 value (level 1 evidence). However, when the alveolar-arterial oxygen gradient is calculated, it is frequently widened. However, a normal alveolar-arterial gradient in the partial pressure of oxygen does not exclude acute pulmonary embolism. A normal $Paco_2$ in a patient with tachypnea suggests increased dead space and, in the appropriate setting, may point to the diagnosis. In severe cases, arterial blood gas measurement may show acidemia, hypoxemia, and hypercapnia.

An elevated level of lactate dehydrogenase (LDH) may be the result of tissue infarction, but this test is insensitive and nonspecific. An elevated level of B-type natriuretic peptide (BNP) is useful in assessing the severity and likelihood of complicating right ventricular failure. If the highly sensitive D-dimer level is normal, it effectively excludes pulmonary thromboembolism if the pretest probability is intermediate or low. However, the D-dimer level may be elevated in patients with unrelated medical conditions, such as congestive heart failure, chronic illness, and connective tissue disorders.

The electrocardiogram may show atrial tachyarrhythmias or evidence of right heart strain as shown by a new right bundle branch block, right ventricular strain pattern, and the $S_I\,Q_{III}\,T_{III}$ pattern (i.e., S wave in lead I, Q wave in lead III, T wave inversion in lead III) that mimics inferior myocardial infarction. The chest radiograph is often normal but may show atelectasis, isolated infiltrates, or a small pleural effusion. Oligemia (Westermark's sign), an abrupt cutoff of pulmonary vessels or enlarged central pulmonary arteries (Fleischner's sign), and a pleural-based area of increased opacity (Hampton's hump) may be seen on the radiograph. In most cases, chest radiographs are not sufficiently sensitive to diagnose a pulmonary embolism.

Three major diagnostic methods are used for the diagnosis of pulmonary embolism: the $\dot{V}/\dot{Q}$ scan, chest CT, and pulmonary arteriography (Fig. 18-1). CT angiography provides a noninvasive and sensitive way to detect pulmonary emboli (E-Fig. 18-5). The Prospective Investigation of Pulmonary Embolism Diagnosis II (PIOPED II) study demonstrated that the best approach is a combination of clinical suspicion, D-dimer determination, CT angiography, and assessment of the lower extremities for deep vein thrombosis DVT by CT or ultrasound. The Christopher study showed that the frequency of a subsequent venous thromboembolism diagnosis in the 3 months after a negative CT angiogram is low (level 1 evidence).

However, for pregnant women or individuals with renal insufficiency or iodinated contrast dye allergy, the $\dot{V}/\dot{Q}$ scan provides an alternative approach. The $\dot{V}/\dot{Q}$ scan compares lung ventilation by radiolabeled tracer gas with lung perfusion by radiolabeled micro-occlusive particles. The usefulness of the $\dot{V}/\dot{Q}$ scan depends greatly on the pretest probability of the disease, which depends on the expertise of the clinician and his or her level of certainty. A *high-probability* $\dot{V}/\dot{Q}$ scan is characterized by lobar or multilobar perfusion defects that coincide with areas of normal or relatively normal ventilation, and it is more than 90% accurate in diagnosing pulmonary embolism. A *normal* $\dot{V}/\dot{Q}$ scan shows no perfusion or ventilation defects and excludes pulmonary embolism in essentially all cases. However, the test is less reliable when interpreted as *low, intermediate,* or *indeterminate* probability. In these circumstances, pulmonary embolism is likely in 4% to 66% of patients, and further testing is necessary for an accurate diagnosis of pulmonary embolism.

Pulmonary arteriography may be considered in patients without contraindications to the procedure when other tests are inconclusive and a high likelihood of pulmonary embolism exists. Although the rate of complications of pulmonary angiography is low with experienced operators, the complications can be significant, ranging from pulmonary hypertension and sudden death to idiosyncratic hypersensitivity reactions to the dye. Pulmonary angiography is now performed infrequently, and operator experience may be limited in certain care settings.

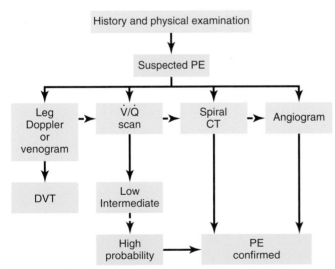

FIGURE 18-1 Tests commonly used in the evaluation of patients who may have pulmonary embolism (PE). Doppler ultrasound or venogram of the leg is useful to evaluate deep vein thrombosis (DVT). Ventilation-perfusion ($\dot{V}/\dot{Q}$) scans are most useful when they are normal or show lesions that suggest an intravascular clot. Unfortunately, these findings are lacking for many patients, who require further investigation. Spiral computed tomography (CT) has high sensitivity and specificity and allows for evaluation of thoracic structures and the vasculature. Angiography is considered the gold standard, but it often is not needed if other noninvasive tests are used alone or in combination.

Treatment

Pulmonary embolism is treated with supportive measures directed at sustaining organ function, such as fluid replacement for hypotension and mechanical ventilation for respiratory failure. Mechanical dislodgement of a pulmonary artery clot, such as by surgical thromboembolectomy, a procedure with a high mortality rate, requires a high level of expertise. Thromboembolectomy is used only for long-standing proximal clots that are complicated by chronic pulmonary hypertension (e.g., group 4 pulmonary hypertension, chronic thromboembolism syndrome) (level 1 evidence).

For acute pulmonary embolism, medical treatments are preferred, and they are used to prevent further clotting or to dissolve an existing clot. Anticoagulation with regular (intravenous) or low-molecular-weight (subcutaneous) heparin (LMWH) is recommended in the acute setting for patients without major contraindications to anticoagulation (e.g., upper gastrointestinal bleeding, hemorrhagic stroke) (level 1 evidence).

For patients with a contraindication to anticoagulation, an inferior vena cava filter should be placed. These filters have been shown to reduce pulmonary embolism occurrence in the setting of proximal deep vein thrombosis in patients also receiving anticoagulation (level 1 evidence). However, the devices carry a long-term risk of increased rates of deep vein thrombosis (level 1), and they do not clearly affect mortality if anticoagulation is also used. The use of thrombolytic medications (e.g., tissue plasminogen activator) is usually reserved for patients at increased risk for death as a result of circulatory collapse caused by obstruction to the flow in large or multiple pulmonary vessels (level 2-2).

Oral anticoagulation therapy with vitamin K antagonists such as warfarin is initiated, overlapping initially with acute heparin or LMWH treatment, and it is continued for at least 3 months to allow resolution of venous clot and to prevent recurrence (level 1 evidence). However, for venous thromboembolism occurring in the setting of active malignancy, LMWH treatment is superior to warfarin in preventing recurrent events (level 1).

Novel oral anticoagulants (i.e., factor Xa inhibitors) have been shown to be noninferior to the combination of heparin and warfarin therapy and to require less testing for safety (level 1 evidence). Patients who have had an unprovoked pulmonary embolism (i.e., pulmonary embolism not associated with a known temporary risk factor such as surgery) have a high rate of recurrence. For these patients, whether therapy should be routinely extended beyond 3 months is unclear, as is the optimal method of anticoagulation, and decisions regarding extended anticoagulation in this setting may be based on clinical factors such as bleeding risk or risk stratification with D-dimer testing.

● PROSPECTUS FOR THE FUTURE

Translational research has markedly enhanced understanding of the pathogenesis of pulmonary hypertensive disorders, and this has resulted in the development of therapies that increase quality of life and improve mortality. There is heightened appreciation of the role of increased vascular cell proliferation in pulmonary vascular remodeling. In particular, abnormal proliferation of pulmonary endothelial cells and development of plexiform lesions have suggested that PAH may be a disease of hyperproliferative pulmonary endothelium.

Little is understood about the adaptive changes of the right ventricle to chronically increased afterload. Future investigations are needed to understand and better treat cor pulmonale. Less information is available about pulmonary thromboembolic disease, although new inhibitors of the coagulation cascade have been developed. Studies are needed in the area of genetic predisposition to thromboembolic disease and vascular dysfunction leading to thrombus formation. The role of thrombolytic therapy outside the setting of shock and the best management strategy after an unprovoked pulmonary embolism need to be clarified.

SUGGESTED READINGS

Barst RJ, Gibbs JS, Ghofrani HA, et al: Updated evidence-based treatment algorithm in pulmonary arterial hypertension, J Am Coll Cardiol 54(Suppl):S78–S84, 2009.

Lansberg MG, O'Donnell MJ, Khatri P, et al: Antithrombotic and thrombolytic therapy for ischemic stroke: antithrombotic therapy and prevention of thrombosis, 9th ed: American College of Chest Physicians Evidence-Based Clinical Practice Guidelines, Chest 141(Suppl):7S–47S, 2012.

Newman JH, Phillips JA III, Loyd JE: Narrative review: the enigma of pulmonary arterial hypertension: new insights from genetic studies, Ann Intern Med 148:278–283, 2008.

Prestion IR: Properly diagnosing pulmonary arterial hypertension, Am J Cardiol 111:2C–9C, 2013.

Stacher E, Graham BB, Hunt JM, et al: Modern age pathology of pulmonary arterial hypertension, Am J Respir Crit Care Med 186:261–272, 2012.

Stein PD, Woodard PK, Weg JG, et al: Diagnostic pathways in acute pulmonary embolism: recommendation of the PIOPED II investigators, Am J Med 119:1048–1055, 2006.

Tapson VF: Acute pulmonary embolism, N Engl J Med 358:1037–1052, 2008.

Wells PS, Anderson DR, Rodger M, et al: Excluding pulmonary embolism at the bedside without diagnostic imaging: management of patients with suspected pulmonary embolism presenting to the emergency department by using a simple clinical model and d-dimer, Ann Intern Med 135:98–107, 2001.

19

Disorders of Respiratory Control

Sharon Rounds and Matthew D. Jankowich

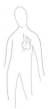

INTRODUCTION

During the transition between wakefulness and sleep, input from the behavioral control system decreases, the hypoxic drive to breathe is reduced, and the ventilatory response to partial pressure of carbon dioxide in arterial blood ($Paco_2$) is diminished. These changes are most dramatic during rapid eye movement (REM) sleep. *Sleep-disordered breathing* refers to a diverse group of conditions in which these physiologic variations are heightened, resulting in abnormal respiratory function and fragmented sleep.

Of the sleep-related disorders, sleep apnea has received the most attention. *Apnea* is the complete cessation of airflow for 10 seconds or longer. *Hypopnea* is a significant decrease in airflow. Occasional episodes of apnea and hypopnea are expected during normal sleep, and their frequency increases with age. However, in patients with sleep apnea, the frequency and duration of the episodes are increased, leading to sleep fragmentation and to hypoxemia and hypercapnia. Upper airway obstruction (i.e., obstructive sleep apnea [OSA]) or decreased central respiratory drive (i.e., central sleep apnea) may be the cause of sleep apnea. Some patients have both disorders.

Some studies suggest that the prevalence of sleep-disordered breathing may be as high as 9% among women and 24% among men, but prevalence levels depend on the definition used. Sleep-disordered breathing is usually defined as a respiratory disturbance index or frequency of abnormal respiratory events that number at least five episodes per hour of sleep. Prevalence estimates are higher for the older adult population, with some studies finding a more than 80% prevalence among older patients. Children are also affected, although less frequently (about 2%).

For a deeper discussion on this topic, please see Chapter 100, "Obstructive Sleep Apnea," in Goldman-Cecil Medicine, 25th Edition.

OBSTRUCTIVE SLEEP APNEA
Definition and Epidemiology

OSA is the most common of the sleep apnea syndromes. It is thought to affect almost 6% of middle-aged and older men; it is less common among women. In these patients, the upper airway relaxation that occurs during sleep produces complete occlusion of the airway and, consequently, cessation of airflow. After various periods of airway occlusion, the patient arouses, reestablishes muscle tone, and opens the airway. This vicious cycle is repeated many times during the night, resulting in recurring episodes of hypoxemia. During airway occlusion, sympathetic tone is increased, resulting in vasoconstriction and hypertension, which persists during the waking hours. OSA is the most common identifiable cause of systemic hypertension (level 1 evidence). With airway occlusion, intrathoracic pressure becomes more negative with inspiration. Episodes of hypoxemia can be associated with cardiac arrhythmias, cardiovascular events, and all-cause mortality (level 1). These events are thought to be linked mechanistically to the increased incidence of stroke and coronary artery disease in patients with OSA.

An important physiologic consequence of airway occlusion is arousal from sleep, resulting in fragmented sleep. Because apneas are more frequent during REM sleep, patients complain of lack of refreshing sleep. Patients with OSA have an increased incidence of motor vehicle crashes, presumably related to somnolence while driving. These patients have an increased incidence of diabetes mellitus and other manifestations of the metabolic syndrome. The cardiovascular complications of OSA appear to be at least partially reversible with treatment of OSA with continuous positive airway pressure (CPAP) (level 2-3 evidence).

Clinical Presentation

The diagnosis of OSA is suggested when patients complain of morning headaches, recurrent awakenings, and daytime somnolence that affects daytime activities, including driving. Complaints of snoring and gasping episodes may be elicited from sleeping partners. Difficulties in maintaining sleep as a result of frequent awakenings may lead to mood effects and decreased quality of life. Recent weight gain, use of sedatives and sleeping pills, or alcohol intake may heighten these symptoms.

The primary risk factors for OSA are obesity (variable) and abnormal upper airway anatomy caused by macroglossia, a long soft palate and uvula, enlarged tonsils, or micrognathia. Patients may have an increased neck diameter (>17 inches in men; >16 inches in women). A narrow oropharynx as a result of a small pharyngeal opening or redundant soft tissue is often observed. Patients may be hypertensive and, in extreme cases, may have right-sided heart failure, which results from prolonged episodes of hypoxemia and pulmonary vasoconstriction that lead to pulmonary hypertension.

Diagnosis and Differential Diagnosis

Chest radiographic images and pulmonary function testing are usually not helpful in the evaluation of patients with sleep apnea. In some cases, OSA is associated with the obesity-hypoventilation syndrome, which is characterized by significant obesity associated with chronic hypoventilation and hypercapnia (i.e., Pickwickian syndrome). In these cases, arterial blood gas determinations show hypoxemia and hypercapnia, and blood cell counts may indicate polycythemia. Although rare, hypothyroidism, acromegaly, and amyloidosis can cause or enhance OSA, and these conditions should be considered.

The diagnosis of OSA requires overnight polysomnography, during which continuous recordings of electrocardiographic and electroencephalographic tracings are made while the patient sleeps. Airflow, oxygen saturation, and respiratory, eye, chin, and limb muscle movements are monitored and recorded. OSA is diagnosed in sleeping patients (confirmed by electroencephalographic tracings) who develop cessations or reductions of airflow despite repeated muscular efforts to breathe (E-Fig. 19-1). These episodes may be accompanied by transient hypoxemia and cardiac arrhythmias. A score (i.e., apnea-hypopnea index) is derived from these data that defines OSA.

Polysomnography can distinguish OSA from central sleep apnea, during which cessation of airflow is associated with halted respiratory movements. Polysomnography is also important to rule out other sleep disturbances caused by insomnia, narcolepsy, parasomnias, and periodic limb movement syndrome. For patients strongly suspected of having OSA, home sleep studies that measure airflow, oxygen saturation, and chest and abdominal muscle movements (with or without an electroencephalogram) are frequently effective in making the diagnosis of OSA (level 1 evidence). However, if the diagnosis is unclear or there is concern about narcolepsy or some other sleep disorder, formal polysomnography in the laboratory is needed.

Treatment

Treatment of sleep apnea includes behavioral and medical approaches. When associated with obesity, significant weight loss (through lifestyle modification or bariatric surgery) results in a reduction in the apnea-hypopnea index (level 1 evidence). Avoidance of sedatives and alcohol are also encouraged (level 3).

Airway obstruction can be prevented with the use of CPAP provided through a tightly fitted mask (level 1 evidence). CPAP maintains positive airway pressure throughout expiration, thereby preventing collapse of the upper airway. The amount of airway pressure can be titrated, and oxygen can be added if necessary. Many patients are begun on autotitrating CPAP; the machine senses apneas and increases CPAP automatically to eliminate them. Autotitrating CPAP is not inferior to a fixed CPAP prescription, based on in laboratory polysomnography (level 1). CPAP is effective in most patients, but compliance with this technique varies.

Surgical removal of obstructing tonsils, adenoids, and polyps or uvulopalatopharyngoplasty may be useful in patients with specific anatomic abnormalities. However, in children with OSA, adenotonsillectomy was not superior to watchful waiting in improving neuropsychological function (level 1 evidence). Mandibular advancement may improve symptoms of OSA in patients who do not tolerate CPAP (level 3). A permanent tracheostomy may be necessary in severe cases after other approaches have failed. However, the surgical approach to this disorder is limited to selected patients only after CPAP has failed. The obesity-hypoventilation syndrome is treated effectively with noninvasive ventilation with bilevel positive airway pressure (level 2-1).

OTHER DISORDERS RELATED TO RESPIRATORY CONTROL

Congenital central hypoventilation syndrome is a rare disorder that usually is diagnosed in infancy. It is caused by mutation in the *PHOX2B* gene (level 1 evidence).

Central sleep apnea is also a rare disorder. It predominates in men and is usually associated with normal body habitus. Patients may complain of daytime sleepiness and insomnia with frequent awakenings. The disorder is caused by apnea or hypopnea resulting from a decreased central respiratory drive. It may be a consequence of central nervous system injury (e.g., structural abnormality of the brain stem), or it may be idiopathic. Affected individuals may hypoventilate even while awake, although they are capable of normal voluntary breaths. During sleep, frequent apnea is common.

In patients with obstructive lung disease, increased work of breathing eventually makes it difficult to maintain sufficient ventilation to maintain normal $Paco_2$ levels. When ventilatory capacity declines, hypoventilation causes $Paco_2$ to increase; the kidneys respond by retaining bicarbonate to keep arterial blood pH at normal levels. These patients appear to have normal ventilatory drive, but they lack the ability to increase minute ventilation to meet increased metabolic demands. This characteristic is observed in certain patients with chronic bronchitis who exhibit the classic signs of the "blue bloater."

Lower brain stem and upper pontine lesions may cause *central hyperventilation*. However, this disorder rarely occurs in the absence of other physiologic or chemical abnormalities. Hepatic cirrhosis and extreme anxiety are causes of central hyperventilation. Pregnancy can also cause hyperventilation due to elevated levels of progesterone and other hormones. *Apneustic breathing* consists of sustained inspiratory pauses, resulting from damage to the midpons, most commonly caused by basilar artery infarction. *Biot respiration* or *ataxic breathing* is a haphazardly random pattern of sleep and is characterized by shallow breaths. A disruption of the respiratory rhythm generator in the medulla causes this sign.

The regular cycling of crescendo-decrescendo tidal volumes, separated by apneic or hypopneic pauses, characterizes Cheyne-Stokes respiration. Patients with this disorder usually have generalized central nervous system disease or congestive heart failure. Heart failure prolongs circulatory times, causing a delay between changes in blood gases at the tissue level and the arrival of those changes at the brain stem chemoreceptors. This delay sets up a cycle of gradual increase to hyperventilation, followed by gradually decreasing ventilation to apnea and then a repetition of the cycle. Studies suggest that OSA and Cheyne-Stokes respiration are consequences of congestive heart failure and contribute to its progression.

> For a deeper discussion on this topic, please see Chapter 86, "Disorders of Ventilatory Control," in Goldman-Cecil Medicine, 25th Edition.

PROSPECTUS FOR THE FUTURE

With more than 5% of the population in the United States suffering from sleep-disordered breathing and with the recognition that these disorders may contribute to systemic illnesses such as hypertension and cardiovascular disorders, interest in the early diagnosis and treatment of disorders of respiratory control is growing. In view of the high incidence and potential health consequences of sleep-disordered breathing, physicians must be on the lookout for this condition. The increased incidence of OSA parallels that of obesity in the United States, a public health problem that has been associated with asthma and increased risk of death. It is highly likely that genetic predisposition to OSA accounts for increased incidence in some families.

SUGGESTED READINGS

Arzt M, Bradley TD: Treatment of sleep apnea in heart failure, Am J Respir Crit Care Med 173:1300–1308, 2006.

Carrillo A, Ferrer M, Gonsalez-Diaz G, et al: Noninvasive ventilation in acute hypercapnic respiratory failure caused by obesity hypoventilation syndrome and chronic obstructive pulmonary disease, Am J Respir Crit Care Med 186:1279–1285, 2012.

Marcus CL, Moore RH, Rosen CL, et al: A randomized trial of adenotonsillectomy for childhood sleep apnea, N Engl J Med 368:2366–2376, 2013.

Qaseem A, Holty JE, Owens DK, et al: Management of obstructive sleep apnea in adults: a clinical practice guideline from the American College of Physicians, Ann Intern Med 159:471–483, 2013.

Rosen CL, Auckley D, Benca R, et al: A multisite randomized trial of portable sleep studies and positive airway pressure autotitration versus laboratory-based polysomnography for the diagnosis and treatment of obstructive sleep apnea: the HomePAP study, Sleep 35:757–767, 2012.

Somers VK, White DP, Amin R, et al: Sleep apnea and cardiovascular disease, J Am Coll Cardiol 52:686–717, 2008.

Yeboah J, Redline S, Johnson C, et al: Association between sleep apnea, snoring, incident cardiovascular events and all-cause mortality in an adult population: MESA, Atherosclerosis 219:963–968, 2011.

Young T, Skatrud J, Peppard PE: Risk factors for obstructive sleep apnea in adults, JAMA 291:2013–2016, 2004.

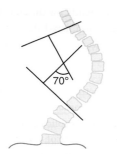
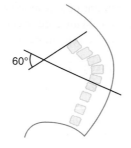

A Posteroanterior   B Lateral

FIGURE 20-2 Schematic depiction of the lines constructed to measure the Cobb angle of scoliosis (**A**) and kyphosis (**B**).

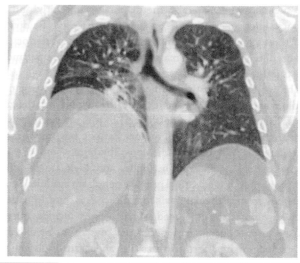

FIGURE 20-3 Computed tomography of a patient with unilateral right hemidiaphragm paralysis and associated right lower lobe atelectasis.

For a given degree of spinal deformity, individuals with kyphoscoliosis due to a neuromuscular disease have more respiratory impairment than those with idiopathic kyphoscoliosis. Factors that contribute to respiratory failure in patients with kyphoscoliosis include inspiratory muscle weakness, underlying neuromuscular disease, sleep-disordered breathing, and airway compression due to distortion of lung parenchyma and twisting of airways.

Treatment consists of general supportive measures such as immunizations against influenza and pneumococci, smoking cessation, maintenance of a normal body weight, supplemental oxygen, and treatment of respiratory infections. It is important to recognize nocturnal hypoventilation because it can be treated with noninvasive positive-pressure ventilation. This is typically delivered through a nasal or full face mask. Indications for instituting noninvasive ventilation include symptoms suggesting nocturnal hypoventilation, signs of cor pulmonale, nocturnal oxyhemoglobin desaturation, or an elevated daytime $Paco_2$.

Obesity

Obesity is a major health problem that affects children and adults throughout the world. Body fat usually constitutes 15% to 20% of body mass in healthy men and 25% to 30% of body mass in healthy women. In cases of obesity, the body fat content may increase by as much as 500% in women and 800% in men. The degree of obesity can be assessed by the body mass index, which is the ratio of body weight (BW) in kilograms to the square of the height (Ht) in meters (BW/Ht^2). Individuals with a BMI between 18.5 and 24.9 kg/m^2 are normal, and those with a BMI greater than 40 kg/m^2 are considered severely or morbidly obese.

Reductions in functional residual capacity and expiratory reserve volume are the most common pulmonary function abnormalities in obesity, whereas vital capacity and total lung capacity may be only minimally reduced. Obesity promotes breathing at low lung volumes, which reduces lung compliance and increases the work of breathing. A subgroup of individuals with obesity hypoventilate and become hypercapnic. When obesity is associated with hypoventilation, it is called the *obesity-hypoventilation syndrome* (i.e., pickwickian syndrome). The mechanism underlying hypoventilation is unknown. Obesity-hypoventilation syndrome may result from factors that reduce respiratory center chemosensitivity, such as hypoxia, sleep apnea, or adipokines such as leptin. The most important consequences of chronic hypoventilation are hypoxemia and pulmonary hypertension.

Nocturnal noninvasive positive-pressure ventilation can help to reverse these abnormalities. Weight loss is the optimal therapy, but it is not always attainable, and long-term weight loss maintenance is even more difficult. Pharmacotherapy or bariatric surgery should be considered for obese individuals who do not achieve weight control with conventional methods (i.e., diet, enhanced physical activity, and behavioral therapy).

Diaphragm Paralysis

The diaphragm separates the thorax from the abdomen and is the major muscle of inspiration. Diaphragm weakness or paralysis can involve one or both hemidiaphragms. Unilateral diaphragm paralysis is more common than bilateral diaphragm paralysis. The most frequent causes of unilateral paralysis include traumatic phrenic nerve injury, herpes zoster infection, cervical spinal disease, and compressive tumors. Patients may be asymptomatic, or the abnormality may be discovered as an incidental finding of an elevated hemidiaphragm on a chest radiograph (Fig 20-3). The diagnosis is confirmed by seeing on fluoroscopy a paradoxical upward motion of the affected diaphragm during a vigorous sniff maneuver. There is no specific treatment for this disorder, but recovery after the initial injury occasionally occurs. When the patient has disabling symptoms and significant elevation of the diaphragm is seen on the chest radiograph, surgical plication of the diaphragm may provide some relief of symptoms.

Bilateral diaphragm paralysis is most often seen in the setting of a disease producing generalized muscle weakness or motor neuron disease such as amyotrophic lateral sclerosis. Pulmonary function test results are associated with severe restrictive impairments. When the patient assumes the supine position, there may be a further reduction ($\leq 50\%$) in vital capacity. It is not surprising that orthopnea is an especially prominent symptom, and patients often have difficulty sleeping in the supine position. Patients also complain of dyspnea when bending or lifting objects.

Bilateral diaphragm paralysis can be difficult to diagnose. Restriction evidenced by pulmonary function test results is non-specific, as is the finding of low lung volumes on chest radiographs. Fluoroscopic sniff testing (i.e., diaphragm fluoroscopy) can yield false-negative and false-positive results. Measurement of transdiaphragmatic pressure is the gold standard, but it is somewhat invasive, requiring placement of catheters in the esophagus and stomach. Alternatively, B-mode ultrasound of the diaphragm in the zone of apposition is a noninvasive means of diagnosing diaphragm paralysis.

Treatment should address the underlying disease, which may or may not be reversible. If paralysis is idiopathic or caused by neuralgic amyotrophy (i.e., brachial plexus neuritis), more than 50% of individuals may recover. Phrenic nerve pacing may be used in patients with spinal cord injuries above C3, and noninvasive positive-pressure ventilation can be used to treat patients with nocturnal hypoventilation. Diaphragm plication is not indicated in patients with bilateral diaphragm paralysis.

⬤ PROSPECTUS FOR THE FUTURE

Numerous advances can be expected in treating individuals with pleural, mediastinal, and chest wall diseases. Progress in pleural fluid analysis using novel biomarkers and nucleic acid amplification tests may lead to more rapid and accurate diagnosis of tuberculous pleural effusions. Assays of pleural fluid tumor markers and chromosome analysis are promising developments for the differentiation of malignant from nonmalignant effusions. Mesothelioma remains resistant to traditional therapeutic approaches, but evolving technology centered on gene therapy may produce a new treatment modality.

Better visualization of mediastinal structures can be achieved as magnetic resonance imaging (MRI) evolves and becomes more routinely applied to examination of the chest. Molecular tracers targeting tumor receptors or proteins may be used with MRI and positron emission tomography imaging techniques to better differentiate malignant from benign mediastinal masses.

Noninvasive nocturnal ventilation remains a cornerstone of therapy for patents with chest wall and neuromuscular diseases, but compliance can be problematic. Continued evolution of techniques to deliver nocturnal noninvasive ventilation may improve compliance with treatment, and application of this technique to patients with obesity-hypoventilation syndrome may reduce morbidity and mortality for them.

Patients with diaphragm paralysis due to high cervical spinal cord lesions may benefit from advances in intramuscular diaphragm pacing. This technique may provide an alternative means of treating respiratory failure in these individuals and others with diaphragm paralysis.

〝 *For a deeper discussion on this topic, please see Chapter 99, "Diseases of the Diaphragm, Chest Wall, Pleura, and Mediastinum," in* Goldman-Cecil Medicine, *25th Edition.*

SUGGESTED READINGS

Brixey AG, Light RW: Pleural effusions occurring with right heart failure, Curr Opin Pulm Med 17:226–231, 2011.

Colice GE, Curtis A, Deslauriers J, et al: Medical and surgical treatment of parapneumonic effusions: an evidence-based guideline, Chest 18:1158–1171, 2000.

Duwe BV, Sterman DH, Musani AI: Tumors of the mediastinum, Chest 128:2893–2909, 2005.

Gottesman E, McCool FD: Ultrasound evaluation of the paralyzed diaphragm, Am J Respir Crit Care Med 155:1570–1574, 1997.

Heffner JE, Klein JS: Recent advances in the diagnosis and management of malignant pleural effusions, Mayo Clin Proc 83:235–250, 2008.

Light RW: The undiagnosed pleural effusion, Clin Chest Med 27:309–319, 2006.

McCool FD, Tzelepis GE: Current clinical aspects of diaphragm dysfunction, N Engl J Med 366:932–942, 2012.

Rahman NM, Maskell NA, West A, et al: Intrapleural use of tissue plasminogen activator and DNase in pleural infection, N Engl J Med 365:518–526, 2011.

Stafanidis K, Dimopolous S, Nanas S: Basic principles and current applications of lung ultrasonography in the intensive care unit, Respirology 16:249–256, 2011.

Summerhill EM, Abu el-Sameed Y, Glidden TJ, et al: Monitoring recovery from diaphragm paralysis with ultrasound, Chest 133:737–743, 2008.

Tzelepis GE, McCool FD: Non-muscular diseases of the chest wall. In Fishman AP, editor: Fishman's pulmonary diseases and disorders, New York, 2007, McGraw-Hill, 2007, pp 1617–1635.

Yusen RD: Medical and surgical treatment of parapneumonic effusions: an evidence-based guideline, Chest 118:1158–1171, 2000.

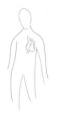

21

Infectious Diseases of the Lung

Narendran Selvakumar, Brian Casserly, and Sharon Rounds

PNEUMONIA

Definition and Epidemiology

Pneumonia is an infection of the lower respiratory tract parenchyma by bacteria, viruses, fungi, or parasites. It should be distinguished from pneumonitis, which is inflammation of the lungs caused by noninfectious causes, including chemicals, blood, radiation, and autoimmune processes. Pneumonia, the leading cause of death of children worldwide and the eighth leading cause of death in the United States, is responsible for 4 to 10 million respiratory infections each year.

Pathology

Microbial agents can be introduced to the lungs through several sources, including normal flora from the sinuses, nasopharynx, or oropharynx and inhalation of dust, liquid, or gases from environmental sources. The most common route is by aspiration of oropharyngeal secretions. Direct inhalation of organisms such as *Legionella* species, mycobacteria, endemic fungi, *Mycoplasma pneumoniae*, *Chlamydophila pneumoniae*, and most viruses can cause pneumonia, resulting in geographic and seasonal clustering of cases.

Much less commonly, pneumonia can arise from hematogenous or embolic spread of infection from infected heart valves or venous clots. The small vessels of the pulmonary circulation act as filters for venous blood carrying small clusters of bacteria from the source. Hematogenous pneumonias are often multifocal with peripheral lesions susceptible to rapid cavitation.

Clinical Presentation

Patients usually exhibit respiratory symptoms, including productive cough, dyspnea, chest pain, and occasionally hemoptysis. Less specific symptoms include fever, general malaise, myalgias, and weight loss. The presentation may be acute (days to weeks), as observed in bacterial pneumonia, or subacute or chronic (weeks to years), as observed with tuberculosis (TB). Immunocompromised patients (e.g., with human immunodeficiency virus [HIV] infection) may be predisposed to specific illnesses, and knowledge of the specific impairment in host defense mechanisms may help to determine the cause of the infection.

The chest radiograph plays an important role. A parenchymal opacity is observed in the patient with pneumonia (E-Fig. 21-1) However, noninfectious disorders can mimic pneumonia, and no radiographic finding is specific for infection.

The initial antibiotic choice may be guided by Gram stain of respiratory secretions. This requires the demonstration of a satisfactory sputum sample (i.e., >25 polymorphonuclear leukocytes and <10 epithelial cells per low-power field) and the presence of a predominant organism (>8 to 10 organisms per high-power field), particularly if the same bacteria are found in white blood cells. However, despite extensive laboratory testing, a causative organism can be identified in only about 50% of all pneumonia cases. Reasons include poor Gram-staining bacteria such as *Legionella pneumophila*, *C. pneumoniae*, absence of a peptidoglycan wall in *M. pneumoniae*, and various difficult-to-culture organisms that give inconclusive results. Table 21-1 lists the most common causative agents of pulmonary infections.

Clinical guidelines have been developed to provide a systematic approach to the diagnosis and management of pneumonia. The initial evaluation should determine whether the pneumonia is community acquired or health care associated.

Differential Diagnosis, Treatment, and Prognosis

Community-Acquired Pneumonia

Community-acquired pneumonia occurs twice as frequently during winter, and those at the extremes of age (<5 years and >65 years) are at increased risk. *Streptococcus pneumoniae* is the most common causative agent. *S. pneumoniae* is a gram-positive, diplococcal bacterium whose encapsulated structure and immunoglobulin A (IgA) protease protects it from host defense.

PATHOGEN	COMMUNITY ACQUIRED INFECTIONS	NOSOCOMIAL INFECTIONS
TABLE 21-1 ORGANISMS CAUSING PULMONARY INFECTIONS		
Bacteria	70-80%	90%
Streptococcus pneumoniae	60-75%	3-9%
Haemophilus influenzae	4-5%	—
Legionella spp.	2-5%	Up to 25%
Staphylococcus aureus	1-5%	10-20%
Gram-negative bacilli	Rare	50
Atypical bacteria	10-20%	Rare
Mycoplasma pneumoniae	5-18%	—
Chlamydia psittaci	2-3%	—
Coxiella burnetii	1%	—
Viruses	10-20%	Rare
Influenza virus	—	8%
Hantavirus	—	Rare

Modified from Modai J: Empiric therapy of severe infections in adults, Am J Med 88:12S–17S, 1990.

Patients may have an antecedent upper respiratory tract infection followed by the sudden onset of fever, shaking chills, dyspnea, and pleurisy. Cough productive of purulent, rust-colored sputum is common. Imaging studies show lobar consolidation. Sputum is gram positive in only 45% of bacteremic cases. The diagnosis is confirmed by culture of the organism from a normally sterile site, such as blood, pleural fluid, or cerebrospinal fluid. In many cases, the diagnosis is presumptive, and recommended antibiotic coverage for community-acquired pneumonia is designed to cover this organism (discussed later).

M. pneumoniae is a slow-growing, facultative anaerobic organism that accounts for 25% to 60% of all atypical pneumonias. *M. pneumoniae* is a common cause of pneumonia in patients between the ages of 5 and 35 years who may initially exhibit upper respiratory tract symptoms, pharyngitis, and bullous myringitis. The clinical presentation includes dry cough and gastrointestinal symptoms in addition to fever, headache, and myalgias. Uncommon complications include cold agglutinin–induced hemolysis, hepatitis, erythema multiforme, hyponatremia caused by the syndrome of inappropriate antidiuretic hormone, pericarditis, myocarditis, and neurologic abnormalities. The chest radiograph may show fine interstitial reticulonodular infiltrates in patients. The diagnosis is based on clinical and epidemiologic features. Acute and convalescent serologic findings are required to confirm the diagnosis, but they are not helpful during the acute illness.

Other common causes of community-acquired pneumonia are *C. pneumoniae* and *Haemophilus influenzae*. Patients with comorbid conditions and those older than 65 years are also at risk for pneumonia from *Legionella* species, *Staphylococcus aureus*, and gram-negative organisms. Anaerobic infection should be considered when large amounts of oropharyngeal secretions are aspirated and in patients with chronic gingivitis.

Viral causes may encompass up to 65% of cases of community-acquired pneumonia in infants and preschool-age children (<5 years). The most common causes include rhinovirus, parainfluenza virus, adenovirus, enterovirus, coronavirus, human metapneumovirus (hMPV), and respiratory syncytial virus (RSV), the most commonly identified pathogen. HMPV is a recent addition to the long list of viral causes that mostly affect the upper and lower respiratory tracts in young children and older adults. It is common in late winter and early spring, when RSV is common, and co-infection with RSV causes severe bronchiolitis in children younger than 2 years of age.

In September 2012, a novel betacoronavirus was isolated from a man in Saudi Arabia. This Middle East respiratory syndrome coronavirus (MERS-CoV) causes severe acute pneumonia, acute respiratory distress syndrome (ARDS), and acute kidney injury. It has since been identified in Europe and other parts of the Middle East. Patients also may have gastrointestinal symptoms, pericarditis, and disseminated intravascular coagulation (DIC). Diagnosis is made by polymerase chain reaction (PCR) assay, and its infectivity is based on antagonizing endogenous interferon (IFN) production in cells. Treatment is supportive with mechanical ventilation or extracorporeal membrane oxygenation (ECMO), but exogenous interferon alfa-2b administration has reduced viral replication in vitro. MERS-CoV has a high mortality rate of 48%, with a median time of survival from clinical presentation of 14 days.

Diagnostic tests for community-acquired pneumonia include a chest radiograph and complete blood count. The role of routine sputum and blood cultures in this setting is controversial. Studies have advocated the use of C-reactive protein and procalcitonin as markers of the inflammatory response to bacterial infection. However, further studies are needed.

The recommended treatment for community-acquired pneumonia is a 7- to 10-day course of a macrolide antibiotic (i.e., erythromycin, clarithromycin, or azithromycin). Azithromycin has been linked to increased risk of cardiovascular death, especially in patients with a high baseline risk of cardiovascular disease. If there are comorbidities such as chronic heart or lung disease, an extended-spectrum fluoroquinolone (i.e., levofloxacin, moxifloxacin, or gemifloxacin) or a β-lactam (e.g., amoxicillin) plus a macrolide should be used. The choice of treatment should be influenced by local antibiotic resistance patterns.

An important decision in the care of community-acquired pneumonia is whether the patient requires hospital admission. This decision should take into consideration the known risk factors of increased mortality from pneumonia, including age 65 years or older; the presence of comorbidities such as diabetes mellitus, renal, or congestive heart failure; altered mental status; tachycardia (>125 beats per minute); tachypnea (>30 breaths per minute); high fever (>38.3° to 40°C); hypotension (systolic blood pressure <90 mm Hg); hypoxia (SaO_2 <90% or PaO_2 <60 mm Hg); multilobar involvement seen on the chest radiograph; and identification of high-risk pathogens such as gram-negative organisms and *S. aureus*.

For hospitalized patients, initial therapy for community-acquired pneumonia usually includes a cephalosporin such as ceftriaxone or cefuroxime with or without a macrolide. Antibiotic treatment should be given as soon as possible because the likelihood of death can increase even after a short delay (>8 hours) in receiving appropriate antibiotics. Sputum and blood cultures should be obtained before instituting antibiotic therapy.

For a deeper discussion on this topic, please see Chapter 289, "Streptococcus Pneumoniae Infections," and Chapter 317, "Mycoplasma Infection," in Goldman-Cecil Medicine, 25th Edition.

Nosocomial Pneumonia

Nosocomial pneumonia is categorized as hospital-acquired pneumonia (HAP), ventilator-associated pneumonia (VAP), and health care–associated pneumonia (HCAP). HAP is pneumonia that occurs 48 hours or more after admission. VAP is a type of HAP that develops more than 48 to 72 hours after endotracheal intubation. HCAP is pneumonia that occurs in a nonhospitalized patient with extensive health care contact. This includes recent hospitalization, residence in a nursing home or other long-term care facility, and recent intravenous therapy. These patients should be considered at high risk for resistant organisms and therefore inappropriate for routine, empirical therapy for community-acquired pneumonia.

Nosocomial pneumonia is the second most common infection among hospitalized patients and the most common infection in the intensive care unit. The pathogenesis of nosocomial pneumonia is based on colonization of the oropharynx and stomach with virulent pathogens and the subsequent aspiration of these organisms into the lower respiratory tract. Gastric colonization by gram-negative organisms is enhanced by neutralization of gastric acidity. In the first 5 days of hospitalization, *H. influenzae*, *S. pneumoniae*, and *S. aureus* are often isolated. After this time, *Pseudomonas aeruginosa*, *S. aureus*, anaerobic microbes, *Acinetobacter* species, and various gram-negative enteric bacilli often are the cause of pneumonia. This finding has important therapeutic implications because these organisms are more commonly associated with multidrug antibiotic resistance.

Treatment depends on combined chemotherapy with β-lactam antipseudomonal penicillin or cephalosporin, together with an aminoglycoside or a quinolone. Vancomycin is added if methicillin-resistant *S. aureus* is suspected. A more definitive identification of organisms and their sensitivity to antibiotics is often sought for these patients using more invasive measures, including endotracheal aspirate in intubated patients or flexible fiberoptic bronchoscopy. However, the best predictor of patient outcome with nosocomial pneumonia appears to be adequacy of the initial empirical antibiotic regimen.

For a deeper discussion on this topic, please see Chapter 282, "Prevention and Control of Health Care–Associated Infections," in Goldman-Cecil Medicine, *25th Edition.*

COMPLICATIONS OF PNEUMONIA

Parapneumonic effusion is a neutrophilic exudative effusion adjacent to a lung with pneumonia (E-Fig. 21-2). It has exudative, fibrinopurulent, and organized stages. Depending on the stage, the effusion can resolve with antibiotics alone or may require drainage in addition to antibiotics. As pneumonia progresses, inflammatory edema leaks into the pleural space, first appearing as an uncomplicated effusion (i.e., exudative stage). At this point, the effusion can resolve with antibiotic therapy alone. During the fibrinopurulent and organized stages, the inflammatory process is marked by anaerobic metabolism, cytokine production, fibrin deposition in the pleural space, and thickening of the pleura.

There is no universally accepted definition of *empyema*, but most clinicians include all pleural effusions that are grossly purulent or contain microorganisms identified by a positive Gram stain or culture. Empyema must always be treated with pleural drainage, usually by a chest thoracostomy tube. Highly inflammatory parapneumonic effusions may behave as if they are infected, although microorganisms are never identified. Effusions described as "complicated" parapneumonic effusions are identified clinically by a pH of less than 7.1, a high serum lactate dehydrogenase (LDH) level, and a glucose level of less than 40 mg/dL. Complicated effusions usually require drainage in addition to antibiotic therapy.

The major risk factor for the development of lung abscess is aspiration resulting in a more indolent, polymicrobial infection, usually involving both aerobes and anaerobes. Conditions predisposing patients to aspiration, such as alcoholism, seizures, or stroke, are associated with an increased incidence of lung abscess. Poor dentition increases the anaerobic bacterial load in the mouth and the likelihood of infection after an aspiration event. In trials of empirical therapy for lung abscess, clindamycin showed superiority over penicillin, probably because the

incidence of penicillin-resistant anaerobes in lung abscesses is 15% to 20%. Antibiotics should be continued for 6 weeks, and drainage should be reserved for very large abscesses or failure to resolve with antibiotics.

MYCOBACTERIUM TUBERCULOSIS INFECTION

Infection with *M. tuberculosis*, an aerobic, nonmotile, acid-fast rod with niacin production, causes TB. In 2011, the World Health Organization (WHO) Global Surveillance and Monitoring Project estimated 8.7 million new cases of TB per year, 13% of whom are co-infected with HIV. Twelve million cases of the disease existed predominately in Asia and Africa. An estimated 1.4 million individuals die of TB each year, and the global case-fatality rate was 23%, with a rate of 50% in some African countries with high HIV rates. In the United States, TB increased at an alarming rate in the early 1990s as a result of the surge of HIV infection, drug abuse, inner-city poverty, and homelessness.

TB infection occurs when aerosolized, contaminated droplets (expectorated by a diseased person) are inhaled by another individual and droplet nuclei reach an alveolus. This is almost always a latent infection, called *latent tuberculosis infection* (LTBI). If the innate immune system of the host fails to eliminate the latent infection, the bacilli proliferate inside alveolar macrophages and kill the cells.

The infected macrophages produce cytokines and chemokines that attract other phagocytic cells, including monocytes, other alveolar macrophages, and neutrophils, which eventually form a nodular granulomatous structure called the *tubercle*. If the bacterial replication is not controlled, the tubercle enlarges, and the bacilli enter the local draining lymph nodes. This leads to lymphadenopathy, a characteristic manifestation of primary TB. The lesion produced by the expansion of the tubercle into the lung parenchyma and lymph node involvement is called the *Ghon complex*.

The bacilli continue to proliferate until an effective cell-mediated immune response develops, usually 2 to 6 weeks after infection. Failure by the host to mount an effective cell-mediated immune response and tissue repair leads to progressive lung injury. Bacterial products, tumor necrosis factor-α, reactive oxygen intermediates, reactive nitrogen intermediates, and the contents of cytotoxic cells (e.g., granzymes, perforin) can contribute to the development of caseating necrosis that characterizes a tuberculous granuloma (E-Fig. 21-3).

If mycobacterial growth is unchecked, the bacilli may spread hematogenously to produce disseminated TB. Miliary TB is a disseminated form with lesions resembling millet seeds. Bacilli can also spread mechanically by erosion of the caseating lesions into the lung airways. It is at this point that the host becomes infectious to others.

Untreated disseminated TB has a mortality rate of 80%, with the remainder developing chronic disease or recovering spontaneously. The chronic disease is characterized by repeated episodes of spontaneous healing with fibrotic changes around the lesions and tissue breakdown. Healing by complete spontaneous eradication of the bacilli is rare.

Reactivation TB results when the persistent bacteria in a host suddenly proliferate. Only 5% to 10% of patients with no underlying medical problems who become infected develop reactivation disease in their lifetimes. Although immunosuppression is clearly associated with reactivation TB, it is not clear what host factors specifically maintain the infection in a latent state for many years and what triggers the latent infection to become overt.

The diagnosis of latent TB infection depends on a positive tuberculin test result, which indicates previous infection but not necessarily active disease. The standard Mantoux test is an intradermal injection of 0.1 mL (5 tuberculin units) of purified protein derivative (PPD) tuberculin in the skin of the forearm. The injection site is evaluated 48 to 72 hours later. The reading is based on the diameter of the indurated or swollen area.

Patients are at high risk for active TB early after tuberculin conversion, and treatment is recommended for LTBI. QuantiFERON-TB Gold (QFT-G) has been approved by the U.S. Food and Drug Administration (FDA) for the diagnosis of LTBI and TB. It uses the enzyme-linked immunosorbent assay (ELISA) for two proteins in *M. tuberculosis* (i.e., ESAT6 and CFP10). Because these proteins are absent from all bacillus Calmette-Guérin (BCG) vaccine strains, this test does not produce false-positive results in people with previous BCG vaccinations. Other advantages to QFT-G are that the results are available within 24 hours without the need for a second visit and without reading biases or errors. However, QFT-G sensitivity for LTBI may be less than the tuberculin skin test (TST). It is also limited in differentiating infection associated with TB disease or LTBI, similar to the TST. Differentiation is based on suggestive symptoms, radiographs, and sputum samples. Negative QFT-G results cannot exclude the absence of infection in patients with TB signs and symptoms, patients who are HIV positive, or those who are severely immunosuppressed.

The risk for active disease is 5% within 2 years of exposure and another 5% per year thereafter. HIV-infected patients are an exception and have a 40% risk for active disease within several months of conversion. The current recommendations about what constitutes a positive PPD test result take into account the degree of clinical suspicion for LTBI (Table 21-2). Typical treatment of LTBI is 5 mg/kg/day to a maximum dose of 300 mg/day of isoniazid for 9 months (Adult).

Treatment of patients suspected of having active disease includes at least four drugs: 5 mg/kg/day of isoniazid, 10 mg/kg/day of rifampin; 15 to 20 mg/kg/day ethambutol; and 15 to 30 mg/kg/day of pyrazinamide. Treatment should be considered before a formal diagnosis is made. Factors suggesting active disease include exposure to active TB, pulmonary symptoms, and cavitary disease seen on imaging studies. If the diagnosis of TB is confirmed, the drugs are continued for 2 months, barring adverse reactions to drug therapy. After 2 months, the regimen can be tailored, depending on drug-sensitivity studies, and continued for another 4 months with at least two active drugs. Rates of drug-resistant TB are increased in certain populations (e.g., recent immigrants from high-prevalence TB areas, homeless people).

Resistance is detected in 9% of patients who have not received previous therapy and in 22.8% of those with prior treatment. In patients with drug-resistant TB, treatment should include at least three drugs that have not been administered before and to which the organism is susceptible in vitro. Treatment should continue

TABLE 21-2 PROPHYLAXIS AGAINST TUBERCULOSIS IN ADULTS

PPD TEST RESULT*	PROPHYLAXIS INDICATED REGARDLESS OF AGE	OTHER INDICATIONS FOR PROPHYLAXIS
≥5 mm	Close contacts recently diagnosed with TB HIV positive or HIV risk factors Fibrotic changes on chest radiograph Patients with organ transplants	No risk factors
≥10 mm	Diabetes mellitus Immunosuppression Hematologic malignancy Injection drug use Renal failure Malnutrition	PPD increased >10 mm within 2 yr Native of high-prevalence country High-risk ethnic minorities Residents and staff of long-term care facilities
≥15 mm	PPD increased >15 mm within 2 yr	No risk factors

HIV, Human immunodeficiency virus; PPD, purified protein derivative of tuberculin; TB, tuberculosis.
*After 48 to 72 hours, evaluation of the injection site is based on the diameter of the indurated or swollen area.

for at least 18 to 24 months. Direct observation of therapy is recommended to ensure compliance.

For a deeper discussion on this topic, please see Chapter 324, "Tuberculosis," in Goldman-Cecil Medicine, *25th Edition.*

PNEUMOCYSTIS PNEUMONIA

Pneumocystis jiroveci pneumonia (PCP), formerly called *Pneumocystis carinii* pneumonia, is an opportunistic fungus that occurs mainly in malnourished, premature infants and in adults with hematologic malignancy undergoing chemotherapy in the era before acquired immunodeficiency syndrome (AIDS). However, its incidence rose significantly in the late 1980s and 1990s in patients with AIDS with low CD4$^+$ lymphocyte counts (<250 cells/mm^3).

Patients may complain of nonproductive cough, fever, dyspnea, and weight loss. The symptoms are slowly progressive over weeks in patients infected with HIV. Oral candidiasis, an increased serum LDH level, an increased A-a oxygen gradient, and a decreased CD4$^+$ count are independent predictors of HIV-related PCP.

The chest radiograph may show diffuse, bilateral interstitial infiltrates, but the chest radiograph may be clear for up to 15% of patients (E-Fig. 21-4). High-resolution computed tomography (HRCT) is more sensitive, with a diagnostic accuracy of 94% for PCP. Other findings include isolated infiltrates, cavitary lesions, nodular masses, pneumothorax, and a miliary pattern. Hilar and mediastinal adenopathy are rare. Identifying the organism in sputum, which is effective in 60% to 85% of patients, helps with diagnosis. Bronchoscopy with bronchoalveolar lavage can increase the yield (86%), especially if a transbronchial biopsy is included (98% to 100%).

Prophylaxis can be provided by oral sulfamethoxazole-trimethoprim or aerosolized pentamidine. For pneumonia, the therapy of choice is sulfamethoxazole-trimethoprim. However, significant adverse effects, including leukopenia, nausea, vomiting, and elevation of liver transaminase levels, are associated with this therapy. Intravenous pentamidine is a reasonable alternative to sulfamethoxazole-trimethoprim, but this therapy may be complicated by hypoglycemia. Less toxic drug regimens are available (e.g., trimethoprim and dapsone, clindamycin and primaquine), but they are recommended only after failure of other medications. Corticosteroids should be considered in patients with severe disease as demonstrated by significant hypoxemia (e.g., PaO_2 <70 mm Hg). Corticosteroids decrease the likelihood of progression to respiratory failure.

> For a deeper discussion on this topic, please see Chapter 341, "Pneumocystis Pneumonia," in Goldman-Cecil Medicine, 25th Edition.

PROSPECTUS FOR THE FUTURE

Lung infections cause high morbidity and mortality rates in the community and in health care settings. A significant portion of these infections affects the extremes of age—young children and older adults. The judicious use of antimicrobial agents helps to prevent emergence of drug resistance. Continued efforts are needed to reinforce vaccination against infectious agents, including influenza and S. pneumoniae.

Co-infection with HIV and TB are significant problems in Africa, where effective HIV therapy is less available. This was highlighted by the identification of extensively drug-resistant TB (XDR-TB), which is caused by a strain of M. tuberculosis that is resistant to many available antimycobacterial agents and is difficult to cure. The potential adverse effects of vaccinations are another area of concern.

New and devastating epidemic infections continue to be recognized. Examples include MERS-CoV and severe acute respiratory syndrome (SARS), a rapidly progressive respiratory illness identified in the Guangdong province of China, Hong Kong, Vietnam, Singapore, and Canada.

There have been four influenza pandemics during the past century, each caused by a novel influenza virus and recently caused by viruses containing components of previous human and avian influenza viruses. Estimates of potential global mortality related to pandemic avian influenza are as high as 62 million deaths, and there is no specific treatment available. In 2009, the H1N1 ("swine") influenza virus emerged in Mexico. It has spread worldwide and has been designated a pandemic by the WHO. At least initially, H1N1 had a relatively low mortality rate, but it may mutate to produce more severe disease in humans. The most recent outbreak of avian influenza A H7N9 in 2013 was limited to China, and most infected patients reported contact with poultry with no evidence of sustained human-to-human transmission.

PCR assay of 16S rRNA genes may provide species-specific signature sequences useful for bacteria identification. The dysbiosis hypothesis states that alterations to microbial communities in terms of structure and stability may result in human disease. Pertinent to the lung, which was previously thought to be sterile, 16S rRNA gene sequencing provides a glimpse into the normal respiratory microbiome. Based on changes in these normal microbial communities, the cause, identification, and management of various diseases may be inferred.

SUGGESTED READINGS

American Thoracic Society, Infectious Diseases Society of America: Guidelines for the management of adults with hospital acquired, ventilator-associated, and healthcare-associated pneumonia, Am J Respir Crit Care Med 171:388–416, 2005.

Blumberg HM, Burman WJ, Chaisson RE, et al: American Thoracic Society/Centers for Disease Control and Prevention/Infectious Diseases Society of America: treatment of tuberculosis, Am J Respir Crit Care Med 167:603–662, 2003.

Kovacs JA, Gill VJ, Meshnick S, et al: New insights into transmission, diagnosis, and drug treatment of Pneumocystis carinii pneumonia, JAMA 286:2450–2460, 2001.

Mandell LA, Wunderink RG, Anzueto A, et al: Infectious Diseases Society of America/American Thoracic Society consensus guidelines on the management of community-acquired pneumonia in adults, Clin Infect Dis 44S:S27–S72, 2007.

Mazurek GH, Villarino ME, CDC: Guidelines for using the QuantiFERON-TB test for diagnosing latent Mycobacterium tuberculosis infection. Centers for Disease Control and Prevention, MMWR Recomm Rep 52:15–18, 2003.

Partinen M, Saarenpää-Heikkilä O, Ilveskoski I, et al: Increased incidence and clinical picture of childhood narcolepsy following the 2009 H1N1 pandemic vaccination campaign in Finland, PLoS ONE 7:e33723, 2012.

Stolz D, Stulz A, Muller B, et al: BAL neutrophils, serum procalcitonin, and C-reactive protein to predict bacterial infection in the immunocompromised host, Chest 132:504–514, 2007.

Tsolia MN, Psarras S, Bossios A, et al: Etiology of community-acquired pneumonia in hospitalized school-age children: evidence for high prevalence of viral infections, Clin Infect Dis 39:681–686, 2004.

Zaki AM, Van Boheemen S, Bestebroer TM, et al: Isolation of a novel coronavirus from a man with pneumonia in Saudi Arabia, N Engl J Med 367:1814–1820, 2012.

22

Essentials in Critical Care Medicine

Narendran Selvakumar, Brian Casserly, and Sharon Rounds

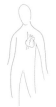

INTRODUCTION

Critical care medicine has evolved dramatically with development of new technologies, and clinical trials have established standards for the management of the critically ill. Since the poliomyelitis epidemic in the 1950s, intensive care units have proved beneficial in treating acute, reversible disorders. However, because of the innovative nature of the technology used and the need for close monitoring and intensive management, the delivery of critical care medicine is expensive, accounting for up to 30% of total hospital costs.

Patients in intensive care units (ICUs) are a heterogeneous population treated for diverse conditions ranging from septic shock and respiratory failure to diabetic ketoacidosis and upper gastrointestinal bleeding. This chapter discusses a few of the most common conditions encountered in the ICU setting. Topics include acute respiratory failure and mechanical ventilation, acute lung injury, and shock.

ACUTE RESPIRATORY FAILURE

Acute respiratory failure results when the lung can no longer accomplish adequate gas exchange, a condition that is fatal if left untreated. Hypoxemic respiratory failure refers to respiratory failure associated with failure to oxygenate (type 1), whereas hypercarbic respiratory failure is the failure to ventilate (type 2). These disorders result from alterations in the arterial partial pressures of oxygen (Pao_2) and carbon dioxide ($Paco_2$), respectively.

Type 1 respiratory failure is hypoxia without hypercarbia that may result from interstitial lung diseases (e.g., pneumonia, emphysema), parenchymal diseases due to ventilation-perfusion ($\dot{V}/\dot{Q}$) mismatch or diseases of vasculature such as pulmonary embolism. Type 2 respiratory failure is the result of inadequate ventilation from various causes, including airway diseases, decreased respiratory drive, and disorders of the chest wall. Inadequate ventilation results in hypoxia and hypercarbia.

The values of Pao_2 and $Paco_2$ that define respiratory failure are somewhat arbitrary, but respiratory compromise is usually evident when the Pao_2 is less than 60 mm Hg or the $Paco_2$ is higher than 45 mm Hg. These values are not synonymous with the need for mechanical ventilation, and they do not preclude the need for mechanical ventilation.

The management of respiratory failure depends on the clinical presentation. Patients with respiratory failure who are awake, cooperative, and hemodynamically stable may tolerate aggressive respiratory therapy without intubation and mechanical ventilation, as long as gas exchange and overall status are continually monitored. Examples include patients with chronic obstructive pulmonary disease (COPD) who can tolerate $Paco_2$ levels as high as 85 mm Hg without severe respiratory acidosis. In contrast, patients in respiratory failure with evidence of severe respiratory distress (e.g., respiratory rate >30 breaths/min), mental deterioration (e.g., impaired judgment, confusion, hallucinations, somnolence), or hemodynamic instability (e.g., bradyarrhythmias, tachyarrhythmias, hypotension) usually require intubation and mechanical ventilation. In the latter circumstances, waiting for arterial blood gas determinations is unnecessary and may dangerously delay therapy. Although arterial blood gas evaluation is crucial when determining the need for mechanical ventilation in the patient with respiratory failure, the patient's clinical status ultimately dictates the course of action.

For a deeper discussion on this topic, please see Chapter 104, "Acute Respiratory Failure," in Goldman-Cecil Medicine, 25th Edition.

MECHANICAL VENTILATION

Modern mechanical ventilation is positive-pressure ventilation. Air is forced into the central airways, increasing central airway pressure. Air follows the pressure gradient from the central airways to the alveoli, inflating the lungs. As the lungs inflate and the device stops forcing air into the central airways, the intra-alveolar pressure increases, and central airway pressure decreases. Exhalation occurs when the air follows the newly reversed pressure gradient from the alveoli to the central airways.

The principal benefits of mechanical ventilation during respiratory failure are improved gas exchange and decreased work of breathing. Mechanical ventilation improves gas exchange by improving $\dot{V}/\dot{Q}$ matching. Improved matching of the $\dot{V}/\dot{Q}$ ratio is primarily a consequence of decreased physiologic shunting. Altered lung mechanics (e.g., increased airway resistance, decreased compliance) and increased respiratory demand (e.g., metabolic acidosis) increase the work of breathing. The ventilatory muscles and diaphragm can tire while trying to maintain the elevated work of breathing, resulting in respiratory failure. Mechanical ventilation can alleviate some or all of the increased work of breathing, allowing recovery of fatigued ventilatory muscles. Deteriorating gas exchange, unresponsive to conservative measures, and respiratory distress are the most common reasons for mechanical ventilation in patients with acute respiratory failure.

Immediate complications of mechanical ventilation include barotrauma causing pneumothorax, pneumomediastinum, or subcutaneous emphysema. Atrophy of the diaphragm and impairment of mucociliary motility may also occur.

Noninvasive Mechanical Ventilation

Although intubation and mechanical ventilation are usually the preferred options in respiratory failure that is considered reversible, noninvasive positive-pressure ventilation (NPPV) is useful in selected patients. NPPV is ventilation delivered through a noninvasive interface (i.e., nasal mask, face mask, or nasal plugs), rather than through an endotracheal tube or tracheostomy. Selecting patients for NPPV requires careful consideration of its indications and contraindications. A trial of NPPV is worthwhile in patients with acute cardiogenic pulmonary edema or hypercapnic respiratory failure due to COPD who do not require emergent intubation and who do not have contraindications to NPPV.

Contraindications to NPPV include cardiac or respiratory arrest; inability to cooperate, protect the airway, or clear secretions; uncontrolled vomiting, hematemesis or hemoptysis; severely impaired consciousness; facial surgery, trauma, or deformity; anticipated prolonged duration of mechanical ventilation; and recent esophageal anastomosis. Early predictors of success include a significant correction in pH (i.e., respiratory acidosis) and a decrease in $Paco_2$ of more than 8 mm Hg.

Invasive Mechanical Ventilation

After the decision to intubate is made, an experienced operator should expeditiously perform intubation. Complications of intubation include prolonged hypoxemia due to delays in the procedure, vomiting and aspiration of gastric contents, trauma to the vocal cords, bleeding, pneumothorax, cardiac arrhythmias, and cardiac arrest. Immediately after insertion, endotracheal location should be confirmed by assessing exhaled carbon dioxide. The endotracheal tube should be secured and its position assessed by examining for breath sounds, followed by chest radiography for confirmation. Direct visualization, such as by bronchoscopy, is occasionally needed for successful intubation.

Initial ventilator settings may vary, but orders should include ventilator mode, fraction of inspired oxygen (Fio_2) of 1.0 (or 100%), respiratory rate set, and tidal volume (discussed later). The adequacy of the ventilator settings is determined with arterial blood gas measurement and clinical evaluation of the patient. After the settings are adjusted to maintain relatively normal levels of arterial blood gases (i.e., pH of 7.3 to 7.45, Pao_2 >60 mm Hg, and $Paco_2$ of 30 to 45 mm Hg), attention should be given to developing a maintenance plan to ensure adequate oxygenation and ventilation until the cause of the respiratory failure is treated and reversed. This plan should include assessment of the need for sedation, appropriate strategy of mechanical ventilation, supportive measures to achieve hemodynamic stability, nutritional assessment, and therapies targeting the initial injurious process that triggered the respiratory failure. Most patients require sedation to diminish discomfort and to decrease the work of breathing, but it should be administered carefully because sedation is often accompanied by a decrease in blood pressure.

Commonly used modes of ventilation are determined by the duration of inspiration, which can be limited by volume, pressure, flow, or time. During volume-limited ventilation, inspiration ends after delivery of a preset tidal volume. Airway pressure varies during volume-limited ventilation and is related to respiratory system compliance, airway resistance, and tubing resistance. Assist control ventilation (ACV), continuous mandatory ventilation (CMV), and synchronized intermittent mandatory ventilation (SIMV) are examples of volume-limited modes of ventilation. CMV has a set rate and set tidal volume that do not allow spontaneous breathing by the patient. Because patient-ventilator asynchrony is a serious problem, CMV is rarely used. ACV is similar to CMV in that there is a set rate and set tidal volume, but this mode allows the patient to initiate machine-delivered breaths. When the machine senses that the patient is attempting to take a breath, it delivers the selected tidal volume. SIMV is similar to ACV in that a set rate and set tidal volume are selected. The patient is also able to generate a spontaneous breath. However, this spontaneous breath may have a very small tidal volume and thereby increase work of breathing. Consequently, this mode of mechanical ventilation is seldom used except when weaning patients from mechanical ventilation.

The pressure control mode of ventilation (PCV) uses machine breaths that are pressure cycled, not volume cycled. With PCV, the pressure to be used for each breath is ordered. If the patient attempts a spontaneous breath, a machine breath at the designated pressure is delivered. This may be helpful in limiting airway pressures in patients with bronchospasm or stiff lungs because it limits the risk for pneumothorax (i.e., barotrauma). Because tidal volumes may vary, PCV must be titrated carefully at the bedside to determine the proper pressure settings. The physician should order the desired minimal tidal volume.

Pressure support ventilation (PSV) is used only for spontaneously breathing patients. The inspiratory and expiratory pressures are selected, and there are no mandatory machine-delivered breaths. Patients find this to be a more comfortable mode of mechanical ventilation. However, PSV should be used only for patients with a stable respiratory drive (i.e., not sedated heavily) and stable lung compliance. PSV is typically used for patients who are weaning from mechanical ventilator support.

Pressure-regulated volume control, airway pressure–release ventilation, and high-frequency ventilation are newer modalities. They are increasingly used in clinical practice.

Settings

Numerous settings need to be considered when mechanical ventilation is initiated. They include tidal volume, respiratory rate, trigger mode and sensitivity, fraction of inspired oxygen, positive end-expiratory pressure (PEEP), flow rate, and flow pattern.

The appropriate initial tidal volume depends on numerous factors, most notably the disease for which the patient requires mechanical ventilation. The tidal volume can then be increased or decreased incrementally to achieve the desired pH and $Paco_2$. Large tidal volumes can cause barotrauma or volutrauma, which increases the risk of ventilator-associated lung injury. The tidal volume should not be increased without considering its effects on airway pressure or the likelihood of ventilator-induced lung injury. In acute respiratory distress syndrome (ARDS), tidal volumes of about 6 mL/kg of ideal body weight are associated with improved mortality (level I evidence).

An optimal method for setting the respiratory rate has not been determined. After the tidal volume has been established, the respiratory rate can be incrementally increased or decreased to achieve the desired pH and $Paco_2$ while monitoring auto-PEEP. Patients who are breathing spontaneously set their own respiratory rates in all modes of ventilation except CMV.

The lowest possible fraction of inspired oxygen (Fio_2) necessary to meet oxygenation goals should be used. This decreases the likelihood that adverse consequences of supplemental oxygen, such as absorption atelectasis, accentuation of hypercapnia, airway injury, and parenchymal lung injury, will develop.

PEEP usually is added to prevent end-expiratory alveolar collapse. This can improve $\dot{V}/\dot{Q}$ matching and arterial oxygenation, and it allows reduction in Fio_2, reducing the risk for oxygen toxicity. However, elevated levels of applied PEEP can have adverse consequences, such as reduced preload (i.e., decreased cardiac output), elevated plateau airway pressure (i.e., increased risk of barotrauma), and impaired cerebral venous outflow (i.e., increased intracranial pressure). The optimal PEEP value enhances oxygenation without lung hyperinflation and decreased blood pressure.

Respiratory therapists typically adjust the inspiratory flow rate, flow pattern, and amount of negative pressure required to trigger a mechanical ventilator breath. If these ventilator settings are not adjusted with due consideration of the patient's respiratory mechanics, two common problems can occur: asynchrony and auto-PEEP.

Patient-ventilator asynchrony occurs if the phases of breaths delivered by the ventilator do not match the breathing pattern of the patient. This can lead to dyspnea, increased work of breathing, and prolonged duration of mechanical ventilation. It is detected by careful observation of the patient and examination of the ventilator waveforms. The abnormality that is most readily apparent is failure of the ventilator to trigger a breath when the patient makes an inspiratory effort.

Auto-PEEP is usually seen when patients do not fully empty their lungs during expiration before the initiation of the next breath. This is called *stacking breaths* or *generating auto-PEEP*. It is particularly worrisome in patients who have exacerbations of COPD or status asthmaticus requiring mechanical ventilation. In ventilated patients, auto-PEEP may cause barotrauma or hemodynamic collapse because of high intrathoracic pressures that prevent blood return to the right ventricle.

Weaning from Mechanical Ventilation

The complications of endotracheal intubation and mechanical ventilation include barotrauma, volutrauma (i.e., acute lung injury caused by high tidal volumes), and ventilator-associated pneumonia. Weaning from mechanical ventilation should be considered on a daily basis, particularly when the original insult that caused respiratory failure has improved. Weaning is most likely to be successful in the awake and cooperative patient without respiratory or hemodynamic instability. Weaning is usually not attempted if requirements for oxygen supplementation remain high (Fio_2 >0.5).

Conventional parameters that determine whether weaning is possible include negative inspiratory force, vital capacity, tidal volume, respiratory rate, and minute ventilation (Table 22-1). However, the strength of these parameters lies in the ability to predict failure to wean rather than in the ability to predict successful spontaneous breathing. A better way to assess weaning capability is to engage the patient in a short weaning trial during which support from the ventilator is diminished. Another strategy is to decrease the pressure generated by the ventilator during a trial of continuous positive airway pressure (CPAP). The patient is monitored for signs of distress or hemodynamic instability, and arterial blood gas levels are measured to determine the effectiveness of spontaneous ventilation. If the patient tolerates the trial, extubation may be indicated, depending on the patient's clinical status, ability to protect the airway, and underlying medical condition.

If the patient fails the weaning trial, attempts should be made to identify the factors responsible for the failure to wean. For very sick patients, all obvious contributory factors might have been identified and corrected, but the patient still requires a more prolonged weaning trial before extubation. The first of two recommended weaning strategies is to engage the patient in spontaneous ventilation trials without positive pressure for 1 hour once or twice each day, with total ventilatory support between trials usually supplied by ACV or PCV. The length of the spontaneous breathing trials can be progressively increased until the patient no longer requires mechanical support. The second strategy uses PSV. The inspiratory pressure is progressively decreased until the patient can breathe spontaneously without ventilatory support.

Both strategies appear to be equally effective, although weaning through PSV may be preferred in patients with chronic lung disease who have been mechanically ventilated for prolonged periods. For patients with prolonged mechanical ventilation, studies have shown that early tracheostomy is beneficial for weaning purposes and facilitates trials of unassisted breathing exercises because it can be easily and repeatedly removed (level II-1 evidence).

For a deeper discussion on this topic, please see Chapter 105, "Mechanical Ventilation," in Goldman-Cecil Medicine, *25th Edition.*

TABLE 22-1	CONVENTIONAL WEANING PARAMETERS	
PARAMETERS	**WEANABLE VALUES**	**NORMAL VALUES**
NIF (cm H_2O)	≤20	≤50
VC (mL/kg)	>10	>65-75
V_T (mL/kg)	<5	>5-7
RR (breaths/min)	<32	12-20
V_E (L/min)	>10	>10
RSBI (RR/V_T)	<105	<40

NIF, Negative inspiratory force; RR, respiratory rate; RSBI, rapid shallow breathing index; VC, vital capacity; V_E, minute ventilation; V_T, tidal volume.

ACUTE LUNG INJURY

Acute lung injury in its most severe form is called *acute respiratory distress syndrome* (ARDS). It typically manifests with dyspnea, cyanosis, tachypnea, tachycardia, diaphoresis, and diffuse crackles detected on examination. ARDS is characterized by increased permeability of the alveolar-capillary membrane, leading to flooding of the alveolar spaces with proteinaceous edema fluid. It is defined by clinical measures of the severity of lung dysfunction (e.g., PaO_2/FIO_2 ratio).

Based on the 2012 revised Berlin definition of ARDS, the severity can be separated into mild, moderate, and severe forms. Mild ARDS requires the Pao_2/FIO_2 ratio to be between 200 and 300 mm Hg on ventilator settings (PEEP or CPAP ≥5 cm H_2O). Moderate or severe ARDS occurs when the PaO_2/FIO_2 ratio is between 100 and 200 mm Hg or 100 mm Hg or less on ventilator settings (PEEP or CPAP ≥5 cm H_2O). Respiratory failure must not be caused by cardiac failure or fluid overload; bilateral opacities representing pulmonary edema on the chest radiograph or CT must be evident; and respiratory symptoms must be of sudden onset due to a known clinical insult (<1 week). Additional criteria include exclusion of cardiogenic pulmonary edema and other causes of acute hypoxemic respiratory failure such as idiopathic pulmonary fibrosis, chronic interstitial lung disease, and diffuse alveolar hemorrhage.

ARDS is triggered by direct injury to the lung, as observed in aspiration pneumonia, smoke inhalation, and near-drowning, or by systemic injury, such as trauma, surgery, sepsis, burns, long bone fractures, pancreatitis, uremia, transfusion therapy, shock, drug intoxication, and cardiopulmonary bypass. About 150,000 cases of ARDS are reported each year in the United States, and aspiration pneumonia and sepsis are the most common associated conditions. The morbidity rate associated with ARDS is high, and 30% to 50% of patients die.

ARDS is the pulmonary manifestation of a systemic disorder that triggers a dysregulated inflammatory response. Uncontrolled inflammation injures the pulmonary vascular endothelium, resulting in increased permeability and allowing extravasation of proteinaceous edema fluid from the intravascular space and its accumulation in the lung interstitium and alveolar spaces (E-Fig. 22-1). Injury to the lung epithelium decreases absorption of water from the alveolar space and causes secretion of abnormal or inadequate quantities of surfactant.

ARDS is often referred to as noncardiogenic or increased permeability pulmonary edema. In the lung, these processes cause right-to-left intrapulmonary shunting of blood that results in refractory hypoxemia and decreased lung compliance that increases the work of breathing. The chest radiograph reveals diffuse bilateral alveolar infiltrates (E-Fig. 22-2). Failure of other organs occurs frequently, and multiorgan failure is common, especially in the setting of sepsis.

Histologically, ARDS is characterized by diffuse alveolar damage with hyaline membranes (E-Fig. 22-3). The damage is further exaggerated by reductions in the quantity and quality of the synthesized surfactant, leading to atelectasis. After a few days, the tissue shows hyperplasia of type II pneumocytes (E-Fig. 22-4) and deposition of connective tissue resulting in fibrosis. These events can be worsened by mechanical ventilation through high tidal volumes, hyperdistention, and hyperoxia.

The diagnosis of ARDS should be considered in patients with a predisposing condition (e.g., sepsis), bilateral pulmonary infiltrates on the chest radiograph, and refractory hypoxemia (i.e., usually a Pao_2/FIO_2 ratio of 200 mm Hg or less) in the absence of significant cardiac dysfunction. Treatment of ARDS relies on supportive measures directed at eradicating the triggering event, sustaining the cardiovascular system, providing nutrition, and avoiding fluid overload. The Fluid and Catheter Treatment Trial (FACTT) conducted by the National Heart, Lung, and Blood Institute Acute Respiratory Distress Syndrome (ARDS) Clinical Trials Network showed that conservative fluid strategy resulted in more ventilator-free (2.5 days) and ICU-free days (2.2 days) than a more liberal fluid management approach (level I evidence). A ventilatory management strategy delivering low tidal volumes (about 6 mL/kg of body weight) increased survival (level I).

Advances in extracorporeal membrane oxygenation (ECMO) and pumpless extracorporeal lung assist (PECLA) have been reported, questioning the previous failures of these devices in patients with acute lung injury. The CESAR trial, which compared conventional ventilatory support with ECMO for severe respiratory failure, showed a significant improvement in survival with decreased disability at 6 months for the patients receiving ECMO (level I evidence). ECMO improved mortality for younger patients with H1N1-induced ARDS (level II-2). Several observational and uncontrolled clinical trials have shown similar improvements in survival rates. However, hemolysis and anticoagulation complications have restricted the use of ECMO.

High-frequency oscillatory ventilation (HFOV) has also been tried in patients with moderate to severe ARDS, but the mortality rate was not reduced, and there were worse outcomes than with conventional positive-pressure ventilation. Corticosteroids, surfactant replacement, and extracorporeal oxygenation have not proved beneficial and are not recommended. Oxygenation can be improved by PEEP and prone ventilation, but these interventions do not improve mortality rates. There was no difference in the 60-day mortality rate or improvement in ventilator-free days between initial trophic and full enteral feeding (EDEN trial, level I evidence). Early and late enteral feeding also showed no difference in mortality rates. Antioxidants, omega-3 fatty acids, and γ-linolenic acid did not improve clinical outcomes in patients with acute lung injury. Because there is no available therapy that lessens acute lung injury or hastens repair, the key to care of patients with ARDS is meticulous supportive care and avoidance of complications such as ventilator-associated pneumonia or catheter-related sepsis.

The lung injury prediction score (LIPS) encompasses various predisposing conditions and risk modifiers that have been found useful as a screening tool (negative predictive value −0.97) in clinical trials (level A evidence). As a result, such prognostic measures in identifying patients at risk of acute lung injury or ARDS on admission may lead to interventions that prevent disease progression or allow for close monitoring of patients for disease progression.

Most patients who survive ARDS do not have significant pulmonary function abnormalities in 12 months. The most common long-term complications in survivors are neuromuscular and psychosocial (level A evidence).

SHOCK

Shock is systemic organ hypoperfusion, usually caused by hypotension, that leads to cell injury and death. Four classifications are provided: cardiogenic shock (i.e., decreased cardiac output as a result of dysfunction), hypovolemic shock (i.e., decreased intravascular volume), septic or redistributive shock (i.e., decreased systemic vascular resistance), and obstructive shock (i.e., decreased cardiac output as a result of obstruction to flow). Anaphylactic shock caused by allergic reaction to a drug or a related insult is not discussed in this textbook.

> For a deeper discussion on this topic, please see Chapter 106, "Approach to the Patient with Shock," 107, "Cardiogenic Shock," and 108, "Shock Syndromes Related to Sepsis," in Goldman-Cecil Medicine, 25th Edition.

When encountering a patient in shock, the strategy is to gain vascular access quickly and to replace volume aggressively while making a careful assessment of the situation. This strategy is particularly appropriate when shock is thought to result from hypovolemia or sepsis. In the case of cardiogenic shock, strategies designed to improve cardiac function should be implemented, including administration of inotropic drugs or, in severe and unresponsive cases, cardiac bypass or cardiac-assist devices. In the case of severe hypovolemia, administration of saline is usually sufficient. Fluid replacement, antibiotic therapy, and drainage of infected spaces are paramount in treating sepsis.

Obstructive shock is the result of obstruction to blood flow, as observed in massive pulmonary embolism or saddle embolus lodged at the bifurcation of the right and left pulmonary arteries. In this setting, it is important to relieve the obstruction mechanically or through other methods (e.g., thrombolysis) or support the patient's circulation until the obstruction subsides.

The management of shock entails monitoring of blood pressure and organ perfusion. A central venous line facilitates the delivery of fluids and assessment of central volume status, and an arterial line allows accurate monitoring of blood pressure. Although the placement of a pulmonary artery catheter (i.e., Swan-Ganz catheter) showed favorable results in initial trails for a selected group of patients, recent studies have shown no beneficial effects (e.g., FACTT study, level I evidence). The catheter allows direct assessment of pressures in the right atrium, right ventricle, and pulmonary artery; measurement of the pulmonary capillary wedge pressure; and assessment of cardiac output.

Concerns have been raised about the true usefulness and benefit-risk ratio associated with catheter placement. Pulmonary artery catheters have been shown to increase complications, primarily nonlethal cardiac dysrhythmias, and to be poor predictors of fluid responsiveness in sepsis. The central venous oxygen saturation ($Scvo_2$) measured from a central venous catheter was shown to be similar to the mixed venous oxygen saturation ($S\bar{v}o_2$). Significant expertise is required for the insertion of these catheters and for adequate interpretation of the data generated.

> For a deeper discussion on this topic, please see Chapters 106, "Approach to the Patient with Shock," and 107, "Cardiogenic Shock," in Goldman-Cecil Medicine, 25th Edition.

SYSTEMIC INFLAMMATORY RESPONSE SYNDROME

The systemic inflammatory response syndrome (SIRS) is a constellation of clinical signs and symptoms triggered by the host response to diverse insults. The most common cause of SIRS is infection, which is called *sepsis*, but SIRS also can be triggered by noninfectious disorders such as pancreatitis and drug intoxication.

The diagnosis of SIRS requires at least two of the following criteria: temperature higher than 38° C or less than 36° C; tachycardia greater than 90 beats per minute; tachypnea greater than 20 breaths per minute; $Paco_2$ less than 32 mm Hg; and white blood cell count greater than 12,000 cells/µL or less than 4000 cells/µL. This systemic response may result in dysfunction of many organs, including the lung, liver, kidneys, heart, and central nervous system, which is called *multiple-organ dysfunction syndrome* or *multiple-organ system failure*. The prognosis worsens as more organs become involved, with mortality rates ranging from 30% for less severe cases to more than 90% for five or more failing organs. Treatment includes aggressive fluid replacement or vasopressors to improve blood pressure and prompt administration of antibiotics after blood and other cultures have been obtained.

> For a deeper discussion on this topic, please see Chapter 108, "Shock Syndromes Related to Sepsis," in Goldman-Cecil Medicine, 25th Edition.

NOXIOUS GASES, FUMES, AND SMOKE INHALATION

Inhalation of certain gases and fumes may cause asphyxia or cellular and metabolic injury (Table 22-2). Carbon monoxide poisoning is a common and frequently unsuspected cause of inhalational injury. It results in tissue hypoxia by competitively displacing oxygen from hemoglobin. Affinity of carbon monoxide for hemoglobin is about 250 times greater than that of oxygen.

The correlation between carbon monoxide levels and symptoms is weak, but patients with levels greater than 30% are usually

TABLE 22-2 TOXIC GASES AND FUMES

INJURIES	AGENTS	OCCUPATIONAL EXPOSURES
Simple asphyxia	Carbon dioxide	Mining, foundries
	Nitrogen	Mining, diving
	Methane	Mining
Cellular hypoxia and oxygen transport	Carbon monoxide	Mining, combustion in closed spaces
	Cyanide	Smoke inhalation
	Hydrogen sulfide	Petroleum refining
Direct tissue injury	Ammonia	Fertilizer, cleaning agents
	Chlorine	Bleaches, swimming pools
	Nitrogen dioxide	Farming, fertilizer, combustion in closed spaces
	Phosgene	Welding, paint removal
	Cadmium, mercury	Welding

symptomatic. Symptoms may range from confusion or fatigue to nausea, headache, tachycardia, and profound coma. The diagnosis is based on clinical grounds and supported by laboratory data. Carbon monoxide intoxication can occur from vehicle exhaust in enclosed automobiles, methylene chloride–based paint strippers, and by exposure to kerosene heaters or charcoal fires in closed spaces.

In suggested cases, arterial blood gas levels should be obtained with measured (not calculated) hemoglobin-oxygen saturation. A carbon monoxide level should be measured in patients with a measured systemic arterial oxygen saturation (Sao_2) lower than the calculated Sao_2 obtained from the arterial oxygen tension. Carbon monoxide does not alter Pao_2, which is a measure of the partial pressure of oxygen dissolved in plasma. Treatment of carbon monoxide poisoning is breathing 100% oxygen. Hyperbaric oxygen may be useful, but this therapy may not be readily available.

Inhalation of caustic substances such as ammonia, chlorine, and hydrogen fluoride causes acute symptoms of eye and upper airway inflammation. Pain, lacrimation, rhinorrhea, and upper airway symptoms usually prompt the individual to flee the environment. Inhalation of nitrogen dioxide (i.e., silo filler's disease) occurs in farmers who work in silos where fermentation of grain produces large quantities of the gas. Most patients recover without sequelae, but a few may develop bronchiolitis obliterans, an irreversible obstruction of small airways.

Metal fume fever causes influenza-like symptoms as a result of the inhalation of metal oxides generated by welding. Inhalation of platinum, formalin, and isocyanates may precipitate asthma. Pneumonitis can be induced by high-intensity inhalation of cadmium and mercury vapors.

Smoke inhalation may cause direct thermal injury that is usually confined to the upper airways, but it may also produce injury to the lower airways if exposure to sufficient steam occurs as a result of the high thermal content of water. Laryngeal edema, airway inflammation, and mucus can lead to airway obstruction, which requires intubation. Anoxia occurs from consumption of oxygen by fire and from cytotoxic injury from gases such as carbon monoxide, cyanide, and oxidants liberated during combustion. The combustion of natural and synthetic polymers often produces aldehydes, acetaldehyde, and acrolein, which also have a high irritant potential.

Cyanide poisoning uncouples oxygen from energy production by binding to cytochrome a,a_3 (i.e., cytochrome c oxidase), preventing electron transfer to oxygen, and it requires prompt treatment with 100% oxygen and sodium thiosulfate. Sodium thiosulfate facilitates the conversion of cyanide to thiocyanate. Recently, the U.S. Food and Drug Administration (FDA) has also approved the use of hydroxocobalamin, which combines with cyanide to form cyanocobalamin (vitamin B_{12}).

The treatment of inhalation injuries is supportive, with close attention to the airway. Oxygen should be provided, and continuous monitoring of cardiac and hemodynamic status is necessary. Sometimes, intubation and mechanical ventilation are needed to overcome airway obstruction and the development of respiratory failure.

 For a deeper discussion on this topic, please see Chapter 110, "Acute Poisoning," in Goldman-Cecil Medicine, *25th Edition.*

DRUG OVERDOSES

Drug overdoses are common causes of admission to the ICU. The presenting complaints and management of the more common overdoses that result in medical emergencies are summarized in Table 22-3.

TABLE 22-3   COMMON DRUG OVERDOSES

DRUG OVERDOSE	CLINICAL SYNDROME	TREATMENT
Acetaminophen (paracetamol)	0.5-24 hr: nausea, vomiting 24-72 hr: nausea, vomiting, right upper quadrant pain; abnormal liver function tests and prothrombin time 72-96 hr: liver necrosis, coagulation, defects, jaundice, renal failure, hepatic encephalopathy 4 days-2 wk: resolution of liver dysfunction	Elimination: gastric lavage (if <1 hr after ingestion); activated charcoal (if <4 hr after ingestion); both longer if sustained-release product Treatment: N-acetylcysteine for toxic ingestion
Amphetamines	Hypertension, tachycardia, arrhythmias, myocardial infarction, vasospasm, seizures, paranoid psychosis, diaphoresis, tachypnea	Elimination: activated charcoal for oral ingestion Agitation or seizures: benzodiazepines Hypertension: control agitation, α-antagonists (phentolamine), vasodilators (nitroglycerin, nitroprusside, nifedipine) Hyperthermia: control agitation, external cooling
Iron	0.5-6 hr: nausea, vomiting, gastrointestinal discomfort, gastrointestinal bleed, drowsiness, hypoglycemia, hypotension 6-24 hr: latency, quiescence (may not occur in severe ingestions) 6-48 hr: shock, coma, seizures, coagulopathy, acidosis, cardiac failure 2-7 days: hepatotoxicity, coagulopathy, metabolic acidosis, renal insufficiency 1-8 wk: gastrointestinal disorders, achlorhydria	Elimination: gastric lavage and/or whole bowel irrigation with polyethylene glycol electrolyte solution, especially after ingestion of tablets containing radiopaque iodinated dye for kidney-ureter-bladder radiography Shock: intravenous fluids and blood (for hemorrhage); vasopressors if needed Antidote: deferoxamine to chelate iron, when iron levels >500 µg/dL or severe ingestion suspected
Tricyclic antidepressants	Wide-complex tachyarrhythmias, hypotension, seizures	Tachyarrhythmias: alkalinize blood (pH 7.5-7.55) with intravenous bicarbonate Seizures: benzodiazepines Hypotension: fluid resuscitation, vasopressors
Salicylate	Respiratory alkalosis (initially), metabolic acidosis (after substantial absorption), pulmonary edema, platelet dysfunction, nausea, vomiting, hearing loss, agitation, delirium	Elimination: activated charcoal, hemodialysis (for severe poisoning), alkalinization of urine Agitation or delirium: alkalinize blood with intravenous bicarbonate

SUGGESTED READINGS

Acute Respiratory Distress Syndrome Network: Ventilation with lower tidal volumes as compared with traditional tidal volumes for acute lung injury and the acute respiratory distress syndrome, N Engl J Med 342:1301–1308, 2000.

ARDS Definition Task Force, Ranieri VM, Rubenfeld GD, et al: Acute respiratory distress syndrome: the Berlin definition, JAMA 307:2526–2533, 2012.

Bernard GR, Sopko G, Cerra F, et al: Pulmonary artery catheterization and clinical outcomes: National Heart, Lung, and Blood Institute and Food and Drug Administration Workshop Report. Consensus statement, JAMA 283(19):2568–2572, 2000.

Dellinger RP, Levy MM, Rhodes A, et al: Surviving sepsis campaign: international guidelines for management of severe sepsis and septic shock: 2012, Crit Care Med 41:580–637, 2013.

Ferguson ND, Cook DJ, Guyatt GH, et al: High-frequency oscillation in early acute respiratory distress syndrome, N Engl J Med 368:795–805, 2013.

Gajic O, Dabbagh O, Park PK, et al: Early identification of patients at risk of acute lung injury: evaluation of lung injury prediction score in a multicenter cohort study, Am J Respir Crit Care Med 183:462–470, 2011.

Griffiths J, Barber VS, Morgan L, et al: Systematic review and meta-analysis of studies of the timing of tracheostomy in adult patients undergoing artificial ventilation, BMJ 330:1243, 2005.

Hill NS: Noninvasive ventilation for chronic obstructive pulmonary disease, Respir Care 49:87–89, 2004.

National Heart, Lung, and Blood Institute Acute Respiratory Distress Syndrome (ARDS) Clinical Trials Network, Wheeler AP, Bernard GR, et al: Pulmonary-artery versus central venous catheter to guide treatment of acute lung injury, N Engl J Med 354:2213–2224, 2006.

National Heart, Lung, and Blood Institute Acute Respiratory Distress Syndrome (ARDS) Clinical Trials Network, Wiedemann HP, Wheeler AP, et al: Comparison of two fluid-management strategies in acute lung injury, N Engl J Med 354:2564–2575, 2006.

Peek GJ, Mugford M, Tiruvoipati R, et al: Efficacy and economic assessment of conventional ventilatory support versus extracorporeal membrane oxygenation for severe adult respiratory failure (CESAR): a multicentre randomised controlled trial, Lancet 374:1351–1363, 2009.

Pham T, Combes A, Rozé H, et al: Extracorporeal membrane oxygenation for pandemic influenza a (H1N1)-induced acute respiratory distress syndrome: a cohort study and propensity-matched analysis, Am J Respir Crit Care Med 187:276–285, 2013.

Rivers E, Nguyen B, Havstad S, et al: Early goal-directed therapy in the treatment of severe sepsis and septic shock, N Engl J Med 345:1368–1377, 2001.

Sehti JM, Siegel MD: Mechanical ventilation in chronic obstructive pulmonary disease, Clin Chest Med 21:799–818, 2000.

Ware LB, Matthay MA: The acute respiratory distress syndrome, N Engl J Med 342:1334–1349, 2000.

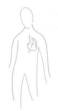

23

Neoplastic Disorders of the Lung

Lauren M. Catalano and Jason M. Aliotta

DEFINITION

Lung cancer is the leading cause of cancer death for men and women in the United States. An estimated 1.3 million people die worldwide of lung cancer each year. Lung cancer causes 28% of all cancer deaths in the United States, more than the next three most common cancers (i.e., colon, breast and prostate) combined.

Most lung cancers are classified as two major types: *small cell lung carcinoma* (SCLC) (E-Fig. 23-1) and *non–small cell lung carcinoma* (NSCLC). NSCLCs are more common and include squamous cell carcinoma (E-Fig. 23-2), adenocarcinoma (E-Fig. 23-3), and large cell carcinoma (E-Fig. 23-4). SCLCs account for less than 20% of all lung cancers.

EPIDEMIOLOGY

Smoking is the leading cause of lung cancer, a cause-effect relationship that was recognized as early as the 1940s. The risk of lung cancer is proportionate to cigarette pack-years smoked (i.e., packs per day multiplied by years smoked), with a peak incidence in the sixth and seventh decades. Compared with never-smokers, men who smoke are 23 times more likely and women 13 times more likely to develop lung cancer. Ex-smokers show a persistent risk of lung cancer throughout life.

Passive smoking is thought to be the cause of lung cancer for a significant percentage of nonsmokers who develop the disease. Nonsmokers who live with smokers have a more than 20% to 30% increased risk of developing lung cancer. However, non-smokers do develop lung cancer that is thought to be unrelated to environmental tobacco exposure; the cause of this phenomenon is poorly understood.

Other risk factors for lung cancer include environmental hazards such as asbestos exposure. Tobacco smoking in the setting of asbestos exposure is thought to have a multiplicative effect on risk. Radon exposure, such as that seen in miners, also increases the risk of lung cancer by approximately 10%. Radon exposure in the home is less significant, but home radon testing is recommended and legally mandated in some states.

PATHOLOGY

The exact mechanisms by which risk factors promote lung cancer remain unclear, but if unopposed, they are likely to cause genetic abnormalities that promote oncogenic transformation of lung epithelial cells. Because of the inherent redundant repair mechanisms available to the lung, however, many genetic insults appear necessary to irreversibly mutate and activate genes such as the *RAS* gene family, *ERBB* gene family, *RB1*, *MYC*, *SRC*, suppressor genes such as *CDKN1A* and *TP53*, and genes encoding growth factors such as gastrin-releasing peptide, insulin-like growth factor, and epidermal growth factor. Epidermal growth factor receptor mutations are prominent in nonsmokers who develop lung cancer and may indicate a unique molecular basis for lung cancer in those patients.

Non–Small Cell Lung Carcinomas

Squamous cell carcinomas arise from the epithelial layer of the bronchial wall as normal columnar epithelial cells undergo metaplasia, eventually being replaced by increasingly atypical squamous epithelial cells. A localized carcinoma, called *carcinoma in situ*, forms and later extends beyond the bronchial mucosa as it becomes invasive. Histologically, squamous cell carcinomas can be distinguished from other NSCLCs by the presence of keratinization, pearl formation, and intercellular bridging.

Adenocarcinomas can form glandlike structures and produce mucus. The tumor cells stain positive for carcinoembryonic antigen (CEA), mucin, and surfactant apoprotein. Slower-growing forms appear to grow and spread along preexisting alveolar walls.

Large cell carcinomas lack the glandular and squamous features typical of other NSCLCs and cytologic features typical of SCLCs. In this respect, it is considered a diagnosis of exclusion.

Small Cell Lung Carcinoma

Small cell carcinoma is strongly associated with cigarette smoking. Tumor cells are of pulmonary neuroendocrine cell origin. Released factors are often associated with paraneoplastic syndromes.

CLINICAL PRESENTATION

Patients may complain of mild cough, dyspnea, increased sputum production, chest pain, and weight loss. Hemoptysis may indicate local airway inflammation or erosion of the neoplasm into surrounding vascular structures. Localized pleuritic chest pain suggests pleural involvement or chest wall invasion (E-Fig. 23-5). Hoarseness is caused by involvement or compression of the left recurrent laryngeal nerve and suggests a mediastinal or hilar mass or significant lymphadenopathy. Dysphagia suggests esophageal involvement or compression by lymph nodes.

A pleural effusion is observed in 9% of patients, is often unilateral, and can be related to direct tumor involvement of the pleura or obstruction of lymph flow from the mediastinal nodes (E-Fig. 23-6). The superior vena cava is involved in less than 5% of patients, but obstruction may result in superior vena cava syndrome, which is characterized by edema of the face and upper extremities due to impaired venous return. Despite its aesthetic and prognostic implications, its involvement typically does not represent a medical emergency.

The physical examination may be normal or may reveal changes in the lung, such as crackles (e.g., postobstructive pneumonia) (E-Fig. 23-7), inspiratory wheeze suggesting airway obstruction, or dullness to percussion as a result of underlying pleural effusion. Lymph node enlargement in the neck or axillary areas suggests metastatic disease (E-Fig. 23-8).

Lung cancers that occur in the apex of the chest and invade apical chest wall structures are known as *superior sulcus* or *Pancoast tumors* (E-Fig. 23-9). The classic description involves a syndrome of radicular-type pain or paresthesias radiating down the arm due to tumor erosion into the brachial plexus. Tumor erosion into the cervical sympathetic chain can result in Horner's syndrome, which is characterized by a triad of physical findings: ptosis, miosis, and anhidrosis over the face and forehead.

Paraneoplastic syndromes are usually neurologic syndromes that are rare and are elicited by a patient's own immune response to neoplastic processes, often originating in the lung. Neurologic symptoms develop over weeks and may include difficulties in walking or swallowing, loss of muscle tone, loss of fine motor coordination, slurred speech, memory loss, vision problems, dementia, sleep disturbances, seizures, and vertigo. Neurologic paraneoplastic syndromes include stiff-person syndrome, encephalomyelitis, cerebellar degeneration, neuromyotonia, and sensory neuropathy. Neuromuscular junction disorders can occur, as observed in the Lambert-Eaton myasthenic syndrome. Myopathies, electrolyte disturbances, and certain visual loss syndromes can also be manifestations of a paraneoplastic syndrome.

DIAGNOSIS AND DIFFERENTIAL DIAGNOSIS
Non–Small Cell Lung Carcinomas

Between 60% and 80% of squamous cell carcinomas tend to be located in central airways (E-Fig. 23-10). The airway lumen may become obstructed, leading to collapse of the lung (i.e., atelectasis) or postobstructive pneumonia. Although necrosis and cavity formation may occur in any lung tumor, this feature is more common with squamous cell carcinomas. Because of their slow rate of growth, these tumors have the lowest propensity for metastasis of all types of lung cancer.

Adenocarcinomas represent the most common type of lung cancer and the most common type in nonsmokers (almost 20% of cases). Adenocarcinomas are most often found in the periphery of the lung (75%) (E-Fig. 23-11). This tumor is frequently associated with malignant pleural effusions (60%) and has a high propensity for distant metastasis.

Previously called *bronchoalveolar cell carcinomas,* it is now understood that these more insidious forms of adenocarcinoma likely exist as a spectrum of disease. In its most benign form, atypical adenomatous hyperplasia (AAH) exhibits mild to moderate nuclear atypia without stromal invasion. A stepwise progression of classification, including adenocarcinoma in situ (AIS), minimally invasive adenocarcinoma, and lepidic pattern adenocarcinoma, describes a gradual progression of invasion. This is the most common form of lung cancer found in nonsmokers and young patients. It can develop as a lung infiltrate or as a solitary nodule, and it can be accompanied by excessive production of secretions.

Large cell carcinomas (giant cell and clear cell subtypes) frequently develop as a peripheral lesion and may be associated with pneumonitis and hilar adenopathy. Patients usually have cough and weight loss. Given the aggressive nature of these tumors, symptoms (e.g., bone pain) are often the consequence of metastatic disease.

Small Cell Lung Carcinomas

SCLC is strongly associated with cigarette smoking. SCLCs typically are found in perihilar locations, frequently originating in the main bronchi, and they often have associated lymphadenopathy (E-Fig. 23-12). These tumors metastasize rapidly, most commonly to the thoracic lymph nodes, bones, liver, adrenal glands, and brain. Approximately 70% of patients have metastatic disease at the time of clinical presentation.

Diagnostic Evaluation

Because lung cancer typically is diagnosed at an advanced stage, when cure is not possible, an effective strategy for detection of lung cancer at an early stage is desirable. Results from the National Lung Screening Trial, sponsored by the National Cancer Institute, have started to support the formation of lung cancer screening guidelines. This was a randomized trial that compared two ways of detecting lung cancer in smokers: low-dose helical computed tomography (CT) and standard chest radiography. More than 50,000 patients were enrolled in this study over a period of 2 years, with a follow-up time of 5 years. Subjects enrolled were between 55 and 74 years old and smoked for a minimum of 30 pack-years. Former smokers enrolled in this study had quit within the preceding 15 years. There was a 20% relative reduction in mortality from lung cancer with low-dose helical CT screening. However, formal recommendations have not been made for the application of these data to larger cohorts given the rate of false positives and concurrent increased rate of invasive procedures (with potential negative outcomes).

When a suspected lung cancer is identified, a tissue diagnosis is essential for most patients. If imaging reveals sites of suspected metastasis, the site of biopsy should be chosen to determine the greatest extent of spread or highest stage of the tumor to prevent patients from undergoing multiple invasive procedures. If the apparent tumor is confined to the chest, bronchoscopy (potentially with endoscopic ultrasound-guided lymph node biopsies) is appropriate for central masses, whereas transthoracic needle aspiration can be performed for more peripheral lesions. An identified pleural effusion should be sampled to assess for malignant cells. In some cases, if the pretest probability is very high that the lung lesion is a primary lung cancer and there is no imaging evidence of disease spread, direct referral for surgical resection may be appropriate. In these cases, equivocal biopsy results should not hamper attempts to remove the lesion. If patients are too debilitated to undergo treatment or insightfully refuse interventions, tissue diagnosis may be deferred with the intention of palliative measures.

After a lung cancer is diagnosed, staging is necessary to determine the treatment and prognosis. For NSCLCs, staging can determine whether the patient may benefit from surgical resection for curative intent or from other treatment modalities such as chemotherapy. Chest CT is useful to delineate the location and size of the primary tumor and to examine for involved mediastinal lymph nodes, pleural disease, and adrenal or liver metastases. However, CT has limited ability to distinguish benign versus malignant lymphadenopathy in the mediastinum. Positron emission tomography (PET) using 18-fluorodeoxyglucose (FDG) is more sensitive and specific than CT for the detection of mediastinal lymph node metastases and may detect unexpected metastases elsewhere in the body. Suspected mediastinal or extrathoracic metastases demonstrated by imaging should be confirmed with tissue sampling before determining whether a patient is an operative candidate. Although rare, multiple primary lung cancers can occur, especially in patients with many cancer risk factors.

Invasive techniques for staging of the mediastinal lymph nodes include endoscopic transbronchial needle aspiration, endoscopic ultrasound-guided needle aspiration, and mediastinoscopy. Mediastinoscopy is frequently performed to exclude mediastinal spread of disease in patients without definite imaging evidence of lymph node involvement before definitive resection of the lung cancer. Head CT with intravenous contrast or magnetic resonance imaging (MRI) is the preferred radiologic study if the clinical history or examination suggests brain metastasis. Bone scans are useful for the investigation of suspected bony metastases if there are corresponding clinical symptoms.

The increased use of CT scan for the work-up other intrathoracic and extrathoracic conditions has led to a marked increase in the incidental diagnosis of solitary and multiple pulmonary nodules. These nodules may be described by their appearance: solid, partially solid, and ground glass. Radiographically, solid nodules demonstrate a soft tissue density. Ground-glass nodules represent alveolar wall inflammation or thickening, with partial air space filling. Radiographically, the nodules appear hazy but do not obscure underlying bronchial and vascular markings of the lung. Mixed nodules contain some combination of the two patterns. These incidental findings pose a conundrum for practitioners when evaluating patients without any other clinical symptoms who may or may not have a smoking history.

Current recommendations were created in 2005 by the Fleischer Society, a multidisciplinary panel of experts in lung cancer. These recommendations provide guidance for radiologic follow-up of incidentally encountered nodules. Patients with these findings are stratified as low risk (i.e., minimal or no history of smoking and other known risk factors) or high risk (i.e., history of smoking with other known risk factors). The recommendations state that nodules less than 4 mm in the greatest dimension require no follow-up in low-risk patients, and if they remain unchanged on a 12-month follow-up CT scan in high-risk patients, no additional scans are warranted. Nodules 4 to 6 mm in the greatest dimension in low-risk patients require a follow-up CT scan at 12 months, and if unchanged, no additional scans are warranted. However, high-risk patients should have a repeat CT scan 6 to 12 months after discovery and then at 18 to 24 months if the situation remains unchanged. This recommendation applies to low-risk patients with nodules between 6 and 8 mm in the greatest dimension. Closer follow-up is recommended for high-risk patients with 6- to 8-mm nodules and all patients with nodules greater than 8 mm in diameter. These patients should have CT scans at 3 to 6, 9 to 12, and 24 months, respectively.

Ground-glass nodules 5 mm or larger seen on thin-slice (1-mm section) chest CT do not warrant further follow-up. Although multiple ground-glass nodules are less likely to represent a neoplastic process, they should be followed to ensure resolution. Ground-glass nodules larger than 5 mm in diameter that persist on a 3-month follow-up CT scan should be monitored by CT scans at 12, 24, and 36 months. If there has been no increase in size after 36 months of observation, follow-up CT scans can be discontinued. Mixed solid and ground-glass nodules that persist on a 3-month follow-up CT scan and have a solid component less than 5 mm in diameter should be followed in a similar fashion. However, nodules with a solid component of 5 mm or larger that persist on a 3-month follow-up CT scan should be biopsied or surgically resected. PET scanning is not helpful in characterizing ground-glass nodules because of the wide variation in radiotracer uptake (from nil to positive). The diagnostic yield of needle biopsy for these lesions varies because operator inexperience and sampling error can affect results.

● TREATMENT

Evidence-based clinical practice guidelines for lung cancer were published by the American College of Chest Physicians (ACCP) in May 2013. These guidelines are based on a comprehensive review of the literature and systematic interpretation of the data to provide management recommendations in a graded fashion.

Management of lung cancer includes preventive strategies, early detection, and treatment. Of these, the most effective approach is prevention. Smoking prevention and cessation strategies are paramount. Individuals who are successful at quitting smoking have a lower long-term rate of lung cancer death than individuals who continue to smoke. Survival differences are seen as early as 5 to 10 years after removal of tobacco exposure. Although cancer risk remains higher in previous smokers than never-smokers, the survival benefit continues to increase as exposure becomes more remote. A diet rich in fruits and vegetables may protect against the development of lung cancer in smokers. Animal studies have suggested that antioxidants contained in these foods might block free radical–induced cell injury, preventing the development of various cancers. However, high-dose supplemental β-carotene, vitamin E, retinoids, and N-acetylcysteine should not be advocated for smokers and former smokers (grade 1A recommendation).

The treatment of lung cancer depends on the stage of disease at the time of presentation. The 7th edition of the International Staging System for Lung Cancer was proposed in 2009 by the International Association for the Study of Lung Cancer and accepted into use in January 2010. Neoplasms of the chest are classified by standardized tumor, node, metastasis (TNM) nomenclature that has been accepted throughout the field of oncology (Table 23-1). The Veterans Administration system of limited-stage versus extensive-stage disease (see Table 23-1) may be used in conjunction with the TNM staging system in the description of SCLC (grade 1B recommendation).

A timely, efficient, multidisciplinary approach using the expertise of a thoracic surgeon, medical and radiation oncologists, and a pulmonologist should be employed to evaluate patients with

TABLE 23-1 LUNG CANCER STAGING SYSTEMS

STAGE	DESCRIPTION
TUMOR, NODE, METASTASIS STAGING SYSTEM FOR NSCLC	
Primary Tumor (T)	
TX	Primary tumor cannot be assessed, or tumor proved by the presence of malignant cells in sputum or bronchial washings but not visualized by imaging or bronchoscopy
T0	No evidence of primary tumor
Tis	Carcinoma in situ
T1	Tumor <3 cm in greatest dimension, surrounded by lung or visceral pleura, without bronchoscopic evidence of invasion more proximal than the lobar bronchus (i.e., not in the main bronchus)
T1a	Tumor <2 cm in greatest dimension
T1b	Tumor >2 cm but <3 cm in greatest dimension
T2	Tumor >3 cm but <7 cm or tumor with any of the following features (T2 tumors with these features are classified T2a if <5 cm): involves main bronchus, >2 cm distal to the carina or invades visceral pleura; associated with atelectasis or obstructive pneumonitis that extends to the hilar region but does not involve the entire lung
T2a	Tumor >3 cm but <5 cm in greatest dimension
T2b	Tumor >5 cm but <7 cm in greatest dimension
T3	Tumor >7 cm or one that directly invades any of the following: chest wall (including superior sulcus tumors), diaphragm, phrenic nerve, mediastinal pleura, parietal pericardium; tumor in the main bronchus <2 cm distal to the carina but without involvement of the carina; associated atelectasis or obstructive pneumonitis of the entire lung; separate tumor nodule(s) in the same lobe
T4	Tumor of any size that invades any of the following: mediastinum, heart, great vessels, trachea, recurrent laryngeal nerve, esophagus, vertebral body, carina; separate tumor nodule(s) in a different ipsilateral lobe
Nodal Involvement (N)	
NX	Regional lymph nodes cannot be assessed
N0	No regional lymph node metastasis
N1	Metastasis in ipsilateral peribronchial and/or ipsilateral hilar lymph nodes and intrapulmonary nodes, including involvement by direct extension
N2	Metastasis in ipsilateral mediastinal and/or subcarinal lymph node(s)
N3	Metastasis in contralateral mediastinal, contralateral hilar, ipsilateral or contralateral scalene, or supraclavicular lymph node(s)
Metastasis (M)	
MX	Distant metastasis cannot be assessed
M0	No distant metastasis
M1	Distant metastasis
M1a	Separate tumor nodule(s) in a contralateral lobe; tumor with pleural nodules or malignant pleural/pericardial effusion
M1b	Distant metastasis
VALG STAGING SYSTEM	
Limited-stage disease (LD)	Tumor confined to the ipsilateral hemithorax and regional lymph nodes, including ipsilateral supraclavicular nodes; can be encompassed within a tolerable radiation therapy port
Extensive-stage disease (ED)	Tumor has spread beyond the boundaries of LD, including malignant pleural or pericardial effusions, contralateral hilar or supraclavicular involvement or distant metastases

Modified from Edge S, Byrd DR, Compton CC, et al, editors: AJCC cancer staging manual, ed 7, New York, 2010, Springer.

NSCLC, Non–small cell lung carcinoma; VALG, Veterans Administration Lung Study Group.

lung cancer for surgical resection, regardless of age (grade 1C recommendation). The presurgical evaluation of patients with lung cancer involves staging, the determination of resectability, and the evaluation of lung function to determine pulmonary reserve. Given the high occurrence of comorbid conditions that increase the likelihood of an adverse perioperative cardiovascular event, a preoperative cardiologic evaluation may be warranted (grade 1C).

A comprehensive respiratory assessment can estimate the preoperative risk from underlying pulmonary disease, such as chronic obstructive pulmonary disease (COPD). Spirometry to ascertain pulmonary function (i.e., forced expiratory volume in 1 second [FEV_1]) is commonly used to assess the suitability of patients with lung cancer for surgery. Patients with an FEV_1 value greater than 2 L (for pneumonectomy), greater than 1.5 L (for lobectomy), or greater than 80% predicted have an average preoperative risk (grade 1C).

Measurement of the lung's carbon monoxide diffusion capacity (D_{LCO}) is necessary for patients with an acceptable FEV_1 value but who have unexplained dyspnea on exertion or evidence of interstitial lung disease on chest imaging. If the measured D_{LCO} is greater than 80% predicted, the patient is still considered to have an average preoperative risk. Radionucleotide perfusion scanning and cardiopulmonary exercise testing may be performed when spirometry and D_{LCO} are borderline, conflicting, or otherwise difficult to interpret and apply to the patient's functional status (grade 1B recommendation).

Non–Small Cell Lung Carcinomas

Surgery is the only curative therapy for NSCLCs, and it is indicated for patients with stage I or II disease who are operative candidates (grade 1B recommendation). Lobectomy is considered superior to wedge resection (grade 1B). Pathologic stage IA or IB disease does not require additional therapies (grade 1B). Adjuvant chemotherapy is appropriate for patients with stage II or greater disease (grade 1A).

For patients with stage IIIA disease, the optimal treatment strategy remains unclear. These patients usually are not candidates for surgery or radiation therapy alone (grade 1A recommendation), and a treatment plan should be individualized in a multidisciplinary setting. For stage IIIB disease, surgery may rarely be indicated for some T4N0-1M0 tumors. A malignant pleural effusion precludes resection. Combined and ideally concurrent chemotherapy and radiation therapy is preferable to radiation therapy alone for patients with stage IIIB disease (grade 1A). For stage IV disease, chemotherapy is recommended because it improves survival and provides palliation for symptoms (grade 1A).

Targeted molecular therapies are emerging as effective lung cancer treatment. Bevacizumab, a humanized monoclonal antibody against vascular endothelial growth factor (VEGF), improves survival when added to a standard platinum-based chemotherapeutic regimen for patients with nonsquamous NSCLC (grade 1A recommendation). However, it was associated with hemoptysis, which was sometimes fatal, in patients with squamous cell carcinoma in an early-stage trial. Erlotinib and gefitinib, tyrosine kinase inhibitors that target the activity of the epidermal growth factor receptor (EGFR), are approved for the first-line treatment of metastatic NSCLCs that have EGFR mutations (grade 1A). Targeting the EGFR seems to have benefit in particular patient groups, such as women, never-smokers, and Asians who harbor these particular receptor mutations.

Small Cell Lung Carcinoma

Most SCLCs are treated with chemotherapy, and common regimens are four to six cycles of platinum-based chemotherapy (cisplatin or carboplatin) plus etoposide or irinotecan (grade 1A recommendation). Thoracic external beam radiation therapy may be useful if disease is limited (grade 2C). Occasionally, SCLCs can be resected if no evidence of metastasis is found (grade 2C). Although chemotherapy and radiation therapy often produce a dramatic response and sometimes are curative for limited disease, relapse is typical, and subsequent treatments usually are less effective.

● PROGNOSIS

The Surveillance, Epidemiology, and End Results (SEER) database, which contains more than 31,000 cases, was used to validate the 2010 TNM staging system, and it provides the most robust prognostic information for lung cancer. Despite persistent advances in the understanding of the biology of lung cancer and the introduction of novel chemotherapeutic agents for its treatment, the overall 5-year survival rate for patients with lung cancer is 15%. Most patients with lung cancer are diagnosed during the advanced stages of the disease, when surgical resection is less likely to be curative.

Non–Small Cell Lung Carcinomas

Patients with stage IA NSCLC have a median survival of 59 months. The median survival for stage IV disease is only 4 months. Approximately 40% of patients experience a recurrence, with a median time to recurrence after surgery of 11.5 months. Average survival after recurrence is about 8 months.

Small Cell Lung Carcinoma

Patients with limited-stage SCLC at the time of presentation have a median survival of 15 to 20 months and a 5-year survival rate of 10% to 13%. Unfortunately, most patients are diagnosed with extensive disease at the time of clinical presentation. Median survival for these patients is only 8 to 13 months, and the 5-year survival rate is 1% to 2%.

SUGGESTED READINGS

Aberle DR, Adams AM, Berg CD, et al: Reduced lung-cancer mortality with low-dose computed tomographic screening, N Engl J Med 365:395–409, 2011.

Detterbeck FC, Boffa DJ, Tanoue LT: The new lung cancer staging system, Chest 136:260–271, 2009.

Detterbeck FC, Lewis SZ, Diekemper R, et al: Executive summary: diagnosis and management of lung cancer, 3rd ed: American College of Chest Physicians evidence-based clinical practice guidelines, Chest 143(Suppl):7S–37S, 2013.

Godoy MC, Sabloff B, Naidich DP: Subsolid pulmonary nodules: imaging evaluation and strategic management, Curr Opin Pulm Med 18:304–312, 2012.

Gustafsson BI, Kidd M, Chan A, et al: Bronchopulmonary neuroendocrine tumors, Cancer 113:5–21, 2008.

MacMahon H, Austin JHM, Gamsu G, et al: Guidelines for management of small pulmonary nodules detected on CT scans: a statement from the Fleischner Society, Radiology 237:395–400, 2005.

Mulshine JL, Sullivan DC: Clinical practice: lung cancer screening, N Engl J Med 352:2714–2720, 2005.

Surveillance Epidemiology and End Results: SEER program (website). http://seer.cancer.gov. Accessed September 2, 2014.

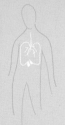

IV

Preoperative and Postoperative Care

24 Preoperative and Postoperative Care
Prashant Vaishnava and Kim A. Eagle

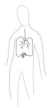

24

Preoperative and Postoperative Care

Prashant Vaishnava and Kim A. Eagle

INTRODUCTION

More than 40 million people undergo noncardiac surgical procedures in the United States annually. It is estimated that the incidence of cardiac complications after noncardiac surgical procedures is between 0.5% and 1% In other words, 200,000 to 400,000 people will experience perioperative cardiac complications annually. Moreover, more than 25% of these patients will die. Patients who survive a postoperative myocardial infarction (MI) are twice as likely to die in the following 2 years as are patients with uneventful surgical procedures. Emerging evidence-based practices dictate that the physician should thoughtfully perform an individualized evaluation of the surgical patient to provide an accurate preoperative risk assessment, risk stratification, and modification of risk parameters that can then provide the framework for optimal perioperative risk reduction strategies. This chapter reviews preoperative and postoperative cardiovascular risk assessment that targets intermediate- to high-risk patients to strategically guide perioperative preventive therapies for optimal outcome.

EVALUATION OF PATIENTS WITH ELEVATED RISK

The preoperative evaluation includes an assessment of the risk associated with the planned surgery or procedure. Historically the risk of procedures has been categorized as low, intermediate, or high. The most recent guidelines from the American College of Cardiology/American Heart Association (ACC/AHA) on perioperative cardiovascular evaluation, however, have simplified the approach by categorizing planned procedures as low or elevated perioperative risk. Low-risk procedures (e.g., colonoscopy, cataract surgery) are associated with a less than 1% risk of major adverse cardiovascular events (MACE) of death or myocardial infarction. Those procedures with a MACE risk of ≥1% are classified as conferring escalated risk. Simple standardized preoperative screening questionnaires have been developed for the purpose of identifying patients at intermediate to high risk who may benefit from a more detailed clinical evaluation (Table 24-1).

Evaluation of such surgical patients should always begin with a thorough history and physical examination including a 12-lead resting electrocardiogram (ECG) in accordance with the ACC/AHA guidelines. A determination of the urgency of the surgery should be included in the history because truly emergent procedures are associated with unavoidably higher rates of morbidity and mortality.

Perioperative risk assessment begins with an assessment of the urgency of the noncardiac surgery; emergency surgery should not be delayed and may not allow for risk stratification. Preoperative testing should be done only for specific clinical conditions based on the history. Healthy patients of any age who are undergoing elective surgical procedures and have no coexisting medical conditions should not need any testing unless the degree of surgical stress could result in unusual changes from the baseline state. The history should focus on symptoms of occult cardiac disease.

PREOPERATIVE CARDIAC RISK ASSESSMENT

During the perioperative risk assessment of patients undergoing noncardiac surgery, there are active cardiac conditions that should be evaluated and treated in accordance with the ACC/AHA guidelines. These conditions include unstable coronary artery disease (CAD), decompensated heart failure, severe

TABLE 24-1	STANDARDIZED PREOPERATIVE QUESTIONNAIRE*

1. Age, weight, and height
2. Are you
   a. Female and 55 years of age or older or male and 45 years of age or older?
   b. If yes, are you also 70 years of age or older?
3. Do you take anticoagulant medications ("blood thinners")?
4. Do you have or have you had any of the following heart-related conditions?
   a. Heart disease
   b. Heart attack within the last 6 months
   c. Angina (chest pain)
   d. Irregular heartbeat
   e. Heart failure
5. Do you have or have you ever had any of the following?
   a. Rheumatoid arthritis
   b. Kidney disease
   c. Liver disease
   d. Diabetes
6. Do you get short of breath when you lie flat?
7. Are you currently on oxygen treatment?
8. Do you have a chronic cough that produces any discharge or fluid?
9. Do you have lung problems or diseases?
10. Have you or any blood member of your family ever had a problem with any anesthesia other than nausea?
    a. If yes, describe
11. If female, is it possible that you could be pregnant?
    a. Perform pregnancy test
    b. Please list date of last menstrual period

From Tremper KK, Benedict P: Paper "preoperative computer," Anesthesiology 92:1212–1213, 2000.

*University of Michigan Health System patient information report. Patients who answer yes to any of questions 2 through 9 should receive a more detailed clinical evaluation.

arrhythmia, and severe valvular disease (including severe aortic stenosis and symptomatic mitral stenosis).

Assessment of exercise tolerance in preoperative risk stratification and precise prediction of in-hospital perioperative risk is most applicable in patients who self-report worsening exercise-induced cardiopulmonary symptoms, patients who may benefit from noninvasive or invasive cardiac testing regardless of the scheduled surgical procedure, and patients with known CAD or with multiple risk factors and the ability to exercise. For the prediction of perioperative events, "poor" exercise tolerance has been defined as inability to walk four blocks and climb two flights of stairs or as inability to meet a metabolic equivalent (MET) level of 4 (Table 24-2). Highly functional symptomatic patients (i.e., those who are able to achieve a functional capacity ≥4 METS without symptoms, as when climbing a flight of stairs or running a short distance) rarely require noninvasive testing or intervention to lower the risk of noncardiac surgery.

If the patient has poor functional capacity or is symptomatic, physicians often use risk indices derived from empirical multivariable predictive models based on clinical assessment of risk factors to identify patients with elevated perioperative cardiac risk. Based on prospective comparison studies, the Revised Cardiac Risk Index (RCRI) is favored by many given its accuracy and simplicity (Table 24-3). A newer predictive model is the National Surgical Quality Improvement Program (NSQIP) risk calculator and is based on multiple clinical predictors. The RCRI relies on the presence or absence of six identifiable predictive factors: high-risk surgery (suprainguinal vascular, intrathoracic, or intraperitoneal surgery), ischemic heart disease, congestive heart failure (CHF), cerebrovascular disease, diabetes mellitus (requiring insulin therapy), and renal failure (with a serum creatinine concentration >2.0 mg/dL). Each of the RCRI clinical predictors, if present, is assigned 1 point. The risk for cardiac events (i.e., MI, pulmonary edema, ventricular fibrillation or primary cardiac arrest, and complete heart block) can then be predicted. A patient with an RCRI score of 0 has an estimated risk of 0.4% to 0.5% for major cardiac complications; the risk is 0.9% to 1.3% for someone with a score of 1, 4% to 6.6% with a score of 2, and 9% to 11% with a score of 3 (Fig. 24-1). Cardiac

risk particularly increases with the presence of two or more predictors and is greatest with three or more. The clinical utility of the RCRI is that it identifies patients who are at higher risk for cardiac complications and helps determine whether they may benefit from further risk stratification with noninvasive cardiac testing or from initiation of preoperative preventive medical management.

Preoperative Noninvasive Cardiac Testing for Risk Stratification

Evidence discourages widespread application of preoperative noninvasive cardiac testing for all patients. Rather, a selective approach based on clinical risk categorization appears to be both effective and cost-effective. No testing is recommended if it might delay surgical intervention for urgent or emergent conditions.

Coronary revascularization offers the potential benefit of identifying asymptomatic but high-risk patients—that is, patients

TABLE 24-3	REVISED CARDIAC RISK INDEX: CLINICAL MARKERS

1. High-risk surgical procedures
2. Ischemic heart disease
   a. History of myocardial infarction
   b. Current angina considered to be ischemic
   c. Requirement for sublingual nitroglycerin
   d. Positive exercise test
   e. Pathologic Q waves on ECG
   f. History of PTCA and/or CABG with current angina considered to be ischemic
3. Congestive heart failure
   a. Left ventricular failure by physical examination
   b. History of paroxysmal nocturnal dyspnea
   c. History of pulmonary edema
   d. S_3 gallop on cardiac auscultation
   e. Bilateral rales on pulmonary auscultation
   f. Pulmonary edema on chest radiography
4. Cerebrovascular disease
   a. History of transient ischemic attack
   b. History of cerebrovascular accident
5. Diabetes mellitus
   a. Treatment with insulin
6. Chronic renal insufficiency
   a. Serum creatinine concentration >2 mg/dL

Modified from Lee TH, Marcantonio ER, Mangione CM, et al: Derivation and prospective validation of a simple index for prediction of cardiac risk of major noncardiac surgery, Circulation 100:1043–1049, 1999.

CABG, Coronary artery bypass grafting; ECG, electrocardiogram; PTCA, percutaneous transluminal coronary angioplasty.

TABLE 24-2	FUNCTIONAL STATUS

EXCELLENT (ACTIVITIES REQUIRING >7 METS)

Carry 24 lb up eight steps
Carry objects that weigh 80 lb
Outdoor work (shovel snow, spade soil)
Recreation (ski, basketball, squash, handball, jog or walk 5 mph)

MODERATE (ACTIVITIES REQUIRING >4 BUT <7 METS)

Have sexual intercourse without stopping
Walk at 4 mph on level ground
Outdoor work (garden, rake, weed)
Recreation (roller-skate, dance, foxtrot)

POOR (ACTIVITIES REQUIRING <4 METS)

Shower/dress without stopping, strip and make bed, dust, wash dishes
Walk at 2.5 mph on level ground
Outdoor work (clean windows)
Recreation (golf, bowl)

Modified from Hlatky MA, Boineau RE, Higginbotham MB, et al: A brief self-administered questionnaire to determine functional capacity (the Duke Activity Status Index), Am J Cardiol 64:651–654, 1989.

MET, Metabolic equivalent.

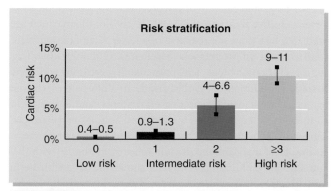

FIGURE 24-1 Bar graph shows the predicted risk for cardiac events during surgery according to a patient's Revised Cardiac Risk Index score.

with acute coronary syndromes, those with left main disease, those with two-vessel coronary disease who have significant proximal left anterior descending artery stenosis and either ischemia on noninvasive testing or reduced left ventricular ejection fraction, and those with three-vessel coronary vessel disease and an ejection fraction of less than 50%. Routine prophylactic coronary revascularization should not be performed in patients with stable CAD before noncardiac surgery. An RCRI score of 3 or higher in a patient with severe myocardial ischemia suggestive of left main or three-vessel disease should lead to consideration of coronary revascularization before noncardiac surgery in appropriate patients.

Noninvasive cardiac testing is most appropriate if it is anticipated that the patient will meet guidelines for initiation of additional medical therapy or coronary angiography and coronary revascularization in the event of a positive test. Noninvasive stress testing of patients with three or more clinical risk factors and poor functional capacity (<4 METS) who require vascular surgery is reasonable, provided that the result might change future management. When feasible, exercise stress testing is the modality of choice and offers the benefit of an objective assessment of functional capacity. Pharmacologic stress tests may be performed instead of exercise tests; they are typically reserved for patients with functional limitations.

Dobutamine echocardiography and nuclear perfusion testing for purposes of identifying patients at risk for perioperative MI or death have excellent negative predictive values (near 100%) but poor positive predictive values (<20%). Therefore, a negative study is reassuring, but a positive study is still only a weak predictor of a "hard" perioperative cardiac event. Which higher-risk patients are most likely to benefit from preoperative noninvasive cardiac testing and treatment strategies to improve outcomes is not well defined.

Choices of Noninvasive Cardiac Testing

The choice among noninvasive tests should be based on the need to assess valvular or ventricular function and on which test is most reliable and available locally. Dobutamine stress echocardiography is often used because it has excellent overall predictive performance and can provide additional information about valvular and left ventricular dysfunction.

In general, poor functional capacity associated with exercise-induced ischemia indicates a higher risk for perioperative cardiac events, and achievement of an excellent workload indicates a lower risk. The ability to attain 75% to 85% of the maximal age-predicted heart rate is predictive of a lower rate of perioperative cardiac events. In patients with baseline ECG abnormalities (e.g., left bundle branch block, left ventricular hypertrophy with repolarization abnormalities, Wolff-Parkinson-White pattern, changes secondary to digoxin therapy, paced rhythms) and in those with an inability to exercise due to comorbid conditions, pharmacologic stress echocardiography or nuclear imaging is preferred.

Studies of myocardial perfusion imaging methods (with thallium 201 and technetium 99m) have shown that reversible perfusion defects, which reflect jeopardized viable myocardium, confer the greatest risk for adverse perioperative outcomes. The uniformly high negative predictive value of a normal myocardial perfusion scan may make this technique particularly useful when

noninvasive testing is pursued. In most studies, fixed perfusion defects do not have significant predictive value for perioperative cardiac events. Coronary vasodilators (e.g., intravenous dipyridamole, adenosine, regadenoson), which induce a "coronary steal" phenomenon, are the preferred pharmacologic agents to use with radionuclide myocardial perfusion imaging.

With dobutamine stress echocardiography, the number of myocardial segments demonstrating wall motion abnormalities or wall motion changes at low dobutamine infusion rates identifies patients who are at higher risk for perioperative cardiac events. Dobutamine should be avoided in patients with significant arrhythmias, and coronary vasodilators are best avoided in those with significant bronchospasm.

Preoperative Invasive Cardiac Testing for Risk Stratification

Recommendations for perioperative coronary angiography are similar to those for patients with suspected or known CAD in general and should conform to the ACC/AHA guidelines for coronary angiography. This procedure should be considered for patients who are at high risk for adverse outcomes based on the presence of unstable angina, angina refractory to medical treatment, high-risk results on noninvasive testing, or a nondiagnostic test in a high-risk patient undergoing high-risk noncardiac surgery. It should be considered on an individual basis for those with extensive ischemia revealed during noninvasive testing, for those at intermediate risk undergoing high-risk surgery for whom test results are nondiagnostic, for those convalescing from MI who require urgent noncardiac surgery, and for those with perioperative MI. In patients who have a high clinical risk (RCRI >3) and high-risk features on noninvasive cardiac testing, diagnostic cardiac catheterization should be considered (see Fig. 24-1).

● PREOPERATIVE RISK MODIFICATION TO REDUCE PERIOPERATIVE CARDIAC RISK
Coronary Revascularization

Retrospective analyses of the Coronary Artery Surgery Study (CASS) registry and the Bypass Angioplasty Revascularization Investigation (BARI), along with prospective study of patients enrolled in the Coronary Artery Revascularization Prophylaxis (CARP) trial, have shown that prophylactic coronary revascularization with either coronary artery bypass grafting (CABG) or percutaneous coronary intervention (PCI) provides no short-term or mid-term benefit for patients without left main disease or multivessel CAD in the presence of poor left ventricular systolic function. Although high-risk patients who have successfully undergone PCI or CABG before elective noncardiac surgery do experience fewer adverse perioperative cardiovascular events compared with similar patients treated with medications alone, the mortality and morbidity associated with PCI or CABG appear to offset the potential benefit of coronary revascularization before any high-risk cardiac surgery (e.g., major vascular surgery). Therefore, evidence is lacking to support elective coronary revascularization as a primary strategy for perioperative risk reduction in intermediate-risk patients undergoing major noncardiac surgery.

Recommendations for PCI are similar to those for patients with suspected or known CAD and should conform to the ACC/AHA guidelines. Recommendations by the AHA/ACC Society for Cardiovascular Angiography and Intervention, the American College of Surgeons, and the American Dental Association Science Advisory Committee are for a 30- to 45-day delay of surgery in patients taking thienopyridine dual antiplatelet therapy after bare-metal coronary stent placement and a 365-day wait after placement of a drug-eluting stent. Some studies indicate that the duration of dual antiplatelet therapy may be shortened to less than 1 year in selected patients receiving newer-generation stents (such as everolimus- or zotarolimus-eluting stents). Individualized decisions about the duration of dual antiplatelet therapy are important, given that recommended timeframes for the use of such therapy are based primarily on expert opinion. If a patient needs to undergo noncardiac surgery within 2 to 6 weeks, drug-eluting stents should not be implanted; balloon angioplasty appears to be a reasonable alternative. If the noncardiac surgery is urgent or emergent, CABG combined with the noncardiac surgery may be considered; however, cardiac risks, the risk for bleeding, and the long-term benefit of coronary revascularization must be weighed.

Currently, studies suggest that optimal medical therapy is the preferred strategy for intermediate- to high-risk patients with RCRI scores of 2 or higher who are without documented severe myocardial ischemia. As stated previously, the CARP trial demonstrated that preoperative coronary revascularization strategies to reduce perioperative cardiovascular risk did not offer significant benefit compared with excellent medical treatment in intermediate- to high-risk patients undergoing vascular surgery. However, high-risk patients with left main coronary stenosis, severe aortic stenosis, left ventricular ejection fraction of 20% or less, or unstable coronary symptoms were excluded from that trial. In many of these patients, coronary or valve surgery may be indicated on its own merit, without factoring in the noncardiac surgery. Therefore, coronary revascularization may be appropriate if diagnostic catheterization reveals left main disease or multivessel disease and depressed ejection fraction.

Using the information obtained from the composite algorithm (Fig. 24-2), a key decision is whether the risk for perioperative cardiac events is sufficiently low to proceed with surgery. For patients identified to be at high cardiac risk who are not candidates for coronary revascularization, the physician may decide to perform a less extensive major plastic reconstruction, consider laparoscopic versus open procedures or alternative palliative procedures, or attempt to modify cardiac risk by additional intraoperative and perioperative therapies.

β-Adrenergic Antagonists

There is uncertainty about the effectiveness and safety of perioperative β-blockade in patients undergoing noncardiac surgery. The ACC/AHA guidelines focusing on recommendations for perioperative β-blocker therapy limit class I recommendations to patients undergoing surgery who are already receiving β-blockers to treat angina, symptomatic arrhythmias, or hypertension. Class IIb recommendations are given for the initiation of β-blocker therapy prior to surgery in those with intermediate- or high-risk myocardial ischemia noted on preoperative noninvasive

stress testing (level of evidence C) and patients with 3 or more RCRI risk factors (level of evidence B). European guidelines make explicit recommendations for the use of atenolol or bisoprolol when oral β-blockade is first introduced in patients undergoing noncardiac surgery.

The Perioperative Ischemic Evaluation (POISE) trial addressed the limitations of perioperative β-blockade. The POISE trial randomized 8351 intermediate- to high-risk patients older than 45 years of age to receive either a long-acting oral metoprolol succinate (metoprolol CR) or placebo. A high starting dose of metoprolol CR was administered: 100 mg was started orally 2 to 4 hours before surgery and continued for up to 6 hours after surgery and then daily for 30 days; alternatively, a slow intravenous infusion of 15 mg every 6 hours was administered until patients were able to receive the drug orally, after which oral administration was continued daily for 30 days. The medication was withheld if systolic blood pressure fell to less than 100 mm Hg or heart rate to less than 50 beats per minute. The results showed that the incidence of cardiac death, nonfatal MI, or cardiac arrest was reduced in the metoprolol group compared with placebo (5.8% versus 6.9%; hazard ratio = 0.84; 95% confidence interval [CI], 0.70 to 0.99; $P = .04$). However, there was an increased incidence of mortality and stroke in the metoprolol group compared with the placebo group (3.1% versus 2.3% [$P = .03$] and 1% versus 0.5% [$P = .005$], respectively,). Therefore, for every 1000 patients treated, metoprolol CR would prevent 11 MIs in intermediate- to high-risk patients undergoing major noncardiac surgery, but at a cost of 8 deaths and 5 disabling strokes. Stroke was associated with perioperative hypotension, bleeding, atrial fibrillation, and a history of stroke or transient ischemic attack. The POISE trialists highlighted the importance of a clear risk and benefit assessment for the initiation of preoperative β-blockers (see Fig. 24-2).

There remains a need for more precise, unambiguous practice recommendations for perioperative β-blockade. Preexisting β-blockade should be continued because withdrawal might increase perioperative mortality. If β-blockers are newly initiated in appropriately selected higher-risk patients undergoing noncardiac surgery, they should be carefully titrated and not abruptly initiated on a high-dose regimen to achieve the desired heart rate.

HMG-CoA Reductase Inhibitors (Statins)

Prospective and retrospective evidence supports the perioperative prophylactic use of 3-hydroxy-3-methylglutaryl–coenzyme A (HMG-CoA) reductase inhibitors (statins) for reduction of perioperative cardiac complications in patients with established atherosclerosis. Statins should be continued in patients who are already on statin therapy and undergoing noncardiac surgery. A class IIa indication is assigned to the use of statins for patients undergoing vascular surgery with or without clinical risk factors.

Calcium Channel Blockers

Evidence is lacking to support the use of calcium channel blockers as a prophylactic strategy to decrease perioperative risk in patients undergoing major noncardiac surgery.

Angiotensin-Converting Enzyme Inhibitors

Angiotensin-converting enzyme (ACE) inhibitors and angiotensin II–receptor antagonists are frequently prescribed for the

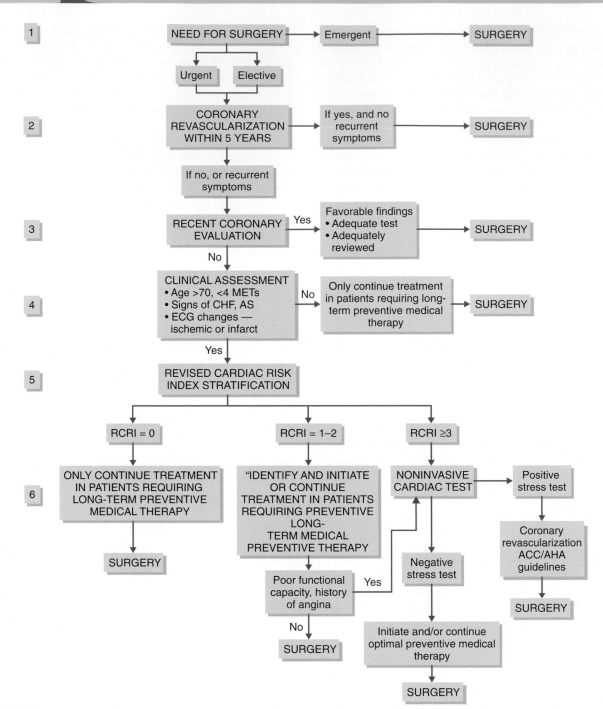

FIGURE 24-2 Stepwise clinical evaluation algorithm for diagnostic cardiac catheterization: (1) emergency surgery; (2) prior coronary revascularization; (3) prior coronary evaluation; (4) clinical assessment; (5) revised cardiac risk index; (6) risk modification strategies. Preventive medical therapy includes β-blocker and statin therapy. ACC, American College of Cardiology; AHA, American Heart Association; AS, aortic stenosis; CHF, congestive heart failure; ECG, electrocardiogram; MET, metabolic equivalent; RCRI, Revised Cardiac Risk Index.

management of hypertension, CHF, chronic renal failure, and ischemic heart disease. Evidence supports the discontinuation of these agents for 24 hours before noncardiac surgery because of adverse circulatory effects after induction of anesthesia in patients on a chronic ACE inhibitor regimen and use of vasopressin agonists for refractory hypotension after induction of anesthesia.

Oral Antithrombotic Agents

Evidence-based recommendations regarding perioperative use of aspirin, clopidogrel, or both to reduce cardiac risk currently lack

clarity. A substantial increase in perioperative bleeding and transfusion requirement in patients receiving dual antiplatelet therapy has been observed. The discontinuation of clopidogrel for 5 days and aspirin for 5 to 7 days before major surgery to minimize the risk of perioperative bleeding and transfusion must be balanced with the potentially increased risk for an acute coronary syndrome, especially in high-risk patients with recent coronary stent implantation. If clinicians elect to withhold aspirin before surgery, it should be restarted as soon as possible postoperatively, especially after vascular graft procedures.

INTRAOPERATIVE STRATEGIES FOR REDUCING PERIOPERATIVE RISK

Anesthetic Management

Epidural anesthesia and analgesia may improve the outcome of major noncardiac surgery through better suppression of surgical stress, a positive effect on postoperative nitrogen balance, more stable cardiovascular hemodynamic response, reduced blood loss, better peripheral vascular circulation, and better postoperative pain control. Overall, there is no preferred myocardium-protective agent, and decisions about anesthetic management should be part of a multidisciplinary effort led by an anesthesiologist. Whereas neuraxial anesthesia (epidural and spinal) may reduce pulmonary and thrombotic complications, its role in lowering cardiac complications is unclear. A technique of combined neuraxial blockade and general anesthesia has merit when indicated to reduce the intraoperative general anesthesia requirements.

Studies have demonstrated that pain management in the perioperative period is crucial for reducing cardiac risk. Adequate pain control reduces catecholamine surges, which are probably responsible for increased myocardial oxygen demand, induction of coronary vasospasm, increased tendency for plaque rupture, and development of a hypercoagulable state.

Intraoperative Pulmonary Artery Catheter

The current evidence on whether the use of a pulmonary artery catheter (PAC) is beneficial for high-risk patients undergoing major noncardiac surgery is controversial. Catheter-guided volume optimization has no clear benefit perioperatively. In a large multicenter randomized trial, Sandham and associates found no benefit for therapy directed by a PAC compared with standard care in elderly, high-risk surgical patients. Nonetheless, a PAC may be considered for patients with signs and symptoms of heart failure preoperatively, who have a very high postoperative incidence of heart failure, and for high-risk patients with limited ventricular reserve who are undergoing procedures that are likely to cause major hemodynamic shifts. Guideline recommendations advocate for evaluation of three parameters—patient disease, surgical procedure (and anticipated intraoperative and postoperative fluid shifts), and practice setting (experience in PAC use)—when considering the intraoperative and postoperative use of a PAC. Regarding practice setting, there is variability in provider understanding of invasive hemodynamic data, and incorrect interpretation of data from a PAC may lead to harm.

Intraoperative Transesophageal Echocardiography

Because ischemia-induced myocardial wall motion abnormalities appear earlier than ischemia-induced electric abnormalities, intraoperative transesophageal echocardiography (TEE) was proposed to be a more sensitive monitor of ischemia than conventional intraoperative 2-lead ECG. Similarly, 12-lead ECG monitoring was also proposed to have greater sensitivity than conventional intraoperative ECG. However, a comparison of intraoperative monitoring using 2-lead ECG versus routine monitoring for myocardial ischemia with TEE or 12-lead ECG during noncardiac surgery failed to provide robust evidence for incremental value in identifying patients at high risk for perioperative ischemic outcomes. Therefore, the routine use of intraoperative TEE is not recommended for monitoring and guiding therapy during noncardiac surgery, except in emergent scenarios in which the cause of an acute persistent and life-threatening hemodynamic instability needs to be determined.

Maintenance of Body Temperature during Noncardiac Surgery

Current ACC/AHA guidelines recommend maintenance of the patient's body temperature in a normothermic range rather than use of hypothermia to provide organ protection during surgical procedures. A retrospective analysis of a prospective randomized controlled trial demonstrated that hypothermia (core temperature $<35°C$) was associated with an increased risk for myocardial ischemia compared with a core temperature greater than or equal to $35°C$. A randomized controlled trial involving 300 high-risk patients undergoing noncardiac surgery in which patients were randomized to active warming or routine care demonstrated that adverse cardiac events (unstable angina, myocardial ischemia, cardiac arrest, and MI) occurred less frequently in the normothermic group than in the hypothermic group (1.4% versus 6.3%; $P = .02$). Furthermore, hypothermia was an independent predictor of adverse cardiac events by multivariable analysis (RR, 2.2; 95% CI, 1.1 to 4.7; $P = .04$), indicating a 55% reduction in risk when normothermia was maintained.

POSTOPERATIVE CARDIAC RISK ASSESSMENT

Monitoring for Myocardial Infarction

Although there are no standard criteria for their diagnosis, most perioperative MIs occur within the first 3 days after noncardiac surgery. A protocol involving ECG evaluation immediately after surgery and on postoperative days 1 and 2 has the highest sensitivity for detection of postoperative MI; routine serial measurements of creatine kinase and its CK-MB fraction led to high false-positive rates and did not increase the sensitivity. Myocardium-specific biomarkers such as troponin I and troponin T have emerged as the most sensitive and specific biochemical markers of myocardial injury and infarction and have been associated with increased risk for cardiac events if elevated in the postoperative period.

While EKG is recommended in the setting of signs or symptoms suggestive of myocardial ischemia, MI, or arrhythmia in the postoperative period, the usefulness of postoperative screening with ECGs is uncertain. Measurement of cardiac biomarkers should be reserved for patients at high risk and for those who demonstrate ECG changes, angina typical of acute coronary syndrome, or hemodynamic evidence of cardiovascular dysfunction.

Postoperative Risk Stratification and Management Strategies

Postoperative patient care involves assessment and treatment of modifiable cardiac risk factors, including hypertension, hyperlipidemia, smoking, obesity, hyperglycemia, and physical inactivity. Patients who sustain a perioperative MI or develop evidence of myocardial ischemia should be carefully investigated because

they are at substantial cardiac risk over the subsequent 5 to 10 years. Noninvasive testing to assess left ventricular function and inducible ischemia should be undertaken to identify patients who may benefit from revascularization or optimization of medical therapy. Postoperative heart failure and pulmonary edema should be treated similar to pulmonary edema in the non-operative setting.

NONCARDIAC SURGERY IN PATIENTS WITH SPECIFIC CARDIOVASCULAR CONDITIONS

Valvular Heart Disease

Special consideration has to be given in preoperative risk assessment for patients with valvular heart disease. All patients undergoing noncardiac surgery should be assessed especially for aortic stenosis by physical examination and by two-dimensional echocardiography for any suspicious murmur. One recent study demonstrated that patients with aortic stenosis have a fivefold increased risk for perioperative mortality and nonfatal MI compared to patients without aortic stenosis. Symptomatic severe represents an active cardiovascular condition that should be evaluated and managed before elective surgery is undertaken. Appropriately selected cases can be managed with valve replacement or valvuloplasty as a bridge to noncardiac surgery.

Less is known about the perioperative risks associated with mitral stenosis and mitral regurgitation in patients undergoing noncardiac surgery. Usually, a preoperative history and physical examination, chest radiograph, or ECG provides clues to the diagnosis, which can be confirmed by echocardiography. Accurate diagnosis may help optimize intraoperative anesthetic strategies, choice of pharmacologic interventions and invasive monitoring, and postoperative medical management. Heart rate should be controlled to ensure a sufficient diastolic filling period and to avoid pulmonary congestion in patients with mild to moderate mitral stenosis. Patients with severe mitral stenosis are likely to benefit from balloon mitral valvuloplasty or surgical intervention before high-risk surgery.

Patients with aortic or mitral valvular regurgitation benefit from volume control and afterload reduction. In aortic insufficiency, it is thought that faster heart rates are better tolerated than slow ones because slow heart rates lead to increased diastolic filling and can exacerbate left ventricular volume overload.

Except for perioperative antibiotic prophylaxis to prevent bacterial endocarditis and the need for effective anticoagulation strategies, perioperative complications in patients with prosthetic heart valves are probably similar to those in patients with comparable degrees of native valvular heart disease. In patients with a mechanical valve prosthesis, the recommendations for anticoagulation are as follows. For patients requiring minimally invasive procedures (i.e., dental procedures, superficial plastic surgery, and biopsies), the international normalized ratio (INR) should be reduced briefly to the low or subtherapeutic range, with the normal dose of oral anticoagulation resumed promptly after the procedure. For those patients in whom the risk of bleeding with oral anticoagulation is high and the risk for thromboembolism without anticoagulation is also high (e.g., mechanical valve in the mitral position, history of thromboembolism while not on anticoagulation, Bjork-Shiley or Starr-Edwards valve, known

hypercoagulability, atrial fibrillation), perioperative unfractionated heparin is recommended. Patients between these two extremes should undergo individual assessment for the risk and benefit of reduced anticoagulation with warfarin versus perioperative heparin initiation and brief interruption perioperatively. The use of low-molecular-weight heparin may be a feasible alternative in appropriately selected patients who require heparin conversion, although there is still controversy about its use for this indication.

Arrhythmias and Conduction Defects

Ventricular and atrial arrhythmias historically are recognized as predictors of perioperative cardiac complications. Therefore, identification of a preoperative arrhythmia warrants a careful evaluation for the presence and severity of underlying ischemic heart disease, cardiomyopathy, or other conditions that may contribute to perioperative complications. In general, asymptomatic arrhythmias or conduction defects warrant only observation and maintenance of an optimal metabolic state. Although new-onset atrial fibrillation raises embolic risk, most cases of postoperative atrial fibrillation resolve within 36 to 48 hours. Short-term rhythm management and anticoagulation may be justified for postoperative atrial fibrillation. Electrical cardioversion is the procedure of choice for supraventricular tachycardia associated with hemodynamic compromise.

Congestive Heart Failure and Left Ventricular Dysfunction

CHF has been identified as a significant marker of cardiac risk in noncardiac surgery. Every effort should be made to identify the etiology of CHF and optimally control it preoperatively because it is a known risk factor for postoperative cardiac complications. However, there are no evidence-based recommendations for optimal perioperative strategy in patients with heart failure undergoing intermediate- to high-risk noncardiac surgery other than making sure that they are taking medications known to improve heart failure in the long-term. Because proper treatment of heart failure depends greatly on its underlying etiology (especially systolic dysfunction versus diastolic dysfunction), characterization of this etiology before elective noncardiac surgery can help in tailoring therapy to each patient. Close monitoring of volume status is needed to avoid perioperative decompensation. Intravenous inotropic agents, vasodilators, or both may be useful for a short duration in the perioperative period to prevent or treat CHF, depending on the situation.

Hypertrophic Cardiomyopathy

Patients with echocardiographically documented hypertrophic cardiomyopathy (HCM) are at risk for exacerbation of dynamic left ventricular outflow tract (LVOT) obstruction during periods of tachycardia, hypotension, or increased inotropy. General anesthesia or neuraxial block can lead to peripheral vasodilation and sympathetic autonomic blockade that may decrease venous return and further exacerbate LVOT obstruction. Observational studies of patients with HCM undergoing noncardiac surgery suggest that for most operations, patients with compensated HCM tolerate the perioperative period well. Perioperative cardiac risk reduction strategies should include avoidance of hypovolemia, vasodilators, phosphodiesterase inhibitors, and β-adrenergic agonists as well as diligent attention to volume repletion and selective use of α-adrenergic agonists. Patients with HCM are at significant risk for development of perioperative hypotension, CHF, and arrhythmias and should be monitored closely.

Congenital Heart Disease

Studies have demonstrated that patients who have left-to-right cardiac shunts with residual hemodynamic abnormalities after surgical repair experience decreased cardiac output in response to stress. Vigorous treatment of ongoing CHF is required for such patients before noncardiac surgery. Patients with a large left-to-right shunt but only a slight increase in pulmonary artery resistance should undergo cardiac repair before noncardiac surgery. Patients with irreversible pulmonary artery hypertension have an extremely high risk associated with noncardiac procedures and should not undergo such procedures unless there is absolutely no alternative. Patients with prior repair of coarctation of the aorta have a significant risk for sudden death during follow-up, caused by residual cardiac defects with CHF, rupture of a major vessel, dissecting aneurysm, or complications arising from severe atherosclerosis. Such patients also have a high incidence of residual hypertension. Therefore, these patients require careful preoperative assessment and close hemodynamic monitoring during the intraoperative and postoperative periods. Patients with tetralogy of Fallot are also prone to sudden cardiac death. Monitoring and aggressive prevention and treatment of life-threatening arrhythmias such as ventricular tachycardia or atrioventricular block are needed for such patients in the perioperative period.

Surgery in patients with cyanotic congenital heart disease and right-to-left shunts poses several unique problems. Most cyanotic patients are polycythemic and therefore prone to thrombotic complications. Use of diuretics should be avoided in such patients because dehydration may increase blood viscosity, which increases the tendency for thrombosis, particularly cerebral thrombosis. Patients with a hematocrit greater than 70% should be considered for plasmapheresis before noncardiac surgery. Phlebotomy is not advisable in this circumstance because it can decrease intravascular blood volume and thus increase cyanosis. Patients with a hematocrit between 55% and 65% should receive intravenous fluids starting the night before the surgery. Patients with congenital heart disease should also receive appropriate prophylaxis for bacterial endocarditis. One retrospective report suggested that, with careful monitoring and precautions as outlined previously, and with careful attention not to introduce air into the vascular system, patients with right-to-left shunts can undergo noncardiac surgery with relatively few complications.

⬤ SUMMARY

CAD accounts for most deaths in patients undergoing noncardiac surgery, and perioperative MI is associated with high mortality rates in these patients. The success of standardized evidence-based preoperative and postoperative cardiac risk reduction strategies in patients undergoing noncardiac surgery depends on collaborative teamwork and sound communication among surgeons, the anesthesiologist, the patient's primary care physician, and the consultant.

The risk for a perioperative cardiac complication varies with the severity of the surgical procedure and with RCRI stratification. A systematic, stepwise approach for preoperative cardiac risk assessment in patients undergoing noncardiac surgery facilitates a decision as to whether the risk for perioperative cardiac events is sufficiently low to proceed with the surgery. Active cardiovascular conditions, including severe aortic stenosis and symptomatic mitral stenosis, may need to be addressed preoperatively. Preoperative noninvasive cardiac testing should be based on a discrete clinical risk categorization, and the choice among noninvasive tests should be based on the need for coronary, valvular, or ventricular function assessment and which test is most reliable and available locally. Preoperative noninvasive cardiac testing should be considered if the results of such testing could inform the decision for angiography or modify management, regardless of the planned surgery.

Although unambiguous practice recommendations for the use of perioperative β-blockade are lacking, preexisting therapy with β-blockers should not be withdrawn, and newly initiated and titrated therapy may be beneficial in appropriately selected higher-risk patients.

Optimal postoperative patient care involves assessment and treatment of modifiable cardiac risk factors, including pain, hypertension, hyperlipidemia, smoking, obesity, hyperglycemia, and physical inactivity. Finally, patients who sustain a nonfatal perioperative MI or develop evidence of ischemia should be carefully investigated because they are at substantial cardiac risk over the subsequent months and years.

> *For a deeper discussion on this topic, please see Chapters 431, "Preoperative Evaluation," and 433, "Postoperative Care and Complications," in* Goldman-Cecil Medicine, *25th Edition.*

SUGGESTED READINGS

Auerbach A, Goldman L: Assessing and reducing the cardiac risk of noncardiac surgery, Circulation 113:1361–1376, 2006.

Boersma E, Kertai MD, Schouten O, et al: Perioperative cardiovascular mortality in noncardiac surgery: validation of the Lee cardiac risk index, Am J Med 118:1134–1141, 2005.

Fleisher LA, Fleischmann KE, Auerbach AD, et al: 2014 ACC/AHA guideline on perioperative cardiovascular evaluation and management of patients undergoing noncardiac surgery: a report of the American College of Cardiology/American Heart Association Task Force on practice guidelines, J Am Coll Cardiol S0735–1097(14)05536–3, 2014.

Hassan SA, Hlatky MA, Boothroyd DB, et al: Outcomes of noncardiac surgery after coronary bypass surgery or coronary angioplasty in the Bypass Angioplasty Revascularization Investigation (BARI), Am J Med 110:260–266, 2001.

Kristensen SD, Knuuti J, Saraste A, et al: 2014 ESC/ESA guidelines on noncardiac surgery: cardiovascular assessment and management: The Joint Task Force on Non-Cardiac Surgery: cardiovascular assessment and management of the European Society of Cardiology (ESC) and the European Society of Anesthesiology (ESA), Eur Heart J 35(35):2382–2431, 2014.

McFalls EO, Ward HB, Moritz TE, et al: Coronary-artery revascularization before elective major vascular surgery, N Engl J Med 351:2795–2804, 2004.

POISE Study Group: Effects of extended-release metoprolol succinate in patients undergoing non-cardiac surgery (POISE trial): a randomized controlled trial, Lancet 371:1839–1847, 2008.

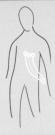

V

Renal Disease

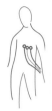

25

Renal Structure and Function

Orson W. Moe and Javier A. Neyra

INTRODUCTION

The kidney maintains the composition and quantity of body fluids, and its failure is manifested by dysfunction of multiple organs. Chronic kidney disease is approaching epidemic proportions worldwide, and acute kidney injury in the inpatient setting affects a very high percentage of hospital admissions with a high mortality rate. The etiologies of these conditions are very diverse. In addition to loss of glomerular filtration, kidney diseases include hypertension, urolithiasis, and a host of electrolyte disorders that do not affect the glomerular filtration rate (GFR) but nonetheless cause significant morbidity and mortality. To understand these conditions, a thorough knowledge of the anatomy and function of the kidney is requisite.

Approximately 25% of the cardiac output is distributed to the kidneys, where the blood is continuously cleansed. In addition to excretion, the kidney is an important metabolic organ and a source of endocrine molecules. Renal failure represents a disruption of all three of these functions. Selected aspects of renal structure and function are reviewed briefly in this chapter to set the foundation for the subsequent chapters that deal with specific renal diseases.

RENAL STRUCTURE

Macroscopic Anatomy

The kidneys are seated against the posterior wall of the abdomen in the retroperitoneal space, making them readily accessible for percutaneous biopsy. The lower poles may be palpable on deep inspiration in a lean individual. Each human kidney weighs about 120 to 170 g; is about 11 cm long, 6 cm wide, and 3 cm thick; and is endowed with approximately 1 million nephrons. There are interindividual variations. The "kidney size" commonly referred to in clinical sonographic reports is actually the cephalocaudal renal length, which is not a perfect surrogate for renal volume and mass.

The kidney is surrounded by a fibrous capsule. The renal arteries enter the kidney and the renal vein and ureters leave the kidney in the renal pelvis. The bisected surface consists of the lighter-colored outer *cortex* and the darker inner *medulla* (Fig. 25-1). A sample from a clinical biopsy typically originates from the cortex in the lower pole. The medulla is divided into outer and inner regions, and the outer medulla is subdivided into outer and inner stripes. The medulla has multiple conical contours, called *pyramids*, with their apices abutting on the renal pelvis as papillae. The contact points of the renal pelvis with the renal papillae are cup-like structures called *calyces*. Interpolated between the pyramids are centripetal extensions of cortical tissue called *columns of Bertin*.

Renal Circulation

Each kidney receives blood from a single renal artery, although supernumerary arteries are present in up to one third of individuals. Just before or after the renal artery enters the kidney, it divides into interlobar arteries that pass between the pyramids of the kidney radially up the columns of Bertin (see Fig. 25-1A). The interlobar arteries further divide into arcuate arteries which arch along the corticomedullary junction (see Fig. 25-1B). Arcuate arteries give rise to cortical ascending arteries, which bring blood to the glomeruli. Afferent arterioles ramify into glomerular capillaries, distributing blood to individual glomeruli. Features of the renal circulation are summarized in Table 25-1.

The glomerular capillary is the site for glomerular ultrafiltration. Even though the efferent arteriole is downstream from the glomerular capillary, it is not a venule because it has arteriolar walls and is upstream of the second capillary system surrounding the tubules. The peritubular capillaries provide oxygen and nutrients for the kidney, collect the fluid and solutes reabsorbed by tubules to return into the circulation, and deliver the solutes to be secreted by tubule into the tubule fluid. The peritubular capillaries surrounding the cortical and juxtamedullary nephrons originate from the efferent arterioles of cortical and juxtamedullary glomeruli, respectively.

The vessels that run parallel to loops of Henle are called *vasa recta* (see Fig. 25-1D) because of their long, straight structures. Blood from the peritubular capillaries is returned to the circulation by a venous system that mirrors the architectural structure of the arterial supply: interlobular vein, arcuate vein, interlobar vein, and renal vein. The parallel countercurrent nature of the vasculature provides the basis for the very high medullar tonicity, which allows urine concentration but also direct arteriovenous diffusion of oxygen, giving rise to the very low oxygen tension in the medulla. This low oxygen tension renders the kidney prone to ischemic injury, which is one of the most common causes of acute kidney injury (see Chapter 31).

Renal Nerves

The capsules of the kidney and the ureters have pain fibers derived from splanchnic nerves. This explains the costovertebral angle pain that occurs when the kidneys are inflamed and during renal colic. The renal parenchyma does not have pain fibers but is richly innervated with sympathetic nerves that enter the renal parenchyma with the renal artery. The sympathetic nerves abut on the arterioles (see Fig. 25-1C), stimulate renin release,

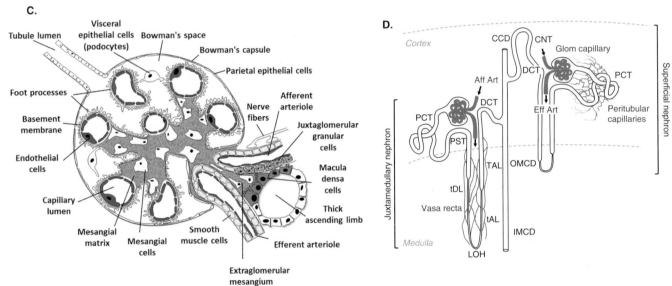

FIGURE 25-1 **A,** Gross anatomy of the kidney. **B,** Schematic representation of the vasculature within a column of Bertin. **C,** Structural components of the glomerulus. **D,** Schematic representation of a superficial and a juxtamedullary nephron based on the location of their glomeruli. The tubules are intimately intertwined with the capillary system. The peritubular capillaries come off the efferent arteriole leaving the glomerular capillary. The capillaries that bathe the long descending and ascending limbs of Henle's loop are called the vasa recta due to their straight nature. The tubular segments are named axially: CCD, Cortical collecting duct; CNT, connecting tubule; DCT, distal convoluted tubule; IMCD, inner medullary collecting duct; LOH, loop of Henle; OMCD, outer medullary collecting duct; PCT, proximal convoluted tubule; PST, proximal straight tubule; TAL, thick ascending limb; tAL, thin ascending limb; tDL, thin descending limb.

TABLE 25-1	CHARACTERISTICS OF THE RENAL CIRCULATION
FEATURE	**IMPLICATIONS**
Few or no anastomoses	Very prone to regional disruption of blood supply
Among the highest blood flow rates per gram of tissue	Lowest oxygen extraction (lowest arteriovenous O_2 difference)
Functional arteriovenous shunts	Solutes and gases (e.g., O_2) can diffuse directly from artery to vein without passing through capillaries
Two capillary systems in tandem	The two capillaries serve completely different functions, in the glomeruli and tubules in sequence

decrease renal blood flow, and promote renal retention of sodium (Na^+). Renal sympathetic denervation has been proposed as a novel treatment of resistant hypertension using radiofrequency energy delivered via an intrarenal arterial catheter radially to disrupt the nerve fibers on the renal artery.

Walk the Nephron

The functional unit of the kidney is the nephron. Each human kidney has approximately 1 million nephrons. Approximately 30% of these have their glomeruli situated deep in the cortex and are referred to as *juxtamedullary nephrons*; the rest are in the outer cortex and are referred to as *superficial nephrons*. Each nephron is a glomerulus followed by a tubule. The surrounding capillaries and the interstitial space are also important functional components of the nephron.

Glomerulus

The glomerulus consists of the glomerular vasculature (arterioles and capillaries) supported by the mesangium (mesangial cells and matrix) inside Bowman's capsule (parietal and visceral epithelial cells) (see Fig. 25-1C). The visceral cells of Bowman's capsule are the podocytes, so named because of their numerous "foot processes." The smooth muscle layers of the afferent and efferent arterioles are critical in determining arteriolar tone. The glomerular capillary contacts the mesangium on one side and is separated from the foot processes of the podocyte on the opposite side by the glomerular basement membrane (GBM). The glomerulus filters large volumes of water and solutes while retaining most of the proteins and all of the cells in the blood. The glomerular filtration barrier is composed of the capillary endothelium, the GBM, and the podocyte slit diaphragm.

Lining the inside of the GBM is a single layer of fenestrated endothelial cells. The fenestrations (50 to 100 nm in diameter) provide a barrier to negatively charged large molecules in the blood. The GBM contains laminin, type IV collagen, nidogen, and proteoglycans that restrict movement of large molecules (e.g., albumin) from the capillary into Bowman's space. The GBM contains dense negative charges due to glycoproteins with sialic acid residues that restrict the passage of anionic plasma solutes. It can be the site of deposition of immunocomplexes that cause glomerulonephritis (e.g., membranous glomerulonephritis, lupus nephritis). Autoantibodies to the GBM cause severe inflammation and loss of filtration. The epithelial layer consists of podocytes and the parietal epithelium, which is flat and squamous with very few organelles. At the vascular pole, the parietal epithelium is contiguous with a completely different epithelium—the proximal convoluted tubule.

On the visceral side of Bowman's space are the podocytes, which constitute the outermost layer of the filtration barrier. These cells have a highly interdigitating system of foot processes that rest against the basement membrane. The podocyte cell bodies lie within the extracellular matrix. The spaces between foot processes are filtration slits approximately 40 nm in diameter; they are bridged by slit diaphragms, which are also negatively charged, contributing to the containment of middle-size negatively charged particles in the capillary. In the last decade, there have been momentous advances in identifying the components of the slit diaphragm complex and understanding their functions. A full discussion is not possible here, but major slit diaphragm–associated proteins include nephrin, podocin, neph-1/2/3, FAT-1, R-cadherin, catenin, CD2AP, ZO-1, and α-actinin 4. Mutations of many of these genes cause congenital nephrotic syndrome (see Chapter 28).

Tubules

The parietal epithelium of Bowman's capsule becomes the renal tubule (see Fig. 25-1D) as it leaves the glomerulus. The renal tubule is a prototypical polarized epithelium. Its salient characteristics are summarized in Figure 25-2. A simple cylinder would not suffice in terms of surface area for transport. In the luminal apical membrane, surface amplification is achieved either by protrusions or by a more extensive form of protrusions called the *brush border* in the proximal tubule. Between cells are structures called *tight junctions*. Although they are called tight junctions, some are truly tight (with high resistance to solute and charge movement), whereas others can be quite leaky to solutes. In addition to resistance, these complexes also regulate whether the junction is more permeable to one ion type compared with another (relative and selective permeability). On the other side of the tight junction is the intercellular space, which is contiguous with the interstitial space. The basolateral cell membrane on the interstitial-capillary side amplifies its surface area by infoldings into the cell and interdigitations between two cells.

The movement of a solute can be through a cell (transcellular transport) or around the cell (paracellular transport) (see Fig. 25-2A). Solute transport is an energy-consuming process that requires metabolic fuels. There are many kinds of transport proteins (see Fig. 25-2B). ATPases directly couple hydrolysis of adenosine triphosphate (ATP) to transport. Cotransporters (symporters) move two solutes in the same direction, and countertransporters (antiporters) move two different solutes in opposite directions. Channels function as protein-lined "holes" that allows specific solutes to permeate. Different transporters can also be coupled together to form a new transport system. Finally, there are proteins that protrude outside the cell in the junctional area to provide a conduit for paracellular transport.

Specialized Structures

Interstitium

The space between the tubules and peritubular capillaries constitutes about 5% to 10% of renal volume and harbors interstitial fibroblasts and dendritic cells. In diseases such as interstitial nephritis (see Chapter 29), the interstitium is full of inflammatory cells, which elaborate cytokines and chemokines that profoundly affect filtration and tubular function. The resident fibroblasts are stellate cells with projections that physically contact tubules and capillaries, provide scaffold support, and secrete and maintain matrix. In pathologic conditions, these cells, when stimulated by cytokines, can transform into myofibroblasts and contribute to interstitial fibrosis. Some specialized fibroblasts in the deep cortex are sensors of oxygen and producers of circulating erythropoietin. The dendritic cells are antigen-presenting cells that express major histocompatibility complex (MHC) class II molecules. They are in intimate communication with the renal parenchyma, constantly sampling and responding to the local antigenic environment. Dendritic cells are involved with innate and adaptive immunity and are major players in immunologic homeostasis and diseases of the renal parenchyma.

Juxtaglomerular Apparatus

A unique feature of the nephron is that each thick ascending limb traverses back to and engages in physical contact with its parent glomerulus. The tubular cell at the point of contact is different from the rest of the thick ascending limb and is called the *macula densa*. The tripartite structure comprising the macula densa, the afferent and efferent glomerular arterioles, and the extraglomerular mesangium, a special part of the mesangium that protrudes

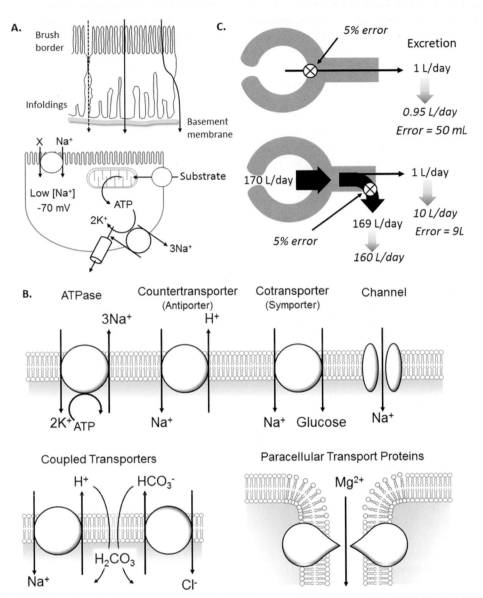

FIGURE 25-2 **A,** *Top,* Transcellular and paracellular transport of solutes. Solute transport is an energy-consuming process that requires metabolic fuels; a sodium cotransporter and a sodium-potassium countertransporter are shown. **B,** Transport proteins. *Top,* Adenosine triphosphatases (ATPases) directly couple ATP hydrolysis to transport. Cotransporters (symporters) move two solutes in the same direction, and countertransporters (antiporters) move two different solutes in opposite directions. Channels function as protein-lined "holes" that allow specific solutes to permeate. *Lower left,* Different transporters can be coupled together to form a new transport system. *Lower right,* Proteins that protrude outside the cell in the junctional area provide a conduit for paracellular transport. **C,** Comparison of a pure filtration (or secretion) design *(top)* and a filtration-reabsorption design *(bottom).* See text for details.

outside the glomerulus, is called the *juxtaglomerular apparatus* (JGA) (see Fig. 25-1C). The JGA is an important structure in the maintenance of GFR by tubuloglomerular feedback and is the site of endocrine renin production.

⬤ RENAL FUNCTION

Excretory Function

Renal excretion of a substance can be mediated and modified by one or a combination of three processes: filtration, secretion, and reabsorption. Figure 25-2C compares two designs—pure filtration (or secretion) and filtration-reabsorption—and their implications in terms of demands on regulation. The

filtration-reabsorption mechanism allows high filtration rates to be achieved, and the coupling with reabsorption prevents loss of valuable fluid and electrolytes. This design also enables economy in transport mechanisms through adaptive targeting of key solutes while allowing the rest to be excreted. However, there is a metabolic price to be paid for this configuration. Consider the excretion of 1 L/day by pure filtration (or secretion). If there is a 5% error (reduction in filtration or secretion), only 0.95 L/day will be excreted—a difference of 50 mL. Compare this to a filtration-reabsorption mechanism wherein 170 L/day is filtered and 169 L/day is reabsorbed, resulting in 1 L/day excretion. A 5% error (reduction) in reabsorption would result in reabsorption of 160 L/day and excretion of 10 L/day, with an absolute error of 9 L. One consequence of a filtration-reabsorption design is that regulation has to have exquisite fidelity, and even small errors are not tolerated.

Filtration

Filtration occurs exclusively at the glomerulus. The GFR, measured as volume per unit time, has been the standard quantitative surrogate for overall kidney function, although there are many disturbances of renal function that are not associated with a decrease in GFR (e.g., nephrotic syndrome, tubulointerstitial disorders, kidney stones). Numerically, GFR can be conceptualized as an equation:

$$GFR = K_f \times (\Delta P - \Delta \Pi)$$

where the ultrafiltration coefficient, K_f, is equal to the surface area for filtration multiplied by the hydraulic permeability; the hydrostatic driving force, ΔP, is the pressure gradient between the glomerular capillary and Bowman's space, which drives fluid to go into Bowman's space to form urine; and the osmotic driving force, $\Delta \Pi$, is the osmotic pressure gradient between the glomerular capillary and Bowman's space, which holds fluid back in the capillary and slows down filtration.

Many renal diseases affect the determinants of GFR. Glomerular disease (see Chapter 28) decreases K_f by affecting both the surface area for filtration and the hydraulic permeability.

Changes in ΔP are commonly involved in diseases that reduce GFR. Changes in renal blood flow and more importantly in afferent and efferent arteriolar resistances can drastically affect ΔP and GFR. Functional changes in ΔP, such as prerenal failure from hypoperfusion or hepatorenal syndrome (see Chapter 31), can radically lower GFR simply by hemodynamic changes without any structural glomerular lesions. Changes in $\Delta \Pi$ also can affect GFR but have not been studied in as much detail.

Reabsorption

High GFR, which is required to maintain a high metabolic rate, can be sustained only if there is high reclamation to maintain intravascular volume and prevent circulatory collapse. Tubular reabsorption thwarts the loss of valuable solutes and allows for finer tuning of the water and solutes not reabsorbed. The resulting tubular contents are excreted. In the mammalian kidney, tubular reabsorption assumes critical roles in the regulation of excretion of many solutes (Table 25-2). A universal mechanism of reabsorption is energy-dependent transepithelial transport, which is mostly Na^+ dependent but can be Na^+ independent. The proximal tubules participate in the reabsorption of all solutes, but some solutes are sequentially reabsorbed by the proximal and distal segments; in these cases, the generic design tends to be high-capacity reabsorption proximally and more of a high-gradient reabsorption for fine tuning distally. The axial difference

TABLE 25-2   SOLUTE EXCRETION

SOLUTE	FILTRATION	REABSORPTION	SECRETION	FE (%)	REGULATION
Water	Yes	Yes	No	0.3-6.0	Responds primarily to body tonicity but also EABV. ADH is the major regulator of collecting duct water permeability.
Na^+	Yes	Yes	No	0.2-2.0	Responds to EABV. Reabsorption is stimulated by sympathetic nerves, angiotensin II, aldosterone; inhibited by atrial natriuretic peptides, dopamine, uroguanylin.
K^+	Yes	Yes	Yes	5-20	Responds to total body potassium status. Secretion is controlled primarily by aldosterone and distal Na^+ delivery.
Ca^{2+}	Yes	Yes	No	2-10	Responds to serum ionized $[Ca^{2+}]$ and body need for calcium. Major calciotropic hormones include parathyroid hormone, vitamin D, and calcitonin. Renal epithelia directly respond to ionized calcium via the calcium sensing receptor.
Mg^{2+}	Yes	Yes	No	3-5	Responds to total body magnesium status and requirements. Paracrine regulation is via epidermal growth factor.
HCO_3^-	Yes	Yes	Yes	0.1-0.5	Most bicarbonate reabsorption is to reclaim the filtered load. Responds to systemic acid-base status which can be mediated by direct sensing by the renal epithelia or via hormonal actions (e.g., angiotensin II, endothelin). Bicarbonate can also be secreted in the collecting duct when alkali excretion is required.
Phosphate	Yes	Yes	No	5-20	Responds to serum phosphate concentration and body phosphate status. Reabsorption primarily resides in the proximal tubule and is regulated by parathyroid hormone and fibroblast growth factor-23.
Glucose	Yes	Yes	No	0.2-0.5	The proximal tubule reclaims almost all filtered glucose except when the filtered load exceeds reabsorptive capacity. The cortical proximal tubule performs gluconeogenesis from other organic substrates.
Uric acid	Yes	Yes	Yes	10-50	Major routes of uric acid clearance are (1) renal excretion and (2) intestinal secretion and uricolysis. Handling of both secretion and reabsorption in the proximal tubule is complex, and regulatory mechanisms are unclear.
Creatinine	Yes	No	Yes	1.0-1.2	Filtered at the glomerulus and secreted by the proximal tubule. The contribution of the tubules to creatinine clearance increases when GFR declines.

ADH, Antidiuretic hormone; EABV, effective arterial blood volume; FE, fractional excretion under normal physiology.

can occur within the same nephron segment (e.g., early vs. late proximal tubule) or across different segments (e.g., proximal vs. distal nephron segments).

Secretion

Secretion is an ancient mode of excretion that is found in lower-order organisms. Although the human nephron is not primarily secretory in nature, a number of solutes are still handled by secretion. For example, the renal excretion of potassium (K^+) and hydrogen (H^+) ions is largely achieved by secretion. Many organic cations and anions are secreted by the proximal tubule, and so are many exogenous toxins such as xenobiotics. The secretion of creatinine by organic cation transporters in the proximal tubule is the reason why creatinine clearance overestimates GFR.

Integrated Models of Excretion

The modes of excretion are well coordinated in a precise, complex, and concerted fashion to effect excretion with exquisite accuracy (see Table 25-2). The kidney is capable of a large range of urinary tonicity (<50 to 1200 mOsm), depending on the need of the organism to excrete or conserve electrolyte-free water. Water is filtered at the glomerulus and is handled isotonically in the proximal tubule. At the lumen of the distal convoluted tubule, urine is maximally dilute as a consequence of low water permeability throughout the thick ascending limb of Henle. The subsequent fate of the urine determines whether there is electrolyte-free water excretion (dilute urine), achieved by low water permeability of the collecting duct, or electrolyte-free water conservation (concentrated urine), effected by the action of antidiuretic hormone (ADH), which renders the collecting tubule permeable to water.

Na$^+$ homeostasis basically occurs via filtration-reabsorption; it is regulated by changes in effective arterial blood volume (EABV) mediated by neurohormonal afferent signals that act directly on tubules. In the proximal tubule, Na$^+$ reabsorption is also regulated by peritubular physical factors. K$^+$ undergoes an interesting sequence in which the filtered load is largely reabsorbed in the proximal tubule and the thick ascending limb; the final determinant of excretion is secretion by the collecting duct, for which aldosterone and distal Na$^+$ delivery are major regulators.

Only Ca^{2+} that is not bound to plasma protein is filtered; it is reabsorbed largely via paracellular pathways in the proximal tubule and thick ascending limb and via transcellular pathways in the distal convoluted tubule.

A massive amount of bicarbonate (HCO_3^-) is filtered and must be reclaimed to forestall catastrophic acidosis. H$^+$ secretion provides the mechanism for HCO_3^- reclamation as well as acid excretion, with the H$^+$ being carried by urinary buffers such as ammonia.

Metabolic Function

The kidney is a major metabolic organ. It consumes a wide range of fuels, regulates plasma levels of metabolic substrates, and is a major source of gluconeogenesis. Metabolic substrates such as amino acids, glucose, organic anions, and fatty acids are converted to ATP, the universal energy unit for all cells (see Fig. 25-2A). ATP is directly hydrolyzed by transport proteins such as Na$^+$/K$^+$-ATPase to create a low intracellular Na$^+$ concentration

($[Na^+]$) and a negative interior cell voltage, thus translating the energy into chemical gradients. About 80% to 90% of the oxygen consumption of the kidney can be attributed to Na$^+$ transport. For example, a protein such as the Na$^+$-glucose cotransporter (see Fig. 25-2B) on the luminal membrane couples the movement of one Na$^+$ ion to one glucose molecule (carrying a net positive charge). The low cell $[Na^+]$ and negative voltage energize glucose uptake, allowing the proximal tubule to capture most of the filtered glucose that otherwise would be lost in the urine. In normal physiology, this glucose reclamation is beneficial.

The amount of filtered organic molecules far exceeds the metabolic consumption by the kidney. Very large amounts of organic metabolic substrates are passively filtered daily; these substrates are not meant to be excreted, but the high GFR and lack of retention at the glomerular capillaries obligate their presence in the glomerular urine. In the proximal tubule, the bulk of the filtered organic molecules are reclaimed from the urine and returned to the systemic circulation. Several thousands of millimoles of amino acids, glucose, and organic cations and anions are retrieved each day by the kidney from the urine.

The kidney rivals the liver as a gluconeogenic organ that sustains circulating blood glucose levels. Although there is no doubt that this is an critical physiologic function, there are no clinical examples of hypoglycemia stemming purely from lack of renal gluconeogenesis.

Endocrine Function

In addition to the prominent and more obvious roles in solute and water balance, the kidney also is an important endocrine organ. The autocrine and paracrine substances elaborated by the kidney are important for both intrarenal and systemic regulation. Although this subject is not addressed fully here, three of these substances are highlighted because they represent important pharmacologic targets (Table 25-3).

Renin

As the initiating component of the renin-angiotensin-aldosterone system (RAAS), renin is important for maintenance of the integrity of the circulation. The RAAS permits the kidney to have a constant GFR in the face of low and fluctuating salt intake, a property that is vital for terrestrial existence. Renin is produced by the JGA (see earlier discussion). Despite the benefits and importance of the RAAS in physiology, its activation in many disease states appears to be maladaptive and contributes to kidney and cardiovascular injury. Pharmacologic blockade of RAAS pathways at various levels has proved beneficial in animal disease models and human clinical studies, and agents to block RAAS signaling are now in clinical use, with others under development (see Table 25-3).

Vitamin D

1α-Hydroxylase (cytochrome P-450 isoenzyme 27B1) is found in the proximal tubule, where the major body defense for maintaining phosphate homeostasis is localized. Lesser expression of the same enzyme is also found in the rest of the nephron segments. The kidney is one of the most important organs for maintaining calcium and phosphate homeostasis, not just as the major controller of external balance but as an elaborator of systemic

TABLE 25-3 SOME ENDOCRINE HORMONES ELABORATED BY THE KIDNEY

HORMONE	SOURCE	FUNCTION	DRUGS
Renin	JGA	Converts angiotensinogen to angiotensin I as an integral part of the renin-angiotensin-aldosterone system	Renin inhibitor ACE inhibitor Angiotensin receptor blocker Mineralocorticoid receptor blocker
$1,25(OH)_2$ vitamin D	Mostly proximal tubule	Converts the precursor 25(OH) vitamin D to its active form, $1,25(OH)_2$ vitamin D	25-Hydroxyvitamin D 1,25-Dihydroxyvitamin D Synthetic vitamin D analogues
Erythropoietin	Renal interstitial cells	Stimulates erythropoiesis in the bone marrow	Recombinant human erythropoietin Glycosylated recombinant human erythropoietin Other "epomimetic" erythropoiesis-stimulating agents

ACE, Angiotensin-converting enzyme; JGA, juxtaglomerular apparatus.

factors such as vitamin D and the Klotho protein. Conversion of the precursor 25(OH)-hydroxyvitamin D to its active form, $1,25(OH)_2$dihydroxyvitamin D, is achieved not exclusively but substantially in the kidney and is mediated by 1α-hydroxylase. Vitamin D deficiency is an important complication in chronic kidney disease. Replacement of vitamin D is efficacious in reducing the complications of chronic kidney disease and may even improve survival.

Erythropoietin

Erythropoietin, which is produced mainly in the kidney, stimulates erythropoiesis. The erythropoietin-producing cells are strategically located in the cortical interstitium to sense the balance between oxygen delivery and consumption. The current model suggests that upregulation of renal erythropoietin production (mainly by anemia and hypoxia) occurs via an increase in the number of latent erythropoietin-producing cells. The mechanism of erythropoietin deficiency in kidney disease is not definitively known, although it does not involve destruction of renal erythropoietin-producing interstitial cells. One possible mechanism is decreased renal oxygen consumption as a consequence of reduced GFR; this results in higher renal tissue oxygen tension and suppression of erythropoietin production. Resetting of the oxygen-sensing mechanism has also been conjectured. Another theory is direct inhibition of the erythropoietin-producing cells by inflammatory cytokines. Others have proposed transdifferentiation of erythropoietin-producing cells into myofibroblasts and a decrease in the number of interstitial cells that can be recruited to produce erythropoietin.

The use of erythropoiesis-stimulating agents (ESAs) has revolutionized the treatment of anemia associated with chronic kidney disease, but because of incomplete understanding of erythropoietin and erythropoietin receptor biology, the clinical outcome is far from ideal due to inability to tailor the optimal hematocrit for individual patients and uncertainty about possible extra-erythropoietic effects of erythropoietin.

SUGGESTED READINGS

Kaissling B, Le Hir M: The renal cortical interstitium: morphological and functional aspects, Histochem Cell Biol 130:247–262, 2008.

Maezawa Y, Cina D, Quaggin SE: Glomerular cell biology, Waltham, 2013, Academic Press, pp 721–757.

Moe OW, Giebisch G, Seldin DW: Logic of the kidney. In Lifton RP, Somio S, Glebisch GH, et al, editors: Genetic diseases of the kidney, New York, 2009, Elsevier, pp 39–73.

Reiser J, Sever S: Podocyte biology and pathogenesis of kidney disease, Annu Rev Med 64:357–366, 2013.

26

Approach to the Patient with Renal Disease

Rajiv Agarwal

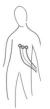

INTRODUCTION

Chronic kidney disease (CKD) may be defined as having an estimated glomerular filtration rate (GFR) of less than 60 mL/min/1.73 m² for at least 3 months. Most of these patients are seen in the outpatient setting, and the focus of their care is on determination of the cause of renal injury, preservation of kidney and cardiovascular function, prevention of the long-term complications of kidney disease, and provision of renal replacement therapy once kidney function deteriorates to the extent that it can no longer sustain an appropriate quality of life. In contrast, most patients with acute kidney injury (AKI) are hospitalized. The focus of their care also starts with accurate determination of the cause of renal failure, but over a period of days to weeks it is important to reverse the kidney failure if possible, replace kidney function if needed, and manage the many potential adverse consequences of AKI.

Because of the widespread use of automated systems for serum chemistry analysis, an elevated serum creatinine concentration is the most common initial manifestation of kidney disease. This test is performed as a screen for renal function abnormalities in most metabolic panels; in most cases, an elevated serum creatinine concentration reflects reduced filtration function of the kidney. After ensuring that intravascular volume is appropriate, the approach to the patient depends on whether renal insufficiency is thought to be acute or chronic. Accordingly, the initial step in evaluating an elevated serum creatinine level is to assess the time course and duration of the changes so as to distinguish AKI from CKD.

A careful history, physical examination, and laboratory evaluation, including imaging studies, are all fundamental to this process. The highest priority is to address acute dehydration, bleeding, and other causes of intravascular volume loss. Evidence of preceding kidney disease may be discovered by searching the records for prior abnormalities of serum creatinine, proteinuria, abnormal urine sediment, or anatomic features such as the presence of multiple cysts in both kidneys. Similarly, a call to the primary care doctor may provide clues to suggest the presence of kidney disease at an earlier time.

Small kidney size, as assessed by ultrasound, can be highly suggestive of CKD. The size of the kidney depends on the height of the patient, but in general, a kidney length on ultrasound images of less than 9 cm in an adult male is considered small. The presence of normal-sized or even large kidneys does not exclude the diagnosis of CKD. In fact, it is common in patients

with diabetic nephropathy for kidneys to be 11 or 12 cm long. Radiography of clavicles or hands is not commonly performed but may demonstrate renal osteodystrophy and suggest the presence of CKD.

Anemia is common in both AKI and CKD and therefore is not a differentiating feature. Rarely, if the initial evaluation is unrevealing, a kidney biopsy may be required to distinguish AKI from CKD and to define the etiology of injury.

APPROACH TO THE PATIENT WITH CHRONIC KIDNEY DISEASE

If the elevated creatinine concentration is thought to be chronic in nature, the history and physical examination should focus initially on detection of diabetes (e.g., diabetic retinopathy) and hypertension, the two most common causes of CKD. In all cases, the evaluation also includes laboratory testing of renal function, serum electrolytes, complete blood count, testing for albuminuria, and microscopic urine sediment analysis. Kidney ultrasound is almost always obtained early in the evaluation to eliminate ureteral or bladder obstruction, a cause of reversible renal failure. In addition, the ultrasound provides important information about kidney size, symmetry, and echogenicity. Kidney biopsy may be needed in some patients, but parenchymal scarring is common in many forms of CKD so the biopsy may not be diagnostic.

Because diabetes and hypertension are common causes of kidney disease, it is important to recognize the associated presentations. To establish a likely diagnosis of diabetic nephropathy, a long-standing history of documented diabetes mellitus is typical, and the presence of diabetic retinopathy, albuminuria, and large kidneys on ultrasound is expected. The urinary sediment is usually unremarkable, so the presence of red blood cell (RBC) casts or a significant number of dysmorphic erythrocytes should initiate a careful evaluation for other causes of CKD. In cases of hypertensive nephrosclerosis, established hypertension typically antedates the diagnosis of renal failure for many years, and the presence of hypertensive retinopathy or cardiovascular disease (e.g., left ventricular hypertrophy) is common. Proteinuria is typically minimal or absent (<2 g/day), and the kidneys are symmetrically small on ultrasound.

In patients with chronic renal failure, it is important not to assume that diabetes and hypertension are the cause. The implication, rather, is that no other identifiable cause of kidney disease is apparent after a thorough evaluation. Notably, in individuals with hypertension, several genes have been identified that appear to be associated with a greater risk of renal disease, and genetic analysis may emerge as one approach to identify those most at risk so that strategies for prevention can be tested in the future.

Once a diagnosis of CKD is established, ongoing evaluation is required, because those with CKD are at increased risk for complications such as hypertension, metabolic bone disease, anemia, hyperkalemia, and metabolic acidosis. Accordingly, the initial diagnosis of CKD may be modified over time, such as by the discovery of RBC casts in a patient with diabetes mellitus. Similarly, if hypertension or volume overload becomes difficult to manage, the dietary intake of sodium can be estimated by 24-hour urine collection as a clue toward more effective management as CKD evolves over time.

History and Examination

The signs and symptoms of CKD depend on the stage at presentation. Early in the clinical course, nonspecific fatigue is typical, and there may be no discernable clues on examination, highlighting the need for laboratory screening. As filtration rate declines, the signs and symptoms of CKD become more common and may include pedal edema, facial puffiness, flank pain, polyuria, nocturia, and hypertension. Symptoms referable to uremia, such as nausea, dysgeusia, and vomiting, tend to occur late and should not be relied on to make a diagnosis of early CKD.

Sometimes the manifestations of the primary disease predominate. For example, the presence of fever, arthralgia, and rash in a young woman with renal failure and active urinary sediment is highly suggestive of lupus nephritis; or a recent history of skin infection or pharyngitis may reveal the presence of postinfectious glomerulonephritis. A family history of deafness can point to the diagnosis of Alport's syndrome; or a history of cerebral hemorrhage due to a ruptured aneurysm may suggest underlying polycystic kidney disease.

Medication history should focus on exposure to nephrotoxins, including long-term use of nonsteroidal anti-inflammatory drugs (NSAIDs), lithium, exposure to cisplatin, and recent escalation of the dose of diuretics. Some nonprescription drugs can lead to CKD (e.g., cocaine-induced glomerulonephritis, Ma Huang–induced ephedrine stones).

Past medical history may reveal diabetes mellitus and its complications (e.g., retinopathy); recurrent urinary tract infection in a patient with renal calculi; or ongoing hepatitis C, infective endocarditis, or Wegner's granulomatosis in patients with glomerular disease. Therefore, knowledge of the past history is important.

Physical examination can reveal the presence of anemia, skin rash (such as in endocarditis, Fabry's disease, Henoch-Schönlein purpura, or cryoglobulinemia), rales, pericardial or pleural friction rub, pedal edema, abdominal bruit, or enlarged kidneys. Retinal examination is of particular importance and may reveal diabetic retinopathy or changes associated with hypertension; in a patient with rapid deterioration of renal function, retinal examination may show cholesterol emboli or septic emboli, pointing to the existence of cholesterol emboli or bacterial endocarditis as possible causes. Rectal examination, and pelvic examination in female patients, may point to clues to urinary tract obstruction such as a tumor or neurogenic bladder. Examination of the

muscle mass is important when interpreting serum creatinine concentration (see later discussion).

The assessment of blood pressure is particularly important. Often, blood pressure is elevated in the clinic but normal at home (*white coat hypertension*). Occasionally, the blood pressure is elevated at home but not in the clinic (*masked hypertension*). In patients who complain of orthostatic symptoms but appear to have normal or high blood pressure in the clinic, home blood pressure measurements or 24-hour ambulatory blood pressure monitoring may be required. The latter may reveal very low blood pressure with orthostatic symptoms, and antihypertensive therapy may need to be modified.

The overall condition of the patient and level of functional status is important in deciding therapies. For example, transplantation may be an option for a patient with correctable cardiovascular disease and dialysis for someone without correctable cardiovascular disease. However, the physician and the patient's family may share the decision to forego renal replacement in an elderly person with advanced dementia and poor functional status.

Assessment of Kidney Function

Knowledge of both the degree and the rate of change in renal function is important in managing CKD. Rapid deterioration of kidney function over a few weeks to a few months may not reflect intrinsic renal function per se; rather, it may reflect superimposed volume depletion (e.g., escalation in the dose of diuretics), exposure to nephrotoxins (e.g., NSAID use), or urinary tract obstruction. Alternatively, progressive renal injury may be associated with malignant hypertension, crescentic glomerulonephritis, microangiopathic hemolytic anemia (thrombotic thrombocytopenic purpura, scleroderma), vasculitides (lupus nephritis, Wegener's granulomatosis), atheroembolic renal disease, or multiple myeloma. In general, a slower course of progression is anticipated in patients with CKD caused by polycystic kidney disease, hypertension, or diabetes mellitus.

Serum creatinine is the standard measure of kidney function. Along with the assessment of albuminuria, it is an important component for staging CKD (Fig. 26-1). If estimated GFR is less than 60 mL/min/1.73 m^2 for 3 months or longer, kidney disease is said to be chronic.

Notably, serum creatinine concentration does not rise to above the population threshold of normal (about 1.3 mg/dL in men and 1.1 mg/dL in women) until approximately 40% of kidney function is lost. In earlier stages of kidney disease, serum creatinine is maintained in the normal range by enhanced tubular secretion of creatinine. This process of creatinine secretion requires cationic transporters; and drugs that compete with creatinine (e.g., cimetidine, triamterene, trimethoprim) may cause elevation of serum creatinine without depressing true GFR. A clue to impaired cationic transport of creatinine is the lack of rise in blood urea nitrogen despite an increase in serum creatinine.

With advanced kidney failure, the changes in serum creatinine may be more rapid. The relationship between serum creatinine and GFR is nonlinear, accelerating as the GFR declines. This means, for example, that an increase in serum creatinine concentration from 3 to 3.5 mg/dL is associated with a lesser decline in GFR than is a change from 1 to 1.5 mg/dL. Specific knowledge

Prognosis of CKD by GFR and Albuminuria Categories: KDIGO 2012			Persistent albuminuria categories Description and range		
			A1	**A2**	**A3**
			Normal to mildly increased	Moderately increased	Severely increased
			<30 mg/g <3 mg/mmol	30–300 mg/g 3–30 mg/mmol	>300 mg/g >30 mg/mmol
GFR categories (ml/min/1.73 m²) Description and range	**G1**	Normal or high	≥90			
	G2	Mildly decreased	60–89			
	G3a	Mildly to moderately decreased	45–59			
	G3b	Moderately to severely decreased	30–44			
	G4	Severely decreased	15–29			
	G5	Kidney failure	<15			

Green: Low risk (if no other markers of kidney disease, no CKD); Yellow: moderately increased risk; Orange: high risk; Red: very high risk.

FIGURE 26-1 Chronic kidney disease (CKD) nomenclature used by the Kidney Disease Improving Global Outcomes (KDIGO) consortium. CKD is defined as abnormalities of kidney structure or function, present for 3 months or longer, with implications for health. CKD is classified on the bases of cause, glomerular filtration rate (GFR), and albuminuria. (From KDIGO: 2012 clinical practice guideline for the evaluation and management of chronic kidney disease, Kid Intl Suppl 3:18, 2013. Available at http://www.kdigo.org/clinical_practice_guidelines/pdf/CKD/KDIGO_2012_CKD_GL.pdf. Accessed June 1, 2014.)

of the baseline level of serum creatinine is important; for example, change from 0.6 to 1.2 mg/dL is still within the normal range in an adult man but actually reflects an approximately 50% loss of GFR.

The relationship between GFR and serum creatinine is best interpreted at steady state and not when the GFR is changing rapidly. For example, bilateral nephrectomy in a patient with previously normal kidney function (as might occur in a patient with renal cell carcinoma) results in drop in GFR from 100 to 0 mL/min. However, serum creatinine would be expected to increase by only about 1 mg/dL/day, and a plateau may not be achieved before 1 week. This delay reflects the fact that the generation of creatinine is insufficient to saturate the volume of distribution of creatinine. A plateau will be reached more rapidly if the rate of creatinine generation is increased, the volume of distribution of creatinine is small, or residual renal function is substantial. Given these variables, it is important to be aware that serum creatinine may be a poor marker of GFR in non–steady-state conditions.

There also are several conditions in which serum creatinine may be falsely low in relation to the GFR. Because creatinine generation is dependent on muscle mass, low creatinine generation occurs in diseases associated with sarcopenia, such as motor neuron diseases (amyotrophic lateral sclerosis), wasting illnesses (advanced cancer, tuberculosis, cardiac cachexia), and even malnutrition. Visual examination of muscle mass (thighs, arms, temporal muscles) may therefore be important in the interpretation of serum creatinine concentrations. Other conditions associated with low creatinine generation include cirrhosis and advanced age. Creatinine generation is reduced in sepsis, and kidney

function may be worse than is detectable by estimation of GFR through measurement of serum creatinine.

At very advanced levels of kidney disease (e.g., GFR <20 mL/min), creatinine is secreted and urea is absorbed by the tubule. Tubular secretion is balanced by tubular reabsorption, making measurements of urea clearance and creatinine clearance useful in estimating true GFR. An average of creatinine and urea clearance closely approximates true GFR in such situations.

At steady state—that is, when the patient is neither gaining or losing weight—the 24-hour urine urea nitrogen measurement can be used to estimate dietary protein intake. In addition to its excretion in urine, nitrogen is lost through the gut, through the skin, and, as non-urea nitrogen, through the kidney in proportion to body weight. It is estimated that 31 mg/kg/day of non-urea nitrogen is excreted in this fashion. Dietary protein intake can be calculated as 6.25 g protein per gram of total daily nitrogen excretion. Accordingly, the formula for dietary protein intake in grams per day is (urine urea nitrogen + 0.031 × body weight in kg) × 6.25.

Although urea by itself is less useful to assess kidney function, it can be helpful in conjunction with the serum creatinine measurement. Urea is reabsorbed by the tubule in sodium-avid states. The normal ratio of urea to creatinine is 10:1. In states of volume depletion such as diuretic use, diarrhea, sweat losses, or third spacing (e.g., ascites), the urea-to-creatinine ratio may be greater than 20:1. Sometimes, ratios greater than 20:1 are also seen in catabolic states (e.g., long-bone fracture, corticosteroid use, burns, sepsis), increased gut protein load (upper gastrointestinal bleeding, high-protein diet), or obstructive uropathy. In contrast, creatinine may rise disproportionally more than urea, for example in advanced cirrhosis, low-protein diets, or states associated with the use of cationic transport inhibitors (e.g., cimetidine).

For many decades, the assessment of creatinine clearance by a 24-hour urine collection has been the mainstay of assessing renal function. However, given that creatinine may be secreted (and not just filtered), this test may overestimate GFR. Furthermore, voiding outside the collection jug is common and may lead to errors in estimating GFR. Although a 24-hour urine collection is not routinely recommended to assess renal function, it may still be useful for estimating GFR in sarcopenic individuals and in those with advanced liver disease. Creatinine clearance can be easily calculated as the urinary flow rate (in mL/min) times the ratio of urinary creatinine to plasma creatinine. A timed collection is needed. Creatinine excretion approximates 15 mg/kg/day. Although this rate is variable (the coefficient of variation from day to day over 28 days on a standard diet varies from 6% to 22%) and depends on meat intake, it can be used to estimate whether urine has been grossly undercollected or overcollected.

Usually, GFR is estimated through the use of equations that account for age in years, race, sex, and serum creatinine. The Modification of Diet in Renal Disease (MDRD) equation uses a creatinine measurement (Scr) that has been calibrated to an isotope dilution mass spectrometry standard:

$$GFR\,[\text{in mL/min/1.73 m}^2] = 175 \times (Scr)^{-1.154} \times (Age)^{-0.203}$$
$$\times\, 0.742\,[\text{if female}] \times 1.212\,[\text{if black}]$$

A newer equation, called the Chronic Kidney Disease Epidemiology Collaboration (CKD-EPI) equation, is less likely to estimate GFR as low if the GFR is higher than 60 mL/min/1.73 m². This equation is more complicated:

$$GFR\,[60\text{ mL/min/1.73 m}^2] = 141 \times min(Scr/\kappa,1)^{\alpha}$$
$$\times\, max(Scr/\kappa,1)^{-1.209} \times 0.993^{Age} \times 1.018\,[\text{if female}]$$
$$\times\, 1.159\,[\text{if black}]$$

where Scr is serum creatinine (in mg/dL), κ is 0.7 for females and 0.9 for males, α is −0.329 for females and −0.411 for males, *min* indicates the minimum of Scr/κ or 1, and *max* indicates the maximum of Scr/κ or 1. Several calculators to estimate GFR using the CKD-EPI equation or the MDRD equation are available on the World Wide Web or as applications for personal devices.

Assessment of Albuminuria

The assessment of albuminuria is fundamental because it may point to the cause of the CKD. Furthermore, greater albuminuria is associated with an accelerated progression of CKD and cardiovascular disease. As a result, albuminuria is now used to stage CKD (see Fig. 26-1).

Albumin excretion rate is normally less than 10 mg/24 hr, and an excretion rate of 30 mg/24 hr or higher is considered abnormal and moderately increased. An albumin excretion rate of 300 mg/24 hr or higher is considered severely increased. Albuminuria can be more conveniently assessed by measuring the ratio of urine albumin and urine creatinine concentrations in a spontaneously voided specimen. Given that the creatinine excretion rate averages 1 g/day, an albumin-to-creatinine ratio of

30 mg/g creatinine or higher is considered abnormal and moderately increased; a ratio of 300 mg/g creatinine is considered severely increased.

An albumin excretion rate higher than 2200 mg/24 hr (corresponding to 3000 mg protein/24 hr) is considered nephrotic. Such a degree of albuminuria/proteinuria is often accompanied by edema, hypoalbuminemia, and hyperlipidemia. The combination of these disorders is referred to as the *nephrotic syndrome*, and the severe proteinuria reflects a profound disorder of glomerular permselectivity. Common causes of nephrotic syndrome in adults are diabetic nephropathy, focal segmental glomerulosclerosis, membranous nephropathy, and amyloidosis. Among children, minimal change nephropathy and focal segmental glomerulosclerosis are important causes of nephrotic syndrome.

Assessment of Blood Pressure

Hypertension is a common accompaniment of CKD, yet the evaluation of hypertension often is performed poorly. Current management of hypertension is directed most often to management of blood pressure measurements obtained during clinic visits. However, blood pressure may be falsely higher in the clinic (*white coat hypertension*) or lower in the clinic (*masked hypertension*) compared with 24-hour ambulatory blood pressure measurements. The latter technique is mostly limited to research or to management in a few difficult cases. However, home blood pressure recordings self-measured by the patient twice daily for about 1 week every month can help diagnose and manage hypertension more effectively. Self-performance of these measurements may promote adoption of a healthier diet and better medication adherence by the patient, as well as reducing therapeutic inertia on the part of the physician.

Assessment of Dietary Sodium Intake

At steady state, when body weight is neither increasing nor decreasing, the dietary sodium intake can be judged by 24-hour urine collection. To establish adequacy of urine collection, the measurement of urine creatinine in 24-hour urine sample is important. The creatinine excretion rate in an adequately collected specimen should approach 1 g/day for women and 1.5 g/day for men. Dietary potassium and protein intake can be monitored similarly. Measurement of urine urea nitrogen in the 24-hour urine sample can reveal the adequacy of dietary protein intake. Dietary sodium restriction can improve blood pressure, can enhance the biologic actions of inhibitors of the renin-angiotensin system, and may protect the heart, blood vessels, and kidneys independent of improvement in blood pressure.

Microscopic Urinalysis

Microscopic urinalysis at initial evaluation and on an ongoing basis can reveal vital information about the health of the kidney. Evaluation should be performed by centrifugation of at least 12 mL of a freshly voided specimen. Cells, casts, crystals, and other elements can corroborate the diagnosis of the cause of CKD. Examples are shown in Figures 26-2 through 26-5.

Renal Imaging

Bladder ultrasonography is a tool that can be used to assess residual urine volume. The wide availability of this tool allows

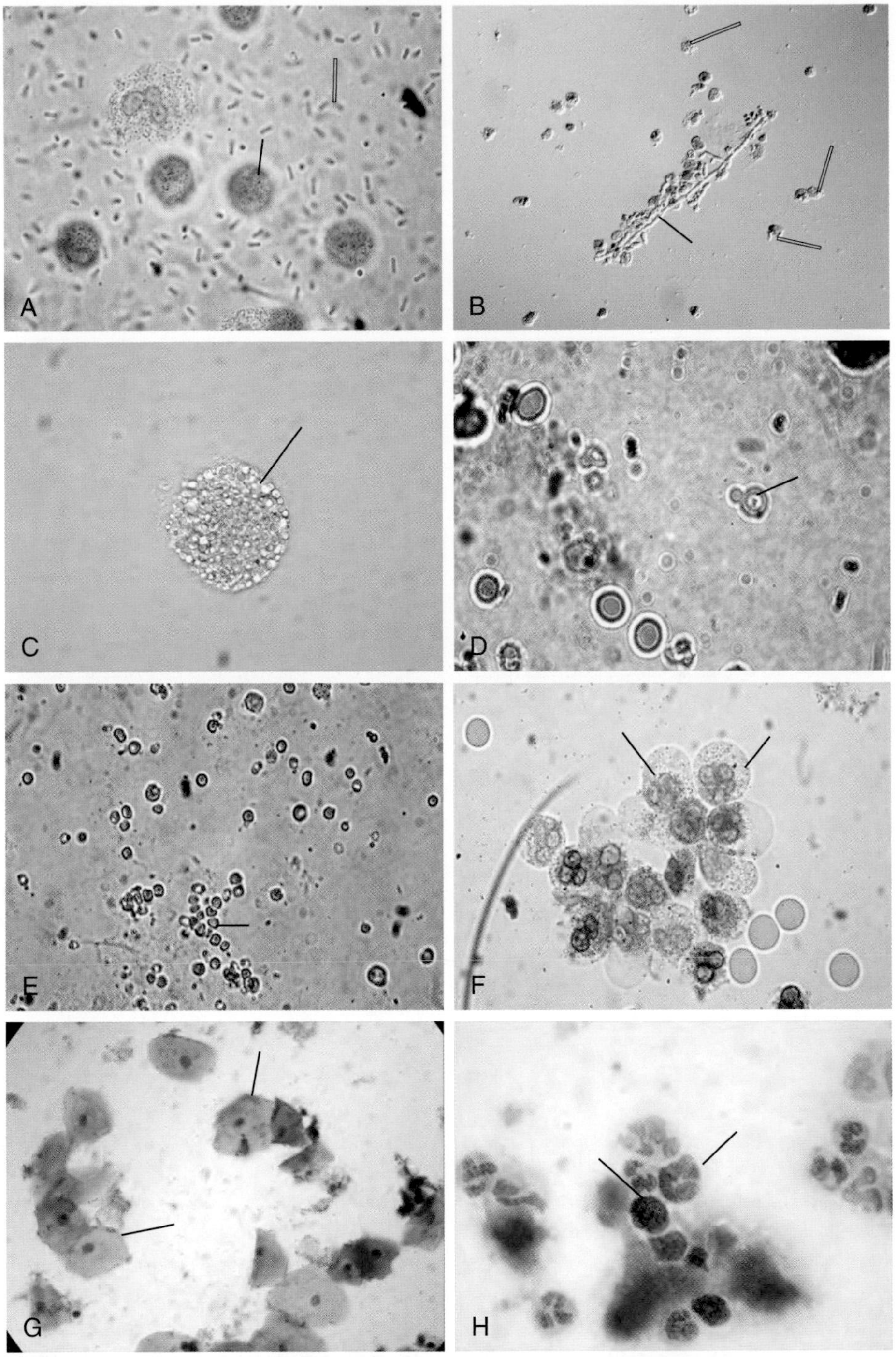

FIGURE 26-2 Cells often found in urine of patients with kidney disease. **A,** Sternheimer-Malbin–stained urine sediment (100× objective) in a patient with urinary tract infection. *Solid line* shows a leukocyte and *hollow line* indicates bacteria. **B,** Sternheimer-Malbin–stained urine sediment (40×) in a patient with fungal urinary tract infection. *Solid line* shows a pseudohypha and *hollow lines* indicate leukocytes. **C,** Unstained urine sediment (40×) shows an oval fat body in a patient with nephrotic syndrome. **D,** Sternheimer-Malbin–stained urine sediment (100×) in a patient with immunoglobulin A (IgA) nephropathy. *Solid line* shows an acanthocyte characterized by outpouching of the red blood cell (RBC) membrane. **E,** Sternheimer-Malbin–stained urine sediment (40×) in a patient with IgA nephropathy shows many acanthocytes *(solid line)*. When acanthocytes constitute more than 5% of the RBCs, their presence is considered significant. **F,** Sternheimer-Malbin–stained urine sediment (100×) in a patient with recovering acute tubular necrosis (ATN). *Solid lines* indicate glitter cells. The granules of these leukocytes have a Brownian motion and appear to glitter under the microscope. These cells can be seen in large numbers during the recovery stage of ATN and in patients with urinary tract infection. **G,** Sternheimer-Malbin–stained urine sediment (40×) shows numerous squamous cells, indicating poor collection technique. **H,** Hansel-stained urine sediment (100×) shows eosinophils that can be seen in patients with allergic interstitial nephritis, cholesterol emboli, or, sometimes, urinary tract infection.

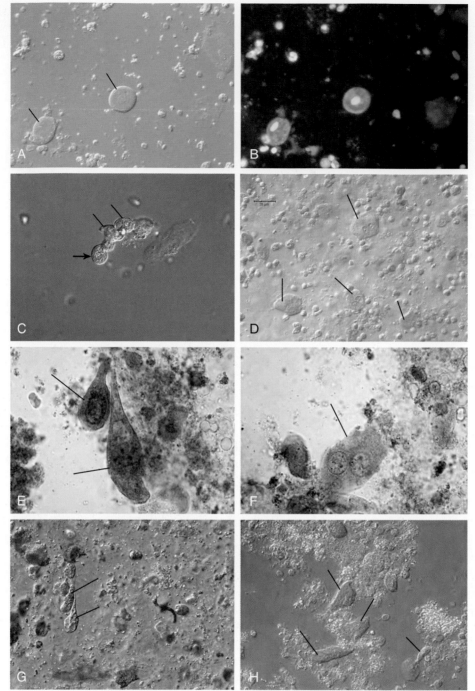

FIGURE 26-3 Tubular cells often found in urine of patients with acute kidney injury. **A,** Unstained urine sediment (40× objective) in a patient recovering from acute tubular necrosis (ATN). *Solid lines* show intact renal tubular epithelial cells. **B,** Same specimen as in **A** but stained with acridine orange-propidium iodide and viewed with a triple excitation band fluorescence filter (triple-cube). Red cells are dead and green cells are live. Both tubular cells appear viable. Smaller cells are leukocytes. **C,** Unstained urine sediment (40×) shows several renal tubular cells that appear monomorphic (as in images **A** and **B**), indicating acute tubular injury. The *arrow* indicates a binucleate tubular cell. **D,** Unstained urine sediment (40×) shows several renal tubular cells *(solid lines)* that appear dysmorphic. Instead of being round, the cells are angular. Furthermore, these cells are multinucleated, indicating failure of the cell to divide. Large numbers of dysmorphic renal tubular cells are often seen if the acute tubular injury is substantial. **E,** Unstained urine sediment (100×) shows two teardrop-shaped dysmorphic renal tubular epithelial cells *(solid lines)*. Because the patient had jaundice, the cells appear to have a color despite lack of staining. **F,** Unstained urine sediment (100×) shows one dysmorphic, binucleate renal tubular epithelial cell *(line)*. This is the same patient as in **E. G,** Unstained urine sediment (40×) shows severe ATN. No dirty-brown granular casts were seen, but the tubular cells were dysmorphic *(lines)*. The large amount of granular debris and absence of casts suggests failure to form Tamm-Horsfall protein and more severe tubular injury. This patient also had jaundice, as is evident from the yellow hue. **H,** Unstained urine sediment (40×) shows dysmorphic renal tubular epithelial cells (triangular, cigar-shaped, and polygonous), often multinucleated as denoted by *lines*.

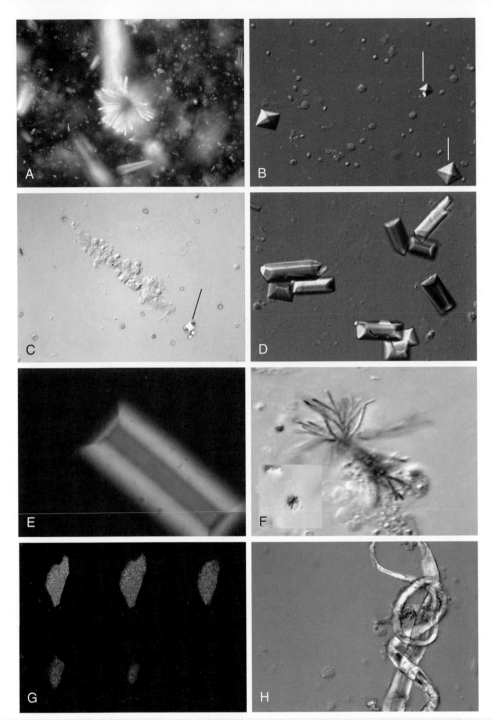

FIGURE 26-4 Crystals commonly found in urine sediment. All images were made with the use of polarized light and a diffusion interference contrast microscope. **A**, Uric acid crystals (40× objective). **B**, Calcium oxalate dihydrate crystals *(white lines)* (40×). Large numbers are seen in patients with ethylene glycol poisoning. **C**, Calcium oxalate monohydrate crystals *(solid line)* (40×). **D**, Magnesium ammonium phosphate crystals, or triple phosphate crystals, are often found in patients with a complicated urinary tract infection (40×). **E**, Coffin-lid appearance of magnesium ammonium phosphate crystals (100×). **F**, Bilirubin crystals in a patient with acute tubular necrosis and obstructive jaundice (100×). Inset shows 40× view of the bilirubin crystals. **G**, Calcium phosphate crystals (40×) in a patient with tumor lysis syndrome. Sequential images *(left to right, top to bottom)* show dissolution of the crystals within a few minutes after urine was acidified by adding 2% perchloric acid. **H**, Fiber artifact in the urine is of no clinical significance.

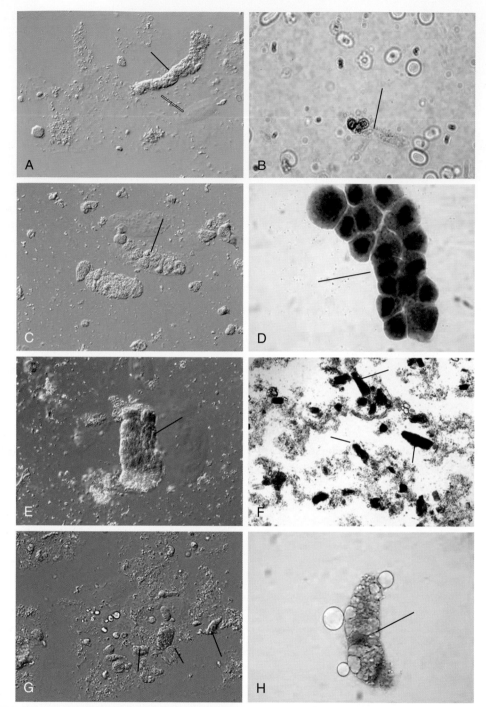

FIGURE 26-5 Casts in urine. **A**, Unstained urine sediment (40× objective) in a patient with glomerulonephritis. *Solid line* shows a granular cast, and *hollow line* shows a hyaline cast. **B**, Sternheimer-Malbin–stained urine sediment (40×). The *solid line* points to an erythrocyte cast in a patient with immunoglobulin A nephropathy. **C**, Unstained urine sediment (40×) shows several renal tubular cells and an epithelial cell cast *(solid line)* indicating acute tubular injury. **D**, Papanicolaou-stained urine sediment *(solid line)* (100×) shows an epithelial cell cast in an otherwise stable patient with diabetic nephropathy. (**E**) Unstained urine sediment (40×) shows bilirubin-stained granular cast *(solid line)* indicating renal inflammation in a patient with liver disease. **F**, Unstained urine sediment (10×) shows dirty-brown granular casts *(solid line)* indicative of acute tubular necrosis (ATN). **G**, Unstained urine sediment (40×) shows severe ATN. No dirty-brown granular casts were seen, but the tubular cells *(solid lines)* were dysmorphic and multinucleated. **H**, Sternheimer-Malbin–stained urine sediment (40×) shows a fatty cast *(solid line)* in a patient with nephrotic syndrome.

diagnosis of bladder outlet obstruction without the need to catheterize the patient.

Renal ultrasonography is the most accurate way of determining kidney size. It is commonly performed to detect renal masses, cysts, and evidence of obstruction characterized by dilatation of the pelvicalyceal system and to evaluate the size and shape of the kidneys. The presence of small kidneys (i.e., <9 cm on both sides) suggests the presence of scarring and therefore CKD. However, kidneys that are larger, typically in the range of 11 to 13 cm, are often seen in conjunction with CKD due to diabetes mellitus, amyloidosis, and multiple myeloma. Therefore, the presence of small kidneys is not needed to make a diagnosis of CKD.

The echogenicity of the kidneys is compared with that of liver parenchyma. Typically, the kidneys are less echogenic than the liver. Increased echogenicity of the kidneys suggests the presence of scarring and therefore CKD. Renal ultrasonography can also easily detect the presence of cysts in the kidneys and therefore is a useful technique to detect polycystic kidney disease. Pulsed Doppler imaging is often used to calculate the resistive index by estimating the systolic and diastolic Doppler velocities in the renal cortex. A resistive index greater than 0.8 suggests that interventional procedures to revascularize the kidney would be unlikely to benefit the patient in terms of improving blood pressure or protecting the long-term decline in kidney function. If the two kidneys differ in size by 1.5 cm, it suggests the presence of renovascular disease in an adult. In children, reflux nephropathy or congenital abnormalities are more common causes.

Computed tomography (CT) of the kidney is often helpful to evaluate complex cysts. In contrast to simple cysts, complex cysts are suspicious for the presence of malignancy, and CT can evaluate them better than ultrasonography. Likewise, CT is important for evaluating renal masses, stones, retroperitoneal conditions (e.g., hemorrhage, tumor, abscess), and renal vein thrombosis. In morbidly obese people, CT is often used to guide kidney biopsy. The use of contrast agents to assess vascular lesions of the kidney may be not be possible if kidney function is compromised due to fear of precipitating AKI. Limiting the volume of the contrast agent and volume repletion before radiocontrast administration may minimize renal injury.

Although intravenous pyelography can image the structures in the kidney, contrast CT has taken the place of classic intravenous pyelography in many centers because of the risk of inducing nephrotoxicity in patients with CKD. In contrast, retrograde pyelography is often used by urologists to define the site and nature of obstruction within the ureter and the pelvis. In addition, during the procedure, ureteric stones can be removed with the use of a basket device.

Magnetic resonance imaging (MRI) is useful for imaging of the vasculature and therefore for the diagnosis of renal vein thrombosis and renal artery stenosis. Gadolinium-based contrast agents are often used for MRI because of their paramagnetic properties. These agents should be avoided if the GFR is less than $30 \text{ mL/min}/1.73 \text{ m}^2$, because in such patients they have been implicated in causing a disabling and untreatable condition called *nephrogenic systemic fibrosis*. Two other MRI contrast agents (one containing iron and another containing manganese) may be used in such patients but are approved by the U.S. Food and Drug Administration only for the evaluation of lesions in the liver. MRI cannot be performed in patients who have metallic implanted devices such as pacemakers, artificial joints, or aneurysmal clips.

After injection of a small amount of radioactive substance, radionuclide imaging can be performed to assess renal perfusion and function of the kidneys. One advantage of this technique is that it can assess kidney function and perfusion simultaneously for each kidney. It therefore allows diagnosis of renal artery stenosis, especially when it is performed before and after administration of angiotensin-converting enzyme (ACE) inhibitors.

Renal arteriography is the reference standard for the diagnosis of renal artery stenosis. It involves direct injection of a radiocontrast dye into the renal arteries. In patients with CKD, contrast injection can be limited and carbon dioxide can be injected to avoid nephrotoxicity. This technique is also useful for assessing vascular malformations in the kidney and for making a diagnosis of polyarteritis nodosa. In the latter condition, renal arteriography can detect the presence of microaneurysms.

APPROACH TO THE PATIENT WITH ACUTE KIDNEY INJURY

The approach to patients with AKI depends on four major factors: (1) the evaluation of risk or susceptibility to renal injury, (2) the nature of the AKI, (3) the severity of injury, and (4) the presence of distant organ effects or consequences. In all cases, it is important to evaluate and optimize intravascular volume early in the course, because this is a readily addressable factor that can prevent or minimize further injury.

The risk factors for AKI include, first and foremost, prior existence of CKD; CKD can easily be detected by a low estimated GFR or the presence of albuminuria. Other common risk factors for AKI include advanced age, diabetes mellitus, hypertension (especially when treated with inhibitors of the renin-angiotensin system), chronic liver disease or cirrhosis, and multiple myeloma.

AKI is a challenging medical problem, and a careful and stepwise approach to evaluation is essential. This approach is guided by knowledge of the causes of injury, which can be divided into five major groups: ischemia, toxins, obstruction, inflammation, and infection.

Ischemia can be caused by volume loss from the gastrointestinal system (vomiting or diarrhea), the skin (sweating, burns), or the kidneys (diuretics, Addison's disease, and solute diuresis). Comparing the body weight of the patient with those weights recorded in the medical record can be valuable. A substantial decrease in body weight may point toward volume depletion as a possible cause of AKI. Third-space fluid losses, as observed patients with ascites, pancreatitis, or ileus, can make the diagnosis of volume depletion challenging because such patients may not have an overall loss in body weight. Ischemia is a common cause of AKI due to poor perfusion associated with significant blood loss or sepsis or both. In the setting of ischemia, glomerular hypoperfusion is aggravated when patients are taking inhibitors of the renin-angiotensin system.

Nephrotoxins can be divided into two major groups: endogenous and exogenous. The endogenous toxins include paraproteins, myoglobin, hemoglobin, uric acid (e.g., in tumor lysis syndrome), and bile acids. Exogenous toxins include contrast dyes, aminoglycosides, chemotherapeutic agents such as cisplatin, and NSAIDs.

Inflammation can involve the glomerular, interstitial, and vascular compartments. Inflammation of these structures produces glomerulonephritis, interstitial nephritis, and vasculitis, respectively.

Infection is an important cause of injury to the nephron. Most often it happens in the intensive care unit, where early sepsis can manifest as a fall in urine output followed by an increase in serum creatinine, confirming AKI. The causes of AKI in the setting of sepsis are multifactorial and include ischemia, direct tubular dysfunction due to sepsis, and concomitant administration of drugs such as nephrotoxic antibiotics (commonly, high doses of vancomycin) and procedures (radiocontrast imaging), often performed to reverse sepsis. Therefore, declines in urine volume, especially in the intensive care unit, should lead to a diligent search for a focus of infection.

Urinary tract obstruction is often a reversible cause of renal injury and therefore important to diagnose. Although urine output is frequently reduced with obstruction, partial obstruction may be associated with an increase in urine output. Renal ultrasound is useful to diagnose hydronephrosis; urinalysis may reveal hematuria, infection, or may be bland. Left untreated renal atrophy may ensue.

In many ways, the severity of injury is best assessed at the bedside. Oliguric renal failure (100-400 mL urine/24 hr) or anuric renal failure (<100 mL urine/24 hr) has a worse prognosis than non-oliguric renal failure (>400 mL urine/24 hr). A low fractional excretion of sodium or, if the patient is taking diuretics, a low fractional excretion of urea may suggest volume depletion as the likely cause. Fractional excretion of any substance is simply calculated as the ratio of the clearance of the analyte in question to the clearance of creatinine. However, a low fractional excretion of urea or sodium may have causes other than volume depletion. For example, because of the heterogeneous nature of nephronal injury, contrast-induced injury, sepsis, or burns often result in a low fractional excretion of sodium despite intrinsic renal failure.

Intrinsic renal injury can be detected by examining the urine sediment. The classic manifestation of acute tubular necrosis (ATN) is the presence of dirty-brown granular casts. However, in severe AKI, there may be a large amount of amorphous granular material without cast formation (see Figs. 26-3 and 26-5). This occurs because severe AKI may result in failure to produce the Tamm-Horsfall protein, leading to no formation of casts. In the absence of dirty-brown granular casts, a diagnosis of acute tubular injury can still be made based on the presence of dysmorphic epithelial cells in the urine. These epithelial cells, under hypoxic conditions, transform from the round, fried-egg appearance of the tubular cell to angular cells taking the shape of triangles or teardrops (see Fig. 26-3). A normal sediment, on the other hand, suggests minimal or no kidney injury.

The severity of injury needs to be assessed, as well as its relationship to the preexisting state of kidney health. Severe injury is required for AKI to be manifested when the kidney is otherwise healthy. Little damage is needed to produce a severe injury if CKD preexists. More important, however, is the response to injury. It remains unclear why do certain individuals have low GFR and others with the same extent of injury do not, but this reflects the protective nature of responses that can result in poor or better GFR.

End-organ manifestations of AKI include pulmonary edema or acute respiratory distress syndrome; uremic encephalopathy as alteration of mental status or asterixis; and uremic pericarditis or pleuritis manifested as pericardial or pleural friction rub. Although pulmonary edema is still a common manifestation of uremia, uremic serositis and encephalopathy are now rare.

The individual elements that can be seen in the urine and may be of diagnostic importance are as follows: dysmorphic RBCs, sterile pyuria manifested by white blood cells (WBCs) in the urine without bacteria, urinary tract infection characterized by both WBCs and bacteria in the urine, dysmorphic tubular cells suggesting ATN, intact renal tubular cells suggesting recovery from AKI, bubble cells, glitter cells, and oval fat bodies (see Figs. 26-2 and 26-3).

Budding yeast in a patient with diabetes may suggest the need to remove a long-standing indwelling catheter. Uric acid crystals in large amount suggest tumor lysis syndrome; calcium oxalate crystals may suggest ethylene glycol poisoning; and magnesium ammonium phosphate (triple phosphate) crystals may suggest infection with urease-positive organisms (see Fig. 26-4).

Casts can occur in various forms, such as RBC, WBC, epithelial cell, granular, hyaline, and dirty-brown granular casts. They can also occur in various shapes, such as broad and narrow casts. Examples of these are demonstrated in Figure 26-5.

For a deeper discussion on this topic, see Chapter 114, "Approach to the Patient with Renal Disease," in Goldman-Cecil Medicine, *25th Edition.*

SUGGESTED READINGS

Agarwal R: Developing a self-administered CKD symptom assessment instrument, Nephrol Dial Transplant 25:160–166, 2010.

Earley A, Miskulin D, Lamb EJ, et al: Estimating equations for glomerular filtration rate in the era of creatinine standardization: a systemic review, Ann Intern Med 156:785–795, 2012.

Gansevoort RT, Matsushita K, van der Velde M, et al: Lower estimated GFR and higher albuminuria are associated with adverse kidney outcomes: a collaborative meta-analysis of general and high-risk population cohorts, Kidney Int 80:93–104, 2011.

Maroni BJ, Steinman TI, Mitch WE: A method for estimating nitrogen intake of patients with chronic renal failure, Kidney Int 27:58–65, 1985.

Perrone RD, Madias NE, Levey AS: Serum creatinine as an index of renal function: new insights into old concepts, Clin Chem 38:1933–1953, 1992.

Pickering TG, Miller NH, Ogedegbe G, et al: Call to action on use and reimbursement for home blood pressure monitoring: a joint scientific statement from the American Heart Association, American Society Of Hypertension, and Preventive Cardiovascular Nurses Association, Hypertension 52:10–29, 2008.

Pickering TG, Shimbo D, Haas D: Ambulatory blood-pressure monitoring, N Engl J Med 354:2368–2374, 2006.

Perazella M, Coca S, Kanbay M, et al: Diagnostic value of urine microscopy for differential diagnosis of acute kidney injury in hospitalized patients, Clin J Am Soc Nephrol 3:1615–1619, 2008.

27

Fluid and Electrolyte Disorders

Biff F. Palmer

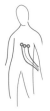

NORMAL VOLUME HOMEOSTASIS
Body Water

In the average adult, total body water is equal to 50% to 60% of body weight: 60% for men and 50% for women because of extra body fat, which is water free. In an average 70-kg man, total body water is 42 kg or 42 L, and for an average 70-kg woman, total body water is 35 kg or 35 L.

Approximately two thirds of total body water is located intracellularly and one third is located extracellularly. One fourth of the extracellular fluid volume (ECF) resides in the intravascular space. In a 70-kg man with 42 L of total body water, 28 L are located intracellularly, 14 L are located in the ECF, and 3.5 L are located in the extracellular intravascular compartment.

ECF volume is determined by the balance between sodium intake and excretion. Under normal circumstances, wide variations in salt intake lead to parallel changes in renal salt excretion, such that ECF volume and total body salt are maintained within narrow limits. This relative constancy of ECF volume is achieved by a series of afferent sensing systems, central integrative pathways, and renal and extrarenal effector mechanisms acting in concert to modulate sodium excretion by the kidney (Table 27-1).

The concentration of salt (i.e., sodium chloride [NaCl]) in the plasma is regulated by renal water handling. Plasma tonicity is maintained by sensing and effector mechanisms that are different from those that regulate volume, although the systems that regulate volume and plasma tonicity do work in concert. For example, if the baroreceptors of the body detect that the ECF volume is low, the kidney responds by retaining NaCl. This transiently leads to an increase in the tonicity of the ECF that stimulates release of arginine vasopressin (AVP), causing renal water retention and expansion of the ECF volume.

Osmolality and Tonicity

Osmolality is the number of particles per kilogram of solution. Plasma osmolality can be directly measured with the use of an osmometer or can be calculated by the following equation:

$$\text{Calculated osmolality} = (Na^+ \times 2) + \text{glucose}/18 + BUN/2.8$$

where Na^+ is the sodium ion concentration and BUN is the blood urea nitrogen level.

The osmolar gap is the difference between the measured and calculated osmolality and is normally less than 10 mOsm/L. A higher value indicates accumulation of an unmeasured substance such as ethanol, methanol, ethylene glycol, or acetone.

It is important to differentiate osmolality from tonicity. *Osmolality* refers to all particles in solution, and *tonicity* describes whether the particles are effective or ineffective osmoles. Effective osmoles such as Na^+, glucose, or mannitol cannot penetrate cell membranes and can lead to changes in cell volume. Ineffective osmoles such as urea and alcohols pass freely into and out of cells and are unable to effect changes in cell volume. As an example, chronic kidney disease patients with BUN levels greater than 100 mg/dL have no cellular shifts of fluid due to the urea. The plasma osmolality is high, but plasma tonicity is normal.

HYPONATREMIA
Definition

Hyponatremia is one the most common electrolyte abnormalities encountered in clinical practice. Increasing age, medications, various disease states, and administration of hypotonic fluids are among the established risk factors for the disorder. Although hyponatremia is most commonly a marker of hypo-osmolality, three causes of hyponatremia are not associated with a hypo-osmolar state (Fig. 27-1). The first is pseudohyponatremia. This condition occurs in the setting of hyperglobulinemia or hypertriglyceridemia, in which plasma water relative to plasma solids is decreased in blood, decreasing the Na^+ concentration in a given volume of blood.

The second cause involves true hyponatremia with elevations in the concentration of an effective osmole. Clinical examples include hyperglycemia as seen in uncontrolled diabetes and infusion of mannitol for the treatment of cerebral edema. Increased plasma glucose concentration raises serum osmolality, which pulls water out of cells and dilutes the serum Na^+ concentration. For every 100-mg/dL rise in glucose or mannitol, the serum Na^+ level quickly falls by 1.6 mEq/L. The increased

TABLE 27-1	SENSORS AND EFFECTORS THAT DETERMINE OSMOREGULATION AND VOLUME REGULATION	
FACTOR	**OSMOREGULATION**	**VOLUME REGULATION**
Sensors	Hypothalamic osmoreceptors	Low- and high-pressure baroreceptors
What is sensed	Plasma osmolality	Effective arterial blood volume
Effectors	Arginine vasopressin (AVP), thirst	Aldosterone, angiotensin II, sympathetic nerves
What is effected	Urine osmolality, thirst	Urine sodium (Na^+) excretion

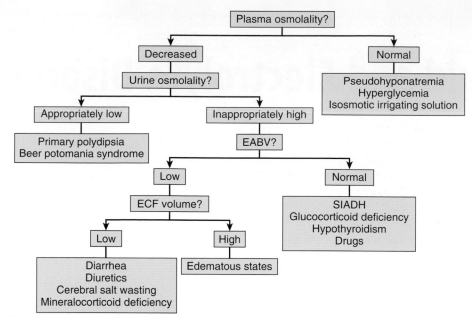

FIGURE 27-1 Approach to the patient with hyponatremia. Assessment of effective arterial blood volume (EABV) is key to understanding the mechanism of renal NaCl retention and whether it is primary or a response to a low EABV. The EABV is the arterial volume sensed by the kidney. If the kidney is working normally and is retaining NaCl, the EABV must be low, and if a normally functioning kidney is excreting large amounts of NaCl, the EABV is large. The physical examination is the most reliable way to assess EABV. Useful findings include the presence or absence of edema and orthostatic changes in blood pressure and pulse. Laboratory tests include collection of a spot urinary sample for sodium (Na^+), chloride (Cl^-), and creatinine to calculate the fractional excretion of Na^+ or fractional excretion of Cl^- using the following equations: FE_{Na} (%) = [(urine Na^+ × plasma creatinine)/(plasma Na^+ × urine creatinine)] × 100 and FE_{Cl} (%) = [(urine Cl^- × plasma creatinine)/(plasma Cl^- × urine creatinine)] × 100. If these parameters are low (<0.5-1%), a low EABV is indicated. Other findings suggesting a low EABV include an increase in the blood urea nitrogen (BUN)/creatinine ratio (>20:1), increased serum uric acid concentration (due to increased proximal tubular reabsorption), and increased hematocrit and serum albumin concentration due to hemoconcentration. SIADH, Syndrome of inappropriate secretion of antidiuretic hormone.

tonicity also stimulates thirst and AVP secretion, both of which contribute to water retention. As the plasma osmolality returns toward normal, the decline in the serum Na^+ level is 2.8 mEq/L for every 100-mg/dL rise in glucose. The net result is a normal plasma osmolality but a low serum Na^+ concentration.

The third cause of hyponatremia in the absence of a hypoosmolar state is the addition of an isosmotic or near-isosmotic, non-Na^+–containing fluid to the extracellular space. This situation typically occurs during transurethral resection of the prostate or during laparoscopic surgery, when large amounts of a nonconducting flushing solution containing glycine or sorbitol are reabsorbed systemically.

Despite these exceptions, hypotonic hyponatremia in most cases implies that water intake exceeds the ability of the kidney to excrete water. Because the normal kidney can excrete 20 to 30 L of water per day, hyponatremia with normal renal water excretion implies that the patient is drinking at least this volume of water. This condition is referred to as *primary polydipsia*. Urine osmolality is less than 100 mOsm/L in this setting. Hyponatremia associated with a maximally dilute urine can also result from more moderate fluid intake combined with extremely limited solute intake, a condition often referred to as *beer potomania syndrome*.

In the absence of primary polydipsia, hypotonic hyponatremia results when water intake exceeds the renal capacity for water excretion due to an inappropriately concentrated urine (>100 mOsm/L). The effective arterial blood volume (EABV) is defined in this setting. Decreased EABV causes baroreceptor

stimulation of AVP secretion and decreases distal delivery of filtrate to the tip of the loop of Henle, accounting for the inability to maximally dilute the urine. If the EABV is low, ECF volume can be low in the volume-depleted patient (i.e., hypovolemic hyponatremia) or can be high in the edematous patient (i.e., hypervolemic hyponatremia). A normal EABV points to the euvolemic causes of hyponatremia (e.g., isovolemic hyponatremia).

Approximately two thirds of diagnosed hyponatremia cases are acquired in the hospital, where the common practices of monitoring daily fluid intake, patient weight, and Na^+ levels normally allow prompt diagnosis. Administration of hypotonic fluids in the postoperative period is a risk factor for acute iatrogenic hyponatremia, especially because AVP levels remain increased several days after surgical procedures. Iatrogenic cases can be prevented by close monitoring of electrolytes and urine output and by fluid restriction and avoidance of solutions with low-Na^+ content; this approach applies particularly to elderly patients.

In neurosurgical patients, the syndrome of inappropriate antidiuretic hormone (SIADH) secretion and cerebral salt wasting are two causes of hyponatremia. Differentiating these disorders can be challenging because there is considerable overlap in the clinical presentation. The primary distinction lies in the EABV assessment. SIADH is a volume-expanded state due to AVP-mediated renal water retention. Cerebral salt wasting is characterized by a contracted EABV resulting from renal salt wasting. Making an accurate diagnosis is important because therapy for these conditions is different. Vigorous salt replacement is indicated for patients with cerebral salt wasting, and fluid restriction is the treatment of choice for patients with SIADH.

Common causes of hyponatremia outside the hospital setting include overhydration, diarrhea, vomiting, central nervous system infection, extreme exercise, liver failure, renal failure, congestive heart failure, drugs, SIADH, and combinations of these and other factors. Thiazide diuretics are the most common cause of drug-induced hyponatremia. Hyponatremia typically develops in the first 2 weeks of drug initiation and is most likely to occur in elderly women and during the summer months because of the increased ingestion of hypotonic fluids when it is hot. Concomitant use of nonsteroidal anti-inflammatory drugs (NSAIDs) and selective serotonin reuptake inhibitors (SSRIs) can further increase the risk of thiazide-induced hyponatremia.

Treatment

Symptoms of hyponatremia include nausea and malaise, which can be followed by headache, lethargy, muscle cramps, disorientation, restlessness, and obtundation. When treating a patient with hyponatremia, the Na^+ concentration should be raised at the rate at which it fell. In patients with chronic hyponatremia (>48 hours' duration), the serum Na^+ concentration has fallen slowly. Neurologic symptoms are minimal, brain size is normal, and the number of intracellular osmoles is decreased. Sudden return of ECF osmolality to normal values produces cell shrinkage and possibly precipitates osmotic demyelination. This complication can be avoided by limiting correction to between 10 and 12 mEq/L in 24 hours and to less than 18 mEq/L in 48 hours. In a patient whose serum Na^+ concentration has decreased rapidly (<48 hours), neurologic symptoms are common, and cerebral edema occurs. In this case, there has not been sufficient time to remove osmoles from the brain, and rapid return to normal ECF osmolality merely returns brain size to normal.

Development of hyponatremia in the outpatient setting is commonly chronic in duration and should be corrected slowly. In contrast, hyponatremia of short duration is more likely to be encountered in hospitalized patients receiving intravenous free water. Use of the illicit drug ecstasy, exercise-induced hyponatremia, or primary polydipsia can cause patients to develop acute hyponatremia, and if symptomatic, they may require rapid correction.

HYPERNATREMIA

Definition

Hypernatremia is a relatively common problem, particularly among the elderly and critically ill. Hypernatremia always indicates hypertonicity and is associated with shrinkage of cells. It is an independent risk factor for mortality in the intensive care unit setting.

The initial approach to any patient with hypernatremia is to determine why there has been inadequate intake of water (Fig. 27-2). Hypernatremia is rare in conscious patients who have free access to water because of the extreme sensitivity of the thirst mechanism. Usually, there is inadequate water intake due to an alteration in the level of consciousness. Patients become unaware of thirst or cannot adequately communicate the need for water, or there is restricted access to water. Rarely, there is a specific lesion of the thirst center. A reduced sensation of thirst occurs in otherwise normal individuals as a feature of increasing age.

The next step is to search for accelerated water loss or Na^+ gain, both of which increase the likelihood of a patient developing hypernatremia. This can best be accomplished by clinical assessment of the EABV. Hypovolemic hypernatremia results from fluid losses in which the Na^+ concentration is less than the plasma concentration. Hypervolemic hypernatremia can result from iatrogenic administration of hypertonic NaCl or hypertonic sodium bicarbonate ($NaHCO_3$) or from mineralocorticoid excess.

Pure water loss, whether from mucocutaneous routes or from the kidneys, causes isovolemic hypernatremia. Because two thirds of pure water loss is sustained from within cells, patients do not become clinically volume depleted unless the water deficit becomes substantial. Insensible losses from the respiratory tract or skin result in concentrated urine. Inappropriate water loss by the kidney, whether from central or nephrogenic diabetes

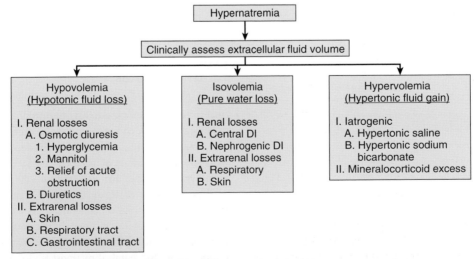

*All are associated with impairment of thirst or access to water.

FIGURE 27-2 Approach to the patient with hypernatremia. DI, Diabetes insipidus.

insipidus, results in dilute urine. Although renal water loss can lead to hypernatremia in patients with impaired thirst or access to water, most patients with diabetes insipidus have neither defect, and they typically have polyuria, polydipsia, and a normal serum sodium concentration at clinical presentation.

Evaluation of Polyuria and Polydipsia

Polyuria can result from osmotic diuresis or water diuresis. Water diuresis may result from inappropriate water loss, as in central or nephrogenic diabetes insipidus, or it may represent appropriate water loss, as in primary polydipsia. The clinical setting and urine osmolality help to differentiate these processes (Fig. 27-3).

Osmotic diuresis causing polyuria is often evident in the clinical setting. Poorly controlled glucose levels in a diabetic, administration of mannitol to a patient with increased intracranial pressure, and high-protein enteral feedings (i.e., urea diuresis) are examples in which polyuria is the result of osmotic diuresis. A urine osmolality value greater than 300 mOsm/L in a polyuric patient suggests a solute or osmotic diuresis.

After excluding osmotic diuresis, the clinician must discriminate between the causes of water diuresis. In patients with central diabetes insipidus, the onset of symptoms is characteristically abrupt, whereas patients with nephrogenic diabetes insipidus usually have a gradual onset of symptoms. Patients with primary polydipsia typically are vague in dating the onset of their symptoms. Nephrogenic and central forms of diabetes insipidus are characterized by severe and frequent nocturia, a feature that is typically absent in patients with primary polydipsia. Patients with central diabetes insipidus seem to have a predilection for ice water, which is not typically described in the other two conditions. A serum Na^+ concentration of less than 140 mEq/L suggests primary polydipsia because the patients tend to have a mildly positive water balance. A value greater than 140 mEq/L suggests central or nephrogenic diabetes insipidus because the patients tend to have a mildly negative water balance.

Urine osmolality increases in response to water deprivation in primary polydipsia but shows no response in diabetes insipidus.

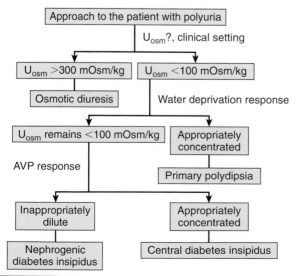

FIGURE 27-3 Approach to the patient with polyuria. AVP, Arginine vasopressin; U, urinary.

Both central and nephrogenic diabetes insipidus are distinguished by the change in urine osmolality after subcutaneous administration of AVP. It is increased in the central type but does not change in nephrogenic diabetes insipidus.

Treatment

Signs and symptoms of hypernatremia include lethargy, weakness, fasciculation, seizures, and coma. Increased ECF osmolality initially causes cell shrinkage in the brain. In response, cells generate intracellular osmoles, which balance the transmembrane osmotic gradient and pull water back into the cells, returning brain size to normal. After this adaptation, if extracellular osmolality is returned rapidly to normal, the additional intracellular osmoles pull water into the brain cells, resulting in cerebral edema. Hypernatremia should be corrected slowly by water administration at a rate that leads to one-half correction in 24 hours. The water deficit can be estimated in men from the following formula:

$$\text{Water deficit} = \text{Current body water} (0.6 \times \text{body weight})$$
$$\times \left(\frac{Na^+_{plasma}}{140} - 1 \right)$$

where $[Na^+]_{plasma}$ is the sodium ion concentration in plasma. The calculation for women uses 0.5 instead of 0.6 as the multiplication factor.

Calculation of the amount of water to give must add insensible losses and ongoing losses from the urinary and gastrointestinal tracts. This formula does not include the volume of isotonic saline required in patients who may be concomitantly volume depleted. Careful monitoring of the serum Na^+ level is required to ensure the rate of correction is appropriate.

⬤ HYPOKALEMIA

Definition

Hypokalemia is a common clinical disorder. Decreases in total body potassium ions (K^+) usually result from gastrointestinal or renal losses, whereas hypokalemia in the setting of normal total body K^+ results from net movement of K^+ into cells. In most cases, the cause can be readily determined by the history, measurement of blood pressure, examination of the acid-base balance, and measurement of urinary K^+ levels.

Cellular Potassium Shift with Normal Total Body Potassium

In the absence of physical and historical evidence of gastrointestinal or renal K^+ losses, a redistribution of K^+ at the cellular level or laboratory error can account for a low serum K^+ concentration. Spurious causes of hypokalemia can be seen in leukemia patients with leukocyte counts of 100,000 to 250,000/m^3, in which the leukocytes extract K^+ from the serum.

The regulation of K^+ distribution between the intracellular and extracellular spaces is referred to as *internal K^+ balance*. Although the kidney is ultimately responsible for maintenance of total body K^+, factors that modulate internal balance are important in the disposal of acute K^+ loads. A large potassium meal, for example, could double extracellular K^+ were it not for the rapid shift of the K^+ load into cells. The kidney cannot excrete

K^+ rapidly enough in this setting to prevent life-threatening hyperkalemia. This excess K^+ must be rapidly shifted and stored in cells until the kidney has successfully excreted the K^+ load. The major regulators of K^+ shift into cells are insulin and catecholamines.

Insulin excess can lower the serum K^+ level when given exogenously to a diabetic patient or when it occurs as an endogenous secretion in a normal person given a high-glucose load. β-Adrenergic agonists used in the treatment of bronchospasm or in treating premature labor can effect similar K^+ shifts. In the setting of an acute myocardial infarction, hypokalemia may result as a sequela of high circulating epinephrine levels and may predispose patients to arrhythmias. Other clinical disorders resulting in an intracellular sequestration of K^+ are treatment of megaloblastic anemia with vitamin B_{12}, hypothermia, and barium poisoning. Hypokalemic periodic paralysis is inherited in an autosomal dominant pattern and is characterized by episodic hypokalemia resulting in muscle weakness. An acquired form of the disorder is seen in thyrotoxic patients, who are often of Japanese or Mexican descent.

Decreased Total Body Potassium

In the absence of a cellular shift, a low serum K^+ level can result from inadequate dietary intake, extrarenal losses through the gastrointestinal tract or skin, or renal losses. The urinary K^+ concentration is a useful guide for deciding among these possibilities. A urine K^+ concentration of less than 20 mEq/L suggests extrarenal losses, whereas a concentration of more than 20 mEq/L suggests renal K^+ losses. Calculation of the transtubular K^+ gradient has also been used for this purpose.

Inadequate dietary intake is an unusual cause of hypokalemia. Clinical situations associated with extreme K^+-deficient diets include anorexia nervosa, crash diets, alcoholism, and intestinal malabsorption. Increased renal K^+ excretion due to magnesium deficiency (which occurs often in these clinical situations) may contribute to the observed hypokalemia.

Extrarenal Potassium Losses

Sweat has a low K^+ concentration and is an unusual cause of K^+ depletion. However, during physical training, sweat losses can become substantial, and K^+ depletion may result. Gastrointestinal syndromes are the most common clinical sources of extrarenal K^+ losses. Diarrhea leads to fecal K^+ wastage and is associated with a normal anion gap acidosis. Acidosis results in K^+ redistribution out of cells, leading to a degree of hypokalemia that is not as severe as the degree of K^+ depletion.

Renal Potassium Losses

Increased distal delivery of Na^+ and water and increased mineralocorticoid activity can each stimulate renal K^+ secretion. Under normal physiologic conditions, these two determinants are inversely regulated by the EABV (Fig. 27-4). Decreased EABV is associated with increased aldosterone secretion but with lower distal delivery of Na^+ and water due to enhancement of reabsorption in the proximal nephron. Renal K^+ excretion is relatively independent of volume status. It is only under pathophysiologic conditions that distal Na^+ delivery and aldosterone become coupled, and in this setting, renal K^+ wasting occurs. The coupling can result from a primary increase in mineralocorticoid activity or a primary increase in distal Na^+ delivery. The term *primary* means that the changes do not depend on changes in the EABV. The causes of hypokalemia, grouped according to the physiologic determinants of renal K^+ excretion, are given in Figure 27-5.

Primary Increase in Mineralocorticoid Activity

Increases in mineralocorticoid activity can result from primary increases in renin or aldosterone secretion, increases in a nonaldosterone mineralocorticoid, or an increased mineralocorticoid-like effect. In these conditions, ECF volume is expanded, and hypertension typically occurs. The differential diagnosis for the patient with hypertension, hypokalemia, and metabolic alkalosis rests on the measurement of plasma renin activity and plasma aldosterone levels.

Primary Increase in Distal Sodium Delivery

Conditions that give rise to primary increases in distal Na^+ delivery are characterized by normal or low ECF volume. Blood pressure is typically normal.

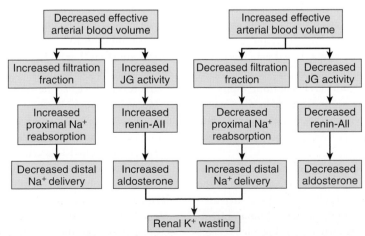

FIGURE 27-4 The relationship between effective arterial volume and distal sodium (Na^+) delivery in determining renal potassium (K^+) excretion. AII, Angiotensin II; JG, Juxtaglomerular.

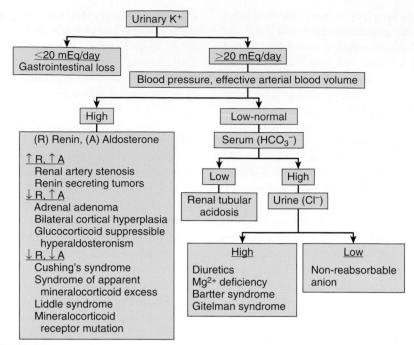

FIGURE 27-5 Approach to the hypokalemic patient. HCO_3^-, Bicarbonate; ↓, decreased; ↑, increased.

Increases in distal Na^+ delivery most frequently result from diuretics that act proximal to the cortical collecting duct. Increased delivery can also be the result of non-reabsorbed anions such as bicarbonate (HCO_3^-), as occurs with active vomiting, or of type II proximal renal tubular acidosis. Ketoanions (i.e., β-hydroxybutyrate and acetoacetate) and the Na^+ salts of penicillin are other examples. The inability to reabsorb these anions in the proximal tubule results in increased delivery of Na^+ to the distal nephron. Because these anions also escape reabsorption in the distal nephron, a more lumen-negative transepithelial voltage develops, and the driving force for K^+ excretion into the tubular fluid is enhanced. Disorders of hypokalemia due to primary increases in distal Na^+ delivery can best be categorized by the finding of metabolic acidosis or metabolic alkalosis.

Clinical Presentation

The most important clinical manifestations of hypokalemia occur in the neuromuscular system. A low serum K^+ concentration leads to cell hyperpolarization, which impedes impulse conduction and muscle contraction. Typically, a flaccid paralysis develops in the hands and feet that moves proximally to include the trunk and respiratory muscles. Death may occur from respiratory insufficiency. Myopathy may also occur, which in its most severe form can lead to frank rhabdomyolysis (i.e., muscle cell lysis) and renal failure. Hypokalemia can also lead to smooth muscle dysfunction, including paralytic ileus.

Changes in the electrocardiogram (ECG) include ST depression, T-wave flattening, and an increase in the amplitude of the U wave. Patients treated with cardiac glycosides are at increased risk for premature ventricular contractions and for supraventricular and ventricular tachyarrhythmia when hypokalemic.

Hypokalemia causes a renal concentrating defect due to a decrease in the medullary gradient and resistance of the cortical collecting tubule to AVP. This leads to polyuria and polydipsia. Prolonged hypokalemia can also lead to tubulointerstitial nephritis and renal failure. Because insulin release is regulated partially by the serum K^+ concentration, hypokalemia can lead to glucose intolerance.

Treatment

The serum K^+ levels can sometimes be misleading about the degree of deficit because a normal or increased K^+ level can occur with significant total body K^+ depletion. In the absence of significant K^+ shifts, a decline in the serum K^+ level from 4 to 3 mEq/L usually is associated with a deficit of 300 to 400 mEq of intracellular K^+ per 70 kg of body weight. A serum K^+ concentration of 2 mEq/L reflects a deficit of roughly 600 mEq. Along with these guidelines, the serum K^+ level should be monitored frequently during replacement therapy.

Supplemental K^+ can be given orally or intravenously as the potassium chloride (KCl) salt. Potassium bicarbonate or citrate can be given if there is concomitant metabolic acidosis. The safest way to administer KCl is orally. KCl can be given in doses of 100 to 150 mEq/day. Liquid KCl is bitter tasting and, like the tablet, can irritate the gastric mucosa. The microencapsulated or wax-matrix forms of KCl are better tolerated.

Intravenous administration of K^+ may be necessary if the patient cannot take oral medications or the K^+ deficit is large and is causing cardiac arrhythmias, respiratory paralysis, or rhabdomyolysis. Intravenous KCl should be given at a maximum rate of 20 mEq/hour and maximum concentration of 40 mEq/L. Higher concentrations result in phlebitis. Replacement of KCl in dextrose-containing solutions can lower the serum K^+ further due to insulin release. Saline solutions are preferred.

Depending on the specific cause, additional therapy for chronic hypokalemia involves the use of K^+-sparing diuretics such as amiloride, spironolactone, or triamterene. Caution is warranted when using these agents in patients with renal insufficiency or other disorders that impair renal K^+ excretion.

HYPERKALEMIA

Definition

As in the hypokalemic disorders, a high serum K^+ concentration can occur in the setting of normal or altered body stores of K^+. The body has a marked ability to protect against hyperkalemia. This includes regulatory mechanisms that excrete excess K^+ quickly and mechanisms that redistribute excess K^+ into cells until it is excreted. All causes of hyperkalemia involve abnormalities in these mechanisms.

Pseudohyperkalemia is an in vitro phenomenon caused by the mechanical release of K^+ from cells during a phlebotomy procedure, specimen processing, or in the setting of marked leukocytosis and thrombocytosis.

Excessive Dietary Potassium Intake

In the setting of normal renal and adrenal function, it is difficult to ingest sufficient K^+ in the diet to produce hyperkalemia. Dietary intake of K^+ as a contributor to hyperkalemia is usually observed in patients with impaired kidney function. Dietary sources particularly enriched with K^+ include melons, citrus juice, and commercial salt substitutes containing KCl.

Cellular Redistribution

Cellular redistribution is a more important cause of hyperkalemia than as a cause of hypokalemia. Tissue damage is probably the most important cause of hyperkalemia due to redistribution of K^+ out of cells. This can be caused by rhabdomyolysis, trauma, burns, massive intravascular coagulation, and tumor lysis (spontaneous or after treatment).

The effect of metabolic acidosis in causing K^+ to exit from cells depends on the type of acid. Mineral acidosis (i.e., ammonium chloride [NH_4Cl] or hydrogen chloride [HCl]), by virtue of the relative impermeability of the chloride anion, results in the greatest efflux of K^+ from cells. In contrast, organic acidosis (lactic or β-hydroxybutyric) results in no significant efflux of K^+.

Increased osmolality, as occurs in uncontrolled diabetics, causes K^+ to move out of cells. The hypertonic state and insulin deficiency account for hyperkalemia often seen in patients with diabetic ketoacidosis who are total body K^+ depleted. β-Adrenergic blocking agents can interfere with the disposal of acute K^+ loads. Other drugs that can result in hyperkalemia include the depolarizing muscle relaxant succinylcholine and digitalis in cases of severe poisoning.

Decreased Renal Excretion of Potassium

Decreased renal excretion of K^+ can occur because of three abnormalities: a primary decrease in distal delivery of salt and water, abnormal cortical collecting duct function, and a primary decrease in mineralocorticoid levels.

Primary Decrease in Distal Delivery of Salt and Water

Acute decreases in the glomerular filtration rate (GFR), as occur in acute kidney injury, may lead to marked decreases in the distal delivery of salt and water, which may secondarily decrease distal K^+ secretion. When acute kidney injury is oliguric, distal delivery of NaCl and volume are low, and hyperkalemia is a frequent problem. When acute kidney injury is nonoliguric, distal delivery is usually sufficient, and hyperkalemia is unusual.

In chronic kidney disease patients, hyperkalemia is unusual until the GFR falls to less than 10 mL/min. Hyperkalemia with a GFR of more than 10 mL/min raises the question of decreased aldosterone levels or a specific lesion of the cortical collecting duct.

Primary Decrease in Mineralocorticoid Activity

Decreased mineralocorticoid activity can result from disturbances that originate at any point along the renin-angiotensin-aldosterone system. These disturbances can be the result of a disease state or various drugs. Hyperkalemia most commonly develops when one of more of these drugs are administered when the renin-angiotensin-aldosterone system is already impaired. A common example is the use of angiotensin-converting enzyme (ACE) inhibitors or angiotensin-receptor blockers (ARBs) in diabetics with hyporeninemic hypoaldosteronism.

Distal Tubular Defects

Certain interstitial renal diseases can affect the distal nephron specifically and lead to hyperkalemia despite mild decreases in the GFR and normal aldosterone levels. Amiloride and triamterene inhibit Na^+ transport, which makes the luminal potential more positive and secondarily inhibits K^+ secretion. A similar effect occurs with trimethoprim and accounts for the development of hyperkalemia after the administration of the antibiotic sulfamethoxazole-trimethoprim. Spironolactone and eplerenone compete with aldosterone and block the mineralocorticoid effect.

Clinical Presentation

Hyperkalemia leads to depolarization of the resting membrane because the potential across cell membranes is in part determined by the ratio of intracellular to extracellular K^+. The heart is particularly sensitive to this depolarizing effect. The progressive changes of hyperkalemia on the electrocardiogram are peaking of T waves, widening of the PR and QRS interval, development of a sine wave pattern, and eventually, ventricular fibrillation and asystole.

ECG changes appear at a serum K^+ level of 6 mEq/L with acute onset of hyperkalemia, whereas the ECG may remain normal up to a concentration of 8 to 9 mEq/L with chronic hyperkalemia. Hyperkalemia can also cause neuromuscular manifestations such as ascending paralysis and flaccid quadriplegia.

Treatment

Acute Hyperkalemia

The immediate treatment for life-threatening hyperkalemia is the administration of calcium usually in the form of calcium gluconate or calcium chloride. ECG changes such as an increasing PR interval or a widening QRS complex warrant treatment with calcium. Glucose and insulin therapy shift K^+ into cells. Acute administration of glucose without insulin can potentially worsen hyperkalemia in diabetics by raising extracellular osmolality and causing K^+ to shift into the extracellular space. Through expansion of the ECF space, $NaHCO_3$ administration results in dilution of the serum K^+ concentration. K^+ also is shifted into cells whenever concomitant metabolic acidosis is corrected. Inhalation of β_2-agonists such as albuterol or parenteral use of salbutamol can effect significant K^+ shifts into cells.

The administration of calcium, HCO_3^-, glucose and insulin, and β_2-agonist therapy provides immediate relief of acute toxicity but does not decrease total body K^+. Measures to reduce total body K^+ include the administration of Na^+ polystyrene sulfonate (Kayexalate) and dialysis.

Chronic Hyperkalemia

After a review the patient's medication profile, drugs that can impair renal K^+ excretion should be discontinued if possible. Prescription or over-the-counter NSAIDs are common offenders. Patients should be placed on a low-K^+ diet with specific counseling against the use of K^+-containing salt substitutes.

Diuretics are particularly effective in minimizing hyperkalemia. In patients with an eGFR >30 mL/min, thiazide diuretics can be used, but for more severe renal insufficiency, loop diuretics are required. In chronic kidney disease patients with metabolic acidosis (HCO_3^- concentration <20 mEq/L), $NaHCO_3$ should be given. Intermittent use of a K^+-binding resin can be tried, but this drug is poorly tolerated when used on a chronic basis and has been associated with gastrointestinal ulceration.

● METABOLIC ACIDOSIS

Metabolic acidosis is diagnosed by a low serum pH, a reduced plasma HCO_3^- concentration, and respiratory compensation resulting in a decrease in the partial pressure of carbon dioxide (P_{CO_2}). A low HCO_3^- concentration alone is not diagnostic of metabolic acidosis because it also results from renal compensation to chronic respiratory alkalosis. Measurement of the arterial pH differentiates these two possibilities. The pH is low in hyperchloremic metabolic acidosis and high in chronic respiratory alkalosis. The clinical approach to a patient with a low serum HCO_3^- concentration is given in Figure 27-6.

After confirming metabolic acidosis, calculation of the serum anion gap is a useful step in determining the differential diagnosis of the disorder. The anion gap is equal to the difference between the plasma concentrations of the major cation (Na^+) and the major measured anions ($Cl^- + HCO_3^-$).

$$\text{Anion gap} = [Na^+] - [Cl^-] - [HCO_3^-]$$

The normal value of the anion gap is approximately 12 ± 2 mEq/L. Most of the unmeasured anions consist of albumin, and the normal anion gap therefore changes in the setting of hypoalbuminemia (i.e., normal anion gap is approximately three times the serum albumin [in g/dL]).

Because the total number of cations must equal the total number of anions, a fall in the serum HCO_3^- concentration must be offset by a rise in the concentration of other anions. If the anion accompanying excess hydrogen ions (H^+) is Cl^-, the decrease in the serum HCO_3^- concentration is matched by an equal increase in the serum Cl^- concentration. The acidosis is

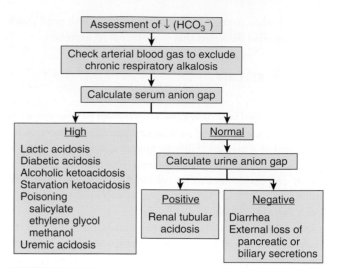

FIGURE 27-6 Approach to the patient with a reduced (↓) serum bicarbonate (HCO_3^-) concentration.

classified as a normal anion gap or hyperchloremic metabolic acidosis. If excess H^+ is accompanied by an anion other than Cl^-, the decrease in HCO_3^- is balanced by an increase in the concentration of the unmeasured anion. The Cl^- concentration remains the same. In this setting, the acidosis is a high anion gap metabolic acidosis.

A useful method for differentiating extrarenal from renal causes of metabolic acidosis is measurement of urinary ammonium ion (NH_4^+) excretion. Extrarenal causes of metabolic acidosis are associated with an appropriate increase in net acid excretion, which is primarily reflected by high levels of urinary NH_4^+ excretion. In contrast, net acid excretion and urinary NH_4^+ levels are low in metabolic acidosis of renal origin. Unfortunately, measurement of urinary NH_4^+ is not a test that is commonly available in clinical medicine. However, the amount of urinary NH_4^+ can be indirectly assessed by calculating the urine anion gap (UAG).

$$UAG = (UNa^+ + UK^+) - UCl^-$$

Under normal circumstances, the UAG is positive, with values ranging from 30 to 50 mEq/L. Metabolic acidosis of extrarenal origin is associated with a marked increase in urinary NH_4^+ excretion, and a large negative value is therefore obtained for the UAG. If the acidosis is of renal origin, urinary NH_4^+ excretion is minimal, and the UAG value usually is positive.

Urine pH cannot reliably differentiate acidosis of renal origin from that of extrarenal origin. For example, an acidic urine pH does not necessarily indicate an appropriate increase in net acid excretion. With a significant reduction in the availability of NH_4^+ to serve as a buffer, only a small amount of distal H^+ secretion leads to a maximal reduction in urine pH. In this setting, the pH of the urine is acidic, but the quantity of H^+ secretion is insufficient to meet daily acid production. Alkaline urine does not necessarily imply a renal acidification defect. In conditions in which availability of NH_4^+ is not limiting, distal H^+ secretion can be massive, but the urine remains relatively alkaline because of the buffering effects of NH_4^+.

Hyperchloremic or Normal Anion Gap Metabolic Acidosis

Hyperchloremic (normal anion gap) metabolic acidosis can have a renal or extrarenal origin. Metabolic acidosis of renal origin is the result of abnormalities in tubular H^+ transport. Metabolic acidosis of extrarenal origin is most commonly caused by gastrointestinal losses of HCO_3^-. Other causes include the external loss of biliary and pancreatic secretions and ureteral diversion procedures. Figure 27-7 provides a clinical approach to metabolic acidosis of renal origin.

Renal Origin of Metabolic Acidosis

Proximal Renal Tubular Acidosis

The diagnosis of proximal renal tubular acidosis (type II RTA) is suspected in a patient with a normal anion gap acidosis, hypokalemia, and an intact ability to acidify the urine to a pH of less than 5.5 while in a steady state. In the steady state, the serum HCO_3^- concentration is usually in the range of 16 to 18 mmol/L. Proximal RTA can be an isolated finding but most commonly is accompanied by generalized dysfunction of the proximal tubule (i.e., Fanconi's syndrome). The UAG is normal.

Proximal RTA is not associated with nephrolithiasis or nephrocalcinosis. However, osteomalacia can develop as a result of chronic hypophosphatemia or deficiency of the active form of vitamin D. Osteopenia may occur as a result of acidosis-induced demineralization of bone.

Treatment of patients with proximal RTA is difficult. Correction of the acidosis is often not possible, even with large amounts of HCO_3^- (3 to 5 mmol/kg/day), because exogenous alkali is rapidly excreted in the urine. This therapy also leads to accelerated renal K^+ losses. Use of a thiazide diuretic to induce sufficient volume depletion to lower the GFR and decrease the filtered load of HCO_3^- may increase the effectiveness of alkali therapy. Potassium-sparing diuretics may limit the degree of renal K^+ wasting. After therapy is initiated, close monitoring is required to guard against severe electrolyte derangements. Topiramate can cause metabolic acidosis due to its inhibitory effects on carbonic anhydrase.

Hypokalemic Distal Renal Tubular Acidosis

The diagnosis of hypokalemic distal RTA (type I RTA) should be considered in a patient with hyperchloremic or normal anion gap acidosis, hypokalemia, and an inability to lower the urine pH maximally. A urine pH greater than 5.5 in the setting of systemic acidosis is consistent with distal RTA. The UAG value is positive. The systemic acidosis tends to be more severe than in patients with a proximal RTA with serum HCO_3^- concentrations as low as 10 mmol/L.

Hypokalemia can be severe and cause musculoskeletal weakness and symptoms of nephrogenic diabetes insipidus. Patients frequently have nephrolithiasis and nephrocalcinosis. The predisposition to renal calcification results from the combined effects of increased urinary calcium ion (Ca^{2+}) excretion due to acidosis-induced bone mineral dissolution, a persistently alkaline urine pH, and low rate of urinary citrate excretion.

Correction of the metabolic acidosis in distal RTA can be achieved by administration of alkali in an amount equal to daily acid production (usually 1 to 2 mmol/kg/day). In patients with severe K^+ deficits, correction of the acidosis with HCO_3^- can transiently cause further lowering of the extracellular K^+ concentration and result in symptomatic hypokalemia. In this setting, the K^+ deficit should be corrected before correcting the acidosis. Potassium citrate is the preferred form of alkali for patients with persistent hypokalemia or with calcium stone disease.

Hyperkalemic Distal Renal Tubular Acidosis

Hyperkalemic distal RTA (type IV RTA) should be suspected in a patient with a normal anion gap (hyperchloremic) metabolic acidosis associated with hyperkalemia. The UAG is slightly positive, indicating little to no NH_4^+ excretion in the urine. Patients in which the disorder is caused by a defect in mineralocorticoid activity typically have a urine pH of less than 5.5, reflecting a

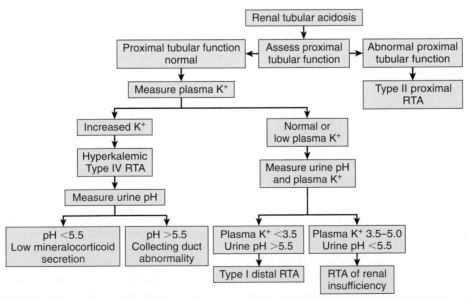

FIGURE 27-7 Approach to the patient with acidosis of renal origin. K^+, Potassium ion; RTA, renal tubular acidosis.

more severe defect in ammonia (NH_3) availability than in H^+ secretion. In patients with structural damage to the collecting duct, the urine pH may be alkaline, reflecting impaired H^+ secretion and decreased urinary NH_4^+ excretion.

The syndrome is most often associated with mild or moderate renal insufficiency. However, the magnitudes of hyperkalemia and acidosis are disproportionately severe for the observed degree of renal insufficiency (Table 27-2).

The primary goal of therapy is to correct the hyperkalemia. In many instances, lowering the serum K^+ level simultaneously corrects the acidosis by restoring renal NH_4^+ production, increasing the buffer supply for distal acidification.

Renal Tubular Acidosis of Renal Insufficiency

Patients with chronic kidney disease initially develop a normal anion gap (hyperchloremic) metabolic acidosis associated with normokalemia as the GFR falls below 30 mL/min. With more advanced chronic kidney disease (GFR <15 mL/min), the acidosis changes to predominately an anion gap metabolic acidosis, reflecting a progressive inability to excrete phosphate, sulfate, and the Na^+ salts of various organic acids. At this stage, the acidosis is commonly referred to as *uremic acidosis*.

Correction of the metabolic acidosis in patients with chronic kidney disease is achieved by treatment with $NaHCO_3$ (0.5 to 1.5 mmol/kg/day), beginning when the HCO_3^- level is less than 22 mmol/L. Metabolic acidosis should be aggressively treated because it can contribute to metabolic bone disease and increase catabolism in chronic kidney disease patients.

Extrarenal Origin of Metabolic Acidosis

Diarrhea

Loss of HCO_3^- in intestinal secretions beyond the stomach leads to development of metabolic acidosis. Volume loss signals the kidney to increase reabsorption of salt. Renal retention of NaCl combined with the intestinal loss of $NaHCO_3$ generates a normal anion gap (hyperchloremic) metabolic acidosis. Net acid excretion markedly increases due to increases in urinary excretion of NH_4^+. Hypokalemia as a result of gastrointestinal losses and the low serum pH stimulate the synthesis of NH_3 in the proximal tubule. Increased availability of NH_3 to act as a urinary buffer allows a maximal increase in H^+ secretion by the distal nephron. Urine pH during chronic diarrheal states may be persistently greater than 6.0 due to the large increase in buffer capacity.

A patient who has hypokalemic hyperchloremic metabolic acidosis with a urine pH greater than 5.5 may have a diarrheal condition or hypokalemic distal RTA (type I RTA). Although the clinical history would be the easiest way to distinguish between these two possibilities, in a patient with surreptitious laxative abuse, it may not be helpful. Determination of the UAG is the best way to differentiate them. In diarrhea, the urine pH is high because of the large amount of NH_4^+ in the urine. This is reflected by a negative UAG value because most of the NH_4^+ is excreted in the urine as NH_4Cl. In hypokalemic distal RTA, the urine pH is high because of the inability to secrete H^+ in the distal nephron. Urinary excretion of NH_3 is very low, and the UAG is positive.

Ileal Conduits

Surgical diversion of the ureter into the intestine may lead to development of a normal anion gap (hyperchloremic) metabolic acidosis due to systemic reabsorption of NH_4^+ and Cl^- from the urinary fluid and exchange of Cl^- for HCO_3^- through activation of the Cl^-/HCO_3^- exchanger in the intestinal lumen. The main determinants for this complication are the length of time urine is in contact with the bowel and the total surface area of bowel exposed to urine.

Anion Gap Metabolic Acidosis

Lactic Acidosis

Lactic acidosis is generated when an imbalance develops between the production and use of lactic acid. Accumulation of a nonchloride anion accounts for the increase in the anion gap. In severe exercise and grand mal seizures, lactic acidosis can develop as a result of increased production. The short-lived nature of the acidosis in these conditions suggests that a concomitant defect in lactic acid use occurs in most conditions of sustained and severe lactic acidosis.

Type A lactic acidosis is characterized by disorders in which there is tissue hypoperfusion or acute hypoxia. These disorders include cardiopulmonary failure, severe anemia, hemorrhage, hypotension, sepsis, and carbon monoxide poisoning. Type B lactic acidosis occurs in patients with a variety of disorders that have in common the development of lactic acidosis in the absence of overt hypoperfusion or hypoxia (Table 27-3).

D-Lactic Acidosis

D-Lactic acidosis is a unique form of metabolic acidosis that can occur in the setting of small bowel resections or in patients with a jejunoileal bypass. These short-bowel syndromes create a situation in which carbohydrates that are normally extensively reabsorbed in the small intestine are delivered in large amounts to the colon. In the setting of colonic bacterial overgrowth, these

---

TABLE 27-2   CAUSES OF HYPERKALEMIC DISTAL (TYPE IV) RENAL TUBULAR ACIDOSIS

I. Mineralocorticoid deficiency
   A. Low renin, low aldosterone levels
      1. Diabetes mellitus
      2. Drugs
         a. Nonsteroidal anti-inflammatory agents
         b. Cyclosporine, tacrolimus
         c. β-Blockers
   B. High renin, low aldosterone levels
      1. Adrenal destruction
      2. Congenital enzyme defects
      3. Drugs
         a. Angiotensin-converting enzyme inhibitors
         b. Angiotensin II receptor blockers
         c. Heparin
         d. Ketoconazole
II. Abnormal cortical collecting duct
   A. Absent or defective mineralocorticoid receptors
   B. Drugs
      1. Spironolactone, eplerenone
      2. Triamterene
      3. Amiloride
      4. Trimethoprim
      5. Pentamidine
   C. Chronic tubulointerstitial disease

TABLE 27-3 CAUSES OF LACTIC ACIDOSIS

I.   Type A (tissue underperfusion and/or hypoxia)
   A.   Cardiogenic shock
   B.   Septic shock
   C.   Hemorrhagic shock
   D.   Acute hypoxia
   E.   Carbon monoxide poisoning
   F.   Anemia
II. Type B (absence of hypotension and hypoxia)
   A.   Hereditary enzyme deficiency (glucose-6-phosphatase)
   B.   Drugs or toxins
      1.   Phenformin, metformin
      2.   Cyanide
      3.   Salicylate, ethylene glycol, methanol
      4.   Propylene glycol
      5.   Linezolid
      6.   Propofol
      7.   Nucleoside reverse transcriptase inhibitors (stavudine, didanosine)
   C.   Systemic disease
      1.   Liver failure
      2.   Malignancy

substrates are metabolized to D-lactate and absorbed into the systemic circulation. Accumulation of D-lactate produces an anion gap metabolic acidosis in which the serum lactate level appears to be normal because the standard test for lactate is specific for L-lactate.

These patients typically seek medical attention after ingestion of a large carbohydrate meal that causes neurologic abnormalities consisting of confusion, slurred speech, and ataxia. Ingestion of low-carbohydrate meals and antimicrobial agents to decrease the degree of bacterial overgrowth are the principal treatments.

Diabetic Ketoacidosis

Diabetic ketoacidosis is a metabolic condition characterized by the accumulation of acetoacetic acid and β-hydroxybutyric acid resulting from insulin deficiency and a relative or absolute increase in the glucagon concentration. The degree to which the anion gap is elevated depends on the rapidity, severity, and duration of the ketoacidosis and the status of the ECF volume. Although an anion gap acidosis is the dominant disturbance in diabetic ketoacidosis, a normal anion gap (hyperchloremic) acidosis often occurs in the earliest stages of ketoacidosis, when the ECF volume is near normal.

Confirmation of ketoacids can be achieved with the use of nitroprusside tablets or reagent strips. However, this test can be misleading in assessing the severity of ketoacidosis because it detects only acetone and acetoacetate, and it does not permit reaction with β-hydroxybutyrate.

Treatment of diabetic ketoacidosis involves the use of insulin and intravenous fluids to correct volume depletion. Deficiencies in K^+, magnesium (Mg^{2+}), and phosphate (PO_4^{3-}) are common, and these electrolytes are typically added to intravenous solutions.

Alcoholic Ketoacidosis

Ketoacidosis develops in patients with a history of chronic ethanol abuse, decreased food intake, and often a history of nausea and vomiting. Alcohol withdrawal, volume depletion, and starvation markedly increase the levels of circulating catecholamines and result in peripheral mobilization of fatty acids that is much larger in magnitude than that typically found with starvation alone. The metabolism of alcohol leads to an increase in the $NADH/NAD^+$ (i.e., balance between the reduced and oxidized forms of nicotinamide adenine dinucleotide), causing a higher ratio of β-hydroxybutyrate to acetoacetate. The nitroprusside reaction may be diminished by this redox shift despite severe ketoacidosis.

Glucose administration leads to the rapid resolution of the acidosis. Stimulation of insulin release leads to diminished fatty acid mobilization from adipose tissue and decreased hepatic output of ketoacids.

Ethylene Glycol and Methanol Poisoning

Ethylene glycol and methanol poisoning are characteristically associated with the development of a severe anion gap metabolic acidosis. Together with the appearance of the anion gap, an osmolar gap manifests and is an important clue to the diagnosis of ethylene glycol and methanol poisoning.

Metabolism of ethylene glycol by alcohol dehydrogenase generates various acids, including glycolic, oxalic, and formic acids. Ethylene glycol is a component of antifreeze and solvents and is ingested by accident or as a suicide attempt. The initial effects of intoxication are neurologic and begin with drunkenness, but they can quickly progress to seizures and coma. If left untreated, cardiopulmonary symptoms such as tachypnea, noncardiogenic pulmonary edema, and cardiovascular collapse may appear. Between 24 and 48 hours after ingestion, patients may develop flank pain and renal failure, which are often accompanied by abundant calcium oxalate crystals in the urine.

Methanol is also metabolized by alcohol dehydrogenase and forms formaldehyde, which is then converted to formic acid. Methanol is found in a variety of commercial preparations such as shellac, varnish, and de-icing solutions. As with ethylene glycol ingestion, methanol is ingested by accident or as a suicide attempt.

Methanol ingestion is associated with an acute inebriation, followed by an asymptomatic period lasting 24 to 36 hours. At this point, abdominal pain is caused by pancreatitis. Seizures, blindness, and coma may develop. The blindness results from the direct toxic effects of formic acid on the retina. Methanol intoxication is also associated with hemorrhage in the white matter and putamen, which can lead to the delayed onset of a Parkinson-like syndrome. Lactic acidosis, which is a feature of methanol and ethylene glycol poisoning, contributes to the elevated anion gap.

In addition to supportive measures, the therapy for ethylene glycol and methanol poisoning centers on reducing the metabolism of the parent compound and accelerating removal of the alcohol from the body. Fomepizole (4-methylpyrazole) is the agent of choice to inhibit the enzyme alcohol dehydrogenase and prevent formation of toxic metabolites.

Salicylate Poisoning

Aspirin (acetylsalicylic acid) poisoning leads to increased lactic acid production. The accumulation of lactic, salicylic, keto, and other organic acids leads to development of an anion gap metabolic acidosis. At the same time, salicylate has a direct stimulatory effect on the respiratory center. Increased ventilation lowers the P_{CO_2}, contributing to the development of respiratory alkalosis. Children primarily have an anion gap metabolic acidosis with toxic salicylate levels, whereas respiratory alkalosis is most evident in adults.

In addition to conservative management, the initial goal of therapy is to correct systemic acidemia and to increase the urine pH. By increasing the systemic pH, the ionized fraction of salicylic acid increases, and there is less accumulation of the drug in the central nervous system. Similarly, an alkaline urine pH favors increased urinary excretion because the ionized fraction of the drug is poorly reabsorbed by the tubule. At serum concentrations greater than 80 mg/dL or in the setting of severe clinical toxicity, hemodialysis can be used to accelerate removal of the drug from the body.

Pyroglutamic Acidosis

Pyroglutamic acidosis is a cause of anion gap metabolic acidosis accompanied by alterations in mental status ranging from confusion to coma. Pyroglutamic acidosis occurs in critically ill patients receiving therapeutic doses of acetaminophen, a setting in which glutathione levels are reduced as a result of acetaminophen metabolism and oxidative stress associated with critical illness. The diagnosis of pyroglutamic acidosis should be considered for patients with unexplained anion gap metabolic acidosis and recent acetaminophen ingestion.

● METABOLIC ALKALOSIS

Definition

The pathogenesis of metabolic alkalosis involves generation and maintenance of the disorder. Metabolic alkalosis is caused by the addition of new HCO_3^- ions to the blood as a result of loss of acid or gain of alkali. New HCO_3^- ions may be generated by renal or extrarenal mechanisms. Because the kidneys have an enormous capacity to excrete HCO_3^-, even vigorous HCO_3^- generation may not be sufficient to produce sustained metabolic alkalosis. To maintain a metabolic alkalosis, the kidney's capacity to correct the alkalosis must be impaired, or the capacity to reclaim HCO_3^- ions must be enhanced.

Metabolic alkalosis is considered by most physicians to be a benign condition. However, a high blood pH can result in a number of effects that decrease tissue perfusion. Increases in blood pH (i.e., alkalemia) cause respiratory depression and decrease tissue oxygen delivery through the Bohr effect and vasoconstriction. Alkalosis should be aggressively corrected in critically ill patients in whom perfusion of the heart and brain is essential.

Treatment

The treatment of metabolic alkalosis is best approached according to the mechanism of maintenance because correction of the mechanism remedies the metabolic alkalosis. If the EABV can be restored with saline, the metabolic alkalosis is easily corrected. Several conditions are poorly responsive to the administration of NaCl. Metabolic alkalosis in these conditions usually is maintained by a combination of increased mineralocorticoid levels along with high distal Na^+ delivery and hypokalemia. The distinction between these entities relies on assessment of the EABV (Table 27-4).

Decreased Effective Arterial Blood Volume and Saline-Responsive Metabolic Alkalosis

Gastrointestinal Acid Loss

Loss of acid, as occurs with vomiting or nasogastric suction, is a common cause of metabolic alkalosis that is maintained by volume contraction. The loss of gastric acid generates a metabolic alkalosis, and the loss of NaCl in the gastric fluid leads to volume contraction. During active vomiting, the plasma HCO_3^- concentration tends to be higher than the threshold for reabsorption in the proximal nephron. The resultant bicarbonaturia leads to increased excretion of $NaHCO_3$ and $KHCO_3$, resulting in further total body Na^+ depletion and development of K^+ depletion. During this active phase, urine Cl^- concentration is less than 15 mEq/L in the setting of high levels of urine Na^+ and K^+ and a urine pH of 7 to 8.

When the patient stops vomiting, equilibrium is established such that bicarbonaturia disappears but a metabolic alkalosis is maintained by volume contraction, K^+ depletion, and reduction

TABLE 27-4 METABOLIC ALKALOSIS CLASSIFICATION

CLASSIFICATION CHARACTERISTIC	TYPES OF METABOLIC ALKALOSIS		
	Decreased EABV, Saline Responsive	Decreased EABV, Saline Resistant	Increased EABV, Saline Resistant
EABV	Low	Low	High
Urine Cl^- concentration (mEq/L)	<15	>15	>15
Response to saline	Corrects (saline responsive)	No correction (saline resistant)	No correction (saline resistant)
Maintenance	Low EABV	Low EABV + high distal Na^+ delivery and mineralocorticoid effect	High distal Na^+ delivery and mineralocorticoid effect
Cause	Gastrointestinal acid loss: Vomiting or nasogastric suction Congenital chloridorrhea Villous adenoma Post-hypercapneic alkalosis Diuretics Non-reabsorbable anions	Primary increase in distal delivery of Na^+: Active diuretic use (loop and thiazide) Mg^{2+} deficiency Bartter syndrome Gitelman syndrome	Primary increase in mineralocorticoid or mineralocorticoid-like effect: Conn syndrome Liddle syndrome Glucocorticoid-suppresible hyperaldosteronism

EABV, Effective arterial blood volume.

in the GFR. Decreased EABV is the main factor in the maintenance of metabolic alkalosis. At this point, urine Na^+ and Cl^- levels are low. Administration of NaCl results in bicarbonaturia, and the metabolic alkalosis is corrected.

Diuretics

Thiazide and loop diuretics are another common cause of metabolic alkalosis. The diuretics produce a metabolic alkalosis that is generated in the distal nephron by the combination of high aldosterone levels and enhanced distal delivery of Na^+. If diuretics are stopped and the patient is maintained on a low-salt diet, the alkalosis is maintained despite the fact that distal delivery is no longer increased. In this setting, patients tend to be volume contracted and K^+ deficient. Contraction of the EABV is the major factor in the maintenance of metabolic alkalosis. Saline infusion in this setting corrects the metabolic alkalosis.

Decreased Effective Arterial Blood Volume and Saline-Resistant Metabolic Alkalosis

In some forms of metabolic alkalosis, the alkalosis is maintained by decreased EABV, but because of other maintenance factors, the alkalosis is not completely saline responsive. In these patients, saline infusions may improve the metabolic alkalosis but do not completely correct it. Patients may have a low EABV but typically do not have a low urine Cl^- level.

Continued use of thiazide or loop diuretics, magnesium deficiency, Gitelman syndrome, and Bartter syndrome can produce this condition. Treatment of the various causes of metabolic alkalosis is summarized in Table 27-5.

Increased Effective Arterial Blood Volume and Saline-Resistant Metabolic Alkalosis

One type of metabolic alkalosis is not maintained by decreased EABV but instead is maintained by K^+ deficiency and high mineralocorticoid levels in the setting of continued distal delivery of Na^+. The most common cause of this saline-resistant alkalosis is a primary increase in mineralocorticoid levels not related to volume contraction. The mechanism of generation of the alkalosis—enhanced Na^+ delivery with high mineralocorticoid activity—is also responsible for maintenance of metabolic alkalosis. The K^+ deficiency that occurs in this setting exacerbates the tendency to produce alkalosis.

The preferred treatment of metabolic alkalosis in patients with volume expansion and primary mineralocorticoid excess is to remove the underlying cause of the persistent mineralocorticoid activity. When this is not possible, therapy is directed at blocking the actions of the mineralocorticoid at the level of the kidney.

🔴 RESPIRATORY ALKALOSIS

Definition

Primary respiratory alkalosis results from hypocapnia and is defined by an arterial partial pressure of carbon dioxide ($Paco_2$) of less than 35 mm Hg in the setting of alkalemia. Primary respiratory alkalosis should be differentiated from secondary hypocapnia, which is a compensatory mechanism in the setting of primary metabolic acidosis.

Respiratory alkalosis is the most frequent acid-base disturbance encountered. It is particularly common in hospitalized patients, for whom it can be the initial clue to gram-negative sepsis. Hepatic failure is a common and important cause of primary hypocapnia. The severity of hypocapnia correlates with the level of blood ammonia and has prognostic significance. Respiratory alkalosis can be an important clue to the existence of salicylate intoxication. High progesterone levels (in pregnancy) can also cause respiratory alkalosis.

Clinical Presentation

Mild respiratory alkalosis causes lightheadedness, palpitations, and paresthesia of the extremities and the circumoral area. Acute hypocapnia decreases cerebral blood flow and causes binding of free calcium to albumin in the blood. At clinical presentation, patients with acute respiratory alkalosis may appear similar to patients with hypocalcemia and have positive Chvostek and Trousseau signs. Patients with ischemic heart disease may occasionally develop cardiac arrhythmias, ischemic electrocardiographic changes, and angina pectoris during acute hypocapnia.

Diagnosis

The diagnosis of respiratory alkalosis is made by evaluating the patient's history, performing a physical examination, and obtaining laboratory data, including a blood gas analysis. Tachypnea or Kussmaul breathing can be detected on physical examination, and it may be the first clue to a primary respiratory alkalosis or a compensatory respiratory mechanism in the setting of primary metabolic acidosis.

Changes in serum electrolytes can aid in the diagnosis of respiratory alkalosis. An acute fall in Pco_2 causes an HCO_3^--Cl^- shift in red blood cells and accounts for the small initial compensatory response in acute respiratory alkalosis in which the

TABLE 27-5 TREATMENT OF SALINE-RESISTANT METABOLIC ALKALOSIS

	DECREASED EABV		INCREASED EABV	
Cause	*Treatment*		*Cause*	*Treatment*
Thiazide and loop diuretics	Discontinue drug, replete EABV		Renin secreting tumor	Remove tumor
Mg^{2+} deficiency	Replete Mg^{2+} deficit		Primary hyperaldosteronism	Remove tumor, spironolactone for BAH
Gitelman syndrome	Amiloride, triamterene, or spironolactone, K^+ supplements, Mg^{2+} supplements		Glucocorticoid-suppressible hyperaldosteronism	Dexamethasone
Bartter syndrome	Amiloride, triamterene, or spironolactone, K^+ supplements, Mg^{2+} supplements in some		Liddle syndrome	Amiloride or triamterene

BAH, Bilateral adrenal hyperplasia; EABV, effective arterial blood volume; K^+, potassium ion; Mg^{2+}, magnesium ion.

TABLE 27-6   COMPENSATION IN ACID-BASE DISORDERS

DISORDER	COMPENSATORY CHANGES
Acute respiratory acidosis	For every 10 mm Hg rise in P_{CO_2}, the HCO_3^- increases by 1 mEq/L
Chronic respiratory acidosis	For every 10 mm Hg rise in P_{CO_2}, the HCO_3^- increases by 3.5 mEq/L
Acute respiratory alkalosis	For every 10 mm Hg fall in P_{CO_2}, the HCO_3^- decreases by 2 mEq/L
Chronic respiratory alkalosis	For every 10 mm Hg decrease in P_{CO_2}, the HCO_3^- decreases by 5 mEq/L
Metabolic acidosis	1.2 mm Hg decrease in P_{CO_2} for each 1 mEq/L fall in HCO_3^- $P_{CO_2} = HCO_3^- + 15$ P_{CO_2} resembles last two digits of pH
Metabolic alkalosis	P_{CO_2} increases by 0.7 mm Hg for each mEq/L HCO_3^-

HCO_3^- concentration falls by 2 mEq/L for every 10 mm Hg decrease in P_{CO_2}. Table 27-6 provides the expected compensatory responses for acid-base disorders.

In chronic respiratory alkalosis, the renal HCO_3^- reabsorptive capacity decreases, and there is a transient HCO_3^- diuresis. This process takes 2 to 3 days to fully manifest. After the new steady state is achieved, the HCO_3^- concentration has decreased by 5 mEq/L for each 10 mm Hg fall in the P_{CO_2}. A higher or lower value for the plasma HCO_3^- concentration suggests an additional metabolic disorder.

To defend ECF volume in the setting of increased urinary loss of $NaHCO_3$, the kidney retains NaCl. These changes are reflected in the serum electrolyte levels of patients with chronic respiratory alkalosis, in whom the Cl^- level is typically increased with respect to the serum Na^+ concentration. Another characteristic finding is an increase of 3 to 5 mEq/L in the serum anion gap. The increased gap results from the greater fixed negative charge on serum albumin and an increase in the serum lactate concentration. Lactate production is increased due to a stimulatory effect of high pH on phosphofructokinase, the rate-limiting step in the glycolytic pathway.

Treatment

Primary respiratory alkalosis is treated by correcting the underlying cause. A patient with anxiety-hyperventilation syndrome should be treated by providing reassurance. Rebreathing into a paper bag or any other closed system causes the P_{CO_2} to increase with each breath taken and leads to partial correction of hypocapnia and improvement of symptoms. In the rare case when there is no response to conservative management, sedatives can be used. In mechanically ventilated patients, the P_{CO_2} can be increased by raising the inspired carbon dioxide tension or by increasing the dead space of the ventilator circuit.

Correction of respiratory alkalosis may prove helpful in correcting arrhythmias in patients with underlying coronary disease. In contrast, caution is warranted in raising the P_{CO_2} in patients with brain injury because cerebral perfusion may increase and worsen intracranial pressure. Respiratory alkalosis frequently develops as a complication of hypoxia. Administration of oxygen or return to lower altitudes can reverse the respiratory alkalosis that develops in this setting.

RESPIRATORY ACIDOSIS

Definition

Respiratory acidosis develops as a result of ineffective alveolar ventilation. This acid-base disorder, which is also called *primary hypercapnia*, should be differentiated from secondary hypercapnia, which develops as a compensatory mechanism in the setting of primary metabolic alkalosis. Primary hypercapnia is clinically recognized by P_{aCO_2} levels greater than 45 mm Hg on arterial blood gas analysis. However, P_{aCO_2} levels of less than 45 mm Hg may still indicate respiratory acidosis if a primary metabolic acidosis is not adequately compensated by alveolar ventilation.

The development of respiratory acidosis is usually multifactorial. Major causes of carbon dioxide retention include diseases of or malfunction in any element of the respiratory system, including the central and peripheral nervous systems, respiratory muscles, thoracic cage, pleural space, airways, and lung parenchyma. Six factors should be considered in the differential diagnosis of acute and chronic respiratory acidosis: inhibition of the medullary respiratory center, disorders of the chest wall and respiratory muscles, airway obstruction, disorders affecting gas exchange across the pulmonary capillary, increased carbon dioxide production, and mechanical ventilation.

Clinical Presentation

Hypercapnic encephalopathy is a clinical syndrome that usually starts with irritability, headache, mental cloudiness, apathy, confusion, anxiety, and restlessness. It can progress to asterixis, transient psychosis, delirium, somnolence, and coma. Papilledema and other manifestations of increased intracranial pressure that are collectively named *pseudotumor cerebri* are occasionally observed in patients with acute or chronic hypercapnia. The increase in intracranial pressure is caused in part due by cerebral vasodilation resulting from acidemia.

Acute respiratory acidosis is typically much more symptomatic than acute metabolic acidosis because carbon dioxide diffuses and equilibrates across the blood-brain barrier much more rapidly than does HCO_3^-, resulting in a more rapid fall in cerebral spinal fluid and cerebral interstitial pH. Severe hypercapnia also can lead to decreased myocardial contractility, arrhythmias, and peripheral vasodilatation, particularly when the blood pH falls to less than 7.1.

Diagnosis

The diagnosis of primary respiratory acidosis is based on the finding of acidemia and hypercapnia on arterial blood gas analysis. Changes in the serum chemistries can aid in the diagnosis of respiratory acidosis.

Acute hypercapnia is associated with a shift of HCO_3^- out of red blood cells in exchange for Cl^-, a process called *red cell HCO_3^--Cl^- shift*. Acutely, the plasma HCO_3^- concentration increases by 1 mmol/L for each 10 mm Hg of elevation in the P_{aCO_2}. After 24 to 48 hours of hypercapnia, proximal tubular cells increase H^+ secretion, resulting in accelerated HCO_3^- reabsorption. The retention of $NaHCO_3$ leads to slight expansion of the ECF compartment and increases renal excretion of NaCl to return the volume level to normal. The net effect is increased serum HCO_3^- and decreased Cl^- concentrations. In chronic respiratory acidosis, there is a 3.5 mEq/L increase in HCO_3^- for each 10 mm Hg elevation in the $PaCO_2$. Higher or lower plasma HCO_3^- concentrations suggest mixed respiratory and metabolic acid-base disorders.

Treatment

The mainstay of treatment in respiratory acidosis is to recognize and treat the underlying cause when possible. Patients with acute respiratory acidosis are primarily at risk for hypoxemia rather than hypercapnia or acidemia. Immediate therapeutic efforts should focus on establishing and securing a patent airway to provide adequate oxygenation. In patients with status asthmaticus, a lower ventilatory rate and peak inspiratory pressure may be required to minimize barotrauma to the lung, but it is achieved at the expense of a persistently higher PCO_2. Small amounts of $NaHCO_3$ can help to prevent excessive decreases in blood pH in this setting. The downside of this therapy is that infusion of $NaHCO_3$ can result in increased carbon dioxide production, causing a further increase in PCO_2 when ventilation cannot be increased.

Excessive oxygen should be avoided in patients with chronic respiratory acidosis because it may lead to worsening hypoventilation. When mechanical ventilation is required, care should be taken to lower the $PaCO_2$ carefully and slowly because there is the risk of overshoot alkalemia due to a high HCO_3^- (i.e., post-hypercapnic metabolic alkalosis). The kidneys must excrete the HCO_3^- to normalize the acid-base status. This excretion does not occur when the EABV is reduced because of salt depletion due to restricted intake or diuretic therapy or because of a salt-retentive state such as heart failure or cirrhosis. Correction of the superimposed metabolic alkalosis can usually be achieved with saline and discontinuation of loop diuretics. In edematous patients with heart failure, this is not possible, and acetazolamide may be needed to correct the alkalosis.

SUGGESTED READINGS

Palmer BF: Managing hyperkalemia caused by inhibitors of the renin-angiotensin-aldosterone system, N Engl J Med 351:585–592, 2004.

Palmer BF: Approach to fluid and electrolyte disorders and acid-base problems, Prim Care 35:195–213, 2008.

Palmer BF: A physiologic based approach to the evaluation of a patient with hyperkalemia, Am J Kidney Dis 56:387–393, 2010.

Palmer BF: A physiologic-based approach to the evaluation of a patient with hypokalemia, Am J Kidney Dis 56:1184–1190, 2010.

Palmer BF: Diagnostic approach and management of inpatient hyponatremia, J Hosp Med 5:S1–S5, 2010.

Palmer BF: Respiratory alkalosis, Am J Kidney Dis 60:834–838, 2012.

Palmer BF: Respiratory acid-base disorders. In Mount D, Sayegh M, Singh Ajay, editors: Core concepts in the disorders of fluid, electrolytes and acid-base balance, New York, 2013, Springer, pp 297–306.

Palmer BF, Alpern RJ: Metabolic alkalosis, J Am Soc Nephrol 8:1462–1469, 1997.

Palmer BF, Alpern RJ: Metabolic acidosis. In Floege J, Johnson RJ, Feehally J, editors: Comprehensive clinical nephrology, ed 4, St Louis, 2010, Elsevier Saunders, pp 155–166.

Palmer BF, Alpern RJ: Normal acid-base balance. In Floege J, Johnson RJ, Feehally J, editors: Comprehensive clinical nephrology, ed 4, St Louis, 2010, Elsevier Saunders, pp 149–154.

Sterns R, Palmer BF: Fluid, electrolyte, and acid-base disturbances, NephSAP 6:210–280, 2007.

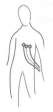

28

Glomerular Diseases

Sanjeev Sethi, An De Vriese, and Fernando C. Fervenza

INTRODUCTION

The glomerulus can be injured in a variety of disorders, and glomerular injury or disease can manifest as hematuria, proteinuria, hypertension, fluid retention, and a reduction in the glomerular filtration rate. Traditionally, glomerular diseases have been classified according to clinical presentation, including asymptomatic microscopic hematuria, the nephritic syndrome, the nephrotic syndrome, and rapidly progressive glomerulonephritis (RPGN). However, great progress has been made in unraveling the molecular causes of glomerular diseases. For instance, autoantibodies against the phospholipase A_2 receptor have been associated with membranous nephropathy, a disease that manifests clinically as nephrotic syndrome. Many glomerular diseases can manifest with more than one constellation of signs and symptoms and show more than one histologic pattern on renal biopsy. In the future, the etiologic approach to the classification of glomerular diseases will undoubtedly be expanded.

CLINICAL PRESENTATION

A detailed history and careful physical examination, with particular attention to the time of symptom onset, help to clarify the differential diagnosis of suspected glomerular disease. Blood pressure and fluid status should be recorded. Urine microscopy is a critical element of this assessment, and it may reveal hematuria, typically with dysmorphic red blood cells and casts. Hematuria due to glomerular disease is painless and often associated with brown or cola-colored urine rather than bright red; clots are rare. Other causes of brown urine include hemoglobinuria, myoglobinuria, and food or drug dyes (e.g., beetroot).

Quantitative evaluation of the degree of urinary protein excretion is essential. In adults, urine total protein excretion is less than 150 mg/24h, and urinary albumin excretion is less than 20 mg/24h. Persistent albumin excretion of 30 to 300 mg/24h reflects high albuminuria (i.e., microalbuminuria), and albumin excretion above 300 mg/24h, the level at which the standard dipstick becomes positive, reflects overt proteinuria. Levels above 3.5 g/24h are considered to be nephrotic-range proteinuria. The principal constituent of the protein excreted by these patients is albumin (up to 98% in some cases).

A 24-hour urine collection remains the gold standard, but it is cumbersome, is often collected incorrectly, and does not provide a rapid result. A protein-to-creatinine ratio measured on a spot urine sample has emerged as a useful alternative. The urine protein concentration (in mg/dL) divided by the urine creatinine concentration (in mg/dL) yields a dimensionless number that approximates the 24-hour protein excretion (in g/24h). The reliability of the protein-to-creatinine ratio is limited in patients who excrete approximately 1 g/24h of creatinine, such as in those who are severely catabolic.

Glomerular proteinuria can be classified as transient or hemodynamic (functional) (e.g., fever, exercise induced, orthostatic) or as persistent (fixed). Although functional proteinuria is benign, fixed nephrotic-range proteinuria is usually results from glomerular diseases. Total proteinuria greater than 1 g/24h in a patient with a negative urine dipstick test result (which detects only albumin) suggests that the proteinuria may be caused by light chains or low-molecular-weight proteins (e.g., retinol-binding protein, α_1-microglobulin).

CLINICAL SYNDROMES

The major clinical syndromes associated with glomerular injury are discussed in this section. In each case, general recognition and management should be pursued in parallel with efforts to define the specific mechanisms of injury.

Nephrotic Syndrome

Nephrotic syndrome is defined as persistent urinary total protein excretion greater than 3.5 g/24h, accompanied by a serum albumin concentration less than 3.5 g/dL. Edema, hyperlipidemia, and lipiduria (i.e., doubly refractile fat bodies) are common but are not required for the diagnosis.

Complications of the nephrotic syndrome include hypogammaglobulinemia, vitamin D deficiency due to loss of vitamin D–binding protein, and iron deficiency anemia due to hypotransferrinemia. Thrombotic complications such as renal vein thrombosis are more common, especially in patients with greater protein loss (>10 g/24h) and serum albumin levels less than 2 g/dL. Patients with severe nephrotic syndrome may also have acute renal failure when there is superimposed volume depletion, sepsis, interstitial nephritis, or use of nephrotoxic agents such as nonsteroidal anti-inflammatory drugs (NSAIDs).

Management of patients with nephrotic syndrome includes diuretics to control edema, regulation of blood pressure (angiotensin-converting enzyme inhibitors [ACEIs] and angiotensin-receptor blockers [ARBs] are preferred), limitation of the intake of protein to between 0.8 and 1 g/kg/day and sodium to less than 4 g/day, and control of lipid levels. Anticoagulation should be considered for patients at increased risk, especially if the nephrotic syndrome is caused by membranous nephropathy or amyloidosis.

Nephritic Syndrome

The nephritic syndrome is defined by oliguria, edema, hypertension, proteinuria (usually <3.5 g/24h), and abnormal urinalysis with dysmorphic red blood cells or casts on microscopic examination.

Rapidly Progressive Glomerulonephritis

RPGN is a clinical syndrome characterized by progressive loss of kidney function with a time course of days to months in a patient with active urinary sediment such as red blood cell casts. Patients may have oliguria. Most of the pulmonary-renal syndromes manifest in this fashion, and the pathologic corollary is often a focal, necrotizing, crescentic glomerulonephritis. When RPGN is suspected, renal biopsy with immunofluorescence studies is extremely helpful.

Linear deposition of immunoglobulin G (IgG) points to Goodpasture disease or anti–glomerular basement membrane (anti-GBM)–mediated glomerulonephritis. Immunoglobulins and complement suggest systemic lupus erythematosus (SLE), cryoglobulinemia, immunoglobulin A nephropathy (IgAN), or postinfectious glomerulonephritis. Negative or weak immunofluorescence (pauci-immune) findings usually indicate an antineutrophil cytoplasmic autoantibody (ANCA) vasculitis (Fig. 28-1).

● GLOMERULAR DISEASES MANIFESTING WITH NEPHROTIC SYNDROME

Minimal Change Disease

In a patient with nephrotic syndrome, minimal change disease (MCD) is defined by a renal biopsy with no significant glomerular abnormalities on light microscopy, negative immunoglobulin and complement deposition on immunofluorescence, and widespread foot process effacement on electron microscopy (Fig. 28-2). MCD is the most common cause of nephrotic syndrome in children and accounts for up to 20% of adults with primary nephrotic syndrome.

The pathogenesis of MCD is unknown. The association with Hodgkin's lymphoma suggests that MCD may be a consequence of T-lymphocyte abnormalities, with T cells producing a lymphokine that is toxic to glomerular epithelial cells. Most cases of MCD are idiopathic, although drugs (e.g., NSAIDs), hematologic malignancies (mainly Hodgkin's lymphoma), and thymoma are well-recognized causes of secondary MCD. Concomitant interstitial nephritis suggests drugs (e.g., NSAIDs) as the likely cause of MCD.

In children, MCD usually manifests with nephrotic syndrome of acute onset. Hematuria, hypertension, or impaired renal function is unusual and suggests another diagnosis. When nephrotic syndrome occurs in a child with normal urinalysis results, the

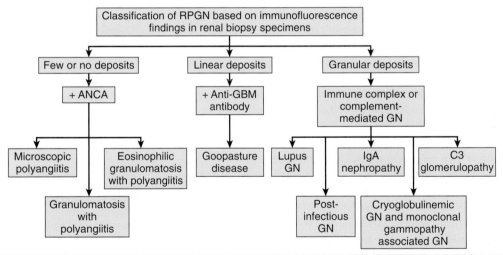

FIGURE 28-1 Rapidly progressive glomerulonephritis (RPGN) is classified according to immunofluorescence microscopy findings in renal biopsy specimens. ANCA, Antineutrophil cytoplasmic autoantibody; GBM, glomerular basement membrane; GN, glomerulonephritis; IgA, immunoglobulin A.

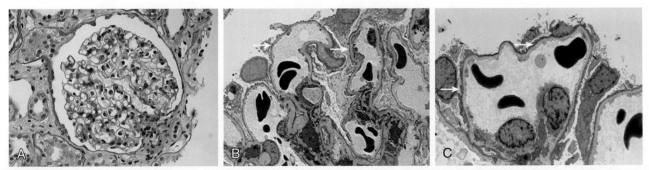

FIGURE 28-2 Minimal change disease. **A,** Light microscopy shows a normal-appearing glomerulus (periodic acid–Schiff, ×40). **B** and **C,** Electron microscopy shows diffuse foot process effacement (arrows) (**B,** ×2500; **C,** ×4200). Immunofluorescence studies were negative for immune deposits.

diagnosis is MCD until proved otherwise, and treatment with high-dose corticosteroid therapy can be started, often without the need of a renal biopsy.

More than 90% of children achieve complete remission after 4 to 8 weeks of treatment. Children who do not respond to corticosteroid therapy should undergo a renal biopsy. Adolescents and adults also respond to high-dose corticosteroids (>80%), but the response is slower, and treatment for 16 weeks or more may be required to achieve remission. Therapy usually is continued for 4 to 8 weeks after remission.

Among patients who have a response to corticosteroids, about 25% have a long-term remission. However, up to 25% of the patients have frequent relapses, and up to 30% become steroid dependent. For these patients, alternative therapies aiming to minimize corticosteroid toxicity include the use of alkylating agents, antimetabolites, and calcineurin inhibitors. Although these agents may allow a lower corticosteroid dose, some patients respond poorly or not all, and use of an agent may be complicated by development of significant side effects. Noncompliance is always a concern, especially in young patients. Rituximab is a chimeric human-murine monoclonal antibody that targets the CD20 antigen expressed on B cells. It has been efficacious in a number of autoimmune diseases and has promise in the treatment of MCD.

Focal Segmental Glomerulosclerosis

Focal segmental glomerulosclerosis (FSGS) is a clinicopathologic syndrome, and the common pathophysiologic element is podocyte injury and depletion leading to glomerular scarring (Fig. 28-3). FSGS accounts for less than 15% of cases of idiopathic nephrotic syndrome in children and up to 25% in adults. FSGS is thought to be the most common form of idiopathic nephrotic syndrome in African Americans; it most likely represents a different disease from FSGS in Caucasians. Hypertension is found in 30% to 50% of patients with FSGS, and microscopic hematuria occurs in 25% to 75% of cases. Up to 30% of those with FSGS have impaired renal function.

The pathogenesis of idiopathic or primary FSGS is unknown. A circulating permeability factor has been demonstrated in some patients. More recently, the soluble urokinase-type plasminogen activator receptor (suPAR) has been identified as a potential marker because levels are elevated in two thirds of cases of primary FSGS and levels are higher in renal transplant recipients with recurrent FSGS. However, suPAR levels do not distinguish primary from secondary FSGS, and serum levels increase with reductions in the glomerular filtration rate. Further research is needed to define the role of serum suPAR in idiopathic FSGS.

Secondary causes of FSGS include genetic mutations in podocyte genes, human immunodeficiency virus (HIV) infection, sickle cell disease, vesicoureteral reflux, obesity, unilateral renal agenesis, remnant kidneys, and aging (Table 28-1). Four histologic variants of FSGS have been described. The cellular or collapsing variant, which has the worst prognosis, is more common in African Americans and patients with HIV infection.

Spontaneous remission of proteinuria is uncommon (<5% of cases). Treatment of the primary forms consists of prolonged (>4 months), high-dose corticosteroid therapy (prednisone, 1 mg/kg/day), but there is no study comparing this approach with other forms of therapy. If patients are going to respond to corticosteroids, proteinuria starts to decrease soon after the start of treatment, and those who show no reduction in proteinuria after 2 to 3 months of prednisone at 1 mg/kg/day are unlikely to respond. For patients who respond to corticosteroids but undergo relapse, alternative therapy includes the use of cytotoxic drugs alone or in combination with corticosteroids, calcineurin inhibitors, and possibly rituximab. For patients with secondary forms of FSGS, treatment should target the cause.

TABLE 28-1   CAUSES OF FOCAL SEGMENTAL GLOMERULOSCLEROSIS

PRIMARY (IDIOPATHIC) FSGS

- Attributed to a circulating permeability factor

SECONDARY FSGS

- Genetic mutations in podocyte genes
- Viral: HIV-associated nephropathy, parvovirus B19, simian virus 40, cytomegalovirus
- Drug induced: heroin, interferon (α, β, γ), pamidronate, sirolimus, calcineurin inhibitors
- Adaptive: reduced nephron mass or glomerular adaptation, unilateral renal agenesis, obesity-related glomerulopathy, basement membrane defects healing phase of focal proliferative glomerulonephritis, body building, sickle cell anemia, hypertensive nephrosclerosis, thrombotic microangiopathy, aging kidney
- Other causes: hemophagocytic syndrome

FSGS, Focal segmental glomerulosclerosis; HIV, human immunodeficiency virus.

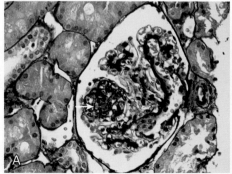 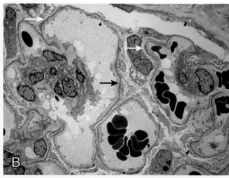

FIGURE 28-3 Focal segmental glomerulosclerosis. **A,** Light microscopy shows segmental sclerosis *(arrow)* with segmental consolidation of the glomerular capillary tufts and visceral epithelial cell hypertrophy over the segmentally sclerosed tufts (silver methenamine, ×40). **B,** Electron microscopy shows diffuse foot process effacement *(arrows)* of the visceral epithelial cells (×1850). Immunofluorescence studies were negative for immune deposits.

In all patients, treatment with an ACEI or ARB, alone or in combination, may substantially reduce proteinuria and prolong renal survival. Patients who have a non–nephrotic-range proteinuria have the best renal survival (>80% at 10 years). In patients who continue to have a high degree of proteinuria (>10 g/day), end-stage renal disease (ESRD) typically develops over 5 to 20 years. Idiopathic FSGS may recur in a transplanted kidney.

HIV-Associated Nephropathy

Patients with HIV infection can have many forms of kidney injury due to sepsis, co-infection with hepatitis B or C virus (HBV or HCV), nephrotoxic drugs, and use of antiretroviral agents. HIV-associated nephropathy (HIVAN) is a clinicopathologic entity characterized by nephrotic-range proteinuria and a collapsing form of FSGS, often with microcystic tubular dilation. On electron microscopy, tubuloreticular inclusions (i.e., interferon fingerprints) may be seen within the glomerular and vascular endothelial cells.

HIVAN occurs almost exclusively in patients of African descent when CD4 levels are low. It is thought to be caused by infection and subsequent expression of HIV viral genes in podocytes. The onset of proteinuria is typically acute. Proteinuria can be greater than 10 g/day, and renal insufficiency can progress rapidly.

Membranous Nephropathy

Membranous nephropathy is the leading cause of nephrotic syndrome in whites. It occurs in persons of all ages and races but is most often diagnosed in middle age, with the incidence peaking during the fourth and fifth decades of life. The male-to-female ratio is about 2 : 1.

Autoantibodies against the phospholipase A_2 receptor in podocytes are found in about 70% of patients with the primary form of the disease. Most patients have nephrotic syndrome, normal renal function, and no hypertension. Microscopic hematuria may be detected in about one third of patients. Secondary membranous nephropathy is caused by autoimmune diseases (e.g., SLE, autoimmune thyroiditis), infection (e.g., HBV, HCV), drugs (e.g., penicillamine, NSAIDs), and solid malignancies (e.g., colon cancer, lung cancer).

On light microscopy, capillary walls may appear thickened, and methenamine silver stain shows subepithelial projections ("spikes") along the capillary walls. Immunofluorescence microscopy shows marked granular deposition of IgG and C3 along the capillary walls, and subepithelial deposits are seen on electron microscopy (Fig. 28-4).

Up to one third of the patients with membranous nephropathy undergo spontaneous remission, and another one third of patients undergo partial remission. Initial therapy should include angiotensin II receptor blockade, a low-salt diet (<4 g/day), a low-protein diet (0.8 to 1 g/kg/day), and lipid control. If spontaneous remission occurs, it usually does so within the first 12 to 24 months.

Patients who remain nephrotic or those with declining renal function are candidates for immunosuppressive therapy, including a combination of corticosteroids and cytotoxic agents or calcineurin inhibitor monotherapy. Rituximab has recently garnered attention as a potential breakthrough in the treatment of membranous nephropathy, and studies are being conducted. The probability of renal survival is more than 80% at 5 years and about 60% at 15 years. Patients with an accelerated course should be evaluated for superimposed anti-GBM disease, acute interstitial nephritis, or renal vein thrombosis.

⬤ GLOMERULAR DISEASES MANIFESTING WITH NEPHRITIC SYNDROME
Infection-Associated Glomerulonephritis

Poststreptococcal glomerulonephritis (PSGN) is a classic form of acute glomerulonephritis that develops 1 to 4 weeks after a pharyngitis or skin infection with specific (nephritogenic) strains of group A β-hemolytic streptococci. It typically occurs in children and usually has a benign course. More recently, however, infection-associated glomerulonephritis has been recognized to have a broader spectrum, including affecting elderly and immunocompromised patients and being associated with different bacteria, particularly staphylococci. Unlike classic PSGN, the variant occurs when the infection is still active and has an unfavorable prognosis.

Infection-associated glomerulonephritis manifests clinically with the abrupt onset of nephritic syndrome. In patients with PSGN, cultures are usually negative, but elevated titers of anti-streptolysin O (ASO), antistreptokinase, antihyaluronidase, and anti-deoxyribonuclease (anti-DNAse B) antibodies may provide evidence of recent streptococcal infection. Activation of the alternative complement pathway is reflected by low C3 complement

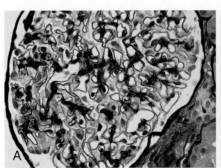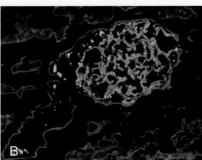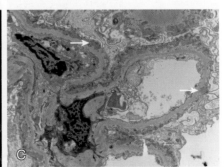

FIGURE 28-4 Membranous nephropathy. **A,** Light microscopy shows thickened glomerular basement membranes (×60). **B,** Immunofluorescence study shows granular immunoglobulin G deposition along the capillary walls (×20). **C,** Electron microscopy shows subepithelial electron-dense deposits *(arrows)* (×15,000).

levels. C4 levels are usually normal or mildly decreased. Other nephrologic conditions associated with low complement are C3 glomerulopathy, lupus nephritis, cryoglobulinemic glomerulonephritis, and cholesterol emboli (Table 28-2).

Renal biopsy typically shows diffuse glomerular hypercellularity and infiltration of polymorphonuclear leukocytes, monocytes, or macrophages on light microscopy. Immunofluorescence shows granular deposition of IgG, C3, and occasionally immunoglobulin M (IgM). On electron microscopy, characteristic dome-shaped subepithelial deposits ("humps") can be seen along the GBM (Fig. 28-5).

Treatment is supportive and aims to minimize fluid overload, optimize blood pressure control, and eradicate ongoing infection. For children, the prognosis is excellent, with most patients recovering renal function in 1 to 2 months. Some patients have persistent microscopic hematuria, proteinuria, hypertension, and renal dysfunction and are said to have *atypical*, *persistent*, or *resolving* PSGN. Some of these patients have mutations or autoantibodies to proteins in the alternative complement cascade.

Immunoglobulin a Nephropathy

IgAN (i.e., Berger disease) is the most common form of a primary glomerulopathy. On light microscopy, mesangial proliferation is

seen along with mesangial deposition of IgA on immunofluorescence and electron-dense deposits in the mesangial cells on electron microscopy (Fig. 28-6).

Patients may have episodes of macroscopic hematuria accompanying an intercurrent upper respiratory tract infection (synpharyngitic) or have asymptomatic hematuria, with or without proteinuria, detected on routine urinalysis. Proteinuria is common, but nephrotic syndrome occurs in less than 10% of cases and raises the possibility of a podocytopathy (e.g., MCD) superimposed on IgAN.

The pathogenesis of IgA nephropathy has been linked to galactose-deficient IgA1 (GD-IgA1) molecules and increased formation of anti–GD-IgA1 autoantibodies, with deposition of IgG or IgA anti–GD-IgA1 immune complexes in the mesangium, resulting in activation of complement and cytokine cascades. Secondary causes of IgAN include chronic liver disease, celiac disease, dermatitis herpetiformis, and ankylosing spondylitis.

In up to 60% of the patients, IgA nephropathy has a benign clinical course, and patients maintain proteinuria of less than 500 mg/24h and preserve renal function. However, progression to ESRD occurs in up to 40% of patients over 10 to 25 years. Clinical predictors of progression include proteinuria greater than 1 g/24h, hypertension, and impaired renal function at diagnosis. Any degree of proteinuria carries a worse prognosis for a patient with IgAN. IgAN frequently recurs after renal transplantation, but loss of the allograft from recurrent disease is uncommon.

The use of angiotensin II system blockade and high-dose corticosteroids has been beneficial in slowing or halting progression of renal disease. Henoch-Schönlein purpura is the systemic form of IgAN. The prognosis is generally good for children but varies for adults.

TABLE 28-2	GLOMERULAR DISEASES ASSOCIATED WITH HYPOCOMPLEMENTEMIA

Acute lupus nephritis
C3 glomerulopathy (C3 glomerulonephritis and dense deposit disease)
Cholesterol emboli
Cryoglobulinemic glomerulonephritis
Postinfectious glomerulonephritis

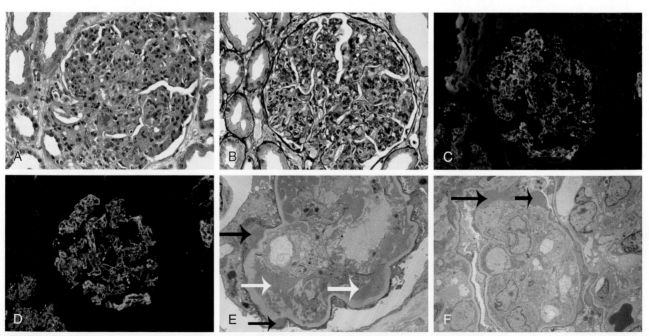

FIGURE 28-5 Postinfectious glomerulonephritis. **A** and **B**, Light microscopy shows diffuse endocapillary proliferative glomerulonephritis. Notice the prominent neutrophil infiltration in the glomerular capillaries (**A**, hematoxylin and eosin; **B**, silver methenamine; both ×40). **C** and **D**, Immunofluorescence studies show granular immunoglobulin G and C3 deposition along the capillary walls (both ×20). **E** and **F**, Electron microscopy shows subendothelial deposits (*white arrows*) and subepithelial humplike deposits (*black arrows*). The subendothelial deposits likely result from circulating immune complexes that are deposited along the glomerular capillary walls and drive the inflammatory response (**E**, ×5800). The subepithelial deposits likely represent in situ immune complex formation (**F**, ×2850).

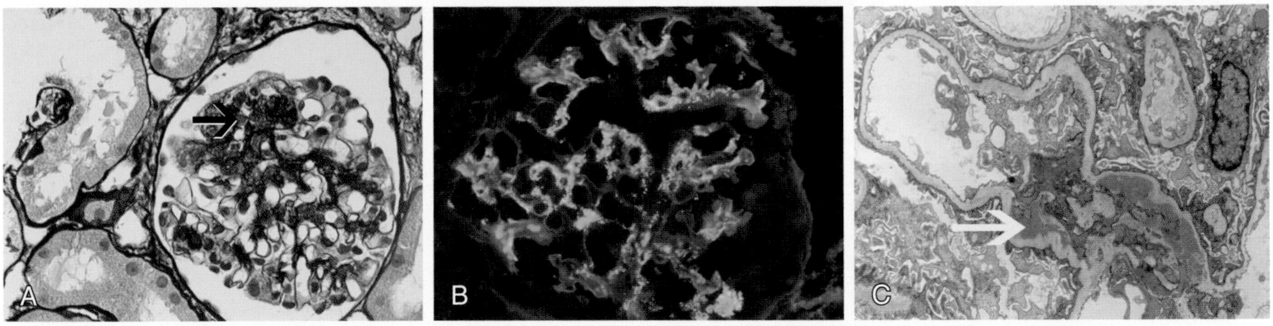

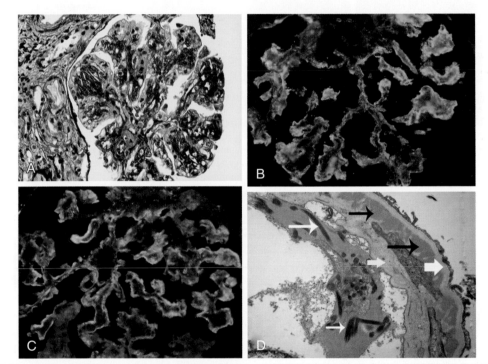

FIGURE 28-6 Immunoglobulin A (IgA) nephropathy. **A,** Light microscopy shows mesangial hypercellularity *(black arrow)* (silver methenamine, ×40). **B,** Immunofluorescence microscopy shows bright mesangial IgA staining. **C,** Electron microscopy shows large mesangial electron-dense deposits *(arrow)* (×7860)

FIGURE 28-7 Immune complex–mediated membranoproliferative glomerulonephritis due to hepatitis C virus infection. **A,** Light microscopy shows a membranoproliferative pattern of injury with mesangial expansion, endocapillary proliferation, double-contour formation along the capillary walls, and lobular accentuation of the glomerular tufts (silver methenamine, ×40). **B** and **C,** Immunofluorescence microscopy shows bright capillary wall staining for immunoglobulin M (**B,** ×40) and for C3 (**C,** ×40). **D,** Electron microscopy shows capillary wall thickening and a double-contour formation due to accumulation of subendothelial electron-dense deposits *(black arrows)*, cellular elements, and new basement membrane formation (i.e., duplication) *(yellow arrow)* that produces the double contour. The *thick white arrow* indicates the old basement membrane, and fibrin tactoids *(white arrows)* in glomerular capillary loops indicate a prothrombotic state (×1350).

In patients with normal renal function, treatment is supportive only. Patients with persistent proteinuria >1 g/24h and/or progressive renal failure should be considered for treatment with high-dose corticosteroids with or without cytotoxic medication.

Membranoproliferative Glomerulonephritis

Membranoproliferative glomerulonephritis (MPGN) is a pattern of glomerular injury resulting from predominantly subendothelial and mesangial deposition of immune complexes or complement factors and their products. On light microscopy, mesangial hypercellularity, endocapillary proliferation, and capillary wall remodeling with double-contour formation are characteristic, and they result in a lobular accentuation of the glomerular tufts.

Immunofluorescence microscopy shows immunoglobulins or complement factors, depending on the underlying cause of MPGN. Electron microscopy typically shows mesangial and subendothelial deposits, and, less commonly, intramembranous and subepithelial deposits (Fig. 28-7).

Based on a recent proposal, MPGN can be classified as immune complex mediated or complement mediated. Immune complex–mediated MPGN shows immunoglobulin and complement factors on immunofluorescence microscopy. Complement-mediated MPGN shows complement factors and a lack of significant immunoglobulin on immunofluorescence microscopy (Fig. 28-8). Immune complex–mediated MPGN results from chronic infections, autoimmune diseases, and monoclonal gammopathies. Complement-mediated MPGN is caused by genetic

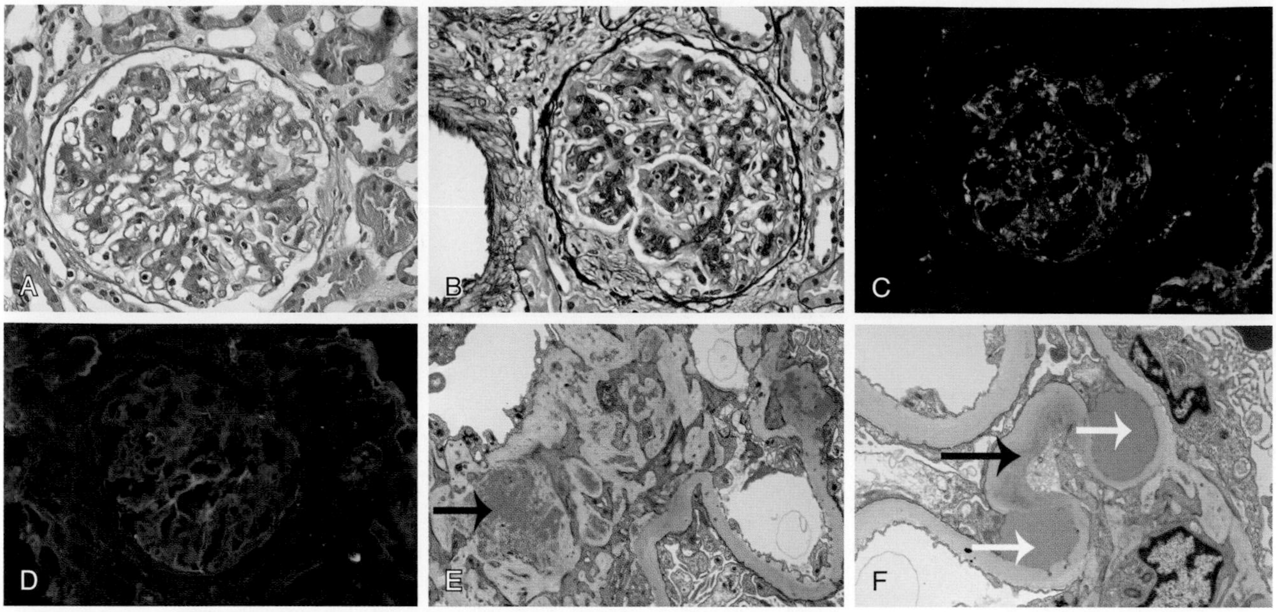

FIGURE 28-8 C3 glomerulonephritis. Light microscopy shows features of mesangial proliferative glomerulonephritis (**A**, periodic acid–Schiff, ×40) and membranoproliferative glomerulonephritis (**B**, silver methenamine stain, ×40) in the same biopsy. Immunofluorescence microscopy shows bright granular mesangial and capillary wall staining for C3 (**C**) and negative staining for immunoglobulin G (**D**). **E,** Electron microscopy shows a large accumulation of smudgy mesangial deposits (*arrow*) (×10,000). **F,** Electron microscopy shows subendothelial deposits (*black arrow*) and subepithelial humplike deposits (*white arrows*) (×150,000). The subepithelial deposits sometimes make it difficult to distinguish C3 glomerulonephritis from postinfectious glomerulonephritis. However, C3 glomerulonephritis may not show Ig (as in this case), and the term *atypical postinfectious glomerulonephritis* sometimes is applied in cases of C3 glomerulonephritis with subepithelial humplike deposits.

or acquired dysregulation of the alternative pathway of complement (C3 glomerulopathy) and can be further sub-classified as C3 glomerulonephritis and dense deposit disease (DDD) based on electron microscopy examination.

Immune complex–mediated MPGN precipitated by an infection is most commonly caused by HCV (i.e., cryoglobulinemic glomerulonephritis). The clinical presentation varies and can include nephrotic and nephritic features. In patients with cryoglobulinemic MPGN, the levels of C3, C4, and CH50 are persistently low, reflecting activation of both complement pathways. Patients with C3 glomerulonephritis or DDD may have a persistently low level of C3 but a normal level of C4. A C3 nephritic factor is found in many cases. C3 nephritic factor is an autoantibody to alternative pathway C3 convertase, resulting in persistent breakdown of C3.

The absence of well-designed studies based on current knowledge of the multiple pathogenic processes that impart a MPGN pattern of injury to the kidney make it impossible to give strong treatment recommendations. From a practical point of view, patients with MPGN due to chronic infections (e.g., HCV, endocarditis), autoimmune disease, and plasma cell dyscrasias should undergo treatment of the underling disease. Patients with normal kidney function, no active urinary sediment, and non–nephrotic-range proteinuria can be treated conservatively with angiotensin II blockade to control blood pressure and reduce proteinuria, because the long-term outcome is relatively benign in this setting. Follow-up is required to detect early deterioration in kidney function. Patients who have advanced renal insufficiency and severe tubulointerstitial fibrosis of renal biopsy are unlikely to benefit from immunosuppressive therapy.

GLOMERULAR DISEASES MANIFESTING WITH RAPIDLY PROGRESSIVE GLOMERULONEPHRITIS

Antineutrophil Cytoplasmic Antibody–Associated Vasculitides

The ANCA-associated vasculitides (AAVs) are a group of three heterogeneous syndromes: granulomatosis with polyangiitis (GPA, formerly Wegener's granulomatosis), microscopic polyangiitis (MPA), and eosinophilic granulomatosis with polyangiitis (EGPA, formerly Churg-Strauss syndrome). The unifying feature is a necrotizing small vessel vasculitis with a predilection for the kidneys, lungs, and peripheral nervous system that occurs in association with autoantibodies against antigens in the cytoplasm of neutrophils (i.e., myeloperoxidase [MPO] and proteinase 3 [PR3]).

Approximately 75% of the patients with GPA are PR3-ANCA positive, and 20% are MPO-ANCA positive, whereas about 50% of patients with MPA are MPO-ANCA positive and about 40% are PR3-ANCA positive. Necrotizing granulomatous inflammation, which affects the upper and lower respiratory tract and frequently precedes other disease manifestations, separates GPA from MPA. EGPA is characterized by asthma and eosinophilia in addition to features of small vessel vasculitis such as mononeuritis multiplex. AAV is the most common cause of a RPGN in patients older than 60 years. AAV is associated with signs and symptoms ranging from limited renal disease to RPGN and pulmonary-renal syndrome (Table 28-3). Renal biopsy is characterized by a focal, necrotizing, and crescentic glomerulonephritis with pauci-immune immunofluorescence (Fig. 28-9).

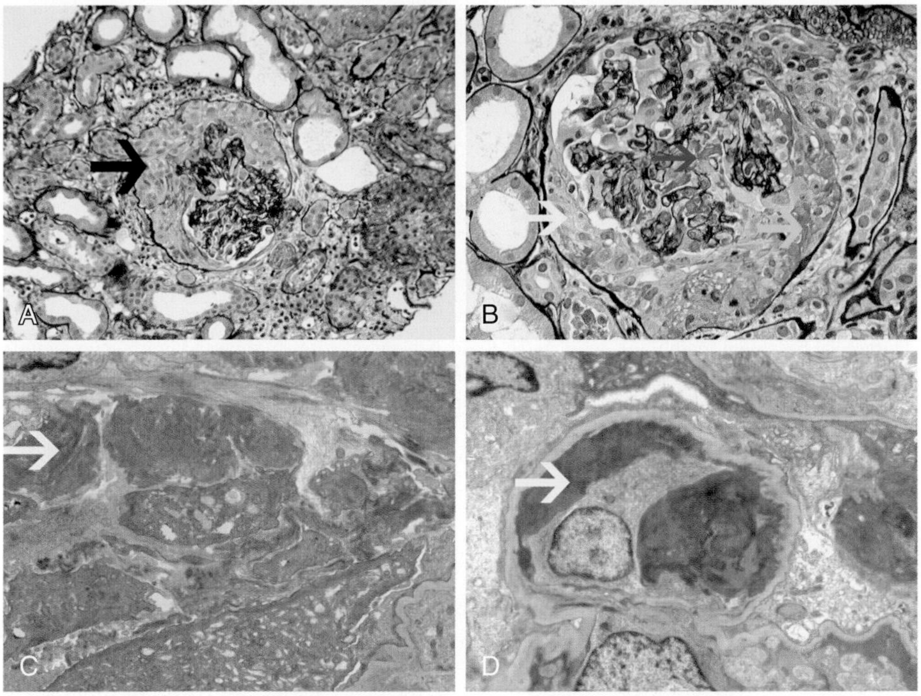

FIGURE 28-9 Crescentic glomerulonephritis. **A** and **B,** Light microscopy and silver methenamine staining show a large cellular crescent *(black arrow)* with fibrinoid necrosis *(blue arrow),* hemorrhage into Bowman's capsule *(yellow arrow),* and collapse of capillary tufts (**A,** ×20; **B,** ×40). **C** and **D,** Electron microscopy shows fibrinoid necrosis (i.e., necrotizing lesion) in Bowman's space *(white arrow)* and capillary loops *(short white arrow)* (both, ×11100).

TABLE 28-3	SIGNS AND SYMPTOMS OF ANTINEUTROPHIL CYTOPLASMIC AUTOANTIBODY VASCULITIS

Abdominal pain and gastrointestinal bleeding
Cutaneous purpura, petechiae, nodules, ulcerations, and necrosis
Facial pain, necrotizing (hemorrhagic) sinusitis, and septal perforation
Hematuria, proteinuria, and renal failure
Hemoptysis and pulmonary infiltrates or nodules
Muscle and pancreatic enzymes in blood
Myalgias and arthralgias
Peripheral neuropathy (mononeuritis multiplex)

Patients with newly diagnosed severe AAV vasculitis can be treated with a combination of high-dose corticosteroids and cyclophosphamide or high-dose corticosteroids and rituximab. Those with pulmonary hemorrhage, respiratory compromise, or severe renal failure (i.e., serum creatinine >5.5 mg/dL) also should undergo plasma exchange. The prognosis for AAV varies. Those with severe renal failure have the worst prognosis; and after successful therapy, AAVs have a relapse rate of 30% to 50% in the first 5 years. In some patients, rising ANCA titers are predictors of relapse. Patients with GPA or who are PR3-ANCA positive or presenting with relapsing disease are at higher risk for future relapses.

Goodpasture Disease: Anti–Glomerular Basement Membrane Antibody–Mediated Glomerulonephritis

Goodpasture disease is a pulmonary-renal syndrome (i.e., Goodpasture syndrome) caused by circulating anti-GBM antibodies. On immunofluorescence staining of biopsy specimens, a linear pattern is seen along the GBM and alveolar basement membrane (Fig. 28-10) using antibodies directed against the α3 chain of type IV collagen (COL4A3 protein). Patients usually have RPGN and various degrees of pulmonary hemorrhage.

The treatment of Goodpasture disease is based on high-dose pulse methylprednisolone (1 g/day for 1 to 3 days) followed by corticosteroids (prednisone, 1 mg/kg/day up to 80 mg daily) in combination with oral cyclophosphamide (2 to 3 mg/kg/day up to 200 mg daily, adjusted for age and creatinine level) and plasma exchange. The prognosis is predicted in part by the percentage of circumferential crescents on the renal biopsy specimen, oliguria, and the need for dialysis. Those with an initial serum creatinine level less than 5.0 mg/dL have a 90% probability of renal survival at 5 years; but those with 100% circumferential crescents and on dialysis do not recover renal function, and immunosuppressive regimens should be avoided except in the case of pulmonary hemorrhage.

Goodpasture disease rarely recurs. Patients with ESRD are candidates for renal transplantation after the antibody has disappeared (6 to 12 months).

Lupus Nephritis

Lupus nephritis occurs in up to 50% to 70% of patients with SLE and is associated with a poor prognosis. Proteinuria is the most common initial manifestation, and it is often in the nephrotic range and accompanied by a decline in renal function. Urinalysis does not always reflect the severity of the glomerular lesion, and kidney biopsy is indicated in those with proteinuria or active urinary sediment, or both, because the type of renal lesion

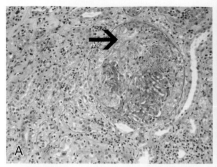
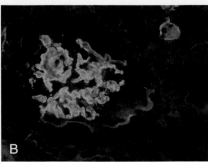
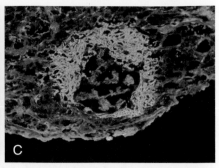

FIGURE 28-10 Anti–glomerular basement membrane–mediated disease. **A,** Light microscopy shows a large, circumferential crescent *(arrow)*, with collapse of the glomerular capillary tufts and many infiltrating neutrophils in the crescent (periodic acid–Schiff, ×20). Immunofluorescence microscopy shows linear staining for anti–immunoglobulin G antibody (**B**) along the glomerular capillary walls and bright staining for fibrinogen in the Bowman's tuft (**C**), indicating crescent formation and fibrinoid necrosis (both, ×40).

TABLE 28-4 ABBREVIATED INTERNATIONAL SOCIETY OF NEPHROLOGY/RENAL PATHOLOGY SOCIETY 2003 CLASSIFICATION OF LUPUS NEPHRITIS

TYPE	MORPHOLOGIC CLASS	RENAL MANIFESTATION
I	Minimal mesangial lupus nephritis	Normal urinary sediment
I	Mesangial proliferative lupus nephritis	Low-grade hematuria and/or proteinuria Normal renal function
III.	Focal lupus nephritis	Active sediment, proteinuria <3 g/1.73 m²/day
IV	Diffuse segmental (IV-S) or global (IV-G) lupus nephritis	Nephritic and nephrotic syndromes Hypertension; progressive renal failure
V	Membranous lupus nephritis	Nephrotic syndrome
VI	Advanced sclerosing lupus nephritis	Inactive urinary sediment Chronic renal failure

Modified from Weening JJ, D'Agati VD, Schwartz MM, et al: The classification of glomerulonephritis in systemic lupus erythematosus revisited, J Am Soc Nephrol 15:241–250, 2004.

influences the therapeutic decisions. The International Society of Nephrology/Renal Pathology Society (ISN/RPS) classification of lupus nephritis recognizes six morphologic classes of renal involvement (Table 28-4). However, patients may migrate from one class to another spontaneously or after treatment.

Immunofluorescence typically shows glomerular deposition of IgG, IgM, IgA, C1q, and C3 (i.e., full-house pattern). On electron microscopy, tubuloreticular inclusions are common within glomerular and vascular endothelial cells. Electron-dense deposits sometimes show fingerprint-like substructures (Fig. 28-11). Histologic lesions correlate with the prognosis; classes III and IV have the worst prognosis (see Fig. 28-11). Other manifestations of SLE include acute and chronic tubulointerstitial nephritis and glomerular capillary thrombi in patients with antiphospholipid antibodies.

Three guidelines for the management of lupus nephritis have been published recently by the American College of Rheumatology, the Kidney Disease-Improving Global Outcomes (KDIGO) working group, and the Joint European League Against Rheumatism and European Renal Association–European Dialysis and Transplant Association (EULAR/ERA-EDTA). For class I lupus

nephritis, the prognosis is excellent, and no immunosuppression is required. Patients with class II lupus nephritis and proteinuria less than 1 g/24h should be treated as dictated by the extrarenal clinical manifestations of lupus. Patients with class II lupus nephritis and proteinuria greater than 3 g/24h should be treated with corticosteroids or calcineurin inhibitors.

Patients with class III or IV lupus nephritis should undergo induction therapy with corticosteroids plus cyclophosphamide or mycophenolate mofetil because both are considered equivalent. Pure class V (membranous) lupus nephritis usually has a benign prognosis, and initial therapy should be supportive. However, patients with progressive or persistent nephrotic-range proteinuria should be treated with corticosteroids plus an additional immunosuppressive agent (e.g., cyclosporine, mycophenolate mofetil). Patients with ESRD should be considered for renal transplantation because there is a low rate of recurrence in the transplanted kidney.

Cryoglobulinemic Glomerulonephritis

Cryoglobulins are immunoglobulins that precipitate at low temperatures and redissolve on rewarming. Cryoglobulinemia usually leads to a systemic inflammatory syndrome with weakness, arthralgias or arthritis, palpable purpura, peripheral neuropathy, and glomerulonephritis. Serum levels of C4 are typically low due to activation of complement by the classic pathway. The disease mainly involves small to medium-sized blood vessels and causes vasculitis due to cryoglobulin-containing immune complexes.

Cryoglobulinemia is classified as type I, II, or III on the basis of immunoglobulin composition. It can be idiopathic or occur in association with autoimmune diseases (see Fig. 26-11B), malignancy, or infection (Table 28-5). Cryoglobulinemia may be associated with chronic HCV infection.

Renal disease occurs in 20% to 60% of patients with cryoglobulinemia and manifests as proteinuria, microscopic hematuria, nephrotic syndrome, or renal impairment. Hypertension is common and may be severe, particularly in the setting of acute nephritic syndrome. The cryocrit values correlate poorly with disease activity. On light microscopy, renal biopsy specimens show an immune complex–mediated membranoproliferative pattern of injury, and on electron microscopy, diffuse, dense subendothelial deposits with a microtubular or crystalline appearance may be seen occluding the capillary loops.

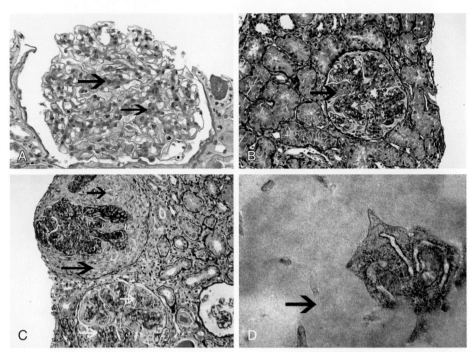

FIGURE 28-11 Light microscopy (**A** to **C**) and electron microscopy (**D**) are used to identify lupus nephritis. **A,** Mild mesangial proliferative glomeru-lonephritis (International Society of Nephrology/Renal Pathology Society [ISN/RPS] class II) has mesangial hypercellularity *(arrows)* (periodic acid–Schiff, ×40). **B,** Diffuse endocapillary proliferation with cryoglobulins in the glomerular capillaries, identified as pale, silver-negative material *(arrow)* (silver methenamine, ×20). **C,** In diffuse proliferative glomerulonephritis (ISN/RPS class IV), the glomerulus on top shows a large cellular crescent *(black arrows),* and the glomerulus at the bottom shows diffuse endocapillary proliferation *(white arrows)* (silver methenamine, ×20). **D,** Electron-dense deposits have fingerprint substructures *(arrow)* (×46,000).

TABLE 28-5	CRYOGLOBULINS AND ASSOCIATED DISEASES	
CRYOGLOBULINEMIA TYPE	**IMMUNOGLOBULIN CLASS**	**ASSOCIATED DISEASES**
I. Monoclonal immunoglobulins	M > G > A > BJP	Myeloma, Waldenström macroglobulinemia
II. Mixed cryoglobulins with monoclonal immunoglobulins	M/G ≫ G/G	Sjögren syndrome, Waldenström macroglobulinemia, lymphoma, essential cryoglobulinemia
III. Mixed polyclonal immunoglobulins	M/G	Infection, SLE, vasculitis, neoplasia, essential cryoglobulinemia

BJP, Bence Jones protein (κ light chain); SLE, systemic lupus erythematosus.

Treatment targets the underlying pathologic process to mini-mize or eliminate the associated cryoglobulinemia. Patients with active HCV infection, for example, should receive antiviral therapy when possible, and those with a monoclonal gammopa-thy should receive appropriate antimyeloma therapy. Immuno-suppressive therapy (including the use of rituximab) with or without plasmapheresis should be considered for patients with a rapidly progressive, organ- or life-threatening course, regardless of the cause of the mixed cryoglobulinemia. Overall, the renal prognosis is usually good, with few patients progressing to ESRD. The long-term outcome reflects the underlying process.

GLOMERULAR DISEASES CAUSED BY PLASMA CELL DYSCRASIAS

Amyloidosis

Amyloidosis is characterized by systemic extracellular deposition of randomly arranged fibrils 8 to 12 nm in diameter that stain positive with Congo red (i.e., green birefringence with polarized light) or thioflavin T. Several processes, including malignancy, genetic mutations, and aging, can produce at least 24

amyloidogenic proteins. With renal deposition, amyloid in biopsy specimens appears as pale, amorphous, extracellular deposits that are periodic acid–Schiff (PAS) and methenamine silver stain negative (Fig. 28-12).

The affinity for kidney compared with other target organs varies according to the type of amyloid protein. Renal manifesta-tions include proteinuria, nephrotic syndrome, and renal failure. Affected patients typically have large kidneys on ultrasound, but the diagnosis depends on demonstration of amyloid deposits. After amyloid is detected, typing should be performed when pos-sible because treatments vary according to the protein involved. The most common approach to amyloid typing involves immu-nofluorescence or immunohistochemistry, but genetic testing and liquid chromatography mass spectrometry are also helpful for high-resolution amyloid typing.

Treatment of amyloidosis depends on the origin of the amy-loidogenic protein. In patients with amyloid light chain (AL) amyloidosis, antimyeloma therapy with high-dose melphalan and autologous stem cell transplantation can be beneficial. In selected cases, bone marrow transplantation has led to resolution of the disease. Secondary amyloid A (AA) amyloidosis is most

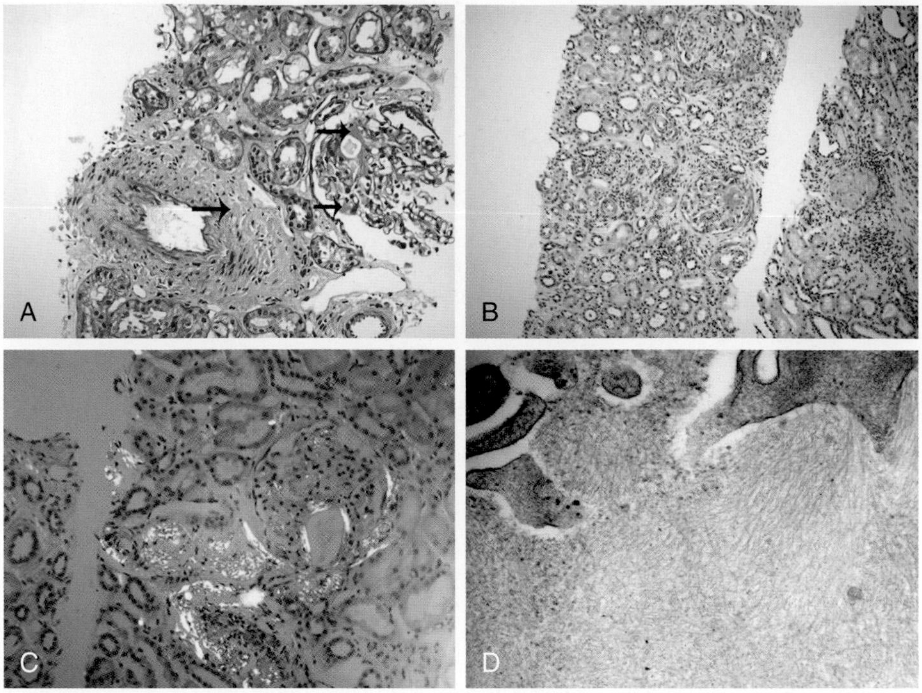

FIGURE 28-12 Amyloidosis. **A,** Light microscopy shows amyloid deposits characterized by mesangial expansion *(small arrows)* with material negative for staining. The material is also seen in vessel walls, where the *arrow* points to vascular deposits (periodic acid–Schiff stain, ×20). **B,** Congo red staining is positive for amyloid and shows reddish brown material in the glomeruli, interstitium, and vessel walls (×10). **C,** Amyloid deposits show apple green to orange-yellow birefringence under polarized light (×20). **D,** Electron microscopy shows randomly oriented amyloid fibrils. The fibrils measured 9 nm thick (×49,000).

common in patients with rheumatoid arthritis, inflammatory bowel disease, chronic infection, or familial Mediterranean fever. Treatment of AA amyloidosis is directed at the underlying inflammatory process with antimicrobials or anti-inflammatory medications.

Light Chain Deposition Disease

Light chain deposition disease is a paraprotein-associated disorder. The peak incidence is in the sixth decade of life, and men are affected more commonly than women. Approximately 30% to 50% of patients with light chain deposition disease have multiple myeloma. Most have a detectable monoclonal protein (usually κ light chain) in the serum or urine, but no hematologic abnormality is identified in about 10% of cases. Renal involvement manifests as proteinuria, and renal insufficiency is the most common initial presentation. Immunoglobulin deposits in other organs may result in myriad associated clinical symptoms.

Renal biopsy specimens show acellular, eosinophilic mesangial nodules that stain strongly positive with PAS, often mimicking diabetes mellitus. The deposited monoclonal proteins do not form fibrils and are Congo red negative. Immunofluorescence microscopic findings are diagnostic, with diffuse linear immunoglobulin light chain deposition (κ in 80% of cases) along the GBM and tubular basement membranes. On electron microscopy, amorphous, noncongophilic, monoclonal immunoglobulin proteins can be seen along the GBM (Fig. 28-13).

Encouraging results have emerged with the use of bortezomib and dexamethasone and with high-dose chemotherapy and autologous stem cell transplantation. Unless remission is achieved after chemotherapy, the disease will recur in the kidney allograft.

GLOMERULONEPHRITIS ASSOCIATED WITH HEPATITIS B VIRUS INFECTION

HBV-mediated glomerular disease usually manifests as membranous nephropathy, especially in children. The diagnosis of HBV-mediated glomerular disease requires detection of the virus in the blood and the exclusion of other causes of glomerular diseases.

HBV-mediated glomerular disease usually has a favorable prognosis, with a high spontaneous remission rate in children, but it is often progressive in adults. Patients with HBV infection and glomerulonephritis should receive treatment with interferon-α and/or with nucleoside analogues as recommended by standard clinical practice guidelines for management of HBV infection. Those with severe vasculitis or RPGN may be candidates for immunosuppressive therapy in combination with antiviral therapy. Rituximab treatment of patients who are positive for HBV has been associated with fatal acute hepatitis.

THROMBOTIC MICROANGIOPATHIES

Thrombotic microangiopathy is characterized by thrombocytopenia, microangiopathic hemolytic anemia, and microvascular occlusion, resulting in various degrees of organ dysfunction. Markers of hemolysis include low haptoglobin levels, increased levels of lactate dehydrogenase and unconjugated bilirubin, and a high reticulocyte count. Schistocytes are seen in peripheral blood smears.

The quintessential forms of thrombotic microangiopathy include hemolytic uremic syndrome (HUS) and thrombotic thrombocytopenic purpura (TTP). Although previously thought to represent different manifestations of the same disease, these disorders are distinct clinically and mechanistically. In adults,

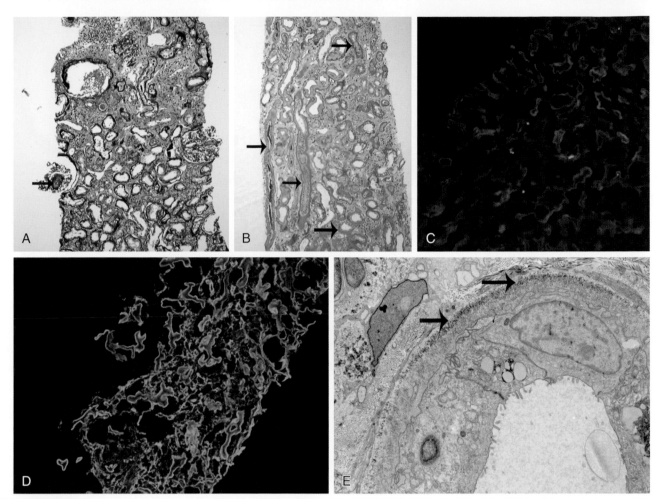

FIGURE 28-13   Light chain deposition disease. **A,** Light microscopy shows glomeruli with silver-positive mesangial nodules *(arrow)* and thickened tubular basement membranes (silver methenamine, ×10). **B,** Periodic acid–Schiff staining shows thickened, wavy tubular basement membranes *(arrow)* (×10). Immunofluorescence studies found negative staining for λ light chains **(C)** and bright staining for κ light chains **(D)** along the tubular basement membranes (both ×10). **E,** Electron microscopy shows granular, punctate, electron-dense deposits *(arrows)* along the tubular basement membranes (×5800).

predominant neurologic involvement suggests a diagnosis of TTP, and predominant renal involvement points to HUS. In most cases, the clinical presentations are very similar, making it difficult to distinguish between HUS and TTP on clinical grounds alone. Other causes of thrombotic microangiopathy include malignant hypertension, drugs (e.g., cocaine, quinidine, ticlopidine), autoimmune diseases (e.g., SLE, scleroderma, antiphospholipid antibody syndrome), malignancy, HIV infection, and antibody-mediated rejection.

Kidney biopsy in HUS and TTP reveals microthrombi in glomerular capillaries and arterioles, and mesangial expansion with loose granular material, called *mesangiolysis*, may be seen in HUS and TTP and in malignant hypertension or autoimmune diseases (Fig. 28-14). Malignant hypertension and autoimmune diseases may also show thickening and intimal fibrosis of arteries and onion-skinning (i.e., laminated deposition of basement membrane–type material) of the vessel walls. Thrombi are common and may occlude the vascular lumen.

Hemolytic Uremic Syndrome

Two subtypes of HUS are recognized: a sporadic or diarrhea-associated form (D+ HUS) and an atypical or non–

diarrhea-associated form (D− HUS). D+ HUS is the most frequently encountered form, and it is linked strongly to ingestion of meat contaminated with enterohemorrhagic *Escherichia coli* or other infectious agents. The bacterium produces a Shiga-like toxin that binds to a glycolipid receptor on renal endothelial cells and triggers activation of the alternative complement cascade, leading to endothelial damage. Therapy for D+ HUS is supportive. Children with D+ HUS have a good prognosis (90% recover renal function), but older patients have increased mortality rates and unfavorable long-term renal survival.

Atypical or D− HUS represents 10% to 15% of the cases of HUS and is more common in adults. The disease results from genetic mutations or autoantibodies against complement factors or complement factors regulating proteins (i.e., C3, factor B, factor H, factor I, MCP, CFHR1, and CFHR3) that control the activity of C3 convertase of the alternative complement pathway. The resulting defective control of C3 convertase leads to widespread activation of the complement cascade.

The complement inhibitor eculizumab has been approved for the treatment of patients with atypical HUS. Eculizumab and plasma infusion may also be considered in the treatment of

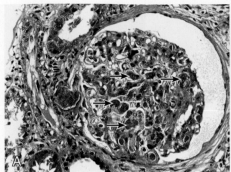
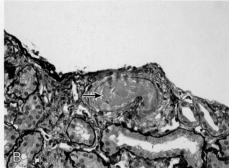

FIGURE 28-14 Thrombotic microangiopathy. **A,** Light microscopy shows multiple, small thrombi *(arrows)* in glomerular capillaries in the setting of hemolytic uremic syndrome (Masson trichrome, ×40). **B,** Light microscopy shows a thrombus *(arrow)* in a small artery in the setting of scleroderma (silver methenamine, ×20).

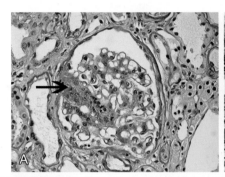
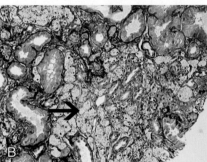
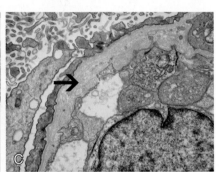

FIGURE 28-15 Alport syndrome. **A,** Light microscopy shows focal segmental glomerulosclerosis *(arrow)* (periodic acid–Schiff, ×40). **B,** Light microscopy shows numerous foam cells *(arrow)* in the interstitium (silver methenamine, ×40). **C,** Electron microscopy shows thickening of the glomerular capillary walls with multiple lamellations of basement membrane material *(arrow)* and formation of the classic basket-weave appearance (×212,000).

children with D+ HUS and severe central nervous system involvement such as seizures, stroke, or coma.

Thrombotic Thrombocytopenic Purpura

TTP results from mutations in the von Willebrand factor (vWF)–cleaving protease (ADAMTS13) or development of an autoantibody against ADAMTS13. ADAMTS13 cleaves large multimers of vWF, and abnormalities or deficiency of ADAMTS13 activity affects vWF function. Patients can have acute or chronic (i.e., relapsing) TTP. Microthrombi rich in large vWF multimers develop in the arterioles and capillaries of the brain and other organs.

Genetic or acquired forms of ADAMSTS13 deficiency can be treated by plasma infusion or exchange to supply functional protease. Plasma exchange should be initiated promptly, based on findings of microangiopathic hemolytic anemia and thrombocytopenia without evidence of other causes of thrombotic microangiopathy (e.g., scleroderma, malignancy, antiphospholipid syndrome). Treatment should not await test results for the levels or activity of ADAMTS13.

● DISEASES WITH GLOMERULAR BASEMENT MEMBRANE ABNORMALITIES

Alport Syndrome

Alport syndrome is an inherited disorder of basement membranes. In more than one half of patients, the disease results from a mutation in the *COL4A5* gene that codes for the α5 chain of type IV collagen (α5[IV]). The mutation in *COL4A5* disables a developmental switch in the GBM collagen that retains its embryonic phenotype and results in a friable GBM.

Alport syndrome is frequently associated with sensorineural hearing loss and ocular abnormalities (e.g., lenticonus of the anterior lens capsule). Patients characteristically have persistent or intermittent hematuria and usually have mild proteinuria, which progresses with age and may reach nephrotic range in up to 30%. The disease is X-linked in approximately 85% of patients, but autosomal recessive and autosomal dominant patterns of inheritance have been described.

In virtually all male patients, the syndrome progresses to ESRD, often before the age of 30 years. The disease is usually mild in heterozygous women, but some develop ESRD, usually after the age of 50 years. The rate of progression to ESRD is fairly constant among affected men within individual families, but it varies markedly from family to family. The degree of deafness correlates with the rate of progression to ESRD.

On light microscopy, the glomerular changes are nonspecific. Diagnostic features are usually seen on electron microscopy. At an early stage, thinning of the GBM may be the only visible abnormality and may suggest thin basement membrane disease. With time, the GBM thickens, and the lamina densa splits into several irregular layers that may branch and rejoin, producing a characteristic basket-weave appearance (Fig. 28-15).

Immunohistochemical studies of type IV collagen show the absence of α3(IV), α4(IV), and α5(IV) chains from the GBM and distal tubular basement membrane. This abnormality occurs only in patients with Alport syndrome and is diagnostic. In families with an unquestionable diagnosis, evaluation of patients with newly diagnosed hematuria can be limited to kidney ultrasound and urinary tract examination in most cases. If a defined mutation has been previously identified, molecular diagnosis of affected men or gene-carrying women is possible. In other cases, confirmation of the diagnosis can be obtained by examination of skin biopsy by immunofluorescence for the expression of the α5(IV) chain. Absence of the α5(IV) chain from epidermal basement membrane is diagnostic of X-linked Alport syndrome and may avoid a renal biopsy. Direct sequencing of the *COL4A5* gene can help to diagnosis patients in whom a clear diagnosis cannot be made based on clinical findings and histologic methods or to identify the carrier state in asymptomatic female members of X-linked Alport syndrome families.

No specific treatment is available for Alport syndrome. Tight control of blood pressure and moderate protein restriction are recommended to retard the progression of renal disease, but the benefit is unproved. Patients with Alport syndrome are phenotypic knockouts for the α3(IV) chain. Consequently, kidney transplantation carries a 5% to 10% risk of subsequent Goodpasture's disease due to the α3(IV) chain (i.e., the Goodpasture antigen) in the transplanted kidney.

Thin Glomerular Basement Membrane Nephropathy

Thin glomerular basement membrane nephropathy, also known as benign familial hematuria, is a relatively common condition characterized by isolated glomerular hematuria and associated with the renal biopsy finding of an excessively thin GBM. It is usually transmitted as an autosomal dominant disease. Heterozygous mutations in the *COL4A3* or *COL4A4* genes have been described in numerous patients with thin glomerular basement membrane nephropathy, indicating a genetically heterogeneous condition.

The usual clinical presentation is isolated, persistent hematuria that is first detected in childhood. In some patients, hematuria is intermittent and may not manifest until adulthood. On light microscopy, glomeruli appear normal, and immunofluorescence microscopy shows no immunoglobulin or complement deposition. Electron microscopy shows diffuse thinning of the GBM (Fig. 28-16). In adults, a GBM thickness less than 250 nm strongly suggests thin GBM disease.

The condition is usually benign and requires no specific treatment. However, a few patients have progressive renal disease that leads to ESRD.

● FABRY DISEASE

Fabry disease is an X-linked recessive inborn error of glycosphingolipid metabolism caused by deficient activity of the lysosomal enzyme α-galactosidase A, which results in the progressive accumulation of neutral glycosphingolipids (predominately globotriaosylceramide, particularly in the vascular endothelial cells of the kidney and heart.

Early manifestations of the disease include angiokeratoma, episodic pain crises, and hypohidrosis. With time, progressive globotriaosylceramide accumulation in the microvasculature in the kidney, heart, and brain leads to clinical manifestations such as proteinuria, renal failure, cardiac arrhythmias, and strokes, resulting in early death during the fourth and fifth decades of life of affected men.

Light microscopy reveals vacuolated glomerular cells, especially podocytes. Electron microscopy shows enlarged podocytes lysosomes filled with osmiophilic, granular to lamellated membrane structures (i.e., zebra bodies) (Fig. 28-17). Enzyme replacement therapy can lead to significant improvement of neuropathic

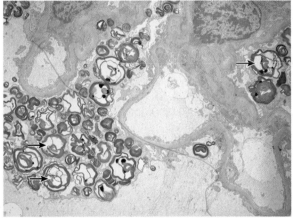

FIGURE 28-17 Fabry's disease. Electron microscopy shows visceral epithelial cells (i.e., podocytes) with numerous multilamellated structures called *myelin bodies* or *zebra bodies (arrows)* that are made of glycosphingolipids (×4800).

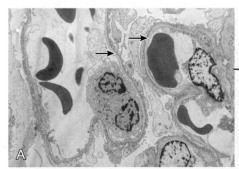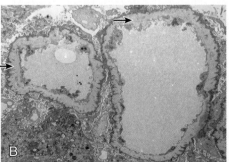

FIGURE 28-16 **A,** In thin glomerular basement membrane nephropathy, electron microscopy shows glomerular basement membranes *(arrows)* that are 198 nm thick (×5800). **B,** In Alport syndrome, electron microscopy shows thickened glomerular capillary walls with lamellations and disorganization of the glomerular basement membranes *(arrows)* and extensive foot process effacement of the visceral epithelial cells (×6000).

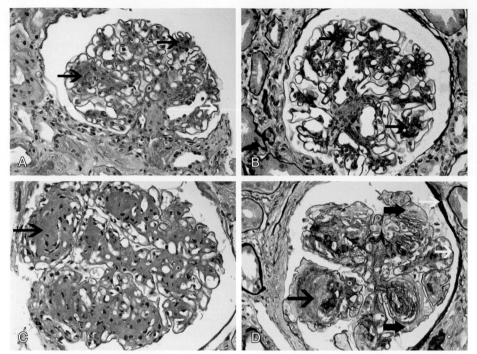

FIGURE 28-18 Light microscopy shows diabetic glomerulosclerosis. **A** and **B,** Early diabetic nodule formation *(arrows).* **C** and **D,** Well-formed Kimmelstiel-Wilson lesions result from mesangial expansion *(thin black arrows).* The nodules are periodic acid–Schiff and silver methenamine positive. The glomerular capillary lumen is distended by formation of small microaneurysms *(thick black arrows).* The glomerular basement membrane and Bowman's capsule *(white arrows)* are thickened (**A** and **C,** periodic acid–Schiff; **B** and **D,** silver methenamine; all ×40).

pain, but the beneficial effects on the severity or progression of other disease manifestations are less clear.

DIABETIC NEPHROPATHY

Diabetic nephropathy accounts for more than 50% of patients on dialysis in the United States. In type 1 diabetes mellitus, nephropathy usually manifests 10 to 15 years after the initial diagnosis; and a similar natural history is likely for patients with type 2 diabetes mellitus. The main risk factors include a positive family history of diabetic nephropathy, hypertension, and poor glycemic control. The risk may be greater in some racial groups (e.g., Pima Indians, African Americans).

The pathogenesis is complex. Increased glycosylation of proteins with accumulation of advanced glycosylation end products that cross-link with collagen and glomerular hyperfiltration with hypertension are important. High albuminuria (i.e., urinary albumin excretion >30 but <300 mg/24h) is the initial manifestation of diabetic nephropathy. With time, high albuminuria may evolve into overt proteinuria (>300 mg/24h), with the degree of proteinuria correlating roughly with the renal prognosis.

After overt proteinuria develops, progression to ESRD is relentless, although rates of decline vary among patients. For patients with type 1 diabetes, there is a strong correlation (95%)

between the development of nephropathy and other signs of diabetic microvascular compromise (e.g., diabetic retinopathy), but the correlation is weaker for patients with type 2 diabetes. Hypertension is almost universal among patients with proteinuria. It is difficult to control and usually requires at least three antihypertensive agents.

On renal biopsy, early signs of diabetic nephropathy include glomerular hypertrophy and thickening of the GBM. As the disease progresses, arteriolar hyalinosis, arteriosclerosis, and progressive mesangial expansion (i.e., diffuse diabetic glomerulosclerosis) and nodular formations (i.e., Kimmelstiel-Wilson nodules) develop (Fig. 28-18). For patients with a history of diabetes longer than 10 years and retinopathy, a renal biopsy may not be necessary. However, renal biopsy is indicated for patients with an atypical course of the disease (e.g., nephrotic syndrome), those with less than 10 years of type 1 diabetes, or patients with rapid loss of renal function.

Treatment with ACEIs or ARBs slows progression of diabetic nephropathy and should be used in all patients with albuminuria, even if normotensive. Tight glycemic control (i.e., glycated hemoglobin <7.0%) may also retard progression of diabetic nephropathy. Target systolic blood pressure should be less than 125 mm Hg, but this may be difficult to achieve and may require multiple medications and a strict low-salt diet.

Major Nonglomerular Disorders of the Kidney

Nilum Rajora, Shani Shastri, and Ramesh Saxena

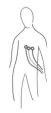

INTRODUCTION

The tubulointerstitial compartment comprises 80% of renal parenchyma, with most of the volume accounted for by renal tubules, interstitial cells, and collagenous matrix. Tubulointerstitial disorders have two common clinical presentations: acute tubulointerstitial nephritis, characterized by sudden onset and a rapid decline in renal function, and chronic tubulointerstitial nephropathy, characterized by a more protracted clinical course. Although primary glomerular and vascular diseases are associated with significant tubulointerstitial changes, the clinical presentations are dominated primarily by injury (see Chapters 28 and 30). Acute tubular injuries are discussed in Chapter 31.

ACUTE INTERSTITIAL NEPHRITIS

Acute interstitial nephritis (AIN), also called *tubulointerstitial nephritis*, is characterized by inflammation and edema of the renal interstitium; glomeruli and vessels are distinctly normal. AIN is associated with an acute, rapid decline in renal function and is a common cause of acute kidney injury, accounting for 15% to 27% of acute kidney injury cases confirmed on biopsy.

On gross examination, the kidneys are pale and swollen. Histologically, the hallmarks of AIN include interstitial edema and infiltration of the interstitium with inflammatory cells comprising lymphocytes, monocytes, plasma cells, eosinophils, and macrophages (E-Figs. 29-1 and 29-2). This inflammation can result in fibrotic changes in 7 to 10 days. Immunofluorescence studies typically are unrevealing, except in cases in which linear or granular immunoglobulin G (IgG) or complement deposits along basement membrane are observed.

In most cases, AIN begins abruptly with a decrease in kidney function within days of exposure to the offending agent. However, AIN may ensue after several weeks of the exposure in some cases. Characteristic clinical manifestations include rash, fever, and eosinophilia. Modest proteinuria (usually <1g/day) or hematuria may be observed, and oliguria is uncommon. A high index of suspicion is required for diagnosis because these features may be absent.

The most common causes of AIN are shown Table 29-1. Frequently used therapeutic drugs merit particular emphasis. They include antibiotics, allopurinol, mesalamine, nonsteroidal anti-inflammatory drugs (NSAIDs), and proton pump inhibitors (PPIs). Other causes of AIN include infections, autoimmune disorders, tubulointerstitial nephritis and uveitis syndrome, snakebite, and herbal supplements.

When evaluating a patient with a recent decline in renal function, the diagnosis of AIN is suggested by a history of exposure to known offending agents coupled with typical clinical features. In addition to identifying elevated serum creatinine levels, a urinalysis can detect the characteristic findings of white blood cells, red blood cells, and white blood cell casts in urine. Identification of eosinophils in urine with Hansel or Wright stains is highly suggestive, but their absence does not rule out AIN. Moreover, eosinophils in urine can be observed in other diseases, including cholesterol embolism, urinary tract infections, parasitic disorders, and glomerulonephritis.

A definitive diagnosis of AIN requires a kidney biopsy, although it is not necessary for management when clinical features are highly suggestive. Treatment of the patients with AIN consists of removal of the offending drug and management of the underlying infection or autoimmune process. Kidney biopsy should be considered when the diagnosis is not obvious. The role of steroids in limiting the inflammatory process is controversial, but early use (within 7 to 14 days) may decrease the duration of

TABLE 29-1	CAUSES OF ACUTE INTERSTITIAL NEPHRITIS	
CAUSE		**EXAMPLES**
Antibiotics		Penicillin Cephalosporin Sulfa drugs Ciprofloxacin Acyclovir
Nonsteroidal anti-inflammatory drugs		Naproxen Ibuprofen Diclofenac Celecoxib
Diuretics		Thiazides Furosemide Triamterene
Other drugs		Cimetidine Omeprazole Phenytoin Allopurinol
Systemic infections		Legionnaires disease Leptospirosis Streptococcal infection Cytomegalovirus infection
Primary kidney infections		Acute bacterial pyelonephritis
Autoimmune disorders		Sarcoidosis Sjögren syndrome

AIN and protect renal function. When indicated, the usual approach includes high-dose intravenous methylprednisolone (250 mg consecutively for 3 days), followed by oral prednisone (1 mg/kg) and tapering over 4 to 6 weeks. Patients who are intolerant or resistant to steroids may benefit from mycophenolate mofetil (500 to 1000 mg twice daily).

Most cases of drug-related AIN resolve after removal of the offending drug. The overall prognosis depends on the duration of the AIN; a longer interval between onset of AIN and drug withdrawal can lead to irreversible kidney damage. Because of the rapid transformation of interstitial cellular infiltrates into fibrosis, up to 40% of patients may not fully recover baseline renal function, and about 10% of the patients may become dialysis dependent.

CHRONIC INTERSTITIAL NEPHRITIS

Chronic interstitial nephritis (CIN) is a clinicopathologic diagnosis. Prolonged exposure to a causative agent initiates an indolent inflammatory process, and chronic interstitial nephritis can lead to permanent renal damage over months to years before it manifests clinically. Patients usually have a gradual decline in renal function. CIN is common and accounts for 15% to 30% of all cases of end-stage renal disease (ESRD).

Histologically, CIN shows tubular atrophy, flattened epithelial cells, tubule dilation, interstitial fibrosis, and areas of mononuclear cell infiltration within the interstitial compartment (E-Fig 29-3). The infiltrates are typically less conspicuous compared with AIN, and there is more interstitial fibrosis. In earlier stages of CIN, glomeruli are usually spared, but with progression, glomerular abnormalities such as segmental and global sclerosis can develop.

Patients with CIN usually have no renal symptoms until they develop overt chronic kidney disease. The features are nonspecific and include fatigue, lack of appetite, nausea, vomiting, hypertension, and sleep disturbances, and other laboratory and clinical findings may develop as listed in Table 29-2. CIN also can cause proximal or distal tubular dysfunction, which can lead to defects in acidification of the urine, partial or complete Fanconi's syndrome, and decreased concentrating ability. Laboratory data for these patients may show elevated levels of creatinine, proteinuria, hematuria, glycosuria, and pyuria. Due to the destruction of erythropoietin-producing interstitial cells, anemia, associated fatigue, and decreased exercise tolerance are common as CIN progresses.

The histologic findings of CIN are nonspecific, and the differential diagnosis can be extensive, as shown in Table 29-3. Repeated injuries from drugs, toxins, radiation nephritis, and reflux nephropathy can result in a similar histologic picture. The most common cause of CIN is chronic NSAID use. Other causes of include infections, immune-mediated disorders, drug reactions, hematologic disorders, chronic urinary tract obstruction, and urinary reflux. Some metabolic disorders and exposure to heavy metals can also lead to CIN. The clinical importance, distinguishing features, causes, and management of several forms of CIN are discussed in the following sections.

Analgesic Nephropathy

Analgesic nephropathy is the prototype CIN, and it occurs commonly worldwide. This disorder is caused by long-term ingestion of aspirin in various combinations with phenacetin, caffeine, or acetaminophen. In its most severe form, analgesic nephropathy is associated with papillary necrosis.

The cumulative amount of phenacetin-acetaminophen combination required to cause chronic interstitial nephritis is estimated to be at least 2 to 3 kg. Although initially thought to be exclusively associated with phenacetin-containing combinations, all analgesics, including acetaminophen, aspirin, and NSAIDs, are capable of inducing CIN.

Analgesic nephropathy is most commonly detected in women in the sixth and seventh decades of life. Patients with analgesic nephropathy have renal insufficiency, modest proteinuria, sterile pyuria, and anemia. Occasionally, patients may have flank pain

---

TABLE 29-2   CLINICAL FINDINGS THAT SUGGEST CHRONIC INTERSTITIAL NEPHRITIS

Hyperchloremic metabolic acidosis (out of proportion to the degree of renal insufficiency)
Hyperkalemia (out of proportion to the degree of renal insufficiency)
Reduced maximal urinary concentrating ability (e.g., polyuria, nocturia)
Partial or complete Fanconi's syndrome (e.g., phosphaturia, bicarbonaturia, aminoaciduria, uricosuria, glycosuria)
Modest proteinuria (<2 g/day)
Anemia
Hypertension

TABLE 29-3   CONDITIONS ASSOCIATED WITH CHRONIC INTERSTITIAL NEPHRITIS

ASSOCIATED CONDITIONS	EXAMPLES
Hereditary diseases	Autosomal dominant polycystic kidney disease
Metabolic disturbances	Hypercalcemia, nephrocalcinosis
	Hyperuricemia
	Hyperoxaluria
	Hypokalemia
	Cystinosis
Drugs and toxins	Analgesics, nonsteroidal anti-inflammatory drugs
	Lead
	Nitrosoureas
	Cisplatin
	Cyclosporine
	Tacrolimus
	Lithium
	Chinese herbs
	Olanzapine
Immune-mediated diseases	Granulomatosis with polyangiitis (Wegener's granulomatosis)
	Sjögren syndrome
	Systemic lupus erythematosus
	Vasculitis
	Sarcoidosis
	Crohn's disease
Hematologic disease or malignancy	Multiple myeloma
	Sickle cell disease
	Lymphoma
Infection	Chronic pyelonephritis
	Xanthogranulomatous pyelonephritis
Obstruction	Tumors
	Stones
	Bladder outlet obstruction
	Vesicoureteral reflux
Miscellaneous disorders	Radiation nephritis
	Hypertensive arterionephrosclerosis
	Renal ischemic disease

and gross hematuria, suggesting papillary necrosis. Diagnosis is supported by a history of heavy analgesic use, and computed tomography (CT) may reveal microcalcifications at the papillary tips.

Treatment of analgesic nephropathy is supportive and includes discontinuation of analgesic use. Long-term follow-up studies are characterized by progression to ESRD requiring dialysis. A high incidence of uroepithelial cancers is also observed in patients with long-term analgesic use.

Chinese Herb Nephropathy and Balkan Endemic Nephropathy

Chinese herb nephropathy (CHN) and Balkan endemic nephropathy (BEN), also called *aristolochic acid nephropathy*, are chronic tubulointerstitial renal diseases associated with urothelial carcinoma. The clinical expression and pathologic lesions observed at different stages of CHN and BEN are strikingly similar except for the higher prevalence of CHN among women and familial clustering of BEN. Both have been linked to exposure to the nephrotoxin and carcinogen aristolochic acid. It has been suggested that *CHN* and *BEN* should be abandoned and replaced by the term *aristolochic acid nephropathy* (AAN).

Aristolochic acid is a major component of *Aristolochia*-containing herbal remedies and is commonly prescribed in China and other Asian countries. AAN was first reported in 1993 in Belgium in young women taking aristolochic acid–containing Chinese herbs for weight reduction, and the finding has been confirmed by many others. BEN was described 50 years ago in farming villages in the Balkan area, where there is dietary exposure to aristolochic acid through the contamination of flour prepared from locally grown wheat.

Unique features of AAN include clustering of the cases among adults in endemic areas and close association with upper urinary tract carcinomas. About 50% of the affected patients develop transitional cell carcinomas; aristolochic acid induces DNA damage with a distinct molecular signature. Unfortunately, no effective specific treatment for AAN is available. Management is supportive with regular monitoring for urothelial malignancy.

Heavy Metals

Heavy metals such as cadmium, lead, and chromium can cause CIN, and exposure usually represents an environmental toxin. Cadmium exposure occurs with tobacco smoke and contaminated water and food. Lead exposure occurs from contact with lead-based paint and lead-contaminated dust and soil. Chromium is used to increase the hardness and corrosion resistance of alloy steel, and chromium exposure can occur when industrial plant employees work with alloy steels, dyes, paints, inks, and plastics. Renal proximal tubules are the principal site of accumulation and injury, but other nephron segments also can be injured.

Heavy metal nephrotoxicity ranges from mild tubular dysfunction to severe renal failure. The extent of renal damage depends on the nature, dose, route, and duration of exposure. With chronic exposure, changes consistent with CIN are observed on kidney biopsy. The best characterized clinical feature of heavy metal renal toxicity is the Fanconi syndrome, which results from proximal tubule damage. These patients have low-molecular-weight proteinuria, aminoaciduria, bicarbonaturia, glycosuria, and phosphaturia. Other clinical findings for lead toxicity include gout from decreased urate excretion in proximal tubules, hemolytic anemia, encephalopathy, and neuropathy.

Other than supportive care, no specific treatment is available for heavy metal–associated renal disease. Chelating agents may be used in acute poisoning, but no randomized clinical trials have proved the efficacy of chelation on clinical outcomes.

Sarcoidosis

Sarcoidosis is a chronic, multisystem, inflammatory disease of unknown origin. It is characterized by noncaseating, epithelioid granulomas in affected organs, leading to organ dysfunction. The severity and diversity of the clinical manifestations related to sarcoidosis depend on the extent of the infiltrating granulomatous lesions. Granulomatous tubulointerstitial nephritis is observed in approximately 20% of patients with sarcoidosis and responds well to steroid therapy. Sarcoidosis is described in details elsewhere.

Steroid therapy is effective in the acute setting and in advanced tubulointerstitial nephritis. Some patients with granulomatous tubulointerstitial nephritis may require long-term treatment with steroids to preserve renal function, although the side effects of steroids limit their use in advanced renal disease. The efficacy of steroid-sparing agents such as mycophenolate mofetil or azathioprine requires further investigation.

Radiation Nephritis

Radiation exposure is a significant cause of chronic kidney disease, and radiation nephritis develops in most patients if they are exposed to more than 2300 cGy. Ionizing radiation directly damages all molecules, including DNA, and initiates cellular synthesis of reactive oxygen species (ROS), which cause secondary tissue damage. Hydroxyl radicals are generated within milliseconds of tissue exposure. Oxidative stress and other factors may play additional roles over time, and patients may develop severe renal injury and impaired function 6 to 12 months (or longer) after exposure.

The diagnosis is based on a history of radiation exposure and the clinical findings of renal injury. Treatment is supportive.

Sickle Cell Disease

Chronic renal insufficiency is relatively common in patients with sickle cell disease, an inherited hematologic disorder characterized by hemolytic anemia and vascular occlusion by sickled red cells. Under normal conditions, the renal medullary zone is characterized by low oxygen tension, acidic pH, and high osmolality, which can predispose to increased blood viscosity and red blood cell sickling. This increases the likelihood of local ischemia and infarction of the renal microcirculation. In the vasa recta, vascular occlusion can interfere with the countercurrent exchange system in the inner medulla, resulting in a defect in the urine-concentrating mechanism.

Patients may have nocturia or polyuria and can develop gross hematuria due to papillary necrosis resulting from medullary ischemia and infarction. The sloughed papillae can obstruct urinary tract outflow, leading to obstructive nephropathy and renal failure. Another renal abnormality associated with sickle cell disease is proteinuria, a consequence of glomerular hyperfiltration that results from reduction in nephron mass.

The treatment of sickle cell nephropathy focuses on primary management of the hematologic disorder. Tubular dysfunction may require potassium and bicarbonate supplementation to treat hypokalemia and acidosis, and those with ESRD are treated with dialysis and renal transplantation.

Lithium

Lithium is a monovalent cation, which is freely filtered through the glomeruli. Up to 80% of filtered lithium is reabsorbed in the proximal tubule, and a small fraction is reabsorbed in the distal nephron through the epithelial sodium channel ($E_{Na}C$). Lithium causes dysregulation of the aquaporin water channel and $E_{Na}C$ expression in the cortical collecting duct. The most common manifestation of renal disease associated with lithium is CIN manifesting as a chronic, insidious decline in renal function. The course of renal disease after discontinuation of lithium is highly unpredictable, with no reliable clinical clues to identify those destined for recovery or progression.

Lithium also is associated with nephrogenic diabetes insipidus, which can occur in up to 40% of patients as early as 8 weeks after lithium initiation. Other tubular dysfunctions associated with lithium include water diuresis, natriuresis, and metabolic acidosis. Lithium-associated nephrogenic diabetes insipidus can be treated with $E_{Na}C$ blockade by amiloride.

Urinary Tract Obstruction

Urinary tract obstruction is a common cause of acute kidney injury and chronic kidney disease. When renal function is normal at baseline, unilateral or partial obstruction anywhere along the urinary tract may be asymptomatic, with no discernable change in renal function or urine output. Bilateral urinary tract obstruction, however, can lead to acute and chronic kidney injury and ESRD. It is important to address this possibility early in the clinical course of unexplained renal insufficiency or uremia.

Obstruction to urine flow causes an increase in ureteral intraluminal pressure. Over time, nephron tubules are injured, and the resulting changes in thromboxane A_2 and angiotensin levels decrease renal blood flow. Tubular damage leads to urinary concentrating defects, renal tubular acidosis, and hyperkalemia. If complete obstruction is not relieved, ischemia and nephron loss decrease the glomerular filtration rate.

The most common causes of obstructive nephropathy are shown in Table 29-4. Among elderly men, benign prostatic hypertrophy is a particular concern. Overall, the clinical presentation depends on the cause, site, and time course of obstruction. Patients with obstructive nephropathy have decreased urine output and are at risk for suprapubic pain (i.e., bladder distention from ureteral obstruction), renal colic (i.e., nephrolithiasis), urinary tract infections, fever, acute kidney injury, hypertension, and hematuria. Pain resulting from stretching of the urinary collecting system is the most common presenting symptom. Acute ureteral obstruction usually results in severe flank pain that typically radiates to the groin and is referred to as *renal colic*. Patients with complete bladder outlet obstruction have acute kidney injury and anuria. Patients with incomplete or intermittent bladder outlet obstruction have urinary hesitancy, dribbling,

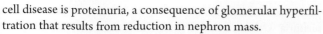

TABLE 29-4 CAUSES OF URINARY OBSTRUCTION

CAUSE	EXAMPLES
Congenital urinary tract malformation	Meatal stenosis Ureterocele Posterior urethral valves Urethral atresia Phimosis Megaureter–prune belly syndrome
Intraluminal obstruction (urethra and bladder outlet)	Phimosis Urethral strictures Benign prostate hyperplasia Pelvic tumor Anticholinergic drugs Neurogenic bladder Tuberculosis Radiation Trauma Calculi Blood clots Papillary necrosis (sickle cell disease, diabetes mellitus)
Extrinsic compression	Pelvic tumors Prostatic hypertrophy Retroperitoneal fibrosis or tumors
Acquired anomalies	Urethral strictures Neurogenic bladder Intratubular precipitates Bladder mass or stones

urgency, decreased urine stream, nocturia, and polyuria. These patients are usually pain free. Tubular injury from obstruction causes decreased urinary concentrating capability leading to polyuria.

The physical examination should include palpation of the kidney and bladder, as well as a rectal, pelvic, and prostate assessment. The patient may have an enlarged and palpable bladder, enlarged prostate, costovertebral tenderness, groin pain, hypertension, or gross hematuria. The mainstays of the initial evaluation include measurement of the postvoid residual volume of the bladder (>125 mL is considered significant and may indicate obstruction) and renal ultrasound to evaluate the kidneys, ureters, and bladder for distention or other abnormalities.

The initial goals of therapy are to manage volume status, electrolyte abnormalities, infection, and other complications of obstructive nephropathy and to relieve the obstruction as soon as possible to prevent further damage to renal parenchyma. If urinary obstruction is suspected, a catheter should be placed in the bladder to address possible bladder outlet obstruction. If a large postvoid residual volume (>125 mL) is detected, the urinary catheter should remain in place while the cause is ascertained. Occasionally, relief of obstruction is associated with a large postobstructive diuresis that may be sufficient in degree to cause volume depletion and hypotension.

If the obstruction is acute, complete recovery of renal function can be expected. If the anatomic site of the urinary tract obstruction is above the bladder, more sophisticated approaches to drainage (e.g., percutaneous nephrostomy tube placement) may be required to relieve obstruction.

CYSTIC KIDNEY DISEASES

Renal cysts are lined by a polarized epithelium and filled with fluid. They result from defects in the structure and the function of renal tubular epithelial cells. Several of the cellular and molecular mechanisms involved in cystogenesis have been identified.

Renal cysts can be acquired, hereditary, or developmental. Acquired conditions include cystic kidney disease that develops in patients with existing ESRD. Cystic kidney diseases also are important causes of ESRD.

The most common inherited cystic kidney diseases are the polycystic kidney diseases (PKDs), including autosomal dominant and autosomal recessive forms of PKD. Other hereditary cystic renal diseases include medullary cystic kidney disease (MCKD), Von Hippel–Lindau disease (VHLD), and tuberous sclerosis. Developmental cystic diseases of the adult kidney include localized renal cystic disease, multicystic dysplastic kidney, and medullary sponge kidney.

In the inherited disorders, several mutations have been associated with cyst formation. Mutation of any of the tubular epithelial–related genes such as *PKD1*, *PKD2*, *MUC1* (formerly *MCKD1*), and *MCKD2* can result in disruption of normal ciliary function, resulting in cyst formation from overproliferation of tubular epithelium and increased fluid secretion. In PKD, the cysts are not connected to the urinary drainage system, and cellular secretion results in cyst enlargement.

Simple Cysts

Widespread use of ultrasonography and CT has resulted in frequent detection of kidney cysts. Simple cysts are most common. They are usually unilateral, solitary, well-defined structures, but they can be multiple and bilateral. They tend to be more common among older adults and are often benign, incidental findings on radiographic imaging. Sonography reveals a thin-walled, fluid-filled cavity with no septations or calcifications. The diameter varies between 0.5 and 1.0 cm, but a few may be as large as 3 to 4 cm in diameter.

Simple cysts are usually asymptomatic but occasionally may result in a palpable abdominal mass, infection, back pain, or hematuria. Differentiation of simple cysts from cysts associated with genetic disorders is based on the cystic pattern, age at detection, and family history.

In the absence of symptoms, no treatment is required for simple cysts. If the kidney cyst becomes infected, causes pain, or leads to renin-mediated hypertension, percutaneous drainage is often the first step in further evaluation and management.

Complex Cysts

Differentiation of simple from complex cysts is usually made radiographically. When in doubt, histologic examination is required to exclude malignancy, but imaging is sensitive and specific, and it suffices in most cases. The distinction between complex and simple cysts is important in monitoring the need for intervention because simple cysts are usually benign, whereas complex cysts have a higher risk of malignancy and other complications.

Initial evaluation includes ultrasonography and triphasic CT to characterize the cyst. If the cyst characteristics of size, nodularity, mural enhancement, or septations change over time, the likelihood of malignancy increases. In a simple cyst, complications resulting from hemorrhage or infection can result in the features

of more complex cysts, including calcification, septa, irregular borders, and multilobularity.

To help with diagnosis and management, the Bosniak classification of renal cyst was introduced in 1996 and revised in 2003. This classification, which includes four categories based on triphasic CT findings, is described in Table 29-5. Category 1 cysts are benign, and category II cysts have a 0% to 5% risk of malignancy. The risk increases to almost 50% for category III cysts. There are also several important subcategories. Category III and IV renal cysts are considered to be renal carcinoma unless proved otherwise, and they should be surgically resected.

POLYCYSTIC KIDNEY DISEASE

Autosomal dominant polycystic kidney disease (ADPKD) is a common cause of cystic renal disease and an important cause of ESRD. The monogenetic, progressive disorder is characterized by multiple cysts in kidneys and other organs, including the liver and pancreas. The incidence of ADPKD is 1 case in 400 to 1000 live births, and between 300,000 and 600,000 Americans are affected by the disease.

Mutations in the *PKD1* and *PKD2* genes are responsible for about 85% and 15% of ADPKD cases, respectively, and there is evidence for important modifier genes. *PKD1* is located on chromosome 14 and encodes the protein polycystin 1 (PC1), which functions as a membrane receptor. *PKD2* is located on chromosome 4 and encodes polycystin 2 (PC2), which functions as a calcium permeable cation channel (E-Fig 29-4). PC1 and PC2 regulate intracellular calcium homeostasis and signaling pathways involved in tubular morphogenesis and cell-cell

TABLE 29-5	**BOSNIAK RENAL CYST CLASSIFICATION SCHEME**
CATEGORY	**DESCRIPTION**
I. Simple cyst	A benign simple cyst with a thin wall and no septa, calcifications, or solid components.
II. Minimally complicated	A benign cystic lesion with a few thin septa. The wall or septa may contain fine calcifications or short segment of a slightly thickened calcification. (This category also includes uniformly high-attenuating lesions that are less than 3 cm in diameter, well marginated, and nonenhancing.)
IIF. Complicated	Well-marginated cysts but more complicated than category II. They have multiple thin septa or minimal smooth thickening of the septa or wall and may contain calcifications that may be thick and nodular. (This category also includes totally intrarenal, nonenhancing high-attenuating lesions that are more than 3 cm in diameter.)
III. Indeterminate	Indeterminate cystic masses that have thickened, irregular, or smooth walls or septa. These lesions are enhancing on computed tomography. Between 40% and 60% of lesions are malignant (e.g., cystic renal cell carcinoma, multiloculated cystic renal cell carcinoma). The remaining lesions are hemorrhagic, chronic, infected cysts or multiloculated cystic nephroma and are benign.
IV. Malignancy	On computed tomography, they have characteristics of category III cysts and contain enhancing soft tissue components that are adjacent to and independent of the wall or septum on the cyst. Between 85% and 100% of lesions are malignant; evaluation and surgical excision are recommended.

interactions. PC1 and PC2 also are integral membrane proteins of cilia, including the primary cilia of renal tubular cells. ADPKD is now classified under the new class of diseases called *ciliopathies*.

In the kidney, increases in cyst size and number over time damage adjacent renal architecture and cause renal insufficiency and renin-mediated hypertension. Total kidney volume increases continuously and is associated with progressive decline of renal function. Higher rates of kidney enlargement are associated with a more rapid decrease in renal function.

ADPKD is a multisystem disease. The clinical presentation may range from no symptoms to an array of multiple renal and extrarenal manifestations. In addition to renal tubules, PC1 and PC2 proteins are found in diverse cell types, including bile ducts, endothelial cells, and neurons. ADPKD patients with mutated PC1 or PC2 proteins often have extrarenal manifestations, including polycystic liver disease, which is detected in about 80% of adults. Cardiac valvular abnormalities and cerebral aneurysms are key noncystic features of ADPKD, and familial clustering of cases occurs. Cerebral aneurysms are observed in about 8% of patients with ADPKD, but the incidence increases to 20% among those with a positive family history of cerebral aneurysm or subarachnoid hemorrhage.

Most patients with ADPKD develop cysts before the age of 30, but renal insufficiency can be delayed to beyond the fourth decade. Patients with the *PKD2* mutation have later onset and slower progression of the disease than patients with the *PKD1* mutation. Renal survival associated with *PKD2* mutations is about 20 years longer than that associated with *PKD1* mutations. Twenty percent of patients with ADPKD can develop uric acid and calcium oxalate nephrolithiasis and may have renal colic, obstructive nephropathy, or urinary tract infection.

ADPKD is usually diagnosed by imaging of the kidneys. The finding of three or more cysts (unilateral or bilateral) in those younger than age 30, two or more cysts in each kidney in those between 40 and 59 years of age, and four or more cysts in each kidney in patients older than 60 years is sufficient to make diagnosis of ADPKD. The absence of more than two cysts in individuals older than 40 years of age makes ADPKD very unlikely. Genetic testing is usually not required for an individual with a positive family history if other diagnostic criteria for ADPKD are met, but other family members should be screened.

No specific treatment is available to prevent the growth of renal or liver cysts. Renin-mediated hypertension is a common complication of ADPKD, and it contributes to an increased incidence of cardiovascular mortality and faster progression to ESRD. The main and most effective therapy remains control of hypertension by angiotensin-converting enzyme inhibitors or angiotensin-receptor blockers to achieve a target blood pressure of less than 125/75 mm Hg.

Renal cyst enlargement can cause pain, and cysts can be complicated by infection or bleeding that warrants specific intervention. Surgical decompression is usually reserved for patients who fail conservative management. If ESRD occurs, patients are treated with renal replacement therapy, including dialysis and renal transplantation. Preemptive management of intracranial aneurysms is important but controversial.

The time of onset and rate of progression of ADPKD varies from patient to patient, even within the same family. Risk factors for progressive renal failure include increases in renal cyst volume, a *PKD1* gene mutation, and uncontrolled hypertension. Other risk factors include male gender, diagnosis of ADPKD before 30 years of age, hypertension before 35 years of age, concurrent diabetes mellitus, and hematuria. About 45% of the patients with ADPKD develop ESRD by 60 years of age, but they have a better prognosis than patients with ESRD from other causes.

● AUTOSOMAL RECESSIVE POLYCYSTIC KIDNEY

Autosomal recessive polycystic kidney disease (ARPKD) also is classified under the ciliopathies. ARPKD is characterized by diffused dilation of the collecting ducts and congenital hepatic fibrosis. The estimated incidence of ARPKD is 1 case in 20,000 live births.

Mutations in the polycystic kidney and hepatic disease 1 gene (*PKHD1*) are responsible for ARPKD. *PKHD1* is a large gene located on chromosome 6. More than 300 mutations have been identified at different loci of the *PKHD1* gene. Fibrocystin (i.e., polyductin) is the product of *PKHD1* gene and is expressed in the primary cilia of the thick ascending limb, in cortical and medullary ducts in the kidney, and in hepatic bile ducts. It has an important role in the terminal differentiation of renal and biliary ductules.

Patients with ARPKD may be diagnosed at different ages, but most are identified in utero or at birth because those with more severe phenotypes develop enlarged kidneys, oligohydramnios, pulmonary hypoplasia, Potter's facies, and deformities of the spine and limb. Neonates usually have renal enlargement and renal failure, and older patients have liver disease, including portal hypertension, hepatosplenomegaly, variceal bleeding, and hepatic fibrosis.

The initial diagnosis is usually suspected on the basis of renal imaging with antenatal ultrasound or after birth. Abdominal ultrasound shows bilateral renal cysts and enlarged kidneys. Fetal imaging shows oligohydramnios, pulmonary hypoplasia, and Potter's syndrome.

No treatment is available for ARPKD, and genetic testing is usually not performed outside of research scenarios. Most deaths occur in utero or at the time of birth, and of those with ARPKD who survive birth, 20% to 30% die within the first year of life. Neonates have more renal manifestations, and older patients have more liver disease manifesting as portal hypertension, hepatosplenomegaly, and bleeding esophageal or gastric varices. The likelihood of patients being alive without ESRD increases with older age at presentation due to their more benign phenotypes.

● JUVENILE NEPHRONOPHTHISIS–MEDULLARY CYSTIC KIDNEY DISEASE COMPLEX

Nephronophthisis and medullary cystic kidney disease (MCKD) are hereditary forms of renal cystic disease. Both produce bilateral cysts at the corticomedullary junction of the kidney and early-onset ESRD. They are clinically and pathologically indistinguishable, and they are separated only by the age of onset and mode of inheritance.

Nephronophthisis is an autosomal recessive cystic kidney disease, and the median age of onset of renal disease is 11.5 years.

MCKD has an autosomal dominant pattern of inheritance, and the median age of onset of renal disease is 28.5 years. Nephronophthisis is more common than MCKD and is the most common cause of ESRD in first 3 decades of life.

Several genes are associated with the nephronophthisis and MCKD phenotypes. Mutations in at least two genes (*MUC1, Uromodulin*) can lead to MCKD. Nephronophthisis is caused by mutations in at least 18 genes: *NPHP1, NPHP2* (now called *INVS*), *NPHP3, NPHP4, NPHP5* (now *IQCB1*), *NPHP6* (now *CEP290*), *NPHP7* (now *GLIS2*), *NPHP8* (now *RPGRIP1L*), *NPHP9* (now *NEK8*), *NPHP10* (now *SDCCAG8*), *NPHP11* (now *TMEM67*), *NPHP12* (now *TTC21B*), *NPHP13* (now *WDR1*), and *NPHP14-18*. Functional defects of any of the proteins associated with these genes can lead to ciliary dysfunction and development of multiple cysts.

The three clinical forms of nephronophthisis are based on the onset of ESRD: an infantile form with a median onset at 1 year of age, a juvenile form with a median onset at 13 years of age, and an adolescent form with a median onset at 19 years of age. In patients with MCKD, ESRD develops between the ages of 50 and 70 years.

The diagnosis of nephronophthisis or MCKD is based mainly on clinical features. Medullary cysts, a low urinary specific gravity, and absence of significant proteinuria may suggest either disease. Genetic testing is available for several gene mutations and can be applied based on the age at presentation. Siblings can be screened by renal ultrasound and urine concentration test results. Renal biopsy is usually not indicated because the findings of interstitial fibrosis and tubular atrophy are nonspecific.

No specific treatment is available for nephronophthisis or MCKD, and treatment is mainly supportive. Sodium supplementation for salt wasting, allopurinol for gout, and dialysis or renal transplantation for ESRD are part of supportive care. The time of onset of ESRD varies between 30 and 60 years, depending on the type of mutation. Nephronophthisis or MCKD does not recur after renal transplantation.

● MEDULLARY SPONGE KIDNEY

Medullary sponge kidney (MSK), also known as Lenarduzzi-Cacchi-Ricci disease, is a relatively uncommon congenital disorder. It usually occurs sporadically, but familial cases have been reported. MSK is characterized by ectasia and cystic dilation of medullary and papillary collecting ducts, resulting in a spongy appearance of the kidney on imaging. MSK is associated with urinary acidification and concentration defects, a high risk of nephrocalcinosis and renal stones, and a moderate risk of urinary infections and renal failure. The prevalence of MSK is 1 case in 5000 persons in the general population, and 15% to 20% of patients with nephrolithiasis have MSK.

No clear genetic basis for MSK has been established. MSK is usually detected between the ages of 30 and 50 years. Most patients with MSK are asymptomatic and may have incidental finding on imaging. The clinical course is benign and is not associated with ESRD.

When suspected, CT urography has replaced intravenous urography as the imaging study of choice for the diagnosis of MSK. There is retention of contrast media in renal pyramids and cystic collecting ducts, giving the appearance of blush or diffused

linear striations. Nephrocalcinosis is common in patients with MSK but is not required to make the diagnosis of MSK. CT imaging may help in excluding papillary necrosis, ADPKD, obstruction, or pyelonephritis.

● RENAL TUMORS

Each year, approximately 65,000 new cases of renal cancer are diagnosed, and 14,000 deaths from renal cell carcinoma (RCC) are reported in the United States. Most cases are sporadic, but there is an association between RCC and VHLD and tuberous sclerosis that has helped to explain the cellular mechanisms involved.

RCC originates from renal epithelial cells and accounts for 85% of renal cancers. Based on histology, the five subtypes are clear cell, papillary (chromophilic), oncocytoma, collecting duct (Bellini's duct), and chromophobe RCC. Clear cell carcinoma is the most common subtype and accounts for about 75% to 80% of all cases.

The classic triad of symptoms of flank pain, hematuria, and a palpable flank mass is uncommon (10%). About 50% of cases are identified as a result of an incidental finding on radiographic imaging. Other clinical symptoms are nonspecific and include fatigue, anemia, and weight loss. Paraneoplastic syndromes associated with RCC include erythrocytosis (i.e., overproduction of erythropoietin), hypercalcemia (i.e., excess parathyroid hormone–related peptide), hepatic dysfunction (i.e., Stauffer's syndrome), and cachexia.

The initial diagnosis of RCC is usually made by imaging. Unlike simple cysts, which are anechoic, round, and smooth walled, RCC is more likely to be a septate, irregular, thick-walled mass. When RCC is suspected, additional evaluation by CT urography or magnetic resonance imaging (MRI) is usually required, along with complete staging and evaluation for metastases (Table 29-6).

When possible, the primary treatment of localized RCC is surgical resection, which usually includes complete or partial nephrectomy. Locally advanced or metastatic RCC is treated medically with chemotherapy and immunomodulatory therapy with interleukin-2. Newer therapies based on molecular targeting of the mammalian target of rapamycin (mTOR), which regulates vascular endothelial growth factor (VEGF), and several tyrosine kinases are promising.

The prognosis for RCC depends primarily on the clinical stage at the time of presentation as assessed by the tumor-node-metastasis (TNM) criteria. TNM stages I through III have a better prognosis than TNM stage IV (metastatic) RCC. With documented metastases, the 1-year survival rate is 12% to 71%, and the 3-year survival rate is 0% to 31%. Other poor prognostic factors include a lower Karnofsky performance status, elevated lactate dehydrogenase level, low hemoglobin level, and hypercalcemia.

● ACQUIRED CYSTIC KIDNEY DISEASE IN RENAL FAILURE

Acquired cystic kidney disease (ACKD) is not associated with hereditary causes of cyst formation but occurs in the setting of chronic kidney disease of many causes. It is defined by three or more cysts per kidney in a patient with chronic kidney disease or

TABLE 29-6 TNM STAGING SYSTEM OF RENAL CELL CARCINOMA

PRIMARY TUMOR (T)

TX	Primary tumor cannot be assessed
T0	No evidence of primary tumor
T1	Tumor <7 cm and limited to the kidney
T1a	Tumor <4 cm and limited to the kidney
T1b	Tumor >4 cm but <7 cm and limited to the kidney
T2	Tumor >7 cm and limited to the kidney
T2a	Tumor >7 cm but <10 cm and limited to the kidney
T2b	Tumor >10 cm and limited to the kidney
T3	Tumor extends into major veins or perinephric tissues but not into the ipsilateral adrenal gland and not beyond Gerota's fascia
T3a	Tumor grossly extends into the renal vein or its segmental branches, or tumor invades perirenal and/or renal sinus fat but not beyond Gerota's fascia
T3b	Tumor grossly extends into the vena cava below the diaphragm
T3c	Tumor grossly extends into the vena cava above the diaphragm or invades the wall of the vena cava
T4	Tumor invades beyond Gerota's fascia, including contiguous extension into the ipsilateral adrenal gland

REGIONAL LYMPH NODES (N)

NX	Regional lymph nodes cannot be assessed
N0	No regional lymph node metastasis
N1	Metastasis in regional lymph node(s)

DISTANT METASTASIS (M)

M0	No distant metastasis
M1	Distant Metastasis

ANATOMIC STAGE/PROGNOSIS GROUPS

Stage I	T1	N0	M0
Stage II	T2	N0	M0
Stage III	T1 or T2	N1	M0
	T3	N0 or N1	M0
Stage IV	T4	Any N	M0
	Any T	Any N	M1

From Edge SB, Byrd DR, Compton CC, et al: AJCC cancer staging manual, ed 7, New York, 2010, Springer Verlag, pp 482–487.

ESRD. The prevalence of ACKD varies from 10% to 100%, and it increases with the duration of dialysis, reaching 87% after 10 years of dialysis. Patients with risk factors of male gender, older age, and a history of heart disease, larger kidneys, and kidney calcifications are more likely to develop ACKD.

Neither the cause of the underlying ESRD nor the mode of dialysis influences the progression of ACKD. It has been postulated that damage to the renal parenchyma in chronic kidney disease increases local growth factors levels that promote hypertrophy and cyst generation in the remaining nephrons. In some cases, increased levels of growth factors and mutated genes (e.g. *ERBB2*) may cause the malignant transformation of cysts, the primary clinical concern for 3% to 7% of ACKD patients.

ACKD-related cyst formation is limited to the kidneys and is an incidental finding on radiographic imaging. Patients with ACKD are usually asymptomatic but may develop infectious or bleeding complications. ACKD can be differentiated from hereditary causes of cystic renal disease by presence of chronic kidney disease or ESRD and the absence of any other clinical findings. Routine screening for ACKD among dialysis patients is contentious but is recommended for patients during their pretransplantation evaluation and after kidney transplantation because of the potential for malignancy.

Patients with ACKD do not require specific treatment. Tumors larger than 3 cm may be considered for nephrectomy. Bilateral nephrectomy is suggested in renal transplant candidates due to the higher risk of subsequent malignant transformation with immunosuppression.

TUBEROUS SCLEROSIS

Tuberous sclerosis complex (TSC) (i.e., Bourneville's disease) is an autosomal dominant genetic disorder that affects adults and children. TSC causes benign tumors to form in multiple organ systems, including the skin, brain, and kidneys. TSC is often characterized by related neurologic disorders such as epilepsy and mental retardation.

The prevalence of TSC in the general population is approximately 1 in 10,000, and 50% to 65% of cases are sporadic. Because TSC has an autosomal dominant pattern of inheritance, there is a 50% risk of siblings being affected. Genetic counseling is important for affected families. The overall diagnosis and management of TSC is discussed in Chapter 115.

TSC is caused by inactivating mutations in the *TSC1* or *TSC2* genes. *TSC1* is located on chromosome 9, and *TSC2* is on chromosome 16, adjacent to the *PKD1* gene. They, respectively, encode the hamartin and tuberin proteins, which together form a complex that regulates specific cellular growth, motility, and migration of cells. Inactivating mutations of the *TSC1* or *TSC2* genes result in disruption of these processes and may cause unrestricted growth of cells and tumorigenesis.

TSC conveys a lifetime risk of 2% to 3% for RCC. Renal tumors are usually bilateral and occur at an early age. More commonly, the tumors are benign. Angiomyolipomas, composed of abnormal, thick-walled vessels, smooth muscle cells, and adipose tissue, are seen in about 80% of patients with TSC by the age of 10 years. These benign renal tumors often require no treatment. However, they can grow, become locally invasive, and cause bleeding, pain, and hypertension.

Conclusive guidelines for surveillance are unavailable, but annual MRI of renal and brain lesions is suggested until the age of 21 years and then every 2 to 3 years to monitor their growth. Patients with progressive lesions should have yearly imaging, and those with tumors larger than 4 cm in diameter are at high risk for spontaneous bleeding and life-threatening hemorrhage. If the angiomyolipomas become locally invasive or cause bleeding, surgical intervention is needed.

Mutations in the *TSC1* or *TSC2* gene cause constitutive activation of mTOR. Everolimus, an inhibitor of mTOR, has been approved for the treatment of patients with TSC-associated subependymal giant cell astrocytomas.

VON HIPPEL–LINDAU DISEASE

VHLD is an autosomal dominant disease that affects multiple organ systems. It is caused by germline mutations in *VHL*, a tumor suppressor gene located on chromosome 3. This mutation predisposes to renal cell carcinoma and to tumor formation in other organs, including the eyes, cerebellum, spinal cord, adrenal glands, epididymis, and pancreas. VHLD affects approximately 1 in 40,000 births, and about 7000 patients are affected in the United States. There is an important association with pheochromocytoma in some patients with VHLD that warrants consideration.

RCC occurs in up to 70% of patients with VHLD. It is usually bilateral and the clear cell type. RCC affects younger patients with a mean age at presentation of 26 years. For a high-risk patient, the diagnosis of VHLD is suggested by central nervous system or retinal hemangioblastoma, RCC, or pheochromocytoma. These patients should be referred for detailed assessment. When indicated, genetic testing can be performed to assess possible mutations of the *VHL* gene.

● NEPHROLITHIASIS
Epidemiology and Pathogenesis

Nephrolithiasis is a common clinical disorder that imposes a substantial burden on human health and resource use. Calcium-containing stones are the most common types, and stones composed of cystine, struvite, and pure uric acid are less common but have high recurrence rates. Based on National Health and Nutrition Examination Survey, the prevalence of kidney stones has increased from 3.2% in the 1976-1980 period to 8.8% in the 2007-2010 period. Diet and lifestyle factors likely play significant roles in the changing epidemiology.

Nephrolithiasis increases with age and is more common in men than in women, except after menopause, when the incidence tends to equalize. The prevalence is higher among white males, intermediate among Hispanics and Asians, and rare among blacks. After the first manifestation, there is a high rate of stone recurrence, approaching about 50% in 5 to 10 years. The risk factors for recurrence include a younger age at initial presentation, a family history of urolithiasis, underlying medical conditions, and recurrent urinary infections.

Stone formation occurs as a result of supersaturation of urinary solutes, expressed as the ratio of solute concentration in urine to its known solubility. A ratio greater than 1 indicates that urine is supersaturated, promoting crystallization. In all cases, low urine volumes increase the probability of urine solute supersaturation and promote stone formation.

Additional factors are involved. Higher urinary calcium and oxalate concentrations promote calcium oxalate stones, whereas alkaline urine and high urinary calcium concentrations promote calcium phosphate crystal formation. Acidic urine is a major determinant of uric acid crystal formation. Normal urine contains substances such as citrate, pyrophosphate, magnesium, Tamm-Horsfall glycoprotein, glycosaminoglycan, osteopontin, and calgranulin that can inhibit aggregation of crystals in urine. Citrate is the only inhibitor that can be modified in clinical settings.

Clinical Presentation and Diagnosis

Patients with nephrolithiasis are often asymptomatic, and calculi are detected as incidental findings on imaging studies. When symptoms occur, flank pain with or without gross hematuria is characteristic. The pain can vary in intensity from mild to severe and is classically abrupt in onset, paroxysmal, and follows a waxing and waning course over hours. Other associated symptoms include dysuria, urgency, nausea, and vomiting. Some patients may pass "gravel" in their urine, a finding more characteristic of uric acid stones. Complications associated with nephrolithiasis include urinary tract obstruction, hydronephrosis, infection, and acute kidney injury from obstructive uropathy in

the setting of bilateral obstruction or unilateral obstruction in the setting of solitary kidney.

A detailed history is crucial for patients with kidney stones and should include age at the first episode, number of stones, bilateral or unilateral occurrence, frequency of stone formation, type of stone if known, type and number of surgical interventions, family history of stone disease, and associated infections. Certain clues elucidated by the history may point toward a systemic cause of nephrolithiasis; for example, patients with malabsorptive states may be predisposed to calcium oxalate stones. The history should include detailed dietary habits, including the amount of fluid intake and dietary levels of sodium, protein, oxalate, and calcium, to determine the potential cause of or contributors to stone formation. Medications that can potentiate stone formation are shown in Table 29-7.

Except during an acute episode of stone passing, most patients have normal physical examination. However, physical examination may sometimes reveal findings suggesting systemic condition such as tophi in patients with hyperuricosuria and uric acid stones.

Laboratory testing includes a complete metabolic profile with attention to calcium, phosphate, and uric acid levels. Hypokalemia and metabolic acidosis suggest renal tubular acidosis, which is associated with a higher incidence of stone formation. A careful urinalysis may identify crystals, and other findings may indicate a specific cause (Table 29-8). When possible, it is important to retrieve stones for chemical analysis. Identification of stone type can guide therapy.

A 24-hour urine collection is the cornerstone of evaluation of most patients with nephrolithiasis and includes quantitation of

TABLE 29-7 MEDICATIONS ASSOCIATED WITH STONE FORMATION

MEDICATION	MECHANISM
Acetazolamide	Hypocitraturia
Vitamin C	Hypocitraturia
Vitamin D	Hypercalciuria
Antacids	Hypercalciuria
Theophylline	Hypercalciuria
Nifedipine	Hypercalciuria
Probenecid, aspirin	Hyperuricosuria
Topamax	Hypocitraturia
Indinavir	Precipitation within the tubule
Acyclovir	Precipitation within the tubule

TABLE 29-8 URINALYSIS AND RADIOGRAPHIC FINDINGS OF RENAL CALCULI

STONE TYPE	URINE MICROSCOPIC FINDINGS	RADIOLOGIC FINDINGS
Calcium oxalate monohydrate	Dumbbell shaped; under polarized light, appear coarse and needle shaped	Opaque, round, multiple calculi
Calcium oxalate dihydrate	Envelope shaped	Opaque
Struvite, magnesium ammonium phosphate	Coffin lid	Opaque, may be staghorn
Uric acid	Pleomorphic, often rhombic plates or rosettes	Radiolucent
Cystine	Hexagonal	Opaque

urine volume, pH, and levels of calcium, uric acid, citrate, oxalate, sodium, urea nitrogen, phosphate, and creatinine to assess the completeness of the collection. Preferably, two collections are performed in outpatient settings while consuming a usual diet. The findings are important for prevention of recurrence.

In the acute setting, noncontrast helical CT has replaced intravenous urography as the test of choice for the diagnosis of renal stones. CT can detect opaque and radiolucent stones with high sensitivity and specificity. Ultrasound can also detect radiolucent and radiopaque stones in kidneys but may miss ureteral stones. Ultrasound has a role in evaluating stones in pediatric and pregnant patients.

Treatment and Prevention

In most cases, small (<4 mm), nonobstructive stones can be managed conservatively because they have a good chance of spontaneous passage. With increases in stone size, the spontaneous passage rate decreases from 55% for stones less than 4 mm in diameter to 35% for stones 4 to 6 mm in diameter and 8% or less for stones greater than 6 mm in diameter.

During an acute episode of renal colic, pain management is essential, and it can be controlled with the use of NSAIDs or narcotics. Patients should be instructed to increase their fluid intake to increase their urine output to at least 2 L/day to hasten stone passage. α_1-Adrenergic receptor blockers and calcium-channel blockers can be used to facilitate stone passage. The α_1-adrenergic receptor blockers decrease ureteral smooth muscle tone and decrease the frequency and force of peristalsis, whereas calcium-channel blockers suppress smooth muscle contraction and reduce ureteral spasm.

Signs of urinary tract infection, inability to take oral fluids, or obstruction of a single functioning kidney warrants hospitalization. In acute kidney injury, anuria, or sepsis with an obstructive stone, urgent urologic consultation should be obtained. Similarly, a urology consultation should be obtained for stones greater than 10 mm in diameter due to the low probability of spontaneous clearance, for failure of conservative management, or for anatomic abnormalities that would prevent passage of the stone.

The type of surgical intervention is determined by stone size, type, and location and by the existence of infection. Shock wave lithotripsy is often recommended as the first-line therapy for non–lower pole renal calculi less than 2 cm in diameter and for lower pole renal calculi less than 1 cm in diameter. Percutaneous nephrolithotomy is suggested for larger stones.

General measures to prevent recurrent stone formation include increases in oral fluid intake to between 2 and 2.5 L/day and limitation of dietary sodium intake to less than 2 g/day and protein intake to 0.8 to 1 g/day. Dietary calcium restriction is not recommended because calcium in food binds to oxalate in the bowel and reduces urinary excretion of the highly lithogenic oxalate. However, calcium supplementation between meals should be avoided in patients with calcium stones.

Types of Renal Stones

Specific treatment modalities can be implemented when the metabolic risk factors for stone formation are identified (Table 29-9).

TABLE 29-9	TREATMENT MODALITIES FOR NEPHROLITHIASIS RISK FACTORS		
URINARY ABNORMALITY	**DIETARY CHANGE**	**MEDICATION**
High calcium	Adequate dietary calcium intake Reduce animal protein intake Reduce sodium intake to <3 g/day	Thiazide
High oxalate	Avoid high oxalate foods Adequate dietary calcium intake	Consider vitamin B_6
High uric acid	Reduce purine intake	Allopurinol
Low citrate	Increase fruit and vegetable intake Reduce animal protein intake	Alkali (potassium citrate)
Low volume	Increase total fluid intake Goal urine output >2 L/day	—

TABLE 29-10	PRINCIPAL RISK FACTORS FOR CALCIUM STONE FORMATION

Low urinary volume
High urinary oxalate
High urinary calcium
Low urinary citrate
Dietary factors
  Low dietary intake of fluids, calcium, phytates, potassium
  High intake of oxalates, sodium, protein, sucrose
Medical conditions: obesity, metabolic syndrome, diabetes mellitus, primary hyperparathyroidism, gout, medullary sponge kidneys

Calcium Stones

Approximately 80% of stones are calcium stones, most of which are composed primarily of calcium oxalate, mixed oxalate, and phosphate, and less often, they are pure calcium phosphate. Calcium oxalate supersaturation is not pH dependent in the physiologic range, whereas alkaline urine promotes calcium phosphate supersaturation. The pathophysiologic mechanisms for calcium kidney stone formation are complex and are associated with several metabolic derangements (Table 29-10).

Hypercalciuria is the most common metabolic abnormality found in recurrent calcium stones formers and is detected in 30% to 60% of adults with nephrolithiasis. It is most often familial or idiopathic. One pathophysiologic mechanism for hypercalciuria is increased intestinal calcium absorption (i.e., absorptive hypercalciuria), which is the most common abnormality. Gut calcium absorption is increased in persons with idiopathic hypercalciuria, but serum calcium values remain unchanged because the absorbed calcium is promptly excreted. A second mechanism is enhanced calcium mobilization from bone (i.e., resorptive hypercalciuria), which leads to urinary loss of bone calcium. This is seen in patients with primary hyperparathyroidism, immobilization, and metastatic tumors. A third mechanism is decreased renal calcium reabsorption (i.e., renal leak), the pathogenesis of which is unclear. It is thought to result from a primary defect in renal tubular of calcium. High-sodium intake decreases proximal sodium reabsorption, and the ensuing urinary sodium excretion causes physiologic increases in calcium excretion, promoting stone formation. Consumption of large amounts of animal protein can increase the acid load, causing calcium release from bones and increased urinary calcium excretion. Acidosis results in decreased tubular calcium reabsorption and depletion of urinary citrate.

Thiazide diuretics are commonly used to decrease urine calcium excretion in recurrent calcium stone formers. They reduce hypercalciuria and stone recurrence regardless of the underlying pathophysiologic mechanism because they promote increased proximal tubule calcium absorption. Thiazides can cause hypokalemia-induced hypocitraturia, and thiazide use should be supplemented with potassium. Potassium citrate has an advantage over other agents because it provides both potassium and citrate.

Hyperoxaluria

Hyperoxaluria (>45 mg/day in women and 55 mg/day in men) is detected in 10% to 50% of calcium stone formers. Hyperoxaluria increases calcium oxalate supersaturation and promotes calcium oxalate stone formation. Hyperoxaluria can result from increased dietary intake, increased gastrointestinal absorption of oxalate, or overproduction of oxalate caused by an inborn error in metabolism.

Dietary issues can be important. Foods known to increase urinary oxalate excretion include rhubarb, spinach, beets, most nuts, chocolate, tea, raspberries, figs, and plums. Enteric hyperoxaluria occurs in patients with malabsorption of fat. Dietary calcium binds to fatty acids in the enteric lumen. The released free oxalate is then available for augmented absorption. Enteric hyperoxaluria is commonly seen in patients with chronic diarrhea, inflammatory bowel diseases, celiac disease, and intestinal resection or after bariatric surgery.

Concomitant risk factors for stone formation include low urine volume, acidic urine, and hypocitraturia. Rarely, hyperoxaluria is caused by inborn errors in metabolism such as primary hyperoxaluria, a rare autosomal recessive genetic disorder of oxalate synthesis. Patients should be advised to avoid excessive vitamin C (>500 mg/day). For patients with enteric hyperoxaluria, measures should be instituted to reduce steatorrhea, such as a low-fat diet, cholestyramine, and administration of medium-chain triglycerides.

Hypocitraturia

Citrate, an endogenous inhibitor of calcium stone formation, is the only inhibitor that is measured and can be modified in clinical settings. Citrate binds to urinary calcium to form a soluble complex and prevent precipitation of calcium with oxalates or phosphates. Citrate also directly inhibits crystal agglomeration. Hypocitraturia can be a consequence of metabolic acidosis, high-protein intake, carbonic anhydrase inhibitors, or hypokalemia, or it may be an idiopathic disorder. Decreases in tubular fluid pH result in conversion of the trivalent citrate anion into the divalent anion, which is more easily reabsorbed by the sodium citrate cotransporter in the luminal membrane. Acidosis results in increased cell citrate use and upregulation of proximal renal tubular reabsorption of citrate, leading to hypocitraturia.

Potassium citrate is more effective in preventing calcium stone formation compared with sodium citrate because the sodium load can worsen hypercalciuria. The usual dose for potassium citrate is 15 to 25 mmol two or three times per day. A potential concern with alkali therapy is the risk of calcium phosphate stone

formation. Among patients with reduced kidney function, serum potassium needs to be monitored closely because of the risk of hyperkalemia.

Calcium Phosphate Stones

Calcium phosphate stone formation is a result of hypercalciuria, hypocitraturia, and persistently alkaline urine. Calcium phosphate stones can be seen in patients with distal renal tubular acidosis, with use of carbonic anhydrase inhibitors such as acetazolamide (which inhibit bicarbonate reabsorption in the proximal tubule), and with use of antiepileptic drugs such topiramate that can inhibit carbonic anhydrase.

Uric Acid Stones

Three major urinary abnormalities causing uric acid precipitation are low urinary pH (urine pH <5.5), low urine volume, and hyperuricosuria. When urinary pH is acidic, changes in physical chemistry result in conversion of more soluble urate into less soluble uric acid, thereby facilitating lithogenesis. Excessive acid loads (e.g., diet high in animal protein) or chronic bicarbonate loss in patients with chronic diarrhea can result in low urinary pH, increasing the propensity for uric acid stone formation. The increased incidence of uric acid stones among patients with insulin resistance and type 2 diabetes mellitus has been linked to impaired ammonia synthesis resulting in reduced urinary pH. Hyperuricosuria also may be seen in certain clinical conditions such as myeloproliferative disorders, tumor lysis syndrome, rare genetic disorders linked to the uric acid synthetic pathway, and mutations in renal uric acid transporters.

Alkaline therapy along with increasing urine volume is the most effective treatment of uric acid stones. Potassium citrate, given as 30 to 80 mmol in divided doses, is prescribed to maintain a urine pH of 6.5 to 7. Further increases in urinary pH to above 7 may result in calcium phosphate precipitation and should be avoided. When marked hyperuricosuria persists (urinary uric acid excretion >600 mg/day in women and 700 mg/day in men) despite dietary animal protein limitation and other measures, xanthine oxidase inhibitors such as allopurinol can be used at doses of 100 to 300 mg/day.

Struvite Stones

Struvite or triple phosphate stones are composed of magnesium ammonium phosphate and calcium carbonate apatite. They can grow rapidly and, if untreated, can fill the entire pelvis, resulting in staghorn calculi. They also can cause chronic kidney disease, including ESRD. Struvite stones result from chronic urinary tract infections with urea-splitting organisms (Table 29-11), which increase urine pH by generating ammonium to produce stones composed of ammonium-magnesium-phosphate.

The mainstay of treatment for struvite stones includes early surgical removal of bacteria-laden stones and eradication of

TABLE 29-11 UREASE-PRODUCING BACTERIA	
Corynebacterium	*Providencia* (most species)
Haemophilus	*Pseudomonas*
Klebsiella	*Serratia*
Proteus (most species)	*Staphylococcus*

associated infection with antibiotics. If other measures are ineffective, acetohydroxamic acid, a urease inhibitor, can be considered, but its use is limited by significant side effects.

Cystine Stones

Cystinuria is the most common of the rare hereditary kidney stone diseases. It is caused by inherited defects of dibasic amino acid transport in the kidney and intestine. Mutations of one of the two subunits of the amino acid transporter in the kidney leads to defective renal tubular reabsorption of dibasic amino acids such as cystine, arginine, lysine, and ornithine. Cystine stones are the main complication of this defect due to the low solubility of cystine in urine. Characteristic hexagonal cystine crystals can be seen on urine sediment analysis.

The diagnosis of cystinuria is based on a family history of stones, stone formation at a young age, mildly radiopaque stones, and measurement of urinary cystine excretion. Patients with cystinuria excrete 250 to 1000 mg of cystine per day (normal is about 30 mg/day).

Treatment must be aimed at decreasing the urinary cystine concentration by increasing urine volume to more than 4 L/day, alkalization of urine (urine pH >6.5) with potassium citrate or sodium bicarbonate, reducing urine cystine excretion by reducing sodium intake and raising urinary pH by decreasing animal protein intake. Thiol derivatives such as D-penicillamine and α-mercaptopropionylglycine split cystine molecules into two cysteines and produce a highly soluble disulfide compound. However, their use may be limited by their side effects.

SUGGESTED READINGS

Badr M, El Koumi MA, Ali YF, et al: Renal tubular dysfunction in children with sickle cell haemoglobinopathy, Nephrology (Carlton) 18:299–303, 2013.

Bosniak MA: The current radiological approach to renal cysts, Radiology 158:1–10, 2012.

Cornec-Le Gall E, Audrezet MP, Chen JM, et al: Type of PKD1 mutation influences renal outcome in ADPKD, J Am Soc Nephrol 24:1006–1013, 2013.

Crino PB, Nathanson KL, Henske EP: The tuberous sclerosis complex, N Engl J Med 355:1345–1356, 2006.

Katabathina VS, Kota G, Dasyam AK, et al: Adult renal cystic disease: a genetic, biological, and developmental primer, Radiographics 30:1509–1523, 2010.

Moe OW: Kidney stones: pathophysiology and medical management, Lancet 367:333–344, 2006.

Moe OW, Pearle MS, Sakhaee K: Pharmacotherapy of urolithiasis: evidence from clinical trials, Kidney Int 79:385–392, 2011.

Perazella MA, Markowitz GS: Drug-induced acute interstitial nephritis, Nat Rev Nephrol 6:461–470, 2010.

Torres VE, Chapman AB, Devuyst O, et al: Tolvaptan in patients with autosomal dominant polycystic kidney disease, N Engl J Med 367:2407–2418, 2012.

Whelan TF: Guidelines on the management of renal cyst disease, Can Urol Assoc J 4:98–99, 2010.

Worcester EM, Coe FL: Calcium kidney stones, N Engl J Med 363:954–963, 2010.

30

Vascular Disorders of the Kidney

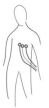

Jeffrey S. Berns

INTRODUCTION

The spectrum of vascular disorders of the kidneys is broad as a result of high renal blood flow and the intimate relationship between blood supply and fundamental glomerular and tubular functions. In this chapter, emphasis is placed on the clinical manifestations of hypertension, chronic kidney disease (CKD), end-stage kidney failure, and the many other causes of acute kidney injury (AKI).

RENAL VASCULAR ANATOMY

The renal arteries arise directly from the aorta and enter the renal hilum. The right renal artery passes anterior to the inferior vena cava (IVC) and is longer than the left renal artery. In up to 30% of the population, accessory renal arteries arise from the aorta to provide blood to portions of one or both kidneys, which may become important when evaluating patients for renovascular hypertension.

The renal arteries give rise to segmental, interlobar, and arcuate arteries (Fig. 30-1). Arcuate arteries course along the corticomedullary junction and give rise to interlobular arterioles, which extend outward into the cortex before branching into afferent arterioles, from which the glomerular capillary tufts arise. The postglomerular efferent arterioles from more superficial glomeruli form a capillary network in the renal cortex, and those extending from glomeruli nearer the cortical-medullary junction (i.e., juxtamedullary glomeruli) form capillaries that extend deeper into the medulla in association with thin, descending and ascending loops of Henle as the vasa recta. The vasa recta provide the sole blood supply for the renal medulla, making this portion of the kidney particularly susceptible to ischemic injury. Venules from the ascending vasa recta and the cortical capillary network empty into the renal veins.

The left renal vein returns to the IVC anterior to the aorta and inferior to the inferior mesenteric artery, which may rarely cause compression of this vein. The left gonadal vein also empties into the left renal vein, and a left varicocele may be evident if the renal vein is occluded by thrombosis or tumor involvement. The right renal vein is much shorter and empties directly into the IVC. The right gonadal vein empties directly into the IVC rather than into the right renal vein.

RENOVASCULAR DISEASE

Any process that narrows the lumen of the main or branch renal arteries sufficiently can elicit a humoral response mediated by increased renin release from the ipsilateral kidney, which leads to increases in circulating angiotensin II and aldosterone levels.

Activation of the renin-angiotensin-aldosterone system increases systemic blood pressure and renal arterial perfusion pressure, renal blood flow, and the glomerular filtration rate (GFR) beyond the stenosis. Hemodynamically significant renal artery stenosis (RAS) requires a reduction in lumen diameter of at least 50% to 60%. The resulting renin-angiotensin-aldosterone system activation leads initially to systemic vasoconstriction mediated by angiotensin II and increased renal sodium and fluid reabsorption, resulting in elevation of systemic blood pressure. If the contralateral kidney has no stenosis, the increased systemic blood pressure increases sodium excretion by that kidney (i.e., pressure natriuresis).

Because hypertension in this setting is maintained by increased vasoconstriction due to angiotensin II, treatment is aimed at blocking the synthesis or effect of the elevated angiotensin II levels with an angiotensin-converting enzyme (ACE) inhibitor

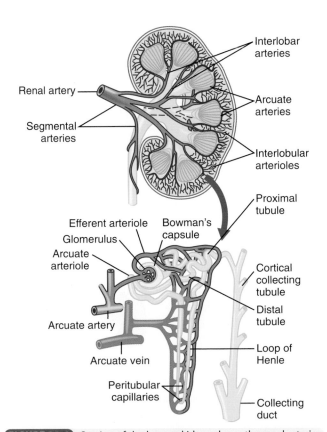

FIGURE 30-1 Section of the human kidney shows the renal arteries and a schematic of the microcirculation of each nephron. (From Guyton AC, Hall JE: Textbook of medical physiology, ed 11, Philadelphia, 2006, Saunders, p 309.)

or angiotensin-receptor blocker (ARB). If the arteries to both kidneys are narrowed, pressure natriuresis does not occur, and hypertension is maintained chronically by the resulting intravascular volume expansion rather than by increased total peripheral resistance. Treatment with diuretics becomes more important in this circumstance. The latter situation also occurs when there is only a single functioning kidney that has stenosis or when an initially normal contralateral kidney suffers microvascular damage from long-standing hypertension (Fig. 30-2).

The pathophysiology of hypertension with RAS is such that its treatment may also compromise kidney function and reduce the GFR. If the kidney contralateral to one with hemodynamically significant RAS is normal, lowering the systemic blood pressure maintains the kidney with the stenosis in a vascularly compromised state. However, this may not be detectable by measurement of the serum creatinine level because of the normally functioning contralateral kidney. A decline in the GFR may be evident if there is underlying renal dysfunction in the contralateral kidney, as is often the case in long-standing hypertension, diabetes, or vascular disease. When a solitary functioning kidney or both kidneys are affected (i.e., bilateral RAS), AKI may result when ACE inhibitor or ARB treatment is initiated.

Atherosclerotic Renovascular Disease

Clinical Presentation

Atherosclerosis is the primary cause of RAS, although any process that narrows one or both renal arteries may cause renal ischemia;

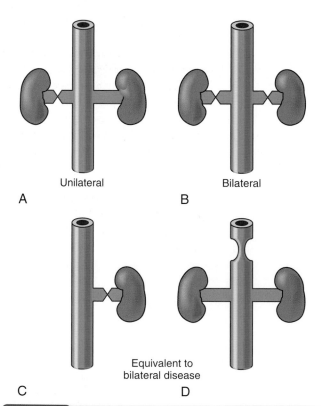

Unilateral   Bilateral

A   B

Equivalent to
bilateral disease

C   D

FIGURE 30-2 Anatomy of renal artery stenosis. Renal artery stenosis may be unilateral (**A**), bilateral (**B**), or unilateral with a solitary kidney (**C**). Aortic disease may serve functionally as bilateral renal artery stenosis (**D**).

others are discussed later in this chapter. Atherosclerotic renovascular disease is a common form of secondary hypertension, affecting up to 5% of patients with hypertension. Atherosclerotic RAS rarely occurs in patients younger than 40 years, and it is more common in men, whites, smokers, diabetics, and patients with atherosclerotic disease in other arterial systems.

RAS should be suspected in patients with refractory hypertension or new-onset hypertension in patients older than 50 years, particularly if they have overt risk factors for atherosclerotic RAS (Table 30-1). Evaluation should always begin with a thorough history and physical examination, including attention to blood pressure and pulse amplitude in each extremity. A significant discrepancy between extremities may indicate peripheral vascular disease and increase the likelihood of RAS. An abdominal bruit is detected in about 50% of subjects but is not specific for RAS. Edema is not typically found unless significant CKD or another edematous condition also exists.

Laboratory evaluation may reveal hypokalemia (K^+ <3.5 mEq/L) or metabolic alkalosis (HCO_3^- >28 mEq/L) due to secondary hyperaldosteronism. A reduced GFR with an elevated serum creatinine concentration may be found, but a normal serum creatinine level does not rule out hemodynamically significant RAS. Plasma renin activity and aldosterone concentrations may be elevated, but their measurement is of limited clinical utility in assessing hypertensive patients for RAS or in making therapeutic decisions. Urinalysis results are usually normal, although low-grade proteinuria (usually <1 g/day) from long-standing hypertension may be seen.

Diagnosis

Standard renal ultrasound imaging provides a limited window into the detection of RAS by revealing a discrepancy in kidney size, which develops only after prolonged ischemia and irreversible renal injury. However, a change in kidney size over time on serial imaging in the setting of known RAS may prompt the clinician to consider treatment with angioplasty and stenting or with surgical revascularization.

Renal ultrasound with pulsed Doppler analysis provides information about flow velocity in the renal arteries that may be helpful in detecting hemodynamically significant RAS. However, renal duplex ultrasonography is technically demanding, particularly in obese patients, and it is best performed by an experienced ultrasonographer at a high-volume center with a proven track record of high diagnostic accuracy. At most centers, the sensitivity, specificity, and positive and negative predictive values of renal

TABLE 30-1	CLINICAL FINDINGS SUGGESTING ATHEROSCLEROTIC RENOVASCULAR DISEASE

Onset of new, severe hypertension or sudden worsening of chronic hypertension at >55 years of age
Accelerated, resistant, or malignant hypertension
Unexplained atrophic kidney or size discrepancy >1.5 cm between kidneys
Sudden, unexplained ("flash") pulmonary edema
Unexplained chronic kidney disease in an individual with atherosclerotic vascular disease elsewhere
Development of acute kidney injury or worsening of chronic kidney disease after starting an ACE inhibitor or ARB

ACE, Angiotensin-converting enzyme; ARB, angiotensin II–receptor blocker.

duplex ultrasonography are unknown, and its clinical utility is probably limited.

Computed tomography (CT) with intravenous iodinated contrast (i.e., CT angiography [CTA]) permits high-resolution evaluation of the arterial vasculature and can be a very useful diagnostic imaging study, particularly in patients with normal or near-normal kidney function. Its use is limited in patients with more significantly impaired kidney function due to the risk of contast-induced AKI. Magnetic resonance angiography (MRA) with intravenous contrast is also useful for detecting RAS. Gadolinium administration to patients with advanced kidney disease (GFR <30 mL/min) may be contraindicated because of the risk of nephrogenic fibrosing dermopathy, although this appears to be much less of a concern or contradiction with the newer gadolinium-containing contrast agents. Overall, CTA and MRA appear to have similarly high sensitivity and specificity in the assessment of patients with possible atherosclerotic RAS.

Nuclear imaging using technetium-99m diethylene triamine pentaacetic acid (^{99m}Tc-DTPA) or technetium-99m mercapto-acetyltriglycine (^{99m}Tc-MAG3) to assess isotopic uptake and excretion in each kidney before and after the administration of a short-acting ACE inhibitor has been used in the past but has fallen out of favor due to limited specificity and lack of sensitivity in patients with bilateral RAS. The most sensitive and specific test—but also the most invasive—is renal arteriography, which remains the gold standard for the detection of RAS.

At some centers, flow measurements can be obtained at the time of arteriography. An added advantage of arteriography is that angioplasty and stenting can be performed during the procedure (discussed later) if appropriate. Because of the frequent occurrence of accessory renal arteries, an aortogram must be performed rather than selective renal angiography to ensure that all vessels are visualized.

Treatment

Patients with atherosclerotic RAS typically have coexistent cerebrovascular, coronary, and peripheral vascular disease as the result of a long history of multiple risk factors such as cigarette smoking and hyperlipidemia. Clinicians should recognize this high cardiovascular risk and understand that long-term outcomes for patients with atherosclerotic RAS are often determined by coexisting nonrenal atherosclerotic disease. The absolute risk of developing end-stage renal disease (ESRD) is increased for patients with atherosclerotic RAS compared with those without RAS, but the risk is much less than the risk of clinically significant coronary artery disease, symptomatic peripheral vascular disease, heart failure, or stroke. As with atherosclerotic disease in other arterial circulations, atherosclerotic RAS should prompt efforts for intensive lipid lowering, use of aspirin, smoking cessation, and control of hypertension and diabetes mellitus.

Intervention for atherosclerotic RAS remains controversial despite several randomized clinical trials designed to investigate the benefits and risks of medical management compared with angioplasty and renal artery stenting. Small clinical studies have suggested that renal artery angioplasty and stenting may improve blood pressure control in selected cases of atherosclerotic RAS, but identifying which patients may benefit has been problematic, and many have little or no improvement in blood pressure or are not able to significantly reduce the number of required antihypertensive medications. Randomized, controlled clinical trials have not demonstrated significant clinical benefit in terms of blood pressure control, kidney function, or mortality for most patients with atherosclerotic RAS.

Renal artery angioplasty and stenting carry a risk of acute worsening of kidney function due to atheroembolic disease, contrast nephropathy, or in-stent thrombosis, among other technical complications, and the procedures may lead to irreversible, progressive kidney dysfunction and ESRD. Decisions to correct atherosclerotic RAS with angioplasty and stenting or surgery must be made on a case-by-case basis, considering underlying kidney function, severity of hypertension, tolerance to antihypertensive medications, unilateral or bilateral RAS, atherosclerotic disease in other vascular beds, and life expectancy based on age and other comorbid conditions. There is no role for angioplasty alone without stenting in most patients with atherosclerotic RAS due to the high risk of recurrent stenosis.

Medical management of hypertension in patients with atherosclerotic RAS must take into consideration other comorbid conditions. Use of ACE inhibitors, ARBs, and diuretics is often very effective, but patients treated with these agents must be monitored closely for further compromise of their kidney function.

Fibromuscular Dysplasia

Fibromuscular dysplasia (FMD) is a nonatherosclerotic, noninflammatory disease that causes RAS. FMD typically affects young women more than other groups. The cause is not established, but it is thought to be a developmental defect. Depending on the population, FMD is responsible for 10% to 25% of all renovascular hypertension and is therefore much less common than atherosclerotic RAS.

FMD most commonly affects the renal arteries (bilaterally in about 35% of affected patients), but carotid and vertebral arteries can also be affected. Although FMD is often thought of as a disease of young women, men and older patients can be affected.

Classification of FMD is based on the histologic layer of the artery involved (i.e., intima, media, or adventitia) (Table 30-2). Medial fibroplasia with a mural aneurysm is the most common cause of FMD in adults (70% of cases). It consists of alternating fibromuscular ridges and aneurysmal segments in the distal two thirds of the renal artery and has a classic string-of-beads appearance on angiography (Fig. 30-3). Perimedial fibroplasia of the outer one half of the media produces severe multifocal stenosis and causes about 15% of FMD in adults.

TABLE 30-2	HISTOLOGIC CLASSIFICATION OF FIBROMUSCULAR DYSPLASIA	
SUBTYPE	**PERCENTAGE OF CASES (%)**	**RADIOLOGIC APPEARANCE**
Medial fibroplasia	60-70	String of beads with aneurysms
Perimedial fibroplasia	15	String of beads without large aneurysms
Medial hyperplasia	5-15	Smooth tubular stenosis
Intimal fibroplasia	1-2	Focal or smooth stenosis
Adventitial fibroplasia	<1	Focal or smooth tubular stenosis

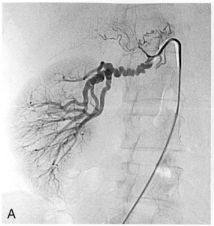
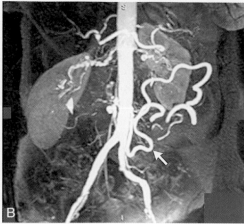

FIGURE 30-3 **A,** Typical medial fibroplasia (i.e., string-of-beads appearance) on an angiogram of a right renal artery. **B,** Gadolinium-enhanced magnetic resonance angiography in the same patient, revealing bilateral medial fibroplasia of the renal arteries and a large marginal artery of Drummond *(arrow)*, indicates that there is disease of the superior mesenteric artery. (From Slovut DP, Olin JW: Fibromuscular dysplasia, N Engl J Med 350:1862–1871, 2004.)

Medial subtypes of FMD usually have a benign course and are responsive to angioplasty. The intimal subtype may have a higher likelihood of ischemic events and multiorgan system involvement. Symptoms are usually precipitated by stenoses, but FMD may rarely cause dissection or macroaneurysms that require intervention. Although CTA or MRA may be useful in the detection of FMD in the main renal arteries and main branch arteries, arteriography is necessary for detection of stenoses in smaller arteries.

Treatment for FMD depends on the severity of complications. Pharmacologic treatment alone may be adequate to control hypertension in many patients. Intervention with angioplasty (with or without stenting) or surgery should be considered for patients with severe or difficult to control hypertension or declining kidney function. Angioplasty without stenting is successful in many patients, but recurrent stenosis is not uncommon, and new stenoses from FMD may develop at other sites. For this reason, regular monitoring of blood pressure and serum creatinine levels is essential, and many patients require imaging studies to detect new or recurrent lesions.

Aortic Dissection

Aortic dissection occurs after disruption of the intimal layer of the aorta and propagation of blood flow that dissects along the wall of the aorta, producing a false lumen and compression of the true aortic lumen. Aortic dissection is classified by the site of origin (i.e., DeBakey classification) or the segment of the aorta involved (i.e., Stanford classification). DeBakey type I and II dissections originate in the ascending aorta, and type III dissections originate in the descending aorta. Stanford type A refers to dissections involving the ascending aorta, and type B refers to all others not involving the ascending aorta.

Major branch vessels of the aorta, including the renal arteries, may become obstructed or occluded as a result of extension of the dissection. Aortic dissection frequently compromises the renal arteries (the left more commonly than the right) when it extends into the abdominal aorta and causes renal failure in approximately 20% of patients with type B dissections. When disease is extensive enough to cause AKI, vascular compromise

to the intestinal and cerebral vasculature and severe aortic regurgitation often contribute to the high mortality rate.

Aortic dissection most frequently affects older patients (>50 years of age) with coexistent vascular risk factors such as hypertension, smoking, and atherosclerosis. Men are affected more commonly than women. Occasionally, a genetic connective tissue defect such as Marfan syndrome or Ehlers-Danlos syndrome type IV (about 5% of cases) causes aortic dissection, and these conditions should be considered in younger patients (<40 years of age).

AKI occurs in about 20% of patients diagnosed with acute type B aortic dissection and is an independent predictor of in-hospital mortality. Trauma or procedures (e.g., aortic catheterization) can also cause dissection of the aorta or renal artery. Isolated, spontaneous renal artery dissection may rarely occur, most commonly in the setting of polyarteritis nodosa or FMD. Segmental arterial mediolysis is another uncommon condition of unknown origin that is characterized by vacuolar degeneration of smooth muscle cells in the arterial media, which leads to disruption of the arterial medial layer, vessel dissection, hemorrhage, and ischemia. Segmental arterial mediolysis can affect abdominal visceral arteries and virtually any other arterial system.

The most frequent symptom during aortic dissection is chest pain, which may be described as a ripping sensation. Isolated loss of pulse in one or more extremities may provide a clinical clue, and the number of arteries involved correlates with the severity of dissection. A common clue to the diagnosis on a routine chest radiograph is a widened mediastinum, with or without a pleural effusion (most often on the left).

After the diagnosis of aortic dissection is established, evaluation of renal artery involvement is best undertaken noninvasively to minimize further vascular injury. Contrast-enhanced CT, magnetic resonance imaging (MRI), or MRA usually provide images capable of confirming or excluding renal involvement, although each modality carries the same limitations as outlined for the evaluation of RAS. Transesophageal echocardiography is useful for establishing the diagnosis of aortic dissection, but it does not provide information about the aorta below the diaphragm. Renal duplex ultrasonography may be useful for evaluating renal perfusion in the setting of aortic dissection, but it is not recommended for the initial investigation of aortic dissection.

Aortic dissection is a hypertensive emergency that requires aggressive reduction of blood pressure; systolic blood pressure should be maintained between 100 and 120 mm Hg. Antihypertensive medications that reduce the rate of increase in blood pressure during the cardiac cycle (dP/dt), such as β-adrenergic receptor blockers, have a theoretical benefit in managing aortic dissection by reducing the rate of progression.

Surgical treatment options for renal involvement due to aortic dissection depend on individual circumstances, and careful evaluation by an experienced vascular surgeon is recommended. Thoracic aortic dissection requires surgical repair due to the high mortality rate if left untreated, but isolated abdominal aortic disease may be medically managed.

Thromboembolic Disease

Systemic arterial emboli, typically originating from the left atrium or left ventricle in patients with atrial fibrillation, infectious endocarditis, cardiac valvular disease, or atrial myxoma, may cause acute obstruction of the renal arteries. Rarely, a paradoxical embolus may occur from the venous system through an atrial septal defect.

Symptoms of acute renal ischemia and infarction include flank pain, gross hematuria, and fever. Laboratory findings are nonspecific but include an elevated level of lactate dehydrogenase (LDH), hematuria, and leukocytosis. A definitive diagnosis can be based on the finding of a focal nonenhancing region on contrast-enhanced CT. Imaging studies are necessary to differentiate renal artery embolic disease from renal artery dissection.

The renal mass affected by a renal artery embolus is usually not large enough to necessitate dialysis, although some worsening of kidney function may be observed. The diagnosis of renal infarction is rarely made early enough to initiate treatment with intraarterial thrombolysis or thrombectomy, and it is questionable whether the risks and marginal benefit of these procedures warrant aggressive treatment. Therapy should instead address the underlying source of renal emboli with symptomatic treatment of pain as necessary. Systemic anticoagulation may be indicated to reduce the risk of further thromboembolic events.

Large and Medium-Sized Vessel Vasculitis

Systemic vasculitides such as temporal (giant cell) arteritis and Takayasu's arteritis affect primarily large and medium-sized arteries. Polyarteritis nodosa and Kawasaki disease affect primarily medium-sized and smaller arteries. These vasculitides are not associated with antineutrophil cytoplasmic antibodies (ANCAs) and do not typically cause glomerulonephritis. They are distinguished from ANCA-associated vasculitides that involve smaller blood vessels and more commonly cause glomerulonephritis.

Takayasu's arteritis and giant cell arteritis are typically associated with a granulomatous vasculitis of the aorta and its branches. Giant cell arteritis typically involves the carotid, vertebral, and temporal arteries, and renal involvement is rare. Both occur much more commonly in women than men. Takayasu's arteritis is usually diagnosed in patients younger than 50 years of age, whereas giant cell arteritis is diagnosed in those 50 years of age or older.

Involvement of the main renal arteries occurs in about 40% of patients with Takayasu's arteritis, producing areas of stenosis with renal ischemia or renal infarction. Common clinical features are constitutional symptoms, claudication, bruits, and hypertension. Pulses are often diminished or absent in one or more extremities, and a blood pressure discrepancy more than 10 mm Hg in the limbs is common. The diagnosis of Takayasu's arteritis is most often made on clinical grounds along with typical angiographic or other imaging findings. Corticosteroids are the primary treatment modality.

Polyarteritis nodosa is a medium-sized or small vessel vasculitis with no gender predilection that predominantly occurs in patients between 40 and 60 years of age. It affects the main renal arteries and renal interlobar arteries (less commonly, the arcuate and interlobular arteries) with a necrotizing vasculitis that typically produces microaneurysms of the intrarenal arteries. They can be seen on arteriograms in 40% to 90% of patients with renal involvement. Renal ischemia leads to loss of kidney function and renin-mediated hypertension. Low-grade proteinuria and hematuria may be seen, but the finding of acute glomerulonephritis indicates some other disorder. Renal infarction may occur, and rarely, a renal artery aneurysm may cause renal artery dissection or rupture.

The diagnosis is made on clinical grounds and by arteriography. There are no confirmatory serologic tests; polyarteritis nodosa is not an ANCA-associated vasculitis. Arteriography appears to be superior for diagnosis compared with CT and MRA. Progressive renal disease is not typical but may occur. Treatment with corticosteroids and immunosuppressive drugs is effective in reducing disease severity and mortality.

Kawasaki disease is an arteritis associated with the mucocutaneous lymph node syndrome that affects mostly medium-sized and small arteries, although the aorta may also be involved. It is primarily a self-limited disease of infants and young children. Renal involvement is extremely rare.

Hypertensive Nephrosclerosis

Chronic hypertension in susceptible individuals may lead to development of proteinuria, CKD, and ESRD. Hypertensive nephrosclerosis is cited as a cause of CKD and ESRD in African Americans at a much higher rate than whites, even with similar levels of blood pressure control and despite good control.

The renal manifestations of chronic hypertension include renal arterial and arteriolar intimal thickening and luminal narrowing with medial hypertrophy and fibroblastic intimal thickening of arteries and deposition of hyaline-like material in the walls of arterioles. Glomeruli show global and focal glomerulosclerosis; the former likely results from glomerular ischemia and the latter from increased intracapillary pressure and compensatory hypertrophy and injury in response to nephron loss. Wrinkled glomerular basement membranes due to glomerular ischemia are seen on electron microscopy. Chronic interstitial nephritis with tubular atrophy and interstitial fibrosis also occurs. These histopathologic changes of hypertensive nephrosclerosis are often found on renal biopsy for patients with other disorders, such as diabetes mellitus, atheroembolic disease, and RAS.

The overall risk of hypertensive nephrosclerosis with progressive CKD is low in the general hypertensive population, and most patients with hypertensive nephrosclerosis have mild hypertension. The risk is greater for those who have had poorly controlled hypertension and for those of African descent, who are at particularly high risk for hypertensive nephrosclerosis. Polymorphisms in the genes that encode for apolipoprotein L1 (*APOL1*) and podocyte nonmuscle myosin heavy chain 9 (*MYH9*) are found more commonly in African Americans compared with European Americans and strongly associate with the risk of hypertensive nephrosclerosis. A diagnosis of hypertensive nephrosclerosis as the cause of otherwise unexplained CKD is much less likely to be made in white patients compared with black patients, particularly in the absence of long-standing, severe hypertension or a history of malignant hypertension.

The diagnosis of hypertensive nephrosclerosis is typically based on a history of long-standing hypertension that precedes development of proteinuria and CKD in the absence of other causes. The urinary sediment is typically bland, with only low-grade proteinuria (<1 g/day). Symmetrical loss of renal cortical thickness is commonly found on renal ultrasound.

Pharmacologic treatment of severe hypertension reduces the risk for progression of CKD to ESRD in many patient populations, providing further evidence for the causative role of hypertension. The optimal blood pressure for patients with hypertensive nephrosclerosis has not been determined. For black patients, this was best addressed by the African American Study of Kidney Disease (AASK) trial, which examined more than 1000 African Americans with long-standing hypertension, slowly progressive CKD, and low-grade proteinuria. Subjects were allocated to treatment with ramipril, metoprolol, or amlodipine to a blood pressure goal of 125/75 mm Hg or 140/90 mm Hg. The mean rate of change in GFR and the rate of other secondary outcomes were similar in the two groups, suggesting that lowering blood pressure to less than 140/90 mmHg does not provide further benefit in slowing CKD progression in black patients with hypertensive nephrosclerosis. However, there was a trend favoring the lower blood pressure goal for patients with higher baseline proteinuria.

Lower blood pressure goals may also be appropriate for patients with other comorbid conditions such as diabetes mellitus. Besides affecting CKD progression, blood pressure control reduces the risk of heart failure and stroke. Most patients with hypertensive nephrosclerosis and CKD require multiple antihypertensive medications to control blood pressure, typically including a thiazide or thiazide-like diuretic (when GFR is well preserved) and a loop diuretic (as the GFR declines to less than 25 to 30 mL/min), along with an ACE inhibitor or ARB, calcium-channel blocker, and β-blocker.

Atheroembolic Disease

Atheroembolic disease is the result of cholesterol embolization from atherosclerotic plaques, most commonly from the aorta and typically dislodged during an invasive arterial procedure such as cardiac catheterization, aortic angiography, cardiac surgery, or surgery on the aorta. Cholesterol emboli may occur spontaneously or may be precipitated by systemic anticoagulation, such as with heparin, or during systemic administration of thrombolytic agents. Because patients must have underlying atherosclerosis, the incidence increases with age,

and atheroembolic disease rarely occurs before 40 years of age.

As the result of systemic embolization from atheromatous plaques, cholesterol crystals lodge in small arterial vessels, including the arcuate or interlobular arteries of the kidneys. Cholesterol emboli frequently involve other organs, and the pattern of organ involvement depends in part on whether disrupted plaque is in the ascending or descending aorta. The extremities are commonly affected with digital ischemia and gangrene, the skin with livedo reticularis, and the gastrointestinal tract with intestinal ischemia, but any organ can be affected. Embolization from the ascending aorta can cause cardiac ischemia, and emboli arising from the ascending aorta or carotid arteries (e.g., after carotid endarterectomy) can cause stroke.

Cholesterol embolization to the eye may be recognized by finding Hollenhorst plaques on funduscopic examination, which are whitish yellow flecks at retinal arteriole bifurcations. They are often asymptomatic but may cause retinal ischemia with usually transient visual field defects.

Patients with atheroembolic disease may have fever, eosinophilia, eosinophiluria, and hypocomplementemia, particularly acutely. Laboratory findings include an elevated erythrocyte sedimentation rate and elevated levels of amylase or liver enzymes. The widespread systemic clinical and laboratory manifestations of atheroemboli can lead to a clinical picture suggesting systemic vasculitis.

The typical pattern of renal atheroembolic disease is a decline in kidney function that first becomes apparent 3 or more days after an inciting procedure or other event. The degree of acute and chronic kidney injury that follows is determined by the magnitude of the embolic burden, whether atheroembolism is a one-time or ongoing process, and the degree of inflammation induced by the plaque material. Many patients have stabilization of the process after the initial insult, whereas others progress with various patterns and tempos to advanced CKD and ESRD. Cholesterol embolization also may cause severe hypertension due to acute renal ischemia leading to renin release.

Diagnosis of renal atheroembolic disease is usually made clinically in the appropriate setting, but for some patients, a kidney biopsy is needed to confirm the diagnosis and exclude others. Because the fixation process washes out the cholesterol crystals from the renal biopsy sample, the pathologic examination reveals a typical needle-shaped disruption in the arterial lumen surrounded by reactive endovascular cells.

There is no specific treatment for cholesterol emboli. Because an inflammatory reaction typically results from the emboli, some physicians advocate corticosteroids, but their use is unproved for preventing further atheroembolism or progression of kidney failure. Avoidance of anticoagulation has been recommended to prevent dissolution and embolization of thrombus that may overlie an atheromatous plaque. Statin therapy is appropriate for most patients for treatment of their underlying atherosclerotic disease, but it has not been shown to influence the renal manifestation of atheroemboli. Treatment with ACE inhibitors or ARBs may be effective for hypertension control in the acute setting, but worsening kidney function may limit their use. Dialysis may be necessary if AKI and ESRD develop.

Preeclampsia

Preeclampsia is characterized by the new onset of sustained hypertension (blood pressure ≥140/90 mm Hg) and proteinuria (>300 mg/day) that develops after 20 weeks' gestation in a previously normotensive woman. Although hypertension and proteinuria are the principal features of preeclampsia, it is a systemic vascular disease that may also cause central nervous system symptoms (e.g., visual disturbances, headache, altered mental status), abdominal pain, nausea and vomiting, liver dysfunction, thrombocytopenia, pulmonary dysfunction, impaired fetal growth, nephrotic-range proteinuria, and AKI. If grand mal seizures develop without other explanation, a diagnosis of eclampsia is made. The HELLP syndrome, characterized by *h*emolysis, *e*levated *l*iver enzymes, and a *l*ow *p*latelet count, may be a manifestation of severe preeclampsia, although some consider it to be a separate disorder. It is also associated with increased maternal and fetal mortality.

Preeclampsia should be distinguished from other hypertensive conditions that can occur during pregnancy, including preexisting hypertension that occurs before 20 weeks' gestation and persists after delivery, preeclampsia superimposed on preexisting chronic hypertension, and gestational hypertension (i.e., new-onset hypertension after 20 weeks' gestation without proteinuria or other related manifestations).

Progress has been made in understanding the pathogenesis of preeclampsia, and maternal and placental or fetal factors have been implicated. Abnormal development of placental vasculature in early pregnancy is thought to lead to some degree of placental hypoperfusion that releases antiangiogenic factors into the maternal circulation, disturbing the delicate balance of angiogenic and antiangiogenic factors. This causes systemic endothelial dysfunction in the mother that leads to hypertension, proteinuria, and other manifestations of the disease.

Soluble FMS-related tyrosine kinase 1 (sFLT1) is a placenta-derived circulating antiangiogenic factor that appears to play a central role in the pathogenesis of preeclampsia. It antagonizes the proangiogenic effects of vascular endothelial growth factor (VEGF) and placental growth factor (PGF) by binding to them and preventing interaction with their receptors. Soluble endoglin (sENG), another antiangiogenic factor that is widely expressed on vascular endothelium, is thought to be an important mediator of preeclampsia. Endothelial dysfunction in preeclampsia is associated with increased sensitivity to vasopressor agents, including angiotensin II, systemic vasoconstriction, and reduced fibrinolytic function.

Kidney biopsy findings include glomerular endothelial cell swelling (i.e., endotheliosis) and occlusion of the capillary lumen with ischemia. These findings are also seen with other microangiopathic disorders, although fibrin thrombi in glomerular capillaries are less commonly seen than with other causes. Foot process effacement is not usually seen.

The only effective treatment for preeclampsia is delivery of the fetus and placenta. The timing of delivery must take into account gestational age, severity of preeclampsia, presence or absence of systemic features, and status of the fetus and mother. Proper obstetric care is essential to balance the risk to the mother against the risk for prematurity of the fetus.

Treatment of mild hypertension in women with preeclampsia should be avoided because it does not treat the underlying disease process, alter the course of disease, or reduce clinical sequelae. In the absence of clinical manifestations other than proteinuria, it is usually unnecessary to start antihypertensive medications unless the systolic blood pressure is greater than 150 mm Hg or the diastolic blood pressure is higher than 100 mm Hg. Labetalol and hydralazine, both of which can be given intravenously or orally, are often recommended as first-line therapy for acute management. For chronic treatment, methyldopa or labetalol are often recommended initially, with extended-release nifedipine added if necessary. Diuretics and dietary sodium restriction usually are avoided unless the patient has pulmonary edema.

The risk profile of these medications is poorly defined in pregnancy. ACE inhibitors, ARBs, and direct renin inhibitors are contraindicated during pregnancy because of the risk of fetal abnormalities. Magnesium sulfate is used in severe cases of preeclampsia to reduce the risk of seizures, but it does not treat other manifestations of the disease or reduce maternal or fetal mortality rates.

Most manifestations of preeclampsia begin to improve shortly after delivery, but in some women, hypertension, proteinuria, and other manifestations may persist for several weeks or months before resolving completely. Because preeclampsia is a risk factor for future hypertension, kidney disease, and cardiovascular events, continued medical follow-up is essential.

Scleroderma Renal Crisis

Systemic sclerosis (i.e., scleroderma) is an idiopathic connective tissue disorder associated with deposition of collagen and other extracellular matrix proteins that produces inflammation and fibrosis of the skin and internal organs. Proliferative endovascular lesions may lead to obliteration of the vascular internal lumina and renal ischemia, with hypertension, increased renin activity, and elevated levels of angiotensin II and aldosterone.

AKI and rapidly worsening hypertension in patients with scleroderma is called *scleroderma renal crisis*. It occurs in approximately 5% to 10% of patients with scleroderma, typically within the first few years after onset and primarily in those with systemic rather than localized cutaneous scleroderma who also have progressive skin and cardiac involvement. Subclinical renal involvement occurs much more frequently. Scleroderma renal crisis occasionally develops before the clinical diagnosis of scleroderma has been made.

Scleroderma renal crisis is often associated with rapid and severe loss of kidney function, oliguria, hypertensive encephalopathy, and heart failure. Microangiopathic hemolytic anemia may also occur. About 10% of patients with scleroderma renal crisis do not have hypertension. This occurs more commonly among patients being treated with ACE inhibitors or high-dose corticosteroids.

Anti–RNA polymerase III antibodies are strongly associated with the risk of scleroderma renal crisis and have been suggested as markers for scleroderma renal crisis. Renal biopsy may reveal interlobular artery involvement with intimal thickening, endothelial cell proliferation, and edema with obliteration of the vessel lumen with concentric onion-skinning of the wall of arterioles. Fibrinoid necrosis occurs in afferent arterioles with intravascular fibrin accumulation extending into the glomeruli, often with ischemic collapse, but without features of glomerulonephritis.

Activation of the renin-angiotensin-aldosterone system appears to play an important role in the progression of the disease. Before the advent of ACE inhibitors and hemodialysis, scleroderma renal crisis was fatal in about 75% of patients at 1 year. ACE inhibitor therapy has reduced this 1-year mortality rate to less than 15%. Captopril is often recommended as the ACE inhibitor of choice due to its short half-life and ease of dose titration. If the diagnosis of scleroderma renal crisis is made before advanced renal failure is established, ACE inhibition may halt or reverse the decline in renal function. Some experts recommend continuing ACE inhibitors even if kidney function declines and temporary dialysis is necessary, citing an increased chance of renal recovery. ACE inhibitors are not useful for prevention of scleroderma renal crisis, and their use in this setting has been associated with a poorer outcome, including greater risk of requiring permanent dialysis if renal crisis occurs. Use of ACE inhibitors rather than ARBs is recommended because of the long track record of success with ACE inhibitors in this disease.

🔵 THROMBOTIC THROMBOCYTOPENIC PURPURA AND HEMOLYTIC-UREMIC SYNDROME

Thrombotic thrombocytopenic purpura (TTP) and hemolytic-uremic syndrome (HUS) manifest with microangiopathic hemolytic anemia (MAHA) and organ dysfunction due to microvascular thrombosis, but each syndrome has distinct clinical, pathophysiologic, and epidemiologic features (Table 30-3).

Although many processes cause microvascular endothelial injury (Table 30-4), renal involvement from these disorders affect the vasculature at different levels. Renal involvement by HUS and TTP primarily affects the glomeruli, whereas scleroderma often extends to the interlobular arteries, and malignant hypertension more often affects the afferent arterioles. However, there is significant overlap and similar histologic features among these diseases, making careful clinical evaluation essential for accurate determination of the cause.

Thrombotic Thrombocytopenic Purpura

TTP is characterized by MAHA and thrombocytopenia. Patients may also have fever, AKI, and neurologic impairment. Purpura is only rarely observed, and it is not necessary to make the diagnosis. TTP occurs with a female-to-male ratio of 3:2 and a peak incidence in the third and fourth decades of life. MAHA and thrombocytopenia manifesting similar to TTP may occur in response to some drugs (e.g., ticlopidine, cyclosporine, tacrolimus), after stem cell transplantation, in association with human immunodeficiency virus (HIV) infection, and in patients with malignant hypertension, sepsis, disseminated intravascular coagulation, or advanced cancers.

TTP may be caused by a deficiency or reduced activity of ADAMTS13 (a disintegrin-like and metalloproteinase with thrombospondin-1–like domains). ADAMTS13 is a plasma protease that normally cleaves von Willebrand factor (vWF) and limits the extent of intravascular thrombosis (Fig. 30-4). Microthrombi composed primarily of platelets and vWF accumulate in the vascular bed of multiple organs, leading to a MAHA. Deficiency in ADAMTS13 may be acquired, caused by

TABLE 30-3   DIFFERENTIATION OF SHIGA TOXIN–RELATED HEMOLYTIC-UREMIC SYNDROME FROM THROMBOTIC THROMBOCYTOPENIC PURPURA

FEATURE	SHIGA TOXIN–RELATED HUS	TTP
Epidemiology	Endemic areas (commonly but not exclusively)	Endemic regions not reported
Similar cases in family	If yes, synchronous	If yes, separated in time and space
Recurrences	Rare	Common
Gastrointestinal prodrome	Painful diarrhea, frequently bloody	Nondiarrheal abdominal symptoms predominate, but not as prodrome
von Willebrand factor profile	Increased degradation to smaller multimers	Ultra-large forms (assay not universally available); depletion of large and ultra-large forms in advanced stage
ADAMTS13 expression	Normal or slightly decreased	Deficient (<0.1 U/mL)
Characteristics of intravascular thrombi	Fibrin predominates	von Willebrand factor predominates
Endothelial cell appearance	Swollen	Not swollen
Response to plasma therapy	Not demonstrated	Yes
Diagnosis	Isolation of STEC; antibody response to *Escherichia coli* O157:H7 LPS antigen	ADAMTS13 activity; inhibitors of ADAMTS13 activity; genetic analysis for mutations of *ADAMTS13* gene

Data from Tarr PI, Gordon CA, Chandler WL: Shiga toxin-producing Escherichia coli and haemolytic uraemic syndrome, Lancet 365:1073–1086, 2005.

ADAMTS3, A disintegrin and metalloproteinase with thrombospondin-1–like domains; HUS, hemolytic-uremic syndrome; LPS, lipopolysaccharide; STEC, Shiga-toxigenic *E. coli*; TTP, thrombotic thrombocytopenic purpura.

TABLE 30-4   DISORDERS ASSOCIATED WITH THROMBOTIC MICROANGIOPATHY

CONDITIONS	EXAMPLES
TTP	ADAMTS13 protease deficiency, acquired (autoantibody), genetic
HUS	Shiga toxin-associated (*E. coli*, others); D+ (typical HUS)
	Complement dysregulation; D− (atypical HUS)
Pregnancy	Preeclampsia, HELLP syndrome
Medications	Cyclosporine, tacrolimus, VEGF inhibitors, chemotherapeutic agents (e.g., mitomycin C), quinine, cocaine, ticlopidine (with anti-ADAMTS13 antibodies), muromonab-CD3 (OKT3), clopidogrel
Transplantation	Allogeneic bone marrow and stem cell transplants, solid organ
Neoplastic diseases	Metastatic cancers
Prothrombotic disorders	Antiphospholipid antibody syndrome
Infectious diseases	Rocky Mountain spotted fever, anthrax, HIV
Other conditions	Malignant hypertension, SLE, scleroderma renal crisis, radiation therapy, DIC, cardiovascular surgery

Data from Tsai HM: Advances in the pathogenesis, diagnosis, and treatment of thrombotic thrombocytopenic purpura. J Am Soc Nephrol 14:1072–1081, 2003.

D+, Positive for diarrhea; D−, negative for diarrhea; DIC, disseminated intravascular coagulation; HIV, human immunodeficiency virus; HELLP, hemolysis, elevated liver enzyme levels, and a low platelet count; HUS, hemolytic uremic syndrome; SLE, systemic lupus erythematosus; TTP, thrombotic thrombocytopenic purpura; VEGF, vascular endothelial growth factor.

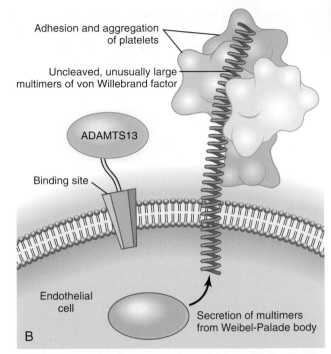

FIGURE 30-4 Relation between ADAMTS13 activity, excessive adhesion and activation of platelets, and thrombotic thrombocytopenic purpura. **A,** In normal subjects, ADAMTS13 (i.e., von Willebrand factor–cleaving metalloprotease) molecules attach to binding sites on endothelial cell surfaces and cleave unusually large multimers of von Willebrand factor as they are secreted by stimulated endothelial cells. The smaller von Willebrand factor forms that circulate after cleavage do not induce the adhesion and aggregation of platelets during normal blood flow. **B,** Absent or severely reduced activity of ADAMTS13 in patients with thrombotic thrombocytopenic purpura prevents timely cleavage of unusually large multimers of von Willebrand factor as they are secreted by endothelial cells. The uncleaved multimers induce the adhesion and aggregation of platelets in flowing blood. (From Moake JL: Thrombotic microangiopathies, N Engl J Med 347:589–600, 2002.)

anti-ADAMTS13 autoantibodies (mostly immunoglobulin G [IgG]), or, much less commonly, genetic.

Other laboratory abnormalities are manifestations of the MAHA and include thrombocytopenia; an elevated LDH concentration, indirect bilirubin concentration, and reticulocyte count; and a low haptoglobin concentration. Coagulation laboratory test results (e.g., prothrombin time, activated partial thromboplastin time, fibrinogen level) are typically normal, although levels of fibrin split products may be elevated. AKI, microscopic hematuria, and low-grade proteinuria are frequently detected.

Without treatment, TTP has a mortality rate of about 90%, with most deaths occurring within 3 months of the onset of symptoms. Treatment with plasma infusion can normalize ADAMTS13 levels, reducing intravascular hemolysis and mortality rates. Plasmapheresis and replacement with fresh-frozen plasma has the advantage of removing inhibitory autoantibodies in addition to normalizing ADAMTS13 levels because of the large volume of plasma that can be infused.

ADAMTS13 activity must be assayed before therapy is initiated to obtain accurate results, but treatment should not be delayed for the results to return. The severity of ADAMTS13 deficiency (<5%) predicts future relapse, although those with severe deficiency are just as likely to respond initially to plasmapheresis as those with a mild deficiency. Patients with MAHA due to other causes not associated with ADAMTS13 deficiency usually do not respond to plasmapheresis or plasma infusion. Patients with HUS do not have abnormalities in ADAMTS13 levels or function.

Hemolytic-Uremic Syndrome

Gastrointestinal tract infection with the Shiga-toxigenic *Escherichia coli* strain O157:H7 produces a diarrheal illness that is complicated in about 15% of cases by a MAHA with intraglomerular thrombosis and AKI, a condition referred to as diarrheal (D+) HUS. *Shigella dysenteriae* serotype 1 or other Shiga toxin–producing strains of *E. coli* may also cause D+ HUS. D+ HUS most commonly affects infants and children, although adults may also be affected. Cases of D+ HUS often cluster because of outbreaks of *E. coli* O157:H7, with peaks occurring in summer and autumn. *E. coli* is endemic in the gastrointestinal tract of cattle, and cases are often tracked to undercooked meat, exposure to bovine fecal matter, animal exposure, or other contaminated food products.

Shiga-toxigenic bacterial strains commonly produce a prodrome of painful, bloody diarrhea, which precedes the development of HUS by 2 to 12 days (median, 3 days). Shiga toxin is directly thrombogenic in the renal vasculature. Although intravascular coagulation in D+ HUS is usually limited to the kidney, the heart, gastrointestinal tract, and central nervous system may also be affected.

Laboratory abnormalities in HUS include elevated creatinine levels, anemia, schistocytes on the peripheral smear, elevated reticulocyte count, and thrombocytopenia. In contrast to disseminated intravascular coagulation, fibrinogen levels are normal or high, and the prothrombin time is normal or only slightly prolonged. Fresh stool should be sent for culture of *E. coli* O157:H7, which can aid in tracing the source of an outbreak.

Stool studies should also be performed for patients without diarrhea because *E. coli* O157:H7 may rarely cause HUS in the absence of intestinal symptoms. If *E. coli* O157:H7 is not detected, culture for other Shiga-toxigenic organisms should be pursued.

The pathologic renal lesions of HUS include vessel wall thickening with endothelial cell swelling and intraglomerular thrombosis with platelet- and fibrin-rich thrombi. Fragmentation of red blood cells may be seen in the renal vasculature and within the vessel wall.

Treatment of D+ HUS is supportive, including adequate volume repletion with isotonic intravenous fluids, transfusion for severe anemia, and avoidance of other nephrotoxic agents (e.g., nonsteroidal anti-inflammatory drugs, aminoglycoside antibiotics, iodinated contrast). Platelet transfusion is not recommended because it may worsen the ongoing microvascular thrombosis. Antibiotic treatment of patients with bloody diarrhea is not recommended because it is not effective in reducing the incidence of HUS and may increase the risk. Corticosteroids, anticoagulation (e.g., aspirin, heparin), thrombolytic agents, and plasma administration have proved ineffective for the treatment of HUS.

With supportive care alone, most patients with D+ HUS recover with normalization of renal function or only mild residual CKD, although about 25% may develop advanced CKD or ESRD over the next 1 to 2 decades of life. Risk for CKD is increased with cortical necrosis and involvement of more than 50% of glomeruli identified on renal biopsy. The risk for complications and death increases with age, with the mortality rate increasing from about 5% to 10% for children to about 30% for adults.

D− HUS (atypical HUS) accounts for about 5% of cases and has a higher likelihood of recurrence, ESRD, or death. Many cases are caused by genetic defects in the complement pathway (e.g., C3, C5, complement H, factor I, CD46). Testing for ADAMTS13 levels, which are normal in D− HUS, can be useful in differentiating atypical HUS from TTP. Specialty laboratories can test for complement cascade abnormalities. Eculizumab is a humanized monoclonal antibody that binds with high affinity to complement protein C5 and prevents the generation of C5a, C5b, and the terminal complement complex C5b-9. In patients with atypical HUS, eculizumab inhibits complement-mediated thrombotic microangiopathy.

● ANTIPHOSPHOLIPID ANTIBODY SYNDROME

Antiphospholipid antibodies (APAs) refer to autoantibodies such as lupus anticoagulants or IgG or immunoglobulin M (IgM) anticardiolipin antibodies that interfere with phospholipid-binding proteins and in vitro phospholipid-dependent clotting assays such as the partial thromboplastin time. Because not all lupus anticoagulants cause prolongation of the partial thromboplastin time, other tests of the coagulation system, such as the dilute Russell viper venom time, may need to be obtained. The diagnosis of antiphospholipid antibody syndrome (APS) is based on the occurrence of arterial or venous clotting events or fetal loss during pregnancy after 10 or more weeks' gestation in the setting of laboratory detection of an APA. Lupus anticoagulant and anticardiolipin antibodies are detectable in up to 10% of healthy populations, and their presence alone is insufficient

for a diagnosis of APS. Apolipoprotein H (apo H, formerly β_2-glycoprotein 1) is the main antigenic target of anticardiolipin antibodies.

In the absence of an underlying autoimmune disease, the syndrome is referred to as primary APS. Secondary APS occurs when associated with other diseases such as systemic lupus erythematosus (SLE). APAs are detectable in 30% to 50% of patients with SLE, and renal involvement is often observed in this setting.

The procoagulant effect of APAs may result from interference with the anticoagulant apo H, inhibition of fibrinolysis, direct endothelial injury, accelerated atherosclerosis, and activation of platelet, monocyte, and endothelial cells. Renal involvement occurs in about 25% of patients with primary APS and can occur in patients with SLE or other causes of APS. Thrombosis may occur throughout the renal vasculature, including main or branch renal arteries, arterioles, glomeruli, and veins. These findings resemble those found in other diseases associated with a thrombotic microangiopathy. Focal atrophy of the cortex in association with interstitial fibrosis may be observed due to resulting ischemia.

The RENAL manifestations of APS vary. Some patients have mild proteinuria with preserved kidney function, and others develop severe hypertension, nephrotic-range proteinuria, and AKI or CKD. Renal arterial thrombosis can cause infarction, acute onset of flank pain, hematuria, and decreased kidney function. Renal vein thrombosis may be silent or, if acute and complete, may manifest with sudden flank pain and reduced kidney function. Pathologic changes seen on renal biopsy of patients with primary APS are small vessel vaso-occlusive disease with fibrous intimal hyperplasia of interlobular arteries, recanalizing thrombi in arteries and arterioles, focal cortical atrophy, and thrombotic microangiopathy. Other manifestations of APS include thrombocytopenia, hemolytic anemia, and a prolonged activated partial thromboplastin time in the absence of heparin therapy.

Long-term warfarin anticoagulation with a target international normalized ratio (INR) between 2 and 3 is indicated for patients with primary or secondary APS and prior deep vein thrombosis, arterial thrombosis, or recurrent spontaneous abortion. Because warfarin is contraindicated during pregnancy, heparin with or without low-dose aspirin (81 mg) is necessary until the end of pregnancy.

Treatment of APA-positive patients in the absence of prior clinical events is controversial because of the high false-positive rate for the tests. Aspirin therapy for primary prevention in patients persistently positive for APAs has been advocated but not proved. Plasmapheresis, prednisone, and hydroxychloroquine have been advocated for the treatment of thrombotic microangiopathy due to APS and should be considered in severe cases.

● RENAL VEIN THROMBOSIS

Renal vein thrombosis (RVT) is uncommon, occurring mostly in association with malignancy, but it also is a consequence of nephrotic syndrome, abdominal surgery or trauma, pancreatitis, and genetic or acquired hypercoagulable states. Most malignancy-associated RVT is caused by renal cell carcinoma with venous invasion, often with spreading to the contralateral kidney, which may cause bilateral renal vein occlusion.

The nephrotic syndrome is associated with a risk for venous thrombosis throughout the circulation, including RVT. The RVT risk in patients with nephrotic syndrome correlates with severity of proteinuria and hypoalbuminemia; patients with a serum albumin concentration of less than 2 g/dL are at particular risk. Some studies have documented an incidence of RVT as high as 30% among patients with nephrotic syndrome, but most cases are not clinically apparent. Patients with membranous nephropathy seem to be at greatest risk for RVT for reasons that are not known, but RVT can also occur with focal segmental glomerular sclerosis, membranoproliferative glomerulonephritis, minimal change disease, and diabetic kidney disease. Hypercoagulability is thought to result from loss of the antithrombotic protein antithrombin III in urine, although other factors such as increased procoagulant factors and platelet activation may also be involved.

RVT may manifest with symptoms attributable to renal cell carcinoma, such as flank pain, gross hematuria, nausea, anorexia, or lower extremity swelling. In male patents, left renal vein occlusion may cause a left varicocele, a result of the venous drainage of the left gonadal vein. In patients without a malignancy, symptoms of RVT depend on the acuity of the thrombosis. Acute, complete thrombosis may manifest with hematuria, flank pain, abdominal distention, and acute renal failure. RVT in adults usually occurs gradually because of collateral venous drainage return; in this setting, symptoms of AKI are uncommon, although proteinuria and creatinine levels may be mildly elevated/

Because patients often do not have symptoms, RVT is likely more common than reported in the literature. Some have suggested CT screening of asymptomatic, high-risk patients, particularly those with membranous nephropathy and severe proteinuria and hypoalbuminemia.

The standard method for diagnosis is renal venography, but because it has a risk of clot dislodgment, bleeding, and iodinated contrast, less invasive methods are commonly used. Contrast-enhanced CT venography appears to have a relatively high sensitivity and specificity, although it carries some risk for contrast nephropathy. MRI using gadolinium-based contrast or time-of-flight sequencing without contrast may also be useful. Renal Doppler ultrasound is useful, but it is operator dependent and has lower sensitivity than CT venography.

Treatment with systemic anticoagulation is recommended in the absence of contraindications. Most clinicians maintain anticoagulation for 6 to 9 months, similar to the approach for non-renal deep vein thrombosis and pulmonary embolism. The long-term recurrence risk is low if the underlying predisposition is successfully treated, and patients are unlikely to require indefinite anticoagulation. Direct intravenous thrombolysis or operative thrombectomy may be considered in severe cases, particularly if the RVT is a source of pulmonary emboli or is causing AKI. Prophylactic anticoagulation in high-risk patients, such as those with severe membranous nephropathy (serum albumin concentration <2.5 g/dL) should be considered for appropriate candidates.

For a deeper discussion on this topic, please see Chapter 125, "Vascular Disorders of the Kidney," in Goldman-Cecil Medicine, 25th Edition.

SUGGESTED READINGS

Barbour T, Johnson S, Cohney S, et al: Thrombotic microangiopathy and associated renal disorders, Nephrol Dial Transplant 27:2673–2685, 2012.

Fattori R, Cao P, De Rango P, et al: Interdisciplinary expert consensus document, on management of type B aortic dissection, J Am Coll Cardiol 61:1661–1678, 2013.

Friedman DJ, Pollak MR: Genetics of kidney failure and the evolving story of APOL1, J Clin Invest 121:3367–3374, 2011.

Furuta S, Jayne DR: Antineutrophil cytoplasm antibody-associated vasculitis: recent developments, Kidney Int 84:244–249, 2013.

Krüger T, Conzelmann LO, Bonser RS, et al: Acute aortic dissection type A, Br J Surg 99:1331–1344, 2012.

Maynard SE, Thadhani R: Pregnancy and the kidney, J Am Soc Nephrol 20:14–22, 2009.

Noris M, Mescia F, Remuzzi G: STEC-HUS, atypical HUS and TTP are all diseases of complement activation, Nat Rev Nephrol 8:622–633, 2012.

Ruiz-Irastorza G, Crowther M, Branch W, et al: Antiphospholipid syndrome, Lancet 376:1498–1509, 2010.

Sadler JE: Von Willebrand factor, ADAMTS13, and thrombotic thrombocytopenic purpura, Blood 112:11–18, 2008.

Scolari F, Ravani P: Atheroembolic renal disease, Lancet 375:1650–1660, 2010.

Shanmugam VK, Steen VD: Renal disease in scleroderma: an update on evaluation, risk stratification, pathogenesis and management, Curr Opin Rheumatol 24:669–676, 2012.

Specks U, Merkel PA, Seo P, et al: Efficacy of remission-induction regimens for ANCA-associated vasculitis, N Engl J Med 369:417–427, 2013.

Textor SC, Misra S, Oderich GS: Percutaneous revascularization for ischemic nephropathy: the past, present, and future, Kidney Int 83:28–40, 2013.

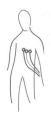

31

Acute Kidney Injury

Mark A. Perazella and Jeffrey M. Turner

DEFINITION

Acute kidney injury (AKI) is a syndrome defined as an abrupt decrease in glomerular filtration rate (GFR) sufficient to promote the retention of nitrogenous waste products (blood urea nitrogen [BUN] and creatinine); disturb the regulation of extracellular fluid volume, electrolyte balance, and acid-base homeostasis; and impair drug excretion. Importantly, even mild abnormalities in kidney structure and function are associated with other end-organ complications and increased mortality.

AKI includes a spectrum of clinical conditions. The numerous causes of AKI vary based on individual comorbidities (and risk for AKI) and whether kidney injury develops in the outpatient setting or in hospital. The incidence of AKI is rising, and its complications include progression to more severe kidney failure, need for renal replacement therapy (RRT), chronic kidney disease (CKD), and death. Several consensus groups have produced definitions and diagnostic criteria for AKI. Table 31-1 describes the diagnostic criteria for the Risk, Injury, Failure, Loss, and End-stage renal disease (ESRD) (RIFLE); Acute Kidney Injury Network (AKIN); and Kidney Disease: Improving Global Outcomes (KDIGO) classifications.

In 2004, the RIFLE classification was put forth to standardize the definition of AKI. Changes in serum creatinine concentration (over 7 days), reductions in estimated glomerular filtration rate (eGFR), and urine output parameters were used in this diagnostic system. The Risk (R), Injury (I), and Failure (F) categories were applicable to AKI, whereas the Loss (L) and ESRD (E) categories were CKD stages. In 2007, the AKIN group modified the RIFLE criteria definition of AKI by adding an absolute increase in serum creatinine of only 0.3 mg/dL, eliminating the eGFR criteria, and changing the time frame for AKI to develop (to 48 hours, compared with the 7 days for RIFLE diagnosis). Focusing on AKI, the AKIN criteria replaced the R, I, and F categories from the RIFLE criteria with stages 1, 2, and 3 and eliminated the L and E categories. In 2012, the KDIGO group combined parts of the RIFLE and AKIN criteria to capture AKI with increased sensitivity.

Understanding of the pathophysiology underlying development of AKI has advanced, and better diagnostic tools have moved the field forward. However, specific directed therapies remain limited for the most common forms of AKI. Although technical advances in RRT and supportive care have improved, patients commonly develop other end-organ disease in the setting of AKI. More concerning is the relatively high mortality rate associated with AKI, particularly when it develops in the hospital setting and requires RRT. E-Table 31-1 shows some of the clinically important outcomes associated with AKI.

ETIOLOGY

In most cases, more than one process contributes to AKI, but for ease of classification, three broad categories (Fig. 31-1) are used: (1) *prerenal AKI*, the result of a decrease in renal blood flow and perfusion of the kidney; (2) *intrinsic AKI*, the result of disease affecting one of the renal parenchymal compartments; and (3) *postrenal AKI*, the result of obstruction to urinary flow anywhere along the urinary tract starting from the renal calyces/pelves and involving the ureters, bladder, or urethra.

The most common form of AKI is due to prerenal physiology, particularly in the outpatient setting, but also in the hospital. Postrenal AKI is more common in elderly men with prostatic

TABLE 31-1 CLASSIFICATION OF ACUTE KIDNEY INJURY

STAGE	SERUM CREATININE INCREASE WITHIN 7 DAYS	URINE OUTPUT
KIDNEY DISEASE: IMPROVING GLOBAL OUTCOMES (KDIGO) CLASSIFICATION (2012)		
1	1.5-1.9 times baseline *or* ≥0.3 mg/dL within 48 hr	<0.5 mL/kg/hr × 6-12 hr
2	2-2.9 times baseline	<0.5 mL/kg/hr × ≥12 hr
3	3 times baseline *or* an increase in the serum creatinine to ≥4 mg/dL with an absolute increase ≥0.3 mg/dL within 48 hr or 1.5 times baseline within 7 days *or* initiation of RRT *or* in patients aged <18 yr, eGFR decreased to <35 mL/min/1.73 m²	<0.3 mL/kg/hr × ≥24 hr
ACUTE KIDNEY INJURY NETWORK (AKIN) CLASSIFICATION (2007)		
1	1.5-1.9 times baseline *or* ≥0.3 mg/dL within 48 hr	<0.5 mL/kg/hr × 6-12 hr
2	2-2.9 times baseline	<0.5 mL/kg/hr × ≥12 hr
3	3 times baseline *or* increase in serum creatinine ≥4 mg/dL with an increase ≥0.5 mg/dL *or* initiation of RRT	<0.3 mL/kg/hr × ≥24 hr *or* anuria ≥12 hr
RIFLE CLASSIFICATION (2004)		
Risk	1.5-1.9 times baseline *or* GFR decrease >25%	<0.5 mL/kg/hr × 6 hr
Injury	2-2.9 times baseline *or* GFR decrease >50%	<0.5 mL/kg/hr × 12 hr
Failure	3 times baseline *or* GFR decrease >75% *or* serum creatinine ≥4 mg/dL with an increase ≥0.5 mg/dL	<0.3 mL/kg/hr × 24 hr *or* anuria × 12 hr
Loss	Complete loss of renal function for >4 wk	
ESRD	End-stage renal disease >3 mo	

eGFR, Estimated glomerular filtration rate; GFR, glomerular filtration rate; RRT, renal replacement therapy.

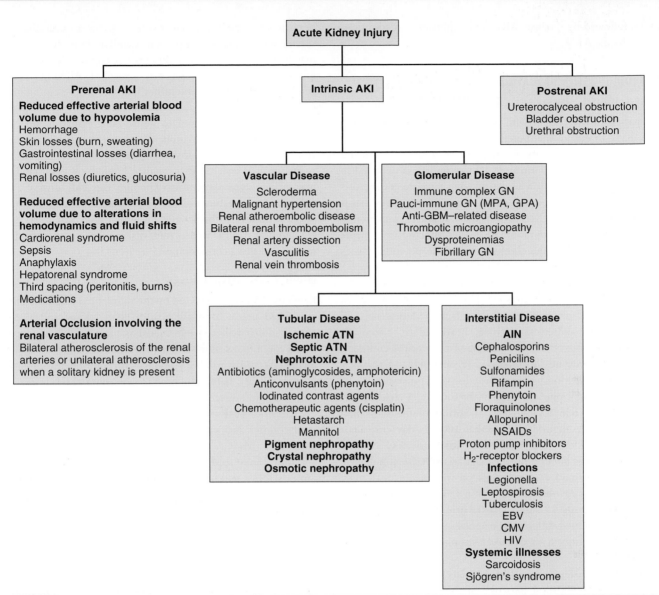

FIGURE 31-1 Common causes of acute kidney injury (AKI). AIN, Acute interstitial nephritis; ATN, acute tubular necrosis; CMV, cytomegalovirus; EBV, Epstein-Barr virus; GBM, glomerular basement membrane; GN, glomerulonephritis; GPA, granulomatosis with polyangiitis; H₂, histamine 2; HIV, human immunodeficiency virus; HUS, hemolytic uremic syndrome; MPA, microscopic polyangiitis; NSAIDs, nonsteroidal anti-inflammatory drugs; TTP; thrombotic thrombocytopenic purpura.

hyperplasia, patients with bladder dysfunction and certain malignancies. Intrinsic AKI may be due to a vascular process, glomerular disease, interstitial disease, or tubular injury. The most common intrinsic AKI is an entity known as *acute tubular necrosis* (ATN), or more recently *acute tubular injury* (ATI), which is histologically more accurate. This is a clinical syndrome characterized by an abrupt and sustained decline in GFR due to an acute ischemic injury, nephrotoxic insult, or a combination of both. The clinical recognition of ATN is based primarily on exclusion of prerenal and postrenal causes of AKI, as well as other causes of intrinsic AKI (glomerulonephritis [GN], acute interstitial nephritis [AIN], and vasculitis). Once other intrinsic causes of AKI are excluded, it is reasonable to conclude ATN is the cause or major contributor to AKI. Although the name *acute tubular necrosis* is not an entirely valid histologic description of the lesion,

the term will be utilized as it is part of the language of clinical medicine.

EPIDEMIOLOGY

AKI occurs more commonly in hospitalized patients as compared to the community setting. Community-acquired AKI defined by various step-wise increases in serum creatinine has an incidence of approximately 1%. Nearly half of the patients involve AKI superimposed on CKD. Prerenal AKI accounts for ~70% of cases, obstructive uropathy ~17%, and intrinsic AKI from various etiologies ~11% of the AKI cases. In contrast, hospital-acquired AKI has an incidence ranging from 4.9% to 7.2%. The incidence of AKI is higher in intensive care unit (ICU) admissions approximating 30%. CKD; older age and other co-morbidities are important risk factors for AKI. Prerenal AKI remains the most common cause, followed by intrinsic AKI from nephrotoxic medications and ischemic ATN.

DIAGNOSTIC EVALUATION

History and Physical Examination

Evaluation of the patient with AKI should be methodical and systematic to ensure that potentially reversible causes are diagnosed and treated expeditiously to preserve kidney function and limit development of permanent kidney injury, as depicted in Table 31-2. Part of the difficulty in arriving at a correct diagnosis is that several potential causes of AKI often coexist. Emphasis is placed on thorough analysis of available data and examination of the sequence of deterioration in kidney function and urine volume in relation to the chronologies of the potential causes of AKI.

Knowledge of the natural history of the various causes of AKI also is critical. The evaluation should include a thorough patient history and chart review to identify risk factors for prerenal AKI (e.g., vomiting, diuretics, diarrhea, heart failure, cirrhosis); potential nephrotoxic drugs (prescribed or over-the-counter); risk factors for prostate disease, cervical cancer, or bladder cancer; and symptoms of urinary tract obstruction (e.g., prostatism, overflow incontinence, anuria). Some of the important chart review data are presented in E-Table 31-2 . The urine volume is less than 400 mL/day with oliguric AKI, less than 100 mL/day with oligo-anuric AKI, and less than 50 mL/day with anuric AKI. Normal urine output does not exclude the diagnosis of AKI: Nonoliguric AKI (>400 mL/day) can be associated with nephrotoxic AKI and partial urinary obstruction. Wide variation in daily urine output also suggests AKI due to partial urinary tract obstruction. Anuria has a limited differential diagnosis, suggesting complete urinary obstruction, a vascular catastrophe, or severe cortical necrosis.

The physical examination should focus on volume status to allow initial classification into one of the broad categories of AKI. Reduced body weight, hypotension, an orthostatic fall in blood pressure (BP), or flat neck veins may be present in patients with prerenal AKI (ischemic AKI) caused by true volume depletion. The presence of edema, pulmonary rales, or an S_3 gallop signals effective volume depletion due to cardiac dysfunction, whereas edema, ascites, and asterixis suggest liver dysfunction

or cirrhosis. If the intravascular volume status is uncertain, measurement of cardiac filling pressures with an indwelling catheter may be useful, but this technique is not commonly used. More often, central venous pressure is measured. Although central venous pressure measurement has limitations, even in monitoring of trends and response to fluid administration or removal, it remains an important tool to guide fluid management. New, noninvasive monitoring tools that more accurately measure volume status are under investigation.

Evidence of systemic disease also should be sought. Findings may include signs of pulmonary hemorrhage indicative of a vasculitis or Goodpasture's disease, skin rash as a manifestation of systemic lupus erythematosus, atheroemboli, vasculitis, cryoglobulins, or AIN, as well as joint disease making lupus or rheumatoid arthritis a consideration.

Basic Laboratory Tests

Laboratory tests are directed by the differential diagnosis that is postulated after a complete history, chart review, and physical examination have been performed. Basic tests include a complete blood count to assess for anemia (microangiopathic or immune-mediated) and thrombocytopenia (thrombotic thrombocytic purpura [TTP], hemolytic-uremic syndrome [HUS], and disseminated intravascular coagulation [DIC]). Other tests to evaluate the cause of AKI include various serologic measurements (antinuclear antibody [ANA], antineutrophil cytoplasmic antibodies [ANCA], anti–glomerular basement membrane antibody [anti-GBM], anti–double-stranded DNA antibodies [anti-dsDNA], and hepatitis B and C viral serologies), complement levels, cryoglobulin levels, blood cultures, serum lactate dehydrogenase (LDH) and haptoglobin measurements, serum and urine immunoelectrophoresis, and serum free light chain assay.

Urinalysis and Urine Microscopy

Urinalysis is a key component of the diagnostic evaluation of AKI, as summarized in Table 31-3. It is important to evaluate urine specific gravity (SG), as well as the presence of blood (or heme), protein, or leukocyte esterase.

A very high urine SG typically suggests prerenal AKI, whereas isosthenuria (SG = 1.010) indicates intrinsic AKI (e.g., ATN). A thorough microscopic examination of the spun urine sediment, with quantification of the urinary elements, adds essential information to the case. Bland urine with no blood or protein and few to no cells or casts favors a diagnosis of prerenal AKI. Vascular causes of AKI have a variable urine tonicity and sometimes hematuria (isomorphic or dysmorphic red blood cells [RBCs]) and granular casts. GN exhibits variable urine tonicity, positive blood and protein on the dipstick, RBCs, and RBC casts. ATN shows isotonic urine with variable protein and variable heme on urine dipstick (heme is positive with rhabdomyolysis and hemolysis), Renal tubular epithelial cells (RTECs), RTEC casts, and fine or coarse pigmented granular casts (sometime muddy brown E-Fig. 31-1) may be present on the sediment examination.

Urine in patients with postrenal AKI is typically isotonic and bland unless there is associated infection (pyuria), nephrolithiasis (hematuria), or concomitant ATN (RTECs, RTEC casts, granular casts).

TABLE 31-2	DIAGNOSTIC APPROACH TO THE PATIENT WITH ACUTE KIDNEY INJURY

1. Record review (see E-Table 31-2); special attention to evidence of recent reduction in glomerular filtration rate and sequence of events leading to deterioration of kidney function to determine possible causative factors
2. Physical examination, including evaluation of hemodynamic status
3. Urinalysis and urine microscopy with thorough sediment examination
4. Determination of urinary indices, including fractional excretion of sodium and urine output
5. Catheterization and measurement of postvoid residual urine volume if outlet obstruction is suspected
6. Fluid challenge in cases of suspected prerenal AKI
7. Radiologic studies, particular as dictated by the clinical setting (e.g., ultrasonography to look for obstruction)
8. Kidney biopsy

AKI, Acute kidney injury.

TABLE 31-3 URINALYSIS AND MICROSCOPIC EXAMINATION OF THE URINE SEDIMENT

TEST	PRERENAL	VASCULITIS	GN	ATN	AIN	POSTRENAL
Specific gravity	High	Normal/high	Normal/high	Isosmotic	Isosmotic	Isosmotic
Dipstick blood	Negative	Positive	Positive	±	±	Negative
Dipstick protein	Negative	Positive	Positive	Negative	±	Negative
Urine sediment examination	Negative, hyaline casts	RBC casts, dysmorphic RBCs	RBC casts, dysmorphic RBCs	Granular casts, RTECs	WBC casts, eosinophils	Negative, sometimes WBCs/RBCs

AIN, Acute interstitial nephritis; ATN, acute tubular necrosis; GN, glomerulonephritis; RBCs, red blood cells; RTECs, renal tubular epithelial cells; WBCs, white blood cells.

With certain processes, crystals may be indicative of the underlying cause of AKI. For example, calcium oxalate crystals may suggest enteric hyperoxaluria or ethylene glycol intoxication, uric acid crystals may point to acute urate nephropathy, and various other crystals may indicate a drug-induced form of AKI.

Urinary Indices

Spot urine chemistry testing (sodium, creatinine, and urea), along with plasma samples (sodium, creatinine, and BUN), has been used to evaluate renal tubular function in the setting of AKI, primarily to distinguish prerenal AKI from ATN. These measures allow the clinician to calculate fractional excretion of sodium (FE_{Na}) and fractional excretion of urea (FE_{Urea}); they are thought to be more accurate indicators than urine sodium concentration, which is less than 10 to 20 mEq/L with prerenal AKI and greater than 20 mEq/L with ATN.

The ratio of the clearance of sodium (Na) to that of creatinine (Cr) is calculated as a percentage:

$$FE_{Na} = (U_{Na}/P_{Na}) \times (P_{Cr}/U_{Cr}) \times 100$$

where U and P are the concentrations in urine and plasma, respectively. Likewise, the ratio of urea clearance to creatinine clearance is

$$FE_{Urea} = (U_{Urea}/P_{Urea}) \times (P_{Cr}/U_{Cr}) \times 100$$

The rationale for the use of these indices is that the ratio of urine to plasma creatinine concentrations (U_{Cr}/P_{Cr}) provides an index of the fraction of filtered water excreted. Assuming that all of the creatinine filtered at the glomerulus is excreted into the urine, any increment in the concentration of creatinine in urine over that in plasma must result from the removal of water.

In prerenal AKI, because the increased stimulus for salt and water retention, U_{Cr}/P_{Cr} typically is considerably greater than it is in ATN; moreover, FE_{Na} is <1%, and urine sodium concentrations are characteristically low. In contrast, in AKI due to ATN, the nephrons excrete a large fraction of their filtered sodium and water, resulting in a lower U_{Cr}/P_{Cr}, higher urine sodium concentrations, and a higher Fe_{Na} (E-Table 31-3). An important clinical exception to this finding is that FE_{Na} can be high (>1 to 2%) with prerenal AKI in the setting of diuretic therapy. To counter this effect, calculation of FE_{Urea} has been used: An FE_{Urea} greater than 35% favors a diagnosis of prerenal AKI, and an FE_{Urea} greater than 50% favors ATN.

Interpretations of these tests, therefore, must be made in conjunction with other assessments of the patient, because clinically important exceptions to these generalizations exist. As an example, prerenal AKI can manifest with an elevated FE_{Na} or FE_{Urea} in the setting of glycosuria, metabolic alkalosis, bicarbonaturia, salt-wasting disorders, or CKD. Similarly, ATN with low FE_{Na} and FE_{Urea} occurs with pigmenturia, sepsis, radiocontrast injury, severe heart or liver failure, and nonoliguric ATN.

Renal Imaging

If either prerenal AKI or ATN is the likely cause of AKI, and if the clinical setting does not require the exclusion of another cause, then no further diagnostic evaluation is required. Further assessment may be necessary if the diagnosis is uncertain, especially if the clinical setting suggests other possibilities (e.g., obstruction, vascular accident); if clinical findings make the diagnosis of prerenal AKI or ATN unlikely; or if oliguria persists without a good reason. When indicated, diagnostic renal imaging is important in the evaluation of AKI. Retroperitoneal ultrasonography of the kidneys, ureters, and bladder is the first test used because it is readily available, noninvasive, free of radiation exposure, and fairly accurate.

Ultrasonography provides information about kidney size (large, normal, or small) and the parenchyma (normal or increased echogenicity), the status of the pelvis and urinary collecting system (normal or hydronephrotic), and the presence of structural abnormalities (e.g., stones, masses, enlarged lymph nodes). In the setting of AKI, this test can rapidly confirm or exclude the presence of hydronephrosis (E-Fig. 31-2) and a diagnosis of obstructive uropathy. Interrogation of the renal arteries by Doppler ultrasonography provides important information about renal blood flow and renal artery stenosis; however, this test is highly operator dependent.

Computed tomography (CT) of the retroperitoneum provides important information about the cause of postrenal AKI (e.g., tumor, stones, retroperitoneal fibrosis) when ultrasound findings are negative or inconclusive. CT angiography can also accurately diagnose renal artery disease and renal infarction, but there is a risk of nephrotoxicity in those patients with underlying acute or chronic kidney disease. Magnetic resonance (MR) imaging does not add much to CT scanning except in the diagnosis of retroperitoneal fibrosis. Gadolinium MR angiography can safely provide important information about renal artery stenosis or thrombosis, but it should be avoided in patients with AKI or stage 4 or greater CKD. Nephrogenic systemic fibrosis can develop in these patients, especially with nonionic or linear gadolinium contrast agents and in the setting of inflammation.

Radionuclide tests are used to assess the presence or absence of renal blood flow, differences in flow to the two kidneys, and excretory (secretory) function. However, these studies have limited utility in AKI and have reduced accuracy in quantitating absolute rates of flow.

Kidney Biopsy

When prerenal AKI, ATN, and obstructive uropathy are unlikely, percutaneous kidney biopsy is sometimes required to determine the cause of AKI and to direct appropriate therapy. Reasonable criteria to support use of kidney biopsy include absence of an obvious cause of AKI such as hypotension or nephrotoxin exposure and prolonged oliguria, usually for more than 2 to 3 weeks. Other potential indications include evaluation for myeloma-related kidney disease in an elderly patient with unexplained AKI; extrarenal manifestations of systemic diseases such as systemic lupus erythematosus, rheumatoid arthritis, or vasculitis; and determination of whether AIN is present in patients receiving a potential culprit drug.

Kidney tissue should be thoroughly examined with the use of light microscopy, immunofluorescence staining, and electron microscopy to facilitate an accurate diagnosis. This ensures a diagnosis of the cause of AKI in most patients. However, kidney biopsy should be employed judiciously to avoid complications such as traumatic renal arteriovenous malformation, severe bleeding requiring transfusion or embolization, other organ injury (liver, spleen, bowel), and nephrectomy for intractable bleeding.

Future Tests for AKI

The limitations of currently available tests to estimate GFR and kidney injury have led to proteomics-based studies to identify novel biomarkers of AKI. The hope is that novel biomarkers will improve the diagnosis and prognosis of AKI. For example, early AKI diagnosis would permit implementation of appropriate preventive strategies and treatment regimens to abrogate permanent loss of kidney function. In patients who develop AKI, biomarker concentrations demonstrate changes earlier than serum creatinine concentrations and appear to distinguish between prerenal AKI, ATN, and other glomerular disorders, which may allow directed interventions and avoidance of potentially harmful therapies. One such example is aggressive intravenous fluid therapy in patients with ATN, which risks volume overload and other end-organ consequences. Finally, biomarkers may allow clinicians to better predict outcomes such as worsening kidney function, RRT requirement, and mortality in patients with hospital-acquired AKI.

● CLINICAL PRESENTATION, DIFFERENTIAL DIAGNOSIS, AND MANAGEMENT OF AKI

Prerenal AKI

Prerenal AKI is primarily the result of inadequate blood flow to the kidneys. Renal blood flow approximates more than 1 L/minute, which is necessary to maintain GFR, preserve oxygen delivery, and sustain ion transport and other energy-requiring processes. Therefore, normal kidney function depends on adequate perfusion; a significant reduction in renal perfusion diminishes filtration pressure and lowers GFR.

Volume Depletion

Both "true" and "effective" hypovolemia activate several neurohormonal vasoconstrictor systems as mechanisms to protect circulatory stability. The substances released include catecholamines from the sympathetic nervous system, endothelin from the vasculature, angiotensin II from the renin-angiotensin system (RAS), and vasopressin. They raise BP through arterial and venous constriction but also can constrict afferent arterioles and reduce GFR, especially when systemic BP is inadequate to maintain renal perfusion pressure.

Structural lesions in the renal arterial and arteriolar tree can also reduce perfusion and promote prerenal AKI. Kidney adaptive responses are stimulated to counterbalance diminished renal perfusion in these circumstances. These adaptive processes include the myogenic reflex, which is activated by low distending pressures sensed in the renal baroreceptors and causes afferent arteriolar vasodilatation. Prostaglandins (e.g., PGE_2, PGI_2), nitric oxide, and products from the kallikrein-kinin system modify the effects of these vasoconstrictors on the afferent arteriole. Importantly, disturbance of the balance between afferent vasodilatation and efferent vasoconstriction can disrupt intrarenal hemodynamics and precipitate AKI.

Medications

The balance of vasoconstricting and vasodilating processes may be altered by medications such as nonsteroidal anti-inflammatory drugs (NSAIDs) and selective cyclooxygenase 2 (COX2) inhibitors. These drugs act to cause prerenal AKI through inhibition of vasodilatory prostaglandins in patients who require prostaglandin effects to maintain renal perfusion. Despite its vasoconstrictor properties, angiotensin II acutely preserves glomerular filtration pressure and GFR in states of reduced renal perfusion by constricting the efferent arteriole more than the afferent arteriole. This salutary effect in part explains the GFR reduction that occurs when a patient who is dependent on angiotensin II to constrict the efferent arteriole is treated with an ACE inhibitor or an angiotensin II receptor blocker (ARB).

Cardiorenal Syndrome

The cardiorenal syndrome (CRS) is an umbrella term that encompasses a number of coexistent cardiac or kidney derangements. Although there are five subtypes of CRS, hospital-acquired AKI due to CRS is most often of the type 1 variety. Reduced cardiac output, arterial underfilling, elevated atrial pressures, and venous congestion, independently or in combination, can impair the renal circulation and reduce GFR, thereby causing a form of prerenal AKI. These processes stimulate neurohumoral adaptations such as activation of the sympathetic nervous system and RAS and increases in vasopressin and endothelin-1, in an attempt to preserve perfusion to vital organs. However, these adaptations enhance salt and water retention and systemic vasoconstriction, which ultimately promote or exacerbate prerenal AKI by two mechanisms: (1) They increase cardiac afterload and further reduce cardiac output and renal perfusion, and (2) they increase central venous pressure, renal venous pressure, and/or intra-abdominal pressure, ultimately lowering GFR.

AKI in patients with heart failure is often caused by CRS type 1, but certainly these patients can also suffer true prerenal AKI from overzealous diuresis or from ischemic or nephrotoxic ATN. Prerenal AKI from true volume depletion is responsive to judicious administration of intravenous fluids and diuretic withdrawal, making it easy to recognize. It is sometimes more difficult to distinguish CRS type 1 from ATN, because the processes often coexist.

Identification of AKI in the setting of heart failure is clinically relevant because reduced GFR is generally associated with a worse prognosis. Therapy is directed at improving cardiac function, especially in patients with low cardiac output, and relieving pulmonary and renal congestion. Loop diuretics are part of the central treatment strategy for relieving venous congestion; however, these agents can directly stimulate maladaptive neurohormonal responses, transiently worsening kidney function after their introduction. Patients with congestive heart failure often have some degree of diuretic resistance. Strategies to overcome this resistance include combination therapy with thiazide diuretics and sometimes device-driven ultrafiltration. With advanced AKI, RRT is required to treat uremia, metabolic complications, and volume overload. Therapies for end-stage cardiac failure include cardiac transplantation and placement of a left ventricular assist device for long-term destination therapy or as a bridge to transplantation.

Hepatorenal Syndrome

A strong physiologic interplay also occurs between liver disease and kidney impairment. Patients with advanced, decompensated cirrhosis or fulminant acute hepatic failure develop a unique form of prerenal AKI called hepatorenal syndrome (HRS). The International Ascites Club diagnostic criteria for HRS include (1) the presence of cirrhosis and ascites, (2) serum creatinine levels higher than 1.5 mg/dL, (3) no improvement in kidney function after at least 48 hours of diuretic withdrawal and volume expansion with albumin, (4) absence of shock, (5) no nephrotoxic drug exposure, and (6) absence of parenchymal kidney disease. There are two subtypes of HRS based on rapidity and severity of kidney impairment. Type 1 HRS is characterized by rapidly progressive renal failure, defined by doubling of the initial serum creatinine concentration (to >2.5 mg/dL in <2 weeks). Type 2 HRS is characterized by moderate kidney failure (serum creatinine increase from 1.5 to 2.5 mg/dL). The hallmark of HRS is profound renal vasoconstriction in the setting of systemic and splanchnic arterial vasodilatation. The hemodynamic changes that occur in HRS are summarized in E-Figure 31-3.

There is no test that is specific for the diagnosis of HRS, and diagnosis requires exclusion of other causes of AKI. The main differential diagnoses of type 1 HRS are prerenal AKI and ATN, which have an acute onset with progressive deterioration of kidney function. Recognition of prerenal AKI is typically easier, because it responds to intravenous fluids (albumin and saline), whereas HRS type 1 and ATN are more difficult to differentiate. Distinguishing ATN from HRS is crucial, because therapies for these two forms of AKI are very different, as are their prognoses and outcomes. For HRS, midodrine and octreotide, vasopressin (or its analogue terlipressin outside of the United States), or norepinephrine is used, whereas ATN requires primarily supportive therapy with initiation of RRT if necessary. Liver (or combined liver-kidney) transplantation is the definitive therapy for HRS.

Intrinsic AKI

Intrinsic AKI reflects kidney injury that arises from a process that damages one of the compartments of the renal parenchyma. To simplify the approach, kidney disease is organized into anatomic sites of injury in the vasculature, glomerulus, tubules, and interstitium.

Vascular Disease

Intrinsic AKI may result from vascular disease in large or medium-sized arteries, small arteries, and arterioles within the renal parenchyma and veins draining the kidneys. Bilateral renal artery thrombosis superimposed on underlying high-grade stenoses, significant cardiac or aortic thromboembolism occluding the renal arteries, or dissection of the renal arteries may cause AKI. With acute presentations, the clinical features often include flank or abdominal pain, fever, hematuria, and oligo-anuria or anuria. Therapy with thrombolytics may reverse acute thrombosis and thromboembolism and restore renal blood flow with early diagnosis. Percutaneous angioplasty with stent placement can noninvasively correct significant underlying renal artery stenosis. Renal artery dissection often requires surgical repair, but at times stent placement may suffice. Vasculitis of large renal vessels (e.g., Takayasu's arteritis, giant cell arteritis) is an extremely rare cause of AKI.

Induction of AKI by renal atheroemboli occurs less commonly than before, perhaps because of improved techniques and use of softer wires during vascular procedures. Cholesterol crystal embolization is caused most often by invasive vascular procedures in patients with atherosclerotic disease that disrupt the fibrous cap on the ulcerated plaque. However, thrombolytic therapy and therapeutic anticoagulation can also precipitate embolization in patients who have a significant burden of renal artery or aortic plaque. When it occurs, atheromatous material may lodge in interlobar, arcuate, or interlobular arteries in the kidneys. In addition to AKI, clinical manifestations include abrupt onset of severe hypertension, livedo reticularis, digital or limb ischemia, abdominal pain from pancreatitis or bowel ischemia, gastrointestinal bleeding, muscle pain, central nervous system symptoms such as focal neurologic deficits, confusion, amaurosis fugax, and retinal ischemic symptoms. Peripheral eosinophilia, hypocomplementemia, elevated sedimentation rate, and eosinophiluria variably accompany the syndrome. Treatment is primarily preventive by avoiding the factors known to precipitate atheroembolization. BP control, treatment with statins, amputation of necrotic limbs, aggressive nutrition, avoidance of anticoagulation (to reduce the risk for further embolization), and RRT for severe AKI may improve the dismal prognosis associated with this syndrome. Steroids and iloprost are sometimes used, but their therapeutic role is uncertain.

AKI from vasculitis involving the medium and small vessels has been described with classic polyarteritis nodosa. It is either idiopathic or secondary to hepatitis B antigenemia and manifests with severe hypertension and AKI. Renal arteriography demonstrating beading in the arterial tree of the kidney (and other organs) is diagnostic. Scleroderma is a disorder characterized by arterial and arteriolar narrowing due to deposition of mucinous material. Scleroderma renal crisis manifests as AKI and severe hypertension, often malignant, in a patient with a disease flare. Urinalysis and urine microscopy may be bland or may show cellular activity. Fibrinoid necrosis with ischemic injury occurs in the kidney. ACE inhibitors effectively control BP and improve AKI.

Rarely, AKI may develop in the setting of renal vein thrombosis, a well-known complication of nephrotic syndrome. Imbalance of anticoagulant substances lost in the urine and procoagulant substances produced by the liver leads to a hypercoagulable state and renal vein thrombosis. AKI is thought to develop from raised intrarenal pressures and reduced kidney perfusion. Therapy includes acute thrombolysis and chronic anticoagulation as well as treatment of the underlying glomerular lesion (often membranous nephropathy) and reduction in proteinuria.

Glomerular Disease

A number of glomerular diseases can cause AKI, and the more common entities are reviewed here. Acute proliferative GN may be broadly classified as (1) immune complex disease, (2) pauci-immune disease, or (3) anti-GBM–related disease. They are all characterized by glomerular cell proliferation and necrosis, polymorphonuclear cell infiltration, and, with severe injury, epithelial crescent formation (E-Fig. 31-4). Acute proliferative GN manifests with hypertension and edema formation and with laboratory results pertinent for hematuria and proteinuria, described as *nephritic sediment*. Examination of the urine sediment classically reveals dysmorphic RBCs and RBC casts. Therapy is directed at the underlying cause, with supportive measures and RRT as necessary.

TTP and HUS are two of the more common causes of thrombotic microangiopathy, which is marked by platelet deposition and endothelial injury with thrombosis of arterioles and glomerular capillaries. AKI results from severe glomerular damage with profound ischemia and necrosis. The thrombotic microangiopathies may manifest with nephritic sediment. Patients with HUS may have severe AKI, or it may be mild, as in patients with TTP. Microangiopathic hemolytic anemia and thrombocytopenia are key features. Therapy often includes modulation of the immune system with plasma exchange or eculizumab, in addition to supportive measures.

The dysproteinemias, which deposit monoclonal immunoglobulin light or heavy chains (or both) in the kidney, may also promote glomerular lesions. The type, metabolism, and packaging of the immunoglobulin determine which type of glomerular lesion develops: light or heavy chain deposition disease, amyloidosis, or one of the fibrillary GNs. The immunoglobulin deposition diseases often manifest with nephrotic proteinuria and AKI, rarely with hematuria.

Light chain deposition disease, heavy chain deposition disease, and light/heavy chain deposition disease cause nodular glomerular lesions. Amyloidosis is also associated with the formation of acellular glomerular nodules. The fibrillary GNs (fibrillary and immunotactoid) may be associated with mesangial expansion or glomerular nodules. More commonly, they appear as a mesangial proliferative, mesangiocapillary, or membranous lesion, sometimes with formation of epithelial crescents. These diseases can be distinguished by electron microscopy. Light and heavy chain diseases produce granular deposits, whereas amyloidosis appears as haphazard fibrils in the 8- to 12-nm size range. Fibrillary GN has fibrils in 20- to 30-nm range, and immunotactoid GN shows fibrils in the 30- to 50-nm range with organized microtubular fibrils.

Tubular Disease

Acute Tubular Necrosis

ATN is the most common form of hospital-acquired intrinsic AKI, accounting for more than 80% of AKI episodes. It is classically divided into ischemic ATN, which makes up almost 50% of the cases, nephrotoxic ATN, and combinations of both. In many instances, ATN results from multiple insults acting together to injure the kidney. The end result of either ischemic or toxic insult is tubular cell injury and death. E-Table 31-4 outlines the important factors underlying the pathogenesis of ATN.

Ischemic ATN

Ischemic ATN is, for the most part, an extension of severe and uncorrected prerenal AKI. Prolonged renal hypoperfusion causes tubular cell injury, which persists even after the underlying hemodynamic insult resolves and may be associated with ischemia-reperfusion injury. Intraoperative and postoperative hypotension impairs renal perfusion and occurs relatively frequently after cardiac and vascular surgical procedures. Ischemic, nephrotoxic, and multifactorial ATN are common on the medical wards and in the ICU. Risk for ischemic ATN is increased by the comorbidities these patients possess. Sepsis and septic shock, severe intravascular volume depletion, cirrhotic physiology, and cardiogenic shock are examples of situations that confer high risk for development of ischemic ATN. Employment of vasopressors to restore BP may further reduce renal perfusion and exacerbate ischemia. In some cases, ischemic ATN is so profound that cortical necrosis (ischemic atrophy of the renal cortex) develops.

Nephrotoxic ATN

Nephrotoxic ATN occurs when exogenous substances injure the tubules, primarily through direct toxic effects but also through perturbations in intrarenal hemodynamics or a combination of these factors. In the past, organic solvents and heavy metals (e.g., mercury, cadmium, lead) were a frequent cause of ATN. Since then, many potentially toxic medications have been synthesized and observed to cause tubular injury by multiple mechanisms.

Aminoglycosides cause proximal tubular injury. AKI rarely develops within the first week of therapy, and injury initially manifests with subtle changes in urine concentrating ability and increased RTECs and granular casts in the urine sediment. The antifungal agent amphotericin B induces AKI through two distinct mechanisms: destruction of cellular membranes through sterol interactions and vasoconstriction-induced tubular ischemia. ATN develops in a dose-dependent fashion and manifests with increasing serum creatinine levels and RTECs and granular casts in the urine. Liposomal and lipid complex formulations are less nephrotoxic but can precipitate AKI in high-risk patients.

Radiocontrast material is a common cause of AKI because it is so widely used with imaging procedures. AKI develops in patients with underlying risk factors such as CKD, especially diabetic nephropathy, "true" or "effective" intravascular volume depletion, advanced age, and exposure to other nephrotoxins. The incidence of AKI may be 25% and approaches 50% in patients with underlying risk factors. ATN occurs from both ischemic tubular injury (prolonged decrease in renal blood flow) and direct toxicity (osmotic cellular injury, oxidative stress, inflammation). Large radiocontrast volumes increase risk, whereas low-osmolar and iso-osmolar radiocontrast agents are less nephrotoxic than high-osmolar material.

The antiviral agents cidofovir and tenofovir, once they have entered the cell from the peritubular blood via the human organic anion transporter 1 on the basolateral membrane, cause AKI through disruption of mitochondrial and other cellular functions. Several chemotherapeutic agents, including the platinum-based drugs, ifosfamide, mithramycin, imatinib, pentostatin, and pemetrexed, cause ATN through direct toxic effects. As with other nephrotoxins, part of their ability to induce ATN resides in the renal handling by the kidneys (transport through tubular cells) as they are being excreted. In addition, zoledronate, the polymixins, high-dose vancomycin, foscarnet, and deferasirox also cause nephrotoxic ATN. AKI prevention is best achieved by judicious prescription of these drugs to high-risk patients, appropriate dose adjustments, avoidance of superimposed volume depletion, and close monitoring with early markers of injury such as urine microscopy.

Pigment Nephropathy

Pigment nephropathy represents the nephrotoxic renal tubular effects of endogenously produced substances. The most common examples are overproduction of heme moieties in serum that are eventually filtered at the glomerulus and excreted in urine. With severe rhabdomyolysis, the heme pigment released from muscle is myoglobin. AKI develops in the setting of myoglobinuria from the combination of direct myoglobin tubular toxicity (in an acid urine), volume depletion, and obstructing myoglobin casts. Therapy includes intravenous fluids (the addition of bicarbonate is questionable), supportive care, and sometimes RRT. Most patients recover kidney function to near-baseline.

Massive intravascular hemolysis from various causes (e.g., immune-mediated, microangiopathic) is associated with hemoglobinuria, which induces tubular injury by promoting the formation of reactive oxygen species and by reducing renal perfusion through inhibition of nitric oxide synthesis. Therapy is directed at the primary cause, with intravenous fluids and supportive care. Most patients ultimately recover kidney function.

Crystal Nephropathy

AKI may result from crystal deposition in distal tubular lumens after massive rises in uric acid or therapy with certain medications. Risk factors for AKI due to crystal deposition are underlying kidney disease and intravascular volume depletion. Acute uric acid nephropathy from urate crystal deposition and tubular obstruction develops in patients with massive tumor lysis syndrome.

Drugs such as sulfadiazine promote intratubular deposition of sulfa crystals in acid urine, whereas acyclovir crystal deposition occurs after large, rapid intravenous doses of the drug, and atazanavir and indinavir crystal deposition occurs in the setting of volume contraction and urine pH higher than 5.5. Ciprofloxacin

can cause AKI due to intratubular crystal deposition when administered in excessive doses, primarily in patients with unrecognized kidney disease and those with alkaline urine. In addition, methotrexate or large doses of intravenous vitamin C (producing oxalate) can cause AKI due to intratubular crystal deposition.

Weight loss therapies such as bariatric surgery with small bowel bypass and orlistat, through induction of malabsorption, cause enteric hyperoxaluria and calcium oxalate crystal deposition, an entity known as acute oxalate nephropathy (E-Fig. 31-5). Sodium phosphate–containing bowel purgatives have also been associated with AKI due to acute phosphate nephropathy, an entity characterized by calcium phosphate intratubular crystal deposition.

Diagnosis of crystal nephropathy is based on a history of exposure to a culprit agent or an underlying disease state associated with excessive crystal production.

Osmotic Nephropathy

Osmotic nephropathy is a little known entity that can promote AKI through the induction of proximal tubular swelling, cell injury, and occlusion of intratubular lumens. The hyperosmolar and unmetabolizable nature of substances such as sucrose, dextran, mannitol, the sucrose excipient of intravenous immune globulin, and hydroxyethylstarch underlies the pathophysiology of this kidney lesion. Cells develop severe swelling with cytoplasmic vacuoles, disturbing cellular integrity and occluding tubular lumens. AKI results from this abnormal tubular process when patients with underlying kidney disease or other risk factors for kidney injury (e.g., intravascular volume depletion, older age) receive these hyperosmolar substances. AKI is dose related and may require RRT. Although most patients recover from AKI, CKD can result. Therapy is primarily supportive, along with avoidance of further exposure to these agents.

Interstitial Disease

Interstitial disease develops in the setting of infection with certain agents, systemic diseases, infiltrative malignancies, and exposure to some medications. Of these, drug-induced disease is by far the most common entity, especially in the hospitalized patient. The syndrome of AIN is characterized by AKI and a variety of clinical findings. The clinical presentation varies based on the offending agent and the host response. As an example, β-lactam antibiotics frequently cause the classic triad of fever, maculopapular skin rash, and eosinophilia. Arthralgias, myalgias, and flank pain may also occur. Aside from causing AKI, NSAIDs can rarely lead to allergic or extrarenal manifestations such as fever, rash, or eosinophilia.

Urinalysis may reveal dipstick-positive (trace to 1+) protein, blood, and leukocyte esterase. Urine microscopy may be bland (~20%), but more often, the urine sediment demonstrates white blood cells (WBCs), RBCs, WBC casts, and granular casts. Wright or Hansel stain may reveal eosinophils in the urine, but neither of these tests is sensitive or specific for AIN.

The diagnosis is best confirmed by kidney biopsy. A cellular infiltrate consisting of lymphocytes, monocytes, eosinophils, and plasma cells is typically present; interstitial edema and fibrosis vary based on the time of drug exposure (E-Fig. 31-6). Tubulitis, or invasion of lymphocytes into the tubular cells, is frequently part of AIN. Granuloma formation and interstitial inflammation occur with certain drugs such as anticonvulsants and sulfonamides, systemic diseases such as sarcoidosis, tubulointerstitial nephritis with uveitis, and idiopathic granulomatous interstitial nephritis. The glomeruli and vasculature are spared until very late in the disease. If kidney biopsy is not possible, gallium scanning or positron emission tomography of the kidneys may help with diagnosis, especially when the differential diagnosis is primarily between AIN and ATN.

Early diagnosis of AIN, coupled with rapid drug withdrawal before advanced tubulointerstitial fibrosis develops, maximizes successful renal recovery. Steroid therapy is controversial but may reduce the duration of AKI and perhaps improve recovery of kidney function in patients with severe AKI if it is used early (within 2 weeks of diagnosis).

Before development of antibiotics and other drugs that have been associated with AIN, interstitial infection was the major cause of tubulointerstitial nephritis. Microbial agents such as staphylococci, streptococci, mycoplasma, diptheroids, and legionella are well-described causes of AIN. Several viral agents including cytomegalovirus, Epstein-Barr virus, human immunodeficiency virus (HIV), Hantaan virus, parvovirus, and rubeola also are associated with AIN. In addition, infectious agents that cause rickettsial diseases, leptospirosis, and tuberculosis also invade the renal interstitium.

The renal interstitium is the target of a number of systemic illnesses. Sarcoidosis causes a lymphocyte-dominant AIN, which can be associated with noncaseating granulomas. AKI and urine sediment containing WBCs and WBC casts point to this disease, along with other systemic findings. Steroids reduce the severity of AIN, but CKD is a potential long-term complication. Systemic lupus erythematosus is more commonly associated with various forms of proliferative GN; AIN may coexist with glomerular disease, or, in rare instances, it may be present in isolation. The interstitial inflammatory lesion is caused by immune complex deposition in the tubulointerstitium. AIN usually responds to the cytotoxic therapy given for lupus nephritis. Sjögren's syndrome also causes a lymphocyte-dominant AIN; it appears to be another immune complex–mediated disease of the renal interstitium.

Patients with HIV infection may develop interstitial disease that appears immune related. Diffuse infiltrative lymphocytosis syndrome (DILS) is a Sjögren-like syndrome associated with multivisceral infiltration of CD8-positive T lymphocytes. DILS appears to be a host-determined response to HIV. Immune reconstitution inflammatory syndrome (IRIS) is another multivisceral disease characterized by an interstitial infiltrate. This disease occurs when combination antiretroviral therapy reconstitutes the immune system in the setting of a previous or occult opportunistic infection. An exuberant immune reaction results in T cell infiltration of several organs, including the kidneys, which develop AIN. Therapy involves treatment of the opportunistic infection. Occasionally, steroids are required to suppress the inflammatory response.

Infiltration of the kidney by cancer is an uncommon cause of AKI. Autopsy studies confirm a high rate of asymptomatic renal infiltration. The malignancies most often associated with interstitial infiltration are the lymphomas and leukemias.

Lymphomatous infiltration of the kidney parenchyma can occur in the form of discrete nodules or diffuse interstitial infiltration. Lymphoma may cause massive kidney enlargement (nephromegaly) and AKI. Leukemic infiltration also causes nephromegaly, AKI, and, rarely, renal potassium wasting from either tubulointerstitial damage or lysozyme production. Successful treatment of the underlying malignancy typically improves the infiltrative lesion; however, irradiation of the kidneys may provide additional benefit. Exclusion of obstructive uropathy from bulky retroperitoneal lymph node disease is also required.

Postrenal AKI

AKI can develop when obstruction to urine flow occurs along the genitourinary system (E-Table 31-5). The process causing postrenal AKI is called *obstructive uropathy*, whereas the dilated urinary collecting system identified on imaging is termed *hydronephrosis*. Tubular defects with AKI that results from urinary obstruction is called *obstructive nephropathy*. AKI can develop only when obstruction is bilateral, involving both ureters or the bladder, or unilateral in a person with a single functioning kidney. Importantly, either complete or partial obstruction can cause AKI. In general, complete obstruction is associated with more severe AKI and hypertension, intravascular volume overload, hyperkalemia, metabolic acidosis, and hyponatremia.

A wide variety of disorders, originating anywhere from the renal calyces to the urethra, can cause AKI due to urinary obstruction. The most common causes of obstructive uropathy in the upper urinary tract are stones and retroperitoneal disease; in the lower tract, at the level of the bladder and below, prostatic hyperplasia and bladder dysfunction most often obstruct urinary flow. Obstructive uropathy should be considered in many patients with AKI, especially those with a history suggesting risk. A history of nephrolithiasis or certain cancers, along with flank pain, suggests upper tract disease; a history of prostate or bladder disease, together with symptoms of prostatism and urinary retention, points to lower tract obstruction. A directed physical examination of the flanks, suprapubic area, and prostate for flank tenderness, a palpable bladder, or prostatic enlargement is required. Large residual urine demonstrated on straight catheterization of the bladder bespeaks lower tract obstruction.

Ultrasonography of the kidneys and retroperitoneum is the most appropriate initial test to evaluate the patient with AKI and possible urinary tract obstruction. The sensitivity and specificity of renal ultrasonography for the detection of urinary obstruction are approximately 90%. Several processes blunt dilatation of the collecting system and the formation of hydronephrosis, including acute obstruction of less than 48 to 72 hours' duration, severe intravascular volume depletion superimposed on obstruction, and retroperitoneal disease involving the kidneys and ureters that encases the collecting system. If ultrasonographic findings are equivocal or negative but high suspicion for urinary obstruction persists, a CT scan may provide more information. One of the major benefits of CT imaging is the ability to detect stones, tumor, enlarged lymph nodes, and other processes causing obstruction despite the absence of hydronephrosis. As last resort, if obstruction as the cause of AKI is still considered likely, retrograde pyelography may provide a diagnosis of upper tract obstruction.

Therapy for AKI due to obstructive uropathy requires rapid diagnosis and intervention to relieve the obstructive process. Delayed interventions, especially in patients with complete obstruction, compromise recovery of kidney function. Upper urinary tract obstruction requires either retrograde ureteral stent placement or nephrostomy tube insertion when it is caused by severe retroperitoneal disease such as ureteral or bladder cancer. Relief of lower tract obstruction with a bladder catheter, a suprapubic tube (rarely), or a nephrostomy tube is the first step in treatment. Electrolyte and fluid management also are required to ensure patient safety in developing postobstructive diuresis. It is a phenomenon that occurs primarily in patients with bilateral, complete obstruction and is characterized by large urine volumes after relief of obstruction. Postobstructive diuresis is physiologic in that excess sodium and water are being excreted from the hypervolemic patient, but impaired tubular function (sodium and water) may lead to excessive diuresis and volume depletion. In this setting, judicious fluid repletion is required to avoid iatrogenic postobstructive diuresis as well as underresuscitation and hypotension.

● COMPLICATIONS OF AKI

Considering the normal functions of the kidneys, it is not surprising that a number of metabolic complications develop in the setting of AKI. Hyperkalemia is a potentially life-threatening complication that often requires urgent intervention. Hyperkalemia disturbs the magnitude of the action potential in response to a depolarizing stimulus. The electrocardiogram (ECG) is a better guide to therapy than a single measurement of potassium concentration. The sequential ECG changes observed in hyperkalemia are peaked T waves, PR prolongation, QRS widening, and a sine wave pattern. The presence of any of these ECG changes mandates prompt therapy.

Metabolic acidosis is common in AKI. However, it is usually well tolerated and does not require therapy unless arterial pH declines to less than 7.1. Hyperkalemia and severe metabolic acidosis not responsive to medical therapy are indications for initiation of RRT. Hypocalcemia is a common but asymptomatic finding and usually does not require therapy. Significant hyperphosphatemia may occur but often can be managed with oral phosphate binders. Anemia typically does not require treatment unless it is severe, is symptomatic, or contributes to cardiac dysfunction. Uremic manifestations of AKI are listed in E-Table 31-6. They may be subtle findings, or they may be obvious and life-threatening, requiring urgent RRT.

Importantly, infectious complications are the main cause of death because of the immune compromise, edema with end-organ dysfunction and skin breakdown, and numerous indwelling catheters in these patients.

● GENERAL MANAGEMENT OF AKI

Management of AKI begins with identification of the cause and pathogenesis of the inciting process. In addition, the complications associated with AKI need to be recognized and rapidly treated to avoid serious adverse events. Prerenal AKI requires optimization of renal perfusion by repletion of intravascular volume in those who are volume depleted and correction of heart failure, liver failure, and other "effective" causes of reduced intravascular volume. Intrinsic AKI requires directed therapy of the disturbed kidney compartment. Management of postrenal AKI mandates early intervention to relieve obstruction and preserve kidney function.

Most consequences of AKI are managed initially with conservative measures. These include interventions to correct hypovolemia or hypervolemia, improvement of hemodynamics, and correction of hyponatremia, hyperkalemia, metabolic acidosis, and hyperphosphatemia. Conversion of patients from oliguric to nonoliguric AKI makes management easier but does not improve outcomes in terms of morbidity or mortality. Manifestations of severe uremia and the other consequences of AKI, as listed in E-Table 31-6, may necessitate RRT if conservative measures are unsuccessful or incompletely reverse the complication.

Hospital-based RRT, which includes primarily acute hemodialysis and continuous renal replacement therapies (CRRTs), is required in certain patients with AKI. Continuous therapies, which can be employed only in the ICU, include continuous venovenous hemofiltration, hemodialysis, hemodiafiltration, slow low-efficiency dialysis, and extended daily dialysis. Emergent indications include severe hyperkalemia, uremic end-organ damage (e.g., pericarditis, seizure), refractory metabolic acidosis, and severe volume overload including pulmonary edema. Although the data do not support a cutoff BUN value to initiate RRT, it is sensible to initiate therapy before severe uremic complications develop. Intractable volume overload with anasarca complicated by skin breakdown is another potential indication. Acute hemodialysis is the modality most commonly employed to treat the consequences of AKI. However, critically ill patients who are hemodynamically unstable benefit most from continuous therapies. CRRT allows more precise control of volume, uremia, acid-base disturbances, and electrolyte disorders with less hemodynamic instability. CRRT also allows aggressive nutritional support. Peritoneal dialysis is rarely used for AKI but is a reasonable modality.

● OUTCOME AND PROGNOSIS OF AKI

Despite the significant advances in supportive care and RRT technology, acute and long-term complications, including mortality, remain common. The mortality associated with AKI in the hospital setting depends on the patient's severity of illness and burden of organ dysfunction. As the number of failed organs increases from 0 to 4, the mortality rate associated with AKI increases from less than 40% to more than 90%. Also, in-hospital mortality increases with AKI that develops in the medical or surgical ICU. Long-term outcomes for patients with AKI include increased risk for death (compared with hospitalized patients without AKI). Furthermore, patients with CKD who have a prehospitalization eGFR lower than 45 mL/min/1.73 m^2 who develop RRT-requiring AKI have a much higher mortality rate than patients with CKD not complicated by AKI. On the whole, all forms of AKI, including the RRT-requiring forms, appear to be associated with an increased risk for development of new CKD, progression of CKD, ESRD, and death.

For a deeper discussion on this topic, please see Chapter 120, "Acute Kidney Injury," in Goldman-Cecil Medicine, *25th Edition.*

SUGGESTED READINGS

Bellomo R, Ronco C, Kellum JA: Acute kidney injury, Lancet 380:756–766, 2012.

Coca SG, Yusuf B, Shlipak MG, et al: Long-term risk of mortality and other adverse outcomes after acute kidney injury: a systematic review and meta-analysis, Am J Kidney Dis 53:961–973, 2009.

Cruz DN, Ricci Z, Ronco C: Clinical review: RIFLE and AKIN—time for reappraisal, Crit Care 13:211, 2009.

Haase M, Bellomo R, Devarajan P, et al: Accuracy of neutrophil gelatinase-associated lipocalin (NGAL) in diagnosis and prognosis in acute kidney injury: a systematic review and meta-analysis, Am J Kidney Dis 54:1012, 2009.

KDIGO: 2012 clinical practice guideline for acute kidney injury. Chapter 2.5: Diagnostic approach to alterations in kidney function and structure, Kid Intl Suppl 2:33–36, 2012.

Mehta RL, Kellum JA, Shah SV, et al: Acute Kidney Injury Network: report of an initiative to improve outcomes in acute kidney injury, Crit Care 11:R31, 2007.

Moreau R, Lebrec D: Acute kidney injury: new concepts, Nephron Physiol 109:73–79, 2008.

Portilla D, Kaushal GP, Basnakian AG, et al: Recent progress in the pathophysiology of acute renal failure. In Runge MS, Patterson C, editors: Principles of molecular medicine, ed 2, Totawa, NJ, 2006, Humana Press, pp 643–649.

Schrier RW, Wang W, Poole B, et al: Acute renal failure: definitions, diagnosis, pathogenesis and therapy, J Clin Invest 114:5–14, 2004.

Uchino S, Kellum J, Bellomo R, et al: Acute renal failure in critically ill patients, JAMA 294:813–818, 2005.

32

Chronic Kidney Disease

Kerri L. Cavanaugh and T. Alp Ikizler

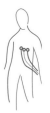

DEFINITION AND EPIDEMIOLOGY

Chronic kidney disease (CKD) is defined as persistent, progressive, and irreversible loss of renal function. The spectrum of CKD includes earlier stages of kidney damage (characterized by proteinuria, electrolyte abnormalities, and elevated serum creatinine) that represent a decrease in the glomerular filtration rate (GFR) and extends to complete loss of kidney function—that is, kidney failure or end-stage renal disease (ESRD). Markers of kidney damage or GFR less than 60 mL/min/1.73 m² must be present to meet the diagnostic criteria of CKD. In addition, these must be present and persistent for at least 3 months to differentiate CKD from acute kidney injury. According to the Kidney Disease: Improving Global Outcomes (KDIGO) 2012 clinical practice guideline, CKD is classified based on the underlying cause of kidney disease, GFR category, and degree of albuminuria. There are six GFR categories, ranging from normal or high (G1, ≥90 mL/min/1.73 m²) to kidney failure (G5, <15 mL/min/1.73 m²), and three albuminuria categories based on severity (Table 32-1).

CKD is a worldwide public health problem of increasing magnitude; in the United States, CKD is estimated to affect 20 million people. Although some have mildly decreased GFR with mild to moderate albuminuria (Fig. 32-1), many people with CKD progress to ESRD and require dialysis or kidney transplantation. The rate of new ESRD patients in the United States has been relatively stable since 2000; however, it was 4% lower (357 per million population) in 2011, as reported by the United States Renal Data System (USRDS) in 2013 (E-Fig. 32-1). Trends in overall prevalence of ESRD suggest a continuing increase in the numbers of patients requiring care, although in 2011 the increase was only 3.4%—the lowest in 30 years (E-Fig. 32-2). Care of the ESRD patient is costly, accounting for $34 billion (6.3%) of the U.S. Medicare budget in 2011. In addition to concern about progression to ESRD, decreased GFR and proteinuria have each been recognized as independent risk factors for cardiovascular disease and death. Therefore, diagnosis of CKD confers risk not only for progressive loss of kidney function but also for decreased survival.

The most common causes of ESRD are diabetes mellitus (45%), hypertension (28%), glomerulonephritis (6-7%), and cystic or congenital conditions (2-3%). During the evaluation of CKD, every attempt should be made to arrive at the specific cause of kidney disease. Renal biopsy is the most specific approach to definitive diagnosis; it also can guide treatment and help to determine suitability for kidney transplantation. However, the procedure has potential complications, and clinical and imaging information may be sufficient to provide a conclusive diagnosis.

PATHOLOGY

After renal injury, surviving nephrons must adjust by increasing their filtration and excretion rates to ensure adequate solute, water, and acid-base balances. Patients with CKD are vulnerable to edema formation and severe volume overload, hyperkalemia, hyponatremia, and azotemia. Initially, sodium balance is maintained by increasing fractional excretion of sodium by the nephrons. Acid excretion is maintained until late stages of CKD (when the GFR falls to less than 30 mL/minute) by increased tubular ammonia synthesis, which provides an adequate buffer for hydrogen in the distal nephron. Later, a significant decrease in distal bicarbonate regeneration results in hyperchloremic metabolic acidosis. Further nephron loss leads to retention of organic ions such as sulfates, which results in an anion gap metabolic acidosis. There is active research to determine whether metabolic acidosis is itself a contributor to progression of CKD and whether its correction by base supplementation is a potential treatment.

Once GFR has decreased below a critical level, CKD tends to progress to ESRD, regardless of the initial insult. Figure 32-2 shows how risk factors may interact with pathophysiologic

TABLE 32-1	CATEGORIES OF GLOMERULAR FILTRATION RATE AND ALBUMINURIA IN CHRONIC KIDNEY DISEASE			

CATEGORY	GFR (mL/min/1.73 m²)	TERMS		
G1*	≥90	Normal or high		
G2*	60-89	Mildly decreased		
G3a	45-59	Mildly to moderately decreased		
G3b	30-44	Moderately to severely decreased		
G4	15-29	Severely decreased		
G5	<15	Kidney failure		

CATEGORY	AER (mg/24 hr)	ACR (mg/g)	ACR (mg/mmol)	Terms
A1	<30	<30	<3	Normal to mildly increased
A2	30-300	30-300	3-30	Moderately increased
A3	>300	>300	>30	Severely increased

Modified from Kidney Disease: Improving Global Outcomes (KDIGO) CKD Work Group: KDIGO 2012 clinical practice guideline for the evaluation and management of chronic kidney disease, Kid Intl Suppl 3:1–150, 2013.

ACR, Albumin-to-creatine ratio; AER, albumin excretion rate; GFR, glomerular filtration rate.

*G1 and G2 alone, without other evidence of kidney damage, do not meet the criteria for chronic kidney disease.

Percentage of US Population by eGFR and Albuminuria Category: KDIGO 2012 and NHANES 1999–2006			Persistent albuminuria categories Description and range			
			A1	**A2**	**A3**	
			Normal to mildly increased	Moderately increased	Severely increased	
			<30 mg/g <3 mg/mmol	30-300 mg/g 3-30 mg/mmol	>300 mg/g >30 mg/mmol	
GFR categories (ml/min/1.73 m²) Description and range	**G1**	Normal or high	≥90	55.6	1.9	0.4	57.9
	G2	Mildly decreased	60-89	32.9	2.2	0.3	35.4
	G3a	Mildly to moderately decreased	45-59	3.6	0.8	0.2	4.6
	G3b	Moderately to severely decreased	30-44	1.0	0.4	0.2	1.6
	G4	Severely decreased	15-29	0.2	0.1	0.1	0.4
	G5	Kidney failure	<15	0.0	0.0	0.1	0.1
				93.2	5.4	1.3	100.0

FIGURE 32-1 Distribution of chronic kidney disease in the United States by glomerular filtration rate (GFR) and albuminuria categories.

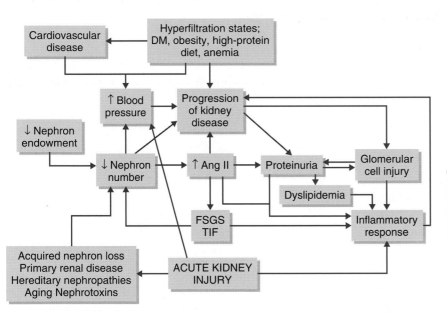

FIGURE 32-2 A simplified depiction of risk factors interacting with pathophysiologic mechanisms to accelerate progression of chronic kidney disease. Ang II, Angiotensin II; DM, diabetes mellitus; FSGS, focal segmental glomerulosclerosis; TIF, tubulointerstitial fibrosis. (Modified from Taal MW, Brenner BM: Predicting initiation and progression of chronic kidney disease: developing renal risk scores, Kidney Int 70:1694–1705, 2006.)

mechanisms to accelerate CKD progression. Detailed studies have elucidated interrelated mechanisms, including glomerular hemodynamic responses to nephron loss, proteinuria, and pro-inflammatory responses. Activation of the renin-angiotensin-aldosterone system (RAAS) pathway and increased production of transforming growth factor-β (TGF-β) also contribute to renal fibrosis. Interventions that reduce intraglomerular pressure, such as protein restriction and the use of angiotensin-converting enzyme (ACE) inhibitors or angiotensin-receptor blockers (ARBs), help attenuate progression of renal disease and further support the importance of glomerular hemodynamics and RAAS in progressive kidney disease.

CLINICAL PRESENTATION
General Features of Uremic Syndrome

Kidney disease commonly manifests first as abnormalities on laboratory or other diagnostic tests. Patients with CKD may not have symptoms until advanced stages, in which the GFR is less than 15 mL/minute. *Uremia* is a systemic syndrome that negatively affects every organ system. Uremic syndrome is likely the consequence of many factors, including retained molecules, deficiencies of important hormones, and metabolic abnormalities, rather than the effect of a single uremic toxin (E-Fig. 32-3). Excess urea can cause symptoms of fatigue, nausea, vomiting, and headaches. Its breakdown product (cyanate) can result in carbamylation of lipoproteins and peptides, leading to multiple organ dysfunctions. Guanidines, byproducts of protein metabolism, are increased and can inhibit α_1-hydroxylase activity within the kidney, leading to secondary hyperparathyroidism. β_2-Microglobulin accumulation in patients with ESRD has been associated with neuropathy, carpal tunnel syndrome, and amyloid infiltration of the joints. Specific roles for other accumulated metabolites are under investigation. The major manifestations of uremia are summarized in Figure 32-3.

Cardiovascular

In addition to hypertension, cardiovascular disorders are common in patients with CKD. More than 60% of patients with ESRD who start dialysis have echocardiographic manifestations of left ventricular hypertrophy, dilation, and systolic or diastolic dysfunction. Metabolic consequences of CKD, including accelerated atherogenesis, contribute to metastatic calcification in the myocardium, cardiac valves, and arteries. Arrhythmias, including those resulting in sudden death, may be caused by electrolyte abnormalities, cardiac structural changes, or ischemic cardiovascular disease. Pericarditis can occur in patients with uremia before they start dialysis or in ESRD patients receiving inadequate dialysis.

Gastrointestinal

Gastrointestinal disturbances are among the earliest and most common signs of the uremic syndrome. Patients describe a metallic taste and loss of appetite. Later, they experience nausea, vomiting, and weight loss, and those with severe uremia may also experience stomatitis and enteritis. Gastrointestinal bleeding caused by gastritis, peptic ulceration, and arterial venous malformations in the setting of platelet dysfunction may be present.

Neurologic

Central nervous system manifestations are frequent in advanced CKD and are characterized predominantly by changes in cognitive function and sleep disturbances. Lethargy, irritability, asterixis, seizures, and frank encephalopathy with coma are late manifestations of uremia and are usually avoided by timely initiation of renal replacement therapy (RRT). Peripheral neurologic manifestations appear as a progressive, symmetrical sensory neuropathy in a glove-and-stocking distribution. Patients have decreased distal tendon reflexes and loss of vibratory perception. Peripheral motor impairment can result in restless legs, footdrop, or wristdrop. Most of these neurologic manifestations reverse with adequate dialysis or kidney transplantation.

Musculoskeletal

Alterations in calcium and phosphate homeostasis, with hyperparathyroidism and disturbance of vitamin D metabolism, also are common. Hypocalcemia and secondary hyperparathyroidism are the result of phosphate retention and lack of α_1-hydroxylase activity in the failing kidney, with consequent deficiency of the most active form of vitamin D. Over time, maladaptive parathyroid hypertrophy leads to bone disease and tissue calcification.

Hematologic and Immunologic

Erythropoietin (EPO), a hormone produced by the kidney that regulates erythrocyte production, becomes progressively

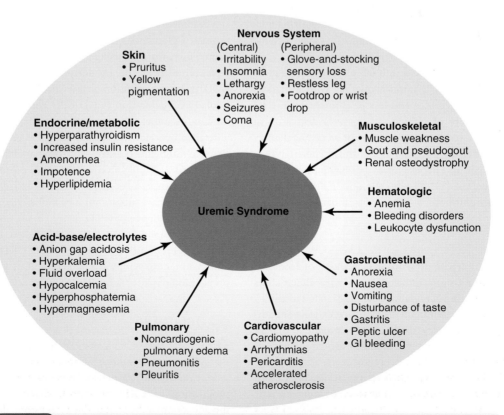

FIGURE 32-3 Diagrammatic summary of the major manifestations of the uremic syndrome. GI, Gastrointestinal.

deficient as CKD progresses. EPO and iron deficiency are common causes of anemia in CKD. Administration of synthetic EPO results in correction of anemia, improved quality of life and anemia-related symptoms, and decreased dependence on blood transfusions. Caution must be exercised, because higher doses of EPO that result in elevations of the serum hemoglobin to more than 12 g/dL may be associated with a higher risk for adverse cardiovascular events. Bleeding disorders, primarily from defects in platelet adherence and aggregation, are common. Bleeding in uremic patients usually can be controlled with cryoprecipitate, 1-deamino-(8-D-arginine)-vasopressin (DDAVP), conjugated estrogens, and dialysis.

Defects occur in both humoral and cellular immune systems in patients with CKD. Although the leukocyte count is typically normal and appropriately responsive in advanced CKD, patients are generally immunosuppressed and susceptible to infections. This may be the result of functional abnormalities of polymorphonuclear leukocytes, lymphocytes, and other cellular host defenses. Additionally, patients with CKD may have a variable immune response to vaccination.

Endocrine and Metabolic

Thyroid function testing may be less reliable in patients with uremia. Common laboratory findings include an increased triiodothyronine (T_3) resin uptake, a low T_3 level resulting from the impaired conversion of thyroxin to T_3 peripherally, and normal thyroxin levels. Thyroid-stimulating hormone levels are usually normal.

A deranged pituitary-gonadal axis can result in sexual dysfunction manifested by impotence, decreased libido, amenorrhea, sterility, and uterine bleeding. Patients have decreased plasma levels of testosterone, estrogen, and progesterone, with normal or increased levels of follicle-stimulating hormone, luteinizing hormones, and prolactin. Pregnancy is uncommon in female patients who have a GFR of less than 30 mL/minute.

Lipid abnormalities are also common in CKD. They are most consistent with type IV hyperlipoproteinemia, with a marked increase in plasma triglycerides and less of an increase in total cholesterol. The activity of lipoprotein lipase is decreased in uremia, resulting in reduced conversion of very-low-density lipoprotein to low-density lipoprotein and thus hypertriglyceridemia. The treatment of choice is the hydroxymethylglutaryl–coenzyme A reductase (HMG-CoA) inhibitor class of drugs because of their pluripotent effects on inflammation and atherosclerosis.

Electrolytes

Hyperkalemia occurs in patients with CKD as a result of decreased renal clearance of potassium, intracellular-to-extracellular shifts of potassium in the setting of metabolic acidosis related to kidney failure, and also the concomitant use of medications such as RAAS blockers. The primary method of treatment is dietary reduction of potassium but may also include use of loop diuretics or potassium-binding medications. Hypokalemia is much less common in CKD but may occur in the setting of very poor nutritional intake or use of high-dose potassium-wasting diuretic medications.

Skin

Uremic hue, a yellowish skin color, is likely the result of retained liposoluble pigments, such as lipochromes and carotenoids. Uremic hue usually responds to dialysis, control of hyperparathyroidism, improved calcium and phosphate balance, and, occasionally, ultraviolet radiation. Calciphylaxis, or calcific uremic arteriolopathy, results in painful skin calcification and is often seen in patients with uncontrolled hyperparathyroidism. Use of warfarin is a risk factor for this condition. Nail findings include the half-and-half nail, characterized by red, pink, or brownish discoloration of the distal nail bed, pale nails, and splinter hemorrhages. Other common signs and symptoms are pruritus and ecchymoses due to disorders of bleeding.

● DIAGNOSIS

Comprehensive care for the patient with kidney disease includes screening, diagnosis, and treatment of CKD to manage complications and prevent further progression (E-Fig 32-4). Screening for CKD is recommended for patients with high-risk comorbid conditions, including diabetes mellitus and hypertension, and also for those with a family history of kidney disease. The diagnosis of CKD requires evidence of kidney damage that has persisted for at least 3 months. Imaging abnormalities are important, but more commonly CKD is detected by the presence of albuminuria or by reductions in the clearance of toxins by the kidney (i.e., elevated serum creatinine or blood urea nitrogen). Albuminuria may be detected in a spot collection of urine and is best reported as an albumin-to-creatinine ratio (ACR). In general, an ACR greater than 30 mg/g confirmed on several samples and without evidence of urinary infection raises concern for a diagnosis of CKD and warrants additional investigation.

Clearance of toxins by the kidney is most often assessed by the estimated glomerular filtration rate (eGFR). Initial assessment should be performed using a serum creatinine–based estimating equation such as the Modification of Diet in Renal Disease (MDRD) study equation or the Chronic Kidney Disease Epidemiology Collaboration (CKD-EPI) equation. Each of these has limitations and cautions regarding application of its results, and a detailed overview can be found in the KDIGO 2012 Clinical Practice Guidelines. The serum biomarker cystatin C may be considered and integrated into another estimating equation for patients who have an eGFR between 45 and 59 mL/min/1.73 m^2 and may not have albuminuria or kidney imaging abnormalities to confirm evidence of CKD.

Once a diagnosis of CKD is established, management goals include (1) prevention of progression of CKD, (2) identification and treatment of symptoms and complications of CKD, and (3) preparation of patients for RRT if appropriate.

● TREATMENT
Prevention of Progression

In addition to treatment of the specific underlying cause of kidney disease, it is important to consider methods to slow the progression of CKD once it is diagnosed. These methods include optimal control of hypertension, diabetes, and other cardiovascular disease risk factors (e.g., tobacco cessation); use of medications that block the RAAS pathway; diet modifications; avoidance of nephrotoxins; and identification of reversible causes of acute kidney injury in the setting of CKD.

Management of Hypertension and Diabetes

Several controlled trials have demonstrated that treatment of hypertension attenuates the rate of progression of kidney disease. The present recommendation is to target blood pressure to lower than 140/90 mm Hg in patients with diabetes or kidney disease. However, the evidence supporting this recommendation in CKD is limited, and there is debate as to whether a higher target may be acceptable. Medications that block the production or effect of angiotensin II further prevent progression of CKD, beyond control of hypertension, in patients with proteinuria. Dihydropyridine calcium channel blockers have not been shown to be as beneficial as ACE inhibitors or ARBs in slowing CKD progression.

For patients with diabetes mellitus, adequate glycemic control also slows progression of CKD. The recommended goal is to maintain glycosylated hemoglobin (hemoglobin A_{1c}) values less than 7%, irrespective of a concurrent diagnosis of CKD, although this level of glycemic control warrants caution due to hypoglycemic risk (see Chapter 66). ACE inhibitors and ARBs may be considered, in patients with diabetes and proteinuria who do not have hypertension, to slow CKD progression.

Diet

Dietary protein restriction is advocated to slow progression of CKD. Several meta-analyses have indicated that reduced-protein diets are modestly beneficial to slow CKD progression, but the largest clinical trial, the MDRD study, did not show a significant benefit. The recommended dietary protein intake in advanced CKD is 0.60 g/kg/day with at least 50% of the protein being of high biologic value. The present consensus is that aggressive dietary management in patients with CKD, including proper restriction of sodium, potassium, phosphorus, and protein intake under the supervision of a dietician, may reduce progression of CKD, albeit to a small extent.

Avoidance of Toxic Drug Effects

Many drugs that are excreted by the kidney should be avoided, or their doses should be reduced, as shown in Table 32-2. Drugs may injure the kidney in many ways, including direct toxicity leading to acute tubular necrosis, induction of interstitial nephritis, and development of urinary crystals that obstruct the kidney. Common classes of medications that injure the kidney include antibiotics, specifically aminoglycosides; nonsteroidal anti-inflammatory drugs, including cyclooxygenase 2 (COX2) inhibitors; and antiretroviral medications. Certain over-the-counter herbal medications, including aristolochic acids, can cause CKD. Others, such as St. John's wort, may interact with kidney transplant medications and should be avoided.

Iodinated radiocontrast agents can cause acute worsening of kidney function, especially in patients with CKD. Iso-osmolar contrast agents are less toxic than high-osmolar agents. Patients who are at high risk for contrast-induced kidney injury should

TABLE 32-2 DRUG DOSAGE ADJUSTMENTS IN CHRONIC KIDNEY DISEASE

MAJOR DOSAGE REDUCTION	MINOR OR NO REDUCTION	AVOID USE
ANTIBIOTICS		
Aminoglycosides	Erythromycin	Nitrofurantoin
Penicillin	Nafcillin	Nalidixic acid
Cephalosporins	Clindamycin	Tetracycline
Sulfonamides	Chloramphenicol	
Vancomycin	Isoniazid, rifampin	
Quinolones	Amphotericin B	
Fluconazole	Aztreonam, tazobactam	
Acyclovir, ganciclovir	Doxycycline	
Foscarnet		
Imipenem		
OTHERS		
Digoxin	Antihypertensives	Aspirin
Procainamide	Benzodiazepines	Sulfonylureas
H_2 antagonists	Quinidine	Lithium carbonate
Meperidine	Lidocaine	Acetazolamide
Codeine	Spironolactone	NSAIDs
Propoxyphene	Triamterene	Phosphate-containing bowel-preparation agents

NSAIDs, Nonsteroidal anti-inflammatory drugs.

receive adequate hydration, and the volume of the contrast agent should be minimized. The magnetic resonance imaging contrast agent gadolinium has been associated with the severe fibrotic skin condition of nephrogenic systemic fibrosis in patients with advanced CKD.

Reversible Causes of Acute Deterioration in Kidney Function

The rate of decline in GFR for individual patients is generally log-linear over time. Accordingly, a plot of the reciprocal of the plasma creatinine concentration against time usually predicts the rate at which a specific patient will reach ESRD (E-Fig. 32-5). When such a patient suddenly shows acute worsening of kidney function, the differential diagnosis should be considered and investigated, as described in Chapter 31 (Acute Kidney Injury).

Care for the Patient with End-Stage Renal Disease

As CKD progresses to kidney failure, preparation is needed for RRT. Patients with moderate CKD should be referred to a nephrologist for comanagement, including evaluation of risk for CKD progression, estimation of timing until kidney failure, and education related to RRT. Late referral (<3 months before ESRD) is associated with a higher risk for death after initiation of RRT.

Renal Replacement Therapies

For those progressing to ESRD, discussions about available RRT options should occur early and should be paired with an assessment of the expectations and values of the patient and other family members. Options include kidney transplantation, dialysis, and medical management without dialysis, sometimes referred to as conservative care. In medically eligible patients, kidney transplantation is encouraged because it allows a better quality of life, increased survival rate, and greater chance for rehabilitation. Kidney transplants may be obtained from deceased or living donors. In the United States in 2011, new kidney transplantations were performed in 15,652 people, although most of these patients (83%) received dialysis before transplantation.

There are two types of dialysis, hemodialysis and peritoneal dialysis. In the United States in 2011, 103,744 patients began hemodialysis, whereas only 7438 (7%) elected peritoneal dialysis. The distribution of patients receiving various modalities differs in other countries. Chronic dialysis is initiated when the patient displays signs of uremia, usually when eGFR is 10 mL/minute or less and there are no apparent reversible causes of kidney failure. However, chronic dialysis may be started at any time when complications of ESRD (e.g., fluid balance, potassium levels) cannot be controlled medically.

Hemodialysis

As illustrated in Figure 32-4, blood is pumped from a vascular access into tubing that leads to a large number of capillary fibers bundled together in a dialyzer (E-Fig. 32-6). These capillaries are made up of semisynthetic materials that are semipermeable and therefore capable of allowing exchange of small molecules between blood and a dialysate solution, permitting countercurrent exchange. The solution contains sodium chloride, bicarbonate, and varying concentrations of potassium. Diffusion through the membrane allows low-molecular-weight substances such as urea and organic acids to move across according to the concentration gradient. Fluid is removed by *ultrafiltration*, which is achieved by applying transmembrane hydrostatic pressure across the dialyzer.

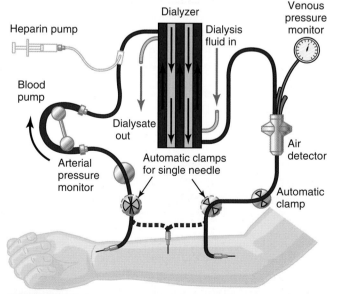

FIGURE 32-4 Essential components of a dialysis delivery system that, together with the dialyzer, make up an *artificial kidney*. In isolated ultrafiltration, no dialysis fluid is used (bypass mode). Also shown is the apparatus for using a single needle for inflow and outflow of blood from the patient. (From Keshaviah PR: Hemodialysis monitors and monitoring. In Maher JF, editor: Replacement of renal Function by dialysis, ed 3, Boston, 1989, Kluwer Academic Publishers.)

In the setting of ESRD, an average patient undergoing *intermittent* chronic hemodialysis requires 4 hours of dialysis three times a week. Common complications include hypotension and muscle cramping. Avoiding excessive fluid weight gain can minimize these complications.

An arteriovenous fistula (AVF) or arteriovenous graft (AVG) is recommended for permanent vascular access for hemodialysis, rather than an indwelling catheter. Although the goal is for more than 74% of prevalent hemodialysis patients to use an AVF or AVG for dialysis access (http://www.healthypeople.gov/2020/), many patients continue to use catheters, especially at the time of initiation of chronic hemodialysis. Temporary catheters are placed into the internal jugular, subclavian, or femoral vein, similar to other central venous lines. Permanent catheters have a cuff around the outer wall of the tubing and tunnel under the chest wall skin for some distance before entering the internal jugular vein. Catheters have a higher rate of infection and a higher risk for mortality compared with AVF or AVG.

Peritoneal Dialysis

In peritoneal dialysis, the peritoneal capillaries act as a semipermeable membrane similar to a hemodialysis dialyzer. This technique has several advantages over hemodialysis: it allows independence from the long time spent in dialysis units; it may not require as stringent dietary restrictions compared with hemodialysis; and it allows more patients to return to full-time employment. In *continuous ambulatory peritoneal dialysis*, dialysate of 2- to 3-L volumes is instilled through a peritoneal catheter (E-Fig. 32-7) into the peritoneal cavity for varying amounts of time and exchanged four to six times daily. In *continuous cyclic peritoneal dialysis*, the patient is connected to a machine, referred to as a *cycler*, that allows inflow of smaller volumes of dialysate with shorter dwell time overnight while the patient sleeps. Modifications to this regimen can be made to fit a patient's lifestyle and still achieve adequate clearance of toxins and removal of fluid. Ultrafiltration is achieved through increasing the dextrose concentration in the dialysate.

Two major drawbacks of peritoneal dialysis are peritonitis and difficulty in achieving adequate clearances in patients with excess body mass. Peritonitis can be treated with intraperitoneal antibiotics. Additionally, a slow deterioration occurs in the permeability of the peritoneal membrane, especially after one or more peritonitis episodes, leading to inadequate dialysis and, ultimately, the need to change the modality of RRT.

Kidney Transplantation

Kidney transplantation is the preferred modality of RRT. The variety of available immunosuppressive drugs, including rapamycin, mycophenylate mofetil, anti–interleukin-2 receptor antibodies, and novel agents such as belatacept have resulted in excellent graft survival.

Types of Kidney Transplants

Kidney transplant donors may be deceased or living and related or unrelated to the patient. The 1-year and 5-year graft survival rates are 91% and 71% with a deceased donor, and 97% and 85%, respectively, with a living donor.

Advantages and disadvantages of deceased versus living donors are listed in Table 32-3. There is an effort to increase living donation because the deceased donor supply is inadequate. The main advantages of a living related donor transplant are less ischemic injury and better histocompatibility matching (Fig. 32-5). However, with procedures to reduce antibodies, including plasmapheresis and pretransplantation immunosuppressive therapy, it is possible to successfully perform kidney transplantations in patients with high levels of antibodies or even ABO blood group incompatibility with the donor.

TABLE 32-3 COMPARISON OF DONOR SOURCES FOR KIDNEY TRANSPLANTATION

ADVANTAGES	DISADVANTAGES
LIVING DONOR	
Better tissue match with less likelihood of rejection	Small potential risk of operation to donor
Smaller doses of drugs for immunosuppression	Requirement of willing, medically suitable family member or other person
Waiting time for transplant reduced	
Sequelae of long-term dialysis avoided	
Elective surgical procedure	
Better early graft function with shorter hospitalization	
Better short-term and long-term success	
DECEASED DONOR	
Availability to any recipient	Tissue match not as similar
Availability of other organs for combined transplants (i.e., kidney-pancreas transplant)	Waiting time variable
Availability of vascular conduits for complex vascular reconstruction	Operation performed urgently
	Early graft function possibly compromised
	Short-term and long-term success not as good as from living donor

Immunosuppressant Drug Therapy

Prophylaxis against and treatment of graft rejection are at the heart of the success of kidney transplantation. All protocols for immunosuppression aim to disrupt the lymphocyte cell cycle, and many include some period of exposure to corticosteroids. The mechanisms of action of commonly used immunosuppressants are illustrated in Figure 32-6.

The hepatic cytochrome P-450 system is essential for metabolism of cyclosporine, tacrolimus, and rapamycin. Significant changes in the levels of these drugs may occur when patients start or discontinue taking any of several drugs that can induce or inhibit this system. Therefore, evaluation for drug-drug interactions is critical to prevent toxic or even subtherapeutic effects of either the immunosuppressant drug or the other prescribed therapy.

Cyclosporine exerts its activity by inhibiting immunocompetent lymphocytes in the G_0 and G_1 phases of the cell cycle. Side effects of cyclosporine include hematologic suppression,

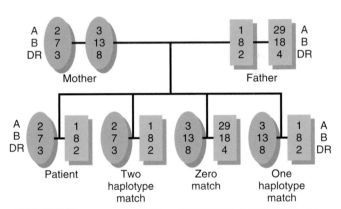

FIGURE 32-5 Diagrammatic representation of possible inheritance of human leukocyte antigen tissue types *(A, B, DR)* in a family with four siblings.

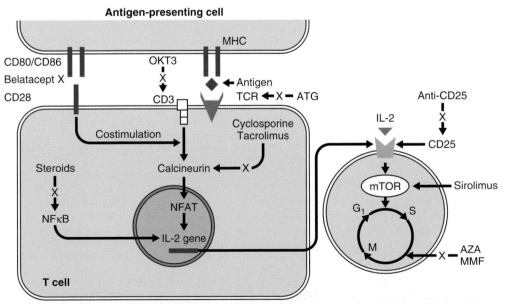

FIGURE 32-6 Pathways of T-cell activation and sites of action of various immunosuppressive agents. ATG, Antithymocyte globulin; AZA, azathioprine; IL, interleukin; MHC, major histocompatibility complex; MMF, mycoplasma membrane fraction; mTOR, mammalian target of rapamycin; NFAT, nuclear factor of activated T cells; NF-κB, nuclear factor-κB; OKT3, anti-CD3 antibody; TCR, T-cell receptor. G_1, S, and M are phases of the cell cycle.

hyperkalemia, seizures, exacerbation of gout, dyslipidemia, and gingival hypertrophy. The most significant of these effects is nephrotoxicity, and this is often related to decreased glomerular blood flow. *Tacrolimus* has a mechanism of action and side-effect profile similar to those of cyclosporine but with the additional problems of hyperglycemia and an increased tendency toward neurotoxicity. Both cyclosporine and tacrolimus can cause calcineurin inhibitor nephrotoxicity, which may contribute to chronic allograft nephropathy and, ultimately, graft loss.

Mycophenolate mofetil (also called *mycophenolic acid*) specifically inhibits proliferation of T and B lymphocytes by interfering with purine synthesis and thus DNA synthesis. Side effects include anemia and leucopenia as well as gastrointestinal symptoms.

Rapamycin is a macrolide antibiotic produced by the fungus *Streptomyces hygroscopicus.* Rapamycin binds to the mTOR (mammalian target of rapamycin) receptor, thus blocking the phosphorylation of p70 S6 kinase (RBS6KB1) and the eukaryotic initiation factor 4E–binding protein 1 (EIF4EBP1, also known as phosphorylated heat- and acid-stable protein regulated by insulin 1 [PHAS-1]). This action leads to the dampening of cytokine and growth factor activity on T, B, and nonimmune cells. The major side effects are thrombocytopenia and dyslipidemia.

Because of the persistence of episodes of rejection and graft loss over time, novel immunosuppressive agents continue to be developed. Most recently, *belatacept,* a fusion protein that inhibits T-cell activation by blocking the CD80 and CD86 sites on antigen-presenting cells. Clinical trials have established its efficacy and demonstrated a side effect profile similar to those of existing immunosuppression options, leading to its approval for use in the United States and other regions.

Acute Rejection

T lymphocytes recognize foreign antigens, especially when they are presented in association with class II major histocompatibility complex (MHC) antigens. This prompts lymphocyte activation. Activated cytotoxic lymphocytes invade the tubular interstitial region of the transplanted kidney, with resulting tubulitis. Clinically, acute rejection is detected by graft tenderness, a rise in serum creatinine levels, oliguria, and, in some instances, fever. Acute humoral rejection involves the intrarenal arteries and leads to vasculitis, carrying a poor prognosis. This type of rejection is often resistant to steroids, necessitating antilymphocyte and possibly plasmapheresis therapy.

Post-transplantation Infection

Infection is second only to cardiovascular disease as the leading cause of mortality in kidney transplant recipients. Prophylaxis therapies are often used immediately after kidney transplantation to prevent infectious diseases that are of particularly high risk, including *Pneumocystis jirovecii* pneumonia, urinary tract infections, and cytomegalovirus infection. In addition to common community-acquired bacterial and viral infections, kidney transplant recipients are susceptible to numerous viral, fungal, and other opportunistic infections that usually do not cause severe illness in an immunocompetent host.

Post-transplantation Malignant Disease

Immunosuppression increases the risk of developing malignant disease; this is thought to be, in part, the result of impaired immune surveillance. Skin cancer (mostly squamous cell) has the highest incidence of any type of malignancy among transplant recipients. With continuous surveillance and aggressive management, metastasis from skin cancers is rare. Transplant recipients are also at high risk for development of non-Hodgkin's lymphoma and Kaposi's sarcoma. In addition to age-appropriate screening, cancer surveillance should be an essential part of post-transplantation care.

PROGNOSIS

The prognosis of CKD varies depending on the underlying cause, severity at presentation, and response to therapy. Moreover, CKD in general is a significant risk factor for cardiovascular disease and death. Mortality from cardiovascular disease in CKD patients, especially those with stage 3 to stage 5 disease, is 3.5 times that of an age-matched population (E-Fig. 32-8), accounting for more than 50% of the deaths in ESRD patients. Research to understand the underlying mechanisms and final pathway, as well as those effects specific to patients with unique characteristics, are necessary to advance efforts to reduce related risks and cure kidney disease.

 For a deeper discussion on this topic, please see Chapter 130, "Chronic Kidney Disease," in Goldman-Cecil Medicine, *25th Edition.*

SUGGESTED READINGS

Abbate M, Remuzzi G: Progression of renal insufficiency: mechanisms. In Massry SG, Glassock RJ, editors: Massry and Glassock's textbook of nephrology, ed 4, Philadelphia, 2001, Lippincott, Williams & Wilkins, pp 1210–1217.

Coresh J, Selvin E, Stevens LA, et al: Prevalence of chronic kidney disease in the United States, JAMA 298:2038–2047, 2007.

Durrbach A, Francois H, Beaudreuil S, et al: Advances in immunosuppression for renal transplantation, Nat Rev Nephrol 6:160–167, 2010.

Kidney Disease: Improving Global Outcomes (KDIGO) CKD Work Group: KDIGO 2012 clinical practice guideline for the evaluation and management of chronic kidney disease, Kid Intl Suppl 3:1–150, 2013.

National Kidney Foundation: K/DOQI clinical practice guidelines and clinical practice recommendations for diabetes and chronic kidney disease, Am J Kidney Dis 49(2 Suppl 2):S12–S154, 2007.

Rubin RH, Marty FM: Principles of antimicrobial therapy in the transplant patient [editorial], Transpl Infect Dis 6:97–100, 2004.

Sarnak MJ, Levey AS, Schoolwerth AC, et al: Kidney disease as a risk factor for development of cardiovascular disease: a statement from the American Heart Association Councils on Kidney in Cardiovascular Disease, High Blood Pressure Research, Clinical Cardiology, and Epidemiology and Prevention, Circulation 108:2154–2169, 2003.

U.S. Renal Data System: USRDS 2013 annual data report: atlas of chronic kidney disease and end-stage renal disease in the United States, Bethesda, Md., 2013, National Institutes of Health, National Institute of Diabetes and Digestive and Kidney Diseases.

Vincenti F, Larsen C, Durrbach A, et al: Costimulation blockade with belatacept in renal transplantation, N Engl J Med 353:770–781, 2005.

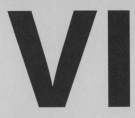

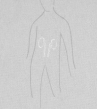
ESSENTIALS

VI

Gastrointestinal Disease

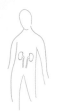

Common Clinical Manifestations of Gastrointestinal Disease

M. Michael Wolfe

A. Abdominal Pain

Charles M. Bliss, Jr. and M. Michael Wolfe

● DEFINITION AND EPIDEMIOLOGY

Abdominal pain is a frequent manifestation of intra-abdominal disease. However, abdominal pain is difficult to localize or grade because the sensation of pain often is colored by emotional and physical factors. Abdominal pain may be classified as acute or chronic. Acute pain occurs suddenly and more often suggests serious physiologic alterations. Chronic pain may be present for several months; although it does not mandate immediate attention, chronic pain may lead to prolonged evaluation. According to a recent report, abdominal pain is the most common symptom in patients presenting to gastroenterology clinics in the U.S., with almost 16 million estimated visits in 2009 alone. Appropriate evaluation of abdominal pain requires knowledge of pain mechanisms, close attention to history and physical examination findings, and recognition of important accompanying symptoms as well as awareness of the strengths and weaknesses of the tests that might be used.

● PHYSIOLOGY

Abdominal pain results from stimulation of receptors specific for thermal, mechanical, or chemical stimuli. Once these receptors are excited, pain impulses travel through sympathetic fibers. Abdominal pain can be characterized as somatic or visceral. Somatic pain originates from the abdominal wall and parietal peritoneum, whereas visceral pain originates in internal organs and from the visceral peritoneum. Two types of neurons carry pain: A fibers, which have rapid conduction, and C fibers, which have slow conduction. Most visceral neurons are of the C type, and the pain resulting from their stimulation tends to be variable with regard to sensation and localization. In contrast, both A and C fibers originate from the parietal peritoneum and abdominal wall, and somatic pain tends to be sharp and distinctly localized.

Because of this pattern of innervation, abdominal viscera are not sensitive to cutting, tearing, burning, or crushing. However, visceral pain results from stretching of the walls of hollow organs or of the capsule of solid organs, as well as from inflammation or ischemia.

● CAUSES OF ABDOMINAL PAIN

Multiple intra-abdominal and extra-abdominal disorders can produce abdominal pain. Distinguishing acute from chronic

symptoms is helpful. The approach varies with each specific cause, but acute abdominal pain usually demands prompt intervention.

● CLINICAL PRESENTATION
History

The differential diagnosis of abdominal pain, whether acute or chronic, requires thorough history taking with regard to pain characteristics, location and radiation, timing, and the presence of any accompanying symptoms. Recognition of characteristic patterns is essential to narrowing the differential diagnosis.

Pain location often indicates the organ responsible for the problem. For instance, epigastric pain is usually typical of peptic ulcer or dyspepsia, whereas right upper quadrant pain is more suggestive of cholecystitis and other biliary disorders. Early in the course of illness, pain may be perceived in one location and subsequently felt in another; this pattern of progression may be suggestive of specific pain syndromes. In acute cases, abdominal pain tends to be sharp and severe. The pain of a perforated viscus is intense, and the pain from a dissecting aneurysm may be described as tearing or crushing. Chronic pain may be less severe; pain from irritable bowel or dyspepsia is constant and dull, and the pain of chronic peptic ulcer is described as gnawing or hunger pain. The pattern of pain relief is helpful for diagnosing some conditions. The physician should also inquire about whether the pain is steady or intermittent and whether it occurs at night. For nocturnal pain, a distinction should be made between pain that awakens the patient and pain that is felt when the patient wakes up for other reasons.

Table 33-1 outlines characteristics, location, and radiation of pain for a few common acute and chronic abdominal conditions.

Physical Examination

Examination of the abdomen provides valuable clues to the diagnosis, but the examination should start with the general appearance of the patient. A patient who is writhing in bed and unable to find a comfortable position may be suffering from obstruction. In contrast, a patient lying with the lower extremities flexed and

TABLE 33-1	KEY ABDOMINAL PAIN SYNDROMES		
CONDITION	**TYPE**	**LOCATION**	**RADIATION**
ACUTE ABDOMINAL PAIN			
Appendicitis	Crampy, steady	Periumbilical, RLQ	Back
Cholecystitis	Intermittent, steady	Epigastric, RUQ	Right scapula
Pancreatitis	Steady	Epigastric, periumbilical	Back
Perforation	Sudden, severe	Epigastric	Entire abdomen
Obstruction	Crampy	Periumbilical	Back
Infarction	Severe, diffuse	Periumbilical	Entire abdomen
CHRONIC ABDOMINAL PAIN			
Esophagitis	Burning	Retrosternal	Left arm, back
Peptic ulcer	Gnawing	Epigastric	Back
Dyspepsia	Bloating, dull	Epigastric	None
IBS	Crampy	LLQ, RLQ	None

IBS, Irritable bowel syndrome; LLQ, left lower quadrant; RLQ, right lower quadrant; RUQ, right upper quadrant.

avoiding any motion may be suffering from peritonitis because movement makes peritoneal pain worse. Abdominal distention indicates obstruction or ascites. Visual inspection for peristalsis is helpful for the diagnosis of small bowel obstruction, but this sign is present only in the early stages. Focal areas of distention may indicate hernias; notice should also be taken of any scars from prior surgeries.

Auscultation should be performed in several areas to evaluate the timbre and pattern of bowel sounds and to search for bruits or hums. Absence of bowel sounds suggests ileus, whereas the presence of hyperactive, high-pitched sounds may indicate obstruction. Multiple bruits alert the examiner to the possibility of significant vascular disease, suggesting ischemia.

The abdomen should be palpated gently, starting in an area away from the pain. The examiner searches for areas of localized tenderness and rebound as well as for masses and enlarged organs. Percussion is performed to identify the size of organs or to determine the presence of ascites. Pain on percussion of the abdomen indicates peritoneal reaction, as does severe rebound tenderness.

A rectal examination is important for identifying a rectal tumor in the case of colon obstruction or tenderness high in the rectum in acute appendicitis. A pelvic examination should be performed in women to rule out pelvic inflammatory disease.

ACUTE ABDOMEN

The evaluation of a patient with an acute abdomen is a challenge in medical practice. The acute abdomen is caused by sudden inflammation, perforation, obstruction, or infarction of an intra-abdominal organ. The urgent question to be answered is whether immediate surgery is needed; a quick but complete evaluation is necessary to avoid undue delay in intervention for patients who require surgery. The physician must assess for abdominal tenderness, rebound, and guarding. Early surgical consultation should be obtained, even in doubtful cases, rather than awaiting confirmation of the diagnosis via laboratory or radiologic studies. However, many extra-abdominal conditions such as pneumonia, myocardial infarction, nephrolithiasis, and metabolic disorders can cause acute abdominal pain.

In some instances of the acute abdomen in its early stages, there are few findings. The examiner should be aware that patients with benign chronic conditions may have severe pain at presentation that is out of proportion to any physical findings. The context provided by the medical history, particularly previous abdominal surgery, is very valuable. Indeed, a patient with sudden crampy pain and abdominal distention may have an intestinal obstruction caused by adhesions or an incarcerated hernia. Therefore, examination of the entire patient, looking for jaundice, skin lesions, evidence of prior surgery, or evidence of chronic liver disease, is important.

In evaluating a patient with acute abdominal symptoms, a complete blood cell count with differential, a urinalysis, and measurements of serum amylase, lipase, bilirubin, and electrolytes are necessary components of the laboratory examination. Additional studies may be done but usually do not aid in the rapid decision making required. An elevated white blood cell count may indicate inflammatory disease, and extremely high values are typical of acute intestinal ischemia. An elevated serum amylase concentration usually indicates acute pancreatitis, although a perforated ulcer or mesenteric thrombosis can also cause hyperamylasemia.

Radiographic examination with an abdominal film is important to reveal the intra-abdominal gas pattern, and an upright film that includes the diaphragm or a left lateral decubitus film may identify intra-abdominal air suggesting perforation of a hollow viscus. Ultrasonography can be helpful in the diagnosis of acute cholecystitis or appendicitis. Computed tomography (CT) scans have become more helpful with technologic improvements in scanners; early CT scans allow prompt diagnosis of sometimes unsuspected abdominal diseases. Examination with a radiopaque medium should be used judiciously, especially if surgery is anticipated. E-Figures 33-1 through 33-4 are CT images of appendicitis, diverticulitis, pancreatitis, and ulcerative colitis, respectively.

CHRONIC ABDOMINAL PAIN

In the evaluation of chronic abdominal pain, it can be challenging to distinguish between organic pain resulting from a specific pathologic process and functional pain. The location and characteristics of pain, as already discussed, serve as important guides, as do other accompanying symptoms. The presence of postprandial nausea and vomiting suggests chronic peptic ulcer, disorders of gastric emptying, or outlet obstruction. Documentation of weight loss mandates the search for an organic cause, such as inflammatory bowel disease or celiac disease. If anorexia accompanies weight loss, particularly in elderly patients, cancer must be excluded. If no cancer can be found and all objective tests are normal, the possibility of chronic depression must be entertained.

The most frequent causes of chronic abdominal pain are functional. Dyspepsia is characterized by chronic intermittent epigastric discomfort, sometimes accompanied by nausea or bloating. These symptoms are not always relieved by acid suppression and may be the result of an underlying motor disorder. Furthermore, when *Helicobacter pylori* is found in a patient with dyspeptic symptoms, its eradication may not necessarily lead to the resolution of symptoms. Controversy exists regarding the most

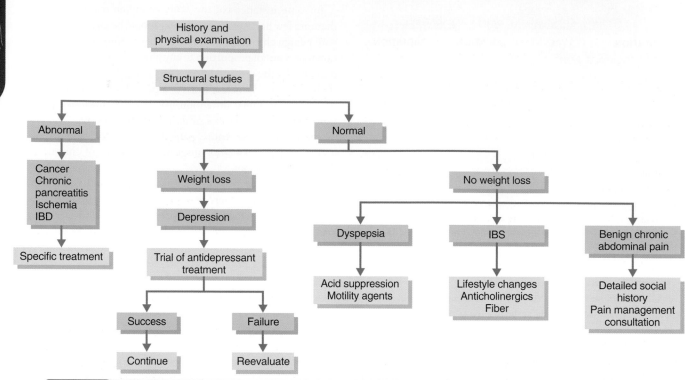

FIGURE 33-1 Approach to the patient with chronic abdominal pain. IBD, Inflammatory bowel disease; IBS, irritable bowel syndrome.

effective strategy for the treatment of dyspepsia when *H. pylori* organisms are found in the absence of peptic ulcer disease.

Irritable bowel syndrome (IBS) is a very common disorder. Estimates are that 15% of Americans suffer from IBS on a regular basis and that 40% to 50% of referrals to gastroenterologists are related to IBS. The syndrome consists of abdominal distention, flatulence, and disordered bowel function. The abdominal pain of IBS tends to be in the left lower quadrant, but it can be located elsewhere or be more generalized. Any patient with weight loss, anemia, nocturnal symptoms, steatorrhea, or onset of symptoms after age 50 years should be evaluated carefully for organic disease because these symptoms are not associated with IBS.

The Rome criteria, developed for research studies, may be helpful in the diagnosis of IBS. These criteria include pain that is associated with change in bowel habits, relieved with defecation, or accompanied by distention or bloating. Patients are reassured, counseled, and treated with anticholinergic agents and stool softeners. Although serotonin (5-HT) agonists such as alosetron and tegaserod showed promise initially, they have been relegated to limited use due to unacceptable side effects. Linaclotide is a new agent for chronic constipation and IBS with constipation (IBS-C). This medication causes increased secretion of chloride and bicarbonate into the intestinal lumen via a cyclic guanosine monophosphate (cGMP) pathway. This pathway also may be responsible for relief of visceral pain in patients with IBS-C.

The more challenging clinical problem is *functional abdominal pain syndrome*. This term describes a condition in which the pain has been present for months or years. The complaints of pain often are not related to eating, defecation, or menses, unlike other causes of chronic pain. The patient is most likely to be a woman who has undergone numerous examinations and diagnostic studies with negative findings and, in many cases, surgical operations without any relief. Lengthy or repeated diagnostic work-ups are counterproductive and only convince the patient that one more test is what is needed to determine the source of the pain. The physician must establish that organic disease is not present and must also realize that the pain is real. These patients are not malingerers despite the fact that the pain does not fit any familiar pattern. Depression may be the result rather than the cause of the pain.

Management of chronic abdominal pain is demanding and requires as much tact, diplomacy, and compassion as scientific knowledge. An effort should be made to inquire about social factors, including history of physical and sexual abuse, particularly in women. Psychiatric evaluation may be necessary, but the suggestion for such a consultation may be interpreted by the patient as evidence that the physician believes "the pain is in my head." Referral to a competent pain management specialist is helpful in some cases. This approach offers the possibility of providing relief with nerve blocks if the pain is localized or with other pain-relieving devices. If this approach fails, referral to a psychologist or psychiatrist may be acceptable to the patient.

The algorithm in Figure 33-1 presents a practical approach to chronic abdominal pain.

For further information, please see Chapter 137, "Functional Gastrointestinal Disorders," in Goldman-Cecil Medicine, *25th Edition.*

B. Gastrointestinal Hemorrhage

D. Roy Ferguson and M. Michael Wolfe

● ACUTE GASTROINTESTINAL HEMORRHAGE

Acute gastrointestinal (GI) bleeding remains a common major medical problem despite recent advances in diagnosis and treatment. Bleeding occurs as a complication of many diverse disease processes, and adequate treatment depends on careful assessment and management that focuses on ensuring hemodynamic stability, determining blood loss, and identifying sources of bleeding. Although advances in medical and surgical intensive care, pharmacologic therapy, and the prompt deployment of endoscopic therapies have significantly decreased the rate of rebleeding, the overall mortality rate from acute bleeding episodes has remained essentially unchanged during the past half-century, at about 5% to 10%, owing to an aging population and an increased prevalence of serious concomitant illnesses.

Clinical Presentation

Significant GI bleeding typically manifests with some combination of weakness, dizziness, lightheadedness, shortness of breath, postural changes in blood pressure or pulse, cramping abdominal pain, and diarrhea. The characteristics of the bleeding may help to localize its source to the upper or lower GI tract. Patients with acute bleeding commonly have one of the following symptoms at presentation.

1. *Hematemesis:* The patient vomits bright red blood or material that resembles coffee grounds, representing partially digested blood. After exclusion of swallowed blood from the nasopharynx or the respiratory tract (hemoptysis), the source of bleeding is likely to be proximal to the ligament of Treitz.
2. *Melena:* Black, tarry, usually foul-smelling stools are most often a manifestation of upper GI bleeding; however, a small bowel or proximal colonic source of bleeding may on occasion lead to melenic stools. Volumes as little as 50 to 100 mL of blood in the stomach can result in melena.
3. *Hematochezia:* The passage of bright-red blood or maroon stools per rectum frequently indicates a lower GI source of bleeding. However, 10% to 15% of patients with acute severe hematochezia have an upper GI source of brisk bleeding. This group of patients commonly displays signs of hemodynamic instability.

Etiology

A major early goal is to distinguish between upper and lower GI sources because the management strategies are different. In addition to the symptoms already described, certain aspects of the history and physical examination, the age of the patient, and results of laboratory studies may be suggestive. However, in many patients, the site of bleeding frequently remains uncertain after the initial evaluation. Common sources of acute GI hemorrhage are listed in Table 33-2.

Approach to the Patient with Acute Gastrointestinal Bleeding

Assessment of Vital Signs and Resuscitation

A simple mnemonic for the approach to gastrointestinal bleeding is *SET:* Stabilization, Evaluation (endoscopy), and Treatment. The first goal in management is to *stabilize the patient* and determine the severity of blood loss (Fig. 33-2). Vital signs with postural changes should be recorded immediately. If the systolic blood pressure drops more than 10 mm Hg or the pulse increases more than 10 beats per minute as the patient changes position from supine to standing, it is likely the patient has lost at least 800 mL (15%) of circulating blood volume. Hypotension, tachycardia, tachypnea, and mental status changes in the setting of acute GI hemorrhage suggest the loss of at least 1500 mL (30%) of circulating blood volume.

The goals of resuscitation are to restore the normal circulatory volume and to prevent complications from red blood cell loss, such as cardiac, pulmonary, renal, or neurologic consequences. Initially, at least two large-bore intravenous catheters are used to administer isotonic solutions (e.g., lactated Ringer's solution, 0.9% NaCl), and blood products if indicated. If the patient is in shock, central venous access should be established. Although the amount of blood to be infused must be individually determined in each case, recent randomized trials and a retrospective review suggest that use of a lower hemoglobin threshold of 7 g/dL, rather than a more liberal level of 9 g/dL, results in improved mortality rates, lower total transfusion requirements, and lower rates of rebleeding in both peptic ulcer bleeding and variceal bleeding in patients in whom early endoscopy (<5 hours) is available. In view of the costs and potential risks of blood transfusion, it is not appropriate to simply transfuse until an arbitrary target hematocrit is achieved. If coagulation studies are abnormal, as is commonly observed in cirrhotic patients, fresh-frozen plasma, platelets, or both may be required to control ongoing hemorrhage.

Initial Evaluation

While resuscitation is underway, the following information should be obtained by history and physical examination to determine the source of bleeding:

1. The nature of the bleeding: melena, hematemesis, hematochezia, or occult blood. A digital rectal examination is essential for determination of stool color and identification of anal fissures or rectal neoplasms.
2. The duration of GI bleeding, which helps dictate the appropriate pace of the evaluation to determine the bleeding source
3. The presence or absence of abdominal pain; for example, hematochezia caused by diverticula or angiodysplasia typically is painless, but hematochezia due to intestinal ischemia it is often accompanied by abdominal pain.

TABLE 33-2 COMMON SOURCES OF ACUTE GASTROINTESTINAL HEMORRHAGE

SOURCE	ASSOCIATED CLINICAL FEATURES	TREATMENTS
UPPER GASTROINTESTINAL TRACT		
Esophagitis	Heartburn, dysphagia, odynophagia	Medication*
		Antireflux surgery or procedures
Esophageal cancer	Progressive dysphagia, weight loss	Chemoradiotherapy, surgery
		Palliative endoscopy procedures
Gastritis, gastric ulcer	Aspirin, NSAID use	Withdraw NSAIDs
Duodenitis, duodenal ulcer	Abdominal pain, dyspepsia, *Helicobacter pylori* infection	Medication†
		Endoscopic therapy for acute bleeding
Gastric cancer	Early satiety, weight loss, abdominal pain	Surgery, chemotherapy
Esophagogastric varices	History of CLD	Variceal banding, sclerotherapy
	Stigmata of CLD on examination	Vasopressin, octreotide
		TIPS or decompressive surgery
Mallory-Weiss tear	History of retching before hematemesis	Supportive (usually self-limited)
		Endoscopic therapy
LOWER GASTROINTESTINAL TRACT		
Infection	History of exposure, diarrhea, fever	Supportive, antibiotics
Inflammatory bowel diseases	History of colitis, diarrhea, abdominal pain, fever	Steroids, 5-ASA, immunotherapy
		Surgery if unresponsive to medication
Diverticula	Painless hematochezia	Supportive
		Surgery for recurrent disease
Angiodysplasia	Painless hematochezia	Endoscopic therapy
	Often in ascending colon	Supportive
	Commonly involves stomach and small bowel as well	Surgery for localized disease
Colon cancer	Change in bowel habit, anemia, weight loss	Surgery
Colon polyp	Usually asymptomatic	Endoscopic or surgical removal
Ischemic colitis	Typically elderly patients	Supportive (self-limited)
	History of vascular disease	
	May produce abdominal pain	
Meckel's diverticulum	Painless hematochezia in young patient Located at distal ileum	Surgery
Hemorrhoids	Rectal bleeding associated with bowel movement	Supportive
		Surgery, banding

CLD, Chronic liver disease; NSAIDs, nonsteroidal anti-inflammatory drugs; TIPS, transjugular intrahepatic shunt; 5-ASA, 5-aminosalicylic acid compounds.

*Proton pump inhibitors or histamine-2 receptor antagonists.

†Proton pump inhibitors or histamine-2 receptor antagonists in the absence of *H. pylori* infection; various combinations of antibiotics, proton pump inhibitors, and bismuth products in the presence of *H. pylori* infection.

4. Other associated symptoms, including fever, urgency or tenesmus, recent change in bowel habits, and weight loss

5. Current or recent medication use, particularly nonsteroidal anti-inflammatory drugs (NSAIDs), including aspirin, which may predispose to ulceration or gastritis (see Chapter 37), anticoagulants, and alcohol. Many over-the-counter products may contain aspirin or NSAIDs.

6. Relevant past medical and surgical history, including a history of prior GI bleeding, abdominal surgery (prior abdominal aorta repair should raise suspicion for an aortoenteric fistula), radiation therapy (radiation proctitis), major organ diseases (including cardiopulmonary, hepatic, or renal disease), inflammatory bowel diseases, and recent polypectomy (postpolypectomy bleeding).

The physical examination must include an assessment of vital signs, cardiac and pulmonary examinations, and abdominal and digital rectal examinations. The initial laboratory examination should include a complete blood cell count, blood typing and cross-matching, and measurements of serum electrolytes, blood urea nitrogen, creatinine, and coagulation factors. The first hematocrit measurement may not reflect the degree of blood loss, but it will decrease gradually to a stable level over 24 to 48 hours.

The initial disposition of the patient must also be considered. Patients older than 60 years of age, those with severe blood loss

or continued bleeding (as reflected by a significant decrease in hematocrit or postural changes in blood pressure or pulse rate), and those with significant comorbid illness are at the greatest risk for complications of GI hemorrhage and are best managed in an intensive care setting until stabilized.

Identification of the Bleeding Source

In 80% to 90% of cases, acute GI hemorrhage resolves spontaneously without recurrence. Nevertheless, it is prudent to localize the bleeding source, especially in those with significant bleeding or comorbidities. Proper identification allows for direct treatment if the bleeding does not spontaneously resolve and for recognition of those patient who are at risk for further bleeding. For example, in a patient with a bleeding gastric or duodenal ulcer, acid suppression with an intravenous proton pump inhibitor may maximize clot stability and enhance platelet aggregation. Proton pump inhibitors, in combination with appropriate endoscopic management, decrease the risks for ulcer rebleeding, need for urgent surgery, and death. Direct visualization of the bleeding site by endoscopy can alter patient management.

Classification systems, such as the Forrest Ulcer Description or the Rockall Scoring System, rely heavily on endoscopic criteria for rebleeding risk stratification. Various stigmata of hemorrhage may be identified within the ulcer crater. Stigmata that carry a high risk for rebleeding include active bleeding (Forrest 1) and the visible presence of a pigmented protuberance (artery) within

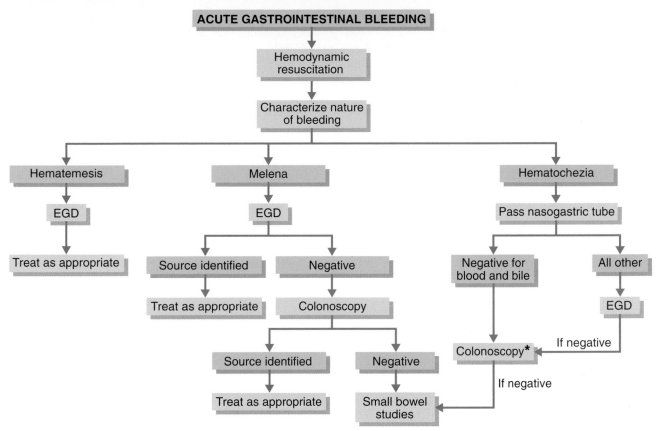

FIGURE 33-2 Approach to the patient with acute gastrointestinal bleeding. EGD, Esophagogastroduodenoscopy. *If severe bleeding prevents endoscopic visualization, arteriography may be performed.

the ulcer crater (Forrest 2). The patient with a "clean base" ulcer exhibiting no such stigmata has an excellent prognosis for cessation of bleeding. Patients found to have high-risk stigmata are likely (~50%) to have continued or recurrent bleeding. In such patients, the site of bleeding may be treated by injection therapy with vasoconstrictors or saline, thermal therapy by electrocautery, or mechanical therapy by placement of endoscopic clips. These endoscopic therapies decrease rates of rebleeding, mortality, need for transfusion, need for surgery, and length of hospital stay. Thermal or mechanical therapy, applied alone or in combination with injection therapy, is more effective than injection therapy alone. Recently developed alternatives, such as hemostatic sprays and cyanoacrylate compounds, offer additional modalities that can be used in such cases.

An overall approach to the patient with acute GI bleeding is outlined in Figure 33-2. Historical points and objective findings often enable localization of the bleeding site to the upper GI tract (proximal to the ligament of Treitz) or to the lower GI tract (distal to that point). For the patient with melena or hematemesis, the upper GI tract should be examined first. Patients with hematochezia more commonly have lower GI bleeding, but when the pace of bleeding is brisk, an upper GI tract lesion may manifest with hematochezia. Placement of a nasogastric tube with aspiration of contents is a reasonable first step. The absence of blood does not by itself rule out the presence of an upper GI source because blood from a duodenal bulb ulcer may not flow back into the stomach to allow sampling by the nasogastric tube. In general, in patients with acute GI hemorrhage who have

significant blood loss, an upper endoscopy should be the initial step in the evaluation.

Once the lower GI tract has been identified as the source of bleeding, sigmoidoscopy or colonoscopy is the test of choice. In cases of lower GI bleeding in which the pace of bleeding is so brisk as to preclude endoscopic visualization of the colon and rectum, scintigraphic erythrocyte scans using technetium-99m (^{99m}Tc)-labeled sulfur colloid or pertechnetate can localize the bleeding site if the rate of blood loss exceeds 0.5 mL/minute. Although the bleeding site identified by scintigraphic examination may not be accurate, it will direct the visceral arteriographic search while minimizing the amount of dye used. The recent description of capsule endoscopy followed by directed push or balloon enteroscopy has provided a possible endoscopic means of delineating and controlling bleeding lesions in the small bowel. There is *no* role for barium studies in the evaluation of acute GI hemorrhage.

CHRONIC GASTROINTESTINAL HEMORRHAGE

Chronic GI bleeding is a diagnostic challenge. It can manifest as self-limited, recurrent episodes of melena or hematochezia, but usually without the degree of hemodynamic compromise discussed earlier. Some patients have no overt evidence of blood loss but rather have persistent anemia and persistent occult blood loss. The evaluation of this condition differs from that of acute GI hemorrhage; the pace of the evaluation is less urgent, and the likely causes of bleeding differ from those associated with acute GI bleeding.

Patients with this condition usually have undergone upper and lower endoscopy at least once without identification of a bleeding source. Therefore, the bleeding must be from a source that is difficult to identify or one that emanates from the small intestine. The small intestine is a difficult area to examine because of its length and configuration. In general, the small intestine is initially evaluated radiographically. The patient may ingest barium, which is followed through the length of the small intestine. To distend the small bowel and provide greater mucosal detail, an enteroclysis tube may be placed with its distal tip near the ligament of Treitz, allowing more forceful administration of barium and air. However, computed tomography and magnetic resonance enterography are rapidly replacing fluoroscopic imaging. All these imaging techniques have limited diagnostic utility. Flat mucosal lesions such as vascular ectasias, a common cause of obscure bleeding, may easily be missed.

If radiographic studies are unrevealing, endoscopic evaluation of the small bowel may be attempted by capsule endoscopy or with push or balloon enteroscopy (see Chapter 34). For the patient with persistent blood loss, no endoscopically identified source of bleeding in the upper GI tract or colon, and negative findings on radiologic studies, the entire small intestine may be examined at laparotomy with endoscopy in the operative suite. In addition, angiographic evaluation of the whole GI tract may reveal the source of chronic blood loss.

C. Malabsorption

Sharmeel K. Wasan, Elihu M. Schimmel, and M. Michael Wolfe

● DEFINITION AND EPIDEMIOLOGY

The main purpose of the gastrointestinal (GI) tract is to digest and absorb major nutrients (fat, carbohydrate, and protein), essential micronutrients (vitamins and trace minerals), water, and electrolytes. Impaired absorption of these nutrients is defined as malabsorption. Under normal conditions, the digestion and absorption of nutrients requires both mechanical and enzymatic breakdown of food. Mechanical processes include chewing, gastric churning, and the to-and-fro mixing in the small intestine. Enzymatic hydrolysis is initiated by intraluminal processes requiring salivary, gastric, pancreatic, and biliary secretions and is completed at the intestinal brush border. The final products of digestion are then absorbed through the intestinal epithelial cells and transported into the portal circulation. The coordinated regulation of gastric emptying, normal intestinal progression, and the presence of adequate intestinal surface area are all important factors. The human gut microbiome, which comprises the communities of microorganisms that inhabit the GI tract, has been recognized to play an important role in nutrient utilization as well. From birth, interactions between the microbiotia and the intestinal mucosa contribute to maturation of the host immune system. Disruptions to the homeostasis between the microbiota and the host immune system can lead to increased inflammation and decreased absorption.

Most dietary components can be absorbed anywhere along the length of the small intestine, but there are important exceptions in which absorption is limited to specific areas (e.g., vitamin B_{12} and cholesterol are absorbed only in the terminal ileum). Diseases associated with diffuse mucosal involvement, such as celiac disease, can lead to impaired absorption of many nutrients, whereas diseases affecting only the terminal ileum can lead to decreased vitamin B_{12} absorption. Bile acids are necessary for fat absorption; they undergo an enterohepatic circulation with release into bile and reabsorption from the terminal small intestine. Diseases interfering with this mechanism deplete the bile acid pool and can lead to fat malabsorption. Water and electrolytes are absorbed primarily by the colon. In addition, there is caloric salvage of much of the carbohydrate from indigestible fiber through bacterial enzymatic activity in the colon. The following sections discuss normal assimilation of the major nutrients and the approach to evaluation of patients with suspected malabsorption.

● DIGESTION AND ABSORPTION OF FAT

Dietary fat is composed predominantly of triglycerides (~95%) with long-chain fatty acids (16- and 18-carbon molecules). In animal fat, the constituent fatty acids are mostly saturated (e.g., palmitic acid, stearic acid), whereas those of vegetable origin are rich in unsaturated fatty acids (i.e., having one or more double bonds in the carbon chain, such as oleic and linoleic acids). Fats are insoluble in water (hydrophobic), and digestion begins with a process of emulsification, wherein larger fat droplets are dispersed in the aqueous medium of the lumen. In the proximal small intestine, bile salts from liver and pancreatic enzymes are released into the intestinal lumen; there, they mix with and bind to the surface of these globules, where colipase activity results in the release of fatty acids and a monoglyceride. These are taken up as mixed micelles with bile salts, and these hydrophobic particles cross the unstirred water layer that overlies the epithelial brush border.

Within the cell, fatty acids are resynthesized into triglycerides, and, together with cholesterol and phospholipids, they are packaged into chylomicrons and very-low-density lipoproteins to be exported via lymphatic channels. Bile salts remain in the intestinal lumen, are recycled into new micelles, and are finally reabsorbed in the terminal ileum with 95% efficiency. Most dietary lipids are absorbed in the jejunum, together with the fat-soluble vitamins A, D, E, and K. It is recommended that dietary fat account for no more than 35% of calories because higher levels are associated with increased risk of cardiac disease, obesity, and some cancers.

● DIGESTION AND ABSORPTION OF CARBOHYDRATES

Most dietary carbohydrates consist of starch (a glucose polymer) and the disaccharides sucrose and lactose, but only monosaccharides are absorbed. Salivary and pancreatic amylases release oligosaccharides from starch. The final hydrolysis to glucose monomers occurs at the brush border and includes disaccharide hydrolysis by sucrase and lactase. Glucose and galactose are actively transported in conjunction with sodium, whereas fructose absorption occurs by facilitated diffusion. About one half of dietary energy is derived from carbohydrate, with a nutritional goal of 55% and an increased component of insoluble fiber (i.e., that which is indigestible by mammalian enzymes but variably broken down by colonic bacteria.)

● DIGESTION AND ABSORPTION OF PROTEINS

Dietary proteins are the major source for amino acids and the only source for the essential amino acids. Digestion starts in the stomach with pepsins secreted by the gastric mucosa, but most of the hydrolysis is accomplished by pancreatic enzymes in the proximal small bowel. The pancreas secretes the proteases trypsin, elastase, chymotrypsin, and carboxypeptidase as inactive proenzymes. Enterokinase (more properly, enteropeptidase) is secreted by the intestinal brush border; it splits trypsinogen to its active form, trypsin, which in turn converts the other proenzymes to their active forms. The products of luminal brush border peptidase digestion consist of amino acids and oligopeptides, which are transported across the epithelial cell. The transfer of most amino acids is sodium dependent and takes place in the proximal small bowel. Dietary requirements for amino acid nitrogen are met with about 15% of calories from protein.

● MECHANISMS OF MALABSORPTION

The term *maldigestion* refers to defective hydrolysis of nutrients, whereas *malabsorption* refers to impaired mucosal absorption. In clinical practice, however, *malabsorption* refers to all aspects of impaired nutrient assimilation. Malabsorption can involve multiple nutrients, or it can be more selective. Therefore, the clinical manifestations of malabsorption are highly variable. The complete process of absorption consists of a *luminal phase*, in which various nutrients are hydrolyzed and solubilized; a *mucosal phase*, in which further processing takes place at the brush border of the epithelial cell with subsequent transfer into the cell; and a *transport phase*, in which nutrients are moved from the epithelium to the portal venous or lymphatic circulation. Impairment in any of these phases can result in malabsorption (Table 33-3).

Luminal Phase

Digestion is accomplished for the most part by pancreatic enzymes, particularly lipase, colipase, and trypsin; the gastric digestive enzymes do not play a major role. As a consequence, chronic pancreatitis can result in malabsorption, particularly for fat and protein. Deficiency in bile salts also contributes to fat malabsorption and may result from cholestatic liver disorders (impaired secretion of bile), bacterial overgrowth (resulting in luminal bile salt deconjugation), or ileal disease or resection with loss of effective enterohepatic circulation of the bile acids. The major part of the luminal phase of digestion occurs in the duodenum and the proximal jejunum.

Mucosal Phase

Mucosal disease is a more common cause of malabsorption. It can result from diffuse small intestinal diseases such as celiac disease or Crohn's disease or from a decrease in surface area (e.g., after surgical resection for small bowel infarction). The net effect is a smaller effective mucosal surface and a relative loss of mucosal absorption. Selective defects in an otherwise normal intestine may result in specific entities such as lactase deficiency or abetalipoproteinemia.

Transport Phase

After absorption, nutrients leave the cells through venous or lymphatic channels. Consequently, malabsorption may be associated with mesenteric venous obstruction, lymphangiectasia, or lymphatic obstruction due to malignancy or infiltrative processes such as Whipple's disease.

TABLE 33-3 PATHOPHYSIOLOGIC MECHANISMS IN MALABSORPTION

LUMINAL PHASE	MUCOSAL PHASE	TRANSPORT PHASE
Reduced nutrient availability	Extensive mucosal loss (resection or infarction)	Vascular conditions (vasculitis; atheroma)
Cofactor deficiency (pernicious anemia; gastric surgery)	Diffuse mucosal disease (celiac disease)	Lymphatic conditions (lymphangiectasia; irradiation; nodal tumor, cavitation, or infiltrations)
Nutrient consumption (bacterial overgrowth)	Crohn's disease; irradiation; infection; infiltrations; drugs: alcohol, colchicine, neomycin, iron salts	
Impaired fat solubilization	Brush border hydrolase deficiency (lactase deficiency)	
Reduced bile salt synthesis (hepatocellular disease)	Transport defects (Hartnup cystinuria; vitamin B_{12} and folate uptake)	
Impaired bile salt secretion (chronic cholestasis)	Epithelial processing (abetalipoproteinemia)	
Bile salt inactivation (bacterial overgrowth)		
Impaired cholecystokinin release (mucosal disease)		
Increased bile salt losses (terminal ileal disease or resection)		
Defective nutrient hydrolysis		
Lipase inactivation (Zollinger-Ellison syndrome)		
Enzyme deficiency (pancreatic insufficiency or cancer)		
Improper mixing or rapid transit (resection; bypass; hyperthyroidism)		

Modified from Riley SA, Marsh MN: Maldigestion and malabsorption. In Feldman M, Scharschmidt BF, Sleisenger MH, editors: Sleisenger and Fordtran's gastrointestinal and liver disease: pathophysiology/diagnosis/management, ed 6, Philadelphia, 1998, WB Saunders, pp 1501–1522.

The absorptive process can be impaired at many stages. For example, patients with subtotal gastrectomy or bariatric surgery often experience malabsorption. There are resultant defects at all phases: impaired gastric churning, premature emptying, and impaired mixing (in the jejunum) of food with bile and pancreatic enzymes. The impaired mixing is a consequence of anatomic changes (gastrojejunostomy bypassing the duodenum) and reduced production of pancreatic enzymes (because cholecystokinin and secretin release is blunted when gastric contents bypass the duodenum). Moreover, stasis may lead to bacterial overgrowth in the afferent loop with changes in the bile acids needed for fat absorption. Another example of manifold mechanisms is diabetes mellitus, which may lead to delayed gastric emptying, abnormal intestinal motility, bacterial overgrowth, and pancreatic exocrine insufficiency.

CLINICAL PRESENTATION

The clinical manifestations of malabsorption are usually nonspecific, particularly in the early stages. A change in bowel movements, usually with diarrhea, and weight loss despite adequate food intake may occur in more severe cases. Usually, however, patients have relatively mild symptoms such as bloating and flatulence. Clinical manifestations related to a specific micronutrient deficiency can occur. For example, iron deficiency anemia may be the only manifestation of celiac disease in some patients. Muscle wasting and edema result from protein malabsorption. Nutritional anemia, caused by deficiencies of iron, folate, and vitamin B_{12}, contributes to fatigue. Bleeding tendency (e.g., ecchymosis) may be attributed to prolonged prothrombin time resulting from vitamin K deficiency related to fat malabsorption. Bulky, oily stools are the hallmark of steatorrhea resulting from fat malabsorption, whereas bloating (abdominal distention) and soft diarrheal movements occur as a result of carbohydrate malabsorption. Signs associated with malabsorption are presented in Table 33-4.

DIAGNOSIS

Malabsorption can be caused by a large number of disorders, and some of the more common of which are listed in Table 33-4. The cause of malabsorption can often be determined by a very detailed patient history. However, because the clinical symptoms are varied, more specific assays of albumin, cobalamin, iron, cholesterol, calcium, folic acid, and prothrombin time are useful to support the diagnosis of malabsorption. These tests are helpful in assessing the severity of malabsorption, but they are not specific for the differential diagnosis. Many tests are available in the work-up of malabsorption; those that have been most useful clinically are discussed in the following sections (Fig. 33-3).

Fecal Fat Analysis

If fat malabsorption is suspected, the simplest qualitative method for detecting fat in stool is microscopic examination with Sudan staining of a drop of stool. Sensitivity is limited, but the test is quick and easy, and it correlates well with the quantitative measurement of fecal fat when moderate to severe steatorrhea is present. To quantify fat, stool is collected for three consecutive days while the patient is on a diet containing 100 g of fat per day,

TABLE 33-4 SIGNS ASSOCIATED WITH MALABSORPTION SYNDROMES

SIGNS	ASSOCIATED SYNDROMES
GASTROINTESTINAL	
Mass	Crohn's disease, lymphoma, tuberculosis, glands
Distention	Intestinal obstruction, gas, ascites, pseudocyst (pancreatic), motility disorder
Steatorrheic stool	Mucosal disease, bacterial overgrowth, pancreatic insufficiency, infective or inflammatory, drug induced
EXTRAINTESTINAL	
Skin	
Nonspecific	Pigmentation, thinning, inelasticity, reduced subcutaneous fat
Specific	Blisters (dermatitis herpetiformis), erythema nodosum (Crohn's disease), petechiae (vitamin K deficiency), edema (hypoproteinemia)
Hair	
Alopecia	Gluten sensitivity
Loss or thinning	Generalized inanition, hypothyroidism, gluten sensitivity
Eyes	
Conjunctivitis, episcleritis	Crohn's disease, Behçet's syndrome
Paleness	Severe anemia
Mouth	
Aphthous ulcers	Crohn's disease, gluten sensitivity, Behçet's syndrome
Glossitis	Deficiencies of vitamin B_{12}, iron, folate, niacin
Angular cheilosis	Deficiencies of vitamin B_{12}, iron, folate, B complex
Dental hypoplasia (pitting, dystrophy)	Gluten sensitivity
Hands	
Raynaud's phenomenon	Scleroderma
Finger clubbing	Crohn's disease, lymphoma
Koilonychia	Iron deficiency
Leukonychia	Inanition
Musculoskeletal	
Monoarthropathy and polyarthropathy	Crohn's disease, gluten sensitivity, Whipple's disease, Behçet's syndrome
Back pain (osteomalacia, osteoporosis, sacroiliitis)	Crohn's disease, malnutrition, gluten sensitivity
Muscle weakness (low potassium, magnesium, vitamin D, generalized inanition)	Diffuse mucosal disease, bacterial overgrowth, lymphoma
Nervous System	
Peripheral neuropathy (weakness, paresthesias, numbness)	Vitamin B_{12} deficiency
Cerebral (seizures, dementia, intracerebral calcification, meningitis, pseudotumor, cranial nerve palsies)	Whipple's disease, gluten sensitivity, diffuse lymphoma

From Riley SA, Marsh MN: Maldigestion and malabsorption. In Feldman M, Scharschmidt BF, Sleisenger MH, editors: Sleisenger and Fordtran's gastrointestinal and liver disease: pathophysiology/diagnosis/management, ed 6, Philadelphia, 1998, WB Saunders, pp 1501–1522.

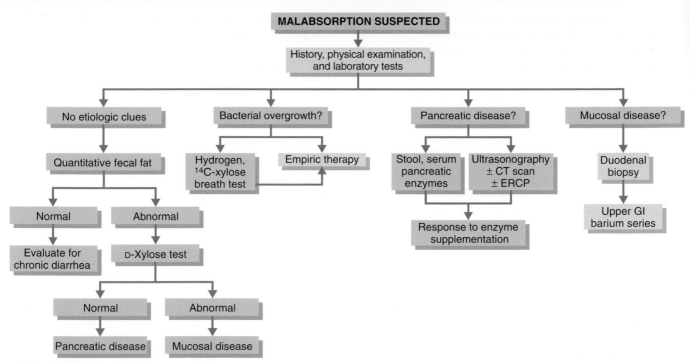

FIGURE 33-3 Approach to the patient with suspected malabsorption. CT, Computed tomography; ERCP, endoscopic retrograde cholangiopancrea-tography; GI, gastrointestinal. (Modified from Riley SA, Marsh MN: Maldigestion and malabsorption. In Feldman M, Scharschmidt BF, Sleisenger MH, editors: Sleisenger and Fordtran's gastrointestinal and liver disease: pathophysiology/diagnosis/management, ed 6, Philadelphia, 1998, WB Saunders, pp 1501–1522.)

and the specimen is analyzed for fat content. Normal fat excretion should not exceed 6 g/day. Although this test is cumbersome and nonspecific, it offers an accurate quantification of fecal fat excretion provided fat consumption is appropriate.

Tests of Pancreatic Exocrine Function

Aspiration of duodenal contents for evaluation of bicarbonate and enzyme output after stimulation of the pancreas may be the best index of pancreatic exocrine function. However, the test is invasive, is time-consuming, and is performed only in a few specialized centers. The measurement of pancreatic enzymes (i.e., fecal elastase 1) in the stool is simple and provides helpful laboratory evidence for the diagnosis of moderate to severe pancreatitic insufficiency. Pancreatic calcifications seen on abdominal films or computed tomography (CT) scans indicate the presence of chronic pancreatitis. Magnetic resonance cholangiopancreatography (MRCP) and endoscopic retrograde cholangiopancreatography (ERCP) can help outline abnormal duct anatomy and may supplement CT scanning for diagnostic purposes to evaluate the sequelae of chronic pancreatitis. However, normal findings on pancreatography do not exclude the presence of pancreatic exocrine insufficiency.

Small Intestinal Biopsy

Whereas the gross appearance of the mucosa during upper GI endoscopy can provide some clues regarding the presence of a disease causing malabsorption, biopsy of the small intestinal mucosal is a key diagnostic test for diseases that affect the cellular phase of absorption. In some diseases, the histologic features are diagnostic; in others, the findings may be highly suggestive (Table 33-5). Several tissue samples should be taken from the

TABLE 33-5 UTILITY OF SMALL BOWEL BIOPSY SPECIMENS IN MALABSORPTION

FINDINGS OFTEN DIAGNOSTIC	FINDINGS ABNORMAL BUT NOT DIAGNOSTIC
Whipple's disease	
Amyloidosis	Celiac disease
Eosinophilic enteritis	Systemic sclerosis
Lymphangiectasia	Radiation enteritis
Primary intestinal lymphoma	Bacterial overgrowth syndrome
Giardiasis	Tropical sprue
Abetalipoproteinemia	Crohn's disease
Agammaglobulinemia	
Mastocytosis	

Data from Trier JS: Diagnostic value of peroral biopsy of the proximal small intestine, N Engl J Med 285:1470, 1971.

duodenal bulb and from the distal duodenum to enhance the diagnostic accuracy.

Imaging Studies

In patients with malabsorption, barium studies of the small bowel are usually nonspecific. Occasionally, however, distinct anatomic changes are seen, such as in jejunal diverticulosis, lymphoma, Crohn's disease, strictures, or enteric fistulas. Also, there may be a distinctive barium pattern of thin-walled, dilated loops suggestive of celiac disease. CT and magnetic resonance enterography provide a more detailed imaging of the small intestine and are more sensitive in identifying abnormalities such as active bowel inflammation, mesenteric stranding and edema, strictures, fibrofatty proliferation of the mesentery, and fistula formation.

Wireless capsule endoscopy is a noninvasive method that permits direct visualization of the small bowel mucosa and can provide a more detailed evaluation of small bowel disease compared with radiographic studies. However, capsule endoscopy should be avoided in patients in whom a stricture is suspected because of the risk of retention. The detection of mucosal lesions by the capsule endoscopy can often be followed by deep enteroscopy (double-balloon endoscopy, single-balloon endoscopy, or spiral enteroscopy), allowing for tissue biopsy, tattoo placement before surgery, balloon dilatation, and foreign body retrieval.

Schilling Test

Vitamin B_{12} is an essential micronutrient, and its absorption requires several steps. First, the ingested vitamin binds to salivary R-factor protein. In the stomach, gastric parietal cells secrete intrinsic factor, which mixes with the ingested meal. In the duodenum, pancreatic trypsin hydrolyzes the R protein, freeing the vitamin to bind with intrinsic factor. The vitamin B_{12}–intrinsic factor complex is then absorbed by specific receptors that are found only on enterocytes in the distal ileum. Malabsorption of vitamin B_{12} can occur because of lack of intrinsic factor (e.g., pernicious anemia, gastric resection), pancreatic insufficiency, bacterial overgrowth, or ileal resection or mucosal disease (e.g., Crohn's disease).

The Schilling test quantifies vitamin B_{12} absorption using radiolabeled vitamin B_{12} as a marker. The test may be expanded to several stages to amplify its diagnostic spectrum. In stage 1, after the injection of 1000 µg of unlabeled vitamin B_{12} to saturate hepatic storage, the patient ingests 0.5 µg of radiolabeled vitamin. Urine is then collected for the measurement of radioactivity; reduced radioactivity suggests B_{12} malabsorption. The test is repeated (stage 2) with the addition of oral intrinsic factor to the ingested vitamin B_{12}. If urinary excretion of the radiolabel is corrected, pernicious anemia is diagnosed. If malabsorption is still present, the patient is given a short course of oral antibiotics (stage 3), and the test is repeated; correction of radiolabeled B_{12} excretion establishes bacterial overgrowth. If the test result remains abnormal, oral pancreatic enzymes are given (stage 4), and the test is repeated; correction of the abnormality at this stage implies pancreatic deficiency. Finally, if all these interventions fail, ileal disease or absence of transcobalamin protein is determined by other diagnostic tests. This long outline serves is merely an example of an algorithm of clinical analysis; the usual routine in clinical settings is to administer parenteral vitamin B_{12} while the etiology is delineated by other modalities.

D-Xylose Test

The D-xylose test serves as an indicator of mucosal absorption in the proximal small bowel and is used to determine whether defects in the epithelium of the intestine are responsible for malabsorption. D-Xylose is a 5-carbon monosaccharide that is transported across the intestinal mucosa largely by passive diffusion. In this test, the subject ingests 25 g of D-xylose, and urine is collected for the next 5 hours. Healthy subjects excrete more than 4.5 g of D-xylose in 5 hours (or ≥20% of the ingested load). Excretion of a lower amount of D-xylose suggests abnormal absorption. However, an abnormally low (false-positive) result may occur in the presence of impaired renal excretory function, gastroparesis, massive peripheral edema, or ascites. Abnormal results can also be seen in the presence of bacterial overgrowth

as a result of bacterial degradation of D-xylose in the lumen, but this "pseudomalabsorption" may be corrected after treatment with antibiotics serving as a therapeutic trial.

Breath Tests

Breath tests rely on bacterial degradation of luminal compounds, which releases metabolic byproduct gases (e.g., hydrogen, methane, carbon dioxide) that can be measured in the exhaled breath. In the case of disaccharidase deficiency, a specific disaccharide (e.g., lactose) that is orally ingested but not properly absorbed in the small intestine is delivered to the colon, where bacterial fermentation liberates metabolites; hydrogen gas is the marker assayed in the breath. In the presence of bacterial overgrowth of the small intestine, orally ingested glucose ferments in the proximal small bowel (instead of being absorbed), resulting in increased hydrogen in the breath; here, the timing of exhaled hydrogen aids in the diagnosis. The measurement of radioactive carbon dioxide in the breath after ingestion of a nutrient labeled with carbon 14 (^{14}C) has been used to estimate the malabsorption of fat or bile acids and for measurement of bacterial overgrowth (^{14}C-xylose). The radioactive tests are cumbersome, and their usefulness in clinical practice is limited.

The overlap of symptoms and the large number of diagnostic tests available for evaluation of malabsorption necessitate the use of a systematic approach and a rational algorithm (see Fig. 33-3). The most accurate test for fat malabsorption remains the 72-hour fecal fat analysis; however, the test is difficult to carry out in clinical practice. Surrogate screening for steatorrhea is done with the qualitative stool fat examination (Sudan stain) and measurement of serum carotene. If the stool fat content is normal, the patient may still have selective impairment of absorption of a specific carbohydrate. This latter condition should be suspected if the primary symptoms are cramps, flatulence, and diarrhea. The most common example of carbohydrate malabsorption is lactose intolerance; specific tests include the oral lactose tolerance test, but measurement of breath hydrogen is more sensitive and more specific.

More generally, an osmotic gap in fecal water suggests a dietary (rather than a secretory) cause of the diarrhea related to luminal short-chain fatty acids or carbohydrates. The osmotic gap is calculated by the following formula:

$$\text{Osmotic gap} = \text{Plasma osmolality} - [2 \times (\text{fecal}[Na^+] + \text{fecal}[K^+])]$$

The osmotic gap is not calculated by directly measuring stool osmolality because it increases with time in the specimen container. In addition, luminal osmolality is equal to serum osmolality because the colon cannot establish a gradient against the serum concentration of solutes.

When fat malabsorption is demonstrated (>6 g/24 hours, or increased qualitative stool fat and decreased serum carotene), a D-xylose absorption-excretion test should be performed next. A normal D-xylose test result makes diffuse mucosal disease unlikely and suggests maldigestion, principally pancreatic enzyme or bile salt deficiency. Clues to chronic pancreatitis include a history of alcohol abuse or previous episodes of pancreatitis. Unusual causes of pancreatic malabsorption, such as cystic fibrosis, microlithiasis, or drug toxicity, require specific testing and a detailed history. Serum enzyme tests and abdominal imaging (plain films or, with much greater sensitivity, abdominal CT scans) can be obtained next to identify pancreatic disease. If the urinary D-xylose excretion is abnormal, the breath hydrogen test may be used to diagnose bacterial overgrowth using glucose for the carbohydrate load. If no bacterial overgrowth is present, a mucosal biopsy should be performed (see Table 33-5). Imaging studies of the small bowel may be helpful on occasion.

If the cause of malabsorption remains unclear, other considerations should include parasitic infection, such *Giardia lamblia*, or ascariasis involvement of the pancreatic duct (more common in undeveloped countries). These diagnoses require a careful stool examination for ova and parasites or fecal antigen studies.

● TREATMENT

The specific treatment of malabsorption depends on identification of the underlying condition. Occasionally, therapeutic trials for treatable conditions should be instituted, such as a gluten-free diet for celiac disease, pancreatic enzyme replacement for pancreatic exocrine malfunction, metronidazole for *G. lamblia* infection, or broad-spectrum antibiotics for suspected bacterial overgrowth. Parenteral nutrition may have a role in maintaining adequate nutritional status. Treatment modalities are discussed in later chapters focusing on specific diseases. Two disorders, celiac disease and bacterial overgrowth, are discussed here as illustrative of the pathophysiology.

Celiac Disease

Celiac disease (also called celiac sprue, nontropical sprue, or gluten-sensitive enteropathy) is characterized by intestinal mucosal injury resulting from gluten-related immunologic damage in persons genetically predisposed to this condition. The prevalence of the disease among relatives of patients with celiac disease is approximately 10%. There is a strong association of celiac disease with human leukocyte antigen (HLA) class II molecules, particularly HLA-DQ2 and HLA-DQ8. The disease is induced by exposure to storage proteins found in grain plants such as wheat (which contains gliadin), barley, and rye and their products. Oats are implicated, not because of gliadin, but because of contamination with wheat during packaging and transportation. The exposure initiates a cellular immune response that results in mucosal damage, particularly in the proximal intestine. Results of investigations suggest that an enzyme, tissue transglutaminase, may be the autoantigen of celiac disease.

Clinical Presentation

Celiac disease can manifest with the classic constellation of symptoms and signs of a malabsorption syndrome. Not uncommonly, however, the manifestation is atypical, with nonspecific GI symptoms such as bloating, chronic diarrhea (with or without steatorrhea), flatulence, lactose intolerance, or deficiencies of a single micronutrient (e.g., iron deficiency anemia). Extraintestinal complaints such as depression, weakness, fatigue, arthralgias, osteoporosis, or osteomalacia may predominate. A number of diseases, including dermatitis herpetiformis, type 1 diabetes mellitus, autoimmune thyroid disease, and selective immunoglobulin A (IgA) deficiency, are found in significant association with celiac disease.

Diagnosis

Celiac disease is a leading consideration in every patient with the malabsorption syndrome, and it should be included as well in the differential of atypical manifestations. Fiberoptic or capsule endoscopy may show the typical features of broad and flattened villi; with the former instrument, tissue can be sampled for histologic analysis. Intestinal biopsy is the most valuable test in establishing the diagnosis. The spectrum of pathologic changes ranges from normal villous architecture with an increase in mucosal lymphocytes and plasma cells (the infiltrative lesion) to partial blunting or total villous flattening. Although abnormal biopsy findings are not specific, they are highly suggestive, particularly because most other conditions that can mimic celiac disease (e.g., Crohn's disease, gastrinoma, lymphoma, tropical sprue, graft-versus-host disease, immune deficiency) may be distinguished clinically. A clinical response to a gluten-free diet establishes the diagnosis and precludes the need, in adults, to document healing by repeated biopsies. Serologic blood tests (antigliadin, antiendomysial, and reticulin antibodies) are helpful in screening of patients with atypical symptoms and asymptomatic relatives of patients with celiac disease.

Treatment

Strict, lifelong adherence to a gluten-free diet is the only treatment for celiac disease. Specific nutritional supplementation should be provided to correct deficiencies, particularly those of iron, vitamins, and calcium. A clinical response may be seen within a few weeks. Patients should be monitored to ensure adequate response and proper adherence to the diet. The long-term prognosis is excellent for patients who adhere to the diet, although there may be a slight increase in the incidence of malignancies, particularly lymphoma.

Bacterial Overgrowth Syndrome

The proximal small bowel normally contains fewer than 10^4 bacteria per milliliter of fluid, with no anaerobic *Bacteroides* organisms and few coliforms. Overgrowth of luminal bacteria can result in diarrhea and malabsorption by a number of mechanisms, including (1) deconjugation of bile salts, which leads to impaired micelle formation and impaired uptake of fat; (2) patchy injury to the enterocytes (small intestinal epithelial cells); (3) direct competition for the use of nutrients (e.g., uptake of vitamin B_{12} by gram-negative bacteria or the fish tapeworm *Diphyllobothrium latum*); and (4) stimulated secretion of water and electrolytes by products of bacterial metabolism, such as hydroxylated bile acids and short-chain (volatile) organic acids.

Conditions Associated with Bacterial Overgrowth

The most important factors maintaining the relative sterility of the upper gut are gastric acidity, peristalsis, and intestinal immunoglobulins (IgA). Conditions that impair these functions can result in bacterial overgrowth. Impaired peristalsis may be caused by motility disorders (e.g., scleroderma, amyloidosis, diabetes mellitus) or by anatomic changes (e.g., surgically created blind loops, obstruction, jejunal diverticulosis). Achlorhydria, pancreatic insufficiency, and hypogammaglobulinemia are also associated with bacterial overgrowth but uncommonly result in clinical steatorrhea.

Diagnosis

Direct culture of jejunal aspirate is the most definitive diagnostic test, but it is invasive, uncomfortable, and costly. The ^{14}C-xylose breath test is an accurate and sensitive laboratory test; measurement of breath hydrogen after an oral challenge with glucose is simpler but not as sensitive or as specific. An empirical therapeutic trial with antibiotics is an acceptable alternative to diagnostic testing.

Treatment

When appropriate, specific therapy, such as surgery for intestinal obstruction, should be provided. More commonly, patients are treated with antibiotics, most appropriately those that are effective against aerobic and anaerobic enteric organisms. Tetracycline, trimethoprim-sulfamethoxazole, or metronidazole, in combination with a cephalosporin or quinolone, are suitable agents. A single course of therapy for 7 to 10 days may be therapeutic for months. In other patients, intermittent therapy (one week of every four) or even an extended period of continuous therapy proves to be most effective.

⬤ MALABSORPTIVE THERAPY

Cardiovascular disease and other consequences of obesity have reached epidemic proportions in the United Sates, and one approach to this problem has been the deliberate induction of malabsorption (primarily of fats) to reduce a patient's lipid levels and body mass index. Medications used for this purpose includes bile acid–binding resins, such as cholestyramine and colestipol, and the lipase inhibitors, orlistsat (Xenical) and ezetimibe (Zetia). Surgical treatment (bariatric operations) usually consists of gastric partition combined with some degree of small intestinal bypass, which induces significant weight loss by several proposed mechanisms, including malabsorption, improved nutrient deposition, and enhanced satiety.

D. Diarrhea

John S. Maxwell and M. Michael Wolfe

⬤ DEFINITION

The average number of bowel movements for the normal adult can range from three per day to three per week. Diarrhea can be defined as increased frequency of stools with decreased consistency and increased volume, but the subjective nature of these complaints and lack of fixed normal values make the definition difficult. The 1997 position statement by the American Gastroenterological Association on chronic diarrhea defines diarrhea as the production of loose stools with or without increased stool frequency. There are also definitions that include fecal weight, which in the United States averages less than 200 g/24 hours but varies according to the type of diet. The 2003 guidelines for the investigation of chronic diarrhea define diarrhea as the abnormal passage of loose or liquid stool more than three times a day or a stool volume greater than 200 g/day or both. Because of the subjective nature of the complaints, a detailed history is needed to arrive at a diagnosis (Table 33-6).

The duration of symptoms is useful in the differential diagnosis of diarrhea and is a part of the necessary history. Acute diarrhea is limited to 2 weeks or less and is usually infectious in origin. Persistent diarrhea persists for longer than 14 days, and chronic diarrhea is considered to last longer than 4 weeks. As time goes on, is etiology is less likely to be infectious.

⬤ PHYSIOLOGY

Approximately 8 to 9 L of fluid enters the small bowel in a 24-hour period. This includes 1 to 2 L from dietary consumption, with the remainder produced by salivary, gastric, biliary, pancreatic, and intestinal secretions. All but 1 to 2 L is absorbed in the small intestine and then enters the colon. Almost all of this fluid is absorbed as it travels through the colon, leaving less than 200 g/day of stool. Disruption of the absorption of ions, solutes, and water or increased secretion of electrolytes results in water accumulation in the lumen and therefore diarrhea.

⬤ ACUTE DIARRHEA

Most cases of acute diarrhea are caused by viral or bacterial infections and are self-limited, resolving without specific therapy. Acute diarrhea in Western countries is common and occurs at a rate of about one episode per person per year. It tends to occur in outbreaks involving food or waterborne contamination or recurrently in specific groups, such as people who care for infants, small children, travelers, and immunocompromised individuals.

TABLE 33-6   CLASSIFICATION OF DIARRHEA

TYPE	PRESENTATION	CAUSE
Acute (duration <2 wk) Chronic (duration >4 wk)	Usually mild; wide range of symptoms	Most commonly infectious
Secretory	Large volume, watery stool No change with fasting	Cholera, neuroendocrine tumors, drugs, nonosmotic laxatives, bile salts, bacterial toxins
Osmotic	Watery stool Stops with fasting	Carbohydrate malabsorption laxatives (Mg, PO$_4$)
Inflammatory	Bloody, mucosy diarrhea Frequent, urgent small stools	Infectious colitis IBD, invasive bacteria
Motility	Soft to watery stools	IBS Bacterial overgrowth Hyperthyroidism Scleroderma
Steatorrhea	Greasy, malodorous	Malabsorption: celiac disease, short bowel syndrome, maldigestion, fistula

IBD, Inflammatory bowel disease; IBS, irritable bowel syndrome.

Most of the deaths associated with acute diarrhea occur in elderly persons because of the physiologic changes of aging that include abnormalities in water homeostasis and decreased thirst perception. Because of volume depletion, elderly patients are at increased risk for falls due to orthostatic hypotension, electrolyte disturbances, and delirium.

Most cases of acute diarrhea are caused by viral infection; studies of acute diarrhea show positive bacterial cultures in only 1.5% to 5.6% of cases. Viruses commonly causing acute infectious diarrhea include noroviruses, rotaviruses, and adenoviruses. The symptoms typically last approximately 48 hours and clear spontaneously.

Bacterial causes of acute infectious diarrhea include *Salmonella, Campylobacter, Shigella,* enterotoxigenic *Escheria coli,* and *Clostridium difficile.* These are the likely causes of most severe cases of acute diarrhea. Among patients with diarrhea lasting longer than 3 days and high outputs, a bacterial cause was found in 87% of cases. Protozoa are infrequent causes of acute diarrhea.

Because of the short duration of symptoms, good prognosis, and high frequency of viral etiologies found in acute diarrhea, clinical investigation is not needed and is not cost-effective in most cases. The indications warranting a complete evaluation involve clinical signs of severe illness: profuse watery diarrhea and hypovolemia; frequent passage of small-volume, bloody stools containing mucus; bloody diarrhea; fever greater than 101° F; illness lasting longer than 48 hours; severe abdominal pain; hospitalization; recent use of antibiotics; age greater than 70 years; immunocompromise; and systemic illness and diarrhea in pregnancy (listeriosis).

Items from the history that might be helpful to the diagnosis include information regarding travel, work exposure, and pets. Fever usually indicates an invasive organism, such as *Salmonella, Shigella, Campylobacter,* certain viruses, *Entamoeba histolytica,* or *C. difficile.* Risk factors include food consumption or preparation involving raw or undercooked meats and dairy products or contaminated fruits and vegetables. Pregnant women have a 20-fold increased risk of developing listeriosis from meat or unpasteurized milk, and this bacterial infection always needs to be considered in a pregnant woman with diarrhea and systemic complaints. Ingestion of preformed bacterial toxins from *Staphylococcus aureus, Bacillus cereus, or Clostridium perfringens* typically causes diarrhea within 6 hours. Acute traveler's diarrhea is most commonly caused by enterotoxigenic *E. coli.*

Infectious agents sometimes can cause mucosal inflammation ranging from mild to severe. These include noroviruses, rotaviruses, and the human immunodeficiency virus (HIV). Bacterial mucosal invasion can be present with *Salmonella,* enteroinvasive *E. coli, Campylobacter jejuni,* and *Yersina enterocolitica*; *E. histolytica, C. difficile, Shigella* spp., *E. coli* O157:H7, *Vibrio,* and *Aeromonas* secrete toxins and invade the mucosa. Patients often relate a history of initially watery diarrhea later progressing to bloody diarrhea.

Noninfectious causes of acute diarrhea are less common. They can include irritable bowel syndrome (IBS), inflammatory bowel disease (IBD), ischemic bowel disease (either ischemic colitis or mesenteric vascular insufficiency), partial bowel obstruction, fecal impaction with overflow diarrhea, and bacterial overgrowth. Most often, these disorders manifest as persistent or chronic diarrhea, but they do have a specific onset. Medications and over-the-counter supplements can be a cause of acute or chronic diarrhea, and the diagnosis may be suggested by introduction of a new medication or an increase in dose. Frequently, oral magnesium replacement, donepezil hydrochloride (Aricept), tube feedings, liquid medications, and chewing gum made with nonabsorbable sugars (e.g., sorbitol) are associated with diarrhea. An accurate medication history (prescription and over-the-counter), including supplements, is necessary.

Evaluation of Acute Diarrhea

Most patients with acute diarrhea do not require a detailed evaluation because their illness is neither severe nor prolonged. There is significant cost involved in laboratory testing, cultures, and procedures, and because a viral infection is responsible for most cases, the results will be unrevealing. These patients typically have watery, nonbloody diarrhea and are not systemically ill. Many patients with traveler's diarrhea have large-volume watery diarrhea due to enterotoxigenic *E. coli.* Some patients who have severity indicators in their history or examination findings, or who are elderly or immunocompromised, should have a laboratory evaluation.

Patients with bloody, frequent, small-volume stools should be evaluated for potential bacterial causes. The same is true for patients who have systemic symptoms (e.g., abdominal pain, fever), fecal leukocytes, an elevated fecal lactoferrin level (a marker for leukocytes), or occult blood in the stool. Stool cultures should be done to look for *Shigella, Samonella, Campylobacter,* and enterohemorrhagic *E coli.* Identification of *Listeria, Yersinia,* and *Vibrio* may require additional testing. Stool should be evaluated for ova and parasites if cultures are negative and if there is persistent diarrhea or a history HIV/AIDS. *Giardia* and *Cryptosporidum* immunoassays and staining for *Microsporidium* are also indicated in these individuals and in patients with a possible exposure history. Because of the risk of community-acquired *C. difficile* infection, testing should be done for the presence of this organism even without a history of antibiotic use.

Finally, if there are no definitive results from the stool studies, endoscopic imaging with either flexible sigmoidoscopy or colonoscopy may be required to evaluate for IBD, ischemic colitis, or cytomegalovirus colitis in immunocompromised patients. Despite an extensive evaluation, no cause can be determined in 20% to 40% of cases.

Treatment

Treatment of acute diarrhea begins with general supportive measures. The most important therapy is hydration, which is best accomplished by the oral route, although intravenous hydration is more frequently used in the United States. Proper oral hydration could decrease the admission rate for children in the United States by at least 100,000 patients per year. Oral hydration solutions are effective because in many small bowel diarrheal illnesses, the intestine remains able to absorb water if glucose and salt are present to allow transport of water from the lumen. The World Health Organization formula that is recommended for oral rehydration consists of the following components:

NaCl 2.6 g (0.092 ounce)

Trisodium citrate dihydrate 2.9 g (0.10 ounce)

KCl 1.5 g (0.053 ounce)

Anhydrous glucose 13.5 g (0.48 ounce) or sucrose 27 g (0.96 ounce)

1 L water

This formula can easily be made and also is commercially available. Drinks made for perspiration replacement, such as Gatorade, are not the same as the hydration fluid but can be used if the individual is not volume depleted.

Antibiotics are not required in most cases but are a consideration in specific circumstances. The inability to obtain immediate results from cultures for enteric pathogens often necessitates a decision regarding empiric antibiotic therapy. In general, empiric antibiotics do not significantly affect the course of acute diarrhea. In one study in which all patients were culture positive, there was a 1-day benefit for those receiving antibiotic treatment compared with nontreatment. Among those who were severely ill, the results were better: 1.5 days for resolution in the treated group compared to 3.4 days in the untreated group.

Antibiotics should be avoided in patients with enterohemorrhagic *E. coli* because no benefit has been demonstrated and there may be an increased risk of hemolytic-uremic syndrome related to increased release of Shiga toxin. These patients often have bloody diarrhea and abdominal pain but no fever. If antibiotics have been started, they should be discontinued if culture results show *E. coli* 0157:H7. There is also no clinical improvement with antibiotic treatment of nontyphoid *Samonella* gastroenteritis, and the clearance of bacteria from the stool may be prolonged.

Symptomatic Therapy

Dietary changes usually do not need to be drastic. The patient should be encouraged to take clear liquids and perhaps soft and low-fiber foods, which will aid in hydration and supply some calories for baseline energy requirements and enterocyte renewal. Milk should be avoided because of possible temporary lactose intolerance due to mucosal injury. Caffeine and ethanol should also be avoided because they stimulate intestinal motility.

In patients with acute diarrhea who do not have bloody diarrhea or fever, loperamide (Imodium), diphenoxylate-atropine (Lomotil), or tincture of opium can decrease the frequency of watery stools. These agents also possess antisecretory properties, and they inhibit intestinal motility, thereby allowing more intestinal absorption. The usual dose of loperamide should not exceed 8 2-mg tablets per day and diphenoxylate should not exceed 8 5-mg tablets per day. Diphenoxylate and tincture of opium have central-acting opioid effects and can cause unwanted side effects, particularly in the elderly. These drugs also are associated with increased risk of hemolytic-uremic syndrome in patients with enterohemorrhagic *E coli* infections. The use of probiotics to repopulate intestinal flora in infectious diarrhea has not been well studied.

● CHRONIC DIARRHEA

The evaluation of chronic diarrhea is more variable, and the establishment of universal guidelines is more difficult, reflecting in part the many potential causes. Diarrhea may result from colonic inflammation, colonic neoplasia, small bowel inflammation, malabsorption due to small bowel mucosal disorders, maldigestion due to pancreatic insufficiency, motility disorders, and functional bowel disorders.

Chronic diarrhea is a common reason for referral to a gastroenterology clinic, but the true incidence is difficult to estimate because of differing definitions and populations. In one study, the estimated prevalence of chronic diarrhea in the elderly population was between 7% and 14%, but that study also included functional bowel disorders. Another estimate excluding abdominal pain placed the prevalence at 4% to 5 % Chronic diarrhea certainly can affect the quality of life, and any clinician who cares for these patients has heard of patients being housebound because of a fear of diarrhea and incontinence.

Evaluation of Chronic Diarrhea

Because of the myriad causes and differing severities, optimal guidelines are not established. Most recommendations are based on expert opinion and may include bias as a result of the types of referrals or regional differences. A thorough history and physical examination are essential. The history should try to establish the likelihood of organic versus functional disorders, to differentiate malabsorptive from inflammatory etiologies, and to determine the cause of the diarrhea. Consequently, important parts of the history include the following:

1. Character of the onset of diarrhea—sudden or gradual
2. Continuous versus intermittent symptoms
3. The presence of nocturnal diarrhea
4. Duration of diarrhea
5. Epidemiology—travel, exposure to contaminated food or water, family members with similar illness
6. Stool characteristics—watery, bloody, greasy
7. Fecal incontinence versus diarrhea or both
8. Abdominal pain—IBD, IBS, mesenteric vascular insufficiency
9. Weight loss—often significant in malabsorption, IBD, ischemia, and neoplasm
10. Aggravating factors—stress, specific foods (e.g., milk)
11. Prior evaluations to avoid repeating tests
12. Mitigating factors—what the patient has tried to control the diarrhea
13. Previous operations, radiation therapy, medications, supplements
14. Factitious diarrhea—always a consideration in eating disorders, malingering, or secondary gain
15. Review of systems—hyperthyroidism, scleroderma, tumor syndromes, diabetes mellitus
16. Risk factors for HIV and other immunosuppressed states

Physical examination rarely provides a specific diagnosis, but it does allow an assessment of fluid status and nutritional status. Some helpful findings include mouth ulcers or perianal disease that suggest the possibility of IBD, rashes or flushing, abdominal mass, and findings of hyperthyroidism.

Some causes are related to socioeconomic status. In contrast to acute diarrhea, infectious causes of chronic diarrhea are unusual in the United States, although they are frequently encountered in developing countries. Infectious causes are a concern in newly arrived immigrants or travelers. Occasionally, persisting infections such as *Giardia, Entamoeba, C. difficile, Aeromonas, Plesiomonas, Cryptosporidium, Tropheryma whipplei* (Whipple's disease), *Blastocystis hominis,* and *Cyclospora* can cause chronic diarrhea. In addition, up to 30% of patients with these infections develop postinfectious IBS as a cause of their chronic diarrhea.

Patients with diarrhea-predominant IBS can have a wide variety of symptoms, but the main complaints are usually chronic abdominal pain and altered bowel movements. These patients complain of small-volume, frequent diarrhea, often with interspersed normal or constipated stools. They may report marked urgency as well as a feeling of incomplete evacuation. Approximately one half of these patients have mucus in the stools. Large-volume diarrhea, bloody diarrhea, nocturnal diarrhea, and greasy stools are not compatible with IBS and raise the probability of organic disease. The Rome III criteria, a consensus statement on functional bowel disorders established for research purposes, may help establish the diagnosis of IBS as well as functional diarrhea. The criteria for IBS are recurrent abdominal pain or discomfort occurring on at least 3 days per month in the last 3 months and associated with two or more of following: (1) improvement of pain with bowel movement; (2) onset associated with a change in frequency of stool; and (3) onset associated with a change in form or consistency of stool.

IBS can be diagnosed based on a typical history and clinical findings and does not usually require an extensive evaluation. If there are potentially serious symptoms that are not consistent with IBS, additional testing is undertaken. Functional diarrhea is defined by the Rome III criteria as continuous or recurrent passage of loose or watery stools without abdominal pain or discomfort, occurring in at least 75% of stools for at least 3 months. This criterion is somewhat ambiguous in guiding the evaluation because it does not help to exclude other causes of chronic diarrhea.

Inflammatory bowel diseases, such as ulcerative colitis and Crohn's disease, are classic causes of chronic diarrhea. Radiation enterocolitis (usually based on the history) and ischemic colitis are more unusual causes. *Crohn's disease* can involve any portion of the GI tract, from the mouth to the anus. Patients with Crohn's disease typically have abdominal pain, diarrhea, weight loss, and fever; gross bleeding is not common with Crohn's disease. There is frequently a delay in presentation and diagnosis of several months from the onset of symptoms to the diagnosis of Crohn's disease. Anemia, leukocytosis, and elevated inflammatory markers are common laboratory findings.

The presentation of *ulcerative colitis* varies a great deal because of variable involvement of the colon. Typically, if the inflammation is limited to the rectum or rectosigmoid region, the symptoms are relatively mild. The onset may be gradual, and there may be episodes of bloody mucus and intermittent diarrhea with fewer than four stools per day. Urgency, mild cramping, and a sensation of incomplete evacuation (tenesmus) are commonly reported, and constipation may also be a complaint. More serious symptoms are often associated with greater involvement of the colon (left-sided colitis or sometimes pancolitis). Patients have frequent loose, bloody stools (up to 10 per day) with mucus. Mild anemia and leukocytosis, mild-to-moderate cramping abdominal pain, and low-grade fever may be present. Weight loss is not common in mild disease. Severe disease with more than 10 bloody stools per day usually indicates pancolitis. There is severe cramping pain, fever, leukocytosis, and anemia, which often requires transfusion. There can be rapid weight loss leading to malnutrition. Overall, approximately one third of these patients have rectosigmoid disease, one third have left-sided disease, and the remainder have pancolitis. Fulminant disease is present in about 10% of patients at presentation. For information regarding the treatment of IBD, see Chapter 37.

Microscopic colitis is most commonly seen in middle-aged women but can be found at all ages and in men as well. It usually manifests with chronic watery diarrhea. There can be mild cramping and weight loss, but dehydration and malnutrition are rare. The name implies that this is a histologic diagnosis, and indeed, the mucosal appearance of the colon at the time of endoscopy is frequently entirely normal, and biopsies are necessary to document its presence. Disease is present throughout the colon but is often more severe on the right side. There are two types of microscopic colitis: lymphocytic and collagenous. Although the underlying cause of the colitis is not known, it is associated with autoimmune disease in up to 50% of cases. Treatment starts with trials of symptomatic pharmacotherapy. Loperamide and cholestyramine may be useful in mild disease; budesonide, a poorly absorbed steroid, may be used, although relapses are frequent after weaning. Mesalamine and sulfasalazine have been used, but there is little information indicating effectiveness.

Malabsorption can result in diarrhea, most commonly from malabsorption of fat and nutrients. The bowel movements are classically described as greasy or oily, foul smelling, and large volume, although not usually watery. There may be associated weight loss. Malabsorption can be congenital, caused by membrane transport defects of small bowel enterocytes, or acquired due to extensive damage or resection of the small bowel resulting in decreased absorptive area. Celiac disease, Crohn's disease, and short bowel syndrome after resection can be causes. The jejunal-ileal bypass procedure, which was performed for patients with morbid obesity in the 1960s and 1970s but is no longer done due to extensive and serious complications, created severe malabsorption resulting in weight loss. Maldigestion resulting from lack of pancreatic enzymes (chronic pancreatitis or, occasionally, pancreatic tumor) and lack of bile salts for fat absorption also can occur.

Laboratory findings depend on the severity of malabsorption and which specific nutrient is deficient. The most common malabsorptive process is lactose intolerance that results in gas, bloating, and diarrhea. Lactose intolerance can be diagnosed by lactose breath testing or the more simple lactose avoidance trial. Celiac disease and tropical sprue can result in a wide spectrum and severity of symptoms, from iron deficiency to calcium and magnesium deficiency, fat-soluble vitamin deficiencies, and weight loss. The rare Whipple's disease can cause not only malabsorption but also systemic findings. Bacterial overgrowth, such as in some gut motility disorders and small bowel diverticula as well as surgically created blind loops, can also result in malabsorption. Breath testing is available for the evaluation of bacterial overgrowth.

Other cases of chronic, but usually self-limited, diarrhea occur in about 10% of patients who have undergone gallbladder removal. The likely cause is the continuous presentation of bile to the intestine that results from the loss of storage capacity in the gallbladder; this continuous flow increases the level of bile salts in the colon, leading to diarrhea. Postcholecystectomy diarrhea usually responds to bile acid–binding agents such as cholestyramine and often resolves over time.

Secretory diarrhea is uncommon and typically manifests with large-volume (>1 L/day), watery diarrhea that occurs both day and night and continues in spite of fasting. Although this diagnosis can usually be established by the history and a trial of stool monitoring while fasting, calculation of the stool osmolar gap from measured stool electrolytes can be helpful (see previous discussion). A secretory diarrhea will have an osmolar gap of less than 50 mOsm/kg, whereas the gap in an osmotic diarrhea will be greater than 125 mOsm/kg. Causes of secretory diarrhea are rarely infectious. They include fairly uncommon but often quite dramatic syndromes such as Zollinger-Ellison syndrome (gastrinoma), vasoactive intestinal peptide–producing tumor (VIPoma), and carcinoid syndrome. For the evaluation of chronic secretory diarrhea, stool cultures should be done. Imaging of the small bowel and colon should be considered, and appropriate testing for hormones and other secretagogues should be based on the history and findings.

SUGGESTED READINGS

A. Abdominal Pain

Camilleri M: Peripheral mechanisms in irritable bowel syndrome, N Engl J Med 367:1626–1635, 2012.

Johnston JM, Kurtz CB, Macdougall JE, et al: Linaclotide improves abdominal pain and bowel habits in a phase IIB trial of patients with irritable bowel syndrome with constipation, Gastroenterology 139:1877–1886, 2010.

Lembo AJ, Schneier HA, Shiff SJ, et al: Two randomized trials of linaclotide in chronic constipation, N Engl J Med 365:527–536, 2011.

Peery A, Dellon ES, Lund J, et al: Burden of gastrointestinal disease in the United States: 2012 update, Gastroenterology 143:1179–1187, 2012.

Sperber AD, Drossman D: The functional abdominal pain syndrome, Aliment Pharmacol Ther 33:514–524, 2011.

B. Gastrointestinal Hemorrhage

Barkun A, Bardou M, Marshall JK: Consensus recommendations for managing patients with nonvariceal upper gastrointestinal bleeding, Ann Intern Med 139:843–857, 2003.

Bounds BC, Friedman LS: Lower gastrointestinal bleeding, Gastroenterol Clin North Am 32:1107–1125, 2003.

Holster IL, Kuipers EJ, Tjwa ET: Hemospray in the treatment of upper gastrointestinal hemorrhage in patients on antithrombotic therapy, Endoscopy 45:63–66, 2013.

Morishita H, Yamagami T, Matsumoto T, et al: Transcatheter arterial embolization with N-butyl cyanoacrylate for acute life threatening gastrointestinal bleeding uncontrolled by endoscopic hemostasis, J Vasc Interv Radiol 24:432–438, 2013.

Ralnek IM, Barkun AN, Bardou M: Management of acute bleeding from a peptic ulcer, N Engl J Med 359:928–937, 2008.

Soulellis CA, Carpentier S, Chen YI, et al: Lower GI hemorrhage controlled with endoscopically applied TC-325 (with videos), Gastrointest Endosc 77:504–507, 2013.

Villavueva C, Colomo A, Bosch A, et al: Transfusion strategies for acute upper gastrointestinal bleeding, N Engl J Med 368:11–21, 2013.

C. Malabsorption

Dye CK, Gaffney RR, Dykes TM, et al: Endoscopic and radiographic evaluation of the small bowel in 2012, Am J Med 125:1228.e1–1228.e12, 2012.

Forsmark CE: Management of chronic pancreatitis, Gastroenterology 144:1282–1291, 2013.

Goulet O, Ruemmele F: Causes and management of intestinal failure in children, Gastroenterology 2(Suppl 1):S16–S28, 2006.

Marth T: New insights into Whipple's disease—a rare intestinal inflammatory disorder, Dig Dis 27:494–501, 2009.

Mueller K, Ash C, Pennisi E, et al: The gut microbiota: introduction, Science 336:1245, 2012.

Rubio-Tapia A, Hill ID, Kelly CP, et al: ACG clinical guidelines: diagnosis and management of celiac disease, Am J Gastroenterol 108:656–676, 2013.

Shepherd SJ, Lomer MC, Gibson PR: Short-chain carbohydrates and functional gastrointestinal disorders, Am J Gastroenterol 108:707–717, 2013.

Swallow DM: Genetics of lactase persistence and lactose intolerance, Ann Rev Genetics 37:197–219, 2003.

D. Diarrhea

American Gastroenterological Association: AGA medical position statement: guidelines for the evaluation and management of chronic diarrhea, Gastroenterology 116:1461–1463, 1999.

Boyce TG, Swederdlow DL, Griffin PM: *Escherichia coli* O157:H7 and the hemolytic uremic syndrome, N Engl J Med 333–364, 1995.

Camilleri M: Chronic diarrhea: a review on pathophysiology and management for the clinical gastroenterologist, Clin Gastroenterol Hepatol 2:198–206, 2004.

Fine KD, Schiller LR: AGA technical review on the evaluation and management of chronic diarrhea, Gastroenterology 116:1464–1486, 1999.

Deshpande A, Lever D, Soffer E: Acute diarrhea. In Carey WD, editor: Cleveland Clinic Disease Management Project in Gastroenterology (online publication), August 1, 2010. Available at: http://www.clevelandclinicmeded.com/medicalpubs/diseasemanagement/gastroenterology/acute-diarrhea/. Accessed August 19, 2014.

Slutsker L, Ries AA, Greene KD, et al: *Escherichia coli* O157:H7 diarrhea in the United States: clinical and epidemiological factors, Ann Intern Med 126:505–513, 1997.

Thomas PD, Forbes A, Green J, et al: Guidelines for the investigation of chronic diarrhea, ed 2, Gut 52(Suppl V):v1–v15, 2003.

Endoscopic and Imaging Procedures

Christopher S. Huang and M. Michael Wolfe

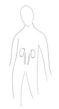

INTRODUCTION

Since Mikulicz first used a prototype esophagoscope to visualize the lumen of the esophagus in 1880, physicians have been attempting to peer into every portion of the gastrointestinal (GI) tract in order to understand disease and to restore their patients to health. This goal has become more achievable than ever as a result of the wide variety of invasive and noninvasive endoscopic and imaging procedures that are currently available. This chapter reviews the various endoscopic and radiographic procedures currently in use, including their indications and basic information regarding their performance.

GASTROINTESTINAL ENDOSCOPY

GI endoscopy is the primary modality for directly visualizing the GI tract and for obtaining tissue samples to establish definitive diagnoses. In addition, a wide variety of therapeutic maneuvers can be performed endoscopically to deal with a host of disease processes, such as hemostasis for bleeding ulcers or varices, resection or ablation of neoplastic tissue, dilation or stenting of strictures, and removal of bile duct stones.

Over the years, endoscopes have evolved from early rigid types with limited capabilities to more sophisticated flexible instruments with advanced imaging capabilities, specialized features for therapeutic maneuvers, and various designs to enable examination of specific areas of the GI tract and biliopancreatic systems. Endoscopes come in varying lengths and in diameters ranging from 3.1 mm to 15 mm (Fig. 34-1). They consist of a control handle, an insertion tube, and a connector section that attaches to the light source and image processing unit. The control handle comprises dials that deflect the scope tip in all directions as well as buttons for suction, air or water insufflation, and image capture. The control handle also includes the entry port to the "working channel," which runs down the length of the insertion tube, through which a wide array of accessories such as biopsy forceps, snares, and balloon dilators can be passed. The tip of the insertion tube houses a charge-coupled device for color image generation, a light guide illumination system, and an objective lens, which may be oriented for forward viewing, side viewing, or oblique viewing, depending on the type of endoscope.

Technologic advances continue to improve the quality of endoscopic imaging. These include the introduction of high-definition instruments, magnification endoscopy (from a baseline of 30× or 35× up to 150×), and enhanced imaging technologies such as narrow band imaging (NBI) and multiband imaging.

GI endoscopy can be performed in dedicated endoscopy suites or at a patient's bedside in emergency situations. After positioning the patient appropriately and providing sedation, if necessary, the endoscopist passes the lubricated endoscope through the intended orifice and advances it manually. The angulations of the GI lumen are navigated by deflecting the endoscope tip and by applying torque to the instrument shaft (i.e., rotating the shaft along the long axis of the instrument). Endoscopy is generally safe, with complications that include bleeding (0.3% to 1% after colonoscopic polypectomy), perforation (0.05% in general, but 0.1% to 0.5% after polypectomy), and sedation-associated hypotension and hypoxia (1% to 5%). Death related to endoscopic procedures is exceedingly rare (0% to 0.01%).

Esophagogastroduodenoscopy

Esophagogastroduodenoscopy (EGD), often referred to as *upper endoscopy*, is performed with a *gastroscope* and allows the

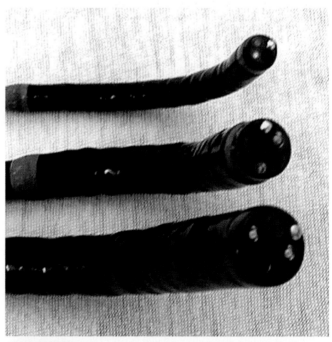

FIGURE 34-1 Endoscopes used for endoscopy of the upper gastrointestinal tract. Endoscopes of varying sizes are available for use in different situations. The uppermost endoscope (6-mm diameter) can be used for unsedated endoscopy. The middle endoscope (9-mm diameter) is used for standard diagnostic endoscopy. The lowermost endoscope (12-mm diameter) is used for therapeutic endoscopy, such as the placement of enteral stents. (Courtesy Brian C. Jacobson, Boston, Mass.)

389

endoscopist to visualize the esophagus, the stomach, and the duodenum as far as its third and sometimes fourth portions (Fig. 34-2). Common indications for EGD include evaluation of upper GI symptoms (e.g., dyspepsia, heartburn, nausea, vomiting, dysphagia, odynophagia), screening for and surveillance of Barrett's esophagus, screening for gastroesophageal varices, evaluation of suspected upper GI bleeding (acute or chronic), and investigation of malabsorptive diarrhea (as in celiac sprue or protein-losing enteropathy). A partial list of the therapeutic interventions that can be performed during EGD includes treatment of esophageal varices; dilation of esophageal strictures, rings, and webs; removal or ablation of neoplastic tissue; hemostasis therapy for upper GI bleeding; and the placement of palliative stents for malignant obstruction of the esophagus, pylorus, or duodenum.

Enteroscopy

Examination of the small intestine beyond the ligament of Treitz is not feasible with a standard gastroscope. Recent advances have allowed direct visualization of the 6 meters or so of the small intestine. *Push* enteroscopy using a long (>200 cm) endoscope allows the endoscopist to both image and biopsy or cauterize lesions in the small intestine. However, because of looping of the endoscope and tortuosity of the small intestine, advancing this instrument beyond the first 50 cm of jejunum can be difficult. Balloon-assisted enteroscopy is a newer technique that provides endoscopic access to most of the small bowel. This method employs balloons, incorporated into overtubes or the endoscope itself, to permit pleating of the small bowel onto the endoscope. By inflating and deflating the balloons in sequence, the enteroscope can be advanced through extremely long stretches of small intestine. With a combined anterograde (through the mouth) and retrograde (through the anus) approach, the entire small intestine can be visualized. Spiral enteroscopy, another novel technique, uses a spiral overtube device that retracts the small bowel over the scope, allowing for deep enteroscopy.

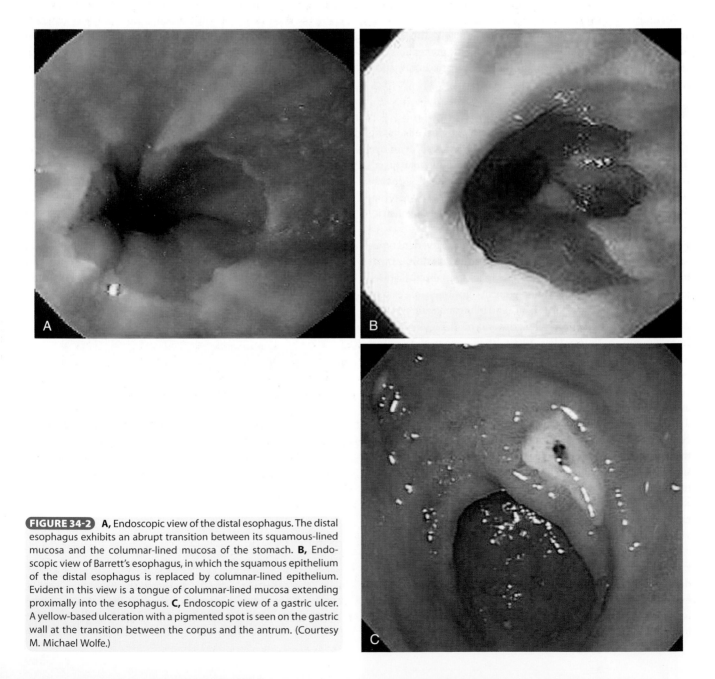

FIGURE 34-2 **A,** Endoscopic view of the distal esophagus. The distal esophagus exhibits an abrupt transition between its squamous-lined mucosa and the columnar-lined mucosa of the stomach. **B,** Endoscopic view of Barrett's esophagus, in which the squamous epithelium of the distal esophagus is replaced by columnar-lined epithelium. Evident in this view is a tongue of columnar-lined mucosa extending proximally into the esophagus. **C,** Endoscopic view of a gastric ulcer. A yellow-based ulceration with a pigmented spot is seen on the gastric wall at the transition between the corpus and the antrum. (Courtesy M. Michael Wolfe.)

The most invasive approach for visualization of the entire small bowel is intraoperative enteroscopy. In this procedure, a surgeon makes an incision in the patient's abdomen and then pleats the small bowel onto the enteroscope while the endoscopist visualizes the lumen. Once a lesion has been identified, the surgeon may elect to proceed directly to a resection of the affected segment of small intestine if the lesion is not amenable to endoscopic treatment.

Video Capsule Endoscopy

The desire to obtain visualization of the GI lumen in the least invasive way has resulted in the development of video capsule endoscopy, in which the patient swallows a pill-sized wireless camera (E-Fig. 34-1; Video 34-1). Capsule endoscopes are now available for evaluation of the esophagus and small intestine, and development of colon capsule endoscopes is underway. Capsules are 11×26 mm and can transmit images wirelessly to a data recorder as they travel through a patient's GI tract, without the need for sedation. At the end of the study, the stored images are uploaded into a computer for viewing while the capsule is ultimately passed in the patient's stool.

The esophageal capsule is helpful in patients being screened for esophageal varices and in those with suspected complications of acid reflux, such as reflux esophagitis or Barrett's esophagus. The small bowel capsule has become the "gold standard" for visualization of the small intestine, most commonly for the purpose of investigating obscure GI bleeding (E-Figs. 34-2 and 34-3; Videos 34-2 and 34-3) or suspected inflammatory bowel disease (E-Figs. 34-4 and 34-5). Retention of the capsule within the small bowel, usually at a site of pathology, occurs rarely but is the main potential complication of capsule endoscopy.

Sigmoidoscopy and Colonoscopy

Flexible sigmoidoscopy allows visualization of the rectum, sigmoid colon, and descending colon to the level of the splenic flexure. Enemas are given before the procedure to clear stool from the distal colon. Because sigmoidoscopy is quick (<10 minutes) and not particularly painful, sedation typically is not necessary, making it a convenient tool for colorectal cancer screening. Sigmoidoscopy may also be useful for evaluating chronic diarrhea and rectal bleeding suspected to arise from the distal colon or rectum and for assessing response to therapy in patients with inflammatory bowel disease involving the rectosigmoid colon.

Colonoscopy allows direct visualization of the entire large bowel and the terminal ileum. Bowel cleansing for colonoscopy requires the ingestion of osmotically active solutions, such as polyethylene glycol, coupled with a clear liquid diet for 24 hours before the procedure. Colonoscopy can be more uncomfortable for the patient than sigmoidoscopy due to stretching and distention of the colon, so sedation and analgesia are typically provided. In recent years, colonoscopy has become widely performed as a first-line colorectal cancer screening test. Other indications for colonoscopy include evaluation of chronic diarrhea, iron deficiency anemia, and overt or occult GI blood loss, as well as assessment of inflammatory bowel disease, including surveillance for dysplasia. Therapeutic interventions that can be performed during colonoscopy include polypectomy, thermal ablation of vascular ectasias, decompression of colonic dilation associated with pseudo-obstruction, stenting of malignant obstruction, and control of lower GI bleeding.

Endoscopic Retrograde Cholangiopancreatography

Endoscopic retrograde cholangiopancreatography (ERCP) is a combined endoscopic and radiographic procedure for imaging the biliary and pancreatic ducts. A *duodenoscope* is an instrument specially designed for use during ERCP that includes an imaging lens oriented on the side of the endoscope's tip, allowing a direct view of the ampulla of Vater on the medial wall of the second portion of the duodenum. An adjustable instrument *elevator* located at the tip of the duodenoscope helps the endoscopist guide a catheter into the duct of interest. Contrast material is then injected through the catheter, filling the duct, and fluoroscopic images are obtained (Fig. 34-3).

Indications for ERCP include evaluation and treatment of bile duct obstruction due to benign or malignant causes (e.g., bile duct stones, strictures, bile duct or pancreatic malignancies), cholangitis, postoperative or traumatic bile leaks and pancreatic duct leaks, drainage of pseudocysts, and evaluation of idiopathic pancreatitis. With the use of a special manometry catheter, sphincter of Oddi pressures can be measured in cases of suspected sphincter of Oddi dysfunction. Therapeutic interventions that are possible during ERCP include sphincterotomy (an incision through the sphincter of Oddi using a catheter with an electrocautery cutting wire), removal of bile duct stones, and placement of biliary or pancreatic duct stents to alleviate signs and symptoms of obstruction or to promote healing of duct leaks. ERCP carries a significant (5%) risk for complications, including pancreatitis, postsphincterotomy bleeding, and perforation. Therefore, ERCP should be performed only if therapeutic benefits are anticipated.

Choledochoscopy and *pancreatoscopy* are techniques in which an endoscope 3 mm or less in diameter is passed through the accessory channel of a duodenoscope and into the bile or pancreatic duct. The use of this small endoscope permits direct visualization of ductal abnormalities, guides electrohydraulic lithotripsy of large stones, and allows for direct sampling of ductal lesions.

Endoscopic Ultrasound

Endoscopic ultrasound (EUS), or endosonography, is performed with an endoscope containing an ultrasound transducer in its tip. Because this transducer can be placed within the GI lumen, high-resolution images of the bowel wall can be obtained, revealing distinct layers that correspond to the mucosa, submucosa, muscularis propria, and serosa (Fig. 34-4). This technique allows the endoscopist to stage tumor depth and determine the layer of origin of a subepithelial mass. In addition, EUS can penetrate the luminal wall, providing sonographic images of adjacent structures within the mediastinum and upper abdomen, including the pancreas, liver, gallbladder, mesenteric vessels, and adrenal glands. High-frequency EUS catheter probes can be passed through the accessory channel of a duodenoscope and into the biliary or pancreatic duct to provide sonographic images of small tumors and stones. They can likewise be used through a standard endoscope to evaluate diminutive subepithelial lesions and to stage obstructing esophageal cancers.

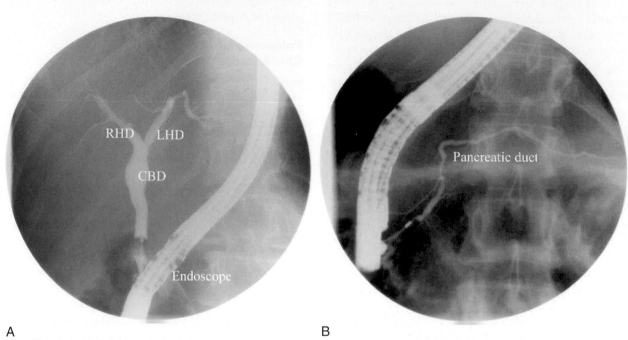

A

B

FIGURE 34-3 Endoscopic retrograde cholangiopancreatography (ERCP). **A,** Normal cholangiogram. Contrast material injected into the biliary tree during ERCP demonstrates the intraductal anatomy of the common bile duct *(CBD)*, right hepatic duct *(RHD)*, left hepatic duct *(LHD)*, and smaller intrahepatic biliary radicals. **B,** Normal pancreatogram. Contrast material injected into the pancreatic duct during ERCP defines the intraductal anatomy throughout the length of the pancreas. (Courtesy Brian C. Jacobson, Boston, Mass.)

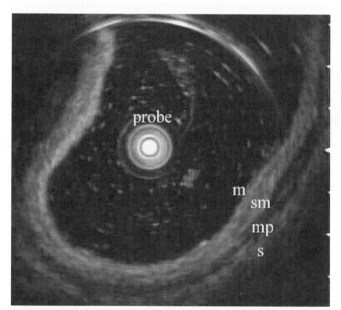

FIGURE 34-4 Endoscopic ultrasound of the gastrointestinal wall. A 12-MHz ultrasound probe, passed through the accessory channel of an endoscope, demonstrates the normal layers of the rectal wall. The mucosa *(m)* appears as a superficial, hyperechoic *(white)* band and a deeper hypoechoic *(black)* band. The submucosa *(sm)* appears as the next hyperechoic layer. The muscularis propria *(mp)* appears hypoechoic, and the serosa *(s)* appears as the outermost, hyperechoic layer. (Courtesy Brian C. Jacobson, Boston, Mass.)

Fine-needle aspiration (FNA) as well as core biopsy can be performed under EUS guidance, and FNA is the preferred approach to obtaining a tissue diagnosis in many circumstances (e.g., pancreatic masses or cysts, subepithelial lesions of the GI tract, intra-abdominal or paraesophageal lymphadenopathy).

Recent advances such as elastography and contrast-enhanced harmonic EUS have further enhanced the diagnostic capability of EUS, particularly in terms of distinguishing malignant from benign processes. However, EUS is more than just a diagnostic modality, and the spectrum of EUS-guided therapies is rapidly expanding. Therapeutic maneuvers that can be performed via EUS guidance include pseudocyst drainage, celiac axis neuroly-sis, fiducial placement into solid tumors to guide stereotactic radiotherapy, drainage of pelvic abscesses, and achievement of bile duct access (when initial attempts at ERCP have failed).

NONENDOSCOPIC IMAGING PROCEDURES

Plain Abdominal Radiographs

Plain abdominal radiographs include upright, supine, and lateral decubitus films obtained with standard radiographic equipment and without the use of contrast agents. Plain films are most useful in the initial evaluation of abdominal pain or nausea and vomiting, particularly when perforation or obstruction is suspected, and they may reveal evidence of a pneumoperitoneum, dilated bowel loops and air-fluid levels, excessive amounts of stool, or displacement of bowel loops. These findings are indicative of a perforation, obstruction or ileus, constipation or fecal impaction, and volvulus or organ enlargement, respectively (Fig. 34-5). Cal-cifications, such as those seen in chronic pancreatitis and gall-stone disease, may also be visible on these radiographs.

Contrast Studies

Contrast agents such as barium or the water-soluble diatrizoate (e.g., Gastrografin) can be administered by mouth or rectum to detect mucosal abnormalities (ulcerations and masses),

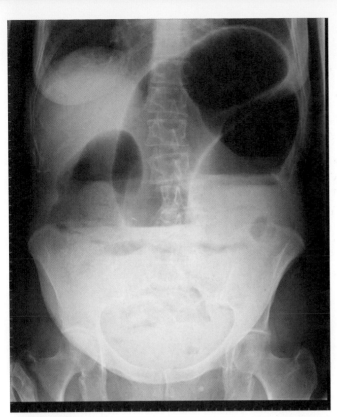

FIGURE 34-5 Upright plain radiograph of the abdomen. Air in dilated loops of colon and air-fluid levels can be seen in this patient with a sigmoid volvulus. (Courtesy Brian C. Jacobson, Boston, Mass.)

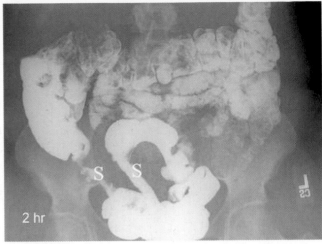

FIGURE 34-6 Small bowel follow-through. Ingested barium defines the contours of the small and large bowel lumen. A long stricture of the terminal ileum (S) can be seen in this patient with Crohn's disease. (Courtesy Brian C. Jacobson.)

strictures, herniations, diverticula, and abnormal peristalsis. Contrast agents can be used alone (single contrast) or along with instillation of air or ingestion of gas-forming agents (double contrast). The former method is more useful for detecting obstructing lesions and motility disturbances, whereas the latter aids in detecting more subtle findings such as small ulcerations or polyps.

A *video esophagogram* (also known as a modified barium swallow) entails the filming of a patient's oral cavity and pharynx during the ingestion of contrast materials of various thicknesses and textures. This imaging modality permits careful assessment of a patient's ability to manipulate a food bolus, swallow effectively, and avoid aspiration events. A video esophagogram is indicated for evaluating patients with oropharyngeal dysphagia and recurrent aspiration pneumonia. A standard *barium esophagogram* (barium swallow) focuses attention on the esophagus during the ingestion of a bolus of contrast material. This study can detect esophageal rings, webs, strictures, and motility problems that endoscopy might miss. A barium esophagogram may be useful for evaluating esophageal dysphagia as well as odynophagia.

An *upper GI series* includes serial radiographic images as an ingested contrast agent travels through the esophagus, stomach, and duodenum. This study can define gastric abnormalities such as masses, ulcerations, and mucosal thickening. It is indicated in the evaluation of abdominal pain and suspected gastric outlet obstruction. If radiographic imaging continues as the contrast agent traverses the jejunum and ileum, the study is called a *small bowel follow-through* (Fig. 34-6). Indications for a small bowel

follow-through include suspected small bowel obstruction or partial obstruction from any cause, suspected small bowel mucosal disease (e.g., Crohn's disease), and obscure GI blood loss. During this more involved procedure, a radiologist obtains multiple films, including *spot films*, or close-up views of regions that appear abnormal. Fluoroscopy can be used to follow a contrast agent during the journey through the small bowel. Attention is paid not only to structural findings but also to the length of time required for the contrast agent to reach and enter the colon. For more detailed small bowel images, *enteroclysis* can be performed. This method requires the infusion of concentrated contrast material directly into the small bowel through a nasojejunal tube placed under fluoroscopic guidance. Because of its invasive nature, enteroclysis is becoming less common in this era of wireless capsule endoscopy.

Single- and double-contrast barium enemas can detect colonic strictures, diverticula, polyps, and colonic ulcerations, and they can be therapeutic in reducing a sigmoid volvulus. Double-contrast barium enema may be used for colorectal cancer screening as a stand-alone test or in conjunction with flexible sigmoidoscopy, or it may be used to visualize the proximal colon when colonoscopy cannot be completed for various reasons. However, it is now infrequently used for these purposes given its relatively poor sensitivity and the availability of computed tomography colography (discussed later). In general, the upper GI series and barium enema have been superseded by upper endoscopy and colonoscopy because the endoscopic procedures offer increased sensitivity for detecting mucosal abnormalities, the ability to obtain mucosal biopsies, and the potential for resection of identified lesions.

Transabdominal Ultrasound

Ultrasonography is often the first imaging study obtained in the evaluation of suspected biliary colic, jaundice, or abnormal liver test results. Its use of sound waves to create an image obviates the need for radiation exposure, and the addition of Doppler techniques permits the assessment of vascular flow. Ultrasound can detect parenchymal abnormalities such as fatty liver or cirrhosis,

focal masses or cysts, ascites, biliary ductal dilation, gallstones, and large vessel thromboses. It may detect thickening of the gut wall and areas of intussusception. Ultrasound is also used to guide needle placement for biopsies or fluid aspiration. Ultrasound cannot penetrate bone or air, preventing its use as a more general diagnostic tool for the GI tract.

Computed Tomographic Methods

Computed tomography (CT) uses computer-aided reconstruction of multiple radiographic images obtained in a circular or helical course around a patient's vertical axis. Internal organs are visualized based on their inherent tissue densities compared with their surroundings. The GI lumen is usually opacified by having the patient drink an oral contrast agent. In addition, intravenous contrast agents can be administered to highlight regions with increased blood flow, thereby improving detection of pathologic lesions such as tumors and areas of active inflammation.

CT can detect parenchymal lesions, such as tumors, cysts, and abscesses, and can define the size, shape, and characteristics of organs such as the liver and spleen. Vascular abnormalities (e.g., perigastric varices, large vessel thromboses) and intra-abdominal fluid (e.g., ascites) can also be seen with CT. The caliber and contour of the GI tract wall are demonstrated by CT, aiding in the diagnosis of inflammatory lesions such as colitis, diverticulitis, and appendicitis. CT may also be used to guide needle biopsies of abdominal masses and to place electrodes into tumors for ablative therapies such as radiofrequency ablation. The use of CT to guide placement of drainage catheters has made possible the percutaneous treatment of intra-abdominal abscesses, pseudocysts, and pancreatic necrosis.

CT enteroclysis and *CT enterography* are two emerging techniques that were developed to provide better images of the small intestine. CT enteroclysis uses a nasojejunal tube to deliver contrast material into the small intestine, whereas CT enterography uses an orally ingested low-density intraluminal contrast agent to distend the lumen and highlight the small intestinal mucosa (Fig. 34-7). With the advancement of this technology and its ability to reconstruct images in multiple planes, both luminal and extraluminal information can be obtained.

CT can also be used to obtain high-resolution images of the colon. CT colography, or *virtual colonoscopy*, makes use of special image reconstruction software to create accurate visualization of the colonic lumen, provided that the patient has completed a bowel-cleansing regimen identical to that used for colonoscopy (although techniques that do not require such preparation are being developed). These CT images are 70% to 90% sensitive for detecting polyps or masses within the colon, helping to determine which patients need therapeutic colonoscopy. Virtual colonoscopy is being used in some centers to complete colonic visualization in the setting of an incomplete colonoscopy.

Magnetic Resonance Methods

Similar to CT, magnetic resonance imaging (MRI) provides multiple cross-sectional images of the abdomen and pelvis. These images are created using powerful field magnets to orient small numbers of nuclei within the body in such a way as to produce a measurable magnetic moment. MRI avoids radiation exposure but requires the patient to lie almost motionless, often within a small enclosed tube, for prolonged periods. MRI can visualize parenchymal lesions such as masses and cysts and may better characterize abnormalities seen on CT, such as hemangiomas, hepatic focal nodular hyperplasia, and fatty liver. MRI is also helpful in better characterizing perirectal abscesses and fistulas in patients with Crohn's disease. Special rectal MRI probes or coils can provide detailed images of rectal cancer used for tumor staging and can evaluate anal sphincters in patients with fecal incontinence.

MRI of the biliary and pancreatic ducts (*magnetic resonance cholangiopancreatography*, or MRCP) is a noninvasive method that can detect ductal dilation, strictures, stones (Fig. 34-8), pancreatic parenchymal changes in chronic pancreatitis, and congenital ductal abnormalities such as pancreas divisum. *Magnetic resonance angiography* is a magnetic resonance method for visualizing blood vessels that serves as an important noninvasive tool in patients with suspected mesenteric ischemia, vasculitis, or other vascular anomalies.

Visceral Angiography

Angiography is an invasive technique whereby a catheter is introduced into a blood vessel and intravascular contrast material is

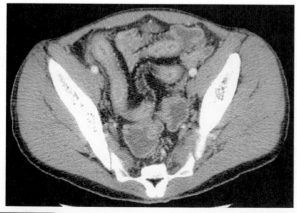

FIGURE 34-7 Computed tomography enterography. A long segment of inflamed terminal ileum is demonstrated in this patient with Crohn's disease. (Courtesy Christopher S. Huang.)

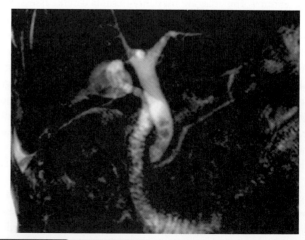

FIGURE 34-8 Magnetic resonance cholangiopancreatography. Several stones are visualized within the common bile duct, appearing as hypointense filling defects on T2-weighted images. (Courtesy Christopher S. Huang.)

injected during fluoroscopic imaging to visualize the vessel's lumen. Visceral angiography is used to evaluate mesenteric vessels in the setting of GI bleeding or suspected mesenteric ischemia. For GI bleeding, angiography is sensitive enough to detect blood loss of as little as 1 to 1.5 mL/minute. Once the site of bleeding has been localized, the radiologist can infuse vasopressin (a vasoconstrictor) or embolize the vessel using tiny coals or gelatin sponges to ensure hemostasis. In the setting of mesenteric ischemia, angiography permits localization of a vascular stenosis or obstruction, followed by possible therapeutic interventions such as balloon angioplasty, stent placement, or infusion of vasodilators and thrombolytics. Other indications for angiography include the placement of transjugular intrahepatic portosystemic shunts (TIPS) in cirrhotic patients with intractable variceal bleeding or refractory ascites and the chemoembolization of liver tumors.

Radionuclide Imaging

Technetium-99m (^{99m}Tc) is currently the major radionuclide used in GI imaging. Its 6-hour half-life and ready availability make it ideal for clinical use. ^{99m}Tc can be used to label various substances for use in several imaging techniques. ^{99m}Tc-sulfur colloid scanning and ^{99m}Tc-labeled red blood cell scanning are two distinct methods that can be used to detect active GI bleeding. The latter uses the patient's own blood cells to carry the radionuclide throughout the body. These methods can detect as little as 0.05 to 0.4 mL/minute of blood loss. However, localization of the site of bleeding is less accurate than with angiography. ^{99m}Tc scans are often performed before angiography to document ongoing bleeding before subjecting a patient to the more invasive, less sensitive study. A ^{99m}Tc-labeled red blood cell scan can also be used to diagnose hepatic hemangioma with an almost 100% positive predictive value.

Cholescintigraphy using ^{99m}Tc-iminodiacetic acid (IDA) analogues is the most commonly performed liver study in nuclear medicine. The radionuclide is taken up by the liver, is excreted into bile, and passes through the biliary tree into the gallbladder and duodenum. Failure to visualize the gallbladder during a hepatobiliary IDA scan may indicate cholecystitis secondary to cystic duct obstruction by a gallstone. Meckel's diverticulum can be a source of abdominal pain and bleeding, but it may be difficult to visualize with standard endoscopic and radiographic imaging. The agent ^{99m}Tc-pertechnetate has a high affinity for gastric mucosa and is therefore used to demonstrate the presence of this congenital anomaly.

Gastric emptying studies are useful for the evaluation of suspected gastroparesis. Patients are given a ^{99m}Tc-sulfur colloid–labeled standardized meal (consisting of liquid egg whites, toast, jam or jelly, and water) and are imaged at 0, 1, 2 and 4 hours after meal ingestion. Gastric retention of more than 10% of contents at 4 hours is highly sensitive and specific for delayed gastric emptying.

PROSPECTUS FOR THE FUTURE

Through continued technologic advances, endoscopic and radiologic image quality and resolution will also continue to improve. In addition, the GI lumen will no longer be regarded as a boundary to therapeutic endoscopy. Examples of expected innovations include the following.

- *The implementation of natural orifice transluminal, endoscopically guided surgical procedures.* With the use of recently introduced instruments, an endoscopist will be able to incise the GI tract wall, advance an endoscope into the peritoneal cavity, and then perform surgical procedures such as cholecystectomy. Endoscopic bariatric procedures for the treatment of obesity are also on the horizon and are likely to be in high demand given the obesity epidemic. A new field of *endosurgery* will develop to accompany these advances and will require training in both surgical principles and gastroenterology.
- *Commercial availability of new endoscopic imaging methods, such as confocal microscopy and fluorescence endoscopy.* Confocal microscopy allows an endoscopist to obtain magnified endoscopic images similar to those seen with a low-power microscope. Fluorescence endoscopy entails the use of special wavelengths of light to excite naturally occurring fluorophores in benign and neoplastic tissue. These fluorophores, such as collagen and nicotinamide adenine dinucleotide plus hydrogen (NADH), then fluoresce in a predictable manner, providing a means of identifying, by endoscopy, otherwise microscopic changes (e.g., dysplasia) without the need for a biopsy.
- *Video capsule endoscopes with advanced diagnostic and possibly therapeutic capabilities.* Through further advances in nanotechnology, video capsule endoscopes will be able to sample GI secretions, measure intraluminal pressures, take biopsy samples, and perhaps even provide focal ablation of lesions using thermal energy or radiofrequency ablation.

For a deeper discussion on this topic, please see Chapter 134, "Gastrointestinal Endoscopy," in Goldman-Cecil Medicine, *25th Edition.*

SUGGESTED READINGS

Byrne MF, Jowell PS: Gastrointestinal imaging: endoscopic ultrasound, Gastroenterology 122:1631–1648, 2002.

DiSario JA, Petersen BT, Tierney WM, et al: Enteroscopes, Gastrointest Endosc 66:872–880, 2007.

Fletcher JG, Huprich J, Loftus EV, et al: Computerized tomography enterography and its role in small-bowel imaging, Clin Gastroenterol Hepatol 6:283–289, 2008.

Gore RM, Levine MS: Textbook of gastrointestinal radiology, ed 2, Philadelphia, 2000, Saunders.

Mishkin DS, Chuttani R, Croffie J, et al: ASGE Technology status evaluation report: wireless capsule endoscopy, Gastrointest Endosc 63:539–545, 2006.

Thrall JH, Ziessman HA: Nuclear medicine: the requisites, ed 2, St. Louis, 2000, Mosby.

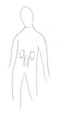

35

Esophageal Disorders

Carla Maradey-Romero, Ronnie Fass, and M. Michael Wolfe

INTRODUCTION

The esophagus appears to be a simple organ with a single function—the transmission of ingested food and fluids to the stomach. This task is achieved, however, by a tightly coordinated pattern of motility, coupled with protective barriers that prevent gastric secretions from entering the esophagus and pharynx. Derangement of these activities can cause a significant number of distressing symptoms that, taken together, are among the most commonly reported gastrointestinal symptoms that are sufficient to cause patients to seek medical care.

NORMAL FUNCTION OF THE ESOPHAGUS

The tubular esophagus begins after the cricopharyngeus muscle and consists of a muscular tube averaging 20 to 22 cm in length (range, 17 to 30 cm). It is composed proximally of skeletal muscle and distally of smooth muscle. Autopsy studies indicate that the proximal 5% or so of tubular esophagus is skeletal muscle, the middle 35% is mixed, and the distal 60% is smooth muscle. The muscular layers are arranged in circular and longitudinal bundles. The esophagus has no serosal layer. Situated between the muscular layers is the myenteric plexus, and between the circular muscle layer and the muscularis mucosa is the submucosal or Meissner's plexus. The ganglia of the myenteric plexus are more prominent in the smooth muscle areas of the tubular esophagus and are thought to integrate messages from the vagus nerve to the muscles of the esophagus.

At the junction of the esophagus and the stomach is a zone of higher resting pressure referred to as the lower esophageal sphincter (LES). This sphincter has no clearly defined anatomic structure, and the current thinking is that it is principally composed of the circular muscle of the distal 2 to 3 cm of the esophagus in conjunction with the oblique muscle fibers running from the lesser curvature to the greater curvature of the stomach (the gastric sling fibers). The right crus of the diaphragm supports the LES in its barrier by physically encircling it and providing mechanical support, particularly during physical exertion.

The process of swallowing is complex and requires fine coordination involving multiple muscle groups. The process begins with the tongue and pharynx, both of which are densely innervated. The pharyngeal musculature is controlled by the trigeminal, facial, glossopharyngeal, vagus, and hypoglossal nerves. Vagal neurons controlling the pharynx and skeletal muscle of the esophagus originate from the nucleus ambiguous. Although the smooth muscle portions of the tubular esophagus are innervated by the vagus nerve—and it is the vagus nerve that controls peristalsis under physiologic conditions—peristalsis in this portion

of the esophagus will continue even if vagal innervation is removed. The neural plexuses of the smooth muscle esophagus control its activity via excitation of circular and longitudinal muscle bundles by muscarinic receptors or via inhibition of the circular muscle layer by nonadrenergic, noncholinergic neurotranmitters: nitric oxide and vasoactive intestinal polypeptide.

Swallowing begins when a food bolus is propelled into the pharynx from the mouth under voluntary muscle control. In rapid sequence and with precise coordination, the larynx is elevated and the epiglottis seals the airway; the upper esophageal sphincter opens; and the bolus is propelled into the tubular esophagus. Peristaltic pressures ranging 40 to 180 mm Hg are generated. The measured pressure tends to be lower in the more proximal portions of the esophagus and greater in the distal smooth muscle portions. The pressures vary not only by location but also by consistency (i.e., solid or highly viscous boluses require greater pressures), volume, and temperature of the bolus itself. Movement through the tubular esophagus is controlled by the vagus nerve, concomitantly with initiation of the swallow. The LES relaxes to gastric baseline and remains relaxed (deglutitive inhibition) as the bolus is propelled distally. Once the bolus has been propelled into the stomach, the LES returns to its state of tonic contraction, preventing movement back into the esophagus.

SYMPTOMS OF ESOPHAGEAL DISEASE

Heartburn (pyrosis) is the most common symptom of esophageal disease, occurring in 44% of Americans at least once a month. About 10% of persons in the United States experience heartburn every day. It is most often described as a burning sensation in the epigastrium that rises into the chest. Patients often move their hand up and down between the xiphoid and sternal angle when describing this symptom. Given that heartburn is a cardinal sign of gastroesophageal reflux, it tends to occur after meals, when the patient is lying supine, or after an increase in intra-abdominal pressure (e.g., bending or lifting). Specific types of food, including fatty or spicy foods and chocolate, may also induce heartburn. Symptoms are often relieved temporarily by antacid preparations. Heartburn may be accompanied by regurgitation of bitter or sour fluid into the back of the throat or by excessive saliva production (so-called *water brash*), which is caused by a vagal reflex.

Dysphagia refers to a sensation of difficulty swallowing; patients report that a food bolus "gets stuck" or "goes down slowly." Although patients may point to their neck or chest when describing where the bolus gets held up, the location to which they point is poorly correlated with the actual level of obstruction. Dysphagia may result from a mechanical obstruction of the esophagus, from inflammation of the esophageal mucosa, or from an abnormality of esophageal motility.

Odynophagia, or pain on swallowing, needs to be differentiated from dysphagia in the patient history because it can be an important clue to the cause of the swallowing disorder. Painful swallowing is most often associated with infectious esophagitis or pill-induced esophageal ulcers but is only rarely present in acid-mediated esophageal disease.

Chest pain may also be a sign of esophageal disease, most often caused by gastroesophageal reflux or esophageal dysmotility. Unfortunately for the clinician, the symptoms of cardiac and esophageal chest pain overlap because of the shared neural pathways mediating pain sensation to these organs. Typical features of angina may occur in reflux-induced chest pain, including radiation to the neck and jaw; relief with nitrates, which modulate esophageal motility; and onset of symptoms with exertion. Chest pain that awakens a patient from sleep, however, is uncommon in true cardiac disease and suggests an esophageal disorder, as does pain that is relieved with antacids or pain that lasts for several hours without associated symptoms. Esophageal chest pain is often thought to occur in response to esophageal spasm, but data suggest that gastroesophageal reflux is responsible for most cases.

⬤ GASTROESOPHAGEAL REFLUX DISEASE

Gastroesophageal reflux disease (GERD) is the most common disorder of the esophagus. It causes occasional heartburn in almost one half of the population and daily symptoms in almost 7% of adult Americans. GERD is responsible for about $10 billion to $12 billion in direct medication costs per year, and related acid antisecretory therapies are among the most commonly prescribed drugs in the United States.

Gastroesophageal reflux is defined as the reflux of gastric contents back into the esophagus. There are three main underlying mechanisms that can result in gastroesophageal reflux. First, in both healthy subjects and those with GERD, reflux of gastric contents occurs primarily in the postprandial period (physiologic reflux) due to transient relaxation of the LES. Two additional mechanisms of gastroesophageal reflux are low baseline LES pressures and stress reflux. The latter indicates an inability to mount sufficient LES pressures to prevent reflux in response to sudden increases in intra-abdominal pressure. Other pathophysiologic mechanisms also bear a role in GERD, including esophageal dysmotility, delayed gastric emptying, duodenogastroesophageal reflux, impaired local defense mechanisms, and decreases in salivation.

Hiatal hernia is another important factor in the pathogenesis of GERD. The size of the hernia tends to correlate with the severity of the reflux. The presence of a nonreducible hiatal hernia disrupts the sphincter mechanism and prolongs esophageal clearance, leading to increased duration of esophageal acid exposure.

Patients with impaired esophageal motility have more severe reflux, slower acid clearance, worse mucosal injury, and more frequent extraesophageal manifestation of GERD. The importance of esophageal dysmotility is best illustrated by scleroderma, in which a hypotensive LES and impaired or absent esophageal peristalsis contribute to reflux that is often severe. Further, many patients with scleroderma have an associated sicca syndrome and therefore have reduced acid-neutralizing capacity as a result of the absence of saliva.

Heartburn is the cardinal clinical feature of GERD, and when it is present, the diagnosis of GERD is made easily. Complaints of bitter regurgitation or water brash add to the diagnostic accuracy, but these features are not always present. In some cases, atypical symptoms dominate in patients with no history of heartburn. Most cases of noncardiac chest pain, which can mimic angina, are thought to be caused by GERD. A significant number of additional symptoms, including chronic cough, asthma, hoarseness, chronic sore throat, and globus sensation, may also result from occult gastroesophageal reflux

Diagnosis

When heartburn is the predominant or sole symptom, gastroesophageal reflux is the cause in at least 75% of individuals, indicating that the presence of heartburn is specific for the diagnosis of GERD. Other GERD-related symptoms include acid regurgitation, belching, water brash, dysphagia, odynophagia, chest pain, globus sensation, chronic cough, hoarseness, and asthma.

A presumptive diagnosis of GERD based on symptoms commonly leads to a trial of empiric antireflux treatment without further diagnostic testing. In first-time health care seekers, more detailed diagnostic evaluation is definitely indicated if alarm symptoms are present (i.e., dysphagia, odynophagia, anorexia, weight loss, or evidence of upper gastrointestinal bleed). Presently, most physicians accept the concept that a marked symptomatic response to antireflux treatment is highly suggestive of GERD as the underlying cause of the patient's symptoms.

Endoscopy has a low sensitivity for diagnosis of GERD, because 50% to 70% of patients with GERD-related symptoms have no evidence of esophageal mucosal injury on endoscopy. However, upper endoscopy remains the "gold standard" for diagnosis of erosive esophagitis, Barrett's esophagus (BE) (E-Fig. 35-1), and other important complications of GERD, such as ulceration and stricture. The test is indicated in patients with alarm symptoms and to exclude BE in those with long-standing symptoms of GERD. Endoscopy is also warranted if there is diagnostic uncertainty (e.g., persistence of symptoms on appropriate empiric therapy).

Presently, pH monitoring is best reserved for patients who are considered to be candidates for antireflux surgery; those who report relapse of GERD symptoms after antireflux surgery; and those with atypical or extra-esophageal symptoms that are poorly responsive to an adequate trial of antireflux therapy. Measurement of esophageal impedance and pH has a role in identifying nonacidic reflux as the case of residual GERD-related symptoms in patients being treated with proton pump inhibitors (PPIs) at least twice daily.

Treatment

For patients with mild or infrequent symptoms, it is reasonable to use antacids and lifestyle modification such as weight loss, cessation of smoking, and elevation of the head of the bed. For patients with more severe reflux symptoms, a definitive treatment is required. Treatment of GERD is summarized in Table 35-1.

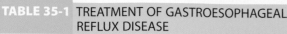

TABLE 35-1	TREATMENT OF GASTROESOPHAGEAL REFLUX DISEASE
Lifestyle modifications	Selective serotonin reuptake
Antireflux medications	inhibitors
Histamine-2 receptor antagonists	Serotonin-norepinephrine
Proton pump inhibitors	reuptake inhibitors
Transient LES relaxation reducers	Antireflux surgery
Baclofen	Endoscopic treatment
Visceral pain modulators	Alternative and complementary
Tricyclic antidepressants	medicines
Trazadone	Acupuncture
	Psychological intervention

LES, Lower esophageal sphincter.

The initial aims of GERD management are confirmation of the diagnosis of GERD, adequate relief of GERD symptoms, and healing of esophagitis, if present. Among patients with mild-to-moderate erosive esophagitis (Los Angeles grades A and B), PPIs are superior to histamine-2 receptor antagonists in providing healing of mucosal erosions and relief of GERD symptoms. For patients with severe erosive esophagitis (Los Angeles grades C and D), PPIs are the sole treatment; in some of these patients, even doubling of the dose of PPI is not infrequently required. Failure of a 4-week course of initial therapy with a PPI should prompt a review of the diagnosis if it is based solely on symptoms. For patients without adequate response to once-daily PPI, addition of a second daily dose before the evening meal is a reasonable next step.

The aims of long-term management of GERD are satisfactory control of reflux symptoms, maintenance of healing of erosive esophagitis, prevention of complications, and improvement of quality of life. Because GERD is predominantly a chronic relapsing disorder, the balance of priorities for long-term care differs from that of initial therapy.

Patients with atypical or extraesophageal manifestations of GERD should be offered double doses of PPI as the initial course of therapy. A response lag of up to 6 months may be encountered.

For patients who are unwilling to take medications for long periods and those who cannot tolerate the side effects of antireflux treatment, surgery is a reasonable alternative, provided that they are fully informed about the risks and possible complications of the procedure (e.g., increased flatulence, dysphagia, diarrhea, early satiety).

⬤ SEQUELAE OF GASTROESOPHAGEAL REFLUX DISEASE

Common complications of GERD include esophagitis, ulceration, and esophageal stricture. Strictures typically produce progressive dysphagia to solids and often require endoscopic dilatation to relieve the obstruction followed by intensive antisecretory therapy to prevent recurrence.

Barrett's Esophagus

BE is defined as a change in the esophageal epithelium of any length that can be recognized at endoscopy and confirmed to involve intestinal metaplasia by biopsy of the tubular esophagus (E-Fig. 35-2A). It is considered to be an acquired condition associated with GERD. Of those individuals undergoing endoscopy for any reason, up to 2% may have BE; among those undergoing

an endoscopy for GERD-related symptoms, 3.5% to 9.6 % are found to harbor this premalignant lesion. Both BE and esophageal adenocarcinoma are much less common in non-Caucasian populations; the reasons are not defined. There are data suggesting that obesity and smoking contribute to the risk of adenocarcinoma arising from BE.

Many authors divide these lesions into short-segment and long-segment BE, based on the length of the metaplastic epithelium (<3 cm and ≥3 cm, respectively). Another approach is the Prague circumference and maximum length criteria: The length: The length of BE is divided to the part (if any) in which the columnar-like epithelium is circumferential (C)and the part that is composed only of metaplastic tongues (M). It is more common to find dysplasia in patients with long-segment BE, and there is a correlation between the length of Barrett's epithelium and the risk of developing dysplasia and adenocarcinoma of the esophagus.

Given the increased risk of adenocarcinoma development, surveillance of patients with known BE is recommended (see E-Fig. 35-2B). The lack of large-scale studies on which to base these recommendations has led to a variety of guidelines based on presumed risk. Because inflammation can mimic the cellular and nuclear changes that are often seen with dysplasia, all patients with BE should be adequately treated with acid suppression therapy (i.e., PPI) before endoscopy. Even if antireflux surgery has been performed, a surveillance program is still warranted.

Under most circumstances, patients with BE without dysplasia should have endoscopic surveillance at 3- to 5-year intervals or if their symptom pattern changes. Multiple biopsies, taken every 2 cm in four quadrants, are recommended. Biopsies should be reviewed by a pathologist familiar with Barrett's metaplasia. If dysplasia of any degree is found, the biopsy specimens should be forwarded to another pathologist who specializes in Barrett's histopathology.

Dysplasia is typically categorized as low-grade, high-grade, or indefinite for dysplasia (see E-Fig. 35-2C). Current recommendations suggest that patients with high-grade or low-grade dysplasia confirmed by an expert pathologist should undergo repeat endoscopy within 6 months. If there is no change, radiofrequency ablation of the Barrett's mucosa is recommended. Various mucosal ablative techniques are available, including photodynamic therapy, radiofrequency ablation, cryoablation, and argon plasma coagulation.

⬤ DYSPHAGIA

Dysphagia means difficulty in swallowing. Dysphagia may result from any alteration of the swallowing process, from bolus entry into the mouth to entry into the stomach. Given the complexity of this process, a wide array of abnormalities may be involved and the symptoms are poorly discriminating. Dysphagia may be divided into abnormalities related to the movement of a food bolus from the mouth to the esophagus (transfer or oropharyngeal dysphagia) and alterations of movement from entry into the esophagus to the stomach (transport or esophageal dysphagia) (Fig. 35-1).

Oropharyngeal Dysphagia

The process of moving a food bolus, particularly liquids, from the mouth to the esophagus, coming as it does in close proximity to

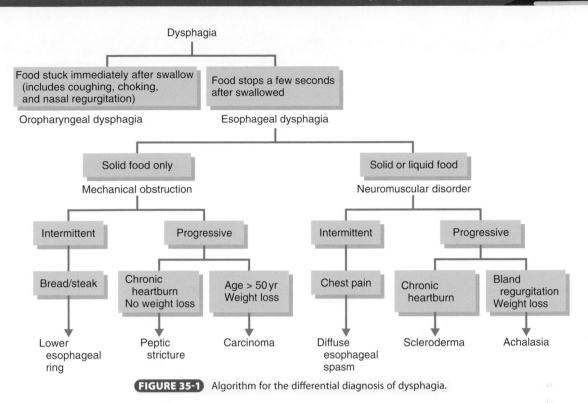

FIGURE 35-1 Algorithm for the differential diagnosis of dysphagia.

the airway, requires a fine coordination of events happening at a very rapid rate. Disruption of this phase of swallowing may be caused by structural defects or, more commonly, by neuromuscular dysfunction. Structural abnormalities that may be encountered in the hypopharynx include cervical osteophytes, hypopharyngeal diverticulum (Zenker's diverticulum), head and neck tumors, radiation injury, and postcricoid webs. In these settings, patients may have difficulty when a solid bolus leaves the mouth and enters the tubular esophagus.

Much more commonly, symptoms of transfer dysphagia result from neuromuscular injury causing disruption of this finely coordinated act of swallowing. In these situations, problems are much more commonly associated with attempts to swallow liquids. Sensory or motor injury may lead to an inability to accomplish the transfer of a bolus from the mouth to the esophagus. Stroke (particularly involving the brain stem) is one of the most common causes of oropharyngeal dysphagia. This scenario is associated with a higher patient mortality rate because of a higher risk of aspiration pneumonia and dehydration.

Essentially, any disease process that affects the brain can result in dysphagia. The more common associations are amyotrophic lateral sclerosis, Parkinson's disease, and brain tumors. Primary muscular diseases may also result in oropharyngeal dysphagia. These include oculopharyngeal muscular dystrophy, myotonic dystrophy, myasthenia gravis, and tardive dyskinesia. Patients with oropharyngeal dysphagia commonly complain that food gets "stuck" immediately upon swallowing; this sensation may be associated with choking, coughing, or nasal regurgitation.

Esophageal Dysphagia

Once the food bolus enters the esophagus, passage may be impeded by structural abnormalities or alterations in esophageal motility. These alterations range from congenital abnormalities to acquired conditions, and they constitute a rather large differential diagnosis. Solid food dysphagia alone is more commonly

seen in patients with mechanical obstruction, whereas solid and liquid dysphagia is typically encountered in esophageal motility disorders such as achalasia. Patients with esophageal dysphagia usually report the onset of symptoms several seconds after initiation of a swallow.

● ESOPHAGEAL MOTILITY DISORDERS

The more common disorders of esophageal motility are achalasia, diffuse esophageal spasm, and scleroderma, and their key features are outlined in Table 35-2.

Primary Motility Disorders

The term *primary motility disorders* refers to a number of conditions in which there is some disruption in the neuromuscular control of esophageal peristalsis.

Achalasia

The prototype of esophageal dysmotility is achalasia. This condition, characterized by loss of esophageal peristalsis and failure of LES relaxation, is the most widely recognized primary motility disorder. A variety of changes have been described in patients with this condition: loss of ganglion cells from the myenteric plexus; degenerative changes in the vagus nerve; degenerative changes in the dorsal motor nucleus of the vagus, including occasional evidence of intracytoplasmic inclusions (Lewy bodies); loss of small intramuscular nerve fibers; and reduction in vesicles of small nerve fibers. The initial site of injury is unknown, and 98% of cases are idiopathic. Achalasia may occur at any age from childhood to late adulthood. The peak occurrence is between the ages of 30 and 60 years.

The hallmark symptom of achalasia is dysphagia, typically for both solids and liquids. Other commonly noted symptoms include regurgitation, chest pain, and what patients describe as "heartburn." Symptoms typically have been present for years before diagnosis, and this may especially be true if patients are

TABLE 35-2	ESOPHAGEAL MOTOR DISORDERS		
FEATURE	**ACHALASIA**	**SCLERODERMA**	**DIFFUSE ESOPHAGEAL SPASM**
Symptoms	Dysphagia Regurgitation of nonacidic material	GERD Dysphagia	Substernal chest pain (angina-like) Dysphagia with pain
Radiographic appearance	Dilated, fluid-filled esophagus Distal "bird-beak" stricture	Aperistaltic esophagus Free reflux Peptic stricture	Simultaneous noncoordinated contractions
CONVENTIONAL MANOMETRIC FINDINGS			
LES	High resting pressure Incomplete or abnormal relaxation with swallow	Low resting pressure	Normal pressure
Body	Low-amplitude, simultaneous contractions after swallowing	Low-amplitude peristaltic contractions or no peristalsis	Some peristalsis Diffuse and simultaneous nonperistaltic contractions, occasionally high amplitude

GERD, Gastroesophageal reflux disease; LES, lower esophageal sphincter.

carefully interviewed. Weight loss may be encountered as well. Achalasia may result in pulmonary symptoms, a complication suggested by the presence of cough resulting from aspiration of esophageal contents. Neuronal denervation is the underlying mechanism of achalasia. This results in failure of esophageal body peristalsis and failure of the LES to relax in response to swallowing.

High-resolution manometry has been used to define three subtypes of achalasia. Each is associated with incomplete LES relaxation. Type 1 (classic achalasia) is devoid of any significant decreases in esophageal pressurization. Type 2 is associated with simultaneous pressurization throughout the esophagus after a swallow. Type 3 (spastic achalasia) is associated with luminal obliterating contractions after a swallow.

When achalasia is identified, its treatment can progress through several stages: (1) medical therapy with nitrates and calcium channel blockers to lower sphincter pressures and with PPIs; (2) botulinum toxin injection to lower LES pressures; (3) pneumatic dilation to facilitate luminal opening; and (4) esophageal myotomy, performed either laparoscopically or in the traditional transthoracic approach (Heller myotomy).

Secondary Achalasia

A number of conditions may result in a syndrome resembling achalasia. The most common and important of these causes is malignancy involving the region of the gastroesophageal junction (e.g., adenocarcinoma of the cardia, gastric lymphoma) or, less commonly, metastatic involvement from a distant primary malignancy (e.g., small cell lung cancer, Hodgkin's lymphoma, hepatocellular carcinoma). The result is a syndrome that radiographically and manometrically resembles primary achalasia. Such involvement is typically seen in older patients in whom the development of dysphagia is rapid. Most of these cases are identified by endoscopic examination. Other diseases that may mimic achalasia include Chagas' disease (South American trypanosomiasis) and intestinal pseudo-obstruction, which may be caused by a host of conditions ranging from familial neuropathies and myopathies to disorders such as muscular dystrophy.

Rings and Webs

Nosology is critical when discussing rings and webs. An esophageal *ring* is a distal esophageal structure that occurs at the esophagogastric junction; it is covered on one side by squamous mucosa

and on the other by columnar mucosa. One exception to this rule is Schatzki's ring, which is typically located radiographically about 2 cm proximal to the esophagogastric mucosal junction, as described later. An esophageal *web* is a ring-like structure along the entire length of the esophagus that is covered entirely by squamous mucosa. Cervical esophageal webs are typically diaphragm-like structures found in the immediate postcricoid area. They may be identified incidentally on radiographic or endoscopic imaging, although they can easily be missed if care is not taken to carefully examine this area of the esophagus. The pathogenesis of cervical webs is unknown. Pathologically, they are composed of normal squamous tissue overlying connective tissue; this bland histology separates these typical cervical webs from those changes found in the proximal esophagus associated with dermatologic diseases (e.g., epidermolysis bullosa, pemphigoid, chronic graft-vs-host disease). Symptomatic patients are more likely to be female. Typically, the symptom complex is intermittent solid food dysphagia. The association between iron deficiency anemia and esophageal webs is referred to as Paterson-Kelly or Plummer-Vinson syndrome.

Treatment of the typical cervical web is usually simple. Most can be disrupted during the performance of endoscopy. Esophageal bougienage may be required in some patients.

A lower esophageal ring (Schatzki's ring) is thought to be the most common cause of dysphagia (E-Fig. 35-3). The history tends to be characteristic. Patients are typically older than 40 years of age and report intermittent, solid food dysphagia occurring early in a meal. The dysphagia is usually transient, and if the bolus passes, the remainder of the meal can be consumed. Patients may go for many weeks without symptoms. The dysphagia is not progressive, and constitutional symptoms such as bleeding or weight loss are absent. Occasionally, patients with Schatzki's ring may have food impaction at presentation.

Rings can be visualized either radiographically or endoscopically, and they cause varying degrees of luminal narrowing. Rings with a luminal diameter of 13 mm or less are more likely to be symptomatic, although other factors, including bolus size and effectiveness of esophageal peristalsis, contribute to the intermittent episodes of dysphagia.

The pathogenesis of esophageal rings is not established. Current research has focused on the likely contribution of acid reflux. Evidence suggests that many patients respond to acid suppression with PPIs, in terms of both increased luminal size of the ring and reduction in symptoms. In some patients, esophageal bougienage or more aggressive endoscopic manipulation (four-quadrant needle knife incision) may be required.

EOSINOPHILIC ESOPHAGITIS

Eosinophilic esophagitis was originally described in the pediatric population, but in the last decade it has been recognized increasingly in adults as well. This inflammatory process is characterized on biopsy by dense eosinophilic infiltration of the submucosa that over time leads to structural abnormalities in most patients. The underlying etiology is proposed to be delayed hypersensitivity reaction to food allergens or immunologic response to allergens outside of the gastrointestinal tract, although identification of a specific allergen is often elusive.

Dysphagia is the most commonly encountered symptom, but patients also may complain of heartburn, chest pain, nausea, and other symptoms. Food impaction may occur, sometimes as a presenting symptom. Endoscopic findings include a uniform small-caliber esophagus, single or multiple corrugations, esophageal mucosal furrows, and stricture formation. Tearing of the esophagus can occur with simple passage of the endoscope, during biopsy, or after dilatation. Diagnosis is established after biopsies from the distal and middle esophagus demonstrate dense infiltrate of 15 to 25 eosinophils per high-power field.

All patients with eosinophilic esophagitis should be treated first with a PPI, possibly twice daily, regardless if there is evidence for GERD. Subsequent treatment relies primarily on swallowed topical steroids. Fluticasone inhalers are used, for example, but the contents are sprayed into the mouth and swallowed to coat the esophagus. This approach has proved to be effective in reducing symptoms and improving histologic findings. If this approach is used, patients should be instructed to wash their mouths out with water after each treatment to prevent the development of oral candidiasis. Budesonide or other oral systemic steroids may be considered in severe cases. All patients with eosinophilic esophagitis should be evaluated for allergic reactions to food or other allergens. The relationship between GERD and eosinophilic esophagitis remains to be elucidated.

ESOPHAGEAL INFECTIONS

Infections of the esophagus are uncommon in immunocompetent individuals. They are, however, a major source of morbidity in those with compromised immunity related to immunosuppression, human immunodeficiency virus (HIV) infection, and other causes of immune suppression. Infectious esophagitis typically manifests with odynophagia as the most common symptom, and dysphagia is common as well. New onset of these symptoms in an immunocompromised individual warrants a detailed evaluation; symptoms do not readily discriminate among the different etiologies, and therapy must be targeted and can be intensive depending on the overall setting.

Candida is perhaps the most common cause of infectious esophagititis. It may or may not be associated with oral thrush, and it tends to produce dysphagia with only mild pain on swallowing. *Candida* has a characteristic appearance on endoscopic examination, and esophageal brushings and biopsies demonstrate fungal hyphae (E-Fig. 35-4). Treatment with oral fluconazole is usually effective.

Herpes simplex virus is associated with more severe odynophagia and causes esophageal ulcers that are often multiple. Acyclovir is the treatment of choice for herpes esophagitis. Cytomegalovirus (CMV) also causes esophageal ulceration and odynophagia. Endoscopic examination usually demonstrates a single large ulcer in the distal esophagus, and biopsies reveal viral inclusions that confirm the diagnosis. Both ganciclovir and foscarnet are effective treatments for CMV esophagitis.

There may be more than one infectious process involved in an individual patient. HIV infection is associated with esophageal ulceration and odynophagia, although much less commonly in the present era of effective antiretroviral therapy. As the overall immune system improves, the esophagitis typically recovers as well.

> *For a deeper discussion on this topic, please see Chapter 138, "Diseases of the Esophagus," in* Goldman-Cecil Medicine, *25th Edition.*

SUGGESTED READINGS

Armstrong D, Bennett JR, Blum AL, et al: The endoscopic assessment of esophagitis: a progress report on observer agreement, Gastroenterology 111:85–92, 1996.

Bogte A, Bredenoord AJ, Oors J, et al: Normal values for esophageal high-resolution manometry, Neurogastroenterol Motil 25:762–766, 2013.

Dellon ES, Gonsalves N, Hirano I, et al: ACG clinical guideline: evidenced-based approach to the diagnosis and management of esophageal eosinophilia and eosinophilic esophagitis (EoE), Am J Gastroenterol 108:679–692, quiz 693, 2013.

Fass R: Therapeutic options for refractory gastroesophageal reflux disease, J Gastroenterol Hepatol 27(Suppl 3):3–7, 2012.

Fass R, Achem SR: Noncardiac chest pain: diagnostic evaluation, Dis Esophagus 25:89–101, 2012.

Kumar AR, Katz PO: Functional esophageal disorders: a review of diagnosis and management, Expert Rev Gastroenterol Hepatol 7:453–461, 2013.

Vakil N, van Zanten SV, Kahrilas P, et al: The Montreal definition and classification of gastroesophageal reflux disease: a global evidence-based consensus, Am J Gastroenterol 101:1900–1920, quiz 1943, 2006.

Wang KK, Sampliner RE: Updated guidelines 2008 for the diagnosis, surveillance and therapy of Barrett's esophagus, Am J Gastroenterol 103:788–797, 2008.

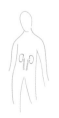

Diseases of the Stomach and Duodenum

Robert C. Lowe and M. Michael Wolfe

INTRODUCTION

The stomach acts as a reservoir for recently ingested food and initiates the process of digestion. By storing large quantities of food (1.5 to 2 L in the adult), the stomach allows intermittent feeding. Once solid particles have been reduced in size to accommodate the much smaller capacity of the duodenum, the gastric contents are released through the pylorus in a controlled fashion. This chapter focuses on the anatomy and physiology of the stomach and duodenum as well as on the most common disease processes that involve these organs.

GASTRODUODENAL ANATOMY

The stomach is in continuity with the esophagus proximally and the duodenum distally. The *lower esophageal sphincter*, a circular smooth muscle structure located at the distal end of the esophagus, creates a high-pressure zone that under normal conditions prevents gastric contents from refluxing into the esophagus. Similarly, the pyloric sphincter, the most distal portion of the stomach, plays an important role in the trituration of solid food particles and ensures the downstream propulsion of the food bolus, preventing duodenogastric reflux. The stomach is divided into four regions (Fig. 36-1; Video 36-1). The cardia is a poorly defined transition from the esophagogastric junction to the fundus. The dome-shaped fundus projects upward above the cardia and is the most superior part of the stomach in contact with the left hemidiaphragm and the spleen. The body, or corpus, located immediately below and continuous with the fundus, is the largest part of the stomach and is characterized by the presence of longitudinal folds known as rugae. The antrum extends from the incisura angularis, a fixed sharp indentation that marks the end of the gastric body, to the *pylorus*, or *pyloric channel*, a tubular structure that joins the stomach to the duodenum.

The mucosa, or inner lining of the stomach, is formed by a layer of columnar epithelium. The submucosa, immediately deep to the mucosa, provides a skeleton of dense connective tissue in which lymphocytes, plasma cells, arterioles, venules, lymphatics, and the myenteric plexus are contained. The third tissue layer, the muscularis propria, is a combination of an inner oblique, middle circular, and an outer longitudinal smooth muscle layer. The serosa, a thin, transparent continuation of the visceral peritoneum, is the final layer of the stomach wall. The autonomic innervation of the stomach stems from both sympathetic and

parasympathetic nervous systems. The anterior and posterior trunks of the vagus nerve provide parasympathetic innervation, whereas the celiac plexus, coursing along the vascular supply of the stomach, provides sympathetic innervation.

The gastric mucosal surface is composed of a single layer of mucus-containing columnar epithelial cells. The surface lining is invaginated by gastric pits, which provide access to the gastric lumen for gastric glands. The gastric glands of different regions

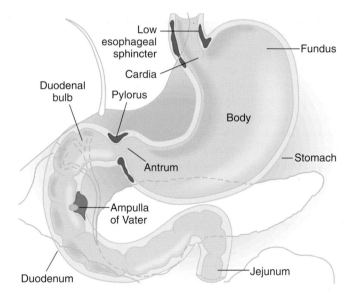

FIGURE 36-1 Anatomic regions of the stomach and duodenum. Agents that affect lower esophageal sphincter (LES) tone and gastroduodenal motility.

① ↑ Increase LES tone
-metoclopramide
-cisapride
-domperidone

↓ Decrease LES tone
-nitroglycerin
-calcium channel blockers
-progesterone
-theophylline
-benzodiazepines
-opioids
-chocolate
-coffee
-peppermint

② Gastric motility + duodenal
↑ Increase
-metoclopramide
-cisapride
-domperidone
-erythromycin

↓ Decrease
-opioids
-anticholinergics
-hyperglycemia
-tricyclic antidepressants

of the stomach are lined with different types of specialized cells. The oxyntic or acid-producing region of the stomach is found in the fundus and body, where gastric glands contain characteristic parietal cells, which secrete both acid and intrinsic factor. These glands also contain zymogen-rich chief cells, which synthesize pepsinogen, and enterochromaffin-like endocrine cells, which secrete histamine. Antral glands have different endocrine cells, including gastrin-secreting G cells and somatostatin-secreting D cells.

The duodenum, the most proximal portion of the small intestine, forms a C-shaped loop around the head of the pancreas and is in continuity with the pylorus proximally and the jejunum distally (see Fig. 36-1 and Video 36-1). Angular changes in course divide the duodenum into four portions. The first part of the duodenum is the duodenal bulb or cap and is characterized by a smooth, featureless luminal surface. The remainder of the duodenum has characteristic circular folds known as the *plica circularis* or *valvulae conniventes*, which increase the surface area available for digestion. Similar to the stomach, the duodenal wall is formed by mucosa, submucosa, muscularis, and serosa layers. The duodenal mucosa is lined with columnar cells forming villi surrounded by crypts of Lieberkühn. The submucosa includes characteristic Brunner glands that produce bicarbonate-rich secretions involved in acid neutralization. The innervation of the duodenum is similar to the stomach.

GASTRODUODENAL MUCOSAL SECRETIONS AND PROTECTIVE FACTORS

Although hydrochloric acid (HCl) is the primary gastric secretion, the stomach also secretes water, electrolytes (hydrogen [H+], sodium [Na+], potassium [K+], chloride [Cl−], and bicarbonate [HCO_3]), enzymes (pepsin and gastric lipase), and glycoproteins (intrinsic factors and mucin) to assist in a wide variety of physiologic functions. The digestion of proteins and triglycerides, as well as the complex process of vitamin B_{12} absorption, begins in the gastric lumen. Gastric acid also prevents the development of enteric microbial colonization and systemic infections. The normal human stomach contains about 1 billion parietal cells that are stimulated to secrete H+ ions by three different pathways: neurocrine, paracrine, and endocrine (Fig. 36-2). The neurocrine pathway involves the vagal release of acetylcholine, which stimulates H+ ion generation through a parietal cell muscarinic M_3 receptor. The paracrine pathway is mediated by release of histamine from mast cells and enterochromaffin-like (ECL) cells in the stomach. Histamine binds to histamine-2 receptors on parietal cells, activating adenylate cyclase, which, in turn, leads to an increase in adenosine 3′,5′-cyclic monophosphate (cAMP) levels and subsequent generation of H+ ions. The secretion of gastrin from antral G cells constitutes the endocrine pathway, which acts both directly on the parietal cell and indirectly by stimulating histamine secretion from ECL cells. The hydrogen-potassium adenosine triphosphatase (H+, K+-ATPase) enzyme, or proton pump, located at the apical surface of the parietal cell, is the final step of acid secretion. A negative feedback loop governs both gastrin release and acid secretion, preventing postprandial acid hypersecretion. Somatostatin, produced by D cells in the gastric corpus and fundus, inhibits release of gastrin from G cells and may also reduce acid secretion from parietal

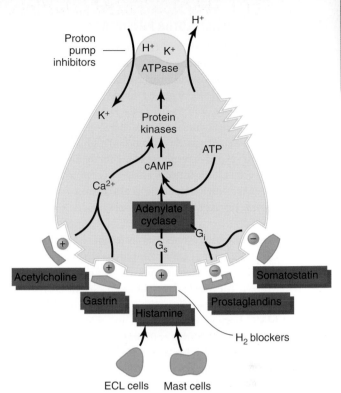

FIGURE 36-2 Schematic representation of acid secretion by the parietal cell. Each transmitter has a specific receptor located on the basolateral surface of the parietal cell. Stimulation of these receptors leads to activation of intracellular second messenger systems. Gastrin and acetylcholine promote the accumulation of intracellular calcium, whereas histamine causes a stimulatory G protein (G_s) to activate adenylate cyclase, which, in turn, generates cyclic adenosine monophosphate (cAMP). These intracellular messengers then activate protein kinases, which activate the proton pump (the H+, K+-ATPase enzyme), located at the apical surface of the parietal cell, to secrete H+ ion in exchange for K+ ions. Prostaglandins and somatostatin inhibit parietal cell function by binding to receptors that act through inhibitory G proteins (G_i) to inhibit adenylate cyclase. *Long arrows* indicate sites of action of various drugs that inhibit acid secretion. ECL, Enterochromaffin-like endocrine cells.

cells and histamine release from ECL cells. Acid is necessary to convert pepsinogen, secreted from gastric chief cells, into pepsin, a proteolytic enzyme that is inactive at a pH greater than 4. Parietal cells also secrete intrinsic factor, a glycoprotein that binds to ingested vitamin B_{12}, allowing its absorption in the terminal ileum.

Several mechanisms are involved in maintaining the protective mucosal barrier. Mucus and HCO_3 constitute the first line of defense. Mucus forms a stable layer that prevents H+ ion back-diffusion and lubricates the mucosa, protecting against mechanical damage and maintaining a significant pH gradient between the gastric lumen and the epithelial cell surface. Endogenous epithelial defensive factors, such as cell migration and proliferation, permit a constant and rapid renewal of the mucosa and ensure the continuity of the epithelium and the integrity of the tight intercellular junctions. Subepithelial defensive factors such as an adequate mucosal blood flow constitute a second line of protection and play a crucial role in maintaining a normal pH environment and thereby the integrity of the gastroduodenal mucosa.

GASTRODUODENAL MOTOR PHYSIOLOGY

Based on electrophysiologic and functional characteristics, the stomach can be divided into two functional compartments. The proximal stomach (fundus and proximal third of the body) acts as a reservoir for recently ingested food, whereas the distal stomach grinds, mixes, and sieves food particles. The smooth muscle of the proximal stomach has a characteristic tonic contraction that allows for gastric accommodation, a process by which the fundus relaxes in response to incoming food and fluid, with little increase in intragastric pressure. In contrast, the distal stomach produces high-amplitude contractions originating from the pacemaker region in the midportion of the greater curvature.

Gastroduodenal motor events vary in response to fasting and food intake. During fasting, gastric motility is characterized by a pattern of phasic contractions known as the migrating motor complex (MMC). The MMC clears the stomach and small intestine of undigested food particles, mucus, and sloughed epithelial cells. The MMC begins in the stomach and migrates down the length of the small bowel with a combined duration of 84 to 112 minutes. Following a meal, irregular contractile activity propels the ingested material distally.

Gastric emptying of a mixed solid and liquid meal involves the coordinated actions of the distinct regions of the stomach with feedback from the small intestine. Although liquids empty from the stomach at a relatively linear rate, solids are propelled forward by gastric contractions toward the antrum, where particles are triturated by high-amplitude contractions. Once solids have been reduced in size to particles of 1 to 2 mm, they are emptied into the pylorus.

A variety of medications and foods that exert significant effects on gastroduodenal motility are described in Figure 36-1 (see Video 36-1). Agents that modify the lower esophageal sphincter and esophageal motility are explained in Chapter 36.

PEPTIC ULCER DISEASE

Definition and Epidemiology

Peptic ulcer disease (PUD) is a common clinical problem characterized by mucosal defects of the stomach or duodenum. The proteolytic enzyme pepsin and gastric acid were initially identified as key factors involved in their pathogenesis, leading to the concept of *no acid, no ulcer*. However, in the past two decades, factors other than acid and pepsin that contribute to the development of ulcers have been recognized. Men and women are at equal risk for developing PUD, and the overall lifetime risk is ~10%. Peptic ulcers are uncommon in children, but the risk increases with age. More than 70% of all ulcer cases occur in individuals between the ages of 25 and 64 years. Whereas the incidence of PUD is decreasing in younger age groups, more persons 65 years of age and older are developing ulcers. These trends are likely related to the overall decrease in the prevalence of *Helicobacter pylori* infection in the general population and the increasing use of NSAIDs by older persons. The most important risk factors for the development of peptic ulcers are infection with *H. pylori* and use of NSAIDs. If neither of these factors is present, an alternative cause must be sought, including

hypersecretory states (e.g., Zollinger-Ellison syndrome [ZES]) or one of the other less common causes of ulcer disease such as Crohn disease, vascular insufficiency, viral infection, radiation therapy, and cancer chemotherapy. Although a significant number of environmental factors, including stress, personality type, occupation, alcohol consumption, and diet, have been linked to the development of ulcers, there is no convincing evidence suggesting that any of these factors by itself can cause PUD.

Pathology

By killing ingested bacteria and other microorganisms, gastric acid prevents the development of enteric colonization and ensures both efficient absorption of nutrients and prevention of systemic infections. Gastric acid is also an important factor in protein hydrolysis and digestion and, under various conditions, may play an etiologic role in inciting gastroduodenal mucosal injury. Postprandial gastric acid secretion is regulated primarily by increases in gastrin expression, which is controlled by a negative feedback loop wherein postprandial gastrin-mediated acid secretion stimulates the release of somatostatin from antral D cells. Somatostatin appears to act by a paracrine mechanism to inhibit further release of gastrin from G cells. Somatostatin produced by D cells in the gastric corpus and fundus may also directly inhibit acid secretion from parietal cells and may suppress histamine release from ECL cells. Although the presence of acid is necessary for the formation of ulcers, acid secretion is normal in nearly all patients with gastric ulcers and is increased in only one third of patients with duodenal ulcers. Therefore, acid is clearly not the only factor involved in the pathogenesis of peptic ulcers, and the balance between aggressive factors that act to injure the gastroduodenal mucosa and defensive factors that normally protect against corrosive agents is also important. When this delicate balance is disrupted for any reason, an ulcer may result.

In addition to the regulation of intragastric acidity, mechanisms involved in maintaining the protective mucosal barrier include mucus and HCO_3^- secretion, mucosal blood flow, cell restitution and repair, and changes in local immune factors. The mucosal defensive properties appear to be mediated to a large extent by endogenous prostaglandins, nitric oxide, and trefoil proteins. When the synthesis of these mediators is diminished, even normal rates of acid secretion may be sufficient to injure the mucosa.

Helicobacter pylori Infection

Helicobacter pylori (*H. pylori*) are curved, flagellated, gram-negative rods found only in gastric epithelium or in regions of gastric metaplasia. It is the most common worldwide cause of microbial infection, involving an estimated 50% of the world's population. *H. pylori* organisms clearly cause histologic gastritis and are found in 50% to 95% of patients with gastroduodenal ulcers. However, only a minority of patients with *H. pylori* gastritis develop peptic ulcer disease (PUD) or gastric cancer. In the Western world, there is a clear age-related prevalence of *H. pylori* infection in healthy individuals, increasing from 10% in those younger than 30 years to 60% in those older than 60 years. The mode of transmission appears to be by the fecal-oral route. Improvements in sanitation and standards of living appear to account for the decline in the rate of infection. *H. pylori* colonization is more common in individuals in lower socioeconomic strata compared with other groups. In the developing world, infection is far more common, with more than 80% of the population being infected by age 20 years. *H. pylori* infection is typically lifelong unless antimicrobial treatment is instituted.

H. pylori organisms reside in the mucus layer overlying gastric epithelium and are characterized as noninvasive organisms. Factors important in the organism's ability to colonize the stomach include its motility, the production of urease, and bacterial adherence. Ammonia generated from urea by *H. pylori* urease neutralizes acid, creating a more hospitable microclimate in which the bacteria can survive. *H. pylori* also have the ability to bind specifically to gastric-type epithelium, which prevents the organisms from being shed during cell turnover, mucus secretion, or gastric motility. Tissue injury is mediated by the production of lipopolysaccharide, leukocyte-activating factors, and vaculolating toxins, which have been associated with cytotoxic effects, inflammation, and cytokine activation. About 65% of *H. pylori* isolates produce a vacuolating toxin. Toxin-producing strains may be more pathogenic than those that do not produce toxins, and their presence correlates with a more intense polymorphonuclear cell infiltration. A cytotoxin-associated gene *(cagA)* is a marker for strains that make the vacuolating toxin, and patients infected with *cagA*-positive strains are more likely to develop ulcers (Fig. 36-3). Colonization causes acute and chronic inflammation consisting of neutrophils, plasma cells, T cells, and macrophages accompanied by varying degrees of epithelial cell injury, all of which resolve after effective treatment.

Although predicting the ultimate outcome of *H. pylori* infection is impossible, the clinical manifestations can be correlated with the distributions of gastric histopathologic states. Antral-predominant *H. pylori* gastritis is associated with duodenal ulcers; individuals infected with *H. pylori* have been shown to have a diminished number of somatostatin-secreting D cells, which decreases the magnitude of the response to luminal acidification. Thus, in patients with *H. pylori* infection limited to the antrum, the negative inhibition of gastrin release is disrupted, resulting in higher postprandial gastrin levels and hypersecretion

of acid. Corporal and fundic colonizations, by contrast, are more likely to cause atrophic gastritis.

Other important factors that may influence the outcomes of the infection include the host response, environmental factors, and age at the time of infection. Virtually all patients with *H. pylori* infection have a chronic superficial gastritis; however, duodenal and gastric ulcers develop in only 20% of infected patients. Patients with *H. pylori* infection and severe atrophic gastritis, corpus-predominant gastritis, or both, along with intestinal metaplasia, are at increased risk for intestinal-type gastric cancer. Finally, the mucosal lymphocytic response to *H. pylori* infection may lead to a monoclonal B-cell proliferation in mucosa-associated lymphoid tissue (MALT). MALT lymphomas, also known as *maltomas*, are rare, with about 1 in 1 million infected patients developing the disease. Complete histologic regression has been demonstrated in 50% to 80% of maltomas following eradication of *H. pylori*. Flat, localized, nonbulky lesions of the distal stomach are associated with greater rates of cure after antibiotic therapy.

Nonsteroidal Anti-inflammatory Drugs

NSAIDs are one of the most widely used classes of drugs. Although generally well tolerated, NSAIDs are associated with a small but significant percentage of adverse gastrointestinal (GI) events. Concepts regarding NSAID-induced gastroduodenal mucosal injury have evolved from a simple notion of topical injury to theories involving multiple mechanisms by which NSAIDs induce both local and systemic effects. According to the dual-injury model, NSAIDs have direct toxic effects on the gastroduodenal mucosa and indirect effects through active hepatic metabolites and decreased synthesis of mucosal prostaglandins. Hepatic metabolites are excreted into the bile and subsequently into the duodenum, where they may cause mucosal damage to the stomach by duodenogastric reflux and to the small intestine by antegrade passage through the GI tract. Prostaglandin inhibition, in turn, leads to reduction in epithelial mucus, decreased secretion of HCO_3, impaired mucosal blood flow, reduced epithelial proliferation, and decreased mucosal resistance to injury. The impairment in mucosal resistance facilitates mucosal injury by endogenous factors, including acid, pepsin, and bile salts.

Prostaglandins are derived from arachidonic acid, which originates from cell membrane phospholipids through the action of phospholipase A_2. The metabolism of arachidonic acid to prostaglandins and leukotrienes is catalyzed by the cyclooxygenase (COX) pathway and the 5-lipoxygenase (LOX) pathway, respectively (Fig. 36-4). Two related but unique isoforms of COX, designated COX-1 and COX-2, have been demonstrated in mammalian cells. Despite their structural similarities, each is encoded by distinct genes that differ with regard to their distribution and expression in tissues; the COX-1 gene is primarily expressed constitutively, whereas the COX-2 gene is inducible. COX-1 appears to function as a housekeeping enzyme in most tissues, including the gastric mucosa, whereas the expression of COX-2 can be induced by inflammatory stimuli and mitogens in many different types of tissue. It is postulated that the anti-inflammatory properties of NSAIDs are mediated through the inhibition of COX-2, whereas adverse effects, such as gastroduodenal ulceration, occur as a result of the effects on COX-1. The discovery of the two COX

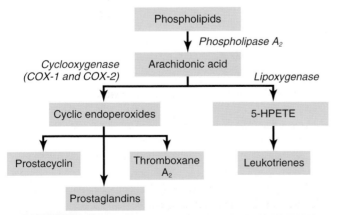

FIGURE 36-3 Mechanisms by which *Helicobacter pylori* may cause gastric ulcers **(A)** and duodenal ulcers **(B)**. IL-8, interleukin-8. (From Peek RM, Blaser MJ: Pathophysiology of *Helicobacter pylori*–induced gastritis and peptic ulcer disease, Am J Med 102:200-207, 1997.)

isoforms led to the development of COX-2–specific inhibitors (e.g., celecoxib, rofecoxib, valdecoxib), drugs that maintain their anti-inflammatory properties while preserving the biosynthesis of protective prostaglandins (Fig 36-5). Unfortunately, adverse cardiovascular effects of COX-2 inhibitors have limited the use of these drugs.

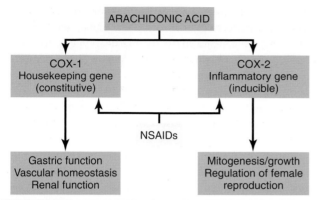

FIGURE 36-4 Biosynthesis of prostaglandins and leukotrienes through the cyclooxygenase and lipoxygenase pathways.

The spectrum of NSAID-related mucosal injury includes a combination of subepithelial hemorrhages, erosions, and ulcerations that is often referred to as *NSAID gastropathy*. Erosions are likely to be small and superficial, whereas ulcers tend to be larger (more than 5 mm in diameter) and deeper. Although no area of the stomach is resistant to NSAID-induced mucosal injury, the most frequently and severely affected site is the antrum. Microscopically, a *reactive* pattern of injury can be found that is characterized by mucin depletion and little or no increase in inflammatory cells. Endoscopic studies have shown a prevalence of gastroduodenal ulcers of 10% to 25% in patients with chronic arthritis treated with NSAIDs, which is 5 to 15 times the expected prevalence in an age-matched healthy population.

In addition, at least 60% of individuals with complicated ulcers (e.g., hemorrhage, perforation) report the use of NSAIDs, including aspirin. NSAID-induced ulceration occurs with all traditional NSAIDs, regardless of enteric coating or delivery as a prodrug formulation. The risk for NSAID-induced ulceration and complications is dose related and increases with age older than 60 years, concurrent corticosteroid use, increasing duration and dose of therapy, anticoagulant therapy, and a history of prior ulcer disease.

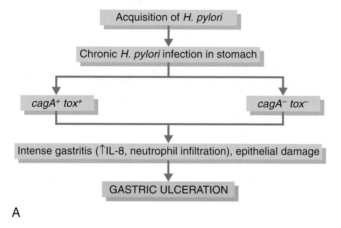

A

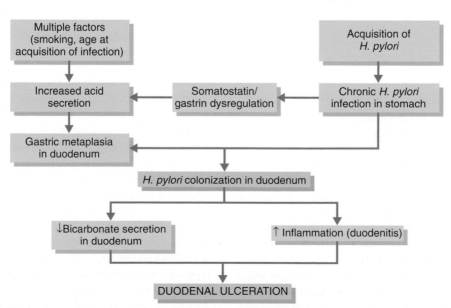

B

FIGURE 36-5 Depiction of the two cyclooxygenase isoenzymes that catalyze the synthesis of tissue prostaglandins from arachidonic acid.

Zollinger-Ellison Syndrome

ZES, an acid hypersecretory state caused by gastrin-secreting tumors, accounts for 0.1% of patients who have PUD and should be considered in patients with ulcers in unusual sites (e.g., distal duodenum, jejunum); multiple, recurrent, or complicated duodenal ulcers; or ulcers associated with chronic diarrhea. This disorder is discussed in detail below.

Clinical Presentation

Peptic ulcer disease can be clinically silent or can exhibit a variety of manifestations ranging from iron deficiency anemia to abdominal pain, obstruction, perforation, and hemorrhage. Symptoms may mimic those of other diseases, including cholecystitis, pancreatitis, gastric cancer, and gastroesophageal reflux. Myocardial ischemia or infarction, especially of the inferior wall, can cause abdominal pain that resembles peptic ulcer. Abdominal pain in PUD is generally epigastric and is usually described as a dull ache but may be sharp or burning. Less than 20% of patients report the hunger-like pain traditionally associated with both gastric and duodenal ulcers. Similarly, the character of the symptoms and their relation with meals, specifically pain relief after food intake for duodenal ulcer and pain worsening for gastric ulcer, do not always correlate with endoscopic diagnosis and are less useful in predicting ulcer location. Nocturnal pain and pain relief with milk or antacids are common with duodenal ulcers but can also occur with gastric ulcers. NSAID-associated ulcers typically produce painless bleeding. Nausea and vomiting are commonly associated with peptic ulcers, being slightly more common with gastric ulcers. Gastric outlet obstruction may be caused by antropyloric or duodenal ulcers but should be differentiated from malignant obstruction resulting from gastric or pancreatic cancer. Weight loss, while suggestive of malignancy, is reported frequently by patients with peptic ulcer disease.

Diagnosis

Because the clinical features of gastroduodenal ulcers may overlap with other disorders, and the physical examination is often not helpful in the diagnosis, imaging studies of the GI tract are required to confirm the presence of peptic ulcers. Although contrast radiology (barium upper GI series) can be used, endoscopy is preferred because, in addition to characterizing the ulcer, it allows tissue sampling to exclude malignancy, assessment of *H. pylori* infection, and, in cases of acute ulcer hemorrhage, delivery of endoscopic therapy for the control of hemorrhage.

Diagnostic Tests for *Helicobacter pylori*

Eradication of *H. pylori* infection is associated with a significant reduction in ulcer recurrence. *H. pylori* testing is thus essential in all patients with PUD, and the diagnostic options and the indications for their use are summarized in Figure 36-6. Immunoglobulin G serologic testing is the noninvasive test of choice for diagnosing *H. pylori* infection in the untreated patient. However, because the antibodies may persist for several years, serologic analysis is not useful as a means to document cure of the infection since positive results may reflect past exposure but not necessarily current infection with *H. pylori*. Another noninvasive approach to detecting *H. pylori* is the ^{13}C- or ^{14}C-labeled urea breath test.

When present, *H. pylori* urease splits the urea, which may be detected as labeled carbon dioxide in the breath of a patient. The urea breath test is more accurate than serologic tests, and although more expensive and less widely available, it is the noninvasive test of choice to document successful *H. pylori* eradication after antibiotic therapy. Patients should not receive PPIs for at least 14 days before administration of breath tests to avoid false-negative results. Stool antigen testing is also available and useful in the initial diagnosis of *H. pylori* infection. If endoscopic examination is performed, the diagnosis is made by the rapid urease test or histologic testing. In the rapid urease test, mucosal biopsies are placed in a urea-containing medium with a pH-sensitive indicator that changes color when ammonia is produced from urea by the urease of the organism. The rapid urease test has high sensitivity and specificity, equivalent to histologic analysis, and is inexpensive. Recent treatment with antibiotics or PPIs, however, may decrease the yield of the test. Histologic analysis is frequently the standard for detecting *H. pylori* infection and can establish the degree, type, and location of inflammation. Gastric biopsy specimens should be taken from both the antrum and the corpus because the bacteria are not uniformly distributed throughout the stomach. The presence of chronic active gastritis is strongly suggestive of *H. pylori* infection, even if bacteria are difficult to identify.

Treatment

Treatment of Peptic Ulcer Disease

Healing Ulcers by Suppressing Acid Secretion

Regardless of the cause, inhibition of gastric acid secretion continues to be the cornerstone of therapy for PUD. Antacids are effective agents for healing ulcers and may provide some symptom relief. However, because of the need to take these drugs multiple times each day, and the associated adverse effects, antacids are now rarely used as initial therapy.

H_2 receptor antagonists reduce acid secretion by competitively and selectively inhibiting histamine receptors on the parietal cell. H_2 receptor antagonists increase intragastric pH and inhibit pepsin activity. In general, H_2 receptor antagonists are safe and well tolerated, although the occurrence of adverse effects is slightly increased with cimetidine because of binding to cytochrome P-450 and hence increased risk for drug interactions. H_2 receptor antagonists heal 90% to 95% of duodenal ulcers and 88% of gastric ulcers after 8 weeks. Given as a single full dose at bedtime, cimetidine (800 mg), ranitidine and nizatidine (300 mg), and famotidine (40 mg) have comparable efficacies for ulcer healing. The recommended duration of treatment is 4 weeks for duodenal ulcers and 8 weeks for gastric ulcers.

Proton pump inhibitors, or PPIs, are the most potent inhibitors of gastric acid secretion available and heal gastroduodenal ulcers more rapidly than H_2 receptor antagonists. However, because they are most effective when the parietal cell is stimulated to secrete acid in response to a meal, PPIs should only be taken before a meal and should not be used in conjunction with H_2 receptor antagonists or other antisecretory agents. Moreover, because acid secretion must be stimulated for maximal efficacy, PPIs are administered before the first meal of the day. These agents are safe and well tolerated; adverse effects are unusual and include headache, diarrhea, and nausea. Single daily doses

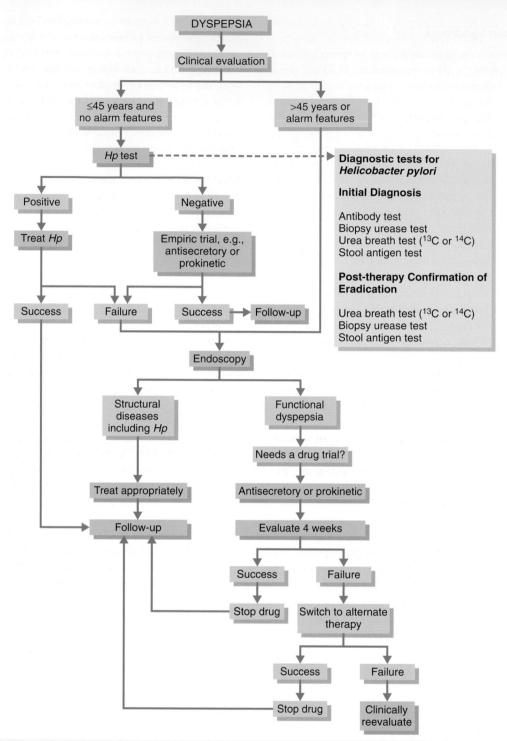

FIGURE 36-6   Diagnostic approach to patients presenting with uninvestigated dyspepsia. Alarm features include weight loss, vomiting, dysphagia, evidence of anemia, gastrointestinal bleeding, or an abdominal mass or lymphadenopathy. *Hp, Helicobacter pylori.* (Modified from American Gastroenterological Association medical position statement: evaluation of dyspepsia, Gastroenterology 114:579-581, 1998.)

of omeprazole (20 mg), pantoprazole (40 mg), rabeprazole (20 mg), lansoprazole (30 mg), or esomeprazole (40 mg), all before breakfast, are effective in healing gastroduodenal ulcers. The recommended duration of treatment is again 4 weeks for duodenal ulcers and 8 weeks for gastric ulcers.

Healing by Enhancing Mucosal Defense

Sucralfate, a complex salt of sucrose sulfate and aluminum hydroxide, appears to be as effective as H_2 receptor antagonists in the treatment of duodenal ulcer disease. The evidence for efficacy in healing of gastric ulcers is less compelling. Sucralfate has little or no effect on acid secretion and acts through several different mucosal protective mechanisms. In the gastroduodenal lumen, sucralfate becomes a gel-like substance that binds to both defective and normal mucosa, acting as a physical barrier to the diffusion of acid, pepsin, and bile acids. The recommended dose is 1 g 4 times daily, which makes it less convenient than other agents for treating PUD.

Although bismuth compounds and prostaglandin analogues have been shown to provide protective effects on the gastroduodenal mucosa and may have some effect on ulcer healing, these agents are not routinely used in the initial treatment of peptic ulcers.

Treatment of *Helicobacter pylori* Infection

Eradication of *H. pylori* should be attempted in all patients with documented current or past PUD and evidence of infection. Successful therapy requires a combination of drugs that prevents the emergence of resistance and effectively reaches the bacteria, and must be of sufficient duration to ensure eradication. Combinations of two antibiotics, plus either a PPI or ranitidine bismuth citrate, are used to maximize the chance of eradication. Current treatment regimens for *H. pylori* are shown in Table 36-1. Factors such as antibiotic resistance and noncompliance with therapy have been identified as predictors of treatment failure. Metronidazole resistance is most common, and both metronidazole and clarithromycin resistance are increasing in frequency, with rates of 37% and 10%, respectively. Because compliance is essential for treatment success, the current regimens offer simpler dosing than earlier options. A failed initial course of antibiotic therapy suggests antibiotic resistance, and it may be assumed that, if the patient received metronidazole or clarithromycin in the original regimen, resistance to that antibiotic is present. When possible, repeat use of the same antibiotic should be avoided. The recommended duration for repeat treatment courses is 14 days. An alternative initial approach involves a shorter, 10-day treatment course with PPI and sequential dosing of amoxicillin and clarithromycin, but further validation studies are needed before this can be recommended as standard therapy.

Maintenance Therapy

Before embarking on long-term maintenance therapy for PUD, careful attention must be paid to eliminating the most important risk factors for ulcer recurrence: *H. pylori* infection and NSAID use. Moreover, hypersecretory states, including gastrinoma, should be excluded in individuals with recurrent ulcers without *H. pylori* infection. Patients with a history of ulcer complications,

frequent ulcer recurrence, continued NSAID use, or *H. pylori*–negative ulcers, and those who fail to clear *H. pylori* infection despite appropriate therapy, should be considered candidates for maintenance antisecretory therapy. However, even patients who have had a complicated ulcer may not require maintenance therapy, provided *H. pylori* infection is cured. Maintenance regimens include an H_2 receptor antagonist at bedtime at one half the dose required for initial healing or a full-dose PPI taken before breakfast.

Treatment and Prophylaxis of NSAID-Induced Ulceration

The optimal treatment of patients with NSAID-induced gastroduodenal ulcers is the discontinuation of the offending agent. If NSAIDs must be continued, therapy with an antisecretory agent should be instituted. Based on their superior safety profile and their ability to heal gastroduodenal ulcers at an accelerated rate whether or not NSAID use is continued, PPIs are preferred over both H_2 receptor antagonists and misoprostol.

Because of the significant rate of serious complications associated with NSAIDs and the poor correlation between dyspeptic symptoms (e.g., abdominal pain, distention, nausea, heartburn) and the presence of gastroduodenal mucosal injury, prevention of ulceration has become the principal goal in the management of NSAID-related GI toxicity. Risk factors for NSAID-related injury include advanced age (>60 years), prior history of PUD or ulcer hemorrhage, concomitant use of anticoagulants or corticosteroids, significant comorbid conditions, and use of high NSAID doses (Table 36-2). Two strategies have been used to prevent ulcers: (1) the concomitant use of medications such as misoprostol or PPIs, and (2) the development of safer anti-inflammatory agents, such as COX-2–specific inhibitors. Misoprostol, a prostaglandin E_1 analogue, significantly reduces the development of both gastric and duodenal ulcers in patients using NSAIDs. By augmenting prostaglandin-dependent pathways, misoprostol reduces gastric acid secretion and enhances mucosal defenses. However, misoprostol is associated with significant adverse effects and a high frequency of therapy discontinuation as a result of these effects, especially when administered 4 times a day. The most frequent symptom is diarrhea, although symptoms such as abdominal pain, nausea, and bloating may also occur. A lower dose of misoprostol (200 mcg 3 times daily) is nearly as effective as 4 times daily dosing for preventing duodenal and gastric ulcers, with a slight reduction in the occurrence of adverse effects.

The second strategy to prevent NSAID-induced ulcers involves the co-administration of an antisecretory agent, usually a PPI, or the substitution of the traditional NSAID with one of the newer

---

TABLE 36-1   TREATMENT REGIMENS FOR *HELICOBACTER PYLORI* INFECTION

Triple therapy (cure rate, 85% to >90%)
BMT triple therapy for 14 days
   Bismuth subsalicylate, 524 mg by mouth 4 times daily
   Metronidazole, 250 mg by mouth 4 times daily
   Tetracycline HCl, 500 mg by mouth 4 times daily + H_2-RA for additional 4 weeks
LAC for 10 or 14 days
   Lansoprazole, 30 mg by mouth twice daily
   Amoxicillin, 1 g by mouth twice daily
   Clarithromycin, 500 mg by mouth twice daily
OAC for 10 or 14 days
   Omeprazole, 20 mg by mouth twice daily
   Amoxicillin, 1 g by mouth two times daily
   Clarithromycin, 500 mg by mouth twice daily
RBC-AC (cure rate, >90%)
   Ranitidine bismuth citrate + amoxicillin + clarithromycin
MOC (cure rate, >90% in the absence of metronidazole resistance)
   Metronidazole + omeprazole + clarithromycin

H_2-RA, histamine-2 receptor antagonist; HCl, hydrochloric acid.

TABLE 36-2   RISK FACTORS FOR DEVELOPMENT OF NSAID-RELATED ULCERS

DEFINITE	POSSIBLE
Advanced age	Concomitant infection with
History of ulcer	*Helicobacter pylori*
Concomitant corticosteroid therapy	Cigarette smoking
Concomitant anticoagulation therapy	Consumption of alcohol
High doses of NSAIDs	NSAIDs, nonsteroidal anti-inflammatory drugs.
Serious systemic disorders	

COX-2–specific inhibitors. According to available evidence, PPIs are superior to H_2 receptor antagonists in preventing gastroduodenal ulceration and improving dyspeptic symptoms during continued NSAID use. Similarly, PPIs provide protection against endoscopic NSAID ulcers at a rate at least comparable with that of misoprostol, with fewer associated GI symptoms. However, misoprostol, but not PPIs, has been shown in a prospective analysis to decrease the prevalence of ulcer complications.

COX-2–specific inhibitors (e.g., celecoxib, rofecoxib, valdecoxib) have suggested an improved GI safety profile with reduced incidence of ulcers and ulcer complications and at least similar effectiveness when compared with traditional NSAIDs. However, recent evidence suggesting an increased risk for cardiovascular events, specifically myocardial infarctions and strokes, associated with the use of selective COX-2 inhibitors, has led to significant public concern with subsequent market withdrawal of some of these agents and restricted use of others. These adverse effects are thought to be related, at least in part, to the inhibition of prostacyclin with the resultant unopposed *thrombogenic* effects of thromboxane A_2. Concern over this issue led to the withdrawal of rofecoxib and valdecoxib from the US market in 2005. Recommendations for the use of nonselective NSAID versus celecoxib and the use of either PPI or misoprostol involve risk stratification of the patient's cardiovascular risk and GI risk by the clinician.

More recent meta-analyses have suggested that concomitant *H. pylori* infection and NSAID use increase the risk for ulcer complications. Therefore, in patients who require chronic NSAID use, the current recommendation is to test for and eradicate *H. pylori*, given that it is a treatable risk factor.

Surgery

Because of the remarkable progress in pharmacologic acid suppression therapy and the recognition that ulcer disease can be cured by eliminating *H. pylori* infection and NSAIDs, surgery now plays a marginal role in treating uncomplicated PUD. Surgical intervention is now mostly reserved for managing the complications of peptic ulcers, especially gastric outlet obstruction and perforation. Some of the different surgical approaches are shown in Figure 36-7.

Complications of Peptic Ulcer Disease

Bleeding

PUD is the leading cause of upper GI bleeding, accounting for about 50% of cases and more than 150,000 hospital admissions annually in the United States. Although bleeding ceases spontaneously in 80% of patients, the mortality rate associated with bleeding ulcers is 5% to 10%. Patients with bleeding ulcers exhibit hematemesis, melena, or hematochezia, often without abdominal pain. The major risk factor for bleeding ulcers is NSAID use. Predictors for an adverse outcome include hemodynamic instability at presentation, bright red blood from the rectum or through the nasogastric tube, age older than 60 years, ongoing transfusion requirements, and an increasing number of underlying medical illnesses. All patients with upper GI bleeding should undergo early upper endoscopic examination, which allows for both therapeutic intervention and the determination of other predictors for rebleeding. Rebleeding rates are about 5% for clean-based ulcers, 10% for ulcers with flat spots, 22% for adherent clots, 43% for nonbleeding visible vessels, and 55% for active oozing or spurting from an ulcer (Fig. 36-8). Patients with large ulcers, greater than 1 to 2 cm in diameter, also have increased rebleeding and mortality rates. Endoscopic therapy with techniques such as multipolar or thermal coagulation, injection with epinephrine, or placement of hemostatic clips, clearly improves the outcome in patients with bleeding ulcers by decreasing mortality, length of hospital stay, number of blood transfusions, and need for emergency surgery.

Because most ulcer bleeding recurs within 3 days of initial presentation, patients with active bleeding or stigmata of hemorrhage, such as raised pigmented spots in an ulcer crater, can be discharged within 2 to 3 days if they are stable. Given the excellent prognosis for patients with clean-based ulcers, discharge within 24 hours of presentation or immediately after endoscopic examination appears to be safe. About 20% of patients rebleed after endoscopic therapy, and 50% of these can be successfully retreated. The remainder may be treated angiographically with either intra-arterial vasopressin or embolization techniques. Surgery is generally reserved for instances in which all other measures have failed. Although endoscopic therapy is the first treatment modality in the management of actively bleeding gastroduodenal ulcers, some evidence also suggests that adjuvant use of acid suppression therapy can reduce recurrent bleeding after initial endoscopic control. A continuous infusion of an intravenous PPI has been shown to reduce the incidence of recurrent ulcer hemorrhage following endoscopic therapy. Thus, patients with significant upper GI bleeding in whom a peptic ulcer is suggested should be treated with an intravenous PPI using a loading dose (80 mg of pantoprazole) followed by a continuous infusion (8 mg per hour of pantoprazole). If at the time of endoscopic

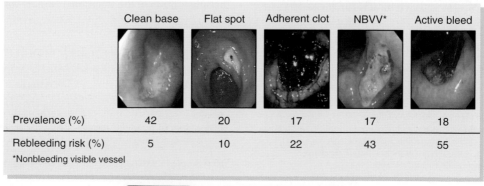

	Clean base	Flat spot	Adherent clot	NBVV*	Active bleed
Prevalence (%)	42	20	17	17	18
Rebleeding risk (%)	5	10	22	43	55

*Nonbleeding visible vessel

FIGURE 36-7 Operations for peptic ulcer disease.

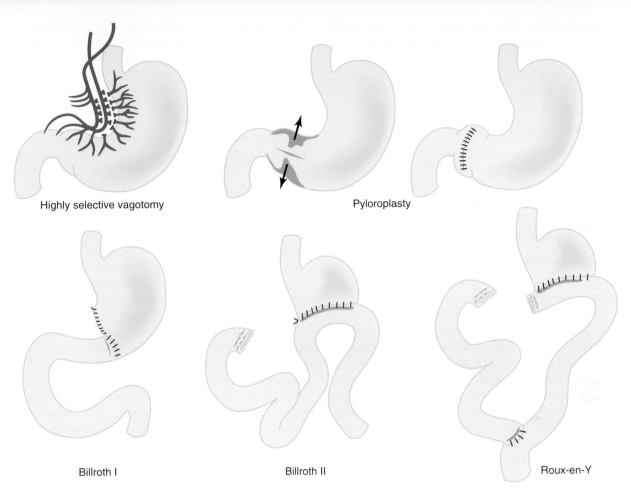

Highly selective vagotomy

Pyloroplasty

Billroth I

Billroth II

Roux-en-Y

FIGURE 36-8 Endoscopic classification of peptic ulcers with prevalence and risk of rebleeding. (From Laine L, Peterson WL: Medical progress: Bleeding peptic ulcer, N Engl J Med 331:717-727, 1994.)

examination, no evidence of recent or active bleeding can be found, and after feeding has been initiated, oral administration can be substituted for the parenteral route.

Perforation

Perforation, which occurs when a peptic ulcer erodes through the full thickness of the stomach or duodenum, is far less common than bleeding. Ulcer perforation usually leads to peritonitis, which, if untreated, may result in sepsis and death. Patients exhibit a sudden onset of severe abdominal pain that typically begins in the epigastrium and radiates throughout the entire abdomen. When peritonitis is present, physical examination is remarkable for abdominal pain, guarding, rebound tenderness, and boardlike rigidity. The clinical suggestion of perforation may be confirmed in most cases by the presence of free intra-abdominal air (pneumoperitoneum) with either an upright chest radiograph or upright and supine abdominal radiographs. In less obvious instances, computed tomography (CT) or an upper GI water-soluble contrast study may be helpful. Perforation mandates surgical intervention. A perforated duodenal ulcer is typically repaired with an omental patch, whereas a perforated gastric ulcer necessitates either an omental patch or a partial resection.

Gastric Outlet Obstruction

In the era before acid suppression and *H. pylori* therapy, PUD accounted for 60% of the cases of gastric outlet obstruction.

More recently, the incidence of both ulcers and obstruction requiring surgery has declined, and estimates indicate that fewer than 5% of patients with duodenal ulcer and less than 1% to 2% with gastric ulcer develop significant gastric outlet obstruction. Gastric outlet obstruction is typically caused by either pyloric channel or duodenal ulcers and may be seen in the setting of acute ulceration, in which edema, spasm, and inflammation lead to obstruction, or as a consequence of chronic ulceration with scarring and fibrosis. Patients usually exhibit symptoms of early satiety, bloating, nausea, vomiting, and weight loss. Endoscopy is the diagnostic test of choice but visualization of the lesion is frequently obscured by the presence of retained food residue. Patients in whom gastric outlet obstruction is suggested should undergo gastric decompression and lavage to remove retained gastric contents before endoscopic examination. Malignancy may now account for 50% of instances of gastric outlet obstruction and should be excluded with adequate biopsy and cytology samples. Occasionally, imaging techniques such as barium upper GI series and radionuclide gastric-emptying scans can also be used to determine the length of the obstructed area and to evaluate gastric emptying. In addition to the correction of fluid, electrolyte, and pH imbalances resulting from persistent vomiting, patients with gastric outlet obstruction should undergo nasogastric decompression for 3 to 5 days. During that time, acid suppression with an intravenous H_2 receptor antagonist or PPI should also be instituted. Adequacy of response may be assessed

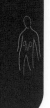

empirically with a trial of refeeding. For patients failing to respond to medical therapy, treatment options include endoscopic balloon dilation and surgery.

● GASTRITIS

Clinical Presentation

Gastritis represents a nonspecific inflammation of the mucosal surface of the stomach. Clinically, the three most common causes of gastritis are *Helicobacter pylori*, nonsteroidal anti-inflammatory drugs (NSAIDs), and stress-related mucosal changes. The approach to *H. pylori* and NSAID induced gastritis is similar to that for PUD, and is detailed above.

Stress-Related Gastric Mucosal Damage

During critical illness, events such as shock, hypotension, and catecholamine release are associated with reduced blood flow to the GI tract and mucosal ischemia. When blood flow to the mucosa is inadequate, the normal mucosal protective mechanisms, including epithelial turnover and mucus and HCO_3 secretion, are altered. In addition, mediators such as cytokines and oxygen-free radicals are released. The combination of these events reduces the mucosal resistance to acid back-diffusion, causing erosions that may progress to ulceration and bleeding. Although mucosal damage develops in most critically ill patients, stress ulcers usually remain superficial and do not erode through the stomach wall to cause perforation. The major problem is blood loss, which is occult in most instances. Although occult stress ulcer bleeding occurs in 20% of patients in long-term intensive care units, gross hemorrhage occurs in only 5%.

Treatment

Aggressive volume resuscitation, control of sepsis, and adequate oxygenation in critically ill patients are important measures that may reduce the occurrence of low-flow states and subsequent mucosal damage. A wide variety of prophylactic strategies are used to prevent GI bleeding in critically ill patients. Pharmacologic agents used in this setting exert their effects through three main mechanisms: (1) acid neutralization, (2) mucosal protection, and (3) inhibition of gastric acid secretion. Acid neutralization with antacids is effective but requires administration every 1 to 2 hours through a nasogastric tube, which is inconvenient and increases nursing time. The side effects of magnesium-containing antacids include diarrhea, hypermagnesemia, and alkalemia, whereas aluminum-based antacids cause hypophosphatemia, constipation, and metabolic alkalosis, as well as potentially toxic plasma aluminum levels in patients with renal insufficiency. Mucosal protective agents such as sucralfate, an aluminum salt of sucrose sulfate, may improve mucosal blood flow through a prostaglandin-mediated mechanism. Sucralfate is well tolerated at doses of 1 g every 4 to 6 hours. Constipation occurs in 2% to 4% of patients, and aluminum toxicity has occurred in patients with chronic renal failure. Prostaglandin analogues (e.g., misoprostol) exert a protective effect on the gastric mucosa but have not been carefully studied for stress ulcer prophylaxis, and their use in this setting cannot be recommended. Antisecretory agents inhibit gastric acid secretion and are

frequently used in the prevention of stress-induced mucosal damage in critically ill patients. Histamine-2 (H_2) receptor antagonists (e.g., cimetidine, ranitidine, famotidine, nizatidine), given either as a continuous infusion or by bolus injection, have been shown to reduce the incidence of clinically significant stress bleeding. An increase in intragastric pH to greater than 4 has been demonstrated with these agents; however, tolerance occurs rapidly and may limit their clinical efficacy. Although H_2 receptor antagonists are considered safe, they do possess both class-specific and individual side-effect potentials. The most prominent class-specific effect is central nervous system toxicity, which occurs more frequently in elderly patients compared with other age groups. Proton pump inhibitors (PPIs) irreversibly block parietal cell H+, K+-ATPase. These agents (e.g., omeprazole, lansoprazole, rabeprazole, pantoprazole, esomeprazole) are prokinetic agents that are normally activated following systemic absorption and localization to the highly acid milieu of the secretory canaliculus of *activated* parietal cells. Activation occurs after a meal, and because critically ill patients are generally fasting, PPIs administered orally or by nasogastric tube are significantly less active in this setting and are thus not recommended. However, in patients receiving enteral feeding, PPIs administered by the enteral route suppressed acid more effectively than intravenous PPIs. Pantoprazole, the first intravenous PPI available in the United States, has shown promising results in several small studies and may prove beneficial in stress bleeding prophylaxis. Intravenous preparations of lansoprazole and esomeprazole have recently become available.

Prophylaxis is recommended in patients with coagulopathy and those with respiratory failure requiring mechanical ventilation for more than 48 hours. Other patients in whom stress bleeding prophylaxis is indicated include those with central nervous system trauma, burns, organ transplantation, a history of PUD with or without bleeding, multiorgan failure, trauma, and major surgery (Table 36-3).

Other Causes of Gastritis

Autoimmune atrophic gastritis exhibits an autosomal-dominant inheritance pattern and is associated with autoantibody formation. Histologically, autoimmune atrophic gastritis is characterized by chronic inflammation, gradual atrophy of glands, and loss of parietal cells. The process is usually confined to the corpus and fundus, where the gastric glands tend to undergo intestinal metaplasia. Loss of parietal cells results in achlorhydria, vitamin B_{12} deficiency, and megaloblastic anemia (pernicious anemia). These patients have an increased risk for carcinoma, seen especially in Scandinavian countries. No overall increased cancer risk has been documented in American patients, and routine surveillance has not been advocated in the United States.

TABLE 36-3	INDICATIONS FOR STRESS BLEEDING PROPHYLAXIS
Coagulopathy	History of peptic ulcer disease with or without bleeding
Respiratory failure	
Central nervous system trauma	Multiorgan failure
Burns	Trauma or major surgery
Organ transplantation	

Lymphocytic gastritis is characterized by a mononuclear infiltration of T cells, usually antral predominant, and is often associated with celiac disease, collagenous and lymphocytic colitis, and Ménétrier disease. *Eosinophilic gastritis* is characterized by an eosinophilic infiltration of the stomach, especially the antrum. All layers of the gastric wall may be affected, but selective predominance of eosinophilic infiltrates may be found in the submucosa, muscle layers, or subserosa, making biopsy diagnosis difficult. Clinical manifestations include delayed gastric emptying or manifestations of anemia from chronic blood loss caused by associated mucosal ulceration. Corticosteroids are used to control symptoms.

Ménétrier disease is a rare disease characterized by giant gastric folds in the fundus and the body of the stomach. Histologically, increased mucosal thickness, glandular atrophy, and an increase in the size of the gastric pits are characteristic findings. Hypochlorhydria and hypoalbuminemia are commonly seen. In children, Ménétrier disease is thought to be caused by cytomegalovirus (CMV), whereas overexpression of a tissue growth factor has been implicated in the adult form of the disease.

In addition to *H. pylori*, a variety of infectious pathogens may involve the stomach. Gastric infections are typically seen in patients who are immunocompromised in the settings of HIV infection, chemotherapy, and organ transplantation. Bacterial infections such as tuberculosis and syphilis rarely involve the stomach. CMV and herpesvirus infection, as well as fungal (e.g., *Candida*, histoplasmosis, mucormycosis, cryptococcosis, aspergillosis), and parasitic infections (e.g., *Cryptosporidium*, *Strongyloides*) are also possible. Other diseases such as sarcoidosis and Crohn disease may involve the stomach. The presence of granulomas on histologic specimens, along with systemic manifestations of the disease, confirms the diagnosis.

The stomach is occasionally involved by acute *graft-versus-host* disease. Gastric erosions or ulcers may be encountered in the investigation of bone marrow transplantation patients with abdominal pain or GI bleeding. Biopsy specimens should be obtained to rule out opportunistic infections (e.g., CMV).

Alcohol, drugs (e.g., cocaine, iron, potassium chloride), and physical agents (nasogastric tubes) are also associated with nonspecific forms of gastritis. Similarly, ischemia as a result of vascular injuries, embolization, vasculitis, and amyloidosis has been described as a cause of gastritis.

● NONULCER DYSPEPSIA

Dyspepsia, defined as pain or discomfort in the upper abdomen, is a common clinical problem and may be seen at some time in 25% to 40% of adults. Though dyspepsia is a classic manifestation of PUD, only 15% to 25% of patients with dyspepsia are found to have a gastric or duodenal ulcer. The remainder of patients have nonulcer or functional dyspepsia, a condition most likely related to an abnormal perception of events in the stomach caused by afferent visceral hypersensitivity. Abnormal gastric motility may also play a role in nonulcer dyspepsia (NUD), and recent evidence suggests that about 40% of patients with NUD have impairment in the fundic accommodation response of the stomach. Dyspeptic symptoms may be chronic, recurrent, or of new onset. The diagnostic evaluation should focus on excluding other causes of dyspepsia such as gastroparesis and gastric cancer.

Management

Three possible strategies for managing patients with NUD have been formulated (see Fig. 36-6). Immediate endoscopic evaluation is indicated for individuals older than 45 years and persons exhibiting alarm features (*red flags*) such as weight loss, recurrent vomiting, dysphagia, GI bleeding, anemia, a strong family history of GI cancer, or an abdominal mass. Urgent endoscopic examination is indicated to exclude a serious underlying disease process, particularly gastric and esophageal carcinoma. If a gastric ulcer is found during endoscopic examination, multiple biopsies and cytologic analysis should be obtained to exclude malignancy. Ulcer treatment is subsequently employed, and ulcer healing should be confirmed with a follow-up endoscopic examination because nonhealing ulcers can occasionally be a manifestation of gastric carcinoma. Barium radiography offers poor sensitivity and specificity and is thus no longer recommended in the evaluation of dyspepsia.

The second option when treating patients younger than 45 years with NUD but without alarm features is an empirical trial of antisecretory therapy for 1 to 2 months. Endoscopy is indicated in patients who fail to respond to this regimen. Avoiding the introduction of long-term drug use in this situation is important, particularly because of the considerable benefit of placebo in such individuals.

The third strategy for managing NUD involves initial noninvasive testing for *H. pylori* followed by antimicrobial therapy in patients with positive tests. This strategy is presumed to heal ulcers if present, eliminate the ulcer diathesis, and save on resources, particularly in patients younger than 45 years without alarm symptoms. The frequency of *H. pylori* infection in the community should also be taken into account because noninvasive tests show decreased accuracy when the prevalence of *H. pylori* is less than 10%. This approach, although advocated by some physicians, has shown variable effectiveness in relieving NUD. Moreover, indiscriminate use of antimicrobial therapy may be associated with altering normal intestinal flora, increasing resistance of *H. pylori* and other bacteria that are not a target of therapy, and producing a series of adverse events such as antibiotic-associated and *Clostridium difficile* colitis.

● ZOLLINGER-ELLISON SYNDROME

Zollinger-Ellison Syndrome (ZES) is characterized by elevated levels of serum gastrin produced by gastrin-secreting tumors that are most often located in the pancreas and duodenum. Hypergastrinemia stimulates hypersecretion of gastric acid and pepsin, which may produce peptic ulcers, duodenojejunitis, esophagitis, and diarrhea. ZES is an uncommon cause of PUD, accounting for less than 1% of the instances. The gastrin-secreting tumor in ZES, referred to as a *gastrinoma*, is frequently located in the *gastrinoma triangle*, an area encompassed by the second and third portions of the duodenum, the junction of the head and neck of the pancreas, and the cystic duct. Seventy-five percent of all gastrinomas are sporadic; the remaining 25% are part of the type I multiple endocrine neoplasia (MEN-I) syndrome, an autosomal-dominant condition with a locus on chromosome 11, typically associated with hyperparathyroidism and pituitary tumors. All patients with sporadic gastrinomas without evidence of liver metastases should be surgically explored with the intent of removing local and regional disease. Unfortunately, despite careful diagnostic testing, no tumor is found in at least 10% of diagnosed instances of ZES.

ZES should be considered in patients with recurrent PUD in the absence of *H. pylori* infection or NSAID use, as well as in patients with multiple duodenal ulcers, ulcers in unusual locations (distal duodenum or jejunum), or severe or refractory diarrhea or gastroesophageal reflux disease. Although peptic ulcer occurs in more than 90% of patients with ZES, as many as 35% of individuals exhibit only diarrhea. The diagnosis of ZES is made when a fasting gastrin concentration of more than 1000 pg/mL exists in the setting of gastric acid hypersecretion. In equivocal cases (e.g., gastrin <1000 pg/mL), a positive secretin provocative test will confirm the diagnosis. The secretin test is positive (≥200 pg/mL increase over the preinjection fasting gastrin level) in about 90% of patients with ZES and moderately elevated gastrin levels. Basal acid output is elevated (>15 mmol per hour without previous gastric acid–reducing surgery and >5 mmol per hour with prior surgery) in more than 90% of patients with ZES. Because gastrinomas constitute a relatively uncommon cause of hypergastrinemia, other causes of an elevated gastrin level should be considered. The most common causes of hypergastrinemia are antrum-dominant *H. pylori* infection or achlorhydria related to either decreased intraluminal acid in the setting of atrophic gastritis or antisecretory therapy with PPIs. Hypergastrinemia may be related to other causes, including retained gastric antrum (after ulcer surgery), massive small bowel resection, chronic gastric outlet obstruction, and chronic renal failure. Therefore, the presence of acid hypersecretion, as documented by gastric acid analysis, may be necessary to establish the diagnosis.

Once hypergastrinemia has been established and obvious causes have been excluded, efforts should focus on localizing and resecting the gastrin-secreting tumor. The single best imaging test for gastrinoma is somatostatin-receptor scintigraphy (SRS), which is more sensitive than conventional imaging studies, including CT, magnetic resonance imaging (MRI), and ultrasonography, although endoscopic ultrasonography (EUS) is equally sensitive for localizing primary tumors of the pancreas. If liver metastasis is present, a CT- or ultrasound-guided liver biopsy should be performed. In patients without liver metastasis, SRS will localize a possible primary tumor in 60% of cases. If the patient is a surgical candidate and SRS is positive for a primary tumor, no additional localization studies are required. If the SRS is negative for a possible primary tumor, the use of MRI, angiography, or EUS will detect a possible primary tumor in an additional 15% of patients. Multiple pancreatic or duodenal tumors are generally detected in patients with MEN-I syndrome, and although the precise role of surgery in these patients is less certain, some physicians recommend surgery if a lesion larger than 3 cm is identified with preoperative imaging techniques to decrease the possibility of hepatic metastasis. However, successful and long-lasting remission of MEN-I syndrome occurs rarely, if at all.

All patients with ZES, whether sporadic or familial, require antisecretory therapy after the diagnosis is established and during initial evaluation as attempts are made to localize the gastrinoma. Patients with ZES should be treated initially with a PPI using twice the dose normally employed to treat common gastroduodenal ulcers. Intravenous PPIs such as pantoprazole in daily doses ranging from 80 to 240 mg can be used in patients who are unable to take medications by mouth, including those undergoing surgery. The goal of therapy is a basal acid output of less than 10 mmol per hour in the hour preceding the next dose of the drug. Chronic therapy with PPIs uniformly results in continued inhibition of acid secretion, good symptom control, complete healing of any mucosal lesions, and few adverse effects.

GASTROPARESIS

Gastroparesis is a syndrome characterized by delayed gastric emptying, resulting in impaired transit of food from the stomach to the duodenum in the absence of mechanical obstruction. Symptoms of gastric stasis include early or easy satiety, bloating, nausea and vomiting, and abdominal discomfort. Because eating exacerbates symptoms, patients frequently exhibit anorexia, weight loss, and nutritional deficiencies. A wide range of clinical disorders is associated with impaired gastric emptying (Table 36-4).

Diabetes mellitus is the most common cause of gastroparesis, and up to 60% of patients with diabetes complain of symptoms consistent with gastric stasis. Although gastroparesis is typically seen in individuals with long-standing (>10 years) type 1 diabetes who have other complications, such as peripheral and autonomic neuropathy, nephropathy, and retinopathy, GI complaints are also common within the first decade of diagnosis. Diabetic gastroparesis appears to occur as a result of permanent neuropathy of autonomic and enteric nerves, transitory variations in glycemic control, or a combination of both. Idiopathic gastroparesis is also common and comprises those instances with no clearly identifiable cause. Up to one third of these patients have virus-induced gastroparesis, with viral infiltration of the myenteric plexus in the stomach. Patients who have undergone gastric

TABLE 36-4	CAUSES OF DELAYED GASTRIC EMPTYING	
MECHANICAL CAUSES	Amyloidosis	
	Pseudo-obstruction	
Peptic ulcer disease, scarred pylorus	Myotonic dystrophy	
Malignancy: gastric cancer, gastric lymphoma, pancreatic cancer	Neuropathy	
	Scleroderma	
Gastric surgery: vagotomy, gastric resection, roux-en-Y anastomosis	Amyloidosis	
	Autonomic neuropathy	
Crohn disease		
ENDOCRINE AND METABOLIC CAUSES	**CENTRAL NERVOUS SYSTEM OR PSYCHIATRIC DISORDERS**	
Diabetes mellitus	Brainstem tumors	
Hypothyroidism	Spinal cord injury	
Hypoadrenal states	Anorexia nervosa	
Electrolyte abnormalities	Stress	
Chronic renal failure	**MISCELLANEOUS**	
Medications		
Anticholinergics	Idiopathic gastroparesis	
Opiates	Gastroesophageal reflux disease	
Dopamine agonists	Nonulcer (functional) dyspepsia	
Tricyclic antidepressants	Cancer cachexia or anorexia	
ABNORMALITIES OF GASTRIC SMOOTH MUSCLE		
Scleroderma		
Polymyositis, dermatomyositis		

surgery, especially those having had preoperative gastric outlet obstruction as a complication of PUD, are also commonly affected by gastroparesis. Finally, Parkinson's disease, rheumatologic disorders, hypothyroidism or hyperthyroidism, chronic intestinal pseudo-obstruction, and a variety of paraneoplastic syndromes can also produce gastroparesis.

The diagnostic evaluation of delayed gastric emptying should focus on excluding structural and metabolic abnormalities. Endoscopy is the preferred initial test to rule out mechanical gastric outlet obstruction, and a CT enterography or capsule endocopic study may be useful to exclude small bowel lesions. Serum electrolytes, blood cell counts, and thyroid studies should also be performed. When these studies are negative, radionuclide scintigraphy (gastric-emptying scan) using a mixed solid-liquid meal can quantitate delayed gastric emptying. Assessment of solid emptying is more clinically relevant than liquid emptying. In especially difficult cases, GI manometry and electrogastrography may help in the diagnosis.

Managing gastroparesis begins with identifying and treating potentially correctable causes. Medications that reduce gastric emptying, such as narcotics, anticholinergics, and tricyclic antidepressants, should be avoided. Because liquids empty easier than solids, and because liquid emptying is often preserved in patients with gastroparesis, simple dietary modifications may be helpful in treatment. The diet should be modified to include blenderized foods and liquid supplements. High-fat and fiber-rich foods should be avoided because they inhibit gastric emptying under normal conditions and are less likely to empty. Medical options are limited and involve the use of prokinetic drugs, which are agents that improve transit in the GI tract.

Metoclopramide is a dopamine-2 receptor antagonist that also facilitates the release of acetylcholine from cholinergic nerve terminals in the gut, thereby accelerating gastric emptying. The efficacy of metoclopramide is inconsistent, and adverse effects and the development of tolerance complicate long-term therapy. Adverse effects occur in up to 20% of patients and include drowsiness, anxiety, fatigue, insomnia, restlessness, agitation, extrapyramidal effects, galactorrhea, and menstrual irregularities. The typical dosage is 10 mg, 20 to 30 minutes before meals and at bedtime, although doses as high as 80 mg or as low as 20 mg may be used daily. Doses should be reduced for patients with renal failure. Domperidone, another dopamine receptor antagonist with prokinetic properties, has similar efficacy to metoclopramide in the treatment of delayed gastric emptying but is currently not available in the United States.

Erythromycin is a macrolide antibiotic that stimulates smooth muscle motilin receptors located at all levels of the GI tract. The prokinetic effects of erythromycin are related to its ability to mimic the effect of the GI peptide motilin to stimulate smooth muscle contraction, which accounts for the acceleration of solid and liquid gastric emptying. Erythromycin may dramatically improve gastric emptying in patients with severe diabetic gastroparesis when given acutely at an intravenous dose of 1 to 3 mg/kg every 8 hours. Long term use of the drug at a dose of 250 to 500 mg orally every 8 hours in patients with gastric stasis is of limited efficacy because of tachyphylaxis and side effects.

Endoscopic botulinum toxin A injection into the pyloric sphincter has also been reported in the treatment of delayed gastric emptying in small studies, but larger clinical trials have not shown this procedure to be effective.

In patients who are refractory to these measures, surgical placement of a jejunal tube, with or without a venting gastrostomy, may be necessary. Total parenteral nutrition is rarely indicated. Surgical gastrectomy should only be considered in patients with refractory postsurgical gastric stasis. Gastric pacemakers and other prokinetics, specifically new serotonin-receptor agonists, are under investigation and may be options in the future.

⬤ RAPID GASTRIC EMPTYING

Rapid gastric emptying is a far less common clinical problem than delayed gastric emptying. *Dumping syndrome* describes the alimentary and systemic manifestations of early delivery of large amounts of osmotically active food to the small intestine. Dumping syndrome is usually seen when the normal reservoir, grinding, and sieving properties of the stomach are disrupted, most commonly following surgery for obesity (Roux-en-Y gastric bypass) or PUD. The accelerated emptying of hypertonic boluses of nutrient material into the small intestine results in splanchnic vasodilation and release of vasoactive peptides. Early dumping symptoms, occurring about 30 minutes after a meal, include epigastric fullness and pain, nausea, vomiting, early satiety, and vasomotor features such as flushing, palpitations, and diaphoresis. Later symptoms, such as diaphoresis, tremulousness, and weakness, occur about 2 hours after a meal and may be caused by hypoglycemia from rebound hyperinsulinemia. Treatment of dumping syndrome involves dietary manipulation to decrease the volume and osmotic load emptied into the intestine. Frequent small feedings of meals low in carbohydrates, separation of liquid and solid intake, and avoidance of hypertonic fluids and lactose are usually helpful. When these measures fail, administration of octreotide at a dose of 25 to 50 mcg subcutaneously 30 minutes before meals may be helpful. Octreotide acts by slowing gastric emptying and intestinal transit as well as by inhibiting the release of insulin. Surgical procedures to slow gastric emptying have limited success.

⬤ GASTRIC VOLVULUS

Gastric volvulus occurs when the stomach rotates within the abdominal or thoracic cavity, compromising its emptying and its vascular supply. This event may be transient, producing few if any symptoms, or may lead to obstruction or even ischemia and necrosis. *Primary gastric volvulus*, seen in one third of the patients, occurs below the diaphragm when the stabilizing ligaments are too lax as a result of congenital or acquired causes. *Secondary gastric volvulus* occurs above the diaphragm in association with paraesophageal hernias or other diaphragmatic defects. Acute gastric volvulus produces sudden, severe pain of the upper abdomen or chest, and persistent retching producing scant vomitus; this is often associated with the inability to pass a nasogastric tube by medical personnel. This combination of symptoms, also known as Borchardt triad, should lead to a strong clinical suggestion of acute gastric volvulus. Chronic gastric volvulus may be associated with mild and nonspecific symptoms, such as epigastric discomfort, heartburn, abdominal fullness or bloating, and borborygmi, especially after meals. The diagnosis of gastric volvulus is made by upper GI series demonstrating an abrupt obstruction at the site of the volvulus. Acute gastric volvulus requires emergency surgical evaluation because of the substantial risk for mortality related to gastric ischemia or perforation. Treatment consists of surgical gastropexy and repair of any associated paraesophageal hernia.

SUGGESTED READINGS

Chan FK, Graham DY: NSAIDs, risks, and gastroprotective strategies: current status and future, Gastroenterology 134:1240–1257, 2008.

Fuccio L, Minardi ME, Rocco MZ, et al: Meta-analysis: duration of first-line proton-pump inhibitor-based triple therapy for *Helicobacter pylori* eradication, Ann Intern Med 147:553–562, 2007.

Olsen KM, Devlin JW: Comparison of the enteral and intravenous lansoprazole pharmacodynamic responses in critically ill patients, Aliment Pharmacol Ther 28:326–333, 2008.

Papatherodoridis GV, Sougioultzia S, Archimandritis AJ: Effects of *Helicobacter pylori* and nonsteroidal anti-inflammatory drugs on peptic ulcer disease: a systematic review, Clin Gastroenterol Hepatol 4:130–142, 2006.

Park MI, Camilleri M: Gastroparesis: clinical update, Am J Gastroeterol 101:1129–1139, 2006.

Vergara M, Catalan M, Gisbert JP, et al: Meta-analysis: role of *Helicobacter pylori* eradication in the prevention of peptic ulcer in NSAID users, Aliment Pharmacol Ther 21:1411–1418, 2005.

Inflammatory Bowel Disease

Hannah L. Miller and Francis A. Farraye

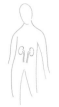

INTRODUCTION

Inflammatory bowel disease (IBD) comprises two disorders: ulcerative colitis and Crohn's disease. The diagnosis of IBD is based on review of clinical, endoscopic, radiologic, and histologic data. Despite the chronic nature of these two diseases and the fact that their causes have not yet been defined, new and emerging targeted anti-inflammatory treatments hold great promise in helping to reduce morbidity and improve the quality of life of individuals with IBD.

DEFINITION AND EPIDEMIOLOGY

Ulcerative colitis (UC) is characterized by inflammatory changes that involve the colonic mucosa in a continuous superficial fashion, typically starting in the rectum and extending proximally. Depending on the extent of the disease, UC can be divided into proctitis (rectum only), proctosigmoiditis (rectum and sigmoid), left-sided colitis (extending to the splenic flexure), and pancolitis (inflammation extends proximal to the splenic flexure). This classification is significant for both prognosis and therapy. Unlike UC, Crohn's disease can involve any segment of the gastrointestinal tract from the mouth to the anus, often in a discontinuous fashion. It is characterized by transmural inflammation, which results in complications such as abscesses, fistulas, and strictures.

In the United States, about 1.4 million individuals have IBD, and the overall annual incidence is about 20 new cases per 100,000 persons years. Although the incidence of UC has remained stable for several decades, the incidence of Crohn's disease has been increasing; it now seems to have plateaued at levels approximately equivalent to those of UC. The prevalence of IBD in the United States is between 249 to 319 per 100,000 persons. A bimodal age at presentation exists, with an initial peak between the second and fourth decades of life and another peak in the sixth decade. The sexes are equally affected.

The incidence and prevalence of IBD reflects the interplay of complex genetic and environmental factors that contribute to these disorders. For example, both diseases are more common in northern climates and among whites, particularly populations with Northern European ancestry such as North Americans, South Africans, and Australians. Individuals of Ashkenazi Jewish descent also have a twofold to eightfold increased risk for these disorders compared with non-Jews. Although incidence rates of IBD are lowest among Hispanics and Asians, IBD can occur in any ethnic or racial group from anywhere in the world. The cause of IBD remains unknown, but it is believed that a combination of genetic, immunologic, infectious, and environmental factors plays a role. In addition, state-of-the-art research points toward a relationship between the human microbiome and dysfunction of the immune system in patients with IBD.

Approximately 5% to 20% of patients with IBD have a first-degree relative with the disease, and first-degree relatives of IBD patients have about a 10- to 15-fold increased risk for developing IBD, predominantly with the same disease as the proband. A positive family history is more frequently observed in patients with Crohn's disease compared with UC, suggesting that genetic factors contribute more significantly in the etiology of Crohn's disease.

Through advances in genome-wide association studies, several susceptibility loci on multiple chromosomes have been linked to IBD, supporting a polygenic cause for these disorders. Polymorphisms in the *NOD2* gene (previously known as *CARD15*), located on chromosome 16, were the first definitive genetic risk factors identified for Crohn's disease. Homozygous mutations of the *NOD2* gene are associated with a greater than 20-fold increase in susceptibility for Crohn's disease. Defects in the NOD2 protein appear to result in abnormal intestinal immune responses to bacterial cell wall components. These gene mutations are estimated to account for 15% to 25% of the cases of Crohn's disease and are linked predominantly to fibrostenotic terminal ileal disease. In addition to *NOD2*, other genes associated with Crohn's disease have been identified that regulate autophagy; they include *ATG16L1*, *IRGM*, and *LRRK*. Genes that regulate the interleukin-17 (IL-17) and IL-23 receptor pathways have been found to increase the risk for both UC and Crohn's disease; they include *IL23R*, *IL12B*, *STAT3*, *JAK2*, and *TYK2*. *IL27* and *TNFSF15* have been implicated only in Crohn's disease. Genes regulating epithelial barrier function have also been discovered for IBD, including members of the *OCTN/IBD5* susceptibility locus (*SLC22A4* and *SLC22A5*), *ECM1*, *CDH1*, *HNF4A*, *LAMB1*, and *GNA12*.

Currently, it is believed that IBD results from an inappropriate, overactive mucosal immune response to commensal intestinal bacteria or the microbiome in genetically susceptible individuals. Profound alterations in mucosal immunology have been demonstrated in patients with IBD. In the normal immunologic state of the intestine, recently activated lymphoid tissue is abundant within the mucosal compartment. This state has been described as controlled or *physiologic* inflammation, and it likely develops in response to constant encounters with antigenic substances (derived from host microbial flora or dietary and environmental sources) that have crossed the epithelial barrier from the luminal environment. Indeed, one of the main functions of the intestinal immune system is to discriminate noxious or harmful substances and organisms from nonharmful ones. As a result, a large and well-maintained network of many different mucosal immune cells exists, including cells involved in reducing immune responses (regulatory cells) and those involved in activating immune responses. In IBD, this homeostatic balance, or immune tolerance, is dysregulated, resulting in overactivation of the immune system.

In Crohn's disease, there is an excessive and persistent CD4-positive helper T lymphocyte subtype 1 (T_H1) immune response to components of commensal bacterial flora. The T_H1 cytokine profile, which includes interferon-γ, IL-2, IL-12, and tumor necrosis factor-α (TNF-α), is elevated in patients with Crohn's disease. Patients with UC demonstrate greater expression of IL-5 and IL-13, cytokines characteristically associated with a T_H2 response. In addition, non-T_H1/T_H2 pathways have been identified as being potentially important in the pathogenesis of IBD. IL-23, for example, has been recognized as an inducer of a subset of proinflammatory T cells (T_H17) that secrete high levels of IL-17 and play an important role in mediating inflammation in murine models of colitis. IL-17 expression has been shown to be upregulated in active IBD, both Crohn's disease and UC.

Environmental factors also are believed to play a role in the pathogenesis of IBD, because the disease is more common in industrialized countries. Moreover, the frequency has tended to increase in countries as they become more industrialized. It has been postulated that poor sanitation, food contamination, and crowded living conditions are associated with helminthic infection, which leads to regulatory T-cell conditioning and stimulation of IL-10 and transforming growth factor-β production by mononuclear cells, thereby preventing intestinal inflammation. However, the only environmental factor clearly associated with IBD is tobacco smoking. Smoking seems to be protective against UC, whereas smoking in Crohn's disease causes a more aggressive disease. No dietary triggers have been found to cause IBD, but elemental diets and diversion of the fecal stream can reduce inflammation in Crohn's disease.

⬤ PATHOLOGY

Mucosal biopsies in IBD reveal acute and chronic inflammation with infiltration by plasma cells, neutrophils, lymphocytes, and eosinophils; focal ulcerations; crypt architectural distortion; and crypt abscesses (Figs. 37-1 and 37-2). In Crohn's disease, the inflammation is transmural and more commonly focal. Granulomas are found in 25% to 30% of histologic specimens in Crohn's disease, but not in UC. The presence of granulomas is not required but can assist in making the diagnosis of Crohn's disease in the right clinical setting (Fig. 37-3). Granulomas are not diagnostic because they can be found in many other diseases, such as Beçhet's disease, tuberculosis, *Yersinia* infection, and lymphoma.

⬤ CLINICAL PRESENTATION
Intestinal Manifestations

UC is characterized by chronic inflammation of the mucosal surface that involves the rectum and extends proximally through the colon in a continuous manner. The extent and severity of the colonic inflammation determine prognosis and presentation

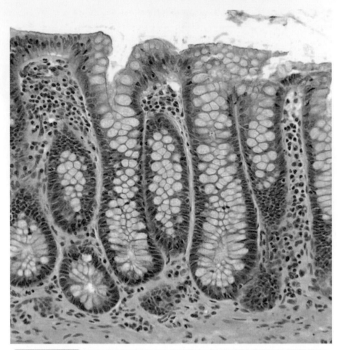

FIGURE 37-1 Normal colonic mucosa (hematoxylin and eosin stain).

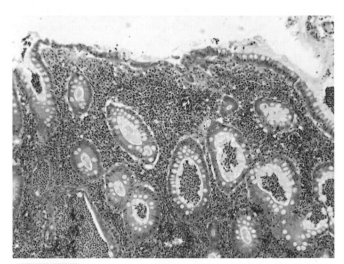

FIGURE 37-2 Mucosal biopsy specimen demonstrates crypt branching and a crypt abscess characteristic of ulcerative colitis (hematoxylin and eosin stain).

(insidious versus acute onset). Most patients initially exhibit diarrhea, abdominal pain, urgency to defecate, rectal bleeding, and the passage of mucus per rectum. At presentation, approximately 40% to 50% of patients have proctitis or proctosigmoiditis, 30% to 40% have left-sided colitis (disease extending to the splenic flexure), and the remaining 20% to 25% have pancolitis. Of the patients who initially present with proctitis or proctosigmoiditis, about 15% develop more extensive disease over time.

The typical clinical course of UC is one of chronic intermittent exacerbations followed by periods of remission. Signs of a worsening clinical course include the development of abdominal pain, dehydration, fever, and tachycardia. Clinical features that have been used to assess severity of UC include bowel frequency, fever, increased heart rate, and hematochezia (blood in the stool), as well as the presence of anemia and an elevated erythrocyte

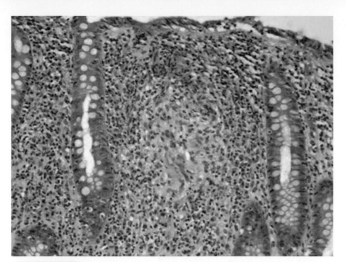

FIGURE 37-3 Colonic biopsy specimen demonstrates a chronic inflammatory infiltrate with a granuloma in a patient with Crohn's colitis (hematoxylin and eosin stain).

TABLE 37-1	EXTRAINTESTINAL MANIFESTATIONS OF INFLAMMATORY BOWEL DISEASE

SKIN	OCULAR
Pyoderma gangrenosum	Uveitis
Erythema nodosum	Episcleritis
Sweet's syndrome	**MISCELLANEOUS**
HEPATOBILIARY	Hypercoagulable state
Primary sclerosing cholangitis	Autoimmune hemolytic anemia
Cholelithiasis	Amyloidosis
Autoimmune hepatitis	
MUSCULOSKELETAL	
Seronegative arthritis	
Ankylosing spondylitis	
Sacroiliitis	

sedimentation rate (ESR) or C-reactive protein (CRP) level. Anemia commonly occurs and is caused by chronic blood loss from the involved colonic mucosa as well as bone marrow suppression from the inflammatory condition. Perforation can occur in patients with severe or fulminant colitis, especially those taking corticosteroids, and in the setting of toxic megacolon. Toxic megacolon is characterized by gross dilation of the large bowel associated with fever, abdominal pain, dehydration, tachycardia, and bloody diarrhea.

The clinical presentation of Crohn's disease depends on the section of gastrointestinal tract involved and the type of inflammation. Crohn's disease can involve any portion of the gastrointestinal tract; the most common site is ileocecal (40% of patients), followed by isolated small bowel disease (30%) and isolated colonic involvement (25%). The remaining sites of Crohn's disease are rare (5%) and include the esophagus, stomach, and duodenum.

Symptoms in Crohn's disease often include right lower quadrant abdominal pain, fever, weight loss, diarrhea, and sometimes a palpable inflammatory mass. Hematochezia is less common than in UC. The disease is often present for months or years before diagnosis, and in children, growth retardation may be the sole presenting sign. In contrast to UC, the inflammation in Crohn's disease is transmural and can result in microperforations and the formation of fistulous tracts. Fistulas may form between different segments of bowel (e.g., enteroenteric, enterocolonic) or between bowel and skin (enterocutaneous), bowel and bladder (enterovesicular), or rectum and vagina (rectovaginal). Over time, as many as 30% to 40% of patients develop disabling perianal involvement with fissures, fistulas, and abscesses.

Chronic inflammation can cause fibrosis and stricture formation, which in turn may result in partial or complete intestinal obstruction, with the patient complaining of abdominal pain, distention, nausea, and vomiting. Strictures can also lead to stasis with subsequent small intestinal bacterial overgrowth. Extensive ileal mucosal disease may lead to malabsorption of vitamin B_{12} (resulting in a megaloblastic anemia and neurologic side effects

if not corrected) and malabsorption of bile salts (resulting in diarrhea induced by unabsorbed bile salts and potential fat-soluble vitamin deficiency). Depletion of the bile salt pool can lead to the formation of gallstones. Weight loss may result from generalized malabsorption caused by loss of absorptive surfaces. Chronic fat malabsorption leads to luminal binding of free fatty acids to calcium; this allows oxalate, which normally is poorly absorbed because it complexes to calcium in the gut lumen, to be absorbed. The increase in oxalate absorption increases the risk for urinary calcium oxalate stone formation. Patients with an ileostomy or chronic volume loss from diarrhea are also at increased risk for uric acid stones.

Extraintestinal Manifestations

Although both UC and Crohn's disease primarily involve the bowel, they are also associated with inflammatory manifestations in other organ systems. This reflects the systemic nature of these disorders (Table 37-1). Extraintestinal manifestations can occur in parallel or independently of colonic activity, and they can become more difficult to treat than the bowel disease itself.

The most common extraintestinal manifestation is arthritis, which is seen in about 9% to 50% of patients and is divided into two major types. The first is a peripheral, large-joint, asymmetrical, seronegative, oligoarticular, nondeforming arthritis that may involve the knees, hips, wrists, elbows, and ankles. This *peripheral arthropathy* usually parallels the course of the large bowel disease and typically lasts for only a few weeks. The second type of IBD-related arthritis is axial in location, consisting of sacroiliitis or ankylosing spondylitis, and does not parallel the activity level of the bowel disease. Ankylosing spondylitis occurs in 5% to 10% of IBD patients and manifests with low back pain and stiffness that is usually worse during the night, in the morning, or after inactivity. Sacroiliitis alone (without ankylosing spondylitis) is common in IBD (up to 20% of patients), but in many cases is asymptomatic.

Liver complications of IBD include both intrahepatic and biliary tract diseases. Intrahepatic diseases include fatty liver, pericholangitis, and chronic active hepatitis. Pericholangitis, also known as small-duct sclerosing cholangitis, is the most common of these diseases. It usually is asymptomatic, identified only by abnormalities in alkaline phosphatase and γ-glutamyl transpeptidase on laboratory tests and histologically by portal tract inflammation and bile ductule degeneration. Small-duct sclerosing cholangitis may progress to cirrhosis.

Biliary tract disease includes an increased incidence of gallstones and of primary sclerosing cholangitis (PSC). PSC is a chronic cholestatic liver disease marked by fibrosis of the intrahepatic and extrahepatic bile ducts; it occurs 1% to 4% of patients with UC and less often in those with Crohn's disease. Overall, about 70% of patients with PSC have UC. Fibrosis leads to strictures of the bile ducts, which in turn may lead to recurrent cholangitis (with fever, right upper quadrant pain, and jaundice) and progression to cirrhosis. In addition, about 10% of patients develop cholangiocarcinoma. Medical or surgical therapy for the IBD does not modify the course of PSC, and most patients progress to cirrhosis and may require liver transplantation.

The two classic dermatologic manifestations of IBD are pyoderma gangrenosum and erythema nodosum. Pyoderma gangrenosum occurs in about 5% of patients and is characterized by a discrete ulcer with a necrotic base, usually on the legs. The ulcer may spread and become large and deep, destroying soft tissues. Pyoderma parallels the bowel activity in 50% of cases. Treatment is usually with systemic or intralesional steroids, or both. Other treatment options include dapsone, cyclosporine, and the anti-TNF agents. Erythema nodosum occurs in 10% of IBD patients, usually with peripheral arthropathy, and produces raised, tender nodules, usually over the anterior surface of the tibia. Erythema nodosum responds to treatment for the underlying bowel disease. A less common dermatologic manifestation of IBD is Sweet's syndrome, or acute febrile neutrophilic dermatosis. This condition is characterized by the sudden onset of fever, leukocytosis, and tender, erythematous, well-demarcated papules and plaques that show dense neutrophilic infiltrates on histologic examination.

Ocular manifestations of IBD, including uveitis and episcleritis, occur in 1% to 5% of patients. Uveitis (or iritis) is an inflammatory lesion of the anterior chamber that produces blurred vision, photophobia, headache, and conjunctival injection. Local therapy includes steroids and atropine. Episcleritis produces burning eyes and scleral injection without vision deficits and is treated with topical steroids.

● DIAGNOSIS AND DIFFERENTIAL DIAGNOSIS

The diagnosis of IBD is based on a constellation of clinical features, laboratory tests, and endoscopic, radiographic, and histologic findings. Laboratory tests are not specific and usually reflect inflammation (leukocytosis) or anemia. Perinuclear antineutrophil cytoplasmic antibody (pANCA) is positive in up to 70% of patients with UC but is rarely positive in patients with Crohn's disease, whereas anti–*Saccharomyces cerevisiae* antibodies (ASCA) are common in Crohn's disease but rarely found in UC (Table 37-2). Additional markers have improved the sensitivity and specificity of serologic testing, including antibodies to OmpC (*Escherichia coli* outer membrane porin C) and antibodies to bacterial flagellins CBir1, FlaX, and A4-Fla2.

Colonoscopy in patients with UC reveals a granular mucosa, decreased vascular markings, decreased mucosal reflection, exudate, and superficial ulcerations (Fig. 37-4). In more severe cases, the mucosa is friable, with deeper ulcerations. Patients with long-standing disease have *pseudopolyps*, which represent islands

	ULCERATIVE COLITIS	CROHN'S DISEASE
TABLE 37-2 DIFFERENTIATING FEATURES OF ULCERATIVE COLITIS AND CROHN'S DISEASE		
Site of involvement	Involves colon only Rectum almost always involved	Any area of the gastrointestinal tract Rectum usually spared
Pattern of involvement	Continuous	Skip lesions
Diarrhea	Bloody	Usually nonbloody
Severe abdominal pain	Rare	Frequent
Perianal disease	No	In 30% of patients
Fistula	No	Yes
Endoscopic findings	Erythematous and friable Superficial ulceration	Aphthoid and deep ulcers Cobblestoning
Radiologic findings	Tubular appearance resulting from loss of haustral folds	String sign of terminal ileum RLQ mass, fistulas, abscesses
Histologic features	Mucosa only Crypt abscesses	Transmural Crypt abscesses, granulomas (about 30%)
Smoking	Protective	Worsens course
Serology	pANCA more common	ASCA more common

ASCA, Anti–*Saccharomyces cerevisiae* antibodies; pANCA, perinuclear antineutrophil cytoplasmic antibody; RLQ, right lower quadrant.

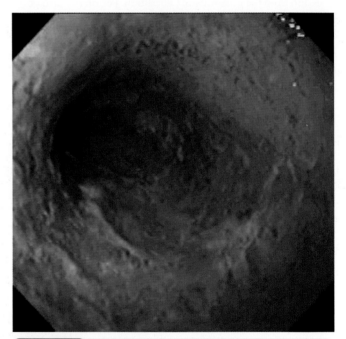

FIGURE 37-4 Endoscopic image of ulcerative colitis demonstrates diffuse inflammation characterized by erythema, edema, friability, and hemorrhage.

of normal tissue in regions of previous ulceration. In Crohn's disease (Fig. 37-5), endoscopic examination may show aphthoid erosions, deep linear or stellate ulcers, edema, erythema, exudate, and friability with intervening areas of normal mucosa (skip lesions). However, a diagnosis of *indeterminate* colitis is occasionally made because of an overlap of findings. For example, colonic Crohn's disease may produce superficial continuous rectal involvement similar to that seen in UC. Similarly, chronic UC can infrequently result in inflammation of the terminal ileum, called *backwash ileitis*. In many patients with indeterminate colitis,

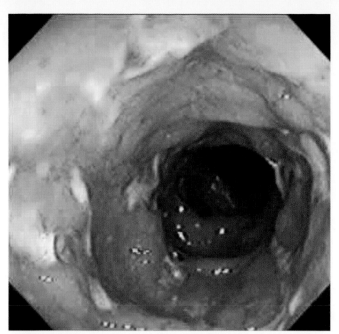

FIGURE 37-5 Endoscopic image of Crohn's disease demonstrates linear ulcers in areas of otherwise normal mucosa.

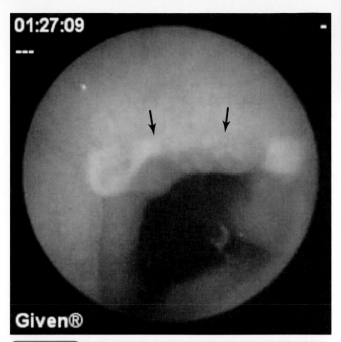

FIGURE 37-6 Video capsule endoscopic image shows ulcerated stenosis in a patient with Crohn's disease *(arrows)*.

repeated examination is necessary, or complications may develop that help identify the disease form.

Several types of radiologic studies can be used to diagnose IBD. In Crohn's disease, the most sensitive test to diagnose small bowel disease is video capsule endoscopy. Small erosions and ulcerations on the mucosa, as well as strictures, can be visualized best on video capsule endoscopy (Fig. 37-6). Patients with known or suspected strictures should be evaluated for risk of capsule retention before undergoing capsule endoscopy. On traditional small bowel radiography, segments of edematous bowel appear thickened next to uninvolved mucosa, a characteristic pattern referred to as *cobblestoning*. Tight, long strictures in the small bowel can be identified and are called a *string sign*. Cross-sectional imaging with computed tomographic (CT) enterography and magnetic resonance enterography has replaced traditional small bowel radiography. Cross-sectional imaging can identify bowel wall thickening with surrounding inflammation, as well as intra-abdominal abscesses and fistulas (Figs. 37-7 and 37-8). A characteristic finding on cross-sectional imaging in Crohn's disease is infiltration of the mesentery with fat, commonly known as *creeping fat*.

The differential diagnosis of IBD includes infectious colitis, ischemic colitis, radiation enteritis, enterocolitis induced by nonsteroidal anti-inflammatory drugs, diverticulitis, appendicitis, gastrointestinal malignancies, and irritable bowel syndrome. In patients with acute onset of bloody diarrhea, infectious causes that must be excluded with stool testing include *Salmonella enteritidis*, *Shigella* species, *Campylobacter jejuni*, *Escherichia coli* O157, and *Clostridium difficile*. Among the infectious causes, *Yersinia enterocolitica* can mimic Crohn's disease because the pathogen causes ileitis, mesenteric adenitis, fever, diarrhea, and right lower quadrant abdominal pain. *Mycobacterium tuberculosis* infection, strongyloidiasis, and amebiasis must be excluded in high-risk populations, because these infections can mimic IBD, and

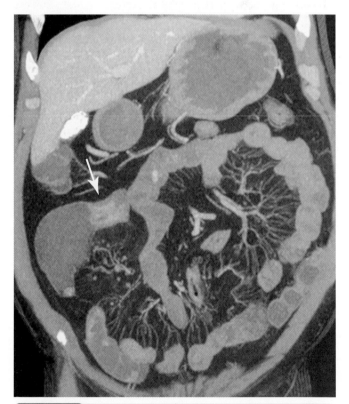

FIGURE 37-7 Computed tomographic enterography shows inflammatory stricture *(arrow)* and small bowel wall thickening in a patient with Crohn's disease.

treatment with corticosteroids can lead to disseminated infection and death.

● TREATMENT

The goal of treatment is induction and maintenance of remission. As part of the initial management of IBD, the clinician must

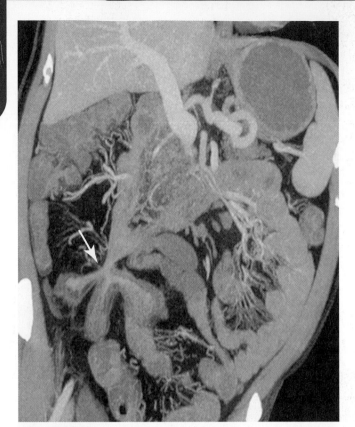

FIGURE 37-8 Computed tomographic enterography shows extensive Crohn's disease with fistula *(arrow)*.

TABLE 37-3 TREATMENT OPTIONS

DISEASE SEVERITY	ULCERATIVE COLITIS	CROHN'S DISEASE
Mild	Oral and topical 5-ASA compounds	5-ASA compounds Antibiotics Elemental diet
Moderate	Oral and topical 5-ASA compounds Oral steroids or budesonide MMX Azathioprine, 6-MP Infliximab, adalimumab, golimumab	5-ASA compounds Antibiotics Oral steroids or budesonide EC Azathioprine, 6-MP Methotrexate Infliximab, adalimumab, certolizumab natalizumab
Severe	Intravenous steroids Cyclosporine Infliximab, adalimumab, golimumab Vedolizumab Surgery	Intravenous steroids Methotrexate Infliximab, adalimumab, certolizumab Natalizumab, vedolizumab Surgery

5-ASA, 5-Aminosalicylic acid; 6-MP, 6-mercaptopurine.

determine the extent and assess the severity of the disease. Patients with mild or moderate disease can be managed as outpatients. Patients with severe or fulminant disease—with abdominal pain, fever, tachycardia, anemia, and leukocytosis—require hospital admission and multidisciplinary team management. Because IBD is a chronic recurrent illness, treatment is centered on controlling the acute attack with induction of remission, followed by maintenance of remission. Treatment options for UC and Crohn's disease are summarized in Table 37-3.

5-Aminosalicylic Acid

The aminosalicylates are given either orally or topically (suppository and enema). They are safe and effective for treatment (i.e., induction of remission) of mild to moderate UC and for maintenance of remission (Level of evidence III, A). The efficacy of the 5-aminosalicylic acid (5-ASA) agents in induction or maintenance of remission in Crohn's disease has not been clearly shown in studies, although they are commonly used off-label for this purpose (level of evidence III, A for induction and III, B for maintenance). This class of anti-inflammatory medications includes sulfasalazine (Azulfidine) at a dose of 4 to 6 g/day in divided doses. This drug consists of 5-ASA linked to a sulfapyridine moiety; the 5-ASA is released after bacterial lysis of an azo bond in the colon.

Side effects, including headache, nausea, and skin reactions, require discontinuation of sulfasalazine in about 30% of patients. Reversible oligospermia may occur, and rare serious side effects include pleuropericarditis, pancreatitis, agranulocytosis, interstitial nephritis, and hemolytic anemia. Patients who take sulfasalazine need folic acid supplementation. Derivatives of oral 5-ASA compounds include mesalamine (Pentasa, 4 g/day in divided doses; Delzicol, 2.4 g/day in divided doses; Asacol HD, 2.4 to 4.8 g/day in divided doses; Lialda, 2.4 to 4.8 g once daily; Apriso, 1.5 g once a day), olsalazine (Dipentum, 1 to 2 g/day in divided doses), and balsalazide (Colazal, 6.75 g/day in divided doses; Giazo 3.3 g/day in divided doses). Topical forms of mesalamine (Canasa suppositories, 1000 mg once daily; Rowasa enemas, 4 g once nightly) are commonly used because of a more favorable side-effect profile. In addition to their use in the primary treatment of IBD, several studies suggest that long-term use of 5-ASA medications may reduce the risk for colorectal cancer in patients with UC.

Corticosteroids

Corticosteroids may be used topically, orally, or intravenously. They are effective for controlling active disease but not for maintaining remission (level of evidence I,A for induction and III, A for maintenance). They are indicated for moderate or severe disease in UC patients for whom treatment with 5-ASA has failed. The most commonly used agent is oral prednisone, started in doses between 40 and 60 mg/day. Patients typically improve rapidly, and the medication is usually tapered down slowly (i.e., by 5 to 10 mg/week until discontinuation. Patients who do not improve after 1 week of oral treatment and those with more severe disease are best treated in the hospital with intravenous corticosteroids, such as intravenous hydrocortisone (300 mg/day), or methylprednisolone (which can be given either by continuous infusion or in three divided doses).

Corticosteroids have numerous side effects with long-term use. Controlled trials have shown that budesonide EC (Entocort EC) is more effective than placebo or oral 5-ASA and has similar efficacy to prednisolone for the induction of remission in Crohn's disease (level of evidence I, A). Entocort EC (9 mg given once daily) undergoes extensive first-pass hepatic metabolism, is available for inducing and maintaining remission of ileal and ileocolonic Crohn's disease (level of evidence III, A), and may offer long-term benefits with decreased corticosteroid side effects. Budesonide MMX (Uceris 9 mg given once daily) has an extended release that targets the colon and is available for the treatment of mild to moderate UC (level of evidence I, A for induction and III, A for maintenance).

Immunomodulators

The immunomodulators used in IBD include azathioprine (Imuran, 2 to 2.5 mg/kg/day) and its active metabolite, 6-mercaptopurine (6-MP) (Purinethol, 1 to 1.5 mg/kg/day), as well as methotrexate and cyclosporine. Azathioprine and 6-MP are effective therapies for maintaining remission in both Crohn's disease and UC and are used primarily as steroid-sparing agents (level of evidence I, A). They have a slow onset of action (weeks to months). Side effects include nausea, abnormal liver enzymes, bone marrow suppression, opportunistic infections, and an increased risk of lymphoma and nonmelanoma skin cancer.

Methotrexate can be used for induction (25 mg subcutaneously once weekly) and maintenance of remission (15 to 25 mg subcutaneously once weekly) in active Crohn's disease (level of evidence IIa, B for induction and I, B for maintenance); the side effect profile is similar but also includes interstitial pneumonitis. Intravenous cyclosporine (2 mg/kg/day given over 24 hours) is used as a rescue medicine and, in severe UC refractory to intravenous steroids, as a *bridge* treatment to one of the above immunomodulators or biologic agents. Given the potential for both short-term and long-term side effects, as well as the need for close follow-up, patients needing these medications are best managed by gastroenterologists.

Biologic Agents

Biologics are a class of medications that target specific aspects of the immune system. The first such agent to be used in IBD was infliximab (Remicade), a chimeric monoclonal antibody to TNF-α, which has been shown to be effective in the treatment of both moderate to severe Crohn's disease, including fistulizing disease, and UC (level of evidence I, A). Because infliximab is a chimeric antibody, its toxicities include infusion reactions, delayed-type hypersensitivity reactions, and formation of autoantibodies (which can reduce its efficacy). Anti-TNF agents that are administered subcutaneously include adalimumab (Humira) and golimumab (Simponi), which are fully human monoclonal antibodies, and certolizumab pegol (Cimzia), which is a humanized anti-TNF antibody Fab fragment. Adalimumab and certulizumab are efficacious in patients with moderate to severe Crohn's disease, whereas adalimumab and golimumab are approved to treat moderate to severe UC.

Natalizumab (Tysabri), a humanized anti–α$_4$-integrin antibody, blocks inflammatory cell migration and adhesion, and has been approved for the treatment of moderate to severe Crohn's disease in patients who have had an inadequate response to, or are unable to tolerate, conventional Crohn's disease therapies including inhibitors of TNF-α (level of evidence IIa, B for induction and IIa, A for maintenance). Vedolizumab (Entyvio), a humanized monoclonal antibody to α4β7 integrin, has been recently approved for the treatment and maintenance of both Crohn's and ulcerative colitis (level of evidence I, A).

Because of the potent effects these biologic agents have on the immune system, careful patient selection and monitoring for complications are necessary. Reactivation of latent tuberculosis and other serious infections have been reported with the anti-TNF agents. Other rare but serious complications include non-Hodgkin's lymphoma, exacerbation of congestive heart failure, abnormal complete blood count (CBC) and liver function test results, and demyelinating disease. Natalizumab has been linked to rare cases of progressive multifocal leukoencephalopathy caused by the human JC virus.

Future biologic agents with alternate mechanisms of action are being discovered and developed. Ustekinumab (Stellara), an IL-12/IL-23 inhibitor already approved for psoriasis, has shown promise and is in clinical trials for Crohn's disease. Tofacitinib, a JAK inhibitor, already approved for rheumatoid arthritis, is now being investigated for Crohn's disease.

Other Agents

Other agents for treatment of IBD include antibiotics, probiotics, antidiarrheals, bile salt resin binders, and nutritional support.

Antibiotics are used primarily in patients with Crohn's disease who have perianal or fistulizing disease. In colonic Crohn's disease, antibiotics can be used in combination with immunosuppressive drugs as an alternate strategy. The role of antibiotics in UC is unclear, and further studies are required. However, intravenous antibiotics are used in the initial treatment of severe, toxic, or fulminant colitis.

Probiotics are viable nonpathogenic organisms that, after ingestion, may prevent or treat intestinal diseases and have been explored in the treatment of IBD. Multiple studies have found them to be effective in treating pouchitis after ileal pouch–anal anastomosis. One probiotic mixture, termed VSL#3, includes four strains of *Lactobacillus* (*L. paracasei*, *L. plantarum*, *L. acidophilus*, and *L. delbrueckii* subsp *bulgaricus*), three strains of *Bifidobacteria* (*B. longum*, *B. breve*, and *B. infantis*), and one strain of *Streptococcus* (*S. thermophiles*). It has been shown in randomized clinical trials to be a safe and effective adjunct modality for achieving clinical response and remission in patients with mild to moderately active UC. So far, none of the probiotics has been shown to be effective in induction or maintenance of remission in patients with Crohn's disease.

Antidiarrheal agents and bile salt resin binders can be used as adjuncts for management of diarrhea in patients with IBD, but antidiarrheal agents should be used cautiously during exacerbations of colitis because they can precipitate toxic megacolon. The main role of antidiarrheal medications involves controlling diarrhea in patients who have undergone previous resections. Patients with Crohn's disease who have had less than 100 cm of terminal ileum removed can develop a bile salt malabsorptive state, during which bile salts enter the colon and cause a secretory diarrhea. Bile salt resin binders such as cholestyramine are an effective treatment in these cases. When patients have undergone one or more extensive resections amounting to more than 100 cm of ileum, the bile salt pool is depleted and fat malabsorption develops. These patients may require a low-fat diet supplemented with medium-chain triglycerides and antidiarrheal agents, but bile salt resin binders should not be used.

Nutritional support is an important adjunctive aspect in the management of IBD. However, the role of nutrition as a primary treatment has been limited to patients with small bowel Crohn's disease. These patients may achieve and maintain remission with total parenteral nutrition or elemental diets after prolonged periods (at least 4 weeks). Many patients with Crohn's disease or UC experience weight loss during exacerbations of their illness and need caloric supplements. Vitamins and minerals can be given orally as a multivitamin with folic acid. Vitamin B_{12} should be supplemented parenterally in patients who have extensive ileal disease or an ileal resection. Patients taking corticosteroids require supplemental calcium and vitamin D, and individuals with extensive small bowel involvement can also develop malabsorption of fat-soluble vitamins (A, D, E, and K), iron, and, rarely, trace minerals. Lactose-free diets and low-fiber diets may be necessary in patients with active disease or strictures.

Surgical Management

Surgical intervention is indicated for patients with severe complications such as obstruction, perforation, massive gastrointestinal hemorrhage, or toxic megacolon not responsive to medical treatment. The other main indication for surgical treatment is the presence of dysplasia or cancer. For patients with UC, regardless of the extent of disease, the entire colon must be removed. Historically, the initial operation for UC was a total proctocolectomy and Brooke ileostomy, but ileal pouch–anal anastomosis has become the procedure of choice in most patients. In this operation, the colon is removed and the small bowel is constructed into a reservoir (ileal pouch) that is anastomosed to the anus, allowing defecation through the anus. Complications include the development of pouchitis, fecal incontinence, reduced fertility, and need for reoperation. Surgery is not curative in Crohn's disease. Many surgical procedures in patients with Crohn's disease are performed to manage complications of the disease, including segmental resection, stricturoplasty, fistulectomy, and abscess drainage.

● PROGNOSIS

The prognosis in a patient with IBD is determined by the relapse rate, the rate of surgery, and the incidence of colon cancer. Approximately two thirds of patients with UC have at least one relapse in the 10 years after their diagnosis. About 20% to 30% of patients with pan-UC will require colectomy within their lifetime. Only 5% of individuals with proctitis undergo colectomy by 10 years after diagnosis. In contrast, more than 60% of Crohn's patients require surgery within the 10 years after their diagnosis. The rate of recurrence in Crohn's disease is high, with 70% of patients having an endoscopic recurrence within 1 year after surgery and 50% having a symptomatic recurrence within 4 years. Predictors of a severe course in Crohn's disease include stricturing or penetrating disease and perianal disease.

The risk for colon cancer is increased in patients with UC, and its magnitude is related to the extent and duration of disease. The colon cancer risk is increased 10- to 20-fold after 8 to 10 years of disease in pancolitis, and after 15 to 20 years in left-sided colitis. The cumulative incidence of colorectal cancer is 2.5% after 20 years and 7.6% after 30 years of disease. Proctitis is not associated with an increased risk of colorectal cancer. In colonic Crohn's disease, the risk of colorectal cancer is equivalent to that in patients with UC of similar extent and duration. Patients with only small bowel Crohn's disease are not thought to be at increased risk for colorectal cancer. The rates of small bowel carcinoma and lymphoma are increased in patients with Crohn's disease.

Screening for dysplasia and colon cancer should be performed by colonoscopy 8 to 10 years after the onset of symptoms. Surveillance examinations are performed every 1 to 3 years. Proctitis does not require endoscopic surveillance. Patients with IBD and PSC appear to have a particularly increased risk for colon cancer, and yearly surveillance is recommended after the initial diagnosis of PSC. It is recommended that a minimum of 33 "random" mucosal biopsy samples be obtained during the colonoscopic examination, in addition to targeted samples of circumscript lesions. The use of chromoendoscopy and other enhanced imaging techniques increases the detection of dysplastic lesions in patients with UC and may replace the performance of random biopsies in the future. Colectomy is indicated in patients with flat high-grade dysplasia, multifocal flat low-grade dysplasia, or evidence of colorectal cancer. Polypoid dysplasia entirely removed by polypectomy without flat dysplasia elsewhere in the colon can be managed with continued surveillance colonoscopy.

As understanding of the etiologic and pathophysiologic aspects of IBD increases, major advances in diagnosis and treatment are anticipated. These will be based on better use of molecular, genetic, and serologic tests to differentiate among the subtypes of disease; earlier and more targeted use of biological agents to manage inflammation; and improvements in the detection and prevention of colorectal cancer in those at risk.

For deeper discussion, see Chapter 141: Inflammatory Bowel Disease in Goldman-Cecil Medicine, 25th edition.

SUGGESTED READINGS

Abraham C, Cho JH: Inflammatory bowel disease, N Engl Med 361:2066–2078, 2009.

Anderson CA, Boucher G, Lees CW, et al: Meta-analysis identifies 29 additional ulcerative colitis risk loci, increasing the number of confirmed associations to 47, Nat Genet 43:246, 2011.

Burger D, Travis S: Conventional medical management of inflammatory bowel disease, Gastroenterology 140:1827–1837, 2011.

Cheifetz AS: Management of active Crohn disease, JAMA 309:2150–2158, 2013.

Cho JH: The genetics and immunopathogenesis of inflammatory bowel disease, Nat Rev Immunol 8:458, 2008.

Danese S, Fiocchi C: Ulcerative colitis, N Engl J Med 365:1713–1725, 2011.

Farraye FA, Odze RD, Eaden J, et al: AGA medical position statement on the diagnosis and management of colorectal neoplasia in inflammatory bowel disease, Gastroenterology 138:738–745, 2010.

Franke A, McGovern DP, Barrett JC, et al: Genome-wide meta-analysis increases to 71 the number of confirmed Crohn's disease susceptibility loci, Nat Genet 42:1118, 2010.

Kornbluth A, Sachar DB: Ulcerative colitis practice guidelines in adults: American College of Gastroenterology, Practice Parameters Committee. [Erratum: Am J Gastroenterol 105:500, 2010.], Am J Gastroenterol 105:501–523, 2010.

Lichtenstein GR, Hanaur SB, Sandborn WJ: Management of Crohn's disease in adults, Am J Gastroenterol 104:465–483, 2009.

Maggiori L, Panis Y: Surgical management of IBD: from an open to a laparoscopic approach, Nat Rev Gastroenterol Hepatol. 10:297–306, 2013.

Talley NJ, Abreu MT, Achkar JP, et al, American College of Gastroenterology IBD Task Force: An evidence-based systematic review on medical therapies for inflammatory bowel disease, Am J Gastroenterol 106(Suppl 1):S2–S25, 2011.

38

Diseases of the Pancreas

David R. Lichtenstein

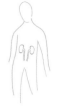

● ACUTE PANCREATITIS

Definition and Epidemiology

Acute pancreatitis is an acute inflammatory process of the pancreas that may also involve peripancreatic tissues and remote organ systems. It is the leading cause of hospitalization of patients with gastrointestinal disorders in the United States, with more than 200,000 admissions annually. This translates into an overall incidence of 1 case per 4000 people in the general population.

Pathology

The pancreas is located in the retroperitoneum and has exocrine and endocrine functions (Fig. 38-1) derived from the pancreatic acinus and the pancreatic islet, respectively. As an exocrine gland, the pancreas participates in normal digestion and nutrient absorption. The enzymes secreted by the pancreas digest starch (i.e., amylase), fats (i.e., lipase), and protein (i.e., trypsin and other proteolytic enzymes). Within acinar cells, proteolytic digestive enzymes are synthesized and packaged separately in the Golgi region into condensing vacuoles and transported in an inactive form referred to as zymogens to the apical portions of the cell. When stimulated, they are discharged into the central ductule of the acinus by exocytosis.

Normal physiology involves secretion of inactive enzymes into the duodenum, where they are converted to an active form by enterokinase, a brush border enzyme secreted by small bowel enterocytes. Trypsinogen conversion to active trypsin is the trigger enzyme that subsequently converts the other zymogens to active enzymes (E-Fig. 38-1).

The pathogenesis of acute pancreatitis remains incompletely understood. Based on experimental models, the initiating event appears to involve intra-acinar activation of trypsin from trypsinogen, resulting in acute intracellular injury, pancreatic autodigestion, and the potential for profound systemic complications after activated enzymes are leaked into the bloodstream. Initiating events may include obstruction of the pancreatic duct (e.g., gallstones, pancreatic tumor), overdistention of the pancreatic duct (e.g., from endoscopic retrograde cholangiopancreatography [ERCP]), reflux of biliary or duodenal juices into the pancreatic duct, changes in permeability of the pancreatic duct, ischemia of the organ, and toxin-induced cholinergic hyperstimulation (Fig. 38-2).

During the initial hospitalization for acute pancreatitis, reasonable attempts to determine the cause are appropriate, particularly those that may affect acute management. The cause of acute pancreatitis is readily identified in 70% to 90% of patients after an initial evaluation consisting of the history, physical examination, focused laboratory testing, and routine radiologic studies. Gallstones account for 45%, alcohol for 35%, miscellaneous causes for 10%, and idiopathic causes for 10% to 20% of acute pancreatitis cases (Table 38-1).

Gallstone Pancreatitis

Among patients with gallstones, the incidence of acute pancreatitis is 0.17% per year. Gallstones increase the relative risk of pancreatitis 25- to 35-fold. It is theorized that gallstone passage causes transient obstruction of the pancreatic duct, precipitating acute pancreatitis. Acute gallstone pancreatitis should be suspected when associated with a transient elevation in liver-associated enzymes, particularly alanine aminotransferase (ALT) levels greater than 150 IU/L. Most stones pass spontaneously from the ampulla and do not require intervention (discussed later).

Alcoholic Pancreatitis

Acute alcoholic pancreatitis is the second most common cause of pancreatitis in the United States. Approximately 10% of chronic alcoholics develop attacks of pancreatitis that are indistinguishable from other forms of acute pancreatitis. Alcoholics with acute pancreatitis most commonly have underlying

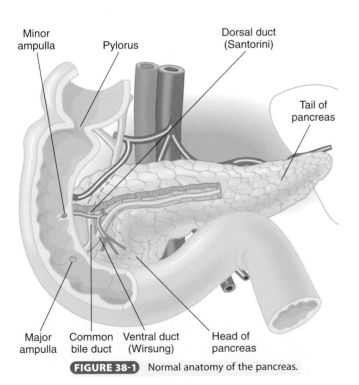

Minor ampulla · Pylorus · Dorsal duct (Santorini) · Tail of pancreas · Major ampulla · Common bile duct · Ventral duct (Wirsung) · Head of pancreas

FIGURE 38-1 Normal anatomy of the pancreas.

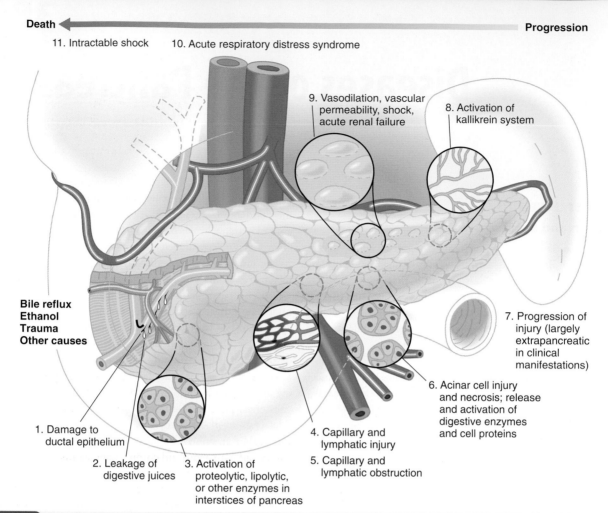

Death ← **Progression**

11. Intractable shock
10. Acute respiratory distress syndrome

9. Vasodilation, vascular permeability, shock, acute renal failure

8. Activation of kallikrein system

7. Progression of injury (largely extrapancreatic in clinical manifestations)

6. Acinar cell injury and necrosis; release and activation of digestive enzymes and cell proteins

Bile reflux
Ethanol
Trauma
Other causes

1. Damage to ductal epithelium

2. Leakage of digestive juices

3. Activation of proteolytic, lipolytic, or other enzymes in interstices of pancreas

4. Capillary and lymphatic injury

5. Capillary and lymphatic obstruction

FIGURE 38-2 The pathophysiology of acute pancreatitis is not fully understood, but as the schematic shows, a cascade of events seems likely, beginning with the release of toxic substances into the parenchyma and ending with shock and death. Damage to the ductal epithelium or acinar cell injury may result from bile reflux, increased intraductal pressure, alcohol, or trauma. (Modified from Grendell JH: The pancreas. In Smith LH Jr, Thier SO, editors: Pathophysiology: the biological principles of disease, ed 2, Philadelphia, 1985, WB Saunders, p 1228.)

chronic disease. However, some have true acute alcoholic pancreatitis because not all patients progress to chronic pancreatitis, even with continued alcohol abuse. The mechanism of pancreatic injury, the genetic and environmental factors that influence its development in alcoholics, and the reason only a small proportion of alcoholics develop pancreatitis are unclear (see Chronic Pancreatitis).

Heredity

Hereditary causes of pancreatitis include mutations in the genes encoding cationic trypsinogen (*PRSS1*), pancreatic secretory trypsin inhibitor (serine protease inhibitor Kazal type 1 [*SPINK1*]), cystic fibrosis transmembrane conductance regulator (*CFTR*), chymotrypsin C (i.e., caldecrin) (*CTRC*), and the calcium-sensing receptor (*CASR*).

The role of genetic testing in idiopathic acute pancreatitis is controversial. Diagnosis of these genetic disorders contributes little to direct management because specific therapy is unavailable. Similarly, inadvertent disclosure of the results of genetic testing protects patients' healthcare insurance but may impact other financial decisions such as disability and life insurance. However, identification of an underlying genetic cause may obviate the need for further testing, allow more informed family planning, and enable better surveillance for complications, including pancreatic cancer. The decision to pursue genetic testing is one that should be made only with the advice and involvement of an experienced counselor.

Neoplasia

Primary pancreatic ductal adenocarcinoma, ampullary tumors, metastasis to the pancreas, and intraductal papillary mucinous neoplasms are uncommon causes of acute pancreatitis. These causes should be considered for patients older than 40 years. Pancreatitis has been reported in up to 10% of patients with pancreatic cancer.

Smoking

Smoking was once thought to be a risk factor due to its synergism with alcohol. However, studies have suggested that cigarette smoking is an independent risk factor for acute and chronic pancreatitis by mechanisms that are unclear.

TABLE 38-1   CAUSES OF ACUTE PANCREATITIS

OBSTRUCTION

Gallstones
Tumors: ampullary or pancreatic tumors
Parasites: *Ascaris* or *Clonorchis* species
Developmental anomalies: pancreas divisum, choledochocele, annular
    pancreas
Periampullary duodenal diverticula
Hypertensive sphincter of Oddi
Afferent duodenal loop obstruction

TOXINS

Ethyl alcohol
Methyl alcohol
Scorpion venom: excessive cholinergic stimulation causes salivation,
    sweating, dyspnea, and cardiac arrhythmias; seen mostly in the West Indies
Organophosphorus insecticides

DRUGS

Definite associations (documented with rechallenges): azathioprine or
    6-mercaptopurine, valproic acid, estrogens, tetracycline, metronidazole,
    nitrofurantoin, pentamidine, furosemide, sulfonamides, methyldopa,
    cytarabine, cimetidine, ranitidine, sulindac, dideoxycytidine
Probable associations: thiazides, ethacrynic acid, phenformin, procainamide,
    chlorthalidone, L-asparaginase

METABOLIC DISORDERS

Hypertriglyceridemia, hypercalcemia, end-stage renal disease

TRAUMA

Accidental: blunt trauma to the abdomen (e.g., car accident, bicycle)
Iatrogenic: postoperative, endoscopic retrograde cholangiopancreatography

INFECTIOUS DISEASES

Parasitic: ascariasis, clonorchiasis
Viral: mumps, rubella, hepatitis A, hepatitis B, hepatitis C, coxsackievirus B,
    echovirus, adenovirus, cytomegalovirus, varicella virus, Epstein-Barr virus,
    human immunodeficiency virus
Bacterial: mycoplasma, *Campylobacter jejuni*, tuberculosis, *Legionella* species,
    leptospirosis

VASCULAR DISORDERS

Ischemia: hypoperfusion (e.g., postcardiac surgery) or atherosclerotic emboli
Vasculitis: systemic lupus erythematosus, polyarteritis nodosa, malignant
    hypertension

IDIOPATHIC DISORDERS

Between 10% and 30% of patients have pancreatitis
Up to 60% have occult gallstone disease (e.g., biliary microlithiasis,
    gallbladder sludge)
Less common causes: sphincter of Oddi dysfunction, mutations in the cystic
    fibrosis transmembrane regulator

MISCELLANEOUS DISORDERS

Penetrating peptic ulcer
Crohn's disease of the duodenum
Pregnancy-associated disorders
Pediatric associations: Reye's syndrome, cystic fibrosis

Autoimmune Pancreatitis

Autoimmune pancreatitis (AIP) is a benign disease with a unique histology of lymphoplasmacytic sclerosing pancreatitis, which is characterized by a periductal lymphoplasmacytic infiltrate, storiform fibrosis, obliterative phlebitis, and abundant immunoglobulin G4 (IgG4) immunostaining (>10 IgG4-positive cells per high-power field).

The most common manifestation of AIP is obstructive jaundice, which closely mimics pancreatic cancer with focal enlargement of the pancreatic head. AIP can also manifest with acute pancreatitis in up to 15% to 30% of individuals, and about 5% of patients evaluated for acute or chronic pancreatitis have AIP. AIP has a peak incidence in the sixth or seventh decades of life and tends to affect men twice as often as women.

Computed tomography (CT) typically demonstrates diffuse enlargement of the pancreas with delayed (rim) enhancement and a diffusely irregular, attenuated main pancreatic duct. More than 60% of individuals have clinical and histologic involvement of other organs, including the biliary tree, retroperitoneum, lacrimal and salivary glands, lymph nodes, periorbital tissues, kidneys, thyroid, lungs, meninges, aorta, breast, prostate, pericardium, and skin. Patients with AIP frequently respond favorably to corticosteroid treatment.

Pancreas Divisum

At approximately 4 weeks' gestation, the dorsal pancreas forms as an evagination from the duodenum, and shortly thereafter, the ventral pancreas forms from the hepatic diverticulum (E-Fig. 38-2). At approximately the eighth intrauterine week of life, the ventral pancreas rotates posterior to the duodenum and comes to rest posterior and inferior to the head portion of the dorsal pancreas with associated fusion of the main ducts. If fusion is incomplete, the duct of Wirsung drains only the ventral pancreas through the major ampulla, and the duct of Santorini drains the bulk of the pancreas (i.e., dorsal pancreas) through the relatively small accessory (minor) ampulla. This anomaly, called *pancreas divisum*, occurs in 5% to 10% of the general population and is associated with acute and chronic pancreatitis.

Theories suggest that pancreatitis results from relative outflow obstruction of the main dorsal duct through the small accessory ampulla. Endoscopic papillotomy and surgical sphincteroplasty are therapeutic maneuvers that may reduce the incidence of recurrent pancreatitis by increasing drainage through the accessory papilla.

Clinical Presentation

The hallmark of acute pancreatitis is persistent abdominal pain. In atypical cases, patients may have unexplained organ failure or postoperative ileus. The onset of pain is typically sudden, severe, and worse when supine. Pain is usually located in the upper abdomen and may radiate to the back, chest, and flanks. Nausea and vomiting are common. Physical examination usually reveals severe upper abdominal tenderness that is sometimes associated with guarding.

Pancreatic enzymes, vasoactive substances (e.g., kinins), and other toxic substances (e.g., elastase, phospholipase A_2), are liberated by the inflamed pancreas and extravasate along fascial planes in the retroperitoneal space, lesser sac, and peritoneal cavity. These materials cause chemical irritation and contribute to the development of ileus, chemical peritonitis, third-space losses of protein-rich fluid, hypovolemia, and hypotension. The toxic molecules may reach the systemic circulation by lymphatic and venous pathways and contribute to subcutaneous fat necrosis and end-organ damage, including shock, renal failure, and respiratory insufficiency (i.e., atelectasis, effusions, and acute respiratory distress syndrome [ARDS]). Grey Turner's sign (i.e., ecchymosis of the flank) or Cullen's sign (i.e., ecchymosis in the periumbilical region) may be associated with hemorrhagic pancreatitis.

Metabolic problems, which are common in severe disease, include hypocalcemia, hyperglycemia, and acidosis. Hypocalcemia is most commonly caused by concomitant hypoalbuminemia. Other mechanisms include complexing of calcium to released free fatty acids, protease-induced degradation of circulating parathyroid hormone (PTH), and failure of PTH to release calcium from bone.

Acute pancreatitis is associated with a variety of local and vascular complications, including local spread of inflammation to contiguous organs. The most common include peripancreatic fluid collections, pseudocyst formation, obstruction of the duodenum or bile duct, and exocrine or endocrine insufficiency. Less common complications include pancreatic fistula formation, vascular thrombosis (i.e., splenic, portal and superior mesenteric veins), colonic necrosis, and development of an arterial pseudoaneurysm. Trypsin can activate plasminogen to plasmin and induce clot lysis. However, trypsin also can activate prothrombin and thrombin and produce thrombosis leading to disseminated intravascular coagulation.

Acute peripancreatic fluid collections are pools of peripancreatic fluid confined by normal peripancreatic fascial planes without a definable wall encapsulating the collection. These fluid collections occur during the first 4 weeks after interstitial pancreatitis. Most remain sterile and are reabsorbed spontaneously during the first several weeks after the onset of acute pancreatitis. When a localized acute peripancreatic fluid collection persists beyond 4 weeks, it is likely to develop into a pancreatic pseudocyst.

Pancreatic pseudocysts (E-Fig. 38-3) are encapsulated fluid collections with well-defined inflammatory walls and are usually located outside the pancreas with minimal or no necrosis. They occur a minimum of 4 weeks after the onset of acute pancreatitis. In symptomatic patients, if the pseudocyst is mature and encapsulated, treatment can involve endoscopic, surgical, or percutaneous drainage. Although most pseudocysts remain asymptomatic, presenting symptoms may include abdominal pain, early satiety, nausea, and vomiting due to compression of the stomach or gastric outlet. Rapidly enlarging pseudocysts may rupture, hemorrhage, obstruct the extrahepatic biliary tree, erode into surrounding structures, and become infected. Indications for pseudocyst drainage include suspicion of infection or progressive enlargement with associated symptoms previously described. Asymptomatic pseudocysts should be followed.

The term *acute necrotic collection* describes a nonorganized accumulation of heterogeneous fluid and necrotic material in the setting of necrotizing pancreatitis. The necrosis may involve the pancreatic parenchyma or peripancreatic tissue, or both. Walledoff pancreatic necrosis is a mature, encapsulated collection of pancreatic or peripancreatic necrosis that usually occurs more than 4 weeks after the onset of necrotizing pancreatitis.

Abdominal compartment syndrome is diagnosed when the intra-abdominal pressure exceeds 20 mm Hg and there are signs of new respiratory, renal, or vascular organ failure. Intraabdominal hypertension typically occurs early and is the result of pancreatic inflammation and fluid third spacing. Abdominal compartment syndrome is associated with mortality rates ranging up to 50% to 75% in various reports. Suggested treatment includes analgesics, sedation, nasogastric tube decompression, and fluid restriction. If these measures do not result in

improvement, percutaneous catheter decompression followed if unsuccessful by a surgical laparotomy is recommended. The ability of this approach to improve outcomes is the focus of ongoing research.

Diagnosis and Differential Diagnosis

The diagnosis of acute pancreatitis is based on a combination of clinical, biochemical, and radiologic factors. A diagnosis of acute pancreatitis requires two of the following three features: abdominal pain characteristic of acute pancreatitis; serum amylase or lipase levels, or both, at least three times the upper limit of normal; and characteristic findings of acute pancreatitis on imaging.

Elevated serum amylase levels may occur in a wide variety of other conditions, including bowel perforation, intestinal obstruction or ischemia, acute appendicitis, cholecystitis, tubo-ovarian disease, and renal failure. Serum amylase levels may be normal in patients with hypertriglyceridemia or alcohol-induced acute pancreatitis. Serum lipase is preferred because it is more sensitive and specific than serum amylase for the diagnosis of acute pancreatitis. The serum lipase level remains normal in some nonpancreatic conditions associated with an elevated serum amylase level, including macroamylasemia (i.e., formation of large molecular complexes between amylase and abnormal immunoglobulins), salivary gland disorders, and tubo-ovarian disease, but it may similarly rise in appendicitis, renal disease, and cholecystitis. The serum lipase concentration is more sensitive than that of amylase because it remains elevated longer and may be diagnostic even for patients seeking medical attention several days after symptom onset. Repeated measurements of serum pancreatic enzymes have little value in assessing clinical progress, and the magnitude of serum amylase or lipase elevation does not correlate with the severity of pancreatitis.

Contrast-enhanced computed tomography (CECT) or magnetic resonance imaging (MRI) of the pancreas should be used for patients whose diagnosis is unclear or who fail to improve within the first 48 to 72 hours after hospital admission. Imaging findings supporting acute pancreatitis include pancreatic enlargement, peripancreatic inflammatory changes, and extrapancreatic fluid collections. Imaging does not exclude the diagnosis of acute pancreatitis because the pancreas appears normal in 15% to 30% of those with mild disease. CECT is also useful for assessing disease severity based on the presence and extent of complications such as pancreatic necrosis and acute peripancreatic fluid collections. Pancreatic imaging should be performed after adequate fluid resuscitation to minimize the risk of contrast-induced nephrotoxicity.

MRI is preferred for patients with a contrast allergy and renal insufficiency because T2-weighted images without gadolinium contrast can similarly diagnose pancreatic necrosis. Early imaging (within 72 hours of symptom onset) can underestimate the existence and extent of pancreatic necrosis. Gallstone pancreatitis should be suspected in patients with transient elevation in liver function test results, particularly a serum ALT level elevated more than threefold. Transabdominal ultrasonography should be performed in all patients with acute pancreatitis when considering a diagnosis of gallstone pancreatitis.

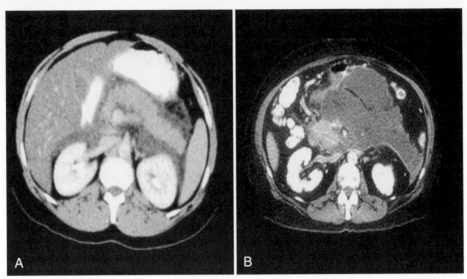

FIGURE 38-3 Contrast-enhanced computed tomography demonstrates interstitial pancreatitis (**A**) and necrotizing pancreatitis (**B**).

Prognosis

The distinction between interstitial and necrotizing acute pancreatitis has important prognostic implications (Fig. 38-3). *Interstitial pancreatitis* is characterized by an intact microcirculation and uniform enhancement of the gland on CECT. *Necrotizing pancreatitis* is characterized by disruption of the pancreatic microcirculation so that large areas (>3 cm or >30%) of pancreatic parenchyma do not enhance on CECT. Approximately 20% to 30% of patients with acute pancreatitis have necrotizing pancreatitis.

The finding of pancreatic necrosis predicts a more severe course, particularly infection in the necrotic pancreatic tissue, also called *infected necrosis*. Infection is a strong determinant of the severity of illness and accounts for a large percentage of the deaths from acute pancreatitis. Infected necrosis develops in 30% to 50% of patients with acute necrotizing pancreatitis but not in those with interstitial disease. Infected necrosis should be suspected in patients with persistent systemic inflammatory response syndrome (SIRS) or organ dysfunction. The diagnosis can be made if extraluminal gas is seen on CECT. More commonly, CT-guided needle aspiration is obtained for Gram stain and culture of necrotic material, or antibiotics are given empirically based on clinical suspicion after appropriate cultures are obtained. Antibiotics that penetrate pancreatic tissue, including cephalosporins, carbapenems, quinolones, and metronidazole, are used for treatment of infected necrosis.

Risk assessment should be performed for all patients to stratify the severity of illness. The current classification includes mild, moderate, and severe forms. Mild acute pancreatitis, the most common form, is characterized by the absence of organ failure and pancreatic necrosis. Mild pancreatitis usually does not require pancreatic imaging, and patients recover within several days with restoration of normal pancreatic function and gland architecture. Patients with mild acute pancreatitis account for 80% of all attacks and less than 5% of the overall mortality rate.

Moderately severe pancreatitis is transient organ failure or local or systemic complications in the absence of organ failure. Local complications include pancreatic necrosis (with or without infection) and acute peripancreatic fluid collections. Death from moderately severe pancreatitis is much less common than in cases of severe pancreatitis.

Severe acute pancreatitis is defined by persistent organ failure extending for more than 48 hours. Severe acute pancreatitis occurs in 15% to 20% of patients. Most individuals with persistent organ failure have underlying necrotizing disease. The respiratory, cardiovascular, and renal systems are most commonly affected. Early deaths (within the first week) are most often the result of multiple organ failure caused by the release of inflammatory mediators and cytokines. Late deaths are more likely to result from local or systemic infection. The risks of infection and death correlate with disease severity and pancreatic necrosis.

Despite the importance of recognizing severe disease, most patients are initially admitted to the hospital without necrosis or organ failure, and methods to predict individuals more likely to progress to severe disease during the initial several days of hospitalization have been defined. A combination of clinical assessment, scoring systems, serum markers, and CECT scanning provides the most useful prognostic information (Table 38-2). Regardless of the prognostic factor chosen, there are significant limitations in predicting disease severity.

Clinical predictors of a poor outcome include severe comorbid illnesses, older age, and obesity. Laboratory findings associated with increased mortality include blood urea nitrogen elevation on admission or a rise during the first 24 hours of admission, hemoconcentration from third spacing of fluids reflected by an elevated hematocrit of 44 or greater on admission, and serum markers reflecting a robust systemic inflammatory response, such as a C-reactive protein level greater than 150 mg/dL (sensitivity of 80%, specificity of 76%, positive predictive value of 67%, and negative predictive value of 86%). Imaging studies predicting a severe outcome include a pleural effusion seen on chest radiography within the first 24 hours or pancreatic imaging identifying necrosis.

Severe pancreatitis is predicted by organ dysfunction, including shock (systolic blood pressure <90 mm Hg), respiratory failure (Pao_2 ≤60 mm Hg), and acute renal injury (creatinine

| TABLE 38-2 PREDICTORS OF SEVERE PANCREATITIS ||
CRITERIA	PROGNOSTIC INDICATORS
Signs*	Heart rate: >90 beats/min Temperature: >38° C or <36° C White blood cell count: >12,000 or <4,000 cells/μL or >10% bands Respiratory rate >20 beats/min or Paco₂ <32 mm Hg
Patient characteristics	Comorbid illnesses Age >55 yr Obesity (BMI >30 kg/m²)
Laboratory values	BUN level of 20 mg/dL or higher and any rise in BUN during the first 24 hr of admission associated with increased mortality Serum creatinine >1.8 mg/dL within first 24 hr Hemoconcentration with Hct ≥44 on admission or failure of Hct to decrease in first 24-48 hr with volume resuscitation predicts severe pancreatitis Serum marker reflecting a systemic inflammatory response, CRP >150 mg/dL
Imaging findings	Pleural effusion Pancreatic necrosis Acute extrapancreatic fluid collections
Scoring systems Ranson's criteria	Eleven prognostic indicators, including five available on admission (age >55 yr, WBC >16,000/mm³, glucose >200 mg/dL, LDH >350 IU/L, AST >250 U/L) and six measured at the end of the first 48 hr (Hct decreased >10, BUN >5 mg/dL, Po₂ <60 mm Hg, base deficit >4 mEq/L, serum calcium <8 mg/dL, estimated fluid sequestration >6 L); mortality rate of 10-20% for three to five signs and >50% for six or more signs
Acute Physiologic and Chronic Health Evaluation (APACHE II) system	Calculated by assigning points based on age, heart rate, temperature, respiratory rate, mean arterial pressure, Pao₂, pH, potassium, sodium, creatinine, Hct, WBC, GCS, and previous health status
Bedside Index for Severity of Acute Pancreatitis (BISAP)	Five variables available in initial 24 hr: BUN >25 mg/dl, impaired mental status (GCS score <15), finding of SIRS, age >60 yr, and pleural effusion on imaging. Each variable adds 1 point to the total score, and scores of 3, 4, and 5 correspond to mortality rates of 5.3%, 12.7%, and 22.5%, respectively.

AST, Aspartate aminotransferase; BMI, body mass index; BUN, blood urea nitrogen; CRP, C-reactive protein; GCS, Glasgow Coma Scale; Hct, hematocrit; LDH, lactate dehydrogenase; SIRS, systemic inflammatory response syndrome; WBC, white blood cells.

*SIRS predisposes to multiple organ dysfunction and pancreatic necrosis. SIRS is defined by two or more of these criteria persisting for more than 48 hours.

>2.0 mg/L after rehydration). SIRS predisposes to multiple organ dysfunction and pancreatic necrosis.

Well-established scoring systems include Ranson's criteria, Acute Physiologic and Chronic Health Evaluation II (APACHE II), and Bedside Index for Severity of Acute Pancreatitis (BISAP). With increasing scores, the likelihood of a complicated, prolonged, and fatal outcome increases.

Treatment

Early steps in the management of patients with acute pancreatitis can decrease severity, morbidity, and mortality (Fig. 38-4). Prevention of complications depends largely on monitoring, vigorous hydration, and early recognition of gancreatic necrosis and choledocholithiasis. Patients with multiorgan dysfunction and those with predicted development of severe disease are at greatest risk for adverse outcomes and should be treated when possible in a care unit with intensive monitoring capability and multidisciplinary input.

Supportive Care

Patients with acute pancreatitis are treated supportively with aggressive intravenous hydration, parenteral analgesics, and bowel rest. Supplemental oxygen is recommended initially for all patients. Nasogastric tube suction is indicated for symptomatic relief in patients with nausea, vomiting, and ileus. No specific treatments are effective in limiting systemic complications. Agents that put the pancreas to rest (e.g., somatostatin, calcitonin, glucagon, H₂-receptor antagonists) and enzyme inhibitors (e.g., aprotinin, gabexate mesylate) have not been shown to lower disease-related morbidity and mortality.

Antibiotics

Antibiotic therapy is no longer recommended for patients with sterile necrosis due to the lack of proven benefit. For patients with suspected infected necrosis, appropriate antibiotics are initiated before the confirmatory diagnosis, with the initial choice taking into consideration the likely pathogenic organisms and the ability of the antimicrobials to penetrate into necrotic pancreatic tissues. After culture results are available, the antibiotics can be tailored appropriately.

Fluid Management

Vigorous fluid resuscitation is important for maintaining the microcirculation and perfusion of the pancreas during the early phase of acute pancreatitis. Early aggressive intravenous hydration translates into a potential benefit of reduced pancreatic necrosis and organ failure. Crystalloid, the preferred intravenous fluid, is administered at an initial rate of 250 to 500 mL/hour with a preceding bolus infusion for individuals with severe volume depletion. Lactated Ringer's solution may be the preferred crystalloid replacement because in one comparative study, it reduced the incidence of SIRS by more than 80% compared with normal saline infusion. Fluids are adjusted every few hours based on the patient's hemodynamic and volume status. Caution must be used for the elderly and those with underlying cardiovascular or renal impairment.

Analgesia

Despite the theoretical concern that narcotic analgesia may result in sphincter of Oddi spasm and worsening pancreatitis, there is no evidence to support withholding narcotics from patients with acute pancreatitis. The physician should consider liberal use of patient-controlled analgesia, although this approach has not been compared prospectively with on-demand analgesia. There is no evidence to indicate superiority of a specific opiate. Patients administered repeated doses of narcotic analgesics should have oxygen saturation monitored due to risks of unrecognized hypoxia.

Nutritional Care

Patients with mild disease may initiate oral intake when pain resolves and appetite returns. Starting with a low-fat solid diet is as safe as a clear liquid diet. For patients with predicted severe pancreatitis or those unlikely to start oral intake within 5 to 7 days, providing supplemental nutrition is important.

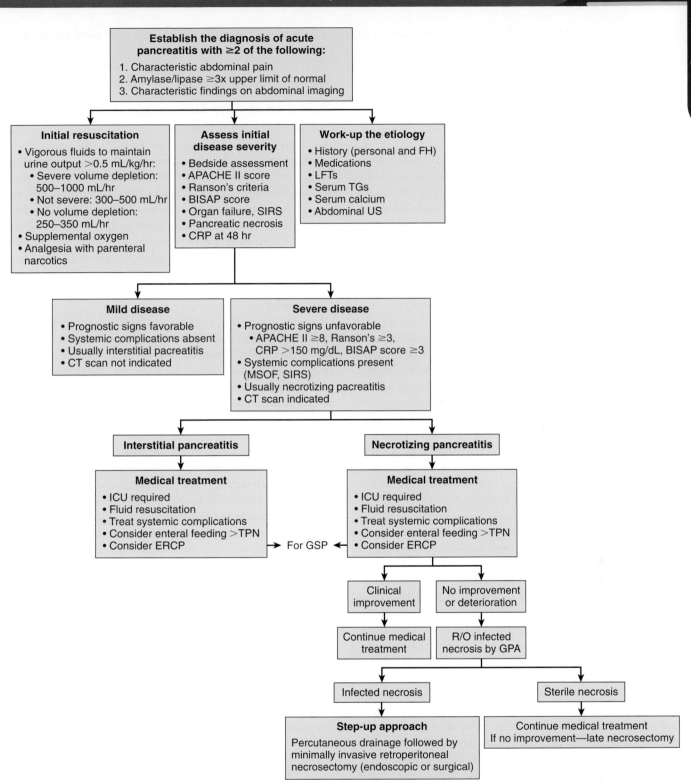

FIGURE 38-4 Management algorithm for acute pancreatitis. Some of the guidelines, such as the diagnostic utility of the C-reactive protein (CRP) level, require further validation. Antibiotic use, including the type and duration of treatment, continues to be examined, and these suggested approaches will likely be modified by the findings of future studies. APACHE II, Acute Physiologic and Chronic Health Evaluation II; BISAP, Bedside Index for Severity of Acute Pancreatitis; CT, computed tomography; ERCP, endoscopic retrograde cholangiopancreatography; FH, family history; GPA, CT-guided percutaneous aspiration; GSP, gallstone pancreatitis; ICU, intensive care unit; LFTs, liver function tests; MSOF, multiple system organ failure; R/O, rule out; SIRS, systemic inflammatory response syndrome; TGs, triglycerides; TPN, total parenteral nutrition; US, ultrasound.

Options include total parenteral nutrition through central venous access or preferably as enteral feeding through a naso-enteric feeding tube. Enteral feeding is safer and less expensive than total parenteral nutrition and is associated with a reduction in systemic infection, need for surgical intervention, organ failure, and mortality. Enteral feeding is usually well tolerated, even by patients with ileus. Nasogastric feeding may offer a safe alternative to nasojejunal feeding because it appears to be equally safe and effective. Parenteral nutrition should be reserved for patients who cannot achieve sufficient caloric intake through the enteral route or those in whom enteral access cannot be maintained.

Management of Recurrence and Necrosis

Gallstone Pancreatitis

The risk of gallstone pancreatitis recurrence is as high as 50% to 75% within 6 months of the initial episode, and cholecystectomy before discharge is recommended for patients with mild attacks of pancreatitis. Cholecystectomy is often delayed in patients with severe pancreatitis to allow for better exposure of the ductal anatomy at the time of surgery. Urgent ERCP (Video 38-1) with identification and clearance of bile duct stones is recommended for patients with evidence of ongoing biliary obstruction, as suggested by imaging and laboratory data. Biliary sphincterotomy leaving the gallbladder in situ is considered an effective alternative for those who are not candidates for cholecystectomy.

Sterile Pancreatic and Extrapancreatic Necrosis

Sterile pancreatic necrosis usually is treated with supportive medical care during the first several weeks, even in patients with multiple organ failure. After the acute pancreatic inflammatory process has subsided and coalesced into an encapsulated structure (e.g., walled-off pancreatic necrosis), débridement may be required for intractable abdominal pain, vomiting caused by extrinsic compression of stomach or duodenum, or persistent systemic toxicity. Débridement is delayed for at least 4 to 6 weeks after the onset of pancreatitis and can be performed by a combination of endoscopic, radiologic, and surgical techniques. Asymptomatic pancreatic necrosis does not warrant intervention, regardless of the extent and location.

Infected Pancreatic and Extrapancreatic Necrosis

Infected pancreatic necrosis is best treated with drainage or débridement, or both. In most cases, the diagnosis of infected necrosis is confirmed by fine-needle aspiration before intervention, but because false-negative results can occur, débridement warrants consideration when infected necrosis is suspected, even if infection is not documented. The consensus is that the best outcomes are achieved when surgery is delayed for a minimum of 4 weeks after the onset of disease to allow liquefaction of necrotic tissues and a fibrous rim to form around the necrosis (i.e., walled-off pancreatic necrosis). Patients with infected necrosis are initially treated with broad-spectrum antibiotics and medical support to allow encapsulation of the necrotic collections, which may facilitate intervention and reduce complications of bleeding and perforation. When there is dramatic clinical deterioration, delay is not feasible, and early intervention is required.

Traditional management of infected pancreatic necrosis has been open surgical necrosectomy with closed irrigation by indwelling catheters, necrosectomy with closed drainage without irrigation, or necrosectomy and open packing. The open surgical approaches are associated with a high morbidity (34% to 95%) and mortality (11% to 39%) rates. A more conservative step-up approach using percutaneous catheter drainage as the initial treatment has gained favor. If the percutaneous approach fails, it is followed by a less invasive, video-assisted retroperitoneal débridement (VARD) or endoscopic transluminal drainage with

or without necrosectomy (Video 38-2), provided expertise is available.

CHRONIC PANCREATITIS

Definition and Epidemiology

Chronic pancreatitis is characterized by inflammation, fibrosis, and irreversible loss of acinar (exocrine) and islet (endocrine) cell function. This disorder contrasts with acute pancreatitis, which is usually nonprogressive. The two conditions may overlap because recurrent attacks of acute pancreatitis may lead to chronic pancreatitis, and individuals with chronic pancreatitis may experience exacerbations of acute pancreatitis. The annual incidence of chronic pancreatitis ranges from 5 to 12 cases per 100,000 people, and the prevalence is about 50 cases per 100,000 people.

Pathology

Chronic pancreatitis can be classified as nonobstructive or obstructive (Table 38-3). The most common cause of the nonobstructive type is chronic alcoholism (70%). Alcohol can cause episodes of acute pancreatitis, but at the time of the initial attack, structural and functional abnormalities often indicate underlying chronic pancreatitis.

Because most alcoholics do not develop pancreatitis, the presumption is that unidentified genetic, dietary, or environmental influences must coexist with alcohol abuse. For example, epidemiologic data have implicated smoking as a causal, dose-dependent cofactor in chronic pancreatitis. The combined effect of smoking and alcohol is synergistic and contributes profoundly to the development and progression of the disease.

If alcoholism is excluded, 20% of U.S. patients have chronic pancreatitis with no immediately demonstrable cause. Gallstone pancreatitis, the major cause of acute pancreatitis, rarely leads to chronic pancreatitis. Calcific pancreatitis is a major cause of chronic pancreatitis in South India and other parts of the tropics. Autoimmune pancreatitis, genetic mutations (*CFTR, SPINK1, PRSS1, CTRC, CASR*), obstruction (e.g., tumors, sphincter of Oddi dysfunction, pancreas divisum), hypertriglyceridemia, and hypercalcemia are potential causes of cases initially labeled idiopathic.

Clinical Presentation

Most patients with chronic pancreatitis experience episodic or continuous pain. Occasionally, patients exhibit exocrine or

TABLE 38-3	CAUSES OF CHRONIC PANCREATITIS
NONOBSTRUCTIVE CAUSES	Metabolic: hypertriglyceridemia, hypercalcemia
Alcohol	
Idiopathic (10%-20% of total cases)	**OBSTRUCTIVE CAUSES**
Tropical	
Genetic (cationic trypsinogen, *CFTR*, chymotrypsin C, *SPINK1*)	Benign obstruction: sphincter of Oddi dysfunction, pancreas divisum, posttraumatic
Traumatic	Neoplastic obstruction: tumors of the ampulla or ductal system
Autoimmune	
Vascular ischemia	

CFTR, Cystic fibrosis transmembrane conductance regulator; SPINK1, serine peptidase inhibitor Kazal type 1.

endocrine insufficiency in the absence of pain. Other patients are asymptomatic and are found to have chronic pancreatitis incidentally on imaging.

The pain of chronic pancreatitis is typically epigastric, often radiates to the back, is occasionally associated with nausea and vomiting, and may be partially relieved by sitting upright or leaning forward. The pain is often worse 15 to 30 minutes after eating. Early in the course of chronic pancreatitis, the pain may occur in discrete attacks; as the condition progresses, the pain tends to become continuous.

The pain of chronic pancreatitis is poorly understood. Possible causes include inflammation of the pancreas, increased intrapancreatic pressure, neural inflammation, and extrapancreatic causes, such as stenosis of the common bile duct and duodenum.

Glucose intolerance occurs with some frequency in chronic pancreatitis, but overt diabetes mellitus usually manifests late in the course of disease. Diabetes in patients with chronic pancreatitis is different from typical type 1 diabetes in that the pancreatic alpha cells, which produce glucagon, are also affected, increasing the risk of hypoglycemia.

Clinically significant endocrine or exocrine insufficiency (i.e., protein and fat deficiencies) does not occur until more than 90% of pancreatic function is lost. Steatorrhea usually occurs before protein deficiencies because lipolytic activity decreases faster than proteolysis. Malabsorption of fat-soluble vitamins (A, D, E, K) and vitamin B_{12} may also occur, although clinically symptomatic vitamin deficiency is uncommon. Because reduced vitamin D absorption can result in osteoporosis, osteopenia, and fractures, periodic assessment of vitamin D levels and bone densitometry are recommended.

Diagnosis and Differential Diagnosis

Because direct biopsy of the pancreas has considerable risk, the diagnosis of chronic pancreatitis is typically based on indirect tests of pancreatic structure and function. Marked structural changes usually correlate with severe functional impairment. In early chronic pancreatitis, however, mild abnormalities of pancreatic function can precede the morphologic changes seen on imaging. Studies of pancreatic structure may remain normal even with advanced deterioration of pancreatic function.

Laboratory evaluations of serum pancreatic enzymes, such as amylase and lipase, are frequently normal in the setting of well-established chronic pancreatitis, even during painful exacerbations. Serum pancreatic enzymes neither confirm nor exclude the diagnosis.

Tests of Function

Function tests assess pancreatic secretory reserve of ductal function capacity for secretion of bicarbonate ions (HCO_3^-) in fluid or acinar function for secretion of digestive enzymes. Direct tests involve stimulation of the pancreas through the administration of hormonal secretagogues. Indirect tests measure the consequences of pancreatic insufficiency, and although more widely available, the results usually are not abnormal until enzyme output has declined by more than 90%. They are insensitive to early pancreatic insufficiency. Clinicians have preferentially relied on noninvasive methods to circumvent the challenges associated with direct pancreatic function tests. Clinically available indirect tests

of pancreatic function include analyses of fecal fat, fecal elastase, and serum trypsin.

The secretin stimulation test takes advantage of the normal response of pancreatic ductular cells to secrete HCO_3^- in response to physiologic and exogenously administered secretin. The observation that HCO_3^- production is impaired early in the course of chronic pancreatitis led to the use of this test to diagnose early-stage disease (sensitivity of 95%). The test involves oral placement of a double-lumen gastroduodenal catheter for aspiration and quantitative measurement of pancreatic enzyme and HCO_3^- production before and after stimulation with intravenous secretin. This quantitative measure of pancreatic secretion and enzyme activity is primarily performed for patients with suspected chronic pancreatitis who have chronic abdominal pain but negative or equivocal results of imaging studies. Peak pancreatic fluid HCO_3^- concentrations of less than 80 mEq/L represent pancreatic insufficiency.

The secretin stimulation test has been infrequently used in clinical practice because the study is labor intensive and is associated with discomfort. Endoscopic collection methods have simplified pancreatic fluid collection and made the test more suitable for clinical use.

The 72-hour fecal fat determination is sometimes used for detection of steatorrhea (fecal fat >7 g/24 hours), but the test is not specific for pancreatic exocrine insufficiency. The test also lacks sensitivity because steatorrhea occurs only in advanced chronic pancreatitis. Because the quantitative fecal fat test is inconvenient, unpleasant for patients, and prone to laboratory error, a qualitative assay is used preferentially in clinical practice to assess for malabsorption.

Determination of fecal elastase is the most commonly used noninvasive test for the diagnosis of pancreatic exocrine insufficiency. Elastase, a protease synthesized by pancreatic acinar cells, is useful for evaluating insufficiency because it is stable in stool, unaffected by pancreatic enzyme replacement, and correlates well with stimulated pancreatic function test results. Mild or severe exocrine insufficiency is based on fecal elastase values of less than 200 or 100 µg/g of stool, respectively.

Low concentrations of serum trypsin are relatively specific for advanced chronic pancreatitis. However, they are not sensitive enough to be helpful for most patients with mild to moderate pancreatic disease.

Tests of Structure

Findings that suggest chronic pancreatitis include ductal abnormalities (e.g., dilation, stones, duct irregularity), parenchymal abnormalities (e.g., calcification, inhomogeneity, atrophy), gland contour changes, and pseudocysts. Imaging studies may be normal or inconclusive in the early stages of disease.

Plain film radiography of the abdomen can detect pancreatic calcifications in approximately 20% of individuals with alcohol-induced chronic pancreatitis. The study should be the first diagnostic test performed when pancreatitis is suspected because it is simple and inexpensive. Calcifications not detected on plain films are more readily apparent by CT (E-Fig. 38-4). CT scans may show supportive findings of pancreatic ductal dilatation, atrophy of the pancreas, and fluid collections (e.g., pseudocysts). Sensitivity and specificity for the diagnosis of chronic pancreatitis are 75% to 90% and 85%, respectively.

ERCP can reliably evaluate structural abnormalities of the pancreatic ductular system. ERCP allows detection of pancreatic duct changes, including ductal dilation, strictures, abnormal side branches, communicating pseudocysts, and ductal stones and leaks. ERCP is highly effective for visualizing these ductal and duct-related findings, with a sensitivity for the diagnosis of chronic pancreatitis of 71% to 93% and a specificity of 89% to 100%. The major limitation of ERCP is the development of procedure-related acute pancreatitis in up to 5% of patients. ERCP should not be used for diagnostic purposes but instead reserved for patients with established chronic pancreatitis when endoscopic therapy is recommended (discussed later).

Magnetic resonance cholangiopancreatography is a noninvasive diagnostic imaging modality that provides visualization of the pancreatic duct with images similar to those of ERCP but without the risk of precipitating acute pancreatitis. However, limited visualization of pancreatic duct side branches makes this test useful only for patients with advanced changes of the main pancreatic duct. A modification of MRI imaging with secretin stimulation enhances side branch visualization, but whether it aids in the diagnosis of chronic pancreatitis remains to be determined.

Endoscopic ultrasound (EUS) as a diagnostic imaging study for chronic pancreatitis relies on quantitative and qualitative parenchymal tissue and ductal findings. EUS appears to be equally or more sensitive than other tests of structure and function. An international consensus panel proposed the Rosemont criteria for diagnosing chronic pancreatitis. Major criteria include hyperechoic foci with shadowing that indicates pancreatic duct calculi and parenchymal lobularity with honeycombing. Minor criteria include cysts, a dilated main duct (≥3.5 mm in diameter), irregular pancreatic duct contour, dilated side branches (≥1 mm in diameter), hyperechoic duct wall, parenchymal strands, non-shadowing hyperechoic foci, and lobularity with noncontiguous lobules. In the absence of any of these criteria, chronic pancreatitis is unlikely, whereas with detection of four or more criteria, the disease is likely, even when other imaging and pancreatic function tests may still be normal.

Treatment

Malabsorption

Treatment of pancreatic exocrine insufficiency is best achieved with pancreatic enzyme supplementation. Most commercial preparations consist of pancreatin, which is the shock-frozen powdered extract of porcine pancreas containing lipase, amylase, trypsin, and chymotrypsin. For most patients, the recommended dose depends on the size and nature of the meal (i.e., fat content), residual pancreatic function, and therapeutic goals (i.e., elimination of steatorrhea, reduction in the abdominal symptoms of maldigestion, or improvement in nutrition).

Approximately 90,000 USP units of lipase per meal are needed for optimal fat absorption. Due to residual pancreatic lipase secretion and physiologic gastric lipase secretion, it is appropriate to begin therapy with at least 50,000 USP units of lipase with each meal and one half of that amount with snacks.

Administration of acid-stable, encapsulated microspheres or microtablets filled with pancreatic enzymes has greatly increased the efficacy of enzyme supplementation.

In cases of gastric hyperacidity, proton pump inhibitors (PPIs) or histamine (H_2)-receptor antagonists should be used to reduce enzyme inactivation. If these methods do not provide improvement, the next step is to decrease dietary fat intake to less than 50 g per day and to substitute medium-chain triglycerides (MCTs), which do not require hydrolysis before absorption. Although clinically effective, patients usually do not like MCT fat because of poor palatability.

Other factors may accentuate steatorrhea, including concomitant small bowel bacterial overgrowth, which can occur in up to 25% of patients with chronic pancreatitis. Bacterial overgrowth may be caused by hypomotility due to inflammatory diseases of the head of the pancreas or chronic use of narcotic analgesics.

Pain

The greatest challenge in treating chronic pancreatitis is controlling abdominal pain. Pain may improve over time, but the course is not predictable, and improvement may take years. Therapy targets the mechanisms responsible for pancreatic pain, including pancreatic hyperstimulation, ischemia, obstruction of ducts, inflammation, and neuropathic hyperalgesia. Pain can develop in the early stages of chronic pancreatitis before morphologic changes can be demonstrated on imaging studies. Patients with chronic pancreatitis are at increased risk for pancreatic cancer, which may cause a change in the pain pattern, and extrapancreatic causes of pain must always be considered.

Pain management should proceed in a stepwise fashion and begin with lifestyle modifications such as alcohol and tobacco abstinence, a low-fat diet, and pancreatic enzyme supplementation, followed by a sequentially more aggressive and invasive approach for symptomatic failures, although it should be recognized that placebo alone is effective for up to 30% of patients. Several approaches can be considered for chronic pain relief.

1. Tobacco and alcohol abstinence. Abstention may decrease the frequency of painful attacks and reduce the likelihood pancreatic function deterioration and development of pancreatic cancer.
2. Nutrition and hydration. Small meals that are low in fat may help to some degree. Although the evidence is anecdotal, encouraging hydration may prevent exacerbations of pancreatitis. Supplementation of dietary fat with MCTs may be of benefit, possibly as a result of antioxidant effects of MCTs or the minimal increases in plasma cholecystokinin (CCK) levels associated with MCTs compared with other sources of dietary fat.
3. Analgesics. Most patients with pain require analgesics. Tramadol, a less potent opioid, is commonly used initially. The risk of addiction to opioids is not known, but studies of opioid use in other chronic pain syndromes suggest rates of less than 20%. Patients with previous addictive behaviors such as substance abuse (alcohol and tobacco included) are at greater risk for analgesic abuse and addiction.
4. Secretion suppression. Oral pancreatic enzyme replacement is thought to blunt pain by reducing endogenous CCK

secretion, which stimulates pancreatic acinar cells. Replacement therapy provides increased trypsin activity in the duodenum, which denatures CCK-releasing peptide, resulting in a reduction in endogenous CCK release and an attendant decrease in pancreatic stimulation and pain. Therapy is initiated with large doses of non–enteric-coated pancrelipases (i.e., pancreatic enzyme preparations) because the enteric-coated preparations theoretically release their enzymes further down the intestine, away from the stimulatory CCK enterocytes. Co-administration of acid suppressive therapy to prevent destruction of the enzymes by gastric acid may be helpful.

5. Neural transmission modification. Gabapentoids, including pregabalin, have been used effectively to treat neuropathic pain disorders, including diabetic neuropathy and neuropathic pain of central origin. Based on the finding that pancreatic pain is accompanied by similar alterations of central pain processing, studies suggest a benefit with pregabalin as an adjuvant treatment to decrease pain associated with chronic pancreatitis. Similarly, tricyclic antidepressants, selective serotonin reuptake inhibitors, and serotonin-norepinephrine reuptake inhibitors can be administered on a trial basis.

6. Antioxidants. Oxidative stress can cause direct pancreatic acinar cell damage through several pathways. Supplementation with antioxidants, such as selenium, vitamins C and E, and methionine, may relieve pain and reduce oxidative stress. In a randomized trial, the reduction in the number of painful days per month was higher for the patients who received antioxidants compared with those who received placebo (7.4 vs. 3.2 days). Patients who received antioxidants also were more likely to become pain free (32% vs. 13%).

7. Endoscopic decompression. Endoscopic decompression of the pancreatic duct is an option for obstruction of the main pancreatic duct caused by strictures, stones, or sphincter of Oddi dysfunction. Endoscopic therapies include pancreatic sphincterotomy, stricture dilation, stone removal with intracorporeal or extracorporeal shock wave lithotripsy, and temporary stent placement. Complete or partial pain relief is reported for approximately 50% to 80% of carefully selected patients during follow-up extending as long as 3 to 4 years.

8. Surgery. Surgical pancreatic ductal drainage, usually with lateral pancreaticojejunostomy (i.e., Puestow procedure), can be offered to those with a dilated (>6 mm in diameter) main pancreatic duct. Pain reduction is reported by approximately 80% of patients. This procedure is safe and has an operative mortality rate of less than 5%; however, only 35% to 60% of patients are free of pain at the 5-year follow-up. Individuals with nonobstructed, nondilated pancreatic ductal systems may be offered resection of focally diseased portions of the gland (i.e., Frey or Beger procedures) or total pancreatectomy with islet cell transplantation.

Management of Complications

The complications of chronic pancreatitis include pseudocysts, pancreatic fistulas, biliary obstruction, pancreatic cancer, small bowel bacterial overgrowth, and gastric varices due to splenic vein thrombosis.

Pancreatic Fistulas

Pancreatic fistulas occur as a result of duct disruption resulting in localized fluid collections, ascites, or pleural effusions. Treatment consists of bowel rest, endoscopic pancreatic duct stenting, and administration of a somatostatin analogue. Surgical intervention may be needed if this conservative approach is unsuccessful.

Vascular Complications

The splenic vein courses along the posterior surface of the pancreas, where it can be affected by inflammation from pancreatitis or malignancy that lead to thrombosis. Splenic vein thrombosis can result in isolated fundal gastric varices. Splenectomy is usually curative for patients who develop bleeding from gastric varices.

Pseudoaneurysm formation is a complication of acute and chronic pancreatitis. Affected vessels, including the hepatic, splenic, pancreaticoduodenal, and gastroduodenal arteries, lie close to the pancreas. CECT or MRI shows the pseudoaneurysm as a cystically dilated vascular structure in or adjacent to the pancreas. EUS with Doppler imaging can show blood flow within the pseudoaneurysm. Mesenteric angiography permits confirmation of the diagnosis and provides a means of therapy because selective embolization of the pseudoaneurysm can be accomplished during the procedure. Surgery for bleeding pseudoaneurysms is difficult and associated with high morbidity and mortality rates.

Biliary and Duodenal Obstruction

Symptomatic obstruction of the bile duct or duodenum, or both, develops in a few patients with chronic pancreatitis. Postprandial pain and early satiety are characteristic of duodenal obstruction, whereas pain and cholestasis (sometimes with resultant cholangitis) suggest a bile duct stricture. These complications most commonly result from inflammation or fibrosis in the head of the pancreas or an adjacent pseudocyst.

Endoscopic stenting may be attempted for bile duct strictures, but they are often refractory and typically require prolonged treatment. Endoscopic failures can be treated with surgical biliary decompression. The importance of decompression is underscored by the observation that it can reverse secondary biliary fibrosis associated with bile duct obstruction.

⬤ CARCINOMA OF THE PANCREAS
Definition and Epidemiology

Carcinoma of the pancreas is the fourth leading cause of cancer-related death in the United States, with approximately 43,000 new cases diagnosed annually. The peak incidence of pancreatic carcinoma occurs in the seventh decade of life. There is a slight male-to-female predominance (relative risk of 1.4 : 1), and blacks have a 30% to 40% higher incidence of pancreatic carcinoma than whites in the United States.

Many environmental factors have been implicated as increasing the risk for pancreatic cancer. Cigarette smoking is the most consistent factor, with the increased risk attributed to the

aromatic amines found in cigarette smoke. Other risk factors include obesity, lack of physical activity, and diabetes mellitus. Studies evaluating the relationship between diet and pancreatic cancer are inconclusive. A Western diet (i.e., high intake of fat and meat, particularly smoked or processed meats) has been linked to the development of pancreatic cancer in many studies. Epidemiologic studies have failed to find a consistent association between alcohol or coffee consumption and the development of pancreatic cancer.

Up to 10% of patients with pancreatic cancer have a family history of the disease, but most cannot be identified with a known genetic disorder. Recognized genetic disorders that predispose to pancreatic cancer include hereditary pancreatitis (*PRSS1* gene), hereditary nonpolyposis colorectal cancer, familial adenomatous polyposis, *BRCA2* germline mutations, Peutz-Jeghers syndrome (*STK11* gene), familial atypical mole melanoma syndrome (*CDKN2A* gene, formerly *MTS1*), ataxia telangiectasia, and the Von Hippel–Lindau syndrome.

Although imaging surveillance of high-risk family cohorts is pursued at some centers, there is no consensus about the optimal methods or frequency of pancreatic cancer screening. Screening has not been shown to improve survival rates.

Pathology

The term *pancreatic cancer* usually refers to ductal adenocarcinoma of the pancreas, representing 85% to 90% of all pancreatic neoplasms. *Exocrine pancreatic neoplasm* is a more inclusive term that includes neoplastic pancreatic ductal and acinar cells and their stem cells and pancreatoblastoma.

More than 95% of malignant neoplasms of the pancreas arise from the exocrine elements. Neoplasms arising from the endocrine pancreas (i.e., islet cell or neuroendocrine tumors) comprise no more than 5% of pancreatic neoplasms. Pancreatic cancers are composed of several distinct elements, including pancreatic cancer cells, tumor stroma, and stem cells. The precursor lesion of pancreatic cancer is pancreatic intraepithelial neoplasia, which progresses from mild dysplasia (PanIN grade 1) to more severe dysplasia (PanIN grades 2 and 3) and eventually to invasive carcinoma.

Clinical Presentation

The clinical manifestations of pancreatic carcinoma may be nonspecific and are often insidious. The tumor has usually reached an advanced stage by the time of diagnosis. Common presenting signs and symptoms of pancreatic cancer include jaundice, weight loss, and abdominal pain. The pain is usually constant, with radiation to the back. Because most cancers begin in the pancreatic head, patients may exhibit obstructive jaundice or a large, palpable gallbladder (i.e., Courvoisier's sign).

Painless jaundice is the most common manifestation in patients with a potentially resectable and curable lesion. Anorexia, nausea, and vomiting may also occur, along with emotional disturbances such as depression. Less common manifestations include superficial thrombophlebitis (i.e., Trousseau's sign), acute pancreatitis, diabetes, ascites, paraneoplastic syndromes (e.g., Cushing's syndrome), hypercalcemia, gastrointestinal bleeding, splenic vein thrombosis, and a palpable abdominal mass.

Diagnosis and Differential Diagnosis

The goal of imaging in the evaluation of suspected pancreatic carcinoma is to establish the diagnosis with a high degree of certainty and to determine resectability in patients who are otherwise candidates for operative resection. The diagnosis of pancreatic cancer is frequently suggested by a pancreatic mass seen on imaging studies. Evidence of a dilated pancreatic duct, hepatic metastases, invasion of vessels, or a dilated common bile duct in the setting of biliary obstruction may also be found. The imaging appearance may be impossible to distinguish from benign causes of pancreatic masses such as focal pancreatitis or autoimmune pancreatitis. Multiphase, multidetector, helical CT is the best initial study to define a mass and assess for liver metastasis or vascular invasion. Compared with CT, MRI, and angiography, EUS is the most accurate diagnostic and staging technique, providing information about tumor location, vascular invasion, and lymph node involvement.

The imaging techniques are highly accurate for recognizing unresectable disease, but they are somewhat limited for identifying resectable disease because occult metastases (<1 cm in diameter) may be on the surface of the liver or peritoneum. Staging laparoscopy is recommended for patients with the highest likelihood of occult metastatic disease: those with tumors of the body or tail of the pancreas who appear to have potentially resectable disease by CT (one half of whom have occult peritoneal metastases), those with large (>3 cm) primary tumors, those for whom imaging suggests occult metastatic disease, and those with a very high initial CA 19-9 level (>1000 units/mL).

The use of tumor markers to diagnose carcinoma of the pancreas has yielded disappointing results. The tumor marker CA 19-9 has a sensitivity of 70% to 80% and a specificity of 85% to 95% for diagnosing selected patients already exhibiting signs and symptoms that suggest pancreatic cancer. However, for early-stage cancers, CA 19-9 has limited sensitivity. Use of CA 19-9 requires the Lewis blood group antigen, which is absent in 5% to 10% of the population. The greatest utility for CA 19-9 is to identify occult metastasis in patients with seemingly resectable tumors, for monitoring patients after apparently curative surgery, and for following those receiving chemotherapy for advanced disease. Rising CA 19-9 levels suggest recurrent disease even in the absence of radiographically detectable lesions.

Unfortunately, only 10% to 20% of carcinomas in the head of the pancreas and rare cancers of the body and tail are resectable for cure. If evaluation is conclusive that a pancreatic tumor is not resectable, the first objective is to confirm the cell type, which can be done accurately by CT- or EUS-guided biopsy.

Treatment

Surgical Resection

The major determinant of operative resectability and long-term survival is vascular invasion or metastatic disease. Although practice varies across institutions, most surgeons consider a pancreatic cancer to be categorically unresectable if there is extrapancreatic involvement, including extensive peripancreatic lymphatic extension, nodal involvement beyond the peripancreatic tissues, or distant metastases (e.g., liver, peritoneum, omentum, extra-abdominal sites). Other indications of unresectability include vascular encasement (i.e., more than one half of the vessel's circumference), occlusion or thrombus of the superior mesenteric vein (SMV) or the SMV–portal vein confluence, or direct involvement of the superior mesenteric artery, inferior vena cava, aorta, celiac axis, or hepatic artery, as defined by the absence of a fat plane between the tumor and these structures on CT. For tumors of the tail of the pancreas, encasement of the splenic vein does not necessarily obviate resectability.

Selective preoperative ERCP with biliary stent placement is recommended for patients with obstructive jaundice when symptoms of intractable pruritus or cholangitis occur or when surgery must be delayed for several weeks. At the time of stent placement, ERCP tissue sampling techniques can confirm a diagnosis of pancreatic malignancy (sensitivity of 30% to 60%), but the sensitivity is lower than that of EUS-guided fine-needle aspiration.

The standard operation for pancreatic cancer of the head or uncinate process is the Whipple procedure (i.e., pancreaticoduodenectomy). Whipple resection consists of removal of the pancreatic head, distal common bile duct, gallbladder, duodenum, proximal jejunum, gastric antrum, and regional lymph nodes. Reconstruction requires pancreaticojejunostomy, hepaticojejunostomy, and gastrojejunostomy. The surgical mortality rate for this procedure is approximately 3% when performed by experienced pancreatic surgeons. Patients who have undergone surgical resection should receive adjuvant treatment using gemcitabine alone or in combination with fluorouracil-based chemoradiation therapy, which improves progression-free and overall survival rates.

The term *borderline resectable* is reserved for cases with focal (less than one half of the circumference) tumor abutment of the visceral arteries or short-segment occlusion of the SMV or SMV–portal vein confluence or hepatic artery. Some centers are performing resection and reconstruction of a short segment of the portal vein or SMV in selected patients. Arterial resection and reconstruction (mostly of the superior mesenteric and hepatic arteries) are performed infrequently, and the morbidity and mortality rates for the operation increase markedly when these arteries are included. The use of preoperative neoadjuvant chemoradiation therapy in an effort to convert patients with unresectable locoregionally advanced disease to a resectable status has increased the overall resection rate, but no difference in survival has been demonstrated.

Palliation

For patients with inoperable cancers or poor performance status, palliative interventions to alleviate jaundice, pain, and intestinal obstruction often become the focus of therapy. When advanced disease is observed operatively, the surgeon must determine whether to perform additional palliative surgery. Biliary bypass is indicated in patients with obstructive jaundice. Duodenal bypass is indicated when features suggest impending gastric outlet obstruction. Alternative palliative endoscopic approaches are available for patients not undergoing exploratory surgery.

Chemoradiation Therapy for Advanced Disease

Systemic chemotherapy provides benefit for patients with advanced pancreatic cancer, improving disease-related symptoms and survival compared with the best supportive care alone. Studies comparing gemcitabine with 5-fluorouracil indicate very low objective response rates for both single agents but superiority for gemcitabine in terms of clinical response based on improvement in symptoms (i.e., pain and weight loss) and performance status. For patients with advanced disease, gemcitabine may be combined with a platinum agent, erlotinib (i.e., epidermal growth factor receptor inhibitor), or a fluoropyrimidine.

Prognosis

Carcinoma of the pancreas accounts for approximately 5% of cancer deaths in the United States. The overall prognosis is poor because less than 20% of patients are alive beyond the first year after diagnosis, and only 1% to 3% are alive beyond the fifth year. Although 15% to 20% of patients have resectable disease at initial diagnosis, most have locally advanced or metastatic cancer. Median survival is 8 to 12 months for patients with locally advanced unresectable disease and 3 to 6 months for those with metastases at diagnosis.

A Whipple resection for pancreatic head cancers is the only chance for cure; however, the median survival after surgery is 15 to 20 months. The overall 5-year survival rate is 10% to 25%, and up to 50% of those who survive 5 years ultimately die of recurrent cancer. Poor prognostic factors include a high tumor grade, a large tumor, high levels of CA 19-9 before and after surgery, tumor-positive surgical margins, and lymph node metastases.

For a deeper discussion of these topics, please see Chapter 144, "Pancreatitis," and Chapter 194, "Pancreatic Cancer," in Goldman-Cecil Medicine, *25th Edition.*

SUGGESTED READINGS

Forsmark CE: Management of chronic pancreatitis, Gastroenterology 144:1282–1291, 2013.
Hidalgo M: Pancreatic cancer, N Engl J Med 362:1605–1617, 2010.
Paulson AS, Cao HS, Tempero MA, et al: Therapeutic advances in pancreatic cancer, Gastroenterology 144:1316–1326, 2013.
Tenner S, Baillie J, DeWitt J, et al: American College of Gastroenterology guideline: management of acute pancreatitis, Am J Gastroenterol 108:1400–1415, 2013.
Van Brunschot S, Bakker OJ, Besselink MG, et al: Treatment of necrotizing pancreatitis, Clin Gastroenterol Hepatol 10:1190–1201, 2012.
Whitcomb DC: Genetic risk factors for pancreatic disorders, Gastroenterology 144:1292–1302, 2013.
Wu BU, Banks PA: Clinical management of patients with acute pancreatitis, Gastroenterology 144:1272–1281, 2013.
Yadav D, Lowenfels AB: The epidemiology of pancreatitis and pancreatic cancer, Gastroenterology 144:1252–1261, 2013.

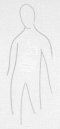

Diseases of the Liver and Biliary System

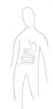

39

Laboratory Tests in Liver Disease

Shaheryar A. Siddiqui and Michael B. Fallon

INTRODUCTION

The liver is the largest solid organ in the body, and it performs many metabolic, secretory, and nutritional functions that are vital to maintenance of a healthy human physiology. The liver is responsible for glucose homeostasis, plasma protein synthesis, lipid and lipoprotein synthesis, bile acid synthesis and secretion (for absorption of fats and vitamins), and vitamin storage (vitamins B_{12}, A, D, E, and K). In addition, the liver is the major site for biotransformation, detoxification, and excretion of a vast array of endogenous and exogenous compounds (e.g., drugs, toxins). As a result of these diverse roles, the clinical manifestations of liver disease are varied and can be quite subtle. Laboratory tests are designed to assess the various functions of the liver, which are then correlated with patient history and physical examination as part of a broader assessment. These tests may be ordered as part of a screening evaluation or to further evaluate clinical signs and symptoms prompting consideration of liver disease, such as hepatomegaly, ascites, jaundice, dark urine, light-colored stool, or gastrointestinal bleeding.

LIVER FUNCTION TESTS

Colloquially, the term *liver function tests* (LFTs) is used quite often when referring to a panel of measurements to assess the "function" of the liver. This panel typically includes measurements of total protein, albumin, aspartate aminotransferase (AST, formerly called serum glutamic-oxaloacetic transaminase or SGOT), alanine aminotransferase (ALT, formerly called serum glutamic-pyruvic transaminase or SGPT), alkaline phosphatase (ALP), γ-glutamyl transpeptidase (GGT), bilirubin (conjugated and unconjugated), and prothrombin time (PT). Unlike tests used to assess function in other organ systems (e.g., arterial blood gases, creatinine clearance), liver function tests do not directly measure hepatic function and may not accurately reflect the cause or severity of liver disease. Rather, they reflect certain patterns or types of liver and biliary cell injury that warrant further evaluation. The most widely available and useful liver function tests are outlined in Table 39-1.

Hepatocellular Injury

AST and ALT are intracellular enzymes that catalyze the transfer of the α-amino group of aspartate or alanine to the α-keto group of ketoglutaric acid, resulting in formation of pyruvate or oxaloacetic acid, respectively. They are important enzymes that participate in gluconeogenesis. With cell injury, AST and ALT are released into the circulation, and higher values are used primarily as markers of liver inflammation. ALT is found predominantly in hepatocytes, and an elevation in ALT is more specific than an elevated AST for liver disease. AST is found in the liver but also in heart, skeletal muscle, brain, kidney, pancreas, and lungs. After injury or death of liver cells, these enzymes are released into the circulation. They are measured indirectly with the use of a spectrophotometer.

In most hepatocellular disorders (e.g., viral hepatitis, acetaminophen toxicity), ALT levels are higher than or equal to AST levels. In alcoholic liver disease, however, the AST usually is more than two-fold higher than the ALT (AST/ALT ratio >2). An AST/ALT ratio greater than 3 is 97% specific for alcohol as the underlying cause. Extremely high transaminase levels (15 times the upper limit of normal) generally indicate acute hepatocellular necrosis from viral or toxic causes such as acetaminophen; less frequently, they indicate acute bile duct obstruction or hepatic ischemia (shock liver).

Patients who have isolated asymptomatic elevations of AST and ALT (usually ALT > AST) may have nonalcoholic fatty liver disease (NAFLD), which is caused by obesity, insulin resistance and diabetes, hyperlipidemia, or excessive alcohol consumption. However, in some cases, the AST is higher than the ALT, mimicking the pattern seen in alcoholic liver disease. A careful history and evaluation are warranted, although the AST/ALT ratio in NAFLD rarely exceeds 2, thus distinguishing it from alcoholic liver disease.

Infiltrative hepatocellular disease (e.g., hemochromatosis) and chronic viral hepatitis are also part of the differential.

Cholestasis

Serum ALP comprises a group of isoenzymes derived from the liver, bone, intestine, and placenta. Hepatic ALP (isoenzyme ALP-1) is present mainly in the mucosal cells lining the bile ducts; the usual flow of bile into the small intestine maintains the normal serum level of ALP. In cholestasis related to biliary obstruction or duct injury, serum ALP levels rise as a result of retention of bile acids in the liver; the bile acids solubilize ALP from the hepatocyte plasma membrane and also stimulate its synthesis. Various other hepatocyte plasma membrane enzymes are simultaneously released, including 5'-nucleotidase (5'-NT) and GGT, confirming that the elevated ALP is caused by hepatobiliary disease. The measurement of ALP is thus correlated with integrity of the biliary system.

Primary biliary cirrhosis (PBC) and primary sclerosing cholangitis (PSC) are examples of obstructive diseases with predominant elevation of ALP. Other conditions, such as bone regeneration, pregnancy, and neoplastic, infiltrative, and granulomatous liver diseases are also associated with elevated ALP levels.

TABLE 39-1　LABORATORY TESTS OF HEPATIC FUNCTION

LIVER ASSAY*	LIVER FUNCTION	ABNORMALITY
Serum albumin (3.5-5.5 g/dL)	Assess the biosynthetic capacity of the liver (days to weeks)	Decreased synthetic capacity Protein malnutrition Nephrotic syndrome Protein-losing enteropathy
Prothrombin time (11-14 sec)	Assess the biosynthetic capacity of the liver (hours to days)	Decreased synthetic capacity (especially factors II and VII) Vitamin K deficiency Consumptive coagulopathy
Serum bilirubin (0.2-1.3 mg/dL) (3.4-22.2 μmol/L)	Extraction of bilirubin from blood; conjugation and excretion into bile	Hemolysis Diffuse liver disease Cholestasis Extrahepatic bile duct obstruction Congenital disorders of bilirubin metabolism
Serum alkaline phosphatase (39-136 units/L)	Present in the cells lining the biliary tree	Bile duct obstruction Cholestasis Infiltrative liver disease (neoplasms, granulomas) Bone destruction, remodeling Pregnancy
γ-glutamyl transpeptidase (7-45 units/L)	Highly sensitive to hepatocyte damage and cholestasis	
5'-nucleotidase (2-17 units/L)	More specific for the liver and for cholestasis than GGT	
Aspartate aminotransferase (AST) or SGOT (5-40 Units/L)	Represent hepatocyte inflammation and damage	Hepatocellular necrosis Cardiac or skeletal muscle necrosis
Alanine aminotransferase or SGPT (5-65 Units/L)	Represent hepatocyte inflammation and damage	Same as AST; however, more specific for liver cell damage

*The reference intervals given here in conventional metric units and in SI units are from several large medical centers. Always use the reference intervals provided by your clinical laboratory, since intervals may be method-dependent.

An isolated elevated ALP level may be the only clue to obstruction of the common bile duct or neoplastic or granulomatous hepatic disease. Elevated serum ALP levels with normal 5'-NT and GGT usually suggests a nonhepatic cause (e.g., bone disease, pregnancy, chronic renal failure, lymphoma, congestive heart failure). Electrophoretic fractionation of ALP isoenzymes may be useful to confirm alternative sources.

Elevated bilirubin levels also are characteristic of cholestasis. Bilirubin is present in the serum in two forms: unconjugated (indirect) and conjugated (direct). Under normal conditions, total serum bilirubin levels are less than 1 mg/dL, with the conjugated fraction representing up to 30% of the total. The serum bilirubin level reflects a balance between bilirubin production and its conjugation and excretion into bile by the liver.

The differential diagnosis for hyperbilirubinemia (see Chapter 42) requires consideration of an extensive list of disorders in which there are alterations of bilirubin production (hematologic disorders with predominantly unconjugated hyperbilirubinemia), hepatic metabolism (congenital abnormalities of bilirubin conjugation, liver disease), or excretion (congenital abnormalities of bilirubin excretion or biliary obstruction with predominantly conjugated hyperbilirubinemia). Hence, an ele-

vated serum bilirubin is not specific but should initiate a more detailed evaluation for more specific causes.

Importantly, individual tests often do not indicate the nature of the underlying liver disease; hence, the common use of the LFT panel of tests. The overall pattern of liver test abnormalities and the relative magnitudes of abnormalities in individual tests often provide significant insights, including categorization as to whether the liver disease is primarily hepatocellular or cholestatic. Figure 39-1 outlines common patterns of liver test abnormalities and common accompanying diagnostic evaluation.

Hepatic Synthetic Function

The serum albumin level and the PT (expressed as the international normalized ratio [INR]) reflect the hepatic capacity for protein synthesis. The PT is dependent on coagulation factors II, V, VII, and X and responds rapidly to altered hepatic function because of the short serum half-lives of factors II and VII (about 6 hours). This makes measurement of PT a useful marker of hepatic synthetic function that can be measured as frequently as daily. However, because serum levels of factors II, VII, IX, and X are dependent on vitamin K, coexistent vitamin K deficiency must be excluded or treated before PT can be used as a measure of intrinsic hepatic function. In contrast, the serum half-life of albumin is 14 to 20 days, and serum levels fall with prolonged liver dysfunction or acute liver impairment. Malnutrition and renal or gastrointestinal losses merit consideration in the evaluation of significant hypoalbuminemia, especially if the PT is relatively well preserved.

QUANTITATIVE TESTS OF LIVER FUNCTION

Quantitative liver tests that depend on the capacity of the liver to transform or transport a test agent have been developed but have not received widespread application. These include indocyanine green clearance, galactose elimination capacity, aminopyrine breath test, antipyrine clearance, monoethylglycinexylidide, and caffeine clearance. They may be superior to conventional biochemical tests in predicting prognosis, but their clinical utility has not been established, and they are limited primarily to research centers.

Specific Disease Markers

Elevations of individual γ-globulins can be suggestive of specific diseases. For example, autoimmune hepatitis is associated with an elevated total immunoglobulin G (IgG) level and the presence of autoantibodies such as antinuclear antibody (ANA), anti–smooth muscle antibody (ASMA), and anti–liver/kidney microsomal antibody type 1 (anti-LKM1). IgG4-related disease is an autoimmune phenomenon in which increased IgG4 levels cause dysfunction in multiple organs, including autoimmune cholangitis and autoimmune pancreatitis. Alcoholic cirrhosis is associated with high IgA levels, and primary biliary cirrhosis is associated with elevated IgM levels.

Viruses are detected by polymerase chain reaction (PCR), enzyme assays, and genotyping. Screening can be performed for specific diseases such as hemochromatosis (iron panels and *HFE* gene mutation testing). Levels of α_1-antitrypsin and serum ceruloplasmin are measured to evaluate patients with liver disease

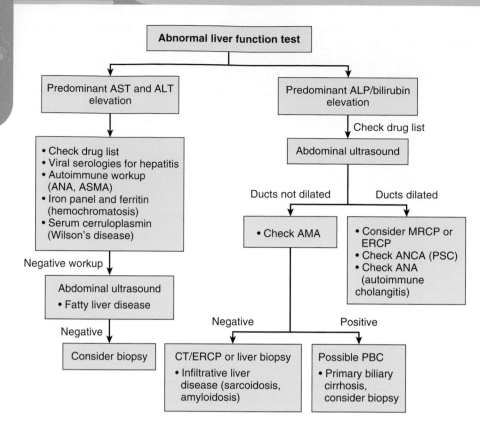

FIGURE 39-1 Diagnostic approach to abnormal liver function test. ACE, Angiotensin-converting enzyme; ALP, alkaline phosphatase; ALT, alanine aminotransferase; ANA, antinuclear antibody; ANCA, antineutrophil cytoplasmic antibody; AMA, antimitochondrial antibody; ASMA, anti–smooth muscle antibody; AST, aspartate aminotransferase; CT, computed tomography; ERCP, endoscopic retrograde cholangiopancreatography; MRCP, magnetic resonance cholangiopancreatography; PBC, primary biliary cirrhosis; PSC, primary sclerosing cholangitis.

for possible α_1-antitrypsin deficiency and Wilson's disease, respectively. Serum ammonia is a poor marker of hepatic function. However, it is used frequently as an aide in the evaluation of possible portosystemic encephalopathy. Carbohydrate-deficient transferrin (CDT) is a marker used to identify chronic alcohol use.

Biomarkers of Liver Histology

Liver biopsy remains the "gold standard" for detection and quantitation of liver cirrhosis, fibrosis, inflammation, steatosis, tumors, and necrosis. Biopsy of the liver is a straightforward procedure that can be performed by either a percutaneous or a transjugular approach. Although it is generally safe, serious complications such as bleeding (1 per 1000) and death (1 per 10,000) may occur. There is also a finite risk of introducing an infection.

Given these potential concerns, noninvasive alternatives to liver biopsy would be attractive if validated. Both noninvasive serum markers and ultrasonographic elastography have been evaluated as potential alternatives to liver biopsy to assess hepatic fibrosis. FibroTest (known as FibroSure in the United States) is the most studied biomarker panel. Other patented biomarker panels include the Enhanced Liver Fibrosis (ELF) test, Hepascore, Fibro Meter, and FIBROSpect by Western blotting. The FibroTest panel incorporates six serum markers: α_2-macroglobulin, haptoglobin, apolipoprotein A-I, GGT, total bilirubin, and ALT. An algorithm is used to calculate a score, represented as a range from F0 to F4, that indicates the probability of fibrosis (F0, no cirrhosis; F4, liver cirrhosis).

Another scoring system, called the NAFLD fibrosis score, uses six variables (age, body mass index [BMI], AST, ALT, platelet count, and serum albumin) to predict advanced fibrosis in patients with NAFLD. The utility of this scoring system in routine clinical practice is not clearly established.

Imaging modalities such as real-time shear wave elastography (SWE) on the Aixplorer ultrasound machine, transient elastography (FibroScan), and acoustic radiation force imaging (ARFI) are sonographic techniques based on the theory that a "shear wave" moves faster in a less elastic liver (i.e., one with more fibrosis and scarring) than in a normal or less fibrotic liver. These imaging modalities have a high specificity in detecting liver fibrosis, comparable to that of serum biomarkers.

Liver Biopsy

Biopsy and histologic examination of liver tissue is still the standard protocol for patients who are undergoing induction therapy for chronic viral hepatitis or are on the transplant list for any other cause of liver failure. Contraindications for biopsy include an uncooperative patient, impaired hemostasis (INR >1.5), thrombocytopenia (fewer than 50,000 to 60,000 platelets per microliter), use of nonsteroidal anti-inflammatory drugs (NSAIDs) within the previous 7 to 10 days, and suspected echinococcal cysts in the liver.

For a deeper discussion on this topic, see Section XIII: Disease of the Liver, Gallbladder, and Bile Ducts in Goldman-Cecil Medicine, *25th Edition.*

SUGGESTED READINGS

Chen J, Liu C, Chen H, et al: Study on noninvasive laboratory tests for fibrosis in chronic HBV infection and their evaluation, J Clin Lab Anal 27:5–11, 2013.
de Lédinghen V, Vergniol J, Gonzalez C, et al: Screening for liver fibrosis by using FibroScan and FibroTest in patients with diabetes, Dig Liver Dis 44:413–418, 2012.

Gangadharan B, Bapat M, Rossa J, et al: Discovery of novel biomarker candidates for liver fibrosis in hepatitis C patients: a preliminary study, PLoS ONE 7(6):e39603, 2012.

Park MS, Kim BK, Cheong JY, et al: Discordance between liver biopsy and FibroTest in assessing liver fibrosis in chronic hepatitis B, PLoS ONE 8(2):e55759, 2013.

Poynard T, De Ledinghen V, Zarski JP, et al: Relative performances of FibroTest, Fibroscan, and biopsy for the assessment of the stage of liver fibrosis in patients with chronic hepatitis C: a step toward the truth in the absence of a gold standard, J Hepatol 56:541–548, 2012.

Poynard T, Munteanu M, Luckina E, et al: Liver fibrosis evaluation using real-time shear wave elastography: applicability and diagnostic performance using methods without a gold standard, J Hepatol 58:928–935, 2013.

Rockey D, Caldwell AH, Goodman ZD, et al: AASLD position paper: liver biopsy, Hepatology 49:1017–1044, 2009.

Sebastiani G, Halfon P, Castera L, et al: Comparison of three algorithms of non-invasive markers of fibrosis in chronic hepatitis C, Aliment Pharmacol Ther 35:92–104, 2012.

Yoneda M, Suzuki K, Kato S, et al: Nonalcoholic fatty liver disease: US-based acoustic radiation force impulse elastography, Radiology 256:640–647, 2010.

Zarski JP, Sturm N, Guechot J, et al: Comparison of nine blood tests and transient elastography for liver fibrosis in chronic hepatitis C: the ANRS HCEP-23 study, J Hepatol 56:55–62, 2012.

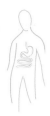

40

Jaundice

Klaus Mönkemüller, Helmut Neumann, and Michael B. Fallon

INTRODUCTION

The term *jaundice* refers to yellow pigmentation of the skin, the conjunctival membranes over the sclera, and other mucous membranes that is caused by elevated serum bilirubin levels (hyperbilirubinemia). The word derives from the French word *jaune*, which means "yellow," and the condition also is known as *icterus* (Greek for "yellow"). Normal serum bilirubin levels range from 0.5 to 1.0 mg/dL, and plasma bilirubin concentrations typically must exceed 2.5 mg/dL before jaundice becomes evident clinically. In most cases, jaundice or hyperbilirubinemia per se is not a pathologic condition but rather a sign of one or more illnesses originating from or affecting the liver and blood. However, there is one notable exception: In newborns, high bilirubin levels can lead to pathologic cerebral changes. In this condition, which is known as *kernicterus* (the word *kern* derives from German and means "nucleus"), sustained high levels of unconjugated bilirubin lead to deposition of unconjugated bilirubin in the cerebral basal ganglia (or nuclei). This process is preventable and treatable and therefore merits special recognition to prevent damage to the developing brain.

BILIRUBIN METABOLISM

Hyperbilirubinemia can be classified based on the three phases of hepatic bilirubin metabolism: uptake, conjugation, and excretion into the bile (the rate-limiting step). In addition, jaundice can be classified into prehepatic, hepatic, and posthepatic causes (Table 40-1). Although the approaches are complementary, we believe that the latter classification is more useful for the practicing clinician.

The main source of bilirubin is the hemoglobin released from senescent red blood cells, and the liver serves as its primary site of metabolism and excretion. Abnormalities at any step—bilirubin production, metabolism, or excretion—can lead to increases in serum bilirubin and clinical jaundice. Under normal conditions, human red blood cells have a life span of about 120 days. As they age, erythrocytes are broken down and removed from the circulation by phagocytes. Most bilirubin (80%) is derived from the breakdown of hemoglobin released from these cells; the remainder is derived from ineffective erythropoiesis and from catabolism of myoglobin and hepatic hemoproteins such as the cytochrome P-450 isoenzymes. The normal rate of bilirubin production is approximately 4 mg/kg body weight per day (E-Fig. 40-1).

TABLE 40-1	CLASSIFICATION OF JAUNDICE AND REPRESENTATIVE CAUSES

PREHEPATIC CAUSES

Predominantly Unconjugated Hyperbilirubinemia

Hemolysis (e.g., sickle cell disease, autoimmune hemolytic anemia, mechanical cardiac valve with accelerated red cell destruction)
Microbe-induced hemolysis (malaria, leptospirosis)
Ineffective erythropoiesis (e.g., megaloblastic anemias)
Hematoma resolution

HEPATIC CAUSES

Unconjugated Hyperbilirubinemia

Decreased hepatic uptake
  Therapeutic drugs that interfere with bilirubin uptake (e.g., rifampin, metformin, methimazole, propylthiouracil, clopidogrel, sulfamethoxazole/trimethoprim)
  Herbal medicines (e.g., *Teucrium viscidum*, kava-kava, chaparral, greater celandine)
  Hyperthyroidism
  Diminished uptake and decreased cytosolic binding proteins (e.g., newborn or premature infants)
  Shunting of blood away from the liver (portal hypertension or surgical shunt)
Decreased conjugation due to limited glucuronyltransferase activity
  Gilbert's syndrome
  Crigler-Najjar syndrome types I and II
  Neonatal jaundice
  Breast-milk jaundice
  Drug-induced inhibition (e.g., chloramphenicol)

Predominantly Conjugated Hyperbilirubinemia

Impaired hepatic excretion
  Familial cholestasis (Dubin-Johnson syndrome, Rotor's syndrome, benign recurrent cholestasis, cholestasis of pregnancy)
  Hepatocellular injury from infiltrative disorders, hemochromatosis, α_1-antitrypsin deficiency, lymphoma, sarcoidosis, extensive metastases)
  Liver cirrhosis
  Hepatitis
  Drug-induced cholestasis (chlorpromazine, erythromycin estolate, isoniazid, halothane, and many others)
  Primary biliary cirrhosis
  Congestive heart failure
  Sepsis

POSTHEPATIC CAUSES

Extrahepatic biliary obstruction
  Common bile duct obstruction from gallstones
  Benign and malignant tumors of the pancreas
  Tumors of bile ducts (cholangiocarcinoma) and ampulla of Vater
  Biliary strictures (postsurgical, gallstone-related, primary sclerosing cholangitis)
  Congenital disorders (biliary atresia, cystic fibrosis)
  Infectious cholangiopathy
  Chronic pancreatitis (fibrosis of the head of the pancreas)

As erythrocytes are destroyed within the reticuloendothelial system, free hemoglobin is ingested by macrophages and then split into heme and globin moieties. The heme ring is cleaved by the enzyme microsomal heme oxygenase to form biliverdin (*verde* = "green"), which is then converted to the tetrapyrol pigment bilirubin by the cytosolic enzyme biliverdin reductase. This unconjugated (or "indirect") bilirubin is released into the plasma, where it is tightly bound to albumin. Because unconjugated bilirubin is insoluble in water, it cannot be excreted in urine or bile. However, it is permeable across lipid-rich environments and therefore can traverse the blood-brain barrier and the placenta.

The unconjugated bilirubin-albumin complex is transported to the liver. Once in the space of Disse, this complex dissociates; unconjugated bilirubin is transported across the basolateral plasma membrane of liver cells and attaches to intracellular binding proteins (ligandins). It is then conjugated with glucuronic acid by the enzyme uridine diphosphate–glucuronyltransferase (UDP-GT) to form bilirubin monoglucuronide and diglucuronide, making the molecule water soluble. This conjugated (or "direct") bilirubin is excreted into bile via active transport across the canalicular membrane by means of a multispecific canalicular transport protein.

If biliary excretion of conjugated bilirubin is impaired, it can exit the basolateral membrane and reenter the circulation, causing an increase in plasma levels. Because conjugated bilirubin is water soluble and less tightly bound to albumin than its unconjugated form, it is readily filtered by the glomerulus and appears in the urine, giving it a dark color (choluria). Once in bile, bilirubin enters the intestine, where bacteria convert it to colorless tetrapyrroles (urobilinogens) that are excreted in feces. Up to 20% of urobilinogen is reabsorbed and undergoes enterohepatic circulation or excretion in urine.

LABORATORY MEASUREMENT OF BILIRUBIN

The *van den Bergh reaction,* which is the most commonly used test for detecting bilirubin in biologic fluids, combines bilirubin with diazotized sulfanilic acid to form a colored compound. The direct-reacting fraction is roughly equivalent to conjugated bilirubin and the indirect-reacting fraction (total minus direct fraction) to unconjugated bilirubin. This characteristic provides a means for classifying jaundice into two categories: unconjugated hyperbilirubinemia and conjugated hyperbilirubinemia.

UNCONJUGATED HYPERBILIRUBINEMIA

Mechanisms that cause unconjugated hyperbilirubinemia include overproduction, impaired hepatic uptake, and decreased conjugation of bilirubin. These disorders are not usually associated with significant hepatic disease.

Etiology of Hyperbilirubinemia

There are many potential causes of hyperbilirubinemia, and the major categories are summarized in Table 40-1. It is helpful to consider them mechanistically as conditions affecting the balance of bilirubin production, liver metabolism, and excretion. The classic cause of bilirubin overproduction is hemolysis, whereas the most common cause of impaired bilirubin uptake and metabolism is cirrhosis or other liver disease. Bile duct obstruction due to cancer, stones, or strictures is the most common cause of obstructive jaundice. Because multiple mechanisms are often involved in an individual patient, the evaluation of jaundice can be complex.

Prehepatic Jaundice

Prehepatic jaundice is associated with excessive bilirubin production (Fig. 40-1), which most often results from hemolysis (intravascular or extravascular), resolution of large hematomas, or mechanical injury to red cells, such as can occur with pulmonary emboli. Certain genetic diseases can lead to increased red cell lysis and therefore to hemolytic jaundice. Sickle cell anemia is the classic cause, but others include glucose 6-phosphate dehydrogenase deficiency and hereditary spherocytosis. Infectious diseases also can cause hemolysis, either directly (e.g., malaria) or indirectly (e.g., autoimmune injury). Jaundice resulting from hemolysis is characteristically mild in degree, and serum bilirubin levels rarely exceed 5 mg/dL in the absence of coexisting hepatic disease. Ineffective erythropoiesis, which may be significantly increased in megaloblastic anemias, also leads to mild jaundice.

Hemolysis should be considered in the evaluation of unconjugated hyperbilirubinemia and evaluated by examination of the peripheral blood smear (and, in some cases, the bone marrow

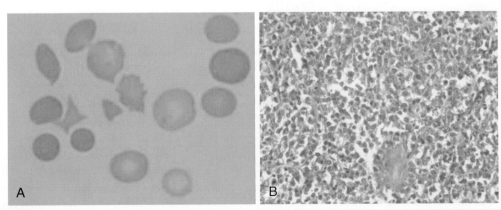

FIGURE 40-1 Hemolytic anemia associated with lymphoma. **A,** Blood smears show the destroyed red blood cells. **B,** Lymphoma.

smear) as well as measurements of the reticulocyte count, haptoglobin, lactate dehydrogenase (LDH), erythrocyte fragility, and Coombs' test as indicated.

Hepatic or Hepatocellular Jaundice

Typically, considerable reserve exists within the liver, so jaundice of hepatocellular origin can be indicative of significant injury or dysfunction. The differential diagnosis is broad because the liver is susceptible to many different forms of injury (Fig. 40-2). The most common categories are viral hepatitis, exposure to toxins (e.g., alcohol, carbon tetrachloride, amanita), prescription or nonprescription drugs, autoimmune disorders (e.g., autoimmune hepatitis, primary biliary cirrhosis [PBC], primary sclerosing cholangitis [PSC]), and liver tumors (mostly metastatic in origin). Impaired hepatic uptake of bilirubin can be a cause of unconjugated hyperbilirubinemia. When present, it is typically caused by competition for bilirubin uptake by drugs such as rifampin. Removal of the competing agent usually leads to resolution of the jaundice.

Impaired Conjugation

Another common cause of unconjugated hyperbilirubinemia is Gilbert's syndrome, a benign disorder that affects up to 7% of the population. This represents a normal variant that is not associated with intrinsic liver disease. Rather, it typically manifests during the second or third decade of life as mild unconjugated hyperbilirubinemia that is exacerbated by fasting or physical stress. Most of those affected have a total bilirubin level of less than 3 mg/dL, mostly of the unconjugated (indirect) fraction. The underlying genetic variant responsible is a homozygous abnormality in the TATAA element of the promoter region of the UDP-GT gene that results in lower enzymatic levels. The diagnosis is strongly suggested by unconjugated hyperbilirubinemia in the setting of normal hepatic enzyme levels, no known liver disease, and no evidence of hemolysis. Liver biopsy usually is not indicated, and therapy is not warranted. However, the bilirubin level does decrease significantly with phenobarbital administration. It is important to be aware of this common cause of unconjugated hyperbilirubinemia so that the patient can be reassured and more costly or invasive tests can be avoided.

Crigler-Najjar syndrome is another cause of unconjugated hyperbilirubinemia in which the bilirubin levels may be much

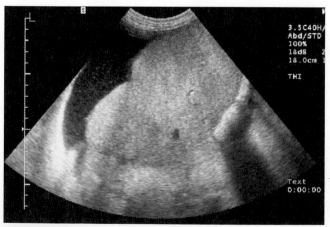

FIGURE 40-2 Ultrasound image shows a cirrhotic liver with atrophy, irregular contours, and ascites.

higher due to a genetically determined decrease or absence of UDP-GT activity. Conjugation may also be impaired by mild, acquired defects of UDP-GT induced by drugs such as chloramphenicol.

NEONATAL JAUNDICE

About 50% of term and 80% of preterm babies develop jaundice, which usually appears 2 to 4 days after birth and resolves spontaneously after 1 to 2 weeks. Most jaundice in newborn infants occurs for two main reasons. First, the enzymatic and transport pathways responsible for bilirubin metabolism are relatively immature and are unable to conjugate bilirubin as efficiently or as quickly as in adults. Second, bilirubin production is increased. Of those two mechanisms, the major defect is in bilirubin conjugation, which may cause mild to moderate unconjugated hyperbilirubinemia between the second and fifth days of life lasting until day 8 in normal births or about day 14 in premature births. This neonatal jaundice is usually harmless, and no specific therapy is required other than close observation.

More severe pathologic unconjugated hyperbilirubinemia can occur in neonates and usually is caused by a combination of hemolysis secondary to blood group incompatibility and defective conjugation. This neonatal jaundice is a serious condition that requires immediate attention because severe hyperbilirubinemia can lead to permanent neurologic damage (kernicterus). Phototherapy provided by conventional lighting or a fiberoptic light is the treatment of choice; it reduces neonatal jaundice (as assessed by serum bilirubin levels) compared with no treatment. Low-threshold compared with high-threshold phototherapy reduces neurodevelopmental impairment and hearing loss and reduces serum bilirubin on day 5 in infants with extremely low birth weight. However, it increases the duration of phototherapy, and it has no effect on mortality or on the rate of exchange transfusion. Close phototherapy, compared with distant light-source phototherapy, reduces the duration of phototherapy in infants with hyperbilirubinemia. If jaundice does not improve with phototherapy, other causes of neonatal jaundice should be assessed.

CONJUGATED HYPERBILIRUBINEMIA

Conjugated hyperbilirubinemia is associated with impaired formation or excretion of *all* components of bile, a situation termed *cholestasis*. The two major mechanisms of conjugated hyperbilirubinemia are defective excretion of bilirubin from hepatocytes into bile (intrahepatic cholestasis) and mechanical obstruction to the flow of bile through the bile ducts.

Impaired Hepatic Excretion (Intrahepatic Cholestasis)

Intrahepatic cholestasis can result from a wide range of conditions, including those that impair canalicular transport (e.g., certain drugs, circulating inflammatory cytokines during sepsis) and those that cause destruction of the small intrahepatic bile ducts. PBC, for example, is a chronic, progressive liver disease that occurs primarily in women and is characterized by the indolent destruction and subsequent disappearance over time of small lobular bile ducts. The gradual decrease in the number of bile ducts leads to progressive cholestasis, portal inflammation, fibrosis, and eventually cirrhosis. A similar loss of intrahepatic ducts can occur as a result of chronic rejection after liver transplantation.

Drug-induced cholestasis is increasingly common, and immune-mediated or idiosyncratic mechanisms predominate. In some cases, there is associated hepatitis with significant cell injury. Representative drugs include, but are not limited to, nitrofurantoin, oral contraceptives, anabolic steroids, erythromycin, cimetidine, gold salts, chlorpromazine, prochlorperazine, imipramine, sulindac, tobutamide, ampicillin, and other penicillin-based antibiotics. Given the broad access to drugs is Western societies and the unpredictable nature of the adverse liver effects, a high index of suspicion for drug-induced cholestasis is required.

Intrahepatic cholestasis of pregnancy (ICP), also known as idiopathic jaundice of pregnancy, is a cholestatic disorder that is characterized by pruritus in the absence of a skin rash and elevation of aminotransferases (often up to 100 IU/L), alkaline phosphatase, 5-nucleotidase, and total and direct bilirubin concentrations. Total levels of bilirubin rarely exceed 6 mg/dL. The levels of γ-glutamyl transpeptidase are normal or only modestly elevated. ICP occurs in the second or third trimester of pregnancy and usually resolves spontaneously within 2 to 3 weeks after delivery. The diagnosis is suggested by the combination of pruritus and abnormal liver function tests with exclusion of other causes such as gallstones or intrinsic liver disease. ICP is associated with a higher risk for adverse perinatal outcome, including preterm birth, meconium passage, and fetal death.

The cause of ICP is not fully defined, but genetic, hormonal, and environmental factors are all likely to be involved. There is a high incidence of ICP in Chile and some other areas, and studies of potential genetic contributors are underway. Because adverse outcomes appear to occur predominantly after 37 weeks' gestation, management by an experienced obstetrics team and consideration of early delivery are warranted. Ursodeoxycholic acid may be effective in ameliorating maternal pruritus and improving liver function test results; however, no medication has yet been shown to reduce the risk to the fetus.

The hemophagocytic syndrome, also known as hemophagocytic lymphohystiocytosis (HLH), is an uncommon hyperinflammatory disorder caused by severe hypercytokinemia. It manifests as fever, splenomegaly, and jaundice, with hemophagocytosis in the bone marrow and other tissues pathologically. Primary or familial HLH, also called familial erythrophagocytic lymphohistiocytosis, is a heterogeneous autosomal recessive disorder that has been found to be more prevalent with parental consanguinity. Secondary HLH is associated with malignancy, immunodeficiency, and infection, especially viral infection. In HLH, there is an inherent defect of natural killer cells and cytotoxic T cells, so they are unable to cope effectively with the infectious agent or antigen. Liver biopsies in HLH reveal sinusoidal dilation with hemophagocytic histiocytosis.

Postoperative jaundice typically occurs 1 to 10 days after surgery and has an incidence of approximately 15% after heart surgery and 1% after elective abdominal surgery. It is multifactorial in origin, with increased bilirubin load from bleeding and blood transfusions as well as impaired bilirubin conjugation and secretion caused by inflammatory cytokines. It typically resolves fully over time. In hepatocellular disease, all three steps of hepatic bilirubin metabolism are impaired. Excretion, the rate-limiting step, is usually most affected, leading to predominantly conjugated hyperbilirubinemia.

Jaundice can be profound in acute hepatitis (see Chapter 41) without adverse prognostic implications. In chronic liver disease, however, persistent jaundice usually implies irreversible decrease in hepatic function and a poor prognosis.

Posthepatic Jaundice

Posthepatic jaundice, also called obstructive jaundice, results from a complete or partial obstruction of intrahepatic or extrahepatic bile ducts (Fig. 40-3 and E-Fig. 40-2). The most common causes are gallstones in the common bile duct and tumors of the pancreatic head. Not infrequently, the first sign of pancreatic cancer is jaundice. Other causes include strictures of the common bile duct resulting from prior surgery or passage of gallstones. Less common causes include congenital biliary atresia, pancreatitis, pancreatic pseudocysts, and parasites such as liver flukes (e.g., *Clonorchis sinensis*, *Dicrocoelium dendriticum*, *Opisthorchis viverrini*).

Mirizzi syndrome is an uncommon cause of posthepatic jaundice observed in 0.7% to 1.4% of patients after cholecystectomy.

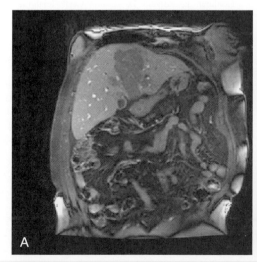
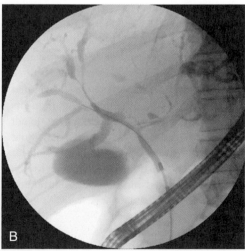

FIGURE 40-3 Hepatocellular carcinoma compressing the bile ducts. **A,** Sagittal view of computed abdominal tomography scan. **B,** Endoscopic retrograde cholangiopancreatography demonstrates multiple strictures of the bile ducts.

This syndrome is caused by extrinsic compression from an impacted stone in the cystic duct that impinges on and obstructs the common bile duct (see Table 40-1). Portal hypertensive biliopathy (or vascular biliopathy) is characterized by anatomic and functional abnormalities of the intrahepatic, extrahepatic, and pancreatic ducts in patients with portal hypertension associated with extrahepatic portal vein obstruction or, less frequently, cirrhosis. These morphologic changes, consisting of dilatation and stenosis of the biliary tree, are caused by extensive venous collaterals that develop in an attempt to decompress the portal venous blockage. The condition is usually asymptomatic until it has progressed to a more advanced stage such as biliary cirrhosis.

Immunoglobulin G4 (IgG4)–related sclerosing disease has recently been recognized as a distinct disease entity that can affect the bile ducts, gallbladder, pancreas, and other sites. Most cases of IgG4-related pancreatobiliary disease are associated with elevated serum IgG4 levels, extensive IgG4-positive plasma cells, and infiltration of lymphocytes into various organs, which leads to fibrosis. Several established systems are used to diagnose IgG4 disease; they rely on a combination of imaging findings of the pancreas, bile duct, and other organs; serologic findings; pancreatic histologic findings; and response to corticosteroid therapy.

● CLINICAL APPROACH TO THE EVALUATION OF JAUNDICE

Because the differential diagnosis of jaundice is broad, a thorough history and physical examination and judicious use of laboratory and imaging studies are needed to define its cause. Jaundice appears as yellowing of the skin and sclera. Other conditions may mimic this presentation (e.g., carotinemia, Addison's disease, quinacrine ingestion), but scleral and mucosal discolorations are absent in these conditions. In hypercarotinemia, for example, the yellowish-orange coloration typically involves only the palms of the hands and soles of the feet.

An elevated serum bilirubin level, usually higher than 3 mg/dL, confirms the clinical impression of jaundice. The most important initial step is to define whether the jaundice is predominately caused by an elevation of unconjugated or of conjugated bilirubin. If jaundice is primarily the result of unconjugated bilirubin, evaluation for hemolysis and other conditions with shortened red blood cell survival is required. In patients with elevated conjugated bilirubin, the clinical challenge lies in determining whether biliary obstruction or impaired hepatic excretion is responsible (see Chapter 39).

In cholestatic jaundice caused by biliary obstruction the alkaline phosphatase level is typically increased to more than three times normal, whereas serum transaminases are usually elevated less than 5-fold to 10-fold (E-Fig. 40-3; see Chapter 39). Patients with cholestasis also may develop pruritus and malabsorption of fat and fat-soluble vitamins (vitamins A, D, E, and K). More specific causes of biliary obstruction are suggested by recurrent abdominal pain and nausea (gallstones) or epigastric pain radiating to the back with weight loss and gallbladder distention

(carcinoma of the pancreatic head). In complete biliary obstruction, conjugated hyperbilirubinemia is prominent and usually peaks at about 30 mg/dL in the absence of renal failure. Eosinophilia may accompany drug-induced jaundice. Inquiry about the use of drugs known to cause cholestasis, serologic testing for antimitochondrial antibody in suspected PBC, and endoscopic retrograde cholangiopancreatography (ERCP) or magnetic resonance cholangiopancreatography (MRCP) to evaluate PSC may be helpful.

In jaundice produced by hepatocellular disease (see Chapters 41 and 43), serum transaminases are characteristically elevated more than 10-fold and alkaline phosphatase levels are less than three times normal. Evidence of hepatocellular damage is commonly associated and includes a prolonged prothrombin time, hypoalbuminemia, and clinical features of hepatic dysfunction (palmar erythema, spider angiomas, gynecomastia, and ascites). A careful evaluation includes inquiry about the use of drugs known to cause hepatocellular injury, alcohol, risk factors for viral hepatitis, and preexisting liver disease. More selected laboratory studies, such as serologic testing for hepatitis, are usually required (see Chapter 41).

A diagnostic approach to jaundice is outlined in E-Figure 40-2. If extrahepatic obstruction is suspected, noninvasive studies such as ultrasound or computed tomography should be used to determine whether bile ducts are dilated. If dilated ducts are found on noninvasive imaging, then direct cholangiography (either endoscopic or radiologic) provides the most reliable approach to management and potential treatment of cholestatic jaundice. If intrahepatic cholestasis is suggested clinically and extrahepatic obstruction is excluded by noninvasive means or by direct cholangiography, then the emphasis is placed on further laboratory testing to define the specific cause. Liver biopsy is sometimes required to define a specific histologic diagnosis, rule out other causes of disease, and assess the degree of injury and fibrosis.

For a deeper discussion on this topic, please see Chapter 147, "Approach to the Patient with Jaundice or Abnormal Liver Tests," in Goldman-Cecil Medicine, *25th Edition.*

SUGGESTED READINGS

Berk PD: Approach to the patient with jaundice or abnormal liver tests. In Goldman L, Ausiello D, editors: Cecil Textbook of Medicine, ed 22, Philadelphia, 2004, Saunders, pp 897–905.

Pathak B, Sheibani L, Lee RH: Cholestasis of pregnancy, Obstet Gynecol Clin North Am 37:269–282, 2010.

Suárez V, Puerta A, Santos LF, et al: Portal hypertensive biliopathy: a single center experience and literature review, World J Hepatol 5:137–144, 2013.

Trauner M, Wagner M, Fickert P, et al: Molecular regulation of hepatobiliary transport systems: clinical implications for understanding and treating cholestasis, J Clin Gastroenterol 39(4 Suppl 2):S111–S124, 2005.

Vlachou PA, Khalili K, Jang HJ, et al: IgG4-related sclerosing disease: autoimmune pancreatitis and extrapancreatic manifestations, Radiographics 31:1379–1402, 2011.

Woodgate P, Jardine LA: Neonatal jaundice, Clin Evid (Online) Epub Sep 15, 2011. Available at: http://www.ncbi.nlm.nih.gov/pubmed/21920055. Accessed September 19, 2014.

41

Acute and Chronic Hepatitis

Jen-Jung Pan and Michael B. Fallon

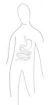

INTRODUCTION

The term *hepatitis* denotes inflammation of the liver. It is applied to a broad category of clinicopathologic conditions that result from the damage produced by viral, toxic, metabolic, pharmacologic, or immune-mediated injury to the liver.

ACUTE HEPATITIS

Acute hepatitis implies a recent-onset inflammatory condition lasting less than 6 months. It can culminate either in complete resolution of the liver damage with return to normal function and structure or rapid progression of the acute injury toward extensive necrosis and a fatal outcome. The most common causes of acute hepatitis are viral hepatitis (hepatitis A through E) and nonviral causes such as drugs (prescription, nonprescription, and illicit), alcohol, toxins, autoimmune hepatitis, and Wilson's disease.

Acute Viral Hepatitis

Five hepatotropic viruses cause acute viral hepatitis (Table 41-1), but other viruses, including cytomegalovirus and herpesviruses, can also cause liver injury. All of the hepatotropic viruses are ribonucleic acid (RNA) viruses except hepatitis B virus (HBV), which has a deoxyribonucleic acid (DNA) genome.

Hepatitis A virus (HAV) is a nonenveloped, single-stranded RNA virus classified in the Piconaviridae family and in the *Hepatovirus* genus. It is stable at moderate temperature and low pH, allowing the virus to survive in the environment and be transmitted by the fecal-oral route. Hepatitis E virus (HEV) belongs to the genus *Hepevirus* in the Hepeviridae family and has four genotypes. HEV1 and HEV2 are restricted to human beings and are

transmitted via contaminated water in developing countries. HEV1 occurs mainly in Asia, whereas HEV2 occurs in Africa and Mexico. HEV3 and HEV4 infect human beings, pigs, and other mammalian species and are responsible for sporadic cases of autochthonous hepatitis E in both developing and developed countries. HEV3 has a worldwide distribution. HEV4 mostly occurs in Southeast Asia.

HBV is a small DNA virus that belongs to the Hepadnaviridae family. Approximately 350 million persons are carriers of HBV worldwide; of these, 75% reside in Asia and the Western Pacific. Hepatitis C virus (HCV) is a single-stranded positive-sense RNA virus that belongs to the Flaviviridae family and has been classified as the sole member of the genus *Hepacivirus*. More than 170 million people are infected with HCV worldwide. HBV has eight genotypes (labeled A through H), and HCV has six genotypes (1 through 6). Both HBV and HCV viruses are transmitted parenterally. HBV is present in virtually all body fluids and excreta of carriers. Transmission occurs most commonly through blood and blood products, contaminated needles, and sexual contact. Historically, HCV was the main cause of post-transfusion hepatitis before 1992. It is currently the most common cause of hepatitis among intravenous drug users. The Centers for Disease Control and Prevention now recommends one-time screening of persons born between 1945 and 1965 for hepatitis C because of the high prevalence of the disease in this birth cohort.

Hepatitis D virus (HDV) is classified in a separate genus of the Deltaviridae family. It is a small, defective RNA virus that can propagate only in an individual who has coexistent HBV infection, either after simultaneous transmission of the two viruses or via superinfection of an established HBV carrier. HDV has at

TABLE 41-1	CHARACTERISTICS OF ACUTE VIRAL HEPATITIDES				
	HEPATITIS A	**HEPATITIS B**	**HEPATITIS C**	**HEPATITIS D**	**HEPATITIS E**
Causative agent	27-28 nm RNA virus Nonenveloped	42 nm DNA virus Enveloped	55-65 nm RNA virus Enveloped	36-43 nm RNA virus Enveloped	27-34 nm RNA virus Nonenveloped
Transmission	Fecal-oral	Blood borne, sexual, percutaneous, perinatal	Similar to HBV; vertical and sexual route uncommon	Similar to HBV	Similar to HAV; transfusion; vertical transmission
Incubation period (days)	15-50	30-180	14-180	Similar to HBV	15-60
Onset	Acute	Acute, insidious	Insidious	Acute, insidious	Acute, insidious
Fulminant disease (%)	0.01-0.5	1	<0.1	5-20	1-2
Chronic hepatitis	No	Yes	Yes	Yes/No	Yes/No
Treatment	Supportive	Nucleos(t)ide analogues; IFN-α	IFN-α + ribavirin ± DAA(s)	IFN-α	Supportive; ribavirin
Prophylaxis	Hygiene; immune globulin, vaccine	Similar to HAV	Hygiene	Hygiene, HBV vaccine	Hygiene, vaccine

DAA, Direct-acting antiviral; HAV, hepatitis A virus; HBV, hepatitis B virus; IFN-α, interferon-α.

least eight genotypes, four of which (genotypes 5 through 8) seem to be of exclusively African origin. Of the 350 million chronic carriers of HBV worldwide, more than 15 million have serologic evidence of exposure to HDV. Like HBV, HDV is transmitted via the parenteral route through exposure to infected blood or body fluids. Because there is evidence for sexual transmission, people with high-risk sexual activity are at increased risk for infection.

Clinical and Laboratory Manifestations

Acute viral hepatitis typically begins with a prodromal phase lasting several days that is characterized by constitutional and gastrointestinal symptoms including malaise, fatigue, anorexia, nausea, vomiting, myalgia, and headache. A mild fever may be present. Clinical manifestations of hepatitis A depend on the age of the host: fewer than 30% of infected young children showed symptomatic hepatitis, whereas about 80% of infected adults had severe acute hepatitis with remarkably elevated serum aminotransferases. Arthritis and urticaria resembling serum sickness, attributed to immune complex deposition, are present in 5% to 10% of cases of acute hepatitis B and C. Taste and smell alterations may also occur. Jaundice soon appears, with bilirubinuria and acholic (pale) stools, which are often accompanied by an improvement in the patient's sense of well-being. The liver is usually tender and enlarged; splenomegaly is found in about one fifth of patients. Notably, many patients with acute viral hepatitis are asymptomatic or have symptoms without jaundice (anicteric hepatitis). In such instances, medical attention often is not sought.

Alanine aminotransferase (ALT) and aspartate aminotransferase (AST) are released from acutely damaged hepatocytes, and serum levels can rise to 20-fold or more above normal. An elevated serum bilirubin level (>2.5 to 3 mg/dL) results in jaundice and is defined as icteric hepatitis. Values higher than 20 mg/dL are uncommon and correlate in a general way with the severity of disease. Elevations in serum alkaline phosphatase (ALP) are usually limited to 3 times normal levels except in cases of cholestatic hepatitis. A complete blood cell count most commonly shows mild leukopenia with atypical lymphocytes. Anemia and thrombocytopenia may also be present. The icteric phase of acute viral hepatitis may last days to weeks and is followed by gradual resolution of symptoms and laboratory values.

Diagnosis

Acute viral hepatitis can be diagnosed either directly, by detecting the nucleic acids of the infecting virus, or indirectly, by demonstrating an immune response in the host (Tables 41-2 and 41-3). Epstein-Barr virus and cytomegalovirus hepatitis are part of the differential diagnosis and also may be diagnosed by the appearance of specific antibodies of the immunoglobulin M (IgM) class.

In acute hepatitis B, hepatitis B surface antigen (HBsAg) and e antigen (HBeAg) are present in serum. Both are usually cleared within 3 months in acute self-limited infection, but HBsAg may persist in some patients with uncomplicated disease for 6 months to 1 year. Clearance of HBsAg is followed after a variable period by the emergence of antibodies against hepatitis B surface antigen (anti-HBs), which confers long-term immunity. Antibodies against hepatitis B core antigen (anti-HBc) and e antigen (anti-HBe) appear in the acute phase of the illness, but neither provides immunity. Uncommonly, during the serologic window period, anti-HBc IgM, a marker of active viral replication suggesting recent infection, may be the only evidence of HBV infection.

Every patient who is HBsAg positive should be tested for antibodies against HDV (anti-HDV IgG), which persist even after the patient has cleared HDV infection. Active HDV infection is now confirmed by the detection of serum HDV RNA with sensitive real-time polymerase chain reaction (PCR) assays. However, because of the variability of the genome sequence, assays of HDV RNA can produce false-negative results. Testing of anti-HDV IgM antibodies still has a role in patients who test negative for HDV RNA but have clinical features of HDV-related liver disease.

Acute hepatitis C can be detected within 2 weeks after exposure with the use of a sensitive PCR assay for HCV RNA. Serum antibodies to HCV develop within 12 weeks after exposure or

TABLE 41-2   SEROLOGIC MARKERS OF VIRAL HEPATITIS

AGENT	MARKER	DEFINITION	SIGNIFICANCE
HAV	Anti-HAV IgM	IgM antibody to HAV	Marker of acute or recent infection
	Anti-HAV IgG	IgG antibody to HAV	Marker of acute or previous infection; post vaccination; confers protective immunity
HBV	HBsAg	Hepatitis B surface antigen	The presence of HBsAg indicates that the person is infectious.
	HBeAg	Hepatitis B e antigen	Transiently positive in acute infection; may persist in chronic infection; reflection of active viral replication and high infectivity
	Anti-HBs	Antibody to surface antigen	Marker of acute self-limited infection; post vaccination; confers protective immunity
	Anti-HBe	Antibody to e antigen	Transiently positive in convalescence; positive in chronic infection before seroconversion; usually a reflection of low infectivity
	Anti-HBc IgM	IgM antibody to core antigen	Marker of acute or exacerbation of chronic infection
	Anti-HBc IgG	IgG antibody to core antigen	Appears at the onset of symptoms in acute infection and persists for life; not seen in vaccinees without prior infection
HCV	Anti-HCV	Antibody to HCV	Marker of acute and chronic infection; does not provide immunity
HDV	Anti-HDV IgM	IgM antibody to HDV	Positive in acute infection, negative in past infection but persists in a large proportion of patients with chronic infection
	Anti-HDV IgG	IgG antibody to HDV	Positive in all individuals exposed to HDV, and persists long-term, even after viral clearance
HEV	Anti-HEV IgM	IgM antibody to HEV	Marker of acute or recent infection*
	Anti-HEV IgG	IgG antibody to HEV	Marker of chronic or previous infection*

HAV, Hepatitis A virus; HBV, hepatitis B virus; HCV, hepatitis C virus; HDV, hepatitis D virus; HEV, hepatitis E virus; IgG, immunoglobulin G; IgM, immunoglobulin M.
*Serologic testing is unreliable, and seroconversion might never occur in immunosuppressed persons.

TABLE 41-3 INTERPRETATION OF DIAGNOSTIC MARKERS IN HEPATITIS B

	HBsAg	HBeAg	ANTI-HBc IgM	ANTI-HBc IgG	ANTI-HBs	ANTI-HBe	BLOOD HBV DNA
Acute infection	+	+	+	+	−	+/−	High
Acute self-limited infection	−	−	+	+	+	+/−	−
Vaccinated	−	−	−	−	+	−	−
Chronic infection							
HBeAg positive	+	+	−	+	−	−	High
HBeAg negative	+	−	−	+	−	+	Low
Immune escape	+	−	−	+	−	+	High
Occult infection	−	−	−	+	−	+/−	Very low
Reactivation of chronic infection	+	+	+/−	+	−	+/−	High

anti-HBc IgG, Immunoglobulin G antibody against hepatitis B core antigen; anti-HBc IgM, immunoglobulin M antibody against hepatitis B core antigen; anti-HBe, antibody against hepatitis B e antigen; anti-HBs, antibody against hepatitis B surface antigen; HBeAg, hepatitis B e antigen; HBsAg, hepatitis B surface antigen; HBV DNA, hepatitis B virus deoxyribonucleic acid.

within 4 to 5 weeks after biochemical abnormalities are discovered. Importantly, these are not neutralizing antibodies and do not indicate immunity. At onset of symptoms, 30% of patients will be missed if checked by serum enzyme immunoassay (EIA) for HCV antibody alone.

Commercial EIAs for hepatitis E to detect both IgM and IgG class antibodies are also available but may lack sensitivity and specificity. Diagnosis of HEV infection should be established by PCR assays in immunosuppressed patients, because serologic testing is unreliable and seroconversion might never occur.

Complications
Cholestatic Hepatitis

In some patients, most commonly during HAV infection, a prolonged but self-limited period of cholestasis occurs that is characterized by marked conjugated hyperbilirubinemia, elevation of ALP, and pruritus. Further investigation may be required to rule out biliary obstruction (see Chapter 40).

Fulminant Hepatitis

Massive hepatic necrosis occurs in fewer than 1% of patients with acute viral hepatitis; it leads to a devastating and often fatal condition called acute liver failure. This condition is discussed in detail in Chapter 42.

Chronic Hepatitis

Hepatitis A does not progress to chronic liver disease, although occasionally it has a relapsing course. Persistence of elevated levels of ALT and AST, viral antigens, or nucleic acids beyond 6 months in patients with hepatitis B or C suggests evolution to chronic hepatitis, although slowly resolving acute hepatitis may occasionally exhibit such test abnormalities for up to 12 months with eventual complete resolution. About 60% of organ transplant recipients infected with HEV fail to clear the virus and go on to develop chronic hepatitis. Chronic hepatitis is considered in detail later in this chapter.

Rare Complications

Acute viral hepatitis may rarely be followed by aplastic anemia, which tends to affect mostly male patients and results in a mortality rate greater than 80%. Pancreatitis, myocarditis, pericarditis, pleural effusion, and neurologic complications including Guillain-Barré syndrome, aseptic meningitis, and encephalitis have also been reported. Cryoglobulinemia and glomerulonephritis

are associated with hepatitis B and C, and polyarteritis nodosa is associated with hepatitis B. These manifestations are more common in patients who fail to clear acute HBV or HCV and develop chronic hepatitis.

Management

Unless complicated by fulminant hepatitis, cases of acute hepatitis A, B, and E are usually self-limited and are managed by supportive care including rest, maintenance of adequate hydration and dietary intake, and avoidance of alcohol use. Hospitalization may be needed for patients who cannot tolerate oral intake and for those with evidence of deteriorated liver function, such as hepatic encephalopathy or coagulopathy.

In general, hepatitis A and E may be regarded as noninfectious after 3 weeks, whereas hepatitis B is potentially infectious to sexual contacts throughout its course, although the risk is low once HBsAg has been cleared. Studies of antiviral therapy in acute hepatitis B have not shown clear benefit, although some experts advocate the use of nucleos(t)ide analogues, specifically in the setting of acute liver failure due to hepatitis B. Treatment of acute hepatitis C is not fully defined because it is often asymptomatic, although early treatment within 12 weeks of diagnosis with pegylated interferon-α–based therapy induces high sustained virologic response rates (>90%) and in responders may prevent the development of chronic infection.

Prevention

In patients with hepatitis A or E, both feces and blood contain virus during the prodromal and early icteric phases. General hygiene measures should include handwashing by contacts and careful handling, disposal, and sterilization of excreta, contaminated clothing, and utensils. HAV vaccination is appropriate for children older than 12 months of age, travelers to endemic areas, individuals with immunodeficiency or chronic liver disease, and those with high-risk behaviors or occupations. Since 2007, HAV vaccination has been preferred over immunoglobulin for postexposure prophylaxis, based on results from randomized trials. With the availability of two candidate vaccines, one of which is already licensed for use in China, HEV prevention through vaccination is now a realistic possibility.

HBV is rarely transmitted by body fluids other than blood; however, it is highly infectious, and strict adherence to universal precautions is mandatory. Efforts at preventing hepatitis B have involved the use of hepatitis B immunoglobulin (HBIG) and recombinant HBV vaccines. Prophylaxis with HBIG after blood or mucosal exposure should be given within 7 days along with HBV vaccine. Preventive vaccination is currently recommended for high-risk individuals—health care professionals, patients undergoing hemodialysis, patients with chronic liver disease, residents and staff of custodial care institutions, and sexually active homosexual men—and is advocated universally for children.

No accepted prevention strategies other than universal precautions are available for HCV, and serum immunoglobulin is not useful for postexposure prophylaxis. The advent of widespread blood product screening for hepatitis C has made such infection after transfusion a rarity.

Alcoholic Liver Disease

Alcohol abuse continues to be a major cause of liver disease in the Western world. The three major pathologic findings resulting from alcohol abuse are fatty liver, alcoholic hepatitis, and cirrhosis. These findings are not mutually exclusive and may all be present in the same patient. The first two conditions are potentially reversible. Alcoholic cirrhosis is discussed in Chapter 43.

Mechanism of Injury

The mechanisms of liver injury caused by alcohol are complex. Ethanol and its metabolites, acetaldehyde and nicotinamide adenine dinucleotide phosphate, are directly hepatotoxic and cause a large number of metabolic derangements. Induction of cytochrome P-450 (i.e., CYP2E1) and cytokine pathways, particularly tumor necrosis factor-α (TNF-α), are also critical in initiating and perpetuating hepatic injury.

Hepatotoxic effects from alcohol vary considerably among individuals. Nevertheless, consumption by men of 40 to 80 g of alcohol per day for 10 to 15 years carries a substantial risk for the development of alcoholic liver disease. Women appear to have a lower threshold of injury than men. Malnutrition and other forms of chronic liver disease may potentiate the toxic effects of alcohol on the liver. Genetic factors contribute to individual susceptibility as well.

Clinical and Pathologic Features

Alcoholic fatty liver may manifest as incidentally discovered hepatomegaly or elevated aminotransferase levels on screening blood tests. Vague discomfort in the right upper quadrant of the abdomen may be the only symptom. Jaundice is rare, and aminotransferases are only mildly elevated (<5 times normal). Liver biopsy shows either diffuse or centrilobular fat occupying most of the hepatocytes.

Alcoholic hepatitis is much more severe and is characterized on liver biopsy by the histologic triad of Mallory bodies, infiltration by polymorphonuclear leukocytes, and a network of interlobular connective tissue surrounding hepatocytes and central veins (pericellular, perivenular, and perisinusoidal fibrosis). Patients with alcoholic hepatitis may be asymptomatic, or they may be extremely ill with hepatic failure. Other common symptoms are anorexia, nausea, vomiting, weight loss, and abdominal pain. For those with fever, infection needs to be ruled out. Jaundice is commonly present and may be pronounced, with cholestatic features that require differentiation from biliary tract disease (see Chapters 40 and 44). Physical examination may reveal cutaneous signs of chronic liver disease, including spider angiomas and palmar erythema. In addition, gynecomastia, parotid enlargement, testicular atrophy, and loss of body hair may be found. The presence of ascites and hepatic encephalopathy suggests cirrhosis. Aminotransferases are only moderately increased (200-400 U/L) in alcoholic hepatitis compared with other forms of acute hepatitis. The ratio of AST to ALT almost always exceeds 2 : 1, in contrast to viral hepatitis, in which the aminotransferases are usually increased in parallel. The white blood cell count may be strikingly increased.

Diagnosis

A history of excessive and prolonged alcohol intake is frequently difficult to obtain from patients with alcoholic liver disease. However, historical, clinical, and biochemical features of alcoholic hepatitis are often sufficient to establish the diagnosis. Many patients suspected or found to imbibe alcohol excessively may have causes in addition to alcohol contributing to liver disease (e.g., chronic viral hepatitis). Therefore, when other causes of liver disease are suggested and alcohol intake is uncertain, appropriate serologic testing and a liver biopsy may be needed to establish a diagnosis.

Treatment

Complete abstinence from alcohol is the most important step. Meticulous supportive care, including tube feeding for those with severe anorexia, is the cornerstone of treatment for acute alcoholic hepatitis. In the absence of contraindications (i.e., infection, gastrointestinal bleeding, or renal failure), some patients with alcoholic hepatitis may benefit from treatment with corticosteroids. A calculated discriminant function (DF) value greater than 32 (where DF = 4.6 × [prothrombin time (in seconds) − control (in seconds)] + total bilirubin [in mg/dL]) may identify a subgroup of patients who are more likely to benefit from the use of corticosteroids, but these patients have advanced liver disease and a high mortality rate. Pentoxifylline, an oral TNF-α antagonist, was shown to reduce the risk of renal failure but not mortality in a single randomized trial.

Complication and Prognosis

Alcoholic fatty liver disease completely resolves with cessation of alcohol intake. Alcoholic hepatitis can also resolve, but it commonly progresses either to cirrhosis, which may already be present at the time of initial diagnosis, or to hepatic failure and death. The development of encephalopathy, ascites, acute kidney injury, and gastrointestinal bleeding from varices often complicates alcoholic hepatitis (see Chapter 43). Patients with a DF greater than 32 have a high risk of death. The Lille model combines six reproducible variables (age, renal insufficiency, albumin, prothrombin time, bilirubin, and evolution of bilirubin at day 7) and is highly predictive of death at 6 months. A score greater than 0.45 predicts a 6-month survival rate of 25%, compared with 85% survival when the score is less than 0.45.

Drug-Induced Liver Injury

Drug-induced liver injury (DILI), also known as hepatotoxicity, refers to liver injury caused by drugs or other chemical agents and represents a special type of adverse drug reaction. More than

1000 medications and supplements are known to cause hepatotoxicity. Antibiotics remain the drugs most commonly responsible for DILI in the United States and Europe; the annual incidence of antibiotic-associated DILI is 1 in 10,000 to 100,000 individuals.

DILI may be classified by the pattern of liver injury observed. *Acute hepatocellular injury* is characterized by elevated levels of serum ALT and minimal elevations of serum ALP. *Cholestatic injury* is characterized by a disproportionately elevated level of ALP, which is synthesized and released by injured bile ducts. Liver injury that has both hepatocellular and cholestatic features is called *mixed liver injury*. DILI can also be classified into two broad categories, predictable and unpredictable, depending on the hepatotoxins involved. Predictable hepatotoxins, such as acetaminophen and carbon tetrachloride, cause dose-dependent liver injury. Acetaminophen is now the leading cause of life-threatening acute liver failure in the United States and Europe. Unpredictable hepatotoxins cause DILI in a so-called idiosyncratic fashion. Idiosyncratic reactions are difficult to predict and are not dose dependent; they occur relatively rarely in individuals with unique genetic and environmental characteristics.

Clinical and Laboratory Manifestations

DILI symptoms are similar to those associated with viral hepatitis and include malaise, anorexia, nausea and vomiting, right upper quadrant abdominal pain, jaundice, acholic stools, and dark (tea-colored) urine. Patients with cholestatic DILI may also have pruritus. Fever and rash, hallmarks of hypersensitivity, may be present with DILI caused by certain drugs such as anticonvulsants and sulfamethoxazole-trimethoprim. Cholestatic or mixed hepatitis related to amoxicillin-clavulanic acid (Augmentin) may develop shortly after the drug has been stopped, usually within 2 to 3 weeks. Nitrofurantoin (Macrobid) characteristically causes a chronic hepatitis after many weeks, months, or even years of therapy and is often associated with the presence of serum antinuclear antibodies (ANA).

Diagnosis

The diagnosis of DILI is challenging because of the lack of specific or uniform clinical features or laboratory tests in the majority of cases. A high level of suspicion for DILI is essential for diagnosis, as is the exclusion of other possible causes of liver injury. The Russel-Uclaf Causality Assessment Method (RUCAM) provides objective and consistent assessment but can be cumbersome for routine clinical use. Moreover, a recent study conducted by Grant and Rockey suggested that expert opinion outperforms RUCAM in making a diagnosis of DILI. There is definitely a need for a simple, accurate, and reproducible method for diagnosing DILI.

Hepatitis E appears to be a small but important alternative diagnosis for suspected DILI. Of 318 patients in the multicenter U.S. Drug-Induced Liver Injury Network (DILIN) with suspected drug hepatotoxicity, 9 (3%) were found to be positive for HEV IgM.

Treatment

The mainstay of management of DILI is withdrawal of the offending agent and supportive care, which is usually sufficient in cases of mild to moderate DILI. Reexposure to the implicated drug should be avoided. Specific therapies are available for some types of DILI. Timely administration of *N*-acetylcysteine (NAC) for acetaminophen overdose can be lifesaving. NAC may also improve outcomes of patients with early acute liver failure from a variety of other causes. Corticosteroids are probably ineffective for DILI from most drugs; however, a short course of steroids is sometimes used for treatment of immune-mediated DILI with the manifestations of rash, fever, and eosinophilia. Ursodeoxycholic acid is safe and may possibly hasten the resolution of jaundice and pruritus.

Complication and Prognosis

With supportive care and discontinuation of the offending drug, mild to moderate DILI usually resolves rapidly. Cholestatic liver injury may take many weeks and even months to completely resolve. Occasionally, cholestatic DILI can evolve into permanent bile duct injury with so-called vanishing bile duct syndrome. Patients who develop acute liver failure manifesting with hyperbilirubinemia, coagulopathy, and hypoalbuminemia may need liver transplantation.

⬤ CHRONIC HEPATITIS

Chronic hepatitis is defined as a sustained inflammatory process in the liver lasting longer than 6 months. On initial presentation, chronic hepatitis can be difficult to differentiate from acute hepatitis on clinical or histologic criteria alone. Except for hepatitis A, acute viral hepatitis, especially that caused by HBV or HCV, can ultimately lead to chronic hepatitis. Nonalcoholic steatohepatitis (NASH) is now the most frequent cause of chronic hepatitis in the United States and Western Europe. Several drugs can cause chronic hepatitis, the best recognized being methyldopa. In contrast to acute hepatitis, an etiologic agent is sometimes difficult to identify in cases of chronic hepatitis. The pathogenesis of these idiopathic forms may represent quiescent autoimmune disease, undetected past DILI or NASH, antibody-negative viral infection, or misdiagnosed cholestatic liver injury (e.g., primary biliary cirrhosis [PBC], primary sclerosing cholangitis [PSC]).

Chronic Viral Hepatitis

In Western countries, acute HBV infection usually occurs in adults; 5% to 10% of patients fail to clear the virus and develop chronic hepatitis. In other areas, childhood acquisition is common, and children who are infected within 2 years of birth have a much higher rate of chronic hepatitis B. HBV infection without evidence of any liver damage may persist, resulting in asymptomatic hepatitis B carriers. In Asia and Africa, many such carriers appear to have acquired the virus from infected mothers during infancy (vertical transmission).

Patients who are HBsAg and HBeAg positive and have high blood HBV DNA (>20,000 IU/mL), coupled with elevated serum aminotransferases, are in a high replicative phase (see Table 41-3). In contrast, patients in a low replicative phase are HBsAg and anti-HBe positive, have low blood HBV DNA (<20,000 IU/mL), and have near-normal or normal aminotransferase levels. Such patients can enter a high replicative phase and exhibit features of acute or chronic hepatitis B. A subgroup of patients with chronic hepatitis B who are HBeAg negative are still in a high replicative phase, as evidenced by high HBV DNA levels in blood. These patients likely have HBV with precore and/or core promoter mutation. Patients infected with HBV in high replicative phase are at high risk for cirrhosis and hepatocellular carcinoma. Such patients and those who have already progressed to early cirrhosis are the primary candidates for antiviral therapy.

Currently, seven drugs are approved for the treatment of adults with chronic hepatitis B in the United States, including interferon-α and its pegylated form and five nucleos(t)ide analogues (lamivudine, telbivudine, adefovir dipivoxil, tenofovir disoproxil, and entecavir). The primary aim of therapy is to eliminate or permanently suppress HBV and thus reduce the activity of hepatitis and slow or limit the progression of liver disease. It is important to start therapy with a nucleos(t)ide analogue that has a high genetic barrier to resistance, such as entecavir or tenofovir, as first-line therapy. Long-term follow-up studies have shown interferon-based therapy increases HBsAg seroclearance over time. HBsAg seroclearance is less common in patients who are treated with nucleos(t)ide analogues rather than interferon-based therapy.

In patients with HBV and HDV coinfection, the fate of HDV is determined by the host response to HBV, which in more than 95% of adults results in viral clearance. By contrast, HDV superinfection of an individual with chronic hepatitis B usually results in chronic HDV infection. Treatment with nucleos(t)ide analogues is not effective in reducing HDV replication. The accepted practice for treatment of chronic HDV infection is weekly pegylated interferon for at least 48 weeks. In patients with a high concentration of HBV DNA, the addition of a potent nucleos(t)ide analogue to inhibit HBV replication is logical, but long-term effectiveness has yet to be defined.

Chronic hepatitis C develops in up to 75% of individuals who are acutely exposed to HCV. Approximately 1.6% of the United States population (4.1 million people) are positive for antibodies to HCV (anti-HCV), and 3.2 million of them have chronic infection. Up to 20% of HCV cases progress to cirrhosis, usually within 20 years after infection. HCV has six major genotypes, of which genotype 1 is the most common in the United States, followed by genotypes 2 and 3. The genotype determines the treatment regimen and duration of therapy. The goal of antiviral therapy is to achieve an sustained virologic response (SVR), defined as undetectable HCV RNA levels (aviremia) 6 months after treatment discontinuation. As many as 80% of patients with genotype 2 or 3 disease achieve SVR after receiving dual therapy consisting of weekly pegylated interferon-α and daily ribavirin for 24 weeks. In contrast, only about 50% of patients with genotype 1 disease can achieve SVR after receiving the dual therapy for 48 weeks. With the addition of direct-acting antivirals (DAA), especially the first generation NS3/4 protease inhibitors boceprevir and telaprevir (both approved in May 2011), to pegylated interferon and ribavirin, up to 70% of patients with genotype 1 hepatitis C can achieve SVR in 24 weeks. However, the addition of a first-generation DAA to interferon- and ribavirin-based treatment for hepatitis C results in increased potential for side effects, drug-drug interactions, and a high pill burden. With the addition of the once daily, second generation protease inhibitor simeprevir (approved in November 2013) and the NS5B polymerase inhibitor sofosbuvir (approved in December 2013) to pegylated interferon and ribavirin, up to 90% of patients with genotype 1 hepatitis C can achieve SVR in as little as 12 weeks. For the first time, patients with genotype 2 and 3 hepatitis C can be treated with an interferon-free regimen consisting of sofosbuvir and ribavirin. Several new DAAs with novel mechanisms of action—such as NS5B polymerase inhibitors, NS5A inhibitors, and new NS3/4 protease inhibitors—are either under review for approval or under development.

Among organ transplant recipients, the consumption of game meat, pork products, or mussels may result in HEV infection, which is most commonly asymptomatic without jaundice. About 60% of such infections become chronic, and up to 10% of patients progress to cirrhosis. Treatment includes careful reduction in immunosuppression, which results in viral clearance in 30% of patients on ribavirin monotherapy.

Autoimmune Hepatitis

Autoimmune hepatitis (AIH) has several clinical forms that share typical histologic findings including significant hepatic inflammation with a preponderance of plasma cells and fibrosis. Type 1, or classic, AIH is characterized by the presence of hypergammaglobulinemia as well as ANA or anti–smooth muscle antibodies (ASMA). Type 2 AIH is characterized by the presence of anti–liver/kidney microsomal antibodies (anti-LKM1) and the absence of ANA and ASMA. The type 1 variant can affect people of any age or gender, whereas the less common type 2 variant primarily affects girls and young women. A third type of AIH with antibodies to soluble liver antigen or liver-pancreas antigen (anti-SLA/LP) is no longer considered a unique entity because these antibodies may be found in type 1 and 2 variants as well. There are also uncommon overlap variants of AIH that have features of both AIH and other liver diseases such as PBC or PSC.

There are no pathognomonic features of AIH, and the diagnosis is made by a combination of factors. A simplified diagnostic algorithm that includes the presence of autoantibodies, hypergammaglobulinemia, typical liver histology, and absence of viral hepatitis has proved useful in identifying patients with AIH. Extrahepatic manifestations such as amenorrhea, rashes, acne, vasculitis, thyroiditis, and Sjögren's syndrome are common. Evidence of hepatic failure and the presence of chronic disease on liver biopsy are often discernable at the time of diagnosis. Indications for treatment include abnormal liver function tests and significant hepatic inflammation on biopsy.

Corticosteroids are the mainstay of treatment, typically in combination with azathioprine as a steroid-sparing agent. This regimen is efficacious in most patients (>80%) and in many instances prolongs survival.

Nonalcoholic Fatty Liver Disease

Nonalcoholic fatty liver disease (NAFLD) has a spectrum of presentations from simple steatosis, which usually does not progress to advanced liver disease, to NASH, which may exhibit or lead to cirrhosis. It is the most common cause of abnormal liver function tests among adults in the United States and western Europe. NAFLD is commonly seen in people with central obesity, hypertension, diabetes, and hyperlipidemia, although it can be observed in persons with normal weight as well. Insulin resistance plays a central role in the pathophysiology of NAFLD. Estimates indicate that about 30 million Americans have NAFLD; of these, 8.6 million have NASH and almost 20% have signs of advanced disease (i.e., bridging fibrosis, cirrhosis) on histologic examination.

Liver biopsy is the "gold standard" for diagnosis of NASH. The procedure is invasive and costly and can cause complications including a small mortality risk (0.01% to 0.1%). Radiologic imaging studies are neither sensitive nor able to distinguish simple steatosis from steatohepatitis. Noninvasive biomarkers are currently under active investigation. The NAFLD Activity Score has been developed and represents the sum of scores for steatosis, lobular inflammation, and hepatocyte ballooning. It ranges from 0 to 8, with a scores of 5 or higher considered diagnostic of NASH.

Currently, no generally accepted medical treatment is available for NASH. However, weight loss and regular exercise are associated with biochemical and histologic improvement and are important components of therapy. Vitamin E and pioglitazone have recently been shown to improve hepatic inflammation in nondiabetic patients with NASH, but they are not routinely recommended because of questions regarding long-term safety.

Genetic and Metabolic Hepatitis

Hemochromatosis is an autosomal recessive genetic disorder that causes defective sensing of iron stores and leads to excessive absorption of iron from the digestive tract. In the United States, about 5 of every 1000 white people have the condition. Elevated ferritin and transferrin saturation values are typically used to screen patients with evidence of chronic liver disease and guide the need for further genetic testing. Most patients with hemochromatosis are homozygous for the C282Y mutation in the *HFE* gene, and a subset of individuals who are heterozygous for both C282Y and the H63D mutation may also develop iron overload. Iron overload is very uncommon among those who are homozygous for the H63D mutation. Genetic mutations in a number of other proteins involving in iron sensing have also been associated with iron overload but are not routinely tested in clinical practice. Hemochromatosis is a systemic disease that can cause skin discoloration, liver cirrhosis and cancer, heart failure, diabetes mellitus, hypogonadism, and arthralgias due to iron deposition in various organs. A high index of suspicion is required to detect the disorder in early stages. The standard treatment for hemochromatosis is therapeutic phlebotomy. For patients who cannot undergo phlebotomy, chelation therapy may be offered.

Wilson's disease is an autosomal recessive genetic disorder that results from mutations in the *ATP7B* gene located on chromosome 13. These mutations result in excessive accumulation of copper in a number of organs, most notably the liver, cornea, and brain. The prevalence of the disease is approximately 1 in 30,000 live births in most populations. Wilson's disease can occur at any age. Measurement of the 24-hour urine copper excretion, slit lamp examination of corneas for Kayser-Fleischer rings, and direct measurement of hepatic copper confirm the diagnosis. Patients should receive lifelong chelation treatment with either penicillamine or trientine. Zinc may be used to maintain stable copper levels in the body.

α_1-*Antitrypsin deficiency* is an autosomal recessive genetic disorder of chromosome 14 that causes retention of α_1-antitrypsin in the liver, resulting in liver damage. The normal gene product is designated as PiM, and the deficiency variants are PiS (50% to 60%) and PiZ (10% to 20%). The most common carrier phenotypes are PiMS and PiMZ, and the disease phenotypes are PiZZ, PiSS, and PiSZ. A low serum α_1-antitrypsin level and diastase-positive staining of hepatocellular α_1-antitrypsin inclusions on liver biopsy support the diagnosis. Phenotypic testing in the serum has been the traditional gold standard for the diagnosis. However, genotypic testing is now available and widely used. Lung disease results from a loss of protective effects in patients with low levels of circulating α_1-antitrypsin. α_1-Antitrypsin replacement therapy is an option for those with lung disease but is not useful for patients with liver disease.

> *For a deeper discussion on this topic, please see Chapters 148, "Acute Viral Hepatitis," and 149, "Chronic Viral and Autoimmune Hepatitis," in* Goldman-Cecil Medicine, *25th Edition.*

SUGGESTED READINGS

Asselah T, Marcellin P: Interferon free therapy with direct acting antivirals for HCV, Liver Int 33(Suppl 1):93–104, 2013.

Grant LM, Rockey DC: Drug-induced liver injury, Curr Opin Gastrointesterol 28:198–202, 2012.

Hughes SA, Wedemeyer H, Harrison PM: Hepatitis delta virus, Lancet 378:73–85, 2011.

Jeong SH, Lee HS: Hepatitis A: clinical manifestations and management, Intervirology 53:15–19, 2010.

Kamar N, Bendall R, Legrand-Abravanel F, et al: Hepatitis E, Lancet 379:2477–2488, 2012.

Kochar R, Sheikh AM, Fallon MB: Andreoli and Carpenter's Cecil essentials of medicine, ed 8, 2010, Saunders, pp 466–475.

Liaw YF: Impact of therapy on the outcome of chronic hepatitis B, Liver Int 33(Suppl 1):111–115, 2013.

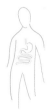

42

Acute Liver Failure

Brendan M. McGuire and Michael B. Fallon

DEFINITIONS

Acute liver failure (ALF) is defined as the onset of encephalopathy within 6 months after the occurrence of jaundice in a patient with hepatic injury but no prior history of liver disease. *ALF* replaces the older term for the same patient population, *fulminant hepatic failure*. Hepatic injury is usually defined as an international normalized ratio (INR) greater than 1.5 times normal with elevations of serum aminotransferases and total bilirubin. Other parameters further define hepatic failure based on the length of time from onset of jaundice to hepatic encephalopathy: *hyperacute hepatic failure* for periods shorter than 7 days, and *late-onset hepatic failure* for periods of 8 to 24 weeks.

PATHOGENESIS

ALF develops as a result of severe, unrelenting hepatocyte necrosis. It is uncommon clinically but represents a medical emergency. ALF may result from infection with hepatitis viruses A, B, C, D, or E (see Chapter 41). Additionally, exposure to hepatotoxins such as acetaminophen, isoniazid, halothane, valproic acid, or mushroom toxins (e.g., those of *Amanita phalloides*) can produce ALF. Reye's syndrome, a disease that predominantly affects children, and acute fatty liver of pregnancy often resemble ALF; they are characterized by microvesicular fatty infiltration and little hepatocellular necrosis. Other rare causes of ALF include Wilson's disease, hepatic ischemia, autoimmune hepatitis, and malignancy (E-Figs. 42-1 and 42-2).

CLINICAL PRESENTATION

The clinical presentation, by definition, includes jaundice and hepatic encephalopathy without clinical evidence of underlying chronic liver disease. Other common but nonspecific symptoms include nausea, vomiting, loss of appetite, right upper abdominal pain from hepatomegaly, fever, fatigue, dark urine, and clay-colored stools. Typically, the features of impaired hepatic synthetic and metabolic function predominate, with portal hypertension much less common than in patients with established cirrhosis.

DIAGNOSIS

The clinical presentation of ALF can be dramatic, with jaundice and advanced systemic manifestations as the first indication of a severe and potentially threatening illness. A complete medical history is essential and should focus on potential exposure to viruses and hepatotoxins, pregnancy, an event associated with hypotension, and clues to suggest autoimmune causes.

Early laboratory testing should focus on assessing the severity of hepatic dysfunction and on detection of possible acetaminophen exposure, for which specific treatment must be initiated in a timely manner. Further specialized laboratory testing is designed to identify particular viral causes—with tests for anti–hepatitis A immunoglobulin M (IgM), hepatitis B surface antigen (HBsAg), anti–hepatitis B core antigen (anti-HBc) IgM, hepatitis D antigen, anti–hepatitis C antibody and/or hepatitis C virus RNA, anti–hepatitis E IgM, anti-varicella IgM, and herpes simplex IgM—or other causes (e.g., pregnancy test in females of child-bearing age, ceruloplasmin level, autoimmune markers).

A negative serum acetaminophen level does not exclude acetaminophen overdose, because the drug is rapidly cleared in the blood. Importantly, acetaminophen overdose accounts for approximately 50% of all cases of ALF and 20% of all cases of presumed indeterminant causes in Western countries. Therefore, careful clinical assessment is essential to determine if an acetaminophen overdose may have occurred.

TREATMENT

Treatment of ALF is largely supportive, because specific treatment for the underlying cause of liver failure is often not available. However, many processes that result in widespread liver cell necrosis and ALF are transient events, and liver cell regeneration with recovery of liver function often occurs if patients survive the initial insult. Acetaminophen toxicity and hypotension with hepatic necrosis are representative. In contrast, ALF resulting from viral hepatitis or idiosyncratic reactions to medications typically has a longer time course and an uncertain prognosis. In either case, meticulous supportive treatment in an intensive care unit setting has been shown to improve survival. Patients with ALF should be treated in centers with experience with this disease and with a liver transplantation program. Numerous complications can result from ALF, and each must be thoroughly identified and treated (Table 42-1). As liver failure progresses, a syndrome of multiorgan failure can result; this can include encephalopathy, coagulopathy, infection, and renal failure in the worst cases.

Hepatic encephalopathy is often the first and most dramatic sign of liver failure. The pathogenesis of hepatic encephalopathy in ALF remains unclear, and it differs from that associated with chronic liver disease or portal hypertension in two important aspects. First, it often responds to therapy only when liver function improves, and second, it is frequently associated with hypoglycemia or cerebral edema, two other potentially treatable causes of coma. Therapy for hepatic encephalopathy in ALF

TABLE 42-1	MANAGEMENT OF SELECTED PROBLEMS IN FULMINANT HEPATIC FAILURE	
COMPLICATION	**PATHOGENESIS**	**MANAGEMENT**
Hepatic encephalopathy	Liver failure	Search for treatable causes (e.g., hypoglycemia, drugs used for sedation, sepsis, gastrointestinal bleeding, electrolyte imbalance, decreased P_{O_2}, increased P_{CO_2}); lactulose
Cerebral edema	Unknown	Elevate head of bed 20-30 degrees; hyperventilate (P_{CO_2}, 25-30 mm Hg); mannitol, 0.5-1 g/kg IV bolus over 5 min; pentobarbital infusion; urgent liver transplantation
Coagulopathy and gastrointestinal hemorrhage	Decreased synthesis of clotting factors Gastric erosions	Vitamin K; fresh-frozen plasma if actively bleeding and for prevention of bleeding; gastric acid suppression
Hypoglycemia	Decreased gluconeogenesis Decreased insulin degradation	IV 10% dextrose, monitor every 2 hr; 30-50% dextrose may be needed
Agitation	May be caused by encephalopathy, intracranial pressure, hypoxemia	Search for treatable causes (e.g., P_{O_2}, skin ulcers, lacerations, abscesses); soft restraints; if severely agitated and injury is a concern, consider sedation along with mechanical ventilation to protect airway
Infection	Liver failure and invasive monitoring	Surveillance cultures and low threshold for empiric antibiotics

P_{CO_2}, Partial pressure of carbon dioxide; P_{O_2}, partial pressure of oxygen.

differs slightly from the principles outlined in Chapter 43. Lactulose may be given orally, through a nasogastric tube, or rectally, but the oral route should not be used if the patient is at risk for aspiration. Lactulose should be discontinued if no improvement is observed after several doses have been administered. Intubation is often necessary to protect the airway from aspiration and to allow ventilation in patients with advanced encephalopathy.

Cerebral edema, the pathogenesis of which is unknown, is a leading cause of death in ALF. Differentiation between cerebral edema and hepatic encephalopathy can be difficult, and computed tomography of the head is often unreliable. Therefore, measurement of the intracranial pressure (ICP) is the standard monitoring tool, although it also can be associated with complications. The goal is to maintain an ICP of less than 20 mm Hg while maintaining a cerebral perfusion pressure (calculated as mean arterial pressure minus ICP) greater than 60 mm Hg. Management includes control of agitation, head elevation of 20 to 30 degrees, hyperventilation, administration of mannitol, barbiturate-induced coma, and urgent liver transplantation.

As hepatic synthetic function deteriorates, *hypoglycemia* can occur as a result of impaired hepatic gluconeogenesis and insulin degradation. All patients at risk should receive 10% glucose IV infusions with frequent monitoring of blood glucose levels. Other metabolic abnormalities commonly occur, including hyponatremia, hypokalemia, respiratory alkalosis, and metabolic acidosis. Therefore, frequent monitoring of blood electrolytes and pH is indicated.

Bleeding occurs frequently and is commonly caused by gastric erosions in the setting of impaired synthesis of clotting factors and prolonged prothrombin times. All patients should receive vitamin K and prophylactic gastric acid suppression. Fresh-frozen plasma should be used if clinically significant bleeding occurs or if major procedures, including ICP monitoring and central line placement, are performed.

Up to 80% of patients with ALF develop infection at some point in their illness; both bacterial (~80% of infections) and fungal (~20% of infections) have been implicated. Patients are at higher risk for infection as a result of impaired immunity resulting from liver failure and the need for invasive monitoring. Severe infection may occur without fever or leukocytosis. Therefore, frequent cultures are recommended, and there should be a low threshold for beginning antibiotic therapy.

Hepatic transplantation (see Chapter 43) has been performed with success in patients with ALF and is the treatment of choice for patients who appear unlikely to recover spontaneously. Because of the urgent need for transplantation, potential candidates should be transferred to transplantation centers before significant complications develop (e.g., coma, cerebral edema, hemorrhage, infection). Transplantation is usually indicated in patients with severe encephalopathy or coagulopathy.

PROGNOSIS

The cause of ALF and the degree of hepatic encephalopathy are important factors in determining prognosis. Patients with ALF resulting from acetaminophen overdose or viral hepatitis A or B have a better survival rate than do patients with Wilson's disease or those without a known cause. The short-term survival rate for patients with ALF in coma is 20% without liver transplantation. The 1-year survival rate of patients with ALF after liver transplantation is 80% to 90%. Patients who survive without transplantation also have an excellent prognosis, because liver tissue usually regenerates normally regardless of the cause of ALF.

SUGGESTED READINGS

Lee WM, Larson AM, Stravitz RT: AASLD position paper: the management of acute liver failure—update 2011. Available at: http://www.aasld.org/practiceguidelines/Documents/AcuteLiverFailureUpdate2011.pdf. Accessed June 23, 2014.

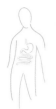

43

Cirrhosis of the Liver and Its Complications

Shaheryar A. Siddiqui and Michael B. Fallon

⬤ LIVER CIRRHOSIS

Definition

Cirrhosis is a slowly progressive disease that is characterized by formation in the liver of fibrous and scar tissue which eventually replaces normal hepatocytes and impairs portal blood flow. Fibrosis can be a self-perpetuating result of many initial processes, including infectious, inflammatory, toxic, metabolic, genetic, and vascular insults that lead to liver damage. Most of the clinical features of cirrhosis develop as a result of portal hypertension, hepatocellular dysfunction, or altered cellular differentiation.

Etiology

Nonalcoholic fatty liver disease (NAFLD), alcoholic liver disease, and hepatitis C virus infection are the most common causes of cirrhosis in industrialized nations; hepatitis B virus is the major cause in Asia and in most of Africa. There are many other significant causes of cirrhosis, including biliary cirrhosis (primary and secondary), autoimmune hepatitis, inherited diseases (e.g., α_1-antitrypsin deficiency), and drug-induced injury, that require specific evaluation. However, a significant number of patients with cirrhosis at presentation have no readily identifiable cause. These cases are referred to as idiopathic or cryptogenic in origin, and it remains a diagnosis of exclusion. Common and uncommon conditions that may lead to cirrhosis are listed in Table 43-1. Chronic active hepatitis, NAFLD, and α_1-antitrypsin deficiency are discussed in Chapter 41.

Pathology

The typical sequence of events that leads to development of cirrhosis involves significant hepatocyte injury followed by ineffective repair that results in hepatic fibrosis. The injury can be acute or chronic in nature, depending on the mechanism. The fibrotic response to injury leads to development of nodules surrounded by fibrous tissue that consist of foci of regenerating hepatocytes, formation of fibrovascular membranes, rearrangement of blood vessels, and finally cirrhosis. This disruption of the normal hepatic lobular architecture distorts the vascular bed and contributes to development of portal hypertension and intrahepatic shunting. On gross morphology, cirrhosis can be referred to as macronodular (>3 mm), commonly seen as a result of chronic active hepatitis, or micronodular (<3 mm) a typical feature of alcoholic cirrhosis or cirrhosis of mixed origin.

Clinical Presentation

Symptoms of liver cirrhosis are often nonspecific in the early stages and include fatigue, malaise, weakness, weight change, anorexia, and nausea. With progression of portal hypertension or loss of hepatocytes, increased abdominal girth, sexual dysfunction, altered mental status, and gastrointestinal bleeding may be noted. Physical findings depend on the stage at presentation. Table 43-2 highlights the pathogenetic mechanisms underlying these diverse signs and symptoms.

Diagnosis

Owing to significant reserves of liver function, patients with cirrhosis are often asymptomatic and the diagnosis is established incidentally at the time of physical examination or laboratory testing. Alternatively, patients abruptly experience specific life-threatening complications of cirrhosis, most notably variceal bleeding, ascites, spontaneous bacterial peritonitis, and hepatic encephalopathy (HE). If cirrhosis is suspected on clinical grounds, the diagnosis can be made reliably by a combination of clinical, laboratory, and radiologic findings in most cases. However, liver biopsy is still considered the "gold standard" for accurate diagnosis. With advances in imaging, biopsy is now done more often to assess the stage and severity of disease, assign prognosis, and monitor the response to treatment.

Laboratory Findings

Hepatocellular dysfunction leads to impaired protein synthesis (hypoalbuminemia), hyperbilirubinemia, low levels of blood urea nitrogen (BUN), and elevated serum ammonia levels. Portal hypertension causes hypersplenism, which results in anemia, thrombocytopenia, and leukopenia. Patients with ascites often develop dilutional hyponatremia as a result of avid renal retention of sodium (Na^+) and water. The liver enzymes alanine aminotransferase (ALT) and aspartate aminotransferase (AST) are good markers of active hepatocyte necrosis, whereas elevations of alkaline phosphatase and bilirubin out of proportion to

TABLE 43-1 COMMON CAUSES OF CIRRHOSIS	
Alcohol abuse	Drug-induced liver injury (DILI)
Nonalcoholic steatohepatitis	Autoimmune hepatitis
Viral hepatitis (chronic hepatitis B, C, and D)	Primary biliary cirrhosis
Cardiac cirrhosis	Hemochromatosis (primary and secondary)
Chronic right-sided heart failure	Wilson's disease
Constrictive pericarditis	α_1-antitrypsin deficiency

TABLE 43-2 CLINICAL FEATURES AND PATHOGENESIS OF CIRRHOSIS

SIGNS AND SYMPTOMS	PATHOGENESIS
CONSTITUTIONAL	
Fatigue, anorexia, malaise, weakness, weight loss	Liver synthetic or metabolic dysfunction
CUTANEOUS	
Spider angiomas, palmar erythema	Altered estrogen and androgen metabolism
Jaundice	Decreased bilirubin excretion
Caput medusae	Porto systemic shunting due to portal hypertension
ENDOCRINE	
Gynecomastia, testicular atrophy, decreased body hair in men	Altered estrogen and androgen metabolism
Decreased libido, virilization, and menstrual irregularities in women	
GASTROINTESTINAL	
Abdominal pain	Hepatomegaly, hepatocellular carcinoma
Abdominal swelling	Ascites due to portal hypertension
Gastrointestinal bleeding	Variceal hemorrhage due to portal hypertension
HEMATOLOGIC	
Anemia, leukopenia, thrombocytopenia	Hypersplenism secondary to portal hypertension
Ecchymosis	Decreased synthesis of coagulation factors
NEUROLOGIC	
Altered sleep pattern, somnolence, confusion, asterixis	Hepatocellular dysfunction: inability to metabolize ammonia to urea

ALT and AST suggest intrahepatic or extrahepatic biliary obstruction.

Radiology

Various radiologic modalities including ultrasound (with and without Doppler imaging of the portal and hepatic venous vasculature), computed tomography, and magnetic resonance imaging have complementary profiles in the evaluation of suspected cirrhosis. Findings supportive of the diagnosis of cirrhosis include relative enlargement of the left hepatic and caudate lobes as a result of right lobe atrophy, surface nodularity, and features of portal hypertension such as ascites, intra-abdominal varices, and splenomegaly.

Transient elastography (Fibroscan) is a newer noninvasive modality that provides an indirect measure of liver fibrosis and cirrhosis by calculating liver stiffness. Abnormal liver stiffness suggests underlying fibrosis; in the presence of clinical and laboratory features of cirrhosis, this finding may obviate the need for diagnostic liver biopsy in some patients. Biopsy is more invasive and is usually reserved for situations in which the results of noninvasive studies are indeterminate or the cause of the liver disease is in doubt.

● COMPLICATION OF CIRRHOSIS

The major sequelae of cirrhosis are illustrated diagrammatically in Figure 43-1 and can be categorized broadly into features of hepatocellular dysfunction and portal hypertension. The pathophysiologic interrelationships among these complications are described in the following sections.

Hepatocellular Dysfunction

The loss of hepatocyte mass that occurs in cirrhosis results in impaired synthesis of many important proteins, which in turn leads to hypoalbuminemia, deficient production of vitamin K–dependent coagulation factors, and diminished capacity for hepatic detoxification (see Chapters 39 and 42 for details). In addition, there is a decline in the capacity for conjugation and excretion of bilirubin.

Portal Hypertension

Under normal circumstances, the portal circulation is a low-pressure system with only small changes in pressure as blood flows from the portal vein, through the liver, and into the inferior vena cava. The hepatic venous pressure gradient (HVPG), which reflects sinusoidal pressure, is the gradient between the wedged hepatic venous pressure and the free hepatic venous pressure measured by direct catheterization. Normal HVPG values range between 3 and 5 mm Hg. In cirrhosis, the distortion of hepatic architecture by fibrous tissue and regenerative nodules, along with an increased intrahepatic vascular tone, leads to increased resistance to portal venous flow and resultant portal hypertension. Portal hypertension is defined as an HPVG greater than 5 mm Hg, and clinically significant complications typically develop at values greater than 10 mm Hg.

Although cirrhosis is the most important cause of portal hypertension, any process that increases resistance to portal blood flow through the presinusoidal, sinusoidal, or hepatic venous outflow tracts may result in portal hypertension (Table 43-3). In addition, cirrhosis is associated with increased cardiac output, which leads to greater splanchnic blood flow, further aggravating portal hypertension. It is important to recognize that the HVPG is reliably increased only in sinusoidal portal hypertension.

With sustained portal hypertension, portosystemic collaterals are formed which have the benefit of decreasing portal pressures at the expense of bypassing the liver. Major sites of collateral formation includes the gastroesophageal junction, retroperitoneum, rectum, and falciform ligament of liver (abdominal and periumbilical collaterals). Clinically, the most important collaterals are those connecting the portal to the azygos vein through the dilated and tortuous vessels (varices) in the submucosa of the gastric fundus and esophagus.

● VARICEAL HEMORRHAGE
Definition and Pathology

Varices are abnormally large veins that are most commonly recognized near the gastroesophageal junction or the stomach wall. Gastroesophageal varices usually develop when the portal pressure gradient (HVPG) exceeds 10 mm Hg, and the risk for variceal rupture increases when the gradient is higher than 12 mm Hg. Bleeding occurs most commonly from large varices in the esophagus when high tension in the walls of these vessels leads to rupture. Among gastric varices, fundal varices have the highest

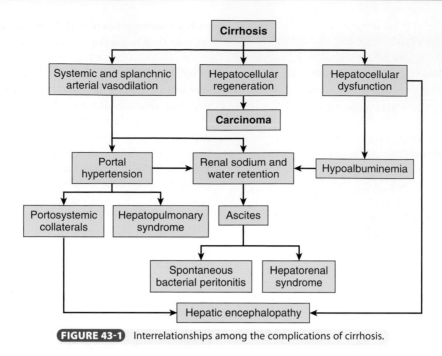

FIGURE 43-1   Interrelationships among the complications of cirrhosis.

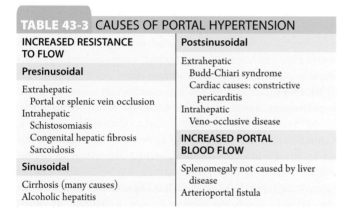

TABLE 43-3 CAUSES OF PORTAL HYPERTENSION	
INCREASED RESISTANCE TO FLOW	**Postsinusoidal**

Presinusoidal	Extrahepatic
	  Budd-Chiari syndrome
	  Cardiac causes: constrictive
	    pericarditis
	Intrahepatic
	  Veno-occlusive disease

Extrahepatic
  Portal or splenic vein occlusion
Intrahepatic
  Schistosomiasis
  Congenital hepatic fibrosis
  Sarcoidosis	

	INCREASED PORTAL BLOOD FLOW
Sinusoidal	Splenomegaly not caused by liver disease Arterioportal fistula
Cirrhosis (many causes) Alcoholic hepatitis	

rate of bleeding and may bleed with portal pressure gradients of less than 12 mm Hg.

Clinical Presentation

Variceal bleeding usually manifests as painless hematemesis, melena, or hematochezia, which typically leads to hemodynamic compromise due to higher portal pressures. Bleeding is further aggravated by impaired hepatic synthesis of coagulation factors and thrombocytopenia from hypersplenism.

Treatment

The management of gastroesophageal varices includes prevention of initial bleeding (primary prophylaxis), treatment of acute variceal hemorrhage, and prevention of rebleeding (secondary prophylaxis) (Fig. 43-2). If varices are large, primary prophylaxis is commonly undertaken with nonselective β-adrenergic receptor blocking (NSBB) agents such as propranolol and nadolol. Carvedilol is a newer NSBB that may improve prevention of initial variceal bleeding. Surveillance for varices using esophagogastroduodenoscopy is advocated on an annual basis in patients with decompensated cirrhosis, every 1 to 2 years in those with compensated cirrhosis, and every 2 to 3 years for cirrhotic

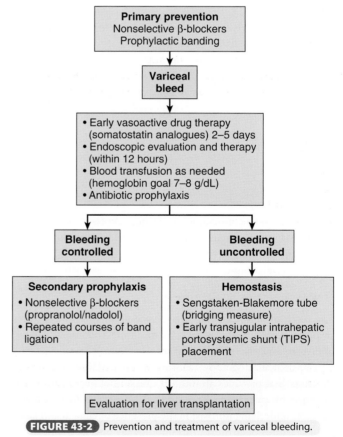

FIGURE 43-2   Prevention and treatment of variceal bleeding.

patients without varices. Periodic endoscopic band ligation (EBL) is also effective if the patient has contraindications or intolerance to β-blockers. Isosorbide mononitrate therapy should not be used for prophylaxis because it has been shown to increase adverse events.

When varices are present, 5% to 15% of patients experience an initial episode of bleeding annually, and this episode carries a significant mortality risk of 7% to 15% at 6 weeks. Management includes stabilization (airway, breathing, and circulation) and blood transfusions to maintain a hemoglobin level of 7 to 8 g/dL. Combined pharmacologic and endoscopic therapy is the current standard for control of bleeding and is superior to either therapy alone. Prophylactic intravenous antibiotics should be administered early because they reduce the risk for infection, rebleeding, and death.

Current pharmacologic therapy consists of octreotide, a somatostatin analogue, which is widely used because of a good safety profile. This agent is best instituted before endoscopic examination. Endoscopic therapy includes EBL or sclerotherapy or both. EBL is the preferred modality given the lower incidence of adverse effects and complications. In patients with gastric variceal hemorrhage, endoscopic variceal ablation with cyanoacrylate glue is superior to EBL, although this therapy is not approved in the United States. Balloon tamponade (Sengstaken-Blakemore tube, Linton tube, or Minnesota tube) is a temporary measure reserved only for cases in which endoscopic therapy has failed in the setting of massive hemorrhage. In these patients, there is evidence that early placement of a transjugular intrahepatic portosystemic shunt (TIPS) for active variceal bleeding improves survival. The most common side effect of the TIPS is postprocedural encephalopathy.

Recommendations for secondary prophylaxis to prevent rebleeding include a combination of nonselective β-blockers (propranolol and nadolol) and variceal obliteration through repeated courses of EBL. In patients who undergo TIPS, the patency must be assessed using Doppler ultrasound on a regular basis.

Prognosis

Overall, the frequency and mortality rates from variceal bleeding appear to be decreasing in the United States over the past 2 decades. However, variceal hemorrhage is life-threatening, and after an initial episode the risk of rebleeding approaches 60% with a mortality rate of approximately 33% if secondary prophylaxis is not instituted.

⬤ ASCITES
Definition and Pathology

Ascites represents the accumulation of excess fluid in the peritoneal cavity. Although cirrhosis is the most common cause of ascites, there are also other important causes (Table 43-4). The precise sequence of events leading to the development of cirrhotic ascites remains debated. The *overflow* theory suggests that portal hypertension and splanchnic vasodilation result in excess renal sodium and water retention and overflow of fluid into the peritoneum. The *underflow* theory suggests that decreased effective circulating blood volume resulting from systemic arterial vasodilation leads to activation of neurohumoral systems and results in sodium and water retention. In any case, avid renal Na^+ retention is characteristic and results in an increase in total body Na^+ and water.

Diagnosis

Physical examination is relatively insensitive for detection of small volumes of ascites, but bulging flanks, shifting dullness, and evidence of portal hypertension (e.g., distended veins over the abdominal wall and caput) become evident with increasing amounts of fluid. Abdominal ultrasound is both sensitive and specific and is widely used in screening. When fluid is present, abdominal paracentesis is the quickest and most direct approach for confirmation of the presence of fluid in the abdominal cavity and initial characterization of the cause. In addition to standard measures such as cell count, the serum-ascites albumin gradient (SAAG), which is proportional to the sinusoidal portal pressure, is calculated as follows:

$$SAAG = (\text{Serum albumin concentration}) - (\text{Ascitic fluid albumin concentration}).$$

An elevated SAAG (>1.1 g/dL) correlates well with portal hypertension as the likely cause of fluid accumulation (see Table 43-4).

Clinical Presentation

Patients usually report increasing abdominal girth, fullness of the flanks, and weight gain with or without peripheral edema. Ascites becomes clinically detectable with fluid accumulation greater than about 500 mL. Shifting dullness to percussion is the most sensitive clinical sign of ascites, but about 1500 mL of fluid must be present for reliable detection.

Treatment

Management of cirrhotic ascites depends on the cause. Patients with high SAAG (>1.1 g/mL), which is used as a surrogate measure for elevated portal pressures, usually respond to salt restriction (<2 g/day) and diuretics to stimulate renal Na^+ loss. The administration of spironolactone, an aldosterone antagonist, supplemented with a loop diuretic (e.g., furosemide), is effective in about 90% of patients. Diuresis should be monitored closely because aggressive diuretic therapy may result in electrolyte disturbances (e.g., hyponatremia, hypokalemia) and hypovolemia, leading to impaired renal function and potentially precipitating HE. Water restriction is implemented when the serum sodium concentration is less than 120 to 125 mEq/L.

Prognosis

Refractory ascites occurs in up to 10% of patients with cirrhosis and is defined as the persistence of tense ascites despite maximal diuretic therapy (spironolactone, 400 mg/day, and furosemide, 160 mg/day) or the development of azotemia or electrolyte disturbances at submaximal doses of diuretics. Treatment includes repeated large-volume paracentesis and colloid volume

TABLE 43-4	CLASSIFICATION OF ASCITES	
SAAG HIGH (>1.1 g/dL)	**SAAG LOW (<1.1 g/dL)**
Cirrhosis	Peritoneal carcinomatosis
Alcoholic hepatitis	Peritoneal tuberculosis
Chronic hepatic congestion	Pancreatic and biliary disease
Right ventricular heart failure	Nephrotic syndrome
Budd-Chiari syndrome	
Constrictive pericarditis	
Massive liver metastases	
Myxedema	
Mixed ascites	

SAAG, Serum-ascites albumin gradient.

expansion with albumin (6 to 8 g/L of fluid removed), TIPS placement in appropriate candidates, and eventually liver transplantation (Fig. 43-3). Peritoneovenous shunts are not commonly used and are reserved for patients who are not candidates for paracentesis, TIPS, or transplantation.

SPONTANEOUS BACTERIAL PERITONITIS

Definition and Pathology

Cirrhotic patients may develop infection of ascitic fluid in the absence of an obvious source of contamination or surgically treatable source, a condition known as acute spontaneous bacterial peritonitis (SBP). The exact mechanism of contamination of the ascitic fluid is unclear. Factors such as bacterial overgrowth, altered motility, and increased intestinal permeability may contribute. The microbiology of SBP includes most commonly *Escherichia coli* and Enterobacteriaceae *(Klebsiella)*. Gram-positive organisms such as *Streptococcus* (viridans), *Enterococcus*, and *Pneumococcus* species may also be found. Anaerobes are uncommon, and a single organism is isolated on culture in most cases; the presence of multiple organisms suggests bowel perforation or other causes of peritonitis.

Clinical Presentation

Clinical features include fever, abdominal pain, and signs of peritoneal irritation. Often, the infection is clinically silent or manifests with worsening of HE, diarrhea, ileus, or renal insufficiency.

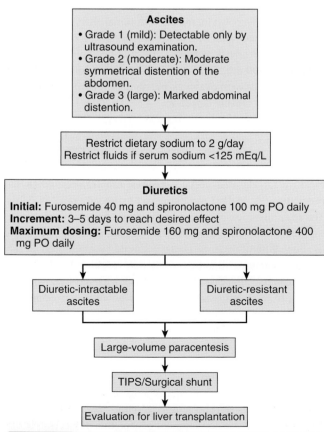

FIGURE 43-3 Management of ascites in cirrhosis. TIPS, Transjugular intrahepatic portosystemic shunt.

Diagnosis

Diagnostic paracentesis should be considered in any patient with cirrhotic ascites who deteriorates clinically. The diagnosis of SBP is highly likely if a high concentration (>250 cells/mm^3) of polymorphonuclear leukocytes (PMNs) is present in the ascitic fluid, and this finding should prompt empiric therapy while blood and ascitic fluid culture results are pending. The use of rapid bedside diagnostic methods such as leukocyte esterase reagent strips is not routinely recommended in view of their low sensitivity.

Treatment

Patients are usually treated with intravenous third-generation cephalosporin (e.g., cefotaxime, 2 g every 8 hours); quinolones are also routinely used, provided that the patient does not have prior exposure and is not in overt shock. Response to treatment is usually seen within 72 hours; therapy is continued for a minimum of 5 days and can extend up to 14 days. Repeat peritoneal fluid analysis may be done if recovery is delayed or to ensure that the ascitic fluid is sterile after treatment. The administration of intravenous albumin on day 1 (1.5 g/kg) and day 3 (1g/kg) has been shown to decrease the incidence of renal dysfunction and to improve short-term survival in SBP.

Prognosis

There is a high rate of recurrence, up to 70% within 1 year, and the 1-year mortality rate with a prior episode of SBP is 50% to 70%. Long-term antibiotic prophylaxis is indicated to reduce the recurrence rate to approximately 20%. Short-term prophylaxis should be considered for patients with cirrhosis and ascites who are hospitalized with upper gastrointestinal bleeding. Common prophylactic regimens for SBP include fluoroquinolones (ciprofloxacin, 750 mg/week; norfloxacin, 400 mg/day) and trimethoprim-sulfamethoxazole (1 double-strength tablet daily). Long-term antibiotic prophylaxis can lead to infection with resistant extended-spectrum β-lactamase (ESBL)-producing organisms or methicillin-resistant *Staphylococcus aureus* (MRSA).

HEPATORENAL SYNDROME

Definition and Pathology

Hepatorenal syndrome (HRS) is a form of functional renal failure that occurs in the presence of significant hepatic synthetic dysfunction and ascites. Three mechanisms of kidney dysfunction have been proposed: splanchnic arterial vasodilation, renal arterial vasoconstriction, and cardiac dysfunction.

Clinical Presentation and Diagnosis

Patients with HRS typically have advanced ascites and other manifestations of cirrhosis but are not otherwise symptomatic. However, some patients may notice decreased urine output or signs of encephalopathy. There is no single laboratory or imaging study that can be used alone to diagnose HRS. However, the 5-year probability of developing HRS in patients with cirrhosis and ascites is 40%, and HRS develops in approximately 30% of cirrhotic patients who are admitted with SBP. Therefore, a high clinical suspicion is warranted along with a systematic approach to diagnosis based on fulfillment of certain criteria.

The diagnostic criteria for HRS as defined by the International Ascites Club Consensus Workshop in 2007 include the following:

1. Cirrhosis with ascites
2. Serum creatinine level higher than 1.5 mg/dL (133 μmol/L)
3. Lack of improvement in the serum creatinine level (to ≤1.5 mg/dL or ≤133 μmol/L) after at least 2 days of diuretic withdrawal and volume expansion with albumin (1 g/kg of body weight per day, up to a maximum of 100 g/day)
4. Absence of shock
5. Lack of current or recent treatment with nephrotoxic drugs
6. Absence of parenchymal kidney disease as indicated by proteinuria of more than 500 mg/day, microhematuria (>50 red blood cells per high-power field), or abnormal renal ultrasonographic findings.

HRS has two types, type 1 and type 2. HRS type 1 is characterized by rapid deterioration of kidney function with doubling of the initial creatinine to greater than 2.5 mg/dL within 2 weeks or less. HRS type 2 produces a more moderate renal failure that is slowly progressive.

An Acute Kidney Injury Network criterion redefines acute renal failure and is generally recognized by criticare specialists and nephrologists. This criterion divides kidney injury into three stages. Stage I is defined as an increase in serum creatinine of more than or equal to 0.3 mg/dL (≥26.4 μmol/L) or urine output of less than 0.5 mL/kg/hour for longer than 6 hours. Stage II is an increase in serum creatinine of more than 2 to 3 folds from baseline or urine output of less than 0.5 mL/kg/hour for longer than 12 hours. Finally stage III is a rise in serum creatinine of more than 3 fold from baseline or serum creatinine of more than or equal to 4.0 mg/dL. This can also be characterized by either oliguria (output <0.3 ml/kg/hour) for 24 hours or anuria for 12 hours. The key is to detect renal failure early and start appropriate therapy promptly in order to prevent progression.

Typically, the kidneys are histologically normal and can regain normal function in the event of recovery of liver function (e.g., after liver transplantation). Severe cortical vasoconstriction has been demonstrated angiographically, and such vasoconstriction reverses when these kidneys are transplanted into patients who do not have cirrhosis.

Treatment and Prognosis

The mortality rate is high in HRS, and so prevention is important. In all patients with cirrhosis, precipitating factors (e.g., diuretics, lactulose, nonsteroidal anti-inflammatory drugs, angiotensin-converting enzyme inhibitors) should be avoided if possible. Patients should be promptly diagnosed and treated for any signs of SBP, and colloid (albumin) should be administered if rising creatinine levels are observed. Prevention of variceal bleeding should also be optimized by primary and secondary prophylaxis.

Studies have shown an increased mortality rate with AKI among hospitalized cirrhotic patients. Several medical therapies are currently under review, including use of terlipressin, a vasopressin V_1 receptor analogue, in combination with albumin for type 1 HRS. Other studies have evaluated the combination of octreotide and midodrine (an α-adrenergic agonist) and intravenous albumin. Placement of TIPS has also been reported to stabilize or even improve renal function, mainly in patients with type 2 HRS. However, a significant limitation of TIPS is the possibility of worsening hepatic function in decompensated cirrhosis. Liver transplantation has become the accepted treatment for HRS because it is the only known therapeutic intervention that reverses the process. It is limited by rapid progression of HRS and lack of available organs.

HEPATIC ENCEPHALOPATHY

Definition

HE is a complex, reversible neuropsychiatric syndrome that occurs in patients with chronic liver disease, portal hypertension, or portosystemic shunting. HE is also seen in patients with acute liver failure. HE develops in about 30% to 45% of cirrhotic patients, and when it is present, the survival probability is approximately 23% at 3 years.

Pathophysiology

The pathogenesis of HE in the setting of cirrhosis is thought to be multifactorial and may differ in acute and chronic liver disease. Contributors include the inadequate hepatic removal of potential endogenous neurotoxins, altered permeability of the blood-brain barrier, and abnormal neurotransmission. Elevation of blood ammonia levels, derived from both amino acid deamination and bacterial hydrolysis of nitrogenous compounds in the gut, has been the best studied factor, but its specific role in the pathogenesis of HE remains uncertain. Many other potential contributors to HE have been investigated, including increased tone of the inhibitory GABAA/benzodiazepine neurotransmitter system, activation of the astrocytic 18-kDa translocator protein (PTBR), production of endogenous benzodiazepine-like compounds, altered cerebral metabolism, zinc deficiency, increase in serotonin levels, up regulation of H1 receptors, altered melatonin production, and deposition of manganese in the basal ganglia.

Clinical Presentation

The clinical features of HE include disturbances of higher neurologic function such as intellectual and personality disorders, dementia, inability to copy simple diagrams (constructional apraxia), disturbance of consciousness, disturbances of neuromuscular function (asterixis, hyperreflexia, myoclonus), and, rarely, a Parkinson-like syndrome and progressive paraplegia. One of the earliest manifestations of overt HE is alteration of the normal sleep-wake cycle

Diagnosis

There is no laboratory or imaging study that allows a specific diagnosis of HE. Rather, it is a clinical syndrome. Blood levels of ammonia are commonly measured, but elevated levels are neither sensitive nor specific for HE. Neuropsychometric and neurocognitive tests such as the Portosystemic Encephalopathy Syndrome Test (PSET) and the earlier Stroop Color-Word Test evaluate the patient's attention, concentration, fine motor skills, and orientation and have been shown to be highly specific for the diagnosis of HE, but they are reasonably labor intensive. Imaging modalities such as magnetic resonance spectroscopy are being used experimentally to assess HE; however, their clinical utility has not been ascertained. It is imperative that reversible causes of neurologic dysfunction, such as hypoglycemia, subdural hematoma, meningitis, and drug overdose, be considered and excluded early in the differential diagnosis of altered mental status in patients with cirrhosis.

Classification of Hepatic Encephalopathy

There are three major types of HE: type A (Acute), which is associated with acute liver failure; type B (Bypass), which is associated with portosystemic shunts in the absence of liver disease; and type C (Cirrhosis), which is associated with liver cirrhosis and is subdivided into episodic, persistent, and minimal types.

HE has been further graded based on the West Haven Criteria from 0 to 4. A new nomenclature, termed the Spectrum of Neurocognitive Impairment in Cirrhosis (SONIC) classification, has been proposed to improve recognition of earlier forms of HE that require specialized testing for detection and to facilitate research studies. Patients are divided into those who are unimpaired, those with covert HE, and those with overt HE (Table 43-5).

Treatment

Treatment of HE starts with identifying and addressing any precipitating factors (Table 43-6), reducing and eliminating substrates for the generation of nitrogenous compounds, and preventing ammonia absorption from the bowel. Protein restriction was considered to be important in preventing excess ammonia production in the past; however, studies have demonstrated that dietary restriction of protein is not of significant benefit. Short-term protein restriction may be considered for patients with severe encephalopathy, but long-term restriction is associated with worsening malnutrition. Treatment with formulas rich in branched-chain amino acids has shown no benefit in improving encephalopathy or mortality.

Nonabsorbable disaccharides (e.g., lactulose) are the mainstay treatment of HE. These agents are fermented to organic acids by colonic bacteria, processes that lower stool pH and trap NH_4^+ in the colon, thereby decreasing absorption. In addition, the cathartic effect of lactulose eliminates ammonia and other nitrogenous compounds. Patients are usually directed to achieve two to three soft stools per day as the goal of lactulose therapy. Reduction and elimination of nitrogenous compound substrates can also be achieved by administering enemas and using nonabsorbable antibiotics such as rifaximin in patients who do not tolerate or respond to lactulose. Rifaximin (Xifaxin), 550 mg PO twice daily, is approved by the U.S. Food and Drug Administration for the treatment of HE and has a favorable side effect profile; however, cost is the limiting factor. Other agents that affect intestinal motility and ammonia generation are being evaluated, including acarbose and probiotics.

TABLE 43-6   HEPATIC ENCEPHALOPATHY: PRECIPITATING FACTORS

Gastrointestinal bleeding
Increased dietary protein
Constipation
Infection
Central nervous system depressant drugs (benzodiazepines, opiates, tricyclic antidepressants)
Deterioration in hepatic function
Hypokalemia: most often induced by diuretics
Azotemia: most often induced by diuretics
Alkalosis: most often induced by diuretics
Hypovolemia: most often induced by diuretics

TABLE 43-5   CLINICAL STAGES OF HEPATIC ENCEPHALOPATHY AS DEFINED BY THE WEST HAVEN CRITERIA AND THE PROPOSED SONIC CLASSIFICATION

	WEST HAVEN CRITERIA		SONIC			
Grade	Intellectual Function	Neuromuscular Function	Classification	Mental Status	Special Tests	Asterixis
0	Normal	Normal	Unimpaired	Not impaired	Normal	Absent
Minimal	Normal examination findings. Subtle changes in work or driving	Minor abnormalities of visual perception or on psychometric or number tests	Covert HE	Not impaired	Abnormal	Absent
1	Personality changes, attention deficits, irritability, depressed state	Tremor and incoordination				
2	Changes in sleep-wake cycle, lethargy, mood and behavioral changes, cognitive dysfunction	Asterixis, ataxic gait, speech abnormalities (slow and slurred)	Overt HE	Impaired	Abnormal	Present (absent in coma)
3	Altered level of consciousness (somnolence), confusion, disorientation, and amnesia	Muscular rigidity, nystagmus, clonus, Babinski sign, hyporeflexia				
4	Stupor and coma	Oculocephalic reflex, unresponsiveness to noxious stimuli				

Modified from Nevah MI, Fallon MB: Hepatic encephalopathy, hepatorenal syndrome, hepatopulmonary syndrome, and systemic complications of liver disease. In Feldman M, Friedman LS, Brandt LJ, editors: Sleisenger and Fordtran's gastrointestinal and liver disease, ed 9, Philadelphia, 2010, Saunders.
   SONIC, Spectrum of Neuro-Cognitive Impairment in Cirrhosis.

HEPATOPULMONARY SYNDROME AND PORTOPULMONARY HYPERTENSION

The effects of cirrhosis and portal hypertension on the pulmonary circulation manifest as two distinct disorders, hepatopulmonary syndrome (HPS) and portopulmonary hypertension (PoPH).

Hepatopulmonary Syndrome

HPS occurs in 5% to 30% of patients with cirrhosis and is a progressive disease. It is characterized by gas exchange abnormalities (increased alveolar-arterial gradient and hypoxemia) resulting from intrapulmonary vascular dilation. The vascular dilation leads to vascular remodeling and angiogenesis, resulting in impaired oxygen transfer from the alveoli to the central stream of red blood cells within capillaries. Usually, this functional intrapulmonary right-to-left shunt significantly improves with the administration of 100% oxygen. HPS also has been reported in cases of hepatic venous outflow obstruction without cirrhosis.

Diagnosis

HPS is diagnosed based on high clinical suspicion and measurement of a widened alveolar-arterial oxygen gradient on room air in the presence or absence of hypoxemia. The gradient is calculated by analyzing arterial blood gases. HPS is graded from mild, in which the arterial partial pressure of oxygen (PaO_2) is greater than 80 mm Hg) to very severe (PaO_2 <50 mm Hg). Intrapulmonary shunting is demonstrated by contrast echocardiography, in which agitated saline is injected into a peripheral vein during the performance of two-dimensional echocardiography. Delayed appearance of microbubbles in the left cardiac chambers (more than three to six cardiac cycles after injection) indicates intrapulmonary vasodilation. Early visualization of microbubbles in the left cardiac chambers indicates intracardiac shunting. Other tests, including chest radiography, computed tomography, and pulmonary function tests, are performed to exclude intrinsic cardiopulmonary disorders.

Clinical Presentation

Clinical features range from subclinical abnormalities in gas exchange to profound hypoxemia causing significant dyspnea. Classically in HPS, the dyspnea is worse on standing and improves when the patient lies down (orthodeoxia and platypnea, respectively). Patients may also have marked nocturnal hypoxemia.

Screening and Treatment

Screening by pulse oximetry typically targets patients with values lower than 96% at rest on room air for further evaluation. However, no generally accepted guidelines exist. Currently, there is no established medical therapy for HPS. Liver transplantation remains the only option and reverses HPS in most patients. The use of TIPS to treat HPS is not established.

Prognosis

HPS carries a mortality rate of up to 40% in 2.5 years.

PORTOPULMONARY HYPERTENSION

PoPH is defined as the presence of pulmonary arterial hypertension in the setting of portal hypertension.

Diagnosis and Pathology

The diagnosis of PoPH is based entirely on results of right heart catheterization. The diagnostic values include a mean pulmonary arterial pressure greater than 25 mm Hg at rest or 30 mm Hg with exercise, a pulmonary capillary wedge pressure lower than 15 mm Hg, and a pulmonary vascular resistance greater than 240 dynes, all in the presence of portal hypertension or liver disease or both. PoPH is graded according to the mean pulmonary artery pressure, from mild (>25 to 35 mm Hg) to moderate (35 to 50 mm Hg) to severe (>50 mm Hg). Patients with mild PoPH do not appear to have increased operative risk. Moderate PoPH carries a high intraoperative risk and should be medically managed before transplantation. Severe PoPH is generally considered a contraindication to surgery. The exact mechanisms of PoPH are poorly understood. Histologically, it has characteristics similar to those of pulmonary hypertension.

Clinical Presentation

The most common symptom of PoPH is dyspnea on exertion, but many cirrhotic patients with PoPH are asymptomatic.

Treatment

In addition to symptomatic treatment (oxygen for dyspnea and diuretics for volume overload), the medical management of PoPH is similar to that for pulmonary arterial hypertension. Small studies have shown benefit for the use of intravenous vasodilator (prostacyclin) therapy, oral treatments including phosphodiesterase inhibitors, and endothelin receptor antagonist.

If moderate PoPH responds to therapy, liver transplantation may be considered. However, it has not been established whether successful liver transplantation reliably reverses PoPH. Liver transplantation is contraindicated in severe PoPH because of high transplant-related morbidity and mortality.

Prognosis

Untreated PoPH carries high rates of morbidity and mortality; the mean survival time from diagnosis is 15 months. A study on the U.S.-based Registry to Evaluate Early and Long-term Pulmonary Arterial Hypertension Disease Management (REVEAL) showed a 5-year survival rate of 40% from the time of diagnosis in patients with PoPH.

HEPATOCELLULAR CARCINOMA
Epidemiology

Liver cancer is the fifth most common cancer in men and the seventh most common in women worldwide; HCC is the most common type of liver cancer. In the United States, approximately 90% of liver cancers are HCC, and cholangiocarcinomas account for most of the rest. In other areas of the world, including sub-Saharan Africa, China, Japan, and Southeast Asia, HCC is one of the most frequent malignancies and is an important cause of mortality, particularly among middle-aged men.

Etiology

HCC often arises from a cirrhotic liver, and it is closely associated with chronic viral hepatitis. Hepatitis B virus DNA has been shown to integrate into the host cell genome, where it may disrupt tumor suppressor genes and activate oncogenes. In areas of high prevalence, vaccination to prevent infection with hepatitis B virus has reduced the incidence of HCC. The exact pathophysiologic mechanisms leading to tumorogenesis in patients with other causes of cirrhosis (e.g., hemochromatosis, alcohol, hepatitis C viral infection) remain poorly understood. Risk factors for the development of HCC and its clinical manifestations are listed in (Table 43-7).

Diagnosis

Table 43-8 lists currently used imaging techniques for detection of HCC and the most common findings. A tissue specimen may be necessary to confirm the diagnosis in some cases, but it is not needed if characteristic clinical and radiologic features are present, especially if they are accompanied by a rise in serum α-fetoprotein levels. Diagnosis of small, treatable tumors is possible with intensive screening programs that employ imaging studies, although the long-term outcomes and cost-effectiveness of these strategies remain unclear.

Staging

Although many staging systems for HCC are in use, the Barcelona Clinic Liver Cancer (BCLC) system is most commonly used.

TABLE 43-7 HEPATOCELLULAR CARCINOMA

ASSOCIATIONS	
Chronic hepatitis B infection	Jaundice
Chronic hepatitis C infection	Hepatic or portal vein obstruction
Hemochromatosis (with cirrhosis)	Metabolic effects
Cirrhosis (alcoholic, cryptogenic)	Erythrocytosis
Aflatoxin ingestion, Thorotrast exposure	Hypercalcemia
α_1-Antitrypsin deficiency	Hypercholesterolemia
Androgen administration	Hypoglycemia
	Gynecomastia
COMMON CLINICAL PRESENTATIONS	Feminization
	Acquired porphyria
Abdominal pain	**CLINICAL AND LABORATORY FINDINGS**
Abdominal mass	
Weight loss	Hepatic bruit or friction rub
Deterioration of liver function	Serum α-fetoprotein >400 ng/mL
UNUSUAL MANIFESTATIONS	
Bloody ascites	
Tumor emboli (lung)	

TABLE 43-8 IMAGING CHARACTERISTICS OF HEPATOCELLULAR CARCINOMA

ULTRASONOGRAPHY

Mass lesion with varying echogenicity but usually hypoechoic

DYNAMIC COMPUTED TOMOGRAPHY

Arterial phase: tumor enhances quickly
Venous phase: quick de-enhancement of tumor relative to parenchyma

MAGNETIC RESONANCE IMAGING

T1-weighted images: hypointense
T2-weighted images: hyperintense
After gadolinium administration, tumor increases in intensity

Treatment

Patients with well-compensated cirrhosis may undergo surgical resection or liver transplantation, with a 5-year survival rate of up to 70%. Nonsurgical options include percutaneous ethanol injection, transarterial chemoembolization (TACE), and radiofrequency ablation. Sorafenib (a receptor tyrosine kinase angiogenesis inhibitor) has been approved for use in patients with unresectable HCC and has been shown to prolong survival in such patients.

Prognosis

In patients with widespread, multifocal disease and in those with vascular invasion, the prognosis is poor, with a 5-year survival rate of 5% to 6%. Accordingly, emphasis is placed on prevention of viral hepatitis and other causes of liver disease and on screening by ultrasound of those who are at higher risk, including patients with known cirrhosis.

⬤ VASCULAR DISEASE OF THE LIVER

Disorders of the hepatic vasculature are uncommon and include portal vein thrombosis (PVT), hepatic vein thrombosis (Budd-Chiari syndrome), and veno-occlusive disease. Affected patients usually have portal hypertension with or without associated liver dysfunction, which may mimic the presentation of cirrhosis.

Portal Vein Thrombosis

Definition and Etiology

Thrombosis of the portal vein may develop after blunt abdominal trauma, umbilical vein infection, neonatal sepsis, intra-abdominal inflammatory diseases (e.g., pancreatitis), or hypercoagulable states, and in association with cirrhosis. Myeloproliferative diseases (including polycythemia vera, essential thrombocytosis, and myelofibrosis) are now being recognized as possible causes of PVT. One study observed that as many as 25% to 65% of patients with splanchnic vein thrombosis in the absence of cirrhosis had a myeloproliferative disease. The Janus kinase 2 (JAK2) mutation is a marker for myeloproliferative disease and is often checked in patients with PVT. The disease produces the manifestations of portal hypertension, but the liver histology is usually normal.

Diagnosis

The diagnosis is established by angiography, but noninvasive imaging modalities such as Doppler ultrasonography, computed tomography, and magnetic resonance imaging may reveal thrombus, collateral circulation near the porta hepatis, and splenomegaly. In long-standing PVT, tortuous venous channels develop within the organized clot, leading to cavernous transformation.

Treatment

In acute PVT, thrombolysis may be attempted, but anticoagulation with warfarin remains the mainstay of therapy. In most patients, recanalization of the thrombus occurs within 6 months after initiation of anticoagulation. Recommendations for duration of anticoagulation after an acute event vary and are usually

3 to 6 months. Long-term anticoagulation may be used in cases of chronic thrombosis, especially when associated with hypercoagulable states.

Concern exists that anticoagulation may precipitate hemorrhage from varices that arise as a consequence of portal hypertension; however, studies have not shown an increased risk for variceal bleeding in anticoagulated patients with chronic PVT. In fact, recent studies suggest a role for prophylactic anticoagulation (Enoxaparin) for prevention of PVT and hepatic decompensation in cirrhosis. If variceal hemorrhage occurs; it is best managed with endoscopic obliteration. Prophylaxis with β-blockers to prevent variceal bleeding may decrease the portal pressure, potentially propagating thrombus, and therefore is not usually recommended. If endoscopic treatment fails, surgical management with portosystemic shunting may be attempted, but this approach is often difficult because of the absence of suitable patent vessels.

Budd-Chiari Syndrome

Definition and Etiology

Occlusion of the major hepatic veins or the inferior vena cava, especially in the intrahepatic and suprahepatic segments, causes Budd-Chiari syndrome. Most cases are associated with hematologic disease (e.g., polycythemia vera, paroxysmal nocturnal hemoglobinuria, essential thrombocytosis, other myeloproliferative disorders), pregnancy, oral contraceptive use, tumors (especially HCC), or other causes of a hypercoagulable state (e.g., factor V Leiden mutation, protein C and S deficiency). Abdominal trauma and congenital webs of the vena cava are also related to Budd-Chiari syndrome. About 20% of cases are idiopathic, but many of these patients prove to have early, subclinical myeloproliferative disease or genetic mutations associated with a hypercoagulable state.

Clinical Presentation

Budd-Chiari syndrome can manifest acutely, possibly in association with acute liver failure, or it can manifest as a subacute or chronic illness. Acute disease produces right upper quadrant abdominal pain, hepatomegaly, ascites, and jaundice, whereas the subacute or chronic form produces primarily portal hypertension. Elevation of serum bilirubin and transaminase levels may be mild, but liver function is often poor, with profound hypoalbuminemia and coagulopathy.

Diagnosis

The diagnosis can be established noninvasively with Doppler ultrasonography, which shows decreased or absent hepatic vein blood flow, and computed tomography, which shows delayed or absent contrast filling of the hepatic veins and hypertrophy of the caudate lobe. Magnetic resonance angiography may also demonstrate these findings. Hepatic venography is especially useful if the results noninvasive imaging are inconclusive. Venography often shows an inability to catheterize and visualize the hepatic veins; the characteristic spiderweb pattern of collateral vessels may also be demonstrated, and the inferior vena cava may appear compressed owing to hepatomegaly or an enlarged caudate lobe. On liver biopsy, centrilobular congestion, hemorrhage, and necrosis (nutmeg liver) are seen, with cirrhosis developing in patients with chronic obstruction.

Treatment

Treatment should be individualized and is dependent on the mode and severity of presentation and the potential cause of the disease. Supportive therapy to relieve ascites and edema (e.g., dietary sodium restriction, diuretics) and chronic anticoagulation may be considered for patients with chronic Budd-Chiari syndrome in whom methods to decompress congestion are not feasible. Thrombolysis followed by anticoagulation is most useful in patients with acute forms of the disease. In selected patients (such as those with venous webs or strictures or single-vessel thrombosis), angioplasty with or without stent placement may be used. Decompressive modalities are most useful before the development of cirrhosis and include transjugular intrahepatic portacaval and side-to-side portacaval shunts. In patients with cirrhosis, liver transplantation followed by continued anticoagulation is often considered the best option.

Veno-Occlusive Disease

Definition and Etiology

Hepatic veno-occlusive disease, also called sinusoidal obstruction syndrome, often occurs after cytoreductive therapy and before bone marrow transplantation but may also follow exposure to other drugs or herbal preparations (e.g., azathioprine, pyrrolizidine alkaloids). Endothelial cell injury leads to obstruction at the level of the hepatic venules and the sinusoids.

Clinical Presentation

The disease is characterized by jaundice, painful hepatomegaly, and fluid retention. Clinical manifestations can be rapidly progressive and lead to multiorgan dysfunction and death in 20% to 25% of patients.

Diagnosis

The diagnosis is clinically suspected when weight gain, epigastric or right upper quadrant abdominal pain, and jaundice develop within the first 3 to 4 weeks after bone marrow transplantation. Laboratory abnormalities include hyperbilirubinemia, elevated transaminases, and, in severe cases, profound synthetic dysfunction. Doppler abdominal ultrasonography may reveal ascites, reversal of portal vein flow, and an elevated hepatic artery resistance index. Liver biopsy is diagnostic and is usually obtained with use of the transjugular approach. The advantages of this approach compared with the percutaneous route include the ability to measure the hepatic venous pressure gradient (which is typically elevated in veno-occlusive disease) and a lower incidence of bleeding.

Treatment

Mild forms of the disease may favorably respond to supportive therapy alone. In moderate to severe disease, treatment has been attempted with tissue plasminogen activator and heparin, antithrombin III, prostaglandin E_1, and glutamine plus vitamin E, although the efficacies of these treatments have not been clearly established. Recently, defibrotide (a mixture of porcine-derived single-stranded phosphodiester oligonucleotides) has been evaluated as a potential treatment option for severe veno-occlusive disease. It is an attractive option because of the lack of severe adverse effects, although convincing evidence for efficacy has not been established.

● LIVER TRANSPLANTATION

MELD Score

The Model for End-stage Liver Disease (MELD) score is calculated based on the serum creatinine concentration, prothrombin time (International Normalized Ratio), and bilirubin level and has been used to predict short-term mortality in cirrhosis and to prioritize patients awaiting liver transplantation. The MELD score ranges from 6 to 40. Higher scores are associated with more advanced disease and increased predicted mortality. Patients are typically considered for liver transplantation when the MELD score reaches 15. The average MELD score nationally at which patients undergo transplantation is 20.

Prognosis

Liver transplantation is a highly successful procedure in patients with progressive, advanced, and otherwise untreatable liver disease. Advances in surgical techniques and supportive care, the use of cyclosporine and tacrolimus for immunosuppression, and careful selection of patients have all contributed to the excellent results of liver transplantation. Between 70% and 80% of patients undergoing liver transplantation survive at least 5 years, usually with good quality of life. The most common indication for liver transplantation in the United States is chronic liver disease resulting from hepatitis C virus infection. Other liver diseases for which transplantation is commonly performed include cirrhosis from alcoholic liver disease, NAFLD, autoimmune hepatitis, primary biliary cirrhosis, and primary sclerosing cholangitis. Patients with hepatitis B are candidates for liver transplantation if they can be given hepatitis B immunoglobulin or nucleoside analogues to help prevent recurrence. Excellent results have also been obtained in selected patients with acute liver failure (see Chapter 42). Liver transplantation for malignant hepatobiliary disease has been less successful because of recurrent disease in the transplanted liver.

> For a deeper discussion on this topic, please see Chapter 153, "Cirrhosis and Its Sequelae," in Goldman-Cecil Medicine, 25th Edition.

SUGGESTED READINGS

Arroyo V: Acute kidney injury (AKI) in cirrhosis: should we change current definition and diagnostic criteria of renal failure in cirrhosis? J Hepatol 59:415–417, 2013.

Garcia-Tsao G, Bosch J: Management of varices and variceal hemorrhage in cirrhosis, N Engl J Med 362:823–832, 2010.

Kamath PS, Kim W: The model for end-stage liver disease (MELD), Hepatology 45:797–805, 2007.

Krowka MJ, Miller DP, Barst RJ, et al: Portopulmonary hypertension: a report from the US-based REVEAL registry, Chest 141:906–915, 2012.

Mehta RL, Kellum JA, Shah SV, et al: Acute Kidney Injury Network: report of an initiative to improve outcomes in acute kidney injury, Crit Care 11(2):R31, 2007.

O'Brien J, Triantos C, Burroughs AK: Management of varices in patients with cirrhosis, Nat Rev Gastroenterol Hepatol 10:402–412, 2013.

Rimola A, Garcia-Tsao G, Navasa M, et al: Diagnosis, treatment and prophylaxis of spontaneous bacterial peritonitis: a consensus document, J Hepatol 32(1): 142–153, 2000.

Runyon BA: Management of adult patients with ascites due to cirrhosis: an update, Hepatology 49:2087–2107, 2009.

Tsien CD, Rabie R, Wong F: Acute kidney injury in decompensated cirrhosis, Gut 62:131–137, 2013.

Valla DC: Thrombosis and anticoagulation in liver disease, Hepatology 47:1384–1393, 2008.

Villa E, Cammà C, Marietta M, et al: Enoxaparin prevents portal vein thrombosis and liver decompensation in patients with advanced cirrhosis, Gastroenterology 143:1253–1260, 2012.

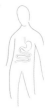

44

Disorders of the Gallbladder and Biliary Tract

Matthew P. Spinn and Michael B. Fallon

INTRODUCTION

The gallbladder and biliary tract transport bile from the liver into the intestines, a process central to digestion of fat and absorption of lipids and fat-soluble vitamins. Gallbladder and biliary tract diseases are among the most common and costly of all digestive disorders. This chapter examines the principal gallbladder and biliary tract disorders, focusing on cholelithiasis. The reader is referred to Chapter 40 for a detailed discussion of bilirubin metabolism and the diagnostic approach to jaundice and to Chapter 34 for a review of the various imaging techniques used to study the biliary tract.

NORMAL BILIARY ANATOMY AND PHYSIOLOGY

Figure 44-1 outlines the basic anatomy of the liver and biliary tract. The liver produces 500 to 1500 mL of bile per day. The secretory product of individual hepatocytes contains bile acids, phospholipids, and cholesterol, which are transported across the apical membrane and into the canalicular space between cells. These canaliculi merge to form larger intrahepatic bile ducts and then the common hepatic duct. During fasting, tonic contractions of the sphincter of Oddi, located in the region of the ampulla of Vater, divert about one half of the bile through the cystic duct into the gallbladder, where it is stored and concentrated by water resorption. Cholecystokinin, which is released after food enters the small intestine, causes the sphincter of Oddi to relax, allowing delivery of a timed bolus of bile into the intestine. Bile acids are present in millimolar concentrations. They are detergent molecules that possess both fat-soluble and water-soluble moieties. Cholesterol is secreted by the liver to the intestine, where it undergoes fecal excretion (see E-Fig. 40-1 in Chapter 40). In the intestinal lumen, bile acids solubilize dietary fat and promote its digestion and absorption. Bile acids are, for the most part, efficiently reabsorbed by the small intestinal mucosa, particularly in the terminal ileum. They are then recycled to the liver for re-excretion, a process termed *enterohepatic circulation*.

GALLBLADDER DISORDERS

Gallstones (Cholelithiasis)

Gallstone formation constitutes a significant health problem, affecting 10% to 15% of the adult population. Complications from gallstones are a leading cause for hospital admissions related to gastrointestinal problems. In the United States, gallstone disease leads to more than 750,000 cholecystectomies annually, making this the most common elective abdominal surgery, with estimated costs of $6.5 billion per year. Gallstones are of two types: 75% are made of cholesterol, and 25% are pigmented stones (black or brown). The latter are composed of calcium bilirubinate and other calcium salts. The risk factors for cholelithiasis are shown in Table 44-1.

Pathogenesis of Cholelithiasis

The three main factors that lead to cholesterol gallstone formation are cholesterol supersaturation of bile, nucleation, and gallbladder hypomotility. The liver is the most important organ in regulating total-body cholesterol stores. Once it is secreted, cholesterol, which is insoluble in water, is solubilized in bile through the formation of mixed micelles with bile acids and phospholipids. In most individuals, there is more cholesterol in bile than can be maintained in stable solution. As bile becomes supersaturated, microscopic cholesterol molecules aggregate into coalescent vesicles that crystallize, a process referred to as *nucleation*. The gradual deposition of additional layers of cholesterol leads to the appearance of macroscopic stones. Factors that influence nucleation include bile transit time, gallbladder contraction, bile composition (concentrations of cholesterol, phospholipids, and bile salts), and presence of bacteria, mucin, and glycoproteins, which can act as a nidus to initiate cholesterol crystal formation. The interplay between *pronucleating* and *antinucleating* factors in the gallbladder may determine whether cholesterol gallstones will form from supersaturated bile. Gallbladder sludge is a superconcentrated mixture of bile acids, bilirubin, cholesterol, mucus, and proteins that exhibits various degrees of fluidity and is prone to precipitate into a semisolid or solid form.

The pathophysiologic factors leading to pigment stone formation are less well understood; however, increased production of bilirubin conjugates (hemolytic states), increased biliary calcium (Ca^{2+}) and bicarbonate (HCO_3^-) levels, cirrhosis, and bacterial deconjugation of bilirubin to a less soluble form are all associated with pigment stone formation. Black pigment stones, which are composed primarily of calcium bilirubinate, are formed in sterile bile in the gallbladder and are common in chronic hemolytic states, in cases of cirrhosis, and in patients with ileal resection. Their brown pigment counterparts, composed primarily of calcium salts, are formed in the bile ducts and are seen in the setting of infection of the biliary tract.

Many of the recognized predisposing factors for cholelithiasis and gallbladder sludge can be understood in terms of the pathophysiologic scheme outlined previously:

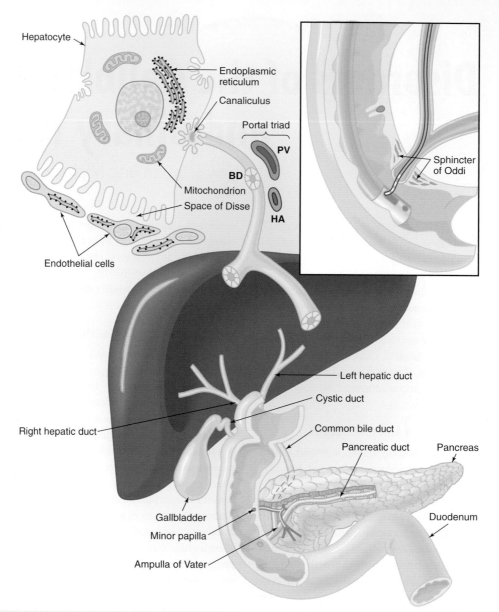

FIGURE 44-1 Normal anatomy and histology of the liver and biliary tract. Materials destined for metabolism or excretion by the liver (such as unconjugated bilirubin) enter the sinusoidal bed and cross the endothelial barrier and the space of Disse. Unconjugated bilirubin is taken up by the hepatocyte, conjugated with glucuronide to become water soluble, and excreted into bile across the canalicular membrane of the hepatocyte. The canaliculi empty into bile ductules (BD), which lead to the interlobular (small), septal (medium), and large intrahepatic bile ducts and finally to the main branches of the common bile duct. The portal areas, or portal triads, are composed mainly of portal vein (PV), hepatic artery (HA), and BD branches. During fasting, tonic contraction of the sphincter of Oddi, located in the region of the ampulla of Vater, diverts about one half of the bile through the cystic duct into the gallbladder, where it is stored and concentrated to be released later during meal times. Disease at any level of the biliary tree can lead to cholestasis and obstructive jaundice.

1. Biliary cholesterol saturation is increased by estrogens, multiparity, oral contraceptives, obesity, rapid weight loss, and terminal ileal disease, which decreases the bile acid pool.

2. Nucleation is enhanced by biliary parasites, recurrent bacterial infection of the biliary tract, and antibiotics such as ceftriaxone, which has a proclivity to concentrate and crystallize with calcium in the biliary tree. Total parenteral nutrition and blood transfusions also promote bile pigment accumulation and *gelfaction* of sludge.

3. Bile stasis is caused by gallbladder hypomotility (resulting from pregnancy, somatostatin, or fasting), bile duct stric-

tures, choledochal cysts, biliary parasites, and total parenteral nutrition.

Clinical Manifestations of Gallstones

Gallstones develop at some point in 10% to 20% of Americans. Between 50% and 60% of these individuals remain asymptomatic, but about one third develop biliary colic or chronic cholecystitis, and 15% develop acute complications. The natural history of gallstone disease is outlined in Figure 44-2. Obstruction of the biliary tract at any level by stones or sludge is the underlying cause of the clinical manifestations of gallstone disease. Obstruction by gallstones can occur at the level of the

TABLE 44-1	RISK FACTORS FOR CHOLELITHIASIS	

PRIMARY	Pregnancy
Age	Diabetes mellitus
Obesity	Low socioeconomic status
Female sex	Sedentary lifestyle
Rapid weight loss	Total parenteral nutrition
Ethnic background (e.g., Native	Hemolysis
American)	Cirrhosis
SECONDARY	Crohn's disease
	Biliary parasites (e.g., *Clonorchis*
Drugs: oral contraceptives,	*sinensis*)
ceftriaxone, octreotide, thiazide	Terminal ileum resection
diuretics	

TABLE 44-2	DIFFERENTIAL DIAGNOSIS OF CHOLELITHIASIS	

Peptic ulcer disease	Nephrolithiasis
Gastroesophageal reflux disease	Pyelonephritis
Nonulcer dyspepsia	Perinephric abscess
Irritable bowel syndrome	Pneumonia
Sphincter of Oddi dysfunction	Angina pectoris
Hepatitis and perihepatitis	Pancreatitis
(Fitz-Hugh–Curtis syndrome)	Ruptured ectopic pregnancy
Hepatic abscess	Appendicitis

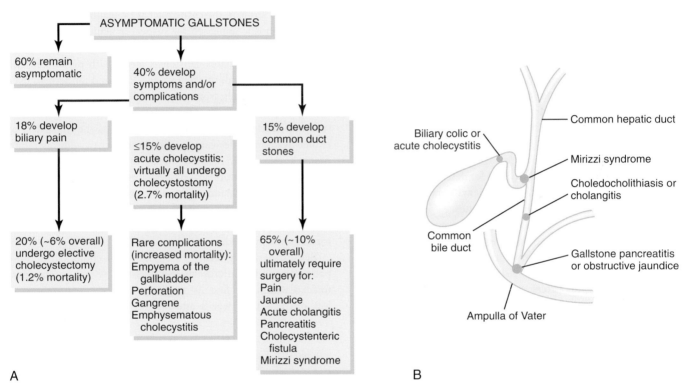

FIGURE 44-2 Natural history of asymptomatic gallstones. **A,** The clinical syndromes associated with gallstones are shown, and the numbers represent the approximate percentage of adults who develop one or more of these symptoms or complications over a 15- to 20-year period. Over this period, about 30% of individuals with gallstones undergo surgery. (The risk for developing complications of gallstones varies considerably among series. The figures shown represent those derived from more recent studies.) **B,** Clinical manifestations of symptomatic gallstones. Locations of blockages associated with various conditions are indicated.

cystic duct, common hepatic duct, common bile duct, or ampulla of Vater (see Figs. 44-1 and 44-2). Symptoms arise from contraction of the gallbladder during transient obstruction of the cystic duct by gallstones, and persistent obstruction of the cystic duct leads to superimposed inflammation or infection of the gallbladder (i.e., acute cholecystitis). Obstruction of the distal common bile duct may result in abdominal pain, cholangitis (infection of the biliary tract), or pancreatitis (resulting from pancreatic duct obstruction). The presence of a large stone in the cystic duct can cause common bile duct obstruction and is referred to as *Mirizzi syndrome*. Common conditions to consider in the differential diagnosis of gallstone disease are listed in Table 44-2.

Asymptomatic Gallstones

Most gallstones are clinically "silent," and they are often uncovered as an incidental finding during abdominal ultrasound performed for another reason. The risk of developing symptoms is low, averaging 2% to 3% per year, 10% at 5 years, and 1% to 2% per year with major complications. Expectant management is an appropriate choice for the general population. Prophylactic cholecystectomy should be considered in those groups who are at increased risk for the development of complications, including (1) patients with diabetes, who have a greater morbidity and mortality from acute cholecystitis; (2) patients with a calcified (porcelain) gallbladder, large gallbladder polyps, or large stones (>3 cm), which are associated with an increased risk for gallbladder carcinoma; (3) patients with sickle cell anemia, in whom hepatic crises may be difficult to differentiate from acute cholecystitis; (4) children with gallstones, because they frequently develop symptomatic disease; and (5) Native Americans, who are predisposed to gallbladder cancer in the setting of gallstones.

Symptomatic Gallstones and Biliary Colic

Symptomatic cholelithiasis is defined by gallbladder pain in the presence of gallstones. *Biliary colic* refers to the constellation of symptoms experienced when the gallbladder contracts against outlet obstruction. Classically, biliary colic starts as a steady ache in the epigastrium or right upper quadrant; it has a sudden onset, reaches a plateau of intensity over a few minutes, and then subsides gradually over 30 minutes to several hours. Referred pain may be felt at the tip of the scapula or right shoulder. Nausea and vomiting may occur, but fever and a palpable mass (signs of acute cholecystitis) are not evident. Other symptoms, such as dyspepsia, fatty food intolerance, bloating and flatulence, heartburn, and belching, may occur in patients with gallstones; however, these symptoms are nonspecific and frequently occur in individuals with normal gallbladders.

Gallstones are best demonstrated by transabdominal ultrasonography, which has become the initial test to evaluate cholelithiasis. The sensitivity and specificity of ultrasound are greater than 90%, but accuracy drops to 20% for visualization of stones within the common bile duct. This limitation has been overcome by endoscopic ultrasonography (EUS) (Video 44-1) and magnetic resonance cholangiopancreatography (MRCP), both of which have an accuracy of 90% to 95% for detecting cholelithiasis and common bile duct stones. Oral cholecystography is no longer used for the routine evaluation of gallstones.

If gallbladder removal is indicated, laparoscopic cholecystectomy has replaced open cholecystectomy as the treatment of choice for recurrent biliary pain. Open cholecystectomy is typically reserved for selected high-risk patients (e.g., prior abdominal surgery with adhesions, obesity, cirrhosis). Laparoscopic cholecystectomy may be accompanied by intraoperative endoscopic retrograde cholangiopancreatography (ERCP) (see Fig. 44-1 and Chapter 34) or transoperative radiologic examination of the common bile duct if concomitant choledocholithiasis is suspected. Factors that may predict the presence of choledocholithiasis include jaundice, pancreatitis, abnormal liver test results, and bile duct dilation.

Cholecystectomy relieves biliary pain in virtually all patients with gallstone disease and prevents the development of future complications. Dissolution of cholesterol gallstones by orally administered chenodeoxycholic acid or ursodeoxycholic acid is successful in highly selected patients but is slow and costly and requires lifelong administration. Alternative methods to eliminate gallstones, including contact dissolution and fragmentation of stones, are used rarely.

Acute Cholecystitis

Acute cholecystitis refers to distention, edema, ischemia, inflammation, and secondary infection of the gallbladder. This typically results from obstruction of the cystic duct by gallstones or, less commonly, from gallbladder cancer or sludge. The clinical hallmark of acute cholecystitis is the acute onset of upper abdominal pain that lasts for several hours. The pain gradually increases in severity and typically localizes to the epigastrium or right hypochondrium with radiation to the right lumbar, scapular, and shoulder area. Nausea and vomiting, anorexia, and low-grade fever are common. Unlike biliary pain, the pain of acute

cholecystitis does not subside spontaneously. The findings on physical examination in patients with acute cholecystitis may include inspiratory arrest on palpation of the right upper quadrant (Murphy's sign), fever, and, less commonly, mild jaundice or a palpable gallbladder.

Complications of acute cholecystitis include emphysematous cholecystitis (in people with diabetes, older adults, and individuals who are immunosuppressed), empyema, gangrene, and perforation of the gallbladder. Gallbladder perforation may occur directly into the peritoneum ("free") or through a cholecystenteric fistula with gallstone migration and bowel obstruction (gallstone ileus). Mirizzi syndrome is the occurrence of profound jaundice resulting from extrinsic compression of the bile duct by an impacted stone in the cystic duct at the gallbladder neck.

The diagnostic approach for suspected acute cholecystitis is similar to that for biliary pain. A transabdominal ultrasound study that demonstrates gallstones, along with pericholecystic fluid, gallbladder wall thickening, and localized tenderness over the gallbladder (ultrasonographic Murphy's sign), provides strong supportive evidence for acute cholecystitis. Ultrasound is safe and widely available and has emerged as the initial test of choice. Radionuclide scanning after intravenous administration of technetium-99m–labeled diisopropyl iminodiacetic acid (DISIDA) or hepatobiliary iminodiacetic acid (HIDA) is also accurate. If the gallbladder fills with the isotope, acute cholecystitis is highly unlikely; if contrast material enters the bile duct and duodenum without gallbladder visualization, acute cholecystitis is strongly supported.

Because of the high risk for recurrent acute cholecystitis, most patients need to undergo cholecystectomy, which is often performed within the first 24 to 48 hours after presentation or, less often, 4 to 8 weeks after an acute episode (Fig. 44-3).

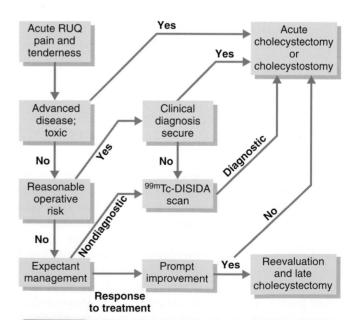

FIGURE 44-3 Algorithm for management of right upper quadrant (RUQ) pain and tenderness in patients with suspected acute cholecystitis. This scheme is based on a policy of early operation (conventional or laparoscopic) for appropriate patients and use of cholecystostomy (operative or percutaneous) for patients who are poor operative risks. 99mTc-DISIDA, Technetium-99m–labeled diisopropyl iminodiacetic acid.

Cholecystostomy may be performed for patients who have a high operative risk. Antibiotics are typically used when fever or leukocytosis is present. Expectant management is reserved for patients with uncomplicated disease who are not good operative candidates and those in whom the diagnosis is not clear.

Acalculous Cholecystitis

Acalculous cholecystitis is an acute inflammatory condition in patients without gallstones. It accounts for approximately 5% of all cases of acute cholecystitis and carries higher morbidity and mortality rates than acute calculous cholecystitis. Acalculous cholecystitis is classically associated with the triad of prolonged fasting, immobility, and hemodynamic instability; such as may occur in critically ill patients, especially if they have required total parenteral nutrition or blood transfusions. Gallbladder ischemia and stasis are considered important in the pathogenesis. It is also seen in patients with AIDS, often in association with cytomegalovirus or *Cryptosporidia* infection. Abdominal pain, fever, and leukocytosis in a patient with the classic triad along with ultrasonographic features of a thickened gallbladder wall and a positive Murphy's sign in the absence of gallstones raises suspicion for this entity. As in acute cholecystitis, the gallbladder is not visualized on HIDA scanning. Management includes administration of antibiotics and cholecystectomy. If the patient is seriously ill, the gallbladder can be drained percutaneously as a temporizing measure.

Chronic Cholecystitis

Chronic cholecystitis is a term used by pathologists to describe chronic inflammatory cell infiltration of the gallbladder on histopathology. Chronic cholecystitis is thought to be an evolving inflammatory process, caused by repeated episodes of low-grade gallbladder obstruction over a period of days to years resulting in recurrent mucosal trauma and inflammation. The symptoms are those of biliary colic without clinical features of acute cholecystitis. Gallstones are the causative agent in most patients. However, there is little correlation between the number of gallstones and the degree of gallbladder wall inflammation. In approximately 12% of patients with chronic cholecystitis, there are no demonstrable stones. The diagnosis is made in a patient with gallstones who has the clinical signs and symptoms with no other obvious cause. Transabdominal ultrasound is the best initial test, and EUS may be used to demonstrate microlithiasis (gallstones ≤3 mm) if gallstones are not seen on initial imaging. The treatment is laparoscopic cholecystectomy, but conversion to open cholecystectomy is required in up to 5% of cases.

Gallbladder Polyps

Gallbladder polyps are outgrowths of the gallbladder mucosal wall that are seen in up to 5% of normal subjects undergoing gallbladder ultrasonography. Most of these lesions are not neoplastic but are hyperplastic or represent lipid deposits (cholesterolosis). The differential diagnosis includes cholesterol polyps, adenomyomatosis, inflammatory polyps, adenomas, and gallbladder cancer. Factors associated with increased risk of malignancy include size greater than 1 cm, presence of gallstones, age greater than 60 years, and increased size on subsequent imaging. Cholecystectomy is indicated if one or more of these

risk factors are present or if the patient has biliary symptoms. Polyps that are smaller than 1 cm should be monitored with periodic ultrasound examination.

Gallbladder Carcinoma

Gallbladder carcinoma is relatively uncommon but has a high case fatality rate. The incidence and mortality are higher in Latin American countries (e.g., Chile) and in Southeast Asia. Carcinoma of the gallbladder often produces advanced disseminated disease with weight loss, jaundice, pruritus, and a large right upper quadrant mass. Symptoms may resemble those of acute or chronic cholecystitis, particularly if the tumor is small. Risk factors include gallbladder polyps, porcelain gallbladder, choledochal cysts, gallstones, and anomalous pancreaticobiliary junction. Although early-stage tumors can be treated surgically, most cases are diagnosed at an advanced stage and are incurable.

Gallbladder Dyskinesia

A disorder caused by abnormal motility or contraction of the gallbladder in the absence of gallstones resulting in symptoms of biliary colic. Laboratory studies and abdominal imaging findings are usually normal. HIDA scanning may show a decreased gallbladder ejection fraction, or there may be reproducible pain with administration of cholecystokinin (CCK). Cholecystectomy commonly shows acalculous cholecystitis.

● BILIARY TRACT DISORDERS

Choledocholithiasis

In Western countries, most stones found in the common bile duct (choledocholithiasis) originate in the gallbladder. Up to 15% of individuals with cholelithiasis develop choledocholithiasis (Fig. 44-4). Less commonly, stones may form de novo in the biliary tree. Common bile duct stones may be asymptomatic (30% to 40%), or they may produce biliary colic and jaundice. Two major complications are acute cholangitis and acute

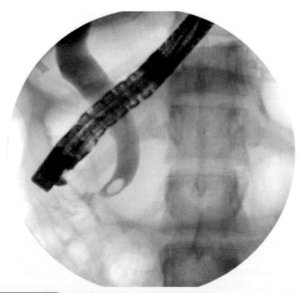

FIGURE 44-4 Cholangiogram obtained on endoscopic retrograde cholangiopancreatography demonstrates a common bile duct stone.

pancreatitis. The diagnosis is supported by the results of liver function tests and abdominal imaging. Transabdominal ultrasound is the initial imaging modality of choice; it has a sensitivity of 20% to 90% for detection of a stone and 55% to 90% for detection of dilation of the common bile duct. EUS and MRCP have replaced ERCP for diagnosis of bile duct stones; the sensitivity and specificity are 94% and 95%, respectively, for EUS and 93% and 94% for MRCP. ERCP is reserved for therapeutic interventions.

Acute Cholangitis

Acute (suppurative) cholangitis is a life-threatening infection of the biliary tract that occurs as a result of choledocholithiasis. The classic clinical manifestations are abdominal pain, jaundice, and fever (Charcot's triad). Clinical findings may be absent or atypical in elderly or immunosuppressed patients. Cholangitis is a medical-surgical emergency that can lead rapidly to sepsis, shock, and death. Diagnosis is based on a compatible clinical and laboratory picture (abnormal liver function test results and leukocytosis) together with radiologic or endoscopic evidence of common bile duct stones.

Treatment of acute cholangitis includes administration of broad-spectrum antibiotics and prompt removal of stones, typically with ERCP and sphincterotomy (Video 44-2). Cholecystectomy is subsequently performed after the patient has been stabilized.

Gallstone Pancreatitis

Biochemical evidence of pancreatic inflammation complicates choledocholithiasis and acute cholecystitis in up to 30% and 15% of patients, respectively. There are two proposed mechanisms by which gallstones may induce pancreatitis: reflux of bile into the pancreatic duct due to transient obstruction of the ampulla and obstruction at the ampulla secondary to stones or edema. Considering that gallstone pancreatitis recurs in 25% of patients, a cholecystectomy should be performed once the patient has recovered clinically from an attack of pancreatitis. If the patient remains jaundiced during an attack, suggesting the presence of a stone in the bile duct, an ERCP with sphincterotomy is performed to extract the stone.

Biliary Neoplasms

Cholangiocarcinoma and cancer of the ampulla of Vater are uncommon in the United States. Cholangiocarcinoma can arise at any level of the biliary system. It is more common in older men, occurring predominantly in men 50 to 70 years of age. Risk factors include primary sclerosing cholangitis (PSC), choledochal cysts, chronic ulcerative colitis, liver flukes, and recurrent pyogenic cholangitis (Oriental cholangiohepatitis). Patients with these cancers usually have unremitting painless jaundice, although necrosis and sloughing of the tumor can cause intermittent biliary obstruction and the appearance of occult fecal blood. Cholangiocarcinoma located at the bifurcation of the extrahepatic bile duct (50% of cases) is known as a *Klatskin tumor* (Fig. 44-5). Surgical cure is possible in only a small proportion of patients with cholangiocarcinoma. If the tumor is unresectable, palliative biliary drainage is undertaken.

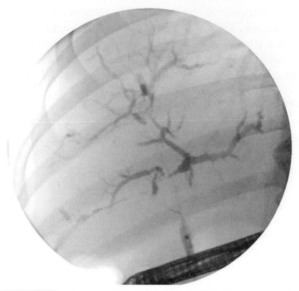

FIGURE 44-5 Cholangiogram obtained on endoscopic retrograde cholangiopancreatography demonstrates a Klatskin tumor at the bile duct bifurcation.

Nonmalignant Causes of Biliary Obstruction
Biliary Strictures

Benign biliary strictures usually result from surgical injury or chronic pancreatitis. Biliary strictures resulting from surgical injury may cause symptoms even years after the initial injury. Early diagnosis is important because strictures that partially obstruct are clinically asymptomatic and can cause secondary biliary cirrhosis. Biliary stricture should be suspected in any patient with a history of surgery of the right upper quadrant or chronic pancreatitis who has persistently elevated levels of serum alkaline phosphatase and γ-glutamyl transpeptidase. Endoscopic balloon catheter dilatation with or without stenting or surgical repair is useful in selected patients.

Other Causes of Biliary Obstruction

Structural abnormalities such as choledochal cysts, Caroli's disease (congenital segmental intrahepatic bile duct dilation), and duodenal diverticula may cause bile duct obstruction, often with secondary choledocholithiasis resulting from bile stasis. Hemobilia, with intermittent bile duct obstruction by blood clots, may be caused by hepatic injury, neoplasms, or hepatic artery aneurysms. Biliary parasites should always be considered as a cause of biliary obstruction in the appropriate epidemiologic setting. *Ascaris lumbricoides* is a common cause of cholangitis and jaundice in South America, Africa, and the Indian subcontinent. *Clonorchis sinensis* is the etiologic agent of Oriental cholangiohepatitis in Korea and Southeast Asia and in immigrants to the United States. The liver fluke *Fasciola hepatica* is a leading cause of biliary strictures and cholangitis worldwide, most commonly in the Bolivian Andes.

Primary Sclerosing Cholangitis

PSC is an idiopathic condition of nonmalignant, nonbacterial, chronic inflammatory fibrosis and obliteration of the intrahepatic and extrahepatic bile ducts. It most commonly occurs in young

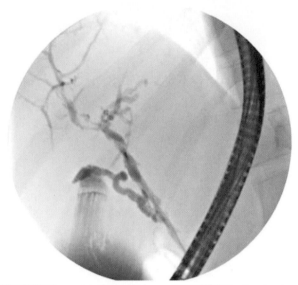

FIGURE 44-6 Cholangiogram obtained on endoscopic retrograde cholangiopancreatography demonstrates the characteristic beading of the intrahepatic and extrahepatic bile ducts in a patient with primary sclerosing cholangitis.

men (two thirds of patients are younger than 45 years of age), often in association with ulcerative colitis. Approximately 70% of patients with PSC have ulcerative colitis. The clinical spectrum of PSC is broad, ranging from asymptomatic patients with abnormal liver enzyme levels (typically an elevated alkaline phosphatase concentration) to patients with recurring episodes of fever, chills, abdominal pain, and jaundice. The diagnosis of PSC is made by MRCP or ERCP, which show characteristic changes (beading) of the intrahepatic and/or extrahepatic bile duct (Fig. 44-6).

No proven therapy exists for PSC, although ursodeoxycholic acid and methotrexate are being used in some centers. Other forms of therapy include prophylactic antibiotics for prevention of recurrent bacterial cholangitis, treatment of pruritus, and repletion of fat-soluble vitamins. Endoscopic dilatation of a dominant biliary stricture during ERCP is an effective treatment of cholestasis in selected patients. Most patients with advanced PSC eventually progress to end-stage liver disease, and evaluation for liver transplantation is appropriate in advanced disease. One third of patients with PSC will develop cholangiocarcinoma; therefore, thorough clinical and laboratory studies (liver function tests and cancer markers such as CA 19-9) and radiologic follow-up are warranted.

Sphincter of Oddi Dysfunction

Sphincter of Oddi dysfunction is a benign motility disorder that leads to noncalculous obstruction of the flow of bile or pancreatic juice at the level of the pancreaticobiliary junction. Patients typically have unexplained biliary-type abdominal pain, with or without elevated results on liver function tests and with or without bile duct dilation. In a selected group of patients, endoscopic or surgical sphincterotomy is of value.

For a deeper discussion of this topic, please see Chapter 155, "Diseases of the Gallbladder and Bile Ducts," in Goldman-Cecil Medicine, 25th Edition.

SUGGESTED READINGS

Attasaranya S, Fogel EL, Lehman GA: Choledocholithiasis, ascending cholangitis, and gallstone pancreatitis, Med Clin North Am 92:925–960, 2008.

Caddy GR, Tham TC: Symptoms, diagnosis, and endoscopic management of common bile duct stones, Best Pract Res Clin Gastroenterol 20:1085–1101, 2006.

Chattopadhyay D, Lochan R, Balupuri S, et al: Outcome of gallbladder polypoidal lesions detected by transabdominal ultrasound scanning: a nine-year experience, World J Gastroenterol 11:2171–2173, 2005.

Elwood DR: Cholecystitis, Surg Clin North Am 88:1241–1252, 2008.

Esteller A: Physiology of bile secretion, World J Gastroenterol 14:5641–5649, 2008.

Shaffer EA: Epidemiology of gallbladder stone disease, Best Pract Res Clin Gastroenterol 20:981–996, 2006.

Stinton LM, Shaffer EA: Epidemiology of gallbladder disease: cholelithiasis and cancer, Gut Liver 6:172–187, 2012.

Tazuma S: Epidemiology, pathogenesis, and classification of biliary stones (common bile duct and intrahepatic), Best Pract Res Clin Gastroenterol 20:1075–1083, 2006.

Venneman NG, van Erpecum KJ: Pathogenesis of gallstones, Gastroenterol Clin North Am 39:171–183, 2010.

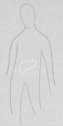
VIII

§ Hematologic Disease

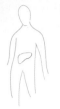

45

Hematopoiesis and Hematopoietic Failure

Eunice S. Wang and Nancy Berliner

⬤ HEMATOPOIESIS

Hematopoiesis is the process of formation and development of blood cells. The constituents of peripheral blood arise by a complex and carefully regulated process of ontogeny. The pluripotent hematopoietic stem cell (HSC) maintains itself by self-renewal and undergoes multilineage differentiation to generate the appropriate numbers and types of cells in the circulating blood compartment (Table 45-1). The hematopoietic system is unique in that it is constantly undergoing this full cycle of maturation by which a primitive cell develops into a variety of highly specialized end-stage cells, all of which have different lifespans and occur in different quantities.

The bone marrow must have the capacity to produce cells to compensate for the normal rapid turnover of hematopoietic cells resulting from senescence, normal use, and migration into tissue spaces. It must have a reserve capacity to produce additional cells in response to unusual demands that arise from bleeding, infection, or other stresses. Understanding the repeated cycle of cellular ontogeny and self-renewal that meets these challenges provides important insights into normal and pathologic mechanisms in hematology.

Hematopoietic Tissues

Hematopoiesis commences in the embryonic yolk sac, in which early erythroblasts in blood islands form the first hemoglobinized cells. After 6 weeks' gestation, the fetal liver begins producing primitive lymphocytoid cells, megakaryocytes, and erythroblasts, and the spleen becomes a secondary site of erythropoiesis. Hematopoiesis then shifts to its definitive long-term site in the bone marrow, the principal site for lifelong hematopoiesis in the normal host.

Early in life, all fetal bones contain regenerative bone marrow, but the marrow becomes progressively replaced by fat with age. In adults, active marrow resides only in the axial skeleton (i.e., sternum, vertebrae, pelvis, and ribs) and in the proximal ends of the femur and humerus. Consequently, bone marrow samples, which are needed for many hematologic diagnoses, are usually obtained from the iliac crest or sternum. Under pathologic conditions that stress the capacity of the marrow space, as seen in diseases associated with marrow fibrosis (e.g., myeloproliferative diseases) or in severe inherited hemolytic anemia (e.g., thalassemia major), extramedullary hematopoiesis may be reestablished in sites of fetal hematopoiesis, especially the spleen.

Stem Cell Theory of Hematopoiesis

All mature hematopoietic cells are hypothesized to originate from a small population of pluripotent stem cells. Comprising less than 1% of all cells in the bone marrow, these cells bear no distinctive morphologic markings and are best defined by their unique functional properties.

Stem cells have two distinctive characteristics. First, they are highly resilient and productive, capable of continuously replenishing huge numbers of granulocytes, lymphocytes, and erythrocytes throughout life. The demand for a continuous, fluctuating supply of blood cells requires a hematopoietic system capable of producing large numbers of selected cells in a short time. For example, overwhelming infection by invading microorganisms triggers the release of neutrophils, whereas hypoxia or acute blood loss leads to increased red blood cell production. Second, HSCs represent a self-renewing cell population that is able to maintain its numbers while providing a continued supply of progenitor cells of many different lineages.

Despite their vast proliferative potential, under normal conditions, most HSCs are quiescent, and few cells undergo expansion or differentiation at any one time. However, their ability to proliferate is striking. Studies with lethally irradiated mice have demonstrated the ability of a few transplanted cells (i.e., spleen colony-forming unit [CFU-S] cells) to regenerate multilineage hematopoiesis.

The signals regulating the differentiation of pluripotent stem cells into committed progenitors are unknown. Data suggest that the first step in lineage commitment is a stochastic (chance)

TABLE 45-1	NORMAL VALUES FOR PERIPHERAL BLOOD CELLS	
CELL TYPE AND SIZE	**MEAN**	**RANGE**
Hemoglobin	Women: 14 g/dL Men: 15.5 g/dL	Women: 12-16 g/dL Men: 13.5-17.5 g/dL
Hematocrit	Women: 41% Men: 47%	Women: 36-46% Men: 41-53%
Reticulocyte count	60,000/μL (1%)	35,000-85,000/μL (0.5-1.5%)
Mean corpuscular volume		80-100 fL
Platelet count	250,000/μL	150,000-400,000/μL
Total white blood cell count	7400/μL	4500-11,000/μL
Neutrophils	4400/μL (40-60%)	1800-7700/μL
Lymphocytes	2500/μL (20-40%)	1000-4800/μL
Monocytes	300/μL (<5%)	200-950 (4-11%)

event; subsequent stages of maturation are hypothesized to occur under the influence of growth factors, or cytokines (Table 45-2). Cytokines act on different cells through specific cytokine receptors. Receptor activation induces signal-transduction pathways that lead to changes in gene transcription and eventual cell proliferation and differentiation. These growth factors also act as survival factors for the developing hematopoietic cells by preventing *apoptosis* (i.e., programmed cell death). This process occurs in the cellular milieu of the bone marrow, where hematopoiesis depends in part on the nonhematopoietic cells (i.e., fibroblasts, endothelial cells, osteoblasts, and fat cells) that make up that microenvironment. Research in HSC biology has focused on how the cells are regulated by growth factors in the bone marrow microenvironment and by unique cell surface ligand interactions between stem cells and the surrounding stromal cells in well-defined sites called *stem cell niches*.

Hematopoietic Differentiation Pathway

Hematopoiesis has been hypothesized to proceed along a tightly regulated hierarchy (Fig. 45-1) governed by effects of intrinsic transcription factors and cytokines in the bone marrow microenvironment. As more primitive cells mature under the influence of specific regulatory cytokines, they undergo several cell divisions and become *progenitor cells* committed to one lineage. They also lose their self-renewal capacity. Morphologically, these cells are transformed from nonspecific blastlike cells into cells that can be identified by their color, shape, and granular and nuclear content. Functionally, they acquire distinguishing cell surface receptors and responses to specific signals.

Maturing granulocytes and erythroid cells undergo several more cell divisions in the bone marrow, whereas lymphocytes travel to the thymus and lymph nodes for further development. Megakaryocytes cease cellular division but continue with nuclear replication. Eventually, these cells are released from the marrow as fully functional erythrocytes, mast cells, granulocytes, monocytes, eosinophils, macrophages, and platelets.

Pluripotent Stem Cells

The pluripotent HSC is morphologically indistinguishable and is best identified by its expression of the cell differentiation antigen, CD34, and by its ability to form pluripotent colonies in vitro. Under the influence of interleukin-1 (IL-1), IL-3, IL-6, FMS-like tyrosine kinase 3 (FLT3), and a specific stem cell factor (KIT ligand [KITLG], or steel factor), this cell matures into a myeloid-lineage stem cell (i.e., granulocyte-erythrocyte-macrophage-megakaryocyte colony-forming unit [CFU-GEMM] cell)

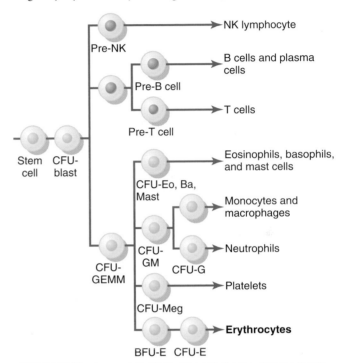

FIGURE 45-1 Development of bone marrow cells. Ba, Basophil; BFU, blast-forming unit; CFU, colony-forming unit; E, erythroid; Eo, eosinophil; G, granulocyte; GEMM, granulocyte-erythrocyte-macrophage-megakaryocyte; GM, granulocyte-macrophage; Meg, megakaryocyte; NK, natural killer.

TABLE 45-2   CYTOKINES AND THEIR ACTIVITIES

ACRONYM	NAME	EFFECTS ON HEMATOPOIESIS
EPO	Erythropoietin	Stimulation of proliferation and maturation of erythroid progenitors; produced by the kidney in response to anemia and hypoxia; important clinically for treatment of anemia associated with low EPO levels (e.g., renal failure, anemia of chronic disease)
G-CSF	Granulocyte colony-stimulating factor	Stimulation of proliferation and maturation of granulocytes; more broad-based effect because also increases release of stem cells in peripheral blood; clinically important for treatment of neutropenia and mobilization of stem cells for transplantation
GM-CSF	Granulocyte-monocyte colony-stimulating factor	Proliferation of granulocyte and monocyte precursors; role unclear in steady-state hematopoiesis because knockout has no hematopoietic phenotype
TPO	Thrombopoietin	Proliferation of megakaryocytes; results disappointing in clinical studies
M-CSF	Monocyte colony-stimulating factor	Proliferation of monocytes
IL-2	Interleukin-2	Proliferation of T cells
IL-3	Interleukin-3 (multi– colony-stimulating factor)	Proliferation of granulocytes, monocytes; broad-based effects, appearing to increase the proliferation of stem cells; not in use clinically
IL-4	Interleukin-4	Proliferation of B cells
IL-5	Interleukin-5	Proliferation of T cells, B cells; proliferation and differentiation of eosinophils
IL-11	Interleukin-11	Proliferation of megakaryocytes; undergoing clinical testing
LIF	Leukemia inhibitory factor	Proliferation of stem cells and megakaryocytes
SCF	Stem cell factor (kit ligand)	Proliferation of progenitor cells; broad-based effects on multiple lineages

or a lymphoid-lineage stem cell. In the presence of granulocyte-macrophage colony-stimulating factor (GM-CSF) and IL-3, the myeloid stem cell further differentiates into daughter cells of its named lineages (see Fig. 45-1). The lymphopoietic stem cell becomes a pre-B cell or a prothymocyte (pre-T cell) and leaves the marrow for further maturation.

Erythroid Lineage

Primitive erythroid precursors arising from the myeloid stem cell are called burst-forming unit–erythroid cells. These cells then differentiate into erythroid colony-forming unit (CFU-E) cells, which are the committed progenitor cells of erythrocytes. CFU-E cells express receptors for erythropoietin (EPO), an 18-kD molecule produced by renal interstitial cells in response to low oxygenation states or anemia. EPO upregulates proliferation of CFU-E cells and promotes their maturation into proerythroblasts and reticulocytes, which begin to synthesize hemoglobin (see Table 45-2).

Granulocyte and Monocyte Lineages

Human GM-CSF acts early in the hematopoietic pathway to regulate maturation of the CFU-GEMM stem cell. Differentiation of this myeloid precursor into specific committed progenitors occurs under the direction of granulocyte CSF (G-CSF) and monocyte CSF (see Table 45-2). Granulocyte CFU cells undergo sequential transformation into easily recognizable myeloblasts, myelocytes, and eventually early polymorphonuclear neutrophils with their characteristic polysegmented nuclei. Monocyte CFU cells, in contrast, retain a single nucleus as they mature from monoblasts to promonocytes to monocytes and sometimes to macrophages.

Other Lineages

Eosinophils and basophils develop from CFU-GEMM cells under the influence of IL-5 and IL-3 plus IL-4, respectively. The acquisition of their specific granular contents helps in distinguishing their precursors from those of early monocytes.

The development of platelets is morphologically distinct from the other lineages. CFU-GEMM cells differentiate into megakaryocyte CFU cells, so named because the cells cease cell division early but not nuclear replication. Megakaryocytes are the only cells in the body with the capacity to double their DNA content (i.e., endomitosis). Over the course of several cell cycles, the maturing megakaryocyte eventually acquires several times the nuclear content of other cells in preparation for its eventual dissolution into platelets with a fraction of the cytoplasm of other hematopoietic cells. Two growth factors, thrombopoietin (TPO) and IL-11, increase platelet counts by promoting megakaryocyte development (see Table 45-2).

Stem Cell Plasticity

Provocative data have challenged the conventional paradigm of hierarchical HSC differentiation. Experts have proposed that HSCs dedifferentiate into more immature progenitors and can cross lineages and transdifferentiate into nonlymphohematopoietic cells such as myocytes, hepatocytes, gastrointestinal epithelial cells, and neurons.

Whether this plasticity of HSCs is an intrinsic property of adult stem cells or is caused by contaminating cells of other populations, fusion of hematopoietic cells with other tissue cells, or artifacts introduced by ex vivo stem cell isolation techniques remains controversial. Nevertheless, the suggestion that adult HSCs may be a dynamic, renewable resource for tissue repair and regeneration holds great promise.

PRIMARY HEMATOPOIETIC FAILURE SYNDROMES

Diseases of the HSC that disrupt the normal regulated pattern of stem cell development can result in underproduction of mature progeny (i.e., aplastic anemia), overproduction of mature progeny (i.e., myeloproliferative disease), or failed differentiation with the production of excess immature forms (i.e., myelodysplasia and acute leukemia). Hematopoietic failure, defined as the inability of HSCs to produce normal numbers of mature blood cells, manifests clinically as peripheral pancytopenia (i.e., decreased production of all blood cell lineages).

Although marrow dysfunction producing pancytopenia can result from several hematologic and nonhematologic causes (Table 45-3), primary bone marrow failure disorders are characterized by a profound impairment of the ability of the HSC to replenish the stem cell pool. Rarely, marrow failure syndromes result from intrinsic HSC defects. In most cases, these disorders are the result of extrinsic damage to normal HSCs. The most common treatment modalities for primary hematopoietic failure disorders are exogenous growth factor administration and stem cell transplantation.

Growth Factors in Clinical Use

Discovery of the factors that influence normal hematopoiesis led to important therapeutic applications for patients with defects in hematopoietic cell production. The finding that committed hematopoietic cells of each lineage can be stimulated to proliferate and differentiate by specific cytokines (see Table 45-2) has been clinically useful.

Advances in DNA technology led to the synthesis and purification of recombinant human (rh) proteins with similar biologic activity in vivo. Administration of these products to patients enabled successful manipulation of mature cells in the peripheral

TABLE 45-3   DIFFERENTIAL DIAGNOSIS OF PANCYTOPENIA

Primary bone marrow disorders
- Aplastic anemia
- Congenital aplastic anemia syndromes
- Fanconi's anemia
- Shwachman-Diamond syndrome
- Congenital dyskeratosis
- Acquired aplastic anemia
- Hypocellular myelodysplastic syndrome
- Myelofibrosis
- Paroxysmal nocturnal hemoglobinuria
- Acute leukemias: acute lymphocytic leukemia, acute myeloid leukemia
- Hairy cell leukemia

Systemic diseases with secondary bone marrow effects
- Metastatic solid tumor to marrow
- Autoimmune disorders: systemic lupus erythematosus, Sjögren's syndrome
- Nutritional deficiencies: vitamin B_{12}, folate, alcoholism
- Infections: overwhelming sepsis from any cause, viruses, brucellosis, ehrlichiosis (mycobacteria)
- Storage diseases: Gaucher's disease, Niemann-Pick disease
- Anatomic defects: hypersplenism

blood. For example, exogenous EPO has become a mainstay in the management of anemia caused by renal failure, chemotherapy, and marrow failure syndromes. The use of G-CSF or GM-CSF in patients with febrile neutropenia and documented infection or sepsis after chemotherapy or radiation therapy has reduced hospital stays and shortened the period of high infection risk. Administration of GM-CSF is thought to improve host immune responses to fungal infections. High-dose G-CSF also is routinely used to mobilize CD34+ marrow stem cells into the peripheral blood for collection before and after stem cell transplantation in patients with delayed stem cell engraftment (discussed later).

Early trials of TPO growth factors to stimulate platelet production were halted because of development of antihuman TPO antibodies in some patients, leading to severe thrombocytopenia. Second-generation thrombopoietic agents bearing no structural resemblance to TPO but designed to bind and activate the TPO receptor are in clinical use. Romiplostim, a recombinant Fc-peptide fusion protein (i.e., peptibody) given as a weekly subcutaneous injection, can increase platelet counts, decrease platelet transfusion requirements, and improve quality of life for patients with refractory chronic immune-mediated thrombocytopenia. Eltrombopag is an orally available, small, organic TPO agonist that increases platelet counts and decreases bleeding in similar patients. The application of TPO agonists for management of thrombocytopenia in other marrow failure syndromes is being investigated.

Hematopoietic Stem Cell Transplantation

Types of Transplantations

Improved understanding of HSC biology has fostered the development of techniques to manipulate these cells for therapeutic purposes. The antitumor effects of most chemotherapeutic drugs and radiation therapy are dose dependent, and both cause the major dose-limiting toxicity of myelosuppression.

Before HSC transplantation, intense myeloablative doses of chemotherapy and total body irradiation are administered to eradicate malignant cells. Stem cells from a donor or the same patient are then infused to replete the ablated marrow. Although historically used in the treatment of primary stem cell disorders such as leukemia, the therapeutic potential of transplantation is also employed for patients with nonmalignant hematologic malignancies (e.g., aplastic anemia, sickle cell anemia, congenital immunodeficiencies), solid tumors (e.g., renal cell carcinoma, melanoma), and nonmalignant autoimmune diseases (e.g., amyloidosis, systemic lupus). Younger patients (<50 years) are considered the best candidates for this intensive therapy, although this is changing in the setting of newer supportive modalities.

Several modes of stem cell transplantation have been developed. In *autologous transplantation*, the patient's bone marrow or peripheral blood stem cells (PBSCs) are collected during remission after high-dose chemotherapy or G-CSF administration. These cells are cryopreserved, thawed, and reinfused. This approach incurs a higher risk of relapse as a result of reinfusion of a stem cell product that may remain contaminated with tumor cells.

In *allogeneic stem cell transplantation,* abnormally functioning hematopoietic bone marrow is eradicated and is replaced with normal bone marrow or stem cells from a compatible source (i.e., related or unrelated donor). High-dose chemotherapy with or without total body irradiation is used to destroy the patient's bone marrow, followed by infusion of new stem cells that engraft and restore normal hematopoiesis. Treatment-related morbidity is significant, and the procedure has a mortality rate of 10% to 30%. However, improvements in supportive care and immunomodulatory therapy designed to suppress graft-versus-host disease (GVHD), an autoimmune phenomenon in which intact lymphocytes in the transplanted marrow attack the host tissues, are continuing to improve outcome.

Donor and patient are tested for compatibility of human leukocyte antigen (HLA) and major histocompatibility complex (MHC) proteins expressed on all cells. Three major HLA class I antigens (i.e., A, B, and C) and three MHC class II antigens (i.e., DP, DQ, and DR) have been developed. The six HLA gene loci are tightly linked on chromosome 6 and are almost always inherited on a single cluster of genes, or *haplotype*. All children are a half-match (i.e., haploidentical) to each of their parents, and full siblings have a 25% probability of being HLA identical to one another. HLA-matched, nonrelated transplants have higher rates of GVHD than transplants from HLA-matched, related donors as a result of other minor HLA incompatibilities. Patients who receive an HLA-mismatched stem cell transplantation risk acute GVHD, marrow rejection, and fatal marrow aplasia. Morbidity and mortality rates associated with non–HLA-compatible transplants can be prohibitive.

Evidence indicates that the excellent response of some patients to HSC transplantation is partly related to the active suppression of the patient's original (residual) or relapsing disease by cells from the newly transplanted donor graft, referred to as the *graft-versus-leukemia effect*. Studies have documented that infusion of donor lymphocytes can restore remission in patients with evidence of relapse after allogeneic transplantation for chronic myelogenous leukemia. Conversely, procedures that minimize the reactivity between donor and host increase disease relapse. For example, there is an increased rate of relapse among patients who undergo syngeneic (identical twin) stem cell transplantation and patients who receive T-cell–depleted marrow in an attempt to reduce GVHD.

The observed effectiveness of donor lymphocyte infusions in controlling chronic myelogenous leukemia led to the conclusion that the immunologic effects of transplanted allogeneic cells might be as important as or more important than cytoreduction for the cure of some hematologic malignancies. To exploit these effects, nonmyeloablative stem cell transplantations are performed. Patients receive conditioning and immunosuppressive regimens in doses sufficient to permit donor stem cell engraftment without aggressive cytoreduction. These mini-transplantations result in chimeric marrows (i.e., part patient and part donor) without significant periods of cytopenias or hematopoietic compromise, although most responding patients convert to a fully donor-derived marrow over time. Although still experimental, these procedures are increasingly being used in patients who are otherwise ineligible for traditional myeloablative transplantation regimens (i.e., age greater than 50 to 55 years, other comorbidities) or in individuals with nonmalignant autoimmune or congenital disorders.

Hematopoietic Stem Cell Sources for Transplantation

Historically, stem cell transplantations have employed allogeneic bone marrow stem cells aspirated from the posterior iliac crest of the donor and intravenously infused into the patient after myeloablation and immunosuppressive therapy. The process of engraftment or reconstitution of normal hematopoietic function takes several weeks. Patients often require almost daily platelet and red blood cell transfusions, and they are hospitalized during this period of prolonged neutropenia to minimize life-threatening bacterial, viral, and fungal infections. Other complications include severe mucositis, hemorrhagic cystitis, GVHD, relapsed disease, and graft failure.

The discovery that high-dose G-CSF treatment mobilizes large numbers of CD34+ hematopoietic progenitor and stem cells from bone marrow sites into circulating blood (i.e., 10-fold to 15-fold increase over baseline levels) led to the use of PBSCs collected by apheresis procedures in place of bone marrow stem cells for allogeneic transplantation. Compared with marrow-derived stem cells, PBSCs engraft more rapidly after myeloablation. Patients receiving allogeneic PBSC transplants have decreased neutrophil recovery time, lower transfusion requirements, fewer inpatient hospital days, and similar rates of acute GVHD and long-term survival outcomes as traditional marrow-transplanted patients. Because PBSC collections often contain threefold to fourfold more CD34+ stem cells and 10-fold more lymphoid cells than harvested marrow grafts, higher rates of chronic GVHD may occur.

Umbilical cord blood (UCB) stem cells are a rich source of immature CD34+ HSCs. The less stringent HLA-compatibility requirements for UCB HSC matches prompted increasing use of these transplants as a therapy for patients lacking fully compatible HLA-matched PBSCs or bone marrow donors. Although still considered experimental, some transplantation centers have reported long-term outcomes after UCB HSC transplants similar to those for conventional marrow or peripheral PBSC transplants for primary hematologic diseases. However, the relatively limited numbers of CD34+ stem cells found in harvested UCB units accounts for a much slower hematopoietic recovery after the procedure and a statistically higher risk for nonengraftment compared with other stem cell sources. For this reason, UCB transplantation procedures have been limited to pediatric patients and smaller adults or to adult patients for whom there is more than one HLA-compatible UCB unit.

Aplastic Anemia

Definition and Epidemiology

Aplastic anemia (AA) is a rare disorder characterized by pancytopenia with a markedly hypocellular bone marrow. This disease was first described in 1888 by Paul Ehrlich, who observed that autopsy bone marrow specimens from a young woman who died of severe anemia and neutropenia were extremely hypoplastic. Later studies demonstrated that patients with severe AA possessed only a fraction of normal pluripotent stem cell numbers despite normal functional marrow stromal cells and normal or even elevated levels of stimulatory cytokines.

The incidence of AA ranges from 1 to 5 cases per million people in the general population. It occurs predominantly in young adults (20 to 25 years old) and older adults (60 to 65 years old). The incidence is threefold higher in developing countries (e.g., Thailand and China) compared with industrialized Western nations (e.g., Europe and Israel), a fact that is not explained by differences in drug or radiation exposure. A few AA cases occur in the context of a congenital bone marrow failure disorder, such as Fanconi's anemia, Shwachman-Diamond syndrome, and dyskeratosis congenita. The most common congenital AA, Fanconi's anemia, is an autosomal recessive disorder arising from mutations in genes encoding DNA repair proteins.

Pathology

The known causes of acquired AA are numerous (Table 45-4) and range from myeloablative radiation exposure to common viruses and medications. Prior bone marrow toxicity from drugs, chemicals (e.g., benzene, cyclic hydrocarbons found in petroleum products, rubber glue, insecticides, chemical dyes), or radiation predisposes to AA because these agents directly injure proliferating and differentiating HSCs by inducing DNA damage. In contrast, cytotoxic chemotherapy (especially with alkylating agents) and radiation therapy target all rapidly cycling cells and often induce reversible bone marrow aplasia. Despite the many causes of acquired AA, most cases are idiopathic.

Acquired and congenital AAs appear to be etiologically linked through abnormal telomere maintenance. Telomeres are repeated nucleotide sequences that cap and protect chromosome ends from degradation. Cell division leads to normal telomere erosion; when telomeres reach a critically short length, cells cease to proliferate, senesce, and undergo apoptosis, often with accompanying DNA damage and genomic instability. Telomerase enzyme in normal HSCs preserves long telomeres and promotes quiescence and a prolonged cellular lifespan. Patients with autosomal dominant dyskeratosis congenita have mutations in the genes for telomerase complexes, predisposing to premature aging and enhanced marrow failure in the setting of accelerated telomere shortening. One third of patients with acquired AA also have short telomeres, likely due to a combination of genetic, environmental, and epigenetic factors.

Autoreactive host lymphocytes can destroy normal hematopoiesis in AA. Bone marrow stromal cells and cytokine levels in patients with AA are normal. The fact that AA also occurs in diseases of immune dysregulation and after viral infections

TABLE 45-4	CAUSES OF ACQUIRED APLASTIC ANEMIA

Drugs (dose related): chemotherapeutic agents, antibiotics (chloramphenicol, trimethoprim-sulfamethoxazole)
Idiosyncratic causes (many unproved): chloramphenicol, quinacrine, nonsteroidal anti-inflammatory drugs, anticonvulsants, gold, sulfonamides, cimetidine, penicillamine
Toxins: benzene and other hydrocarbons, insecticides
Viral infection: hepatitis, Epstein-Barr virus, human immunodeficiency virus (HIV)
Immune disease: graft-versus-host disease in immunodeficiency, hypogammaglobulinemia
Paroxysmal nocturnal hemoglobinuria (PNH)
Radiation exposure
Pregnancy

further suggests an immune-mediated mechanism for the disease. One hypothesis is that drug or viral antigens presented to the immune system trigger cytotoxic T-cell responses that persist and destroy normal stem cells. Only 1 in 100,000 patients develops severe AA as an idiosyncratic drug reaction. Whether these individuals have a genetically predisposed sensitivity to common exposures (e.g., nonsteroidal anti-inflammatory drugs, sulfonamides, Epstein-Barr virus) is unknown.

Clinical Presentation

The clinical onset of AA can be insidious or abrupt. Patients often complain of symptoms related to their cytopenias: weakness, fatigue, dyspnea, or palpitations resulting from anemia; gingival bleeding, epistaxis, petechiae, or purpura caused by low platelet counts; or recurrent bacterial infections caused by low or nonfunctioning neutrophils. Results of the physical examination are often normal except in patients with congenital AA, who may have various abnormalities.

Diagnosis and Differential Diagnosis

Diagnostic confirmation of AA requires bone marrow biopsy to confirm hypocellularity and to rule out other marrow processes. Normal bone marrow cellularity ranges from 30% to 50% up to age 70 years and is less than 20% after 70 years of age (E-Fig. 45-1A). In contrast, bone marrow cellularity in patients with AA usually ranges from 5% to 15%, with increased fat accumulation and few or no hematopoietic cells (primarily plasma cells and lymphocytes) (see E-Fig. 45-1B).

In AA, hematopoietic progenitor and precursor cells are morphologically normal but number less than 1% of normal levels, and they are markedly dysfunctional, with a decreased ability to form differentiated progenitor cell colonies in vitro. Evidence of increased blasts, dysplastic hematopoietic cells (e.g., pseudo-Pelger-Huët abnormalities, micromegakaryocytes) (E-Fig. 45-2), and clonal cytogenetically abnormal cells in the peripheral blood or marrow are diagnostic of acute leukemia or myelodysplasia but not AA, even in the setting of a hypocellular marrow.

In young patients, a diagnosis of Fanconi's anemia is made by demonstrating enhanced sensitivity of cultured cells to mitomycin or diepoxybutane-induced chromosomal damage. Although patients with AA typically have a low reticulocyte count from low red blood cell production and a paucity of blood cells (E-Fig. 45-3A) and macrocytic red cells (see E-Fig. 45-3B) on the peripheral smear, patients with other primary marrow disorders may exhibit similar findings.

Treatment and Prognosis

Treatment of AA is based on the severity of disease. Patients with mild cytopenias can be monitored expectantly. However, patients with severe AA based on peripheral blood cells counts (i.e., neutrophil count <500/μL, platelet count <20,000/μL, anemia with corrected reticulocyte count <1%, and marrow cellularity of 5% to 10%) have a poor median survival of 2 to 6 months without treatment. Because most of these patients die of overwhelming infections, supportive care with broad-spectrum antibiotics, antifungal agents, and antiviral agents is warranted for those with advanced neutropenia. Red blood cell and platelet transfusions can help patients who are profoundly symptomatic, along with care given to patients eligible for transplantation.

Current therapeutic approaches to AA focus on replacing the defective HSCs by stem cell transplantation or controlling an overactive immune response. All young patients with severe AA and an HLA-compatible bone marrow donor should be considered for allogeneic bone marrow transplantation, which offers the best chance for definitive cure. Although long-term survival is excellent for patients younger than 30 years transplanted from a sibling donor (75% to 90%), morbidity due to the transplant itself and the management of long-term complications are continuing problems. Outcomes for patients older than 40 years or patients without an HLA-matched related donor are poor.

The presumed immune mechanisms for drug-induced aplasia have encouraged immunosuppressive approaches to the treatment of AA in older patients, in patients who are unable to find a compatible HSC donor, and in those who are otherwise ineligible for stem cell transplantation. Treatment with a combination of antithymocyte globulin (ATG) and cyclosporine (a specific T-cell inhibitor) restores marrow function (i.e., independence from red blood cell or platelet transfusions) in 70% to 80% of patients, and responders have a 5-year survival rate of 90%. Side effects of ATG include anaphylaxis and serum sickness as a result of foreign antigens in the antisera, but these adverse effects usually are self-limited.

Patients often relapse, and recurrence of disease may warrant retreatment with ATG, androgens, and newer immunosuppressive agents. Alemtuzumab, a humanized monoclonal antibody directed against the CD52 protein found on lymphocytes and which has efficacy in other autoimmune diseases, has been as effective as rabbit ATG and cyclosporine in relapsed and refractory severe AA. Eltrombopag, an oral TPO mimetic drug that stimulates platelet production by binding to MPL receptors on megakaryocytes, is an exciting agent for the treatment of severe AA patients. Almost one half of patients treated with eltrombopag exhibited clinically significant responses in all three hematopoietic lineages, with normalization of bone marrow cellularity and trilineage hematopoiesis.

Treatment of AA with traditional chemotherapy such as high-dose cyclophosphamide usually has proved too toxic. Because endogenous cytokine production is usually high in patients with AA, the routine use of growth factors such as G-CSF, EPO, or stem cell factor typically is ineffective. However, in patients with refractory disease, long-term administration of combination cytokines may have some effect in sustaining blood cell counts. Patients who survive initial treatment of AA remain at increased risk for the emergence of other primary hematologic disorders, such as myelodysplasia, leukemia, and paroxysmal nocturnal hemoglobinuria (PNH) for unknown reasons.

Paroxysmal Nocturnal Hemoglobinuria

Definition, Epidemiology, and Pathology

PNH is an uncommon disease characterized by intravascular hemolysis, venous thrombosis, and bone marrow failure. The disease arises from expansion of pluripotent HSCs containing a somatic mutation in the phosphatidylinositol glycan complementation class A (*PIGA*) gene. Loss of *PIGA*, which codes for a membrane lipid moiety (i.e., glycosyl phosphatidylinositol [GPI]), produces abnormal hematopoietic cells deficient in dozens of proteins that are normally attached to the cell surface by the GPI anchor. Disease manifestations of PNH result from lack of the GPI-linked proteins (CD55 and CD59) that usually protect red blood cells and platelets from complement-mediated attack. Loss of CD55 or CD59 leads to increased immune destruction of blood cells.

Blood cells arising from abnormal PNH clones can have complete (type III cells) or partial (type II cells) GPI deficiency. The degree of GPI deficiency is associated with the severity of the clinical symptoms. GPI-deficient cells typically coexist in the marrow with various populations of normal GPI-expressing cells (type I cells). Small numbers of abnormal PNH clones in patients with AA or myelodysplastic syndrome (MDS) suggest significant overlap in the causes of these three diseases. This led to reclassification of PNH as classic PNH disease and PNH in the setting of another specified bone marrow disorder. Suppression of normal hematopoiesis by the host immune system directly or indirectly by a preceding or coexistent disorder appears to provide a marrow environment favoring selective expansion of PNH stem cell clones and their deficient blood cell progeny over normal hematopoiesis.

Clinical Presentation

Patients are typically younger individuals with chronic complaints of abdominal pain, dysphagia, erectile dysfunction, and intense lethargy due to smooth muscle dystonia resulting from depletion of circulating nitric oxide levels by free hemoglobin. Acute exacerbations may occur intermittently or frequently and are difficult to manage.

Diagnosis and Differential Diagnosis

The diagnosis of PNH is made by identification of complete or partial GPI protein deficiency on red cells and granulocytes, which usually is determined by the loss of CD59, CD55, CD16, or CD24 expression in a clonal population. Laboratory tests reveal ongoing, low-grade intravascular hemolysis with increased lactate dehydrogenase levels correlating with severity of hemolysis and symptoms. Cytopenias, particularly anemia, often render patients transfusion dependent with ongoing hemoglobinuria due to the release of free plasma hemoglobin from intracellular compartments. About 15% of PNH patients have spontaneous resolution of disease without long-term sequelae, suggesting that *PIGA* mutations may appear transiently and disappear spontaneously in normal hematopoietic cell populations for unknown reasons.

Treatment

Treatment of PNH ranges from supportive care with transfusions and iron and folic acid supplementation to allogeneic stem cell transplantation in selected patients for curative intent. Documented venous thrombosis is treated with lifelong full anticoagulation.

Eculizumab is a humanized monoclonal antibody that binds with high affinity to the complement protein C5, preventing terminal complement-mediated intravascular hemolysis in PNH patients. Eculizumab therapy decreases hemolysis and

hemoglobinuria, reduces requirements for red blood cell transfusions, improves chronic renal failure, and is associated with significant improvement in quality of life and survival for PNH patients. The incidence of life-threatening thrombotic events is decreased by more than 80%, likely contributing to the significant improvement in overall survival. Although this agent is associated with a theoretical increased risk for meningococcal infections due to complement-mediated blockade, the long-term safety and efficacy of sustained eculizumab therapy administered for more than 5 years appear to outweigh the potential risks of prolonged treatment.

Prognosis

Despite advances in treatment and adequate anticoagulation, PNH remains a life-threatening disease. Venous thrombosis involving the cerebral and intra-abdominal veins occurs in about one half of patients and is the cause of death for up to one third, although the cause of the increased thrombotic risk is not entirely understood. Other causes of morbidity and mortality are side effects of progressive AA and a 5% long-term risk for leukemic transformation. Historically, the median survival from diagnosis is 10 to 15 years, with one third of patients dying within 5 years of the diagnosis. Whether long-term eculizumab therapy can change the natural history of disease is unknown and is the goal of an international registry of PNH patients.

Myelodysplastic Syndrome
Definition and Epidemiology

MDS is a heterogeneous group of blood disorders characterized by ineffective and disordered hematopoiesis in one or more of the major myeloid cell lines: erythroid cells, neutrophils and their precursors, and megakaryocytes. Patients have one or more cytopenias despite normal or increased numbers of hematopoietic cells in the bone marrow. Disordered maturation is accompanied by increased intramedullary apoptosis, which contributes to the decreased release of mature cells into the periphery.

Primary MDS is predominantly a disease of elderly persons and occurs in about 1 of 500 patients between the ages of 60 and 75 years. Most cases are idiopathic. Although often considered a preleukemic disease, the overall risk of MDS transformation to acute myeloid leukemia (AML) is only 25% to 30%. However, identification of characteristic gene deletions (5q−) and translocations diagnostic of MDS and AML subtypes (see Chapter 46) underlines the likelihood of similar mechanisms of clonal myeloid stem cell injury in both disorders.

Pathology

Persons with prior exposure to radiation therapy, chemotherapy, and organic chemicals (e.g., benzene) are at increased risk for secondary MDS. This disorder may occur at any age and comprises 10% to 15% of all diagnosed MDS cases. MDS arising months to years after prior chemotherapy (involving any cytotoxic agent but particularly alkylating agents and anthracyclines), ionizing radiation, radiolabeled antibody therapy, or stem cell transplantation for cancer is called *therapy-related MDS*. Because therapy-related MDS typically evolves swiftly to more aggressive disease, these cases have been reclassified with therapy-related AML and treated accordingly (see Chapter 46).

Clinical Presentation

Most patients with MDS are referred for evaluation of an incidental finding of peripheral cytopenias. Symptomatic patients usually exhibit findings related to the secondary effects of cytopenias: bleeding and bruising caused by thrombocytopenia, infection caused by leukopenia, or fatigue and dyspnea related to anemia. Physical examination is usually unremarkable, although 25% or more of patients may have splenomegaly. In some patients with MDS, development of skin lesions with fever (i.e., acute febrile neutrophilic dermatosis [Sweet's syndrome]) may herald the transformation of MDS into acute leukemia.

The disease course of MDS varies widely. Some patients may live normal lifespans, but most die prematurely of cytopenia-related complications, marrow failure, or evolution to AML. Median survival is usually less than 2 years.

Diagnosis and Differential Diagnosis

Dysplasia of myeloid hematopoietic cells is evident in the blood and marrow of MDS patients. Review of the peripheral blood smear may show characteristic morphologic abnormalities in addition to cytopenias. Erythroid cells are usually macrocytic, often with basophilic stippling. Neutrophils are often hypogranular and hypolobulated, with a characteristic bilobed nuclear morphology called *pseudo-Pelger-Huët abnormality*. This anomaly should be anticipated when automated differential cell counts report unusually large numbers of bands.

The bone marrow in MDS is usually normocellular or hypercellular, although 10% of patients may have a hypocellular marrow. Dysplastic changes usually occur in all three cell lines. Erythroid cells appear megaloblastic, with multinucleated cells or asynchronous nuclear-cytoplasmic development. Extremely small micromegakaryocytes and agranular megakaryocytes also may be seen. The myeloid series shows poor maturation with a left shift to earlier hypogranulated myeloid forms. Although elevated numbers of myeloid blasts are common, increasing blast numbers indicate progression to acute leukemia. Electron microscopy of the marrow shows cellular changes (i.e., prominent nuclear chromatin, cytoplasmic vacuoles, and blebs) characteristic of increased apoptosis (see E-Fig. 45-4).

The natural history and treatment of some MDS subtypes correlate with specific cytogenetic abnormalities, and careful molecular studies of the marrow should be performed during the initial evaluation. For example, MDS cases associated with deletion of the short arm of chromosome 7 (7p−) or complex cytogenetic abnormalities such as monosomy 7 or trisomy 8 often have poor clinical outcomes. MDS with an isolated deletion in the long arm of chromosome 5 (i.e., 5q− syndrome) can have a well-characterized clinical course. Patients are predominantly older women with a refractory macrocytic anemia, normal or elevated platelet counts, and an overall better clinical prognosis. These patients often live for several years with intermittent red blood cell transfusions and have a low risk of leukemic transformation. Multiple or complex cytogenetic aberrations carry a worse prognosis.

Although one third to one half of patients with cytopenia and myeloid dysplasia have diagnostic clonal cytogenetic abnormalities in marrow cells, the marrow karyotype is normal in many cases. For these patients, the diagnosis of MDS should be one of exclusion after other potential causes of marrow failure and pancytopenia have been evaluated (see Table 45-3). MDS should never be diagnosed in acute disease states, during chronic hospitalization, or within 6 months of known myelotoxic therapy (e.g., irradiation, chemotherapy). Causes such as vitamin B_{12} or folate deficiency, alcohol use, and human immunodeficiency virus (HIV) infection should be considered. A patient with possible MDS and hypocellular bone marrow must be evaluated for AA. Consistent cytopenia in one or more myeloid lineages, no other obvious causes, and dysplasia of at least 10% of myeloid marrow cells or 5% to 19% of blast cells should be considered MDS.

In the past, MDS was classified based on dysplastic marrow morphology and percentage of blasts as one of five subtypes: refractory anemia (RA), refractory anemia with ringed sideroblasts (RARS), refractory anemia with excess blasts (RAEB), refractory anemia with excess blasts in transformation (RAEBT), and chronic myelomonocytic leukemia (CMML). Later, these five subtypes were expanded to eight subtypes, with recognition of multilineage dysplasia as an important feature (e.g., refractory cytopenia with multilineage dysplasia, refractory cytopenia with multilineage dysplasia and ringed sideroblasts) and the reclassification of CMML as myeloproliferative-myelodysplastic syndrome (Table 45-5). MDS with an isolated 5q− cytogenetic abnormality was established as a distinct clinical syndrome. Evidence of marrow dysplasia after prior chemotherapy, radiation therapy, or other myeloablative therapy is considered therapy-related AML. Although MDS patients with refractory anemia and excess blasts or refractory cytopenias with multilineage dysplasia usually fare poorly, morphologic classification of MDS correlates only approximately with overall survival.

Treatment

Insights into the pathophysiology of ineffective hematopoiesis characterizing MDS has led to several therapeutic options for this disease. Individualized therapy is based on the patient's preference, performance status, disease biology, and prognostic risk category.

Transfusions and Growth Factors

Most patients with MDS are elderly individuals who may not tolerate or desire aggressive intervention without hope of cure. Asymptomatic individuals who have disease at low risk for disease transformation or progression and are transfusion independent are typically observed expectantly. Those with symptomatic anemia and thrombocytopenia can often be treated supportively with chronic red blood cell and platelet transfusions to maintain quality of life.

One complication of chronic transfusion therapy is iron overload caused by the delivery of between 200 and 250 mg of iron with each unit of transfused red blood cells. Excess iron is stored in macrophages and eventually accumulates in the hepatic parenchyma, myocardium, skin, and the pancreas, leading to secondary hemochromatosis or transfusional iron overload. Clinical symptoms include liver dysfunction, heart failure, hyperpigmentation, and diabetes mellitus. To prevent these symptoms, patients who develop marked elevations in transferrin saturation or serum ferritin levels should undergo iron chelation therapy with deferoxamine or an oral agent (e.g., deferiprone).

Chronic administration of recombinant EPO reduces the transfusion needs of some MDS patients, particularly those with low endogenous serum EPO levels and few transfusion requirements. Individuals with recurrent or refractory neutropenic infections often receive G-CSF and GM-CSF treatment alone or in addition to EPO and antibiotic regimens. These treatments are supportive and do not affect overall survival.

Immunosuppressive Therapy

Certain MDS disease subgroups appear to have hematopoietic failure mediated in part by autoimmune cells selectively targeting the destruction of normal HSCs. These disease subsets exhibit significant overlap with AA and PNH. For instance, some young patients with low-risk MDS disease and an HLA-DR15 haplotype have demonstrated a 30% to 50% improvement in counts after T-cell immunosuppressive therapy with ATG or cyclosporine. MDS patients with isolated trisomy 8 or demonstrated PNH clones, or both, have responded to treatment with immunosuppressive agents.

Stem Cell Transplantation

As in other hematologic stem cell disorders, the only curative therapy for MDS patients remains allogeneic stem cell transplantation, ideally performed at complete remission. All MDS patients younger than 40 years with an available HLA-matched sibling donor should be offered transplantation at diagnosis. Long-term, disease-free survival rates for patients with low-risk disease are greater than 50%. However, the high transplantation-related mortality, morbidity, and relapse rates associated with mismatched or unrelated donor transplants or with transplantation in older MDS patients have limited the use of these forms of transplantation to patients with high-risk disease.

Patients with intermediate-2 or high-risk MDS (i.e., MDS with cytogenetic abnormalities predisposing to leukemic transformation or high levels of circulating blasts with International Prognostic Scoring System [IPSS] scores of intermediate-2 or higher) (Table 45-6) may be offered acute leukemia-based chemotherapy regimens (see Chapter 46) designed to eradicate rapidly proliferating blast cells, not dysfunctional MDS cells. These therapies for MDS patients are associated with a high relapse rate within 12 to 18 months and no significant prolongation of overall survival, even for patients who achieve remission.

Targeted Therapeutic Agents

Although not curative, a panoply of novel therapeutic agents targeting the unique biologic features of MDS have improved outcomes for many MDS patients ineligible for or unwilling to pursue stem cell transplantation or supportive care. Administered largely in the outpatient setting, these agents have induced disease remissions, retarded leukemia evolution, and for the first time, prolonged overall survival of MDS patients.

TABLE 45-5 WORLD HEALTH ORGANIZATION CLASSIFICATION OF MYELODYSPLASTIC SYNDROMES

CLASS	DEFINITION
Refractory anemia	Blood: anemia, no or rare blasts BM: erythroid dysplasia only, <5% blasts, and <15% ringed sideroblasts
Refractory anemia with ringed sideroblasts (RARS)	Blood: anemia, no blasts BM: ≥15% ringed sideroblasts, erythroid dysplasia only, <5% blasts
Refractory cytopenia with multilineage dysplasia (RCMD)	Blood: cytopenias (bicytopenia or pancytopenia), no or rare blasts, <1 × 10^9/L monocytes BM: dysplasia in ≥10% of the cells of two or more myeloid cell lines, <5% blasts, no Auer rods, <15% ringed sideroblasts
Refractory cytopenia with multilineage dysplasia and ringed sideroblasts (RCMD-RS)	Blood: cytopenias (two or more), no or rare blasts, no Auer rods, and <1 × 10^9/L monocytes BM: dysplasia in ≥10% of the cells of two or more myeloid cell lines, <5% blasts, ≥15% ringed sideroblasts, no Auer rods
Refractory anemia with excess blasts type 1 (RAEB-1)	Blood: cytopenias, <5% blasts, no Auer rods, <1 × 10^9/L monocytes BM: unilineage or multilineage dysplasia, 5-9% blasts, no Auer rods
Refractory anemia with excess blasts type 2 (RAEB-2)	Blood: cytopenias, 5-19% blasts, Auer rods ± <1 × 10^9/L monocytes BM: unilineage or multilineage dysplasia, 10-19% blasts, ± Auer rods
Myelodysplastic syndrome–unclassified (MDS-U)	Blood: cytopenias, no or rare blasts, no Auer rods BM: unilineage dysplasia in one myeloid line, <5% blasts, no Auer rods
MDS associated with isolated del(5q)	Blood: anemia, usually normal or increased platelet count, <5% blasts BM: normal to increased megakaryocytes with hypolobulated nuclei, <5% blasts, isolated cytogenetic abnormality of deletion 5q, no Auer rods

BM, Bone marrow.

TABLE 45-6 WORLD HEALTH ORGANIZATION CLASSIFICATION-BASED PROGNOSTIC SCORING SYSTEM (WPSS) FOR MYELODYSPLASTIC DISORDERS

FACTOR	SCORING*			
	0	1	2	3
WHO category	RA, RARS, 5q−	RCMD, RCMD-RS	RAEB-1	RAEB-2
Karyotype[†]	Good	Intermediate	Poor	—
Transfusion requirement[‡]	No	Regular	—	—

MDS, Myelodysplastic syndrome; RA, refractory anemia; RARS, refractory anemia with ringed sideroblasts; RCMD, refractory cytopenia with multilineage dysplasia; RCMD-RS, refractory cytopenia with multilineage dysplasia and ringed sideroblasts; RAEB-1, refractory anemia with excess of blasts type 1; RAEB-2, refractory anemia with excess of blasts type 2; 5q−, myelodysplastic syndrome with isolated del(5q) and marrow blasts less than 5%; WHO, World Health Organization.

*Risk groups were determined as follows: very low (total score = 0), low (1), intermediate (2), high (3 to 4), and very high (5 to 6).

[†]Karyotype was as follows: good: normal, −Y, del(5q), del(20q); poor: complex (≥3 abnormalities), chromosome 7 anomalies; and intermediate: other abnormalities.

[‡]Red blood cell (RBC) transfusion dependency was defined as having at least one RBC transfusion every 8 weeks over a period of 4 months.

The recognition that epigenetic modifications of the abnormal HSC clones in MDS affect cell growth and apoptosis and are central to disease pathogenesis led to the therapeutic application of two DNA methyltransferase inhibitors (i.e., 5-azacytidine and decitabine) to the disease. These agents are hypothesized to reverse the abnormal hypermethylation and gene silencing in abnormal HSCs.

5-Azacytidine delays the time to leukemic transformation in two thirds of patients with transfusion-dependent MDS, decreases transfusion requirements, and improves quality of life compared with transfusion support alone. This agent is the only drug shown to significantly prolong overall survival of MDS patients, largely by delaying (but not preventing) the time of onset of acute leukemic transformation in a phase III clinical trial comparing 5-azacytidine with conventional care regimens for higher-risk MDS patients. These results are the first to demonstrate that any therapy can alter the natural history of this disease and renders 5-azacytidine the standard of care for transfusion-dependent MDS patients.

Decitabine is a compound related to 5-azacytidine and represents an alternative treatment option for patients with high-risk MDS. Decitabine therapy induces remission and reduces transfusion needs compared with supportive care and historical controls; however, the survival benefit of decitabine use in MDS has not been demonstrated.

A unique feature of DNA methyltransferase inhibitor therapy with either hypomethylating agent is that most therapeutic responses occur 4 to 6 months after treatment initiation. Moreover, MDS patients treated with 5-azacytidine who did not achieve a defined complete remission in the marrow still survived significantly longer than patients treated with supportive care alone. These data suggest that (unlike AML) the best treatment for MDS is not cytotoxic-mediated eradication of abnormal HSC clones but chronic (epigenetic) modification of cells resulting in restoration of normal hematopoiesis. It remains to be seen whether achievement of remission after hypomethylation modulation in MDS equates with long-term disease control.

Lenalidomide

Patients with lower-risk MDS characterized by deletions in the long arm of chromosome 5 (5q– aberration) typically have anemia with preserved platelet counts. Many have a disease subtype that is extraordinarily sensitive to therapy with lenalidomide, an immunomodulatory agent that exerts antigrowth effects on MDS cells and their surrounding marrow microenvironment. Complete and durable responses after lenalidomide therapy occur in up to 66% of 5q– syndrome MDS patients and are accompanied by disappearance of the abnormal cytogenetic clone in the marrow in some patients. Defects in ribosomal protein function, specifically the ribosomal subunit protein RPS14, have been identified as the cause of 5q– syndrome MDS, paralleling findings implicating a different ribosomal subunit (RPS19) in the congenital bone marrow syndrome Diamond-Blackfan anemia.

Studies have suggested that lenalidomide targets aberrant signaling pathways caused by haploinsufficiency of specific genes in a commonly deleted region on chromosome 5 (i.e., *SPARC*, *RPS14*, *CDC25C*, and *PPP2CA*). The agent specifically targets del(5q) clones while also promoting erythropoiesis and repopulation of the bone marrow in normal cells. Lenalidomide induces responses in up to one third of non-5q– MDS patients, demonstrating a specific defect in erythroid differentiation on gene expression profiling.

Prognosis

Formulation of MDS prognostic categories remains a work in progress. In 1998, the IPSS was developed by an international working group to better predict clinical outcomes in MDS. The IPSS divides patients with MDS into three prognostic categories based on cytogenetic abnormalities, cytopenias, advanced age, and percentage of bone marrow blasts, and it provides median survival and time to leukemic transformation for each IPSS stage (Table 45-7).

Based on criticism that the IPSS relies only on characteristics of patients at disease onset and includes cases now considered to be AML by the World Health Organization (WHO) criteria, a new WHO classification–based prognostic scoring system (WPSS) was devised emphasizing WHO morphology, karyotype, and transfusion dependence at any time during the MDS disease course. Division of MDS patients into five new risk categories was validated to predict for overall survival and leukemic evolution for MDS at any follow-up time (see Table 45-6).

Combined data from multiple international databases, including 7012 MDS patients, were statistically analyzed and used to generate a new prognostic classification system for untreated MDS patients, the Revised International Prognostic Scoring System (R-IPSS). This model retained marrow cytogenetics (including several novel karyotypic abnormalities), marrow blast percentage, and cytopenias as clinically prognostic markers but divided patients into five, rather than three, prognostic categories (Table 45-8). Despite the advances made in predicting outcomes for MDS patients, all of these prognostic models are limited by their exclusion of molecular features, specifically gene mutations.

Modern genomic sequencing technologies have revolutionized biomedical investigation by allowing parallel assessment of

TABLE 45-7	INTERNATIONAL PROGNOSTIC SCORING SYSTEM FOR MYELODYSPLASTIC DISORDERS				
SCORE	BLASTS	KARYOTYPE	CYTOPENIAS*	OVERALL SCORE	MEDIAN SURVIVAL (YR)
0	<5%	Normal, −Y, 5q–, 20q–	0-1 cytopenias	0	5.7
0.5	5-10%	All other abnormalities	2-3 cytopenias	0.5-1.0	3.5
1.0		Abnormal 7, >3 abnormalities		1.5-2.0	1.2
1.5	11-20%			2.5 or higher	0.4
2.0	21-30%				

*Cytopenias are defined as hemoglobin <10 g/dL, neutrophils <1500/μL, platelets <100,000/μL.

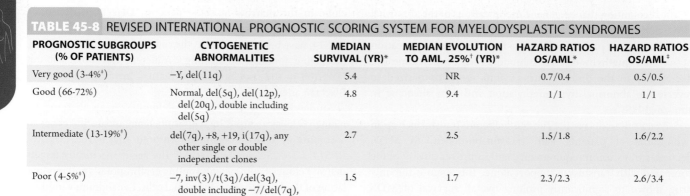

TABLE 45-8 REVISED INTERNATIONAL PROGNOSTIC SCORING SYSTEM FOR MYELODYSPLASTIC SYNDROMES

PROGNOSTIC SUBGROUPS (% OF PATIENTS)	CYTOGENETIC ABNORMALITIES	MEDIAN SURVIVAL (YR)*	MEDIAN EVOLUTION TO AML, 25%[†] (YR)*	HAZARD RATIOS OS/AML*	HAZARD RATIOS OS/AML[‡]
Very good (3-4%[‡])	−Y, del(11q)	5.4	NR	0.7/0.4	0.5/0.5
Good (66-72%)	Normal, del(5q), del(12p), del(20q), double including del(5q)	4.8	9.4	1/1	1/1
Intermediate (13-19%[‡])	del(7q), +8, +19, i(17q), any other single or double independent clones	2.7	2.5	1.5/1.8	1.6/2.2
Poor (4-5%[‡])	−7, inv(3)/t(3q)/del(3q), double including −7/del(7q), complex: 3 abnormalities	1.5	1.7	2.3/2.3	2.6/3.4
Very poor (7%[‡])	Complex: >3 abnormalities	0.7	0.7	3.8/3.6	4.2/4.9

AML, Acute myeloid leukemia; NR, not reached; OS, overall survival.

*Multivariate analysis, $N = 7012$; data from patients in the International Working Group for Prognosis in MDS (IWG-PM) database.

[†]AML, 25% indicates time for 25% of patients to develop AML.

[‡]$N = 2754$; Data from Schanz J, Tüchler H, Solé F, et al: New comprehensive cytogenetic scoring system for primary myelodysplastic syndromes and oligoblastic AML following MDS derived from an international database merge, *J Clin Oncol* 30:820–829, 2012.

hundreds of thousands of genes, pathways, and biologic processes in cancer samples. Whole-genome sequencing of untreated MDS samples has revealed that at least 78% of patients carry one or more oncogenic mutations. Although more than 40 genes are recurrently mutated in MDS, most are altered in less than 5% of MDS patients, reflecting the enormous biologic heterogeneity of this disorder. Genes implicated in MDS are involved in cell signaling, DNA methylation, chromatin regulation, and most importantly, RNA splicing. Several studies have shown that several individual gene mutations, including *EZH2, DNMT3A, SF3B1, TET2, NRAS, TP53, RUNX1,* and *ASXL1,* predict MDS outcomes independent of IPSS classification and can improve on prognostication based on clinical features alone.

Comprehensive genomic screening of diagnostic MDS samples occurs largely in academic centers. However, as technology advances, it is likely that novel prognostic models incorporating these mutational signatures will be adopted into the clinical care of patients.

PROSPECTUS FOR THE FUTURE

The field of stem cell biology is rapidly changing. The study of HSC function in marrow failure syndromes provides hints of specific molecular pathways disturbed in many diseases of hematopoietic and nonhematopoietic stem cells. These observations are furthering our knowledge about the complex interplay among AA, PNH, and MDS. Understanding stem cells' plasticity and regulatory roles promises new therapeutic avenues for a wide array of diseases.

UCB stem cells represent a potential source of donor cells for allogeneic stem cell transplantation in patients with primary hematologic diseases lacking other HLA-matched marrow donors. Nonmyeloablative stem cell transplantations (i.e., mini-transplantations) employing low-dose conditioning and immunosuppressive regimens represent another emerging treatment option for older patients with primary marrow failure syndromes.

The TPO agonist eltrombopag and the anti-CD52 antibody alemtuzumab show promise in restoring normal hematopoiesis

in refractory AA patients. Novel agents targeting the unique biologic features of ineffective hematopoiesis in marrow failure syndromes have improved outcomes for many patients over the past few years: eculizumab in PNH; 5-azacytidine in transfusion-dependent MDS; immunosuppressive drugs in AA and MDS subsets; lenalidomide in 5q− MDS.

Discoveries elucidating the complex genomic landscape of MDS have revealed that almost 80% of cases are characterized by at least one oncogenic mutation, and more than 40 unique genes are recurrently mutated in this disorder. Much research remains to be done to determine how best to incorporate this vast amount of information into the clinical care of MDS patients and to tailor therapeutic options for these unique biologic signatures.

For a deeper discussion of these topics, please see Chapter 156, "Hematopoiesis and Hematopoietic Growth Factors," in Goldman-Cecil Medicine, 25th Edition.

SUGGESTED READINGS

Bejar R, Stevenson KE, Caughey BA, et al: Validation of a prognostic model and the impact of mutations in patients with lower-risk myelodysplastic syndromes, J Clin Oncol 30:3376–3382, 2012.

Hillmen P, Muus P, Roth A, et al: Long-term safety and efficacy of sustained eculizumab treatment in patients with paroxysmal nocturnal haemoglobinuria, Br J Haematol 162:2–73, 2013.

Marsh JC, Kulasekararaj AG: Management of the refractory aplastic anemia patient: what are the options? Blood 122:3561–3567, 2013.

Olnes MJ, Scheinberg P, Calvo KR, et al: Eltrombopag and improved hematopoiesis in refractory aplastic anemia, N Engl J Med 367:11–19, 2012.

Papaemmanuil E, Gerstung M, Malcovati L, et al: Clinical and biological implications of driver mutations in myelodysplastic syndromes, Blood 122:3616–3627, 2013.

Risitano AM: Paroxysmal nocturnal hemoglobinuria and the complement system: recent insights and novel anticomplement strategies, Adv Exp Med Biol 735:155–172, 2013.

Scheinberg P, Nunez O, Weinstein B, et al: Activity of alemtuzumab monotherapy in treatment-naive, relapsed, and refractory severe acquired aplastic anemia, Blood 119:345–354, 2012.

46

Clonal Disorders of the Hematopoietic Stem Cell

Eunice S. Wang and Nancy Berliner

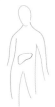

● INTRODUCTION

Malignant transformation involves combined defects in cellular maturation and differentiation. The multistep theory of oncogenesis suggests that these defects are often separable and contribute to a stepwise progression from a normal to a fully transformed cell. The continuous cycling of hematopoietic cells provides a milieu for the development of clonal genetic abnormalities that supports the multistep model. Clonal defects of the hematopoietic stem cell give rise to an array of preleukemic and leukemic disorders. Primary defects of maturation give rise to the myelodysplastic disorders (see Chapter 45), whereas loss of normal control of proliferation results in myeloproliferative disease. All of these disorders are preleukemic, with a variable but definite rate of transformation to acute leukemia.

● MYELOPROLIFERATIVE NEOPLASMS

Definition and Pathology

Myeloproliferative neoplasms (MPNs), also known as chronic myeloproliferative diseases (MPDs), are clonal stem cell disorders characterized by leukocytosis, thrombocytosis, erythrocytosis, splenomegaly, and bone marrow hypercellularity. The hallmark of MPNs is the failure of a transformed multipotent stem cell to respond to normal feedback mechanisms regulating hematopoietic cell mass. Stem cells from patients with MPNs demonstrate clonal colony growth in vitro when they are grown in serum without the addition of exogenous cytokines, and this technique has been used as a diagnostic test for MPNs.

MPNs have traditionally been divided into four classic disorders based on the predominant hyperproliferative cell type: polycythemia vera (PV), essential thrombocytosis (ET), primary myelofibrosis (PMF; i.e., idiopathic myelofibrosis or agnogenic myeloid metaplasia), and chronic myelogenous leukemia (CML). Hypereosinophilic syndrome (HES), mast cell disease, and other less common diseases are also included (Table 46-1).

Complications of MPNs arise from the overproduction of one or more lineages in the blood. All can be associated with clonal evolution and blastic transformation to acute leukemia, although with the exception of CML, this is an infrequent and late complication. In most patients with MPNs, the pathogenesis of disease is attributed to dysfunctional kinases.

In CML, a reciprocal translocation between chromosomes 9 and 22 (i.e., Philadelphia chromosome or translocation) results in an Abelson (ABL) leukemia virus–breakpoint cluster region

(BCR) fusion protein (BCR/ABL) with constitutive kinase activity. In PV, PMF, and ET, a mutation involving the substitution of a valine for phenylalanine at position 617 (V617F) in the Janus kinase 2 (JAK2) has been identified in most patients and may account for the abnormal growth properties that characterize these stem cell disorders.

Identification of somatic JAK2 mutations in all MPNs has led to clinical development and testing of orally bioavailable small-molecule inhibitors that selectively target dysfunctional JAK2 for the treatment of MPNs. Results from these trials are eagerly awaited.

● POLYCYTHEMIA VERA

Definition and Epidemiology

PV, a term meaning increased numbers of red blood cells in the blood, is a syndrome of increased red blood cell mass in the peripheral blood resulting from a clonal multipotent hematopoietic stem cell defect. PV occurs in 1 to 3 of 100,000 people, with a median age at diagnosis of 65 years.

Clinical Presentation

PV is a primary clonal stem cell disorder of unknown origin that is characterized by predominant erythrocytosis associated with other hematopoietic abnormalities. Although one half of patients

TABLE 46-1	WORLD HEALTH ORGANIZATION 2008 CLASSIFICATION OF MYELOID NEOPLASMS

1. Acute myeloid leukemia
2. MDS
3. MPNs
   a. Chronic myelogenous leukemia
   b. Polycythemia vera
   c. Essential thrombocythemia
   d. Primary myelofibrosis
   e. Chronic neutrophilic leukemia
   f. Chronic eosinophilic leukemia, not otherwise categorized
   g. Hypereosinophilic syndrome
   h. Mast cell disease
   i. MPNs, unclassifiable
4. MDS, MPN
5. Myeloid neoplasms associated with eosinophilia and abnormalities of PDGF-RA, PDGF-RB, or FGF-R1

FGF-R1, Fibroblast growth factor receptor 1; MDS, myelodysplastic syndrome; MPN, myeloproliferative neoplasm; PDGF-RA, platelet-derived growth factor receptor-α polypeptide; PDGF-RB, platelet-derived growth factor receptor-β polypeptide.

have concurrent leukocytosis or thrombocytosis, erythrocytosis is the hallmark and the cause of the most serious clinical complications of this disease. Typically, patients complain of headache, visual problems, mental clouding, and pruritus after bathing. Occlusive vascular events such as stroke, transient ischemic attacks, myocardial ischemia, and digital pain, paresthesias, or gangrene are common. Pulmonary, deep vein, hepatic, and portal vein thromboses may occur. Paradoxically, patients are also predisposed to hemorrhagic events, which are presumably caused by abnormal platelet function, and they may exhibit gastrointestinal bleeding. Physical examination often shows retinal vein occlusion, ruddy cyanosis, and splenomegaly.

Diagnosis and Differential Diagnosis

When patients are first diagnosed with an elevated hemoglobin concentration per unit volume (i.e., erythrocytosis), the initial evaluation should focus on whether this increase reflects an enhanced red cell mass (i.e., absolute erythrocytosis or polycythemia) or a normal red cell mass in the setting of a decreased plasma volume (i.e., relative erythrocytosis caused by dehydration or other causes). The latter condition is not true polycythemia (Table 46-2). Polycythemia or absolute erythrocytosis is an absolute increase in red cell mass caused by increased red blood cell production.

Under normal conditions, the body's ability to increase red blood cell production in states of hypoxemia, anemia, hemolysis, and acute blood loss ensures continuous oxygen delivery to tissues. In response to physiologic stimuli, pluripotent stem cell precursors are activated by erythropoietin (EPO) to differentiate into erythroid progenitor cells and eventually into hemoglobin-carrying erythrocytes. When numbers of mature red blood cells are adequate, a negative feedback mechanism suppresses further EPO production, and the serum hemoglobin level remains normal.

Diagnosis of PV was formerly one of exclusion based on an elevated red cell mass, splenomegaly, thrombocytosis, leukocytosis, lack of hypoxemia and other secondary causes of polycythemia, and elevated levels of leukocyte alkaline phosphatase and serum vitamin B_{12}–binding protein levels. More information about the disease pathophysiology led to new diagnostic criteria (Table 46-3) based on the discovery of *JAK2* gene mutations in 97% of patients with PV. A suspected diagnosis of PV can now be confirmed by testing for a *JAK2* mutation, and identification of low serum EPO levels and EPO-independent erythroid colony growth have become secondary diagnostic criteria.

Peripheral blood often appears microcytic, with or without iron deficiency. Bone marrow examination shows a hypercellular marrow with pronounced hyperplasia of erythroid lineage cells. Cytogenetic features at the time of diagnosis are usually normal. The development of clonal cytogenetic abnormalities heralds transformation in the later stages of disease.

Treatment and Prognosis

Early recognition and treatment of PV are important because untreated patients with PV suffer significant morbidity and mortality from thromboembolic complications involving the cerebral, coronary, and mesenteric circulations. Twenty percent of patients show symptoms of arterial and venous thrombosis, and thrombosis remains the most common cause of death. Without treatment, one half of patients with PV die of thrombotic complications within 18 months of diagnosis. With therapy, PV is a chronic, progressive disease. The risk of transformation to acute myeloid leukemia (AML) is 2.3% at 10 years and 5.5% at 15 years. Patients with advanced age (>60 years), prior history of thrombosis, leukocytosis, and high hematocrit values are at high risk for subsequent vascular events. The JAK2 V617F mutation and clinical cardiovascular factors are also associated with an increased risk of thrombosis.

Intermittent phlebotomy is the mainstay of treatment and usually results in iron deficiency anemia, which further reduces the rate of red blood cell production. Cytoreductive therapy is indicated for patients who cannot tolerate or fail phlebotomy, those with a history of or risk factors for thrombosis, and those with symptomatic splenomegaly. Cytoreductive therapies include hydroxyurea (i.e., low-dose cytotoxic agent that does not appear to increase leukemic risk), interferon-α (i.e., for young

---

TABLE 46-2   CAUSES OF ERYTHROCYTOSIS

I. Relative or spurious erythrocytosis (normal red cell mass)
  A. Hemoconcentration due to dehydration (e.g., diarrhea, diaphoresis, diuretics, water deprivation, emesis, ethanol, hypertension, preeclampsia, pheochromocytoma, carbon monoxide intoxication)
II. True or absolute erythrocytosis
  A. Polycythemia vera
  B. Primary congenital polycythemia
  C. Secondary erythrocytosis due to
    1. Congenital causes (e.g., activating mutation of erythropoietin receptor)
    2. Hypoxia caused by carbon monoxide poisoning, high oxygen affinity hemoglobin, high-altitude residence, chronic pulmonary disease, hypoventilation syndromes such as sleep apnea, right-to-left cardiac shunt, neurologic defects involving the respiratory center
    3. Nonhypoxic causes with pathologic erythropoietin production
      a. Renal disease (e.g., cysts, hydronephrosis, renal artery stenosis, focal glomerulonephritis, renal transplantation)
      b. Tumors (e.g., renal cell cancer, hepatocellular carcinoma, cerebellar hemangioblastoma, uterine fibromyoma, adrenal tumors, meningioma, pheochromocytoma)
    4. Drug-associated causes
      a. Androgen therapy
      b. Exogenous erythropoietin growth factor therapy

Modified from Hoffman R, Benz EJ, Shattil SJ, et al, editors: Hematology: basic principles and practice, ed 2, New York, 1995, Churchill Livingstone.

TABLE 46-3   WORLD HEALTH ORGANIZATION 2008 DIAGNOSTIC CRITERIA FOR POLYCYTHEMIA VERA

Major criteria*
1. Hemoglobin (Hgb) >18.5 g/dL (men), >16.5 (women); *or* Hgb or hematocrit (Hct) >99% reference range for age, sex, or altitude of residence; *or* Hgb >17 g/dL (men), >15 g/dL (women) if associated with a sustained increase of ≥2g/dL from baseline that cannot be attributed to correction of iron deficiency; *or* elevated red cell mass (>25% above mean normal predicted value)
2. Presence of *JAK2* V617F or similar mutation
Minor criteria
1. Bone marrow trilineage myeloproliferation
2. Subnormal serum erythropoietin level
3. Endogenous erythroid colony formation in vitro

*Both major criteria and one minor criterion *or* the first major criterion and two minor criteria must be met for the diagnosis of polycythemia vera.

patients and women during pregnancy), and anagrelide (i.e., megakaryotoxic agent for treating refractory thrombocytosis).

The typical goal of therapy is maintenance of hematocrit values less than 45% in men and less than 42% in women. In a multicenter, prospective clinical trial, adult PV patients randomized to a therapeutic hematocrit target of less than 45% using hydroxyurea, phlebotomy, or both modalities had a significantly lower rate of cardiovascular death (2.7% vs. 9.8%) and major thrombosis than those with a hematocrit target between 45% and 50%.

Low-dose chemotherapeutic agents (e.g., chlorambucil, busulfan) may be used to treat leukocytosis and thrombocytosis not responding to hydroxyurea, but they are associated with increased toxicity and risk of secondary AML. As with all myeloproliferative disorders, initiation of cytoreductive therapy may precipitate hyperuricemia that results in secondary gout and uric acid stones, warranting treatment with allopurinol.

Low-dose aspirin and treatment of asymptomatic thrombocytosis decrease thromboembolic events in low- and high-risk PV patients and are especially important in older patients with significant cardiovascular risk factors. In younger patients, nonsteroidal anti-inflammatory drugs and antiplatelet agents should be used judiciously because of the risk of gastrointestinal hemorrhage.

With effective therapy, the long-term survival of PV patients is excellent. Clinical trials of novel agents targeting constitutively active JAK2 signaling pathways are being conducted (primarily in patients failing prior hydroxyurea therapy), and it remains to be seen whether this class of drugs will improve outcomes and/or quality of life for PV patients.

● ESSENTIAL THROMBOCYTHEMIA
Definition and Epidemiology

ET (i.e., primary thrombocythemia) is a pluripotent stem cell disorder resulting in elevated levels of platelets and white blood cells. Platelet function and length of survival remain normal. ET is an uncommon disorder, with an increasing number of cases found among patients who are asymptomatic on routine laboratory testing. Although the median age at diagnosis is 60 to 65 years, 10% to 25% of patients are younger than 40 years.

Clinical Presentation

Up to two thirds of patients are symptomatic. Vasomotor symptoms include headache, dizziness, visual changes, and erythromelalgia (i.e., burning pain and erythema of feet and hands). Serious arterial thrombotic complications such as transient ischemic attacks, strokes, seizures, angina, and myocardial infarctions may occur. Patients may rarely have purpuric skin lesions or hematomas. The risk for gastrointestinal bleeding is less than 5%.

Diagnosis and Differential Diagnosis

Elevated platelet counts (i.e., thrombocytosis) can result from other causes (e.g., bacterial infections, sepsis, iron deficiency, autoimmune diseases, malignant diseases), which must be excluded before a diagnosis of ET is considered. The diagnosis requires a platelet count exceeding $450,000 \times 10^9/L$ with a JAK2 V617F mutation or no evidence of reactive thrombocytosis.

Bone marrow histology displays predominant proliferation involving the megakaryocytic lineage with increased mature megakaryocytes and little or no granulocytic or erythroid proliferation. Marrow immunohistochemical and cytogenetic studies are essential to exclude myelodysplasia, myelofibrosis, or the Philadelphia chromosome, which are diagnostic of CML (Table 46-4).

Although no genetic or biologic marker is 100% specific for ET, the JAK2 V617F mutation is found in more than one half of samples from patients with ET. Unlike other MPNs, bone marrow cells from patients with ET frequently do not show factor-independent colony growth, and the precise cause of this disease and its relation to JAK2 mutational status are under intense investigation.

Treatment and Prognosis

Patients with ET typically have long-term survival rates similar to those of age-matched control patients. Similar to PV, shortened overall survival is associated with increased age (>60 years), a history of thrombosis, and leukocytosis. The risk of leukemic transformation is extremely low (3% to 4%) compared with other MPNs. However, morbidity from recurrent hemorrhagic and thrombotic complications is high and cannot be reliably predicted from the platelet count or platelet function abnormalities.

Because treatment requires lifelong administration for disease control, assessment of risk factors and a history of clinical signs and symptoms dictate therapeutic choices. All patients benefit from aggressive management of cardiovascular risk factors (e.g., smoking, hypertension, obesity, hypercholesterolemia). Although low-dose enteric aspirin may be used in all patients to relieve neurologic symptoms and carries a minimal risk for bleeding, excessive thrombocytosis (platelet count >1000 × 10^9/L) can be associated with excessive bleeding due to acquired von Willebrand syndrome. Although young and pregnant patients are often not treated until they become symptomatic, older patients (>60 years) and those with a history of thrombosis, long disease duration, or significant cardiovascular risk factors are likely to benefit from the addition of platelet-lowering agents.

Hydroxyurea, an oral cytotoxic, myelosuppressive agent, is the most common first-line agent, and it usually is well tolerated and has low long-term leukemogenic risks. Anagrelide, an oral antiplatelet agent that inhibits platelet aggregation and megakaryocyte maturation, is also used, primarily as a second-line agent

---

TABLE 46-4 WORLD HEALTH ORGANIZATION 2008 DIAGNOSTIC CRITERIA FOR ESSENTIAL THROMBOCYTHEMIA

Major criteria*
1. Platelet count $\geq 450 \times 10^9/L$
2. Megakaryocyte proliferation with large and mature morphology; no or little granulocytic or erythroid proliferation
3. Not meeting WHO criteria for CML, PV, PMF, MDS, or other myeloid neoplasm
4. Demonstration of JAK2 V617F mutation or other clonal marker or no evidence of reactive thrombocytosis

CML, Chronic myelogenous leukemia; MDS, myelodysplastic syndrome; PMF, primary myelofibrosis; PV, polycythemia vera; WHO, World Health Organization.
*Diagnosis of essential thrombocytopenia requires meeting all four major criteria.

after hydroxyurea failure. This agent is associated with acute side effects (e.g., fluid retention, palpitations), hemorrhage (i.e., with concomitant aspirin use), and an increased risk of transformation to myelofibrosis. Both agents are known teratogens and therefore cannot be used in the significant fraction of patients with ET who are young women of childbearing age. Because patients with ET have a high incidence of fetal wastage, interferon-α (i.e., cytokine that alters the biologic mechanisms of the malignant clone but does not cross the placenta) with heparin or aspirin has been recommended to improve pregnancy outcomes in these patients.

⬤ PRIMARY MYELOFIBROSIS

Definition and Epidemiology

PMF (i.e., idiopathic myelofibrosis or agnogenic myeloid metaplasia) is a clonal stem cell disorder characterized by abnormal excessive marrow fibrosis leading to marrow failure. PMF is a rare chronic disease that usually is seen in elderly persons. The annual incidence of PMF is 0.5 cases per 100,000 people.

Pathology

An abnormal myeloid precursor is thought to give rise to dysplastic megakaryocytes that produce increased levels of angiogenic and fibroblast growth factors. These cytokines act on normal fibroblasts and other stromal cells, a process that stimulates excessive proliferation and collagen deposition. Over time, increasing fibrosis of the bone marrow leads to premature release of multipotent hematopoietic precursors into the periphery. These cells then migrate and reestablish themselves in other sites, thereby shifting hematopoiesis out of the bone marrow and into other tissues, especially the spleen and liver. This process is called *extramedullary hematopoiesis*.

Diagnosis and Differential Diagnosis

Early in the disease, patients may be asymptomatic, with incidental findings of abnormal blood counts on routine laboratory tests. Although low blood counts may occur, overall platelet and red blood cell numbers at diagnosis may be increased or normal depending on the degree of compensatory extramedullary hematopoiesis. Review of the peripheral blood profile commonly reveals leukoerythroblastic changes characterized by teardrop-shaped erythrocytes, giant platelets, and nonleukemic immature myeloid, erythroid, and leukocyte cells.

Diagnosis of PMF is made by demonstration of bone marrow fibrosis with markedly increased reticulin or collagen fibers (see E-Fig. 46-1) or increased marrow cellularity. Other underlying causes of neoplastic and non-neoplastic bone marrow fibrosis (Table 46-5) should be ruled out. Testing for *JAK2, BCR/ABL*, or other diagnostic mutations and cytogenetic markers should be performed before a diagnosis of PMF is made (Table 46-6).

Clinical Presentation

Although many patients are asymptomatic at diagnosis, most complain over time of progressive fatigue and dyspnea related to anemia or early satiety and left upper quadrant pain associated with splenomegaly and splenic infarction. More than one half of these patients develop massive hepatosplenomegaly due to extramedullary hematopoiesis. Patients with more advanced disease

TABLE 46-5	CAUSES OF BONE MARROW FIBROSIS

I. Neoplastic causes
  a. Chronic myeloproliferative disorders: chronic idiopathic myelofibrosis, chronic myelogenous leukemia, polycythemia vera
  b. Acute megakaryoblastic leukemia (FAB M7)
  c. Myelodysplasia with myelofibrosis
  d. Hairy cell leukemia
  e. Acute lymphoblastic leukemia
  f. Multiple myeloma
  g. Metastatic carcinoma
  h. Systemic mastocytosis
II. Non-neoplastic causes
  a. Granulomatous diseases: mycobacterial infections, fungal infections, sarcoidosis
  b. Paget's disease of bone
  c. Hypoparathyroidism or hyperparathyroidism
  d. Renal osteodystrophy
  e. Osteoporosis
  f. Vitamin D deficiency
  g. Autoimmune diseases: systemic lupus erythematosus, systemic sclerosis

FAB M7, French-American-British acute myeloid leukemia classification subtype 7.

TABLE 46-6	WORLD HEALTH ORGANIZATION 2008 DIAGNOSTIC CRITERIA FOR PRIMARY MYELOFIBROSIS MAJOR CRITERIA

Major criteria*
1. Megakaryocyte proliferation and atypia accompanied by reticulin and/or collagen fibrosis, *or* in the absence of reticulin fibrosis, the megakaryocytic changes must be accompanied by increased marrow cellularity, granulocytic proliferation, and often decreased erythropoiesis (i.e., prefibrotic primary myelofibrosis)
2. Not meeting World Health Organization criteria for chronic myelogenous leukemia, polycythemia vera, myelodysplastic syndrome, or other myeloid neoplasm
3. Demonstration of *JAK2* V617F mutation or other clonal marker or no evidence of reactive marrow fibrosis

Minor criteria
1. Leukoerythroblastosis
2. Increased serum lactate dehydrogenase level
3. Anemia
4. Palpable splenomegaly

*Diagnosis of primary myelofibrosis requires meeting all three major criteria and two minor criteria.

may have constitutional symptoms such as fever, weight loss, night sweats, cachexia, pruritis, and bone pain.

As bone marrow failure evolves, complications of neutropenia, thrombocytopenia, and anemia develop as a result of ineffective hematopoiesis. Bleeding from occult disseminated intravascular coagulation is a risk. Extramedullary hematopoiesis in the peritoneal and pleural cavities and in the central nervous system (CNS) may also cause symptoms.

Treatment and Prognosis

Median survival of patients with PMF is poor, ranging from 2 to 5 years after diagnosis. The most commonly accepted adverse prognostic factors at onset include age greater than 65 years, hemoglobin concentration of less than 10 g/dL, leukocyte count of more than 25×10^9/L, a high percentage of circulating blasts (≥1%), and constitutional symptoms. Other important clinical factors are leukopenia, thrombocytopenia (platelets <100 × 10^9/L), massive hepatosplenomegaly, red cell transfusion needs, and unfavorable cytogenetic abnormalities.

Over time, the disease may progress from a chronic phase to an accelerated phase, with acute leukemic transformation in 8% to 20% of patients. Treatment of PMF-related AML is usually ineffective. Other causes of nonleukemic death include heart failure, infection, intracranial hemorrhage, and pulmonary embolism.

Medical therapy for PMF is predicated on the risk category of patients. Low-risk, asymptomatic patients may be treated expectantly. All patients with symptomatic anemia benefit from palliative transfusions and administration of recombinant EPO, androgens (e.g., danazol), or low-dose thalidomide to maintain red blood cell levels. Symptoms caused by excess thrombocytosis and leukocytosis or progressive extramedullary hematopoiesis may be managed with hydroxyurea as a first-line agent or interferon-α in younger or pregnant patients. Symptomatic splenomegaly is best managed with hydroxyurea because open splenectomy is associated with significant operative morbidity and mortality and splenic irradiation is poorly tolerated except as a palliative approach. Young patients with intermediate- to high-risk PMF and possible HLA-matched donors should be considered for potentially curative allogeneic stem cell transplantation (SCT) at academic medical centers.

Although not all patients with PMF have the JAK2 V617F mutation, almost all have constitutive activation of the JAK1 and JAK2 signaling pathways, rendering them potentially responsive to treatment with novel JAK1/2 inhibitors. Ruxolitinib is an oral JAK inhibitor approved for the treatment of patients with intermediate- or high-risk myelofibrosis, including PMF, and myelofibrosis arising from prior PV or ET independent of JAK2 mutational status.

In two prospective, randomized, phase III clinical trials, ruxolitinib therapy for myelofibrosis patients was compared with placebo (COMFORT-I trial) and with best available therapy (COMFORT-II trial). Patients receiving ruxolitinib had significantly greater spleen volume reduction and symptom improvement (e.g., abdominal pain, early satiety, night sweats, muscle pain), which correlated with overall improvement in quality of life. Updates from both trials have demonstrated significantly prolonged overall survival and improvements in bone marrow fibrosis in the ruxolitinib-treated patients compared with control arms.

Many other JAK2 inhibitors are in active clinical development as single agents and in combination with ruxolitinib. Preliminary results of these trials suggest that even more effective therapies for PMF are on the horizon.

CHRONIC MYELOGENOUS LEUKEMIA
Definition, Epidemiology, and Pathology

CML is the most common MPN, accounting for 15% to 20% of all leukemias and occurring in 1 of 100,000 people. The median age at diagnosis is 53 years, but patients of any age may be affected. CML is characterized by a predominant increase in the granulocytic cell line associated with concurrent erythroid and platelet hyperplasia. It is unique among the MPNs in its natural history, including an inevitable transformation to acute leukemia.

CML was the first malignant hematologic disease shown to be associated with a specific chromosomal abnormality. More than 95% of patients with CML have a clonal expansion of a stem cell that has acquired the Philadelphia chromosome, which is a balanced translocation between chromosomes 9 and 22 that is designated t(9;22)(q34;q11). The translocation juxtaposits the ABL gene from chromosome 9 (region q34) to the BCR gene on chromosome 22 (region q11) and generates the oncogenic BCR/ABL fusion gene. The gene product, the BCR/ABL protein, is a deregulated, constitutively active cytoplasmic tyrosine kinase that induces a leukemic phenotype in hematopoietic stem cells. Expression of the BCR/ABL fusion protein activates multiple downstream signal transduction pathways that permits proliferation independent of cytokine and stromal regulation and renders cells resistant to chemotherapy and normal programmed cell death (i.e., apoptosis).

Diagnosis and Differential Diagnosis

Laboratory tests for CML patients typically demonstrate a markedly elevated white blood cell count (median, 170×10^9/L), with low leukocyte alkaline phosphatase levels, high uric acid and lactate dehydrogenase levels, and thrombocytosis. Review of the peripheral smear in chronic phase CML demonstrates a full complement of myeloid cells in all stages of granulocytic development, including immature myeloblasts (usually <5%), myelocytes, metamyelocytes, basophils, eosinophils, bands, and neutrophils. In contrast, the peripheral blood smear in reactive granulocytic hyperplastic states (i.e., leukemoid reaction) caused by acute infection or sepsis consists predominantly of mature neutrophils and bands with few myelocytes, basophils, or eosinophils.

The bone marrow in CML is densely hypercellular, with an overwhelming predominance of myeloid cells at all developmental stages and reticulin fibrosis (see E-Fig. 46-2). The differential diagnosis of CML includes reactive leukocytosis (e.g., in active infection or sepsis with a profound neutrophilic response) and other MPNs (e.g., myelofibrosis).

Detection of the Philadelphia chromosome on standard cytogenetic studies and abnormal BCR/ABL transcripts using reverse transcriptase–polymerase chain reaction (RT-PCR) or fluorescent in situ hybridization (FISH) analysis is required for the diagnosis of CML. Assessment of the BCR/ABL fusion gene by the same methods is used to monitor disease and response to therapy. Exquisitely sensitive and quantitative RT-PCR procedures allow detection of up to a single BCR/ABL-positive cell in 10^5 to 10^6 peripheral cells and permit measurement of disease status in peripheral blood and marrow samples.

A subset of patients with CML lacking a detectable Philadelphia chromosome was found to possess detectable BCR/ABL fusion products by RT-PCR, indicating a subchromosomal translocation resulting in the same pathologic gene product. Responses to treatment regimens for CML are defined as hematologic (i.e. restoration of normal peripheral blood cell counts), cytogenetic (i.e., loss of the Philadelphia chromosome determined by normal karyotypic or FISH analysis), and molecular (i.e., a three log or greater reduction of detectable BCR/ABL transcripts below a standard baseline by RT-PCR) remissions.

Clinical Presentation

Up to 40% of newly diagnosed CML patients are initially asymptomatic. Other patients exhibit fatigue, lethargy, shortness of breath, weight loss, easy bruising, and early satiety. Physical examination usually detects splenomegaly.

The natural history of CML is characterized by chronic, accelerated, and blastic phases. Patients are typically diagnosed during the chronic phase of CML, an indolent stage lasting 3 to 5 years. Peripheral white blood cell counts are elevated, with eosinophilia and basophilia (>20%) but few blasts (<5%). With control of peripheral blood cell counts, patients are essentially asymptomatic during this period.

Eventually, the disease enters the accelerated phase, which is characterized by fever, weight loss, worsening splenomegaly, and bone pain related to rapid marrow cell turnover. Despite therapy, the white blood cell count rises with increased numbers of circulating blasts (between 10% and 19%). The increased percentage of peripheral blood basophils (>20%) results in histamine production, with symptoms of pruritus, diarrhea, and flushing. During the accelerated phase of CML, patients may develop increasing splenomegaly, persistent thrombocytopenia, or thrombocytosis and leukocytosis, with new clonal cytogenetic abnormalities found in marrow cells.

The CML blast crisis phase marks the evolution to acute leukemia, in which marrow is replaced by 20% or more blasts, with accompanying loss of normal mature cellular elements in the marrow and periphery and extramedullary blast proliferation. Death occurs in a few weeks to months. Two thirds of patients develop AML, whereas the others develop acute lymphocytic (lymphoblastic) leukemia (ALL), a finding confirming that the initial neoplastic cell is an early stem cell capable of multilineage differentiation.

Treatment

Historically, oral chemotherapeutic agents such as hydroxyurea and busulfan were used to reduce myeloid cell numbers in patients during the chronic phase of CML. Although these drugs decreased the rate of acute disease complications, they did not alter the long-term prognosis or prevent progression to blast crises.

Treatment with interferon resulted in hematologic remissions in 60% to 80% of patients with chronic phase CML and was the first agent to induce cytogenetic responses in 20% to 30% of these patients. Achievement of cytogenetic remissions using interferon-α was associated with prolonged survival, and higher response rates were obtained by combining chemotherapy with interferon. Although most patients treated with interferon still possessed cells with a detectable BCR/ABL translocation by PCR and remained at risk for disease relapse, many remained in hematologic and cytogenetic remission for several years. Unfortunately, patients with accelerated or blast crisis CML did poorly with interferon, and high-dose chemotherapy regimens induced only transient responses, with durations of less than 6 months.

Imatinib mesylate (Gleevec, formerly known as STI-571) for the treatment of CML was heralded as the first successful targeted therapy for cancer. Imatinib is a rationally designed competitive inhibitor of multiple tyrosine kinases, including ABL, BCR/ABL, platelet-derived growth factor receptor (PDGFR), and KIT. Inhibition of phosphorylation of BCR/ABL results in blockade of downstream signaling and growth pathways and induces apoptosis of BCR/ABL-positive cells. Preclinical studies demonstrated that imatinib potently inhibited the growth of BCR/ABL-expressing CML cell lines and progenitor cells in vitro and prolonged survival in animal tumor models.

Initial clinical trials of this orally active drug were begun in 1998 in CML patients who had failed interferon-α. Imatinib was well tolerated and had manageable side effects., In the treatment arm, 96% of patients receiving a dose greater than 300 mg per day for 4 weeks achieved hematologic remissions, and 33% obtained cytogenetic remissions after 8 weeks. Imatinib was subsequently shown to be superior to interferon-α and cytarabine in untreated patients with newly diagnosed chronic phase CML and to induce complete cytogenetic responses in almost 90% of patients with chronic phase CML, with an estimated overall survival rate of 89%. Based on this study, imatinib was the first rationally designed biologically targeted drug approved for the treatment of cancer.

Despite these results, imatinib has not cured chronic phase CML. Similar to interferon-α treatment, most patients achieving cytogenetic responses on imatinib demonstrate persistence of BCR/ABL-positive leukemic CML stem cells by sensitive molecular testing. Lifelong imatinib therapy may be required to control disease, and even patients with excellent control of chronic phase CML on imatinib therapy remain at risk for eventual disease progression and therapy failure. It is estimated that up to one third of chronic phase CML patients initiated on imatinib therapy will eventually discontinue drug due to long-term intolerance of drug-induced side effects (e.g., nausea, vomiting, gastrointestinal issues, peripheral and periorbital edema) or development of imatinib resistance.

To address these issues, four newer tyrosine kinase inhibitors (TKIs) of BCR/ABL have been developed for the treatment of chronic phase CML: dasatinib (Sprycel), nilotinib (Tasigna), bosutinib (Bosulif), and ponatinib (Iclusig). All display increased in vitro potency against the BCR/ABL kinase compared with imatinib.

Imatinib, dasatinib, and nilotinib are approved for the initial therapy of chronic phase CML. After the diagnosis, patients are typically started on one of these three TKIs along with careful interim monitoring for toxicities and clinical response. Standardized RT-PCR assays for BCR/ABL are used to measure disease response on a molecular level at 3, 6, and 12 months after therapy initiation. In two randomized clinical trials comparing dasatinib with imatinib or nilotinib with imatinib in newly diagnosed CML patients, both second-generation TKIs outperformed imatinib, as reflected by significantly higher numbers of patients treated with these agents achieving complete cytogenetic and molecular responses at the specific time points compared with imatinib-treated individuals. However, whether these results translate into long-term overall survival benefit for either agent over imatinib remains to be seen.

CML patients resistant to or intolerant of first-line TKI therapy are usually switched to another agent. Up to one half of CML patients who develop resistance to imatinib have cancer cells carrying single-nucleotide mutations in the BCR/ABL gene. These mutations result in conformational changes of the BCR/ABL kinase, altering drug binding and inhibitory effects. For this reason, it is recommended that patients requiring second-line therapy or beyond undergo testing for identification of mutations as a potential guide to therapy. CML patients with disease associated with a mutation at T315I are known to be resistant to imatinib, nilotinib, dasatinib, and bosutinib, but not to ponatinib, a third-generation BCR/ABL inhibitor.

Omacetaxine mepesuccinate is a natural alkaloid product with proven antitumor activity and efficacy in CML patients failing multiple TKIs or carrying the T315I mutation, or both. Its mechanisms of action are distinct from the TKIs and involve inhibition of protein synthesis and induction of apoptosis in tumor cells. Several clinical trials have confirmed the activity of this agent in this patient population. A major drawback is the need for subcutaneous injections administered twice daily for 7 to 14 days of every 28 days per month.

Unfortunately, although treatment with the newer BCR/ABL inhibitors can induce transient hematologic and cytogenetic responses in patients with accelerated or blast phase CML, these responses are short lived. The treatment modality known to result in eradication of all detectable BCR/ABL-expressing cells remains allogeneic SCT. Before the advent of targeted BCR/ABL kinase inhibitor therapy, young patients with an HLA-matched donor were routinely offered potentially curative allogeneic bone marrow transplantation at the time of diagnosis of chronic phase CML. Evidence indicated that the excellent response (50% to 75%) of CML patients to SCT was partly related to the active suppression of the disease by the newly transplanted graft, called the *graft-versus-leukemia effect*.

In the face of the excellent control and low overall toxicity of long-term BCR/ABL inhibitors for chronic phase CML, together with the known 20% to 30% mortality and morbidity rates after SCT, transplantation is viewed as an option only for patients with accelerated or blast phase disease or chronic phase CML failing multiple lines of prior therapy. Transplantation remains the only known curative therapy for these patients. Blast phase CML patients often undergo induction chemotherapy with acute leukemia regimens followed by BCR/ABL inhibition and allogeneic SCT.

Prognosis

Overall, the transformation of CML from a progressively fatal cancer to one in which almost 90% of patients are alive with stable disease on oral kinase therapy after 5 years remains one of the crowning achievements in cancer therapy in the past decade. The median overall survival for chronic phase CML patients has risen dramatically from a few months to a few years in the first half of the 20th century to 6 years for interferon-treated patients. In the era of BCR/ABL inhibition therapy, it is expected to be almost normal for most patients on long-term TKI therapy.

The standard of care for CML patients who are responding optimally to treatment is to continue TKI therapy indefinitely. However, ongoing studies are examining the impact of discontinuing TKI in selected individuals whose disease has responded particularly well to therapy based on molecular criteria. Despite many therapeutic advances, a true cure for CML disease remains elusive and presents a therapeutic challenge for the years ahead.

ACUTE LEUKEMIAS
Definition and Epidemiology

The acute leukemias are clonal hematopoietic diseases that arise from the malignant transformation of an early hematopoietic stem cell. Leukemias occur in 8 to 10 of 100,000 people (compared with 42 of 100,000 for prostate cancer and 62 of 100,000 for breast cancer). Acute leukemias are classified by cell lineage as AML or ALL based on morphology, cytogenetics, cell surface and cytoplasmic markers, and molecular studies. Between 80% and 90% of adult leukemia diagnoses are AML (others are ALL), whereas most childhood leukemias are ALL (10% are AML).

Pathology

The pathogenesis of acute leukemia is under intense investigation. Many patients with acute leukemia have detectable characteristic clonal chromosomal abnormalities, but the role of all but a few of these aberrations in malignant transformation is unknown. Unregulated proliferation of immature cells incapable of further differentiation (i.e., blasts) results in marrow replacement and hematopoietic failure.

Known risk factors for leukemia are high-dose radiation exposure and occupational exposure to benzene. Patients with secondary AML after prior chemotherapy have usually received alkylating agents (e.g., chlorambucil, melphalan, nitrogen mustard) or topoisomerase II inhibitors (e.g., epipodophyllotoxins). Patients with chromosomal instability disorders such as Bloom's syndrome, Fanconi's anemia, Down syndrome, and ataxia telangiectasia also have an increased incidence of leukemia.

Diagnosis and Differential Diagnosis

The distinction between AML and ALL is crucial diagnostically, therapeutically, and prognostically. AML can be distinguished from ALL by cell morphology and the finding of Auer rods, which are formed by the aggregation of myeloid granules (E-Fig. 46-2). Further immunophenotyping of blast cells using cell surface antigens, cytochemistry, and immunohistochemistry confirms cells as having a myeloid or lymphoid origin (Table 46-7). Morphologic subgroups of ALL and AML were originally defined by the French-American-British (FAB) classification and then by the World Health Organization (WHO) classification, which incorporated newer biologic information (Table 46-8).

Clinical Presentation

Patients exhibit clinical evidence of bone marrow failure similar to other hematopoietic disorders. Complications of disease include anemia, infection, and bleeding from peripheral cytopenias. Proliferating blasts infiltrating the bone marrow may cause bone pain. Blasts also invade other organs and lead to peripheral, mediastinal, and abdominal lymphadenopathy, hepatosplenomegaly, skin infiltration, and meningeal involvement.

Treatment

Therapy for acute leukemias is divided into several stages. *Induction therapy* is directed at reducing the number of leukemic blasts to an undetectable level and restoring normal hematopoiesis (i.e.,

TABLE 46-7   LABORATORY AIDS TO DIFFERENTIATE AML FROM ALL

CHARACTERISTIC	AML	ALL
Morphology of blasts	Granules in cytoplasm Auer rods* Multiple nucleoli	Agranular basophilic cytoplasm Regular, folded nucleolus
FAB subclassification	L1-L3	M1-M7
Histochemistry	Myeloperoxidase positive	Myeloperoxidase negative, PAS positive
Cytoplasmic markers	—	TdT positive
Surface markers (% of cases)	—	B-cell markers (5%) T-cell markers (15-20%): CD2, CD3, or CD5 CALLA (50-65%): CD10
Cytogenetic and oncogenetic profile	M3: t(15;17) M5: t(9;11)	L3: t(8;14) Abnormal ALL: *BCR/ABL* fusion gene (Philadelphia translocation)

ALL, Acute lymphoblastic leukemia; AML, acute myeloblastic leukemia; CALLA, common acute lymphoblastic leukemia antigen; FAB, French-American-British classification system; PAS, periodic acid–Schiff stain; TdT, terminal deoxynucleotidyl transferase.

*Auer rods are a linear coalescence of cytoplasmic granules that stain pink with Wright's stain.

complete remission). At complete remission, however, significant subclinical disease persists, requiring further therapy.

Subsequent *consolidation therapy* involves continuing chemotherapy with the same agents to induce elimination of additional leukemic cells. With development of a wider range of effective agents, *intensification therapy* has been introduced. It involves the use of high-dose therapy with different non–cross-reactive drugs to eliminate cells with potential primary resistance to the induction regimen.

Maintenance therapy employs low-dose, intermittent chemotherapy given over a prolonged period to prevent subsequent disease relapse. The goal of therapy is to induce remission (>5% blasts in the bone marrow and recovery of normal peripheral blood counts).

Prognosis

Adverse clinical prognostic factors for AML and ALL are similar despite widely different treatment approaches. In both leukemias, cytogenetic abnormalities represent the best independent predictor of overall survival (Tables 46-9 and 46-10). Clinical factors that predict a poor outcome include age exceeding 35 years for ALL or 60 years for AML, secondary or therapy-related disease, antecedent hematologic disorder, high initial leukocyte count (50 to 100 × 10⁹/L), and prolonged time (>4 weeks) to achieve a response to initial treatment.

● ACUTE MYELOID LEUKEMIA
Definition and Epidemiology

AML represents a biologically heterogeneous group of neoplasms with widely divergent clinical outcomes. Long-term cure rates (survival >5 years) range from 5% to 60% after chemotherapy alone, with an overall cure rate of 20% to 30%. AML occurs primarily in older adults, with a median age at diagnosis of 65 years.

TABLE 46-8   FRENCH-AMERICAN-BRITISH AND WORLD HEALTH ORGANIZATION CLASSIFICATIONS OF ACUTE LEUKEMIA

FAB CLASSIFICATION OF ACUTE MYELOID LEUKEMIA (AML)

M0: Acute myelocytic leukemia with minimal differentiation
M1: Acute myelocytic leukemia without maturation
M2: Acute myelocytic leukemia with maturation (predominantly myeloblasts and promyelocytes)
M3: Acute promyelocytic leukemia
M4: Acute myelomonocytic leukemia
M5: Acute monocytic leukemia
M6: Erythroleukemia
M7: Megakaryocytic leukemia

FAB CLASSIFICATION OF ACUTE LYMPHOBLASTIC LEUKEMIA (ALL)

L1: Predominantly small cells (twice the size of normal lymphocyte), homogeneous population; childhood variant
L2: Larger than L1, more heterogenous population; adult variant
L3: Burkitt-like large cells, vacuolated abundant cytoplasm

WHO 2001 CLASSIFICATION OF ACUTE LEUKEMIA

I. AML
  A. AML with recurrent genetic abnormalities
    1. AML with t(8;21)(q22;q22)
    2. AML with abnormal bone marrow eosinophils, inv(16) (p13;q22) or t(16;16)(p13;q22); (CBFB/*MYH11*)
    3. Acute promyelocytic leukemia (AML with t[15;17][q22;q12] [PML/RARA]) and variants
    4. AML with 11q23 (MLL) abnormalities
  B. AML with multilineage dysplasia
  C. AML and MDS, therapy related, alkylating agent related, topoisomerase II inhibitor related
  D. AML not otherwise defined
    1. AML minimally differentiated
    2. AML without maturation
    3. AML with maturation
    4. Acute myelomonocytic leukemia
    5. Acute monoblastic and monocytic leukemia
    6. Acute erythroid leukemia
    7. Acute megakaryoblastic leukemia
    8. Acute basophilic leukemia
    9. Acute panmyelosis with myelofibrosis
    10. Myeloid sarcoma
  E. Acute leukemia of ambiguous lineage
    1. Undifferentiated acute leukemia
    2. Bilineal acute leukemia
    3. Biphenotypic acute leukemia
II. Acute lymphocytic leukemia
  A. Precursor B-lymphoblastic leukemia/lymphoblastic lymphoma
  B. Precursor T-lymphoblastic leukemia/lymphoblastic lymphoma

CBF, Core binding factor; ETO, eight twenty-one; FAB, French-American-British; MDS, primary myelodysplastic syndrome; MLL, mixed-lineage leukemia; *MYH11*, myosin heavy chain gene; PML, promyelocytic leukemia; RARA, retinoic acid receptor-α; WHO, World Health Organization.

TABLE 46-9   POOR PROGNOSTIC CLINICAL FACTORS IN ACUTE MYELOID LEUKEMIA

Age >60 yr (median age for acute myeloid leukemia, 65 yr)
Therapy related or with antecedent hematologic disorder (e.g., myelodysplastic syndrome, myeloproliferative neoplasm, aplastic anemia)
Poor performance status
White blood cell count >20,000-30,000/mm³
Extramedullary disease sites

Clinical Presentation

Patients most often have complications related to progressively severe cytopenia, such as infection due to leukopenia, shortness of breath or fatigue due to anemia, or bleeding due to thrombocytopenia. AML patients may also have unique acute clinical emergencies requiring immediate stabilization.

TABLE 46-10	PROGNOSTIC FACTORS IN ACUTE LYMPHOBLASTIC LEUKEMIA	
FACTOR	**FAVORABLE**	**UNFAVORABLE**
Age	2-10 yr	<2 yr or >10 yr
White blood cell count at diagnosis	<30,000/μL	>50,000/μL
Phenotype	Precursor B	Precursor T
Chromosome number	Hyperdiploidy	Pseudo/hypodiploidy, near tetraploidy
Chromosome abnormality	t(12;21)	MYC alterations: t(8;14), t(2;8), t(8;22) mixed-lineage leukemia alterations (11q23) Philadelphia chromosome: t(9;22), creating BCR-ABL
Central nervous system disease at diagnosis	No	Yes
Sex	Women	Men
Ethnicity	White	African American, Hispanic
Time to remission	Short (7-14 days)	Prolonged time to remission or failure to achieve remission

Leukostasis (i.e., hyperleukocytosis syndrome) caused by high levels of circulating blasts (>80,000 to 100,000) leads to diffuse pulmonary infiltrates and acute respiratory distress. Blast cells may also injure surrounding vasculature, causing life-threatening CNS bleeding and thromboses. High blast cell numbers result in the release of cellular breakdown products (i.e., tumor lysis syndrome), leading to hypokalemia, acidosis, and hyperuricemia with resultant renal failure.

Treatment of leukostasis should be instituted as soon as possible for all patients with white blood cell counts in excess of 100 to 200 $\times 10^9$/L. Treatment consists of leukapheresis, hydroxyurea, and initiation of induction chemotherapy to inhibit further production of circulating tumor cells. Hydration, urine alkalinization to reduce urine crystallization, allopurinol, or rasburicase, or a combination, should be initiated as indicated. Red blood cell transfusions are often contraindicated in patients with high numbers of circulating blast cells because of the risk of further increases in blood viscosity. CNS complications such as intracranial bleeding, cranial nerve invasion, and leukemic meningitis are treated with emergency whole brain irradiation or radiation directed to affected sites.

Laboratory evaluation of patients with AML typically shows white blood cell counts ranging from neutropenic levels (<1 × 10^9/L) to extreme leukocytosis (>100,000 × 10^9/L). Severe thrombocytopenia, normocytic anemia, and circulating peripheral blasts are common. Bone marrow aspirate and biopsy typically show a profusion of myeloblasts (20% to 100%) and depressed production of normal mature cells.

Diagnosis

Diagnostic marrow aspirates are typically evaluated using morphology, flow cytometry, cytogenetic, and molecular analyses to distinguish between AML and ALL and to determine AML disease subsets for therapeutic purposes. In the past, AML subsets were classified based largely on morphologic criteria and immunohistochemical staining as FAB subtypes M0 through M7, which are defined by the stage of cellular differentiation of the abnormal cells (see Table 46-8 and E-Fig. 46-3).

Some FAB subsets correlate with specific clinical syndromes, which helps to determine treatment approaches and prognosis. The most common FAB subtype of adult AML is M2. Patients with AML M3 (i.e., acute promyelocytic leukemia) often exhibit spontaneous bleeding from disseminated intravascular coagulation (discussed later). Patients with AML M4 or M5 disease (i.e., acute monocytic-myelomonocytic leukemias) have high levels of circulating white blood cells and may have swollen gums resulting from tissue infiltration with leukemic blasts. Patients with megakaryoblastic leukemia (AML M7) have significant marrow fibrosis and usually exhibit organomegaly and pancytopenia similar to those seen in patients with myelofibrosis and myeloid metaplasia.

In 2008, AML was reclassified as new subtypes defined primarily by unique karyotypic abnormalities—specifically t(8;21), inv(16), and t(15;17)—and gene mutations in a dysplastic bone marrow, independent of the number of marrow blasts. Because finding these specific cytogenetic abnormalities is crucial for the diagnosis, therapy, and prognosis for AML patients, karyotypic analysis is considered essential for any suspected AML diagnosis. Evidence of marrow dysplasia after prior chemotherapy, irradiation, or other myeloablative therapy is considered therapy-related AML rather than myelodysplastic syndrome (MDS), independent of the blast count (see Table 46-8).

Treatment and Prognosis

Chemotherapy for AML involves induction chemotherapy (administered in the inpatient setting) followed by two to four cycles of consolidation chemotherapy administered over 4 to 6 months. Standard induction regimens employing cytosine arabinoside (i.e., cytarabine) with high-dose anthracycline (i.e., daunorubicin or idarubicin) lead to complete remission in 60% to 80% of younger adults with de novo AML. Lower remission rates are achieved for older adults (>60 years) and in patients with antecedent hematologic diseases evolving into AML.

After achieving complete remission after induction, patients may be offered additional consolidation chemotherapy or treatment with allogeneic or autologous SCT (see Chapter 45). Patients whose AML fails to respond to initial induction therapy have a grim overall prognosis and may be retreated with experimental agents or with non–cross-reactive chemotherapy drugs such as epipodophyllotoxins, or both, to obtain remission.

Given the biologic heterogeneity of this disease, the AML risk category constitutes the most crucial determinant of an appropriate therapeutic strategy for individual patients. In the past, AML outcome could be predicted to some degree by clinical factors such as patient age, disease manifestation (i.e., white blood cell count), and history of antecedent hematologic or therapy-related disease (see Table 46-9). In the current era, AML risk is defined by diagnostic AML cytogenetics and molecular abnormalities and is typically divided into three categories: favorable, intermediate, and poor risk.

AML characterized by t(8;21), inv(16) or del(16q), or t(15;17) aberrations is unusually responsive to induction chemotherapy followed by two to four cycles of high-dose cytosine arabinoside consolidation. Long-term 5-year survival rates of 55% to 60% can be obtained.

AML subtypes associated with a poor prognosis include those with known deletions in chromosome 5 or 7, 11q23 aberrations other than t(9;11), inv(3q), t(3;3), t(6;9), t(9;22) (i.e., Philadelphia chromosome), monosomal karyotype, or three or more karyotypic abnormalities (i.e., complex karyotype). Remission rates for these AML subtypes are low; if remission is achieved, patients remain at high risk for AML relapse with chemotherapy-refractory disease. Overall survival rates for poor-prognosis AML are 5% to 15%.

The remaining AML patients have intermediate-risk cytogenetics, which is defined as a normal karyotype, trisomy 8, t(9;11), or other cytogenetic abnormalities not included in the other groups. These patients have a 30% to 45% long-term survival rate with standard chemotherapy (see Table 46-10).

Large-scale genomic analyses of AML samples have revealed the vast molecular complexity of this disease and identified myriad gene mutations capable of further refining AML prognosis in conjunction with karyotype. For instance, up to one third of patients with normal-karyotype AML have constitutive activation of the FMS-like tyrosine kinase 3 (FLT3) receptor as a result of point mutations or internal tandem duplications (ITDs) not seen on routine karyotypic testing) in FLT3 kinase. FLT3 ITDs in AML patients predict low remission rates, high relapse rates, and shorter overall survival compared with FLT3-negative AML patients. Mutations that predict improved overall survival after chemotherapy include biallelic mutations in the transcription factor CCAAT/enhancer binding protein-α (CEBPA) and nucleophosmin 1 (NPM1) in the absence of FLT3 ITDs (Table 46-11).

After remission is achieved after induction, AML patients are offered additional therapy in the form of consolidation chemotherapy and autologous or allogeneic SCT. Decisions about the best time to perform SCT in patients are most often guided by clinical risk factors and prognostic risk category (see Tables 46-9 and 46-10). Although clinical outcomes are improved when patients undergo SCT after initial induction chemotherapy (i.e., during the first complete remission) rather than after disease relapse, chemotherapeutic regimens are also more effective in the first remission than they are after transplantation, and they may be better tolerated than SCT, which carries an overall mortality rate of 25% to 30%.

Allogeneic SCT is recommended for and represents the best chance for long-term cure of patients with poor-risk AML such as disease associated with unfavorable cytogenetic and molecular features, antecedent hematologic disease, or therapy-related or primary refractory disease. Poor-risk AML patients younger than 60 years undergoing allogeneic bone marrow transplantation from a matched donor have long-term overall survival rates of 40% to 60%, compared with cure rates after conventional chemotherapy of only 5% to 20%. AML patients with favorable disease features potentially responsive to high-dose cytarabine chemotherapy are encouraged to delay SCT until the time of relapse.

Intermediate- to high-risk AML patients (based on clinical or cytogenetic data) who are ineligible for allogeneic transplantation because of advanced age, other medical issues, or lack of HLA-compatible donors may be offered chemotherapy or autologous SCT instead. Whether autologous transplantation improves AML outcomes compared with chemotherapy alone is a matter of debate. However, the long-term survival rates after autologous transplantation range from 20% to 40% and are at least equivalent to consolidation chemotherapy regimens for these patients.

Because the median age at diagnosis of AML is 65 years, a sizable proportion of AML patients are elderly individuals with major comorbidities or antecedent hematologic or malignant diseases, rendering them poor candidates for standard induction chemotherapeutic regimens or myeloablative SCT. Infectious complications remain the major cause of morbidity and mortality during intensive inpatient chemotherapy despite advances in prophylactic growth factor support, antibiotics, and antifungal agents. The low expected remission rates (30% to 50%) and high mortality and morbidity rates associated with induction are additional reasons for many patients to decline aggressive therapy. For these patients, therapeutic options include supportive therapy with hydroxyurea, transfusion support alone, and hospice.

Patients unfit for and those who choose not to receive intensive therapy are increasingly being treated with low-dose chemotherapy regimens. Low-dose subcutaneous cytarabine is associated with remission rates of about 18%. Alternatively, hypomethylating agents (e.g., 5-azacytidine, decitabine) have been well tolerated in older AML patients and result in complete remission rates ranging from 20% to 47% in some studies. Individuals treated with these drugs also experience hematologic improvement and disease stabilization associated with prolonged overall survival, even in absence of complete remissions.

AML patients with relapsed or refractory disease after standard therapy should be considered for allogeneic SCT and clinical trials. Experimental therapies for AML, particularly nonmyeloablative SCT (see Chapter 45), have resulted in durable long-term remissions in a proportion of older AML patients and should be pursued based on patient preference, overall health status, and availability of an appropriate HLA-matched donor.

TABLE 46-11	PROGNOSIS OF ACUTE MYELOID LEUKEMIA BASED ON CYTOGENETIC AND MOLECULAR ABNORMALITIES	
RISK STATUS	CYTOGENETICS	MOLECULAR ABNORMALITIES
Favorable	inv(16) or t(16;16) t(8;21), t(15;17)	Normal cytogenetics: *NPM1* mutation in the absence of *FLT3* ITDs or isolated biallelic *CEBPA* mutation
Intermediate	Normal cytogenetics +8 alone, t(9;11) Other undefined	t(8;21), inv(16), or t(16;16) in the presence of *KIT* mutation
Poor	Complex (≥3 aberrations) Monosomal karyotype −5, 5q−, −7, 7q− 11q23: non-t(9;11) inv(3), t(3;3), t(6;9), t(9;22)	Normal karyotype with *FLT3* ITDs

ITDs, Internal tandem duplications.

There has been much interest in the clinical development of TKIs blocking mutant FLT3 signaling pathways for the treatment of FLT3 mutant AML, similar to BCR/ABL inhibitors in CML. The most effective FLT3 inhibitor, AC220 (quizartinib), resulted in a composite complete remission rate of approximately 50% in relapsed or refractory FLT3 ITD mutant AML in the phase II setting. However, multiple signaling pathways in AML cells and rapid proliferation of AML clones likely contribute to the rapid development of drug resistance. The results of additional studies examining the efficacy of FLT3 inhibitors combined with chemotherapy for relapsed and newly diagnosed FLT3-positive AML patients are eagerly awaited.

● ACUTE PROMYELOCYTIC LEUKEMIA

Definition, Epidemiology, and Pathology

Acute promyelocytic leukemia (APL), formerly known as the FAB M3 subtype of AML (see Table 46-8), is a rare malignancy that represents 10% to 15% of adult AML. The incidence is increased among younger patients (median age, 40 years). The annual incidence in the United States ranges from 600 to 800 cases.

APL is different from other acute leukemias because of its unique disease biology. Morphologically, APL blasts are distinctive immature promyelocytic cells containing large granules and typically high numbers of Auer rods diagnostic of AML. APL is characterized by a chromosomal translocation—t(15;17) (q22;q12)—involving the promyelocytic leukemia gene (PML) on chromosome 15 and the retinoic acid receptor-α gene (RARA) on chromosome 17. Sequestration of the resulting PML/RARA fusion protein with other proteins produces a complex that represses the gene transcription essential for granulocytic differentiation, effectively arresting differentiation of leukemia cells at the promyelocytic stage.

Clinical Presentation

Clinically, patients with APL often exhibit life-threatening bleeding caused by disseminated intravascular coagulation related to high levels of procoagulant factors released from APL granules. Bleeding complications in the CNS and other sites can be rapidly fatal if the disease is not recognized and treated as a medical emergency. All patients suspected of having APL should be started empirically with all-*trans*-retinoic acid (ATRA) therapy (discussed later) and treated aggressively with transfusions of fresh-frozen plasma, fibrinogen, and platelets until resolution of coagulopathy and disease confirmation.

Unlike patients with other AML subsets, APL patients typically have cytopenias rather than leukocytosis. High-risk APL patients are defined as those with white blood cell counts greater than 10×10^9/L.

Treatment and Prognosis

Treated appropriately, APL is the most curable acute leukemia in adults. The centerpiece of APL treatment is the use of agents that induce the terminal differentiation of leukemic promyelocytes followed by senescence and spontaneous apoptosis. ATRA is an oral derivative of vitamin A shown to overcome growth arrest and permit differentiation of immature APL blast cells into neutrophils by altering the configuration of PML/RARA to allow normal gene transcription.

Patients initiated on ATRA must be closely observed for development of retinoic acid or APL differentiation syndrome, which is life-threatening acute cardiopulmonary distress characterized by bilateral pulmonary effusions and infiltrates. This serositis-like disorder is attributed to adhesion of differentiating neoplastic cells to the pulmonary vasculature and carries a 5% to 10% mortality rate. Treatment consists of early initiation of corticosteroids and aggressive diuresis. In severe cases, ATRA should be temporarily withheld.

Although ATRA alone induces clinical remissions in up to 90% of patients with APL, high relapse rates observed after monotherapy led to the practice of combining ATRA with anthracycline with or without cytarabine chemotherapy in initial induction regimens. Using this approach, complete remission rates for APL rose to between 90% and 95%, and more than two thirds of patients with APL treated with standard ATRA-containing induction, consolidation, and maintenance chemotherapy regimens achieved long-term remission.

Relapsed APL patients were treated with arsenic trioxide, a naturally occurring compound used both as a poison and a drug in many countries. Low-dose arsenic therapy promotes APL cell differentiation and apoptosis and induces remission rates in up to 90% of relapsed APL cases. APL differentiation syndrome and prolongation of the QT interval are common side effects of arsenic therapy. Based on its tolerability and non-overlapping cytotoxicities with conventional cytotoxic drugs, arsenic was successfully used for consolidation therapy in APL patients and improved clinical outcomes.

Although highly effective, combination ATRA and chemotherapy regimens for newly diagnosed APL patients were associated with an overall mortality rate of 10% to 20% during the first month of treatment. Most deaths resulted from uncontrolled hemorrhage, differentiation syndrome, and complications of prolonged myelosuppression after cytotoxic therapy, particularly in older individuals. To address these concerns, a phase III trial randomized lower-risk APL patients to dual-differentiation therapy with ATRA and arsenic only (without cytotoxic chemotherapy) or to standard ATRA and chemotherapy during induction and consolidation. The trial results demonstrated that ATRA plus arsenic treatment was not inferior to ATRA plus chemotherapy and was not associated with increased toxicity.

The trial results led to establishment of differentiation therapy alone as the standard of care for lower-risk APL patients. Patients with residual PML/RARA-positive cells after standard induction and consolidation therapy containing ATRA and arsenic should be considered for autologous or allogeneic SCT.

● ACUTE LYMPHOBLASTIC LEUKEMIA

Definition, Epidemiology, and Pathology

ALL is a neoplasm of immature lymphoblasts expressing markers of B-cell or T-cell lineage. ALL is predominantly a pediatric malignancy, with most cases occurring in children younger than 6 years. The prior FAB classification system divided ALL into three subtypes (i.e., L1, L2, and L3) based on the morphology of malignant cells (E-Fig. 46-3). The WHO system reclassified the disease as precursor B-cell or T-cell ALL based on the lineage of specific cell surface antigens found on these cells during normal maturation (see Table 46-7). T-cell ALL represents 15% to 25% of ALL diagnoses. More than 50% of T-cell ALL cases have activating mutations in NOTCH1, a key regulator of T-cell fate. One third of adult and 20% of pediatric B-cell ALL cases are associated with detection of the Philadelphia chromosome, t(9;22).

Clinical Presentation

Clinical and biologic features, particularly cytogenetics, at diagnosis have been identified as important prognostic factors (see Table 46-10).

Treatment

Treatment of ALL is lengthy and involves multiple chemotherapeutic agents given over 2 to 3 years. Induction chemotherapy typically includes vincristine, corticosteroids, and L-asparaginase with the addition of an anthracycline, cytarabine, or cyclophosphamide (or a combination) for adult patients. Given the propensity of ALL cells to reside in the CNS and testes (so-called sanctuaries for leukemia cells because standard systemic chemotherapy does not penetrate into these sites), most ALL patients undergo lumbar puncture at the time of diagnosis, followed by routine administration of intrathecal methotrexate or whole brain irradiation, or both, as a necessary adjunct to systemic induction and consolidation chemotherapy. Complete remission rates are 97% to 99% for children and 75% to 90% for adults.

After normal hematopoiesis returns, patients undergo consolidation and intensification therapy with multiple drugs to eradicate disease. For unknown reasons, ALL tends to relapse several months to years after initial remission. Studies have shown that the frequency of relapse is reduced by maintenance chemotherapy given for 2 to 3 years after initial remission achievement. Prolonged treatment may eliminate slow-growing leukemic clones, prevent further transformation, or destroy occult disease in other sites, particularly the CNS.

Progress in the understanding and treatment of this disease in the 1990s led to cure rates of up to 90% for children with ALL. Despite this success, only 20% to 40% of adult patients with ALL achieve cure. The poorer outcomes for adults are attributed to differences in the biologic mechanisms of disease in the different age groups and the inability of older patients to tolerate the intensive chemotherapy or transplantation procedures required to achieve long-term responses. Moreover, Philadelphia chromosome–expressing ALL, which is much more common in older individuals, is notoriously chemoresistant, has an increased risk of CNS involvement, and has an overall 5-year survival rate of less than 10%. Patients with Philadelphia chromosome–positive ALL routinely receive therapy with the oral BCR/ABL TKIs (i.e., imatinib and dasatinib) used in CML in addition to conventional chemotherapy. High-risk young patients with B-cell ALL may benefit from anti-CD20 antibodies (i.e., rituximab) directed against B-cell antigens on abnormal lymphoblasts.

In ALL, as in AML, the worse the prognosis, the earlier transplantation should be offered. Studies have shown that high-risk ALL patients (i.e., as older patients, Philadelphia chromosome–positive disease, high white blood cell count at presentation, or prolonged time to first remission) clearly benefit from SCT, preferably from an HLA-matched sibling, during the first remission. Early transplantation in adults has achieved 5-year survival rates of 40% to 44%, compared with 20% with other therapies.

Unfortunately, outcomes for high-risk ALL patients without an available HLA-matched donor are poor, and these individuals should pursue HLA-matched unrelated donor allogeneic SCT or experimental therapies. No significant benefit has been seen with autologous transplantation over standard chemotherapy for these patients. Standard-risk ALL patients, particularly pediatric patients, with high long-term remission rates after conventional chemotherapy and maintenance need not undergo allogeneic SCT unless disease recurs.

Most ALL relapses arise within 2 years of the initial diagnosis, with recurrence of leukemic cells in the bone marrow, CNS, or testes. Although relapsed disease may respond to further chemotherapy and local irradiation, the duration of second remissions is usually less than 6 months. All patients with relapsed ALL should be considered for allogeneic SCT (which represents the only known cure for disease) or experimental treatment. Autologous SCT for refractory or relapsed ALL is not routinely recommended because ALL blasts appear to be more chemoresistant, and failure rates after treatment are higher.

For relapsed ALL patients not eligible for SCT, several novel therapeutic approaches are available. The newest BCR/ABL inhibitor, ponatinib, is being investigated in combination with chemotherapy for Philadelphia chromosome–positive ALL. Toxin-containing antibodies targeting the B-cell markers CD19 and CD52 in relapsed ALL patients are also being explored. Marqibo, a liposomal formulation of vincristine and a standard chemotherapy drug used in initial ALL therapy, has induced clinical responses in 35% of refractory or relapsed ALL patients as a single agent with tolerable toxicities.

Perhaps the most exciting strategies for ALL therapy involve technologies specifically exploiting patient host immune responses to affect long-term cure. Blinatumomab (BiTE) is a bispecific single-chain antibody that binds the T-cell receptor CD3 on T cells and the B-cell antigen CD19 expressed by malignant lymphoblasts. Dual binding of CD3 and CD19 by BiTE brings reactive T cells close to tumor cells, redirects T cell lysis, and eliminates disease. Administration of BiTE to ALL patients in clinical remission but with evidence of minimal residual disease after standard chemotherapy resulted in eradication of detectable persistent disease in 76% of patients. Ongoing trials evaluating BiTE in relapsed or refractory ALL patients with much higher tumor burdens and in combination with chemotherapy regimens are ongoing.

An alternative approach has been to genetically modify autologous T cells from ALL patients with CD19-expressing chimeric antigen receptors, effectively reprogramming them to recognize and destroy CD19-expressing tumor cells. Reinfusion of these cells after lymphodepleting chemotherapy resulted in the complete eradication of ALL disease in 80% to 90% of individuals and some long-term disease control alone and when followed by SCT. Whether these engineered T-cell strategies will be broadly applicable for most patients with ALL outside of clinical trials at major academic centers remains to be determined.

⬤ PROSPECTUS FOR THE FUTURE

Molecular understanding of the pathogenesis of MPNs and acute leukemia is progressing rapidly. It is already promoting development of novel therapeutic approaches that promise to transform the clinical approach to these diseases in the coming years.

Myeloproliferative Disease

The importance of the spectacular success of imatinib as targeted therapy for CML cannot be overstated. As the first successful therapy based on an understanding of pathogenesis, imatinib has become emblematic of the translation of an understanding of disease pathogenesis into tangible innovations in clinical care. Because second- and third-generation TKIs with activity against imatinib-resistant CML are available, SCT is now only rarely offered to patients with CML.

Similarly, the discovery of JAK2 mutations in non-CML myeloproliferative diseases opened new avenues for targeted intervention in diseases for which previous therapy was largely supportive. Treatment with the JAK2 inhibitor, ruxolitinib, has decreased splenomegaly and improved constitutional symptoms in higher-risk myelofibrosis patients independent of JAK2 mutation status. Moreover, provocative results demonstrating that ruxolitinib potentially prolongs overall survival and reduces marrow fibrosis in myelofibrosis patients offer hope that JAK2 inhibitors, like BCR/ABL inhibitors in CML, may eventually alter the natural history of disease.

Acute Leukemia

An understanding of the molecular pathogenesis of acute leukemia has led to important therapeutic advances in the treatment of disease. The discovery of the link between the retinoic acid receptor and the origins of APL provided important insights into the unique sensitivity of this disease to ATRA therapy and paved the road for successful implementation of dual differentiation therapy with ATRA and arsenic. This regimen marks the first time that any acute leukemia can be cured without cytotoxic chemotherapy or SCT.

Oral BCR/ABL kinase inhibitors have become a routine part of the treatment of Philadelphia chromosome–positive ALL. Advances in novel immunotherapeutic approaches that effectively reprogram host T cells to seek out and destroy ALL cells in patients have begun to prove their worth in the clinic and await further clinical validation.

In AML, identification of FLT3 kinase mutations in normal-karyotype AML has led to ongoing clinical trials of targeted inhibitors of this pathway in newly diagnosed and relapsed patients and offer hope for this subset of patients, who historically respond poorly to standard chemotherapy. Similar approaches may soon provide therapeutic entry points into the treatment of other acute leukemias associated with pathognomonic chromosomal translocations and genetic and molecular aberrations. Development of low-dose chemotherapy and reduced intensity SCT strategies has allowed older AML patients the opportunity to live longer and, in some cases, to be cured of their disease.

SUGGESTED READINGS

Aifantis I, Raetz E, Buonamici S: Molecular pathogenesis of T-cell leukemia and lymphoma, Nat Rev Immunol 8:380–390, 2008.

Baxter EJ, Scott LM, Campbell PJ, et al: Acquired mutation of the tyrosine kinase JAK2 in human myeloproliferative disorders, Lancet 365:1054–1061, 2005.

Byrd J, Mrozek K, Dodge R, et al: Pretreatment cytogenetic abnormalities are predictive of induction success, cumulative incidence of relapse, and overall survival in adult patients with de novo acute myeloid leukemia, Blood 100:4325–4336, 2002.

Harrison CN, Campbell PJ, Buck G, et al: Hydroxyurea compared with anagrelide in high-risk essential thrombocythemia, N Engl J Med 353:33–45, 2005.

Landolfi R, Marchioli R, Kutti J, et al: Efficacy and safety of low-dose aspirin in polycythemia vera, N Engl J Med 350:114–124, 2004.

Maziarz RT: Who with chronic myelogenous leukemia to transplant in the era of tyrosine kinase inhibitors?, Curr Opin Hematol 15:127–133, 2008.

Pullarkat V, Slovak ML, Kopecky KJ, et al: Impact of cytogenetics on the outcome of adult acute lymphocytic leukemia: results of the Southwest Oncology Group 9400 study, Blood 111:2563–2572, 2008.

Tefferi A, Vardiman JW: Classification and diagnosis of myeloproliferative neoplasms: the 2008 World Health Organization criteria and point-of-care diagnostic algorithms, Leukemia 22:14–22, 2008.

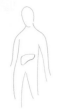

47

Disorders of Red Blood Cells

Michal G. Rose and Nancy Berliner

NORMAL RED BLOOD CELL STRUCTURE AND FUNCTION

The red blood cells (RBCs), or erythrocytes, deliver oxygen to all the tissues in the body and carry carbon dioxide back to the lungs for excretion. The erythrocyte is uniquely adapted to these functions. It has a biconcave disk shape that maximizes the membrane surface area for gas exchange, and it has a cytoskeleton and membrane structure that allow it to deform sufficiently to pass through the microvasculature. Passage through capillaries whose diameter may be one fourth the resting diameter of the erythrocyte is made possible by interactions between proteins in the membrane (band 3 and glycophorin) and underlying cytoplasmic proteins that make up the erythrocyte cytoskeleton (spectrin, ankyrin, and protein 4.1).

The mature RBC contains no nucleus and is dependent throughout its life span on proteins synthesized before extrusion of the nucleus and release of the cell from the bone marrow into the peripheral circulation. About 98% of the cytoplasmic protein of the mature erythrocyte is hemoglobin. The remainder is mainly enzymatic proteins, such as those required for anaerobic metabolism and the hexose monophosphate shunt.

Defects in any of the intrinsic structural features of the erythrocyte can result in hemolytic anemia. Abnormalities of the membrane or cytoskeletal proteins are the causes of alterations in erythrocyte shape and flexibility. Inborn defects in the enzymatic pathways for glucose metabolism decrease the resistance to oxidant stress, and inherited abnormalities of hemoglobin structure and synthesis lead to polymerization of abnormal hemoglobin (sickle cell disease) or to the precipitation of unbalanced hemoglobin chains (thalassemia). All of these changes result in decreased erythrocyte survival.

Oxygen is transported by hemoglobin, a tetramer composed of two α chains, two β-like (β, γ, or δ) chains, and four heme molecules, each of which is composed of a protoporphyrin molecule complexed with iron. In fetal life, the main hemoglobin is fetal hemoglobin (HbF: α_2, γ_2); the switch from HbF to adult hemoglobin (HbA: $\alpha_2\beta_2$) occurs in the perinatal period. By 4 to 6 months of age, the level of HbF has fallen to about 1% of total hemoglobin. HbA$_2$ ($\alpha_2\delta_2$) is a minor adult hemoglobin, representing about 1% of adult hemoglobin (Table 47-1).

CLINICAL PRESENTATION

Anemia, defined as a reduction in RBC mass, is an important sign of disease. It may reflect decreased production of erythrocytes that reflects nutritional deficiencies, primary hematologic disease, or a response to systemic illness. Alternatively, anemia may reflect increased blood loss or cellular destruction from hemolysis. Hemolysis may occur as a result of intrinsic abnormalities of the RBC, immune-mediated RBC destruction, or a systemic vascular process. The investigation of anemia is a critical component of the evaluation of the patient and commonly provides valuable insight into systemic illness. Figure 47-1 provides an overview of the differential diagnosis of anemia.

The symptoms of anemia reflect both the severity and the rapidity with which the reduction in erythrocyte mass has occurred. Patients with acute hemorrhage or massive hemolysis may exhibit symptoms of hypovolemic shock. However, most patients develop anemia more slowly and have few symptoms. Usual complaints are fatigue, decreased exercise tolerance, dyspnea, and palpitations. In patients with coronary artery disease, anemia may precipitate angina. On physical examination, the major sign of anemia is pallor. Patients may be tachycardic and often have audible flow murmurs. Patients with hemolysis often exhibit jaundice and splenomegaly.

LABORATORY EVALUATION

The key components of the laboratory evaluation of anemia are the reticulocyte count, the peripheral blood smear, erythrocyte indices, nutritional studies, and the bone marrow aspirate and biopsy.

The *reticulocyte count* allows the critical distinction between anemia arising from a primary failure of RBC production and anemia resulting from increased RBC destruction or bleeding. Erythrocytes newly released from the marrow still contain small amounts of RNA; these cells, termed *reticulocytes,* can be detected with the use of automated counters and fluorescent nucleic acid–binding dyes or manually by staining of the peripheral blood smear with methylene blue or other supravital stains. In response to the stress of anemia, erythropoietin (EPO) production increases, promoting the production and release of increased numbers of reticulocytes. The number of reticulocytes in the

TABLE 47-1	STRUCTURE AND DISTRIBUTION OF HUMAN HEMOGLOBINS	
NAME OF HEMOGLOBIN (Hb)	**DISTRIBUTION**	**STRUCTURE**
A	95-98% of adult Hb	$\alpha_2\beta_2$
A$_2$	1.5-3.5% of adult Hb	$\alpha_2\delta_2$
F	Fetal, 0.5-1.0% of adult Hb	$\alpha_2\gamma_2$
Gower 1	Embryonic	$\zeta_2\varepsilon_2$
Gower 2	Embryonic	$\alpha_2\varepsilon_2$
Portland	Embryonic	$\zeta_2\gamma_2$

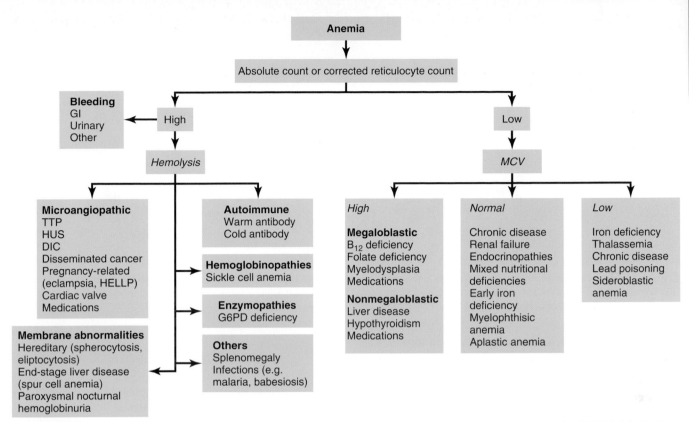

FIGURE 47-1 Overview of the differential diagnosis of anemia. DIC, Disseminated intravascular coagulation; G6PD, glucose-6-phosphate dehydrogenase; GI, gastrointestinal; HELLP, hemolysis, elevated liver enzyme levels, and low platelet count; HUS, hemolytic-uremic syndrome; MCV, mean corpuscular volume; TTP, thrombotic thrombocytopenic purpura.

peripheral blood therefore reflects the response of the bone marrow to anemia.

The reticulocyte count can be expressed either as a percentage of the total number of RBCs or as an absolute number. In patients without anemia, the normal reticulocyte count is 0.5% to 1.5% of RBCs or 20,000 to 75,000/µL. When the anemia is caused by decreased RBC survival, the appropriate marrow response results in a reticulocyte count greater than 2%, with an absolute count of more than 100,000/µL. If the reticulocyte count is not elevated, a cause of failure of RBC production should be sought. Reticulocyte counts that are expressed as a percentage of total RBCs must be corrected for anemia because decreasing the number of circulating cells increases the reticulocyte percentage without any increase in release from the marrow. The *corrected reticulocyte count* is calculated by multiplying the reticulocyte count by the ratio of the patient's hematocrit to a normal hematocrit. The advantage of using the absolute reticulocyte count is that this correction is not necessary.

Evaluation of the *peripheral blood smear* may provide important clues to the cause of anemia. Erythrocyte morphologic examination is especially critical in the evaluation of anemia associated with reticulocytosis, wherein an examination of the smear is essential to distinguish between immune hemolysis (which results in spherocytes) and microangiopathic hemolysis (which causes schistocytes or erythrocyte fragmentation). Changes associated with other causes of anemia include sickle and target cells that are characteristic of hemoglobinopathies, teardrop cells

and nucleated RBCs associated with myelofibrosis and marrow infiltration, intracorpuscular parasites in malaria and babesiosis, and pencil-shaped deformities associated with severe iron deficiency. Examination of myeloid cells and platelets may also be helpful. Hypersegmented neutrophils and large platelets support the diagnosis of megaloblastic anemia, and the presence of immature blast forms may be diagnostic of leukemia. Figure 47-2 presents some common peripheral blood smear findings in patients with anemia.

In patients with anemia and an elevated reticulocyte count, the vigorous production of new erythroid cells suggests that marrow function is normal and is responding appropriately to the stress of the anemia. Bone marrow examination in this situation is rarely indicated because the marrow will simply show erythroid hyperplasia, usually without revealing any primary pathologic anomaly of the marrow. Evaluation in these cases should be focused on determining whether the cause of RBC consumption is bleeding or hemolysis. In contrast, bone marrow examination is often required for the evaluation of hypoproliferative anemia. After common abnormalities such as iron deficiency and other nutritional deficiencies have been ruled out, marrow aspiration and biopsy are indicated to search for abnormalities such as marrow infiltration, marrow involvement with granulomatous disease, marrow aplasia, or myelodysplasia.

The *mean corpuscular volume* (MCV) is an extremely helpful tool in the diagnosis of anemia with a low reticulocyte count (hypoproliferative anemia). The size of the RBCs (measured in femtoliters per cell) is used to characterize the anemia as

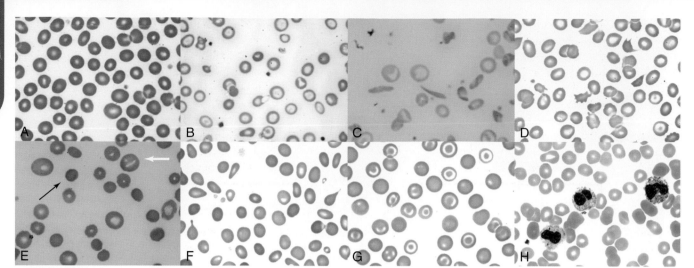

FIGURE 47-2 Peripheral blood smears in patients with anemia. **A,** Normal red blood cells. **B,** Iron deficiency anemia. **C,** Sickle cell anemia. **D,** Microangiopathic hemolytic anemia. **E,** Spherocytosis *(black arrow)* and reticulocytosis *(white arrow)* in autoimmune hemolytic anemia. **F,** Teardrops in myelofibrosis. **G,** Target cells. **H,** Pseudo-Pelger-Huet anomaly in myelodysplasia.

microcytic (MCV <80), normocytic (MCV 80 to 100), or macrocytic (MCV >100).

● EVALUATION OF HYPOPROLIFERATIVE ANEMIAS

Microcytic Anemias

The differential diagnosis of microcytic anemia is outlined in Table 47-2. Microcytosis and hypochromia are the hallmarks of anemias caused by defects in hemoglobin synthesis, which can reflect either failure of heme synthesis or abnormalities in globin production. The leading cause of microcytic anemia is iron deficiency, in which lack of heme synthesis results from the absence of iron to incorporate into the porphyrin ring (see later discussion). Up to 30% of patients with anemia of chronic inflammation have microcytosis. Lead poisoning blocks the incorporation of iron into heme, also resulting in a microcytic anemia.

Sideroblastic anemias arise from failure to synthesize the porphyrin ring, usually as a result of inhibition of the heme synthetic pathway enzymes. Congenital sideroblastic anemia may respond to pyridoxine, a cofactor for several of the heme synthetic pathway enzymes. A more common cause of acquired sideroblastic anemia is alcohol abuse; ethanol inhibits most of the enzymes in the heme synthetic pathway. Failure of globin synthesis occurs in thalassemic syndromes (see Hemolgobinopathies). All these disorders lead to decreased mean corpuscular hemoglobin concentration, resulting in hypochromia and a decrease in RBC size (i.e., low MCV).

Iron Deficiency Anemia

Iron deficiency is the leading cause of anemia worldwide. Although the presentation of classic iron deficiency anemia is linked with a microcytic anemia, early iron deficiency is associated with a normocytic anemia. Consequently, iron deficiency should be considered in all patients with anemia, and iron indices should be a part of the evaluation of any patient with hypoproductive anemia, regardless of the MCV.

Iron is acquired in the diet from heme sources (i.e., meat) and from nonheme sources (e.g., vegetables such as spinach). Iron

TABLE 47-2	DIFFERENTIAL DIAGNOSIS OF ANEMIA WITH LOW RETICULOCYTE COUNT
MICROCYTIC ANEMIA (MCV <80 fL/cell)	**Nonmegaloblastic Macrocytosis**
Iron deficiency	Liver disease
Thalassemia minor	Hypothyroidism
Anemia of chronic inflammation	Reticulocytosis
Sideroblastic anemia	**NORMOCYTIC ANEMIA (MCV 80-100 fL/cell)**
Lead poisoning	
MACROCYTIC ANEMIA (MCV >100 fL/cell)	Early iron deficiency
	Aplastic anemia
Megaloblastic Anemias	Myelophthisic disorders
	Endocrinopathies
Folate deficiency	Anemia of chronic inflammation
Vitamin B_{12} deficiency	Anemia of renal failure
Drug-induced megaloblastic anemia	Mixed nutritional deficiency
Myelodysplasia	

MCV, Mean corpuscular volume.

from heme is better absorbed than nonheme iron. Iron absorption is increased in iron deficiency, hypoxia, ineffective erythropoiesis, and hereditary hemochromatosis (most commonly caused by mutations in the *HFE* gene). Iron is absorbed from the proximal small intestine; it is transported in the cell bound to ferroportin and through the plasma bound to transferrin. Its uptake into the RBC precursors is mediated through the transferrin receptor. Iron absorption from the intestine is further regulated by hepcidin (see Anemia of Chronic Inflammation). Iron outside hemoglobin-producing cells is stored in ferritin. Men and women have total-body iron concentrations of 50 mg/kg and 40 mg/kg, respectively. Between 60% and 75% of the iron is found in hemoglobin. A small amount (2 mg/kg) is found in heme and nonheme enzymes, and 5 mg/kg is found in myoglobin. The remainder is stored in ferritin, which resides primarily in liver, bone marrow, spleen, and muscle. The capacity for excreting iron is limited, and iron overload occurs in patients with excessive absorption from the gastrointestinal tract (as a result of ineffective erythropoiesis or congenital hemochromatosis) and in those with chronic transfusions. Iron overload leads to increased iron deposition in these tissues and secondary deposition in endocrine organs, resulting in liver dysfunction, diabetes, and other endocrine abnormalities.

The most frequent cause of iron deficiency is occult blood loss. All men and postmenopausal women who are found to be iron deficient should have an evaluation for a source of gastrointestinal blood loss, regardless of the detection of occult blood. In premenopausal women, iron deficiency is most frequently related to loss of iron with menstruation (about 15 mg per month) and during pregnancy (about 900 mg per pregnancy). *Helicobacter pylori* infection can cause iron deficiency even in the absence of intestinal bleeding. Dietary deficiency of iron is most commonly seen in multiparous women of childbearing age, in young children whose growth outstrips their intake of iron, and in babies who drink mostly milk at the expense of an intake of iron-containing foods.

Laboratory Evaluation

As previously stated, early iron deficiency does not exhibit the hallmark microcytosis and hypochromia that characterize classic iron deficiency. Evaluation of the blood smear in advanced iron deficiency often demonstrates hypochromic RBCs, target cells, and pencil-shaped elongated cells. Iron deficiency is frequently associated with reactive thrombocytosis.

The mainstay of the diagnosis of iron deficiency is the peripheral blood iron indices. These include iron concentration, total iron-binding capacity (TIBC), transferrin saturation, and ferritin concentration. The transferrin saturation is the ratio of serum iron to transferrin concentration; it is normally at least 20%. Iron deficiency results in a decrease in serum iron and an increase in iron-binding capacity, decreasing this ratio to less than 10%. Chronic inflammatory conditions (e.g., infection, inflammation, malignancy) often decrease both iron and TIBC, but the transferrin saturation usually remains above 20%. The ferritin level is a reflection of total-body iron stores. The liver synthesizes ferritin in proportion to total-body iron, and a level of less than 12 ng/mL strongly supports a diagnosis of iron deficiency. Unfortunately, ferritin is an acute phase reactant, and levels rise in the setting of fever, inflammatory disease, infection, or other stresses. However, ferritin levels in response to stress do not often rise above 100 ng/mL, and levels higher than 100 ng/mL usually rule out iron deficiency.

If the indirect measurement of iron indices does not definitively confirm or refute a diagnosis of iron deficiency, a therapeutic trial of iron supplementation may be considered. Alternatively, a bone marrow examination can be performed to provide a direct assessment of marrow iron stores. Presence of iron in the marrow excludes iron deficiency anemia because marrow iron stores will be depleted before there is any fall in RBC production resulting from iron deficiency; conversely, complete absence of marrow iron confirms the diagnosis of iron deficiency.

Treatment

Oral iron supplementation, with administration of ferrous sulfate or ferrous gluconate two or three times daily, is the treatment for iron deficiency. Patients should be educated about the potential gastrointestinal side effects, including diarrhea or constipation, and some may benefit from a gradual increase in the dose based on tolerance. Iron should be administered for several months after resolution of anemia to allow for the reconstitution of iron stores.

In patients with malabsorption, a complete inability to tolerate oral iron, or iron demands that outstrip replacement with oral supplements, parenteral iron may be administered. The parenteral administration of iron, especially iron dextran, has been associated with anaphylaxis. However, newer preparations such as sodium ferric gluconate, iron sucrose, ferumoxytol, and ferric carboxymaltose are significantly safer. As previously stated, all male patients and postmenopausal women with iron deficiency require evaluation for a source of gastrointestinal bleeding.

Macrocytic Anemias

Two categories of hypoproductive macrocytic anemias exist: megaloblastic anemias and nonmegaloblastic macrocytic anemias. Megaloblastic anemias arise from a failure of DNA synthesis and result in lack of synchrony between the maturation of the nucleus and the cytoplasm of hematopoietic cells. Nonmegaloblastic macrocytic anemias usually reflect membrane abnormalities resulting from defects in cholesterol metabolism and are most commonly found in patients with advanced liver disease or severe hypothyroidism. Reticulocytosis greater than 10% causes an elevated MCV on automated blood counts because reticulocytes are larger than mature RBCs.

Megaloblastic Anemias

Megaloblastic anemias result from a block in the synthesis of critical nucleotide precursors of DNA, which leads to a cell cycle arrest in S phase. Cytoplasmic maturation occurs, but maturation of the nucleus is arrested. Cells take on a bizarre appearance, with large immature nuclei surrounded by more mature-appearing cytoplasm. Interference with DNA synthesis affects all rapidly dividing cells, so patients with megaloblastic syndromes often have pancytopenia and gastrointestinal symptoms such as diarrhea and malabsorption. In women, megaloblastic changes of the cervical mucosa occur and may cause abnormal results on Papanicolaou smears. The most common causes of megaloblastic anemia are deficiencies of vitamin B_{12} or folate, medications that inhibit DNA synthesis or that block folate metabolism, and myelodysplasia.

Cobalamin Deficiency

Cobalamin (vitamin B_{12}) is absorbed from animal protein in the diet. The process of cobalamin absorption and metabolism is complex because cobalamin is always bound to other proteins. In the stomach, protein-bound vitamins are released by digestion with pepsin and are bound to haptocorrin (transcobalamin I). Within the proximal duodenum, pancreatic proteases digest cobalamin away from haptocorrin, and cobalamin binds to intrinsic factor (IF), also known as transcobalamin III. IF is secreted by the parietal cells of the stomach and mediates absorption of cobalamin through the cubam receptor in the distal ileum. Within the ileal mucosal cell, the IF-cobalamin complex is again digested, and cobalamin is released into the plasma bound to haptocorrin and transcobalamin II.

Within the cell, cobalamin is a cofactor for two intracellular enzymes, L-methylmalonyl–coenzyme A (CoA) mutase and homocysteine-methionine methyltransferase (Fig. 47-3).

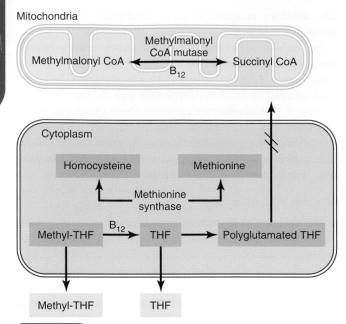

FIGURE 47-3 Metabolic pathways of folic acid and cobalamin. CoA, Coenzyme A; THF, tetrahydrofolate.

TABLE 47-3 CAUSES OF COBALAMIN DEFICIENCY	
Malabsorption of Vitamin B_{12}	Tapeworm infection
Pernicious anemia	Nutritional (vegans)
Partial or total gastrectomy	Congenital deficiency of intrinsic
Pancreatic insufficiency	factor or haptocorrin
Bacterial overgrowth	
Diseases of the terminal ileum	

TABLE 47-4 CAUSES OF FOLATE DEFICIENCY	
DIETARY INSUFFICIENCY	**MALABSORPTION**
INCREASED FOLATE REQUIREMENTS	Sprue
	Crohn's disease
	Short bowel syndrome
Pregnancy	**ANTIFOLATE MEDICATIONS**
Lactation	
Hemolysis	Chemotherapy agents (e.g.,
Exfoliative dermatitis	methotrexate, pemetrexed)
Malignancy	Sulfa drugs

Methylmalonyl-CoA mutase is a mitochondrial enzyme that functions in the citric acid cycle to convert methylmalonyl-CoA to succinyl-CoA. The cytoplasmic enzyme homocysteine-methionine methyltransferase is necessary for the transfer of methyl groups from N-methyltetrahydrofolate to homocysteine to form methionine. Demethylated tetrahydrofolate is necessary as a carbon donor in the conversion of deoxyuridine to deoxythymidine. Absence of cobalamin results in a *trapping* of tetrahydrofolate in its methylated form, which blocks the synthesis of thymidine 5′-triphosphate for incorporation into DNA. The megaloblastic changes induced by cobalamin deficiency are mediated through this functional folate deficiency, which explains the similarity in the hematologic abnormalities induced by cobalamin and folate deficiency.

Causes of Cobalamin Deficiency
The most common cause of cobalamin deficiency is pernicious anemia, an autoimmune disease associated with gastric parietal cell atrophy, defective gastric acid secretion, and absence of IF. Antiparietal cell and anti-IF antibodies are frequently found in patients with pernicious anemia and other autoimmune conditions such as type 1 diabetes, vitiligo, Graves' disease, Addison's disease, and hypoparathyroidism. Many other lesions in the gastrointestinal tract can interfere with absorption of cobalamin (Table 47-3). Gastrectomy causes loss of parietal cell function and IF secretion. Pancreatic insufficiency interferes with digestion of the haptocorrin-cobalamin complex, thus hindering the binding of cobalamin to IF and ileal absorption. Resection of the terminal ileum prevents vitamin B_{12} absorption, as do diseases that affect ileal mucosal function, such as Crohn's disease, sprue, intestinal tuberculosis, and lymphoma. Because the body stores of cobalamin are large and daily loss of cobalamin is low, the stores of cobalamin are adequate for 3 to 4 years if intake stops abruptly; signs of cobalamin deficiency do not develop until defective absorption has occurred for several years. Nutritional cobalamin deficiency is rare and is seen only in individuals who have been on strict vegan diets that exclude all animal products for many years. Infants born to vegan mothers who are breastfed are also at risk for development of cobalamin deficiency.

Folate Deficiency
Folate is widely present in foods such as leafy vegetables, fruits, and animal protein. However, because it is destroyed by prolonged cooking, fresh fruits and vegetables are the most reliable sources of folate. Consequently, nutritional folate deficiency is common in malnourished individuals who eat very little fresh fruits and vegetables. Folate deficiency can also be caused by increased demand, as occurs with pregnancy, hemolysis, or exfoliative dermatitis, and by increased losses, which occur with dialysis (Table 47-4). Folate is absorbed in the proximal small intestine, and malabsorption of folate can also lead to folate deficiency.

Other Causes of Megaloblastic Anemia
Drugs and toxins are common causes of megaloblastic anemia. Some drugs, such as methotrexate and sulfa drugs, act as direct folate antagonists and mimic folate deficiency. Purine and pyrimidine analogue chemotherapeutic agents (e.g., azathioprine, 5-fluorouracil) are direct DNA-synthesis inhibitors. Antiviral agents cause megaloblastic changes by unclear mechanisms. Alcohol interferes with folate metabolism, increasing the effect of frequent concomitant nutritional folate deficiency. Myelodysplasia commonly appears as a macrocytic anemia, with megaloblastic changes primarily in the erythroid series.

Clinical Manifestations of Megaloblastic Anemia
The development of megaloblastic anemia is usually gradual, allowing adequate time for concomitant plasma expansion to prevent hypovolemia. Consequently, patients are frequently severely anemic at presentation. They may have yellowish skin as the result of a combination of pallor and jaundice. Some patients have glossitis and cheilosis. With severe anemia, patients usually have an MCV greater than 110 fL/cell, although concomitant iron deficiency, caused by malabsorption secondary to

megaloblastic changes in the intestinal tract, may decrease the macrocytosis. Patients frequently have pancytopenia.

A peripheral smear demonstrates large, oval cells (macro-ovalocytes), hypersegmented neutrophils, and large platelets. The bone marrow is hypercellular, with megaloblastic changes and abnormally large precursors. In addition, intramedullary destruction of erythrocytes (ineffective hematopoiesis) causes elevated concentrations of bilirubin and lactate dehydrogenase.

Cobalamin deficiency is associated with neurologic abnormalities that are not seen with other causes of megaloblastic anemia. The neurologic signs may range widely, from a subtle loss of vibratory sensation and position sense caused by demyelination of the dorsal columns to frank dementia and neuropsychiatric disease. The neurologic changes may be present without anemia, especially if a patient with cobalamin deficiency is treated with folate, which may correct the hematologic manifestations of megaloblastic anemia but does not treat the neurologic abnormalities. The neurologic manifestations of cobalamin deficiency are thought to be secondary to loss of function of the mitochondrial enzyme methylmalonyl-CoA mutase. One proposed explanation is that the failure to metabolize odd-chain fatty acids, which results in their improper incorporation into myelin, causes the neurologic dysfunction. This explains why these findings are uniquely seen in patients with cobalamin deficiency and are not seen in those with the megaloblastic anemias caused by abnormalities in the folate pathway.

Serum levels of both cobalamin and folate should be measured in patients with megaloblastic anemia because megaloblastic changes in the gut mucosa can cause concomitant malabsorption of folate in the presence of cobalamin deficiency and vice versa. RBC folate levels better reflect the body folate stores and should be measured if a deficiency is clinically suggested but the serum folate levels are normal. Recent studies have shown, however, that many patients with pernicious anemia may have normal serum cobalamin levels. Homocysteine levels are elevated in cobalamin and folate deficiency, and methylmalonic acid levels are elevated in cobalamin deficiency. These levels should be measured if cobalamin deficiency is suggested but serum cobalamin levels are in the normal range. Anti-IF and anti–parietal cell antibodies may help determine the cause of cobalamin deficiency.

Treatment of Megaloblastic Anemia

For patients with cobalamin deficiency, both high-dose oral and parenteral cobalamin administration have been shown to be effective. The oral dose should be at least 1000 μg daily. Patients with neurologic abnormalities or medication noncompliance and those who have not responded to oral therapy should receive parenteral therapy with 1000 μg subcutaneously or intramuscularly several times per week for four to eight doses. Maintenance therapy should then be instituted with 1000 μg parenterally monthly. Therapy with cobalamin should be accompanied by folate therapy because concomitant secondary folate deficiency may develop when RBC production increases with the availability of cobalamin. Treatment of pernicious anemia should be continued for life.

Patients with folate deficiency should receive replacement with 1 to 5 mg per day of oral folate. As previously stated, it is critical to be certain that patients are not cobalamin deficient: Replacement of folate may correct the hematologic parameters in patients with cobalamin deficiency, but it will not improve the neurologic sequelae.

After treatment of megaloblastic anemia, a rapid response usually occurs. Reticulocytosis is seen as early as 2 days after therapy and peaks within 7 to 10 days. Despite rapid resolution of neutropenia, hypersegmentation of neutrophils may persist for several days. During this period, rapid cellular proliferation and turnover occur, which may precipitate hypokalemia, hyperuricemia, or hypophosphatemia. Patients should also be monitored for the development of iron deficiency, which may occur in the face of increased hematopoiesis. Anemia and other cytopenias should respond completely within 1 to 2 months, but the neurologic manifestations of cobalamin deficiency improve slowly and may be irreversible.

Normocytic Anemias

The differential diagnosis of a normocytic hypoproductive anemia is extensive. Most nutritional anemias that cause microcytosis or macrocytosis begin as a normocytic anemia. Patients with combined nutritional deficiencies may also have a normal MCV. The measurement of EPO levels may be helpful in the diagnosis of anemia resulting from renal failure, and many of the anemias associated with chronic inflammation and endocrinopathies exhibit a depressed EPO level. However, interpretation of EPO levels can be difficult in patients with mild anemia because the levels do not usually rise above the normal range until the hematocrit is depressed below 30%. Even with a hematocrit level of 30%, the EPO level is often in the normal range, but such levels are inappropriately low in the setting of anemia. An elevated EPO level suggests an inadequate marrow response to anemia and increases the likelihood of myelophthisis or primary bone marrow failure. In patients for whom the diagnosis is not clear after routine nutritional and endocrine studies, a bone marrow examination is indicated to rule out primary pathologic conditions of the marrow.

Anemia of Chronic Inflammation

The anemia of chronic inflammation (previously called anemia of chronic disease) occurs in patients with chronic inflammatory, infectious, malignant, or autoimmune disorders. Patients have low-serum iron levels, but in contrast to the iron indices in iron deficiency anemia, the iron-binding capacity is also reduced, and the transferrin saturation is usually greater than 10%. Ferritin levels are often elevated, both as an acute phase reactant and as a reflection of decreased iron incorporation. These patients have inappropriately high levels of hepcidin, an acute phase reactant that facilitates the metabolism of ferroportin and reduces both intestinal iron absorption and iron mobilization from macrophages. Cytokines, including tumor necrosis factor, the interleukins, and interferon, also play a role in the anemia of chronic inflammation, both by inducing hepcidin and by directly increasing EPO resistance in erythroid progenitors. Patients have an absolute or relative EPO deficiency, poor iron incorporation into developing erythrocytes, and shortened erythrocyte survival time. The prevalence of anemia of inflammation increases with age; most likely, this is related to age-related comorbidities and mediated through an increase in inflammatory cytokines and a relative EPO resistance.

Treatment of Normocytic Anemias

The mainstay of therapy for the anemia of chronic inflammation is treatment of the underlying condition and correction of nutritional deficiencies. Iron supplementation should be offered to all patients with a ferritin level lower than 100 ng/mL. Erythroid-stimulating agents (ESAs) have been shown to reduce transfusion needs in many of these patients. However, randomized studies and meta-analyses have shown that their use is associated with an increased incidence of arterial and venous thromboembolic events, an increased risk of mortality from cancer, and a reduced survival time. ESA should be avoided in cancer patients if they are being treated with curative intent, and in all other patients with cancer they should be offered only after a careful discussion of the risks and benefits (grade 1B recommendation).

Anemia of Chronic Kidney Disease

Most patients who have a glomerular filtration rate of less than 30 mL/min have anemia related primarily to low EPO levels. ESAs can help prevent transfusions in this population; however, their use has been associated with an increased risk of stroke, access thrombosis, hypertension, and even mortality in some studies, especially when the hemoglobin levels were normalized. Therefore, most guidelines recommend a target hemoglobin concentration of 10 to 11.5 g/dL when using ESA in patients with chronic kidney disease (grade IB). As in the management of anemia of chronic inflammation, nutritional deficiencies should be corrected before the use of ESAs. The evaluation and treatment of primary marrow failure syndromes and hematologic malignancies are discussed in Chapters 45 and 46, respectively.

⬤ EVALUATION OF ANEMIA WITH RETICULOCYTOSIS

An elevated reticulocyte count in the setting of anemia signals a compensatory response by a normal marrow to premature loss of erythrocytes. Hemolysis is the premature destruction of RBCs in the reticuloendothelial system (extrinsic hemolysis) or in blood vessels (intrinsic hemolysis). The only other condition that causes anemia with reticulocytosis is acute bleeding. The differential diagnosis of hemolytic anemia is outlined in Table 47-5.

Whereas examination of the peripheral blood smear is helpful in characterizing any anemia, it is absolutely critical in the evaluation of hemolytic anemia. Morphologic examination of the erythrocytes is helpful in distinguishing immune hemolysis from microangiopathic hemolytic anemia. In addition, other RBC morphologic abnormalities are characteristic for specific diseases such as sickle cell disease (sickled cells), enzyme defects (*bite* cells), and erythrocyte membrane abnormalities (spherocytes and elliptocytes).

Immune Hemolytic Anemia

Immune-mediated hemolysis results from coating of the erythrocyte membrane with antibodies or complement, or both. It may be mediated by immunoglobulin G (IgG) antibodies (*warm* antibody) or by IgM antibodies (*cold* antibody). The designations *warm* and *cold* denote the temperature at which maximal

TABLE 47-5	DIFFERENTIAL DIAGNOSIS OF HEMOLYTIC ANEMIA

IMMUNE HEMOLYTIC ANEMIA

Immunoglobulin G (warm antibody)–mediated hemolysis
Immunoglobulin M (cold antibody)–mediated hemolysis

HEMOLYSIS FROM CAUSES EXTRINSIC TO THE ERYTHROCYTE

Microangiopathic Hemolysis

Disseminated intravascular coagulation
Thrombotic thrombocytopenic purpura
Preeclampsia, eclampsia, HELLP syndrome
Drugs (mitomycin, cyclosporine, gemcitabine)
Valvular hemolysis

Splenomegaly

Infection (e.g., malaria, babesiosis)

HEMOLYTIC ANEMIA CAUSED BY DISORDERS OF THE ERYTHROCYTE MEMBRANE

Inherited Membrane Abnormalities

Hereditary spherocytosis
Hereditary elliptocytosis
Hereditary pyropoikilocytosis

Acquired Membrane Abnormalities

Paroxysmal nocturnal hemoglobinuria
Spur cell anemia

HEMOLYSIS CAUSED BY ERYTHROCYTE ENZYMOPATHIES

Glucose-6-phosphate dehydrogenase deficiency
Other enzyme deficiencies

HEMOGLOBINOPATHIES

Sickle cell disease
Other sickle syndromes
Thalassemia

HELLP, Hemolysis, elevated liver enzymes, and low-platelet count in association with preeclampsia.

antibody binding takes place, and the clinical syndromes caused by the two types of antibodies are distinct.

The diagnosis of hemolytic anemia is based on the direct and indirect antiglobulin (Coombs) tests. To perform a direct Coombs test, the patient's erythrocytes are mixed with antisera or monoclonal antibodies directed against human immunoglobulins and human complement. The cells are then monitored for agglutination, the presence of which confirms the presence of antibody or complement on the patient's RBCs. The indirect Coombs test is performed by mixing the patient's serum with ABO-compatible erythrocytes and then combining this mixture with antisera against IgG; the indirect Coombs tests allows for the evaluation of antibody in the patient's serum.

IgG-Mediated (Warm) Hemolytic Anemia

Classic autoimmune hemolytic anemia (AIHA) is caused by IgG antibody directed against erythrocyte antigens. Warm type hemolysis may be primary (idiopathic) or associated with autoimmune disease, lymphoproliferative disorders, or drugs. Patients exhibit acute anemia, jaundice, and an elevated reticulocyte count. Some patients have splenomegaly. The peripheral blood smear demonstrates spherocytes (see Fig. 47-2E). Laboratory analysis confirms the presence of IgG on the erythrocyte membrane, as demonstrated by a positive Coombs test; in some patients, the erythrocytes are also coated with complement.

Some patients do not have reticulocytosis; in them, the antibody may be destroying both reticulocytes and mature erythrocytes.

The mainstay of therapy for AIHA is corticosteroids. Patients are usually treated with 1 to 2 mg/kg of prednisone, and in responding patients, doses are tapered slowly over several months. Patients who fail to respond to prednisone or cannot be tapered off the prednisone can be treated with other immunosuppressive agents, such as cyclophosphamide, azathioprine, chlorambucil, or rituximab. Some patient respond to intravenous immunoglobulin. Splenectomy is effective in many patients who are steroid refractory or steroid resistant, and it is associated with greater sustained response rates than other immunosuppressive therapies in steroid-resistant patients. However, patients who do not respond and who have ongoing hemolysis after splenectomy are at high risk for secondary thromboembolic events.

Warm antibodies mediate *drug-induced hemolysis*. Several mechanisms exist through which drugs may induce AIHA (Table 47-6). Penicillin produces hemolysis by binding to erythrocytes and acting as a hapten; the antibody is directed against the drug, and hemolysis occurs only in the presence of the drug. Type 2 hemolysis is caused by the formation of an antibody-drug complex that binds to the erythrocyte membrane and activates complement. Drugs associated with this type of hemolysis include quinidine, quinine, and rifampin. Still other drugs, including methyldopa and procainamide, cause hemolysis by inducing the production of *true* antierythrocyte antibodies directed against Rh and other RBC antigens. Antibody may persist in the absence of the drug, but not all patients with a positive Coombs test have evidence of hemolysis.

IgM-Mediated (Cold) Hemolytic Anemia

Cold-type immune hemolysis is usually postinfectious. The most common associated infectious agents are *Mycoplasma pneumoniae* and Epstein-Barr virus (EBV). IgM antibodies are produced that are directed against the RBC antigen I (*Mycoplasma*) or i (EBV). The antibodies bind at lower temperatures, present in fingers and toes, and bind complement. During the return to the central circulation, the IgM falls off the RBC, leaving complement bound. The Coombs test is negative for IgG and IgM but positive for complement. Hemolysis is self-limited, is rarely severe, and resolves with supportive therapy. In cases of severe hemolysis requiring transfusion, the patient should be kept warm, and blood should be administered through a blood warmer to minimize further hemolysis.

Cold agglutinin disease is a chronic IgM antibody–mediated hemolysis that is usually seen in association with lymphoproliferative disease. Hemolysis is usually low grade; if severe, it responds poorly to steroids and splenectomy. Acute severe IgM-mediated hemolysis may respond to plasmapheresis. Supportive therapy includes avoidance of exposure to the cold. In the setting of lymphoproliferative disease, patients may respond to immunotherapy with rituximab.

Hemolysis from Causes Extrinsic to the Erythrocyte

Microangiopathic Hemolysis

Microangiopathic hemolytic anemia (MAHA) is caused by traumatic destruction of RBCs as they pass through small vessels. The leading causes of MAHA include thrombotic thrombocytopenic purpura and hemolytic-uremic syndrome (TTP/HUS) (see Table 47-5 and Fig. 47-1). Other causes include pregnancy-related syndromes such as preeclampsia, eclampsia, and the HELLP syndrome (*h*emolysis, *e*levated *l*iver enzyme levels, and *l*ow *p*latelet count); drugs; and metastatic cancers. A similar hemolytic picture can be seen in traumatic hemolysis on a damaged cardiac valve.

The finding of schistocytes (fragmented erythrocytes) on the peripheral blood smear confirms the diagnosis of MAHA (see Fig. 47-2D). The presence of normal prothrombin and partial thromboplastin times supports a diagnosis of TTP/HUS over that of disseminated intravascular coagulation. Diagnosis and management are described further in Chapter 51.

Infection

Hemolysis can be caused by direct infection of RBCs by parasites, as seen in malaria, babesiosis, and bartonellosis. Severe, overwhelming hemolysis can be seen in clostridial sepsis, in which bacterial toxins directly damage the membrane.

TABLE 47-6 DRUG-INDUCED AUTOIMMUNE HEMOLYTIC ANEMIA

TYPE	MECHANISM	COMMON DRUGS IMPLICATED	DIRECT COOMBS TEST	INDIRECT COOMBS TEST
1	Hapten mediated	Penicillin Cephalothin	IgG positive Complement positive or negative	Positive only in the presence of drug
2	Immune complex mediated	Quinine Quinidine Phenacetin Rifampin Isoniazid Tetracycline Chlorpromazine	IgG negative Complement positive	Positive only in the presence of drug
3	True anti-RBC antibody	Methyldopa Levodopa Procainamide Ibuprofen Interferon-α	IgG positive Complement negative	Positive also in absence of drug

IgG, Immunoglobulin G; RBC, red blood cell.

Hemolytic Anemias Caused by Disorders of the Erythrocyte Membrane

Inherited Membrane Abnormalities

Hereditary spherocytosis (HS) is caused by heterogeneous congenital abnormalities in proteins of the erythrocyte cytoskeleton (Table 47-7). Most patients with HS have dominantly inherited mutations in spectrin or ankyrin. HS is characterized by hemolytic anemia, splenomegaly, and the presence of prominent spherocytes in the peripheral blood. Spherocytes are the result of *conditioning* of the erythrocytes in the spleen, during which reticuloendothelial cells remove portions of the abnormal membrane that are caused by the disordered cytoskeleton. Spherocytes reflect membrane loss that decreases the membrane-to-cytoplasm ratio. Because a high membrane-to-cytoplasm ratio is responsible for the flexible, biconcave shape of the normal erythrocyte, the erythrocyte loses its biconcave morphologic characteristics and assumes a spherocytic shape with loss of membrane. Spherocytes are less flexible and may be destroyed in the microvasculature. The laboratory finding characteristic of HS is increased osmotic fragility, which is caused by the loss of distensibility associated with a decrease in surface membrane. HS is usually a mild disorder with well-compensated hemolysis. Patients typically have exacerbations during infections or when given marrow-suppressing medication. Patients with significant hemolysis should receive folate supplementation. Many patients require cholecystectomy for pigment stones. Severe, symptomatic anemia is treated with splenectomy.

Hereditary elliptocytosis (HE) is caused by dominantly inherited mutations affecting the interactions between membrane proteins and underlying cytoplasmic proteins. The most common abnormalities affect the interactions with spectrin and protein 4.1, which causes the RBCs to assume an elliptical shape. As in HS, patients usually have mild hemolysis and splenomegaly.

Hereditary pyropoikilocytosis (HPP) is a rare recessive disorder that is frequently caused by the inheritance of two different membrane disorders (e.g., one allele for HS and one for HE). Patients have severe hemolysis with microspherocytes and elliptocytes on the smear. As with HS, treatment for symptomatic anemia in HE and HPP is splenectomy.

> *More information on hemolytic anemias caused by inherited membrane disorders can be found in Chapter 161, "Hemolytic Anemias: Red Cell Membrane and Metabolic Defects," in* Goldman-Cecil Medicine, *25th Edition.*

TABLE 47-7	CONGENITAL RED BLOOD CELL MEMBRANE ABNORMALITIES	
CONDITION	**ABNORMAL MEMBRANE PROTEINS**	**INHERITANCE**
Spherocytosis	Spectrin, ankyrin, band 3, protein 4.2	Autosomal dominant Recessive (rare)
Elliptocytosis	Spectrin, protein 4.1	Autosomal dominant Recessive (rare)
Pyropoikilocytosis	Spectrin	Recessive
Stomatocytosis	Sodium channel permeability defect	Autosomal dominant

Acquired Membrane Abnormalities

Paroxysmal Nocturnal Hemoglobinuria

Paroxysmal nocturnal hemoglobinuria (PNH) is an acquired clonal disease that is associated with an abnormality of complement regulation. Normal erythrocytes are protected from complement-mediated cell lysis by the presence of membrane proteins, including delay-accelerating factor (DAF or CD55) and membrane inhibitor of reactive lysis (MIRL or CD59). Both these proteins are members of a family of proteins that are anchored to the membrane by a glycosyl phosphatidylinositol (GPI) anchor. Patients with PNH have clonal mutations in phosphatidyl inositolglycan A (PIG-A), the enzyme required for synthesis of GPI. These mutations arise in the hematopoietic stem cell, and all hematopoietic cells lack GPI-anchored proteins. Absence of GPI-anchored proteins from erythrocytes renders them susceptible to complement-mediated lysis. The diagnosis can be made by flow cytometric documentation of the absence of CD55 or CD59 on the surface of RBCs or leukocytes.

PNH is a clonal stem cell disorder with several unique characteristics. Patients suffer from episodic acute intravascular hemolysis with a release of free hemoglobin that results in the hemoglobinuria for which the disease is named. Patients are also susceptible to venous thrombotic complications, including Budd-Chiari syndrome, portal vein thrombosis, cerebrovascular thrombosis, and peripheral veins. The disease is associated with a risk for development of myelodysplasia, myelofibrosis, acute leukemia, or aplastic anemia. Furthermore, patients with aplastic anemia who respond to immunosuppressive therapy frequently develop PNH-like clones. In the past, treatment has been largely supportive. However, treatment with eculizumab, a monoclonal antibody that binds to the C5 component of complement, has been shown to reduce hemolysis, transfusion requirements, and thromboembolic events in this disease. Young patients should be considered for allogeneic stem cell transplantation.

Spur Cell Anemia

Spur cells (acanthocytes) are cells with abnormal membrane morphology found in patients with advanced liver disease, severe malnutrition, malabsorption, or asplenia. The membrane acquires protrusions as a result of the presence of abnormal lipids. The changes may be associated with mild hemolysis, although in patients with advanced liver disease, it is difficult to distinguish hemolysis from hypersplenism. Similar changes may be observed in patients with abetalipoproteinemia.

Hemolytic Anemias Caused by Disorders of Erythrocyte Enzymes

Glucose-6 Phosphate Dehydrogenase Deficiency

Glucose-6-phosphate dehydrogenase (G6PD) is a critical enzyme in the hexose monophosphate shunt pathway. By maintaining intracellular stores of reduced glutathione, it protects erythrocytes from membrane and hemoglobin oxidation (Fig. 47-4). The gene for G6PD resides on the X chromosome, and therefore almost all patients with G6PD deficiency are male. Most G6PD mutations are found in African and Mediterranean populations, most likely because they confer resistance to malaria.

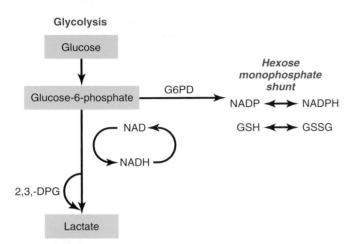

FIGURE 47-4 Metabolism of the red blood cell. 2,3-DPG, 2,3-Diphosphoglycerate; G6PD, glucose-6-phosphate dehydrogenase; GSH, reduced glutathione; GSSG, reduced and oxidized glutathione; NAD, nicotinamide adenine dinucleotide; NADH, reduced form of NAD; NADP, nicotinamide adenine dinucleotide phosphate; NADPH, reduced form of NADP.

The African form of G6PD deficiency is relatively mild, whereas the Mediterranean form is severe.

Absence of G6PD renders erythrocytes sensitive to oxidative stress. In the setting of infection, acidosis, or oxidant drugs, hemoglobin may precipitate within the cells, causing hemolysis. Many drugs are associated with hemolysis in the setting of G6PD deficiency, including sulfonamides, antimalarials, dapsone, aspirin, and phenacetin. The diagnosis should be considered in male patients of African American or Mediterranean extraction who have evidence of hemolysis in the setting of acute infection or recent exposure to oxidant drugs. Patients with the Mediterranean variant of G6PD deficiency may develop hemolysis on exposure to fava beans (favism). Cells with precipitated hemoglobin contain Heinz bodies that can be visualized with crystal violet staining of the peripheral blood smear. These inclusions are removed in the spleen, resulting in the additional finding of bite cells in the blood smear. The diagnosis can be confirmed with measurement of G6PD levels in the peripheral blood. However, reticulocytes and young RBCs in patients with G6PD deficiency have a higher enzyme level; consequently, if the diagnosis is probable, the patients with a normal G6PD level should be retested at a time removed from the acute episode, when the percentage of young RBCs is high. The mainstay of preventing hemolysis in these patients is avoidance of oxidative stress, especially drugs implicated in causing hemolysis. Splenectomy is recommended only for patients with severe episodic or chronic hemolysis.

Other Enzyme Deficiencies

Enzyme deficiencies as rare causes of hemolytic anemia have been reported involving almost all of the enzymes of the glycolytic pathway. The most common of these is pyruvate kinase deficiency. Autosomal genes encode these enzymes, and the pattern of inheritance is therefore autosomal recessive.

More information on hemolytic anemias caused by inherited enzyme deficiencies can be found in Chapter 161,

TABLE 47-8	CLINICAL MANIFESTATIONS OF SICKLE CELL DISEASE	
ACUTE MANIFESTATIONS	**CHRONIC MANIFESTATIONS**
Vaso-occlusive crisis	Chronic renal disease
Painful crisis	Isosthenuria
Acute chest syndrome	Chronic renal failure
Priapism	Chronic pulmonary disease
Cerebrovascular events	Sickle hepatopathy
Thrombotic stroke	Proliferative retinopathy
Hemorrhagic stroke	Avascular necrosis
Aplastic crisis	Skin ulcers
Splenic sequestration	
Osteomyelitis	

"Hemolytic Anemias: Red Cell Membrane and Metabolic Defects," in Goldman-Cecil Medicine, *25th Edition.*

Hemoglobinopathies

Hemoglobinopathies are disorders caused by mutations that result in the synthesis of quantitatively or qualitatively abnormal hemoglobins. The most common of these are the sickle syndromes and the thalassemias, which, like G6PD deficiency, arose in areas of the world with endemic malaria.

Sickle Cell Disease

Sickle cell disease, the most common of the sickle syndromes, arises from a point mutation that causes a substitution of valine for glutamic acid in the sixth amino acid of the β-globin gene. It has arisen as an independent mutation in diverse populations in Africa, India, the Mediterranean, and the Middle East. The substitution of a hydrophobic for a hydrophilic residue renders the deoxygenated sickle hemoglobin (HbS) less soluble and therefore susceptible to polymerization and precipitation. The rate of precipitation of HbS is exquisitely sensitive to the intracorpuscular concentration of deoxygenated hemoglobin. Sickling is therefore increased in settings in which that concentration is increased, either by changes in cellular hydration (dehydration) or by changes in the oxygen dissociation curve (e.g., hypoxia, acidosis, high altitude).

Acute Manifestations

Most of the acute complications of sickle cell disease are related to vaso-occlusion (Table 47-8). Painful crises, secondary to occlusions of the microvasculature and ischemia of organs and tissues, can occur anywhere, with pain most commonly experienced in the extremities, chest, abdomen, and back. Painful crises are commonly precipitated by infections, dehydration, rapid changes in temperature, and pregnancy. Often, however, no obvious precipitating cause is found for an acute painful crisis.

Vaso-occlusion in the pulmonary circulation can be a particularly ominous complication of sickle cell disease. It results in the *acute chest syndrome*, which is characterized by chest pain, hypoxemia, and pulmonary infiltrates. The roles of infection, infarction, and in situ thrombosis in the acute chest syndrome are indistinguishable, but all patients should receive antibiotics for presumed pneumonia. Because hypoxemia predisposes to further sickling and increasing respiratory compromise, the acute chest syndrome is life-threatening and is an indication for emergent exchange transfusion.

Neurologic events are a major cause of morbidity in patients with sickle cell disease. Acute large-vessel occlusions occur in children, with a recurrence rate of 70% if untreated; such strokes are an indication for long-term exchange transfusion, which has been shown to decrease the rate of repeated occlusions. For reasons that are poorly understood, such large-vessel occlusions rarely occur in adults. Adults may suffer hemorrhagic strokes as a result of aneurysmal dilation of proliferative vessels that form in response to repeated micro-occlusions in the cerebral vessels.

Any toxic or infectious insult that transiently suppresses bone marrow activity can cause an *aplastic crisis*. The shortened survival time of the RBC in sickle cell disease renders patients highly dependent on vigorous ongoing marrow activity, and short intervals of decreased reticulocyte formation can cause profound anemia. Most dramatic are infections associated with parvovirus B19, which directly infects erythroid precursors. Supportive care is usually all that is required. However, some patients go on to develop bone marrow necrosis, with a leukoerythroblastic picture; this development may be further complicated by bone marrow embolization to the lungs.

Certain vascular beds are especially prone to complications of sickle cell disease. The renal medulla is highly susceptible to damage by vaso-occlusion because its high tonicity and low oxygen tension both significantly increase the concentration of HbS. All patients with sickle cell disease develop defects in the ability to concentrate urine, and by adulthood, they are uniformly isosthenuric. Acute episodes of hematuria secondary to papillary necrosis are common.

The spleen is another site in which recurrent sickling uniformly occurs. By adulthood, all patients have become functionally asplenic from repeated infarctions of the microvasculature. This contributing factor increases the susceptibility of patients with sickle cell disease to infections with encapsulated organisms. Acute infection remains a significant cause of death. For unclear reasons, patients with sickle cell disease are particularly prone to osteomyelitis, and there is an unusually high incidence of *Salmonella* as the responsible organism.

Chronic Manifestations

Sickle cell disease used to be a disease of childhood. As more patients survive to adulthood, it has become clear that repeated episodes of vaso-occlusion lead to damage to almost every end organ (see Table 47-8). Renal failure and pulmonary failure are leading causes of death in adult patients with sickle cell disease. Other long-term complications include chronic skin ulcers, retinopathy, and liver dysfunction. In addition, most patients require cholecystectomy for pigment stones.

Treatment

Treatment of sickle cell disease remains largely supportive. Painful crises are treated with fluid, oxygen supplementation, and analgesics. Patients with any indication of infection should receive antibiotics. Patients with symptomatic anemia should be transfused. Exchange transfusion is indicated for chest syndrome, stroke, bone marrow necrosis, and priapism. More controversial indications for exchange transfusion include intractable pain and slow response to other supportive measures. The goal of exchange transfusion is to achieve a level of 30% to 40% HbS. As previously mentioned, patients who have sustained a thrombotic large-vessel stroke should undergo chronic exchange transfusion.

Treatment with hydroxyurea, an agent that increases the concentration of HbF in patients with sickle cell disease, reduces the incidence of vaso-occlusive crises. The efficacy of hydroxyurea in patients with recurrent crises has been demonstrated in a randomized study, and follow-up studies have revealed a survival advantage for patients treated with hydroxyurea.

Other Sickle Syndromes

Hemoglobin C

Hemoglobin C (HbC) is caused by another substitution, glutamic acid to lysine, in the sixth position of the β-globin chain. Homozygous HbC causes very mild symptoms of anemia and is usually clinically silent. Patients with hemoglobin S-C (HbSC) are compound heterozygotes for HbS and HbC. These patients are symptomatic, although the clinical manifestations are milder than in patients with homozygous HbS (HbSS). They have a higher hematocrit, and the higher viscosity increases the degree of retinopathy. They do not sustain splenic infarctions; unlike patients with HbSS, they usually have splenomegaly. Consequently, they occasionally have episodes of acute splenomegaly associated with profound decreases in hemoglobin concentration and hematocrit (splenic sequestration crisis). Although such crises also occur in children with HbSS, functional asplenia prevents this complication in adults with HbSS.

Sickle Cell β-Thalassemia

Patients who are double heterozygotes for HbS and β-thalassemia have a spectrum of disease dependent on the level of β-globin that they produce. Sickle cell β^+-thalassemia is a milder disease than HbSS, probably because of the decreased intracorpuscular concentration of HbS. Patients with sickle cell β^0-thalassemia (see discussion that follows) produce no normal β chains and have essentially the same phenotype as patients with HbSS.

Thalassemia

The thalassemic syndromes (Table 47-9) are a heterogeneous group of disorders associated with decreased or absent synthesis of either α- or β-globin chains. Severe thalassemic syndromes are associated with severe hemolytic anemia and are diagnosed in early childhood. However, mild forms of thalassemia minor frequently cause mild microcytic anemia with little or no evidence of hemolysis. These syndromes are often confused with iron deficiency because of the decreased MCV.

β-Thalassemia

Over 100 mutations have been described that lead to β-thalassemia, causing a decrease or absence of expression from the β-globin locus. The decreased expression of β-globin can be caused by structural mutations in the coding region of the gene, which result in nonsense mutations, truncated messenger RNA (mRNA), and no expression of intact globin from the affected allele (β^0-thalassemia). However, a large number of mutations that result in decreased transcription or translation or altered splicing of the β-globin mRNA result in reduction but not elimination of globin-chain expression from the affected allele (β^+-thalassemia).

TABLE 47-9 THALASSEMIC SYNDROMES

DISORDER	GENOTYPIC ABNORMALITY	CLINICAL PHENOTYPE
β-THALASSEMIA		
Thalassemia major (Cooley's anemia)	Homozygous β^0-thalassemia	Severe hemolysis, ineffective erythropoiesis, transfusion dependency, iron overload
Thalassemia intermedia	Compound heterozygous β^0- and β^+-thalassemia	Moderate hemolysis, severe anemia, but not transfusion dependent; iron overload
Thalassemia minor	Heterozygous β^0- or β^+-thalassemia	Microcytosis, mild anemia
α-THALASSEMIA		
Silent carrier	$\alpha-/\alpha\alpha$	Normal complete blood count
α-thalassemia trait	$\alpha\alpha/--$ (α-thalassemia 1) *or* $\alpha-/\alpha-$ (α-thalassemia 2)	Mild microcytic anemia
Hemoglobin H	$\alpha-/--$	Microcytic anemia and mild hemolysis; not transfusion dependent
Hydrops fetalis	$--/--$	Severe anemia, intrauterine anasarca from congestive heart failure; death in utero or at birth

Defective globin-chain synthesis in β-thalassemia causes both decreased normal hemoglobin production and the production of a relative excess of α chains. The decrease in normal hemoglobin synthesis results in a hypochromic anemia, and the excess α chains form insoluble α-chain complexes and cause hemolysis. In mild thalassemic syndromes, the excess α chains are insufficient to cause significant hemolysis, and the primary finding is a microcytic anemia. In severe forms of thalassemia, hemolysis occurs both in the periphery and in the marrow, with intense secondary expansion of the marrow production of RBCs. The expansion of the marrow space causes severe skeletal abnormalities, and the ineffective erythropoiesis also provides a powerful stimulus to absorb iron from the intestine.

The clinical spectrum of β-thalassemia reflects the heterogeneity of the molecular lesions causing the disease (see Table 47-9). β-Thalassemia major results from homozygous β^0-thalassemia, leading to severe hemolytic anemia; such patients are diagnosed in infancy and are transfusion dependent from birth. Patients with β-thalassemia intermedia also have two β-thalassemia alleles, but at least one of them is a mild β^+ mutation. These patients have severe chronic hemolytic anemia but do not require transfusions. Because of ineffective erythropoiesis, they patients chronically hyperabsorb iron and may develop iron overload in the absence of transfusions. β-Thalassemia minor is usually caused by heterozygous β-thalassemia, although it may reflect the inheritance of two mild thalassemic mutations. These are the patients in whom iron deficiency is often misdiagnosed. Iron studies show normal to increased iron with normal iron saturation. Documentation of a compensatory increase in HbA_2 and HbF on hemoglobin electrophoresis confirms the diagnosis.

α-Thalassemia

α-Thalassemia is almost always caused by mutations that delete one or more of the α-chain loci on chromosome 16. Four α-chain loci exist with two, almost identical, copies of the α-globin gene on each chromosome. The spectrum of α-thalassemia therefore reflects the lack of one, two, three, or all four α-globin genes (see Table 47-9). In general, the clinical manifestations of α-thalassemia are milder than those of β-thalassemia for two reasons. First, the presence of four α-chain genes allows for adequate α-chain synthesis unless three or four loci are deleted. Second, β-chain tetramers are more soluble than their α-chain counterparts and do not cause hemolysis. Patients with the loss of a single α-chain gene are silent carriers and have a normal hematocrit and MCV. Patients with deletion of two α chains, either on the same chromosome ($--/\alpha\alpha$, called α-thal 1) or on different chromosomes ($\alpha-/\alpha-$; α-thal 2), are microcytic and mildly anemic. Patients who inherit one α-thal 1 allele and one α-thal 2 allele ($--/\alpha-$) have hemoglobin H disease. Hemoglobin H is the product of excess β-chain production, specifically β_4; it causes mild hemolytic anemia and minimal or no intramedullary erythrocyte destruction. Inheritance of the homozygous α-thal 2 allele results in no functional α-chain loci and is incompatible with life. The fetus is unable to make any functional hemoglobin beyond embryonic development because HbF also requires α chains. Free γ chains form tetramers, termed *hemoglobin Barts*. Hemoglobin Barts have an extremely high oxygen affinity, and failure to release oxygen in peripheral tissues results in severe congestive heart failure and anasarca, a clinical picture termed *hydrops fetalis*. Affected fetuses are stillborn or die soon after birth.

More information on the thalassemias, sickle cell disease, and other hemoglobinopathies can be found in Chapter 162, "The Thalassemias," and Chapter 163, "Sickle Cell Disease and Other Hemoglobinopathies," in Goldman-Cecil Medicine, *25th Edition.*

● PROSPECTUS FOR THE FUTURE

Anemia is increasingly recognized as a marker of increased morbidity and mortality in adults with a wide range of medical conditions, including renal failure, malignancy, cardiac disease, inflammatory conditions, and other chronic diseases. Advances in understanding the pathophysiology of anemia of chronic inflammation are contributing to knowledge of iron metabolism and the roles cytokines play in hematopoiesis. These developments are paving the way for the development of new therapies for patients with anemia and iron overload. Ongoing progress in stem cell transplantation will contribute to the ability to treat the thalassemic syndromes and other hemoglobinopathies.

SUGGESTED READINGS

Andrews NC: Forging a field: the golden age of iron biology, Blood 112:219–230, 2008.

Bain BJ: Diagnosis from the blood smear, N Engl J Med 353:498–507, 2005.

Bennett CL, Silver SM, Djulbegovic B, et al: Venous thromboembolism and mortality associated with recombinant erythropoietin and darbepoetin administration for the treatment of cancer-associated anemia, JAMA 299:914–924, 2008.

Finberg KE: Unraveling mechanisms regulating systemic iron homeostasis, Hematology Am Soc Hematol Educ Program 2011:532–537, 2011.

Kidney Disease: Improving Global Outcomes (KDIGO): Anemia Work Group: KDIGO clinical practice guidelines for anemia in chronic kidney disease, Kidney Int Suppl 2:279–335, 2012.

Marks PW: Approach to anemia in the adult and child. In Hoffman R, Benz EJ, Silberstein LE, et al, editors: Hoffman: hematology—basic principles and practice, ed 6, New York, 2013, Saunders, pp 418–426.

Stabler SP: Vitamin B12 deficiency, N Engl J Med 368:149–160, 2013.

48

Clinical Disorders of Neutrophils

Michal G. Rose and Nancy Berliner

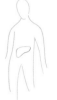

INTRODUCTION

Leukocytes provide the main defense against bacterial infection. Monocytes and granulocytes are phagocytic cells that can kill ingested bacteria through the generation of reactive intermediates. Monocytes also release inflammatory mediators that increase the activity of lymphocytes. Lymphocyte function is discussed in Chapter 49.

NORMAL GRANULOCYTE DEVELOPMENT, STRUCTURE, AND FUNCTION

Neutrophils

Neutrophils (i.e., polymorphonuclear leukocytes) are the predominant white blood cell in the peripheral blood. They are morphologically recognizable by their characteristic segmented nucleus. Neutrophils also contain cytoplasmic granules that give them a characteristic appearance and are functionally important (Fig. 48-1).

Neutrophils achieve intracellular killing of bacteria through chemotaxis, adhesion, and phagocytosis (Fig. 48-2). *Chemotaxis* is the ordered movement of the cell toward an attracting stimulus, such as bacterial formyl peptides or complement fragments (i.e.,

C3b and C5a). Neutrophils adhere to endothelial cells by interaction of neutrophil surface glycoproteins (i.e., CD11b/CD18) with endothelial adhesion molecules (i.e., intracellular adhesion molecule 1 and endothelial leukocyte adhesion molecule 1), a process called *margination*. In response to a chemotactic stimulus, the adherent neutrophils move toward the target along the endothelial surface.

The syndrome of leukocyte adhesion deficiency underscores the importance of neutrophil adhesion as the first step in bacterial killing. This rare congenital disease is caused by the absence of surface expression of the CD11b/CD18 complex on neutrophils. Neutrophils fail to adhere to endothelium, are unable to undergo chemotaxis, and do not phagocytose or kill bacteria. Patients have severe, life-threatening bacterial infections despite high levels of circulating neutrophils.

Phagocytosis requires recognition of target bacteria or debris by the neutrophil. Targets are opsonized by the surface binding of immunoglobulin or complement factor C3b. The neutrophil has surface receptors for C3b and the Fc portion of immunoglobulin G, which allows recognition and binding to the opsonized target. The target then becomes engulfed in a phagocytic vacuole, which fuses with neutrophil granules inside the cell.

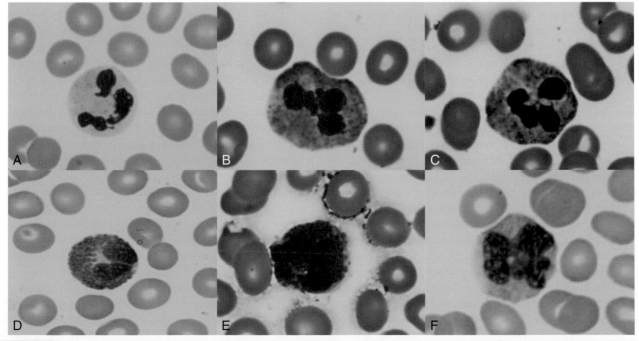

FIGURE 48-1 Normal granulocytes and monocytes in peripheral blood. **A** to **C**, Neutrophils (i.e., polymorphonuclear cells). **D**, Eosinophils. **E**, Basophils. **F**, Monocytes. (Courtesy Robert J. Homer, MD, PhD, Yale School of Medicine, New Haven, Conn.)

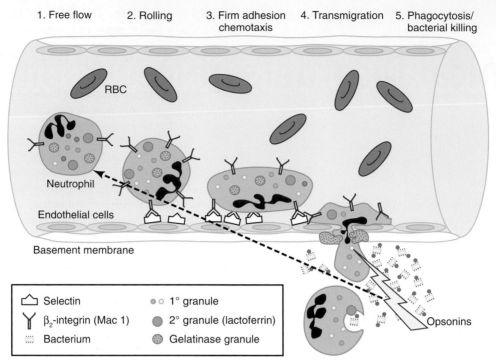

1. Free flow   2. Rolling   3. Firm adhesion   4. Transmigration   5. Phagocytosis/
                                    chemotaxis   bacterial killing

RBC

Neutrophil

Endothelial cells

Basement membrane

☐ Selectin   ⊙ ○ 1° granule
Y β₂-integrin (Mac 1) ⦿ 2° granule (lactoferrin)
⫴ Bacterium   ⦿ Gelatinase granule

Opsonins

FIGURE 48-2 Sequence of neutrophil activation shows the process of rolling, engagement with the vessel wall, attachment, diapedesis, and phagocytosis. Mac 1, Macrophage antigen 1 (CDl lb/CD18); RBC, red blood cell.

Intracellular killing occurs by oxygen-dependent and oxygen-independent mechanisms. Contents of the primary granules, including cathepsin G, defensins, and lysozyme, break down the bacterial cell wall and kill the target organism. However, the major mechanism of bacterial killing is the *respiratory burst*. Stimulation of the neutrophil activates a membrane-bound oxidase complex, which generates superoxide through the transfer of an electron from reduced nicotinamide-adenine dinucleotide phosphate (NADPH). The interaction of superoxide with water generates hydroxyl ions. Myeloperoxidase catalyzes the formation of hypochlorite ion from hydrogen peroxide and chloride. The NADPH oxidase is a multisubunit enzyme. Absence or decreased activity of any one subunit impairs bacterial killing and results in chronic granulomatous disease, a congenital illness in which patients are predisposed to life-threatening bacterial infections.

Neutrophil granules give neutrophils their characteristic appearance and have important functions in neutrophil-mediated activation and killing. *Primary granules* arise early in myeloid differentiation and are found in neutrophils and monocytes. They contain a large number of proteins, including myeloperoxidase, acid hydrolases, and neutral proteases. These granules fuse with the phagocytic vacuole and aid in the digestion of ingested bacteria. *Secondary granules* arise later in the differentiation pathway and give the neutrophil its characteristic granular (electron-dense) appearance. These granules contain lactoferrin, transcobalamin, and the matrix-modifying enzymes collagenase and gelatinase. On neutrophil stimulation, the granules are released into the extracellular space. Lactoferrin and transcobalamin act as antibacterial proteins by sequestering iron and vitamin B_{12} away from bacteria, and collagenase and gelatinase break down connective tissues at the site of inflammation.

Abnormalities in neutrophil granules have been described in rare clinical syndromes. Absence of myeloperoxidase produces surprisingly mild symptoms and may be associated with defects in control of fungal infections. Secondary granule deficiency is rare and is associated with a slight increase in the risk of bacterial infections.

For a deeper discussion of these topics, please see Chapter 169, "Disorders of Phagocyte Function," in Goldman-Cecil Medicine, *25th Edition.*

Eosinophils and Basophils

Eosinophils and basophils arise from myeloid precursors in the bone marrow. They transit rapidly from the marrow to the blood and into the peripheral tissues, where they play a role in allergic and inflammatory reactions. Like neutrophils, they have secondary granules that give them a characteristic appearance and are functionally important. Both cell types occur in small numbers under normal conditions.

Although eosinophils are capable of phagocytosis, most of the activity of these cells is mediated through the release of granule contents. The eosinophil numbers are elevated in parasitic and helminthic infections, in which these cells are thought to play a role in the allergic response to those organisms. Cell numbers are also elevated in allergic reactions and in collagen vascular diseases, linking their function to immunomodulation. Hypereosinophilic syndromes, in which extremely high levels of eosinophils can be seen, are rare, and hypereosinophilia can be associated with damage to the lung, peripheral nervous system, and endocardial tissues. The differential diagnosis of eosinophilia is outlined in Table 48-1.

TABLE 48-1	DIFFERENTIAL DIAGNOSIS OF EOSINOPHILIA
CAUSES	**COMMENTS**
Infection*	Especially parasites; less commonly mycobacteria
Allergic diseases*	Drugs, asthma, allergic rhinitis, atopy, urticaria
Pulmonary diseases*	Churg-Strauss disease, Löffler's pneumonia, pulmonary infiltrates with eosinophilia
Drug reactions*	Usually disappears when drug discontinued
Malignancy*	Paraneoplastic, angioimmunoblastic T-cell lymphoma, Hodgkin's and non-Hodgkin's lymphoma
Connective tissue diseases*	Rheumatoid arthritis, eosinophilic fasciitis, vasculitis
Primary hypereosinophilic syndrome	More than 6 months of >1500 eosinophils/μL with no other apparent cause

*Reactive forms.

Basophils appear to play a role in immediate hypersensitivity reactions and chronic inflammatory conditions. Their levels are increased in chronic myeloid leukemias.

Monocytes

Monocytes arise from a common myeloid precursor along with granulocytes under the influence of granulocyte-macrophage colony-stimulating factor (GM-CSF) and macrophage colony-stimulating factor (M-CSF). Most circulating monocytes are marginated along the walls of blood vessels. They migrate from the vessels into tissues, where they develop into macrophages.

The monocyte-macrophage lineage has many diverse functions. These phagocytic cells perform chemotaxis, phagocytosis, and intracellular killing in much the same manner as neutrophils. They are especially important in killing infectious mycobacterial, fungal, and protozoal species.

Monocytes interact with other components of the immune system. They are antigen-presenting cells for T lymphocytes, they are capable of cellular cytotoxicity, and they secrete certain cytokines. The macrophages (i.e., differentiated monocytes) that process antigens and present them to T lymphocytes take on different forms in different tissues: Langerhans cells in the skin, interdigitating cells in the thymus, and dendritic cells in the lymph nodes. Antigen-presenting cells are nonphagocytic, and the process by which they internalize antigen is not fully understood. Protein antigens are partially digested and expressed on the cell surface in association with major histocompatibility complex class II (Ia) antigens. This feature permits interaction with and activation of helper T cells. Other macrophages, such as Kupffer cells of the liver and alveolar macrophages of the lung, play an important role in removing particulate and cellular debris and senescent erythrocytes from the circulation.

Monocytes are capable of antibody-dependent and antibody-independent cytotoxicity against tumor cells. Cytotoxicity is increased by tumor necrosis factor, interleukin-1, and interferon, which are secreted by monocytes. Monocytes secrete large numbers of immunomodulatory proteins (e.g., tumor necrosis factor, interleukin-1, interferon), cytokines (e.g., granulocyte colony-stimulating factor [G-CSF], GM-CSF), coagulation proteins, cell adhesion proteins, and proteases.

DETERMINANTS OF PERIPHERAL NEUTROPHIL NUMBERS

Most granulocyte precursors are in the bone marrow, where maturation occurs over 6 to 10 days. Marrow precursors represent 20% of the granulocyte mass, and the storage pool represents 75% of the granulocyte mass. Peripheral neutrophils represent only 5% of the total granulocyte mass.

Neutrophils circulate in transit between the marrow and peripheral tissues. More than one half of the circulating neutrophils adhere to the vascular endothelium (margination). The half-life of a neutrophil in the circulation was thought to be 6 to 12 hours, but in vivo studies suggest it may be as long as 3 to 4 days. After neutrophils migrate into tissues, they survive another 1 to 4 days. The peripheral neutrophil count therefore represents a sampling of less than 5% of the total granulocyte pool and is taken during a very short interval of the total neutrophil lifespan.

The peripheral white cell count is a poor reflection of granulocyte kinetics. Abnormalities in neutrophil number can occur rapidly and may reflect a change in marrow granulocyte production or a shift among various cellular compartments. An elevated peripheral white cell count may result from increased marrow production, or it may reflect mobilization of neutrophils from the marginated pool or release from the marrow storage pool. Similarly, a low granulocyte count may reflect decreased marrow production, increased margination or sequestration in the spleen, or increased destruction of peripheral cells.

The *total peripheral white cell count* represents the sum of lymphocytes and granulocytes. The significance of an elevated or depressed leukocyte count depends on the nature of the cellular elements that are increased or decreased. *Leukocytosis* is a nonspecific term that may denote an increase in lymphocytes (i.e., lymphocytosis) or neutrophils (i.e., granulocytosis). In rare cases, increases may reflect excessive numbers of monocytes or eosinophils. Leukocytosis related to an elevation in the neutrophil count is called *neutrophil leukocytosis* or *neutrophilia*.

Extreme elevation of the white blood cell count to more than 50,000 cells/μL of blood with the premature release of early myeloid precursors is called a *leukemoid reaction,* which may be associated with inflammation and infection. It requires consideration of a diagnosis of myeloproliferative disease, especially chronic myelogenous leukemia (CML). Evaluation of the peripheral blood smear may reveal characteristic changes that provide clues to the underlying disorder. A leukoerythroblastic smear shows immature granulocytes, teardrop-shaped erythrocytes, nucleated erythrocytes, and increased platelets. These changes reflect marrow infiltration (i.e., myelophthisis) by fibrous tissue, granulomas, or neoplasm. As with leukocytosis, leukopenia may reflect lymphopenia or neutropenia. Neutropenia is defined by an absolute neutrophil count of less than 1500 cells/μL.

NEUTROPHILIA

Neutrophilia (i.e., leukocytosis) usually results from other processes, and it rarely indicates a primary hematologic disorder

(Table 48-2). However, patients with a persistently elevated neutrophil count, especially associated with an elevated hematocrit or platelet count, should be evaluated to rule out a primary myeloproliferative disorder. Peripheral blood evaluation for the BCR/ABL fusion product can be performed to rule out CML, and assays for JAK2 and calreticulin mutations can help to rule out non-CML myeloproliferative neoplasms. A leukocyte alkaline phosphatase assay was formerly used to rule out CML because the result was 0 in chronic phase CML, but with the advent of BCR/ABL testing, it has become obsolete.

Neutrophilia related to acute infection, stress, or acute steroid administration primarily reflects demargination and is usually transient. Persistent neutrophilia usually reflects chronic bone marrow stimulation. Nevertheless, a bone marrow aspirate and biopsy are rarely indicated in the work-up of neutrophilia. The exception is for patients who demonstrate leukoerythroblastic changes, for which a bone marrow examination and culture may be indicated to rule out tuberculosis or fungal infection, marrow infiltration with tumor, or marrow fibrosis. Cytogenetic and molecular studies should be performed to help eliminate the diagnosis of marrow malignancies, and the marrow should be cultured for mycobacteria and fungi.

NEUTROPENIA
Differential Diagnosis

Neutropenia (i.e., leukopenia) may reflect decreased production, increased sequestration, or peripheral destruction of neutrophils (Table 48-3). Patients should first be evaluated for splenomegaly to rule out the possibility of sequestration.

For patients who are completely asymptomatic and for whom previous studies are unavailable, the possibility of constitutional or cyclic neutropenia should be entertained and can be evaluated by serial peripheral blood counts. The normal neutrophil count varies among ethnic groups and is lower in American blacks (i.e., constitutional neutropenia) than it is in whites. Cyclic neutropenia is a relatively benign disorder, in which cyclical changes occur in all hematopoietic cell lines but are most dramatic in the neutrophil lineage. At the nadir of the neutrophil counts, patients may have infections, but the disease is often clinically silent. In contrast, patients with congenital agranulocytosis or severe congenital neutropenia (SCN) exhibit profound neutropenia and infections in the perinatal period. Kostmann's syndrome is a subset of SCN that was described 50 years ago as an autosomal

recessive disorder; later studies demonstrated that SCN might be autosomal dominant, autosomal recessive, X-linked, or sporadic and that the causes were also heterogeneous.

About 50% of autosomal dominant SCN and almost 100% of cyclic neutropenia cases are associated with inherited mutations in the neutrophil elastase gene. The mutations are thought to produce a misfolded neutrophil elastase protein, which accumulates in the endoplasmic reticulum and activates the unfolded protein response. This complex cellular stress response coordinates the degradation of misfolded protein in the endoplasmic reticulum and can trigger cellular apoptosis if the stress is severe. Later studies have established that autosomal recessive SCN (i.e. Kostmann's syndrome) is caused by mutations in the HAX1 gene, which encodes a mitochondrial protein that is required for stabilization of the mitochondrial membrane. Absence of HAX1 results in loss of the mitochondrial membrane potential and induction of apoptosis.

Until G-CSF became available, most patients with SCN died in early childhood, but the availability of cytokine therapy has prolonged survival. However, SCN is also associated with a significantly increased incidence of acute leukemia, a complication that has become apparent as patients survive longer. Up to 30% of patients with SCN develop acute myelogenous leukemia over 10 years. Acute myelogenous leukemia in these patients is often associated with truncation mutations in the G-CSF receptor. These acquired somatic mutations may contribute to the pathogenesis of leukemia but do not contribute to the congenital neutropenia. The role of the G-CSF receptor mutations in the pathogenesis of leukemic transformation is controversial, as is the relationship between G-CSF therapy and the acquisition of these mutations.

Neutropenia may occur during or after viral, bacterial, or mycobacterial infections. Postviral neutropenia is especially common in children and probably reflects increased neutrophil consumption and a viral suppression of marrow neutrophil production. Neutropenia may be seen as a complication of overwhelming sepsis and is associated with a poor prognosis.

Drug-induced neutropenia may reflect dose-dependent marrow suppression or an idiosyncratic immune response. The former is one of the most common complications of chemotherapeutic drugs and is also common with antibiotics such as sulfamethoxazole-trimethoprim. Chloramphenicol causes

TABLE 48-2	DIFFERENTIAL DIAGNOSIS OF NEUTROPHILIA	
PRIMARY HEMATOLOGIC DISEASE	Cytokine stimulation (e.g., granulocyte colony-simulating factor)
Congenital neutrophilia	Chronic inflammation
Leukocyte adhesion deficiency	Malignancy
Myeloproliferative disorders	Myelophthisis
DUE TO OTHER DISEASE PROCESSES	Marrow hyperstimulation
	Chronic hemolysis, immune thrombocytopenia
Infection (acute or chronic)	Recovery from marrow suppression
Acute stress	After splenectomy
Drugs (e.g., steroids, lithium)	Smoking

TABLE 48-3	DIFFERENTIAL DIAGNOSIS OF NEUTROPENIA
DECREASED PRODUCTION OF NEUTROPHILS	**INCREASED PERIPHERAL DESTRUCTION**
Congenital and/or constitutional cause	Overwhelming infection
Constitutional neutropenia	Immune destruction
Benign chronic neutropenia	Drug related
Kostmann's syndrome	Associated with collagen vascular disease
Benign cyclic neutropenia	Isoimmune (in newborns)
Postinfectious cause	Large granular lymphocyte leukemia
Nutritional deficiency (B_{12}, folate)	Hypersplenism and/or sequestration
Drug-induced cause	
Primary marrow failure	
Aplastic anemia	
Myelodysplasia	
Acute leukemia	

dose-dependent marrow suppression, although its more ominous complication is the rare idiosyncratic reaction that gives rise to marrow aplasia. Drugs that are most commonly associated with neutropenia include clozapine, sulfasalazine, ticlopidine, and the thionamide antithyroid agents. Most drug-induced neutropenias respond rapidly to discontinuation of the offending agent. The administration of G-CSF speeds recovery.

Autoimmune neutropenia may be seen as a primary disease or as a secondary manifestation of systemic autoimmune disease or lymphoproliferative disease. Primary autoimmune neutropenia is a disorder of infants and young children that resolves spontaneously in more than 90% of patients within 2 years. Secondary autoimmune neutropenia is a common accompaniment to systemic lupus erythematosus. Although not usually clinically severe, neutropenia is often a marker of disease activity.

Neutropenia in rheumatoid arthritis is associated with splenomegaly (i.e., Felty's syndrome) and is part of the spectrum of large granular lymphocyte (LGL) leukemia. LGL leukemia is a clonal expansion of suppressor T cells. Patients who develop LGL in association with rheumatoid arthritis share a common HLA-DR4 haplotype with patients with Felty's syndrome, suggesting that they are in a common spectrum of disease. LGL is also a relatively common cause of acquired neutropenia in elderly patients in the absence of rheumatoid arthritis. Recent data have linked LGL to mutations in the STAT3 gene.

Laboratory Evaluation

Unless the diagnosis of benign or cyclic neutropenia is likely, the evaluation of the patient with neutropenia should include stopping all potentially offending drugs and performing serologic studies to rule out collagen vascular disease. Unlike the evaluation of patients with leukocytosis, bone marrow examination is indicated early for those with neutropenia and is frequently diagnostic. Neutropenia often reflects primary hematologic disease, and bone marrow examination enables the physician to diagnose marrow failure syndromes, leukemia, and myelodysplasia. In the absence of bone marrow failure, other causes of neutropenia may give a characteristic bone marrow picture. All patients undergoing bone marrow examination should have cytogenetic studies performed to aid in the diagnosis of myelodysplasia.

Sudden onset of agranulocytosis that does not affect platelets or erythrocytes typically is attributable to drug or toxin exposure. Bone marrow examination is rarely necessary. If performed, drug-induced neutropenia produces a characteristic maturation arrest of myeloid cells. Rather than actual inhibition of neutrophil maturation, this feature reflects the immune destruction of myeloid precursors that leaves only the earliest cells behind.

Treatment

The therapeutic approach to patients with neutropenia depends on the degree of depression of the neutrophil count. Neutrophil counts between 1000 and 1500 cells/µL are not usually associated with significant impairment of the host response to bacterial infection and require no intervention beyond that demanded for diagnosis and treatment of the underlying cause. Patients with neutrophil counts between 500 and 1000 cells/µL should be alerted to their slightly increased risk of infection, although serious problems are rarely encountered in patients with functional neutrophils and counts higher than 500 cells/µL.

Patients with neutrophil counts lower than 500 cells/µL are at significant risk for infection. They should be instructed to notify the physician at the first sign of infection or fever, and they must be managed aggressively with intravenous antibiotics regardless of the documentation of a source or infecting organism. Patients with a significantly depressed neutrophil count may exhibit few signs of infection because much of the inflammatory response at the site of infection is generated by the neutrophils themselves.

In patients with severe immune-mediated neutropenia, steroids and intravenous immunoglobulin may be helpful in elevating the neutrophil count and in preventing infectious complications. G-CSF may increase the peripheral white cell count and may help resolve infections in neutropenia induced by drugs, including chemotherapy. It has been efficacious for some patients with immune-mediated neutropenia and those with myelodysplasia.

For a deeper discussion of these topics, please see Chapter 167, "Leukocytosis and Leukopenia" in Goldman-Cecil Medicine, *25th Edition.*

PROSPECTUS FOR THE FUTURE

Significant progress has been made in elucidating the molecular pathogenesis of severe congenital neutropenia and cyclic neutropenia. Compounds that modulate the unfolded protein response may play a role in the treatment of these disorders. Other studies of the molecular basis of myeloid differentiation are establishing the importance of transcription factor function in neutrophil maturation and are providing insights into the pathogenesis of leukemia and myelodysplasia. Their findings may delineate pathways with entry points for therapeutic intervention in myeloid malignancies.

SUGGESTED READINGS

Aktari M, Curtis B, Waller EK: Autoimmune neutropenia in adults, Autoimmun Rev 9:62–68, 2009.

Andres E, Maloisel F: Idiosyncratic drug-induced agranulocytosis and acute neutropenia, Curr Opin Hematol 15:15–21, 2008.

Baehner R: Normal phagocyte structure and function. In Hoffman R, Benz EJ, Shattil SJ, editors: Hematology: basic principles and practice, ed 4, New York, 2005, Churchill Livingstone, pp 737–762.

Beekman R, Touw IP: G-CSF and its receptor in myeloid malignancy, Blood 115:5131–5136, 2010.

Berliner N: Lessons from congenital neutropenia: 50 years of progress in understanding myelopoiesis, Blood 111:5427–5432, 2008.

Berliner N: Leukocytosis and leukopenia. In Goldman L, Schafer AI, editors: Goldman's Cecil medicine, ed 24, Philadelphia, 2011, Elsevier Saunders.

Glogauer M: Disorders of phagocyte function. In Goldman L, Schafer AI, editors: Goldman's Cecil medicine, ed 24, Philadelphia, 2011, Elsevier Saunders.

Pillay J, den Braber I, Vrisekoop N, et al: In vivo labeling with 2H2O reveals a human neutrophil lifespan of 5.4 days, Blood 116:625–627, 2010.

Xia J, Link DC: Severe congenital neutropenia and the unfolded protein response, Curr Opin Hematol 15:1–7, 2008.

Zhang R, Shah MV, Loughran TP Jr: The root of many evils: indolent large granular lymphocyte leukaemia and associated disorders, Hematol Oncol 28:105–117, 2010.

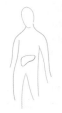

49

Disorders of Lymphocytes

Jill Lacy and Stuart Seropian

● INTRODUCTION

The central cell of the immune system is the lymphocyte. Lymphocytes mediate the adaptive immune response, providing specificity to the immune system by responding to specific pathogens and conferring long-lasting immunity to reinfection. Lymphocytes are derived from pluripotent hematopoietic stem cells that reside in the bone marrow and give rise to all of the cellular elements of the blood. The two major functional classes of lymphocytes—B lymphocytes (B cells) and T lymphocytes (T cells)—are distinguished by their site of development, antigenic receptors, and function.

The major disorders of lymphocytes include neoplastic transformations of specific subsets of lymphocytes that result in an array of lymphomas or leukemias, congenital or acquired defects in lymphocyte development or function with resultant immunodeficiency syndromes, and physiologic responses to infection or antigenic stimulation that may lead to lymphadenopathy, lymphocytosis, or lymphocytopenia.

● LYMPHOCYTE DEVELOPMENT, FUNCTION, AND LOCALIZATION

B Cells

B cells are characterized by cell surface immunoglobulins (i.e., antibodies). Their major function is to mount a humoral immune response to antigens by producing antigen-specific antibodies.

B cells develop in the bone marrow in a series of highly coordinated steps that involve sequential rearrangement of the heavy- and light-chain immunoglobulin genes and expression of B-cell–specific cell surface proteins (Fig. 49-1). Rearrangement of the immunoglobulin genes results in generation of a large repertoire of B cells that are each characterized by an immunoglobulin molecule with unique antigenic specificity. Mature B cells

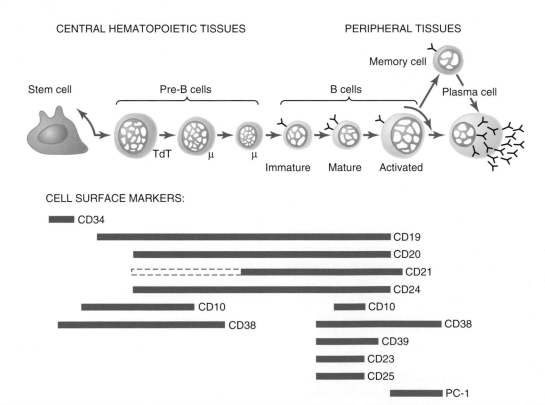

FIGURE 49-1 The maturation of B lymphocytes. *Top*, The changes in immunoglobulin production and maturation. *Bottom*, The appearance and disappearance of surface markers. TdT, Terminal deoxynucleotidyl transferase. (Modified from Ferrarini M, Grossi CE, Cooper MD: Cellular and molecular biology of lymphoid cells. In Handin RI, Lux SE, Stossel TP, editors: Blood principles and practice of hematology, Philadelphia, 1995, JB Lippincott, p 643.)

migrate from the bone marrow to lymphoid tissue throughout the body and are readily identified by cell surface immunoglobulin and antigens that are B cell specific, including CD19, CD20, and CD21.

In response to antigen binding to cell surface immunoglobulin, mature B cells are activated to proliferate and undergo differentiation to end-stage plasma cells, which lose most of their B-cell surface markers and produce large quantities of soluble antibodies. Neoplastic disorders of B cells arise from B cells at different stages of development, and B-cell lymphomas can have highly varied morphology and cell surface expression of B-cell antigens (i.e., immunophenotype).

T Cells

T cells perform an array of functions in the immune response, including those that are regarded as classic cellular immune responses. T-cell precursors migrate from the bone marrow to the thymus, where they differentiate into mature T-cell subsets and undergo selection to eliminate autoreactive T cells that respond to self-peptides. In the thymus, T-cell precursors undergo a coordinated process of differentiation that involves rearrangement and expression of the T-cell receptor (TCR) genes and acquisition of cell surface proteins that are unique to T cells, including CD3, CD4, and CD8.

As T cells mature in the thymus, they ultimately lose the CD4 or CD8 protein. Mature T cells are composed of two major groups: CD4$^+$ and CD8$^+$ cells. After T-cell maturation and selection in the thymus, mature CD4$^+$ and CD8$^+$ T cells migrate to lymph nodes, spleen, and other sites in the peripheral immune system. Mature T cells constitute about 80% of peripheral blood lymphocytes, 40% of lymph node cells, and 25% of splenic lymphoid cells.

Mature CD4$^+$ and CD8$^+$ T-cell subsets mediate distinct immune functions. CD8$^+$ cells kill virus-infected or foreign cells and suppress immune functions; CD8$^+$ cells are called *cytotoxic T cells*. CD4$^+$ cells activate other immune response cells such as B cells and macrophages by producing cytokines and through direct cell contact; CD4$^+$ cells are caled *helper T cells*.

Similar to B cells, T cells express unique TCR molecules that recognize specific peptide antigens. In contrast to B cells, T cells respond only to peptides that are processed intracellularly and bound to (or presented by) specialized cell surface antigen-presenting proteins, designated major histocompatibility complex (MHC) molecules. CD4$^+$ and CD8$^+$ T cells are MHC class restricted in their response to peptide-MHC complexes. CD4$^+$ cells recognize antigenic peptide fragments only when they are presented by MHC class II molecules, and CD8$^+$ cells recognize antigenic peptide fragments only when they are presented by MHC class I molecules. Binding of the TCR by a specific peptide-MHC complex triggers activation signals that lead to the expression of gene products that mediate the wide diversity of helper functions of CD4$^+$ cells or cytotoxic effector functions of CD8$^+$ cells. A detailed discussion is provided in Chapter 45.

Lymphoid System

Lymphocytes localize to the peripheral lymphoid tissue, which is the site of antigen-lymphocyte interaction and lymphocyte activation. The peripheral lymphoid tissue is composed of lymph nodes, the spleen, and mucosal lymphoid tissue. Lymphocytes circulate continuously through these tissues through the vascular and lymphatic systems.

The lymph nodes are highly organized lymphoid tissues that are sites of convergence of the lymphatic drainage system, which carries antigens from draining lymph to the nodes, where they are trapped. A lymph node consists of an outer cortex and an inner medulla (Fig. 49-2). The cortex is organized into lymphoid follicles composed predominantly of B cells. Some of the follicles contain central areas or germinal centers, where activated B cells undergo proliferation after encountering a specific antigen, that are surrounded by a mantle zone. The T cells are distributed more diffusely in paracortical areas surrounding the follicles.

The spleen traps antigens from blood rather than from the lymphatic system and is the site of disposal of senescent red cells. The lymphocytes in the spleen reside in the areas described as the white pulp, which surround the arterioles entering the organ. As in lymph nodes, the B and T cells are segregated into a periarteriolar lymphoid sheath that is composed of T cells and flanking follicles composed of B cells. The mucosa-associated lymphoid tissues (MALTs) collect antigen from epithelial surfaces and include the gut-associated lymphoid tissue (i.e., tonsils, adenoids, appendix, and Peyer's patches of the small intestine) and more diffusely organized aggregates of lymphocytes at other mucosal sites.

Lymphocytes circulate in the peripheral blood and represent 20% to 40% of peripheral blood leukocytes in adults; the proportion is higher in newborns and children. Between 80% and 90% of peripheral blood lymphocytes are T cells, and the remaining lymphocytes are largely B cells. A small percentage of peripheral blood lymphoid cells represents a third category of lymphoid cells that are referred to as natural killer (NK) cells. These cells

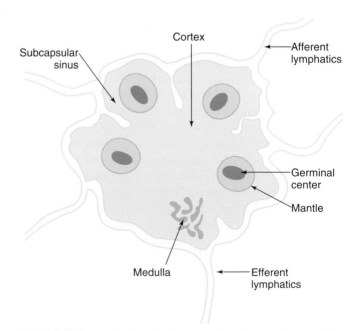

FIGURE 49-2 Structure of the normal lymph node. The cortical area contains the follicles, which consist of a germinal center and a mantle zone. The medulla contains a complex of channels that lead to the efferent lymphatics.

do not bear the characteristic cell surface molecules of B or T cells, and their immunoglobulin or TCR genes have not undergone rearrangement. Morphologically, the cells are large, with abundant cytoplasm containing azurophilic granules, and they are often called *large granular lymphocytes*. Functionally, they are part of the innate immune system, responding nonspecifically to a wide range of pathogens without requiring prior antigenic exposure.

NEOPLASIA OF LYMPHOID ORIGIN

Malignant transformation of lymphocytes leads to a diverse array of neoplasms of lymphoid origin, including tumors that arise from T cells, B cells, or NK cells. Lymphoid malignancies usually involve lymphoid tissues, but they can arise in or spread to any site. The major clinical groupings of lymphoid malignancies include non-Hodgkin's lymphomas (NHLs), Hodgkin's lymphoma, lymphoid leukemias, and plasma cell dyscrasias.

Non-Hodgkin's Lymphomas

Definition and Epidemiology

The NHLs comprise a heterogeneous group of lymphoid malignancies that have different histologic appearances, cells of origin and immunophenotypes, molecular biologic factors, clinical features, prognoses, and outcomes with therapy. According to the Surveillance, Epidemiology, and End Results (SEER) database, the NHLs are the seventh most common cancer type, with 70000 cases occurring in 2013 and 19,000 patients succumbing to these diseases. The NHLs occur at a median age of 66 and are more common in men and in whites. The rate of NHLs increased slowly between 2000 and 2010 by 0.5% per year, but the annual death rate declined during the same time period.

Pathology

In view of the heterogeneity of NHLs, classification systems have been devised to identify specific pathologic subtypes that correlate with distinct clinical entities. These systems have evolved steadily over the past 50 years as correlations between histopathologic and biologic behavior have emerged. Pathologic classification schemes have attempted to correlate malignant NHL subtypes with normal cellular counterparts. The World Health Organization (WHO) classification (Table 49-1) is the most current and incorporates morphologic features, immunophenotype, and cytogenetic characteristics to describe NHL subtypes. The most common NHLs encountered in the United States are diffuse large B-cell lymphoma (DLBCL), follicular lymphoma, small lymphocytic lymphoma or leukemia (i.e., chronic lymphocytic leukemia [CLL]), and mantle cell lymphoma.

The cause of most NHLs is unknown. In most patients with NHL, no apparent genetic predisposition or epidemiologic or environmental factor can be identified. Many of the NHL subtypes carry pathognomonic chromosomal translocations that often involve an immunoglobulin locus (or TCR locus in T-cell–derived NHLs) and an oncogene or growth regulatory gene. The cause of these aberrant chromosomal rearrangements is unknown.

Patients with congenital immunodeficiency syndromes or autoimmune disorders are at increased risk for NHL. Oncogenic human viruses play a causal role in some of the less common

TABLE 49-1	WORLD HEALTH ORGANIZATION CLASSIFICATION OF LYMPHOID NEOPLASMS*

B-CELL NEOPLASMS

Precursor B-cell neoplasm
Precursor B-lymphoblastic leukemia/lymphoma (precursor B-cell acute lymphoblastic leukemia)
Mature (peripheral) B-cell neoplasms
B-cell chronic lymphocytic leukemia/small lymphocytic lymphoma
  B-cell prolymphocytic leukemia
  Lymphoplasmacytic lymphoma
  Splenic marginal zone B-cell lymphoma (± villous lymphocytes)
  Splenic B-cell lymphoma/leukemia, unclassifiable
  Hairy cell leukemia
Plasma cell myeloma/plasmacytoma
Extranodal marginal zone B-cell lymphoma of MALT type
  Nodal marginal zone B-cell lymphoma of MALT type
  Primary cutaneous follicle center lymphoma
Follicular lymphoma
Mantle cell lymphoma
Diffuse large B-cell lymphoma
  Mediastinal large B-cell lymphoma
  Primary effusion lymphoma
Burkitt's lymphoma/Burkitt cell leukemia

T-CELL AND NK-CELL NEOPLASMS

Precursor T-cell neoplasm
Precursor T-lymphoblastic lymphoma/leukemia (precursor T-cell acute lymphoblastic leukemia)
Mature (peripheral) T-cell neoplasms
  T-cell prolymphocytic leukemia
  T-cell granular lymphocytic leukemia
  Aggressive NK-cell leukemia
  Adult T-cell lymphoma/leukemia (HTLV-1 positive)
  Extranodal NK-cell or T-cell lymphoma, nasal type
  Enteropathy-type T-cell lymphoma
  Hepatosplenic gamma-delta T-cell lymphoma
  Subcutaneous panniculitis-like T-cell lymphoma
Mycosis fungoides/Sézary syndrome
  Anaplastic large cell lymphoma, T-cell/null cell, primary cutaneous type
Peripheral T-cell lymphoma, not otherwise characterized
Angioimmunoblastic T-cell lymphoma
Anaplastic large cell lymphoma, T-cell/null cell, primary systemic type

HTLV-1, Human T-cell leukemia virus type 1; MALT, mucosa-associated lymphoid tissue; NK, natural killer.

*Only major categories are included, and common entities are shown in bold type. B-cell and T-cell/NK-cell neoplasms are grouped according to major clinical presentations: predominantly disseminated or leukemic, primary extranodal, and predominantly nodal.

NHL variants. Epstein-Barr virus (EBV) is associated with several biologically aggressive NHLs, including acquired immunodeficiency syndrome (AIDS)–related diffuse, aggressive lymphomas, the lymphoproliferative disorders that arise in patients who are immunosuppressed after organ transplantation, and the form of Burkitt's lymphoma that is endemic in Africa. Human T-cell lymphotropic virus type 1 (HTLV-1) is causally linked with adult T-cell leukemia/lymphoma, which is endemic in areas of Japan and the Caribbean basin. The human herpesvirus 8 (HHV-8) of Kaposi's sarcoma has been implicated in a variant of diffuse, aggressive NHL that arises in serosal cavities and is encountered almost exclusively in patients infected with human immunodeficiency virus (HIV).

Several indolent lymphomas have been linked to infectious agents that appear to indirectly promote lymphomagenesis through chronic antigen stimulation, resulting in B-lymphocyte proliferation. *Helicobacter pylori* infection is linked to gastric MALT lymphomas in this manner, and eradication of infection with antibiotics is often associated with regression of the lymphoma.

Clinical Presentation

Although numerous subtypes of NHL are recognized, most disease entities may be viewed conceptually as clinically indolent (i.e., low grade) or aggressive (i.e., high grade). Indolent lymphomas typically grow slowly, do not always require therapy, and have a long natural history. A clinical history of recurring and regressing adenopathy may be elicited. Aggressive lymphomas are more likely to manifest with symptoms and are associated with limited survival in the absence of therapy.

Most patients with NHL exhibit painless lymphadenopathy involving one or more of the peripheral nodal sites. NHL can involve extranodal sites, and patients can exhibit a variety of symptoms that reflect the site of involvement. Common sites of extranodal disease include the gastrointestinal tract, bone marrow or focal bone lesions, liver, skin, and Waldeyer's ring in the nasopharynx and oropharynx, although virtually any site can be involved. Aggressive subtypes of NHL are more likely than indolent lymphomas to involve extranodal sites.

Central nervous system involvement, including leptomeningeal spread, rarely occurs with the indolent subtypes but does occur with the aggressive variants. The most aggressive NHLs (i.e., Burkitt's and lymphoblastic lymphomas) have a particular propensity to spread to the leptomeninges.

Constitutional symptoms such as fever, weight loss, or night sweats occur in about 20% of patients with NHL at the time of onset. These symptoms are more common in patients with aggressive subtypes of NHL.

Diagnosis and Differential Diagnosis

Many causes of lymphadenopathy exist in addition to lymphoid malignancies (Table 49-2). A thorough history and careful physical examination are important before performing a lymph node biopsy. The investigation of lymphadenopathy can be organized according to the location of the enlarged nodes (i.e., localized or generalized) and clinical symptoms.

Cervical lymphadenopathy is most often caused by infections of the upper respiratory tract, including infectious mononucleosis syndromes, viral syndromes, and bacterial pharyngitis. Unilateral axillary, inguinal, or femoral adenopathy may be caused by skin infections involving the extremity, including cat-scratch fever. Generalized lymphadenopathy may be caused by systemic infections (e.g., HIV, cytomegalovirus), drug reactions, autoimmune diseases, or one of the systemic lymphadenopathy syndromes. If the cause of persistent lymphadenopathy is not apparent after a thorough evaluation, an excisional lymph node biopsy should be undertaken. An enlarged supraclavicular lymph node strongly suggests malignancy and should always be sampled.

The accurate diagnosis of lymphoma requires excisional biopsy of a lymph node or generous biopsy of involved lymph tissue. Fine-needle aspiration or needle biopsy is rarely sufficient. Analysis of the pathologic specimen should include routine histologic examination and immunophenotyping. Immunophenotyping can determine the cell of origin (i.e., B cell, T cell, NK cell, or nonlymphoid cell), and the pattern of cell surface antigens aids subclassification of lymphomas. In the case of B-cell NHLs,

TABLE 49-2 CAUSES OF LYMPHADENOPATHY
INFECTIOUS DISEASES
Viral: infectious mononucleosis syndromes (cytomegalovirus, Epstein-Barr virus), acquired immunodeficiency syndrome, rubella, herpes simplex, infectious hepatitis
Bacterial: localized infection with regional adenopathy (streptococci, staphylococci), cat-scratch disease (*Bartonella henselae*), brucellosis, tularemia, listeriosis, bubonic plague (*Yersinia pestis*), chancroid (*Haemophilus ducreyi*)
Fungal: coccidioidomycosis, histoplasmosis
Chlamydial: lymphogranuloma venereum, trachoma
Mycobacterial: scrofula, tuberculosis, leprosy
Protozoan: toxoplasmosis, trypanosomiasis
Spirochetal: Lyme disease, syphilis, leptospirosis
IMMUNOLOGIC DISEASES
Rheumatoid arthritis
Systemic lupus erythematosus
Mixed connective tissue disease
Sjögren syndrome
Dermatomyositis
Serum sickness
Drug reactions: phenytoin, hydralazine, allopurinol
MALIGNANT DISEASES
Lymphomas
Solid tumors metastatic to lymph nodes: melanoma, lung, breast, head and neck, gastrointestinal tract, Kaposi's sarcoma, unknown primary tumor, renal, prostate
ATYPICAL LYMPHOID PROLIFERATIONS
Giant follicular lymph node hyperplasia
Transformation of germinal centers
Castleman's disease
MISCELLANEOUS DISEASES AND DISEASES OF UNKNOWN CAUSE
Dermatopathic lymphadenitis
Sarcoidosis
Immunoglobulin G4 (IgG4) Lymphadenopathy
Amyloidosis
Mucocutaneous lymph node syndrome (Kawasaki disease)
Sinus histiocytosis (Rosai-Dorfman syndrome)
Multifocal Langerhans cell (eosinophilic) granulomatosis
Lipid storage diseases: Gaucher's and Niemann-Pick diseases

immunophenotyping can also reveal whether the process is monoclonal in origin (i.e., neoplastic) by determining whether the surface immunoglobulin is restricted to the κ or λ light chain. In some cases, cytogenetic analysis or molecular studies of immunoglobulin or TCR gene rearrangement may be required to determine the pathologic subtype of lymphoma or to establish a monoclonal (i.e., malignant) process. If a lymph node biopsy is nondiagnostic and unexplained lymph node enlargement persists, the biopsy should be repeated.

For patients with bone marrow and peripheral blood involvement, such as in small lymphocytic lymphoma or CLL, the diagnosis may be made based on immunophenotyping of peripheral blood lymphocytes by flow cytometry. Care must be taken to exclude the possibility of aggressive lymphoma manifesting with involved lymph nodes or extranodal sites in a patient harboring a low-grade or chronic indolent lymphoma such as small lymphocytic lymphoma that is confined to the blood or bone marrow.

Treatment

After a lymphoma has been diagnosed, patients should undergo a complete staging evaluation (Table 49-3). Staging determines

TABLE 49-3　STAGING EVALUATION FOR LYMPHOMAS

REQUIRED EVALUATION PROCEDURES

Biopsy of lesion with review by an experienced hematopathologist
History with attention to the presence or absence of B symptoms
Physical examination with attention to node-bearing areas (including Waldeyer's ring) and size of liver and spleen
Standard blood work:
　Complete blood count
　Lactate dehydrogenase and β_2-microglobulin
　Evaluation of renal function
　Liver function tests
　Calcium, uric acid
Bone marrow aspirate and biopsy
Radiologic studies, including:
　Chest radiograph (posteroanterior and lateral)
　Chest, abdomen, and pelvic CT scans
　PET scan (in Hodgkin's and intermediate- and high-grade lymphomas)

PROCEDURES REQUIRED UNDER CERTAIN CIRCUMSTANCES

Plain bone radiographs of symptomatic sites or abnormal areas on bone scan
Brain or spinal CT or MRI if neurologic signs or symptoms
Serum and urine protein electrophoresis
Lumbar puncture with cerebrospinal fluid cytology (Burkitt's and lymphoblastic lymphoma)

B symptoms, Fever, sweats, and weight loss >10% of body weight; CT, computed tomography; MRI, magnetic resonance imaging; PET, positron emission tomography.

TABLE 49-4　LYMPHOMA STAGING SYSTEM

STAGE*	DESCRIPTION
I	Involvement of a single lymph node region or structure (I) or a single extralymphatic site (IE)
II	Involvement of two or more lymph node regions on the same side of the diaphragm (II) or localized involvement of a contiguous extralymphatic site and lymph node region (IIE)
III	Involvement of lymph node regions on both sides of the diaphragm (III), which may be accompanied by localized involvement of one extralymphatic site (IIIE) or spleen (IIIS) or both (IIISE)
IV	Diffuse or disseminated involvement of one or more extralymphatic organs with or without associated lymph node involvement

*Presence or absence of symptoms should be documented with each stage designation: A (asymptomatic) or B (fever, sweats, and weight loss >10% of body weight).

the extent of involvement, provides prognostic information, and may influence the choice of therapy. The modified Ann Arbor staging classification is used to stage patients with NHL and Hodgkin's disease (Table 49-4).

A variety of ancillary tests may be performed in specific situations. For example, a test for HTLV-1 or HIV should be performed if adult T-cell leukemia/lymphoma is suspected. Patients with a clinical history suggesting immunodeficiency or behavioral risk factors should be tested for HIV infection. A gastrointestinal series or endoscopic evaluation may be warranted for patients with gastrointestinal symptoms or patients at risk for gastrointestinal tract involvement (i.e., mantle cell lymphoma and other lymphomas involving Waldeyer's ring). The choice of therapy for NHLs is guided by stage, specific subtype, and clinical considerations such as age and the general medical condition of the patient.

Lymphoma Subtypes

Indolent Non-Hodgkin's Lymphomas

The common low-grade or indolent histologic conditions include follicular lymphoma, small lymphocytic lymphoma (which is identical to CLL and discussed later), and marginal zone lymphomas.

Follicular lymphoma accounts for one third of all lymphomas and is the most common indolent lymphoma. It is a mature clonal B-cell neoplasm that histologically retains nodular architecture in the lymph node, which is infiltrated by small, mature-appearing lymphocytes. The immunophenotype is positive for surface markers (CD10, CD19, CD20, CD21) and negative for CD5. Follicular lymphomas are characterized cytogenetically by the t(14;18) translocation that juxtaposes the immunoglobulin heavy chain *(IGH)* locus with the antiapoptotic B-cell CLL/lymphoma 2 gene *(BCL2)*; the BCL2 protein is uniformly overexpressed in follicular lymphomas, immortalizing affected cells.

Follicular lymphoma is a low-grade, indolent neoplasm with a long natural history (median survival approaches 10 years), but 80% to 90% of patients have advanced-stage (III/IV) disease at diagnosis, often with bone marrow involvement, and they cannot be cured with standard treatment modalities. For up to one half of patients with follicular NHL, the disease eventually transforms to a more aggressive lymphoma, characterized pathologically by a diffuse large cell infiltrate and clinically by rapidly expanding nodes or other tumor masses, rising lactate dehydrogenase (LDH) levels, and the onset of disease-related symptoms.

Management of follicular lymphomas is influenced by the stage. For the few patients with early-stage (I/some nonbulky II) disease after clinical staging, the appropriate treatment is radiation therapy. With the use of subtotal or total lymphoid irradiation, more than one half of patients with early-stage disease achieve a durable remission or cure.

For patients with advanced-stage disease, the management is more controversial. Although advanced-stage indolent NHL is responsive to a variety of treatment modalities, the incurability and the long natural history have led to the practice of deferring treatment until the patient develops symptoms. This strategy is referred to as the *watch and wait approach*. Indications for treatment include cosmetic or mechanical problems caused by enlarging lymph nodes, high tumor burden, constitutional symptoms, and evidence of marrow compromise.

Available treatment options include monoclonal antibody therapies, chemotherapeutic agents, and radiolabelled antibodies. For most patients, the appropriate treatment typically includes the chimeric anti–B-cell monoclonal antibody rituximab with or without systemic chemotherapy. The addition of rituximab to chemotherapy regimens has increased response rates, duration of remission, and in some studies, overall survival (level I evidence).

The choice of chemotherapy to employ in combination with rituximab may be influenced by the patient's age and medical condition. Multiple options are available, and no regimen has proved superior with regard to overall survival. The combination of bendamustine, a unique agent with properties similar to alkylating agents and purine analogues, plus rituximab appeared advantageous compared with the CHOP regimen (i.e., cyclophosphamide, hydroxydaunorubicin [doxorubicin], Oncovin [vincristine], and prednisone) plus rituximab in a randomized trial with regard to toxicity, response rate, and progression-free survival (level 1 evidence).

Most patients respond to treatment, and at least one third achieve a clinical complete remission that may last 1 to 3 years. Treatment with cytotoxic agents is typically discontinued when the maximum response has been achieved, but rituximab may be continued on an intermittent schedule to maintain remission. It has been shown to prolong remission times in randomized studies (level 1 evidence). Risk of recurrence and cost considerations may influence the use of this therapy because rituximab may also be used at the time of recurrence with similar outcomes.

After a patient relapses, subsequent remissions may be achieved but are often less durable compared with the first remission. Therapeutic options for patients who relapse include retreatment with chemotherapy, often with a different drug or combination than that used initially. Patients in relapse can also be treated with rituximab as a single agent. Two radioactively labeled anti-CD20 antibodies, ibritumomab tiuxetan (yttrium labeled) and tositumomab (iodine 131 labeled), are also used for patients with relapsed or refractory follicular lymphoma, and they have been associated with a high response rate. For patients who have clinical or pathologic evidence of transformation to a higher grade of lymphoma, treatment that is appropriate for a diffuse, aggressive histology should be offered (discussed later).

High-dose chemotherapy with autologous or allogeneic stem cell transplantation for follicular NHLs may be appropriate for selected patients with recurrent or refractory disease. Long-term follow-up of patients undergoing allogeneic transplantation suggests that some patients are cured with this modality, but the morbidity associated with allogeneic transplantation has limited its widespread use for refractory indolent lymphomas.

In addition to the follicular NHLs, the MALT lymphomas and closely related marginal zone lymphomas are considered low-grade, indolent subtypes. Given the excellent prognosis, localized nature, and long natural history of the MALT lymphomas, they usually are managed conservatively with local treatment modalities (i.e., irradiation or surgery) and avoidance of systemic chemotherapy. The monoclonal antibody rituximab has activity against MALT lymphomas and may be used when systemic therapy is desired. The gastric MALT lymphomas are highly associated with *H. pylori* infection, and remissions can often be achieved with eradication of this infection. Antibiotic therapy is the first-line treatment for early *H. pylori*–positive gastric MALT lymphoma.

Aggressive Non-Hodgkin's Lymphomas

Aggressive NHLs include DLBCL, anaplastic large cell lymphoma, peripheral T-cell lymphomas, and the high-grade lymphomas, Burkitt's lymphoma and lymphoblastic lymphoma (see High-Grade Non-Hodgkin's Lymphomas). Most of the diffuse, aggressive large cell lymphomas are B cell in origin; aggressive T-cell lymphomas are managed similarly but have an overall worse prognosis compared with their B-cell counterparts.

DLBCL accounts for up to 40% of all NHL subtypes. In contrast to patients with low-grade follicular NHLs, all patients with diffuse, aggressive histology should be offered immediate therapy because these lymphomas are life-threatening but potentially curable. The standard initial therapy for all patients with diffuse, aggressive NHL, regardless of stage, is a multidrug chemotherapy regimen that includes an anthracycline in combination with the anti-CD20 monoclonal antibody rituximab.

For DLBCL, CHOP is the most widely used chemotherapy regimen. Patients with early-stage disease (I/nonbulky II) may be treated with local radiation therapy after a minimum of three cycles of CHOP plus rituximab if there is a need to limit exposure to chemotherapy. Patients with advanced-stage disease require six cycles of CHOP plus rituximab; the role of local radiation to sites of bulky disease in the setting of advanced-stage disease is not established. Complete remissions can be achieved with CHOP plus rituximab or similar regimens, and more than 50% of patients are cured.

Patients who experience relapse after achieving a remission may be cured with high-dose chemotherapy with autologous peripheral blood stem cell transplantation, particularly if their relapsed disease remains responsive to standard doses of chemotherapy. High-dose chemotherapy with autologous stem cell transplantation is superior to standard doses of salvage chemotherapy and is considered standard therapy for patients with chemosensitive diffuse, aggressive NHL that has relapsed.

Mantle Cell Lymphoma

Mantle cell lymphoma accounts for 5% to 8% of all NHLs and is most common in older male patients. Mantle cell lymphomas are mature B-cell neoplasms that appear to arise in the mantle zone of the lymphoid follicle and display a highly characteristic immunophenotype, expressing the CD5 antigen and other B-cell markers, but CD23 expression is absent, in contrast to CLL. Mantle cell lymphomas are also characterized by a pathognomonic t(11;14) chromosomal translocation that juxtaposes the immunoglobulin heavy chain gene (14q32 locus) with the *BCL1* gene, which encodes the growth-promoting protein cyclin D1. Demonstration of the translocation or expression of cyclin D1 protein by immunohistochemistry allows a definitive diagnosis in most cases. Pathologic classification as a blastoid or pleomorphic subtype and a high proliferation rate are features associated with more aggressive behavior and a poor outcome.

Mantle cell lymphomas are in many ways similar to indolent lymphomas in that patients usually have advanced-stage disease with frequent bone marrow involvement. These lymphomas have a peculiar propensity to involve the Waldeyer ring and gastrointestinal tract. As with the low-grade follicular lymphomas, mantle cell lymphomas are treatable but not typically curable. However, in contrast to the indolent lymphomas, these neoplasms may be biologically aggressive, with a median survival of only 3 years.

Patients are usually treated with systemic chemotherapy combined with rituximab at diagnosis, but durable remissions are difficult to achieve. High-dose chemotherapy and autologous stem cell transplantation are often applied during first remission for younger patients and have been associated with more durable remissions (level II-1 evidence). Multiple agents and regimens are available for those who are not candidates for transplantation and patients with recurrent disease.

The proteosome inhibitor bortezomib is a novel nonchemotherapeutic agent with activity against mantle cell NHL. The Bruton tyrosine kinase inhibitor ibrutinib is a novel compound for the treatment of recurrent mantle cell lymphoma, and it represents a new class of targeted agents available for NHL treatment.

High-Grade Non-Hodgkin's Lymphomas

The two high-grade subtypes, Burkitt's lymphoma and lymphoblastic lymphoma, are rare in the adult population. Nonetheless, these subtypes are important because they are potentially curable with appropriate therapy and often require urgent, inpatient treatment at the time of diagnosis due to their highly aggressive nature, rapid growth, and tendency to develop tumor lysis on initiation of therapy.

Lymphoblastic lymphoma in adults is an aggressive lymphoma that is usually considered the lymphomatous counterpart of acute T-cell lymphocytic leukemia. B-cell lymphoblastic lymphoma is less common. Lymphoblastic lymphoma usually afflicts young adult men and involves the mediastinum and bone marrow, with a propensity to relapse in the leptomeninges.

Burkitt's lymphoma is a rare B-cell lymphoma in adults that is highly aggressive, with a propensity to involve the bone marrow and central nervous system. Burkitt's lymphoma is characterized cytogenetically by the pathognomonic t(8;14) translocation that moves the *MYC* oncogene from chromosome 8 to a location close to the enhancers of the antibody heavy-chain genes (*IGH* locus) on chromosome 14. In central Africa, where Burkitt's lymphoma is endemic in children, it is usually associated with EBV. However, in the United States, it is uncommon for sporadic Burkitt's lymphoma to be EBV positive.

Burkitt's lymphoma and lymphoblastic lymphomas require treatment with intensive multiagent chemotherapy, including intrathecal chemotherapy to prevent leptomeningeal relapse. These lymphomas undergo rapid tumor lysis on initiation of chemotherapy, and all patients must receive prophylaxis against tumor lysis syndrome before and during their first course of chemotherapy. Prophylaxis includes hydration, alkalinization of the urine, allopurinol, and consideration of rasburicase therapy for rapid lowering of elevated uric acid levels.

Prognosis

A variety of prognostic variables have been identified for NHL, and specific prognostic schemes have been devised for common diseases, including DLBCL, follicular NHL, and mantle cell lymphomas. The predictors for poor survival for most subtypes of NHL include advanced stage (III/IV) at onset, involvement of multiple extranodal sites of disease, elevated LDH levels, B symptoms (e.g., fever, night sweats, weight loss), and poor performance status.

The International Prognostic Index (IPI) stratifies patients based on age, performance status, stage, and number of extranodal sites. The likelihood of cure and long-term, disease-free survival ranges from more than 75% for patients with one or no adverse factors to less than 50% for patients with four or more adverse factors.

Factors associated with shortened survival in follicular NHL include older age, advanced stage, anemia, multiple lymph node sites (more than four), and elevated LDH levels. Patients with three or more of these factors have a median survival of 5 years, roughly one half of that of patients with zero or one risk factor. Aggressive T-cell lymphomas usually fare more poorly than B-cell NHL, and patients are typically considered candidates for investigational studies and transplantation therapies.

For a deeper discussion of these topics, please see Chapter 185, "Non-Hodgkin's Lymphomas," in Goldman-Cecil Medicine, *25th Edition.*

Hodgkin's Lymphoma

Hodgkin's lymphoma is a node-based lymphoid malignancy characterized by the neoplastic Reed-Sternberg (RS) cell in an inflammatory background. Hodgkin's lymphoma accounts for 10% of lymphomas, with about 9000 new cases diagnosed in the United States annually, and it is the most common lymphoma among young adults. The age distribution in industrialized countries is bimodal, with the larger peak occurring between the ages of 15 and 35 and a smaller peak seen in patients older than 50 years.

The cause of Hodgkin's lymphoma remains enigmatic. Risk factors include a history of infectious mononucleosis, high socioeconomic status, immunosuppression (e.g., HIV infection, allograft transplantion, immunosuppressive drugs), and autoimmune disorders. Although EBV is frequently detected in patients, a direct casual role has not been established.

Pathology

Hodgkin's lymphoma is diagnosed by identifying the RS cell in involved lymphoid tissue. The classic RS cell is large and binucleate, with each nucleus containing a prominent nucleolus, suggesting the appearance of owl eyes. Although the cellular origin of the RS cell was debated for decades, molecular studies have confirmed that RS cells are B cells with clonal rearrangement of the germline *IG* locus. Unlike NHL, the bulk of the infiltrate in lymph nodes involved with Hodgkin's lymphoma is usually composed of benign reactive inflammatory cells, and the RS cells often can be difficult to find. Immunophenotyping of classic RS cells reveals that they are CD30 (Ki-1) and CD15 positive and are negative for CD20, CD45, and cytoplasmic or surface immunoglobulin. EBV is identified in the RS cells in about 50% of cases.

The pathologic subtypes of classic Hodgkin's lymphoma include four variants—nodular sclerosing (NS), mixed cellularity (MC), lymphocyte depleted (LD), and lymphocyte rich (LR)—and the nonclassic variant, nodular lymphocyte-predominant (NLP). The NS form is the most common variant (60% to 80%) and is characterized by fibrous bands separating the node into nodules and by the lacunar type of RS cells. It is the predominant type encountered in adolescents and young adults and typically involves the mediastinum and supradiaphragmatic nodal sites. In the MC type (15%), band-forming sclerosis is absent, and RS cells are easily identified in a diffuse inflammatory infiltrate that is more heterogeneous than that seen in the NS variant. The LR variant (5%) is characterized by classic RS cells in a background composed predominantly of small lymphocytes. LD is a rare variant (<1%) that is associated with advanced age, HIV infection, and low socioeconomic status. The pathologic hallmarks of LD Hodgkin's lymphoma include a notable paucity of inflammatory cells and sheets of RS cells.

The NLP variant has emerged as a distinct entity that is more closely related to indolent NHL than to classic Hodgkin's lymphoma. The NLP form is characterized by a nodular growth pattern with variants of RS cells that have polylobated nuclei (i.e., popcorn cells); classic RS cells are usually absent. The immunophenotype of these variant cells is distinct from classic RS cells, with expression of B-cell antigens (CD19 and CD20) and CD45 and absence of CD15 and CD30. The existence of CD20 allows the therapeutic use of rituximab, an agent not typically employed in classic Hodgkin's lymphoma. The NLP variant accounts for 5% of Hodgkin's lymphoma cases, has a strong male preponderance, and tends to involve peripheral nodes but spare the mediastinum. The prognosis is excellent, although late relapses are more common than they are in classic Hodgkin's lymphoma.

Clinical Presentation

Hodgkin's lymphoma arises in lymph nodes, most commonly in the mediastinum or neck, and spreads to adjacent contiguous or noncontiguous nodal sites, including retroperitoneal nodes and the spleen. As the disease progresses, it spreads hematogenously to involve extranodal sites, including bone marrow, liver, and lung. Unlike NHL, Hodgkin's lymphoma rarely arises in extranodal sites, although it can involve extranodal sites by contiguous spread from an adjacent lymph node (e.g., vertebrae from retroperitoneal lymph nodes, pulmonary parenchyma from hilar nodes).

Hodgkin's lymphoma usually produces painless enlargement of lymph nodes, most often in the neck. Mediastinal adenopathy may be found incidentally in an asymptomatic patient on routine chest radiography. Massive mediastinal or hilar adenopathy, with or without adjacent pulmonary involvement, may cause respiratory symptoms such as cough, shortness of breath, wheezing, or stridor. At clinical presentation, about one third of patients have constitutional symptoms of fever, night sweats, or weight loss (i.e., B symptoms). Generalized pruritus is associated with the NS subtype, and patients may give a history of troubling pruritus for months to years before the diagnosis.

If left untreated, the natural history is one of inexorable, albeit often slow, progression to involve multiple nodal sites, followed by hematogenous spread to the bone marrow, liver, and other viscera. As the disease advances, patients experience B symptoms, malaise, cachexia, and infectious complications. Patients with progressive disease ultimately die of complications of bone marrow failure or infection.

Accurate staging of patients with newly diagnosed Hodgkin's lymphoma is important for treatment planning, prognosis, and assessing response to therapy. A modification of the Ann Arbor classification is used (see Table 49-4), and the suffix A or B is appended to denote the absence or presence, respectively, of B symptoms. The staging work-up of a newly diagnosed patient is similar to that for patients with NHL (see Table 49-3) and includes a history and physical examination; complete blood work, including erythrocyte sedimentation rate (ESR) and HIV serology; computed tomography (CT) scan of the chest, abdomen, and pelvis; positron emission tomography (PET)

scan; and in selected cases, a bone marrow aspirate and biopsy. Additional radiographic tests (e.g., bone films, spinal magnetic resonance imaging [MRI]) should be obtained only if symptoms suggest involvement of these structures. Patients also require evaluation of cardiac and pulmonary function before administration of chemotherapy and testing for hepatitis B due to the risk of reactivation during chemotherapy. The information derived from this noninvasive work-up defines the clinical stage of a patient with Hodgkin's lymphoma.

Diagnosis and Differential Diagnosis

The diagnosis requires an adequate biopsy of the involved nodal tissue. Immunophenotyping is routinely performed to confirm the diagnosis made on routine light microscopy and to differentiate Hodgkin's lymphoma from morphologically similar NHLs (e.g., T-cell–rich large B-cell lymphoma, anaplastic large cell lymphoma).

Treatment

Hodgkin's lymphoma is highly curable; the cure rate exceeds 80% with the use of current treatment modalities. The optimal treatment, including the duration of chemotherapy and the use and dose of radiation therapy, is determined by the stage (i.e., early stage [I/II] vs. advanced stage [III/IV]), and additional prognostic features. Because most patients are young adults and experience long-term, disease-free survival, the emphasis during the past 3 decades has shifted to using therapies that minimize treatment-related morbidity and mortality without sacrificing curative potential. Primary radiation therapy is rarely used because of its delayed toxicities, which include a substantial risk of secondary solid tumors within the radiation field a decade or more after treatment, including a particularly high risk of breast cancer. Additional long-term sequelae of standard doses of chest irradiation include thyroid dysfunction (usually hypothyroidism) and accelerated coronary artery disease.

Most patients with early-stage (I/II) Hodgkin's lymphoma are treated with the ABVD chemotherapy regimen (i.e., doxorubicin [Adriamycin], bleomycin, vinblastine, and dacarbazine) followed by a course of low-dose radiation (<30 Gy) to involved lymph node sites, which has not been associated with an increased risk of secondary solid tumors. The duration of chemotherapy and the dose of radiation depend on whether the patient has favorable or unfavorable early-stage disease. The definition of favorable disease usually incorporates the absence of a large mediastinal mass, a limited number of involved nodal sites, absence of B symptoms, younger age, and a low ESR. Patients with favorable early-stage disease typically receive two to four cycles (months) of ABVD followed by 20 Gy of radiation, whereas four to six cycles of ABVD and 30 Gy of radiation are required for patients with unfavorable disease (level I evidence).

Patients with advanced-stage (III/IV) Hodgkin's lymphoma are treated primarily with chemotherapy. The ABVD regimen is the most widely used initial treatment in the United States. ABVD is more effective and less toxic than the older MOPP regimen (i.e., nitrogen mustard, vincristine [Oncovin], procarbazine, and prednisone), and it does not cause the long-term sequelae of sterility, infertility, or treatment-induced leukemias associated with MOPP (level I evidence). Roughly 60% of patients with stage III or IV disease are cured with six cycles (months) of ABVD.

The intensive regimen of BEACOPP (i.e., bleomycin, etoposide, Adriamycin, cyclophosphamide, vincristine, prednisolone, and procarbazine) has been associated with higher rates of complete response and freedom from treatment failure compared with ABVD-based regimens used for patients with advanced disease, although overall survival has not been increased in all studies (level I evidence). BEACOPP is used increasingly in selected patients with high-risk features. Gonadal toxicity with permanent infertility is common after BEACOPP, and an increased risk of secondary leukemia has been reported. Late sequelae and acute toxicities must be considered when choosing this regimen.

Radiation therapy in combination with chemotherapy is typically not used to treat advanced-stage disease. However, in patients with bulky mediastinal disease, consolidative irradiation to the mediastinum after completion of chemotherapy has decreased the rate of relapse.

Evaluating the response to therapy involves repetition of the staging evaluation (i.e., physical examination, CT, and PET) during and at the completion of treatment. A mid-treatment PET scan after two cycles of ABVD for advanced disease is prognostically informative because persistent metabolic activity seen on PET highly correlates with resistance or subsequent relapse of disease. Conversely, patients may be cured despite the finding of a residual abnormality on CT (e.g., enlarged nodes, residual mediastinal mass) when residual disease is not found on PET imaging. A persistently positive PET scan after treatment of patients with residual radiographic abnormalities is associated with a high rate of subsequent relapse, and these patients should be monitored closely or considered for immediate repeat biopsy or salvage therapy. Most patients destined to relapse do so within 2 years; relapses after 5 years are rare except for patients with the NLP variant.

Patients who relapse or fail to respond after initial therapy should be offered salvage therapy because many can be cured if treated with high-dose chemotherapy and autologous hematopoietic cell transplantation (level I evidence). Patients who relapse after autologous transplantation usually are incurable, although a subset of young and medically fit patients can be considered for potentially curative allogeneic transplantation.

Palliation of refractory Hodgkin's lymphoma can be achieved with radiation therapy, salvage chemotherapy regimens, or with brentuximab vedotin, an immunotoxin composed of a CD30-directed antibody linked to an antitubulin agent. The latter agent is associated with high response rates, including complete responses in more than 30% of patients with relapsed disease after autologous transplantation (level II-1 evidence).

Prognosis

Approximately 80% of patients with Hodgkin's lymphoma are cured. Prognostic factors that influence risk of relapse or survival include MC or LD histology, male sex, large numbers of involved nodal sites, age older than 40 years, B symptoms, high ESR, and bulky disease (i.e., mediastinum widening by more than one third or a mass larger than 10 cm). The International Prognostic Score, based on seven variables at diagnosis, is a validated predictor of outcome in advanced disease.

Lymphoid Leukemias

Acute Lymphocytic Leukemias

The acute lymphocytic leukemias that arise from precursor B or T cells are described in detail in Chapter 48.

Chronic Lymphocytic Leukemia and Small Lymphocytic Lymphoma

Definition and Epidemiology

B-cell CLL is a malignant disorder of lymphocytes characterized by expansion and accumulation of small lymphocytes of B-cell origin. CLL is essentially identical to B-cell small lymphocytic lymphoma but represents the leukemic form of the disease. CLL is the most common form of leukemia in the United States and affects twice as many men as women. Although it can occur at any stage of life, the incidence increases with age, and more than 90% of cases are diagnosed in adults older than 50 years of age.

The cause of CLL is unknown. Familial clustering of CLL suggests a genetic basis in some cases. Radiation and common carcinogen exposures have not been associated with an increased risk of CLL.

Pathology

The common form of CLL is a clonal proliferation of mature B cells expressing characteristic mature B-cell markers and low levels of surface immunoglobulin M (IgM) that is light chain restricted, reflecting the clonal origin of this malignancy. Smears of the bone marrow or peripheral blood reveal a predominance of small lymphocytes with inconspicuous nucleoli; ruptured cells (i.e., smudge cells) are often observed. Examination of involved lymph nodes reveals a diffuse infiltrate of small lymphocytes ablating the normal architecture.

The diagnostic immunophenotype of CLL is unique, with expression of CD5 and CD23 along with the mature B-cell markers CD19, CD20 (dim expression), and CD21. Although a pathognomonic chromosomal abnormality has not been identified in CLL, 30% to 50% of patients have cytogenetic abnormalities, more so if sensitive assays such as fluorescence in situ hybridization (FISH) are employed. The most frequent abnormalities involve chromosome 12 (often trisomy 12), 13, and 14. Cytogenetic abnormalities of chromosomes 17 and 11 are associated with a very poor prognosis.

Diagnosis and Differential Diagnosis

The diagnosis of CLL is often made incidentally on a routine blood cell count that shows a leukocytosis with a predominance of small lymphocytes. Flow cytometric analysis of peripheral blood or a bone marrow aspirate reveals the characteristic clonal B-cell population that is CD5 and CD23 positive.

CLL must be distinguished from reactive causes of lymphocytosis and other forms of lymphoma or leukemia. Mantle cell lymphoma may appear similar morphologically and with a similar immunophenotype, although CD23 is typically absent and cyclin D1 expression is detected. An absolute lymphocytosis of more than 5000 cells/μL is required for the diagnosis of CLL.

Patients with characteristic clonal CLL cells in the blood to a lesser degree as an isolated abnormality are thought to have monoclonal B-cell lymphocytosis and may be observed.

Clinical Presentation

CLL cells accumulate in bone marrow, peripheral blood, lymph nodes, and spleen, resulting in lymphocytosis, lymphadenopathy, splenomegaly, and ultimately decreased bone marrow function. CLL is also frequently associated with immune dysregulation, exhibited as hypogammaglobulinemia with an increased risk of bacterial infections and autoimmune phenomena such as Coombs-positive hemolytic anemia or immune thrombocytopenia. Some patients exhibit lymphadenopathy, symptoms related to cytopenias, or occasionally, recurrent infections. As the disease progresses, patients develop generalized lymphadenopathy, hepatosplenomegaly, and bone marrow failure. Death often results from infectious complications or bone marrow failure after patients have become refractory to treatment. In about 5% of cases, CLL transforms to a highly malignant diffuse large cell lymphoma, which is usually rapidly fatal. This transformation is commonly referred to as Richter's syndrome.

Treatment

CLL is a low-grade leukemia or lymphoma that is typically characterized by a long natural history with slow progression over years or decades. Median survival is in excess of 6 years. The extent of disease (stage) at onset is the best predictor of survival. In the absence of immune phenomena, anemia and thrombocytopenia are signs of advanced-stage disease associated with poor survival.

Because standard therapy is not curative and CLL may have an asymptomatic phase lasting years, specific treatment is often withheld until signs of disease progression or development of symptoms (e.g., bulky lymphadenopathy, constitutional symptoms such as fevers, cytopenias caused by bone marrow infiltration). The rate of rise of the white blood cell count may also be used to predict development of symptoms and the need for therapy.

When treatment is required, multiple options for therapy are available. The patient's age, medical condition, and cytogenetic abnormalities may influence the choice of therapy. Active chemotherapeutic agents include several alkylating agents (e.g., chlorambucil, cyclophosphamide), the nucleoside analogue fludarabine, or the novel agent bendamustine. The monoclonal anti-CD20 antibody rituximab has activity against CLL, but it is most effectively employed in combination with chemotherapeutic agents.

Most patients respond to therapy with significant reductions in tumor burden. Fludarabine-based therapies are typically associated with a higher rate of complete remissions compared with other therapies, but they may carry higher risks of infections or marrow stem cell injury. Patients with recurrent or refractory disease may respond to a growing list of monoclonal antibodies. Alemtuzumab, a humanized monoclonal antibody to the CD52 molecule, which occurs on most lymphocytes, is efficacious, including in patients with a 17p deletion, a group for whom conventional chemotherapy works poorly. Additional agents include the anti-CD20 antibodies ofatumumab and obinutuzumab,

which was shown to improve remission duration in previously untreated patients when administered in combination with chlorambucil (level I evidence).

Patients with poor-risk cytogenetic abnormalities are more likely to demonstrate resistance to standard therapies and have shortened survival. These patients may be candidates for allogeneic transplantation, which appears to exert a therapeutic effect through a strong immune or graft-versus-leukemia phenomenon. Patients who develop autoimmune phenomena require treatment with corticosteroids, and intravenous gamma globulin may be used to reduce the frequency of infections in patients who have developed hypogammaglobulinemia. The development of a rapidly enlarging mediastinal mass, constitutional symptoms, and high serum LDH level suggests transformation of the disease to a diffuse large cell lymphoma (i.e., Richter's syndrome), which is associated with a poor prognosis.

Plasma Cell Disorders

The plasma cell disorders, or dyscrasias, are a group of clonal B-cell diseases that are related to each other by virtue of their production and secretion of monoclonal immunoglobulin (or part of an immunoglobulin molecule), called the *M protein*. The laboratory hallmark of plasma cell dyscrasias is a homogeneous immunoglobulin molecule (whole or part) that can be detected in the serum or urine by protein electrophoresis. Clinically, these disorders may be characterized by the systemic effects of the M protein and by the direct effects of bone and bone marrow infiltration. Primary amyloidosis, for instance, results in tissue injury through deposition of light chains produced by a clonal population of plasma cells in the absence of an observable proliferation of the plasma cell clone. Waldenström's macroglobulinemia is a disorder with features of NHL and plasma cell disorders. It is discussed in this section because of the distinct clinical effects of the IgM paraprotein produced in this disease.

The most common plasma cell dyscrasia is *monoclonal gammopathy of uncertain significance* (MGUS), followed by multiple myeloma and the closely related plasmacytoma, which is a solitary myeloma of bone or extramedullary soft tissue. Less common plasma cell dyscrasias include osteosclerotic myeloma (i.e., polyneuropathy, organomegaly, endocrinopathy, monoclonal gammopathy, and skin abnormalities [POEMS syndrome]), heavy-chain disease, and primary amyloidosis.

When an M protein found on serum protein electrophoresis is from individuals with no apparent associated disease and in the absence of any other laboratory or clinical evidence of a plasma cell disorder, it is designated as a MGUS. MGUS is defined by low serum levels of M protein (<3 g/dL), no urinary Bence Jones protein, less than 10% clonal bone marrow plasma cells, and absence of anemia, hypercalcemia, renal failure, and lytic bone lesions. MGUS is more common than myeloma and increases in frequency with aging, occurring in 3% of the population older than 50 years. MGUS is considered a premalignant condition, and patients are at increased risk (sevenfold) for overt myeloma or related malignant plasma cell dyscrasias compared with the general population. Nonetheless, progression of MGUS to a frank plasma cell neoplasm occurs only in about 1% of patients per year.

Distinguishing patients with stable, nonprogressive MGUS from patients in whom multiple myeloma will eventually develop is difficult. The risk of progression is greater among patients with IgA- or IgM-type M proteins, in patients with initial concentrations of M protein in excess of 1.5 g/dL, and in patients with an abnormal free κ-to-λ light-chain ratio. Although no definitive evidence has been found that monitoring patients with the diagnosis of MGUS improves survival, it is recommended that patients undergo annual evaluation, including serum electrophoresis, to detect progression to multiple myeloma before the onset of overt symptoms or complications.

M proteins can be found in benign and malignant conditions other than the plasma cell dyscrasias (Table 49-5). About 10% of patients with CLL have detectable levels of monoclonal IgG or IgM in their sera. M proteins can also be detected in a variety of autoreactive or infectious disorders.

TABLE 49-5   CLASSIFICATION OF DISORDERS ASSOCIATED WITH MONOCLONAL IMMUNOGLOBULIN (M PROTEIN) SECRETION

DISORDER	M PROTEIN PATTERN
PLASMA CELL NEOPLASMS	
Multiple myeloma	IgG > IgA > IgD; ± free light chain or light chain alone (κ > λ)
Solitary myeloma of bone	IgG > IgA > IgD; ± free light chain or light chain alone (κ > λ)
Extramedullary plasmacytoma	IgA > IgG > IgD; ± free light chain or light chain alone (κ > λ)
Waldenström macroglobulinemia	IgM ± free light chain (κ > λ)
Heavy-chain disease	γ, α, or μ heavy chain or fragment
Primary amyloidosis	Free light chain (λ > κ)
Monoclonal gammopathy of unknown significance	IgG > IgM > IgA, usually without urinary light-chain secretion
OTHER B-CELL NEOPLASMS	
Chronic lymphocytic leukemia	M protein occasionally secreted; IgM > IgG
B-cell non-Hodgkin's lymphomas; Hodgkin's disease	M protein occasionally secreted; IgM > IgG
NONLYMPHOID NEOPLASMS	
Chronic myelogenous leukemia	No consistent patterns
Carcinomas (e.g., colon, breast, prostate)	No consistent patterns
AUTOIMMUNE OR AUTOREACTIVE DISORDERS	
Cold agglutinin disease	IgM κ most common
Mixed cryoglobulinemia	IgM or IgA
Sjögren syndrome	IgM
MISCELLANEOUS INFLAMMATORY, STORAGE, OR INFECTIOUS DISORDERS	
Lichen myxedematosus	IgG λ
Gaucher's disease	IgG
Cirrhosis, sarcoid, parasitic diseases, renal acidosis	No consistent pattern

Modified from Salmon SE: Plasma cell disorders. In Wyngaarden JB, Smith LH Jr, editors: Cecil textbook of medicine, ed 18, Philadelphia, 1988, WB Saunders, p 1026.
Ig, Immunoglobulin.

Multiple Myeloma

Definition and Epidemiology

Multiple myeloma is a malignant plasma cell disorder characterized by neoplastic infiltration of the bone marrow and bone and by monoclonal immunoglobulin or light chains in the serum or urine. The cause of myeloma is uncertain.

The disease is more common in men than women and in American backs than whites. Myeloma risk increases with age, with a median age of 69 years at diagnosis (SEER data). Myeloma risk is increased for patients with first-degree relatives with a plasma cell dyscrasia. Associations have been described with occupational exposures to organic solvents, pesticides, petroleum products, and ionizing radiation, but these risk factors are rarely seen in affected individuals.

Pathology

The tumor cell of these disorders exhibits features of a differentiated plasma cell that is adapted to synthesize and secrete immunoglobulin at a high rate. Biopsies of bone marrow or targeted bone biopsies of tumor sites reveal infiltration by plasma cells with light-chain restriction, defining clonality. Cell surface markers useful in identifying and enumerating plasma cells include CD38, CD 138, and immunoglobulin light chains; the B-cell marker CD20 is typically absent and aids in distinguishing other lymphoproliferative disorders from myeloma.

Genetic aberrations are détectable in most patients with myeloma if adequately sensitive tests are applied. Standard karyotyping and FISH are perfomed routinely on marrow samples to determine abnormalities of prognostic significance, including translocations involving the immunoglobulin heavy-chain locus on chromosome 14, hyperploidy, or délétions of chromosomes 1, 13, or 17.

Diagnosis and Differential Diagnosis

Myeloma must be distinguished from related disorders, including MGUS and plasmacytoma. The diagnosis of multiple myeloma is made by identifying some combination of an increase (>10%) in the number of plasma cells in the bone marrow, a serum M protein other than IgM exceeding 3 g/dL, or a clonal protein in the urine. Asymptomatic myeloma (i.e., stage I myeloma or "smoldering myeloma") is diagnosed when clonal plasma cells are found in more than 10% of the bone marrow or monoclonal protein occurs in an amount greater than 3 g/dL in the absence of end-organ–related injury, or both.

Patients with disease-related organ dysfunction (e.g., anemia, lytic bone lesions, hypercalcemia, renal dysfunction) are considered to have symptomatic myeloma, for which therapy is indicated. Recurrent infection with hypogammaglobulinemia is also considered a criterion for symptomatic myeloma. Solitary plasmacytoma is diagnosed when a single clonal plasma cell tumor is identified in bone or soft tissue in the absence of bone marrow involvement or other end organ–related injury.

Evaluation of the patient with suspected myeloma includes bone marrow biopsy; measurement of hemoglobin, calcium, renal function, and the serum free κ-to-λ light-chain ratio; serum or urine protein electrophoresis; immunoelectrophoresisimmunoelectrophoresis; and a skeletal survey.

PET and MRI are considered to further evaluate bone disease and may be necessary for patients with oligosecretory or non-secretory disease to define disease and evaluate after therapy. Conventional bone scans are less useful due to the osteolytic nature of myeloma.

About 20% of patients with multiple myeloma do not have detectable serum M protein by standard electrophoresis but have circulating free light chains that may be detectable by serum free light-chain assays. Free light chains may appear in the urine (i.e., Bence Jones protein) and can also be detected in a 24-hour urine collection by urine protein electrophoresis. In rare cases, patients with nonsecretory myeloma have neither detectable serum nor urine M protein. Free light-chain assays are quite sensitive and may provide measurement of clonal protein in patients thought to have nonsecretory disease by other methods. Free light chains have a relatively short half-life (2 to 6 hours) in the circulation compared with weeks for intact immunoglobulin molecules and may therefore be used to obtain a more rapid assessment of disease response for patients on therapy.

Clinical Presentation

The clinical manifestations of multiple myeloma are the direct effects of bone marrow and bone infiltration by malignant plasma cells, the systemic effects of the M protein, and the effects of the concomitant deficiency in humoral immunity that occurs in this disease. The most common symptom in multiple myeloma is bone pain. Bone radiographs typically show pure osteolytic punched-out lesions, often in association with generalized osteopenia and pathologic fractures. Bony lesions can show as expansile masses associated with spinal cord compression. Hypercalcemia caused by extensive bony involvement is common in myeloma and may dominate the clinical picture. Anemia occurs in most patients as a result of marrow infiltration and suppression of hematopoiesis and causes fatigue; granulocytopenia and thrombocytopenia are less common.

Patients with myeloma are susceptible to bacterial infections because of impaired production and increased catabolism of normal immunoglobulins. Gram-negative urinary tract infections are common, as are respiratory tract infections caused by *Streptococcus pneumoniae*, *Staphylococcus aureus*, *Haemophilus influenzae*, and *Klebsiella pneumoniae*.

Renal insufficiency occurs in about 25% of patients with myeloma. The cause of renal failure is often multifactorial; hypercalcemia, hyperuricemia, infection, and amyloid deposition can contribute. However, direct tubular damage from light-chain excretion invariably occurs. Because of their physicochemical properties, M proteins can cause a host of diverse effects, including cryoglobulinemia, hyperviscosity, amyloidosis, and clotting abnormalities resulting from interaction of the M protein with platelets or clotting factors.

Several staging or classification systems exist for myeloma. The International Staging System (ISS) for myeloma identifies three stages with distinct prognoses based on only two variables: β_2-microglobulin and albumin levels (Table 49-6).

Treatment

Most patients with myeloma exhibit symptomatic, advanced-stage disease and require therapy. Patients with stage I disease or

TABLE 49-6 INTERNATIONAL STAGING SYSTEM FOR MULTIPLE MYELOMA

STAGE	CRITERIA	SURVIVAL TIME (mo)
I	B2M <3.5 mg/L Albumin ≥3.5 g/dL	62
II	Not stage I or III	44
III	B2M >5.5 mg/L	29

Greipp PR, San Miguel J, Durie BG, et al: International staging system for multiple myeloma, *J Clin Oncol* 23:3412–3420, 2005.
B2M, β_2-Microglobulin.

asymptomatic myeloma may have an indolent course and do not always require immediate therapy. Disease progression occurs at a rate of 5% to 10% per year, and patients should be monitored for disease progression by serial quantification of the M protein and evaluation for disease-related signs or symptoms. For patients with solitary bone or extramedullary plasmacytomas, particularly in the head and neck region, local radiation therapy can induce long-term remissions and is the treatment of choice. Patients with a solitary plasmacytoma of bone are often found on routine MRI of the spine to have asymptomatic bone disease and are at higher risk for progression to myeloma.

Patients with symptomatic myeloma require systemic therapy and meticulous supportive care. Although myeloma is not a curable malignancy, systemic therapy can prolong survival and dramatically improve quality of life. Options for treatment have expanded in the past decade to include multiple compounds in two broad classes of agents, the immunomodulatory drugs (IMIDs) and proteosome inhibitors. These agents may be used as single agents or in combinations for more intensive therapy. They are typically administered in combination with high doses of dexamethasone, which is a potent antimyeloma therapy. The IMIDS include thalidomide, lenalidomide, and pomalidomide. Proteosome inhibitors include bortezomib and carfilzomib. These agents have largely supplanted traditional chemotherapeutic agents as the cornerstone of initial and secondary therapies because they are efficacious and usually well tolerated. Multiple combination regimens have been devised that also incorporate chemotherapeutic agents in modest doses.

Thalidomide is the first-in-class IMID and was initially used as a sedative in the United Kingdom in the 1960s, but it was found to cause birth defects when used to combat nausea during pregnancy. The antiangiogenic properties of thalidomide subsequently led to its development as an anticancer agent. Although the mechanism of action of the IMIDs is unclear, they are now thought to exert antitumor effects primarily through stimulation of immune effectors. The IMIDs are typically used in combination with dexamethasone, and when used as initial therapy, they have good tolerability and result in high response rates.

Toxicity related to thalidomide includes peripheral neuropathy, constipation, somnolence, and rash. Later-generation IMIDs have a more favorable side effect profile. Myelosuppression is more likely, but neuropathy and constitutional symptoms occur less frequently. The second-generation IMID lenalidomide is more commonly used in North America due its favorable tolerability. A troublesome and unique side effect of the IMID-steroid combination programs is development of deep vein thrombosis in up to 25% of patients, and some form of preventative therapy is typically prescribed.

Bortezomib is the first-in-class proteosome inhibitor and is a favored therapy for patients with adverse cytogenetic risk factors. Bortezomib is typically administered subcutaneously and may cause thrombocytopenia, asthenia, and neuropathy.

Most patients respond to initial therapy with a reduction in bone pain, hypercalcemia, and anemia in association with a decline in the M protein level. The selection of initial therapy depends on stage, cytogenetic risk, and candidacy for high-dose chemotherapy and autologous stem cell transplantation. The use of high-dose chemotherapy with alkylating agents followed by autologous peripheral stem cell infusion during first or second remission has improved survival and quality of life compared with standard doses of chemotherapy. Although this approach is not curative, it does represent an important treatment option for some patients and has an acceptable toxicity profile, even in older patients. The relative value of autologous stem cell transplantation compared with ongoing therapy with the newer agents is unknown and is an area of active clinical investigation. Allogenic stem cell or bone marrow transplantation may be associated with durable remission in selected patients, but it carries a much higher near-term risk of morbidity and mortality. Patients who experience relapse after standard therapy or transplantation may be treated with alternate chemotherapy regimens or with novel combination therapies, including newer agents and chemotherapy drugs.

Supportive care directed toward anticipated complications of myeloma is an important aspect of the management of this disease. Bone resorption can be reduced with regular injections of the diphosphonates zoledronic acid or pamidronate, reducing pain and pathologic fractures. Bony lesions, particularly those involving weight-bearing bones, may require palliative irradiation for controlling pain and preventing pathologic fractures. Vertebral bony lesions may lead to spinal cord compression, with increasing back pain and neurologic symptoms. Symptoms suggesting cord compression require prompt evaluation with spinal MRI and, if necessary, local irradiation of involved areas.

Avoidance of nephrotoxins, including intravenous dyes, is important to prevent renal failure. All patients should receive pneumococcal and *H. influenzae* vaccines, and intravenous gamma globulin may be useful in preventing recurrent infections in patients with profound hypogammaglobulinemia. Use of erythropoietin may alleviate anemia and decrease the need for blood transfusions.

Prognosis

Multiple myeloma is considered incurable, but the overall survival of these patients has improved considerably with the widespread use of autologous stem cell transplantation and development of newer agents. For example, median survival reported by the Mayo Clinic has increased from 29 to 44 months.

The prognosis depends on the stage of disease and cytogenetic profile. Patients with an adverse karyotype, including t(14;16) and 17p deletion, have a less favorable prognosis and are considered for more intensive therapies or clinical investigation. Adverse factors also include advanced stage, impaired renal function, elevated LDH levels, abnormal bone marrow cytogenetics,

depressed serum albumin levels, and elevated β_2-microglobulin levels.

Waldenström Macroglobulinemia

Waldenström macroglobulinemia is a malignancy of plasmacytoid lymphocytes that secrete large quantities of IgM. It is a chronic disorder affecting elderly patients (median age of 64 years) that shares features of the low-grade lymphomas and myeloma. Unlike myeloma, Waldenström macroglobulinemia is associated with lymphadenopathy and hepatosplenomegaly, and although bone marrow involvement invariably occurs, lytic lesions and hypercalcemia are rare.

The major clinical manifestations of Waldenström macroglobulinemia include symptomatic anemia and the hyperviscosity syndrome caused by the physical properties of IgM. In contrast to IgG, IgM remains largely confined to the intravascular space, and as IgM levels rise, plasma viscosity increases. Epistaxis, retinal hemorrhages, dizziness, confusion, and congestive heart failure may occur as a result of the hyperviscosity syndrome. About 10% of IgM proteins have properties of cryoglobulins, and patients show symptoms of cryoglobulinemia or cold agglutinin syndrome demonstrated as acrocyanosis, Raynaud's phenomenon, and vascular symptoms or hemolytic anemia precipitated by exposure to cold. Some patients with Waldenström macroglobulinemia may develop a peripheral neuropathy that may antedate the appearance of the neoplastic process.

The approach to and treatment of Waldenström macroglobulinemia are similar to those of other low-grade B-cell lymphomas. The use of nucleoside analogues such as fludarabine or an alkylating agent, alone or in combination with prednisone, is effective in decreasing adenopathy and splenomegaly and controlling the M spike, but it is not curative. Rituximab has activity against Waldenström macroglobulinemia, as has the proteosome inhibitor bortezomib. The use of rituximab may be complicated by initial worsening of hyperviscosity in patients with high IgM burdens. Plasmapheresis is highly effective in acutely decreasing serum IgM levels and is often needed initially to treat hyperviscosity. Although complete remissions are rare, patients who respond to therapy have median survivals of 4 years, and some patients survive more than a decade.

Rare Plasma Cell Disorders

Heavy-chain disease is a rare lymphoplasmacytoid neoplasm characterized by production of a defective heavy chain of the γ, α, or μ type. The clinical manifestations vary with the type of heavy chain secreted. The γ-type heavy-chain disease is associated with lymphadenopathy, Waldeyer's ring involvement with palatal edema, and constitutional symptoms. The α-type heavy-chain disease, also known as Mediterranean lymphoma, is characterized by lymphoid infiltration of the small intestine with associated diarrhea and malabsorption. The μ-type heavy-chain disease is associated with CLL.

Primary amyloidosis is a systemic illness characterized by deposition of immunoglobulin light chains in organs and tissue, resulting in an array of symptoms caused by organ dysfunction. Congestive heart failure, bleeding diathesis, nephrotic syndrome, and peripheral neuropathy are common complications. Patients with primary amyloidosis may respond to selected treatments similar to therapy for myeloma. The combination of bortezomib, cyclophosphamide, and dexamethasone is effective in some patients. Selected patients may respond well to high-dose chemotherapy and autologous stem cell support, but there are increased risks of morbidity and mortality if significant end-organ dysfunction such as cardiomyopathy occurs.

POEMS syndrome is a rare disorder characterized by polyneuropathy, sclerotic bone lesions, endocrinopathy, monoclonal gammopathy, and skin lesions. The cause of POEMS syndrome is unknown, but the disease may be progressive, causing severe disability, third spacing of fluid, and elevated vascular endothelial growth factor (VEGF) levels. Monoclonal λ light chains are typically elevated. Limited bone disease may be treated with radiotherapy. High-dose therapy and autologous stem cell transplantation is effective in patients with extensive disease.

For a deeper discussion of these topics, please see Chapter 187, "Plasma Cell Disorders," and Chapter 188, "Amyloidosis," in Goldman-Cecil Medicine, *25th Edition.*

CONGENITAL AND ACQUIRED DISORDERS OF LYMPHOCYTE FUNCTION

Several congenital disorders affect lymphocyte maturation or function, resulting in immunodeficiency disorders. Acquired disorders of lymphocyte function are far more common than congenital disorders. HIV infection is the most important infectious cause of acquired immunodeficiency (see Chapter 109). Patients with HIV infection are at increased risk for NHL. NHLs that occur in the setting of HIV have the diffuse, aggressive B-cell histology and include DLBCL and Burkitt's lymphoma, and they are frequently associated with EBV infection and are often advanced stage (III or IV) at diagnosis, with extranodal sites of involvement.

Patients with HIV-associated NHL are potentially curable with the multidrug chemotherapy regimens used for treating the NHL subtypes found in the general population. Treatment of the underlying HIV infection with highly active antiretroviral therapy (HAART) has improved the outcome and prognosis of patients with HIV-associated NHL.

Patients who have undergone allogeneic organ transplantation require potent immunosuppressive drugs (e.g., cyclosporine, tacrolimus, mycophenolate, corticosteroids, methotrexate) to prevent graft-versus-host disease in the case of bone marrow transplantation or allograft rejection in the case of solid organ transplantation. These medications can cause profound defects in T-cell function with an associated acquired immunodeficiency state, and transplant recipients are susceptible to a host of viral and protozoal infections.

Patients who receive potent immunosuppressive drugs are at risk for a lymphoproliferative disorder (i.e., post-transplantation lymphoproliferative disorder [PTLD]) that can behave clinically as an aggressive lymphoma. PTLD is an EBV-associated lymphoproliferative disorder characterized by a polymorphous or monomorphous population of B cells that can be monoclonal or polyclonal. Patients who develop PTLD are treated by reducing the doses of immunosuppressive drugs whenever possible. Patients with polymorphous disease early after organ transplantation may respond well to this approach. Patients who are not candidates for withdrawal of immunosuppression because of allograft rejection or who develop late monophorphic disease may respond better to treatment with rituximab alone or in combination with chemotherapy.

SUGGESTED READINGS

Canellos GP, Anderson JR, Propert KJ, et al: Chemotherapy of advanced Hodgkin's disease with MOPP, ABVD, or MOPP alternating with ABVD, N Engl J Med 327:1478–1484, 1992.
Coiffier B, Lepage E, Briere J, et al: CHOP chemotherapy plus rituximab compared with CHOP alone in elderly patients with diffuse large-B-cell lymphoma, N Engl J Med 346:235–242, 2002.
Engert A, Plütschow A, Eich HT, et al: Reduced treatment intensity in patients with early-stage Hodgkin's lymphoma, N Engl J Med 363:640–652, 2010.
Fisher RI, Gaynor ER, Dahlberg S, et al: Comparison of a standard regimen (CHOP) with three intensive chemotherapy regimens for advanced non-Hodgkin's lymphoma, N Engl J Med 328:1002–1006, 1993.
Geisler CH, Kolstad A, Laurell A, et al: Long-term progression-free survival of mantle cell lymphoma after intensive front-line immunochemotherapy with in vivo purged stem cell rescue: a nonrandomized phase 2 multicenter study by the Nordic Lymphoma Group, Blood 112:2687–2693, 2008.
Hasenclever D, Diehl V: A prognostic score for advanced Hodgkin's disease. International Prognostic Factors Project on Advanced Hodgkin's Disease, N Engl J Med 339:1506–1514, 1998.
Kyle RA, Therneau TM, Rajkumar SV, et al: A long-term study of prognosis in monoclonal gammopathy of undetermined significance, N Engl J Med 346:564–569, 2002.
Maloney DG, Grillo-Lopez AJ, White CA, et al: IDEC-C2B8 (rituximab) anti-CD20 monoclonal antibody therapy in patients with relapsed low-grade non-Hodgkin's lymphoma, Blood 90:2188–2195, 1997.
McSweeney PA, Niederwieser D, Shizuru JA, et al: Hematopoietic cell transplantation in older patients with hematologic malignancies: replacing high-dose cytotoxic therapy with graft-versus-tumor effects, Blood 97:3390–3400, 2001.
National Cancer Institute: SEER cancer statistics fact sheets: myeloma, Bethesda, Md, 2013. Available at: http://seer.cancer.gov/statfacts/html/mulmy.html. 2013. Accessed October 3, 2014.
National Cancer Institute: SEER cancer statistics fact sheets: non-Hodgkin lymphoma, Bethesda, Md., 2013. Available at: http://seer.cancer.gov/statfacts/html/nhl.html. Accessed October 3, 2014.
Philip T, Guglielmi C, Hagenbeek A, et al: Autologous bone marrow transplantation as compared with salvage chemotherapy in relapses of chemotherapy-sensitive non-Hodgkin's lymphoma, N Engl J Med 33:1540–1545, 1995.
Rummel MJ, Niederle N, Maschmeyer G, et al: Bendamustine plus rituximab versus CHOP plus rituximab as first-line treatment for patients with indolent and mantle-cell lymphomas: an open-label, multicentre, randomised, phase 3 non-inferiority trial, Lancet 381:1203–1210, 2013.
Singhal S, Mehta J, Desikan R, et al: Antitumor activity of thalidomide in refractory multiple myeloma, N Engl J Med 341:1565–1571, 1999.
Swerdlow S, Campo E, Harris N, et al: World Health Organization classification of tumours of hematopoietic and lymphoid tissues, ed 4, Lyon, 2008, IARC Press.
Wang ML, Rule S, Martin P: Targeting BTK with ibrutinib in relapsed or refractory mantle-cell lymphoma, N Engl J Med 369:507–516, 2013.

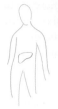

50

Normal Hemostasis

Alexa J. Siddon, Henry M. Rinder, and Christopher A. Tormey

INTRODUCTION

Hemostasis is the physiologic balance of procoagulant and anticoagulant forces that maintains both liquid blood flow and the structural integrity of the vasculature. Vascular damage results in initiation of clotting that produces a *localized* platelet-fibrin plug to prevent blood loss; this action is followed by processes that lead to clot containment, wound healing, clot dissolution, tissue regeneration, and remodeling. In healthy persons, all these reactions occur continuously and in a balanced fashion so that bleeding is contained while blood vessels simultaneously remain patent to deliver adequate organ blood flow. If any of these processes are disrupted because of inherited defects or acquired abnormalities, disordered hemostasis may result in either bleeding or thromboembolic complications.

Blood flow in the arterial system is different from that in the venous system and imposes different needs on the coagulation system. In the pressurized arteries, relatively minor vascular damage can rapidly result in massive blood loss; therefore, the procoagulant response in arteries must rapidly arrest bleeding. Platelets are critical to this arterial response; they initially contain the blood loss and then provide an active surface for soluble coagulation factors to both localize and accelerate formation of fibrin and, ultimately, clot formation. By contrast, the slower flow rates in the venous circulation produce slower bleeding, a feature that makes platelets less critical; instead, the balance of venous hemostasis is most dependent on the rate of thrombin generation. These differences are underscored clinically by the anticoagulant agents used in these distinct settings: antiplatelet agents such as aspirin and clopidogrel to prevent coronary and cerebral artery thrombus, whereas interventions that inhibit thrombin, including the heparins and warfarin, are used for treatment and prophylaxis of venous thromboembolic disease. Recently, new anticoagulants have been introduced, including direct thrombin inhibitors (e.g., dabigatran etexilate) and Xa inhibitors (e.g., rivaroxaban); they selectively inhibit activated coagulation factors for prophylaxis against systemic embolism from atrial fibrillation and from venous thromboembolism, respectively.

This chapter briefly details the physiologic and interdependent mechanisms of vascular hemostasis, including the normal balance of procoagulant and anticoagulant functions of the blood vessel wall, platelet physiologic factors and receptor-ligand interactions that are critical for hemostasis, and the highly complex, interwoven pathways that represent the coagulation cascade.

VASCULAR WALL PHYSIOLOGY

Vascular endothelial cells (ECs) are capable of orchestrating both procoagulant and anticoagulant events depending on circumstances. When the vasculature is intact, healthy ECs exert tonic anticoagulant activity, helping to maintain blood fluidity. In part, they provide a passive barrier function, separating the blood from subendothelial procoagulants such as collagen and tissue factor (TF). In addition, healthy ECs actively regulate the hemostatic balance of activity in their microenvironment through their secreted products (Table 50-1). These include prostacyclin and nitric oxide, both of which induce vascular smooth muscle relaxation and reduced shear when released in an abluminal direction. When secreted into the blood, they promote the generation of platelet cyclic adenosine monophosphate (cAMP), thus inhibiting platelet activation and aggregation. ECs also secrete adenosine diphosphatase, which degrades extracellular platelet-released adenosine diphosphate (ADP), thereby inhibiting platelet recruitment into the growing platelet clot. Soluble coagulation factors are also regulated by ECs in both tonic and inducible fashion. Tissue factor pathway inhibitor (TFPI) in its nascent circulating form blunts the initiation of coagulation; TFPI is subsequently primed for increased activity by exposure to small amounts of factor Xa. Quiescent thrombomodulin and tissue plasminogen activator are localized at the EC extracellular matrix, ready to be activated by local formation of thrombin and fibrin, respectively, to carry out their anticoagulant and fibrinolytic functions.

When ECs are physically damaged or become activated, their balance of coagulant properties is shifted to favor a procoagulant state. This function is mediated both by the ECs themselves and by the underlying subendothelial matrix that is exposed by vascular injury. ECs that have become activated (e.g., by toxins or

TABLE 50-1	PROPERTIES OF ENDOTHELIAL CELL COAGULANTS	
PROCOAGULANT		**ANTICOAGULANT**
Collagen		Vasodilation
Factor VIII		Adenosine diphosphatase
Fibronectin		Heparan sulfates
Integrins		Nitric oxide
Platelet-endothelial cell adhesion molecule-1 (PECAM-1)		Prostacyclin
Selectins (E and P)		Thrombomodulin
Vasoconstriction		Tissue factor pathway inhibitor
von Willebrand factor		Tissue plasminogen activator

secreted factors) express adhesive ligands on their surface, including the selectins (both E-selectin and P-selectin), β_1 and β_2 integrins, platelet endothelial cell adhesion molecule-1 (PECAM-1), and von Willebrand factor (vWF) multimers (see Table 50-1). On the EC surface, vWF multimers localize and promote platelet adhesion, whereas integrins mediate adhesion and subsequent transendothelial migration of leukocytes into the tissues. After EC damage, exposed subendothelial matrix also binds vWF multimers (Fig. 50-1A) to localize platelet adhesion. Subendothelial procoagulant proteins, including thrombospondin, fibronectin, and collagen, function both as ligands to capture platelets and as activators of adherent platelets. Collagen, in particular, is both a platelet ligand and a strong platelet agonist. The latter capability causes platelets to undergo dense granule release and to express conformationally active ligands such as glycoprotein IIb/IIIa (GPIIb/IIIa; see later discussion). Another critical procoagulant mediator exposed by EC damage is TF, which is constitutively expressed by subendothelial smooth muscle cells and fibroblasts. As outlined later, TF is the major initiator of the soluble coagulation system which, along with activated platelets, results in the formation of a definitive platelet-fibrin clot (Fig. 50-2).

● PLATELET PHYSIOLOGY

The platelet functions as the cellular-based platform for hemostasis. Platelet surface receptors mediate primary hemostasis and allow platelets to bind directly to endothelium and subendothelium at sites of damage (see Fig. 50-1B). Platelet interactions with their ligands cause transmembrane signaling through surface receptors to induce platelet activation and promote procoagulant function through various pathways, including translocation of additional receptors to the membrane surface, receptor conformational change to active forms, release of granule contents that recruit platelet adhesion, and exposure of procoagulant membrane phospholipids. The procoagulant surface of the platelet then serves as a platform for enhanced assembly of the coagulation cascade to generate thrombin. Thrombin feeds back on platelets and the clotting cascade to amplify the procoagulant response and also produces fibrin to provide secondary, long-lasting hemostasis. Finally, the platelets assist thrombin in clot consolidation and in protection from fibrinolysis by contributing factor XIII and platelet factor 4, respectively, to the clot milieu (Table 50-2).

Platelet Hemostasis

Platelets are anucleate cells between 2 and 4 μm in diameter with a volume between 6 and 11 fL. Platelets are derived from the megakaryocyte cytoplasm after a maturation time of about 4 days, with each megakaryocyte contributing 1000 to 3000 circulating platelets in its lifetime. When platelets are released into the circulation, they survive for 7 to 10 days; platelets leave the circulation through a combination of senescence and the normal maintenance of vascular structural integrity. For the latter, very few platelets are needed; approximately 7100 platelets/μL are required for hemostasis per day if vascular structures are intact (e.g., no recent surgery or trauma) and if there is no increase in normal platelet consumption (e.g., sepsis).

The normal platelet count ranges between 150,000 and 450,000/μL, depending on the population used to establish the reference range. With platelet counts in the normal range and normal platelet function, the bleeding time, an in vivo measure of platelet function, is typically less than 8 minutes. However, if the number of normal functioning platelets is less than 100,000/μL, the bleeding time is prolonged. Therefore, in the presence of thrombocytopenia, the bleeding time cannot be used to determine whether bleeding is caused by abnormal platelet function or by connective tissue disease. The bleeding time is an operator-dependent, highly variable in vivo assay that can leave scars; many laboratories have therefore switched to a so-called in vitro bleeding time test such as the Platelet Function Analyzer-100 (PFA-100), which uses anticoagulated whole blood to examine "closure time" (details on the PFA-100 and other platelet function platforms are provided in Chapter 51). However, the PFA-100 and other like-minded tests are similar to the bleeding time test in that they are unable to distinguish between thrombocytopenia and abnormal platelet function when platelet counts are lower than 100,000/μL.

Shear-Induced Adhesion

The interaction between platelets and the vessel wall has been well characterized at the high flow velocities of the arterial circulation. The interaction between the vasculature and flowing blood, as shown on the left side of Figure 50-1A, creates parallel planes of blood moving at different velocities; the blood closest to the vessel wall moves more slowly than blood that is closer to the center of the vessel. These different velocities create shear stress that is greatest at the vessel wall and least at the center of the vessel. Shear rate therefore changes inversely with the vessel diameter, with levels estimated to vary between 500 s^{-1} in larger arteries and 5000 s^{-1} in the smallest arterioles. Shear rates at the surface of atherosclerotic plaques with modest (50%) stenosis reach 3000 to 10,000 s^{-1}, with even greater shear in more clinically significant stenoses. The high-velocity aspect of arterial blood flow actually opposes the tendencies to clot by (1) limiting the time available for procoagulant reactions to occur and (2) disrupting cells and proteins that are not tightly adherent to the vessel wall. However, once the vessel wall is damaged and bleeding occurs, platelets can rapidly and decisively respond to the loss of endothelial integrity while they simultaneously resist the tendency to be swept downstream.

One of the forces enhancing platelet readiness for wall adhesion in the arterial circulation is radial dispersion, the tendency of larger cells (erythrocytes and leukocytes) to stream in the center of the vessel, where shear is lowest. This process effectively pushes the smaller platelets toward the vessel wall and optimally positions them to respond to hemostatic challenges. This size-dependent flow may also explain the seemingly paradoxical ability of red blood cell transfusions to slow or stop bleeding in patients with thrombocytopenia or consumptive coagulopathy (see Chapter 51). This effect also underscores the importance of platelets in arterial hemostasis; reductions in platelet number or function may be associated with severe arterial hemorrhage after surgery or trauma. By contrast, the lesser shear forces experienced in the venous circulation permit more random cell movement and greater time for coagulation reactions to occur; for this reason, the minimum requirements for platelet number and function in venous hemostasis are less stringent.

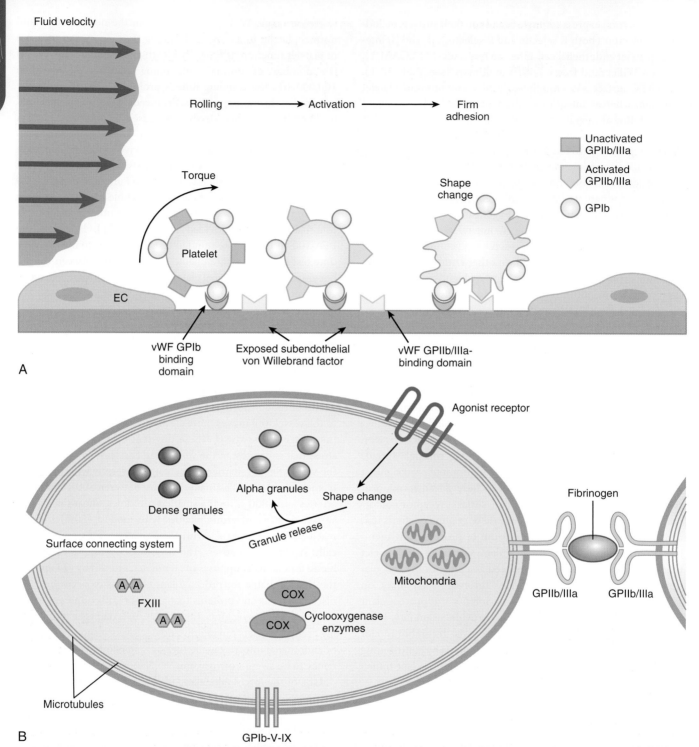

Fluid velocity

Rolling ⟶ Activation ⟶ Firm adhesion

Torque

Unactivated GPIIb/IIIa

Activated GPIIb/IIIa

GPIb

Platelet

Shape change

EC

vWF GPIb binding domain

Exposed subendothelial von Willebrand factor

vWF GPIIb/IIIa-binding domain

A

Agonist receptor

Alpha granules

Shape change

Dense granules

Granule release

Surface connecting system

Fibrinogen

Mitochondria

GPIIb/IIIa   GPIIb/IIIa

FXIII

COX

COX   Cyclooxygenase enzymes

Microtubules

B

GPIb-V-IX

FIGURE 50-1   **A,** The adhesive interactions that produce stable platelet attachment to subendothelial von Willebrand factor (vWF). The initial attachment between platelet glycoprotein Ib (GPIb) and its binding domain on vWF is rapid but has a short half-life, and the result is a rolling movement caused by torque generated by flowing blood. The vWF-GPIb interaction produces transmembrane signaling that activates the platelet to change shape and simultaneously transforms GPIIb/IIIa into an activated conformation capable of binding to a distinct arginine-glycine-aspartate domain on vWF. This secondary adhesion causes the platelet to firmly adhere to the exposed subendothelial vWF. **B,** The internal and external anatomy of a platelet. The platelet consists of several important external, transmembrane, and internal components that help to promote platelet activation, adhesion, aggregation/agglutination, and general coagulation factor–based hemostasis. The most important and most clinically relevant aspects of platelet anatomy are shown. Details regarding the steps leading to platelet activation and release of granules and cytosolic contents are discussed in the text. A, A subunits of Factor XIII; COX, Cyclooxygenase; EC, Endothelial cell; FXIII, factor XIII; GP, glycoprotein complex.

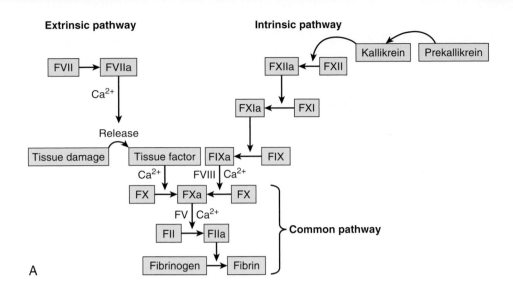

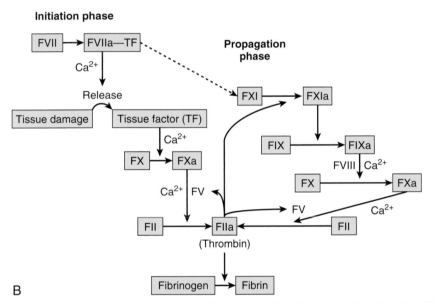

FIGURE 50-2   **A,** The classic view of the coagulation cascade. The laboratory-defined *extrinsic* and *intrinsic* pathways allow monitoring of anticoagulation by serial measurements of the prothrombin time (PT) and partial thromboplastin time (PTT), respectively. The PT primarily monitors factor VII activity, whereas the PTT is the best measure of XI and the hemophilic factors IX and VIII; both assays will detect deficiency of the common pathway factors (X, V, and II). **B,** In the more modern view of the coagulation cascade, initiation of clotting begins with exposure to tissue factor (TF), which combines with small amounts of circulating factor (F)VIIa to form the extrinsic tenase (Xase) complex and generate FXa. FXa forms the prothrombinase complex with FVa and FII, generating small amounts of thrombin (FIIa), which begins to cleave fibrinogen into weak fibrin monomers in the initiation phase of coagulation. Thrombin's ability to activate factors, especially on the activated platelet surface, is responsible for propagation of the coagulant response. Thrombin generates FXIa, which, in turn, activates FIX; the TF-VIIa complex (before it is shut down by TFPI) also generates FIXa. Thrombin-activated FVIIIa then combines with IXa to form the intrinsic Xase complex, generating large amounts of FXa and prothrombinase complex on the platelet surface to further amplify thrombin generation. The large amounts of thrombin now generate enough fibrin monomers to form stable polymers and fibrin clot. HMWK, High-molecular-weight kininogen; PK, prekallikrein; TFPI, tissue factor pathway inhibitor.

In the setting of high-velocity blood flow at an arterial bleeding site, platelets must activate and adhere to the injured vessel almost instantaneously (see Fig. 50-1A). Two molecules that are present in the subendothelium are critical for this process: vWF and collagen. Control of bleeding in vessels under the highest shear stresses absolutely depends on the presence and function of vWF. vWF is a large molecule synthesized as multimeric *strings* in ECs and megakaryocytes, and multimeric vWF is both constitutively secreted into blood and stored in Weibel-Palade bodies of ECs. The *ultralarge* vWF multimers are the most active at binding platelets, particularly when *unfolded*, either by shear stress or after tethering to the vessel surface. The multimeric forms of vWF, which are immobilized by adherence to exposed subendothelial collagen, bind to the GPIb-IX-V complex on the platelet surface when normally cryptic loci are exposed by high shear stress. This binding is extremely rapid but has low affinity; therefore, the platelets are slowed at this interface, but they are left only weakly adherent to subendothelial vWF. With platelets no longer streaming by, but instead tumbling or sliding over the subendothelium, the high shear stress in tandem with

TABLE 50-2	PROCOAGULANT PROPERTIES OF PLATELETS

RECEPTOR-LIGAND INTERACTIONS PROMOTING ADHESION

*GPIb-IX-V-vWF
†GPIIb/IIIa-fibrinogen and GPIIb/IIIa-vWF
‡GPIa/IIa-collagen
§P-selectin–P-selectin glycoprotein ligand-1

RECEPTOR-LIGAND INTERACTIONS MEDIATING ACTIVATION

GPV-thrombin
GPVI-collagen

SECRETED ALPHA-GRANULE PROTEINS

Ligands (fibrinogen, fibronectin, thrombospondin, vitronectin, von Willebrand factor)
Enzymes (α_2-antiplasmin; factors V, VIII, and XI)
Antiheparin (platelet factor 4)

SECRETED DENSE-GRANULE AGONISTS

Adenosine diphosphate, serotonin

COMPONENTS AND FUNCTIONS OF PLATELETS WHICH PROMOTE COAGULATION

Thromboxane A_2 formation, phosphatidylserine expression

GP, Glycoprotein.
   *GPIb-IX-V complex is also known as CD42.
   †GPIIb/IIIa (integrin $\alpha_{2b}\beta_3$) complex is also known as CD41.
   ‡GPIIa is also known as CD29.
   §P-selectin is also known as CD62P and P-selectin glycoprotein ligand-1 as CD162.

transmembrane signaling produced by the GPIb-V-IX-vWF interaction results in loss of the normal platelet discoid shape and conformational change in another platelet receptor, GPIIb/IIIa (see Fig. 50-1A).

Ligands

The activated GPIIb/IIIa receptor then binds either to fibrinogen or to the larger vWF multimers at a site distinct from the GPIb-IX-V binding site. This secondary adhesion is a higher-affinity interaction, and it secures the platelets firmly to the subendothelium (see Fig 50-1B). At shear rates that approximate arterial occlusion, platelet adhesion to vWF multimers can be mediated entirely through GPIb-V-IX-vWF binding without platelet activation. One important regulator of this process of platelet binding and activation through vWF is the circulating vWF-cleaving protease in plasma; this is a disintegrin and metalloproteinase with a thrombospondin type 1 motif, member 13 (ADAMTS-13). ADAMTS-13 modulates the activity of vWF by cleaving the ultralarge multimers into smaller fragments that have reduced overall affinity for platelet binding. Besides directly activating platelets, thrombin causes proteolysis of ADAMTS-13, thereby promoting the persistence of large vWF multimers and enhanced platelet recruitment into areas of vessel injury. Congenital or acquired pathologic loss of the ADAMTS-13 cleaving protease activity results in unchecked platelet adhesion to ultralarge vWF multimers and widespread microvascular thrombosis (see the discussion of *thrombotic thrombocytopenic purpura* in Chapter 52).

At more moderate shear rates, GPIb-V-IX-vWF adhesion is supplemented by platelet binding to subendothelial collagen, an adhesive moiety that is capable of arresting the platelet by binding to GPIa/IIa (see Table 50-2). Thus, subendothelial vWF and collagen act cooperatively to initiate platelet adhesion, with the former predominating at higher shear. Collagen is unique in that

it can anchor platelets at one locus by binding to platelet GPIa/IIa and activate platelets at a second locus by binding to platelet GPVI; both platelet receptors are critical for physiologic platelet function. Indeed, the congenital absence of any of the critical platelet adhesion receptors—GPIIb/IIIa, GPIb/IX-V, GPVI, or GPIa/IIa—results in a significant hemostatic defect, correctable only by platelet transfusion. This finding is further reinforced by the fact that the α chain of GPIb normally serves as a cofactor for thrombin activation of platelets through both the GPV receptor and the protease-activated receptor (PAR). Like defects in platelet receptors, decreases in the vWF ligand, especially the larger multimeric forms, can lead to bleeding.

Once a layer of platelets is adherent to the site of injury, vWF bound to GPIb-IX-V on the luminal side of the adherent platelets serves to recruit additional platelets from the flowing blood into the growing platelet plug. Platelet recruitment is further enhanced by platelet activation and release of serotonin and ADP, which serve to activate and adhere platelets from the circulation to the growing platelet clot (see Fig. 50-1B and Table 50-1). Platelet activation is actually a series of interdependent processes with five major effects: (1) local release of ligands essential to stabilization of the platelet-platelet matrix, (2) continued recruitment of additional platelets, (3) vasoconstriction of smaller arteries to slow bleeding, (4) localization and acceleration of platelet-associated fibrin formation, and (5) protection of the clot from fibrinolysis.

The basis of the platelet plug is a platelet-ligand-platelet matrix with fibrinogen, fibronectin, and vWF serving as bridging ligands (Fig. 50-3). Both fibrinogen and vWF are endocytosed from plasma and stored in alpha granules inside the resting platelet, and both are released with activation. Fibrinogen plays the predominant role of binding to a GPIIb/IIIa receptor on each of two platelets, thereby linking them. Some data suggest that vWF is capable of a similar role. As mentioned earlier, platelet GPIIb/IIIa undergoes a calcium-dependent conformational change that allows it to bind to a locus containing the amino acid sequence arginine-glycine-aspartate (RGD) on fibrinogen, fibronectin, or vWF. Each fibrinogen molecule has two RGD sites on its polar ends, and the larger vWF multimers have several RGD sites, all capable of binding to conformationally altered GPIIb/IIIa and creating the platelet-ligand-platelet matrix. GPIIb/IIIa is the most abundant glycoprotein on the platelet surface, with about 50,000 copies on the *resting* platelet and additional GPIIb/IIIa receptors within the platelet cytosol that are mobilized to the surface after activation.

Activation

Platelets are also recruited into the platelet plug by local agonists (collagen, epinephrine, and thrombin) and by platelet release of agonists into the local microenvironment (see Fig. 50-1B). Both collagen (as noted previously) and thrombin interact with their specific platelet receptors to activate platelets strongly; although epinephrine alone is not a powerful platelet agonist, stimulation of the α-adrenergic receptor on platelets primes them for synergistic activation by even relatively weak agonists such as ADP. Activating compounds released directly from the platelet include thromboxane A_2 (TXA_2), which is formed in the platelet cytosol after cyclooxygenase 1 (COX1)–mediated

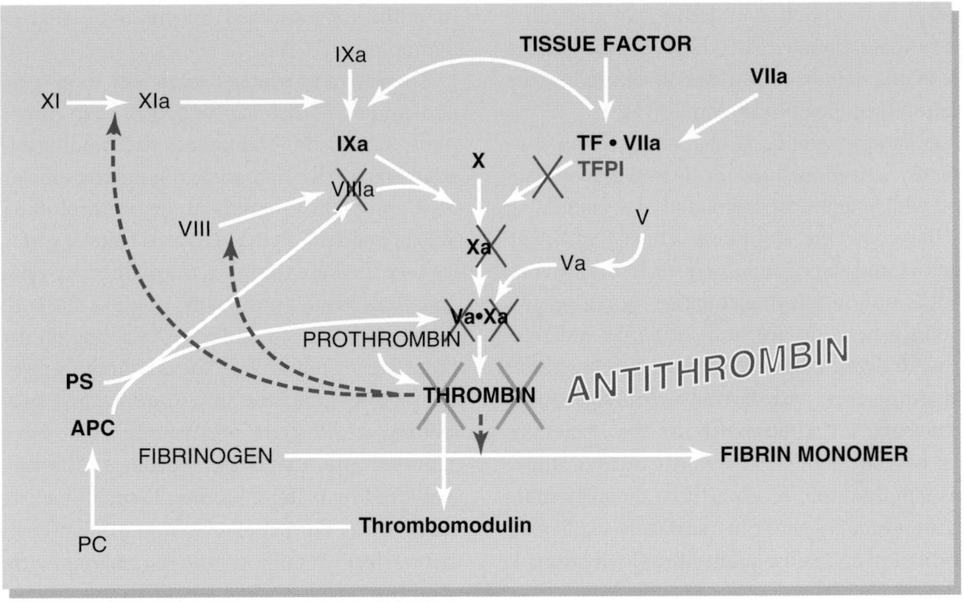

FIGURE 50-3 Endogenous anticoagulant pathways. Tissue factor pathway inhibitor (TFPI) shuts off tissue factor (TF) stimulation and blocks the TF-VIIa-X complex; in addition, the clotting cascade is further downregulated by the natural anticoagulants. This inhibition is partly generated by thrombin, which activates thrombomodulin. Circulating antithrombin inhibits thrombin activity and Xa generation of thrombin. The complex of thrombin and thrombomodulin activates protein C (PC) to become activated protein C (APC), which combines with protein S (PS) to cleave and inactivate VIIIa and Va, further blocking thrombin generation.

cleavage of arachidonic acid and then released into the clot milieu. TXA_2 is both a platelet agonist and a vasoconstrictor, and it is rapidly degraded to its inert byproduct, thromboxane B_2.

Platelet COX1 activity is *irreversibly* inhibited by aspirin, which blocks TXA_2 formation for the lifetime of that platelet. Aspirin irreversibly and covalently binds to a specific serine residue on COX1 and causes steric hindrance of the active site, a tyrosine molecule across from the serine residue. Nonsteroidal anti-inflammatory drugs (NSAIDs) do not covalently bind through acetylation at serine. Instead, they reversibly and competitively bind at the active, catalytic tyrosine site. Therefore, in contrast to aspirin, the antiplatelet effects of NSAIDs are dependent on the continual presence of plasma levels of the NSAID.

COX2 is an induced isoform within leukocytes that mediates inflammation and pain. Because mature platelets do not appear to possess COX2 activity, one rationale for development of the highly selective COX2 inhibitors for inflammatory diseases was to avoid the bleeding caused by platelet dysfunction by not affecting platelet COX1 activity. However, it appears that vascular ECs use COX2 activity to synthesize the antithrombogenic compound, prostacyclin (see Table 50-1 and Chapter 50). Downregulation of EC prostacyclin, coupled with preserved platelet prothrombotic function, may tip the hemostatic balance in favor of clot formation, and large-scale clinical trials have now shown that some highly selective COX2 inhibitors increase the likelihood of hypertension and vascular arterial events, including myocardial infarction and stroke.

Other platelet agonists are liberated into the extracellular fluid by fusion of the dense granules and alpha granules with the platelet canalicular membrane, and the result is extrusion of granule contents (see Fig. 50-1B). The dense granules contain serotonin, which, like TXA_2, is both a platelet agonist and a vasoconstrictor.

Another dense granule constituent, ADP, acts purely as a platelet agonist through the G protein–linked P2RY12 receptor and has no vasoactive properties (see Table 50-2). The importance of TXA_2- and serotonin-induced vasoconstriction is not entirely clear. However, by decreasing the vessel diameter, vasoconstriction may increase shear stress and thereby facilitate recruitment of platelets to the injured site.

The importance of dense-granule release to the maintenance of hemostasis is underscored by the severe bleeding seen in patients with congenital dense-granule deficiencies (e.g., Hermansky-Pudlak syndrome). Platelet activation therefore serves to amplify platelet adhesion and to optimize the platelet surface for interaction with soluble coagulation factors, resulting in the explosive generation of thrombin and fibrin (see later discussion). Finally, other components present in platelets, such as cytosolic factor XIII, are also released into the vascular space on activation. In this case, factor XIII serves as a clot stabilizer, once again reflecting the additional role that activated platelets play in promoting hemostasis.

● SOLUBLE COAGULATION

Coagulation Models

The classic "cascade" model of soluble coagulation (see Fig. 50-2A), as first described more than 40 years ago, features two starting points that converge to a common pathway leading to thrombin and fibrin generation. This model allowed great strides to be made in identifying the proteolytic reactions that culminate in fibrin clot, and it dovetailed well with the prothrombin time (PT) and activated partial thromboplastin time (aPTT) assays that guide warfarin and heparin dosing, respectively. Although the model is workable for some clinical scenarios, bleeding in a disease such as hemophilia contradicts its prediction that when one of these pathways is dysfunctional, activity of the other should be sufficient to maintain adequate clot formation. More recent models have made significant strides in clarifying the dynamics of coagulation (see Figs. 50-2B and50-3).

Regulation of coagulation proteins is characterized by continuous low-grade factor activation and coordinated assembly of enzyme complexes, which are downregulated by circulating inhibitor proteins. These enzyme complexes consist of serine proteases, their cofactors, and zymogen substrates. In the absence of overt blood vessel disruption, enzyme complex formation and the resultant thrombin generation are both minimal and relatively slow; circulating anticoagulants are sufficient to inactivate these procoagulant complexes and prevent clot formation. However, once a procoagulant stimulus occurs that generates significant amounts of activated factors, formation of these enzyme complexes is rapidly amplified—partly by their assembly on a favorable membrane (phospholipid) surface—leading to intense thrombin formation and subsequent fibrin formation.

Clot Initiation

Coagulation in vivo occurs after exposure of the blood to a source of TF, typically on the surface of a fibroblast coming into contact with blood through a break in the vessel wall. The intrinsic or contact pathway of coagulation has no role in the earliest events in clotting. TF-initiated coagulation has two phases: an *initiation* phase and a *propagation* phase (see Fig. 50-2B). The initiation phase begins as the exposed TF binds to factor VIIa, picomolar amounts of which are present in the circulation at all times. This VIIa-TF complex catalyzes the conversion of very small amounts of factor X to Xa, which in turn, generates nanomolar amounts of thrombin. The seemingly trivial amount of thrombin formed during the initiation phase sparks the inception of the propagation phase, successful completion of which culminates in explosive thrombin generation and, ultimately, fibrin deposition.

Clot Propagation

Thrombin generated during the initiation phase is a potent platelet activator, supplying the developing clot with an activated platelet surface membrane and abundant platelet-released factor V. More than 96% of the total thrombin that is generated during clotting occurs during the propagation phase. Factor V is then promptly activated to Va by thrombin. Factor VIII, conveniently brought to the bleeding site by its carrier, vWF, is also activated by thrombin, a step that causes its release by vWF. VIIIa then complexes with the picomolar amounts of factor IXa generated by the TF-VIIa complex during the initiation phase to create the VIIIa-IXa complex. The formation of this complex on the platelet surface heralds the switch of the primary path of Xa generation from the TF-VIIa complex (the extrinsic Xase) to the intrinsic Xase (the VIIIa-IXa complex). This switch is of significant kinetic advantage, with the intrinsic Xase complex exhibiting 50-fold higher efficiency than the extrinsic Xase. The bleeding diathesis associated with hemophilia is testament to the physiologic importance of the exuberant thrombin generation engendered by the switch from extrinsic to intrinsic Xase. The aPTT, which measures the initiation phase of clotting begun by an artificial in vitro stimulant, is prolonged by severe deficiencies of either VIII or IX, but it is thrombin generation during the propagation phase, a

function not evaluated by the aPTT, that is most impaired in hemophilia.

The activated platelet expresses receptors for VIIIa and IXa, and binding of these active proteases in complex with membrane phosphatidylserine enhances the binding of the enzyme's substrate, factor X, increasing the kinetic efficiency of the intrinsic Xase complex. Assembly of the prothrombinase complex is similarly dependent on the activated platelet surface for optimal activity. Like the Xase complex, the membrane-bound prothrombinase complex activates prothrombin with a rate enhancement 300,000-fold higher than that of free Xa acting on prothrombin in solution. Platelet-bound Xa is the rate-limiting enzyme in prothrombin cleavage for both the initiation and the propagation phases of clotting; its substrate, prothrombin, binds to GPIIb/IIIa on both activated and unactivated platelets. The net kinetic advantage conferred by platelet binding is such that assembly of the entire reaction on the platelet membrane increases the catalytic efficiency by 13 million–fold compared with proteases free in solution.

What roles do other intrinsic pathway factors play in coagulation? Evidence is growing that factor XI further amplifies the propagation phase of coagulation. Factor Xa is particularly rate-limiting once the switch to the intrinsic Xase has been made. Although small amounts of IXa are generated by the TF-VIIa complex, IXa generation in this manner is limited by TFPI. To generate Xa in amounts sufficient to fuel the propagation phase, a kinetically superior source of IXa is required. Factor XI is another zymogen activated by very small amounts of initiation phase–generated thrombin, but this activation is restricted to the activated platelet surface. Platelet-bound XIa activates IX on the platelet surface, thereby favoring assembly of the intrinsic Xase complex. Moreover, binding to the platelet surface protects XIa from its inhibitor, protease nexin 2. In summary, XIa generation on the activated platelet is instrumental for providing IXa in amounts sufficient to maintain peak Xa generation through the efficient intrinsic Xase complex.

Limiting Soluble Coagulation

Endogenous anticoagulants can either inactivate formed thrombin or prevent thrombin generation (see Fig. 50-3). The most important natural anticoagulant that inactivates thrombin is antithrombin (AT). AT is physiologically present at more than twice the concentration (3.2 μmol/L) of the highest local thrombin concentration (1.4 μmol/L) that can be reached during clotting, and AT activity against thrombin is potentiated 1000-fold by endogenous EC-associated heparan sulfate proteoglycans. Platelet surface membranes and platelet-released platelet factor 4 protect thrombin from inactivation at the clot. However, any thrombin that escapes into the circulation is immediately (<1 minute) inhibited by plasma AT, and in the microenvironment of healthy ECs that bind about 60,000 molecules of AT per cell, free thrombin is neutralized almost instantaneously. Therefore, early thrombin generation is critically dependent on protection by the activated platelet membrane to allow sufficient time to make the transition from the initiation to the propagation phase.

Among endogenous anticoagulants that target thrombin generation, the earliest in the coagulation process is TFPI, which inactivates factor Xa and the TF-VIIa complex. TFPI is constitutively released by ECs into the microvasculature. Under normal conditions, TFPI is largely localized to the endothelial surface by binding to EC-associated glycosaminoglycans, but it can be displaced by heparin. Nascent TFPI has direct activity only against Xa, but after exposure to Xa, TFPI acquires activity against the TF-VIIa complex. During the initiation phase, platelet-bound Xa is protected from inactivation by both TFPI and AT. Preservation of the small amounts of Xa that are generated during this early stage of coagulation is critical to formation of the nanomolar amounts of thrombin needed to begin the propagation phase of clotting.

Activated protein C (APC) has anticoagulant, anti-inflammatory, and profibrinolytic properties that make it an important regulator of both thrombosis and inflammation. Like TFPI, protein C becomes activated only after coagulation is underway. Formed thrombin binds to thrombomodulin, a proteoglycan associated with endothelial and monocyte cell surfaces. Thrombomodulin-bound thrombin loses its ability to activate platelets and instead activates protein C. On the EC surface, nascent protein C binds to endothelial cell protein C receptor (EPCR), which positions it for activation by the adjacent thrombomodulin-bound thrombin. In a reaction that is enhanced by EPCR and protein S, APC inactivates factors VIIIa and Va, (components of the Xase and prothrombinase complexes, respectively), thereby limiting procoagulant self-amplification (Fig. 50-4). As with other coagulation factors, the activated platelet membrane protects VIIIa and Va from APC inactivation. In addition to its effects on thrombin generation, APC neutralizes plasminogen activator inhibitor-1 (PAI-1) to enhance clot remodeling. APC has anti-inflammatory properties as well; recombinant APC reduces production of tumor necrosis factor-α after endotoxin challenge, and protein C–deficient mice (heterozygotes) exhibit higher levels of proinflammatory cytokines with systemic endotoxemia.

The liver is the major site of synthesis of all coagulation factors. Factor VIII levels are not usually diminished in liver disease because VIII is also produced by EC and the reticuloendothelial system. The subset of coagulation factors that depend on vitamin K for synthesis include prothrombin (II), VII, IX, and X and the anticoagulants, protein C and protein S. Post-translational modification (through a vitamin K–dependent carboxylase) of the amino-terminal domain of these proteins adds 10 to 12 γ-carboxyglutamate residues; these residues are critical for calcium binding and for determining the functional three-dimensional structure of the proteins and their proper orientation for binding to membrane surfaces. Warfarin blocks vitamin K epoxide reductase and thereby decreases generation of vitamin K (from vitamin K epoxide) in the vitamin K cycle.

CLOT VIABILITY AND MATURATION

Evidence is growing that initial formation of a thrombus does not ensure sustained hemostasis. Events initiated during generation of both fibrin-rich clots in the venous circulation and platelet-rich clots in the arterial circulation that are critical to clot stability operate after the clot is formed.

Fibrin Clot Architecture

The architecture of a fibrin clot is surprisingly variable. Although genetic factors unquestionably play a role in determining clot structure, two dominant factors are the local concentrations of thrombin and fibrinogen, whose reactions yield the fibrin strands. A thrombin-rich microenvironment typically results in thinner, more tightly cross-linked fibers, making the overall fibrin clot virtually impermeable to lytic enzymes. In thrombin-poor locations, the fibrin strands are thicker and the structure is more porous, making the clot vulnerable to thrombolysis. Similarly, high fibrinogen concentrations are associated with large thrombi whose tight, rigid meshwork makes them less deformable and more resistant to lysis. Low fibrinogen concentrations produce a less compact clot that is highly lysis prone.

Fibrin Cross-Linking by Factor XIIIa

Factor XIII also plays a critical role in stabilization of the forming clot. Factor XIII circulates in the plasma and is also stored within platelets; indeed, fully 50% of the total fibrin-stabilizing activity in blood resides in the platelet and is released by activation. In plasma, factor XIII is a tetrameric molecule consisting of two α subunits, which contain the active site of the enzyme, and two β

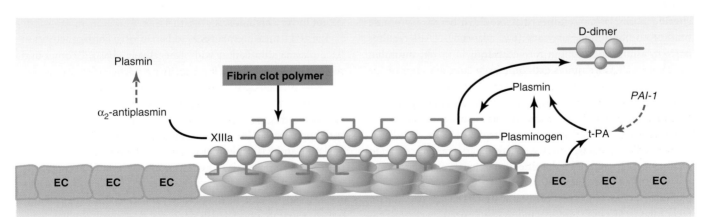

FIGURE 50-4 Balanced fibrinolysis limits the platelet-fibrin clot. The platelet plug and fibrin matrices are strengthened by incorporation of factor XIIIa into the fibrin clot. Factor XIIIa also binds α₂-antiplasmin to the clot to protect it from plasmin-mediated fibrinolysis. At the same time, nearby intact endothelial cells (ECs) secrete tissue plasminogen activator (t-PA). t-PA that evades plasminogen activator inhibitor-1 (PAI-1) converts clot-bound plasminogen to plasmin and leads to fibrin clot degradation and release of soluble fibrin peptides and D-dimer. Therefore, detection of circulating D-dimer usually indicates active fibrinolysis.

subunits, which increase the zymogen's plasma half-life but must be dissociated for full enzyme activity. Platelet factor XIII, by contrast, is a dimer that contains only the two α subunits. Both forms of the zymogen require thrombin cleavage and fibrin as a cofactor, but plasma factor XIII activation proceeds at a considerably slower rate owing to the need for dissociation of the β subunits. Thrombin-activated factor XIIIa binds to fibrin and cross-links the fibrin units, thereby rendering them less permeable and more resistant to lysis. Furthermore, factor XIIIa cross-links the major plasmin inhibitor, α_2-antiplasmin, directly to fibrin, positioning it for neutralization of any invading plasmin.

Fibrinolysis

The fibrinolytic system operates to prevent fibrin from occluding healthy vessels. During clot formation, Xa and thrombin stimulate healthy ECs to release tissue-type plasminogen activator (t-PA) and urokinase-type plasminogen activator (u-PA), both of which are capable of cleaving plasminogen into plasmin. The vast excess of plasminogen in the plasma dictates that under normal circumstances, the concentration of these enzymes is rate-limiting for plasmin formation. The kinetic efficiency of t-PA is improved by at least an order of magnitude by the presence of fibrin. This helps to keep t-PA most active in the microenvironment of the clot. By contrast, u-PA appears to require binding to activated platelets for its ability to liberate plasmin.

Acting to contain fibrinolysis are plasma mediators that either inactivate formed plasmin (such as α_2-antiplasmin and possibly α_2-macroglobulin) or block plasmin formation. Foremost among the latter is PAI-1. PAI-1 is present in several-fold molar excess in the plasma and is also released by activated platelets, thereby protecting clots from premature lysis. Plasma levels of PAI-1 can be highly variable, in part because of its circadian pattern of secretion, but also because of polymorphisms of the PAI-1 gene. The 4G promoter region polymorphism of PAI-1 is associated with higher PAI-1 levels and a higher risk for thromboembolic disease (see Chapter 52).

Another mediator that limits fibrinolysis in the vicinity of the clot is thrombin activator fibrinolysis inhibitor (TAFI). TAFI is synthesized in an inactive form by the liver and circulates in the plasma, possibly in a complex with plasminogen. TAFI cleaves specific fibrin lysine residues that would otherwise promote binding of fibrinolytic enzymes (e.g., plasmin). TAFI requires either plasmin or thrombin for activation; however, thrombin activation of TAFI requires extraordinarily large amounts of *free* thrombin. By contrast, EC-associated thrombomodulin increases thrombin-induced TAFI activation 1250-fold, making this an essential cofactor and one that is predominantly available only at the interface between the blood and the vessel wall.

In addition to the EC surface, macrophages are also critical to fibrinolysis. Macrophages degrade fibrin clot through lysosomal proteolysis by a plasmin-independent mechanism. The macrophage binds to fibrin and fibrinogen through its surface integrin receptor, CD11b/CD18; this binding is followed by internalization of the complex into the lysosome, where fibrin and fibrinogen are degraded.

Tissue repair and regeneration are the physiologic end points of clotting, and they eventually lead to dissolution of the fibrin-based clot. Besides t-PA and urokinase, the intrinsic pathway

activators kallikrein, XIIa, and XIa also generate active plasmin from plasminogen. Plasminogen binding to cell surface receptors promotes its own activation to plasmin by placing it in proximity to t-PA and fibrin clot and protects plasmin from inactivation by circulating (not clot-bound) α_2-antiplasmin (see Fig. 50-4). Plasmin eventually dissolves the fibrin matrix to produce soluble fibrin peptides and D-dimer; it also activates metalloproteinases that further degrade damaged tissue. Fibroblasts and leukocytes migrate into the wound, the latter mediated by selectin binding, and these inflammatory cells act in concert with growth factors secreted by leukocytes and activated platelets (e.g., transforming growth factor-β) to enhance vascular repair and tissue regeneration.

Laboratory Testing of Coagulation

For purposes of laboratory testing, the coagulation cascade is artificially divided into extrinsic and intrinsic pathways, measured as PT and PTT, respectively. These converge to form a common pathway that leads to thrombin and fibrin generation (see Fig. 50-2A). In the laboratory, the *extrinsic* pathway (PT) is assessed by measuring the interaction of circulating VIIa with exogenously added TF (also known as *thromboplastin*). The PT is highly sensitive to deficiencies of factors II, VII, V, and X, all of which are associated with significant bleeding. Because II, VII, and X are also vitamin K dependent factors, with VII having the shortest circulating half-life, the PT is currently the best test for monitoring warfarin (Coumadin) therapy. The PT is unaffected by intrinsic pathway deficiencies of XII, XI, IX, or VIII. The degree of prolongation of the PT by warfarin depends on the strength of the particular thromboplastin (based on its international sensitivity index [ISI]) and the specific coagulation instrument used for the assay. The international normalized ratio (INR) takes these factors into account to standardize among laboratories for variations in prolongation of the PT induced by warfarin. The INR is calculated for each patient as follows: (patient PT/mean control PT)^{ISI}. Therapeutic INRs with warfarin allow for global application of anticoagulant recommendations; these vary according to the specific disease indication and are covered in Chapter 51. In contrast, the PT is relatively insensitive to therapeutic anticoagulation with unfractionated heparin except in very high doses.

The aPTT measurement is based on in vitro contact activation (e.g., plasma stimulation with a negatively charged compound such as kaolin). The aPTT is sensitive to deficiencies of contact factors—prekallikrein (PK), high-molecular-weight kininogen (HMWK), and factor XII—and to deficiencies of coagulation factors of the intrinsic pathway (XI, IX, and VIII) and the common pathway (V, X, and prothrombin). Deficiencies of PK, HMWK, and XII prolong the aPTT but do not result in clinical bleeding, implying that these factors are irrelevant to physiologic hemostasis. By contrast, severe deficiencies of XI, and especially IX and VIII, cause significant bleeding. The aPTT is also highly sensitive to unfractionated heparin and is used to monitor therapeutic heparin anticoagulation. Compared with the INR for anticoagulation with warfarin, the range for therapeutic aPTT levels with unfractionated heparin is much wider and not as easily standardized. Therapeutic unfractionated heparin levels can be measured by sensitive assays of anti-Xa activity; therapeutic levels of

0.3 to 0.7 anti-Xa U/mL typically correspond to aPTT values between 1.8 and 2.5 times greater than the patient's baseline PTT (before starting heparin) or the mean PTT of a control population.

Most of the commonly used laboratory tests of soluble coagulation measure the kinetics of the initiation phase only. The PT and PTT have as their end points the first appearance of fibrin gel, which occurs when less than 5% of the total reaction has been completed and when only minimal levels of prothrombin have been activated. The PT and PTT are very sensitive for detecting congenital abnormalities associated with severe factor deficits (e.g., hemophilia) and for guiding heparin and warfarin therapy. However, these tests fail to give information relevant to thrombin generation during the propagation phase, which determines whether a persistent clot forms or the endogenous anticoagulants and fibrinolytic regulators constrain it from excess growth.

In surgical settings and in intensive care units, there is a need for immediate turnaround in coagulation testing. One specific point-of-care test used for coagulation testing is thromboelastometry (TEG). TEG uses whole blood to detect hyperfibrinolysis and can also assess for platelet dysfunction. As the whole blood begins to solidify in the presence of a prothrombotic agent (e.g., kaolin) a detector collects information about the speed and strength of clot formation.

SUGGESTED READINGS

Bauer KA: Recent progress in anticoagulant therapy: oral direct inhibitors of thrombin and factor Xa, J Thromb Haemost 9:12–19, 2011.

Cosemans JMEM, Angelillo-Scherrer A, Mattheij NJA, et al: The effects of arterial flow on platelet activation, thrombus growth, and stabilization, Cardiovasc Res 99:342–352, 2013.

Gorlinger K, Shore-Lesserson L, Dirkmann D, et al: Management of hemorrhage in cardiothoracic surgery, J Cardiothorac Vasc Anesth 27:20–34, 2013.

Monroe DM, Hoffman M: The clotting system: a major player in wound healing, Haemophilia 18:11–16, 2012.

Monroe DM, Hoffman M: The coagulation cascade in cirrhosis, Clin Liver Dis 13:1–9, 2009.

Tripodi A: The laboratory and the direct oral anticoagulants, Blood 121:4032–4035, 2013.

Whelihan MF, Mann KG: The role of the red cell membrane in thrombin generation, Thromb Res 131:377–382, 2013.

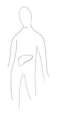

51

Disorders of Hemostasis: Bleeding

Christopher A. Tormey and Henry M. Rinder

INTRODUCTION

The approach to an individual with a bleeding disorder considers whether bleeding has been a lifelong issue (i.e., congenital) or has recently become a problem (i.e., acquired). The approach also considers the underlying pathophysiology, such as defects in the vasculature, platelets, or coagulation factor proteins that predispose the patient to bleeding. This chapter explores clinical concepts and tools that should aid the development of an appropriate framework for evaluating and treating patients with hemostatic defects.

CLINICAL AND LABORATORY EVALUATION OF BLEEDING

The evaluation of bleeding requires a careful history, physical examination, and laboratory evaluation. The patient's history should include a description of bleeding (e.g., epistaxis, menorrhagia, hematoma formation), the circumstances in which bleeding occurs (e.g., trauma, surgery, dental procedures), and whether blood products (and what kind) were required to staunch the bleeding. The temporal addition of medications such as aspirin can be associated with bleeding, as can concomitant medical illnesses such as infection or liver disease. Determining a family history of bleeding is important, and the physician may need to question several generations and second-degree relations (e.g., maternal uncles) if hemophilia is suggested in the proband.

The physical examination may yield some clues as to the origin of bleeding by differentiating small vessel bleeding, such as petechial (pinpoint) hemorrhage, from larger vessel bleeding, which usually produces hematomas and purpura (i.e., large bruises). Small vessel bleeding in the skin, mucous membranes, or gastrointestinal (GI) tract tends to occur more often in patients with thrombocytopenia (i.e., decreased platelet counts), qualitative platelet defects, vascular abnormalities, or von Willebrand disease (vWD). In women, menorrhagia may be the only symptom of a bleeding disorder, and it should never be attributed solely to a gynecologic cause. Large vessel bleeding in organs, joints, deep tissue, or muscles is more commonly associated with factor deficiencies (e.g., hemophilia).

Screening laboratory assays are useful in the initial assessment of the bleeding patient (Table 51-1) and should include blood cell counts (especially the platelet count) and examination of a peripheral blood smear; prothrombin time (PT), which is highly sensitive to defects in vitamin K–dependent coagulation factors (particularly factor VII); and activated partial thromboplastin time (aPTT), which detects deficiencies in factors VIII, IX, and

XI (Fig. 51-1). Abnormalities of factors X, V, I (fibrinogen), and II (prothrombin) elevate the PT and aPTT. If the PT or aPTT is prolonged, a mixing study should be performed: The patient's plasma is combined with normal plasma and the clotting time study is repeated. The mixing study distinguishes between factor deficiency (i.e., PT or aPTT corrects to the normal range) and the presence of a circulating inhibitor (i.e., clotting time remains prolonged). Another readily available test for the patient with bleeding is the thrombin time, which assays the functional fibrinogen level. The physiology of the coagulation cascade is explained in Chapter 52.

Platelet function traditionally has been assessed by the in vivo bleeding time, an invasive measure of the time required to halt bleeding in a skin incision (see Chapter 52). The bleeding time is prolonged by qualitative platelet defects and by rare connective tissue disorders. The bleeding time test depends on the expertise of the technician performing the test. Its poor reproducibility and the difficulty of performing the test in infants and neonates have limited its use.

	TABLE 51-1 SCREENING ASSAYS FOR HEMOSTASIS	
LABORATORY TEST	**ASPECT OF HEMOSTASIS TESTED**	**CAUSES OF ABNORMALITIES**
Blood counts and peripheral blood smear	Platelet count and morphologic features	Thrombocytopenia, thrombocytosis, gray platelet and giant platelet syndromes
Prothrombin time	Factor VII–dependent pathways	Vitamin K deficiency and warfarin, liver disease, DIC, factor deficiency (VII, V, X, II), factor inhibitor
Partial thromboplastin time	Factor XI–, IX–, and VIII–dependent pathways	Heparin, DIC, lupus anticoagulant,* vWD, factor deficiency (XI, IX, VIII, V, X, II), factor inhibitor
Thrombin time	Fibrinogen	Heparin, hypofibrinogenemia, dysfibrinogenemia, DIC
Platelet function analysis	Platelet and vWF function	Aspirin, vWD, storage pool disease
Mixing study	Factor inhibitors or deficiencies	Abnormal clotting time corrects for a deficiency; does not correct for an inhibitor

DIC, Disseminated intravascular coagulation; vWD, von Willebrand disease; vWF, von Willebrand factor.
*Lupus anticoagulant is not associated with bleeding.

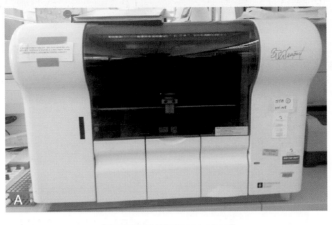

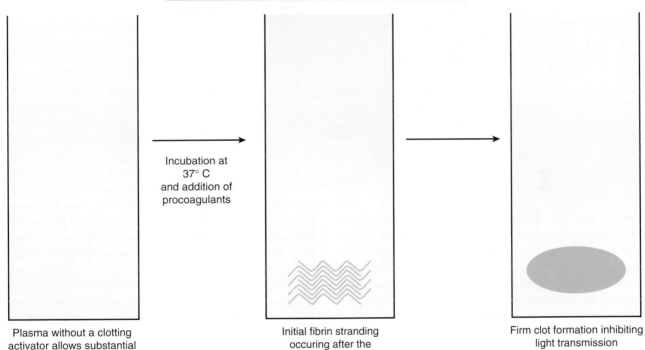

| Plasma without a clotting activator allows substantial light transmission | Incubation at 37° C and addition of procoagulants → Initial fibrin stranding occuring after the addition of the procoagulant | → Firm clot formation inhibiting light transmission |

B

FIGURE 51-1   Basic methodology underlying measurement of prothrombin (PT) and activated partial thromboplastin time (aPTT). **A,** Typical laboratory instrument used to perform basic and complex coagulation assays. **B,** Plasma specimens are incubated at 37° C and then mixed with tissue factor and phospholipid (PT) or a surface activator and phospholipid (aPTT). The time it takes for clot formation to block light passage through the specimen is measured and compared with a reference range. Prolongation of the PT or aPTT clotting time can be associated many congenital or acquired coagulation factor defects. Abnormal PT or aPTT values are typically followed by more specific coagulation factor assays, depending on the type of prolongation and the suspected underlying clinical disease.

Several instruments use phlebotomized whole blood for in vitro assessment of platelet function. One that delivers an in vitro bleeding time is the Platelet Function Analyzer-100 (PFA-100). Citrate-anticoagulated whole blood is passed through a small orifice in a cartridge impregnated with platelet activators such as collagen, adenosine diphosphate (ADP), and epinephrine. As the platelets become activated and adhere, the orifice gradually becomes obstructed, and the time needed for complete occlusion by the platelet plug is measured as the closure time (Fig. 51-2). The closure time is prolonged by qualitative platelet defects such as those caused by aspirin and vWD. Although thrombocytopenia (<100,000 platelets/μL) obviates use of the closure time (similar to the in vivo bleeding time), these in vitro tests are gradually supplanting the measurement of bleeding time.

Another laboratory study for evaluation of a prolonged aPTT, especially in the inpatient setting, is use of the aPTT with an added substance (e.g., hexadimethrine bromide [Polybrene], protamine, heparinase) to neutralize any contaminating heparin resulting from drawing of the blood through an intravenous line. A prolonged aPTT that does not correct in the mixing study may also be observed in patients with a lupus anticoagulant, often in the context of thrombosis. The diagnosis of a lupus anticoagulant can be confirmed by documenting the correction of the aPTT with the addition of excess phospholipid and with other specific tests for lupus anticoagulant (see Antiphospholipid Antibody Syndrome in Chapter 54).

A rapid approach to identifying possible causes of bleeding (Fig. 51-3) considers several major disease categories: (1) vWD,

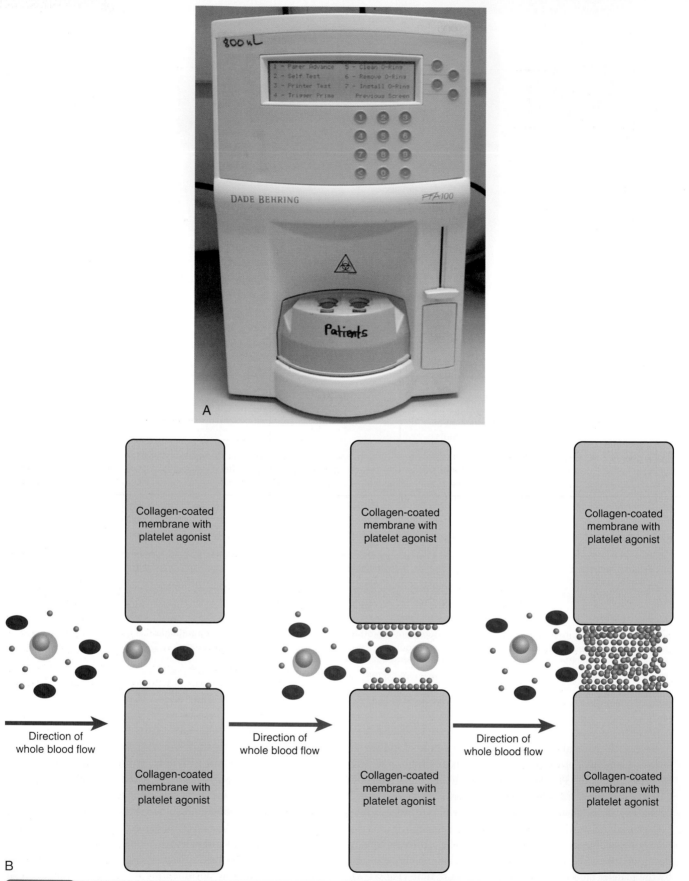

FIGURE 51-2 Methodology underlying the Platelet Function Analyzer-100 (PFA-100). **A,** Whole blood platelets are streamed toward a collagen-based aperture. The membrane is infused with a potent platelet agonist (i.e., adenosine diphosphate or epinephrine). **B,** Streaming the platelets through the instrument channels induces shear-based activation, which in conjunction with the agonists, should yield an initial wave of platelet adhesion and aggregation. Over time, activated platelets continue to aggregate, closing off the aperture to whole blood flow. The time it takes for aperture closing is measured in seconds and compared with a reference range. Abnormally prolonged closure times can be associated with von Willebrand disease due to the reliance on adhesion in this assay or with a platelet functional defect due to the reliance on aggregation for complete aperture closure.

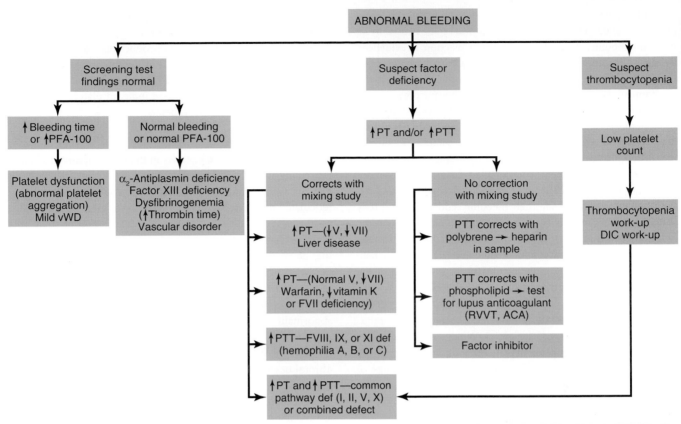

FIGURE 51-3 Algorithm for the evaluation of bleeding. Screening laboratory tests for platelet and factor deficiencies are used to narrow the work-up for bleeding, followed by specific factor and other coagulation studies (e.g., mixing studies, D-dimer) to confirm the diagnosis. ACA, Anti-cardiolipin antibody; DIC, disseminated intravascular coagulation; FVIII, factor VIII; PFA-100, Platelet Function Analyzer-100; PT, prothrombin time; PTT, partial thromboplastin time; RVVT, Russell viper venom time; vWD, von Willebrand disease; ↑, increased; ↓, decreased.

thrombocytopenia, or abnormal platelet function; (2) low levels of multiple coagulation factors resulting from vitamin K deficiency, liver disease, or disseminated intravascular coagulation (DIC); (3) single-factor deficiency (usually inherited); and, more rarely, (4) an acquired inhibitor to a coagulation factor such as factor VIII. The laboratory evaluation is most efficient when it is performed in this context.

BLEEDING CAUSED BY VASCULAR DISORDERS

Vascular purpura (i.e., bruising) is defined as bleeding caused by intrinsic structural abnormalities of blood vessels or by inflammatory infiltration of blood vessels (i.e., vasculitis). Although vascular purpura usually causes bleeding in the setting of normal platelet counts and normal coagulation study results, vasculitis and vessel damage may be severe enough to cause secondary consumption of platelets and coagulation factors.

Collagen breakdown and thinning of the subcutaneous tissue that overlies blood vessels is often observed in older patients (i.e., senile purpura), and similar atrophic skin changes are a common effect of steroid therapy. Another acquired cause of vascular purpura is scurvy (i.e., defeicney of vitamin C [ascorbic acid]). Patients with scurvy have bleeding around individual hair fibers (i.e., perifollicular hemorrhage) and corkscrew-shaped hairs. Bruising occurs in a classic saddle pattern over the upper thighs. The bleeding gums are caused by gingivitis and not by the subcutaneous tissue defect. Edentulous patients with scurvy do not have bleeding gums, and scurvy should not be excluded on this basis.

Congenital defects of the vessel wall can cause bruising. These rare syndromes include pseudoxanthoma elasticum, a defect of the elastic fibers of the vasculature that is associated with severe GI and genitourinary bleeding, and Ehlers-Danlos syndrome, which is characterized by abnormal collagen molecules in blood vessels and subcutaneous tissue. Both syndromes cause bruising in the skin, but only patients with pseudoxanthoma elasticum develop significant GI bleeding.

Another inherited vessel wall defect associated with GI bleeding is hereditary hemorrhagic telangiectasia (i.e., Osler-Weber-Rendu syndrome). This disorder is characterized by degeneration of the blood vessel wall that results in angiomatous lesions resembling blood blisters on mucous membranes, including the lips and GI tract. The frequency of bleeding caused by breakdown of these lesions increases with age, and GI lesions commonly cause significant chronic bleeding, often resulting in iron deficiency.

The sudden onset of palpable purpura (i.e., localized, raised hemorrhages in the skin) associated with rash and fever may be caused by aseptic or septic vasculitis. Septic vasculitis can be caused by meningococcemia and other bacterial infections and is often accompanied by thrombocytopenia and prolongation of clotting times. One cause of aseptic vasculitis in young children and adolescents is Henoch-Schönlein purpura, a vasculitis of the skin, GI tract, and kidneys that is usually accompanied by abdominal pain from bleeding into the bowel wall. This syndrome may occur after a viral prodrome and appears to be caused by an immunoglobulin A (IgA) hypersensitivity reaction, as evidenced by serum IgA immune complexes and renal histopathologic features resembling IgA nephropathy. For example, hypersensitivity to allopurinol can produce extensive cutaneous purpura.

The therapy for bleeding from vascular disorders is straightforward. Senile purpura and steroid-induced purpura do not usually require treatment. Scurvy is corrected by vitamin C supplementation. In congenital disorders, including Ehlers-Danlos syndrome, hereditary hemorrhagic telangiectasia, and pseudoxanthoma elasticum, patients should avoid medications (e.g., aspirin) that may aggravate their bleeding tendencies, and they should receive supportive therapy (e.g., iron supplementation, red blood cell transfusion). Systemic administration of estrogen to patients with hereditary hemorrhagic telangiectasia may help to decrease epistaxis by inducing squamous metaplasia of the nasal mucosa, which protects lesions from trauma.

Treatment of septic vasculitis focuses on appropriate antibiotic therapy. In the case of aseptic vasculitis, steroids and immunosuppressive agents are most effective. When vasculitis is severe enough to cause consumption of platelets and coagulation factors (see Disseminated Intravascular Coagulation), transfusions of platelets, cryoprecipitate, or fresh-frozen plasma (FFP) may be indicated.

🔴 BLEEDING CAUSED BY THROMBOCYTOPENIA

Thrombocytopenia (<150,000 platelets/μL) is one of the most common problems in hospitalized patients. The initial diagnostic approach to thrombocytopenia involves classifying whether the low platelet count is caused by decreased platelet production, increased platelet sequestration, or increased platelet destruction (Fig. 51-4).

Evaluation of the number and morphologic features of marrow megakaryocytes has been the traditional diagnostic test for differentiating decreased platelet production from peripheral sequestration (e.g., splenomegaly) or destruction (e.g., immune thrombocytopenic purpura [ITP]). The reticulated platelet count is used as a peripheral blood index of platelet kinetics in the evaluation of thrombocytopenia.

Decreased Marrow Production of Platelets

Decreased production of platelets in the bone marrow is characterized by decreased or absent megakaryocytes on the bone marrow aspirate and biopsy and a low percentage of circulating reticulated platelets. Suppression of normal megakaryocytopoiesis occurs after marrow damage and destruction of stem cells (such as occurs with cytotoxic chemotherapy); destruction of the normal marrow microenvironment and replacement of normal stem cells by invasive malignant disease, aplasia, infection (e.g., miliary tuberculosis), or myelofibrosis; specific but rare intrinsic defects of the megakaryocytic stem cells; and metabolic abnormalities affecting megakaryocyte maturation.

Drug- and Nutrition-Associated Thrombocytopenia

Thrombocytopenia may result from cytotoxic or immunosuppressive chemotherapy for malignant or autoimmune disease. The pathophysiology of decreased platelets is typically directly attributable to the toxicity of the drug or metabolite, or both. For example, myeloablative chemotherapy drugs inhibit stem cell proliferation, leading to megakaryocyte death in the bone marrow and reduced circulating mature platelets. Other commonly used drugs such as thiazide diuretics, alcohol, and estrogens may damage bone marrow megakaryocytes in a similar fashion.

Although the diagnosis of these disorders can be complex, it frequently is made by withdrawing the offending drug.

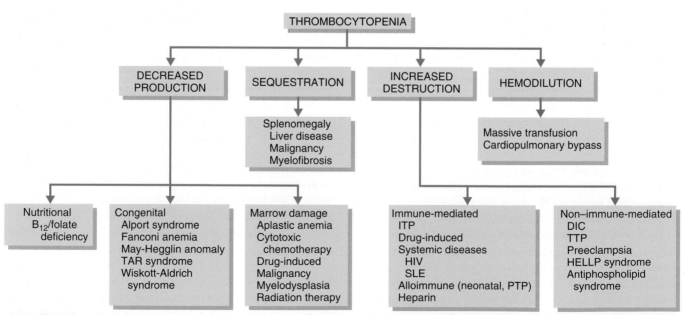

FIGURE 51-4 Differential diagnosis of thrombocytopenia. Disorders resulting in a decreased circulating platelet number can be classified by four main pathophysiologic mechanisms: hypoproduction, sequestration, peripheral destruction, and hemodilution. The history, physical examination, and bone marrow evaluation usually narrow the range of possible causes. DIC, Disseminated intravascular coagulation; HELLP, hemolysis, elevated liver enzymes, and low-platelet count in association with pregnancy; HIV, human immunodeficiency virus; ITP, immune thrombocytopenic purpura; PTP, post-transfusion purpura; SLE, systemic lupus erythematosus; TAR, thrombocytopenia-absent radius syndrome; TTP, thrombotic thrombocytopenic purpura.

Other helpful assays measure the reticulated platelet count and immature platelet fraction. In principle, RNA-rich immature platelet elements should be readily identifiable in peripheral blood. In the setting of thrombocytopenia, the normal compensatory response of a healthy bone marrow is to increase platelet production, and increased production correlates with increased numbers of immature platelets. However, in the setting of marrow-suppressive drug therapy, immature platelet counts are typically low, indicating hypoproliferative megakaryocytes. A decreased reticulated platelet fraction in the setting of a known offending drug can help to confirm the diagnosis.

Drug-associated thrombocytopenia is usually reversible, and platelet production rebounds as megakaryocytic stem cells eventually recover and regenerate after cessation of the toxic therapy. However, repeated or intensive chemotherapy (e.g., stem cell transplantation) may permanently damage the megakaryocytic stem cells and supporting stromal environment and cause chronic thrombocytopenia. This condition may be accompanied by leukopenia and anemia.

Similar to drug-related marrow suppression, nutritional disorders, especially alcoholism and abnormal folate or cobalamin (vitamin B_{12}) metabolism, are commonly associated with thrombocytopenia. Like destructive drug therapy, the lack of essential nutrients such as vitamin B_{12} or folate paralyzes normal megakaryocyte development, resulting in decreased mature platelet production. The diagnosis of a nutritional deficiency can be confirmed by testing vitamin B_{12} and folate levels in peripheral blood. Platelet counts should respond to abstinence from alcohol and to appropriate multivitamin replacement therapy for deficient nutrients.

Malignancy-Associated Thrombocytopenia

Platelet production is suppressed by intrinsic malignant diseases of the bone marrow (e.g., leukemia, multiple myeloma) and by malignant diseases that secondarily invade the bone marrow (e.g., non-Hodgkin's lymphoma, small cell lung cancer, breast and prostate cancers). The pathophysiology often is attributable to the toxic nature of the bone marrow milieu; normal megakaryocyte development is frequently suppressed by scores of abnormal bone marrow elements or invasive tumors.

The diagnosis of malignancy-associated thrombocytopenia is typically based on a bone marrow aspirate, which characteristically shows decreased megakaryocytes and occasionally shows malignant cells. Bone marrow biopsy has a much higher yield for diagnosing malignant involvement of the marrow. Flow cytometric evaluation for clonal B cells in the marrow aspirate is also highly sensitive for detecting monoclonal B-cell lymphoproliferative disease (e.g., non-Hodgkin's lymphoma). Definitive treatment of the thrombocytopenia relies on aggressively treating the underlying disease process.

Although not strictly an invasive cellular process, myelofibrosis (i.e., increase in reticulin fibers and sometimes collagen) of the marrow may lead to thrombocytopenia or pancytopenia. Myelofibrosis occurs most commonly in myeloproliferative disorders, mastocytosis, and mycobacterial and other infections involving the marrow. It is occasionally seen in patients with myelodysplasia or acute megakaryocytic leukemia and rarely occurs on a congenital basis (i.e., osteogenesis imperfecta).

Like pure malignancy-associated forms of decreased platelet production, myelofibrosis is diagnosed by bone marrow studies. Treating the underlying disorder is the best approach to addressing myelofibrotic thrombocytopenia.

Congenital Thrombocytopenia Syndromes

Thrombocytopenia in children can result from congenital defects of megakaryocyte production, as seen in thrombocytopenia–absent radii syndrome, congenital amegakaryocytic thrombocytopenia (i.e., mutation in the thrombopoietin receptor), and Fanconi's anemia (i.e., congenital aplastic anemia with renal hypoplasia and skin hyperpigmentation). Other disorders that are intrinsic to the bone marrow include the May-Hegglin anomaly and related myosin heavy chain 9 gene (*MYH9*) diseases, characterized by giant platelets and Döhle bodies (i.e., basophilic inclusions in leukocytes and platelets).

Thrombocytopenia with small platelets is characteristic of Wiskott-Aldrich syndrome, an X-linked disorder with eczema and immunodeficiency that can be diagnosed by the lack of CD43 expression on T lymphocytes. When accompanied by nerve deafness and nephritis, congenital hypoproductive thrombocytopenia is called *Alport's syndrome*.

The defects and detailed approaches to the diagnosis of decreased platelet production associated with the previously described conditions are outside the scope of this chapter. Nonetheless, the definitive treatment for many of the congenital thrombocytopenia problems is allogeneic stem cell transplantation, in which the abnormal, endogenous progenitor cell elements are eliminated and replaced by normal precursors capable of producing typical levels of functioning, mature platelets.

Platelet Sequestration

Up to 30% of circulating platelets are normally sequestered within the spleen at any time. Thrombocytopenia due to sequestration is common in advanced liver disease, myeloproliferative disorders accompanied by splenomegaly (e.g., chronic myelogenous leukemia, chronic idiopathic myelofibrosis), and malignant disease involving the spleen. In each of these conditions, increased trapping of platelets in the splenic system decreases platelet counts to between 50,000 and 100,000/μL, although rarely lower.

The diagnosis of platelet sequestration may be suspected by physical examination findings or imaging studies demonstrating splenomegaly. The reticulated platelet counts or immature platelet fractions may be normal or slightly elevated, and bone marrow studies typically reveal normal megakaryocyte numbers and morphology. Given the lack of specific tests for platelet sequestration, the diagnosis often is one of exclusion of other causes of hypoproliferative and destructive thrombocytopenia.

Treatment of thrombocytopenia due to splenomegaly frequently depends on the underlying cause for increased spleen size. Splenectomy may be indicated in some conditions such as myeloproliferative disease, but it is rarely used to treat thrombocytopenia resulting from portal hypertension. The decision to perform splenectomy for thrombocytopenia in patients with myeloproliferative syndromes must be individualized and weighed against the possibilities of surgical complications, loss of the spleen's extramedullary hematopoietic ability, and rebound thrombocytosis. Medications that help to control underlying disorders (e.g., chemotherapy for malignancy) or actions such as

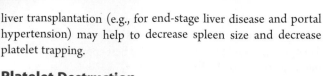

liver transplantation (e.g., for end-stage liver disease and portal hypertension) may help to decrease spleen size and decrease platelet trapping.

Platelet Destruction

One of the first major considerations in thrombocytopenia believed to be caused by platelet destruction is whether such destruction is due caused by immune mechanisms (e.g., antibody-mediated platelet clearance) or nonimmune mechanisms (e.g., microangiopathic processes). This division is important because the pathophysiology, diagnosis, and treatment of these two types of platelet destruction are widely divergent.

Immune-Mediated Platelet Destruction

Immune platelet destruction typically refers to antibody-mediated clearance. Platelet destruction can be further divided into autoimmune forms (i.e., antibody against self-antigens) and alloimmune forms (i.e., antibody against nonself-antigens). Autoimmune thrombocytopenia is the most commonly encountered form of immune-mediated platelet destruction. It may be a primary disorder directed only at platelets or a secondary complication of another autoimmune disease, such as systemic lupus erythematosus. Alloimmune-mediated platelet destruction is rare and is usually encountered only in neonates as a result of maternal antibodies formed against fetal platelet antigens or in chronically transfused individuals, who form alloantibodies against foreign platelet antigens.

In autoimmune and alloimmune thrombocytopenia, immune platelet destruction is caused by increased levels of polyclonal antiplatelet antibodies directed against platelet membrane glycoprotein receptors, most often cryptic neoepitopes of glycoprotein IIb/IIIa (GPIIb/IIIa) and less commonly glycoprotein Ib (GPIb) or human leukocyte antigens (HLAs). Coating of the platelet with these antibodies leads to opsonization of platelets by Fc receptors on cells of the reticuloendothelial system (RES). Antibody-coated platelets are cleared by the spleen and, to a lesser extent, by the liver.

These disorders involve a dramatic increase in marrow platelet production reflected by increased numbers of marrow megakaryocytes. The younger platelets produced have relatively high granule contents, providing increased hemostatic function. Bone marrow examination for increased or normal megakaryocyte numbers is the traditional means of distinguishing platelet destruction from decreased production. However, increased percentages of reticulated platelets are associated with destructive, especially immune-mediated, thrombocytopenia and may be sufficient for diagnosing platelet destruction.

Thrombocytopenia resulting from immune clearance may be severe, and platelet survival is often reduced from the normal 7 to 10 days to less than 1 day. Despite severe thrombocytopenia, serious bleeding or hemorrhagic death is uncommon, partly because the function of young platelets is increased and partly because the number of circulating platelets required to maintain vascular integrity is relatively low, estimated at 7100/μL per day.

Immune Thrombocytopenic Purpura

In children, acute ITP is often preceded by a viral infection such as varicella. Patients with ITP exhibit petechial hemorrhage and mucosal bleeding, and platelet counts are often lower than 20,000/μL. The blood smear shows large platelets but no other abnormal cells such as blasts, which accompany childhood leukemia. The bone marrow has increased or occasionally normal numbers of megakaryocytes. The diagnosis of ITP is partly made by exclusion. Fever, organomegaly, pancytopenia, lymphadenopathy, or abnormal peripheral blood cells should prompt an evaluation for malignant disease, such as leukemia, neuroblastoma, Wilms' tumor, or other bone marrow disorders.

Laboratory tests may complement the clinical evaluation but are not required to make the diagnosis of ITP. Tests may demonstrate an increased percentage of reticulated platelets in the peripheral blood or detect platelet autoantibodies in serum or on the platelet (i.e., platelet-associated immunoglobulin). Assays of platelet-associated antibodies, although sensitive, are not specific for ITP because levels of immunoglobulins that bind nonspecifically to platelets are often increased in patients with thrombocytopenia due to liver disease or human immunodeficiency virus (HIV) infection. Techniques that measure serum antibodies to specific platelet glycoproteins have greater specificity but are relatively insensitive. An increase in mean platelet volume is also a relatively insensitive indicator of destructive thrombocytopenia, in part because of the wide range of normal values. An increase in the reticulated platelet percentage is consistent with increased platelet destruction but cannot distinguish between ITP and other causes of platelet destruction such as heparin-induced thrombocytopenia (HIT) and thrombotic thrombocytopenic purpura (TTP) (see Chapter 54).

Acute ITP in children can resolve without therapy, but clinicians may prefer to treat children with steroids or intravenous immunoglobulin (IVIG), particularly in severe or complex cases. IVIG therapy for ITP is thought to work by three mechanisms. First, high immunoglobulin G (IgG) concentrations block Fc receptors on phagocytes of the RES and on cellular effectors of antibody-dependent cytotoxicity. Second, infusion of IgG increases the fractional rate of IgG catabolism and thereby increases the destruction of antiplatelet IgG in direct proportion to its concentration. Third, clearance of antiplatelet immunoglobulin may increase through anti-idiotypic effects (i.e., generating an immunologic response to the ITP antibodies).

More than 80% of children with acute ITP have a rapid remission, and ITP does not recur. A subset of 10% to 20% of children eventually develops recurrent thrombocytopenia (i.e., chronic ITP); however, more than 70% of them respond completely to splenectomy. For those with chronic courses after splenectomy, episodic IVIG, Rh immunoglobulin, and in severe cases, immunotherapy with rituximab (Rituxan) are used. Hemorrhagic deaths are rare in acute childhood ITP (<2%), but mortality rates of 2% to 5% are associated with chronic, refractory ITP.

The diagnosis of ITP in adults, as in children, is made largely by exclusion, but acute ITP in adults rarely remits spontaneously, and it evolves to chronic ITP in more than 50% of cases. Petechial hemorrhage and mucosal bleeding are accompanied by platelet counts commonly lower than 20,000/μL and often as low as 1000 to 2000/μL. Fewer than 10% of adults with ITP die of hemorrhage.

ITP in adults may be associated with diseases such as HIV or hepatitis C infection. ITP may be the initial manifestation of HIV infection, whereas thrombocytopenia in more advanced stages of HIV infection is often caused by bone marrow failure resulting from megakaryocyte infection with HIV, mycobacterial infection of the bone marrow, and nutritional deficiencies of end-stage HIV disease.

ITP occurs in patients with autoimmune disorders such as systemic lupus erythematosus, inflammatory bowel disease, and nonviral hepatitis. In some patients, ITP is accompanied by autoimmune hemolytic anemia, also called *Evans' syndrome.* The direct Coombs test is usually positive, indicating a warm-reactive autoantibody against erythrocytes. Initial treatment may not be significantly different from that for ITP alone, but chronic Evans' syndrome is thought to respond poorly to splenectomy, unlike ITP alone.

In the setting of systemic lupus erythematosus, ITP may result from factors associated with the autoimmune disease itself, including immune complex deposition on the platelet surface and active vasculitis, both of which may lead to increased platelet clearance and low counts. Therapy for ITP and the underlying autoimmune disorder is usually complementary. When the lupus anticoagulant or anticardiolipin antibody is associated with systemic lupus erythematosus and thrombocytopenia, the diagnosis of secondary antiphospholipid antibody syndrome is made, and this entity most commonly has thromboembolic complications (see Chapter 54).

The first-line treatment of acute ITP in adults is steroids, usually 1 to 2 mg/kg of prednisone per day. Studies have suggested that high-dose dexamethasone given in pulses every 14 or 28 days for six to eight doses may result in superior control of disease. Platelet transfusions typically are not used in ITP because transfused-platelet survival is brief and bleeding complications are uncommon. However, in patients with significant bleeding or who require surgery, platelet transfusions have been safely used and may transiently increase the platelet count, although usually for less than 24 hours.

In patients with acute ITP with severe thrombocytopenia (<5000/μL) or with life-threatening bleeding, high-dose methylprednisolone (1 g/day for 3 days) may be administered alone or in combination with IVIG (1-2 g/kg in divided doses over 2 to 5 days) and platelet transfusion. For recurrent ITP, chronic steroid treatment is often necessary but is usually accompanied by significant side effects. High-dose pulse dexamethasone given for 4 days every 2 weeks is associated with prolonged responses in about two thirds of patients with chronic ITP.

Children and adults with chronic ITP who initially respond to IVIG therapy usually respond well to splenectomy, whereas those who do not respond to IVIG are less likely to have disease remission after splenectomy. More than 50% of chronic ITP patients have some degree of disease remission after splenectomy. If ITP does recur after splenectomy, an accessory spleen must be ruled out, usually by liver and spleen scanning, because Howell-Jolly bodies may still be found.

Recurrent disease often is episodic, especially after viral infections, and these patients can be treated with IVIG. Alternatively, patients who are positive for the blood group Rh(D) antigen can be treated with Rh immunoglobulin (RhoGAM), a preparation of IgG class anti-Rh(D) antibodies. Anti-D induces red cell hemolysis (usually mild), presumably causing Fc receptor blockade of the RES and decreased platelet uptake by the spleen and liver.

Some patients with ITP, especially those with HIV infection, have significant, even fatal, hemoglobinemia or hemoglobinuria after anti-Rh(D) therapy, which should be carefully monitored. Rh immunoglobulin is usually ineffective in patients who have undergone splenectomy. In patients who fail to respond to splenectomy, steroid administration may be avoided by the addition of a combination of IVIG, vincristine, and anti-Rh(D) with danazol and immunosuppressive therapy (e.g., azathioprine).

Some patients with chronic ITP have responded to infusions of the anti-CD20 monoclonal antibody rituximab. Chronic ITP with normal marrow cellularity can respond to stimulation of thrombopoiesis using thrombopoietin mimetics and agonist antibodies, which have shown promise in experimental trials and clinical practice. However, because many patients with chronic ITP never achieve normal platelet counts, the goal for therapy is often to keep platelet counts higher than 30,000/μL to avoid significant bleeding. About 5% of adults with ITP die of chronic, refractory disease and the complications of its therapy.

Drug-Induced Platelet Destruction

Immune-mediated platelet destruction associated with specific drugs is an often overlooked cause of thrombocytopenia. Unlike some of the drugs mentioned earlier (e.g., chemotherapeutic agents) that act by directly suppressing megakaryocyte production, drugs in this category of thrombocytopenia induce an immune response against platelet antigens.

Drugs may induce an autoimmune response by several mechanisms. One is the development of an antibody response against soluble drug molecules. When soluble drugs bind to the platelet membrane, drug-induced antibodies act to destroy circulating platelets through the RES. Other mechanisms of drug-induced thrombocytopenia include formation of an immunogenic neoantigen through drug-platelet interactions (hapten response) with autoantibodies directed against drugs that cross-react with platelet antigens. Occasionally, immune complexes that include the drug and circulating platelets are formed.

Historically, quinidine or quinine-based formulations were among the first classes of drugs to be associated with platelet antibodies. The antibodies can be detected by tests using a drug coupled to a carrier protein. As awareness of drug-induced thrombocytopenia has grown, scores of drugs, including antibiotics, anticonvulsants, psychotropic drugs, and antiplatelet agents, have been reported to mediate platelet destruction (Table 51-2).

Heparin also induces thrombocytopenia, but unlike other drugs, this reaction paradoxically leads to a prothrombotic state. The mechanism of heparin-induced thrombocytopenia and its prothrombotic effects are discussed in greater detail in Chapter 54.

When eliciting the medical history from patients with acute-onset thrombocytopenia, a careful review of all medications, particularly those initiated just before the development of low platelet counts, may help to deduce the cause and reverse the platelet count decline. Regardless of the mechanism of induction, development of thrombocytopenia is temporally related to exposure to the drug and is usually rapid. Discontinuation of the offending drug usually results in an equally rapid rise in the platelet count. For some patients with prolonged thrombocytopenia after drug removal, immunosuppression with agents such as IVIG (2 g/kg in two to three divided doses) or steroids may restore baseline platelet counts.

Although confirmation of drug-induced thrombocytopenia can often be made by testing for antibodies with drug specificities, these tests are usually routinely performed only by specialty reference laboratories. When drug-induced thrombocytopenia is suspected, clinicians should not wait for specific antibody testing results before discontinuing potential offending agents.

Fetal and Neonatal Alloimmune Thrombocytopenia

Fetal and neonatal alloimmune thrombocytopenia (FNAIT) occurs when a mother is homozygous for an uncommon platelet alloantigen, most often human platelet antigen 1b (HPA-1b) on the platelet GPIIIa receptor, and a child expresses the HPA-1a haplotype inherited from the father. The pathogenesis of alloimmune thrombocytopenia is analogous to the mechanism by which Rh(D) sensitization induces hemolytic disease of the newborn. The mother is exposed to the HPA-1a antigen during a first pregnancy, and during that or subsequent pregnancies, she produces high-titer IgG antibody against HPA-1a. These antibodies cross the placenta, react with HPA-1a–positive fetal platelets, and cause peripheral-platelet destruction through the RES.

A diagnosis of FNAIT is frequently suspected when in utero fetal bleeding is observed by imaging studies or when an otherwise healthy newborn has unexpected bleeding associated with thrombocytopenia (typically with platelet counts of 50,000 to 75,000/µL or lower). A maternal history of FNAIT is a strong predictor of its occurrence during future pregnancies.

After a diagnosis of FNAIT is suspected, it may be confirmed by examining maternal sera for anti-HPA alloantibodies. Although bleeding may be severe in cases of FNAIT, the antibody does not necessarily predict whether bleeding will occur in utero, at delivery, or in the first days of life, and it is used primarily for confirmatory purposes.

Transfusion of washed maternal platelets (or random platelets lacking the HPA-1a antigen) and IVIG are useful for treating bleeding and restoring the platelet count. For newborns who recover from bleeding, there are few long-lasting deficits from FNAIT after circulating maternal antibodies are cleared from the circulation.

Post-transfusion Purpura

Alloimmune thrombocytopenia can occur in adults after transfusion (i.e., post-transfusion purpura [PTP]). As in neonates, this condition is based on exposure to a common platelet alloantigen that is not present on the patient's native platelets. For instance, PTP can occur after transfusion of a blood product in an individual who lacks HPA-1a and who has been previously alloimmunized to this antigen during a prior pregnancy or transfusion. Because more than 95% of blood donors express HPA-1a and the antigen is shed by platelets, any blood product can contain HPA-1a. Although not clearly understood, some investigators have speculated that soluble HPA antigens are deposited onto endogenous platelets, resulting in their rapid clearance by anti-HPA alloantibodies.

The diagnosis of PTP can be confirmed by demonstrating anti-HPA antibodies in the serum of an affected individual. Patients are typically treated with IVIG, and additional transfusions must be derived from donors lacking the implicated HPA. Although HPA-1a is the most common cause of alloimmune thrombocytopenia, other platelet alloantigens can cause this clinical syndrome (Table 51-3).

TABLE 51-2 COMMONLY USED DRUGS ASSOCIATED WITH IMMUNE THROMBOCYTOPENIA

DRUG CLASS	EXAMPLES
Antibiotics	Penicillins
	Cephalosporins (cephalothin, ceftazidime)
	Vancomycin
	Sulfonamides (sulfisoxazole)
	Rifampin
	Linezolid
	Quinine
Antiepileptics, antipsychotics, and sedative-hypnotics	Benzodiazepines (diazepam)
	Haloperidol
	Carbamazepine
	Lithium
	Phenytoin
Antihypertensives	Diuretics (chlorothiazide)
	Angiotensin-converting enzyme inhibitors (ramipril)
	Methyldopa
Analgesics and anti-inflammatories	Acetaminophen
	Ibuprofen
	Naproxen
Antiplatelet agents	Abciximab
	Tirofiban
Anticoagulants	Heparin
	Low-molecular-weight heparin

TABLE 51-3 MOLECULAR BASIS FOR ALLOIMMUNE THROMBOCYTOPENIA

GLYCOPROTEIN	ALLELES (ALLOANTIGENS)	PHENOTYPE/ FREQUENCY	AMINO ACID AND LOCATION
IIIa	HPA-1a/1b	0.98/0.25	Leucine/proline; 33
Ib	HPA-2a/2b	0.99/0.14	Threonine/methionine; 145
IIb	HPA-3a/3b	0.91/0.70	Isoleucine/serine; 843
IIIa	HPA-4a/4b	0.99/0.01	Arginine/glutamine; 143
Ia	HPA-5a/5b	0.99/0.21	Glutamic acid/lysine; 505
IIIa	HPA-6a/6b	NA	Proline/glutamic acid; 407
IIIa	HPA-7a/7b	NA	Proline/glutamic acid; 407
IIIa	HPA-8a/8b	NA	Arginine/cystine; 636

HPA, Human platelet antigen; NA, data not available.

Non–Immune-Mediated Platelet Destruction

Disseminated Intravascular Coagulation

One of the most common and potentially life-threatening causes of nonimmune platelet destruction is DIC, which is associated with sepsis, malignancy, advanced liver disease, and other disorders that trigger endotoxin release or cause severe tissue damage (Table 51-4). In DIC caused by bacterial sepsis, circulating endotoxin induces expression of tissue factor on circulating monocytes and endothelial cells, a process leading to overwhelming thrombin and fibrin generation. Deposition of fibrin occurs throughout the vasculature, with relatively inadequate concurrent fibrinolysis leading to a thrombotic or microangiopathic vasculopathy and subsequent organ damage. Thrombin activation of platelets and circulating factors eventually overwhelms the bone marrow and liver synthetic capability, respectively, resulting in thrombocytopenia and prolongation of the PT and aPTT.

Although the primary lesion of DIC is thrombin and clot generation, the clinical end point is usually a consumptive coagulopathy with depletion of platelets and coagulation factors. Mucosal bleeding, especially in the GI tract, and oozing from intravenous puncture sites are early signs of DIC.

Fibrinogen levels are usually low but may be normal in DIC because the acute phase reaction to sepsis or the underlying disorder may increase fibrinogen secretion. DIC should not be ruled out because fibrinogen is in the normal range. Fibrinolysis in DIC is triggered by fibrin clot formation and the action of tissue-type plasminogen activator. Laboratory testing shows increased levels of fibrin split products to more than 40 μg/mL (i.e., cleavage of fibrin monomers) and D-dimer to more than 0.5 mg/mL (i.e., cleavage of fibrin-fibrin bonds). Although levels of fibrin split products are usually elevated in patients with DIC, this finding is nonspecific. An elevated D-dimer level is more specific for DIC and is often used to confirm or replace the fibrin split product screening assay. The blood smear may also help in the diagnosis of DIC by showing significant numbers of schistocytes, but this result is not specific for DIC and is found in other microangiopathies such as TTP (see Chapter 54).

Chronic DIC may be triggered by consumption of platelets and factors in large clots associated with aneurysms, hemangiomas, and mural thrombi. Another cause of chronic DIC is malignant disease, often adenocarcinoma or acute promyelocytic leukemia. Malignant cells in these disorders promote thrombin formation through secretion of tissue factor, elaboration of cysteine proteases that activate factor X, induction of platelet-ligand binding, and upregulation of endothelial cell plasminogen activator inhibitor-1 (PAI-1) or cyclooxygenase 2 (COX2). Chronic DIC associated with malignancy usually causes enough factor consumption that the PT and aPTT are prolonged. Clinically, patients exhibit migratory thrombophlebitis (i.e., Trousseau's syndrome) or nonbacterial thrombotic (marantic) endocarditis.

Therapy for DIC should be aimed at (1) treatment of the underlying disorder, such as antibiotics for sepsis or chemotherapy for malignant disease; (2) supportive hemostatic therapy, including platelets, cryoprecipitate (for fibrinogen), and FFP; and (3) disruption of the activation of coagulation factors and platelets. For the last approach, anticoagulation is usually not indicated unless the balance of procoagulant with anticoagulant activity actively favors clotting, such as arterial thromboemboli with mural thrombus or migratory thrombophlebitis with Trousseau's syndrome. These thrombotic complications of chronic DIC are often resistant to warfarin therapy and usually require more intensive anti-Xa therapy with unfractionated or low-molecular-weight heparin. In DIC precipitated by sepsis, use of pharmacologic activated protein C has significantly decreased mortality.

Thrombocytopenia with Pregnancy-Induced Hypertension

Mild thrombocytopenia in pregnant women is related to hemodilution, a normal physiologic response of pregnancy that can bring platelet counts into the range of 100,000 to 150,000/μL; these counts are not associated with maternal or fetal complications. However, pregnancy-induced hypertension can result in platelet counts of less than 100,000/μL, and these conditions can be associated with complications.

The spectrum of pregnancy-induced hypertension includes hypertension progressing to proteinuria and renal dysfunction (i.e., preeclampsia) and to cerebral edema and seizures (i.e., eclampsia). Thrombocytopenia may appear as a late finding accompanying pregnancy-induced hypertension, often occurring at the time of delivery or late in the third trimester. The HELLP syndrome in pregnancy (characterized by *h*emolysis, *e*levated *l*iver enzymes, and *l*ow *p*latelet counts) is occasionally associated with hypertension. The thrombocytopenia associated with pregnancy-induced hypertension or HELLP may result from abnormal vascular prostaglandin metabolism or placental dysfunction that leads to platelet consumption, vasculopathy, and microvascular occlusions. Both disorders are usually reversed by delivery of the fetus and placenta. Occasionally, IVIG or plasmapheresis has been required when the disorder does not resolve after delivery.

Other conditions sometimes associated with pregnancy that mediate nonimmune platelet destruction include TTP, hemolytic-uremic syndrome (HUS), and antiphospholipid syndrome. However, these platelet-consumptive processes usually yield a thrombotic state rather than a bleeding tendency, despite the associated thrombocytopenia. These medical problems associated with thrombocytopenia are discussed in Chapter 54.

TABLE 51-4	CAUSES OF DISSEMINATED INTRAVASCULAR COAGULATION	
SEPSIS OR ENDOTOXIN	**PRIMARY VASCULAR DISORDERS**
Gram-negative bacteremia	
TISSUE DAMAGE	Vasculitis
	Giant hemangioma (Kasabach-Merritt syndrome)
Trauma	Aortic aneurysm
Closed-head injury	Cardiac mural thrombus
Burns	
Hypoperfusion or hypotension	**EXOGENOUS CAUSES**
MALIGNANT DISEASE	Snake venom
	Activated-factor infusions
Adenocarcinoma	(prothrombin-complex
Acute promyelocytic leukemia	concentrate)

Consumption and Dilutional Thrombocytopenia

In addition to sequestration, hypoproductive, and destructive causes of thrombocytopenia, low platelet counts occasionally result from consumption and hemodilution. The pathophysiology of thrombocytopenia in these cases is directly attributable to the underlying cause of the bleeding, frequently large-scale trauma.

Overwhelming hemorrhage causes the consumption of endogenous platelets in an attempt to curb bleeding, and platelets are consumed faster than they can be released by the spleen or generated in the bone marrow. Resuscitative efforts after trauma, including infusion of massive volumes of intravenous solutions, red blood cells, and FFP, result in the dilution of circulating platelet numbers. The combination of platelet consumption and dilution during trauma can have catastrophic consequences and historically has been a leading cause of death in this setting. In addition to identifying the source of a large bleed, aggressive platelet transfusions in the setting of trauma may provide the greatest benefit in overcoming the effects of consumption and dilution (discussed later).

⬤ BLEEDING CAUSED BY PLATELET FUNCTION DEFECTS

The ability of platelets to adhere to damaged vasculature and to recruit additional platelets into the clot is essential for primary hemostasis, especially when patients are challenged by trauma or surgery. Unlike bleeding caused by thrombocytopenia, individuals with platelet function defects bleed because their platelets cannot adhere or aggregate appropriately in response to in vivo stimuli.

These qualitative platelet disorders are most frequently encountered in individuals with normal or near-normal platelet counts. Evaluation often relies on tests that assess the function (rather than the number) of circulating platelets. From an epidemiologic standpoint, acquired qualitative platelet defects are much more frequently encountered than their congenital counterparts.

Acquired Causes of Platelet Dysfunction

Aspirin and Antiplatelet Therapy

The patient's history and preoperative screening should assess whether patients are taking medications that interfere with platelet function, such as aspirin. Aspirin irreversibly blocks normal arachidonic acid metabolism, and all exposed platelets are irreversibly affected and do not respond to stimulation even after aspirin is discontinued. The characteristic aspirin-induced platelet aggregation pattern is shown in Table 51-5 and Figure 51-5.

Nonsteroidal anti-inflammatory drugs (NSAIDs) (e.g., indomethacin) reversibly inhibit COX, and platelet function is restored within 24 to 48 hours after discontinuing the drug. Bleeding after most surgical procedures that is associated with aspirin or NSAIDs is usually mild, and aspirin may not need to be discontinued before surgery, especially because aspirin-induced platelet dysfunction is desirable in patients at risk for stroke or myocardial infarction.

The aspirin effect is restricted to COX1, and various NSAIDs have different relative affinities for COX1 and COX2. COX2 is an inducible enzyme that is synthesized in endothelial cells in response to inflammatory cytokines. Suppression of COX2 reduces synthesis of endothelial cell prostaglandin I_2 (i.e., prostacyclin), a molecule that exhibits antithrombotic effects through inhibition of platelet aggregation. The net effect of nonselective NSAIDs on the prothrombotic or antithrombotic balance favors bleeding because NSAID-induced COX1 inhibition means that thromboxane A_2 production in platelets is blocked. In contrast, the increased cardiovascular risk with administration of more selective COX2 inhibitors is probably attributable to the COX2-induced lack of endothelial cell prostacyclin production, coupled with intact platelet function (i.e., no inhibition of thromboxane A_2 by COX2 blockade). Recent data show that NSAIDs given before aspirin compete for COX1 binding sites and diminish aspirin's antiplatelet effect, another possible factor in the coagulant balance of concomitant use of NSAIDs and aspirin.

Another category of antiplatelet agents acts independently of the COX1/2 pathways. These drugs are P2Y12 receptor antagonists (e.g., clopidogrel; prasugrel). They disrupt function by irreversibly binding to the surface receptor for the platelet agonist, ADP. P2Y12 receptor antagonists are primarily used as adjunctive anticoagulant therapy for individuals at risk for thrombosis associated with coronary artery disease and stroke. If an individual taking a P2Y12 receptor antagonist experiences bleeding, these drugs can inhibit platelet activation at the site of injury, not unlike the effect in an individual taking aspirin.

Regardless of the type of agent used, discontinuing an antiplatelet drug is a reasonable first step for a patient who has moderate to severe bleeding while on the therapy. Discontinuation of the drug has no effect on anticoagulated platelets given for

	RESPONSE TO AGONIST				
DISORDER	*Epinephrine*	*ADP*	*Collagen*	*Arachidonic Acid*	*Ristocetin*
Aspirin and NSAIDs	PW	PW	NL, ↓*	↓	NL
Glanzmann disease	Absent	Absent	Absent	Absent	PW
Bernard-Soulier syndrome	NL	NL	NL	NL	Absent
Storage pool disease	↓	PW	↓	NL, ↓	PW
Hermansky-Pudlak syndrome	↓	PW	↓	NL	PW
Gray platelet syndrome	↓	↓	↓	NL	NL
von Willebrand disease	NL	NL	NL	NL	↓, NL†

TABLE 51-5 DISORDERS CAUSING ABNORMAL PLATELET AGGREGATION

ADP, Adenosine diphosphate; NL, normal; NSAIDs, nonsteroidal anti-inflammatory drugs; PW, primary wave aggregation only; ↓, decreased.
*Aspirin results in decreased aggregation with most collagen doses.
†In von Willebrand disease type 2B, patients have increased aggregation with low-dose ristocetin and decreased or normal aggregation with standard doses of ristocetin.

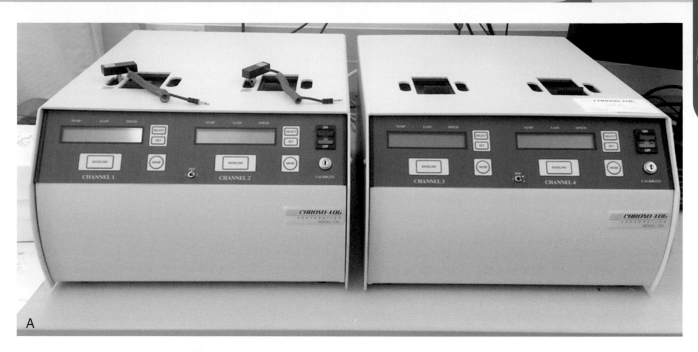

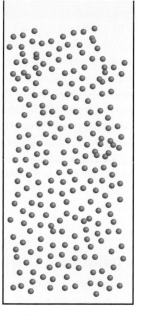

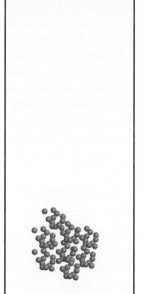

Platelet density yields little-to-no light transmission

Addition of platelet agonist

Platelet aggregate formation yields a large increase in light transmission

B   Platelet-rich plasma   Platelet aggregates

FIGURE 51-5 Methodology underlying light transmission aggregometry. **A,** Typical laboratory light transmission aggregometer. **B,** Platelet function is directly proportional to light transmission in this assay. Platelet-rich plasma, which prevents light transmission, is exposed to various agonists (i.e., adenosine diphosphate, epinephrine, collagen, arachidonic acid, and ristocetin). As platelets begin to aggregate or agglutinate, light transmission increases over time and is typically reflected as a primary or secondary wave of aggregation for most agonists. Low or no increase in light transmission typically correlates with diminished platelet function.

irreversible inhibitors, but this action should allow newly produced platelets to be free of drugs effects and to function appropriately at the site of an injury.

Beyond stopping the offending drug, bleeding caused by aspirin or other antiplatelet agents may be addressed by infusion of 1-deamino-(8-D-arginine)-vasopressin (DDAVP). This agent has been effective in decreasing the bleeding time of platelet anticoagulated patients. Occasionally, platelet transfusion is appropriate. In most cases, a single platelet transfusion of 4 to 6 random donor units (or one apheresis unit) contributes enough normal platelets (>10% of total circulating number) to restore primary hemostasis. Platelet dysfunction and bleeding caused by other drugs is similarly treated by discontinuing the drug and providing platelet transfusions when needed (Table 51-6).

Uremic Platelet Dysfunction

Renal insufficiency can be associated with the accumulation of toxic proteins such as guanidinosuccinic acid, which induces high levels of nitric oxide formation by vascular endothelial cells to inhibit platelet function. The uremic state can also suppress platelet secretory pathways and platelet adhesion to exposed endothelium through mechanisms that are not well understood.

TABLE 51-6 DRUGS AFFECTING PLATELET FUNCTION

STRONG INHIBITORS	
Abciximab (and other anti-GPIIb/ IIIa or anti-RGD compounds)	Dextran
	Fibrinolytics
Aspirin (often contained in over-the-counter medications)	Heparin
	Hetastarch
Clopidogrel, ticlopidine (ADP-receptor blockers)	**WEAK INHIBITORS**
Nonsteroidal anti-inflammatory drugs	Alcohol
	Nitroglycerin
MODERATE INHIBITORS	Nitroprusside
Antibiotics (penicillins, cephalosporins, nitrofurantoin)	

ADP, Adenosine diphosphate; GP, glycoprotein; RGD, arginine-glycine-aspartate.

Nonetheless, the uremic state does put an individual at risk for platelet dysfunction–related bleeding. Because no formal tests are available, the diagnosis should be suspected in individuals with acute or chronic renal failure who demonstrate platelet-like bleeding disorders.

Short-term treatment of uremic platelet dysfunction includes administration of DDAVP and cryoprecipitate. Both increase circulating von Willebrand antigens, which can help to overcome some of the uremia-associated platelet deficits. Conjugated estrogens are of some benefit for long-term treatment. Platelet transfusions may be marginally useful in patients with life-threatening bleeding and acute renal failure, but the effect of this treatment is short lived because the transfused platelets rapidly acquire the uremic defect. Platelet transfusion should not be considered as a first-line therapy for most forms of uremic bleeding.

Congenital Causes of Platelet Dysfunction

Platelet Glycoprotein Defects

Inherited qualitative platelet defects include abnormalities of platelet receptors and granules. Two rare but well-characterized platelet receptor disorders are Bernard-Soulier syndrome and Glanzmann's thrombasthenia.

Bernard-Soulier syndrome is caused by decreased surface expression of platelet GPIb (i.e., primary von Willebrand factor [vWF] receptor) and less commonly by diminished GPIb function. The syndrome is characterized by mild thrombocytopenia, increased bleeding time, large platelets, and mild to moderate bleeding symptoms. The diagnosis is usually made in children, but some may not show symptoms until adulthood. Laboratory testing for Bernard-Soulier syndrome shows an absent platelet aggregation response to ristocetin (see Table 51-5 and Fig. 51-5) despite adequate vWF levels and function, such as normal ristocetin cofactor (Rcof) activity.

Glanzmann's thrombasthenia is characterized by an increased bleeding time and abnormally low levels of expression of platelet GPIIb/IIIa (i.e., receptor for vWF and fibrinogen) or, less commonly, normal expression but absent GPIIb/IIIa function. Patients usually exhibit bleeding in childhood. In cases of Glanzmann's thrombasthenia, platelet aggregation testing confirms an absent or diminished response to all agonists except ristocetin (see Table 51-5 and Fig. 51-5).

Platelet transfusions correct the bleeding in Bernard-Soulier syndrome and Glanzmann's thrombasthenia. However, because of the high risk for alloimmunization with frequent platelet transfusions (i.e., patients lack GPIb or GPIIb/IIIa), this therapy should be used sparingly and only as clinically needed.

Platelet Granule or Secretory Defects

Inherited platelet granule disorders are defined by the type of granule that is absent or defective. Storage pool disease is characterized by a relative decrease or absence of dense granules and correspondingly moderate to severe mucosal bleeding. Release of dense granule constituents that recruit and activate platelets is impaired. Storage pool disease has a diminished or absent secondary wave of aggregation in response to most agonists (see Table 51-5 and Fig. 51-5).

Hermansky-Pudlak syndrome is a dense granule deficiency associated with oculocutaneous albinism and mild thrombocytopenia. Patients have significant bleeding, which may occur spontaneously but more often occurs with surgical procedures.

Chédiak-Higashi syndrome is a rare granule disorder characterized by mild bleeding, partial albinism, and recurrent pyogenic infections. Large, irregular, gray-blue inclusions are seen in neutrophils and monocytes.

Gray platelet syndrome is characterized by colorless or gray platelets that lack normal staining on the peripheral smear, and electron microscopy confirms the loss of α-granules or their contents. Patients with gray platelet syndrome have a history of mild bleeding, and aggregation testing detects diminished responses to epinephrine, ADP, and collagen.

All the platelet granule disorders are successfully treated by avoiding aspirin and other antiplatelet drugs and by hormonal control of menses in women. Platelet transfusions are used when bleeding occurs.

Platelet Transfusion Therapy

Standard Platelet Therapy

Platelet transfusions derived from the whole blood of healthy donors can be used to stop or prevent bleeding. The two broad categories of platelet transfusion support are based on the conditions previously discussed: prophylactic platelet transfusions for thrombocytopenia in nonbleeding patients and platelet transfusion for acute bleeding.

For the nonbleeding thrombocytopenic patient, several triggers can prompt platelet transfusion in the absence of frank hemorrhage. Patients receiving chemotherapy may be severely thrombocytopenic and should be transfused when their platelet counts are less than 10,000/μL to prevent spontaneous bleeding. This is a safe and appropriate threshold for patients with relatively uncomplicated clinical pictures without fever, sepsis, or GI bleeding. The threshold of 10,000/μL, which was rigorously established through several prospective, randomized, controlled trials, significantly decreases the frequency of platelet transfusion and thereby reduces risks associated with multiple blood product exposures. If the patient has complicating circumstances or is being treated on an outpatient basis, prophylactic transfusions may be given when platelet counts are lower than 20,000/µL, although this threshold is not rigorously based on clinical trial evidence.

For patients undergoing invasive procedures (e.g., surgery) or those with trauma, it is reasonable to transfuse platelets when counts are lower than 50,000/µL. Higher platelet counts are suggested for patients undergoing neurologic or ophthalmologic operations; platelet counts greater than 100,000/µL are recommended, if possible, because of the catastrophic nature of bleeding in these anatomic locations. The thresholds of 50,000 and 100,000/µL are based primarily on experience and nationally published guidelines, and clinical trials are lacking in these settings.

For the acutely bleeding patient, the decision to transfuse platelets depends on several factors, of which thrombocytopenia is the most straightforward and useful criterion. Platelet counts higher than 50,000/µL are a reasonable goal for most cases of acute bleeding, whereas counts higher than 100,000/µL may be necessary for neurologic bleeding.

Congenital or acquired platelet dysfunction must be considered for acutely bleeding patients. Those with significant bleeding who have taken an antiplatelet drug such as aspirin may benefit from platelet transfusion regardless of baseline counts. Another consideration is the volume of blood products and fluids received. Trauma patients may receive more than 10 units of transfused red blood cells in addition to plasma, volume expanders, and saline. Resuscitation with large fluid volumes (≥10 units transfused) reduces the platelet count to less than 50% of baseline, resulting in a significant dilutional coagulopathy. In these scenarios, repeated platelet counts must be obtained and platelets liberally transfused to maintain adequate hemostasis.

When the decision to transfuse platelets has been made, platelet units can be requested from the blood bank or transfusion service. Blood banks provide random-donor pooled platelets and apheresis platelets (E-Fig 51-1). Random-donor pooled platelets consist of platelet concentrates from four to six donors combined (pooled) into one large dose. For the adult patient with uncomplicated thrombocytopenia, a single random-donor platelet concentrate unit typically raises the platelet count by about 8000 to 10,000/µL. Between 4 and 6 units pooled together can be expected to raise counts by 30,000 to 60,000 platelets/µL. Apheresis platelets are collected from one donor using automated apheresis instruments. The dose of these *single-donor platelets* is almost equivalent to that of a 6-unit platelet pool and is estimated to increase platelet counts by up to 50,000/µL in the uncomplicated patient.

Based on the expected increments and typical transfusion goals outlined previously, one random-donor platelet pool or one apheresis platelet product should sufficiently raise platelet counts to correct thrombocytopenia and prevent spontaneous bleeding. These doses should also be sufficient to stop or prevent bleeding associated with thrombocytopenia in the setting of invasive procedures, mild to moderate trauma, or bleeding associated with platelet dysfunction. For the complicated patient (e.g., thrombocytopenia with intracranial hemorrhage, massive trauma), additional platelet doses may be necessary over time to achieve adequate hemostasis.

Platelet Transfusion Failure and Platelet Refractoriness

Platelet transfusions in thrombocytopenic patients are not successful in all cases. Uremia causes an acquired dysfunction of transfused platelets, limiting their hemostatic capabilities in vivo. Patients who are thrombocytopenic due to conditions such as ITP usually do not show increased platelet counts after transfusion because circulating autoantibodies cause rapid destruction of both endogenous and infused platelets. This phenomenon, known as *platelet transfusion refractoriness*, can be caused by many other recipient problems, including fever, sepsis, splenomegaly, and DIC. Although the pathophysiology of refractoriness is well understood for conditions such as ITP or DIC (in which platelets are cleared from the circulation), few data are available to suggest why individuals with conditions such as fever or infection have an inappropriate response to platelet transfusion.

When approaching a patient with platelet transfusion refractoriness, the physician should consider whether it is mediated by nonimmune or immune factors. Immune refractoriness indicates antibody-mediated clearance. For nonimmune-mediated refractoriness, as in the setting of fever or DIC, the underlying conditions usually decrease transfused platelet survival over time but do not affect immediate platelet recovery.

A standard diagnostic approach to platelet refractoriness involves measuring the platelet count 10 minutes to 1 hour after completion of the platelet transfusion. The patient with non–immune-mediated refractoriness typically shows an initial but blunted increase in the platelet count 1 hour after transfusion, with a subsequent decline at a steeper rate than expected because of the underlying disorder. For patients with this type of platelet refractoriness, addressing the underlying illness often increases the effectiveness of platelet transfusions.

For patients with immune-mediated platelet refractoriness, there is virtually no increase in the platelet count, even minutes after completion of a transfusion. The antiplatelet antibodies are most frequently encountered in individuals who have been chronically transfused. Repeated exposures to transfused products can induce alloantibodies, most commonly to HLA antigens. Over time and with multiple transfusion exposures, the titer of alloantibodies can increase sharply and cause rapid clearance of incompatible platelets after infusion.

For the alloimmunized patient, immunosuppression fails to decrease platelet alloantibodies, and efforts to improve platelet recovery after transfusion are focused on finding compatible platelet units. The first step in managing transfusion of the alloimmunized patient is to provide ABO antigen–matched platelets to minimize clearance caused by naturally occurring ABO antibodies; this is often helpful because platelets express A and B antigens on their surface. If this step fails to yield increases in platelet counts, donor platelets that lack target antigens for the detected alloantibodies should be pursued. One strategy is to use the patient's serum to crossmatch platelet donor units, with selection of those units demonstrating compatibility for subsequent transfusion.

If crossmatch-compatible platelets fail to induce adequate platelet recovery, blood banks should provide platelets that are matched to the recipient's HLA system in the hope of evading

HLA-based antibodies. HLA-matched platelets are collected from compatible donors using apheresis at frequent intervals until the patient's platelet count recovers, and they are no longer transfusion dependent. Many blood banks and transfusion services have attempted to address the problem of platelet HLA alloimmunization through prevention They provide blood products that have undergone filtration to reduce their white blood cell content, a process called *leukoreduction*. Because contaminating leukocytes are the primary sources of exposure to HLAs, their removal can be quite effective in preventing subsequent alloimmunization, even in chronically transfused patients.

BLEEDING CAUSED BY VON WILLEBRAND DISEASE

Disorders of the functional ligands for platelet adhesion to the vasculature cause bleeding that clinically resembles the bleeding associated with platelet or vascular disorders (e.g., epistaxis, GI bleeding). vWF is synthesized in endothelial cells and megakaryocytes and functions in plasma to mediate platelet adhesion to the damaged site (see Fig. 51-1). vWF is a large, multimeric protein; the largest multimers contain the greatest number of adhesive sites and confer greater hemostatic ability than smaller vWF molecules. In patients with low vWF levels, platelet adhesion to damaged vessels is delayed and results in mucosal bleeding and a prolonged bleeding time. vWF is also the carrier protein for factor VIII, and deficiency of vWF or abnormal vWF-VIII binding leads to rapid clearance of factor VIII, decreased factor VIII levels, and a prolonged aPTT.

vWD can manifest clinically with bleeding that resembles a platelet defect and a coagulation factor defect. The many mutations in the *VWF* gene have been phenotypically grouped into three major subtypes of vWD (E-Table 51-1).

Type 1 von Willebrand Disease

Most patients have type 1 vWD, a mild to moderate quantitative decrease in all vWF multimers. This condition is commonly caused by a heterozygous mutation and has a dominant pattern of inheritance. Type 1 vWD is characterized by equivalent decreases in factor VIII, vWF antigen, and Rcof activity. Rcof measures the ability of the patient's plasma (which contains vWF) to agglutinate normal platelets in the presence of ristocetin. Patients with type 1 vWD usually have mild to moderate bleeding, often only in relation to surgery or dental procedures.

Patients with type 1 vWD are treated with DDAVP, which stimulates endothelial cells to release stored vWF and leads to an increase in plasma vWF antigen, Rcof, and factor VIII levels. DDAVP, given subcutaneously at a dose of 0.3 µg/kg, usually yields excellent results. However, tachyphylaxis to DDAVP occurs because endothelial cells require time to synthesize new vWF after repeated DDAVP administration.

vWF concentrates must sometimes be used in patients with more severe type 1 vWD or in those who are undergoing a more prolonged hemostatic challenge. Bleeding in type 1 vWD during pregnancy is rare. Because the vWF level rises significantly in pregnancy, vWF antigen and Rcof levels usually normalize during the second or third trimester and eliminate the bleeding risk at that time. Most pregnant women with type 1 vWD have no bleeding complications with delivery and do not require therapy during pregnancy or in the early postpartum period.

Type 2 von Willebrand Disease

Type 2 vWD is characterized by heterozygous mutations of variable penetrance that produce a qualitative defect in the vWF molecule. The most common type 2 disorders have a relative lack of the larger vWF multimers (see E-Table 51-1). High-molecular-weight vWF multimers are absent in type 2A disease, and these patients show disproportionately low Rcof activity compared with the vWF antigen level.

The molecular defect is related to mutations in the A2 domain of vWF that render the molecule more susceptible to the vWF-cleaving protease (i.e., ADAMTS13). Patients with type 2A vWD respond to vWF concentrate and less commonly to DDAVP.

The abnormal vWF molecule in type 2B vWD has an increased affinity for platelets, which causes the loss of high-molecular-weight multimers from the circulation and often produces thrombocytopenia. Platelet aggregometry in type 2B vWD (see E-Table 51-1) shows an abnormal increase in low-dose ristocetin-induced platelet agglutination; in the laboratory, the addition of the patient's vWF to normal platelets similarly increases ristocetin-induced platelet agglutination and confirms the abnormal vWF. DDAVP induces release of the abnormal vWF in patients with type 2B vWD, causing thrombocytopenia and is therefore contraindicated. vWF concentrate should be used instead.

Type 2M vWD has laboratory findings similar to those in type 2A, but it has high-molecular-weight multimers. The defect in this rare type of vWF is most often a mutation in the vWF that reduces binding to its platelet ligand GPIbα. Some patients with type 2M vWD respond to DDAVP, but most require vWF concentrate.

In type 2N vWD, the abnormal vWF molecule has decreased binding affinity for factor VIII, which decreases factor VIII survival and produces a bleeding phenotype similar to hemophilia A. The low factor VIII levels do not respond to high-purity factor VIII infusions, unlike true hemophilia A, but they improve with vWF concentrate. Rcof and vWF antigen levels are normal in type 2N vWD because the mutation in the factor VIII binding site does not affect vWF function or survival. The diagnosis of type 2N vWD should be considered in females who have hemophilia A. Tests for vWF binding to factor VIII are available in reference laboratories.

Type 3 von Willebrand Disease

The rare patient with type 3 vWD has a complete deficiency of vWF, often as a result of the inheritance of two abnormal vWF alleles (i.e., compound heterozygote). Patients with type 3 vWD have no or extremely low levels of Rcof and vWF antigen and factor VIII levels of 3% to 10% of normal, and they usually have severe bleeding that may mimic hemophilia. Type 3 vWD does not respond to DDAVP and requires vWF concentrates to treat bleeding.

Acquired von Willebrand Disease

The acquired form of vWD usually appears as a severe, type 2A–like defect without larger vWF multimers in a patient with no history of bleeding. Acquired vWD is caused by abnormal clearance of the larger vWF multimers and is associated with monoclonal gammopathies, lymphoproliferative disorders, myeloma, and other malignant and myeloproliferative diseases characterized by thrombocytosis. In these cases, acquired vWD has been successfully treated with IVIG and therapy for the underlying disease.

Another cause of abnormal vWF multimer clearance resulting in acquired vWD is critical aortic stenosis. It is corrected with successful surgical repair.

● BLEEDING CAUSED BY COAGULATION FACTOR DISORDERS

Normal platelet hemostasis initiates plugging of vascular lesions and maintains mucosal integrity. Because of abnormalities of coagulation factors, the initial platelet plug is not solidified by secondary hemostasis, and the effects are clot breakdown and bleeding. This bleeding is different from platelet-type bleeding. Coagulation factor deficiencies lead to bleeding in deep tissues and joints, and milder deficiencies result in bleeding in a delayed fashion after surgery.

Most patients with significant factor deficiencies have abnormal screening laboratory test results (E-Table 51-2; see Fig. 51-1), although patients with mild deficiencies can have bleeding and only borderline-abnormal coagulation factor values. Like other hemostasis abnormalities previously discussed, coagulation factor problems can be classified as congenital deficiencies and those acquired from medications or underlying medical conditions.

Congenital Factor Deficiencies
Hemophilia A and B

The X-linked deficiencies of factor VIII (i.e., hemophilia A) and factor IX (i.e., hemophilia B) are the most common factor deficiencies after vWD. Hemophilia A is about six times more common than hemophilia B.

About 50% or more of cases of severe hemophilia A arise as a result of an inversion of a major portion of the gene that results in complete loss of activity. Other mutations tend to result in milder disease. Most patients with hemophilia B have mutations that result in a functionally abnormal factor IX with no activity. The combined results of antigenic and functional assays can resolve whether a deficiency results from a loss of the protein or loss of its normal function.

Both hemophilia A and hemophilia B are categorized by their factor levels. Severe deficiency is characterized by less than 1% of factor VIII or IX, whereas patients with moderate and mild hemophilia have factor levels of 1% to 5% and more than 5%, respectively.

Symptoms and signs of severe hemophilia A and hemophilia B develop in childhood with bleeding into muscles, joints, and soft tissue. Because they are X-linked disorders, they are observed primarily in male patients; the mother of an affected male patient is a carrier, and 50% of maternal uncles have the disease. However, about 25% to 30% of cases of hemophilia result from new mutations and have no relevant family history. In rare instances, a female carrier with extremely skewed X-inactivation may have a mild bleeding disorder with factor levels lower than 30%.

Bleeding in severe hemophilia is often spontaneous and is common after any type of surgery or even mild trauma. Hemorrhage in this condition frequently manifests as hemarthrosis (i.e., bleeding into joints) or retroperitoneal bleeding, or both. Hematuria and mucosal or intracranial bleeding can also occur. Patients with moderate hemophilia have less spontaneous bleeding, but they are still at significant risk for hemorrhagic complications of surgery or trauma. Patients with mild hemophilia may be undiagnosed into adulthood and then only because of bleeding after major surgery.

The complications of hemophilia stem from chronic bleeding into joints and muscles, which leads to severe deformities, arthritis, muscle atrophy, and contractures. These complications require intensive physical therapy and orthopedic care, often culminating in joint replacement. Patients with hemophilia who received pooled-factor concentrates before the era of viral inactivation have complications related to transfusion-transmitted infections, including HIV and hepatitis B and C. Current therapy uses factor concentrates that are virally inactivated or recombinant.

Non–hemophilia A or B Congenital Factor Deficiencies

Inherited bleeding disorders caused by deficiencies of coagulation factors V, VII, X, and XI (see E-Table 51-2) are much less common than hemophilia A and B. Patients with factor V deficiency usually lack plasma factor V and platelet factor V and have joint and muscle bleeding similar to patients with hemophilia. Some patients who are plasma factor V deficient are asymptomatic until they are challenged with the stress of surgery or trauma, and these patients are thought to have normal platelet factor V levels. Rarely, patients inherit factor deficiencies in tandem, such as combined factors V and VIII deficiencies.

Patients with factor XI deficiency usually have a milder bleeding disorder (even with factor XI levels <5%) than patients with hemophilia A or B, whereas factor X deficiency is usually more severe. Factor XI deficiency is an autosomal recessive disorder seen with increased frequency among Ashkenazi Jews, often manifesting late in adulthood and in the clinical settings of increased fibrinolysis, such as after prostate surgery. Acquired factor X deficiency can occur in patients with amyloidosis, a condition in which the abnormal circulating light chains adsorb to and clear factor X, producing low levels and occasional bleeding.

Fibrinogen (factor I) functions as a bridging ligand for the platelet receptor GPIIb/IIIa in the platelet-platelet matrix at sites of vascular damage. Fibrinogen also functions in the final steps of the coagulation cascade to form the fibrin clot. Congenital hypofibrinogenemias and afibrinogenemias are rare. Patients with these disorders produce very low amounts of fibrinogen. Alternatively, some individuals produce an abnormally functioning fibrinogen, which is typically associated with genetic mutations affecting fibrin cross-linking and polymerization. These disorders are referred to as *congenital dysfibrinogenemias*.

Because of fibrinogen's dual role in promoting platelet and coagulation factor hemostasis, patients with congenital fibrinogen disorders can have moderate to severe bleeding problems from early in life. It is not uncommon for patients to have the mucosal membrane bleeding associated with platelet disorders and the deep tissue or joint bleeding classically associated with coagulation factor deficiencies.

The diagnosis of congenital afibrinogenemia or dysfibrinogenemia can be established by screening assays (see E-Table 51-2), laboratory assays to measure fibrinogen levels, and tests such as the thrombin time that are designed to measure fibrinogen function. Treatment depends on replacement of fibrinogen by infusion of cryoprecipitate or a fibrinogen concentrate (discussed later).

Acquired Coagulation Factor Disorders

Factor Inhibitors in Congenital Factor Deficiencies

About 25% of patients with hemophilia A develop alloantibodies to transfused factor VIII. An inhibitor acts functionally and can be measured in the laboratory as Bethesda units (BU); 1 BU is defined as the amount of inhibitor that neutralizes 50% of factor activity. High-level inhibitors (>10 BU) completely neutralize the activity of infused factor concentrates, negating their effectiveness in bleeding episodes.

Bleeding requires therapeutic regimens with factor VIII inhibitor bypass activity (FEIBA) or recombinant factor VIIa. For long-term treatment, suppression of an inhibitor is accomplished by a combination of IVIG, immunosuppressive therapy, plasmapheresis, and induction of immune tolerance using high-dose concentrate infusions. Patients with hemophilia B have a lower incidence of inhibitors (2% to 6%), but bleeding in the setting of these inhibitors is treated in a similar fashion with high-dose FEIBA or recombinant VIIa; similar strategies for long-term suppression of the antibody are typically employed.

Acquired Factor Inhibitors

Acquired inhibitors to factor VIII (and rarely to other coagulation factors) occasionally are found in patients (usually older) who do not have a history of bleeding. In contrast to the antibodies in patients with severe congenital hemophilia, acquired inhibitors are typically autoantibodies.

Acquired factor VIII inhibitor titers can be extremely high and are sometimes associated with pregnancy, autoimmune disorders, and malignant diseases, especially lymphoproliferative disorders. Association with these underlying disorders implies some form of immune dysregulation, but the mechanisms underlying acquired factor inhibitors remain poorly understood.

The diagnosis of an acquired inhibitor can be made by laboratory techniques similar to those detailed for patients with congenital hemophilia. For the treatment of bleeding, patients with acquired inhibitors to factor VIII are administered factor VIIa or FEIBA to promote hemostasis. Intensive immunosuppressive therapy with rituximab, an anti-CD20 agent, has become the mainstay of successful treatment and should be started as soon as possible to eradicate the inhibitor.

Vitamin K Deficiency

Bleeding in inpatients and outpatients who are severely ill may be caused by acquired coagulation factor deficiencies resulting from nutritional deficiencies. Foremost among these is vitamin K deficiency, which has several causes. Biliary tract disease can interfere with enterohepatic circulation, leading to decreased absorption of vitamin K. Drugs, especially antibiotics, can sterilize the gut and reduce bacterial sources of vitamin K or other drugs (e.g., cholestyramine) that directly block vitamin K absorption; this category also includes cephalosporins, which interfere with intrahepatic metabolism of fat-soluble vitamin K. Vitamin K deficiency also may reflect poor nutritional status due to malabsorption, chronic disease, or reduced oral intake in patients who are acutely ill.

Factors II, VII, IX, and X are vitamin K–dependent procoagulant factors, as are the natural anticoagulants proteins C and S. In addition to disease-associated vitamin K deficiency, the anticoagulant warfarin blocks vitamin K–dependent γ-carboxylation of factors II, VII, IX, and X and causes an acute decrease in functional factor VII levels because factor VII has the shortest half-life (6 hours) of all vitamin K–dependent factors in vivo. Individuals who experience bleeding while on warfarin may be treated by repletion of vitamin K.

Dilutional Coagulopathy

As with platelets, coagulation factors can be depleted through the dilutional effects of a pure red blood cell transfusion or with the administration of massive amounts of volume expanders or saline solutions. For every 10 units of red cells acutely transfused, there is a concomitant increase in the international normalized ratio (INR) to greater than 2. This also occurs in conjunction with depletion and consumption of circulating coagulation factors due to acute bleeding.

In the setting of trauma, it is important to maintain adequate coagulation factor activity through plasma transfusion. Evidence from the trauma literature suggests that transfusion ratios of red cells to plasma should approach 1 : 1 to optimize hemostasis. The effects of dilutional coagulopathy should be monitored by repeated testing of PT and aPTT with a liberal plasma transfusion strategy.

Liver Disease

Unlike patients with vitamin K deficiency or those receiving warfarin, patients with liver disease have low levels of most factors, not just the vitamin K–dependent factors; the exception is factor VIII. Although liver transplantation increases factor VIII levels in patients with hemophilia, factor VIII levels are usually normal or increased with liver disease, a finding corresponding to RES and megakaryocytic sources of factor VIII production. If factor VIII levels are decreased in patients with liver disease, consideration should be given to superimposed DIC.

When a prolonged PT is evaluated for its cause, measurement of factor VII and a non–vitamin K–dependent factor, such as factor V, is useful. In vitamin K deficiency, the level of factor VII is low, and that of factor V is normal; levels of both factors are low in patients with generalized liver disease. The PT is a sensitive measure of liver function and becomes prolonged in patients with even mild liver disorders; elevation precedes a significant decrease in the albumin or prealbumin levels and is usually coincident with transaminase changes. In patients with mild to moderate liver disease, the PT is prolonged, but the aPTT usually remains within the normal range. In severe liver disease, the PT becomes even more prolonged, and the aPTT also becomes abnormal.

Other causes of bleeding in liver disease include decreased clearance of fibrin split products or associated DIC, inhibition of platelet function, and increased levels of tissue plasminogen activator. Treatment of bleeding associated with liver disease is based primarily on replacement of coagulation factors by plasma transfusions, although they only temporarily correct abnormalities. Liver transplantation is the only definitive treatment for these synthetic defects.

Fibrinogen Loss or Acquired Defects

Low fibrinogen levels are most commonly seen with consumptive disorders such as DIC, the pathophysiology of which was described earlier. Dysfibrinogenemia, which is occasionally a congenital disorder, is much more often acquired with liver disease. In this setting, diseased hepatocytes produce abnormal fibrinogen molecules arising from defects in post-translational modifications. The abnormal fibrinogen molecules cannot undergo normal cross-linking or polymerization, resulting in bleeding disorders.

The PT and aPTT are prolonged by abnormalities of fibrinogen quantity or function (see E-Table 51-2). A prolonged thrombin time is diagnostically more specific for a low fibrinogen level or abnormal molecule, although inhibitors such as heparin and fibrin split products also prolong the thrombin time. The reptilase time, which is insensitive to heparin, can be used to eliminate the possibility of an increased thrombin time resulting from heparin contamination of the sample and can help to confirm a diagnosis of dysfibrinogenemia.

⬤ BLEEDING IN PATIENTS WITH NORMAL LABORATORY VALUES

Some patients with factor- or platelet-dependent bleeding disorders do not exhibit any abnormalities in screening laboratory assays (e.g., PT, aPTT). Vascular purpuras and other bleeding variants follow this pattern. Patients with bleeding caused by mild vWD may have a normal aPTT, but additional studies usually show mild decreases in factor VIII, vWF antigen, or vWF Rcof. Multimeric analysis may demonstrate abnormal levels in patients with mild type 2A vWD. Similarly, mild deficiencies of factor II, V, VII, VIII, IX, or XI may not prolong the PT or aPTT, but specific-factor assays demonstrate levels lower than the normal range.

Mild bleeding, often with a delayed onset after surgery or trauma, may occur in patients with clot instability resulting from factor XIII deficiency or dysfibrinogenemia. In neonates, factor XIII deficiency manifests with late umbilical stump bleeding. Factor XIII deficiency is diagnosed in the laboratory by screening for increased clot solubility in urea; if the clot dissolves abnormally quickly in 8 mol/L of urea, an enzyme-linked immunosorbent assay for the precise XIII level should be performed. Factor XIII deficiency is treated with cryoprecipitate transfusion or an approved factor XIII concentrate. Because of the long half-life of factor XIII, prophylactic therapy for severe deficiency need be provided only in single doses on a 3- to 4-week recurring schedule.

Plasma and Coagulation Factor Transfusion Therapy

For patients with one or multiple defects in coagulation proteins, there are several options for replacement therapy. The most widely used product for replacement of coagulation factors is FFP (E-Fig 51-2). It is collected from the whole blood of healthy donors and is frozen within 8 hours of collection. It contains normal (i.e., therapeutic) levels of all coagulation factors necessary to maintain hemostasis. FFP is the best choice for replacement of coagulation factors for many conditions, including liver failure and deficiencies of factors II, V, X, and XI.

FFP is commonly used with vitamin K therapy for the reversal of warfarin therapy before invasive procedures or with the onset of bleeding. The appropriate dose of FFP is weight based and does not depend on the extent of prolongation in coagulation studies alone. Administration of FFP at 10 to 15 mL/kg should be sufficient to replace deficient coagulation factors and correct abnormal coagulation values. Assuming a volume of about 200 mL per unit of FFP, a reasonable dose for a 70-kg individual is 3 to 4 units of FFP. Administration is time sensitive because coagulation factors degrade at standard half-lives on infusion, and FFP should be provided immediately before an intended procedure to ensure adequate hemostasis.

In some cases, patients may not be able to tolerate the infusion of the large volumes of FFP required to reverse coagulopathic states, and other treatment modalities are available. Prothrombin complex concentrate (PCC) quickly reverses prolonged PTs without the need for large volumes of FFP. PCC is a concentrated, lyophilized, human-derived concentrate containing factors II, VII, IX, and X that can be reconstituted in small volumes and provided by intravenous bolus injection. A true four-factor PCC was approved for clinical use in 2013 by the U.S. Food and Drug Administration (FDA). A variant, human-derived PCC, FEIBA, contains factors II, IX, and X and factor VII that has been modified to be in its active form; FVIIa is the major difference between FEIBA and standard PCC. FEIBA is typically administered in doses of 50-100 U/kg every 8 to 12 hours.

PCC is a good alternative to FFP for bleeding in the setting of warfarin anticoagulation, and FEIBA is primarily used to overcome bleeding in the setting of a coagulation factor inhibitor. Vitamin K should also be considered as an alternative to plasma infusion. Oral or parenteral replacement of vitamin K (1 to 10 mg/day for 3 days) restores coagulation factor synthesis in patients with normal liver function and the vitamin deficiency.

For patients with hemophilia A or B, several virally inactivated, human-derived or recombinant factor VIII and IX concentrates are available. These products were developed because of the high morbidity and mortality rates caused by HIV and hepatitis virus contamination of the pooled products used during the 1980s.

For hemophilia, factor replacement is the key to effective therapy. Patients with severe hemophilia often infuse themselves with low doses of prophylactic factor on a regular basis (25 to 40 U/kg three times per week) and boost their dose or frequency of infusion when they sense internal bleeding, sustain trauma, or undergo dental procedures (E-Table 51-3). Patients with mild hemophilia A may not need factor infusions for minor surgery. Their disease often is managed with ε-aminocaproic acid, an antifibrinolytic agent, using 4 g every 4 to 6 hours with or without infusions (0.3 μg/kg) of DDAVP.

Most patients with hemophilia require factor infusions prophylactically or at times of surgery or trauma. Factor VIII products are infused every 8 to 12 hours, and 1 U/kg of factor VIII concentrate raises plasma factor VIII activity by 2%; 50 U/kg of factor VIII theoretically yields 100% factor VIII activity in a patient with severe hemophilia A. Factor IX has a longer half-life and is infused every 18 to 24 hours; factor IX requires 2 U/kg for a 2% increase in factor IX activity (i.e., 100 U/kg for 100% activity). Major surgery in patients with hemophilia requires intensive factor therapy to achieve normal factor levels (>80%) in the intraoperative period and the early postoperative period to prevent wound hematoma formation. The dose of factors (see E-Table 51-3) is adjusted downward from this intensity, depending on the severity of the insult, the patient's response to previous factor infusions, and whether factor inhibitors have developed.

Patients with severe hemophilia A or B can develop alloantibodies (inhibitors) directed against factor VIII or IX. Standard doses of factor do not reverse the coagulopathy because administered factors are rapidly cleared and bleeding persists. Several therapies have been developed to bypass the intrinsic pathway of coagulation, thereby eliminating the need for active factor VIII or IX in the coagulation cascade. FEIBA has been employed for this purpose at doses of 50 to 100 U/kg.

Another widely used bypass agent is activated factor VII (f VIIa), a recombinant factor protein. For a patient with hemophilia A or B and a strong factor inhibitor who has bleeding, f VIIa is usually administered at 90 μg/kg every 2 hours until the bleeding is controlled. This agent has been quite successful at controlling bleeding in hemophilia inhibitor populations, in patients with congenital factor VII deficiency, and those with acquired coagulation factor inhibitors. Based on its success in treating bleeding associated with hemophilia, trials of f VIIa have been performed for non–hemophilia-associated bleeding. Because of their limited success, the FDA has approved the use of f VIIa only in the setting of factor VII deficiency (15 to 30 μg/kg) or for treatment of bleeding associated with a factor inhibitor or Glanzmann's thrombasthenia.

Several virally inactivated, intermediate-purity factor VIII concentrate products (not recombinant or monoclonal antibody purified) are available. These factors usually contain large amounts of vWF (e.g., Humate-P) and are particularly useful for bleeding or prophylaxis in moderate to severe vWD, as effective replacement immediately before major invasive procedures, or in vWD patients who have failed or do not qualify for DDAVP therapy.

Cryoprecipitate Transfusion Therapy

Cryoprecipitated antihemophiliac factor (i.e., cryoprecipitate or cryo) is an often overlooked but important blood product for the treatment of a variety of bleeding disorders. Cryoprecipitate is prepared by thawing frozen plasma at very cold temperatures and removing the precipitated portion. It contains a narrow array of coagulation factors, but fibrinogen, fibronectin, factor VIII, vWF, and factor XIII occur in high concentrations. A major advantage

of cryoprecipitate is that the average single unit is only 10 to 20 mL (E-Fig 51-3).

Based on its contents and small volume, cryoprecipitate is useful for the replacement of fibrinogen in DIC or in patients with hypofibrinogenemia or dysfibrinogenemia. The product may be helpful for isolated factor XIII deficiency or factor XIII consumption in DIC. Mounting evidence suggests that the vWF and factor VIII in cryoprecipitate can be used to overcome bleeding in uremia by enhancing the adhesive properties of circulating platelets.

Cryoprecipitate is most frequently administered for hypofibrinogenemia, and appropriate dosing should take into account a patient's total plasma volume, baseline fibrinogen levels, and goal fibrinogen levels. For most bleeding associated with hypofibrinogenemia, a concentration of more than 100 mg/dL of fibrinogen is reasonable. For a 70-kg adult with a fibrinogen level less than 100 mg/dL, a 10-unit pool (total volume of about 150 to 200 mL) should be sufficient to provide adequate fibrinogen and enhance other hemostatic properties. For more advanced dosage protocols, such as for children, large patients, or those with extreme hypofibrinogenemia, consultation with the transfusion service is strongly recommended for specific calculations.

PROSPECTUS FOR THE FUTURE

Novel modalities continue to be developed for the diagnosis of patients with bleeding disorders. For instance, assays measuring thrombin generation offer a quantitative view of coagulation that may provide greater insight into the source of abnormal bleeding than current tests. Alternatives and improvements in transfusion are also being developed, including cells harvested from induced progenitor cells that can be customized for specific needs and fibrin-coated albumin particles that can evade immune-mediated platelet destruction while yielding important therapeutic impact. Progress continues to be made in the development and application of human-derived and recombinant coagulation factors for the treatment of hemophilia, with a focus on preparation of factors that are less immunogenic and therefore less prone to induce the development of significant inhibitors.

SUGGESTED READINGS

Altomare I, Wasser J, Pullarkat V: Bleeding and mortality outcomes in ITP clinical trials: a review of thrombopoietin mimetics data, Am J Hematol 87:984–987, 2012.

Branchford BR, Di Paola J: Making a diagnosis of VWD, Hematology Am Soc Hematol Educ Program 2012:161–167, 2012.

Favaloro EJ, Franchini M, Lippi G: Biological therapies for von Willebrand disease, Expert Opin Biol Ther 12:551–564, 2012.

Ferreira J, DeLosSantos M: The clinical use of prothrombin complex concentrate, J Emerg Med 44:1201–1210, 2013.

Hayward CP, Moffat KA, Liu Y: Laboratory investigations for bleeding disorders, Semin Thromb Hemost 38:742–752, 2012.

Hedges SJ, Dehoney SB, Hooper JS, et al: Evidence-based treatment recommendations for uremic bleeding, Nat Clin Pract Nephrol 3:138–153, 2007.

Hod E, Schwartz J: Platelet transfusion refractoriness, Br J Haematol 142:348–360, 2008.

Holbrook A, Schulman S, Witt DM, et al: Evidence-based management of anticoagulant therapy: antithrombotic therapy and prevention of thrombosis, ed 9, American College of Chest Physicians Evidence-Based Clinical Practice Guidelines, Chest 141(Suppl):e152S–e184S, 2012.

Kenney B, Stack G: Drug-induced thrombocytopenia, Arch Pathol Lab Med 133:309–314, 2009.

Levy JH, Greenberg C: Biology of factor XIII and clinical manifestations of factor XIII deficiency, Transfusion 53:1120–1131, 2013.

Peddinghaus ME, Tormey CA: Platelet-related bleeding: an update on diagnostic modalities and therapeutic options, Clin Lab Med 29:175–191, 2009.

Peterson JA, McFarland JG, Curtis BR, et al: Neonatal alloimmune thrombocytopenia: pathogenesis, diagnosis and management, Br J Haematol 161:3–14, 2013.

Peyvandi F, Bolton-Maggs PH, Batorova A, et al: Rare bleeding disorders, Haemophilia 18(Suppl 4):148–153, 2012.

Poon MC, Card R: Hemophilia management in transfusion medicine, Transfus Apher Sci 46:299–307, 2012.

Roback JD, Caldwell S, Carson J, et al: Evidence-based practice guidelines for plasma transfusion, Transfusion 50:1227–1239, 2010.

Rydz N, James PD: Why is my patient bleeding or bruising?, Hematol Oncol Clin North Am 26:321–344, viii, 2012.

Salles II, Feys HB, Iserbyt BF, et al: Inherited traits affecting platelet function, Blood Rev 22:155–172, 2008.

Sborov DW, Rodgers GM: How I manage patients with acquired haemophilia A, Br J Haematol 161:157–165, 2013.

Seligsohn U: Treatment of inherited platelet disorders, Haemophilia 18(Suppl 4):161–165, 2012.

Scott DW, Pratt KP, Miao CH: Progress toward inducing immunologic tolerance to factor VIII, Blood 121:4449–4456, 2013.

Slichter SJ: Platelet transfusion therapy, Hematol Oncol Clin North Am 21:697–729, 2007.

Stasi R: Immune thrombocytopenia: pathophysiologic and clinical update, Semin Thromb Hemost 38:454–462, 2012.

Theusinger OM, Madjdpour C, Spahn DR: Resuscitation and transfusion management in trauma patients: emerging concepts, Curr Opin Crit Care 18:661–670, 2012.

Wada H, Matsumoto T, Hatada T: Diagnostic criteria and laboratory tests for disseminated intravascular coagulation, Expert Rev Hematol 5:643–652, 2012.

52

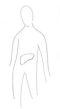

Disorders of Hemostasis: Thrombosis

Richard Torres and Henry M. Rinder

PATHOLOGY OF THROMBOSIS

The Virchow triad defines the pathologic mechanisms underlying thrombosis: diminished blood flow, damage to the vascular wall, and an imbalance favoring procoagulant over anticoagulant factors. The first two factors are clearly localized to specific vascular beds; although the last element of the triad may be systemic, data show at least partial regulation of the hemostatic balance by anatomic region. For example, congenital deficiency of AT, protein C, or protein S typically leads to venous thromboembolism (VTE) of the lower extremities. In contrast, the inherited hypercoagulable disorders associated with the factor V Leiden and prothrombin G20210A mutations not only produce lower extremity VTE but also are associated with thrombosis of the cerebral veins and sinuses.

This hemostatic regulation in vascular tissues is mediated by multiple factors that include (1) microenvironmental signals, such as shear stress resulting from turbulence in the disrupted flow of damaged vessels, that affect endothelial cell (EC) expression of thrombomodulin, tissue factor, and nitric oxide synthase as well as platelet activation; (2) EC subtype–specific signaling (e.g., shear stress upregulates aortic, but not pulmonary artery, nitric oxide synthase); (3) differences in EC transcriptional regulation of proteins such as von Willebrand factor (vWF) and its cleaving protease, ADAMTS-13; and (4) the increasingly appreciated important link between inflammation and thrombosis that is mediated in both physiologies by selectin and integrin ligands.

Atherothrombosis

This section briefly discusses hematologic factors that predispose to thrombosis in the setting of atherosclerotic plaque (atherothrombosis); the pathophysiologic mechanisms of atherogenesis are discussed in Chapter 8.

Atherothrombosis and Fibrinolysis

In addition to EC-directed regulation of hemostasis, the interaction of EC with the fibrinolytic system is important in the development of atherothrombotic disease because it affects the degree of clot propagation. The breakdown of stable fibrin polymers into fibrin split products, including the D-dimer segments that are routinely measured in the laboratory to detect recent thrombosis, is mediated by plasmin. Plasmin is converted from its inactive form, plasminogen, by tissue-type plasminogen activator (t-PA), the activity of which is regulated by plasminogen activator inhibitor-1 (PAI-1). Abnormal levels of both t-PA and PAI-1 are epidemiologically associated with an increased risk for arterial thrombosis, but the degree to which absolute levels contribute to arterial thrombosis remains controversial. For this reason, the current clinical utility of t-PA and PAI-1 measurements is limited.

The fact that it is high t-PA levels (rather than high PAI-1 levels) that are associated with higher rates of atherothrombosis, specifically acute myocardial infarction and stroke, is a curious phenomenon. It may be a manifestation of upregulation of t-PA serving as a surrogate marker for high de novo PAI-1 levels, although a direct correlation of PAI-1 levels and overall arterial thrombosis rates remains weak. Notably, PAI-1 is markedly increased in generalized inflammation. The strong association between abnormal hemostasis and high PAI-1 levels in patients with the metabolic syndrome or vascular disease in type 2 diabetes may be related to inflammatory roles for PAI-1, emphasizing the importance of the thrombosis-inflammation interplay. Relatedly, the risk for acute myocardial infarction is elevated in the subset of patients with angina pectoris who have increased PAI-1 activity levels, and there is evidence for a direct contribution of PAI-1 levels to the risk of stent restenosis after angioplasty. From a genetic risk standpoint, the 4G isoform of PAI-1 (compared with the 5G form) results in higher levels of PAI-1 but only a small increase in relative risk for arterial thrombosis. By contrast, t-PA polymorphisms and plasminogen levels do not correlate with atherothrombotic risk.

Hyperhomocysteinemia in Arterial Disease

Increased levels of plasma homocysteine (HCY) are linked to atherothrombosis. The rare congenital syndromes (e.g., cystathionine β-synthase deficiency) that are characterized by homocysteinuria and hyperhomocysteinemia are associated with both VTE and premature atherosclerosis. Elevated HCY induces EC dysfunction and apoptosis, triggering normal coagulation pathways designed to respond to EC damage but without the corresponding upregulation of EC-dependent anticoagulant function (e.g., activated protein C [APC]). Even moderate elevations in HCY may thus contribute to coronary, peripheral, and cerebral arterial disease. Mildly elevated HCY levels are associated with the thermolabile form of the methylene tetrahydrofolate reductase (MTHFR) enzyme, which results from a polymorphism (C677T) in the coding region of the MTHFR binding site. This isoform occurs in 30% to 40% of the general population and introduces a higher set point for regulation of HCY concentration (the substrate for MTHFR), particularly when a relative folate deficiency exists. In fact, deficiency of any of the vitamin cofactors of HCY metabolism (folate, vitamin B_6, and vitamin B_{12}) may lead to mild hyperhomocysteinemia.

Reduction in HCY levels by supplementation with vitamin B_6, vitamin B_{12}, and folate is probably the most effective means of reducing modest HCY elevations, but such supplementation does not decrease atherothrombotic risk, regardless of the cause of hyperhomocysteinemia or the presence of the MTHFR polymorphism. Therefore, the origin of the connection between high HCY and thrombosis remains incomplete, and the search for associated factors that link HCY and hypercoagulability continues.

Role of Platelets in Atherothrombosis

Although EC-associated abnormalities clearly influence hemostasis, platelet activation and adhesion are also critical to the development of atherothrombosis, especially in patients with acute coronary syndrome or ischemic stroke. Antiplatelet therapies are the primary modalities for maintaining short- and long-term patency in arteries, especially after coronary revascularization. Antiplatelet therapy can be targeted against specific platelet functions, including cyclooxygenase-mediated formation of thromboxane A_2, interaction of adenosine diphosphate (ADP) with its platelet receptor, and binding of the glycoprotein IIb/IIIa complex (GPIIb/IIIa) to fibrinogen for aggregation (Table 52-1).

Aspirin has long been a mainstay in the treatment of myocardial infarction, angina, and stroke because of its irreversible inhibition of platelet cyclooxygenase, a process that blocks the release of thromboxane A_2. Aspirin effectively prevents platelet aggregation to weak physiologic agonists (see Table 51-5 in Chapter 51) over the lifetime of a platelet (7 to 10 days); however, aspirin poorly inhibits platelet stimulation by thrombin and other strong agonists such as collagen. Therefore, blockade of other platelet activation pathways is important for patients who are at risk for arterial thrombosis.

Some drugs used to treat stroke or coronary disease (i.e., clopidogrel and prasugrel) specifically block platelet P2RY12, the ADP receptor, from interaction with ADP in the clot milieu, thereby decreasing platelet recruitment by preventing locally released ADP from activating additional platelets. Clopidogrel is effective in combination with aspirin for preventing ischemic stroke and for blocking stent thrombosis after revascularization; however, a significant proportion (up to one third) of patients demonstrate functional platelet resistance to clopidogrel. Under such circumstances, clopidogrel is poorly metabolized to its active form because of the presence of polymorphisms in the cytochrome P-450 gene, *CYP2C19*, that cause loss of function.

The more potent inhibitor, prasugrel, is not affected by cytochrome P-450 genotypes, although nongenetic factors such as platelet turnover, absorption, and compliance also play important roles in response variability.

Antiplatelet therapy with aspirin and a P2RY12 inhibitor (clopidogrel, prasugrel, or ticagrelor) reduces the risk of stent thrombosis and subsequent cardiovascular events after percutaneous coronary intervention and should be administered for 12 months unless the patient is at high risk for bleeding. In acute coronary syndrome, prasugrel and ticagrelor further reduce cardiovascular ischemic events compared with clopidogrel, although they are associated with higher bleeding risk. This effect occurs because drug interactions and variant cytochrome genotypes do not significantly affect production of the active metabolites of prasugrel and ticagrelor; the result is greater and more rapid inhibition of P2RY12 receptor–mediated platelet aggregation in most patients.

A third avenue for blocking platelet activation targets GPIIb/IIIa, the primary platelet receptor for binding to fibrinogen and vWF. Abciximab, a modified monoclonal antibody, prevents GPIIb/IIIa from binding to fibrinogen and blocks platelet aggregation after angioplasty, stent placement, or pharmacologic thrombolysis. Abciximab has been shown to reduce the incidence of recurrent acute ischemic events after percutaneous coronary revascularization in patients with myocardial infarction or unstable angina, mainly by decreasing the incidence of platelet-mediated thrombosis within the infarct-related vessel during and after the procedure. Other GPIIb/IIIa blockers, including eptifibatide (Integrilin) and tirofiban (Aggrastat), interfere with the GPIIb/IIIa arginine-glycine-aspartate (RGD) binding sites; they are used acutely for parenteral administration in patients with acute coronary syndrome or to maintain coronary patency after percutaneous coronary intervention. Thrombocytopenia is an uncommon (<2%) complication of all the GPIIb/IIIa inhibitors; it is most likely related to exposure of neoepitopes on the receptor and immune-mediated platelet destruction. Clearance of the drug typically resolves the thrombocytopenia within 1 week. Platelet transfusion should be considered only if there is significant thrombocytopenic bleeding because of the association of this procedure with a high incidence of stent thrombosis after stent implantation.

Additional novel strategies for mediating platelet activity include inhibition of cyclic nucleotide phosphodiesterases (e.g., dipyridamole, cilostazol) and blockade of proteinase-activated receptor 1 (PAR-1). Phosphodiesterase inhibitors most likely have multiple mechanisms of action. They result in decreased signal transduction within platelets, which impairs their responsiveness. PAR-1 is one of two principal recognized targets for thrombin stimulation of platelets, the other being PAR-4. The potential benefit of adding phosphodiesterase or PAR-1 inhibitors to aspirin and/or clopidogrel (e.g., prevention of restenosis in atherothrombosis) is being evaluated.

Venous Thromboembolism: Inherited Risk Factors

The balance between thrombin formation and anticoagulant pathways has been extensively studied in patients with inherited deficiencies of naturally occurring anticoagulants (Table 52-2).

TABLE 52-1 ANTIPLATELET THERAPIES	
INHIBITORS OF CYCLOOXYGENASE	**PHOSPHODIESTERASE INHIBITORS**
Aspirin	Dipyridamole
Nonaspirin NSAIDs (not COX2 selective)	Prostacyclin
	GPIIB/IIIA BLOCKERS
P2RY12 ANTAGONISTS	Abciximab
Prasugrel	Integrilin
Ticagrelor	Tirofiban
Clopidogrel	

COX2, Cyclooxygenase 2; GPIIb/IIIa, glycoprotein IIb/IIIa complex; NSAIDs, nonsteroidal anti-inflammatory drugs.

TABLE 52-2 PREVALENCE AND THROMBOTIC RELATIVE RISK ASSOCIATIONS OF LABORATORY FINDINGS*

PREVALENCE IN GENERAL POPULATION	VENOUS RR	ARTERIAL RR
Hyperhomocysteinemia (25%)	1-2	1.16
Activated protein C resistance (5%)		
Heterozygous FVL	7	1
Homozygous FVL	20-80	
Prothrombin G20210A mutation (1-2%)		
Heterozygous	2-5	1
Homozygous	>5	1
Platelet GPIIb/IIIa HPA-lb homozygosity (2-3%)		4 (MI in men)
Protein C deficiency (0.2-0.5%)	7	1
Protein S deficiency (0.1%)	8.5	1
AT deficiency (0.02-0.05%)	8	1
Dysfibrinogenemia (rare)	~1	1.5

AT, Antithrombin; FVL, factor V Leiden; GPIIb/IIIa, glycoprotein IIb/IIIa complex; HPA-1b, human platelet antigen-1b; MI, myocardial infarction; RR, relative risk.

*Data on prevalence and relative risk vary widely, often with conflicting results. This information represents an interpretation of data collected from various sources, mainly meta-analyses.

These patients are predisposed to VTE, which includes deep vein thrombosis (DVT) and pulmonary embolism (PE).

Factor V Leiden

The most common inherited disorder leading to VTE is the FVL mutation. About 5% of individuals with European ancestry are heterozygous for FVL. The FVL mutation increases VTE risk by decreasing the susceptibility of factor Va to APC-mediated inactivation and by impairing the APC-cofactor activity of factor V in factor VIIIa inactivation, all of which lead to increased thrombin generation. APC resistance can be demonstrated by specialized clotting tests in which the addition of APC fails to inhibit thrombin generation. About one fourth of patients with their first VTE are heterozygous for FVL, and this percentage increases to almost 60% among those with recurrent VTE or a strong family history of VTE.

Heterozygous FVL conveys a seven-fold increased risk for VTE. However, at 50 years of age, only 25% of persons with heterozygous FVL have had VTE, compared with much higher percentages in other inherited thrombophilias. It is with concomitant *acquired* risk factors such as immobilization, pregnancy, or oral contraceptive use that the risk for VTE in persons with FVL becomes more significant. The prothrombin G20210A mutation demonstrates a synergistic effect with FVL, but the MTHFR mutation does not. Homozygous FVL individuals have a 20- to 80-fold increased risk for VTE. APC resistance *without* the FVL mutation occurs rarely. Factor V Cambridge, although much less common than FVL, has a similar mutation at an APC cleavage site (Arg306) and is associated with APC resistance and thrombosis. Other minor alleles of factor V, including the 6755 A/G (D2194G) R2 haplotype, may enhance APC resistance. When this haplotype is on a different chromosome than the FVL mutation, it diminishes normal factor V transcription and increases the ratio of FVL to normal factor V.

Prothrombin G20210A

Another mutation associated with inherited thrombophilia is the prothrombin G20210A mutation, which occurs in the 3'-untranslated region of the prothrombin gene. This mutation leads to higher than normal prothrombin levels and a two-fold increased risk for VTE. The heterozygous mutation is present in about 3% of European-derived populations but is identified in about 15% of patients with VTE. Patients homozygous for prothrombin G20210A are rare, but their relative risk for VTE is thought to be about 10-fold. Exactly how the prothrombin mutation affects thrombus development has not been fully defined, but changes in polyadenylation of the prothrombin messenger RNA (mRNA) during transcription appear to be involved. Diagnosis of the G20210A genotype is made by examination of the patient's DNA for this specific mutation; no screening or functional assays are available.

Inherited Deficiency of Natural Anticoagulants

Deficiencies in the natural anticoagulant proteins (AT, protein C, and protein S) are less common than FVL or prothrombin G20210A, but they are more likely to produce symptomatic VTE at an earlier age. Only about one half of the cases of VTE occurring in patients with these deficiencies are associated with acquired risk factors such as pregnancy, surgery, or immobilization. Deficiencies of AT, protein C, or protein S are detected by functional or antigenic assays because some mutations cause a quantitative decrease in the factor, whereas others produce a dysfunctional protein. Many gene mutations have been associated with these deficiencies, but none is predominant. Deficiencies of AT, protein C, and protein S in the aggregate account for fewer than 5% to 10% of all patients with VTE.

AT is a naturally occurring anticoagulant that complexes with endogenous heparan sulfates to inhibit both formed thrombin and factor Xa. Heterozygous AT deficiency leads to AT activity levels less than 70% of normal and a 20-fold increase in the risk for VTE; VTE usually occurs by the age of 25 years in 50% of such patients. More than 200 associated mutations are known. Homozygous mutations are very rare, likely because of lethality in utero. Rare homozygous mutations show mild impairment in heparin binding or thrombin inhibition.

Acquired causes of AT deficiency are more common. Because AT has a low molecular weight, it is lost in the proteinuria of nephrotic syndrome. Acquired AT deficiency (as well as protein C deficiency) may also be associated with severe hepatic veno-occlusive disease after stem cell transplantation; AT and protein C may be excessively consumed in the damaged hepatic microvasculature. Low levels of AT are also associated with poorer outcomes in severely ill patients. Successful treatment of symptomatic patients with heterozygous AT deficiency has included short-term replacement with fresh-frozen plasma or recombinant AT protein, usually coupled with unfractionated heparin (UFH) anticoagulation; long-term therapy for congenitally deficient patients has consisted primarily of warfarin.

The complex of thrombin and thrombomodulin on the EC surface activates protein C; APC coupled with its cofactor, protein S, cleaves and inactivates factors Va and VIIIa. These actions downregulate the prothrombinase and tenase complexes, respectively, to slow the rate of thrombin generation. Like AT deficiency, heterozygous protein C and protein S deficiencies are observed with venous, and occasionally arterial, thrombosis at in younger patients (median age at occurrence, 20 to 40 years).

The rare homozygous protein C deficiency manifests in the neonate as *purpura fulminans* with widespread VTE and skin necrosis. A similar clinical presentation has been reported in heterozygous protein C–deficient adults after institution of warfarin therapy without simultaneous heparinization; this is called *warfarin-induced skin necrosis*. About one third of these patients are deficient in protein C on a hereditary basis, whereas the rest appear to have acquired protein C deficiency, possibly associated with vitamin K deficiency. Warfarin is a vitamin K antagonist that inhibits production of vitamin K–dependent protein C synthesis; and because of its short half-life, protein C levels rapidly fall before a decline in the levels of the procoagulant factors II, IX, and X. This imbalance shortly after starting warfarin favors a procoagulant state and may result in widespread microvascular thrombosis. Therefore, patients with active VTE should be fully anticoagulated with UFH or low-molecular-weight heparin (LMWH) before concurrent warfarin therapy is begun. UFH/ LMWH should be continued until warfarin is therapeutic for at least 48 hours.

Inherited deficiency of protein S has similarly been implicated in warfarin-induced skin necrosis. Protein S deficiency is commonly acquired in acute illness. Protein S circulates in a free form and is bound by complement 4b (C4b)-binding protein; only free protein S is active as a cofactor for protein C. Because C4b-binding protein is an acute phase reactant, its increase with severe illness can decrease the level of free protein S. A similar effect is seen in normal pregnancy.

Short-term therapy for homozygous protein C deficiency or for doubly heterozygous protein C or S deficiency, especially in the setting of neonatal purpura fulminans, has included plasma or protein C concentrate with full-dose UFH anticoagulation. Functional and antigenic levels of AT, protein S, and protein C can be assessed to define whether functional deficiency is caused by a dysfunctional protein or by diminished synthesis. As with AT deficiency, initial heparin therapy followed by long-term treatment with warfarin has been successful in heterozygous protein C or S deficiency. As expected, both protein C and protein S levels are decreased during warfarin therapy; therefore, for adequate evaluation of protein C and S, the patient must not be taking warfarin when tested.

Venous Thrombosis: Acquired Risk Factors

Surgery and Medical Hospitalization

Medical and surgical illnesses convey increased thrombotic risk; these *acquired* risk factors are well accepted, even though the pathophysiologic features favoring thrombosis may be uncertain (Table 52-3). Stasis of blood flow is a clear risk factor for thrombus formation (e.g., VTE in immobilized inpatients). Other high-risk situations, including surgery (especially orthopedic) and trauma, are similarly associated with immobilization and stasis of lower extremity blood flow. When evidence of thrombosis is thoroughly sought, both surgery and trauma can be shown to be associated with extremely high (>50%) incidences of VTE. Fat embolism and tissue damage may also contribute to the risk for VTE with surgery and trauma, particularly in closed head injuries that result in massive tissue factor release. Prophylactic permanent or temporary inferior vena cava (IVC) filters are often

TABLE 52-3	ACQUIRED RISK FACTORS FOR THROMBOSIS
MEDICAL AND SURGICAL ILLNESSES	Immobilization Malignancy Myeloproliferative disorders with thrombocytosis Nephrotic syndrome Orthopedic procedures Pregnancy Trauma, fat embolism
Antiphospholipid antibody, lupus anticoagulant Artificial heart valves Atrial fibrillation (nonvalvular) Congestive heart failure Hemolytic anemias (autoimmune hemolysis, sickle cell, thrombotic thrombocytopenic purpura, paroxysmal nocturnal hemoglobinuria) Hyperlipidemia	**MEDICATIONS** Heparin-induced thrombocytopenia Oral contraceptives, hormone replacement therapy Prothrombin complex concentrates

placed in trauma patients to protect against PE, especially in high-risk patients for whom anticoagulation is contraindicated because of the increased risk for bleeding.

All hospitalized medical patients should be considered for venous thromboprophylaxis with LMWH. Bleeding risk attributes that argue against anticoagulation include thrombocytopenia, coagulopathy (with or without liver disease), and recent hemorrhage. Risk factors that most argue for prophylaxis include malignancy, prior VTE, immobilization, and thrombophilic conditions.

Pregnancy and Fetal Loss

Pregnancy is a hypercoagulable state associated with venous stasis; the risk for VTE during pregnancy and in the postpartum period for women with identified thrombophilia is about five-fold higher than it is for nonpregnant women. Pregnancy increases procoagulant proteins, including fibrinogen, vWF, and factors VII, VIII, and X, and decreases anticoagulants such as protein S and AT as well as fibrinolytic inhibitors such as PAI-1 and thrombin activator fibrinolysis inhibitor (TAFI). VTE can occur at any time during pregnancy or the puerperium. The risk of postpartum VTE is significantly higher in women with any of the following conditions: stillbirth, pre-term delivery, obstetric hemorrhage, caesarean procedure, medical comorbidities, or a prepregnancy body mass index greater than 30 kg/m^2.

Inherited maternal thrombophilia can compound the procoagulant state of pregnancy and predispose to both fetal loss and VTE in the mother. The principal inherited associated risk factors for fetal loss are FVL, the G20210A prothrombin mutation, AT deficiency, and protein C or protein S deficiency. The relative risk for fetal loss is markedly higher in those mothers with a history of prior VTE, although this particular risk appears to be restricted to the period after 9 weeks of gestation. In fact, inherited thrombophilia may be protective against fetal loss during the first 9 weeks, possibly by limiting oxygen toxicity to the early embryo. Therefore, recommended indications for evaluating the inherited thrombophilia risk in women seeking to become pregnant are a history of VTE or recurrent fetal loss after 9 weeks of gestation when no other specific cause (e.g., antiphospholipid syndrome) can be identified. Both AT deficiency and hyperhomocysteinemia have also been associated with placental abruption.

In the absence of an identified inherited thrombophilia or a diagnosis of antiphospholipid syndrome (discussed later), no role has been identified for prophylactic anticoagulant therapy with recurrent pregnancy loss.

Oral Contraceptives and Hormone Replacement

Oral contraceptive use conveys an increased risk for VTE, and a similar increased risk is seen early after institution of hormone replacement therapy in postmenopausal women. Concomitant heterozygosity for FVL synergistically increases the risk for VTE in women who take oral contraceptives or hormone replacement therapy. Cigarette use in women using oral contraceptives also increases the risk of thrombosis, possibly through increased platelet reactivity mediated by increased thromboxane synthesis. On the arterial side, epidemiologic evidence clearly points to smoking as the main cardiovascular risk factor. Paradoxically, most data suggest a protective role for hormone replacement therapy in cardiovascular disease. As discussed previously, acquired APC resistance and decreases in the levels of both free and functional protein S occur with oral contraceptive use.

Other Prothrombotic Disease States

As described earlier, thrombosis in nephrotic syndrome is associated with loss of AT through the kidneys. Hemolysis is a general prothrombotic state that appears to be mediated through blood cell destruction, perhaps through increased exposure to procoagulant membrane phospholipids; hemolysis with thromboembolic complications has been observed in patients who have artificial heart valves, sickle cell disease, and other hemolytic anemias, including Coombs-positive autoimmune hemolytic anemia. In the case of paroxysmal nocturnal hemoglobinuria (PNH), complement activation may directly mediate platelet activation, and therapy with the complement inhibitor eculizumab has significantly decreased the rate of thromboembolic disease in PNH.

Platelet activation and clearance appear to be the primary prothrombotic manifestations of heparin-induced thrombocytopenia (HIT) and thrombotic thrombocytopenic purpura (TTP). Although chronic disseminated intravascular coagulation (DIC) is classically associated with certain malignancies such as mucinous adenocarcinoma and promyelocytic leukemia, in that setting, known as Trousseau syndrome, there is an increased risk in malignancy for VTE that is not related to DIC. Indeed, VTE occurs in a wide spectrum of malignancies, including lung, breast, gastrointestinal, and any metastatic solid tumor. However, when idiopathic VTE occurs in a cancer-free individual, an intensive work-up to find an occult malignancy is not warranted and has not been shown to improve subsequent cancer-related morbidity or mortality. However, once a cancer diagnosis is established in patients with prior VTE, they are at increased risk for subsequent VTE events, especially if the FVL or G20210A prothrombin mutation is present. LMWH prophylaxis after malignancy-associated VTE achieves superior prevention compared to warfarin, possibly because of better maintenance of an anticoagulated state. In the special case of myeloproliferative disorders (e.g., essential thrombocythemia), abnormal platelet physiologic mechanisms causing hyperaggregability are often present and require platelet-specific inhibition (See Hypercoagulability and Platelet Disorders).

Antiphospholipid Antibody Syndrome

Another acquired prothrombotic disorder is the antiphospholipid antibody syndrome (APS). APS is a primary disorder, unlike the occasional association of lupus anticoagulant or antiphospholipid antibodies with other autoimmune diseases such as systemic lupus erythematosus (SLE). The etiologic connection with SLE has not been fully defined, but replacement of the host immune system after hematopoietic stem cell transplantation for refractory SLE has the potential to eradicate the lupus anticoagulant and thromboembolic risk. All of the manifestations of APS are related to hypercoagulability, including recurrent venous or arterial thrombosis, thrombocytopenia caused by microcirculatory platelet clearance, and recurrent fetal loss resulting from placental vascular insufficiency. Serologic markers of APS include *anticardiolipin antibodies, anti–β$_2$-glycoprotein I antibodies*, and *lupus anticoagulants*. The Sydney Consensus Criteria for Antiphospholipid Syndrome is the current standard for diagnosis of APS. Diagnosis requires both the clinical criterion of radiologically or pathologically confirmed thrombosis or thrombosis-related fetal loss and the laboratory criterion of positive tests on two or more occasions at least 12 weeks apart. Anticardiolipin and anti-glycoprotein antibodies are detected by enzyme-linked immunosorbent assay (ELISA), whereas lupus anticoagulants are defined by correction of prolonged phospholipid-dependent clotting tests (most commonly hexagonal phase partial thromboplastin time [PTT] or Russell viper venom clotting time), with addition of excess phospholipid. Therefore, *lupus anticoagulant* is a misnomer; its presence predisposes the patient to clotting rather than to bleeding, and the risk for thrombosis is highest when a lupus anticoagulant is detectable. Another misleading aspect of this nomenclature is that phospholipid-reactive antibodies are actually directed against phospholipid-binding proteins in plasma (e.g., β$_2$-glycoprotein I antibody, annexin V, prothrombin). Anti–β$_2$-glycoprotein I antibody is detected by immunoassay, and high titers of this marker are also correlated with thromboembolic risk.

In patients with recurrent pregnancy loss in the context of APS, LMWH during pregnancy can help reduce further miscarriages.

Hypercoagulability and Platelet Disorders

Essential thrombocythemia and polycythemia vera are clonal myeloproliferative disorders associated with mutations in the *JAK2* gene. They are wholly (essential thrombocythemia) or partially (polycythemia vera) characterized by thrombocytosis, and patients with these disorders are at increased risk for thrombosis. Platelet aggregometry in these disorders often shows abnormal responses, especially to epinephrine and ADP; however, the abnormal aggregation does not correspond to either bleeding or thrombosis risk. Patients with polycythemia vera in particular have a high incidence of thrombosis in the mesenteric, portal, and hepatic venous circulation.

Thrombotic complications, both arterial and venous, occur in essential thrombocythemia, even in young patients. The risk of arterial thrombosis in essential thrombocythemia (and probably also in primary myelofibrosis and polycythemia vera) is most increased by a history of previous thrombosis or the presence of the *JAK2* V617F mutation. Therefore, prophylaxis with low-dose aspirin is probably justified in patients with high-risk essential thrombocythemia and other myeloproliferative disorders.

Increased platelet turnover in thrombocytosis is also associated with thromboembolic complications, but this does not necessarily involve high platelet counts, as has been demonstrated by radioactive platelet survival studies and an increase in reticulated (young) platelets in thrombotic essential thrombocytopenia. Moreover, successful treatment of symptomatic patients with aspirin increases platelet survival by decreasing platelet clearance. Concomitant therapy to prevent thrombotic complications of thrombocytosis includes lowering the platelet count with hydroxyurea. Evidence suggests that patients with essential thrombocythemia who are at high risk for arterial thrombosis are most effectively treated with the combination of hydroxyurea and low-dose aspirin. Patients with reactive (secondary) thrombocytosis resulting from iron deficiency anemia, chronic infection, rheumatoid arthritis, or the postsplenectomy state do not generally have increased thrombotic risk and do not require aspirin prophylaxis.

Heparin-Induced Thrombocytopenia

HIT must be distinguished from other drug-induced forms of immune thrombocytopenia because of its potentially catastrophic *thrombotic* complications and its unique pathophysiologic features. Almost 25% of patients who are exposed to UFH develop antibodies (detected by ELISA) that recognize the complex of heparin and platelet factor 4 (PF4), the latter being released from activated platelets. When such patients receive heparin again, between 5% and 10% develop HIT, most with platelet counts between 50,000 and 100,000/μL. HIT rarely occurs in patients who have not been previously exposed to heparin (0.3% incidence).

Surgery is a specific risk factor for HIT; the incidence of HIT in surgical patients is about 2.6%, compared with 1.7% in medical patients. HIT antibodies occur with high frequency in patients undergoing either cardiac surgery with cardiopulmonary bypass or an orthopedic procedure such as hip replacement. The incidence of HIT in patients who have received only LMWH is far lower, only about one-tenth the rate seen with UFH. However, the mechanism of thrombocytopenia for both UFH and LMWH appears to be similar: Platelet Fc-receptor binding of the heparin-PF4 antibody complex causes signal transduction and platelet activation with enhanced thrombin generation on the platelet surface.

The diagnosis is predominantly clinical (e.g., using the 4Ts algorithm for scoring HIT—magnitude of thrombocytopenia, timing of platelet fall, thrombotic sequelae, and ruling out other causes of thrombocytopenia), but the rapid ELISA test will detect heparin-PF4 antibodies in serum. The main drawback of ELISA is that it does not indicate whether the antibody complex is a functional activator of platelets; therefore, it is sensitive but not specific for HIT. The serotonin release assay is the functional test for HIT; it detects platelet activation after exposure to serum antibody in the presence of a therapeutic heparin level. However, a low probability for HIT based on the 4Ts score can be used to exclude the HIT diagnosis.

The thrombin-based procoagulant response in HIT incorporates platelets into microcirculatory clots, leading to thrombocytopenia; about 30% of HIT patients have overt thromboembolic complications, which can be severe or life-threatening. Thromboembolic events can occur before, concurrent with, and after development of thrombocytopenia in HIT, with about equal frequency. Although thrombosis is more frequent in patients with both HIT and concomitant cardiovascular disease and in those receiving full-dose heparin, any heparin dose (even heparin flushes) can result in thrombosis in HIT. Arterial and venous thromboembolic disease can occur even weeks after heparin has been discontinued, an effect perhaps mediated by EC glycosaminoglycan binding to PF4, which serves as a target for circulating HIT antibodies.

Discontinuation of all heparin is critical; moreover, although the antibody may have been induced by treatment with UFH, more than 80% of these antibodies cross-react with LMWH. Therefore, the preferred therapy for short-term anticoagulation in patients with HIT is a direct thrombin inhibitor (DTI), such as argatroban or bivalirudin, which is not a target for the heparin-PF4 antibodies. Indeed, because the event rate for subsequent thrombosis, limb amputation, and death is increased in patients with HIT even if they do not have thrombosis at presentation, DTI therapy is mandated after discontinuation of heparin. The choice of DTI may be dictated by other clinical conditions; for example, renal insufficiency slows bivalirudin clearance, increasing the bleeding risk, whereas argatroban is cleared by hepatic metabolism. For patients who develop HIT after warfarin has already been started, in addition to substituting a DTI, one should administer vitamin K to correct protein C levels. Although it has not been approved by the U.S. Food and Drug Administration (FDA) for this clinical scenario, the Xa inhibitor fondaparinux has the advantages of once-daily subcutaneous administration without need for laboratory monitoring and of having no affect on the international normalized ratio (INR).

DTI therapy should be continued until the platelet count is higher than 100-150,000/μL. Warfarin can then be added, and the two therapies should overlap for at least 5 days and with the INR at a therapeutic level for at least 48 hours. Because DTIs prolong the INR, a therapeutic warfarin level after 5 days may result in a supratherapeutic INR (usually >4); gradual downward titration of the DTI as the INR increases is a logical management strategy. Once DTIs are stopped, it is essential to repeat the INR measurement after 4 to 6 hours to confirm that it remains within the therapeutic range.

If there is no thrombosis with HIT, the total duration of anticoagulation should be 4 weeks; if thrombosis is present, anticoagulation should be continued for 3 to 6 months. Warfarin should never be used primarily to treat HIT, and it should not be instituted without simultaneous DTI coverage because it may induce acquired protein C deficiency leading to venous limb gangrene. One hallmark of protein C depletion in HIT is a sudden rise in the INR (to >3.5) after a single warfarin dose; in that circumstance, warfarin should be discontinued and the patient repleted with vitamin K. Patients with a history of HIT who need surgery requiring cardiopulmonary bypass can be safely reexposed to brief systemic UFH if ELISA testing is negative for the antibody at least 100 days after the previous UFH exposure.

Thrombotic Thrombocytopenic Purpura

Another cause of thrombocytopenia resulting from platelet activation and clearance is TTP. In patients with congenital or familial TTP, mutations in the vWF-cleaving protease, ADAMTS-13 (a *d*isintegrin *a*nd *m*etalloproteinase with *t*hrombospondin type 1 motif, member 13), abrogate its activity. Patients with acquired TTP usually have an antibody that blocks the normal function of vWF-cleaving protease to less than 10% of normal. Ultralarge vWF multimers released by EC normally anchor to EC through P-selectin and form long strings that adhere and aggregate platelets in the microcirculation. ADAMTS-13 downregulates the size of these multimers by docking to the A1/A3 vWF domains and cleaving within the A2 site. Deficient cleaving protease function in TTP leads to an increase in the larger, highest-molecular-weight vWF multimers, which are most effective in anchoring and activating platelets. These, in turn, cause increased platelet adhesion and clearance *without* activating the coagulation cascade. Therefore, both the prothrombin time (PT) and the PTT are normal in TTP, unlike in DIC.

TTP after chemotherapy (mitomycin C) or in association with pregnancy, stem cell transplantation, lupus, or HIV infection appears to have a similar pathogenic mechanism of thrombosis. Thrombocytopenia (often severe) is accompanied by microangiopathy with schistocytes on smear and increased serum lactate dehydrogenase. Microvascular occlusions in multiple organs cause symptoms, especially in the kidney and brain. The classic pentad (fever, thrombocytopenia, microangiopathic hemolysis, neurologic symptoms, and renal insufficiency) is present in fewer than 25% of patients with TTP. The diagnosis is typically made based on the clinical assessment of thrombocytopenia and microangiopathic hemolytic anemia; assays for ADAMTS-13 activity and inhibitor do not have a rapid turnaround time in most laboratories.

Treatment of familial TTP is based on replenishment of cleaving protease activity with plasma transfusion; acquired TTP additionally requires removal of the antibody. The latter is accomplished by plasma exchange, whereby patient plasma is removed (plasmapheresis) and replaced with fresh-frozen plasma, which often had been made "cryo-poor" to reduce ultralarge vWF multimers in transfused plasma. Steroids and antiplatelet drugs (e.g., aspirin, dipyridamole) are often administered simultaneously, but any added benefit to plasma exchange remains unclear. Platelet transfusions are relatively contraindicated in TTP because of the risk of thrombosis, and they should not be given for thrombocytopenia in the absence of significant bleeding. When plasma exchange fails to remit acquired TTP or when early relapse occurs, immunosuppressive therapy with anti-CD20 may be successful. The mortality rate associated with severe TTP (defined as undetectable ADAMTS-13 activity) is still significant, almost 10% at 18 months after therapy with plasma exchange. Replacement of ADAMTS-13, which is present in fresh-frozen plasma and in cryoprecipitate, is a potential treatment.

The *hemolytic-uremic syndrome* (HUS) is part of the TTP spectrum of disease and also is associated with microvascular platelet thrombi. However, the hemolytic anemia and renal failure of HUS are not usually accompanied by neurologic impairment, and HUS usually does not produce the same degree of thrombocytopenia or microangiopathy as TTP. Moreover, fewer than 3% of HUS cases are associated with decreased vWF-cleaving protease activity. Unlike TTP, HUS is primarily diagnosed in children (and less commonly in adults) who have hemorrhagic colitis caused by Shiga-like, toxin-producing bacteria, especially the *Escherichia coli* O157:H7 serotype. Atypical HUS (i.e., without diarrhea or Shiga-like toxin) is rarely associated with other bacterial infections or with complement dysregulation due to mutations or polymorphisms in factors H, I, and B. These mutations increase platelet activation through complement (C3) deposition on the platelet surface. Atypical HUS cases are those that are clinically consistent with HUS but are not associated with toxin-producing bacteria. Some HUS cases, particularly atypical forms, may respond to plasmapheresis with plasma exchange along with maintenance hemodialysis until renal function recovers. Data increasingly suggest that anti-C5a complement therapy can help prevent the complement-mediated damage associated with this disease.

⬤ CLINICAL EVALUATION OF THROMBOSIS

The approach to patients with thromboembolism is defined by the clinical history, results of laboratory studies, and even physical findings. Events that trigger VTE disease include immobilization, orthopedic and other surgical procedures, use of oral contraceptives, and pregnancy. VTE that is recurrent (thrombophilia) may manifest at an early age or at unusual thrombotic sites (e.g., cerebral vessels) and may be accompanied by a family history of VTE suggesting an inherited disorder. Acquired VTE risk may be associated with systemic disorders such as hemolysis (e.g., PNH, autoimmune hemolytic anemia), collagen vascular disorders (e.g., lupus), or various malignant diseases (e.g., adenocarcinoma). In contrast, arterial thromboembolic disease is more commonly superimposed on ruptured atherosclerotic plaque (e.g., coronary artery disease) or on atheroembolic disorders (e.g., ischemic stroke, peripheral arterial disease). Arterial vascular disease is mainly associated with metabolic risk factors including hypertension, hypercholesterolemia, and diabetes. The clinical approach to thrombotic disease is tailored to the location of the disease (arterial versus venous and the specific vascular bed) and whether there are abnormalities of the vascular endothelium, platelets, or soluble coagulation factors that predispose the patient to thromboembolic risk.

Laboratory Diagnostics

Recurrent VTE is a strong indication for laboratory testing for causes of thrombophilia, especially in patients younger than 50 years of age, in those with unexplained VTE, and in those with a family history of VTE. Any risk factors that may predispose these individuals to recurrence must be defined, as well as any inherited disorders that may necessitate family counseling or avoidance of additional environmental risks. The current work-up for VTE thrombophilia includes the following: (1) APC resistance, (2) genotyping for prothrombin G20210A, (3) lupus anticoagulant assay and anticardiolipin and anti–β_2-glycoprotein I antibody serologies, (4) functional AT and protein C levels, and (5) free protein S (Table 52-4). Genotyping for the FVL mutation can substitute for APC resistance and also determines whether the

TABLE 52-4	LABORATORY EVALUATION OF VENOUS THROMBOSIS
Activated protein C resistance, factor V Leiden	Prothrombin G20210A mutation
Lupus anticoagulant	Antithrombin activity
Anticardiolipin, anti–β_2-glycoprotein I antibody serology	Protein C activity
	Free protein S level
Homocysteine level: fasting or after methionine load	

patient is heterozygous or homozygous, although it may miss rare variants of APC resistance.

The utility of laboratory testing in the setting of atherothrombosis and arterial thromboembolism is unclear. In the setting of a myeloproliferative disorder, the platelet count and platelet function (e.g., aggregation and closure times) can justify hydroxyurea and/or aspirin therapy. In patients with unusual or recurrent arterial disease, other assays can be justified, including testing for t-PA and PAI-1 levels and for dysfibrinogenemia (thrombin time and antigen : activity ratio), all of which should be performed in consultation with specialists in hemostasis.

THERAPY FOR VENOUS THROMBOEMBOLISM

Once VTE has been diagnosed, immediate therapy is required. In most patients, anticoagulation is accomplished on a short-term basis with heparin compounds and on a long-term basis with warfarin. Thrombolytic therapy is indicated for patients with extensive proximal venous clots or PE. IVC filters are used in patients with contraindications to anticoagulation, complications of anticoagulation (usually active bleeding), or failure of anticoagulation (recurrent PE). IVC filters clearly decrease the incidence of early PE, but their use is also associated with thrombosis at the insertion site and late complications of IVC thrombosis as well as a 10% to 20% incidence of postphlebitic syndrome. Temporary IVC filters are often used in trauma patients and appear to be most efficacious when they are placed for fewer than 7 to 10 days.

UFH is often the anticoagulation therapy of choice for inpatients because of its short half-life and reversibility, but LMWH is increasingly used for this indication. UFH is begun as a bolus intravenous infusion of 80 U/kg, followed by a continuous infusion of 18 U/kg/hour; UFH doses in excess of 30,000 U/day have been shown to be most efficacious at preventing recurrent VTE. UFH is monitored by the PTT, and the therapeutic PTT range determined by each hospital corresponds to anti-Xa levels of 0.3 to 0.7 U/mL. All hospitals have established protocols for adjustment of UFH infusion based on the patient's weight and PTT monitoring.

UFH should be continued for at least 4 days (longer in patients with extensive clots) and may be discontinued after the patient has been fully anticoagulated with warfarin (INR ≥2 for 2 consecutive days). Some patients receiving large doses of heparin (usually >40,000 U/day) do not develop a therapeutic PTT. This *heparin resistance* can be caused by a variety of mechanisms, including increased heparin-binding proteins, counteracting medications (e.g., protamine), and decreased AT. An *apparent* heparin resistance is often seen in patients with coexistent inflammatory disease with high plasma levels of factor

VIII and fibrinogen; direct monitoring of anti-Xa levels is indicated.

LMWH is an excellent alternative to UFH in the treatment of thromboembolism and acute coronary events. The small controlled-size elements of LMWH stimulate AT activity that is more restricted to factor Xa compared with UFH, which has effects on thrombin, factor IX, and factor XI, in addition to others. The practical advantages of LMWH over UFH include increased plasma half-life, more predictable dose response allowing for intermittent fixed dosing, a lower de novo incidence of HIT (10% to 20% of the rate for UFH), and significantly reduced monitoring requirements. LMWH levels are prolonged in renal failure and in those circumstances may need to be monitored and adjusted based on anti-Xa levels. Peak anti-Xa levels (0.5 to 1 U/mL for twice-daily dosing and 1 to 2 U/mL for once-daily dosing) typically occur between 3 and 5 hours after subcutaneous LMWH injection. As with UFH, switching from LMWH to warfarin for long-term management can be accomplished after therapeutic INR values have been present for at least 2 days.

Warfarin and LMWH are used for long-term prophylaxis of VTE. Warfarin should be begun during the first 24 hours after presentation with VTE, concurrent with heparin treatment. The PT is prolonged within hours by warfarin because of a rapid decrease in factor VII levels; however, therapeutic warfarin anticoagulation does not occur until other vitamin K–dependent factors (II, IX, and X) also decrease. Therapeutic warfarin anticoagulation is usually achieved within 4 to 5 days with adequate warfarin dosing; UFH or LMWH may be discontinued after the INR has been greater than 2 for at least 2 consecutive days. One long-standing problem with warfarin anticoagulation is the interindividual variability in INR response; at least 50% of this variability in sensitivity to warfarin may be explained by polymorphisms in the *CYP2C9* and *VKORC1* genes. Although these have been incorporated into models for predicting safe and therapeutic warfarin dosing, most clinicians simply begin dosing and adjust therapy as needed based on periodic monitoring.

The therapeutic INR range depends on the condition predisposing the patient to thromboembolism. Prophylaxis after uncomplicated VTE in a patient without known risk factors requires an INR between 2 and 3; in contrast, warfarin prophylaxis for patients with APS and recurrent VTE may require INR values between 3 and 4 (Table 52-5).

The duration of warfarin or LMWH prophylaxis varies depending on the circumstances of the VTE, the risk for bleeding, and the potential for recurrence. In general, the longer the period of anticoagulation with warfarin, the less the chance of recurrence. Short-term warfarin (6 weeks) is less effective at preventing recurrence that longer courses (6 months). Patients with definite transient risk factors such as orthopedic surgery have low recurrence rates, even with short-term therapy; still, prolonged thromboprophylaxis (>21 days) after total hip replacement is more efficacious than shorter therapy (7 to 10 days). It is not clear that oral Xa inhibitors and dabigatran provide any benefit over LMWH for thromboprophylaxis after total hip or knee replacement (Table 52-6).

In contrast, patients with "unprovoked" VTE (i.e., outside the setting of trauma, surgery, immobilization, pregnancy, or cancer) have significant recurrence rates, even after 3 to 6 months of

TABLE 52-5 THERAPEUTIC INTERNATIONAL NORMALIZED RATIO (INR) RANGES FOR WARFARIN

PATIENT SUBGROUP	INR RANGE
VENOUS THROMBOSIS	
Treatment	2.0-3.0
Prophylaxis	1.5-2.5
ARTIFICIAL HEART VALVES	
Tissue	2.0-2.5
Mechanical	3.0-4.0
ATRIAL FIBRILLATION (NONVALVULAR)	
Prophylaxis	1.5-2.5
LUPUS ANTICOAGULANT	
Treatment, prophylaxis	2.0-3.0
Refractory thromboembolism	3.0-4.0

TABLE 52-6 NEW ORAL ANTICOAGULANTS (NOAC) AND THEIR INDICATIONS

NOAC	INDICATIONS
Dabigatran	Direct thrombin inhibitor for nonvalvular atrial fibrillation (to prevent stroke and non-CNS embolism)
Rivaroxaban	Anti-Xa for nonvalvular atrial fibrillation (to prevent stroke and non-CNS embolism); treatment of VTE and subsequent prophylaxis; and prophylaxis of VTE after hip or knee replacement
Apixaban	Anti-Xa for nonvalvular atrial fibrillation (to prevent stroke and non-CNS embolism)
Edoxaban	Anti-Xa for prevention of VTE in surgical patients; prevention of embolism in atrial fibrillation
Ticagrelor	Platelet P2RY12 inhibitor for prevention of thrombosis in acute coronary syndromes

CNS, Central nervous system; VTE, venous thromboembolism; Xa, activated factor X.

TABLE 52-7 GUIDELINES FOR DURATION OF PROPHYLACTIC ANTICOAGULATION AFTER VTE

CONDITION	DURATION OF THERAPY
Distal or superficial vein thrombus	3-12 wk
FIRST PROXIMAL VTE	
No risk factors	3-6 mo*
Correctable risk factor (e.g., surgery, trauma)	3-6 mo
Malignancy	Long-term[†]
Antiphospholipid syndrome	Long-term
Inherited risk factor[‡]	>6 mo
Recurrent VTE/PE	Lifelong

PE, Pulmonary embolism; VTE, venous thromboembolism (includes deep vein thrombosis, pulmonary embolism, and sinus or cerebral thrombosis).

*Evaluation of D-dimer after 3-6 mo may assist in the decision to stop prophylaxis.

[†]Long-term therapy must be adjusted individually according to presence of other diseases, risks for bleeding, presence of transient risk factors, and ease of compliance.

[‡]Inherited risk factors include factor V Leiden; prothrombin 20210A; deficiencies of antithrombin, protein C, or protein S.

TABLE 52-8 DRUGS THAT AFFECT WARFARIN LEVELS

INCREASED WARFARIN LEVELS: PROLONGED INR	DECREASED WARFARIN LEVELS: SUBTHERAPEUTIC INR
↓ Warfarin clearance	↑ Hepatic metabolism of warfarin
Disulfiram	Barbiturates
Metronidazole	Rifampin
Trimethoprim-sulfamethoxazole	↓ Warfarin absorption
↓ Warfarin-protein binding	Cholestyramine
Phenylbutazone	
↑ Vitamin K turnover	
Clofibrate	

↑, Increased; ↓, decreased; INR, international normalized ratio.

warfarin therapy. Because the risk for recurrence in patients with unprovoked proximal VTE or PE is relatively low when D-dimer levels are normal 3 weeks after cessation of anticoagulation, this measure may help providers decide whether anticoagulation past 3 to 6 months is necessary.

Evidence also indicates that inherited hypercoagulable disorders (e.g., FVL) probably confer a lifelong increased risk for VTE or PE. Some studies have shown that the bleeding risks incurred by long-term, low-intensity warfarin use are favorably balanced by the decreased incidence of recurrent thrombosis. Therefore, the presence of inherited thrombophilia may warrant continuation of warfarin therapy for a longer period, depending on the patient's other medical illnesses and whether transient circumstances may have predisposed the patient to VTE. Patients who develop recurrent VTE after discontinuation of warfarin should receive long-term anticoagulation regardless of whether they have a defined cause of thrombophilia. Patients with APS and a first episode of VTE are at very high risk for recurrent VTE (up to 50% per year) after anticoagulation is discontinued, clearly supporting the rationale of testing for antiphospholipid. Table 52-7 suggests broad guidelines for the duration of warfarin therapy in specific patient subgroups. Because warfarin is a teratogen, effective contraception should be used concurrently in women of childbearing age.

Supratherapeutic INR levels commonly occur with warfarin therapy, with or without bleeding. In patients with moderately elevated INR values (>5) and little or no bleeding, temporary discontinuation of warfarin and reinstitution of the drug at a lower maintenance dose may be sufficient. Patients with higher INR values (5 to 9) who are without serious bleeding should have warfarin withheld and should receive low doses (1 to 2.5 mg/day) of oral vitamin K to reach therapeutic INR levels; parenteral vitamin K may be given if gastrointestinal function is problematic. If serious active bleeding occurs with high INR values, especially if surgery is required to correct the bleeding, a combination of vitamin K and transfusion of plasma (see Chapter 51) will rapidly correct the INR. The INR can become elevated as a result of concurrent use of drugs that increase free warfarin levels (Table 52-8). Whenever bleeding occurs as a complication of anticoagulation, serious consideration must be given to future bleeding risks and to whether the patient requires placement of an IVC filter for prophylaxis.

Antithrombotic Therapy during Pregnancy

Heparins, both UFH and LMWH, are the safest therapy for venous thrombosis during pregnancy. Heparin does not cross the placenta, unlike warfarin, which causes a characteristic fetal embryopathy. Warfarin also causes fetal hemorrhage and placental abruption and should be avoided during pregnancy. VTE or PE during pregnancy should be treated with intravenous UFH for 5 to 10 days, followed by an adjusted-dose regimen of subcutaneous UFH, starting with 20,000 U every 12 hours and adjusted to achieve a PTT higher than 1.5 times baseline at 6 hours after injection. An attractive alternative to UFH during pregnancy is LMWH, which can be given subcutaneously once or twice daily and does not require monitoring. Suprarenal IVC filters have also been used successfully during pregnancy without significant morbidity. In women with APS who become pregnant, therapy is critical to prevent fetal loss; aspirin (160 mg) is combined with prophylactic doses of either subcutaneous UFH (10,000 to 15,000 U/day in divided doses) or LMWH (to achieve an anti-Xa level of 0.1 to 0.3 U/mL). When such women have a history of thromboembolic disease, therapeutic doses of LMWH or UFH plus aspirin are employed.

Heparin should be discontinued at the time of labor and delivery, although the risk for hemorrhage is not high during delivery, especially if anti-Xa levels are less than 0.7 U/mL. One concern with residual anticoagulation at delivery is the risk for spinal hematoma with epidural anesthesia; this concern has been reported with both UFH and LMWH. The anti-Xa level that is safe for an epidural procedure is not known. Protamine sulfate can be used to neutralize UFH if the PTT is prolonged during labor and delivery; however, LMWH is only partially (10%) reversed by protamine.

Anticoagulation during the postpartum period can be carried out with heparin or warfarin; neither drug is contraindicated during breast-feeding. Women receiving long-term warfarin therapy (e.g., for valvular heart disease) who wish to become pregnant need to be switched to a fully anticoagulating dose of UFH or LMWH; warfarin treatment may be restarted after delivery.

Perioperative Anticoagulation

A common clinical problem is the management of anticoagulation in patients who require surgery. The principles of care in this situation reflect the need for adequate hemostasis during and immediately after surgical procedures as well as the critical importance of restarting anticoagulation as soon as possible postoperatively, especially because surgery itself represents a relative hypercoagulable state. The perceived risk for thromboembolism in patients with atrial fibrillation clearly affects the management of perioperative anticoagulation; in this clinical situation, the CHADS-2 score (cardiac failure, hypertension, age, diabetes, and stroke) may estimate postoperative stroke risk and thus dictate the need for bridging anticoagulation with UFH/LMWH when stopping vitamin K antagonist. For patients with VTE who are anticoagulated on a short-term basis (<1 month), elective surgical procedures should be postponed; if such patients must undergo surgery, discontinuation of anticoagulation and placement of a temporary IVC filter may be the best option. In most patients receiving long-term anticoagulation for VTE, preoperative heparin is not typically used; vitamin K antagonist should be discontinued for at least 4 days preoperatively to allow the INR to decrease gradually to less than 1.5, a level that is safe for surgery. Postoperatively, intravenous heparin (or SC LMWH) can be safely used for anticoagulation until therapeutic INR levels are reached after warfarin has been restarted. As with all guidelines, individual patient circumstances may dictate changes. For example, institution of heparin immediately after a major surgical procedure may be contraindicated because of the high risk for hemorrhage; reinstitution of anticoagulation may need to be delayed for 12 to 24 hours postoperatively.

For a deeper discussion on this topic, please see Chapter 171, "Approach to the Patient with Bleeding and Thrombosis," in Goldman-Cecil Medicine, *25th Edition.*

SUGGESTED READINGS

Adam SS, McDuffie JR, Lachiewicz PF, et al: Comparative effectiveness of new oral anticoagulants and standard thromboprophylaxis in patients having total hip or knee replacement, Ann Intern Med 159:275–284, 2013.

Barbui T, Finazzi G, Carobbio A, et al: Development and validation of an international prognostic score of thrombosis in World Health Organization-essential thrombocythemia (IPSET-thrombosis), Blood 120:5128–5133, 2012.

Beer PA, Erber WN, Campbell PJ, et al: How I treat essential thrombocythemia, Blood 117:1472–1482, 2011.

Brilakis ES, Patel VG, Banerjee S: Medical management after coronary stent implantation, JAMA 310:189–198, 2013.

Cattaneo M: The platelet P2Y12 receptor for adenosine diphosphate: congenital and drug-induced defects, Blood 117:2102–2112, 2011.

Cuker A, Gimotty PA, Crowtheer MA, et al: Predictive value of the 4Ts scoring system for heparin-induced thrombocytopenia, Blood 120:4160–4167, 2012.

Dobromirski M, Cohen AT: How I manage venous thromboembolism risk in hospitalized patients, Blood 120:1562–1569, 2012.

Douketis JD: Perioperative management of patients who are receiving warfarin therapy: an evidence-based and practical approach, Blood 117:5044–5049, 2011.

Sobieraj DM, Lee S, Coleman CI, et al: Prolonged versus standard-duration venous thromboprophylaxis in major orthopedic surgery, Ann Intern Med 156:720–727, 2012.

Sultan AA, Tata LJ, West J, et al: Risk factors for first venous thromboembolism around pregnancy: a population-based cohort study from the United Kingdom, Blood 121:3953–3961, 2013.

Tosetto A, Iorio A, Marcucci M, et al: Predicting disease recurrence in patients with previous unprovoked venous thromboembolism: a proposed prediction score (DASH), J Thromb Haemost 366:1019–1025, 2012.

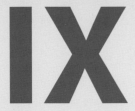

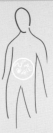
Cecil
ESSENTIALS

IX

Oncologic Disease

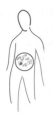

53

Cancer Biology

Aram F. Hezel

INTRODUCTION

Cancer is a complex genetic disease that is defined by the transition of a normal cell, governed by processes that control its replication and behavior, into a cancer cell that is typified by unrestrained proliferation and dissemination, leading ultimately to a state of disease and/or death. The underlying landscape of cancer genetics is now fully defined for many cancers, aided by the evolving technologies in gene sequencing. Many therapeutic advances of the last decade have successfully focused on targets identified by the study of genetic mutations. Whereas genetic changes, usually acquired by cells over time, are at the ontologic core of cancer, many other patient factors affect its formation and the course of disease, including concurrent disease of the target organ, the immunologic response, and the underlying metabolic state. This chapter reviews the essential elements of cancer biology and key underlying genetic alterations driving this biology.

HALLMARKS OF CANCER

Cancer has many effects on the human body. This heterogeneity of clinical behaviors results from the various organs and tissues affected and the different ways in which cancers can alter normal physiologic function, and it is mirrored in the appearance of different cancers at the microscopic and genetic levels. Even among cancers originating from the same organ or cell type, there is wide diversity of behaviors. More than 100 types of cancer have been identified, and they are separated into categories based on the organ and tissue from which they arose and the histologic appearance. However, with further investigations into genetic subtypes of tumors, we may come to appreciate thousands of different diseases in years to come.

Despite the clinical, histologic, and genetic diversity of cancers, they tend to share common abilities and traits. Hanahan and Weinberg first defined the acquired capabilities that are essential for tumor growth in 2000 and then updated their conceptual framework for understanding cancer through the addition of "emerging hallmarks" and "enabling characteristics" (Table 53-1).

Normal cellular division is controlled both by the restriction of growth and division signals to times of tissue injury and repair and by the presence of inhibitors of cell division and growth. In contrast, tumor cells universally are *self-sufficient in growth signals* and *insensitive to anti-growth signals*. *Resistance to apoptosis* (programmed cell death) also allows cancers to bypass another evolutionarily conserved mechanism that restrains cell survival. In addition, normal cells undergo only a set number of divisions, limiting their growth potential. Tumor cells, in contrast, are immortalized and have *limitless replicative potential*. Beyond factors inherent in the tumor cells themselves are two capabilities in the environment. *Angiogenesis*, or the establishment of a blood supply, provides tumors with the oxygen and nutrients needed to grow beyond a size of 1 to 2 mm. *Invasion and metastasis* allow tumor cells to escape their primary sites and establish colonies at new sites. Metastatic disease is the cause of death in more than 90% of cancer patients.

Recent research has redirected attention to areas of cancer biology that are important for cancer prevention and treatment. Emerging hallmarks include the *distinct metabolic requirements* of cancer cells, with a growing number of metabolic genes (e.g., *IDH1/2, FH,* and *SDHB*) identified as mutated in cancers. Also recognized as essential is the tumor's capacity to *evade the body's immune response,* which is reflected in the clinical efficacy of drugs targeting the immune-modulating molecule PD1.

Enabling characteristics of cancer include *genomic instability,* which is important for the development of cancers as well for the resistance to treatments that can emerge during systemic therapy. Tumor-promoting inflammation probably accounts for the stepwise progression of tumors and may sustain cancers by providing an inflammatory environment.

In many instances, identification of these hallmark cancer traits has led to novel therapeutic approaches. Examples include drugs that target growth-stimulating proteins and pathways by means of inhibitors developed against epidermal growth factor receptor (EGFR) in lung and colon cancer, HER2/neu (ERBB2) in breast cancer, and RAF and MEK in melanoma. Similarly, drugs that block angiogenesis (e.g., vascular endothelial growth factor [VEGF]) are now used in cancer therapy.

THE GENETICS OF CANCER

Cancers falls along a spectrum, ranging from minor genetic derangements in some malignancies (e.g., *BCR-ABL* transloca- tion in chronic myelogenous leukemia [CML]) to a genetically complex, multistep process in others (e.g., in colon, pancreas, and breast cancer). A cell that is undergoing malignant transforma- tion acquires a growth or survival advantage relative to normal

TABLE 53-1 THE CANCER PHENOTYPE	
HALLMARKS OF CANCER	**EMERGING HALLMARKS**
Self-sufficiency in growth signals	Immune evasion
Insensitivity to anti-growth signals	Metabolic dysregulation
Evasion of apoptosis	
Limitless replicative potential	**ENABLING CHARACTERISTICS**
Induction of angiogenesis	Genomic instability
Tissue invasion and metastasis	Inflammation

cells. Most invasive cancers develop only after multiple genes are mutated, and they seem to retain genetic flexibility or a mutator phenotype. Mutations can occur on exposure to environmental carcinogens, in the setting of dysregulated DNA repair, as a consequence of random replication errors during cell turnover and normal aging, or, occasionally, in families with hereditary germline mutations in a cancer gene. Mutations in cancer are classified into three categories depending on the functional consequence of the mutation: oncogenes, tumor suppressor genes, and stability or caretaker genes. However, there are newly discovered mutations that do not fall neatly into one of these categories. Table 53-2 shows the clinical consequences of selected mutations.

Oncogenes

Oncogene mutations convert a normal cell into a cancerous cell; they include chromosomal translocations, gene amplifications, and intragenic mutations. Oncogenes often activate pathways that are important for cancer. For example, CML occurs when the proto-oncogene *ABL* from chromosome 9 translocates to the *BCR* gene on chromosome 22. The new protein formed by expression of the combined gene *BCR-ABL* sends unchecked growth-promoting signals to the nucleus. An activating mutation in one allele of an oncogene is usually sufficient to promote tumorigenesis (e.g., in *KRAS*).

Because oncogenes activate pathways that drive cancer growth, their discovery has led to specifically designed drugs that target the products of these genes and the pathways they control. For example, among patients with breast cancer, HER2 amplification serves as a biomarker that identifies those who will

benefit from treatment with the anti-HER2 monoclonal antibody, trastuzumab. Similarly, activating mutations in EGFR serve to identify patients with non–small cell lung cancer who will improve with the use of drugs that specifically inhibit the mutated form of EGFR. Another example is BRAF mutations in melanoma. This paradigm—identify a mutated oncogene, find a specific drug that inhibits the activated mutant protein, and treat patients who have the specific mutation with a drug that affects the mutated protein—has repeatedly been proven to be a successful approach.

Tumor Suppressor Genes

Tumor suppressor genes control cellular replication and growth. Point mutations or deletions of tumor suppressor genes give cells harboring these mutations a growth advantage. Inactivation of tumor suppressor genes may lead to diminished activity of the protein product by several mechanisms: silencing or inactivating point mutations, large DNA deletions or rearrangements, or methylation and chromatin remodeling of the regions harboring the gene. In contrast to oncogene activation, inactivation of both alleles of a tumor suppressor gene is required for tumorigenesis. For instance, an inherited mutation in a single retinoblastoma gene (*RB1*, a tumor suppressor gene) may not, by itself, cause retinoblastoma in a young child. However, a "second hit" after birth (i.e., an *RB1* somatic mutation) can result in multiple tumors including bilateral retinoblastomas. The tumor suppressor gene *TP53* is the most commonly mutated gene in sporadic human cancers. Deletion of this gene can be inherited, and families with inherited mutations have higher rates of a variety of cancers, including breast and brain tumors, leukemia, and sarcoma, a pattern termed the *Li-Fraumeni syndrome*.

Stability Genes

Mutations in stability or caretaker genes can also promote tumorigenesis. These genes are responsible for the repair of errors in normal DNA replication. They include mismatch repair genes, base-excision repair genes, and nucleotide-excision repair genes. Mutations in stability genes lead to increased errors in DNA replication. Eventually, DNA replication errors (mutations) are introduced in oncogenes and tumor suppressor genes, resulting in malignant transformation. Lynch syndrome, also called hereditary nonpolyposis colon cancer, is an inherited syndrome of defects in DNA mismatch repair genes. Colon and endometrial cancers are commonly observed in families with this syndrome, and rates of many gastrointestinal cancers are also higher in these families.

● THE ORIGINS OF CANCER
Steps Toward Cancer

Many malignancies, including colon, breast, pancreas, and liver cancers, develop in a stepwise progression from normal to cancerous cells that is driven by a cascade of genetic events. This model was first articulated in colon cancer, where precancerous polyps were found to harbor some of the same mutations found in advanced cancers. This type of progression provides the genetic and biologic basis for the efficacy of many cancer screening and prevention programs that focus on identifying

TABLE 53-2	CANCERS ASSOCIATED WITH SELECTED GENETIC MUTATIONS	
GENE	**ASSOCIATED HEREDITARY SYNDROME**	**MAJOR TUMOR TYPES**
ONCOGENES		
KRAS	–	Pancreatic, lung, bladder, and colon cancers
BCR-ABL translocation		Chronic myelogenous leukemia
BCL2	–	Chronic lymphocytic leukemia
KIT, PDGFRA	Familial gastrointestinal stromal tumors	Gastrointestinal stromal tumors
TUMOR SUPPRESSOR GENES		
TP53 (p53)	Li-Fraumeni syndrome	Breast, sarcoma, adrenal, brain, multiple others
APC	Familial adenomatosis polyposis	Colon, stomach, intestine
VHL	Von Hippel–Lindau syndrome	Kidney
SMAD4	Juvenile polyposis/hereditary hemorrhagic telangiectasia syndrome	Colon, gastric, and pancreatic cancer
CDKN2A (p16)	Familial atypical multiple mole melanoma syndrome	Melanoma, pancreatic adenocarcinoma, non–small cell lung cancer
STABILITY GENES		
BRCA1, BRCA2	Hereditary breast cancer	Breast, ovary
MSH2, MLH1	Lynch syndrome	Colon, uterus, stomach

and treating preneoplastic lesions to prevent progression to malignancy. Well-known examples of such approaches include colonoscopy for colon cancer and Papanicolaou (Pap) smears for cervical cancer.

Cancer Stem Cells

The concept of cancer stem cells has gained traction in some malignancies. Observations of a hierarchy of cells within a malignancy, wherein some cells retain a proliferative self-renewing capacity and others do not, support this concept. These populations of cells may be responsible for treatment resistance.

For a deeper discussion on this topic, please see Chapter 181, "Cancer Biology and Genetics," in Goldman-Cecil Medicine, 25th Edition.

SUGGESTED READINGS

Cancer Genome Atlas Network: Comprehensive molecular characterization of human colon and rectal cancer, Nature 487:330–337, 2012.

Hanahan D, Weinberg RA: Hallmarks of cancer: the next generation, Cell 144:646–674, 2011.

Jordan CT, Guzman ML, Noble M: Cancer stem cells, N Engl J Med 355:1253–1261, 2006.

Vander Heiden MG, Cantley LC, Thompson CB: Understanding the Warburg effect: the metabolic requirements of cell proliferation, Science 324:1029–1033, 2009.

Vogelstein B, Kinzler KW: Cancer genes and the pathways they control, Nat Med 10:789–799, 2004.

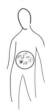

54

Cancer Epidemiology

Gary H. Lyman and Nicole M. Kuderer

INTRODUCTION

Globally, more than 11 million individuals are diagnosed with cancer and some 7 million die from the disease annually. At the same time, it is estimated that there are more than 22 million cancer survivors worldwide, and their number is increasing dramatically each year. In the United States in 2014, it was estimated that 1.7 million individuals would be diagnosed with cancer, for an age-adjusted incidence rate of 470 per 100,000 population. At the same time, it was estimated that more than 585,000 individuals would die of cancer, for an age-adjusted death rate of 176 per 100,000. Cancer is the leading cause of mortality among both women and men between the ages of 40 and 80 years, and it is the second leading cause of death for most other age groups, including children between 1 and 14 years of age.

The leading types of new invasive cancer cases and cancer-specific deaths are shown in Figure 54-1. Although breast cancer in women and prostate cancer in men are the most common noncutaneous forms of cancer, lung cancer is now the leading cause of cancer-specific mortality, accounting for almost 30% of cancer deaths in both genders. Mortality rates for gastric and cervical cancers have decreased steadily for decades, and overall cancer death rates have decreased some 20% since their height in the early 1990s, with the greatest declines observed for colorectal, prostate, and lung cancers in men and colorectal and breast cancer in women (Fig. 54-2). Death rates over the last decade have also declined by more than 8% for chronic myeloid leukemia and more than 3% for non-Hodgkin's lymphoma. Cancer mortality rates in developed countries are consistently higher among those from racial and ethnic minority groups, especially African Americans in the United States, and among those from lower socioeconomic strata. Greater mortality rates among racial and ethnic minorities are not fully explained by differences in the stage at diagnosis. Socioeconomic factors, access to appropriate treatment, and comorbidities represent additional determinants of greater cancer mortality.

CANCER EPIDEMIOLOGY METHODS

Epidemiologists study disease variation among populations and the factors that influence such variation. The proportion of individuals with disease in the population at a given point in time is the *prevalence*. *Incidence and mortality rates* represent the number of events in a population over a defined period of time (e.g., cancers per 100,000 per year). To facilitate comparisons among populations, rates are often adjusted for age, sex, race, or other demographic characteristics.

The association between a characteristic or exposure and cancer risk is typically assessed in either cohort or case-control studies. Cohort studies are usually prospective and evaluate disease experience in exposed and unexposed individuals. Case-control studies assess the exposure experience of individuals with and without the disease of interest. The *relative risk* (RR) is a measure of association between exposure and disease, with estimates greater than 1.0 representing an increase in risk. In case-control studies, RR is estimated by the *odds ratio* (OR), because the sizes of the exposed and unexposed populations are often not known. The larger the study population, the more precise is the estimate of association between exposure and disease. However, proper interpretation of the results must explore whether any systematic error or bias was introduced during the study design or analysis.

Confounding factors may obscure or weaken a true association or create a false association (i.e., because of an association between the factor itself and both exposure and disease). Confounding can be evaluated and adjusted for in stratified or multivariate analysis if the potential confounder is recognized and has been properly measured in the data. It is usually not safe to assume that all possible confounding factors have been considered. Therefore, causal inference is seldom justified on the basis of a single study but evolves gradually with study repetition and consideration of other information, including results from animal and other laboratory findings, the strength of the association, and a careful consideration of likely confounding factors.

Interventions for cancer prevention and screening are typically studied in randomized controlled trials that require large numbers of participants, close monitoring for adherence to the intervention, long-term follow-up, and appropriate ascertainment of disease and disease-free status.

RISK FACTORS
Genetic

Risk factors for cancer can be grouped as either genetic (inherited) or acquired. Although they are important for understanding carcinogenesis, only a small proportion of cancers are inherited in a mendelian fashion. Neoplasms inherited in an autosomal dominant manner include retinoblastomas, multiple endocrine neoplasia syndromes, and polyposis coli. Several additional preneoplastic conditions demonstrate mendelian inheritance with variable penetrance. Some common malignancies demonstrate familial risk patterns with low penetrance, including breast cancer and colorectal cancer. Genetic testing and potential preventive measures are available for some inherited cancer syndromes

Estimated New Cases

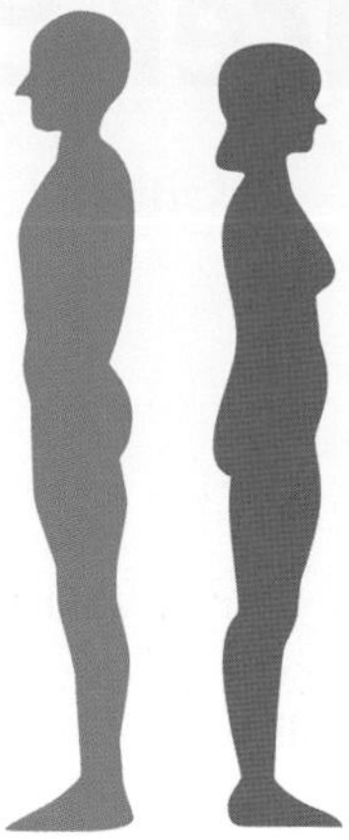

			Males	Females			
Prostate	238,590	28%		Breast	232,340	29%
Lung and bronchus	118,080	14%		Lung and bronchus	110,110	14%
Colorectum	73,680	9%		Colorectum	69,140	9%
Urinary bladder	54,610	6%		Uterine corpus	49,560	6%
Melanoma of the skin	45,060	5%		Thyroid	45,310	6%
Kidney and renal pelvis	40,430	5%		Non-Hodgkin lymphoma	32,140	4%
Non-Hodgkin lymphoma	37,600	4%		Melanoma of the skin	31,630	4%
Oral cavity and pharynx	29,620	3%		Kidney and renal pelvis	24,720	3%
Leukemia	27,880	3%		Pancreas	22,480	3%
Pancreas	22,740	3%		Ovary	22,240	3%
All Sites	**854,790**	**100%**		**All Sites**	**805,500**	**100%**

Estimated Deaths

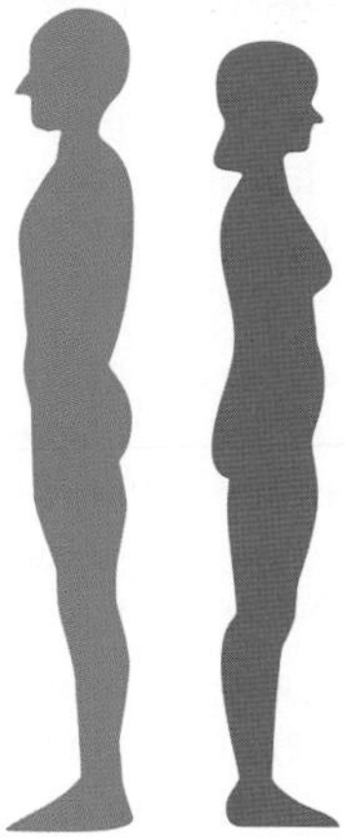

			Males	Females			
Lung and bronchus	87,260	28%		Lung and bronchus	72,220	26%
Prostate	29,720	10%		Breast	39,620	14%
Colorectum	26,300	9%		Colorectum	24,530	9%
Pancreas	19,480	6%		Pancreas	18,980	7%
Liver and intrahepatic bile duct	14,890	5%		Ovary	14,030	5%
Leukemia	13,660	4%		Leukemia	10,060	4%
Esophagus	12,220	4%		Non-Hodgkin lymphoma	8,430	3%
Urinary bladder	10,820	4%		Uterine corpus	8,190	3%
Non-Hodgkin lymphoma	10,590	3%		Liver and intrahepatic bile duct	6,780	2%
Kidney and renal pelvis	8,780	3%		Brain and other nervous system	6,150	2%
All Sites	**306,920**	**100%**		**All Sites**	**273,430**	**100%**

FIGURE 54-1 U.S. cancer statistics, 2013: estimated new cases and deaths. Estimates are rounded to the nearest 10 and exclude basal cell and squamous cell skin cancers and in situ carcinoma except urinary bladder. (Modified from Siegel R, Naishadham D, Jemal A: Cancer statistics, 2013. CA Cancer J Clin 63:11–30, 2013 [Figure 1]. Available at http://onlinelibrary.wiley.com/doi/10.3322/caac.21166/full#fig1. Accessed June 27, 2014.)

(Table 54-1). Although genetic testing is available for several identified cancer susceptibility genes, care must be taken in selecting individuals for such testing. Genetic testing requires a reasonable understanding of cancer genetics as well as the target population along with relevant ethical, economic, and societal issues.

Acquired somatic mutations are universally identified in malignant cells, and some clearly drive the development and progression of cancer. Although random genetic mutations occur frequently, proto-oncogenes involved in cell growth and proliferation, tumor suppressor genes involved in regulation of cellular proliferation, and mismatch repair genes associated with chromosomal instability play critical roles in carcinogenesis, tumor growth, progression, invasion, and metastasis. Because the spontaneous mutation rate is relatively low, more than one mutational event is usually necessary for complete carcinogenic transformation resulting in a malignancy.

Lifestyle

Acquired risk factors for cancer include lifestyle factors as well as occupational and other environmental exposures to carcinogenic substances. Major lifestyle risk factors include tobacco, alcohol and other dietary factors, and lack of physical activity (Table 54-2).

Tobacco

Tobacco products are, by far, the single greatest contributor to cancer incidence and mortality worldwide. Cigarette smokers have a 20-fold or greater risk for developing cancer compared with nonsmokers, and smoking is the single largest cause of lung cancer. Tobacco accounts for one third of all cancers in the United States. Worldwide, more than 1 million people are estimated to die from tobacco-induced cancers every year. The vast majority of lung cancers are attributable to cigarette smoking, and exposure to secondhand smoke increases the risk for lung cancer

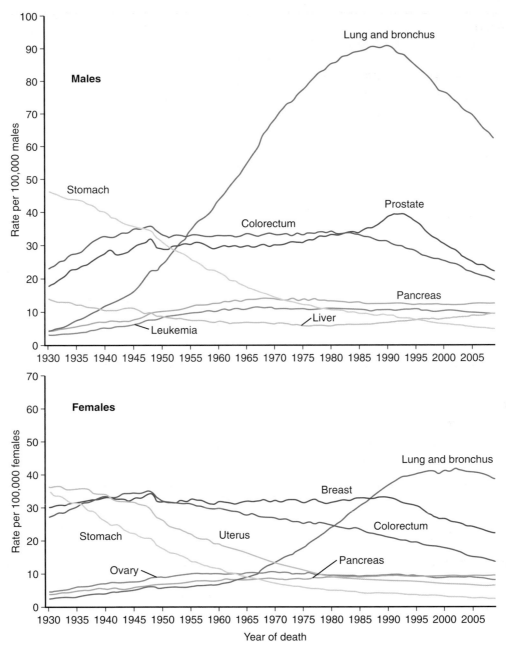

FIGURE 54-2 U.S. cancer mortality rates, 1930-2009. (Modified from Siegel R, Naishadham D, Jemal A: Cancer statistics, 2013. CA Cancer J Clin 63:11–30, 2013 [Figures 4 and 5]. Available at http://onlinelibrary.wiley.com/doi/10.3322/caac.21166/full#fig1. Accessed June 27, 2014.)

in nonsmokers. Cigarette and cigar smoking and tobacco chewing are major risk factors for head, neck, mouth, and esophageal cancers. Although tobacco use has declined in the United States over the last 2 decades, it remains unacceptably high, especially among younger women, and continues to increase in many parts of the developing world.

Nutrition

Diet and body weight appear to play an important role in cancer causation. Excess alcohol use is clearly a significant risk factor for cancers of the liver, head and neck, esophagus, and breast. Obesity and dietary fat intake are associated with colon and breast cancers, but the exact nature of the relationship is still under investigation. Central or visceral adiposity in both men and women is associated with increased incidence and mortality from a number of cancers, including those of the endometrium, breast (in postmenopausal women), kidney, gallbladder, pancreas, esophagus, colon, and prostate.

Infection

Several chronic infections have been associated with an increased risk of different types of cancer, including bacterial, viral, and parasitic infections. In certain parts of the developing world, infection with *Schistosoma haematobium* is a major cause of squamous cell carcinoma of the bladder. Viruses associated with human malignancies include the Epstein-Barr virus (EBV,

TABLE 54-1   GENETIC TESTING FOR SELECTED HEREDITARY CANCER SYNDROMES

TYPE OF CANCER AND INVOLVED GENES	PREVENTION MEASURES
BREAST	
BRCA1, BRCA2	Prophylactic mastectomy
PTEN, STK11, TP53	Selective estrogen receptor modulators
	Lifestyle measures
	Increased intensity of screening, including breast MRI
LOBULAR BREAST CANCER AND GASTRIC CANCER	Prophylactic gastrectomy
	Prophylactic mastectomy
CDH1 (E-cadherin)	Increased intensity of screening, including breast MRI
	Selective estrogen receptor modulators
OVARIAN	
BRCA1, BRCA2	Prophylactic oophorectomy
	Oral contraceptives
COLON	
Familial adenomatous polyposis (FAP)	Prophylactic colectomy
	NSAIDs
APC	Lifestyle measures
Hereditary nonpolyposis colon cancer (HNPCC)	Lifestyle measures
	NSAIDs
MLH1, MSH2	Increased surveillance
MSH6, PMS2	Prophylactic total abdominal hysterectomy and oophorectomy
MYH-associated polyposis	Lifestyle measures
MYH	NSAIDs
	Prophylactic colectomy
UTERINE	
PTEN, MLH1, MSH2, MSH6, PMS2	Prophylactic hysterectomy
	Increased surveillance

MRI, Magnetic resonance imaging; MYH, mutY homologue; NSAIDs, nonsteroidal anti-inflammatory drugs.

TABLE 54-2   CANCER RISK FACTORS

LIFESTYLE FACTOR	ASSOCIATED CANCERS
Tobacco	Lung, bronchus, esophagus, head and neck, stomach, pancreas, kidney, bladder, cervix
High alcohol consumption	Liver, rectum, breast, oral cavity, pharynx, larynx, esophagus
Obesity, high dietary fat	Colon, breast, endometrium, kidney, pancreas, esophagus, prostate
Low dietary fiber	Colon
Sedentary lifestyle	Colon, breast
Environmental exposures	
Human papillomavirus: types 16, 18	Cervical
Hepatitis B and C viruses	Liver and hepatocellular cancers
Asbestos	Mesothelioma and other types of lung cancer
Radon	Lung
Ultraviolet radiation	Melanoma, basal and squamous cell carcinomas
Ionizing radiation	Leukemia, thyroid, lung, breast

anogenital squamous cell carcinoma. Chronic hepatitis B and C viral infections have been linked with the development of hepatocellular carcinoma. Human papillomaviruses 16 and 18 have been linked with cervical cancer, and vaccines against these virus strains and those causing genital warts are now on the market.

Radiation

Non-ionizing Radiation

Ultraviolet (UV) radiation is unquestionably associated with an increase risk of skin cancers, including basal and squamous cell carcinomas as well as cutaneous melanoma, with observed rates increasing directly with the amount of daily sunlight exposure. Most of the harmful effects from sun exposure are related to direct DNA damage associated with exposure to intermediate-wavelength UVB. The use of tanning beds and frequent exposure to sunlight are of particular concern given the rapid increase in rates of melanoma among younger individuals.

Ionizing Radiation

Ionizing radiation is an extensively studied carcinogen; it is unequivocally associated with an increased risk for both hematologic malignancies and various solid tumors in humans. Radiation-induced malignancies including leukemia and solid tumors have been most extensively studied in occupational settings among radiation workers and miners, among survivors of the atomic weapons used in Hiroshima and Nagasaki in World War II, and among those exposed to radiation for medical indications. Excess cancer risk from radiation exposure has a latency period ranging from a few years (leukemia) to decades (solid tumors) and correlates with the cumulative exposure dose. As the survivors of the atomic bombing of Japan age, estimates of the associated risk of cancer have continued to increase.

Natural sources account for at least 80% of human exposure to radiation, most notably from radon. Radon exposure is estimated to be the second leading cause of lung cancer due to widespread low-level exposure in the residential setting. In the occupational setting, there is a strong interaction between smoking and radon, such that most radon-induced lung cancers occur among smokers. Medical exposure accounts for most of the remaining average annual radiation exposure in the United States. Repeated exposure to radiation from multiple imaging studies (e.g., CT scans), especially at a young age, is associated with an increased risk of cancer later in life.

Chemicals

Various pharmacologic agents have been associated with an increased risk for specific cancers. As with radiation, these agents may be used in the occupational setting, for diagnostic or therapeutic medical use, and for various purposes in the home setting. Organic and inorganic chemical compounds linked to human cancers include benzene (leukemia), benzidine (bladder), arsenic, soot and coal tars (lung and skin), and wood dusts (nasal). Arguably, asbestos is the most common cause of occupational cancer because of its link with the development of mesothelioma and other types of lung cancer. Almost all mesotheliomas diagnosed in the United States are associated with prior asbestos

with nasopharyngeal cancer and Burkitt's lymphoma) and human T-cell leukemia virus type I (HTLV-I). Patients with the acquired immunodeficiency syndrome, which is associated with the human immunodeficiency virus (HIV), are at increased risk for Kaposi's sarcoma, non-Hodgkin's lymphoma, and exposure. A strong interaction exists between asbestos exposure and cigarette smoking leading to lung cancer.

A range of medications are associated with increased cancer risk, including the alkylating agents, anthracyclines, and other classes of cancer chemotherapy agents and immunusuppressants. Estrogen use in postmenopausal women increases the risk of endometrial cancer; the rates drop when estrogen is combined with progesterone. Synthetic estrogens, such as diethylstilbestrol (DES), administered to mothers during pregnancy increase the risk of vaginal cancer in offspring. Lifestyle exposures to carcinogenic chemicals include multiple carcinogens in tobacco products and dietary factors, including aflatoxins, in many parts of the world.

⬤ CANCER PREVENTION

Cancer prevention strategies are either primary or secondary based on whether they reduce risk of exposure or detect cancer at an early stage when intervention can change the natural history of the disease. Primary prevention strategies include reductions in lifestyle risks (e.g., smoking cessation; use of sunscreen; adherence to a low-fat, high-fiber diet), avoidance of occupational or environmental risks, and chemoprevention (see Table 54-2).

Lifestyle Changes

Smoking cessation is unquestionably the most direct and effective cancer prevention strategy available. More than 1 million people die from tobacco-induced cancers globally each year, and tobacco accounts for one third of all cancer diagnoses in the United States. Although tobacco prevention and control programs have resulted in a decline in smoking prevalence in the United States, tobacco use continues to be high and has been increasing in a number of countries. There is also evidence from epidemiologic studies that other lifestyle changes, including regular exercise and dietary modification, may also reduce the risk of cancer. Central adiposity is associated with increased incidence of and mortality from a number of cancers, including breast and endometrial cancers. Sufficient dietary intake of fruits and vegetables appears to reduce the risk for gastric and esophageal cancers. Avoidance of excessive sun exposure and artificial tanning devices may reverse the recent upward trend in cutaneous malignancies. Reduction in exposures to known carcinogenic agents is an important goal in both occupational and domestic settings. Evidence for an association between air pollution and lung cancer incidence illustrates how difficult such reductions may be. However, limiting the use of potentially carcinogenic chemicals and of radiation in the medical setting is sensible.

Chemoprevention

Chemopreventive agents are drugs, vaccines, or micronutrients (e.g., minerals, vitamins) that prevent the development of cancer. Both randomized trials and epidemiologic studies suggest that a number of strategies can reduce the risk of some common types of cancer. Daily aspirin use may reduce the risks of colon cancer and melanoma. Hepatitis B vaccination may reduce the incidence of hepatocellular cancer. The vaccine directed against specific strains of the human papillomavirus (HPV) promises to prevent cervical cancer.

⬤ CANCER SCREENING

Cancer screening programs should detect premalignant states or early-stage cancers before the onset of symptoms with relatively high sensitivity. For cancer screening to be useful, there must be a treatment available that improves the outcome for patients with premalignant or early-stage disease. Ideally, such screening programs should also be noninvasive, inexpensive, and associated with high specificity (i.e., low rate of false-positive results). Identification of high-risk individuals assists in genetic counseling and testing as well as in cancer screening efforts.

Proper interpretation of the results of cancer screening studies must consider both *lead-time bias* and *length-time bias*. Lead time is the time between detection of disease by screening and the actual appearance of symptomatic disease. If screening leads to early diagnosis, it may appear that the patient lived longer than would have been the case without screening even when the survival of the patient from the onset of disease has not been altered. Length-time bias occurs when subsets of the cancer under study have different growth rates. Screening is more likely to detect cancers that grow slowly because of the greater prevalence of asymptomatic people with slow-growing tumors than those with fast-growing tumors. Patients with cancer that is detected by screening may appear to have longer survival times as a result of screening when in fact the longer course of their disease results from the behavior of the tumor itself. Although randomized controlled trials of cancer screening programs require large numbers of participants and take years to complete, such trials are needed to quantitate the value of screening and to address both lead-time and length-time bias.

Screening tests may also be associated with false-negative and false-positive results. False-negative results fail to identify a proper diagnosis and patients therefore are not provided the opportunity for effective early treatment. False-positive results may also cause harm by leading to unnecessary testing and treatment and by contributing to patient costs and emotional stress.

Currently, recommended cancer screening tests include clinical examination and mammography to detect breast cancer, Papanicolaou smears and HPV DNA tests to detect cervical dysplasia or cancer, colonoscopy to detect polyps or colon cancer, and digital rectal examination and serum prostate-specific antigen (PSA) measurement to detect prostate cancer. Although issues remain to be resolved, low-dose computed tomographic scanning to screen appropriate high-risk individuals for lung cancer has recently been recommended based on results from the National Lung Cancer Screening Trial.

▬ SUGGESTED READINGS

Colditz GA, Sellers TA, Trapido E: Epidemiology: identifying the causes and preventability of cancer, Nat Rev Cancer 6:75–83, 2006.

Detterbeck FC, Mazzone PJ, Naidich DP, et al: Screening for lung cancer: diagnosis and management of lung cancer, 3rd ed. American College of Chest Physicians evidence-based clinical practice guidelines, Chest 143:e78S–92S, 2013.

Kushi LH, Doyle C, McCullough M, et al: American Cancer Society guidelines on nutrition and physical activity for cancer prevention: reducing the risk of cancer with healthy food choices and physical activity, CA Cancer J Clin 62:30–67, 2012.

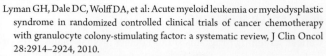

Lyman GH, Dale DC, Wolff DA, et al: Acute myeloid leukemia or myelodysplastic syndrome in randomized controlled clinical trials of cancer chemotherapy with granulocyte colony-stimulating factor: a systematic review, J Clin Oncol 28:2914–2924, 2010.

Raaschou-Nielsen O, Andersen ZJ, Beelen R, et al: Air pollution and lung cancer incidence in 17 European cohorts: prospective analyses from the European Study of Cohorts for Air Pollution Effects (ESCAPE), Lancet Oncol 14:813–822, 2013.

Schottenfeld D, Beebe-Dimmer J: Alleviating the burden of cancer: a perspective on advances, challenges and future directions, Cancer Epidemiol Biomarkers Prev 15:2049–2055, 2006.

Siegel R, Naishadham D, Jemal A: Cancer statistics, 2013, CA Cancer J Clin 63:11–30, 2013.

Siegel R, Zou Z, Jemal A: Cancer Statistics, 2014, CA Cancer J Clin 64:9–29, 2014.

Smith RA, Brooks D, Cokkinides V, et al: Cancer screening in the United States, 2013: a review of current American Cancer Society guidelines, current issues in cancer screening, and new guidance on cervical cancer screening and lung cancer screening, CA Cancer J Clin 63:88–105, 2013.

55

Principles of Cancer Therapy

Davendra P.S. Sohal and Alok A. Khorana

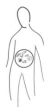

INTRODUCTION

The treatment of cancer is evolving rapidly. Chemotherapy is the mainstay of systemic treatment, but the explosive increase in knowledge of cancer biology has allowed research efforts to focus on the development of more specific "targeted" agents. The annual number of new drugs approved for cancer treatment has increased several-fold since the 1990s. In addition, almost 400 anticancer agents are in clinical trials, more than for any other class of medicine. Surgery and radiation therapy are safe and effective treatments for localized cancers, and techniques continue to be refined. However, cancer remains the second leading cause of death in the United States, requiring that resources be devoted to palliative care as well. The treatment of cancer requires various specialists, including surgeons and medical and radiation oncologists, to work in an integrated fashion to deliver optimal care to the patient. This chapter reviews the principles of surgical, radiation, and medical approaches to cancer treatment; it also considers diagnosis and staging as well as supportive care interventions that are integral to the care of patients with cancer.

DIAGNOSIS AND STAGING

Definitive treatment for cancer usually requires an adequate histologic diagnosis. This typically involves performance of an invasive biopsy to obtain sufficient material to evaluate the morphology and invasiveness of the tumor and the expression of various molecular markers. Noninvasive tests such as radiologic imaging are seldom substitutes for tissue diagnosis. There are some exceptions, such as an elevated α-fetoprotein level along with imaging evidence, which can be used to make a diagnosis of hepatocellular carcinoma.

Once the diagnosis of cancer has been made, the next step is to systematically determine the extent of tumor spread, a process called *staging*. Tumor staging can be clinical or pathologic. *Clinical staging* involves physical examination and imaging studies, including targeted ultrasound, computed tomography scans, magnetic resonance imaging, whole-body positron-emission tomography scans, radionuclide scans, or a combination thereof. The choice of studies for particular tumors depends on their propensity to spread to particular organs. *Pathologic staging* is more definitive and follows the tumor-node-metastasis (TNM) method developed by the American Joint Committee on Cancer and the International Union against Cancer. This system requires a careful evaluation of the primary resection specimen for three measurements: (1) the size and extent of invasion of the primary tumor (the T score), (2) the number and location of histologically involved regional lymph nodes (the N score), and (3) the

presence or absence of distant metastases (the M score). The M score is based on information derived from both clinical and pathologic staging. TNM scores are then grouped into a pathologic stage, from I through IV, reflecting an increasing burden of disease. The final TNM stage has both prognostic and therapeutic implications. For instance, a resected colon cancer that invades the muscularis propria, involves 2 of 16 lymph nodes, but shows no evidence of distant metastases is staged as a T2 N1 M0 (stage III) colon cancer. The likelihood of tumor recurrence is 40% to 50%; a patient receives 6 months of chemotherapy after surgery. On the other hand, if no lymph nodes are involved (T2 N0 M0, stage I), the likelihood of recurrence is less than 10%, and chemotherapy is not recommended.

Biomarkers provide additional prognostic information, such as the absence of hormone receptors or expression of HER2 in breast cancer, which are indicative of a poor prognosis. Such markers can also be predictive; for instance, overexpression of HER2 in breast cancer predicts response to trastuzumab. Similarly, *KRAS* mutations in colorectal cancer predict lack of response to antibodies (e.g., cetuximab, panitumumab) that are directed against the epidermal growth factor receptor (EGFR). Both prognostic and predictive biomarkers provide important information in addition to the formal TNM stage. Gene expression signatures also provide additional prognostic or predictive information. A 21-gene signature is commonly used for clinical decision making regarding adjuvant therapy in patients with certain estrogen receptor–positive breast cancers. For certain tumors, measurement of serum levels of tumor markers (e.g., carcinoembryonic antigen in colon cancer, α-fetoprotein in testicular and liver cancers) can also be of prognostic importance. All of this information is compiled into a final assessment of whether the cancer is curable or not.

The next step is to evaluate the patient's overall clinical condition with respect to comorbidities affecting major organ function and the patient's functional ability, termed *performance status*. Performance status is assessed with the use of various history-based methods, such as the Eastern Cooperative Oncology Group or Karnofsky performance score. Patients with poor performance status or major comorbid conditions may not derive a benefit from cancer-directed therapy and are at greater risk for adverse events. This comprehensive assessment—diagnosis, stage, prognostic and predictive markers, and patient condition—dictates the management plan: either curative or palliative.

PRINCIPLES OF CANCER SURGERY

Surgery can prevent cancer by removal of precancerous lesions or organs that are at high risk for cancer (e.g., bilateral mastectomy in those with hereditary defects that can lead to breast cancer). Surgery can also make the diagnosis of cancer by biopsy; assist in staging by sampling lymph nodes; provide definitive treatment by removing the primary tumor; reconstruct the limb or organ sacrificed; and provide palliative treatment of cancer (e.g., intestinal bypass for obstruction, spinal cord decompression, or orthopedic procedures to prevent or treat pathologic fractures). Invasive procedures, such as biopsies and the insertion of various access devices, tubes, stents, catheters, and drains, are also performed by interventional specialists, including radiologists, gastroenterologists, and pulmonologists.

When a solid organ cancer is localized, surgery is the most effective curative treatment available. The intent is to completely remove the tumor, regional lymph nodes, and adjacent involved tissue, along with a safe margin of normal tissue. At surgery, the tumor is isolated and is almost never opened during the procedure. Refinements in cancer surgery include increasing use of laparoscopic procedures in selected cancers and the identification of a sentinel lymph node by injection of a dye during surgery, which avoids a full lymph node dissection if the sentinel node is uninvolved by cancer.

🔴 PRINCIPLES OF RADIATION THERAPY

Many cancer patients receive radiation therapy at some point during the course of their disease. Radiation therapy can sometimes be used as definitive treatment, either alone or in combination with chemotherapy. Unlike surgery, local or regional treatment with radiation can preserve organ structure and function, improving quality of life for patients. For example, use of radiation with chemotherapy for treatment of localized laryngeal cancer has outcomes similar to those of surgery but allows preservation of the larynx. Radiation therapy is also effective in the palliative setting, where it is used to control various cancer-related problems such as pain, dysphagia, and bleeding.

Ionizing radiation damages cellular DNA directly or indirectly through free radical intermediates. Cells are most susceptible to radiation during the M and G_2 phases of the cell cycle. The aim of radiation therapy is to deliver the highest dose possible to the tumor with minimal toxicity to adjacent normal tissues. Dividing the total planned radiation dose into small daily fractions takes advantage of the difference in repair capability between normal and malignant tissue and improves the tolerance of normal tissue. The biologic effects of radiation can be modified by numerous factors, including the amount of oxygen in the irradiated tissue and the use of chemotherapy for sensitizing tissue to radiation.

The goal of treatment planning for radiation therapy is to precisely define the dose and volume to be irradiated. The dose of radiation is measured in units of absorbed dose, Gray (Gy), which has replaced the older unit, rad (1 Gy = 100 rad). Conventional radiation treatments deliver 1.8 to 2 Gy/day on 5 days per week, over a period of 5 to 6 weeks. For palliative treatment, higher doses per fraction may be used to deliver an effective dose over a shorter period.

Ionizing radiation can be administered as external-beam therapy with the use of a linear accelerator to generate electrons or high-energy x-rays. Electrons have a limited depth of penetration and are useful for superficial tumors. High-energy x-rays

	TABLE 55-1	ACUTE AND LATE EFFECTS OF RADIATION THERAPY	
ORGAN	**ACUTE**	**LATE**	**DOSE (GY) ASSOCIATED WITH ADVERSE EFFECTS**
Bone marrow	Aplasia	Leukemia, myelodysplasia	25
Spinal cord	None	Myelopathy	45
Heart	None	Pericarditis, cardiomyopathy, coronary artery disease	45
Rectum	Diarrhea, tenesmus	Stricture, obstruction	60
Eye	Conjunctivitis	Retinopathy	55
Lung	Pneumonitis	Chronic pneumonitis	25

deliver the radiation deep into the body while reducing the dose to the skin as they enter. Brachytherapy uses radioactive sources to deliver ionizing radiation (gamma rays) directly to the tumor. An example is the implantation of iodine-125 seeds into the prostate as definitive therapy for early prostate cancer. Current approaches to improving radiation therapy include the use of advanced technology that allows delivery of a higher dose of radiation to specific areas of the tumor and sparing of normal tissue (conformal and intensity-modulated radiation therapy).

Injury to normal tissue from radiation therapy can be either acute or late (Table 55-1). Acute effects occur within days to weeks after irradiation and are seen primarily in rapidly proliferating tissues such as skin and gastrointestinal mucosa. The severity depends on the total dose, but the damage can usually be repaired. Late effects, such as necrosis, fibrosis, or organ failure, appear months or years after irradiation and are dependent on fraction size. Another late complication of radiation therapy is the development of secondary malignancies (e.g., after radiation for breast cancer or Hodgkin's disease).

🔴 PRINCIPLES OF MEDICAL THERAPY

The term *chemotherapy* refers to the use of cytotoxic agents, singly or in combination, for the systemic treatment of cancer. Most such agents are general antiproliferative agents that are more effective against rapidly growing tumors and have significant adverse effects on normal tissues that also divide rapidly, such as bone marrow and digestive tract mucosa. Newer agents, including monoclonal antibodies and signal transduction inhibitors, are directed against targets that are relatively specific to tumor cells and therefore may have less toxicity. These drugs are classified separately from chemotherapy as *targeted therapy* agents.

Mechanisms of Chemotherapy

Chemotherapeutic agents can be cell cycle specific or cell cycle nonspecific. Cell cycle–nonspecific agents have a greater effect on cells traversing the cell cycle but also affect noncycling cells; cell cycle–specific agents affect only cycling cells. Chemotherapy agents are further classified according to their mechanism of action into alkylating agents, antimetabolites, antitumor antibiotics, and mitotic spindle inhibitors (Table 55-2). Most chemotherapy agents suppress the bone marrow, leading to infections

TABLE 55-2 COMMONLY USED CHEMOTHERAPY AGENTS

DRUG	CANCERS TREATED	SPECIFIC CLASS OR MECHANISM OF ACTION	COMMON SIDE EFFECTS
CELL CYCLE SPECIFIC			
5-Fluorouracil	Gastrointestinal, head and neck, breast	Antimetabolite, inhibits thymidylate synthase	Myelosuppression, mucositis, diarrhea
Gemcitabine	Pancreas, lung, breast, bladder	Antimetabolite, deoxycytidine analogue	Myelosuppression, nausea, emesis
Methotrexate	ALL, choriocarcinoma, bladder, lymphoma	Antimetabolite, folic acid antagonist	Myelosuppression, mucositis, acute renal failure
Doxorubicin	Breast, lung, NHL	Anthracycline, intercalates into DNA	Myelosuppression, nausea, emesis, cardiomyopathy
Irinotecan	Colorectal, lung	Camptothecin, topoisomerase I inhibitor	Myelosuppression, diarrhea
Paclitaxel	Breast, lung, Kaposi sarcoma, ovarian	Plant alkaloid, inhibits microtubule formation	Myelosuppression, hypersensitivity reaction, neuropathy
Vincristine	ALL, lymphomas, myeloma, sarcoma	Plant alkaloid, disrupts microtubule assembly	Peripheral neuropathy, constipation
CELL CYCLE NONSPECIFIC			
Cyclophosphamide	Breast, NHL, CLL, sarcoma	Alkylating agent, cross-links DNA	Myelosuppression, hemorrhagic cystitis, nausea, emesis
Cisplatin	Lung, bladder, ovarian, testicular, head and neck	Alkylating agent, cross-links DNA	Nephrotoxicity, nausea, emesis, ototoxicity, sensory neuropathy

ALL, Acute lymphoblastic leukemia; CLL, chronic lymphocytic leukemia; NHL, non-Hodgkin's lymphoma.

from neutropenia and life-threatening bleeding from thrombocytopenia. For most drugs, treatment schedules give successive doses every 2 to 4 weeks. This interval between successive doses, the *cycle* of chemotherapy, allows recovery of blood counts and other side effects before administration of the next dose. The concept of *dose intensity* is also important. Cellular killing with chemotherapy follows first-order kinetics: A given dose of drug kills only a fraction of tumor cells. The dose-response curve for chemotherapy drugs is steep. Therefore, the greater the dose administered, the greater the kill: A 2-fold increase in dose can lead to a 10-fold increase in tumor cell kill. This also means that dose reductions may adversely affect the eventual cure rate. Arbitrary reductions in doses of chemotherapy to spare patients toxicity should be avoided. Shortening of the duration of cycles of chemotherapy using growth factor support—a "dose-dense" approach—has been shown to improve survival in selected patients when compared with traditional chemotherapy for breast cancer.

Single chemotherapy agents seldom cure cancer. Combination chemotherapy regimens have therefore been developed for a variety of cancers. Combination therapy provides maximal cell kill and broader coverage of resistant cells; it may also prevent or slow the development of resistant cells. Drugs used in a combination are chosen because they have known efficacy as single agents but have differing mechanisms of action and non-overlapping toxicity profiles. These regimens are commonly referred to by acronyms, such as CHOP (cyclophosphamide, doxorubicin, vincristine, and prednisone) for lymphoma or FOLFOX (5-fluorouracil, leucovorin, and oxaliplatin) for colorectal cancer.

Indications for Chemotherapy

Chemotherapy for localized or advanced cancers is summarized in (Table 55-3). *Adjuvant* chemotherapy refers to its use after the primary tumor has been resected. Here, chemotherapy is directed against presumed systemic micrometastases in patients who are at high risk for recurrence. In the example of stage III colon cancer (described earlier), 6 months of adjuvant

TABLE 55-3 EFFICACY OF MEDICAL THERAPY IN SELECTED CANCERS

CURE POSSIBLE IN ADVANCED SETTING

Testicular cancer
Acute leukemia: lymphocytic, promyelocytic, selected myelocytic
Lymphomas: Hodgkin's lymphoma, selected non-Hodgkin's lymphomas
Childhood solid tumors: rhabdomyosarcoma, Ewing's sarcoma, Wilms' tumor
Choriocarcinoma
Small cell lung cancer

CURE POSSIBLE IN ADJUVANT SETTING

Breast cancer
Colorectal cancer
Osteosarcoma
Non–small cell lung cancer

INCREASED SURVIVAL AND PALLIATION IN ADVANCED DISEASE

Colorectal cancer
Breast cancer
Ovarian cancer
Head and neck cancer
Bladder cancer
Small cell lung cancer
Hepatocellular cancer
Renal cancer
Multiple myeloma

chemotherapy after colonic resection can reduce the patient's likelihood of developing recurrent cancer from 50% to 25%. Adjuvant chemotherapy has been shown to increase cure rates in other cancers.

Neoadjuvant or *preoperative* chemotherapy refers to the use of chemotherapy before surgery, sometimes in combination with radiation therapy. If successful, neoadjuvant therapy can reduce the size of the tumor and consequently permit less removal of normal tissue, such as a lumpectomy instead of a mastectomy in breast cancer or limb-sparing surgery instead of amputation in extremity sarcoma. In certain tumor sites, such as the larynx or the anal canal, neoadjuvant therapy can obliterate the tumor and avoid the need for surgery altogether.

Chemotherapy is most often employed in the treatment of metastatic disease for which surgery or radiation therapy is ineffective. Chemotherapy can sometimes be curative, (e.g., in certain lymphomas or testicular cancers). Even when it is not curative, chemotherapy often extends survival and improves cancer-related symptoms and quality of life.

Limitations of Chemotherapy

Chemotherapy is curative only under certain circumstances, because it is inherently limited by side effects (i.e., the dose ceiling). There are several reasons for the inability of standard doses of chemotherapy to cure cancer. First, tumor cell kinetics naturally protect against chemotherapy. When chemotherapy was initially developed, it was believed that tumors contained a percentage of cells traversing the cell cycle. However, most human tumors display Gompertzian growth kinetics—that is, the rate of tumor cell doubling *slows* progressively as tumor size increases. Therefore, the growth fraction of tumors is greatest when a tumor is clinically undetectable. Be the time the patient is symptomatic and has clinically evident disease, the growth fraction of tumors can be less than 5%. Chemotherapy can be successful in the adjuvant setting (when the burden of disease is minimal), but it rarely results in cure in the metastatic setting.

Second, cancer cells can be resistant to chemotherapy. One of the most important forms of resistance is intrinsic and is mediated by an evolutionarily conserved cell membrane efflux pump called *P-glycoprotein*. Resistance can also be acquired after a period of exposure to chemotherapy agents by a variety of mechanisms; for example, tumor cells can decrease the uptake of methotrexate by decreasing the expression of the folate transporter, or they can amplify expression of the target enzyme thymidylate synthase when treated with 5-fluorouracil.

Third, mutations in the *TP53* gene are common in various cancers. The TP53 protein causes cell-cycle arrest and mediates apoptosis when DNA damage occurs. In the absence of a functioning TP53, cancer cells are protected from chemotherapy-induced apoptosis.

Stem Cell Transplantation

One way of overcoming the limitations of chemotherapy is to increase the dose given to patients. However, delivery of higher doses can lead to life-threatening complications as a result of bone marrow suppression and other end-organ damage. Stem cell transplantation is a procedure whereby patients are given myeloablative doses of chemotherapy (sometimes with radiation therapy) and then "rescued" with infusions of peripheral blood or bone marrow stem cells that reconstitute the ablated bone marrow. The source of stem cells can be the patients themselves (*autologous* transplantation) or a human leukocyte antigen–matched related or unrelated donor (*allogeneic* transplantation). Stem cell transplantation improves survival in selected patients with chronic myelogenous leukemia (CML), relapsed Hodgkin's and non-Hodgkin's lymphoma, refractory acute myelogenous leukemia, or multiple myeloma.

Allogeneic transplantations are more successful in inducing cures than autologous transplantations, owing to the immunologic response mounted by the donor cells, termed *graft-versus-tumor* effect. Newer approaches to stem cell transplantation take advantage of this phenomenon by using lower, nonmyeloablative doses of chemotherapy and relying on the graft-versus-tumor effect to achieve tumor remissions. However, allogeneic transplantations can be offered only to a minority of patients because of the limited availability of matched donors (particularly in ethnic minority populations) and the inability of older patients and those with comorbid illnesses to tolerate this procedure. To increase the availability of donors, umbilical cord blood is being studied as a source of stem cells.

The complications of stem cell transplantation are primarily related to the toxicity of chemotherapy and radiation therapy to vital organs, including lungs and liver. Long-term morbidity and mortality after allogeneic transplantation can result from *graft-versus-host disease* and from complications of immunosuppressive agents used to treat it.

Endocrine Therapy

Cancers originating from tissues that are regulated by hormones, such as breast and prostate tissues, may to be susceptible to hormonal control mechanisms even when metastatic. Endocrine therapy includes the use of both hormonal and anti-hormonal agents that work as antagonists or partial agonists.

Many patients with metastatic breast cancer express hormone receptors (estrogen or progesterone) in tumor cells. More than 60% of these patients respond either to tamoxifen, an estrogen receptor modulator, or to aromatase inhibitors (letrozole, anastrozole, or exemestane), which inhibit adrenal steroid production. Similar responses are observed in men with metastatic prostate cancer treated with the luteinizing hormone–releasing hormone agonists leuprolide or goserelin, which decrease testosterone to castrate levels.

In selected breast and prostate cancer patients, metastatic disease can be controlled for years with only endocrine therapy. Tamoxifen and the aromatase inhibitors are also highly effective adjuvant treatment after breast cancer resection. Furthermore, tamoxifen has been shown to reduce the incidence of breast cancer by 50% in healthy women who are at high risk for developing breast cancer.

Targeted Therapy

The limitations of chemotherapy, coupled with a greater understanding of cancer cell biology, have led to the development of a new class of drugs directed against targets that are relatively specific to cancer cells: growth factors and signaling molecules that are essential for proliferation of tumor cells; cell-cycle proteins; regulators of apoptosis; and molecules mediating host-tumor interactions such as angiogenesis and tumor immunity (Fig. 55-1). These agents include monoclonal antibodies directed against cell surface antigens or growth factors, specific or multi-targeted receptor tyrosine kinase inhibitors, specific pathway signal transduction inhibitors, antisense oligonucleotides, and gene therapies. Additional agents are under development. The usual side effects of chemotherapy, such as myelosuppression, nausea, emesis, diarrhea, and alopecia, are not observed with these drugs. However, other toxicities require careful monitoring and management (Table 55-4).

The best-known targeted therapy agent is imatinib, which inhibits both BCR-ABL, the constitutively active fusion product

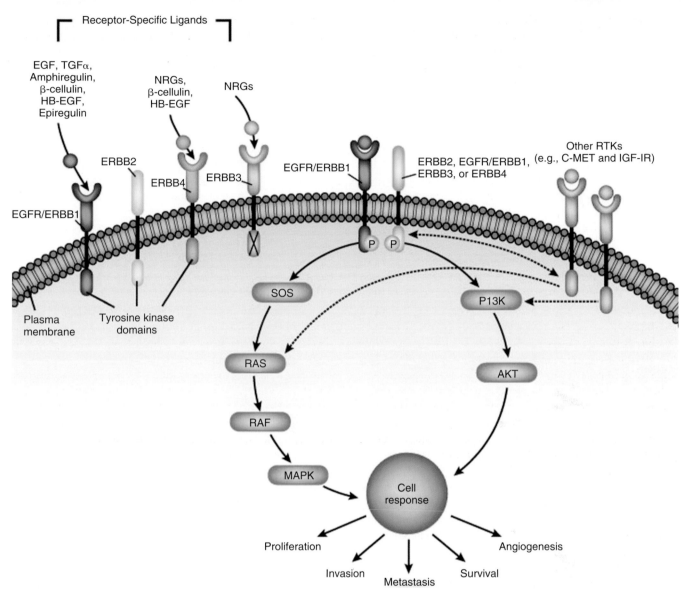

FIGURE 55-1 The epidermal growth factor receptor (EGFR) pathway and related therapeutic targets. This figure depicts the transmembrane receptors of the EGFR family and the molecules involved in downstream signal transduction that ultimately lead to control of key proteins affecting cell survival, growth, and proliferation. Approved therapeutic agents targeting these molecules include cetuximab and panitumumab (EGFR); erlotinib and gefitinib (EGFR tyrosine kinases); trastuzumab, pertuzumab, and lapatinib (ERBB2); and sorafenib and vemurafenib (RAF). Several other agents are currently in clinical development, including those targeting PI3K, AKT, MAPK, and ERBB3. HB-EBF, Heparin-binding EGF-like growth factor; IGF-IR, insulin-like growth factor-I receptor; NRGs, neuregulins; P, elemental phosphorus; RTKs, receptor tyrosine kinases; TNF-α, tumor necrosis factor-α. (Modified from Doebele RC, Oton AB, Peled N, et al: New strategies to overcome limitations of reversible EGFR tyrosine kinase inhibitor therapy in non-small cell lung cancer. Lung Cancer 69:1–12, 2010.)

arising from the Philadelphia chromosome of CML, and KIT (c-kit, CD117), which is overexpressed in gastrointestinal stromal tumors (GIST). The daily oral administration of imatinib results in complete hematologic responses in more than 90% of patients in chronic-phase CML and partial responses in more than 50% of patients with metastatic GIST. Although imatinib is a major advance, it is not considered curative in most patients. Cancer cells rapidly evolve to escape cell kill from targeted therapies by employing new mutations and redundant intracellular pathways. Multiple parallel clones evolve within a given tumor, and some are resistant to the targeted therapy. Drug resistance to imatinib occurs in the form of a mutation in the kinase domain of *ABL* that leads to poor binding of the drug.

The success of imatinib as a single agent is unlikely to be replicated in many other malignancies, in which multiple redundant signaling pathways are dysregulated. Increasingly, tyrosine kinase inhibitors with multiple (as opposed to specific) targets are being studied. Sorafenib and sunitinib are two examples of such agents that inhibit various pathways, including vascular endothelial growth factor (VEGF), platelet-derived growth factor (PDGF), and KIT. Studies have shown these drugs to be effective in renal and liver cancers.

Targeted therapy drugs can increase the efficacy of chemotherapy through various mechanisms. For instance, bevacizumab, an anti-angiogenic agent directed against the pro-angiogenic VEGF, increases both response and survival rates when

TABLE 55-4 COMMONLY USED TARGETED THERAPY AGENTS

DRUG	CANCERS TREATED	TARGETS	COMMON SIDE EFFECTS
MONOCLONAL ANTIBODIES			
Alemtuzumab	CLL	CD52	Myelosuppression, fever, rash
Bevacizumab	Colorectal, renal, lung	VEGF	Hypertension, proteinuria, bleeding, thromboembolism
Cetuximab	Colorectal	EGFR	Rash
Ipilimumab	Metastatic melanoma	CTLA4	Cytokine release storm
Ofatumumab	CLL	CD20	Rash, diarrhea, respiratory tract infections
Panitumumab	Colorectal	EGFR	Rash
Pertuzumab	Breast	HER2	Rash, diarrhea
Rituximab	NHL	CD20	Infusional reaction, skin reactions
Trastuzumab	Breast	HER2/Neu	Infusional reaction, congestive heart failure
SIGNAL TRANSDUCTION INHIBITORS			
Axitinib	Renal	VEGF, PDGF, KIT	Hypertension, hand-foot syndrome, diarrhea
Crizotinib	Lung	EML4-ALK	Edema, diarrhea
Dasatinib	CML	BCR-ABL	Myelosuppression, pleural effusions
Imatinib	CML, GIST	BCR-ABL	Diarrhea, fluid retention, myelosuppression
Erlotinib	Lung, pancreas	EGFR tyrosine kinase	Rash, diarrhea
Gefitinib	Lung	EGFR tyrosine kinase	Rash, hypertension
Lapatinib	Breast	HER2, EGFR	Rash, diarrhea
Regorafenib	GIST, colorectal	VEGF	Hypertension, hepatotoxicity, dysphonia
Sunitinib	Renal, GIST	VEGF, PDGF, KIT	Rash, diarrhea, fatigue
Sorafenib	Liver, renal	VEGF, PDGF, KIT	Hypertension, fatigue, diarrhea, hand-foot syndrome
Vandetanib	Medullary thyroid	VEGF, EGFR, RET	Rash, abdominal pain, diarrhea
Vemurafenib	Melanoma	BRAF	Rash, skin lesions, arthralgia
OTHERS			
All-*trans*-retinoic-acid	Acute promyelocytic leukemia	Differentiating agent	Vitamin A toxicity, retinoic acid syndrome, hyperlipidemia
Azacitidine	Myelodysplasia	Hypomethylating agent	Myelosuppression, injection site reactions
Bortezomib	Lymphoma, myeloma	Proteasome inhibitor	Rash, nausea, emesis, neuropathy
Everolimus	Renal, breast, neuroendocrine	mTOR inhibitor	Hyperglycemia, diarrhea, fatigue

CLL, Chronic lymphocytic leukemia; CML, chronic myelogenous leukemia; CTLA4, cytotoxic T lymphocyte–associated protein 4; EGFR, epidermal growth factor receptor; GIST, gastrointestinal stromal tumor; mTOR, mammalian target of rafampin; NHL, non-Hodgkin's lymphoma; VEGF, vascular endothelial growth factor.

combined with standard chemotherapy in advanced colorectal cancer. Similarly, the EGFR antagonists, cetuximab and panitumumab, increase the efficacy of irinotecan-based chemotherapy in colorectal cancer and that of definitive radiation therapy in oropharyngeal cancers. The availability of these agents has increased the number of drug combinations that can be used in particular cancers. For example, multiple combinations of chemotherapy and targeted therapy are now available for the treatment of advanced colon cancer. Correspondingly, the median survival time of patients with this disease has doubled.

Biologic and Immunologic Therapy

Cytokines that use host immunomodulatory effects as their primary mechanism of action are classified as *biologic response modifiers* or *biologic agents*. Monoclonal antibodies are sometimes classified as biologic agents, although here they have been reviewed under targeted therapy (see earlier discussion). Interferons are commonly used in CML, although they are not as successful as imatinib in inducing responses. Interferons are also used for the treatment of hairy cell leukemia, Kaposi's sarcoma, and selected melanomas and renal cell carcinomas. Interleukin-2 (IL-2) functions as a T-cell growth factor and induces lymphokine-activated and natural killer cell activity. IL-2 can induce responses in 10% to 20% of patients with metastatic melanoma or renal cell carcinoma. In a minority of these patients, responses are complete and last for years. However, IL-2 has toxicity—in particular, a capillary leak syndrome that leads to hypotension, edema, renal insufficiency, and even death.

Immunotherapy agents act by altering the host immune response to the tumor. Cancer vaccines, such as the dendritic cell vaccine sipuleucel-T for prostate cancer, are primed to target cells with specific tumor antigens. Molecules that achieve immune checkpoint blockade have some benefit in melanoma. These agents block T-cell inhibitory molecules such as cytotoxic T lymphocyte–associated protein 4 and programmed cell death 1, thereby releasing T-cells to actively target cancer cells.

Personalized Medicine

The field of oncology is rapidly moving toward an era in which individual patient biospecimens can be evaluated using advanced techniques to reveal specific molecular aberrations that can then be targeted with precise therapeutic agents. Such an approach is referred to by various names, including *precision* or *personalized medicine* and *genomics-driven therapeutics*. The time and costs involved in analyzing the whole genome from a patient's tumor are now much reduced and continue to fall rapidly. In addition to DNA, whole transcriptome (RNA), epigenome (DNA methylation), and single-nucleotide polymorphism (SNP array) analyses can also be performed. Several cancers have already been sequenced completely. Such work creates "reference libraries" against which a patient's tumor can be tested. Based on findings from such analyses, specific drugs or regimens can be recommended for individual patients. Currently used assays include a 21-gene expression profile in breast cancer, *KRAS* in colorectal cancer, *EGFR* and *EML4-ALK* in lung cancer, and *BRAF* in melanoma. Such evaluation of tumor tissues allows patients to participate in clinical trials of targeted therapies, which may ultimately identify agents that further improve clinical outcomes.

EVALUATION OF RESPONSE

The efficacy of cancer-directed therapies is gauged by various methods and has been granted its own vocabulary. In patients with metastatic disease, all known sites of disease are monitored by physical examinations and serial radiologic imaging. Responses are judged according to the internationally accepted Response Evaluation Criteria in Solid Tumors (RECIST) rules. Disappearance of all known lesions is called a *complete response*, whereas a 30% or greater reduction in size is called a *partial response*. Appearance of new lesions or an increase in the size of known lesions by 20% is termed *progression of disease* and implies failure of treatment. A tumor that is neither responding nor progressing is termed *stable disease*.

The percentage of patients who experience a response is called the *response rate* to the agent or agents being administered. New drugs are often evaluated on the basis of response rates. However, a "response" does not imply cure. Even a drug with a 100% response rate is not curative if all patients relapse. Therefore, the "gold standard" for measuring the efficacy of a drug is considered to be an improvement in *survival*, or its surrogate, *disease-free survival*—the time interval during which the patient is alive without disease. The use of effective second-line therapies may minimize the survival differences between two treatments prescribed as initial therapy, and in this context, disease-free survival can serve as an important end point in evaluating new regimens. Increasingly, quality-of-life end points such as use of pain medications or patient-reported outcomes are being used to assess the efficacy of drugs in palliation. In patients receiving adjuvant therapy, response rates cannot be measured because there is no clinically evident disease: Disease-free survival and overall survival are the only end points of efficacy in this setting. Serial measurement of tumor markers can also be useful in identifying recurrence of cancer and monitoring response to therapy in patients with some cancers.

SUPPORTIVE CARE

Supportive care interventions can improve the safety and tolerability of cancer treatments. Many drugs can moderate chemotherapy-related side effects. Serotonin receptor antagonists and neurokinin-1 receptor antagonists, in combination with older antiemetic drugs, may control chemotherapy-induced nausea and vomiting. Granulocyte colony-stimulating factor (filgrastim) and granulocyte-macrophage colony-stimulating factor (sargramostim) stimulate the proliferation and differentiation of myeloid progenitor cells and can prevent or minimize the duration of chemotherapy-induced neutropenia and reduce the likelihood of neutropenic fever. These agents are also used to mobilize and collect stem cells for transplantation. Filgrastim can shorten the duration of cycles of chemotherapy, permitting the dose-dense approach in adjuvant treatment of breast cancer (see earlier discussion). Recombinant human keratinocyte growth factor (palifermin) reduces chemotherapy- and radiation therapy–induced mucositis.

Supportive care is an integral part of the treatment of cancer, particularly in noncurative settings. Palliative aspects of treating cancer address not only physical symptoms, in particular pain syndromes, but also psychosocial and spiritual concerns. Chemotherapy and radiation therapy are often used with palliative intent and can improve quality of life.

Acknowledgments

Dr. Khorana is supported by grants from the National Cancer Institute (K23 CA120587), the National Heart, Lung and Blood Institute (R01HL095109), and the V Foundation and would like to acknowledge the Sondra and Stephen Hardis Endowed Chair in Oncology for research support.

SUGGESTED READINGS

Aparicio S, Caldas C: The implications of clonal genome evolution for cancer medicine, N Engl J Med 368:842–851, 2013.

DeVita VT, Rosenberg SA: Two hundred years of cancer research, N Engl J Med 366:2207–2214, 2012.

Garraway LA: Genomics-driven oncology: framework for an emerging paradigm, J Clin Oncol 31:1806–1814, 2013.

Vogelstein B, Papadopoulos N, Velculescu VE, et al: Cancer genome landscapes, Science 339:1546–1558, 2013.

Yap TA, Omlin A, de Bono JS: Development of therapeutic combinations targeting major cancer signaling pathways, J Clin Oncol 31:1592–1605, 2013.

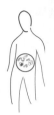

56

Lung Cancer

Patrick C. Ma

● DEFINITION AND EPIDEMIOLOGY

Lung cancer is the second most common cancer in both women and men; however, it is the leading cause of cancer death in both genders in the United States, and an estimated 1 million people die worldwide of lung cancer each year. Despite recent advances in understanding of the biology and genetics of lung cancer and the advent of novel therapeutic agents for its treatment, the 5-year survival rate for patients with lung cancer is only about 15%. The relatively poor rate of long-term survival partly stems from the fact that most patients with lung cancer have an advanced stage of the disease at the time of diagnosis.

There are two major types of bronchogenic carcinoma: *small cell* carcinoma (SCLC) (E-Fig. 56-1) and *non–small cell* carcinoma (NSCLC). NSCLCs are more common and include adenocarcinoma (32%) (E-Fig. 56-2), squamous cell carcinoma (30%) (E-Fig. 56-3), large cell carcinoma (10%) (E-Fig. 56-4), and some more poorly differentiated histologic subtypes not otherwise specified (NOS). SCLCs account for fewer than 20% of all bronchogenic carcinomas.

A current or prior cigarette smoking history remains the leading known risk factor for the development of lung cancer, although up to 15% of newly diagnosed NSCLC cases, often of the adenocarcinoma subtype, are seen in nonsmokers. It has been estimated that 1 in 5 adults is a current everyday cigarette smoker, implying that lung cancer will continue to be a major public health burden in the coming decades. SCLC is predominantly correlated with cigarette smoking, which plays a key pathogenic role in the disease, whereas NSCLC is commonly diagnosed in never-smokers or in those with only a light-smoking history. In recent years, it has been recognized that lung cancer in smokers is a different disease from lung cancer in nonsmokers at both the molecular and the genetic/genomic levels.

The risk for lung cancer is generally proportionate to number of cigarette pack-years smoked (packs per day × years smoked), and the incidence peaks in the sixth and seventh decades. Ex-smokers show a persistent risk for lung cancer throughout life. Passive smoking also contributes as a cause of lung cancer in a portion of nonsmokers who develop the disease. Nonsmokers who live with smokers have a more than 30% increased risk of developing lung cancer. Other risk factors for lung cancer include environmental hazards such as asbestos and petroleum exposure. Smoking is considered an important cofactor of lung cancer in the setting of asbestos exposure. Radon exposure also increases the risk for lung cancer (see Chapter 54).

Understanding of the underlying pathogenic mechanisms of lung cancer has evolved to recognize the disease as a genetic or even genomic disease. An ever-growling list of oncogenic alterations identified in both proto-oncogenes and tumor suppressor genes is accumulating as a result of the genomic analysis effort in recent years, including The Cancer Genome Atlas (TCGA) project sponsored by the National Institutes of Health (NIH) in the United States (see later discussion).

Unique molecular-genomic subgroups of lung cancer have been recognized, including those harboring (1) mutated epidermal growth factor receptor (*EGFR/ERBB1*), (2) mutated Kirsten rat sarcoma viral oncogene homolog (*KRAS*), and (3) anaplastic lymphoma kinase (*ALK*) 2p23 chromosomal rearrangement, more commonly as *EML4-ALK,* a fusion with echinoderm microtubule-associated protein-like 4 (*EML4*). Importantly, these oncogenic genomic alterations provide therapeutic windows of opportunity, especially in the context of oncogenic addiction resulting from these alterations in the tumor cells.

Several targeted therapies have been approved by the U.S. Food and Drug Administration (FDA) for treatment of advanced NSCLCs containing mutated *EGFR* (erlotinib, afatinib, and gefitinib) or the *ALK* 2p23 rearrangement (crizotinib). Lung cancers with *EGFR* mutations are more frequently identified in never-smokers or in those with a light-smoking history, are more often of the adenocarcinoma subtype, and are more often, but not exclusively, diagnosed in females and in patients of East Asian ethnicity. *KRAS*-mutated lung cancers are found primarily in patients with heavier smoking exposure. Lung cancers with mutated *EGFR* and those with the *ALK* 2p23 rearrangement are typically seen in younger patient populations, with the median age at diagnosis being approximately 55 years.

● PATHOLOGY

Histologic Subgroups

Non–Small Cell Lung Carcinomas

Most lung cancers fall under the major histologic subgroup of NSCLCs. Of these, *adenocarcinomas* and *squamous cell carcinomas* are the most common.

Adenocarcinomas

Adenocarcinoma is the most commonly diagnosed subtype of lung cancer, accounting for approximately 40% of lung cancer diagnoses and 65,000 deaths each year in the United States. It is the histologic subtype most commonly diagnosed in nonsmokers. Primary lung adenocarcinomas are usually found in the periphery of the lung (75%) (E-Fig. 56-5), in contrast to squamous cell carcinomas.

Pathologically, adenocarcinomas typically form glandular structures and produce mucus. *EGFR* mutations are more commonly associated with nonmucinous lung adenocarcinoma, whereas the mucinous subtype is more commonly associated with mutated *KRAS*. The tumor cells typically stain positive for cytokeratin 7 (CK7), thyroid transcription factor 1 (TTF-1), carcinoembryonic antigen (CEA), mucin, and surfactant apoprotein and negative for cytokeratin 20 (CK20). Adenocarcinomas respond poorly to therapy and have a poor prognosis.

Bronchoalveolar cell carcinomas (BAC), a subset of adenocarcinomas, are the most common form of lung cancer found in nonsmokers and young patients. They manifest as lung infiltrates or as a solitary nodule and can be accompanied by bronchorrhea. BAC cells can grow in a lepidic (scaly) pattern and spread along alveolar walls.

Squamous Cell Carcinomas

Squamous cell carcinomas arise from the epithelial layer of the bronchial wall. Normal columnar epithelial cells undergo metaplasia, dysplasia, and then localized carcinoma (*carcinoma in situ*) formation; this can then further extend and invade beyond the bronchial mucosa as it acquires a full malignant invasive phenotype (carcinoma). Because most squamous cell carcinomas arise within central airways (E-Fig. 56-6), the airway lumen may become obstructed, leading to collapse of the lung (atelectasis) or postobstructive pneumonia. Although necrosis and cavity formation can occur in any lung tumor, this feature is more common in squamous cell carcinomas. Because of their slow rate of growth, these tumors have the lowest propensity for metastasis of all types of lung cancer. Pathologically, squamous cell carcinomas can be distinguished from other NSCLCs by the presence of keratinization, pearl formation, and intercellular bridging.

Adenosquamous Carcinomas

Adenosquamous carcinomas constitute between 0.4% and 4% of cases and may have a worse prognosis. They have components of both adenocarcinoma and squamous cell carcinoma, each comprising at least 10% of the tumor.

Large Cell Carcinomas

Large cell carcinomas frequently develop as a peripheral lesion and may be associated with pneumonitis and hilar adenopathy. The two main subtypes are *giant cell carcinoma*, an anaplastic tumor that has a median survival time of less than 1 year; and *clear cell carcinoma*, a tumor that resembles renal cell carcinoma and has fewer malignant features.

NSCLC Not Otherwise Specified

Despite one's best efforts in defining subtype differentiation of a NSCLC through histology and immunophenotyping, there may remain poorly differentiated tumors that defy such classification. These are designated NSCLC-NOS.

Small Cell Lung Carcinoma

SCLC cells are of pulmonary neuroendocrine cell origin and are often associated with paraneoplastic syndromes (Table 56-1). SCLCs typically are perihilar in location, not infrequently

TABLE 56-1	PARANEOPLASTIC SYNDROMES ASSOCIATED WITH LUNG CANCER	
SYNDROME	**CELL TYPE**	**MECHANISM**
Hypertrophic pulmonary osteoarthropathy and clubbing	All except small cell	Unknown
Hyponatremia	Small cell most common; may be any type	SIADH, ectopic antidiuretic hormone production by tumor
Hypercalcemia	Usually squamous cell	Bone metastases, osteoclast-activating factor, parathyroid hormone–like hormone, prostaglandins
Cushing syndrome	Usually small cell	Ectopic ACTH production
Eaton-Lambert myasthenic syndrome	Usually small cell	Voltage-sensitive calcium channel antibodies in >75%; affects presynaptic neuronal calcium channel activity
Other neuromyopathic disorders	Small cell most common; may be any type	Antineuronal nuclear antibodies, also known as anti-Hu; others unknown
Thrombophlebitis	All types	Unknown

ACTH, Adrenocorticotropic hormone; *SIADH*, syndrome of inappropriate secretion of antidiuretic hormone.

originate in the main bronchi, and often have associated malignant adenopathy (E-Fig. 56-7). These tumors have a high propensity for metastasis, most commonly to the thoracic lymph nodes, bones, liver, adrenal glands, and brain. Most patients are already affected with metastatic disease at the time of presentation. SCLC has traditionally been staged as *limited disease* (confined to one hemithorax) or *extensive disease* (distant metastases); although a TNM staging system has recently been suggested. SCLC is an aggressive lung tumor; without treatment, the median survival time of patients with this cancer is less than 5 months. The overall survival at 5 years is 5% and has not improved over the past several decades.

Molecular-Genomic Subtypes

Lung cancer is now increasingly regarded as a disease with collections of often very distinct and heterogeneous molecular and genomic subclasses or disease subgroups (Table 56-2). Many of these molecular-genomic alterations can inform the use of targeted therapeutics and predict responses.

Mutant *EGFR*

EGFR mutation testing and targeting therapy are part of routine clinical care of patients with NSCLC worldwide. Specific somatic *EGFR* gene kinase domain–activating mutations, predominantly occurring in lung adenocarcinoma, predict sensitivity and clinical response to the EGFR inhibitors gefitinib and erlotinib. These mutations are usually found in never-smokers or female light smokers with adenocarcinoma. *EGFR* mutations are more prevalent in Asian patients (30%, compared with 7-10% in Caucasians). Molecular tumor selection by profiling is superior to clinical selection.

ALK 2p23 Rearrangement

The *EML4-ALK* fusion in NSCLC is an oncogenic driver fusion-kinase. Oncogenic *ALK*-rearrangements occur in 3% to 7% of NSCLCs, in light smokers (<10 pack-years) or never-smokers. In

TABLE 56-2 MOLECULAR-GENOMIC SUBTYPES OF NSCLC

ONCOGENE	CLASS OF MOLECULAR-GENOMIC ALTERATIONS	CHARACTERISTICS
EGFR-mutant	Somatic missense mutations (most common with L858R in exon 21) and exon 19 deletions	More frequent in Asians, females, never-smokers or light smokers; most frequently adenocarcinoma subtype Sensitizing to EGFR inhibitors erlotinib, gefitinib, and afatinib T790M mutation in EGFR is resistant to the inhibitors.
EML4-ALK	ALK 2p23 chromosomal translocation	3-7% of NSCLCs More common in light smokers (<10 pack-years) or never-smokers Sensitizing to ALK inhibitor crizotinib
KRAS-mutant	Somatic mutations	Found in 15-25% lung adenocarcinomas Less common but can be present in squamous cell carcinomas More commonly seen in former or current cigarette smokers No effective targeted treatment at present
PIK3CA-mutant	Somatic mutations	The PIK3CA gene encodes the $p110\alpha$, one of the catalytic subunits, of PI3K, which belongs to a family of lipid kinases involved in many cellular processes, including cell growth, proliferation, survival and motility. Mutated in 1-3% of all NSCLCs More common in squamous cell carcinoma PIK3CA shows significant potential as a candidate for targeted therapy
BRAF-mutant	Somatic mutations	Belong to a family of serine-threonine protein kinases Identified in 1-3% of cases Sensitizing to a mutated BRAF–specific inhibitor, vemurafenib, which has been approved by the FDA for treatment in V600E-BRAF–mediated cutaneous melanoma
HER2	Amplification, mutations, small insertions	HER2 alterations were identified in ~2% to 4% of NSCLCs In the selected population of EGFR/KRAS/ALK-mutation–negative patients, HER2 mutations can reach up to 6% Predominantly found in females, nonsmokers; predominantly adenocarcinoma subtype May be associated with sensitivity to HER2-targeting drugs (trastuzumab, lapatinib, pertuzumab, and T-DM1) used in breast cancer
LKB1	Inactivating mutations, deletion	A tumor suppressor gene also known as STK11 Mutational frequency about 17-35% of NSCLCs in Caucasians but only 3-7% in the Asian population
RET-fusion	Chromosomal translocations	Recently found in some lung adenocarcinomas (1-2%)
ROS1-fusion	Chromosomal translocations	ROS1 is a receptor tyrosine kinase of the insulin receptor family ROS1-fusions were identified in ~2% of NSCLCs More commonly found in younger people, more likely in never-smokers, and Asian patients are overrepresented ROS1-positive status may be associated with response to the kinase inhibitor crizotinib (ALK/MET inhibitor)
FGFR1	Amplification and mutations	Gene belongs to the family of FGFR TK members that includes FGFR types 1, 2, 3 and 4. Genomic alterations of FGFR1 have been identified predominantly in the squamous subtypes of lung cancer, raising the possibility of targeted therapy in this unique cancer subtype
MET	Alternative spliced variant, mutations, amplification, receptor overexpression	The MET proto-oncogene is a key invasive signaling axis. MET gene amplification can be found in 2-4% of NSCLCs, whereas overexpression of its receptor protein is much more common MET overexpression has been correlated with poor prognosis. A number of MET-targeting therapeutic agents have entered clinical trial studies. MET high expression may be a predictive biomarker of treatment response.
BCL2	Amplification, receptor overexpression	BCL2 overexpression is more common in SCLC than in NSCLC. Various BH3 mimetics have been developed to target the mitochondrial antiapoptotic marker BCL2 in human cancers (e.g. SCLC, CLL).

CLL, Chronic lymphocytic leukemia; EGFR, epithelial growth factor receptor; FDA, U.S. Food and Drug Administration; FGFR, fibroblast growth factor receptor; NSCLC, non–small cell lung cancer; PI3K, phosphatidyl 3-kinase; SCLC, small cell lung cancer; TK, tyrosine kinase.

most cases, EML4-ALK fusions do not overlap with other oncogenic mutations of EGFR or KRAS.

Mutant KRAS

KRAS gene mutations are uncommon in squamous cell carcinomas but are present in 15% to 25% of lung adenocarcinomas. KRAS mutations are more commonly seen in former or current cigarette smokers than in never-smokers or light smokers. There is currently no effective targeted treatment for mutated KRAS.

The Lung Cancer Genome

In the last decade, the TCGA project in comprehensive genomic analysis of human cancers has brought forth a renewed understanding of lung cancer at the genomic level.

The TCGA analysis mapped the hallmarks of lung adenocarcinoma and identified a relatively high exonic somatic mutation rate (mean, 12.0 events per megabase), similar to the rate found in squamous cell lung carcinoma. These lung cancer types also have similar copy number profiles. Three distinct expression subtypes of lung adenocarcinoma were identified from RNA-sequencing data: bronchioid, magnoid, and squamoid. In addition, multiple gene fusions were found to be expressed in lung adenocarcinomas, and multiple mechanisms for CDKN2A inactivation were uncovered.

For squamous cell NSCLCs, a most unexpected finding in the TCGA study was the identification of loss-of-function mutations in the HLA-A gene, which encodes a major histocompatibility complex that plays an important immune regulatory role on the tumor cell surface in antigen presentation and immune recognition. This is regarded as the first evidence of somatic cancer genome alterations evading the immune system by changing their surface antigens. Potential therapeutic targets were identified in most tumors, offering new therapeutic avenues of investigation for targeted therapy in lung cancer.

CLINICAL PRESENTATION

Initial symptoms of lung cancer are usually nonspecific—cough, dyspnea, sputum production, chest pain, and weight loss—and are often attributed to bronchitis or pneumonia. The cancer has often invaded adjacent structures or metastasized when first recognized, causing symptoms that reflect the site of involvement, such as hemoptysis, pleuritic chest pain, and pleura or chest wall invasion; hoarseness (left recurrent laryngeal nerve); pleural effusion related to direct tumor involvement of the pleura or obstruction of lymph flow from the mediastinal nodes (E-Fig. 56-8); dysphagia (esophageal involvement); *malignant pericardial effusion,* which can progress to *cardiac tamponade; spinal cord compression;* and brain metastasis. A malignant pleural effusion precludes resection. Superior vena cava obstruction may result in the *superior vena cava syndrome,* with edema of the face and upper extremities due to impaired venous return.

The Physical examination can be normal but may reveal changes in the lungs that reflect the effect of the tumor, such as crackles (e.g., postobstructive pneumonia [E-Fig. 56-9]); inspiratory wheezes, suggestive of airway obstruction; dullness to percussion at the lung bases from underlying pleural effusion; and lymph node enlargement in the supraclavicular (E-Fig. 56-10) or cervical and axillary (distant) areas. The most common sites of metastases are the lymph nodes, liver (E-Fig. 56-11), brain, adrenal glands, kidneys, and lungs.

Lung cancers that occur in the apex of the chest and invade apical chest wall structures are known as *superior sulcus* or *Pancoast tumors* (E-Fig. 56-12). The classic description involves a syndrome of pain radiating down the arm due to tumor erosion into the brachial plexus. Tumor erosion into the cervical sympathetic chain causes *Horner syndrome,* with ptosis, miosis, and anhydrosis over the face and forehead.

DIAGNOSIS AND DIFFERENTIAL DIAGNOSIS
Diagnostic and Staging Work-Up

When possible lung cancer is identified, either incidentally or because of symptoms, a tissue diagnosis is essential unless the patient is not eligible for treatment because of comorbidity. After assessment for metastases, the site of biopsy should be chosen to determine the greatest extent of spread or highest stage of the tumor, if this is feasible. If the apparent tumor is confined to the chest, bronchoscopy is appropriate for central masses, and a transthoracic needle aspiration would be suitable for peripheral lesions. Pleural effusion should be sampled to assess for malignant cells, which would indicate metastatic-stage disease (M1a).

Solitary Pulmonary Nodule

A *solitary pulmonary nodule* (SPN) is a single, rounded lesion in the lung that is 3 cm in diameter or smaller. Although these lesions are commonly lung cancers in certain patient populations, the differential diagnosis of SPN includes many other malignant and benign etiologies. In addition to primary lung cancer (adenocarcinoma; see E-Fig. 56-5), other possible causes include bronchial carcinoid tumors and metastases from extrapulmonary malignancies (e.g., malignant melanoma, sarcoma, colon, kidney, breast, and testicle). Benign etiologies include benign tumors of the lung (hamartomas) (E-Fig. 56-13), infectious granulomas (from fungal diseases including histoplasmosis and coccidioidomycosis as well as mycobacterial disease), lung abscess, vascular abnormalities (arteriovenous malformation), rounded atelectasis, and pseudotumor (pleural fluid trapped within a fissure).

Accurate and early determination is essential and can potentially lead to cure in the case of a malignant tumor. In a benign nodule, it may preclude surgery with its associated risks and complications. Diagnostic evaluation should consider the patient's age, gender, smoking history, family history of lung and other types of cancer, and other relevant risk factors.

Radiographic features of an SPN can be helpful diagnostically. Larger lesions are more likely to be malignant. Lesions 4 to 7 mm in diameter in patients without a history of cancer have a 0.9% chance of being malignant; this probability rises to 18% for lesions 8 mm to 2 cm in diameter, and 50% for those larger than 2 cm. Benign tumors tend to have smooth and discrete borders, whereas irregular and spiculated borders are more likely in malignant SPNs. A benign tumor tends to have a diffuse, central, laminated (onion-skin), or popcorn calcification pattern. Conversely, lesions with peripheral or eccentric (asymmetrical) calcifications are more likely to be malignant. It is important to assess the rate of occurrence of an SPN and its stability by comparing imaging studies with previous scans whenever available. An SPN that has not changed in size for more than 2 years is unlikely to be malignant.

Once a diagnosis of lung cancer is established, staging is necessary for prognostication and treatment. Staging in NSCLC determines whether surgical resection for cure or chemotherapy or radiation therapy is indicated. The tumor-node-metastasis (TNM) system is used (Table 56-3). For staging of SCLC, the Veterans Administration Lung Study Group designations of limited-stage (confined to one hemithorax) and extensive-stage (beyond one hemithorax) are used. Combined chemoradiation therapy with curative intent is considered for the former, but palliative chemotherapy is the treatment of choice for the latter.

Chest computed tomography (CT), including images of the abdomen, is useful to delineate the location and size of the primary tumor and to examine for mediastinal lymph nodes, pleural disease, and adrenal or liver metastases. However, CT has limited ability to distinguish benign from malignant lymphadenopathy in the mediastinum. Positron emission tomography (PET) using 18-fluorodeoxyglucose (FDG) is more sensitive and more specific than CT in the detection of mediastinal lymph node metastases and may also detect unexpected metastases elsewhere. In principle, any suspected mediastinal or extrathoracic metastases identified by imaging alone should be confirmed with tissue sampling before the patient is excluded from being considered an operative candidate. Techniques for invasive staging of the mediastinal lymph nodes include bronchoscopic transbronchial needle aspiration and mediastinoscopy. Mediastinoscopy can also assess mediastinal spread of disease in patients

TABLE 56-3   TNM STAGING SYSTEM FOR LUNG CANCER (2010)

T (PRIMARY TUMOR)

TX	Primary tumor cannot be assessed, or tumor proven by the presence of malignant cells in sputum or bronchial washings but not visualized by imaging or bronchoscopy
T0	No evidence of primary tumor
Tis	Carcinoma in situ
T1	Tumor ≤3 cm in greatest dimension, surrounded by lung or visceral pleura, without bronchoscopic evidence of invasion more proximal than the lobar bronchus (i.e., not in the main bronchus)*
T1a	Tumor ≤2 cm in greatest dimension
T1b	Tumor >2 cm but ≤3 cm in greatest dimension
T2	Tumor >3 cm but ≤7 cm or tumor with any of the following features (T2 tumors with these features are classified T2a if ≤5 cm):
	Involves main bronchus, ≥2 cm distal to the carina
	Invades visceral pleura
	Associated with atelectasis or obstructive pneumonitis that extends to the hilar region but does not involve the entire lung
T2a	Tumor >3 cm but ≤5 cm in greatest dimension
T2b	Tumor >5 cm but ≤7 cm in greatest dimension
T3	Tumor >7 cm or one that directly invades any of the following: chest wall (including superior sulcus tumors), diaphragm, phrenic nerve, mediastinal pleura, parietal pericardium; or tumor in the main bronchus (<2 cm distal to the carina* but without involvement of the carina; or associated atelectasis or obstructive pneumonitis of the entire lung or separate tumor nodule(s) in the same lobe
T4	Tumor of any size that invades any of the following: mediastinum, heart, great vessels, trachea, recurrent laryngeal nerve, esophagus, vertebral body, carina, separate tumor nodule(s) in a different ipsilateral lobe

N (REGIONAL LYMPH NODES)

NX	Regional lymph nodes cannot be assessed
N0	No regional lymph node metastases
N1	Metastasis in ipsilateral peribronchial and/or ipsilateral hilar lymph nodes and intrapulmonary nodes, including involvement by direct extension
N2	Metastasis in ipsilateral mediastinal and/or subcarinal lymph node(s)
N3	Metastasis in contralateral mediastinal, contralateral hilar, ipsilateral or contralateral scalene, or supraclavicular lymph node(s)

M (DISTANT METASTASIS)

MX	Distant metastasis cannot be assessed
M0	No distant metastasis
M1	Distant metastasis
M1a	Separate tumor nodule(s) in a contralateral lobe; tumor with pleural nodules or malignant pleural (or pericardial) effusion†
M1b	Distant metastasis

From Edge S, Byrd DR, Compton CC, et al, editors: AJCC Cancer Staging Manual, ed 7, New York, 2010, Springer.

*The uncommon superficial spreading tumor of any size with its invasive component limited to the bronchial wall, which may extend proximally to the main bronchus, is also classified as T1a.

†Most pleural (and pericardial) effusions with lung cancer are due to tumor. In a few patients, however, multiple cytopathologic examinations of pleural (pericardial) fluid are negative for tumor, and the fluid is nonbloody and is not an exudate. Where these elements and clinical judgment dictate the effusion is not related to the tumor, the effusion should be excluded as a staging element and the patient should be classified as M0.

without definite imaging evidence of lymph node involvement before definitive resection of the lung cancer. PET scanning is limited in its ability to detect brain lesions, and magnetic resonance imaging (MRI) of the brain with intravenous contrast (or CT scanning if MRI cannot be done) should be performed if brain metastasis is suspected. Bone scans are useful for suspected symptomatic bony metastases.

Metastatic disease is now subdivided into those lesions that occurred with "local intrathoracic spread" (M1a)—malignant pleural/pericardial effusion or separate tumor nodule(s) in the contralateral lung—and those that already have "disseminated (extrathoracic) disease" (M1b) in liver, bone, brain, or adrenal gland. M1a disease has a better prognosis than M1b disease.

● TREATMENT

Prevention by avoiding or stopping smoking is a responsibility of all physicians (Chapter 54). The United States Preventive Services Task Force (USPSTF) supports lung cancer screening for the high-risk populations: current and former smokers, aged 55 to 80 years, with a smoking history equivalent to 1 pack per day for 30 years or 2 packs per day for 15 years. The recommendation for screening includes those who have quit within the past 15 years.

Small Cell Lung Cancer

SCLCs can occasionally be resected if no evidence of metastasis is found, but most SCLCs are treated with chemotherapy for systemic disease. SCLC is staged as limited-stage, for which definitive treatment using combination chemoradiation with curative intent is pursued, and extensive-stage, for which chemotherapy with palliative intent is the mainstay of treatment. Combinations of cisplatin/carboplatin and etoposide constitute the standard front-line chemotherapeutic regimen. Topotecan is used for salvage therapy during disease relapse. SCLC responses to both chemotherapy and radiation therapy and long-term survival are possible. However, relapse with progressive therapeutic resistance is usual despite initial treatment response. Prophylactic cranial irradiation enhances overall survival in both limited-stage disease after completion of chemoradiation and extensive disease with response to chemotherapy.

Non–Small Cell Lung Cancer
Early-Stage Disease (Stages I and II)

Surgery is potentially curative for early-stage NSCLC and is indicated for patients with stage I or II disease who are eligible as operative candidates. Lobectomy (or greater) is considered unless the patient has medical comorbidities or is of advanced age. Wedge resection may be considered as an alternative to lobectomy, but patients also may be offered local ablative radiation therapy techniques such as stereotactic body radiation therapy (SBRT) or CyberKnife radiosurgery.

Locally Advanced Disease (Stages IIIA and IIIB)

Patients with stage III disease are heterogeneous, and the optimal treatment strategy is unclear. For stage IIIA disease, curative surgery, in combination with neoadjuvant chemotherapy and radiation, may be offered. Most patients with stage IIIB NSCLC are not surgical candidates, and 5-year survival is poor for this group. Concurrent chemotherapy and radiotherapy are preferable to radiotherapy alone.

Advanced Metastatic Disease (Stage IV)

Chemotherapy improves survival and provides palliation for symptoms in stage IV disease. Patients with high performance often receive doublet chemotherapy, combining a platinum agent (cisplatin or carboplatin) and a second agent (e.g., paclitaxel, pemetrexed, gemcitabine). Histology-specific personalized therapy is now becoming possible; for the adenocarcinoma subtype, pemetrexed is used, and for the squamous cell subtype, gemcitabine.

Genomics-Guided Precision Therapy

Mutational analysis and genomic profiling hold promise for "precision therapy" or "personalized targeted therapy." For example, NSCLC, especially adenocarcinoma, can be viewed as having distinct subgroups of mutated oncogenes, some known to be "actionable" or "targetable" with novel treatment (E-Fig. 56-14). In *EGFR*-mutant lung cancer, the EGFR inhibitor gefitinib or erlotinib improved the progression-free survival rate better than chemotherapy treatment did. An era in which "molecular profiling" trumps profiling by clinical parameters has arrived.

Targeted therapy in lung cancer has already made an impact in terms of a treatment paradigm shift and in clinical outcome. The major obstacle in fully unleashing the power of targeted therapy lies in the invariable development of acquired drug resistance, which ultimately leads to disease progression and death of the patient. The predominant mechanism in erlotinib resistance is the emergence of *EGFR* T790M mutation in exon 20, which accounts for about half of all resistant cases. Other novel mechanisms of acquired erlotinib resistance have come to light more recently, including *MET* amplification or the RTK activation, *PIK3CA* mutation, *EGFR* amplification, *AXL* upregulation, and even histologic SCLC transformation. Various mechanisms of resistance against crizotinib in *ALK*-genotype specific targeted therapy are also being uncovered at a rapid pace.

Currently, a number of Clinical Laboratory Improvement Amendments (CLIA)-certified genomics laboratories perform tumor genomic profiling, but what constitutes the best lung cancer genomic profiling method remains uncertain.

PROGNOSIS

The most important prognostic factor in lung cancer is the TNM stage of the disease at the time of presentation. Poor performance status and weight loss are also negative prognostic factors for survival of patients with lung cancer.

For a deeper discussion on this topic, please see Chapter 191, "Lung Cancer and Other Pulmonary Neoplasms," in Goldman-Cecil Medicine, 25th Edition.

SUGGESTED READINGS

Hirsch FR, Jänne PA, Eberhardt WE, et al: Epidermal growth factor receptor inhibition in lung cancer: status 2012, J Thorac Oncol 8:373–384, 2013.

Imielinski M, Berger AH, Hammerman PS, et al: Mapping the hallmarks of lung adenocarcinoma with massively parallel sequencing, Cell 150:1107–1120, 2012.

National Lung Screening Trial Research Team, Aberle DR, Adams AM, et al: Reduced lung-cancer mortality with low-dose computed tomographic screening, N Engl J Med 365:395–409, 2011.

Rosell R, Bivona TG, Karachaliou N: Genetics and biomarkers in personalization of lung cancer treatment, Lancet 382:720–731, 2013.

Sequist LV, Waltman BA, Dias-Santagata D, et al: Genotypic and histological evolution of lung cancers acquiring resistance to EGFR inhibitors, Sci Transl Med 3(75):75ra26, 2011.

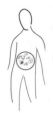

57 Gastrointestinal Cancers

Davendra P.S. Sohal and Alok A. Khorana

● INTRODUCTION

Cancers arising in the gastrointestinal system are among the most common cancers worldwide. Every year, they account for more than 2.7 million deaths globally and approximately 145,000 deaths in the United States. Gastrointestinal cancers are typically epithelial malignancies—carcinomas—with well-defined pathologic patterns of neoplastic transformation. Risk factors and presentations are site specific, and management usually involves multimodality therapy including surgery, chemotherapy, and radiation therapy. Additional contributors to morbidity from these cancers are the complications of malignancy, including intestinal or biliary obstruction and impaired nutrition due to anatomic and physiologic alteration of the digestive system. Therefore, interventions to palliate symptoms and maintain adequate nutrition are an important component of care.

● ESOPHAGEAL CANCER

Epidemiology

Population trends of esophageal cancer are slowly evolving. In the United States, the incidence of esophageal squamous cell carcinoma is declining but the incidence of esophageal adenocarcinoma is rising. These changes mirror the demographic trends in risk factors: prevalence of tobacco and alcohol use, linked to the former, is declining, whereas obesity, reflux disease, and metabolic syndrome, associated with the latter, are increasing.

Pathology

Squamous cell carcinoma is commonly seen in the upper esophagus; it develops, like head and neck cancer, from chronic mucosal injury caused by carcinogens in tobacco smoke and exacerbated by alcohol use. Adenocarcinoma usually arises in the setting of chronic acid reflux and from a background of Barrett's esophagus, involving epithelial metaplasia in the distal esophagus or the gastroesophageal junction. People with Barrett's esophagus have an annual risk of 0.12% of developing this disease, an 11-fold elevation over the general population.

Clinical Presentation

The cardinal symptom of esophageal cancer is dysphagia. Longstanding gastroesophageal reflux disease is often present in adenocarcinoma. Unintentional weight loss due to limited oral intake and other factors is a common clinical association.

Diagnosis

Endoscopy remains the preferred diagnostic test. Visualization for masses and mucosal irregularities yields a quick clinical diagnosis; biopsy of suspicious areas provides histologic confirmation. Endoscopic ultrasound is a useful modality in assessing the T and N components of staging (i.e., depth of tumor invasion into the esophageal wall and beyond, and surrounding lymph node involvement, respectively). Fine-needle aspiration of suspicious lymph nodes can further improve N-staging. Imaging for systemic disease (M-staging) is performed before the therapeutic plan is finalized, preferably with contrast-enhanced computed tomography (CT).

Treatment

If esophageal cancer is diagnosed early (stage I), surgical resection is the treatment of choice. The esophagectomy can be performed with a transthoracic (Ivor-Lewis) or a transhiatal technique, with comparable clinical outcomes. For locally advanced disease (stages II and III), multimodality therapy is required. This consists of chemotherapy, radiation therapy, and surgery. Combined chemoradiation using 5-fluorouracil (5-FU) and cisplatin remains the standard of care for squamous cell cancer; in this setting, surgery may be foregone, especially for cervical esophagus tumors, because chemoradiation can provide good disease control. For adenocarcinomas of the distal esophagus and gastroesophageal junction, there are competing standards of care, including perioperative chemotherapy using epirubicin, cisplatin, and 5-FU; preoperative chemoradiation using paclitaxel and carboplatin; or surgery followed by adjuvant chemotherapy and radiation using 5-FU–based regimens.

For advanced disease (stage IV), combination chemotherapy can improve survival. Trastuzumab is a monoclonal antibody directed against human epidermal growth factor receptor 2 (HER2), a cell surface receptor that signals cellular proliferation. The addition of this agent to standard chemotherapy is of benefit in adenocarcinomas of the gastroesophageal junction that exhibit overexpression of HER2. Supportive care and palliative interventions for dysphagia, such as local irradiation and placement of a feeding tube, can improve quality of life.

Prognosis

Early-stage (stage I) esophageal cancer is curable. Rates of cure for locally advanced (stage II or III) disease are lower, and metastatic disease (stage IV) remains incurable. Five-year survival rates with appropriate treatment are 70%, 40%, 30%, and 5% for stages I, II, III, and IV, respectively.

GASTRIC CANCER

Epidemiology

Gastric adenocarcinoma is one of the rare malignancies that has shown a remarkable decline in incidence and mortality in the United States over the 20th century. Much of this decline can be attributed to refrigeration, which obviated the use of food preservatives that harbor carcinogenic nitrites and nitrosamines. Improved hygiene and sanitation also lowered the prevalence of *Helicobacter pylori* infection, which is associated with gastric cancer. However, this disease remains common in Asian countries (China, Japan, and Korea), in the Middle East, and in Eastern Europe, placing it among the five most common cancers worldwide.

Pathology

Traditionally, two main histologic subtypes exist: diffuse and intestinal. The diffuse type is associated with younger age, poor differentiation, signet ring cells, an increasing incidence, and a worse prognosis. Carriers of inactivating mutations in the E-cadherin gene (*CDH1*), such as those with hereditary diffuse gastric cancer syndrome, are prone to such cancers. The intestinal type is seen in older patients, is differentiated with a background of intestinal metaplasia, and has a declining incidence and a somewhat better prognosis. In many cases, however, this histologic distinction is not possible and does not alter management.

Clinical Presentation

The classic triad is anemia, anorexia, and asthenia. Early satiety (linitis plastica), dysphagia (gastroesophageal junction or cardia tumors), epigastric pain, nausea, vomiting, and gastrointestinal bleeding are also commonly seen. Metastatic spread causing peritoneal carcinomatosis can lead to ascites.

Diagnosis

Esophagogastroduodenoscopy is the preferred diagnostic test. Biopsies to confirm disease should follow, and then metastatic disease assessment by CT. If linitis plastica is suspected, blind biopsies may be needed, because overt mucosal lesions are often not evident. Screening endoscopy is recommended in high-incidence countries such as Japan.

Treatment

Surgery remains the cornerstone of treatment for nonmetastatic disease. The extent of dissection is debated. In high-incidence countries such as Japan and Korea, extended surgery (D2 dissection) to remove the stomach, all surrounding lymph nodes, and the spleen is performed and is associated with clinical benefit. However, this benefit has not been seen in the Western population. For locally advanced disease, in addition to surgery, either perioperative chemotherapy with epirubicin, cisplatin, and 5-FU or postoperative chemoradiation with 5-FU is an acceptable approach. For metastatic disease, first- and second-line palliative chemotherapy can improve outcomes, including survival. For patients with HER2-overexpressing tumors, the addition of trastuzumab to chemotherapy further extends survival.

Prognosis

Clinical outcomes depend on the stage at diagnosis. Early-stage cancer can be cured; 5-year survival rates are 65%, 40%, 15%, and 5% for stages I, II, III, and IV, respectively. Survival outcomes in Japan and Korea are better than in most Western countries; this disparity may be attributable to routine screening endoscopies or to differences in disease biology.

PANCREATOBILIARY CANCERS

Epidemiology

The incidence and mortality of pancreatic ductal adenocarcinoma are slowly but steadily increasing. It is the tenth most common cancer but the fourth leading cause of cancer-related death in the United States. Smoking and chronic pancreatitis are established clinical risk factors. Pancreatic cancer risk increases with inherited mutations in *BRCA1*, *BRCA2*, and *PALB2* and with familial syndromes such as the Peutz-Jeghers and Lynch syndromes. Pancreatic neuroendocrine tumors are uncommon malignancies that originate from the endocrine cells in the pancreas. They may be nonfunctional, or they may secrete hormones such as insulin (insulinoma), gastrin (gastrinoma), glucagon (glucagonoma), or vasoactive intestinal peptide (VIPoma).

Cholangiocarcinoma, defined as cancer arising from the biliary epithelium, comprises intrahepatic and extrahepatic cholangiocarcinoma and gallbladder cancer. It is an uncommon malignancy. Established risk factors include conditions that cause chronic inflammation of the biliary system, such as primary sclerosing cholangitis, cholelithiasis, and infection with liver flukes (*Clonorchis*, *Opsithorcis*), and anatomic abnormalities of the biliary tree (e.g., Caroli's disease, choledochal cysts). Gallbladder cancer is particularly prevalent in Chile and northern India.

Pathology

Pancreatic adenocarcinoma develops with an accumulation of mutations in the pancreatic duct epithelium; the affected genes are *KRAS*, followed by *CDKN2A (p16)*, *TP53*, *SMAD4 (DPC4)*, and others. Histologic progression occurs in various stages of pancreatic intraepithelial neoplasia, leading to invasive adenocarcinoma. Desmoplastic reaction—the production of abundant fibrotic stroma—is often seen in pancreatic cancer.

Clinical Presentation

Painless jaundice is a frequent presenting symptom and is caused by biliary obstruction. Epigastric pain radiating through to the back and new-onset type 2 diabetes mellitus in an adult older 50 years of age without overt obesity-related risk factors should raise suspicion for pancreatic cancer. Constitutional symptoms include anorexia, unintentional weight loss, and malaise. Steatorrhea occurs because of exocrine pancreatic insufficiency. Venous thromboembolism, seen with various malignancies, is most associated with pancreatic cancer and can be a presenting feature. Gallbladder cancer is sometimes an incidental finding during the evaluation of histologic specimens after cholecystectomy, which is commonly performed for presumed cholelithiasis or cholecystitis. Secretory pancreatic neuroendocrine tumors can cause symptoms related to excess hormone production, including hypoglycemia (insulinoma), Zollinger-Ellison syndrome (gastrinoma), hyperglycemia (glucagonoma), and diarrhea with electrolyte disturbances (VIPoma).

Diagnosis

Imaging of the pancreatobiliary system using ultrasound, CT, or magnetic resonance imaging (MRI) can identify lesions. However, small intrapancreatic, periampullary, and biliary system lesions causing pancreatobiliary obstruction may not be evident on imaging. If a malignancy is suspected, endoscopic ultrasound and endoscopic retrograde cholangiopancreatography are very useful tests. During these procedures, lesions can be visualized better, obstruction can be relieved by stent placement, and histologic confirmation can be obtained by biopsies, fine-needle aspirations, and bile duct brushings. Somatostatin-receptor scintigraphy can be helpful in localizing occult neuroendocrine tumors.

Treatment

Pancreatobiliary malignancies are some of the most difficult cancers to treat. Their anatomic locations make them poor candidates for resection: Pancreatic cancer frequently involves the celiac arterial axis and superior mesenteric artery, and biliary cancers can obstruct the entire biliary outflow (Klatskin tumors). Aggressive surgeries such as the Whipple procedure (pancreatoduodenectomy), radical cholecystectomy (resection of the gallbladder, porta hepatis, liver segments IV and V), and segmental liver resection with biliary tree reconstruction (for cholangiocarcinoma) can be attempted. However, the 5-year overall survival rate after pancreatic adenocarcinoma resection is less than 20%.

Recent studies with multiagent regimens such as a combination of 5-FU, irinotecan, and oxaliplatin, or combined gemcitabine and nab-paclitaxel, have demonstrated improved overall survival for metastatic pancreatic cancer. Gemcitabine with cisplatin has emerged as a standard for cholangiocarcinoma. Octreotide, a somatostatin analogue, is useful in the management of neuroendocrine tumors. Recent studies in neuroendocrine tumors have also shown improvement in outcomes with targeted agents such as everolimus and sunitinib. Palliation of symptoms is a large component of care. Opioid analgesics and celiac nerve plexus blocks for pain; biliary stents and percutaneous tubes for obstructive jaundice; palliative surgeries for gastric outlet and biliary obstruction; appetite stimulants such as olanzapine, megestrol, and dronabinol for anorexia; and supplemental pancreatic enzymes for malabsorption are all interventions that can improve patients' quality of life.

Prognosis

Pancreatobiliary malignancies have some of the worst outcomes; the 5-year overall survival rate remains less than 10%. Survival has not improved significantly over the last few decades, in contrast to several other cancers.

● HEPATOCELLULAR CARCINOMA
Epidemiology

Hepatocellular carcinoma (HCC), or primary liver cancer, is a common disease around the world. It is the second most common cause of cancer-related death in men, worldwide.

Pathology

Most HCCs arise in the setting of underlying cirrhosis, with alcohol use, hepatitis B, and hepatitis C being the most common causes. Other diseases causing cirrhosis are also contributory, such as hemochromatosis, primary biliary cirrhosis, and α_1-antitrypsin deficiency. Cirrhosis involves chronic hepatocyte injury and ensuing cell regeneration, which provides the substrate for cancer development: inflammatory cytokine stress, constant cell cycling, and aberrant cell development and differentiation.

Clinical Presentation

HCC is frequently masked by the underlying liver disease. Abdominal distention from ascites, fatigue, muscle wasting, anorexia, and encephalopathy are features of cirrhosis. Acute hepatic decompensation or right upper quadrant pain may herald the development of HCC. HCC can also be an incidental finding during routine surveillance by screening ultrasound for patients with cirrhosis.

Diagnosis

HCC is one of those rare malignancies for which a diagnosis can be made without histologic confirmation. Nonhistologic criteria for diagnosis include underlying cirrhosis, elevated α-fetoprotein level (>400 ng/mL), and a characteristic appearance on contrast-enhanced CT or MRI (arterial enhancement and rapid washout). In the absence of underlying cirrhosis, a tissue diagnosis must be obtained. For patients with cirrhosis, a surveillance program incorporating regular measurements of α-fetoprotein and ultrasound imaging can detect early lesions.

Treatment

For small lesions, surgical resection can be curative. Preoperative assessment of liver function to ensure that the patient is an appropriate candidate for partial liver resection is critical. Liver transplantation is an option that can treat HCC as well as the underlying cirrhosis. Strict criteria, such as the Milan criteria (i.e., single tumor ≤5 cm, or up to three tumors each <3 cm, and no vascular invasion), are used to determine which patients are eligible for transplantation. For those who are ineligible for surgical approaches, radiofrequency ablation, transarterial chemoembolization, yttrium-90 embolization, and percutaneous ethanol injection can provide local control. Sorafenib, a multikinase inhibitor that targets RAF kinases (CRAF, BRAF), vascular endothelial growth factor receptors (VEGFR-1, VEGFR-2, VEGFR-3), and other cell surface kinase receptors (PDGFR-β, KIT, FLT3, and RET), has been shown to improve clinical outcomes for metastatic disease.

Prognosis

The 5-year survival rate approaches 50% with complete surgical resection or liver transplantation. For advanced HCC, the median overall survival time with sorafenib therapy remains less than 1 year. It is important to note that prognosis in HCC is often determined by the severity of the underlying liver disease.

COLORECTAL CANCER

Epidemiology

Colorectal cancer is the third most common cancer as well as the third most common cause of cancer-related death in the United States, with approximately 150,000 new cases diagnosed each year. Worldwide, it is a growing problem and is one of the most common cancers. There appears to be an increased association with high dietary fat, red meat consumption, low dietary fiber, obesity, and alcohol use. Conversely, increased physical activity and use of supplemental estrogen, folate vitamin, aspirin, and nonsteroidal anti-inflammatory drugs appear to be protective. A history of inflammatory bowel disease is a risk factor for colorectal cancer.

Pathology

Adenocarcinoma of the colon progresses from normal epithelium to frank cancer in a stepwise fashion, as illustrated in Figure 57-1. Most colon cancers arise in polyps. Typically, hamartomatous polyps are non-neoplastic, serrated, and hyperplastic; they have low neoplastic potential, whereas adenomatous polyps can progress to cancer. Sporadic colon cancers arise by one of three major molecular pathways:

1. The classic adenoma-carcinoma sequence, accounting for about 75% of all colon cancers, is initiated by a somatic mutation of the adenomatous polyposis coli *(APC)* gene. This leads to dysregulation of the *WNT* signaling pathway through release of β-catenin and subsequent upregulation of *MYC* and *CCND1 (Cyclin D1)*, two key cell proliferation genes, causing adenoma formation. As disease progresses, chromosomal instability and mutations in other genes, such as *KRAS*, *TP53*, and *SMAD2/4* accumulate, leading to eventual development of adenocarcinoma.
2. In the DNA mismatch repair pathway, mutations accumulate, leading to the formation of "microsatellites." This condition, termed *microsatellite instability*, is associated with 15% of all colon cancers. Increased methylation of tandem repeats of cytosine and guanine, called CpG islands, in the promoter region of various genes in this pathway (e.g., *MLH1*), promote

carcinogenesis. *BRAF* mutations are commonly seen in association with this pathway.
3. Promoter methylation, in the absence of microsatellite instability, can also lead to colon cancer formation. These tumors also develop *KRAS*, but not *BRAF*, mutations. Such cases account for about 5% of all colon cancers.

Inherited abnormalities in many of the genes mentioned earlier lead to a genetic predisposition to colon cancer. Such syndromes are responsible for 3% to 5% of all colon cancers. They can be divided into syndromes associated with underlying polyps and those without polyps. Classic familial adenomatous polyposis (FAP) is caused by an autosomal dominant mutation in the *APC* gene. The colon is full of polyps—hundreds to thousands—that start forming during adolescence, leading to development of cancer in early adulthood. Patients with attenuated FAP have fewer polyps and later development of malignancy. *MYH*-associated polyposis is caused by an autosomal recessive mutation in the *MYH* gene, and the phenotype mimics that of attenuated FAP. Peutz-Jeghers syndrome, juvenile polyposis, and Cowden's syndrome are other uncommon conditions that are associated with an inherited predisposition to colorectal polyps leading to cancer.

The classic nonpolyposis syndrome is hereditary nonpolyposis colorectal cancer, also called Lynch syndrome. Germline recessive mutations in genes involved in the mismatch repair pathway (*MSH2, MSH3, MSH6, MLH1, MLH3, PMS1, PMS2*) lead to adenocarcinoma. These cases are indistinguishable from sporadic cases associated with defective mismatch repair except for the family history of colon and other associated cancers in the inherited syndrome.

Clinical Presentation

Hematochezia and altered bowel habits are the classic symptoms of colon cancer. Early cases are essentially asymptomatic and are typically identified by screening. Advanced cases can manifest with bowel obstruction or perforation, frank rectal bleeding, weight loss, abdominal pain, and ascites due to hepatic or peritoneal metastases. Cancers associated with the mismatch repair pathway have certain typical features: They are right-sided, occur

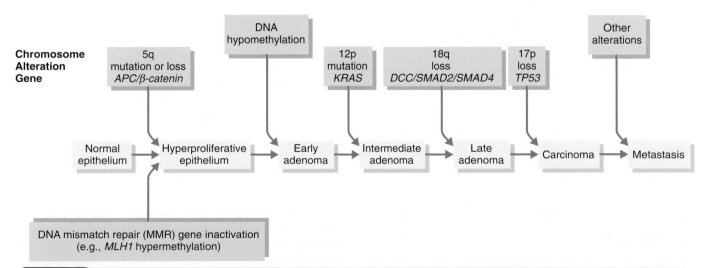

FIGURE 57-1 Model of colorectal carcinogenesis. Several genes are involved in the stepwise progression from normal colonic epithelium to adenocarcinoma.

in younger patients, are more common in women, are poorly differentiated, and are locally advanced but without significant lymph node spread.

Diagnosis

Screening for colorectal cancer is an important public health tool. Screening methods include fecal occult blood testing, imaging (barium enema, CT-guided colonography), and endoscopy (flexible sigmoidoscopy, colonoscopy). The resource setting, patient preference, and risk assessment (personal and family medical history) should guide the choice of screening method. Colonoscopy is the "gold standard" for visual confirmation and histologic diagnosis. In addition, colonoscopy aids in cancer prevention because it allows removal of adenomatous polyps that could progress to cancer if left untreated. Once a cancer diagnosis is established, staging is performed with the use of CT scans to evaluate for distant disease.

Treatment

For patients with resectable disease, surgical resection is the treatment of choice. Removal of the involved segment of the colon, along with the associated mesentery containing all draining lymph nodes, is recommended. Such procedures are being increasingly performed with the use of laparoscopic techniques, resulting in decreased perioperative morbidity. Decisions regarding chemotherapy after surgery (i.e., adjuvant chemotherapy) are based on the pathologic findings. For stage I disease (T1 or T2, N0), no chemotherapy is recommended. For stage III disease (any T, N+), chemotherapy is strongly recommended. A combination of a fluoropyrimidine (5-FU, capecitabine) with oxaliplatin, administered for 6 months, is the standard of care. For stage II disease (T3 or T4, N0), data are controversial. A careful risk-benefit evaluation for each patient is recommended to determine whether adjuvant chemotherapy is appropriate. Rectal cancer is associated with a high rate of local recurrence that can lead to significant morbidity. To improve outcomes, preoperative chemotherapy and radiation therapy are used, and surgery should include total mesorectal excision.

For metastatic colorectal cancer, treatment options include chemotherapy agents such as fluoropyrimidines, oxaliplatin, and irinotecan. The advent of targeted therapies has improved clinical outcomes. These therapies include anti-angiogenic agents (bevacizumab, ziv-aflibercept), anti–epidermal growth factor receptor antibodies (cetuximab, panitumumab), and multikinase inhibitors (regorafenib). Colon cancer is one of the few malignancies in which some cases of metastatic disease can also be cured with aggressive systemic therapy and surgery. Therefore, close surveillance after treatment of the initial cancer is recommended to detect recurrences early. Surveillance should include regular physical evaluation, CT scanning, and measurement of serum levels of carcinoembryonic antigen (CEA), a protein synthesized disproportionately by malignant epithelial cells. Increased physical activity and dietary modifications (reduced red meat and fat; increased fruits, vegetables, and fiber) have been associated with improved outcomes. Another important component of colorectal cancer care is family risk assessment, because this is a common disease, with up to 7500 cases each year in the United States being attributable to heritable

syndromes. Referral for genetic counseling should be made if such a syndrome is suspected.

Prognosis

Among gastrointestinal cancers, colorectal cancer has the best overall prognosis. For nonmetastatic disease, the 5-year survival rate ranges from 50% to 95%, depending on the extent of lymph node involvement. For metastatic disease, newer therapies, given in succession, can achieve a median overall survival time of more than 2 years. The key remains early detection by screening, which can improve population-level outcomes.

● ANAL CANCER

Epidemiology

Anal cancer is an uncommon malignancy, with about 7000 cases reported annually in the United States. It is strongly associated with human papillomavirus (HPV) infection. It is also more common in patients with human immunodeficiency virus (HIV) infection and in those who engage in anal-receptive sexual intercourse, most likely because of poor host immunity and increased transmission of HPV, respectively. Condyloma acuminata are precursor lesions for this cancer.

Pathology

The histology is typical of a squamous cell carcinoma, with sheets of hyperproliferative keratinized cells. HPV, especially types 16 and 18, causes inactivation of the tumor suppressor genes *TP53* and *RB1* via the viral proteins E6 and E7, predisposing to eventual development of carcinoma. Chronic local inflammation due to inflammatory bowel disease or recurrent anal fissures and fistulas can also lead to anal cancer.

Clinical Presentation

Local symptoms, such as perianal pruritus or pain, bleeding, discharge, and a mass-like sensation, are common presentations. In cases of chronic underlying disease such as Crohn's disease, the presence of a nonhealing anal or perianal lesion despite good disease control elsewhere should raise suspicion for malignancy.

Diagnosis

Physical examination is adequate to identify suspicious lesions. A biopsy should be obtained to confirm the diagnosis. Evaluation for distant spread should include CT scans of the chest, abdomen, and pelvis. Special attention should be paid to examination of inguinal lymph nodes, because they are common sites of early spread.

Treatment

Anal cancer is one of the few solid tumor malignancies that are curable without surgical resection. For very small, early lesions, complete excision may suffice. However, for most cases, combined chemotherapy with 5-FU and mitomycin, together with radiation therapy, is the standard curative modality. This regimen has significant short-term toxicities that should be managed carefully. This treatment can obviate the need for a large operation that would result in a permanent colostomy.

Prognosis

More than 70% of cases can be cured with chemoradiation. Relapsed disease is usually treated with surgical excision (if local) or systemic chemotherapy (if distant). Widespread vaccination against HPV and better prevention and treatment of HIV infection should lower the incidence of anal cancer.

Acknowledgments

Dr. Khorana is supported by grants from the National Cancer Institute (K23 CA120587), the National Heart, Lung and Blood Institute (R01HL095109), and the V Foundation and would like to acknowledge the Sondra and Stephen Hardis Endowed Chair in Oncology for research support.

For a deeper discussion on this topic, please see Chapters 192, "Neoplasms of the Esophagus and Stomach," 193, "Neoplasms of the Large and Small Intestine," 194, "Pancreatic Cancer," and 196, "Liver and Biliary Tract Tumors," in Goldman-Cecil Medicine, *25th Edition.*

SUGGESTED READINGS

Bang YJ, Van Cutsem E, Feyereislova A, et al: Trastuzumab in combination with chemotherapy versus chemotherapy alone for treatment of HER2-positive advanced gastric or gastro-oesophageal junction cancer (ToGA): a phase 3, open-label, randomised controlled trial, Lancet 376:687–697, 2010.

Conroy T, Desseigne F, Ychou M, et al: FOLFIRINOX versus gemcitabine for metastatic pancreatic cancer, N Engl J Med 364:1817–1825, 2011.

Grothey A, Van Cutsem E, Sobrero A, et al: Regorafenib monotherapy for previously treated metastatic colorectal cancer (CORRECT): an international, multicentre, randomised, placebo-controlled, phase 3 trial, Lancet 381:303–312, 2013.

Hvid-Jensen F, Pedersen L, Drewes AM, et al: Incidence of adenocarcinoma among patients with Barrett's esophagus, N Engl J Med 365:1375–1383, 2011.

Neoptolemos JP, Moore MJ, Cox TF, et al: Effect of adjuvant chemotherapy with fluorouracil plus folinic acid or gemcitabine vs observation on survival in patients with resected periampullary adenocarcinoma, JAMA 308:147–156, 2012.

Valle J, Wasan H, Palmer DH, et al: Cisplatin plus gemcitabine versus gemcitabine for biliary tract cancer, N Engl J Med 362:1273–1281, 2010.

van Hagen P, Hulshof MC, van Lanschot JJ, et al: Preoperative chemoradiotherapy for esophageal or junctional cancer, N Engl J Med 366:2074–2084, 2012.

Yao JC, Shah MH, Ito T, et al: Everolimus for advanced pancreatic neuroendocrine tumors, N Engl J Med 364:514–523, 2011.

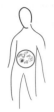

58

Genitourinary Cancers

Robert Dreicer, Jorge Garcia, Timothy Gilligan, and Brian Rini

RENAL CELL CARCINOMA

Definition and Epidemiology

Renal cell carcinoma (RCC) represents 2% to 3% of all malignancies. It is the fifth most common cancer in men and the seventh most common cancer in women, with approximately 65,000 new cases diagnosed in the United States in 2013. Most patients do not have an identifiable risk factor. Smoking is an established risk factor for RCC, with a relative risk of two-fold greater than that of nonsmokers. Less certain risk factors include obesity and hypertension. RCC is also more common in patients with end-stage renal failure or polycystic kidney disease. A small number (3%) of cases of RCC are inherited.

The most recognized inherited RCC is von Hippel-Lindau (VHL) syndrome, an autosomal dominant disorder that is characterized by the development of multiple vascular tumors including clear cell RCC. The genetic event underlying VHL syndrome (inactivation of the *VHL* gene) also occurs in sporadic (noninherited) clear cell tumors, leading to RCC characterized by reliance on blood vessels for growth. Research into this syndrome has led to modified treatment options for advanced disease (see later discussion).

Pathology

The histologic subtypes of RCC are characterized by distinct genetic characteristics, histologic features, and clinical phenotypes. Clear cell RCC (75% of all RCCs) is the most common subtype and is characterized by *VHL* gene inactivation. Less common are the papillary, chromophobe, and unclassified subtypes and medullary RCC, which occurs almost exclusively in patients with sickle cell trait. Although these RCC subtypes are biologically distinct, the current surgical and medical approaches are uninfluenced by subtype.

Diagnosis and Differential Diagnosis

Masses in the kidney may be benign or malignant, with an increasing likelihood of malignancy with increasing size. Most clear cell RCC tumors are distinguishable based on their contrast enhancement. Other considerations for renal masses include benign tumors (e.g., oncocytoma), metastatic disease from another primary site (rare), angiomyolipoma, a lipid-containing benign tumor (most commonly occurring in young females), and infectious processes. The diagnosis is made on the basis of a biopsy or at the time of nephrectomy, although the radiographic appearance of each of the differential diagnoses is often characteristic.

Clinical Presentation

RCC is more common in males $(2:1)$, and the median age at presentation is approximately 65 years. Most contemporary presentations are asymptomatic and incidental (identified on imaging studies ordered for other indications). Classic signs and symptoms include hematuria, flank pain, and a palpable abdominal mass. Systemic symptoms occur with metastatic disease or paraneoplastic syndromes. A renal mass is discovered, usually on computed tomography (CT) scanning, and has an appearance that is characteristic of RCC (i.e., highly vascular). Subsequently, a full staging work-up is performed, including CT scanning of the chest; CT head and bone scans are performed only as symptoms dictate. Diagnosis is usually made at the time of nephrectomy, although a biopsy of the renal mass may be indicated, such as in a patient with distant metastases in whom nephrectomy is not pursued or in a patient with a small renal mass that may be initially observed.

Treatment

Renal Masses

Some renal masses (approximately 20%) are not cancerous, so a diagnostic biopsy is indicated if the radiographic appearance is not classically consistent with RCC. One option for renal masses, even if proven to be RCC, is initial observation. Retrospective series have defined this approach in a select group of patients with renal masses smaller than 4 cm in diameter for whom surgery is not preferred. The growth rate is approximately 3 mm/year, and the reported incidence of development of metastases is very low. If surgery is pursued, then removal of either part of the kidney (partial nephrectomy) or the entire kidney (radical nephrectomy) is the standard of care, depending on factors such as the extent and anatomy of the tumor, native renal function, and surgical skill. Cancer outcomes are equivalent, although renal function is better preserved with partial nephrectomy. Another management option for renal masses is exposure to temperature extremes: freezing (cryotherapy) or burning (radiofrequency ablation). This approach is usually pursued in patients with contraindications to surgery. The long-term outcome awaits further data. To date no clinical trial evidence has demonstrated improvement in patient outcome, either before (neoadjuvant) or after (adjuvant) nephrectomy, regardless of risk of recurrence, despite l clinical trials.

Surgery in Metastatic RCC

Removal of the primary renal tumor in the face of metastatic disease (i.e., debulking or cytoreductive nephrectomy) is pursued in patients with good performance status, limited extrarenal disease, and low comorbidities. Two randomized trials have shown an overall survival benefit in these circumstances. In addition, surgical removal of solitary metastatic sites is associated with disease control in up to 30% of highly selected patients.

Systemic Therapy for Metastatic RCC

The initial treatments for metastatic RCC—hormone therapy and chemotherapy—produced only minimal benefits (Table 58-1). Immunotherapy has yielded modest benefits, majority of benefit realized in highly selected patients who have a durable complete response to high-dose interleukin-2. The major treatment advance in metastatic RCC was the discovery of the reliance of the cancer on the vascular endothelial growth factor (VEGF) pathway, which results from *VHL* gene inactivation. This led to the clinical development of a number of VEGF pathway inhibitors, as outlined in Table 58-1. In general, 70% to 75% of patients who receive these drugs have some reduction or stabilization of tumor burden. Periods of disease control typically last for some months, although they can extend to several years in a small minority of patients. Combinations of existing agents are more toxic and no better than monotherapy. The current standard of care is a sequence of monotherapies with agents targeted to VEGF and/or mammalian target of rapamycin (mTOR).

Prognosis

The prognosis of localized kidney cancer is determined largely by the stage and grade of the primary tumor. Other systems have been based on other features, such as tumor necrosis, symptoms at presentation, or performance status. In metastatic disease, established schema associated with prognosis use performance status, time from diagnosis to metastatic disease, and laboratory values (lactate dehydrogenase [LDH], hemoglobin, calcium, neutrophils, and platelets).

⬤ BLADDER CANCER
Definition and Epidemiology

Urothelial carcinoma of the bladder (UCB) represents 4% of all malignancies and about 3% of cancer-related deaths in the United States. It is more common in developed countries and is the fourth most common cancer among men and ninth among women in the Western world. Smoking is an established risk factor for bladder cancer; the incidence rate is four times higher for smokers than for nonsmokers. Occupational exposures from a range of agents that contain aromatic amines, as chlorinated hydrocarbons and polycyclic aromatic hydrocarbons, are believed to account for up to 20% of all bladder cancers. Genetic susceptibility is increasingly recognized as an important risk factor. The risk of bladder cancer is doubled in first-degree relatives of patients with bladder cancer. Inherited genetic factors, such as the slow acetylator *N*-acetyltransferase 2 (NAT2) variants and the glutathione *S*-transferase Mu 1 (GSTM1)–null genotypes, are established risk factors.

Pathology

Transitional cell carcinoma is the predominant histologic subtype in the United States and Europe, where it accounts for 90% of all bladder cancers. Adenocarcinoma, squamous cell carcinoma, and small cell cancers account for most of the remaining 10%, although there are parts of the world where nonurothelial carcinomas are more common. The bladder wall consists of four layers: urothelium (the innermost epithelial lining), lamina propria, muscularis propria (detrusor muscle), and adventitia (serosa).

Clinical Presentation

UCB is more common in males (4 : 1), and the median age at presentation is 73 years. Approximately 75% of newly diagnosed cases of UCB are not muscle invasive; the remaining 25% exhibit de novo invasion of the muscle wall of the bladder at presentation.

Patients with bladder cancer typically have painless hematuria at presentation, although irritative voiding symptoms (frequency, urgency, and dysuria) can be the initial manifestation. Patients with more advanced disease may have progressive flank or pelvic pain from direct extension of disease or as a consequence of ureteral obstruction.

Diagnosis and Differential Diagnosis

The initial evaluation typically involves an office-based cystoscopic evaluation, with the collection of urine for cytology. Subsequently, patients undergo a transurethral resection of bladder tumor (TURBT) under anesthesia to obtain tissue for histologic

TABLE 58-1 SUMMARY OF THERAPEUTIC APPROACHES IN METASTATIC RCC

AGENT	OBJECTIVE RESPONSE RATE	PFS (mo)	COMMENTS
Hormonal therapy	2%	N/A	Limited, palliative role in the treatment of metastatic RCC
Chemotherapy	5-6%	N/A	Not generally used
Interleukin-2	~20-25% (high dose)	3.1	Durable complete response rate of 7-8%
Interferon alfa	10-15%	4.7	Modest improvement in overall survival compared with inactive therapy
VEGF inhibitors*	Approximately 30%	9-11	Common toxicity includes fatigue, mucositis, hand-foot syndrome, diarrhea, hypertension, and hypothyroidism
mTOR inhibitors†	2% (treatment refractory) to 9% (treatment naive)	4-7	Increased overall survival of temsirolimus monotherapy vs IFN monotherapy in poor-risk patients Toxicity includes fatigue, mucositis, rash and hypertriglyceridemia/hyperglycemia/hypercholesterolemia

IFN, Interferon; mTOR, mammalian target of rapamycin; N/A, not applicable; PFS, progression-free survival; RCC, renal cell carcinoma; VEGF, vascular endothelial growth factor.
*VEGF inhibitors: sorafenib, sunitinib, pazopanib, axitinib.
†mTOR inhibitors: temsirolimus, everolimus.

diagnosis. Inclusion of muscle in the pathologic specimen is necessary to exclude muscle invasion. Additional evaluation includes CT scanning of the abdomen and pelvis (or CT urogram). For patients with muscle-invasive disease, CT imaging of the chest is indicated; and in patients with bone pain, bone scintigraphy. Most new cases of UCB are staged as Ta (involvement of epithelial lining), T1 (invasion of lamina propria), or carcinoma in situ (CIS); these are typically grouped and considered as non–muscle-invasive bladder cancer (NMIBC).

Patients with low-grade, low-stage bladder cancer remain at high risk for non–muscle-invasive recurrence, whereas patients with higher-grade, higher-stage disease are at increased risk for both recurrence and progression to muscle-invasive disease. Secondary involvement of the bladder with other cancers (e.g., lymphoma, sarcoma) is uncommon.

Treatment

Organ-Confined Disease

Low-grade, low-stage, non–muscle-invasive UCBs are typically managed with TURBT and intravesically administered cytotoxic agents. Multifocal, low-grade recurrent disease or high-risk NMIBC (high-grade T1 or CIS) is managed with intravesically administered bacillus Calmette-Guérin (BCG) or cystectomy.

Muscle-invasive bladder cancer is optimally managed with radical cystectomy and bilateral pelvic lymphadenectomy. For patients who are deemed poor surgical candidates or who refuse cystectomy, external beam radiotherapy and TURBT are alternative management options.

Cisplatin-based multiagent chemotherapy administered before cystectomy (i.e., neoadjuvant chemotherapy) has been shown by level I evidence to improve survival. Although it has not been prospectively evaluated in the neoadjuvant setting, the regimen of gemcitabine plus cisplatin (GC) is widely substituted for the older combination of methotrexate, vinblastine, doxorubicin, and cisplatin (M-VAC).

Metastatic Disease

Level I evidence from a series of phase III trials provides evidence that cisplatin-based chemotherapy (i.e., M-VAC or GC) in patients with de novo metastatic disease leads to median survival times in the range of 14 to 15 months, with 5% to 15% of patients likely to be cured. The latter group is made up primarily of patients with nodal metastatic disease.

Between 30% and 50% of patients with advanced UCB are ineligible for cisplatin because of concomitant renal insufficiency, typically as a consequence of age-related renal comorbidity or disease-related extrinsic obstruction. Although there have been no completed randomized phase III trials comparing cisplatin-based chemotherapy with carboplatin-based therapy in patients with advanced UCB, multiple randomized phase II trials have reported superior activity with cisplatin-based regimens.

The management of disease progression after front-line therapy (either perioperative or in the metastatic setting) is primarily palliative. Currently, there is no level I evidence that systemic therapy yields meaningful improvement in progression-free or overall survival. A large number of chemotherapeutic agents have been studied in the "salvage" setting, and there is no evidence that multiagent therapy is more effective than single-agent therapy in palliating disease-related symptoms.

Prognosis

Patients with low-grade, low-stage NMIBC typically do not progress to muscle-invasive disease. Their disease does not alter life expectancy but is associated with morbidity and use of health care resources and requires long-term follow-up. Patients with muscle-invasive disease who undergo cystectomy are at risk for systemic failure based on the T stage and extent of nodal involvement. Patients with organ-confined disease without nodal involvement have cure rates greater than 50%. Patients with metastatic disease have median survival times in the range of 14 to 16 months with systemic therapy, and only a small subset (5% to 15%) are long-term survivors.

🔴 PROSTATE CANCER

Definition and Epidemiology

Prostate cancer is the most common malignancy among men in the United States; more than 239,000 cases were expected to be diagnosed in 2013. Biologically, prostate cancer is a heterogeneous disease with a diverse but often long natural history. Although the lifetime risk of developing prostate cancer is approximately 1 in 6, most men do not die of the disease. The promiscuous use of prostate-specific-antigen (PSA) measurement as a screening tool has affected the incidence of prostate cancer. Despite a recent transient decline, incidence rates remain high compared with the pre-PSA era.

Multiple risk factors, including age, race, dietary factors, and genetic factors, have been linked to prostate cancer. The median age at diagnosis is 65 years, and younger men (<40 years) rarely develop prostate cancer. African American men have a greater risk of developing prostate cancer compared with white or Hispanic men. Genetic mutations such as *BRCA1/2*, Lynch syndrome, and, more recently, abnormalities in homeobox B13 (*HOXB13*) have been linked to prostate cancer. A man with first-degree relatives affected by prostate cancer has a five-fold to ten-fold increased risk of prostate cancer. Whereas high animal fat intake has been linked to prostate cancer, no association between a diet rich in antioxidants, lycopene, fruit, or vegetables and prostate cancer has been identified.

Recently, a large chemoprevention trial (SELECT) demonstrated that intake of selenium and vitamin E does not reduce the risk of prostate cancer. Two studies evaluating the 5α-reductase inhibitors, finasteride and dutasteride, demonstrated a 23% to 25% reduction in relative risk of prostate cancer. Despite these benefits, the use of these agents remains low, primarily because of side effects such as erectile dysfunction, lack of libido, and gynecomastia.

Pathology

Prostate cancer is typically diagnosed by transrectal ultrasound and biopsy, often performed after an abnormal PSA level or digital rectal examination result. In patients undergoing radical prostatectomy, the entire prostate, including seminal vesicles and lymph nodes (if present), is analyzed. Prognosis and treatment depend on tumor volume, the presence of perineural invasion, extraprostatic extension, Gleason score, margin status, and involvement of seminal vesicles. Adenocarcinoma accounts for more than 95% of all prostate cancers. The remaining histologic subtypes include small cell carcinoma and sarcoma. Neuroendocrine differentiation and papillary features carry a poor prognosis.

The Gleason scoring system is pivotal in the management of prostate cancer, but its interpretation requires expertise in pathology. The score is based on growth pattern and degree of differentiation and ranges from 1 to 5 (5 being the least differentiated). The composite Gleason score is derived by adding together the numerical values for the two most prevalent differentiation patterns. For instance, if a specimen comprises primarily a grade 3 pattern and secondarily a grade 4 pattern, the score is reported as 7 (3 + 4). Scores of 8 to 10 represent poorly differentiated cancers, which are associated with poorer outcomes.

Diagnosis and Differential Diagnosis

With the exception of men with metastatic disease at presentation, most patients are diagnosed with the use of extended core biopsies (12 cores). A negative prostate biopsy result does not rule out prostate cancer. For men with metastatic disease, lymph node or bone biopsies can be performed. If the disease is confined to the prostate, imaging studies (bone scans and CT scans of the abdomen and pelvis) are obtained only in high-risk patients (i.e., high Gleason score, high PSA level). After diagnosis, risk stratification based on PSA level, Gleason score, and clinical stage becomes crucial to define management. Other important features determining treatment include age, comorbidities, patient preferences, and life expectancy.

Clinical Presentation

Because prostate cancer can be detected in small subsets even with very low PSA levels (i.e., <1 ng/mL) there is no "normal" PSA value. PSA values can be affected by rectal examination, ejaculation, infection, and urinary obstruction. PSA screening has been used extensively in the United States, but there is no evidence for a consequent reduction in mortality from prostate cancer.

Most men with early disease have no symptoms; however, urinary frequency, urgency, nocturia, and hesitancy do occur. The presence of hematuria or hematospermia should prompt consideration of prostate cancer. An abnormal rectal examination result (asymmetric mass/nodule) is also suggestive of cancer.

Treatment

Available treatment options for localized prostate cancer include radical prostatectomy, radiation therapy (either external beam radiation or brachytherapy), and active surveillance. For men with very-low-risk prostate cancer, active surveillance is appropriate. The selection between radical prostatectomy and radiation therapy is based on risk stratification and patient preferences. Surgery carries risks of urinary incontinence and erectile dysfunction. Radiation therapy has fewer local complications but can cause myelosuppression fatigue and a 3% to 5% lifetime risk of a secondary malignancy. Primary radiation therapy for intermediate- and high-risk patients is often given in combination with androgen deprivation therapy.

Once patients develop advanced disease, androgen deprivation therapy is widely used, although the appropriate timing remains unknown. For men with metastatic disease, continuous therapy with leutenizing hormone releasing hormone (LHRH) agonist with or without anti-androgen is the most common form of treatment, but intermittent androgen deprivation therapy is an effective alternative for patients whose only sign is a rising PSA level. In the setting of de novo metastatic disease, achievement of an undetectable PSA level at 6 months with androgen deprivation therapy predicts good outcome. Androgen deprivation therapy also has major side effects, including night sweats, hot flashes, erectile dysfunction, weight gain, loss of muscle mass, fatigue, bone loss, and metabolic syndrome.

Bone health is a significant problem in men with prostate cancer. Osteoporosis and skeletal-related events from metastases are both common. Two agents are available to prevent these complications: zoledronic acid, a bisphosphonate, and denosumab, a RANK-ligand inhibitor.

All patients with metastatic prostate cancer eventually develop castrate-resistant prostate cancer (CRPC), defined by serologic, clinical, or objective progression in the setting of a castrated testosterone level. Although the mechanism of CRPC is not well understood, several treatment options are now available. Sipuleucel-T, an autologous cell product capable of prolonging survival, and abiraterone acetate, a novel CYP17A1 (C17,20-lyase) inhibitor, are often used in the prechemotherapy setting. Two additional agents, cabazitaxel (a novel chemotherapy agent) and the androgen receptor inhibitor enzalutamide, have become a standard of care after docetaxel-based chemotherapy.

Prognosis

Many patients with favorable-risk, organ-confined disease are cured with surgery or radiotherapy. Most patients who have evidence of PSA recurrence after therapy will eventually manifest metastatic disease, but the natural history is variable. Patients with metastatic disease at presentation typically live for 3 to 5 additional years.

⬤ TESTICULAR CANCER
Definition and Epidemiology

The incidence of testis cancer varies widely among racial groups and geographic regions. In the United States, it is the most common cancer diagnosed in men aged 20 to 40 years of age, but it is rarely diagnosed before age 15 or after age 55. It is five times more common in whites than in blacks. The incidence has increased by more than 50% since 1975. Currently, a U.S. male faces a 0.37% lifetime risk of testis cancer and a 0.02% risk of dying from it. Risk factors include cryptorchidism and a personal or family history of testis cancer. Orchiopexy for cryptorchism before puberty reduces the risk of testis cancer.

Pathology

Approximately 95% of testis cancers are germ cell tumors; the others are mostly lymphomas, sex-cord stromal tumors, and adenocarcinomas of the rete testis. Germ cell tumors are divided into two broad categories: seminomas and nonseminomas (i.e., nonseminomatous germ cell tumors, or NSGCTs). Seminomas by definition are 100% seminoma, whereas most NSGCTs are a mixture of two or more of the five types of germ cell tumors: seminoma, embryonal carcinoma, teratoma, yolk sac tumor, and choriocarcinoma. A tumor that contains any elements of embryonal carcinoma, teratoma, yolk sac tumor, or choriocarcinoma is considered to be an NSGCT even if most of the tumor is seminoma. Because seminomas do not produce α-fetoprotein (AFP), patients who have an elevated AFP level have a NSGCT by definition regardless of the histopathology.

Diagnosis and Differential Diagnosis

Whenever a testis tumor is suspected, transscrotal ultrasound should be performed; if a mass suspicious for cancer is seen, the standard diagnostic procedure is an inguinal orchiectomy. Transscrotal orchiectomy or biopsy is contraindicated because of the risk of seeding the tumor in the scrotum and altering the pattern of spread. Differential diagnosis includes testicular lymphoma, torsion, epididymo-orchitis and other benign scrotal lesions.

Clinical Presentation

Testis cancer most often manifests as testicular enlargement, mass, or induration. It may or may not be painful or tender, and the presence of pain does not exclude a diagnosis of cancer. Testicular atrophy, gynecomastia, back pain, and thromboembolic disease are less common presentations.

Staging the cancer requires measuring postorchiectomy levels of serum AFP, human chorionic gonadotropin (β-HCG), and LDH as well as assessing for nodal and organ metastases, which should be done with a CT scan of the abdomen and pelvis and either chest CT or a chest radiography. The testes drain to the retroperitoneal lymph nodes, and retroperitoneal nodal spread constitutes stage II disease. In practice, testis cancer is divided into three categories: stage I (localized), with no evidence of spread to lymph nodes or beyond; stage II (regional), with enlarged retroperitoneal lymph nodes but no distant metastases; and disseminated disease. Disseminated disease includes stage I or II disease in which serum AFP and/or β-HCG levels are persistently elevated after orchiectomy, bulky stage II disease, and all stage III disease. Metastases to other organs or to pelvic or other nonretroperitoneal lymph nodes represents stage III disease, as does spread to retroperitoneal nodes in the setting of highly elevated serum tumor markers. Disseminated disease is divided into three categories: good-risk, intermediate-risk, and poor-risk disease; treatment differs for the different risk groups.

Treatment

Stage I seminomas and NSGCTs are usually managed with surveillance after surgery. The risk of relapse is about 18% for seminomas and 30% for NSGCTs. Alternatives to surveillance are single-agent carboplatin chemotherapy or radiation therapy for seminomas and bleomycin and etoposide and cisplatin (BEP) chemotherapy or retroperitoneal lymph node dissection (RPLND) for NSGCTs. Long-term disease-specific survival for stage I disease is 99% regardless of which of these approaches is used.

Stage II seminomas are usually treated with radiation, but chemotherapy (with bleomycin, etoposide, and cisplatin [BEP]

or etoposide plus cisplatin [EP]) is used when the disease bulk is greater than 5 cm and sometimes for less bulky tumors. Management of stage II NSGCTs depends on the disease bulk and the levels of serum AFP and β-HCG. If either marker is elevated, then chemotherapy is preferred regardless of disease bulk. If no nodes are bigger than 2 cm and there are fewer than six enlarged nodes, then RPLND or close observation is appropriate. For bulkier disease, chemotherapy is administered, although RPLND may be used in carefully selected cases.

Treatment of stage III disease depends on the sites of metastases and the levels of serum tumor markers. For good-risk disease, the treatment is three cycles of BEP or four cycles of EP chemotherapy. For intermediate- and poor-risk disease, the treatment is four cycles of BEP chemotherapy (or etoposide, ifosfamide, and cisplatin [VIP] chemotherapy). In NSGCT, all residual masses should be resected after chemotherapy if feasible. In cases of seminoma, residual masses are typically observed unless they show increased uptake on 8-fluorodeoxyglucose (FDG) positron emission tomography (PET scan). Patients with pure seminomas and residual masses after chemotherapy are the only testis cancer patients who should be considered for PET scans.

Relapsed disease after chemotherapy is treated with salvage chemotherapy given either at standard doses or at high doses with hematopoietic stem cell support.

Prognosis

Overall, the long-term disease-specific survival rate for testis cancer is 95%. By stage, the survival rates are 99% for stage I, 96% for stage II, and 73% for stage III. By disseminated disease risk category, survival is about 90% for good-risk disease, about 80% for intermediate-risk disease, and about 50% for poor-risk disease.

For a deeper discussion on these topics, please see Chapters 197, "Tumors of the Kidney, Bladder, Ureters, and Renal Pelvis," 200, "Testicular Cancer," and 201, "Prostate Cancer," in Goldman-Cecil Medicine, 25th Edition.

SUGGESTED READINGS

Alva A, Hussain M: The changing natural history of metastatic prostate cancer, Cancer J 19:19–24, 2013.

Burger M, Oosterlinck W, Konety B, et al: ICUD-EAU international consultation on bladder cancer 2012: non–muscle-invasive urothelial carcinoma of the bladder, Eur Urol 63:36–44, 2012.

Calabrò F, Albers P, Bokemeyer C, et al: The contemporary role of chemotherapy for advanced testis cancer: a systematic review of the literature, Eur Urol 61:1212–1220, 2012.

Cooperberg MR, Carroll PR, Klotz L, et al: Active surveillance for prostate cancer: progress and promise, J Clin Oncol 29:3669–3676, 2011.

de Bono JS, Logothetis CJ, Molina A, et al: Abiraterone and increased survival in metastatic prostate cancer, N Engl J Med 364:1995–2005, 2011.

Gakis G, Efstathiou J, Lerner S, et al: ICUD-EAU international consultation on bladder cancer 2012: radical cystectomy and bladder preservation for muscle-invasive urothelial carcinoma of the bladder, Eur Urol 63:45–57, 2013.

Galsky M, Hahn N, Rosenberg J, et al: Treatment of patients with metastatic urothelial cancer "unfit" for cisplatin-based chemotherapy, J Clin Oncol 29:2432–2438, 2011.

Howlader N, Noone AM, Krapecho M, et al: SEER Cancer Statistics Review, 1975-2011, Bethesda, Md., 2014, National Cancer Institute. Available at: http://seer.cancer.gov/csr/1975_2011/. Accessed July 9, 2014.

James N, Hussain S, Hall E, et al: Radiotherapy with or without chemotherapy in muscle-invasive bladder cancer, N Engl J Med 366:1477–1478, 2012.

National Comprehensive Cancer Network: NCCN clinical practice guidelines in oncology: prostate cancer, version 2, 2013. Available at: www.NCCN.org. Accessed July 7, 2014.

Rini BI, Campbell SC, Escudier B: Renal cell carcinoma, Lancet 373:1119–1132, 2009.

Scher HI, Fizazi K, Saad F, et al: Increased survival with enzalutamide in prostate cancer after chemotherapy, N Engl J Med 367:1187–1197, 2012.

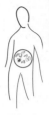

59

Breast Cancer

Nicole M. Kuderer and Gary H. Lyman

EPIDEMIOLOGY

Breast cancer is the most common cancer in women other than skin cancer, and it represents the second leading cause of cancer death after lung cancer among women in the United States. An estimated 232,340 women will be diagnosed with invasive breast cancer, and almost 40,000 will die of the disease in 2013. Although breast cancer is far less common in males, more than 2000 men are diagnosed with breast cancer annually in the United States. Whereas reported breast cancer incidence rates have continued to rise, breast cancer mortality has declined by more than 2% annually since 1990 (Figs. 59-1 and 59-2).

Breast cancer is a disease of aging with an increasing incidence throughout most of adult life. Other risk factors for breast cancer include a family history of breast cancer, early menarche, late menopause, nulliparity or initial pregnancy after 25 years of age, prolonged use of exogenous estrogen, exposure to ionizing radiation, and obesity. Women with a history of breast cancer are also at increased risk for breast cancer in the contralateral breast. Although only 5% of patients with breast cancer have the breast cancer susceptibility genes, *BRCA1* and *BRCA2*, genetic counseling and possible testing for *BRCA1* and *BRCA2* should be offered, especially to patients with multiple affected family members and those with a personal or family history of male breast cancer, bilateral breast cancer, breast cancer at a young age (before age 45 to 50 years), ovarian cancer, or certain high-risk ethnicities (e.g., Ashkenazi Jewish).

SCREENING, INITIAL PRESENTATION, AND STAGING

Breast cancer is most often diagnosed through screening mammography or after a patient or her physician notices a palpable mass. Mammographic screening has been shown to reduce breast cancer mortality in both average- and high-risk populations. Although there is some variability among the major breast cancer screening guidelines, most recommend annual screening by mammography with or without physical examination between the ages of 50 to 74 years. Younger women might consider annual or biannual mammographic screening beginning at age 40. Screening with magnetic resonance imaging (MRI) of the breast is recommended in addition to mammography for women with a substantially increased predisposition, especially a strong family history or other genetic predisposition. A palpable breast mass warrants full evaluation even in the absence of diagnostic changes on mammography or breast MRI.

Breast cancer staging requires removal of the primary tumor and assessment of the ipsilateral axillary lymph nodes. Increasingly, lymphatic mapping with sentinel lymph node assessment is being used to evaluate the axilla, with complete lymph node dissection performed only for those with a positive sentinel node biopsy. A subset of women with a good prognosis and only a few positive lymph nodes may be able to forgo lymph node dissection altogether. Women with tumors larger than 5 cm and those with positive axillary lymph node involvement require additional staging imaging: a bone scan

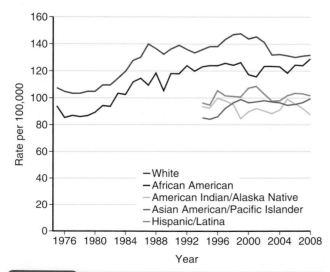

FIGURE 59-1 Breast cancer incidence rates by race and ethnicity. (Modified from DeSantis C, Siegel R, Bandi P, et al: Breast cancer statistics, 2011, CA Cancer J Clin 61:409–418, 2011.)

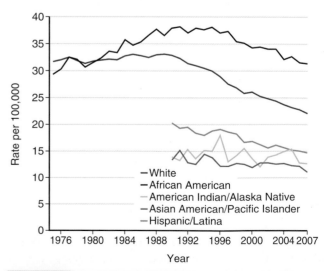

FIGURE 59-2 Breast cancer mortality rates by race and ethnicity. (Modified from DeSantis C, Siegel R, Bandi P, et al: Breast cancer statistics, 2011, CA Cancer J Clin 61:409–418, 2011.)

and computed tomographic (CT) scanning of the chest and abdomen. In the absence of signs or symptoms suggestive of metastatic disease, patients with smaller tumors and negative lymph node involvement usually do not require further imaging. Fewer than 10% of women have metastatic breast cancer at diagnosis.

PATHOLOGY

Because of the increasing utilization and sophistication of breast cancer screening, ductal carcinoma in situ (DCIS) is being reported more frequently; however, it is infrequently invasive. Most invasive breast cancers are infiltrating ductal carcinomas, and a smaller proportion are infiltrating lobular carcinomas. Tubular and mucinous carcinomas, a subtype of infiltrating ductal cancers, are associated with a better prognosis. Inflammatory breast cancer is on the other end of the spectrum, frequently denoting a poor prognosis. Inflammatory breast cancer remains a clinical diagnosis: it is recognized by breast skin changes such as edema and erythema of the skin (peau d'orange), often in the absence of a palpable mass.

At the time of breast biopsy and definitive surgery, the estrogen and progesterone receptor status of the primary tumor should be routinely assessed. Overexpression of the human epidermal growth factor receptor HER2/neu or its gene amplification is critical for treatment selection and prognosis and should also be assessed. So-called triple-negative tumors—those that are negative for the estrogen and progesterone receptors and for amplification of the HER2 [ERBB2] oncogene—are associated with a poorer prognosis and offer fewer treatment options. Triple-negative tumors are more commonly found in women who have the BRCA breast cancer susceptibility gene. In women with hormone receptor–positive tumors, gene expression assays may provide additional prognostic information to guide treatment decision making.

TREATMENT

The appropriate care of patients with early-stage breast cancer is multidisciplinary, involving a radiologist, pathologist, surgeon, medical oncologist, radiation oncologist and often others. Breast-conserving therapy with lumpectomy followed by radiation therapy represents the current standard of care for most women with small invasive breast cancers. Women with large tumors may be considered for mastectomy with or without breast reconstruction. Currently, many such patients are considered for neoadjuvant (preoperative) chemotherapy; this may allow breast conservation in these women who would otherwise not be able to undergo a lumpectomy, and it also provides an objective assessment of tumor response to systemic therapy. Women who have had previous radiation to the breast for breast cancer or another malignancy, are usually treated with mastectomy. Frail patients with hormone receptor–positive tumors may be considered for primary hormonal therapy rather than radiation therapy; surgical treatment is usually indicated for these patients.

Adjuvant therapy with chemotherapy and hormonal therapy following definitive surgery improves relapse-free and overall survival rates in premenopausal and postmenopausal women. Subsequent adjuvant therapy for 1 year with the monoclonal antibody trastuzumab improves disease-free survival in patients with tumors that demonstrate overexpression of the HER2 oncoprotein or amplification of its HER2 (ERBB2) oncogene. DCIS is treated with either lumpectomy followed by radiation therapy or with mastectomy alone. Women with larger or multifocal DCIS should have assessment of their lymph node status to exclude lymph node involvement associated with occult invasive cancer. In the absence of invasive disease, adjuvant chemotherapy is not indicated for DCIS.

The risks and benefits associated with tamoxifen for chemoprevention in patients with higher risk features should be discussed. Women with the BRCA1 or BRCA2 breast cancer susceptibility genes should be offered prophylactic bilateral mastectomy and oophorectomy given their high risk for development of invasive breast cancer as well as ovarian cancer at a relatively young age. Close surveillance with breast clinical examinations as well as screening mammography and breast MRI should be offered to those patients with BRCA susceptibility genes who elect a nonsurgical approach. Oophorectomy or antiestrogen therapy can help decrease the risk of breast cancer in these women and others at high risk for the disease.

Breast cancer most commonly recurs with metastases in the bone, liver, lung, and central nervous system, but it can recur in any organ system. Rates of breast cancer recurrence and mortality are greater among African American women than white women; those of other ethnicities have lower mortality rates (see Fig. 59-2). Although women with metastatic breast cancer have an average life expectancy of years rather than months, the disease remains incurable. The decision to offer systemic therapy in women with metastatic breast cancer is based on extent and sites of disease, severity of symptoms, patient physical functioning, previous treatment, comorbid conditions, and especially the tumor molecular characteristics of hormone receptor and HER2 status. Although tumor hormonal status and HER2 status may change over the treatment course in a patient with metastatic breast cancer, life expectancy is typically longer in women with hormone-responsive (receptor-positive) disease and when the sites of metastases are lymph nodes or bone rather than liver, lung, or central nervous system. Patients with hormone-responsive metastatic breast cancer may live for many years, often responding to hormonal therapy for years before requiring chemotherapy for disease control.

In patients with HER2-positive tumors, trastuzumab may be used in combination with chemotherapy or hormonal therapy. Several novel anti-HER2 therapies have been developed that are changing and expanding the therapeutic options and improving the prognostic outlook of these patients. Many chemotherapeutic agents (singly or in combination), including the anthracyclines, taxanes, alkylating agents, fluoropyrimidines, vinca alkaloids, gemcitabine, and epithilones, demonstrate activity against breast cancer. Bisphosphonates, such as zoledronate and pamidronate, are given intravenously to decrease the pain associated with bone metastases and the risk for fracture in women with skeletal metastases.

PROGNOSIS

Most women with early-stage breast cancer survive for many years after their initial diagnosis and treatment, and many enjoy a normal life expectancy. The survival of patients with breast cancer has continued to improve over the last several decades because of improved early detection and more effective therapy (see Fig. 59-2). The rapidly increasing number of breast cancer survivors necessitates consideration of a number of important issues, including monitoring for cancer recurrence and management of the delayed and long-term physical and emotional effects of cancer and cancer treatment. Local disease recurrence should be detected early and treated with curative intent. Patients with a prior history of breast cancer are at increased risk for a second primary breast cancer in the ipsilateral or contralateral breast. However, there is no evidence that additional laboratory or imaging procedures (beyond a careful history and physical examination and appropriate screening imaging recommendations) provide further benefit in asymptomatic breast cancer survivors. Patients previously treated with chemotherapy, especially anthracyclines and alkylating agents, are at increased risk for acute myeloid leukemia or myelodysplastic syndrome, although these sequelae are uncommon. Anthracyclines and trastuzumab therapy also increase the risk for congestive heart failure.

The most common symptoms in longer-term breast cancer survivors are fatigue, depression, and sexual dysfunction. Fatigue appears to be the most common post-treatment symptom but is often underreported. Patients with fatigue should be evaluated for early signs of congestive heart failure due to prior therapy with anthracyclines or trastuzumab. Likewise, menopausal symptoms with hot flashes due to ovarian suppression from chemotherapy or the direct effects of endocrine therapy may contribute to fatigue.

Breast cancer survivors should be encouraged to follow a healthy lifestyle including an appropriate low fat diet, regular exercise, and limited alcohol consumption. Recently updated guidelines from the American Society of Clinical Oncology for breast cancer follow-up recommend regular history taking and physical examination every 3 to 6 months for 3 years after the initial diagnosis, followed by annual or biannual follow-up for 2 years and annual follow-up thereafter. It is also appropriate for many lower-risk patients to consider transitioning to a specialized survivorship program or primary care follow-up after the first year.

Improved understanding of the underlying biology of breast cancer along with the complexity of available diagnostic, prognostic, and therapeutic interventions has resulted in a compelling need for close coordination and integration of multiple specialty fields for the optimal care of patients with breast cancer. As efforts to detect breast cancer early and therapeutic interventions continue to improve, increasing importance must be placed on the most appropriate strategies for monitoring and managing the long-term consequences of breast cancer and its treatment in order to provide patients with the best chance for living a long and successful life as breast cancer survivors.

For a deeper discussion on this topic, please see Chapter 198, "Breast Cancer and Benign Breast Disorders," in Goldman-Cecil Medicine, 25th Edition.

SUGGESTED READINGS

DeSantis C, Siegel R, Bandi P, et al: Breast cancer statistics, 2011, CA Cancer J Clin 61:409–418, 2011.

Holmes MD, Chen WY, Feskanich D, et al: Physical activity and survival after breast cancer diagnosis, JAMA 293:2479–2486, 2005.

Khatcheressian JL, Hurley P, Bantug E, et al: Breast cancer follow-up and management after primary treatment: American Society of Clinical Oncology clinical practice guideline update, J Clin Oncol 31:961–965, 2013.

Lyman GH, Baker J, Geradts J, et al: Multidisciplinary care of patients with early-stage breast cancer, Surg Oncol Clin N Am 22:299–317, 2013.

Lyman GH, Benson AB, Bosserman L, et al: Sentinel lymph node biopsy for patients with early-stage breast cancer, American Society of Clinical Oncology clinical practice guideline update, J Clin Oncol 32:1365–1383, 2014.

Lyman GH, Sparrenboom A: Chemotherapy dosing in overweight and obese patients with cancer, Nat Rev Clin Onc 10:451–459, 2013.

Peto R, Davies C, Godwin J, et al: Comparisons between different polychemotherapy regimens for early breast cancer: meta-analyses of long-term outcome among 100,000 women in 123 randomised trials, Lancet 379:432–444, 2012.

60

Other Solid Tumors

Michael J. McNamara

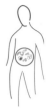

INTRODUCTION

Head and neck cancer, melanoma, sarcoma, and carcinoma of unknown primary site are distinct malignancies each with its own epidemiology, histopathology, treatment, and prognosis. Head and neck cancer and melanoma are relatively common, but sarcomas and unknown primary carcinoma are rare. Recent advances in understanding of the molecular biology of cancer and the interaction between the immune system and malignancy have improved therapeutic options for patients with these diseases.

HEAD AND NECK CANCER

Definition and Epidemiology

Head and neck cancers are squamous cell carcinomas that arise from the mucosal lining of the oral cavity, oropharynx, nasopharynx, hypopharynx, and larynx (Fig. 60-1). Other malignancies arising from structures within the head and neck, such as salivary gland tumors or thyroid cancers, differ in regard to biology, presentation, natural history, pathology, and response to therapy.

Head and neck cancer accounts for 3.2% of new cancer diagnoses in the United States. In 2013, there were expected to be 53,640 patients diagnosed with this disease and 11,520 deaths. Chronic exposure to tobacco smoke and alcohol have been considered the strongest risk factors for developing this disease, but in recent decades human papilloma virus (HPV) has been responsible for a dramatic increase in the incidence of oropharyngeal squamous cell carcinoma. Patients with HPV-associated oropharyngeal cancer are typically younger than patients with HPV-negative disease and often have minimal history of tobacco or alcohol use. Rather, these patients share a history of high-risk sexual behaviors, including earlier age at first intercourse and a large number of partners. Nasopharyngeal squamous cell carcinoma is relatively uncommon in the United States and is distinct from other head and neck cancers, given its association with Epstein-Barr virus (EBV) infection.

Pathology

Approximately 95% of all cancers arising from the squamous epithelium of the upper aerodigestive tract are squamous cell carcinomas. Mucosal melanomas, adenocarcinomas, and neuroendocrine tumors are also encountered. Squamous cell carcinomas are subdivided into well differentiated, moderately well differentiated, and poorly differentiated types based on their degree of resemblance to normal squamous epithelium. Poorly differentiated disease is more aggressive and has a worse prognosis. Nasopharyngeal carcinomas are also classified as either keratinizing or nonkeratinizing, the latter strongly associated with EBV infection.

The increasingly common HPV-associated oropharyngeal cancer differs in molecular profile from alcohol- and smoking-related squamous cell carcinoma. For example, head and neck cancer related to alcohol and tobacco smoke is frequently associated with mutations in the tumor suppressor gene *TP53* and decreased expression of the cell cycle regulatory protein p16-INK4a. Conversely, HPV-associated oropharyngeal cancer displays wild-type TP53 with increased expression of p16-INK4a. Immunohistochemistry results demonstrating p16-INK4a establishes a diagnosis of HPV-related disease.

Clinical Presentation

The presentation of patients with head and neck cancer depends on the location of the primary tumor and the extent of local disease. Disease dissemination to distant sites is uncommon at the time of diagnosis, so patients rarely have signs or symptoms of metastatic disease at presentation. Tumors of the nasopharynx often block the Eustachian tube or cause epistaxis. Oral cavity tumors may manifest with a painful, ulcerated lesion. HPV-associated oropharynx cancer usually manifests with cervical lymphadenopathy; the primary tumors are often small and asymptomatic. Cancer of the hypopharynx manifests with dysphagia and that of the larynx with hoarseness.

Metastases develop late in the course of this disease, commonly in lung or bone. Patients may also develop hypercalcemia as a paraneoplastic syndrome related to ectopic production of parathyroid hormone–related protein.

Diagnosis and Differential Diagnosis

The diagnosis of squamous cell carcinoma requires biopsy. Staging is accomplished by a combination of imaging and careful inspection of the upper aerodigestive tract. Second primary cancers are common in patients with a history of heavy alcohol and tobacco abuse. CT, MRI, and positron emission tomography (PET) can detect nodal involvement not appreciated on physical examination as well as distant metastases. Patients with squamous cell carcinoma who have cervical lymphadenopathy and no apparent primary site at presentation require random biopsies of the base of the tongue and surrounding tissues, in combination with an ipsilateral tonsillectomy, to identify the occult primary site.

Treatment and Prognosis

The prognosis of head and neck cancer depends on tumor stage. The American Joint Committee on Cancer (AJCC) TNM staging

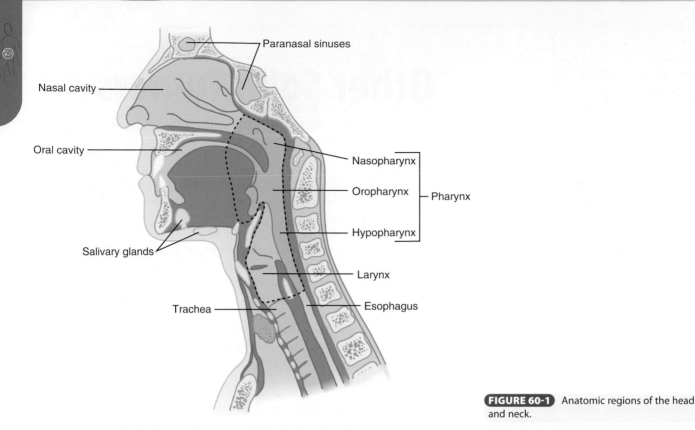

FIGURE 60-1 Anatomic regions of the head and neck.

system is used. Patients with early-stage disease have an excellent prognosis, with 5-year survival rates approaching 90%. However, only a minority of patients are diagnosed with early-stage disease; cancer is usually locally advanced at the time of diagnosis, with large, invasive primary tumors or regional lymph node metastases. Cure is possible with multimodality therapies, but the aggregate outcome is less favorable.

The prognosis for patients with HPV-associated oropharyngeal cancer is better than for those whose cancer is related to tobacco smoke and alcohol abuse. Both the biology of the disease and medical comorbidities contribute to the poorer prognosis. Furthermore, these patients are at high risk for development of second primary cancers of the upper aerodigestive tract, including lung cancer and esophageal cancer—so-called *field cancerization*: the entire upper aerodigestive epithelium is at increased risk for malignant transformation.

Both surgery and radiotherapy are potentially curative in patients with head and neck cancer. Chemotherapy alone is not a curative treatment, but chemotherapy given simultaneously with radiotherapy, termed *chemoradiotherapy*, may enhance the cytotoxic effects of radiation. Chemoradiotherapy is more efficacious but more toxic than radiotherapy alone. The choice of treatment is based on the location of the primary tumor and the extent of disease. Surgery or radiotherapy alone can cure early-stage disease. Patients with locally advanced cancers require more aggressive management, either chemoradiotherapy or a combination of chemoradiotherapy and surgery.

Radiation-based treatment may be used instead of surgery for disease for which tumor resection could cause cosmetic deformity or loss of organ function. For example, chemoradiotherapy may be used to treat locally advanced laryngeal cancer without the

need to sacrifice the larynx. Although chemoradiotherapy may permit organ preservation, it has both acute and chronic toxicity.

Metastatic disease is incurable, and therapy is palliative. Chemotherapy may mitigate cancer-related symptoms and produce a modest improvement in the median survival time compared with supportive care alone.

MELANOMA

Definition and Epidemiology

Melanoma, a malignant disorder of melanocytes, differs from other common skin cancers by its aggressive behavior and proclivity for regional and distant metastasis. The incidence of melanoma is increasing; it is now the fifth most common cancer in the United States. There were expected to be 76,690 new diagnoses and 9,480 deaths from melanoma in 2013. Melanoma is more common in fair-skinned individuals who tend not to darken with sun exposure. Although there are multiple risk factors for melanoma, sun exposure is the most important. Intense and intermittent sun exposure, especially during childhood and early adulthood, is the strongest risk factor for development of this disease. Chronic or occupational sun exposure does not confer the same degree of risk but may contribute to the development of melanoma on sun-exposed areas such as the head and neck. Other risk factors for melanoma include a family or personal history of this disease, multiple typical nevi, and the presence of atypical nevi.

Pathology

Melanocytes are derived from neural crest cells that have migrated to the epidermis. They occupy the basal layer of the epidermis and function in part to produce and transfer melanin to keratinocytes, thereby determining the color of skin and hair. There are also benign proliferative disorders of melanocytes, including the common acquired nevus (mole).

Melanoma has four major clinicopathologic subtypes. The most common subtype is superficial spreading melanoma, which can occur anywhere on the body but has a predilection for the torso and legs. Lentigo maligna melanoma manifests typically as a tan macule on chronically sun-exposed areas in older individuals. Nodular melanoma is associated with vertical growth into the dermis and manifests as a dark, nodular lesion. Acral lentiginous melanoma is an uncommon variant found on the palmar and plantar surfaces as well as subungual areas. This subtype is the most common form of melanoma in dark-skinned individuals. Other variants have also been described. Although this classification, which dates from the 1960s, captures the clinical heterogeneity of melanoma, it does not provide prognostic information or help determine clinical management.

Pathologic features that have prognostic relevance include the depth of invasion, the presence of ulceration, and the presence and number of mitotic figures. All of these features are incorporated into the AJCC TNM staging system of malignant melanoma. Increasing depth of invasion predicts a poor prognosis. The risk of lymph node metastasis, distant metastasis, and death, exists on a continuum with increasing tumor thickness. Therefore, patients with thin melanomas ($\leq$1 mm thickness) generally have favorable outcomes, whereas patients with thick melanomas (>4 mm thickness), even in the absence of nodal disease, have a 5 year survival rate often less than 50% (Table 60-1).

Clinical Presentation

Most patients with cutaneous melanoma have early-stage disease at presentation. Approximately 15% of patients have clinically apparent regional adenopathy or radiographic evidence for metastatic disease at the time of diagnosis. A number of benign lesions share morphologic features with melanoma, making identification by physical examination challenging. Because survival for patients with limited disease is excellent, early detection is important.

Features favoring malignancy are suggested by the *ABCDE* rule: *a*symmetry, irregular *b*orders, variable *c*olor, *d*iameter greater than 6 mm, and *e*volving lesion. A lesion that is changing in shape, size, or color should be considered suspicious.

Melanoma typically disseminates to regional lymph nodes. Regional lymph nodes should be examined. Metastatic disease also occurs in the liver, lung, skin, bone, and brain. Symptoms of advanced disease are highly variable.

In contrast to cutaneous melanoma, mucosal melanoma is often advanced at the time of diagnosis. This disease is rare, and the sites include the head and neck, anorectum, and vulvovaginal areas. Presenting symptoms are similar to those of the more common malignant diseases of these regions.

Diagnosis and Differential Diagnosis

The diagnosis of melanoma requires histologic evaluation of a biopsy specimen. In general, pigmented lesions suspicious for melanoma should undergo an excisional biopsy. This allows adequate assessment of tumor thickness, which informs decisions regarding the need for a sentinel lymph node biopsy and the width of subsequent local excision. If an excisional biopsy cannot be performed, a full-thickness punch biopsy is recommended. So-called shave biopsies of suspicious lesions make subsequent determination of tumor thickness difficult and may provide insufficient material for diagnosis. The histologic diagnosis is based on characteristic morphology and on immunohistochemical staining for markers such as S100, HMB45, and MART1.

In general, imaging investigations for staging purposes are not required for patients with thin or intermediate-thickness melanoma. The likelihood of demonstrating metastatic disease is low. Patients with thick melanomas or lymph node metastasis detected on clinical examination or by sentinel lymph node biopsy are at high risk for disease dissemination and need radiographic staging by CT of the chest, abdomen, and pelvis. Further imaging depends on the clinical context. For example, patients with clinically advanced melanoma and new, diffuse bone pain should undergo a bone scan; those with neurologic symptoms should undergo brain imaging.

Treatment and Prognosis

The prognosis of melanoma can be accurately estimated using the AJCC TNM staging system. Overall survival depends on the thickness of the primary tumor and the presence and number of regional lymph node metastases. Tumor ulceration and high mitotic rate are associated with a poor prognosis. Metastatic disease is incurable, and the clinical course depends on the pattern and extent of dissemination. An elevated serum lactate dehydrogenase (LDH) level is an independent poor prognostic factor for patients with metastases.

Surgery with wide margins is the cornerstone of curative therapy for nonmetastatic disease. The optimal margin depends on the depth of invasion and the location of the primary lesion but is typically between 1 and 2 cm. Patients with tumors larger than 1 mm in thickness and a negative physical examination should also undergo regional lymph node biopsy to evaluate for metastasis. Patients with melanoma in the initial node or nodes merit lymph node dissection for more accurate staging and to remove any residual disease.

TABLE 60-1	ESTIMATED OVERALL SURVIVAL FOR PATIENTS WITH MELANOMA BASED ON THE DEPTH OF INVASION AND NUMBER OF INVOLVED REGIONAL LYMPH NODES.	
DEPTH OF PRIMARY TUMOR INVASION (mm)	**AJCC T STAGE**	**5-YR OVERALL SURVIVAL (%)**
$\leq$1	T1	95
1.01-2.0	T2	85
2.01-4.0	T3	70
>4.0	T4	55
NUMBER OF INVOLVED REGIONAL LYMPH NODES	**AJCC N STAGE**	**5-YR OVERALL SURVIVAL (%)**
1	N1	65
2-3	N2	55
$\geq$4	N3	35

Data from Edge S, Byrd DR, Compton CC, et al: AJCC Cancer Staging Manual, ed 7, New York, 2010, Springer.
AJCC, American Joint Committee on Cancer.

Adjuvant therapy with high-dose interferon may be considered for patients with a high risk of recurrence after complete resection—that is, those with a primary tumor larger than 4 mm or lymph node metastasis. Adjuvant interferon is administered over the course of 1 year; it has substantial morbidity. The improvement in outcome is modest, and the effect on overall survival remains unclear.

For patients with metastatic disease, new agents have been developed based on the molecular biology of the disease and the immune response to malignancy. Ipilimumab, for example, is a monoclonal antibody which targets cytotoxic T-lymphocyte antigen 4 (CTLA-4), an immune regulatory molecule that inhibits T cell activation. The immunomodulatory effects of ipilimumab result in an immune response against tumor antigens, improving the survival of patients with metastatic disease (level A evidence).

Approximately 45% of cutaneous melanomas have activating mutations of the proto-oncogene *BRAF*, a component of the mitogen-activated protein kinase (MAPK) signaling pathway. Vemurafenib and dabrafenib are oral BRAF inhibitors that improve the survival of patients with metastatic disease who harbor specific *BRAF* mutations (level A evidence). Trametinib is an orally active agent that targets MEK, another component of the MAPK pathway downstream of BRAF. This agent has also demonstrated activity in patients with *BRAF*-mutant metastatic melanoma.

⬤ SARCOMA

Definition and Epidemiology

Sarcomas are heterogeneous solid tumors of mesenchymal origin. These tumors are broadly categorized as sarcomas of bone or sarcomas of soft tissue, with several distinct clinicopathologic subtypes. There were expected to be 11,410 new diagnoses of soft tissue sarcoma and 3,010 new diagnoses of bone sarcoma in the United States in 2013. Overall, sarcomas account for fewer than 1% of all new cancer diagnoses.

Most sarcomas are sporadic, but risk factors include prior radiation exposure, chemical carcinogens, and genetic predisposition (familial adenomatous polyposis [FAP], Li-Fraumeni syndrome). Moreover, human herpesvirus 8 (HHV-8) infection is associated with the development of Kaposi's sarcoma.

Soft tissue sarcomas can be further classified by their anatomic site of origin: head and neck, visceral, retroperitoneal, intra-abdominal, and extremity. This categorization is useful for staging, assessing prognosis, and establishing a therapeutic approach. The most common soft tissue sarcomas are gastrointestinal stromal tumors (GISTs), pleomorphic sarcoma, liposarcoma, leiomyosarcoma, and synovial sarcoma. The most commonly encountered sarcomas of bone are the Ewing's family of sarcomas, chondrosarcomas, and osteosarcomas.

Clinical Presentation

Given the heterogeneity of this group of diseases, including differences in tumor biology and in anatomic site of origin, the clinical presentation is variable. Soft tissue sarcomas of the extremities and of the head and neck usually manifest as a progressively enlarging, often painless, mass. Visceral and intra-abdominal sarcomas including GISTs are often found incidentally and are not symptomatic until they are locally advanced. Symptoms are often nonspecific but may include early satiety, abdominal fullness, bloating, or discomfort.

Bone sarcomas, such as Ewing's sarcoma and osteosarcoma, typically manifest with pain. The most frequently involved locations are the femur, tibia, and humerus. The physical examination may reveal a palpable mass, which is often tender to palpation. Symptoms may be present for several months before diagnosis. Most patients have locally confined disease at diagnosis; the lungs and bone are the most common sites of metastatic spread.

Diagnosis and Differential Diagnosis

The diagnosis of sarcoma can be established only by obtaining histologic confirmation, for which a biopsy is required. This disease must be distinguished from more common malignancies such as lymphoma, melanoma, and poorly differentiated carcinoma. The diagnosis of sarcoma is based on characteristic morphology but may be aided by the use of immunohistochemical and molecular studies. For example, Ewing's sarcoma is often associated with a characteristic reciprocal translocation between chromosomes 11 and 22, t(11:22). Several other molecular derangements have been identified and are helpful in establishing the specific diagnosis.

For bone sarcomas, plain films often demonstrate a mixture of lytic and blastic components with associated soft tissue edema. For osteosarcoma, the periosteal reaction produces a "sunburst" appearance as new bone forms at right angles to the tumor, as opposed to the "onion peel" appearance caused by layering of reactive bone, which is more commonly associated with Ewing's sarcoma.

Treatment and Prognosis

Surgery is the primary therapy for locally confined disease. Radiotherapy before or after surgery may decrease the likelihood of local recurrence. Chemotherapy patients with certain histologic subtypes of sarcoma (Ewing's sarcoma, osteosarcoma) may improve local control, decrease the risk of distant recurrences, and improve overall survival.

Patients with metastatic sarcoma may occasionally benefit from surgical extirpation of their disease. However, once metastatic dissemination has been detected, the intent of therapy is palliative. Chemotherapy can reduce the overall tumor burden and minimize cancer-related symptoms; doxorubicin, ifosfamide, and gemcitabine are used.

Targeted therapies have revolutionized the management of GISTs. The small-molecule tyrosine kinase inhibitor, imatinib, is highly active in patients with GISTs. It rapidly reduces tumor burden with sustained benefit. Imatinib is currently administered to patients with GISTs in the perioperative and advanced/metastatic settings (level A evidence).

⬤ CANCER OF UNKNOWN PRIMARY SITE
Definition and Epidemiology

Malignancies for which there is no apparent site of origin after a thorough history, physical examination, imaging investigations, and appropriate diagnostic procedures are referred to as *cancers of unknown primary site* (CUP). CUP accounts for approximately 2% of all new cancer diagnoses in the United States, with 31,860 new cases anticipated in 2013. CUPs are heterogeneous with a highly variable clinical presentation and prognosis. Although the primary site rarely becomes evident during the course of the disease, molecular profiling suggests that CUP is frequently a result of occult lung, kidney, bladder, or pancreaticobiliary cancer.

Clinical Presentation

Most patients with CUP have nonspecific complaints. Constitutional symptoms such as anorexia, weight loss, and fatigue are typical of advanced disease and are commonly present at the time of diagnosis. Pain at the time of presentation is more variable but is frequently experienced by patients with bone metastasis. Less common presenting signs and symptoms include epidural spinal cord compression, hypercalcemia, isolated brain metastasis, ascites, and venous thromboembolic disease.

However, many patients have very few symptoms initially, such as progressive lymphadenopathy only. Occasionally, the diagnosis is arrived at incidentally, during evaluation for an unrelated condition.

Pathology

CUPs are categorized based on histologic evaluation. Most CUPs demonstrate adenocarcinoma histology. However, squamous cell carcinoma, neuroendocrine carcinoma, and poorly differentiated carcinoma are also commonly encountered. Poorly differentiated carcinoma must be distinguished from melanoma, lymphoma, and sarcoma, because the treatments differ by disease.

Immunohistochemistry may disclose the site of origin. For example, in the case of poorly differentiated tumors, the presence of S100 and HMB45 supports a diagnosis of melanoma, whereas CD45 supports a diagnosis of lymphoma. Chromogranin and synaptophysin suggest neuroendocrine differentiation. Cytokeratin 5 (CK5) and CK6 are strongly expressed by squamous cell carcinomas, whereas the expression pattern of CK7 and CK20 can limit the differential diagnosis of adenocarcinomas.

Molecular tumor profiling studies suggest that gene expression profiles can identify the primary site in 60% to 80% of patients. However, it remains unclear whether gene expression profiling improves patient outcomes.

Treatment and Prognosis

CUP confers a median survival time of 8 to 11 months. Therapy is almost always offered with palliative intent. Chemotherapy can mitigate cancer-related symptoms and improve overall survival. However, there are several clinical presentations for which the prognosis is more favorable and therapy can be curative. For example, a woman presenting with adenocarcinoma isolated to unilateral axillary lymph nodes should be evaluated and treated as for a locally advanced breast cancer, regardless of whether imaging investigations demonstrate a primary breast malignancy. Likewise, a patient with squamous cell carcinoma isolated to cervical lymph nodes at presentation should receive therapy for locally advanced head and neck cancer, again regardless of whether a primary lesion can be identified. In both these circumstances, therapy may prove curative. Another clinical scenario for which specific therapy is beneficial is that of a young man with a poorly differentiated midline tumor: A favorable response to a chemotherapy regimen for germ cell cancers may be beneficial.

Assays that provide a molecular tumor profile, which may more accurately identify the primary site than standard clinicopathologic variables, are currently available.

For a deeper discussion on this topic, please see Chapters 190, "Head and Neck Cancer," 202, "Sarcomas of Soft Tissue and Bone, and Other Neoplasms of Connective Tissues," 203, "Melanoma and Nonmelanoma Skin Cancers," and 204, "Cancer of Unknown Primary Origin," in Goldman-Cecil Medicine, *25th Edition.*

SUGGESTED READINGS

Chapman PB, Hauschild A, Robert C, et al: Improved survival with vemurafenib in melanoma with BRAF V600E mutation, N Engl J Med 364:2507–2516, 2011.

Fletcher CDM, Unni KK, Mertens F: World Health Organization classification of tumors: pathology and genetics of tumors of soft tissue and bone, Lyon, 2002, IARC Press.

Hainsworth JD, Rubin MS, Spigel DR, et al: Molecular gene expression profiling to predict the tissue of origin and direct site-specific therapy in patients with carcinoma of unknown primary site: a prospective trial of the Sarah Cannon Research Institute, J Clin Oncol 31:217–223, 2012.

Rajendra R, Pollack SM, Jones RL: Management of gastrointestinal stromal tumors, Future Oncol 9:193–206, 2013.

Robert C, Thomas L, Bondarenko I, et al: Ipilimumab plus decarbazine for previously untreated metastatic melanoma, N Engl J Med 364:2517–2526, 2011.

Siegel R, Naishadham D, Jemal A: Cancer statistics, 2013, CA Cancer J Clin 63:11–30, 2013.

Wisco OJ, Sober AJ: Prognostic factors for melanoma, Dermatol Clin 30:469–485, 2012.

Zandberg DP, Bhargava R, Badin S, et al: The role of human papillomavirus in nongenital cancers, CA Cancer J Clin 63:57–81, 2013.

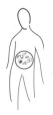

61

Complications of Cancer and Cancer Treatment

Bassam Estfan and Alok A. Khorana

INTRODUCTION

Patients with cancer can experience various complications as a direct result of their disease or its treatment. Cancer complications can be localized or systemic (Table 61-1). Cancer treatments, especially chemotherapy and radiation therapy, have potentially significant side effects and complications; most are temporary, but some, such as peripheral neuropathy, can become permanent (Table 61-2). The significance of complications of cancer and its treatment goes beyond quality of life; cancer outcomes can be affected by resulting treatment delay or cessation, dose reduction, and hospitalization. Frequently, the management of cancer complications requires a multidisciplinary approach. This chapter highlights some important complications of cancer and its treatment.

CANCER-ASSOCIATED THROMBOSIS

Epidemiology

Patients with cancer are at increased risk for both venous and arterial thromboembolism; thromboembolic events are the second leading cause of death among patients with cancer.

TABLE 61-1 COMPLICATIONS OF CANCER

LOCALIZED	SYSTEMIC
Brain metastases	Anorexia/cachexia
Cancer-related pain	Cancer-associated thrombosis
Cord compression/cauda equina syndrome	Cancer-related anemia
Malignant effusions	Cancer-related fatigue
Pathologic fractures	Hypercalcemia
Superior vena cava syndrome	Paraneoplastic syndromes
Visceral obstruction	Tumor lysis syndrome

TABLE 61-2 COMPLICATIONS OF CANCER TREATMENT

Alopecia
Central line thrombosis/infections
Cytopenias
Febrile neutropenia
Hot flashes
Hypertension
Nausea and vomiting
Peripheral neuropathy
Secondary malignancies
Skin toxicity
Stomatitis
Tumor lysis syndrome

Pathology

The hypercoagulable state in patients with cancer is a result of activation of the coagulation system by neoplastic cells. Certain cancers such as pancreas, stomach, lung, lymphoma, and brain are particularly associated with venous thromboembolism. Cancer treatments including chemotherapy, anti-angiogenic agents, and hormonal therapy further increase the risk. Other risk factors include central venous catheters, obesity, and prior history of thrombosis and use of erythropoiesis-stimulating agents. Biomarkers, including elevated platelet and leukocyte counts, have also been shown to be predictive. However, risk cannot be determined on the basis of single risk factors alone, because the etiology is multifactorial. The Khorana Score is a validated risk that incorporates five simple clinical and laboratory variables has been endorsed by various guidelines for risk assessment.

Clinical Presentation

Clinical suspicion should be high in cancer patients whose presenting symptoms include dyspnea, cough, wheezing, chest pain, tachycardia, upper abdominal pain, or extremity swelling. Thrombosis remains a consideration even in ambulatory patients and those already receiving adequate anticoagulation. Incidental pulmonary embolisms may be identified on imaging studies conducted for staging of cancer; they are also associated with adverse outcomes and should be treated appropriately.

Treatment

Venous thromboembolism can be prevented with the use of prophylaxis in hospitalized cancer patients. Unfractionated heparin, low-molecular-weight heparins (LMWHs), and fondaparinux are safe and effective. Prophylaxis is being investigated in the ambulatory setting and appears to be beneficial in highly selected patients.

Established thrombosis should be treated with anticoagulation. Oral anticoagulation with warfarin is frequently complicated by interactions with chemotherapeutic agents, variable nutritional status, and relative resistance. In a randomized clinical trial, the LMWH dalteparin, given for up to 6 months, was more effective than warfarin in preventing recurrent thrombosis, and this class of anticoagulants is preferred for first-line therapy.

Vena caval interruption using filters should be considered only if anticoagulation is clearly contraindicated (e.g., in the presence of active bleeding) or after failure of LMWHs. Novel oral antico-agulants have not yet been studied in the cancer setting.

SPINAL CORD COMPRESSION

Epidemiology

Spinal cord compression is the second most common neurologic complication of cancer after brain metastasis; it is estimated that 2.5% of cancer patients will suffer from cord compression. Breast, lung, and prostate cancers and multiple myeloma are the most common etiologies.

Pathology

Most cases (60% to 70%) occur at the level of the thoracic spine, followed by the lumbar and cervical spine. The conus medullaris terminates at the level of the L1 or L2 vertebral body; epidural disease below that level is associated instead with a cauda equina syndrome. Most spinal metastases affect the vertebral body; compression results from posterior extension of the tumor to the thecal sac. This leads to obstruction of the epidural venous circulation and vasogenic edema of the white and gray matter.

Clinical Presentation

Cord compression usually manifests with gradually worsening back pain around the level of involvement. Sudden positional back pain should raise the suspicion for vertebral compression fracture instead. Pain can become radicular and is usually worsened by the Valsalva maneuver. Sensorimotor neurologic deficit is a sign of advanced cord compression. Motor weakness is more common at presentation (up to 85% of patients); it is usually symmetric, but radicular motor weakness may be noticed with lateral vertebral metastases. Sensory deficit is less common and can manifest as paresthesia or lack of sensation. Bowel and bladder incontinence and urinary retention are usually late findings.

Diagnosis

Cord compression should be suspected clinically with any new back pain in the setting of cancer and rapidly investigated with spinal imaging. Plain radiographs of the vertebrae can reveal abnormalities such as lytic lesions or vertebral fractures, but magnetic resonance imaging (MRI) is the preferred diagnostic imaging modality. MRI of the full spine should be obtained even with localized symptoms, because multiple vertebral levels may be affected.

Treatment

The magnitude of the neurologic deficit before treatment is a good predictor of response and outcome. On diagnosis, pain management is important to allow better ambulation. Glucocorticoids have been used, while definitive therapy is awaited, at doses between 16 and 96 mg/day with both symptomatic and functional relief. There is no proven advantage to higher doses, which can be associated with more side effects. Surgical decompression and radiation are the two main treatment modalities.

In a phase III trial, 101 cancer patients with spinal cord compression were randomly assigned to receive radiation alone

(30 Gy in ten fractions) or surgical decompression followed by the same radiation regimen. More people in the surgical arm were ambulatory at interim analysis (84% versus 57%), and more people in that group regained the ability to walk (10/16 versus 3/16). Radiation therapy alone is useful for palliation of symptoms and local control; it is usually reserved for patients with spinal cord compromise without neurologic deficit or for those with an expected shorter survival time. Initial chemotherapy can be used in highly chemosensitive malignancies such as certain lymphomas or small cell lung carcinoma. Patient age, overall prognosis, and other comorbidities should be considered in treatment decision making.

SUPERIOR VENA CAVA SYNDROME

Definition

Superior vena cava syndrome in malignancy is the result of flow obstruction by either external compression or intravascular thrombosis. The superior vena cava is thin walled and therefore easily compressed. The most common malignant causes are lung cancer and lymphoma.

Clinical Presentation

Presentation depends on the rate of obstruction. Slow compression allows for the development of collaterals from the azygos, internal mammary, paraspinous, lateral thoracic, and esophageal venous systems. The azygos vein is the most important of these, and obstruction below its level is not well tolerated. Symptoms can be sudden or insidious. Most patients experience dyspnea (60% to 70%) and facial or neck swelling (50%). Cough, pain, arm swelling, and dysphagia are less common. Symptoms are frequently exacerbated by leaning forward or lying down. Physical findings may include venous distention of neck and chest wall, facial edema, plethora, cyanosis, and upper extremity edema.

Diagnosis

Plain chest radiographs are usually abnormal; mediastinal widening (64%) and pleural effusion (26%) are the most common findings. The diagnosis is best established with contrast-enhanced computed tomographic scanning of the chest. It demonstrates the location and size of masses, the presence of intravascular thrombosis, and collateral venous drainage. When superior vena cava syndrome is the initial manifestation of malignancy, pathologic diagnosis is the first step in establishing the proper initial treatment modality.

Treatment

The goals of treatment are to alleviate symptoms urgently and to treat the underlying malignancy. General supportive measures include head elevation and administration of glucocorticoids and diuretics. It is essential not to start radiation or glucocorticoids before obtaining a biopsy, because they could mask the diagnosis. Specific management depends on the underlying pathology. Chemotherapy is the preferred first line of therapy for chemosensitive malignancies such as lymphoma, small cell lung cancer, or germ cell tumors. For non–small cell lung cancers and other less chemosensitive tumors, initial radiation therapy may be preferred.

Symptomatic relief can occur within 2 weeks but is often temporary; therefore, systemic management should be initiated when indicated. Some tumors require surgical treatment. Persistent symptoms not relieved by chemotherapy or irradiation and those severe enough to warrant intervention before diagnosis can be successfully managed with endovascular stent placement with or without balloon angioplasty. For catheter-related thrombosis, anticoagulation is indicated; the decision regarding catheter removal should be individualized.

HYPERCALCEMIA

Epidemiology

Hypercalcemia complicates cancer in up to 10% of cases, occurring in both hematologic and solid malignancies. The most common etiologies are multiple myeloma, breast cancer, and squamous cell carcinoma.

Pathology

Mechanisms leading to hypercalcemia include osteolysis due to bony involvement and tumor production of parathyroid hormone–related protein (PTHrP), calcitriol, or cytokines. Even in the presence of cancer, primary hyperparathyroidism should be ruled out. Many cancer patients have low albumin and calcium levels that should be corrected.

Clinical Presentation

Early symptoms of hypercalcemia include constipation, polydipsia, polyuria, nausea, vomiting, and bradycardia. Most patients have signs of dehydration. Altered mental status is often a presenting symptom. The severity of symptoms depends on the time course over which hypercalcemia has developed rather than the absolute calcium level.

Treatment

Calcium supplements, vitamin D, and diuretics should be stopped. Aggressive fluid resuscitation with normal saline at 200 to 300 mL/hour should be started to maintain a high urine output. This should be done carefully in patients with compromised cardiac or renal function. These measures may be adequate for mild hypercalcemia, but moderate and severe hypercalcemias require further interventions.

Bisphosphonates are the preferred agents for management. They inhibit osteoclasts and bone resorption. Intravenous pamidronate and zoledronic acid are the two most commonly used bisphosphonates. In a pooled analysis, zoledronic acid was associated with a higher rate of calcium normalization and longer control. Calcium response to bisphosphonates can take a few days; therefore, if a rapid reduction is required for acute hypercalcemia, subcutaneous calcitonin (4 units/kg) can be given 2 to 4 times daily. Calcitonin works by increasing calcium renal excretion and reducing bone resorption. Other agents less commonly used in the management of hypercalcemia include gallium nitrate and glucocorticoids. Management should eventually include control of the underlying disease. Frequently, new or recurring hypercalcemia indicates disease progression or treatment resistance, which should be addressed with systemic therapy.

FEBRILE NEUTROPENIA

Definition

Febrile neutropenia is a common complication of chemotherapy. It is defined as a temperature of 100.4° F (38° C) in the setting of a neutrophil count lower than 500/μL (or lower than 1000/μL with a predicted decrease to less than 500/μL in the next 48 hours). The risk of febrile neutropenia increases with the intensity of the chemotherapy regimen and the severity and duration of neutropenia. It can lead to treatment delays or interruptions, prolonged hospitalizations, decreased quality of life, and increased morbidity and mortality.

Treatment

Although most cases are managed in the hospital, low-risk patients may occasionally be successfully managed as outpatients. The American Society of Clinical Oncology (ASCO) has published guidelines for outpatient management that are based on a risk-stratified scoring system. All patients should have a history and physical examination to identify possible focal sources of infection. Attention should be given to the presence of mucositis and to swelling or induration and erythema around indwelling catheters as possible sources of infection. The initial workup should include a full chemistry profile, complete blood count with differential, blood cultures with at least one from each existing catheter tip, urinalysis, and chest radiography.

Once the diagnosis is established and cultures have been obtained, empiric treatment with broad-spectrum antibiotics must be initiated. Frequently, organisms are not identified on cultures. Therapy is usually directed to coverage of gram-negative bacteria with cefipime or piperacillin-tazobactam. If line infection or mucosal or skin infection is suspected, vancomycin is indicated. Prolonged neutropenia increases the risk of fungal infections, and antifungal agents should be considered. The duration of antimicrobial treatment is determined on an individual basis, but it should continue at least until there is evidence of bone marrow recovery (usually a neutrophil count >500). Prophylaxis with myeloid growth factors such as filgrastim or pegfilgrastim can reduce the risk of febrile neutropenia from chemotherapy and is used in high-risk settings.

CHEMOTHERAPY-INDUCED NAUSEA AND VOMITING

Definition

Nausea and vomiting are perhaps the most feared adverse effects of chemotherapy. Chemotherapy agents are stratified according to risk of emetogenicity (Table 61-3). Nausea and emesis are typically categorized as acute, delayed, or anticipatory. Acute nausea and vomiting occurs during the first 24 hours of treatment, whereas delayed nausea occurs 2 to 5 days after treatment initiation. Patients with high levels of anxiety or prior poor control of nausea may also suffer symptoms in anticipation of starting treatment. The risk of chemotherapy-induced nausea and vomiting is greater in younger patients and in women. A history of increased alcohol consumption is associated with lower risk.

TABLE 61-3 NAUSEA AND VOMITING RISK WITH CANCER THERAPY

EMETIC RISK	PERCENTAGE OF PATIENTS AFFECTED	REPRESENTATIVE AGENTS	RECOMMENDED PREVENTIVE ANTIEMETIC
High	>90	Cisplatin, high-dose cyclophosphamide	NK1 antagonist + dexamethasone + 5HT3 antagonist
Moderate	30-90	Oxaliplatin, doxorubicin, irinotecan	5HT3 antagonist + dexamethasone
Low	10-30	Paclitaxel, etoposide, gemcitabine	Dexamethasone or 5HT3 antagonist or dopamine antagonist
Minimal	<10	Vincristine, bleomycin	Not needed

5HT3, Serotonin receptor; NK1, neurokinin 1.

Pathology

The mechanism is not completely understood but involves an effect of chemotherapy on the gastrointestinal mucosa and central nervous system, such as the chemoreceptor trigger zone (area postrema). The neurotransmitters that are involved include dopamine, serotonin, and substance P.

Treatment

The best approach for treatment is prevention. The prophylactic antiemetic protocol depends on the chemotherapy regimen and emetic risk (see Table 61-3). Randomized clinical trials have established that the combination of a neurokinin 1 (NK1) receptor antagonist (aprepitant or fosaprepitant), a 5HT3 serotonin receptor antagonist, and dexamethasone is the regimen of choice for highly emetogenic chemotherapy. For moderately emetogenic chemotherapy, a 5HT3 antagonist with dexamethasone is usually adequate. All patients should be given a dopamine or 5HT3 receptor antagonist as rescue therapy for intermittent nausea.

Dexamethasone is the preferred treatment for delayed nausea and vomiting in highly and moderately emetogenic chemotherapy. Other agents with proven efficacy include olanzapine for the prevention of both acute and delayed nausea and vomiting. Anticipatory nausea or vomiting is best treated with proper control of symptoms in the initial cycles. When it occurs, it is best treated with a benzodiazepine before chemotherapy.

⬤ DERMATOLOGIC TOXICITY

Many chemotherapeutic and targeted agents are associated with dermatologic toxicity, which can lead to patient morbidity, alter quality of life, and affect therapeutic dosing.

Clinical Presentation

Acneiform eruptions are observed with agents targeted against epidermal growth factor receptor (EGFR) in 70% to 80% of patients. The rash is usually erythematous with pustulopapular eruptions over the face, scalp, and upper trunk.

Palmar-plantar erythema, or so-called hand-foot syndrome, is seen with chemotherapeutic agents such as 5-fluorouracil and capecitabine or with tyrosine kinase inhibitors such as sorafenib, sunitinib, and regorafenib. Manifestations can differ slightly between classes of drugs, but they usually involve symmetrical redness of the palms or soles. Tingling and pain may accompany erythema. With progression, painful blistering or skin peeling may occur. Symptoms are frequently observed at pressure areas, such as on the soles of the feet after prolonged standing or running.

Treatment

Treatment of skin rash associated with anti-EGFR therapies is tailored to the severity of the rash and may include topical steroids, oral antibiotics (minocycline or doxycycline), and dose modification or cessation. Sunscreens, reduced sun exposure, and lotions for dry skin should be used for prevention. For hand-foot syndrome, preventive measures such as sunscreens and routine application of lotion to hands and feet are helpful. The most effective treatment is a brief treatment break (typically for several days, until complete resolution occurs), followed by resumption but with a reduced dose of the inciting agent.

⬤ TUMOR LYSIS SYNDROME

Definition

Tumor lysis syndrome occurs in malignancies with a high proliferative rate (such as aggressive lymphoma or leukemia), usually after the initiation of cytotoxic chemotherapy. It is an oncologic emergency. Rarely, it can occur spontaneously.

Pathology

Massive tumor cell lysis causes the release of large amounts of potassium, phosphate, and nucleic acids into blood. This leads to rapidly increased production of uric acid, which can precipitate in the renal tubules, causing acute renal insufficiency.

Diagnosis

Tumor lysis syndrome should be suspected in the presence of hyperuricemia, hyperkalemia, hyperphosphatemia, and hypocalcemia. Elevated creatinine can occur with renal damage from uric acid precipitation.

Treatment

In the appropriate clinical setting, tumor lysis syndrome should be anticipated and prevented. An international panel has developed a risk stratification scheme. Aggressive hydration is key to preventing this syndrome and should continue until the tumor burden is largely resolved. Allopurinol at a dose of 150 mg—or, in high-risk cases, rasburicase at a dose of 0.2 mg/kg—can be used for prophylaxis. Rasburicase may also be used to treat severe hyperuricemia and to prevent renal insufficiency.

For a deeper discussion on this topic, please see Chapters 176, "Hypercoagulable States," Chapter 179, "Tumor Lysis," Chapter 245, "Hypercalcemia," and Chapter 400, "Spinal Cord Compression" in Goldman-Cecil Medicine, 25th Edition.

SUGGESTED READINGS

Bayo J, Fonseca PJ, Hernando S, et al: Chemotherapy-induced nausea and vomiting: pathophysiology and therapeutic principles, Clin Trans Oncol 14:413–422, 2012.

Connors JM: Prophylaxis against venous thromboembolism in ambulatory patients with cancer, N Engl J Med 370:2515–2519, 2014.

Cooper KL, Madan J, Whyte S, et al: Granulocyte colony-stimulating factors for febrile neutropenia prophylaxis following chemotherapy: systematic review and meta-analysis, BMC Cancer 11:404, 2011.

Flowers CR, Seidenfeld J, Bow EJ, et al: Antimicrobial prophylaxis and outpatient management of fever and neutropenia in adults treated for malignancy: American Society of Clinical Oncology clinical practice guideline, J Clin Oncol 31:794–810, 2013.

Howard SC, Jones DP, Pui CH: The tumor lysis syndrome, N Engl J Med 364:2011, 1844-1854.

Huang V, Anadkat M: Dermatologic manifestations of cytotoxic therapy, Dermatol Ther 24:401, 2011.

LeGrand SB: Modern management of malignant hypercalcemia, Am J Hosp Palliat Care 28:515–517, 2011.

Lepper PM, Ott SR, Hoppe H, et al: Superior vena cava syndrome in thoracic malignancies, Respir Care 56:653–666, 2011.

Loblaw DA, Mitera G, Ford M, et al: A 2011 updated systematic review and clinical practice guideline for the treatment of malignant extradural spinal cord compression, Int J Radiat Oncol Biol Phys 84:312–317, 2012.

Lyman GH, Khorana AA, Kuderer NK, et al: Venous thromboembolism prophylaxis and treatment in patients with cancer: American Society of Clinical Oncology practice guideline update, J Clin Oncol 31:2189–2204, 2013.

Patchell RA, TIbbs PA, Regine WF, et al: Direct decompressive surgical resection in the treatment of spinal cord compression caused by metastatic cancer: a randomized trial, Lancet 366:643–648, 2005.

Roila F, Herrstedt J, Aapro M, et al: Guideline update for MASCC and ESMO in the prevention of chemotherapy- and radiotherapy-induced nausea and vomiting: results of the Perugia consensus conference, Ann Oncol 21(Suppl 5):v232–v243, 2010.

Wu PA, Balagula Y, Lacouture ME, et al: Prophylaxis and treatment of dermatologic adverse events from epidermal growth factor receptor inhibitors, Curr Opin Oncol 23:343–351, 2011.

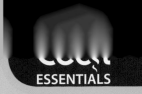

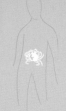

ESSENTIALS

X

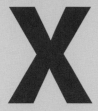

Endocrine Disease and Metabolic Disease

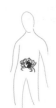

Hypothalamic-Pituitary Axis

Kawaljeet Kaur and Diana Maas

ANATOMY AND PHYSIOLOGY

The pituitary gland sits in the skull base in a bony structure called the sella turcica. It weighs approximately 600 mg and is composed of three lobes, the adenohypophysis (anterior lobe), the neurohypophysis (posterior lobe), and the intermediate lobe. The infundibular stalk, which contains the portal plexus circulation, connects the hypothalamus to the pituitary gland. The pituitary gland is surrounded by important structures that can be compromised by its enlargement, including the optic chiasm, located superior to the gland, and the cavernous sinuses, located on both sides of the gland. The cavernous sinuses each contain the internal carotid artery and cranial nerves III, IV, V1, V2, and VI. (Fig. 62-1).

The anterior pituitary gland produces six hormones that are produced by specific cell types within the gland: adrenocorticotropic hormone (ACTH), follicle-stimulating hormone (FSH), luteinizing hormone (LH), growth hormone (GH), prolactin, and thyroid-stimulating hormone (TSH or thyrotropin). These hormones are regulated by stimulatory and inhibitory peptides produced within the ventral hypothalamus and are transported to the anterior pituitary gland by the infundibular portal system. The posterior pituitary gland makes up about 20% of the total pituitary mass and stores and secretes two major peptide hormones: vasopressin (AVP or antidiuretic hormone) and oxytocin. These neurohypophyseal hormones are synthesized by the supraoptic and paraventricular nuclei of the hypothalamus and transported to the posterior lobe in neurosecretory granules along the supraopticohypophyseal tract. (Table 62-1) The intermediate lobe regresses in humans at about 15 weeks gestation and is absent in the adult normal pituitary gland.

On imaging studies, the normal adult pituitary gland has a flat superior border and a vertical height of approximately 8 to 10 mm. The anterior pituitary is homogeneous in signal on magnetic resonance imaging (MRI), the preferred imaging method, and enhances homogeneously after intravenous administration of a contrast agent (see Fig. 62-1). During periods of increased hormonal activity, most notably during pregnancy, the pituitary gland can increase in size and change shape. The posterior pituitary lobe is distinguished from the anterior lobe on T1-weighted MRI as a bright spot in the posterior aspect of the gland, best seen on a sagittal view. The bright appearance is thought to result from the presence of AVP and/or phospholipid vesicles within the normal neurohypophysis.

PITUITARY TUMORS

Pituitary tumors account for approximately 10% to 15% of intracranial tumors. They are the most commmon tumors in

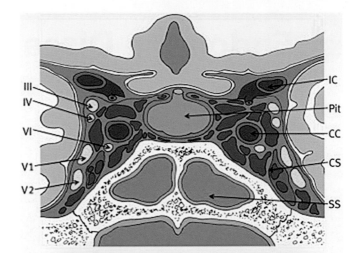

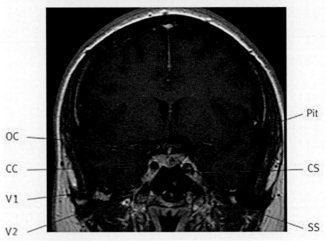

FIGURE 62-1 Coronal section and corresponding magnetic resonance imaging scan of the pituitary gland and surrounding structures, including cranial nerves III (oculomotor), IV (trochlear), V1 (trigeminal, ophthalmic branch), V2 (trigeminal, maxillary branch), and VI (abducens). CC, Carotid artery (intracavernous); CS, cavernous sinus (left); IC, internal carotid artery; OC, optic chiasm; Pit, pituitary gland; SS, sphenoid sinus. (From Jesurasa A, Kailaya-Vasan A, Sinha S: Surgery for pituitary tumors, Surgery 29:428–433, 2011, Figure 1.)

the sella, accounting for more than 90% of masses that develop in that area, and they are usually benign. Their true incidence is difficult to determine because they are often asymptomatic, but the prevalence is about 10% to 20% in radiologic studies. Most pituitary tumors are slow growing, but some have higher growth rates and can be invasive. Pituitary carcinomas are very rare and are defined by the presence of a metastasis that is noncontiguous with the original tumor or cerebrospinal fluid dissemination.

TABLE 62-1 PITUITARY–TARGET ORGAN HORMONE AXIS

HYPOTHALAMIC HORMONE	PITUITARY TARGET CELL	PITUITARY HORMONE AFFECTED	PERIPHERAL TARGET GLAND	PERIPHERAL HORMONE AFFECTED
STIMULATORY				
Anterior Lobe of Pituitary Gland				
Thyrotropin-releasing hormone (TRH)	Thyrotroph	Thyroid-stimulating hormone (TSH)	Thyroid gland	Thyroxine (T₄) Triiodothyronine (T₃)
Growth hormone-releasing hormone (GHRH)	Somatotroph	Growth hormone (GH)	Liver	Insulin-like growth factor-I (IGF-I)
Gonadotropin-releasing hormone (GnRH)	Gonadotroph	Luteinizing hormone (LH)	Ovary Testis	Progesterone Testosterone
		Follicle-stimulating hormone (FSH)	Ovary Testis	Estradiol Inhibin
Corticotropin-releasing hormone	Corticotroph	Adrenocorticotrophic hormone (ACTH)	Adrenal gland	Cortisol
Posterior Lobe of Pituitary Gland				
Vasopressin (AVP)			Kidney	
Oxytocin			Uterus	
			Breast	
INHIBITORY				
Somatostatin	Somatotroph	GH	Thyroid	
	Thyrotroph	TSH	Liver	
Dopamine	Lactotroph	Prolactin	Breast	

Pituitary tumors are classified by size and functionality or secretory capacity. Tumors that are smaller than 10 mm in diameter are called *microadenomas*, whereas lesions 10 mm or larger are called *macroadenomas*. Hormone-producing tumors are called *secretory adenomas,* and those that do not secrete a hormone are known as *nonsecretory adenomas.* Pituitary tumors may be composed of any of the anterior pituitary cell types, with multiple cell types forming plurihormonal tumors or nonsecretory tumors. Prolactin-secreting pituitary tumors are the most common type. Table 62-2 reviews the prevalence of the various pituitary tumors, and Table 62-3 describes the screening tests used to determine the secretory status of a new pituitary tumor.

The clinical manifestations of pituitary tumors are usually signs and symptoms caused by hormone overproduction or underproduction or mass effect. Common clinical features of pituitary mass effect include headaches, visual field defects, and cranial nerve palsies. Superior extension of a tumor compresses the optic chiasm, causing bitemporal hemianopsia; lateral

TABLE 62-2 PREVALENCE OF PITUITARY TUMORS

TUMOR	PREVALENCE (%)
Prolactinomas	40-45
Somatotroph adenomas	20
Corticotroph adenomas	10-12
Gonadotroph adenomas	15
Null cell adenomas	5-10
Thyrotroph adenomas	1-2

extension into the cavernous sinuses results in ophthalmoplegia, diplopia, or ptosis due to compression of cranial nerves III, IV, or VI or facial pain due to compression of V1 or V2. Compromise of normal pituitary tissue by a tumor can cause hormone loss or hypopituitarism. Screening tests for pituitary hormone deficiency are shown in Table 62-3; typically, a destructive pituitary lesion causes loss of pituitary hormones in the following progression: first GH, then FSH and LH, then TSH, and finally ACTH.

Disorders of Anterior Pituitary Hormones

 PROLACTIN

Definition and Epidemiology

The mature prolactin polypeptide contains 199 amino acids and is formed after a 28-amino acid signal peptide is proteolytically cleaved from the prolactin prohormone (pre-prolactin). Prolactin synthesis and secretion by pituitary lactotrophs is under tonic inhibitory control by hypothalamic-derived dopamine, which keeps prolactin at its basal levels. Factors stimulating prolactin synthesis and secretion, in addition to reduced dopamine availability to the lactotrophs, include

thyrotropin-releasing hormone (TRH), estrogen, vasoactive intestinal polypeptide (VIP), AVP, oxytocin, and epidermal growth factor.

Prolactin levels physiologically increase during pregnancy. After delivery, prolactin induces and maintains lactation of the primed breast. Once lactation has been initiated by these elevations in prolactin, prolactin falls to basal levels and lactation is maintained by the infant's suckling reflex. Hyperprolactinemia, regardless of the etiology, can cause hypogonadism through its inhibitory effect on gonadotropin release, infertility, galactorrhea, and/or bone loss from the hypogonadism.

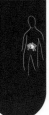
TABLE 62-3	SCREENING TESTS FOR PITUITARY DISORDERS		
DISORDER	**TESTS**	**DISORDER**	**TESTS**
PITUITARY TUMOR		**HYPOPITUITARISM**	
Acromegaly	IGF-I	GH deficiency	IGF-I
	OGTT: measure blood sugar and GH (0, 60, 120 min)		GH provocative test: ITT
Prolactinoma	Basal serum prolactin		Arginine-GHRH
ACTH-secreting	24-hr urine-free cortisol and creatinine level		Glucagon stimulation test
tumor	1-mg overnight dexamethasone suppression test	Gonadotropin	Women: basal estradiol, LH, FSH
	11 PM salivary cortisol	deficiency	Men: 8 AM fasting testosterone (total; free), LH, FSH
	Serum ACTH	TSH deficiency	Serum TSH, free T_4
	Dexamethasone-CRH test	ACTH deficiency	ACTH
	Bilateral inferior petrosal sinus sampling		Provocative test: ITT
TSH-secreting tumor	Serum TSH, FT4, FT3		Metyrapone test
Gonadotropin-	FSH, LH, alpha subunit		Cosyntropin-stimulation test (1 µg and 250 µg)
secreting tumor			

ACTH, Adrenocorticotropic hormone; CRH, corticotropin-releasing hormone; FSH, follicle-stimulating hormone; GH, growth hormone; GHRH, growth hormone–releasing hormone; IGF-I, insulin-like growth factor-I; ITT, insulin tolerance test; LH, luteinizing hormone; OGTT, oral glucose tolerance test; T_4, thyroxine; TSH, thyroid-stimulating hormone; TFT, thyroid function test.

Prolactinomas and hyperprolactinemia are more common in women, with a peak prevalence between 25 and 35 years of age. The mean prevalence of patients medically treated for hyperprolactinemia is approximately 20 per 100,000 in men and approximately 90 per 100,000 in women. Prolactinomas are rare in childhood or adolescence.

Clinical Presentation

The clinical presentation of a prolactinoma varies with the age and gender of the patient. Typically, the patient is a young woman with menstrual irregularities, galactorrhea, and infertility. Galactorrhea occurs in 50% to 80% of affected women. Men may report a decrease in libido and erectile dysfunction as result of hypogonadism caused by reduced secretion of LH and FSH. Typically, however, their tumors are diagnosed after symptoms of tumor compression appear, including headache, neurologic deficits, and vision changes. Galactorrhea and gynecomastia are rare in men. Because of the early presentation of menstrual irregularities in women, microprolactinomas are more common in women; macroprolactinomas are more frequent in men and in postmenopausal women.

Diagnosis and Differential Diagnosis

Hyperprolactinemia is diagnosed by a single measurement of serum prolactin; a level above the upper limit of normal confirms the diagnosis. For prolactinomas, serum prolactin levels typically parallel tumor size. A prolactin level greater than 250 ng/mL usually indicates the presence of a prolactinoma. Dynamic testing is not needed to diagnose hyperprolactinemia.

Two types of artifacts can occur during the standard measurement of prolactin: the presence of macroprolactin and the hook effect. When a patient with mild hyperprolactinemia does not have the expected clinical features of hyperprolactinemia (e.g., galactorrhea, menstrual disturbance, infertility), one should consider the presence of macroprolactin. Although 85% of circulating prolactin is monomeric, serum also contains the macroprolactin, a polymeric form of prolactin that is biologically inactive. Most commercially available prolactin assays do not detect macroprolactin, but it can be detected inexpensively in the serum by polyethylene glycol precipitation. The estimated incidence of macroprolactin accounting for a significant proportion of hyperprolactinemia is 10% to 20%. The hook effect should be

considered whenever a patient has a very large pituitary mass but only a mild elevation in prolactin. The hook effect is an assay artifact that occurs when very high serum prolactin concentrations saturate antibodies in the standard two-site immunoradiometric assay, resulting in falsely lower levels. This artifact can be overcome by repeating the prolactin measurement on a 1 : 100 serum sample dilution.

Physiologic increases in prolactin occur with pregnancy, physical or emotional stress, exercise, and chest wall stimulation. Other causes for hyperprolactinemia include some drugs, such as metoclopramide and risperidone, that can increase prolactin to greater than 200 ng/mL. Mild to moderate hyperprolactinemia (25 to 200 ng/mL) in the presence of a larger pituitary mass is more likely to be caused by a non–prolactin-secreting tumor with infundibular stalk compression and inhibition of dopamine transport to the lactotroph. Other causes include hypothalamic-pituitary disorders, systemic disorders, and neurogenic and idiopathic etiologies.

Treatment and Prognosis

Medical management with a dopamine agonist—bromocriptine or cabergoline—is the recommended treatment. The dopamine agonists normalize prolactin, decrease tumor size, and restore gonadal function in more than 80% of patients with prolactinomas. Because of the rapidity and efficacy of the dopamine agonists in treating these tumors, they are also the initial treatment for macroprolactinomas that have caused compromise in vision, neurologic deficits, or pituitary dysfunction.

Cabergoline, the newer agent, is preferred to other dopamine agonists because it has higher efficacy in normalizing prolactin levels and shrinking tumor size and has fewer side effects. The most common side effects seen with dopamine agonists are nausea, vomiting, orthostatic lightheadedness, dizziness, and nasal congestion. Because of the concern for cabergoline-related cardiac valvulopathy that was reported in patients who had Parkinson's disease treated with high doses of cabergoline and the possible long-term need for treatment, bromocriptine could be used in young patients if it is tolerated. Transsphenoidal resection of the tumor is indicated for patients who cannot tolerate the dopamine agonists or who do not respond to medical treatment. No treatment is required for patients who have microprolactinomas that are asymptomatic.

Recent studies have shown that dopamine agonists may be safely withdrawn in patients who have maintained normal prolactin levels for 2 years and who have no visible tumor remnant on tapering doses of dopamine agonist. Once the dopamine agonist is discontinued, prolactin levels should be checked every 3 months for 1 year and then annually. An MRI should be obtained only if the prolactin level becomes elevated again. Recurrence risk after drug withdrawal ranges from 26% to 69% and is predicted by the initial prolactin level and tumor size.

🔴 GROWTH HORMONE

Definition

GH is a single-chain polypeptide hormone consisting of 191 amino acids that is synthesized, stored, and secreted by the anterior pituitary somatotrophs. GH secretion is regulated by two factors derived from the hypothalamus: growth hormone–releasing hormone (GHRH) and somatostatin. GHRH stimulates somatotroph GH release, and somatostatin inhibits it. GH stimulates secretion of insulin-like growth factor-I (IGF-I) by the liver. IGF-I circulates in the blood attached to binding proteins; although there are six binding proteins in serum, more than 80% of IGF-I is bound to a protein called IGFBP3. Postnatally and through puberty, GH and IGF-I are critical in determining longitudinal skeletal growth, skeletal maturation, and acquisition of bone mass. In adulthood, they are instrumental in the maintenance of skeletal architecture and bone mass. GH also has effects on the metabolism of carbohydrates, lipids, and proteins by antagonizing insulin action, increasing lipolysis and free fatty acid production, and increasing protein synthesis.

Growth Hormone Deficiency

Epidemiology

Childhood-onset GH deficiency is most commonly idiopathic, but it may be genetic or associated with congenital anatomic malformations in the brain or sellar region. The most common cause of GH deficiency in adults is a pituitary macroadenoma and its treatment; deficiency of one or more pituitary hormones occurs in 30% to 60% of such cases. The incidence of hypopituitarism 10 years after irradiation of the sellar region is approximately 50%.

Clinical Presentation

Children with GH deficiency exhibit growth retardation, short stature, and fasting hypoglycemia. Manifestations of adult GH deficiency include reduced bone mineralization, decreased muscle strength and exercise performance, decreased lean body mass with increase in fat mass and abdominal adiposity, glucose intolerance and insulin resistance, abnormal lipid profile including elevated low-density lipoprotein and triglyceride levels with decreased high-density lipoprotein, depressed mood, and impaired psychosocial well-being.

Diagnosis and Differential Diagnosis

Because of the pulsatile nature of pituitary GH secretion, a single random measurement of serum GH is not helpful to diagnose GH deficiency. In adults with GH deficiency due to a pituitary tumor and concomitant hypopituitarism involving any three

other pituitary hormones, a low IGF-I level is sufficient to diagnose GH deficiency, and provocative testing is not warranted. Falsely low IGF-I levels are also seen in malnutrition, acute illness, celiac disease, poorly controlled diabetes mellitus, liver disease, and estrogen ingestion. In children, there tends to be greater variation in IGF-I levels that do not correspond to the true GH status, so provocative testing is required.

The historical "gold standard" stimulatory test is insulin-induced hypoglycemia (insulin tolerance test or ITT). Symptomatic hypoglycemia with a serum glucose level lower than 45 mg/dL is a potent stimulus for GH secretion; the normal GH response is greater than 10 ng/mL in children and greater than 5 ng/mL in adults. Because of the unavailability in the United States of GHRH, which is as sensitive and specific as the ITT in stimulating GH secretion, glucagon stimulation is being used, especially in adults with ischemic heart disease or seizures. A normal response with the glucagon stimulation test is defined as a GH peak greater than 3 ng/mL.

Treatment and Prognosis

Recombinant human growth hormone (hGH) is administered to promote linear growth in short children. The U.S. Food and Drug Administration (FDA) has approved GH treatment for conditions involving complete absence of GH associated with severe growth retardation or partial GH deficiency resulting in short stature. Short stature is defined as height more than 2.5 standard deviations below the mean for age-matched normal children, growth velocity less than the 25th percentile, delayed bone age, and predicted adult height less than the mean parental height. The conditions approved by the FDA to use GH include GH deficiency, idiopathic short stature, Turner's syndrome, Prader-Willi syndrome, chronic kidney disease, AIDS-associated muscle wasting, *SHOX* gene deficiency, Noonan's syndrome, and children born small for gestational age. Combined clinical evaluations, along with an inadequate pituitary GH response to provocative testing, are used in the assessment of childhood GH deficiency. Higher doses of GH are recommended for children without GH deficiency disorders or with partial GH deficiency.

In adults, GH is administered as a daily subcutaneous injection starting at 0.1 to 0.3 mg, with dose increases at 6-week intervals based on clinical response, side effects, and IGF-I levels. Absolute contraindications to GH therapy in adults include active neoplasm, intracranial hypertension, and proliferative diabetic retinopathy; uncontrolled diabetes and untreated thyroid disease are relative contraindications. Side effects of GH therapy are usually transient and include arthralgias, fluid retention, carpal tunnel syndrome, and glucose intolerance. Additional side effects in children include slipped capital femoral epiphysis and hydrocephalus.

Acromegaly or Growth Hormone Hypersecretion

Definition and Epidemiology

Acromegaly is literally translated as abnormal enlargement of the extremities of the skeleton. It is caused by hypersecretion of GH in adulthood. In children, excessive GH secretion before closure of the epiphyseal growth plate leads to gigantism. In both cases, the cause is almost always a GH-secreting pituitary tumor.

Approximately, 30% of GH-secreting pituitary adenomas are plurihormonal and also secrete prolactin. The incidence of acromegaly is about 2 to 4 per million population, and the mean age at diagnosis is 40 to 50 years.

Pathology

GH-secreting tumors are caused by a clonal expansion of pure somatotrophs or mixed somatomammotrophs. A variety of genetic abnormalities can be found in GH-secreting pituitary adenomas. GH hypersecretion due to somatotroph hyperplasia and adenomas is also seen in patients with McCune-Albright syndrome, which is caused by a G protein–activating mutation. There are also familial syndromes associated with GH-secreting pituitary adenomas, including multiple endocrine neoplasia type 1, Carney complex (myxomas, skin pigmentation, and testicular, adrenal, and pituitary tumors) and mutations in AIP (aryl hydrocarbon receptor interacting protein).

Clinical Presentation

Acromegaly is a rare disease, and the rate of change of symptoms and signs is slow and insidious. The usual period from earliest onset of symptoms and signs to diagnosis is 8 to 10 years, during which time many patients undergo medical and surical treatments for many of the metabolic abnormalities and morbidities caused by GH excess. Characteristic clinical findings of this disease include physical changes of the bone and soft tissue and with multiple endocrine and metabolic abnormalities (Table 62-4).

Diagnosis and Differential Diagnosis

Measurement of serum IGF-I can be used to diagnose excess GH in most patients with acromegaly. An alternative is an oral glucose tolerance test using a 100-g glucose load. Normally, glucose suppresses GH levels to less than 1 ng/mL after 2 hours; in patients with acromegaly, GH levels may paradoxically increase, remain unchanged, or decrease but not below 1 ng/mL. Most acromegalic patients have GH-secreting pituitary tumors, and

TABLE 62-4 CLINICAL FEATURES OF ACROMEGALY

CHANGE	MANIFESTATIONS
SOMATIC CHANGES	
Acral changes	Enlarged hands and feet
Musculoskeletal changes	Arthralgias
	Prognathism
	Malocclusion
	Carpal tunnel syndrome
	Proximal myopathy
Skin changes	Sweating
Colon changes	Polyps
	Carcinoma
Cardiovascular symptoms	Cardiomegaly
	Hypertension
Visceromegaly	Tongue
	Thyroid
	Liver
ENDOCRINE-METABOLIC CHANGES	
Reproduction	Menstrual abnormalities
	Galactorrhea
	Decreased libido
Carbohydrate metabolism	Impaired glucose tolerance
	Diabetes mellitus
Lipids	Hypertriglyceridemia

approximately 70% of cases of acromegaly are caused by pituitary macroadenomas. Rarely, GH hypersecretion is caused by ectopic GHRH-secreting tumors, including hypothalamic hamartomas and gangliocytomas, pancreatic islet cell tumors, small cell carcinoma of the lung, carcinoid, adrenal adenomas, and pheochromocytomas. Ectopic GH secretion has also been reported in pancreatic, lung, and breast cancers.

Treatment and Prognosis

Treatment of acromegaly requires both treatment of the tumor and normalization of GH and IGF-I levels, along with management of the comorbidities and metabolic abnormalities caused by the excess GH. Treatment often requires the use of multiple modalities to achieve adequate control of the disease. Primary therapy is almost always transsphenoidal surgery, with the cure rate being directly proportional to tumor size. Patients with intrasellar microadenomas have a 75% to 95% cure rate with surgery. Even in patients with noninvasive macroadenomas, surgical removal results in normalization of IGF-I in 40% to 68% of patients.

Approximately 40% to 60% of tumors are not controlled with surgery alone because of cavernous sinus invasion or intracapsular intra-arachnoid invasion. Additional treatment options include primary medical therapy or primary surgical debulking of the tumor followed by medical therapy for hormonal control and/or radiation therapy for treatment of residual tumor. Conventional radiotherapy can normalize GH and IGF-I levels in more than 60% of patients, but the maximum response takes 10 to 15 years to achieve. Focused single-dose gamma knife radiotherapy has a 5-year remission rate of 29% to 60%. Hypopituitarism is seen in more than 50% of patients within 5 to 10 years after radiotherapy.

Currently, three drug classes are used to treat acromegaly: dopamine agonists, somatostatin receptor ligands (SRLs) such as octreotide and lanreotide, and GH receptor antagonists. SRLs work mainly through the somatostatin receptor subtypes 2 and 5, causing a decrease in tumor GH secretion. In acromegaly, SRLs are indicated for first-line treatment when there is low probability of surgical cure, after a failed surgical cure of GH hypersecretion, preoperatively to improve severe comorbidities that prevent or could complicate immediate surgery, and to provide GH and IGF-I control or partial control while waiting for radiotherapy to achieve its maximum effect. SRLs reduce GH and IGF-I levels to normal in 40% to 65% of patients and shrink tumor size in approximately 50% of cases. Side effects of SRLs include diarrhea, abdominal cramping, flatulence, and cholelithiasis (15%).

Pegvisomant is the only GH receptor antagonist available. It works by blocking the peripheral action of GH through blockade of the GH receptors located on the liver. Pegvisomant is indicated for patients who have persistent elevation in IGF-I even with maximum doses of SRLs. This drug is highly effective in the treatment of acromegaly and normalizes IGF-I levels in 97% of patients; transient elevation in liver function enzymes is seen in 25% of those treated, and tumor growth in fewer than 2%.

Cabergoline is the most efficacious of the dopamine agonists for treatment of acromegaly, but it is effective in fewer than 10% of patients.

Thyroid-Stimulating Hormone

TSH is a glycoprotein secreted from the thyrotroph cells of the anterior pituitary. It is composed of alpha and beta subunits. Its release is regulated by TRH (stimulatory) and somatostatin (inhibitory). In addition, it is subject to the negative feedback of thyroid hormones released from the thyroid gland.

Evaluation

Assessment of the pituitary-thyroid axis requires checking levels of TSH as well as thyroid hormones released by the thyroid gland (i.e., thyroxine [T_4] and triiodothyronine [T_3]). Dynamic testing using TRH is no longer available.

Deficiency of TSH
Definition and Epidemiology

Deficiency of TSH leads to secondary hypothyroidism: The diminished secretion of TSH from the pituitary provides inadequate stimulation to the thyroid gland for thyroid hormone release. The estimated prevalence of TSH deficiency is about 1 in 80,000 to 120,000 individuals.

Pathology

Hypopituitarism due to encroachment of a tumor on the normal pituitary can cause deficiency of one or more pituitary hormones. Radiation treatment of the pituitary gland can also cause hypopituitarism over time.

Clinical Presentation

The usual signs and symptoms of hypothyroidism are weight gain, fatigue, cold intolerance, and constipation. If the condition is caused by an underlying sellar tumor, symptoms of mass effect may also be present, depending on the size of the tumor.

Diagnosis and Differential Diagnosis

Secondary hypothyroidism is characterized by low levels of free T_4 along with low or inappropriately normal TSH. The differential diagnosis includes euthyroid sick syndrome, which is often seen in the setting of an acute illness. This syndrome does not require any intervention, and the laboratory results normalize on repeat testing after resolution of the acute illness.

Treatment and Prognosis

Management focuses on replacement of the thyroid hormones, as in primary hypothyroidism. However, measurement of free T_4, rather than TSH, is used as a guide to adjust therapy. Underlying adrenal insufficiency should always be excluded and treated before treatment of secondary hypothyroidism to avoid precipitating an adrenal crisis.

TSH-Secreting Pituitary Tumors
Definition and Epidemiology

TSH-secreting pituitary tumors are rare and are characterized by inappropriate release of TSH that is refractory to the negative feedback mechanism of the thyroid hormones released by the thyroid gland. The prevalence of TSH-secreting pituitary adenomas is 1 to 2 cases per million in the general population.

Pathology

The pathogenesis of TSH-secreting pituitary tumors is unknown.

Clinical Presentation

The most common age of presentation is in the early fifth decade, and there is no gender bias. Presenting symptoms can be the result of a mass effect of the tumor or, most commonly, there are symptoms and signs of hyperthyroidism, including weight loss, tremors, heat intolerance, and diarrhea. Diffuse goiter is observed in up to 80% of patients. Many times, these tumors are initially misdiagnosed as primary hyperthyroidism and patients are mistakenly treated with radioactive iodine. Sometimes, the TSH produced by these tumors is biologically inactive and the tumors are diagnosed as an incidental finding on imaging studies.

Diagnosis and Differential Diagnosis

The diagnosis is made in the setting of elevated or inappropriately normal TSH along with elevated levels of thyroid hormones (free and total T_4 and T_3). The differential diagnosis includes genetic resistance to thyroid hormone and euthyroid hyperthyroxinemia, which is characterized by normal TSH, high total T_4, normal free T_4, and elevated thyroxine-binding globulin levels. Imaging studies (MRI) should be done only after biochemical confirmation because of the high incidence of incidental pituitary tumors.

Treatment and Prognosis

Surgery (transsphenoidal resection) is the first-line treatment and should be performed by an experienced neurosurgeon. Radiotherapy can be used if surgery is declined or contraindicated. Medical therapy with somatostatin analogues (e.g., octreotide, lantreotide) may also be used for persistent hyperthyroidism after surgery. Most patients do well and achieve control of symptoms of thyrotoxicosis as well as reduction in tumor burden.

⬤ ADRENOCORTICOTROPIC HORMONE

ACTH is a 39-amino-acid peptide hormone that is formed from a precursor molecule, pro-opiomelanocortin (POMC) and is synthesized and secreted by corticotrophs in the anterior pituitary. It is stimulated by hypothalamic corticotropin-releasing hormone (CRH). ACTH, in turn, stimulates release of glucocorticoids and androgens from the adrenal cortex.

ACTH Deficiency
Definition and Pathology

ACTH deficiency causes secondary adrenal insufficiency leading to decreased cortisol and adrenal androgens. Aldosterone secretion from the adrenal glands is not impaired because it is maintained via the renin-angiotensin axis. ACTH deficiency can result from a large pituitary tumor impinging on the normal pituitary. Secondary or tertiary adrenal insufficiency is most commonly iatrogenic, caused by the use of steroids for other disease processes.

Clinical Presentation

Both primary and secondary adrenal insufficiency are characterized by weight loss, fatigue, muscle weakness, orthostatic symptoms, nausea, vomiting, diarrhea, and abdominal pain. Biochemical abnormalities include hyponatremia, azotemia, eosinophilia, and anemia. Importantly, hyperpigmentation of the skin and hyperkalemia are seen only with primary adrenal insufficiency, not with ACTH deficiency.

Diagnosis and Differential Diagnosis

The gold standard for diagnosis of secondary adrenal insufficiency has been an insulin tolerance test. The test is contraindicated in elderly patients and in those with a history of seizures, cardiovascular disease, or cerebrovascular disease. A safer test is an 8 AM fasting rapid ACTH stimulation test. This test measures the cortisol response to synthetic ACTH or cosyntropin. ACTH and cortisol levels are measured at baseline, followed by cortisol levels at 30 and 60 minutes. An 8 AM cortisol level of less than 5 μg/dL suggests adrenal insufficiency. A peak plasma cortisol level higher than 18 to 20 μg/dL is considered a normal response.

Treatment

Glucocorticoid replacement therapy in the form of hydrocortisone (10 mg in AM and 5 mg in PM) or prednisone (5 to 7.5 mg/day) should be initiated. Patient education regarding stress dosing of steroids is important. Mineralocorticoids are usually not needed in patients with central adrenal insufficiency.

ACTH-Secreting Pituitary Tumors (Cushing's Disease)

Definition and Epidemiology

ACTH-secreting pituitary tumors (by definition, Cushing's disease) account for about 80% of the cases of Cushing's syndrome; they are usually microadenomas. There is a female preponderance (female-to-male ratio, about 3 : 1).

Pathology

The chronic stimulation by excessive ACTH causes simple diffuse hyperplasia of the bilateral adrenal glands or sometimes multinodular hyperplasia, both leading to excessive cortisol production.

Clinical Presentation

Signs and symptoms of Cushing's disease are related to the hypercortisolism and include central obesity, hirsutism, facial plethora, violaceous striae, supraclavicular and dorsocervical fat pads, and muscle weakness (Fig. 62-2). Additional manifestations of Cushing's disease are type 2 diabetes mellitus, hypertension, dyslipidemia, osteoporosis, and hypogonadism.

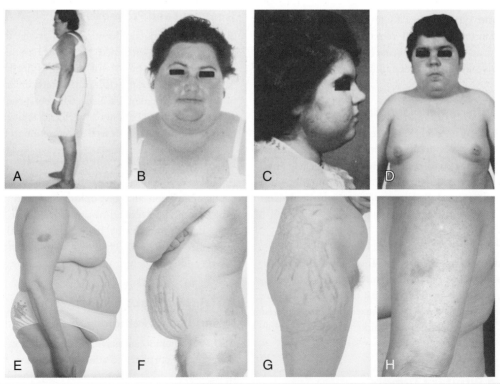

FIGURE 62-2   Clinical features of Cushing's syndrome. **A,** Centripetal and some generalized obesity and dorsal kyphosis in a 30-year-old woman with Cushing's disease. **B,** Moon facies, plethora, hirsutism, and enlarged supraclavicular fat pads in the same woman as in **A. C,** Facial rounding, hirsutism, and acne in a 14-year-old girl with Cushing's disease. **D,** Central and generalized obesity and moon facies in a 14-year-old boy with Cushing's disease. Typical centripetal obesity with livid abdominal striae in a 41-year-old woman **(E)** and a 40-year-old man **(F)** with Cushing's disease. **G,** Striae in a 24-year-old patient with congenital adrenal hyperplasia treated with excessive doses of dexamethasone as replacement therapy. **H,** Typical bruising and thin skin of a patient with Cushing's disease. In this case, the bruising has occurred without obvious injury. (From Larsen PR, Kronenberg H, Melmed S, et al: Williams Textbook of Endocrinology, ed 10, Philadelphia, 2003, Saunders.)

Diagnosis and Differential Diagnosis

Three different tests are performed in combination to assess for endogenous hypercortisolism. A 24-hour urine collection may show an elevated cortisol level, but this test is not reliable in patients with renal dysfunction. A second test, the 1-mg dexamethasone suppression test, measures an 8 AM fasting cortisol level after a dose of 1 mg dexamethasone given at 11 PM the night before. Cortisol suppression to less than 1.8 µg/dL is considered a normal response. Another diagnostic test is the late-night salivary cortisol measurement, using saliva collected at 11 PM on two consecutive nights. The test relies on a normal sleep cycle. Individuals who are using inhaled or topical steroids are not good candidates because of a high rate of false-positive results. A single positive finding is not sufficient to make this diagnosis and must be repeated and confirmed by doing additional tests. Because of the potential of cyclic ACTH overproduction by these tumors, repeat testing is recommended for individuals with high clinical suspicion but negative initial testing.

Pathologic hypercortisolism should be differentiated from physiologic activation of the hypothalamic-pituitary-adrenal axis, which can be observed in conditions such as critical illness, eating disorders, alcoholism, pregnancy, severe neuropsychiatric illness, and poorly controlled diabetes. Further, pathologic hypercortisolism can be ACTH dependent or independent. Once the diagnosis of ACTH-dependent hypercortisolism is established, a pituitary MRI should be performed, because most of these patients have a corticotroph adenoma; however, 40% to 45% of ACTH-secreting pituitary tumors are not seen even with MRI scanning. In those cases, patients with ACTH-dependent Cushing's syndrome should have inferior petrosal sinus sampling (IPSS) for ACTH with CRH stimulation; this differentiates between pituitary and ectopic ACTH overproduction by demonstrating a pituitary-to-peripheral ACTH gradient.

Treatment and Prognosis

The treatment involves removal of the pituitary tumor by an experienced neurosurgeon. Options after a failed resection include reoperation, bilateral adrenalectomy, radiotherapy, or pharmacotherapy. Pharmacotherapeutic agents include ketoconazole, metyrapone, mitotane, cabergoline, pasireotide, and mifepristone. In severe cases, intravenous etomidate may be used to stabilize patients for surgery. Long-term remission after resection of a pituitary microadenoma ranges from 69% to 98%, with a recurrence rate of 3% to 19%.

⬤ GONADOTROPINS

The two gonadotropins, LH and FSH, are glycoprotein hormones that are synthesized and secreted by gonadotrophs in anterior pituitary. They are both composed of an alpha and a beta subunit, the latter of which gives each its specific biologic function. These hormones bind to the receptors in the gonads (ovaries and testes) and modulate gonadal function. Secretion is regulated both by gonadotropin-releasing hormone (GnRH) from the hypothalamus and by feedback from circulating sex steroids (estrogen and testosterone).

Gonadotropin Deficiency (Hypogonadotropic Hypogonadism)

Definition

Hypogonadotropic hypogonadism is characterized by decreased or absent secretion of LH and FSH, which causes reduced secretion of the sex steroids (estrogen and testosterone).

Clinical Presentation

Signs and symptoms depend on the time of onset and the extent of gonadotropin deficiency. If deficiency occurs during fetal life, it can cause ambiguous genitalia. If deficiency occurs after birth but before puberty, it can cause delayed or absent sexual development. Onset after puberty often causes insidious changes and may remain undiagnosed for years, especially in men. The usual presentation after puberty includes symptoms of hypogonadism as well as infertility.

Diagnosis and Differential Diagnosis

The diagnosis is made by the presence of low or inappropriately normal FSH and LH levels along with low sex steroids (estrogen or testosterone). Causes of gonadotropin deficiency can be congenital (Kallman's syndrome, Prader-Willi syndrome, septo-optic dysplasia) or acquired, as in hemochromatosis, hyperprolactinemia, sellar tumors, cranial irradiation, and inflammatory and infiltrative disorders.

Treatment

For women, replacement therapy in the form of oral or transdermal estrogen should be continued until the age of natural menopause. Progesterone addition to induce withdrawal bleeding is essential in women with an intact uterus to prevent endometrial hyperplasia. For men, testosterone replacement is available in multiple forms, including an intramuscular injection product, several gels, and a patch. Fertility treatment requires additional therapy with recombinant FSH and LH in women or human chorionic gonadotropin (hCG) and FSH in men.

Gonadotropin-Secreting Pituitary Tumors

Definition and Epidemiology

Gonadotropin-secreting pituitary tumors are usually large and typically manifest with signs and symptoms of mass effect. Patients can also have symptoms of hypogonadism and other pituitary hormone deficiencies. These tumors can secrete FSH, LH, and/or alpha subunit.

Diagnosis and Differential Diagnosis

Hormonal evaluation reveals elevated FSH, LH, and/or alpha subunit in the absence of low estrogen or testosterone. Immunoperoxidase staining on surgical specimens is also needed to establish the diagnosis, especially in the case of postmenopausal women.

Treatment

Primary treatment is transsphenoidal surgical removal. Radiation therapy may be used as an adjunct treatment because of the size and more aggressive nature of these tumors, compared with true nonsecretory pituitary tumors.

Disorders of Posterior Pituitary Hormones

AVP and oxytocin are the two hormones that are produced in the hypothalamus and stored in and released from the posterior pituitary.

● DIABETES INSIPIDUS

Definition

Diabetes insipidus (DI) is characterized by AVP deficiency and excretion of large volumes of dilute urine.

Pathology

Central DI can be familial due to an autosomal dominant mutation in the vasopressin gene that affects the functioning of the AVP-producing neurons. It can also be acquired secondary to intrasellar and suprasellar tumors, infiltration of the hypothalamus and posterior pituitary, infection, trauma or surgery, or as part of an autoimmune condition. Table 62-5 gives a more extensive list of causes of diabetes insipidus.

Clinical Presentation

Polyuria (defined as excretion of more than 3 L of urine per day) and polydipsia are the clinical hallmarks of DI.

Diagnosis and Differential Diagnosis

DI can be central, caused by AVP deficiency, or nephrogenic, caused by resistance to AVP. As long as access to free water is maintained and the thirst mechanism is intact, patients with DI are usually able to maintain normal serum sodium levels

TABLE 62-5   CAUSES OF DIABETES INSIPIDUS
CENTRAL DIABETES INSIPIDUS
Idiopathic
Familial
Hypophysectomy
Infiltration of hypothalamus and posterior pituitary
Langerhans cell histiocytosis
Granulomas
Infection
Tumors (intrasellar and suprasellar)
Autoimmune
NEPHROGENIC DIABETES INSIPIDUS
Idiopathic
Familial
V_2 receptor gene mutation
Aquaporin-2 gene mutation
Chronic renal disease (e.g., chronic pyelonephritis, polycystic kidney disease, or medullary cystic disease)
Hypokalemia
Hypercalcemia
Sickle cell anemia
Drugs
Lithium
Fluoride
Demeclocycline
Colchicine

and osmolality. The water deprivation test is the primary test used to make the diagnosis and to differentiate the cause of DI. In patients with DI, the serum sodium level and osmolality increase in response to water deprivation. The response to a synthetic analogue of vasopressin is analyzed if the normal rise in urine osmolality and decrease in urine volume are not seen. Patients with central DI respond to the synthetic analogue by increasing urine osmolality and decreasing urine volume. In contrast, patients with nephrogenic DI do not respond to the synthetic vasopressin. Patients with partial central DI may have a limited response.

Primary polydipsia is characterized by increased water intake without a deficiency or resistance to AVP. Patients with primary polydipsia concentrate their urine without the need for synthetic vasopressin.

Treatment

Replacement therapy with desmopressin (DDAVP), an analogue of AVP, is available in oral, parenteral, and intranasal forms. Aqueous vasopressin is a shorter-acting analogue of AVP that can be given subcutaneously in the immediate postoperative period. Additional AVP analogues include DDAVP, which is available in subcutaneous, intranasal, and intravenous forms, and desmopressin, the only tablet form. Because of the transient nature of DI and a possible shift to a transient syndrome of inappropriate secretion of antidiuretic hormone (SIADH) phase in the patient who has undergone pituitary surgery, AVP is given cautiously and not as a scheduled medication to avoid hyponatremia.

● SYNDROME OF INAPPROPRIATE SECRETION OF ANTIDIURETIC HORMONE

SIADH is covered in the discussion of hyponatremia in Chapter 27.

▣ SUGGESTED READINGS

Biller BM, Grossman AB, Stewart PM, et al: Treatment of adrenocorticotropin-dependent Cushing's syndrome: a consensus statement, J Clin Endocrinol Metab 93:2454–2462, 2008.

Fleseriu M, Petersenn S: Medical management of Cushing's disease: what is the future? Pituitary 15:330–341, 2012.

Freda P, Beckers A, Katznelson L, et al: Pituitary incidentaloma: an Endocrine Society clinical practice guideline, J Clin Endocrinol Metab 96:894–904, 2011.

Melmed S: Medical progress: acromegaly, N Engl J Med 355:2558–2573, 2006.

Melmed S, Casanueva F, Hoffman A, et al: Diagnosis and treatment of hyperprolactinemia: an Endocrine Society clinical practice guideline, J Clin Endocrinol Metab 96:273–288, 2011.

Melmed S, Colao A, Barkan A, et al: Guidelines for acromegaly management: an update, J Clin Endocrinol Metab 94:1509–1517, 2009.

Nieman L, Biller B, Findling J, et al: The diagnosis of Cushing's syndrome: an Endocrine Society clinical practice guideline, J Clin Endocrinol Metab 93:1526–1540, 2008.

Swearingen B, Biller B: Diagnosis and management of pituitary disorders, New York, 2008, Humana Press.

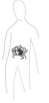

Thyroid Gland

Theodore C. Friedman

INTRODUCTION

The thyroid gland secretes thyroxine (T_4) and triiodothyronine (T_3), both of which modulate energy utilization and heat production and facilitate growth. The gland consists of two lateral lobes joined by an isthmus (E-Fig. 63-1). The weight of the adult gland is 10 to 20 g. Microscopically, the thyroid is composed of several follicles that contain colloid surrounded by a single layer of thyroid epithelium. The follicular cells synthesize thyroglobulin, which is stored as colloid. Biosynthesis of T_4 and T_3 occurs by iodination of tyrosine molecules in thyroglobulin.

THYROID HORMONE PHYSIOLOGY

Thyroid Hormone Synthesis

Dietary iodine is essential for synthesis of thyroid hormones. Iodine, after conversion to iodide in the stomach, is rapidly absorbed from the gastrointestinal tract. After active transport from the bloodstream across the follicular cell basement membrane, iodide is enzymatically oxidized by thyroid peroxidase, which also mediates the iodination of the tyrosine residues in thyroglobulin, to form monoiodotyrosine and diiodotyrosine. The iodotyrosine molecules couple to form T_4 (3,5,3′,5′-tetraiodothyronine) or T_3 (3,5,3′-triiodothyronine). Once iodinated, thyroglobulin containing newly formed T_4 and T_3 is stored in the follicles. Secretion of free T_4 and T_3 into the circulation occurs after proteolytic digestion of thyroglobulin, which is stimulated by thyroid-stimulating hormone (TSH). Deiodination of monoiodotyrosine and diiodotyrosine by iodotyrosine deiodinase releases iodine, which then re-enters the thyroid iodine pool (E-Fig. 63-2).

Thyroid Hormone Transport

T_4 and T_3 are tightly bound to the serum carrier proteins thyroxine-binding globulin (TBG), thyroxine-binding prealbumin, and albumin. The unbound or free fractions are the biologically active fractions; they represent only 0.04% of the total T_4 and 0.4% of the total T_3.

Peripheral Metabolism of Thyroid Hormones

The normal thyroid gland secretes T_4, T_3, and reverse T_3, a biologically inactive form of T_3. Most of the circulating T_3 is derived from deiodination of circulating T_4 in the peripheral tissues. Deiodination of T_4 can occur at the outer ring (5′-deiodination), producing T_3 (3,5,3′-triiodothyronine), or at the inner ring (5-deiodination), producing reverse T_3 (3,3,5′-triiodothyronine).

Control of Thyroid Function

Hypothalamic thyrotropin-releasing hormone (TRH) is transported through the hypothalamic-hypophyseal portal system to the thyrotrophs of the anterior pituitary gland, stimulating synthesis and release of TSH (Fig. 63-1). TSH, in turn, increases thyroidal iodide uptake and iodination of thyroglobulin, releases T_3 and T_4 from the thyroid gland by increasing hydrolysis of thyroglobulin, and stimulates thyroid cell growth. Hypersecretion of TSH results in thyroid enlargement (goiter). Circulating T_3 exerts negative feedback inhibition of TRH and TSH release.

Physiologic Effects of Thyroid Hormones

Thyroid hormones increase the basal metabolic rate by increasing oxygen consumption and heat production in several body tissues. Thyroid hormones also have specific effects on several organ systems (Table 63-1). These effects are exaggerated in hyperthyroidism and lacking in hypothyroidism, accounting for the well-recognized signs and symptoms of these two disorders.

THYROID EVALUATION

A careful thyroid examination is essential in evaluating a patient with thyroid disease (Video 63-1). Thyroid gland function and structure can be evaluated by (1) determining serum thyroid hormone levels, (2) imaging thyroid gland size and architecture, (3) measuring thyroid autoantibodies, and (4) performing a thyroid gland biopsy by fine-needle aspiration (FNA).

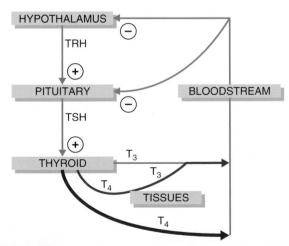

FIGURE 63-1 Hypothalamic-pituitary-thyroid axis. T_4 is converted to T_3 in peripheral tissues. T_3, Triiodothyronine; T_4, thyroxine; TRH, thyrotropin-releasing hormone; TSH, thyroid-stimulating hormone.

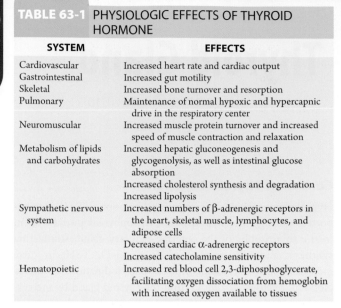

TABLE 63-1 PHYSIOLOGIC EFFECTS OF THYROID HORMONE

SYSTEM	EFFECTS
Cardiovascular	Increased heart rate and cardiac output
Gastrointestinal	Increased gut motility
Skeletal	Increased bone turnover and resorption
Pulmonary	Maintenance of normal hypoxic and hypercapnic drive in the respiratory center
Neuromuscular	Increased muscle protein turnover and increased speed of muscle contraction and relaxation
Metabolism of lipids and carbohydrates	Increased hepatic gluconeogenesis and glycogenolysis, as well as intestinal glucose absorption
	Increased cholesterol synthesis and degradation
	Increased lipolysis
Sympathetic nervous system	Increased numbers of β-adrenergic receptors in the heart, skeletal muscle, lymphocytes, and adipose cells
	Decreased cardiac α-adrenergic receptors
	Increased catecholamine sensitivity
Hematopoietic	Increased red blood cell 2,3-diphosphoglycerate, facilitating oxygen dissociation from hemoglobin with increased oxygen available to tissues

TABLE 63-2 HIGH-RISK FACTORS FOR MALIGNANCY IN A THYROID NODULE

HISTORY

Head and neck irradiation
Exposure to nuclear radiation
Rapid growth
Recent onset
Young age
Male sex
Familial incidence (medullary and about 5% of papillary carcinomas)

PHYSICAL EXAMINATION

Hard consistency of nodule
Fixation of nodule
Lymphadenopathy
Vocal cord paralysis
Distant metastasis

LABORATORY AND IMAGING STUDIES

Elevated serum calcitonin
Cold nodule on technetium scan
Ultrasonography:
    Presence of microcalcifications
    Presence of nodule hypoechogenicity compared with the normal thyroid parenchyma
    Presence of increased nodular vascularity
    Presence of irregular infiltrative margins
    Nodule taller than wide on transverse view
    Absent halo
    Suspicious cervical lymphadenopathy
    Partially cystic nodule
    Spongiform appearance, defined as an aggregation of multiple microcystic components in >50% of the nodule volume

Tests of Serum Thyroid Hormone Levels

Measurements of total serum T_4 and total T_3 indicate the total amount of hormone bound to thyroid-binding proteins by radioimmunoassay. Total T_4 and T_3 levels are elevated in hyperthyroidism and low in hypothyroidism. Increased production of TBG (as with pregnancy or estrogen therapy) increases the total T_4 and T_3 levels without actual hyperthyroidism. Similarly, total T_4 and T_3 are low despite euthyroidism in conditions associated with low levels of thyroid-binding proteins (e.g., congenital decrease, protein-losing enteropathy, cirrhosis, nephrotic syndrome). Therefore, further tests to assess the free hormone levels, which reflect biologic activity, must be performed. Free T_4 and free T_3 levels can be measured directly or by dialysis or ultrafiltration.

Serum TSH is measured by a third-generation immunometric assay that accurately discriminates between normal TSH levels and levels below the normal range. Thus, the TSH assay can diagnose clinical hyperthyroidism (elevated free T_4 and free T_3 and suppressed TSH) and subclinical hyperthyroidism (normal free T_4 and free T_3 and suppressed TSH). In hyperthyroidism, the free T_3 may be elevated in the presence of a normal free T_4. In primary (thyroidal) hypothyroidism, serum TSH is supranormal because of diminished feedback inhibition. The TSH is usually low but may be normal in secondary (pituitary) or tertiary (hypothalamic) hypothyroidism.

Serum thyroglobulin measurements are useful in the follow-up of patients with papillary or follicular carcinoma. After thyroidectomy and iodine-131 (^{131}I) ablation therapy, thyroglobulin levels should be less than 0.5 μg/L while the patient is on suppressive levothyroxine treatment. Levels in excess of this value indicate the possibility of persistent or metastatic disease.

Calcitonin is produced by the C cells of the thyroid and has a minor role in calcium homeostasis. Calcitonin measurements are invaluable in the diagnosis of medullary carcinoma of the thyroid and for monitoring the effects of therapy for this entity.

Thyroid Imaging

Technetium-99m (^{99m}Tc) pertechnetate is concentrated in the thyroid gland and can be scanned with a gamma camera, yielding information about the size and shape of the gland and the location of the functional activity in the gland (thyroid scan). The thyroid scan is often performed in conjunction with a quantitative assessment of radioactive iodine (^{123}I) uptake by the thyroid. Functioning thyroid nodules are called *warm* or *hot* nodules; *cold* nodules are nonfunctioning. Malignancy is usually associated with a cold nodule; 16% of surgically removed cold nodules are malignant.

Thyroid ultrasound evaluation is useful in the differentiation of solid nodules from cystic nodules. It also may be used to guide the clinician during FNA of a nodule (E-Fig. 63-3), and ultrasound characteristics of thyroid nodules may be helpful to distinguish those that are more likely to be malignant (Table 63-2).

Thyroid Antibodies

Autoantibodies to several different antigenic components in the thyroid gland, including thyroglobulin (TgAb), thyroid peroxidase (TPO Ab, formerly called *antimicrosomal antibodies*), and the TSH receptor, can be measured in the serum. A strongly positive test for TPO Ab indicates autoimmune thyroid disease. Elevated TSH receptor antibody occurs in Graves' disease (see later discussion).

Thyroid Biopsy

FNA of a nodule to obtain thyroid cells for cytologic evaluation is the best way to differentiate benign from malignant disease.

FNA requires adequate tissue samples and interpretation by an experienced cytologist.

⬤ HYPERTHYROIDISM

Thyrotoxicosis is the clinical syndrome that results from elevated levels of circulating thyroid hormones. Clinical manifestations of thyrotoxicosis result from the direct physiologic effects of the thyroid hormones as well as the increased sensitivity to catecholamines. Tachycardia, tremor, stare, sweating, and lid lag are all caused by catecholamine hypersensitivity.

Signs and Symptoms

Table 63-3 lists the signs and symptoms of hyperthyroidism. Thyrotoxic crisis, or *thyroid storm*, is a life-threatening complication of hyperthyroidism that can be precipitated by surgery, radioactive iodine therapy, or severe stress (e.g., uncontrolled diabetes mellitus, myocardial infarction, acute infection). Patients develop fever, flushing, sweating, significant tachycardia, atrial fibrillation, and cardiac failure. Significant agitation, restlessness, delirium, and coma frequently occur. Gastrointestinal manifestations may include nausea, vomiting, and diarrhea. Hyperpyrexia out of proportion to other clinical findings is the hallmark of thyroid storm.

Differential Diagnosis

Thyrotoxicosis usually reflects excess secretion of thyroid hormones resulting from Graves' disease, toxic adenoma, multinodular goiter, or thyroiditis (Table 63-4 and Fig. 63-2). However, it may be the result of excessive ingestion of thyroid hormone or, rarely, thyroid hormone production from an ectopic site (as in struma ovarii).

Graves' Disease

Graves' disease, the most common cause of thyrotoxicosis, is an autoimmune disease that is more common in women, with a peak incidence between 20 and 40 years of age. One or more of the following features are present: (1) goiter; (2) thyrotoxicosis; (3) eye disease ranging from tearing to proptosis, extraocular muscle paralysis, and loss of sight as a result of optic nerve involvement; and (4) thyroid dermopathy, usually observed as significant skin thickening without pitting in a pretibial distribution (pretibial myxedema).

Pathogenesis

Thyrotoxicosis in Graves' disease is caused by overproduction of an antibody that binds to the TSH receptor. These thyroid-stimulating immunoglobulins increase thyroid cell growth and thyroid hormone secretion. Ophthalmopathy results from inflammatory infiltration of the extraocular eye muscles by lymphocytes with mucopolysaccharide deposition. The inflammatory reaction that contributes to the eye signs in Graves' disease may be caused by sensitization of lymphocytes to antigens that are common to the orbital muscles and the thyroid.

Clinical Presentation

The common manifestations of thyrotoxicosis (see Table 63-3) are characteristic features of younger patients with Graves' disease. In addition, patients may exhibit a diffuse goiter or the eye signs characteristic of Graves' disease. Older patients often do not have the florid clinical features of thyrotoxicosis, and the condition termed *apathetic hyperthyroidism* is exhibited as flat affect, emotional lability, weight loss, muscle weakness,

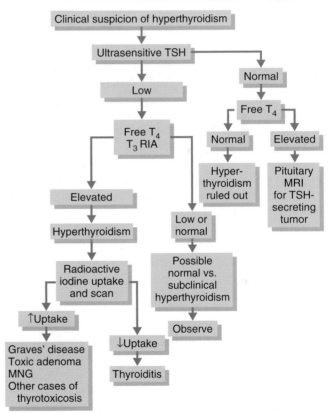

FIGURE 63-2 Algorithm for differential diagnosis of hyperthyroidism. MNG, Multinodular goiter; MRI, magnetic resonance imaging; RIA, radioimmunoassay; T₃, triiodothyronine; T₄, thyroxine; TSH, thyroid-stimulating hormone.

TABLE 63-3	SIGNS AND SYMPTOMS OF HYPERTHYROIDISM
SYMPTOMS	**SIGNS**
Palpitations	Tachycardia
Nervousness	Atrial fibrillation
Shortness of breath	Wide pulse pressure
Heat intolerance	Brisk reflexes
Fatigue and weakness	Fine tremor
Increased appetite	Proximal limb-girdle myopathy
Weight loss	Chemosis (swelling of conjunctiva)
Oligomenorrhea	Thyroid bruit (Graves' disease)

TABLE 63-4	CAUSES OF THYROTOXICOSIS	
COMMON CAUSES	Thyrotoxicosis factitia
Graves' disease	Postpartum thyroiditis (probably variant of silent thyroiditis)
Toxic adenoma (solitary)	
Toxic multinodular goiter	**RARE CAUSES**
LESS COMMON CAUSES	Struma ovarii
	Metastatic thyroid carcinoma
Subacute thyroiditis (de Quervain's or granulomatous thyroiditis)	Hydatidiform mole
	TSH-secreting pituitary tumor
Hashimoto's thyroiditis with transient hyperthyroid phase	

TSH, Thyroid-stimulating hormone.

congestive heart failure, and atrial fibrillation resistant to standard therapy.

Eye signs associated with Graves disease may also occur as a nonspecific manifestation of hyperthyroidism from any cause (e.g., thyroid stare). In Graves' disease, a specific inflammatory infiltrate of the orbital tissues leads to periorbital edema, conjunctival congestion and swelling, proptosis, extraocular muscle weakness, or optic nerve damage with visual impairment (E-Fig. 63-4).

Pretibial myxedema (thyroid dermopathy) (E-Fig. 63-5) occurs in 2% to 3% of patients with Graves' disease and results in a thickening of the skin over the lower tibia without pitting. Onycholysis, characterized by separation of the fingernails from their beds, often occurs in patients with Graves' disease. Thyroid acropachy, or clubbing, may also occur.

Diagnosis

Elevated total or free T_4 or T_3 (or both) and a suppressed TSH confirm the clinical diagnosis of thyrotoxicosis. Thyroid-stimulating immunoglobulin is usually elevated, and its measurement may be useful in patients with eye signs who do not have other characteristic clinical features. Increased uptake of ^{123}I differentiates Graves' disease from early subacute or Hashimoto's thyroiditis, in which uptake is low in the presence of hyperthyroidism. Magnetic resonance imaging or ultrasonography of the orbit usually shows orbital muscle enlargement, whether or not clinical signs of ophthalmopathy are observed.

Treatment

Three treatment modalities are used to control the hyperthyroidism of Graves' disease: antithyroid drugs, radioactive iodine therapy, and surgery.

Antithyroid Drugs

The thiocarbamide drugs propylthiouracil, methimazole, and carbimazole block thyroid hormone synthesis by inhibiting thyroid peroxidase. Propylthiouracil also partially inhibits peripheral conversion of T_4 to T_3. Medical therapy is usually administered for a prolonged period (1 to 3 years), with the dose gradually reduced until spontaneous remission occurs. One approach is to gradually decrease the dose while maintaining T_4 and T_3 in the normal range. After cessation of medication, 40% to 60% of patients remain in remission. Those who experience relapse can either resume therapy with thiocarbamide drugs or undergo definitive surgery or radioactive iodine treatment. Side effects of the thiocarbamide regimen include pruritus and rash (in about 5% of patients), elevated liver function enzymes, cholestatic jaundice, acute arthralgias, and, rarely, agranulocytosis (<0.5% of patients).

Methimazole is less toxic to the liver than propylthiouracil and has now become the preferred medical treatment for hyperthyroidism. Patients must be instructed to discontinue the medication and consult a physician if they develop fever or sore throat, because those symptoms may indicate agranulocytosis. At the onset of treatment during the acute phase of thyrotoxicosis, β-adrenergic receptor blockers are used to help alleviate tachycardia, hypertension, and atrial fibrillation. As the thyroid hormone levels return to normal, the treatment with β-blockers is tapered.

Radioactive Iodine

In terms of cost, efficacy, ease, and short-term side effects, radioactive iodine has a better benefit profile than either surgery or antithyroid drugs; however, 80% to 90% of patients become hypothyroid after radiotherapy and require lifelong thyroid hormone replacement. ^{131}I is often the treatment of choice in adults with Graves' disease. It is contraindicated in women who are pregnant, but it does not increase the risk of birth defects in offspring conceived after ^{131}I therapy. Patients with severe thyrotoxicosis, very large glands, or underlying heart disease should be rendered euthyroid with antithyroid medication before receiving radioactive iodine, because ^{131}I treatment can cause a release of preformed thyroid hormone from the thyroid gland that could precipitate cardiac arrhythmias and exacerbate symptoms of thyrotoxicosis.

After administration of radioactive iodine, the thyroid gland shrinks; patients become euthyroid and later hypothyroid over a period of 6 weeks to 3 months. Serum free T_4 and TSH levels should be monitored, and replacement with levothyroxine should be instituted when hypothyroidism occurs. Hypothyroidism always occurs after surgical total thyroidectomy, frequently after subtotal thyroidectomy or administration of radioactive iodine, and in a smaller percentage of patients after antithyroid medication; therefore, lifelong monitoring of all patients with Graves' disease is mandated.

Surgery

Either subtotal or total thyroidectomy is the treatment of choice for patients with very large glands and obstructive symptoms, those with multinodular glands, and sometimes in those who desire pregnancy within the next year. It is essential that the surgeon be experienced in thyroid surgery. Preoperatively, patients receive 6 weeks of treatment with antithyroid drugs to ensure that they are euthyroid at the time of surgery. Two weeks before surgery, oral saturated solution of potassium iodide is administered daily to decrease the vascularity of the gland. Permanent hypoparathyroidism and recurrent laryngeal nerve palsy occur postoperatively in fewer than 2% of patients.

Graves' orbitopathy can be treated with glucocorticoids, orbital radiotherapy, or surgery. It was recently found that selenium is effective for Graves' orbitopathy.

Toxic Adenoma

Solitary toxic nodules, which are usually benign, occur more frequently in older patients. The clinical manifestations are those of thyrotoxicosis. Physical examination shows a distinct solitary nodule. Laboratory investigation shows suppressed TSH and significantly elevated T_3 levels, often with only moderately elevated T_4. Thyroid scan shows a hot nodule in the affected lobe with partial or complete suppression of the unaffected lobe. Solitary toxic nodules are usually treated with radioactive iodine. Euthyroidism results if the unaffected lobe has suppressed uptake on a thyroid scan, and often hypothyroidism occurs if the unaffected lobe does not have suppressed uptake. For large nodules, unilateral lobectomy after the administration

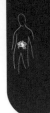

of antithyroid drugs to render the patient euthyroid may be required.

Toxic Multinodular Goiter

Toxic multinodular goiter occurs in older patients with long-standing multinodular goiter, especially in patients from iodine-deficient regions when they are exposed to increased dietary iodine or receive iodine-containing radiocontrast dyes. The presenting clinical features are frequently tachycardia, heart failure, and arrhythmias. Physical examination shows a multinodular goiter. The diagnosis is confirmed by laboratory features of suppressed TSH, elevated T_3 and T_4, and a thyroid scan showing multiple functioning nodules. The treatment of choice is often ^{131}I ablation. It is especially effective in patients with small glands and a high degree of radioactive uptake. Larger glands may require surgery.

Subclinical Hyperthyroidism

In subclinical hyperthyroidism, total or free T_4 and T_3 levels are normal and TSH is suppressed. The causes of this condition include early presentation of any form of hyperthyroidism (e.g., Graves' disease, toxic adenoma, toxic multinodular goiter). Because these patients, especially those who are older, are at an increased risk for cardiac dysrhythmias, many patients with a persistently suppressed TSH should be treated with thiocarbamide drugs or radioactive iodine. A decreased bone mineral density is another indication for treatment.

Thyroiditis

Thyroiditis may be classified as acute, subacute, or chronic. Although thyroiditis may eventually result in clinical hypothyroidism, the initial presentation is often that of hyperthyroidism as a result of acute release of T_4 and T_3. Hyperthyroidism caused by thyroiditis can be readily differentiated from other causes of hyperthyroidism by suppressed uptake of radioactive iodine in the thyroid gland, reflecting decreased hormone production by damaged cells.

A rare disorder, acute suppurative thyroiditis, is caused by infection, usually bacterial. Patients exhibits high fever, redness of the overlying skin, and thyroid gland tenderness; the condition may be confused with subacute thyroiditis. If blood cultures are negative, FNA should identify the organism. Intensive antibiotic treatment and, occasionally, incision and drainage are required.

Subacute Thyroiditis

Subacute thyroiditis (also known as de Quervain's thyroiditis or granulomatous thyroiditis) is an acute inflammatory disorder of the thyroid gland that probably is caused by a viral infection and resolves completely in 90% of cases. Patients with subacute thyroiditis complain of fever and anterior neck pain. The patient may have symptoms and signs of hyperthyroidism. The classic feature on physical examination is an exquisitely tender thyroid gland. Laboratory findings vary with the course of the disease. Initially, the patient may be symptomatically thyrotoxic with elevated serum T_4, depressed serum TSH, and low radioactive iodine uptake on the thyroid scan. Subsequently, the thyroid status fluctuates through euthyroid and hypothyroid

phases and may return to euthyroidism. An increase in radioactive iodine uptake on the scan reflects recovery of the gland. Treatment usually includes high-dose aspirin or other nonsteroidal anti-inflammatory drugs, but a short course of prednisone may be required if pain and fever are severe. During the hypothyroid phase, replacement therapy with levothyroxine may be indicated.

Postpartum thyroiditis resembles subacute thyroiditis in its clinical course. It usually occurs within the first 6 months after delivery and goes through the triphasic course of hyperthyroidism, hypothyroidism, and then euthyroidism, or it may develop with only hypothyroidism. Some patients have underlying chronic thyroiditis.

Chronic Thyroiditis

Chronic thyroiditis (Hashimoto's or lymphocytic thyroiditis), caused by destruction of the normal thyroidal architecture by lymphocytic infiltration, results in hypothyroidism and goiter. Riedel's struma is probably a variant of Hashimoto's thyroiditis; it is characterized by extensive thyroid fibrosis resulting in a rock-hard thyroid mass. Hashimoto's thyroiditis is more common in women and is the most common cause of goiter and hypothyroidism in the United States. Occasionally, patients with Hashimoto's thyroiditis have transient hyperthyroidism with low radioactive iodine uptake owing to the release of T_4 and T_3 into the circulation. Chronic thyroiditis can be differentiated from subacute thyroiditis in that, in the former, the gland is nontender to palpation and antithyroid antibodies are present in high titer. TPO Ab is usually present early and typically remains present for years. Presence of TgAb does not reflect Hashimoto's thyroiditis and does not provide additional information beyond the TPO Ab finding. Serum T_3 and T_4 levels are either normal or low; when they are low, the TSH is elevated. FNA of the thyroid shows lymphocytes and Hürthle cells (enlarged basophilic follicular cells). Hypothyroidism and significant glandular enlargement (goiter) are indications for levothyroxine therapy. Adequate doses of levothyroxine are administered to normalize TSH levels and shrink the goiter.

Thyrotoxicosis Factitia

Patients with thyrotoxicosis factitia ingest excessive amounts of thyroxine, often in an attempt to lose weight, and exhibit typical features of thyrotoxicosis. Serum T_3 and T_4 levels are elevated and TSH is suppressed, as is the serum thyroglobulin concentration. Radioactive iodine uptake is absent. Patients may require psychotherapy.

Rare Causes of Thyrotoxicosis

Struma ovarii occurs when an ovarian teratoma contains thyroid tissue that secretes thyroid hormone. A body scan confirms the diagnosis by demonstrating uptake of radioactive iodine in the pelvis.

Hydatidiform mole is caused by proliferation and swelling of the trophoblast during pregnancy, with excess production of chorionic gonadotropin, which has intrinsic TSH-like activity. The hyperthyroidism remits with surgical and medical treatment of the molar pregnancy.

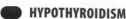

HYPOTHYROIDISM

Hypothyroidism is a clinical syndrome caused by deficiency of thyroid hormones. In infants and children, hypothyroidism causes retardation of growth and development and may result in permanent motor and mental retardation. Congenital causes of hypothyroidism include agenesis (complete absence of thyroid tissue), dysgenesis (ectopic or lingual thyroid gland), hypoplastic thyroid, thyroid dyshormogenesis, and congenital pituitary diseases. Adult-onset hypothyroidism results in a slowing of metabolic processes and is reversible with treatment. Hypothyroidism is usually primary (thyroid failure), but it may be secondary (hypothalamic or pituitary deficiency) or rarely the result of resistance at the thyroid hormone receptor (Table 63-5).

In adults, autoimmune thyroiditis (Hashimoto's thyroiditis) is the most common cause of hypothyroidism. This condition may be isolated, or it may be part of polyglandular failure syndrome type II (Schmidt's syndrome), which also includes insulin-dependent diabetes mellitus, adrenal insufficiency, pernicious anemia, vitiligo, gonadal failure, hypophysitis, celiac disease, myasthenia gravis, and primary biliary cirrhosis. Iatrogenic causes of hypothyroidism include ^{131}I therapy, thyroidectomy, and treatment with lithium or amiodarone. Iodine deficiency or excess can also cause hypothyroidism.

Clinical Presentation

The clinical presentation of hypothyroidism (Table 63-6) depends on the age at onset and the severity of the thyroid deficiency. Infants with congenital hypothyroidism (also called *cretinism*) may exhibit feeding problems, hypotonia, inactivity, an open posterior fontanelle, and edematous face and hands. Mental retardation, short stature, and delayed puberty occur if treatment is delayed.

Hypothyroidism in adults usually develops insidiously. Patients often complain of fatigue, lethargy, and gradual weight gain for years before the diagnosis is established. A delayed relaxation phase of deep tendon reflexes (*hung-up* reflexes) is a valuable clinical sign that is characteristic of severe hypothyroidism. Subcutaneous infiltration by mucopolysaccharides, which bind water, causes the edema; this condition, termed *myxedema*, is responsible for the thickened features and puffy appearance of patients with severe hypothyroidism.

Severe untreated hypothyroidism can result in myxedema coma, which is characterized by hypothermia, extreme weakness, stupor, hypoventilation, hypoglycemia, and hyponatremia and is often precipitated by cold exposure, infection, or psychoactive drugs.

Diagnosis

Laboratory abnormalities in patients with primary hypothyroidism include elevated serum TSH and low total and free T_4. A low or low-normal morning serum TSH level in the setting of hypothalamic or pituitary dysfunction characterizes secondary hypothyroidism. Often, the serum total and free T_4 levels are at the lower limits of normal.

Hypothyroidism is often associated with hypercholesterolemia and elevated creatine phosphokinase skeletal muscle (MM) fraction (the fraction representative of skeletal muscle). Anemia is usually normocytic and normochromic but may be macrocytic (with vitamin B_{12} deficiency resulting from associated pernicious anemia) or microcytic (caused by nutritional deficiencies or menstrual blood loss in women). Because TPO Ab is usually positive in Hashimoto's thyroiditis, the major cause of hypothyroidism in adults, its measurement is helpful in deciding whether levothyroxine treatment is appropriate in patients with subclinical hypothyroidism (discussed later).

Differential Diagnosis

Because the initial manifestations of hypothyroidism are subtle, early diagnosis demands a high index of suspicion in patients with one or more of the signs and symptoms (see Table 63-6). Early symptoms that are often overlooked include menstrual irregularities (usually menorrhagia), arthralgias, and myalgias.

Laboratory diagnosis may be complicated by the finding of a low total T_4 level in euthyroid states associated with low TBG, such as nephrotic syndrome, cirrhosis, or TBG deficiency. TSH and free T_4 levels are normal in these instances. A low total T_4 level may also be found with nonthyroidal illness (*euthyroid sick syndrome*), a condition occurring in acutely ill patients. In such patients, total and occasionally free T_4 levels are low' the serum TSH level is usually normal but may be mildly elevated. This condition can be differentiated from primary hypothyroidism by absence of a goiter, negative antithyroid antibodies, and elevated serum reverse T_3 levels as well as by the clinical presentation.

TABLE 63-5 CAUSES OF HYPOTHYROIDISM

PRIMARY HYPOTHYROIDISM	Hypoplastic thyroid
Autoimmune	Biosynthetic defects
Hashimoto's thyroiditis	**SECONDARY HYPOTHYROIDISM**
Part of polyglandular failure syndrome, type II	**Hypothalamic Dysfunction**
Iatrogenic	Neoplasms Tuberculosis Sarcoidosis
^{131}I therapy Thyroidectomy	Langerhans cell histiocytosis Hemochromatosis
Drug-Induced	Radiation treatment
Iodine deficiency Iodine excess	**Pituitary Dysfunction**
Lithium Amiodarone Antithyroid drugs	Neoplasms Pituitary surgery Postpartum pituitary necrosis Idiopathic hypopituitarism
Congenital	Glucocorticoid excess (Cushing's syndrome)
Thyroid agenesis Thyroid dysgenesis	Radiation treatment to the pituitary

TABLE 63-6 CLINICAL FEATURES OF HYPOTHYROIDISM

CHILDREN	Weight gain
Learning disabilities Mental retardation Short stature Delayed bone age Delayed puberty	Constipation Menstrual irregularities Dry, coarse, cold skin Periorbital and peripheral edema Delayed reflexes Bradycardia
ADULTS	Arthralgias, myalgias
Fatigue Cold intolerance	

The thyroid hormone levels return to normal with resolution of the acute illness, and patients do not require levothyroxine therapy.

Treatment

Hypothyroidism should be treated initially with synthetic levothyroxine. Administration of levothyroxine results in physiologic levels of bioavailable T_3 and T_4. Levothyroxine has a half-life of 8 days; consequently, it needs to be given only once a day. The average replacement dose of levothyroxine for adults is 75 to 150 μg/day. In healthy adults, 1.6 μg/kg/day is an appropriate starting dose. In some older patients and patients with cardiac disease, levothyroxine should be increased gradually, starting at 25 μg/day and increasing the dose by 25 μg every 2 weeks; however, most patients can safely be started on a full replacement dose. The therapeutic response to levothyroxine therapy should be monitored clinically and with measurement of serum TSH levels 6 weeks after a dose adjustment. TSH levels between 0.5 and 2 mU/L are optimal. Because TSH measurements are not a useful guide in patients with secondary hypothyroidism (pituitary or hypothalamic dysfunction), these patients should be given levothyroxine until their free T_4 is in the mid-normal range.

Recent studies have suggested that a percentage of patients treated with levothyroxine for hypothyroidism continue to have hypothyroid symptoms despite normalization of TSH. Furthermore, a large study found that more than 20% of athyreotic patients treated with levothyroxine replacement did not maintain free T_3 or free T_4 values in the normal range despite normal TSH levels. This reflects the inadequacy of peripheral deiodination to compensate for the absent T_3 secretion. Because of these studies, there is renewed interest (accompanied by a large amount of controversy) in treating hypothyroid patients who have not had an adequate clinical response to levothyroxine replacement with a combination of levothyroxine and liothyronine, or with desiccated thyroid preparations that contain levothyroxine and liothyronine.

In patients with myxedema coma, 500 to 800 μg of levothyroxine is administered intravenously as a loading dose, followed by 100 μg/day of levothyroxine, hydrocortisone (100 mg IV intravenously three times daily), and intravenous fluids. Steroids should be given before thyroxine in autoimmune conditions. The underlying precipitating event should be corrected. Respiratory assistance and treatment of hypothermia with warming blankets may be required. Although myxedema coma carries a high mortality rate despite appropriate treatment, many patients improve in 1 to 3 days.

Subclinical Hypothyroidism

In subclinical hypothyroidism, T_4 and T_3 levels are normal or low-normal, and TSH is mildly elevated. Some of these patients develop overt hypothyroidism. The decision as to when to treat patients who have a mildly elevated TSH level is controversial. It is frequently recommended that patients should be treated with levothyroxine if they have a TSH level greater than 5 mU/L on two occasions and either positive anti–TPO Ab test results or a goiter. If the patient does not have an appreciable goiter and has negative anti–TPO Ab test results, many experts suggest that levothyroxine should be given only if the TSH level is greater than 10 mU/L on two occasions. Other experts suggest treatment at lower TSH levels depending on the presence of TPO antibody.

GOITER

Enlargement of the thyroid gland is called a *goiter*. Patients with goiters may be euthyroid (simple goiter), hyperthyroid (toxic nodular goiter or Graves' disease), or hypothyroid (nontoxic goiter or Hashimoto's thyroiditis). Thyroid enlargement (often focal) may also be the result of a thyroid adenoma or carcinoma. In nontoxic goiter, inadequate thyroid hormone synthesis leads to TSH stimulation with resultant enlargement of the thyroid gland. Iodine deficiency (endemic goiter) was once the most common cause of nontoxic goiter. Since the widespread availability of iodized salt, endemic goiter is less common in North America.

Goitrogens are agents that can cause a goiter, and iodine and lithium are the two chemicals or drugs that frequently cause a goiter. Natural goitrogens include thioglucosides found in vegetables such as cabbage, broccoli, brussel sprouts, turnips, cauliflower, kale, and other greens. Other foods that are goitrogens include soybeans and soybean products, peanuts, spinach, sweet potatoes, and fruits (e.g., strawberries, pears, and peaches). Thyroid hormone biosynthetic defects can cause goiter associated with hypothyroidism (or, with adequate compensation, euthyroidism).

A careful thyroid examination coupled with thyroid hormone tests can reveal the cause of the goiter. A smooth, symmetrical gland, often with a bruit, and hyperthyroidism are suggestive of Graves' disease. A nodular thyroid gland with hypothyroidism and positive antithyroid antibodies is consistent with Hashimoto's thyroiditis. A diffuse, smooth goiter with hypothyroidism and negative antithyroid antibodies may be indicative of iodine deficiency or a biosynthetic defect. Goiters can become very large, extending substernally and causing dysphagia, respiratory distress, or hoarseness. An ultrasound evaluation or radioactive iodine scan delineates the thyroid gland, and measurement of the TSH level determines the functional activity of the goiter.

Hypothyroid goiters are treated with thyroid hormone at a dose that normalizes TSH. Previously, euthyroid goiters were treated with levothyroxine therapy; however, regression with levothyroxine therapy is unlikely and is no longer recommended. Surgery is indicated for nontoxic goiter only if obstructive symptoms develop or substantial substernal extension is present.

SOLITARY THYROID NODULES

Thyroid nodules are common. They can be detected clinically in about 4% of the population and are found in about 50% of the population at autopsy. Benign thyroid nodules are usually follicular adenomas, colloid nodules, benign cysts, or nodular thyroiditis. Patients may have one prominent nodule on clinical examination, but thyroid ultrasound evaluation may reveal multiple nodules. Although most nodules are benign, a small percentage are malignant. Fortunately, most thyroid cancers are low-grade malignancies. History, physical examination, and laboratory tests can be helpful in differentiating benign from malignant lesions (see Table 63-2). For example, lymph node involvement or hoarseness is strongly suggestive of a malignant tumor.

The major etiologic factor for thyroid cancer is childhood or adolescent exposure to head and neck radiation. Previously, radiation was used to treat an enlarged thymus, tonsillar disease, hemangioma, or acne. More recently, exposure to radiation from nuclear plants (e.g., Chernobyl, Ukraine) contributed to an increased incidence of thyroid cancer. Patients with a history of irradiation should have a baseline thyroid ultrasound study, and careful palpation of their thyroid every 1 to 2 years.

A dominant nodule (>1 to 1.5 cm) or nodules with ultrasound features compatible with neoplasia should undergo FNA, which is a safe procedure that has reduced the need for surgical excision. An expert cytologist can identify most benign lesions (75% of all biopsies). In addition, malignant lesions (5% of biopsies), such as papillary, anaplastic, and medullary carcinomas, can be specifically identified. Follicular neoplasms, however, cannot be diagnosed as benign or malignant by FNA; a cytology report of follicular neoplasia, along with "suspicious" cytology, requires surgical excision. Molecular testing can now be performed on FNA specimens to help determine whether follicular lesions have molecular characteristics of malignancy and should be removed. If the patient has a follicular lesion and a suppressed TSH level, a thyroid scan should be performed, because hot nodules are rarely malignant.

Although in the past benign thyroid nodules were treated with levothyroxine suppression, this is no longer recommended because it is uncommon for thyroid nodules to shrink substantially with levothyroxine.

● THYROID CARCINOMA

The types and characteristics of thyroid carcinomas are presented in Table 63-7. Papillary carcinoma is associated with local invasion and lymph node spread. Indicators of poor prognosis include thyroid capsule invasion, size greater than 2.5 cm, age at onset older than 45 years, tall cell or Hürthle cell variant, and lymph node involvement. Follicular carcinoma is slightly more aggressive than papillary carcinoma and can spread by local invasion of lymph nodes or hematogenously to bone, brain, or lung. Many tumors show both papillary and follicular cell types. Patients may exhibit metastases before diagnosis of the primary thyroid lesion. Anaplastic carcinoma tends to occur in older individuals, is very aggressive, and rapidly causes pain, dysphagia, and hoarseness.

Medullary thyroid carcinoma is derived from calcitonin-producing parafollicular cells and is more malignant than papillary or follicular carcinoma. It is multifocal and spreads both locally and distally. It may be either sporadic or familial. When familial, it is inherited in an autosomal dominant pattern and is part of multiple endocrine neoplasia type IIA (medullary carcinoma of the thyroid, pheochromocytoma, and hyperparathyroidism) or multiple endocrine neoplasia type IIB (medullary carcinoma of the thyroid, mucosal neuromas, intestinal ganglioneuromas, marfanoid habitus, and pheochromocytoma). Elevated basal serum calcitonin levels confirm the diagnosis. Evaluation for *RET* proto-oncogene mutations should be performed in patients with medullary carcinoma; if mutations are present, all first-degree relatives should be examined.

Treatment

Lobectomy may be performed for isolated papillary microcarcinoma. However, larger papillary tumors and most follicular tumors require thyroidectomy with a central compartment lymph node dissection, as well as a modified neck dissection if evidence of lateral lymph node metastases is found. After surgery, patients with low-risk, small carcinomas may be administered doses of levothyroxine sufficient to keep the TSH level in the low-normal or slightly suppressed range and monitored with serum thyroglobulin determinations and neck ultrasound examinations. Patients with large lesions and those at high risk for persistence or metastatic disease should be treated with radioactive iodine. Sufficient levothyroxine is then administered to suppress serum TSH to subnormal levels. Frequent clinical and ultrasound neck examinations for masses should be accompanied by measurement of serum thyroglobulin levels.

Thyroid cancer patients are considered to have no residual disease if neck ultrasound imaging studies are negative and serum thyroglobulin is suppressed after recombinant TSH stimulation. Recurrence and metastases are also evaluated by ^{131}I whole body scans carried out under conditions of TSH stimulation, which increase ^{131}I uptake by the thyroid tissue. Elevated TSH levels can be achieved by withdrawal of thyroxine supplementation for 6 weeks or by treatment with recombinant human TSH administered while the patient maintains therapy with thyroid hormone replacement. The latter avoids symptomatic hypothyroidism. A rise in serum thyroglobulin levels suggests recurrence of thyroid cancer. Local or metastatic lesions that take up ^{131}I on whole body scanning can be treated with radioactive iodine after the patient has stopped thyroid hormone replacement, whereas those that do not take up ^{131}I can be treated with surgical excision or local x-ray therapy. Conventional chemotherapy has limited efficacy in the treatment of differentiated thyroid cancer, but newer biologic agents targeting the molecular pathogenesis of these tumors appear promising.

TABLE 63-7	CHARACTERISTICS OF THYROID CANCERS			
TYPE OF CANCER	**PERCENTAGE OF THYROID CANCERS**	**AGE AT ONSET (YR)**	**TREATMENT**	**PROGNOSIS**
Papillary	80	40-80	Thyroidectomy, followed by radioactive iodine ablation	Good
Follicular	15	45-80	Thyroidectomy, followed by radioactive iodine ablation	Fair to good
Medullary	3	20-50	Thyroidectomy and central compartment lymph node dissection	Fair
Anaplastic	1	50-80	Isthmusectomy followed by palliative x-ray treatment	Poor
Lymphoma	1	25-70	X-ray therapy or chemotherapy or both	Fair

Medullary carcinoma of the thyroid requires total thyroidectomy with removal of the central lymph nodes in the neck. Completeness of the procedure and monitoring for recurrence are determined by measurements of serum calcitonin.

Anaplastic carcinoma is treated with isthmusectomy to confirm the diagnosis and to prevent tracheal compression, followed by palliative x-ray treatment. Thyroid lymphomas are also treated with x-ray therapy or chemotherapy or both.

The prognosis for well-differentiated thyroid carcinomas is good. The patient's age at the time of diagnosis and sex are the most important prognostic factors. Men older than 40 years of age and women older than 50 years of age have higher recurrence and death rates than do younger patients. The 5-year survival rate for invasive medullary carcinoma is 50%, whereas the mean survival time for anaplastic carcinoma is 6 months.

For a deeper discussion on this topic, please see Chapter 226, "Thyroid," in Goldman-Cecil Medicine, *25th Edition.*

SUGGESTED READINGS

Abraham P, Avenell A, McGeoch SC, et al: Antithyroid drug regimen for treating Graves' hyperthyroidism, Cochrane Database Syst Rev CD003420, 2010.

Alexander EK, Kennedy GC, Baloch ZW, et al: Preoperative diagnosis of benign thyroid nodules with indeterminate cytology, N Engl J Med 367:705–715, 2012.

Cooper DS, Doherty GM, Haugen BR, et al: Revised American Thyroid Association management guidelines for patients with thyroid nodules and differentiated thyroid cancer, Thyroid 19:1167–1214, 2009.

Franklyn JA: The thyroid—too much and too little across the ages: the consequences of subclinical thyroid dysfunction, Clin Endocrinol (Oxf) 78:1–8, 2013.

Gharib H, Papini E, Paschke R, et al: American Association of Clinical Endocrinologists, Associazione Medici Endocrinologi, and European Thyroid Association Medical guidelines for clinical practice for the diagnosis and management of thyroid nodules: executive summary of recommendations, Endocr Pract 16:468–475, 2010.

Gullo D, Latina A, Frasca F, et al: Levothyroxine monotherapy cannot guarantee euthyroidism in all athyreotic patients, PLoS ONE 6:e22552, 2011.

Wiersinga WM: Do we need still more trials on T4 and T3 combination therapy in hypothyroidism?, Eur J Endocrinol 161:955–959, 2009.

Adrenal Gland

Theodore C. Friedman

PHYSIOLOGY

The adrenal glands (Fig. 64-1) lie at the superior pole of each kidney and are composed of two distinct regions: the cortex and the medulla. The adrenal cortex comprises three anatomic zones: the outer *zona glomerulosa*, which secretes the mineralocorticoid aldosterone; the intermediate *zona fasciculata*, which secretes cortisol; and the inner *zona reticularis*, which secretes adrenal androgens. The adrenal medulla, lying in the center of the adrenal gland, is functionally related to the sympathetic nervous system and secretes the catecholamines epinephrine and norepinephrine in response to stress.

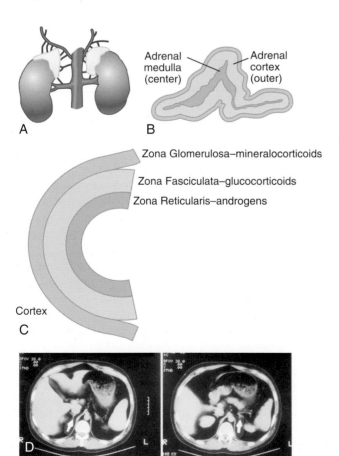

FIGURE 64-1 **A,** Anatomic location of the adrenal glands. **B,** Distribution of adrenal cortex and medulla. **C,** Zones of the adrenal cortex. **D,** Magnetic resonance images of the abdomen showing the position and relative size of the normal adrenal glands *(arrows)*. (**D,** From Nieman LK: Adrenal cortex. In Goldman L, Schafer AI, editors: Cecil-Goldman medicine, ed 24, Philadelphia, 2012, Saunders, Figure 234-1.)

The synthesis of all steroid hormones begins with cholesterol and is catalyzed by a series of regulated, enzyme-mediated reactions (Fig. 64-2). Glucocorticoids affect metabolism, cardiovascular function, behavior, and the inflammatory and immune responses (Table 64-1). Cortisol, the natural human glucocorticoid, is secreted by the adrenal glands in response to adrenocorticotropic hormone (ACTH), a 39-amino-acid neuropeptide that is regulated by corticotropin-releasing hormone (CRH) and vasopressin (AVP) produced in the hypothalamus (see Chapter 62). Glucocorticoids exert negative feedback on CRH and ACTH secretion. The brain hypothalamic-pituitary-adrenal (HPA) axis (Fig. 64-3) interacts with and influences the functions of the reproductive, growth, and thyroid axes at many levels, with major participation of glucocorticoids at all levels.

The renin-angiotensin-aldosterone system (Fig. 64-4) is the major regulator of aldosterone secretion. Renal juxtaglomerular cells secrete renin in response to a decrease in circulating volume or a reduction in renal perfusion pressure or both. Renin is the rate-limiting enzyme that cleaves the 60-kD angiotensinogen molecule, synthesized by the liver, to produce the bioinactive decapeptide angiotensin I. Angiotensin I is rapidly converted to the octapeptide angiotensin II by angiotensin-converting enzyme in the lungs and other tissues. Angiotensin II is a potent vasopressor; it stimulates aldosterone production but does not stimulate cortisol production. Angiotensin II is the predominant regulator of aldosterone secretion, but plasma potassium concentration, plasma volume, and ACTH level also influence aldosterone secretion. ACTH also mediates the circadian rhythm of aldosterone, and as a result, the plasma concentration of aldosterone is highest in the morning. Aldosterone binds to the type I mineralocorticoid receptor. In contrast, cortisol binds to both the type I mineralocorticoid receptor and type II glucocorticoid receptors. The intracellular enzyme 11β-hydroxysteroid dehydrogenase (11β-HSD) type II, which catabolizes cortisol to inactive cortisone, limits the functional binding to the former receptor. The availability of cortisol to bind to the glucocorticoid receptor is modulated by 11β-HSD type I, which interconverts cortisol and cortisone. Binding of aldosterone to the cytosol mineralocorticoid receptor leads to sodium (Na^+) absorption and potassium (K^+) and hydrogen (H^+) secretion by the renal tubules. The resultant increase in plasma Na^+ and decrease in plasma K^+ provide a feedback mechanism for suppressing renin and, subsequently, aldosterone secretion.

Adrenal androgen precursors include dehydroepiandrosterone (DHEA) and its sulfate and androstenedione. These are synthesized in the zona reticularis under the influence of ACTH and other adrenal androgen-stimulating factors. Although they

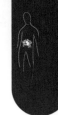

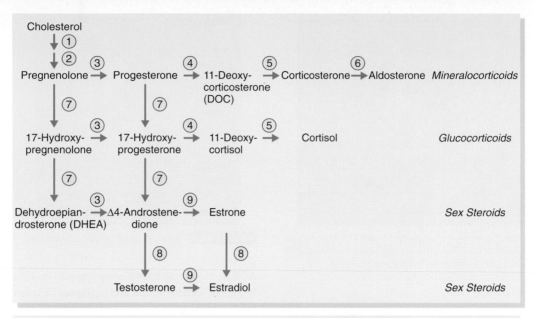

Enzyme Number	Enzyme (Current and Trivial Name)
1	StAR; Steroidogenic acute regulatory protein
2	CYP11A1; Cholesterol side-chain cleavage enzyme/desmolase
3	3β-HSD II; 3β-Hydroxylase dehydrogenase
4	CYP21A2; 21α-Hydroxylase
5	CYP11B1; 11β-Hydroxylase
6	CYP11B2; Corticosterone methyloxidase
7	CYP17; 17α-Hydroxylase/17, 20 lyase
8	17β-HSD; 17β-Hydroxysteroid dehydrogenase
9	CYP19; Aromatase

FIGURE 64-2 Pathways of steroid biosynthesis.

have minimal intrinsic androgenic activity, they contribute to androgenicity by their peripheral conversion to testosterone and dihydrotestosterone. In men, excessive levels of adrenal androgens have no clinical consequences, but in women they result in acne, hirsutism, and virilization. Because of gonadal production of androgens and estrogens and the secretion of norepinephrine by sympathetic ganglia, deficiencies of adrenal androgens and catecholamines are not clinically recognized.

SYNDROMES OF ADRENOCORTICAL HYPOFUNCTION
Adrenal Insufficiency

Glucocorticoid insufficiency can be primary, resulting from destruction or dysfunction of the adrenal cortex, or secondary, resulting from ACTH hyposecretion (Table 64-2). Autoimmune destruction of the adrenal glands (Addison's disease) is the most common cause of primary adrenal insufficiency in the industrialized world, accounting for about 65% of cases. Usually, both glucocorticoid and mineralocorticoid secretions are diminished in this condition which, if left untreated, can be fatal. Isolated glucocorticoid or mineralocorticoid deficiency may also occur, and it is becoming apparent that mild adrenal insufficiency (similar to subclinical hypothyroidism, discussed in Chapter 63) should also be diagnosed and, in some cases, treated. Adrenal medulla function is usually spared. About 70% of patients with Addison's disease have antiadrenal antibodies.

Tuberculosis used to be the most common cause of adrenal insufficiency. However, its incidence in the industrialized world

has decreased since the 1960s, and it now accounts for only 15% to 20% of patients with adrenal insufficiency; calcified adrenal glands can be observed in 50% of these patients. Rare causes of adrenal insufficiency are listed in Table 64-2. Many patients with human immunodeficiency virus (HIV) infection have decreased adrenal reserve without overt adrenal insufficiency.

Addison's disease may be part of two distinct autoimmune polyglandular syndromes. The triad of hypoparathyroidism, adrenal insufficiency, and mucocutaneous candidiasis characterizes type I polyglandular autoimmune syndrome, which usually manifests in childhood. Other, less common manifestations include hypothyroidism, gonadal failure, gastrointestinal malabsorption, insulin-dependent diabetes mellitus, alopecia areata and totalis, pernicious anemia, vitiligo, chronic active hepatitis, keratopathy, hypoplasia of dental enamel and nails, hypophysitis, asplenism, and cholelithiasis. Type II polyglandular autoimmune syndrome, also called *Schmidt's syndrome*, is characterized by Addison's disease, autoimmune thyroid disease (Graves' disease or Hashimoto's thyroiditis), and insulin-dependent diabetes mellitus. Other associated diseases include pernicious anemia, vitiligo, gonadal failure, hypophysitis, celiac disease, myasthenia gravis, primary biliary cirrhosis, Sjögren's syndrome, lupus erythematosus, and Parkinson's disease. This syndrome usually develops in adults.

Common manifestations of adrenal insufficiency are anorexia, weight loss, increasing fatigue, occasional vomiting, diarrhea, and salt craving. Muscle and joint pain, abdominal pain, and postural dizziness may also occur. Signs of increased pigmentation

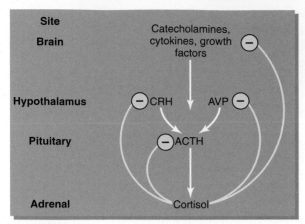

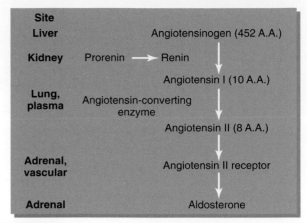

FIGURE 64-3 Brain hypothalamic-pituitary-adrenal axis. Minus signs indicate negative feedback. ACTH, Adrenocorticotropic hormone; AVP, arginine vasopressin; CRH, corticotropin-releasing hormone.

FIGURE 64-4 Renin-angiotensin-aldosterone axis. A.A., Amino acids.

TABLE 64-1	ACTIONS OF GLUCOCORTICOIDS

METABOLIC HOMEOSTASIS

Regulate blood glucose level (permissive effects on gluconeogenesis)
Increase glycogen synthesis
Raise insulin levels (permissive effects on lipolytic hormones)
Increase catabolism, decrease anabolism (except fat), inhibit growth hormone axis
Inhibit reproductive axis
Stimulate mineralocorticoid receptor by cortisol

CONNECTIVE TISSUES

Cause loss of collagen and connective tissue

CALCIUM HOMEOSTASIS

Stimulate osteoclasts, inhibit osteoblasts
Reduce intestinal calcium absorption, stimulate parathyroid hormone release, increase urinary calcium excretion, decrease reabsorption of phosphate

CARDIOVASCULAR FUNCTION

Increase cardiac output
Increase vascular tone (permissive effects on pressor hormones)
Increase sodium retention

BEHAVIOR AND COGNITIVE FUNCTION

Daytime fatigue
Nocturnal hyperarousal
Decreased short-term memory
Decreased cognition

EUPHORIA OR DEPRESSION

IMMUNE SYSTEM

Increase intravascular leukocyte concentration
Decrease migration of inflammatory cells to sites of injury
Suppress immune system (thymolysis; suppression of cytokines, prostanoids, kinins, serotonin, histamine, collagenase, and plasminogen activator)

(initially most significant on the extensor surfaces, palmar creases, and buccal mucosa) often occur secondary to the increased production of ACTH and other related peptides by the pituitary gland (E-Fig. 64-1). Laboratory abnormalities may include hyponatremia, hyperkalemia, mild metabolic acidosis, azotemia, hypercalcemia, anemia, lymphocytosis, and eosinophilia. Hypoglycemia may also occur, especially in children.

Acute adrenal insufficiency is a medical emergency, and treatment should not be delayed pending laboratory results. In a critically ill patient with hypovolemia, a plasma sample for cortisol,

ACTH, aldosterone, and renin should be obtained, and then treatment with hydrocortisone (100 mg IV bolus) and parenteral saline administration should be initiated. Sepsis-induced adrenal insufficiency is recognized by a basal cortisol level lower than 10 μg/dL or a change in cortisol of less than 9 μg/dL after administration of 0.25 mg ACTH (1-24) (cosyntropin). In severe illness, albumin and cortisol-binding globulin (CBG) are low, resulting in a low level of total cortisol but not free cortisol; therefore, a low total cortisol level may not be diagnostic of adrenal insufficiency in this setting.

In a patient with chronic symptoms suggestive of adrenal insufficiency, a basal morning plasma cortisol measurement or a 1-hour cosyntropin test, or both, should be performed. In the latter test, 0.25 mg of cosyntropin is given intravenously or intramuscularly, and plasma cortisol is measured after 0, 30, and 60 minutes. A normal response is a plasma cortisol concentration higher than 20 μg/dL at any time during the test. A patient with a basal morning plasma cortisol concentration lower than 5 μg/dL and a stimulated cortisol concentration lower than 18 μg/dL probably has adrenal insufficiency and should receive treatment. A basal plasma morning cortisol concentration between 10 and 18 μg/dL in association with a stimulated cortisol concentration lower than 18 μg/dL probably indicates impaired adrenal reserve and a requirement for receiving cortisol replacement under stress conditions (see later discussion).

Once the diagnosis of adrenal insufficiency is made, the distinction between primary and secondary adrenal insufficiency needs to be established. Secondary adrenal insufficiency results from inadequate stimulation of the adrenal cortex by ACTH (see Chapter 62). Hyperpigmentation does not occur. In addition, because mineralocorticoid levels are normal in secondary adrenal insufficiency, symptoms of salt craving, as well as the laboratory abnormalities of hyperkalemia and metabolic acidosis, are not present, although hyponatremia may be observed. Hypothyroidism, hypogonadism, and growth hormone deficiency may also be present. To distinguish primary from secondary adrenal insufficiency, a basal morning plasma ACTH value should be obtained, along with a standing (upright for at least 2 hours) serum aldosterone level and a measurement of plasma renin activity (PRA). A plasma ACTH value greater than 20 pg/mL (normal, 5 to 30 pg/mL) is consistent with primary adrenal insufficiency, whereas a value lower than 20 pg/mL probably represents

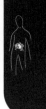

TABLE 64-2	SYNDROMES OF ADRENOCORTICAL HYPOFUNCTION

PRIMARY ADRENAL DISORDERS

Combined Glucocorticoid and Mineralocorticoid Deficiency

Autoimmune
   Isolated autoimmune disease (Addison's disease)
   Polyglandular autoimmune syndrome, type I
   Polyglandular autoimmune syndrome, type II
Infectious
   Tuberculosis
   Fungal
   Cytomegalovirus
   Human immunodeficiency virus
Vascular
   Bilateral adrenal hemorrhage
   Sepsis
   Coagulopathy
   Thrombosis, embolism
   Adrenal infarction
Infiltration
   Metastatic carcinoma and lymphoma
   Sarcoidosis
   Amyloidosis
   Hemochromatosis
Congenital
   Congenital adrenal hyperplasia
   21-Hydroxylase deficiency
   3β-ol Dehydrogenase deficiency
   20,22-Desmolase deficiency
   Adrenal unresponsiveness to ACTH
   Congenital adrenal hypoplasia
   Adrenoleukodystrophy
   Adrenomyeloneuropathy
Iatrogenic
   Bilateral adrenalectomy
   Drugs: metyrapone, aminoglutethimide, trilostane, ketoconazole, o,p'-DDD, mifepristone, pasireotide

Mineralocorticoid Deficiency without Glucocorticoid Deficiency

   Corticosterone methyl oxidase deficiency
   Isolated zona glomerulosa defect
   Heparin therapy
   Critical illness
   Angiogensin-converting enzyme inhibitors

SECONDARY ADRENAL DISORDERS

Secondary Adrenal Insufficiency

Hypothalamic-pituitary dysfunction
Exogenous glucocorticoids
After removal of an ACTH-secreting tumor

Hyporeninemic Hypoaldosteronism

Diabetic nephropathy
Tubulointerstitial diseases
Obstructive uropathy
Autonomic neuropathy
Nonsteroidal anti-inflammatory drugs
β-Adrenergic drugs

ACTH, Adrenocorticotropic hormone; o,p'-DDD, o,p'-dichlorodiphenyldichloroethane (mitotane).

secondary adrenal insufficiency. An upright PRA value greater than 3 ng/mL/hour in the setting of a suppressed aldosterone level is consistent with primary adrenal insufficiency, whereas a value lower than 3 ng/mL/hour probably represents secondary adrenal insufficiency. The 1-hour cosyntropin test is suppressed in both primary and secondary adrenal insufficiency.

Secondary adrenal insufficiency occurs commonly after the discontinuation of glucocorticoids. Alternate-day glucocorticoid treatment, if feasible, results in less suppression of the HPA axis than does daily glucocorticoid therapy. Complete recovery of the HPA axis can take 1 year or more, and the rate-limiting step appears to be recovery of the CRH-producing neurons.

Under stress, cortisol secretion is increased. Therefore, the concept of adrenal fatigue, proposed by some alternative providers, has no biologic validity.

After stabilization of acute adrenal insufficiency, patients with Addison's disease require lifelong replacement therapy with both glucocorticoids and mineralocorticoids. Many patients are overtreated with glucocorticoids and undertreated with mineralocorticoids. Because overtreatment with glucocorticoids results in insidious weight gain and osteoporosis, the minimal cortisol dose that can be tolerated without symptoms of glucocorticoid insufficiency (usually joint pain, abdominal pain, or diarrhea) is recommended. An initial regimen of 15 to 20 mg hydrocortisone first thing in the morning plus 5 mg hydrocortisone at about 3:00 PM mimics the physiologic dose and is recommended; a third dose is occasionally needed. Whereas glucocorticoid replacement is fairly uniform in most patients, the requirement for mineralocorticoid replacement varies greatly. The initial dose of the synthetic mineralocorticoid fludrocortisone should be 100 μg/day (often in divided doses), and the dosage should be adjusted to keep the standing PRA value between 1 and 3 ng/mL/hour.

Under the stress of a minor illness (e.g., nausea, vomiting, fever >100.5°F), the hydrocortisone dose should be doubled for as short a period as possible. An inability to ingest hydrocortisone pills may necessitate parenteral hydrocortisone administration. Patients undergoing a major stressful event (e.g., surgery necessitating general anesthesia, major trauma) should receive 150 to 300 mg parenteral hydrocortisone daily (in three divided doses) with a rapid taper to normal replacement during recovery. All patients should wear a medical information bracelet and should be instructed in the use of intramuscular emergency hydrocortisone injections.

Hyporeninemic Hypoaldosteronism

Mineralocorticoid deficiency can result from decreased renin secretion by the kidneys. Resultant hypoangiotensinemia leads to hypoaldosteronism with hyperkalemia and hyperchloremic metabolic acidosis. The plasma sodium concentration is usually normal, but total plasma volume is often deficient. PRA and aldosterone levels are low and unresponsive to stimuli, including hypokalemia. Diabetes mellitus and chronic tubulointerstitial diseases of the kidney are the most common underlying conditions leading to impairment of the juxtaglomerular apparatus. A subset of hyporeninemic hypoaldosteronism is caused by autonomic insufficiency and is a frequent cause of orthostatic hypotension. Stimuli such as upright posture or volume depletion, mediated by baroreceptors, do not cause a normal renin response. Administration of pharmacologic agents such as nonsteroidal anti-inflammatory agents, angiotensin-converting enzyme inhibitors, and β-adrenergic antagonists can also produce conditions of hypoaldosteronism. Salt administration often with fludrocortisone and the $α_1$-receptor agonist midodrine are effective in correcting the orthostatic hypotension and electrolyte abnormalities caused by hypoaldosteronism.

Congenital Adrenal Hyperplasia

Congenital adrenal hyperplasia (CAH) refers to autosomal recessive disorders of adrenal steroid biosynthesis that result in glucocorticoid and mineralocorticoid deficiencies and compensatory increase in ACTH secretion (see Fig. 64-2). Five major types of CAH exist, and the clinical manifestations of each type depend on which steroids are in excess and which are deficient. 21α-Hydroxylase (CYP21) deficiency is the most common of these disorders and accounts for about 95% of patients with CAH. In this condition, there is a failure of 21-hydroxylation of 17-hydroxyprogesterone and progesterone to 11-deoxycortisol and 11-deoxycorticosterone, respectively, with deficient cortisol and aldosterone production. Cortisol deficiency leads to increased ACTH release, resulting in adrenal hyperplasia and overproduction of 17-hydroxyprogesterone and progesterone. Increased ACTH production also leads to increased biosynthesis of androstenedione and DHEA, which can be converted to testosterone. Patients with 21-hydroxylase deficiencies can be divided into two clinical phenotypes: classic 21-hydroxylase deficiency, which usually is diagnosed at birth or during childhood, and late-onset 21-hydroxylase deficiency, which develops during or after puberty. Two thirds of patients with classic 21-hydroxylase deficiency have various degrees of mineralocorticoid deficiency (salt-losing form); the remaining one third have the non–salt-losing type (simple virilizing form). Both decreased aldosterone production and increased concentrations of precursors that are mineralocorticoid antagonists (progesterone and 17-hydroxyprogesterone) contribute to salt loss.

Late-onset 21-hydroxylase deficiency represents an allelic variant of classic 21-hydroxylase deficiency and is characterized by a mild enzymatic defect. This deficiency is the most common autosomal recessive disorder in humans and is present at high frequency in Ashkenazi Jews. The syndrome usually develops at the time of puberty with signs of virilization (hirsutism and acne) and amenorrhea or oligomenorrhea. This diagnosis should be considered in women who have unexplained hirsutism and menstrual abnormalities or infertility.

The most useful initial measurement for the diagnosis of classic 21-hydroxylase deficiency is that of plasma 17-hydroxyprogesterone. A value greater than 200 ng/dL is consistent with the diagnosis. The diagnosis of late-onset 21-hydroxylase deficiency is based on the finding of an elevated level of plasma 17-hydroxyprogesterone (>1500 ng/dL) 30 minutes after administration of 0.25 mg of synthetic ACTH (1-24).

The aim of treatment for classic 21-hydroxylase deficiency is to replace glucocorticoids and mineralocorticoids, suppress ACTH and androgen overproduction, and allow for normal growth and sexual maturation in children. A proposed approach to treating classic 21-hydroxylase deficiency recommends physiologic replacement with hydrocortisone and fludrocortisone in all affected patients. Virilizing effects can be prevented by the use of an antiandrogen (flutamide) and an aromatase inhibitor (testolactone). Although the traditional treatment for late-onset 21-hydroxylase deficiency is dexamethasone (0.5 mg/day), the use of an antiandrogen such as spironolactone (100 to 200 mg/day) or flutamide (125 mg/day) is probably equally effective and has fewer side effects. Mineralocorticoid replacement is not needed in late-onset 21-hydroxylase deficiency.

11β-Hydroxylase (CYP11B1) deficiency accounts for about 5% of patients with CAH. In this syndrome, the conversions of 11-deoxycortisol to cortisol and 11-deoxycorticosterone to corticosterone (the precursor to aldosterone) are blocked. Affected patients usually have hypertension and hypokalemia because of increased amounts of precursors with mineralocorticoid activity. Virilization occurs, as with 21-hydroxylase deficiency, and a late-onset form manifesting as androgen excess also occurs. The diagnosis is made from the finding of elevated plasma 11-deoxycortisol levels, either basally or after ACTH stimulation.

Rare forms of CAH are 3β-HSD type II deficiency, 17α-hydroxylase (CYP17) deficiency, and steroidogenic acute regulatory protein (StAR) deficiency.

SYNDROMES OF ADRENOCORTICAL HYPERFUNCTION

Hypersecretion of the glucocorticoid hormone cortisol results in Cushing's syndrome, a metabolic disorder that affects carbohydrate, protein, and lipid metabolism. Hypersecretion of mineralocorticoids such as aldosterone results in a syndrome of hypertension and electrolyte disturbances.

Cushing's Syndrome

Pathophysiology

Increased production of cortisol is seen in both physiologic and pathologic states (Table 64-3). Physiologic hypercortisolism occurs with stress, during the last trimester of pregnancy, and in persons who regularly perform strenuous exercise. Pathologic conditions of elevated cortisol levels include exogenous or endogenous Cushing's syndrome and several psychiatric states, such as depression, alcoholism, anorexia nervosa, panic disorder, and alcohol or narcotic withdrawal.

Cushing's syndrome may be caused by exogenous administration of ACTH or glucocorticoid or by endogenous overproduction of these hormones. Endogenous Cushing's syndrome is either ACTH dependent or ACTH independent. ACTH dependency accounts for 85% of patients and includes pituitary sources of ACTH (Cushing's disease) and ectopic sources of ACTH. Pituitary Cushing's disease accounts for 90% of patients with ACTH-dependent Cushing's syndrome. Ectopic secretion of ACTH occurs most commonly in patients with small cell lung carcinoma. These patients are older, usually have a history of smoking, and primarily exhibit signs and symptoms of lung cancer rather than those of Cushing's syndrome. Patients with the clinically apparent ectopic ACTH syndrome, in contrast, have mostly intrathoracic (lung and thymic) carcinoids. ACTH-independent causes account for 15% of patients with Cushing's syndrome and include adrenal adenomas, adrenal carcinomas, micronodular adrenal disease, and autonomous macronodular adrenal disease. The female-to-male ratio for noncancerous forms of Cushing's syndrome is 4 : 1.

Clinical Presentation

The clinical signs, symptoms, and common laboratory findings of hypercortisolism observed in patients with Cushing's syndrome are listed in Table 64-4 (see also Fig. 64-2). Patients with

TABLE 64-3	SYNDROMES OF ADRENOCORTICAL HYPERFUNCTION

STATES OF GLUCOCORTICOID EXCESS	STATES OF MINERALOCORTICOID EXCESS
Physiologic States	**Primary Aldosteronism**
Stress	Aldosterone-secreting adenoma
Strenuous exercise	Bilateral adrenal hyperplasia
Last trimester of pregnancy	Aldosterone-secreting carcinoma
	Glucocorticoid-suppressible
Pathologic States	hyperaldosteronism
Psychiatric conditions (pseudo-Cushing's disorders)	**Adrenal Enzyme Deficiencies**
Depression	11β-Hydroxylase deficiency
Alcoholism	17α-Hydroxylase deficiency
Anorexia nervosa	11β-Hydroxysteroid dehydrogenase
Panic disorders	type II deficiency
Alcohol and drug withdrawal	
ACTH-dependent states	**Exogenous Mineralocorticoids**
Pituitary adenoma (Cushing's disease)	Licorice
Ectopic ACTH syndrome	Carbenoxolone
Bronchial carcinoid	Fludrocortisone
Thymic carcinoid	
Islet cell tumor	**Secondary Hyperaldosteronism**
Small cell lung carcinoma	Associated with hypertension
Ectopic CRH secretion	Accelerated hypertension
ACTH-independent states	Renovascular hypertension
Adrenal adenoma	Estrogen administration
Adrenal carcinoma	Renin-secreting tumors
Micronodular adrenal disease	Without hypertension
	Bartter's syndrome
Exogenous Sources	Sodium-wasting nephropathy
	Renal tubular acidosis
Glucocorticoid intake	Diuretic and laxative abuse
ACTH intake	Edematous states (cirrhosis, nephrosis, congestive heart failure)

ACTH, Adrenocorticotropin hormone; CRH, corticotropin-releasing hormone.

TABLE 64-4	SIGNS, SYMPTOMS, AND LABORATORY ABNORMALITIES OF HYPERCORTISOLISM

FEATURE	PERCENTAGE OF PATIENTS
Fat redistribution (dorsocervical and supraclavicular fat pads, temporal wasting, centripetal obesity, weight gain)	95
Menstrual irregularities	80 (of affected women)
Thin skin and plethora	80
Moon facies	75
Increased appetite	75
Sleep disturbances	75
Nocturnal hyperarousal	75
Hypertension	75
Hypercholesterolemia and hypertriglyceridemia	70
Altered mentation (poor concentration, decreased memory, euphoria)	70
Diabetes mellitus and glucose intolerance	65
Striae	65
Hirsutism	65 (of affected women)
Proximal muscle weakness	60
Psychological disturbances (emotional lability, depression, mania, psychosis)	50
Decreased libido and erectile dysfunction	50 (of affected men)
Acne	45
Osteoporosis and pathologic fractures	40
Easy bruisability	40
Poor wound healing	40
Virilization	20 (of affected women)
Edema	20
Increased infections	10
Cataracts	5

Cushing's syndrome often have some, but not all, of the signs and symptoms discussed here. Typically, the obesity is centripetal, with a wasting of the arms and legs, which is distinct from the generalized weight gain observed in idiopathic obesity. Rounding of the face (called *moon facies*) and a dorsocervical fat pad (*buffalo hump*) may occur in obesity not related to Cushing's syndrome, whereas facial plethora and supraclavicular filling are more specific for Cushing's syndrome. Patients with Cushing's syndrome may have proximal muscle weakness; consequently, the inability to stand up from a squat or to comb one's hair can be revealing. Sleep disturbances and insomnia, hyperarousal in the evening and night, mood swings, and other psychological abnormalities are frequently seen. Cognitive dysfunction and severe fatigue are often present. Menstrual irregularities often precede other cushingoid symptoms in affected women. Patients of both sexes complain of a loss of libido, and affected men frequently complain of erectile dysfunction. Adult-onset acne or hirsutism in women could also suggest Cushing's syndrome. The skin striae observed in patients with Cushing's syndrome are violaceous (i.e., purple or dark red) with a width of at least 1 cm. Thinning of the skin on the top of the hands is a specific sign in younger adults with Cushing's syndrome. Old pictures of patients are extremely helpful for evaluating the progression of the physical stigmata of Cushing's syndrome.

Associated laboratory findings in Cushing's syndrome include elevated plasma alkaline phosphatase levels, granulocytosis, thrombocytosis, hypercholesterolemia, hypertriglyceridemia, and glucose intolerance and/or diabetes mellitus. Hypokalemia or alkalosis usually occurs in patients with severe hypercortisolism as a result of the ectopic ACTH syndrome.

Diagnosis

If the history and physical examination findings are suggestive of hypercortisolism, then the diagnosis of Cushing's syndrome can usually be established by collecting urine for 24 hours and measuring the urinary free cortisol (UFC). This test is extremely sensitive for diagnosis of Cushing's syndrome because in 90% of affected patients, the initial UFC level is greater than 50 μg/24 hours (Fig. 64-5).

The overnight dexamethasone suppression test has been widely used as a screening tool to evaluate patients who may have hypercortisolism. Dexamethasone, 1 mg, is given orally at 11:00 PM or midnight, and plasma cortisol is measured the following morning at 8:00 AM. A morning plasma cortisol level greater than 1.8 μg/dL suggests hypercortisolism. This test produces a significant number of both false-positive and false-negative results, but it is still recommended in the 2008 Endocrine Society consensus guidelines.

Cortisol is normally secreted in a diurnal manner: The plasma concentration is highest in the early morning (between 6:00 and 8:00 AM) and lowest around midnight. Most patients with Cushing's syndrome have blunted diurnal variation. Nighttime plasma cortisol values greater than 50% of the morning values are

Diagnosis

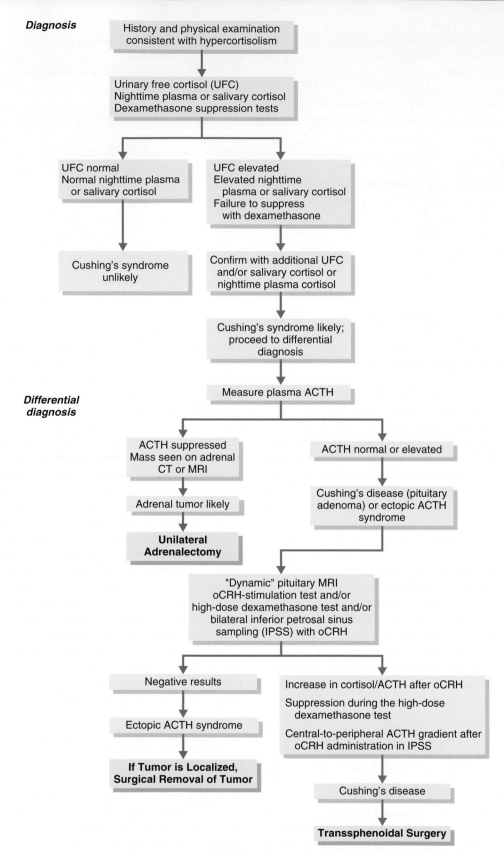

Differential diagnosis

FIGURE 64-5 Flowchart for evaluation of a patient with possible Cushing's syndrome. ACTH, Adrenocorticotropic hormone; CT, computed tomography; MRI, magnetic resonance imaging; oCRH, ovine corticotropin-releasing hormone.

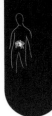

considered to be consistent with Cushing's syndrome. Because of the difficulty of obtaining nighttime plasma cortisol levels, measurement of late-night salivary cortisol has been developed to assess hypercortisolism. This test appears to have a high degree of sensitivity and specificity for diagnosis of Cushing's syndrome. Multiple measurements of UFC or salivary cortisol may be needed either diagnose or exclude Cushing's syndrome, especially in subjects with suggestive signs and symptoms of hypercortisolism.

Differential Diagnosis

Once the diagnosis of Cushing's syndrome is established, the cause of the hypercortisolism needs to be ascertained by biochemical studies that evaluate the feedback regulation of the HPA axis; this can be accomplished by venous sampling and imaging procedures. The initial approach is to measure basal ACTH levels, which are normal or elevated in Cushing's disease and the ectopic ACTH syndrome but are suppressed in primary adrenal Cushing's syndrome. Patients with a suppressed ACTH level can proceed to adrenal imaging studies. To distinguish between Cushing's disease and the ectopic ACTH syndrome, the high-dose or 8-mg overnight dexamethasone suppression test, the ovine CRH (oCRH) test, and bilateral simultaneous inferior petrosal sinus sampling (IPSS) are used.

In the dexamethasone suppression test (Liddle test), 0.5 mg of dexamethasone is given orally every 6 hours for 2 days (low dose), followed by 2 mg of dexamethasone every 6 hours for another 2 days (high dose). On the second day of high-dose dexamethasone, the UFC level will be suppressed to less than 10% of the baseline collection value in patients with pituitary adenomas but not in patients with the ectopic ACTH syndrome or adrenal cortisol-secreting tumors. The Liddle test has some methodologic drawbacks, and results should be interpreted cautiously; other confirmatory tests should be performed before surgery is recommended.

An overnight high-dose dexamethasone suppression test is helpful in establishing the cause of Cushing's syndrome. In this test, a baseline cortisol level is measured at 8:00 AM, and then 8 mg of dexamethasone is given orally at 11:00 PM. At 8:00 AM the following morning, a plasma cortisol measurement is obtained. Suppression, which occurs in patients with pituitary Cushing's disease, is defined as a decrease in plasma cortisol to less than 50% of the baseline level.

The oCRH test can also be used to establish the cause of Cushing's syndrome, but this test was not available in the United States in 2014.

Bilateral IPSS is an accurate and safe procedure for distinguishing pituitary Cushing's disease from the ectopic ACTH syndrome. Venous blood from the anterior lobe of the pituitary gland empties into the cavernous sinuses and then into the superior and inferior petrosal sinuses. Venous plasma samples for ACTH determination are obtained from both inferior petrosal sinuses, along with a simultaneous peripheral sample, both before and after intravenous bolus administration of oCRH. Significant gradients at baseline and after oCRH stimulation between petrosal sinus and peripheral samples suggest pituitary Cushing's disease. In baseline measurements, an ACTH concentration gradient of 1.6 or more between a sample from either of the petrosal sinuses and the peripheral sample is strongly suggestive of

pituitary Cushing's disease, whereas patients with the ectopic ACTH syndrome or adrenal adenomas have no ACTH gradient between their petrosal and peripheral samples. After oCRH administration, a central-to-peripheral gradient of more than 3.2 is consistent with pituitary Cushing's disease. The use of oCRH has enabled complete distinction of pituitary from nonpituitary Cushing's syndrome. An ACTH gradient ipsilateral to the side of the tumor is found in 70% to 80% of pituitary Cushing's disease patients sampled. Although this procedure requires an radiologist who is experienced in IPSS, it is available at many tertiary care facilities.

Magnetic resonance imaging (MRI) with gadolinium is the preferred procedure for localizing a pituitary adenoma. In many centers, a *dynamic* MRI is performed; the pituitary is visualized as the gadolinium enters and leaves the gland. Because about 10% of normal individuals are found to have a nonfunctioning pituitary adenoma on pituitary MRI, pituitary imaging should not be the sole criterion for the diagnosis of pituitary Cushing's disease.

Treatment

The preferred treatment for all forms of Cushing's syndrome is appropriate surgery or, in some cases, radiation therapy (see Chapter 62). A more appealing option for patients with Cushing's disease who remain hypercortisolemic after pituitary surgery is bilateral adrenalectomy followed by lifelong glucocorticoid and mineralocorticoid replacement therapy.

In patients with the ectopic ACTH syndrome, the goal is to localize the tumor by appropriate scans so it can be removed surgically. A unilateral adrenalectomy is the treatment of choice in patients with a cortisol-secreting adrenal adenoma. Cortisol-secreting adrenal carcinomas initially should also be managed surgically; however, the prognosis is poor, with only 20% of patients surviving more than 1 year after diagnosis.

Medical treatment for hypercortisolism may be needed to prepare patients who are undergoing or have undergone pituitary irradiation and are awaiting its effects before surgery as well as those who are not surgical candidates or elect not to have surgery. Ketoconazole, o,p′-DDD (mitotane), metyrapone, aminoglutethimide, mifepristone, and trilostane are the most commonly used agents for adrenal blockade and can be used alone or in combination. The somatostatin analogue, pasireotide, which decreases ACTH and may decrease tumor size, is a recently FDA-approved drug for treating Cushing's disease.

Primary Mineralocorticoid Excess
Pathophysiology

The causes of primary aldosteronism (see Table 64-3) are aldosterone-producing adenoma (75%), bilateral adrenal hyperplasia (25%), adrenal carcinoma (1%), and glucocorticoid-remediable hyperaldosteronism (<1%). Adrenal enzyme defects (11β-HSD type II, 11β-hydroxylase, and 17α-hydroxylase deficiencies) and apparent mineralocorticoid excess (from ingestion of licorice or carbenoxolone, which inhibit 11β-HSD type II, or from a congenital defect in this enzyme) are also states of functional mineralocorticoid overactivity. Secondary aldosteronism (see Table 64-3) results from an overactive renin-angiotensin system.

Primary aldosteronism is usually recognized during evaluation of hypertension or hypokalemia and represents a potentially curable form of hypertension. Up to 5% of patients with hypertension have primary aldosteronism. These patients are usually between the ages of 30 and 50 years, and the female-to-male ratio is 2 : 1.

Clinical Presentation

Hypertension, hypokalemia, and metabolic alkalosis are the main clinical manifestations of hyperaldosteronism; most of the presenting symptoms are related to hypokalemia. Symptoms in patients with mild hypokalemia are fatigue, muscle weakness, nocturia, lassitude, and headaches. If more severe hypokalemia exists, polydipsia, polyuria, paresthesias, and even intermittent paralysis and tetany can occur. Blood pressure can range from minimally elevated to very high. A positive Trousseau or Chvostek sign may occur as a result of metabolic alkalosis.

Diagnosis and Treatment

Initially, hypokalemia in the presence of hypertension must be documented (Fig. 64-6). The patient must have adequate salt intake and discontinue diuretics before potassium measurement. A morning plasma aldosterone level (measured in ng/dL) and a

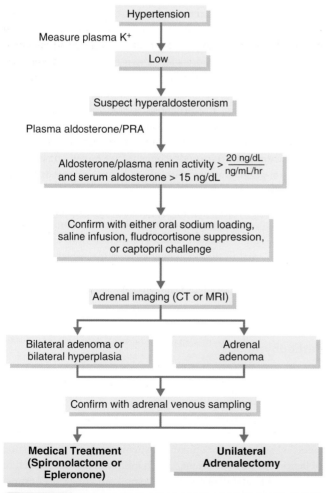

FIGURE 64-6 Flowchart for evaluation of a patient with probable primary hyperaldosteronism. Plasma aldosterone is measured in ng/dL, and plasma renin activity (PRA) is measured in ng/mL/hour. CT, Computed tomography; MRI, magnetic resonance imaging.

PRA value (in ng/mL/hour) should be obtained. A ratio of serum aldosterone to PRA greater than 20 with a serum aldosterone level greater than 15 ng/dL suggests the diagnosis of hyperaldosteronism. Confirmatory tests for hyperaldosteronism should be performed, such as oral sodium loading, saline infusion, fludrocortisone suppression, or captopril challenge.

Once the diagnosis of primary aldosteronism has been demonstrated, it is important to distinguish between an aldosterone-producing adenoma and bilateral hyperplasia, because the former is treated with surgery and the latter is treated medically. A computed tomography (CT) scan of the adrenal glands should be performed to localize the tumor. The patient should undergo unilateral adrenalectomy if a discrete adenoma is observed in one adrenal gland and the contralateral gland is normal. Patients in whom biochemical and localization study findings are consistent with bilateral hyperplasia should be treated medically with a potassium-sparing diuretic, usually eplerenone or spironolactone. Hyperaldosteronism and hypertension secondary to activation of the renin-angiotensin system can occur in patients with accelerated hypertension, in those with renovascular hypertension, in those receiving estrogen therapies, and, rarely, in patients with renin-secreting tumors. Hyperaldosteronism without hypertension occurs in patients with Bartter's syndrome, sodium-wasting nephropathy, or renal tubular acidosis, as well as those who abuse diuretics or laxatives.

⬤ ADRENAL MEDULLARY HYPERFUNCTION

The adrenal medulla synthesizes the catecholamines norepinephrine, epinephrine, and dopamine from the amino acid tyrosine. Norepinephrine, the major catecholamine produced by the adrenal medulla, has predominantly α-agonist actions, causing vasoconstriction. Epinephrine acts primarily on the β-receptors, having positive inotropic and chronotropic effects on the heart and causing peripheral vasodilation and increasing plasma glucose concentrations in response to hypoglycemia. The action of circulating dopamine is unclear. Whereas norepinephrine is synthesized in the central nervous system and sympathetic postganglionic neurons, epinephrine is synthesized almost entirely in the adrenal medulla. The adrenal medullary contribution to total body norepinephrine secretion is relatively small. Hypofunction of the adrenal medulla has little physiologic effect, whereas hypersecretion of catecholamines produces the clinical syndrome of pheochromocytoma.

Pheochromocytoma

Pathophysiology

Although pheochromocytomas can occur in any sympathetic ganglion in the body, more than 90% arise from the adrenal medulla. Most extra-adrenal tumors occur in the mediastinum or abdomen. Bilateral adrenal pheochromocytomas are present in about 5% of the cases and may occur as part of familial syndromes. Pheochromocytoma occurs as part of multiple endocrine neoplasia type IIA or IIB. The former (Sipple's syndrome) is marked by medullary carcinoma of the thyroid, hyperparathyroidism, and pheochromocytoma; the latter is characterized by medullary carcinoma of the thyroid, mucosal neuromas, intestinal ganglioneuromas, marfanoid habitus, and pheochromocytoma. Pheochromocytomas are also associated with neurofibromatosis, cerebelloretinal hemangioblastosis (von Hippel–Lindau disease), and tuberous sclerosis.

Clinical Presentation

Because most pheochromocytomas secrete norepinephrine as the principal catecholamine, hypertension (often paroxysmal) is the most common finding. Other symptoms include the triad of headache, palpitations, and sweating as well as skin blanching, diarrhea, anxiety, nausea, fatigue, weight loss, and abdominal and chest pain. Emotional stress, exercise, anesthesia, abdominal pressure, or intake of tyramine-containing foods may precipitate these symptoms. Orthostatic hypotension can also occur. Wide fluctuations in blood pressure are characteristic, and the hypertension associated with pheochromocytoma usually does not respond to standard antihypertensive medicines. Cardiac abnormalities, as well as idiosyncratic reactions to medications, may also occur.

Diagnosis and Treatment

Although measurements of fractionated catecholamine and metanephrine levels in the urine are often used as screening tests, plasma free metanephrine and normetanephrine levels are the best tests for confirming or excluding pheochromocytoma. A plasma free metanephrine level greater than 0.61 nmol/L and a plasma free normetanephrine level greater than 0.31 nmol/L are consistent with the diagnosis of a pheochromocytoma. If these levels are only mildly elevated, a clonidine suppression test can be performed. In patients with pheochromocytoma, levels are unchanged or increased. Once the diagnosis of pheochromocytoma is made, a CT scan of the adrenal glands should be performed. Most intra-adrenal pheochromocytomas are readily visible on this scan and enhance with contrast. If the CT scan is negative, then extra-adrenal pheochromocytomas can often be localized by iodine 131–labeled metaiodobenzylguanidine (^{131}I-MIBG), positron emission tomography, octreotide scan, or abdominal MRI. Pheochromocytomas show high signal intensity on T2-weighted images.

The treatment of pheochromocytoma is surgical if the lesion can be localized. Patients should undergo preoperative α-blockade with phenoxybenzamine 1 to 2 weeks before surgery. β-Adrenergic antagonists should be used before or during surgery. About 5% to 10% of pheochromocytomas are malignant. ^{131}I-MIBG or chemotherapy may be useful, but the prognosis is poor. α-Methyl-*p*-tyrosine, an inhibitor of tyrosine hydroxylase, the rate-limiting enzyme in catecholamine biosynthesis, may be used to decrease catecholamine secretion from the tumor.

Incidental Adrenal Mass

Clinically inapparent adrenal masses may be discovered inadvertently in the course of diagnostic testing or treatment for other clinical conditions not related to the signs and symptoms of adrenal disease; they are commonly known as *incidentalomas* (E-Fig. 64-2). Some of these tumors secrete a small amount of excess cortisol, leading to a condition called *subclinical Cushing's syndrome*. A morning plasma ACTH level and an overnight 1-mg dexamethasone test are recommended for patients with an adrenal incidentaloma. Patients with hypertension should also undergo measurement of serum potassium, plasma aldosterone concentration, PRA, and urine or plasma free metanephrines. Surgery should be considered for all patients with functional adrenal cortical tumors that are hormonally active or larger than 4 cm. Tumors not associated with hormonal secretion that are smaller than 4 cm can be monitored with repeated imaging and hormonal assessment.

Primary Adrenal Cancer

Primary adrenal carcinomas are rare, with an incidence of 1 to 5 per 1 million persons. The female-to-male ratio is 2.5 : 1, and the mean age at onset is 40 to 50 years. About 25% of patients have symptoms, including abdominal pain, weight loss, anorexia, and fever. Eighty percent of primary adrenal carcinomas are functional, with secretion of glucocorticoid alone (45%) or glucocorticoid plus androgens (45%) being most common.

At presentation, metastatic spread is evident in 75% of cases. An incidentally discovered adrenal mass that is large is more likely to be malignant. Resection is recommended for tumors larger than 6 cm and often for those larger than 4 cm. In patients who do not have a known cancer, most adrenal masses that turn out to be malignant are primary adrenocortical carcinomas, whereas in patients with a known malignancy, an adrenal mass is likely to be a metastasis in about 75% of cases.

The treatment of adrenocortical carcinomas is surgery. These cancers are usually resistant to radiation and chemotherapy, but the adrenolytic compound mitotane has been shown to improve survival. Adrenocortical carcinomas carry a poor prognosis, with overall 5-year survival rates of less than 20%.

For a deeper discussion on this topic, please see Chapter 227, "Adrenal Cortex," in Goldman-Cecil Medicine, *25th Edition.*

SUGGESTED READINGS

Annane D: Adrenal insufficiency in sepsis, Curr Pharm Des 14:1882–1886, 2008.

Neary N, Nieman L: Adrenal insufficiency: etiology, diagnosis and treatment, Curr Opin Endocrinol Diabetes Obes 17:217–223, 2010.

Nieman LK, Biller BM, Findling JW, et al: The diagnosis of Cushing's syndrome: an Endocrine Society clinical practice guideline, J Clin Endocrinol Metab 93:1526–1540, 2008.

Vassiliadi DA, Tsagarakis S: Endocrine incidentalomas: challenges imposed by incidentally discovered lesions, Nat Rev Endocrinol 7:668–680, 2011.

Young WF Jr: Adrenal causes of hypertension: pheochromocytoma and primary aldosteronism, Rev Endocr Metab Disord 8:309–320, 2007.

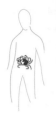

Male Reproductive Endocrinology

Glenn D. Braunstein

INTRODUCTION

The testes are composed of Leydig (interstitial) cells, which secrete testosterone and estradiol, and the seminiferous tubules, which produce sperm. They are regulated by the luteinizing hormone (LH) and follicle-stimulating hormone (FSH), which are secreted by the anterior pituitary under the influence of the hypothalamic decapeptide gonadotropin-releasing hormone (GnRH) (Fig. 65-1). LH stimulates the Leydig cells to secrete testosterone, which feeds back in a negative fashion at the level of the pituitary and hypothalamus to inhibit further LH production. FSH stimulates sperm production through interaction with the Sertoli cells in the seminiferous tubules. Feedback inhibition of FSH is through gonadal steroids, as well as through inhibin, a glycoprotein produced by Sertoli cells.

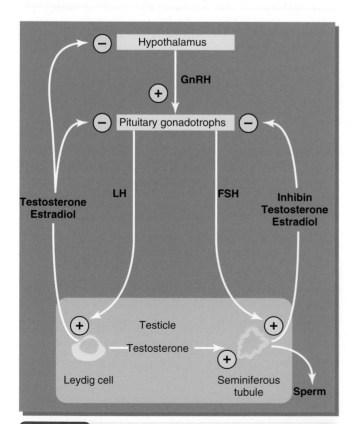

FIGURE 65-1 Regulation of the hypothalamic-pituitary-testicular axis. The *plus* (+) and *minus* (–) symbols indicate positive and negative feedback, respectively. FSH, Follicle-stimulating hormone; GnRH, gonadotropin-releasing hormone; LH, luteinizing hormone.

Biochemical evaluation of the hypothalamic-pituitary-Leydig axis is carried out by measurement of serum LH and testosterone concentrations, whereas a semen analysis and serum FSH determination provide an assessment of the hypothalamic-pituitary-seminiferous tubular axis. The ability of the pituitary to release gonadotropins can be tested dynamically through GnRH stimulation, and the ability of the testes to secrete testosterone can be evaluated through injections of human chorionic gonadotropin (HCG), a glycoprotein hormone that has biologic activity similar to that of LH.

HYPOGONADISM

Either testosterone deficiency or defective spermatogenesis constitutes *hypogonadism*. Often both disorders coexist. The clinical manifestations of androgen deficiency depend on the time of onset and the degree of deficiency. Testosterone is required for development of the wolffian duct into the epididymis, vas deferens, seminal vesicles, and ejaculatory ducts, as well as for virilization of the external genitalia through the major intracellular testosterone metabolite, dihydrotestosterone (DHT). Consequently, early prenatal androgen deficiency leads to the formation of ambiguous genitalia and to male pseudohermaphroditism. Androgen deficiency occurring later during gestation may result in micropenis or *cryptorchidism*, the unilateral or bilateral absence of testes in the scrotum resulting from the failure of normal testicular descent.

During puberty, androgens are responsible for male sexual differentiation, which includes growth of the scrotum, epididymis, vas deferens, seminal vesicles, prostate, penis, skeletal muscle, and larynx. Additionally, androgens stimulate the growth of axillary, pubic, facial, and body hair and increase sebaceous gland activity. They are also responsible through conversion to estrogens for the growth and fusion of the epiphyseal cartilaginous plates, clinically seen as the *pubertal growth spurt*. Prepubertal androgen deficiency leads to poor muscle development, decreased strength and endurance, a high-pitched voice, sparse axillary and pubic hair, and the absence of facial and body hair. The long bones of the lower extremities and arms may continue to grow under the influence of growth hormone; this condition leads to eunuchoid proportions (i.e., arm span exceeding total height by ≥5 cm) and greater growth of the lower extremities relative to total height. Postpubertal androgen deficiency may result in a decrease in libido, impotence, low energy, fine wrinkling around the corners of the eyes and mouth, and diminished facial and body hair.

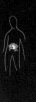

Male hypogonadism may be classified into three categories according to the level of the defect (Table 65-1). Diseases directly affecting the testes result in *primary* or *hypergonadotropic hypogonadism*, which is characterized by oligospermia or azoospermia and low testosterone levels but exhibits elevations of LH and FSH because of a decrease in the negative feedback regulation on the pituitary and hypothalamus by androgens, estrogens, and inhibin. In contrast, hypogonadism from lesions in the hypothalamus or pituitary gives rise to *secondary* or *hypogonadotropic hypogonadism*; the low testosterone level or ineffective spermatogenesis results from inadequate concentrations of the gonadotropins. The third category of hypogonadism is the result of defects in androgen action.

Hypothalamic-Pituitary Disorders

Panhypopituitarism occurs congenitally from structural defects or from inadequate production or release of the hypothalamic-releasing factors. The condition may also be acquired through replacement by tumors, infarction from vascular insufficiency, infiltrative disorders, autoimmune diseases, trauma, and infections.

Kallmann syndrome is a form of hypogonadotropic hypogonadism that is associated with problems in the ability to discriminate odors, either incompletely (*hyposmia*) or completely (*anosmia*). This syndrome results from a defect in the migration of the GnRH neurons from the olfactory placode into the hypothalamus. Therefore, it represents a GnRH deficiency. Patients remain prepubertal, with small, rubbery testes, and they develop eunuchoidism (E-Fig. 65-1).

Hyperprolactinemia may result in hypogonadotropic hypogonadism because prolactin elevation inhibits normal release of GnRH, decreases the effectiveness of LH at the Leydig cell level, and also inhibits some of the actions of testosterone at the level of the target organ. Normalization of prolactin levels through withdrawal of an offending drug, by surgical removal of the pituitary adenoma, or with the use of dopamine agonists reverses this form of hypogonadism.

Weight loss or systemic illness in male patients can cause another form of secondary hypogonadism, *hypothalamic dysfunction*. Weight loss or illness induces a defect in the hypothalamic release of GnRH and results in low levels of gonadotropin and testosterone. This condition is commonly observed in patients with cancer, AIDS, or chronic inflammatory processes.

Primary Gonadal Abnormalities

The most common congenital cause of primary testicular failure is *Klinefelter's syndrome*, which occurs in about 1 of every 600 live male births and is usually caused by a maternal meiotic chromosomal nondisjunction that results in an XXY genotype. At puberty, clinical findings include the following: a variable degree of hypogonadism; gynecomastia; small, firm testes measuring less than 2 cm in the longest axis (normal testes, 3.5 cm or greater); azoospermia; eunuchoid skeletal proportions; and elevations of FSH and LH (E-Fig. 65-2). Primary gonadal failure is also found in patients with another congenital condition, *myotonic dystrophy*, which is characterized by progressive weakness; atrophy of the facial, neck, hand, and lower extremity muscles; frontal baldness; and myotonia.

About 3% of full-term male infants have *cryptorchidism*, which spontaneously corrects during the first year of life in most cases; consequently, by 1 year of age, the incidence of this condition is about 0.75%. When the testes are maintained in the intra-abdominal position, the increased temperature leads to defective spermatogenesis and oligospermia. Leydig cell function usually remains normal, resulting in normal levels of adult testosterone.

Bilateral anorchia, also known as the vanishing testicle syndrome, is a rare condition in which the external genitalia are fully formed, indicating that ample quantities of testosterone and DHT were produced during early embryogenesis. However, the testicular tissue disappears before or shortly after birth, and the result is an empty scrotum. This condition is differentiated from cryptorchidism by an HCG stimulation test. Patients with cryptorchidism have an increase in serum testosterone level after an injection of HCG, whereas patients with bilateral anorchia do not.

Acquired gonadal failure has numerous causes. The adult seminiferous tubules are susceptible to a variety of injuries, and seminiferous tubular failure is found after infections such as mumps, gonococcal or lepromatous orchitis, irradiation, vascular injury, trauma, alcohol ingestion, and use of chemotherapeutic drugs, especially alkylating agents. The serum FSH concentration may be normal or elevated, depending on the degree of damage to the seminiferous tubules. The Leydig cell compartment may also be damaged by these same conditions. In addition, some men experience a gradual decline in testicular function as they age, possibly because of microvascular insufficiency. Patients with decreased testosterone production may clinically exhibit lowered libido and potency, emotional lability, fatigue, and vasomotor symptoms such as hot flushes. The serum LH concentration is usually elevated in this situation.

Defects in Androgen Action

When either testosterone or its metabolite, DHT, binds to the androgen receptor in target cells, the receptor is activated and binds DNA; the resulting stimulation of transcription, protein synthesis, and cell growth collectively constitutes androgen

TABLE 65-1	CLASSIFICATION OF MALE HYPOGONADISM

HYPOTHALAMIC-PITUITARY DISORDERS (SECONDARY HYPOGONADISM)

Panhypopituitarism
Isolated gonadotropin deficiency
Complex congenital syndromes
Hyperprolactinemia
Hypothalamic dysfunction

GONADAL DISORDERS (PRIMARY HYPOGONADISM)

Klinefelter's syndrome and associated chromosomal defects
Myotonic dystrophy
Cryptorchidism
Bilateral anorchia
Seminiferous tubular failure
Adult Leydig cell failure
Androgen biosynthesis enzyme deficiency

DEFECTS IN ANDROGEN ACTION

Testicular feminization (complete androgen insensitivity)
Incomplete androgen insensitivity
5α-Reductase deficiency

action. An absence of androgen receptors causes the syndrome of *testicular feminization*, a form of male pseudohermaphroditism. These genetic males have cryptorchid testes but appear to be phenotypic females. Because androgens are inactive during embryogenesis, the labial-scrotal folds fail to fuse, and a short vagina results. The fallopian tubes, uterus, and upper portion of the vagina are absent because the testes secrete müllerian duct inhibitory factor during early fetal development. At puberty, these patients have breast enlargement because the testes secrete a small amount of estradiol and the peripheral tissues convert testosterone and adrenal androgens to estrogens. Axillary and pubic hair does not grow because androgen action is required for their development. The serum testosterone concentrations are elevated as a result of continuous stimulation by elevated concentrations of LH. LH is high because of the inability of the testosterone to act in a negative feedback fashion at the hypothalamus. Patients may have incomplete forms of androgen insensitivity caused by point mutations affecting the androgen receptor gene, and clinically these patients show varying degrees of male pseudohermaphroditism.

Patients who lack the 5α-reductase enzyme that is required to convert testosterone to DHT are born with a *bifid scrotum*, which reflects abnormal fusion of the labial-scrotal folds, and *hypospadias*, in which the urethral opening is in the perineal area or in the shaft of the penis. At puberty, androgen production is sufficient to partially overcome the defect; the scrotum, phallus, and muscle mass enlarge, and these patients appear to develop into physiologically normal men.

Diagnosis

Figure 65-2 illustrates an algorithm for the laboratory evaluation of hypogonadism in a phenotypic man. Serum concentrations of LH, FSH, and testosterone should be obtained, and a semen analysis should be performed. A low testosterone level with low concentrations of gonadotropins indicates a hypothalamic-pituitary abnormality, which needs to be evaluated with serum prolactin determination and radiographic examination. Elevated concentrations of gonadotropins with a normal or low testosterone level reflect a primary testicular abnormality. If no testes are palpable in the scrotum and careful *milking* of the patient's lower abdomen does not bring retractile testes into the scrotum, an HCG stimulation test should be performed. A rise in serum testosterone concentrations indicates the presence of functional testicular tissue, and a diagnosis of cryptorchidism can be made. Absence of a rise in testosterone suggests bilateral anorchia. Small, firm testes in the scrotum are highly suggestive of

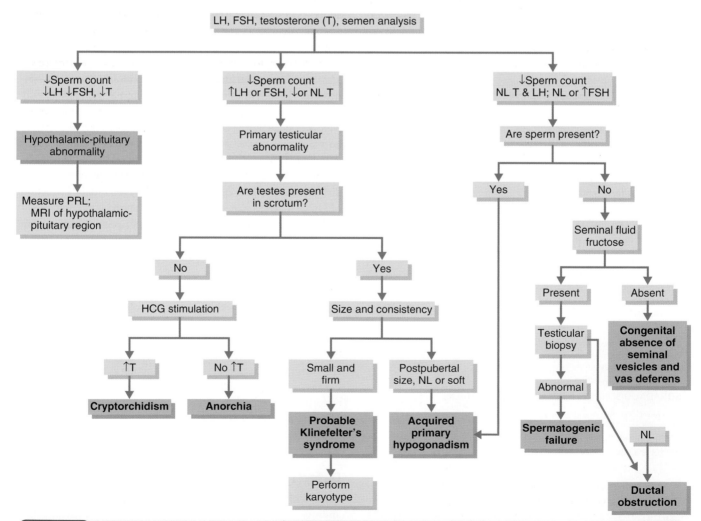

FIGURE 65-2 Laboratory evaluation of hypogonadism. ↑, Elevated; ↓, decreased or low; FSH, follicle-stimulating hormone; HCG, human chorionic gonadotropin; LH, luteinizing hormone; MRI, magnetic resonance imaging; NL, normal; PRL, prolactin.

Klinefelter's syndrome; this diagnosis needs to be confirmed with a chromosomal karyotype. Testes that are more than 3.5 cm in longest diameter and that are either of normal consistency or are soft indicate postpubertal acquired primary hypogonadism.

If the major abnormality is a deficient sperm count with or without an elevation of FSH, differentiation between a ductal problem and acquired primary hypogonadism must be made. If spermatozoa are present, at least the ducts emanating from one testicle are patent; this condition indicates an acquired testicular defect. If the patient has no sperm in the ejaculate, a primary testicular or ductal problem may be responsible. The seminal vesicles secrete fructose into the seminal fluid. Therefore, the presence of fructose in the ejaculate should be followed by a testicular biopsy to determine whether the defect results from spermatogenic failure or from an obstruction of the ducts leading from the testes to the seminal vesicles. Absence of seminal fluid fructose indicates a congenital absence of the seminal vesicles and vas deferens.

Male Infertility

Infertility affects about 15% of couples, and male factors appear to be responsible in about 40% of cases. Female factors account for another 40%, and a couple factor is present in about 20% of cases. In addition to the defects in spermatogenesis that occur in patients with hypothalamic, pituitary, testicular, or androgen action disorders, hyperthyroidism, hypothyroidism, adrenal abnormalities, and systemic illnesses can result in defective spermatogenesis, as can microdeletions of genetic material on the Y chromosome. Disorders of the vas deferens, seminal vesicles, and prostate may also lead to infertility, as may diseases affecting the bladder sphincter that result in *retrograde ejaculation*, in which the sperm passes into the bladder rather than through the penis. Anatomic defects of the penis (as observed in patients with hypospadias), poor coital technique, and the presence of antisperm antibodies in the male or female genital tract also are associated with infertility.

Therapy for Hypogonadism and Infertility

Treatment of androgen deficiency in patients who have hypothalamic-pituitary or primary testicular abnormalities is best accomplished with exogenous testosterone administration—either intramuscular injection of intermediate-acting testosterone esters or transdermal testosterone patches or gel. Testosterone therapy increases libido, potency, muscle mass, strength, athletic endurance, and hair growth on the face and body. Side effects include acne, fluid retention, erythrocytosis, benign prostate hyperplasia, and, rarely, sleep apnea. This therapy is contraindicated in patients with cancer of the prostate.

If fertility is desired, patients with hypothalamic abnormalities may develop virilization and spermatogenesis with the use of GnRH delivered in a pulsatile fashion subcutaneously by an external pump. Direct stimulation of the testes in patients with hypothalamic or pituitary abnormalities may be accomplished with the use of exogenous gonadotropins, which increase testosterone and sperm production. If primary testicular failure is present and the patient has oligospermia, an attempt can be made to concentrate the sperm for intrauterine insemination or in vitro fertilization. If the azoospermia is caused by ductal obstruction,

repair of the obstruction may be undertaken or aspiration of sperm from the epididymis may be accomplished for in vitro fertilization.

GYNECOMASTIA

Gynecomastia refers to a benign enlargement of the male breast that results from proliferation of the glandular component. This common condition is found in as many as 70% of pubertal boys and in about one third of adults 50 to 80 years old. Estrogens stimulate and androgens inhibit breast glandular development; gynecomastia results from an imbalance between estrogen and androgen actions at the breast tissue level. This condition may result from an absolute increase in free estrogens, a decrease in endogenous free androgens, androgen insensitivity of the tissues, or enhanced sensitivity of the breast tissue to estrogens. Table 65-2 lists the common conditions associated with gynecomastia.

Gynecomastia must be differentiated from fatty enlargement of the breasts without glandular proliferation and from other disorders of the breasts, especially breast carcinoma. *Male breast cancer* usually manifests as a unilateral, eccentric, hard or firm mass that is fixed to the underlying tissues. It may be associated with skin dimpling or retraction or with crusting of the nipple or nipple discharge. In contrast, gynecomastia occurs concentrically around the nipple and is not fixed to the underlying structures. Although physical examination is usually sufficient to differentiate gynecomastia from breast carcinoma, mammography may be required.

Painful and tender gynecomastia in a pubertal adolescent should be monitored with periodic examinations because, in most patients, pubertal gynecomastia disappears within 1 year. Incidentally discovered, asymptomatic gynecomastia in an adult requires a careful assessment for alcohol, drug, or medication

TABLE 65-2	CONDITIONS ASSOCIATED WITH GYNECOMASTIA

PHYSIOLOGIC CONDITIONS

Neonatal
Pubertal
Involutional

PATHOLOGIC CONDITIONS

Neoplasms
   Testicular
   Adrenal
   Ectopic production of human chorionic gonadotropin
Primary gonadal failure
Secondary hypogonadism
Enzyme defects in testosterone production
Androgen insensitivity syndromes
Liver disease
Malnutrition with refeeding
Dialysis
Hyperthyroidism
Excessive extraglandular aromatase activity
Drugs
   Estrogens and estrogen agonists
   Gonadotropins
   Antiandrogens or inhibitors of androgen synthesis
   Cytotoxic agents
   Efavirenz
Alcohol
Human immunodeficiency virus infection
Idiopathic

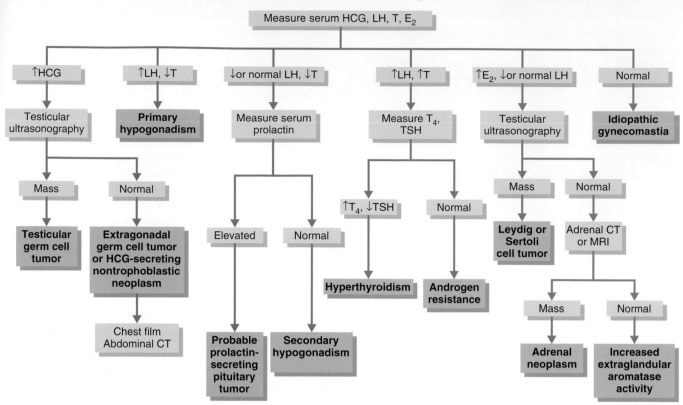

FIGURE 65-3 Diagnostic evaluation for causes of gynecomastia based on measurements of serum human chorionic gonadotropin (HCG), luteinizing hormone (LH), testosterone (T), and estradiol (E_2). ↑, Increased; ↓, decreased; CT, computed tomography; MRI, magnetic resonance imaging; T_4, thyroxine; TSH, thyroid-stimulating hormone. (From Braunstein GD: Gynecomastia, N Engl J Med 328:490–495, 1993.)

use; liver, lung, or kidney dysfunction; and signs and symptoms of hypogonadism or hyperthyroidism. If these conditions are not present, only follow-up is required. In contrast, in an adult with recent onset of progressive painful gynecomastia, thyroid, liver, and renal function should be determined. If test results are normal, serum concentrations of HCG, LH, testosterone, and estradiol should be measured. Further evaluation should be carried out according to the schema outlined in Figure 65-3.

Removal of the offending drug or correction of the underlying condition causing the gynecomastia may result in regression of the breast glandular tissue. If the gynecomastia persists, a trial of antiestrogens (e.g., tamoxifen) may be given for 3 months to see whether regression occurs. Gynecomastia that has been present for longer than 1 year usually contains a fibrotic component that does not respond to medications. In these cases, correction usually requires surgical removal of the tissue.

For a deeper discussion on this topic, please see Chapter 236, "Reproductive Endocrinology and Infertility," in Goldman-Cecil Medicine, 25th Edition.

SUGGESTED READINGS

Bhasin S, Basaria S: Diagnosis and treatment of hypogonadism in men, Best Pract Res Clin Endocrinol Metab 25:251–270, 2011.

Dickson G: Gynecomastia, Am Fam Physician 88:716–722, 2012.

Mathers MJ, Sperling H, Rubben H, et al: The undescended testis: diagnosis, treatment and long-term consequences, Dtsch Arztebl Int 106:527–532, 2009.

Palermo GD, Neri QV, Monahan D, et al: Development and current applications of assisted fertilization, Fertil Steril 97:248–260, 2012.

Shamlaul R, Ghanem H: Erectile dysfunction, Lancet 381:153–165, 2013.

Stahl PJ, Stember DS, Goldstein M: Contemporary management of male infertility, Annu Rev Med 63:525–540, 2012.

Wikstrom AM, Dunkel L: Klinefelter syndrome, Best Pract Res Clin Endocrinol Metab 25:239–250, 2011.

Diabetes Mellitus, Hypoglycemia

Robert J. Smith

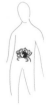

DIABETES MELLITUS

Definition and Diagnostic Criteria

Diabetes mellitus is not a single disease but a group of disorders that develop as a consequence of absolute or relative deficiency of the hormone insulin. Inadequate actions of insulin in stimulating the uptake of glucose by body tissues and regulating the metabolism of carbohydrate, fat, and protein result in *hyperglycemia*. Other metabolic disturbances in addition to hyperglycemia typically occur in uncontrolled diabetes, including altered lipoprotein dynamics and elevated free fatty acid levels. These abnormalities contribute to the acute and chronic clinical consequences of diabetes.

The criteria used to diagnose diabetes mellitus in nonpregnant individuals are summarized in Table 66-1. The diagnosis can be made on the basis of a fasting blood glucose level of 126 mg/dL or higher, a random blood glucose concentration (i.e., determined at any time in association with meals or fasting) of 200 mg/dL or higher, or a 2-hour glucose level of 200 mg/dL or higher as part of a 75-g oral glucose tolerance test. Alternatively, diabetes can be diagnosed if the hemoglobin A_{1c} (HbA_{1c}) level is 6.5% or higher. HbA_{1c}, a measure of the percentage of hemoglobin in circulating erythrocytes that is glycosylated, correlates with mean circulating glucose levels. HbA_{1c} provides an index of the average blood glucose level over the preceding 2 to 3 months. Because HbA_{1c} accumulates progressively throughout the lifespan of an erythrocyte, spurious values may occur in states of altered erythrocyte turnover (e.g., with various anemias) or with certain hemoglobinopathies that increase or decrease the susceptibility of hemoglobin to glycosylation. In patients with marked elevations in blood glucose or HbA_{1c} and coincident symptoms typical for hyperglycemia (e.g., polyuria and polydipsia), the

diagnosis can be made based on a single test result. With less marked glucose elevations in the absence of symptoms, the diagnosis should be confirmed by repeat testing on a separate day.

Patients who have mild elevations in plasma glucose levels that do not reach the threshold for diagnosis of diabetes (e.g., HbA_{1c} levels between 5.7% and 6.4%) are at increased risk for progression to diabetes and therefore are considered to have *prediabetes*. Prediabetes patients with fasting blood glucose levels between 100 and 125 mg/dL are more specifically labeled as having *impaired fasting glucose*, and those with 2-hour postprandial plasma glucose levels between 140 and 199 mg/dL (most reliably measured after a standardized 75-g oral glucose load) have *impaired glucose tolerance* (see Table 66-1). Although not all individuals with prediabetes will become diabetic, the mean progression rate to overt diabetes is approximately 6% per year. There also is evidence from observational studies that the prediabetic state is associated with an increased risk of cardiovascular disease.

Gestational diabetes mellitus (GDM) is a term applied to diabetes first recognized during pregnancy. The most widely accepted thresholds for diagnosis of GDM are a fasting plasma glucose level of 92 mg/dL or higher at any gestational stage and values on a 75-g oral glucose tolerance test at 24 to 28 weeks' gestation of 92 mg/dL or higher fasting, 180 mg/dL or higher at 1 hour, or 153 mg/dL or higher at 2 hours after glucose loading (Table 66-2). Untreated diabetes in pregnancy is associated with increased fetal malformations, problems in delivery, and possibly more frequent diabetes complications in the mother.

Etiologic Classification

Once the diagnosis is made based on elevated blood glucose or HbA_{1c} values, it is important to establish the specific subtype of diabetes based on a combination of clinical and molecular pathophysiologic features Table 66-3.

TABLE 66-1 CRITERIA FOR THE DIAGNOSIS OF DIABETES MELLITUS

MEASUREMENT	NORMAL	PREDIABETES	DIABETES MELLITUS
Plasma glucose (mg/dL)			
Fasting*	<100	100-125[†]	≥126
2-hr Postload[‡]	<140	140-199[§]	≥200
Random[‖]			≥200
Hemoglobin A_{1c} (%)	≤5.6	5.7-6.4	≥6.5

Data from the American Diabetes Association clinical practice recommendations 2013, Diabetes Care 36(Suppl 1):S11–S66, 2013.
*Fasting: no caloric intake for ≥8 hr.
[†]Impaired fasting glucose.
[‡]Postload: Following a standardized 75-g oral glucose load or after a meal.
[§]Impaired glucose tolerance.
[‖]Random: any time of day, unrelated to meals.

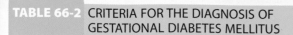

TABLE 66-2 CRITERIA FOR THE DIAGNOSIS OF GESTATIONAL DIABETES MELLITUS

MEASUREMENT	DIAGNOSTIC THRESHOLD (mg/dL)
Plasma glucose	
Fasting*	≥92
After 75-g oral glucose load	
1 hr	≥180
2 hr	<153

Data from the American Diabetes Association clinical practice recommendations 2013, Diabetes Care 36(Suppl 1):S11–S66, 2013.
　*Fasting: no caloric intake for ≥8 hr.

TABLE 66-3 ETIOLOGIC CLASSIFICATION OF DIABETES MELLITUS

TYPE 1 DIABETES MELLITUS

Immune-mediated (type 1a)
Idiopathic (type 1b)

TYPE 2 DIABETES MELLITUS

OTHER SPECIFIC TYPES

Genetic defects of beta-cell function
　Maturity-onset diabetes of the young (MODY) and other disorders
Genetic defects in insulin action
　Insulin receptor mutations and other disorders
Diseases of the exocrine pancreas
Endocrinopathies
　Cushing's syndrome, acromegaly, and other disorders
Drug- or chemical-induced
　Glucocorticoids most common
Infections
Uncommon forms of immune-mediated diabetes
　Insulin receptor–blocking antibodies and other disorders
Other genetic syndromes sometimes associated with diabetes

GESTATIONAL DIABETES MELLITUS

Data from the American Diabetes Association clinical practice recommendations 2013, Diabetes Care 36(Suppl 1):S67–S74, 2013.

Type 1 diabetes (T1DM) is characterized by extensive destruction of the insulin-producing beta cells within the islets of Langerhans in the pancreas and dependence on insulin therapy for survival. In previous medical literature, the terms *juvenile-onset diabetes* or *insulin-dependent diabetes* were used for T1DM. This terminology is no longer used, because T1DM not uncommonly has its onset in adulthood, and multiple other forms of diabetes often require treatment with insulin. T1DM accounts for 5% to 10% of all diabetes in the United States. In most patients, it involves autoimmune mechanisms leading to beta cell destruction (the *type 1A* form). Rare individuals have no markers for autoimmunity and are classified as having *type 1B (idiopathic) diabetes*. Most patients with T1DM progress to marked insulin deficiency over a period of several weeks to months after initial presentation. A smaller number of individuals with evidence of beta cell autoimmunity but much slower disease progression have a variant form of T1DM that is designated *latent autoimmune diabetes of adulthood* (LADA).

In patients with marked elevations in glucose and accompanying ketoacidosis, particularly if they are young and nonobese, the diagnosis of T1DM is highly probable. This can be confirmed by measuring autoantibodies, often as a panel including insulin, anti-IA2 (anti–tyrosine phosphatase), anti-insulin, and glutamic acid decarboxylase (GAD or GAD65) antibodies, and also by a clinical course demonstrating an ongoing need for insulin to control hyperglycemia. A fasting C-peptide level can be measured later in the disease to confirm marked deficiency in insulin secretion. C-peptide is a fragment of the insulin precursor proinsulin, which is cleaved during the synthesis of insulin. It is secreted and circulates in proportion to endogenous insulin production but is absent from injected exogenous insulin preparations.

Type 2 diabetes (T2DM) is a heterogeneous, clinically defined subtype that accounts for more than 90% of all diabetes in the United States. It typically has a gradual onset with progression over multiple years or even decades. There is often prolonged preservation of at least partial insulin secretory capacity together with evidence of insulin resistance. Most patients have associated obesity (80% to 90%), although a subset of patients with a clinical picture otherwise typical for T2DM are nonobese. T2DM usually can be presumptively distinguished from T1DM by its indolent course in the presence of risk factors such as obesity and by the milder hyperglycemia and absence of ketoacidosis due to residual insulin secretion. If there is clinical suspicion of T1DM based on earlier age at onset, degree of hyperglycemia, absence of obesity, or presence of ketoacidosis, an autoantibody panel (which should be negative) and a C-peptide level (which should be positive) can be measured.

An expanding number of diabetes etiologies distinct from T1DM and T2DM are classified under a broad category designated *other specific types*. Although these forms of diabetes are uncommon (1% to 2% of all diabetes), it is important to recognize them in clinical practice. They include a group of inherited, autosomal dominant disorders historically designated *maturity-onset diabetes of the young (MODY)*; many of these patients have clinical features similar to those of T2DM but onset typically before 25 years of age. Patients with MODY3 (hepatocyte nuclear factor-1alpha mutations) are particularly sensitive to sulfonylureas, whereas those with MODY2 (glucokinase mutations) have mild, nonprogressive blood glucose elevations and often require no treatment except during pregnancy. For this reason, patients with early-onset diabetes, lack of autoimmune markers, and family histories suggestive of autosomal dominant inheritance should be considered for MODY gene sequencing.

Much less common genetic defects include mutations in insulin receptors or various other genes involved in insulin action. Exocrine pancreatic disease from causes such as chronic pancreatitis or surgery results in loss of the glucagon-producing islet alpha-cells as well as the insulin-producing beta cells. These patients often exhibit greater sensitivity to insulin and more of a propensity for hypoglycemia than T1DM patients because of the absent insulin counter-regulatory effects of glucagon. Endocrine disorders with excess production of hormones that counteract insulin, such as growth hormone in acromegaly or glucocorticoids in Cushing's syndrome, are important to recognize as causes of diabetes because removal of the source of excess hormone can lead to resolution of the diabetic state. Many drugs have been associated with diabetes, most notably glucocorticoids.

The category GDM includes any woman in whom diabetes is first recognized during pregnancy and usually represents T2DM.

Type 1 Diabetes

Epidemiology and Pathology

The principal features of T1DM, contrasted with T2DM, are summarized in Table 66-4. The peak incidence occurs between the ages of 6 and 14 years, but onset in approximately half of patients with T1DM occurs after the age of 20. The role of genetic factors in T1DM risk is supported by an observed increased incidence of T1DM among family members of affected patients: approximately 5% in siblings, 6% in offspring of a diabetic father, and 2% in offspring of a diabetic mother. On a background of genetic risk factors, it is hypothesized that the immune destruction of beta cells is precipitated by environmental factors that still are not well understood but may include microbial, chemical, or dietary triggers (Fig. 66-1). The operation of a combination of genetic and environmental factors is thought to explain the high but not absolute concordance observed in monozygotic twins (30% to 50%).

The prevalence of T1DM varies substantially in different populations; for example, it is relatively high in northwestern Europe and much lower in parts of Asia. The overall prevalence in the United States is approximately 2.4 cases per 1000 population. The frequent onset before age 20 makes T1DM one of the most common chronic, serious childhood diseases. It is the most common subtype of diabetes in childhood, accounting for approximately 70% of all cases, with T2DM accounting for most of the remainder. LADA, a variant form of autoimmune T1DM, is characterized by onset in adulthood and a more prolonged waxing and waning course than is typical for T1DM.

The onset of overt T1DM follows a preclinical phase of variable duration (typically extending from months to years) during which there is specific destruction of beta cells resulting predominantly from cell-mediated immune mechanisms (mononuclear cells; mainly CD8+ T lymphocytes). It is believed that the autoantibodies (to islet cells, insulin, GAD, and tyrosine phosphatases) are generated for the most part in response to exposure of beta cells and islets and are not themselves mediators of the destructive process. Demonstration of one or more autoantibodies also represents the most sensitive and useful way to establish preclinical disease in patients at risk (e.g., first-degree relatives of patients with T1DM).

The complement of islets in a healthy individual normally provides enough excess beta cell secretory capacity to maintain blood glucose levels until 80% to 90% of beta cells have been lost. In some patients, the subclinical loss of beta cells may be unmasked, resulting in hyperglycemia during the course of an intercurrent illness such as an incidental upper respiratory tract infection. Hyperglycemia and even ketogenesis can result from a lack of adequate insulin, decreased glucose excretion due to hypovolemia, accelerated gluconeogenesis, increased insulin resistance, and hepatic ketogenesis. After diagnosis and institution of insulin and other therapy, stress-induced insulin resistance resolves, and there may be some degree of recovery of beta cell function. Some patients revert to a state in which no insulin is required. This phenomenon, designated the *honeymoon* period, lasts for several weeks to as long as 1 year. Patients generally should continue insulin administration at doses low enough to be tolerated during this interval, because progressive beta cell function can be expected eventually to result in recurrent hyperglycemia and, potentially, diabetic ketoacidosis (DKA).

Screening for T1DM is not a part of standard medical care. Screening for autoantibody determinations in individuals at risk is not clinically useful.

Clinical Presentation

T1DM most often manifests clinically with symptoms resulting from hyperglycemia and consequent osmotic diuresis. Patients typically have a history extending over days to weeks of worsening polyuria, plus polydipsia (as a compensatory response to

TABLE 66-4 GENERAL COMPARISON OF THE TWO MOST COMMON TYPES OF DIABETES MELLITUS

	TYPE 1	TYPE 2
Previous terminology	Insulin-dependent diabetes mellitus, type I; juvenile-onset diabetes	Non–insulin-dependent diabetes mellitus, type II; adult-onset diabetes
Age at onset	Usually <30 yr, particularly childhood and adolescence, but any age	Usually >40 yr, but increasingly at younger ages
Genetic predisposition	Moderate; environmental factors required for expression; 35-50% concordance in monozygotic twins; multiple candidate genes proposed	Strong; 60-90% concordance in monozygotic twins; many candidate genes proposed
Human leukocyte antigen associations	Linkage to DQA and DQB, influenced by DRB3 and DRB4 (DR2 protective)	None known
Other associations	Autoimmune; Graves' disease, Hashimoto's thyroiditis, vitiligo, Addison's disease, pernicious anemia	Heterogeneous group, ongoing subclassification based on identification of specific pathogenic processes and genetic defects
Precipitating and risk factors	Largely unknown; microbial, chemical, dietary, other	Age, obesity (central), sedentary lifestyle, previous gestational diabetes
Findings at diagnosis	85-90% of patients have one and usually more autoantibodies to ICA512, IA-2, IA-2β, GAD$_{65}$, IAA	Possibly complications (microvascular and macrovascular) caused by significant hyperglycemia in the preceding asymptomatic period
Endogenous insulin levels	Low or absent	Usually present (relative deficiency), early hyperinsulinemia
Insulin resistance	Only with hyperglycemia	Mostly present
Prolonged fast	Hyperglycemia, ketoacidosis	Euglycemia
Stress, withdrawal of insulin	Ketoacidosis	Nonketotic hyperglycemia, occasionally ketoacidosis

GAD, Glutamic acid decarboxylase; IA-2, IA-2β, insuloma-associated protein 2 and 2β (tyrosine phosphatases); IAA, insulin autoantibodies; ICA, islet cell antibody; ICA512, islet cell autoantigen 512 (fragment of IA-2).

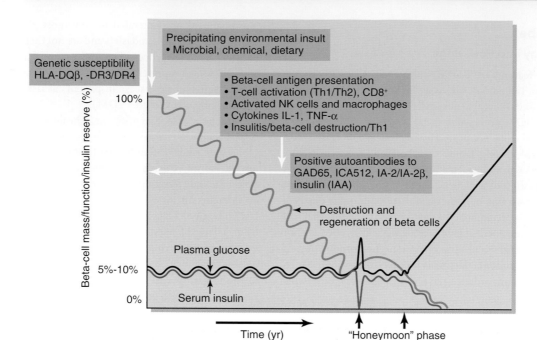

FIGURE 66-1 Natural history of type 1 diabetes mellitus. The honeymoon period with temporary improvement in beta-cell function occurs with the initiation of insulin therapy at the time of clinical diagnosis. GAD, Glutamic acid decarboxylase; HLA, human leukocyte antigen; IA-2, IA-2β, tyrosine phosphatases; ICA, islet cell antibody; ICA512, islet cell autoantigen 512 (fragment of IA-2); IL-1, interleukin-1; NK, natural killer; Th1, subset of CD4+ helper T cells responsible for cell-mediated immunity; Th2, subset of CD4+ helper T cells responsible for humoral immunity; TNF-α, tumor necrosis factor-α.

hypovolemia and increased serum osmolality). The polyuria may be evident as bed wetting or daytime incontinence in children and as nocturia in adults. There typically also is weight loss, and patients often describe low energy and lethargy. Approximately 25% of patients with T1DM have progressed to DKA by the time of clinical presentation.

Treatment

The management of T1DM involves immediate treatment at the outset to correct hyperglycemia, fluid deficits, and DKA, if present, plus attention to possible precipitating or complicating factors such as infection. The initial treatment of T1DM should be coupled with education of patients and their family members (appropriate to the patient's age) concerning the needed skills to manage insulin administration, blood glucose testing, nutrition, and exercise. This often is best accomplished by a team involving the physician, educators (typically specially trained nurses or pharmacists), and a dietician. Medical advice, patient education, and psychological support should be provided on an ongoing, long-term, individualized basis. The primary goal of glucose management is to minimize the degree of hyperglycemia, and its attendant risks of long-term complications of diabetes, while avoiding the acute and chronic risks of hypoglycemia. Medical care also should include attention to control of lipid levels, blood pressure, and other factors that affect the risks of long-term diabetes complications. Routine assessments of foot care, peripheral nerve function, retinal status, and renal function should be used to detect incipient diabetes complications and enable early treatment interventions. Other sources should be consulted for

information on specific issues related to T1DM management in children and adolescents.

Blood Glucose Control

Patients with T1DM have an absolute requirement for exogenous insulin. The Diabetes Control and Complications Trial (DCCT) and other studies have established that improved glycemic control in patients with T1DM decreases long-term microvascular complications (retinopathy, nephropathy, and neuropathy). A follow-up study of the same patients (the Epidemiology of Diabetes Interventions and Complications [EDIC] study) further demonstrated lower cardiovascular morbidity and mortality with intensive insulin management. Based on these and other studies, the most generally accepted target goal for HbA$_{1c}$ in T1DM is 7.0%. For patients who have difficulty sensing hypoglycemia or who have other factors complicating blood glucose management (e.g., renal failure), it is appropriate to set an individualized HbA$_{1c}$ goal of 8.0% or even higher.

Many preparations of insulin are available. They differ in rapidity of onset, degree of peaking of blood levels, and duration of action after subcutaneous injection (Table 66-5). The different kinetics of recombinant human insulin preparations derive from their specific complexing with proteins and zinc. Additionally, multiple analogues of human insulin are available that have rapid or slow kinetics as a consequence of altered solubility at subcutaneous injection sites. Most insulin preparations are provided at a concentration of 100 U/mL (U-100). Self-monitoring of blood glucose (SMBG) by patients using glucose meters is critical to the implementation of an effective insulin regimen. Ideally,

TABLE 66-5	TYPES OF INSULIN*						
INSULIN TYPE	**GENERIC NAME**	**PREPRANDIAL INJECTION TIMING (HR)**	**ONSET (HR)**	**PEAK (HR)**	**DURATION (HR)**	**BG NADIR (HR)**
Rapid-acting	Lispro†	0-0.2	0.1-0.5	0.5-2	<5	2-4
	Aspart‡	0-0.2	0.1-0.3	0.6-3	3-5	1-3
	Glulisine§	0-0.25 (15 min before a meal or within 20 min after starting a meal)	0.15-0.3	0.5-1.5	1-5.3	2-4
Short-acting	Regular	0.5-1	0.3-1	2-6	4-8	3-7
Intermediate-acting	NPH	0.5-1	1-3	6-15	16-26	6-13
Long-acting	Glargine‖**	Once daily§ or twice daily (approx 12 hourly)	1.1-4	Little or no peak	10.8->24	Before next dose
	Detemir**	Once daily§ or twice daily (approx 12 hourly)	1.1-4	Little or no peak	12-24	Before next dose
HUMAN PREMIXED						
NPH/regular	70/30	0.5-1	0.5-1	2-12	14-24	3-12
NPH/regular	50/50	0.5-1	0.5-1	2-5	14-24	3-12
INSULIN ANALOGUE PREMIXED						
NPL/lispro	75/25	0.25	0.15-0.25	1	14-24	—
NPA/aspart	70/30	0.25	0.15-0.3	2-4	24	—
NPL/lispro	50/50	0.25	0.15-0.25	1	14-24	—

BG, Blood glucose; NPA, neutral protamine aspart; NPH, neutral protamine Hagedorn; NPL, neutral protamine lispro.

*Time profiles depend on several factors, including dose, anatomic site of injection, method (profiles in this table are for subcutaneous injections), duration of diabetes, type of diabetes, degree of insulin resistance, level of physical activity, presence of obesity, and body temperature. Some time ranges are wide to include data from several separate studies. Preprandial injection timing depends on premeal BG values and insulin type. If BG is low, it may be necessary to inject insulin and eat immediately (carbohydrate portion of meal first). If BG is high, it may be necessary to delay the meal after insulin injection and the eat the carbohydrate portion last.

†Insulin analogue with reversal of lysine and proline at positions 28 and 29 on the B chain of the insulin molecule.

‡Insulin analogue with substitution of aspartic acid for proline at position 28 on the B chain of the insulin molecule.

§Insulin analogue with substitution of lysine for asparagine at position 3 on the B chain and glutamic acid for lysine at position 29 on the B chain of the insulin molecule.

‖Insulin analogue with substitution of glycine for asparagine at position 21 on the A chain and addition of two arginines to the carboxyl terminus of the B chain of the insulin molecule.

§Administer at same time each day, unrelated to meals. Morning administration may result in greater glucose lowering and less nocturnal hypoglycemia.

**Do not mix glargine or detemir with other insulins.

SMBG should be performed as frequently as practicable: fasting, preprandial, 2 hours postprandial, at bedtime, and occasionally at 2:00 to 3:00 AM. Values and times are saved in most meters for subsequent review. It is helpful for patients to manually record these data on a flow chart, and it is also possible to download meter data to a computer. SMBG records are most useful when annotated with relevant details on food intake, exercise, or the occurrence of symptoms. HbA₁c determinations should be obtained every 3 months.

Most cases of T1DM should be managed with an *intensive insulin therapy regimen* involving multiple (three or more) daily subcutaneous injections or continuous subcutaneous insulin infusion (CSII) using an insulin pump. Multiple-injection regimens, also termed *basal-bolus therapy,* typically involve injections of a long-acting insulin analogue (such as glargine or detemir) once or twice daily to establish a stable basal insulin level. Regular insulin or a rapid-acting insulin analogue is additionally injected three or more times daily (before each meal and sometimes before snacks) to provide appropriate post-meal peaks in insulin levels. Usually, once glucose levels are stabilized on a regimen, the doses of long-acting insulin are kept constant from day to day. The rapid-acting insulin doses can be kept constant with efforts to ingest a fixed amount of carbohydrate and total calories at each meal. Alternatively, better control and greater flexibility can be achieved if rapid-acting insulin doses are adjusted according to the blood glucose level (measured before each meal) and the carbohydrate calories ingested with the meal. The long-acting insulin glargine and detemir analogues cannot be mixed in a single syringe with other insulins; for

this reason, basal-bolus regimens often require four or more daily injections.

For patients newly diagnosed with T1DM, a typical starting dose of insulin is a total of 0.2 to 0.4 U/kg/day, with the expectation that this will be increased to 0.6 to 0.7 U/kg/day over time. Approximately half of the total dose should be given as basal insulin. Depending on individual patient blood glucose responses, the basal glargine or detemir insulin may be administered as a single daily dose (in the morning or at bedtime), or two equally divided doses may be required. For a neutral protamine Hagedorn (NPH) basal regimen, two thirds of the dose should be given in the morning and one third at bedtime. This decreases the risk of nocturnal hypoglycemia and times the maximum NPH peak to approximately match the midday meal. The rapid-acting component of the daily insulin dose is distributed before meals according to meal size and content.

An insulin pump (CSII) represents the preferred method of insulin administration for many T1DM patients. These small, wearable devices contain a reservoir of rapid-acting insulin that is infused via an easily placed subcutaneous catheter. A microprocessor-controlled pump provides the basal insulin infusion and can be programmed to adjust basal rates at multiple points during the day according to predetermined patient needs. The patient further instructs the pump to make bolus insulin injections to cover meals, snacks, or needed corrections in hyperglycemia. Controlled studies have shown that modestly better blood glucose control can be achieved with CSII, compared to basal-bolus regimens with multiple daily injections. When used appropriately, CSII represents the most flexible means of managing insulin doses, with options for dose adjustments and supplementation that do not require separate injections. Limitations include need for greater patient involvement, lack of a long-acting pool, and pump failure. Newly diagnosed T1DM should be managed for a period of time (at least 6 to 12 months) with intermittently injected insulin before transition to a pump is considered. During the transition from intermittent insulin injections to CSII in a patient with well-controlled blood glucose levels (HbA$_{1c}$ ≤7.0%), the total daily insulin dose typically is decreased by 10% to 20% initially.

Many CSII patients require a slightly higher basal infusion rate in the early morning hours to accommodate the *dawn phenomenon*, a period of decreased insulin sensitivity secondary to circadian changes in secretion of insulin counter-regulatory hormones such as growth hormone. Adjustments in the basal rate may also be needed at other times of day because of changes in insulin sensitivity that may occur (e.g., after exercise). Premeal insulin boluses are calculated to include a correction dose if needed, based on the premeal blood glucose level, plus a meal coverage dose calculated from the patient's predetermined individual carbohydrate/insulin ratio. It often is most effective for a patient to be seen in a specialty setting during transition to CSII, so that an experienced educator (often a specially trained RN) can assist with needed patient education. Devices are available that provide continuous glucose monitoring (CGM), either as a separate device or integrated with an insulin pump. Because of concern about their consistent accuracy, insulin infusion rates are not adjusted automatically in response to the measured glucose levels by current devices; rather, patient intervention is required to make changes.

Intensive insulin therapy is not appropriate for all T1DM patients. Some patients are unwilling or unable to manage the required frequent glucose monitoring, diet adherence, and multiple insulin boluses. In other patients, the tight blood glucose control and low HbA$_{1c}$ targets that are the goals of intensive insulin therapy may not be feasible. For example, there may be an increased risk of hypoglycemia because of autonomic neuropathy and inability to sense hypoglycemia, or gastrointestinal neuropathy may cause gastroparesis resulting in unpredictable variations in nutrient digestion and absorption. Under such circumstances, simpler approaches to insulin therapy and blood glucose management, previously termed *conventional insulin therapy*, may be appropriate. Such a regimen may be based, for example, on two injections per day of intermediate-acting insulin with or without short- or rapid-acting insulin. As one example, a *split-mixed regimen* uses NPH/regular or NPH/lispro (or aspart or glulisine) formulations twice daily. Initially, two thirds of the estimated total daily dose is given before breakfast and one third before dinner; at each of these times, two thirds of the insulin is given as NPH and one third as regular or a rapid-acting insulin. The amount of each insulin type at each of the injection times is then adjusted according to measured blood glucose levels, with the expectation that the peak of the morning NPH will cover lunch, the rapid-acting insulins will cover the other meals, and the NPH will otherwise ensure adequate basal blood glucose control. Two daily injections are made possible by mixing the intermediate- and rapid-acting insulins in a single syringe. Premixed insulin

preparations, such as 70% NPH plus 30% rapid-acting insulin or 50% NPH plus 50% regular insulin, also are available for injection with syringes or with preloaded insulin pens. Premixed insulins provide greater ease of use but are less likely to achieve good glycemic control.

Hypoglycemia Management

Irrespective of the specific treatment regimen, patients with T1DM need to learn how to manage hypoglycemia. Patients usually experience adrenergic symptoms (e.g., sweating, anxiety, tremulousness) as blood glucose levels decrease below the normal range (<50 to 70 mg/dL). If glucose levels decrease markedly enough, patients may experience central nervous system (CNS) symptoms ranging from difficulty thinking clearly to confusion, obtundation, and loss of consciousness. If low blood glucose is confirmed (e.g., <70 mg/dL), 10 to 15 g of rapidly absorbed carbohydrate should be ingested. For a glucose level lower than 50 mg/dL, 20 to 30 g of carbohydrate is advisable. This can be provided as orange juice or crackers, or patients can carry glucose tablets or squeeze tubes of glucose solution (obtainable over-the-counter from pharmacies) for use in treating hypoglycemia. The blood glucose level should be retested after 15 minutes, and the treatment should be repeated as needed until hypoglycemia is resolved. An alternative is to inject glucagon. For patients who have a history of hypoglycemia severe enough (including loss of consciousness) to require assistance from others, it often is helpful for a family member to be trained in glucagon injection. With severe hypoglycemia, there is a risk of injury, such as from a fall or automobile accident, as well as neurologic damage if hypoglycemia is sustained.

Nutritional Management

Appropriate nutritional management is an essential component of an effective T1DM treatment program. This ideally should be individualized to the patient's lifestyle, exercise regimen, eating habits, culture, and financial resources. Many expert panel recommendations allow individualized decisions regarding the relative amounts of carbohydrate, fat, and protein consumed within a general set of guidelines. For example, the American Diabetes Association (ADA) recommends the following:

- Fat intake, less than 7% of total calories with minimal amounts of trans-fats
- Total cholesterol intake, less than 200 mg/day
- Dietary protein intake, 15% to 20% of total calories in the absence of renal failure
- Fiber intake, at least 14 g per 1000 total calories
- Reduced sodium intake (1500 mg/day), especially in the context of even mild hypertension.

Patients should work with a medical professional who is trained in diabetes care to establish nutritional goals.

Most diets focus on measuring and controlling the amounts rather than the sources of carbohydrates. Patients can be taught to estimate the grams of carbohydrate in a meal (*carbohydrate counting*) as a means of ensuring that a consistent amount of carbohydrate is ingested. Alternatively, they can use carbohydrate counting with each meal as part of a strategy that enables day-to-day variations in consumption with adjustments of mealtime insulin doses according to a predetermined, patient-specific *insulin/carbohydrate ratio*. It is advisable to avoid foods that contain supplemental fructose as a sweetener because of the potential adverse effects of fructose on lipid metabolism. Alcohol consumption in moderation is acceptable (one drink or less for women and two drinks or less for men per day).

Because of the contribution of excess body weight to increased cardiovascular risk, a fundamental goal of nutritional management should be to maintain normal body weight or to achieve weight reduction in overweight or obese patients. Eating disorders including binge eating, anorexia nervosa, and bulimia are relatively common in T1DM, especially among younger female patients.

Exercise

Regular physical exercise should be encouraged for its beneficial effects on weight control, risks of long-term complications, and overall quality of life. The general recommendation of several expert panels is 30 minutes or more of moderate-intensity physical exercise on at least 5 days per week. Physical exercise burns calories in proportion to its duration and intensity and also may result in increased insulin sensitivity after exercise (sometimes lasting for many hours). It often is most effective for patients to schedule regular exercise periods with a consistent temporal relationship to meals and insulin injections. Blood glucose should be tested before and after exercise, and exercise should not be undertaken if the initial blood glucose level is low (because of increased risk of hypoglycemia) or if it is higher than 250 mg/dL (because of risk of inducing further blood glucose elevation and development of ketosis). Patients with T1DM should be encouraged to pursue age- and overall health-appropriate athletic interests, including competitive sports, but this should be done only with careful attention to blood glucose monitoring and appropriate adjustments in insulin regimen and diet.

Type 2 Diabetes

Epidemiology and Pathology

T2DM is an extraordinarily common disorder, affecting 8% to 10% of the population in the United States and with a similar prevalence in most other developed or developing countries. Many patients with T2DM are undiagnosed, and many additional individuals (approximately 6% of the U.S. population) have a prediabetic state. T2DM is characterized by varying degrees of insulin resistance and insulin deficiency, which are believed to result from the impact of environmental factors on a background of genetic risk. The principal features of T2DM, contrasted with T1DM, are summarized in Table 66-4. The prevalence of T2DM has increased more than 10-fold over the past 50 years, driven primarily by increased calorie intake, decreased exercise, and resulting obesity. More than 80% of patients with T2DM are obese. The peak incidence of T2DM occurs in the fifth and sixth decades; however, T2DM now accounts for up to 30% of childhood diabetes in some populations. The lifetime risk of developing T2DM is approximately 40% among the offspring of a single affected parent, and approximately 70% if both parents are affected. The incidence of T2DM in the United States is higher in Hispanic/Latino populations, among African Americans, and in some east Asian populations, compared to populations of northern and western European ancestry. This is thought to result in part from effects of socioeconomic and cultural factors (e.g., differences in consumption of low-cost, calorie-dense foods) but also from genetic differences among these populations. The genetic predisposition in all populations that have been studied is thought to reflect the combined influence of more than 40 genes. No single gene or small group of genes with dominant influence on diabetes risk in any population has been identified.

T2DM is typically preceded by a prolonged preclinical or prediabetic phase during which there is a gradual deterioration in glucose tolerance (Fig. 66-2). This process occurs over a decade or more on average, with marked individual variation in the rate of progression. Most patients are insulin resistant during the preclinical phase but are able to compensate by producing more insulin (hyperinsulinemia) to maintain euglycemia. With time, there is progressive deterioration in the capacity to compensate for the insulin resistance. This is associated with a decrease in beta cell mass during the preclinical phase of T2DM, but substantial residual beta cells (typically 40% to 50% of the normal complement) are still present at the time that overt hyperglycemia develops. Therefore, there is compromised function as well as a reduced number of beta cells in T2DM. As blood glucose levels rise, the hyperglycemia itself may contribute to progression of the diabetic state by further decreasing insulin secretion and insulin resistance through mechanisms that are not well understood (referred to as *glucotoxicity*).

Screening of certain high-risk populations for T2DM and prediabetes by determination of a fasting or random plasma glucose measurement is considered cost-effective. More than 30% of people with T2DM and an even higher percentage of those with prediabetes are undiagnosed. Expert panel recommendations from the ADA for screening based on age, lifestyle factors, family history, and ethnicity are summarized in Table 66-6. Because of the insidious nature of T2DM, patients have a high risk for development of complications by the time of clinical diagnosis (see later discussion).

Clinical Presentation

Many patients are asymptomatic and are diagnosed on routine blood glucose testing. Blood glucose levels that rise high enough to exceed the renal threshold for glucose reabsorption (>170 mg/dL) induce an osmotic diuresis, resulting in the typical presenting symptoms of polyuria and polydipsia, as well as blurred vision secondary to osmotic shifts in the lens. Patients may also have weight loss or bacterial urinary tract or cutaneous fungal infections at presentation. Osmotic diuresis secondary to hyperglycemia may lead to electrolyte abnormalities and even occasionally to a severe hyperosmolar state associated with clinical symptoms and signs including fatigue, weakness, and ultimately compromised mental status that can range from confusion to coma (see later discussion). This most frequently occurs in elderly patients who may have compromised baseline renal function. In contrast to patients with T1DM, those with T2DM usually have enough

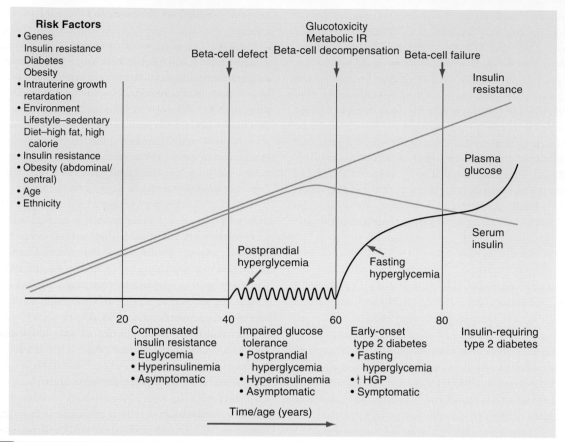

Risk Factors
- Genes
  Insulin resistance
  Diabetes
  Obesity
- Intrauterine growth
  retardation
- Environment
  Lifestyle–sedentary
  Diet–high fat, high
  calorie
- Insulin resistance
- Obesity (abdominal/
  central)
- Age
- Ethnicity

Glucotoxicity
Metabolic IR
Beta-cell defect   Beta-cell decompensation   Beta-cell failure

Insulin
resistance

Plasma
glucose

Serum
insulin

Postprandial
hyperglycemia

Fasting
hyperglycemia

20	40	60	80
Compensated insulin resistance	Impaired glucose tolerance	Early-onset type 2 diabetes	Insulin-requiring type 2 diabetes
• Euglycemia	• Postprandial hyperglycemia	• Fasting hyperglycemia	
• Hyperinsulinemia	• Hyperinsulinemia	• ↑ HGP	
• Asymptomatic	• Asymptomatic	• Symptomatic	

Time/age (years)

FIGURE 66-2 Natural history of type 2 diabetes mellitus. The numbers for time/age markers in years for the different phases of beta-cell decompensation toward overt diabetes and an insulin-requiring state are approximate guides. Certain groups are more insulin sensitive and require a greater loss of beta-cell function to precipitate diabetes, compared with obese insulin-resistant people, who develop diabetes after small declines in beta-cell function. Use of insulin in patients with type 2 diabetes varies considerably and is not age dependent. HGP, Hepatic glucose production; IR, insulin resistance.

residual insulin activity to partially suppress lipolysis, and this protects them from developing DKA. In a subset of T2DM patients, DKA can develop, possibly reflecting individual variations in the degree of suppression of insulin secretion by glucotoxicity.

As a consequence of prolonged exposure to hyperglycemia and associated metabolic disturbances, patients with T2DM may already have developed long-term microvascular or macrovascular complications of diabetes by the time of diagnosis. Therefore, patients may experience a cardiovascular event, such as acute myocardial infarction, and then incidentally be found to have T2DM.

The Metabolic Syndrome

Susceptibility to cardiovascular disease is further increased by the frequent association of insulin resistance, prediabetes, and T2DM with other cardiac risk factors, including abdominal or visceral obesity, dyslipidemia, and hypertension. The term *metabolic syndrome* has been applied to patients who have a combination of these cardiovascular risk factors. Different but overlapping diagnostic criteria for the metabolic syndrome have been proposed by various expert panels. The National Cholesterol Education Program Adult Treatment Panel III (ATP III) defines this syndrome as the presence of any three of the following five characteristics:

1. Fasting blood glucose level ≥100 mg/dL or drug treatment for elevated blood glucose
2. High-density lipoprotein (HDL)-cholesterol <40 mg/dL in men or <50 mg/dL in women or drug treatment for low HDL-cholesterol
3. Plasma triglycerides ≥150 mg/dL or drug treatment for elevated triglycerides
4. Abdominal obesity (waist ≥102 cm in men or ≥88 cm in women
5. Blood pressure ≥130/85 mm Hg or drug treatment for hypertension.

There is debate about whether the metabolic syndrome represents a discrete pathologic entity, but its recognition does draw attention to the frequent clustering of cardiovascular risk factors.

Treatment

Patients with T2DM should receive nutrition counseling starting at the time of diagnosis. This should include efforts at weight loss in overweight or obese patients. Adjustments in diet, especially reductions in calorie intake, can rapidly improve blood glucose levels in many patients independent of other interventions. Weight reduction by as little as 10% to 20% of body weight can have marked beneficial effects on insulin resistance and glycemia in some patients.

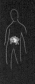

TABLE 66-6 SCREENING CRITERIA FOR DIABETES IN ASYMPTOMATIC ADULTS

1. Testing for diabetes should be considered in all persons ≥45 yr of age; if normal, the test should be repeated at 3-yr intervals.
2. Testing should be considered at a younger age (<30 yr) or performed more frequently in individuals who
   a. Are overweight (BMI ≥25) or who have central obesity with normal BMI (18.5-24.9)
   b. Have an habitually sedentary lifestyle
   c. Have a first-degree relative with diabetes (i.e., parent or sibling)
   d. Are members of a high-risk ethnic population (e.g., African American, Latino/Hispanic American, Native American, Asian American, Pacific Islander)
   e. Have delivered a baby weighing >9 lb (4 kg), have experienced unexplained perinatal death of a child, or have been diagnosed with gestational diabetes
   f. Are hypertensive (≥140/90 mm Hg)
   g. Have an HDL cholesterol level <35 mg/dL (0.9 mmol/L) and/or a triglyceride level >250 mg/dL (2.82 mmol/L)
   h. Had, on previous testing, impaired glucose tolerance (plasma glucose ≥140 mg/dL [7.8 mmol/L] but <200 mg/dL [11.1 mmol/L] 2 hr after 75-g oral glucose tolerance test), impaired fasting glucose (plasma glucose 100-125 mg/dL [5.6-6.9 mmol/L]), or HbA_{1C} ≥5.7%
   i. Have other clinical conditions associated with insulin resistance (e.g., PCOS, acanthosis nigricans)
   j. Have a history of cardiovascular disease

Modified from the American Diabetes Association Clinical Practice Recommendations 2013, Diabetes Care 36(Suppl 1):S11–S66, 2013.

BMI, Body mass index (weight [kg]/height [m²]); HbA_{1C}, glycosylated hemoglobin; HDL, high-density lipoprotein; PCOS, polycystic ovary syndrome; T1DM, type 1 diabetes mellitus; T2DM, type 2 diabetes mellitus.

Depending on initial blood glucose levels, the presence or absence of symptoms related to hyperglycemia, and the presence of other complicating medical conditions, a decision can be made on whether to treat the patient initially with diet alone or to also start medication. Patients with marked hyperglycemia, fluid deficits, altered mental status related to hyperosmolar state, and DKA should be hospitalized for acute treatment (see later discussion).

For most patients, treatment of T2DM can be conducted on an outpatient basis. Useful and frequently updated guidelines are available on line from the ADA and the European Association for the Study of Diabetes. Most expert panels recommend starting with one or two oral glucose-lowering medications (depending on the degree of hyperglycemia) with progression to a third oral agent or insulin if this proves ineffective. In patients with marked hyperglycemia (>300 mg/dL or HbA_{1c} >9.0% to 9.5%), consideration should be given to starting insulin from the outset. There typically is gradually progressive loss of beta cell function in T2DM, extending sometimes over many years, and this results in a need over time for increased doses or additional glucose-lowering agents and often, ultimately, the use of insulin. As for T1DM, the overall management of T2DM should include not only the treatment of hyperglycemia but also interventions that assess, decrease the risks for, and treat long-term microvascular and macrovascular complications.

Blood Glucose Control

The United Kingdom Prevention of Diabetes Study (UKPDS) and other randomized, controlled trials have established that improved blood glucose control lowers the risk of microvascular long-term complications (retinopathy, nephropathy, and neuropathy) in T2DM. The risk appears to increase progressively, starting with any increment above normoglycemia. Randomized clinical trial data have not convincingly demonstrated improved macrovascular (i.e., cardiovascular disease) outcomes in T2DM. HbA_{1c} goals therefore should be developed on an individualized basis, such that the benefits of improving microvascular complications are balanced against the risks of hypoglycemia. T2DM patients, particularly those who are older or have complicating comorbid conditions, may have limited capacity to manage a tight blood glucose control regimen and also increased susceptibility to adverse effects of hypoglycemia. Whereas an HbA_{1c} of 7.0% or less is an appropriate target for younger T2DM patients, 8.0% or less may be an acceptable and safer target for older patients with complicating medical conditions and limited life expectancy. Patients or their caregivers should perform regular glucose monitoring (SMBG) to assess ongoing blood glucose control, identify potential hypoglycemia, and detect marked increases in blood glucose that may occur during an intercurrent illness. HbA_{1c} determinations provide important supplemental information about blood glucose control and should be performed at intervals of 3 to 6 months.

Non-Insulin Pharmacologic (Antidiabetic) Agents in T2DM

Non-insulin pharmacological agents from many different drug classes are available for treatment of T2DM, some taken orally and others by injection (Table 66-7). When non-insulin pharmacologic agents are appropriate, metformin is first-line therapy because of its glucose-lowering efficacy, absence of weight gain and hypoglycemia, favorable safety and tolerability profile based on many years of clinical experience, and low cost. For patients who are unable to tolerate metformin, a sulfonylurea is a reasonable choice, again based on efficacy, tolerability, and low cost. Sulfonylureas have the disadvantages of inducing modest weight gain in many patients, and they carry a risk of causing hypoglycemia. Agents in other drug classes can be considered for first-line therapy, but there is less knowledge or more concern about their long-term safety profiles, and they have higher cost.

If a single drug is tolerated but does not adequately control blood glucose levels, the usual practice is to continue that drug and add a second. Drug combinations often are selected from classes with complementary mechanisms of actions. For example, the combination of an insulin sensitizer such as metformin and an insulin secretagogue such as a sulfonylurea has theoretical appeal in providing greater potential for additive or synergistic actions. Patients with marked hyperglycemia that is not judged severe enough to merit insulin treatment may be started on two agents from the outset. This has the potential advantage of more rapidly achieving blood glucose control but the disadvantage of exposing patients to the potential side effects of taking two drugs simultaneously. Many combination preparations are available for administration of more than one drug; these are more convenient for patients and sometimes less expensive than taking the multiple drugs separately.

Available non-insulin antidiabetic agents are summarized here and in Table 66-7. Current manufacturer information should be

TABLE 66-7 NON-INSULIN ANTIDIABETIC AGENTS BY DRUG CLASS*

DRUG CLASS	AVAILABLE AGENTS (GENERIC NAME)	ROUTE OF ADMINISTRATION	MODE OF ACTION
Biguanides	Metformin	Oral	Insulin sensitizer
Sulfonylureas	Glipizide, glyburide, glimeperide, gliclazide, chlorpropamide, tolazamide	Oral	Insulin secretagogue
Meglitinides	Repaglinide, nateglinide	Oral	Insulin secretagogue
Thiazolidinediones	Pioglitazone, rosiglitazone	Oral	Insulin sensitizer
GLP-1 analogues	Exenatide, liraglutide, albiglutide	Subcutaneous injection	Incretin mimetic
DPP-4 inhibitors	Sitagliptin, saxagliptin, linagliptin, alogliptin	Oral	Incretin amplifier
α-Glucosidase inhibitors	Acarbose, miglitol	Oral	Delay carbohydrate digestion/absorption
Amylin mimetics	Pramlintide	Subcutaneous injection	Delay gastric emptying, suppress glucagon
SGLT2 inhibitors	Canagliflozin, dapagliflozin, empagliflozin	Oral	Increase urinary glucose excretion

DPP-4, Dipeptidyl peptidase-4; GLP-1, glucagon-like peptide-1; SGLT2, sodium glucose transport protein subtype 2.
*Consult current manufacturer information for details on available combinations, prescribing, and safety.

consulted before prescribing these drugs to ensure updated and adequately detailed information on available single and combination agents and their effective and safe use.

Metformin

Metformin is an oral agent in the biguanide class that produces its most prominent effects by decreasing gluconeogenesis and thus reducing hepatic glucose production. This insulin-sensitizing effect is associated with a low risk of hypoglycemia. It has been in use for more than 30 years and is available in inexpensive generic form. The usual starting dose is 500 mg once or twice daily with incremental advancement at several-week intervals to a usual maximum of 2000 mg daily in two or three divided doses. Metformin typically decreases HbA_{1c} by about 1.5%. Further benefits include modest weight loss (approximately 3 kg on average) and a small improvement in plasma lipid profile (decrease in low-density lipoprotein [LDL]-cholesterol and triglycerides and increase in HDL). Adverse reactions include gastrointestinal effects and, rarely, lactic acidosis. The drug should be avoided in patients with renal insufficiency.

Sulfonylureas

Sulfonylureas stimulate endogenous insulin secretion by binding and activating potassium channels in beta cells. In patients with adequate residual beta cell function, they can lower HbA_{1c} levels by 1% to 2%. Drugs in this class have been in clinical use for more than 40 years, and many inexpensive, generic sulfonylureas are available that differ in duration of action, metabolism, and mode of clearance. Because they can increase insulin secretion even in the absence of hyperglycemia, they have significant potential to cause hypoglycemia. Patients need to be instructed how to recognize and treat hypoglycemia before starting a sulfonylurea. Factors that increase the risk for hypoglycemia with sulfonylureas include advanced age, poor nutrition, alcohol ingestion, and hepatic and renal insufficiency. Other disadvantages of this drug class are a tendency to cause weight gain and a loss of effectiveness over time.

Meglitinides

Repaglinide and nateglinide activate beta cell potassium channels and thus stimulate endogenous insulin secretion through a mechanism similar to that of sulfonylureas, although they generally result in less reduction in blood glucose than sulfonylureas. They have rapid action and have less tendency to cause hypoglycemia

than sulfonylureas. Their use has been limited by high cost and lack of advantage over the sulfonylureas.

Thiazolidinediones

The thiazolidinediones (TZDs) activate the nuclear peroxisome proliferator-activated receptor-γ (PPAR-γ), which leads to changes in transcription rates of multiple genes. The net effect is reduced insulin resistance, and the resulting augmented actions of insulin lead to increased glucose uptake in peripheral tissues and reduced hepatic glucose production. Pioglitazone typically lowers HbA_{1c} by 0.5% to 1.4% and carries a low risk of hypoglycemia. Potential side effects include weight gain and hepatotoxicity.

Glucagon-Like Peptide-1 Analogues

Glucagon-like peptide-1 (GLP-1) is one of several hormones produced in the small intestine (designated *incretins*) that modify gastrointestinal motility and insulin secretion. The GLP-1 analogues, exenatide, liraglutide, and albiglutide, bind to GLP-1 receptors and improve blood glucose control by enhancing insulin-dependent insulin secretion, slowing gastric emptying, suppressing postprandial glucagon production, and decreasing food intake through enhanced satiety. This results in decreases in HbA_{1c} by 0.5% to 1.5% and modest weight loss (in the range of 3 kg). They are administered via injection with prefilled pens—exenatide twice daily or once weekly in long-acting form, liraglutide once daily, and albiglutide once weekly. The most common side effects are nausea and sometimes diarrhea, likely related to the drugs' effects on gastrointestinal motility. GLP-1 analogue use is tempered by the inconvenience of injection, relatively high cost, and a lack of long-term data on durability of weight loss or other outcome benefits. They most often are used as second-line agents in conjunction with other glucose-lowering drugs or insulin.

Dipeptidyl Peptidase-4 Inhibitors

The dipeptidyl peptidase-4 (DPP-4) inhibitors—sitagliptin, saxagliptin, linagliptin, and alogliptin—block the deactivation of GLP-1 (described in the previous section) and glucose-dependent insulinotropic peptide (GIP), peptide hormones that are important in the regulation of glucose homeostasis. Some of the effects of DPP-4 inhibitors may overlap with those of administered GLP-1 analogues, but they likely have additional actions by increasing levels of hormones other than GLP-1. DPP-4

commonly, usually manifesting as a bilaterally symm
distal, primarily sensory polyneuropathy (with or withou
involvement) in a *glove-and-stocking* distribution. Pain,
ness, hyperesthesias, and paresthesias progress to sens
This condition, together with loss of proprioception, ca
an abnormal gait with repeated trauma and potential for f
of the tarsal bones, sometimes resulting in the develop
Charcot joints. These changes lead to abnormal pressure
feet that, together with the soft tissue atrophy related to
eral arterial insufficiency, result in foot ulcers that may
to osteomyelitis and gangrene. Detailed, regular ne
examination of all patients is essential to elicit the earl
light touch (using a size 5.07/10-g monofilament), refle
vibratory sensation.

A second common form of diabetic neuropathy is au
neuropathy, which may develop in concert with or separ
distal polyneuropathy. Resulting symptoms can be deb
including postural hypotension leading to falls or sync
troparesis, enteropathy with constipation or diarrhea, and
outflow obstruction with urinary retention. Diabetic au
neuropathy together with vascular disease is a contri
erectile dysfunction in males. Gastrointestinal dysfunct
autonomic neuropathy can complicate efforts to achiev
glucose control by causing variable absorption of food
pected diagnosis of autonomic neuropathy can be stren
by demonstrating loss of normal variability in heart r
deep respirations or the Valsalva maneuver.

Other, less common manifestations of diabetic ne
include thoracic and lumbar nerve root *polyradiculopath*
vidual peripheral and cranial nerve *mononeuropath*
asymmetrical neuropathies of multiple peripheral nerves
neuropathy multiplex). Diabetic amyotrophy causing
atrophy and weakness most often involving the anteri
muscles and pelvic girdle is an uncommon form of diab
ropathy that often resolves after several months.

The primary approach to all diabetic neuropathies
of efforts to improve blood glucose control. Clinical tr
shown decreased development of distal polyneuropa
improved glycemia in T1DM. It also is particularly i
for patients with neuropathies to receive regular foot car
ing daily self-inspection of the feet, regular physician
tions, and early interventions for developing callouses, i
or other foot lesions. Painful polyneuropathies cause su
morbidity and are difficult to treat. First-line drugs
amitriptyline, venlafaxine, duloxetine, and pregaba
patients who do not respond adequately to one drug,
tion therapy with two drugs of different classes can b
Alternative treatments that may be effective in some
include topical capsaicin cream, lidocaine patch,
acid, isosorbide dinitrate topical spray, and transcutane
trical nerve stimulation (TENS). *Gastroparesis* seco
autonomic neuropathy may improve symptomatica
metoclopramide or domperidone (dopamine D2 ant
erythromycin (motilin agonist) for bacterial overgro
apride (cholinergic agonist), or mosapride (selective
5-HT4 receptor agonist). Diarrhea may respond to lo
or diphenoxylate and atropine. Orthostatic hypotensi
treated by attention to mechanical factors such as ele

inhibitors are taken orally and result in decreased HbA_{1c} in the range of 0.5% to 1.0%. They can be used as monotherapy or in combination with one or more other agents and have favorable side effect profiles.

α-Glucosidase Inhibitors

The α-glucosidase inhibitors, acarbose and miglitol, are oral agents that improve glycemia by inhibiting the enzymatic breakdown of complex carbohydrates within the lumen of the small intestine. They have modest glucose-lowering effects, decreasing HbA_{1c} in the range of 0.5% to 0.8%. Their use is limited by the frequent occurrence of flatulence and diarrhea as a consequence of undigested carbohydrates reaching lower intestinal regions.

Pramlintide

Pramlintide is a stable analogue of the beta cell peptide, amylin, which has actions that include slowing of gastric emptying, satiety effects that decrease food intake, and decrease in postmeal glucagon. It is not widely used because of required multiple injections and limited efficacy in lowering HbA1c.

SGLT2 Inhibitors

Canagliflozin, dapagliflozin, and empagliflozin are recently approved oral agents that function by inhibiting the subtype 2 sodium glucose transport protein (SGLT2). SGLT2 mediates more than 90% of glucose reabsorption in the renal tubules, and the drug lowers blood glucose levels by promoting excretion of glucose in the urine. This results in a decrease in HbA_{1c} in the range of 0.5% to 1.0% and modest weight loss. Concerns about potential side effects of increased cardiovascular events, increased LDL-cholesterol, urinary and genital infections, hypotension, and hypoglycemia are under investigation.

Insulin Treatment in T2DM

For patients who have inadequate glycemic control with oral agents, insulin may be started as a basal supplement to the oral regimen. Frequently used choices include glargine (once daily), detemir (once or twice daily), or NPH (once daily at bedtime) (see later discussion and Table 66-5 for more details on different types of insulin). Starting doses are typically in the range of 10 U (or can be more specifically calculated as 0.2 U/kg), with increases of 2 to 4 U at intervals of 3 days or longer. Oral agent regimens commonly are simplified at the time of starting insulin (e.g., shifting from multiple agents to a single oral agent). For patients who do not achieve adequate control with basal insulin, mealtime coverage is provided by a rapid-acting insulin. Often, under this circumstance, all oral agents are discontinued, and blood glucose control is achieved with the use of exogenous insulin alone. Compared to patients with T1DM, those with T2DM may not require as tight a match of carbohydrate to insulin doses at meals, perhaps because of some residual insulin secretion. For this reason, insulin pumps are only rarely used in T2DM.

Nutritional and Weight Management

Patients should receive counseling from a dietician and be assisted in developing a nutritional plan that is individualized to their lifestyle, exercise, culture, and financial resources.

Guidelines from many current expert panels allow flexibility in the relative amounts of carbohydrate, fat, and protein. Nutritional management in T2DM often has a major focus on achieving reductions in calorie intake and weight loss. Achieving weight loss may be made more difficult by a tendency of some oral antidiabetic agents and also insulin to induce a degree of weight gain.

An important goal of nutritional management should be to balance the timing and quantities of ingested macronutrients with medications and exercise to help achieve targets for blood glucose control without periods of hypoglycemia.

For overweight or obese patients, it often is practical to set an initial goal of losing 5% to 10% of body weight. This may significantly improve diabetes control and increase the patient's motivation to then set goals for further weight loss (see Chapter 67).

Bariatric surgical procedures represent a method for achieving weight loss and potentially dramatic improvements in glycemia and risk factors for long-term complications in T2DM. Patients typically have improvements in glycemic control and lower requirements for antidiabetic medications within days after undergoing the Roux-en-Y gastric bypass procedure. This is thought to reflect changes in gut hormones and metabolic factors independent of weight loss. Beneficial effects on glucose control develop more gradually after the placement of an adjustable gastric band or sleeve gastrectomy. Randomized trials comparing bariatric surgery with medical nutrition therapy alone for weight loss have shown greater efficacy in achieving HbA_{1c} goals with surgery, and some studies have shown dramatic rates of remission, with 75% of patients or more becoming normoglycemic off all antidiabetic agents (see Chapter 67).

Exercise

Physical exercise should be encouraged in T2DM as an important component of weight loss regimens and also for its beneficial effects in decreasing the risks of long-term complications. The general recommendation of several expert panels is 30 minutes or more of moderate-intensity physical exercise on at least 5 days per week, but the regimen needs to be highly individualized according to a patient's capabilities and limitations imposed by other medical conditions such as cardiovascular disease. Patients who are unwilling or unable to undertake significant aerobic exercise should be encouraged to do daily walking or other physical activities within their limitations.

Standards of Care in T1DM and T2DM in Addition to Blood Glucose Control

A number of assessments and interventions should be performed at intervals in patients with T1DM or T2DM. These include blood pressure measurement and examination of the feet at each physician visit. Patients who smoke should receive counseling at each visit about the importance of and strategies for discontinuing. A dilated eye examination should be performed annually, or more often in patients with diabetic eye disease. A dental examination also should be performed at least annually. Starting 5 years after disease onset in T1DM and at the time of diagnosis in T2DM, patients should have annual measurement of their urinary albumin/creatinine ratio with confirmation if elevated (>30 mg albumin per gram of creatinine). A fasting lipid profile should be obtained annually. Aspirin (75 to 162 mg daily) is

and patients may be vulnerable to development of mo...
hyperglycemia and volume deficits over this extended p...

HHS is associated with infections (40%), diuretic use...
40%), and residency in nursing homes (25% to 30%...
precipitating and complicating factors may include i...
obstruction, mesenteric thrombosis, pulmonary emboli...
toneal dialysis, subdural hematoma, and an extensive list...
cations. The overall mortality rate exceeds that of DKA...
40%), with higher mortality rates associated with age o...
70 years, nursing home residency, and higher osmolality...
Na+ concentration. Clinically, patients have evidenc...
marked fluid and electrolyte deficits and tend to have mo...
inent neurologic abnormalities than those with DKA, i...
confusion, obtundation, and coma.

Therapy for HHS follows the same general principle...
for DKA, with a greater volume replacement required (...
8 to 12 L in fully developed HHS). Restoration of...
and electrolyte deficits should proceed more slowly...
DKA, ideally over 36 to 72 hours. Insulin therapy s...
started only after rehydration is in progress. There i...
for K+ replacement, but less than in DKA. Patients w...
may be more sensitive to insulin than those with D...
may require lower insulin doses. In view of the severe...
tion and predisposition to vascular thrombosis, hep...
phylaxis usually should be provided. Despite the very...
hyperglycemia of HHS, patients may be able to retur...
treatment eventually.

Chronic Complications of Diabetes

Chronic complications of T1DM and T2DM are si...
include microvascular complications (nephropathy, ret...
and neuropathy) and macrovascular or cardiovascular c...
tions (coronary artery disease, peripheral vascular dis...
cerebrovascular disease). The long-term complications...
tes result in substantial morbidity and shorten the ave...
span by 10 years. Candidate mechanisms for microvas...
macrovascular complications include activation of th...
pathway (with accumulation of sorbitol), formation o...
proteins and advanced glycation end products (cross-li...
cated proteins), abnormalities in lipid metabolism,...
oxidative damage, hyperinsulinemia, hyperperfusion o...
tissues, hyperviscosity, platelet dysfunction (increased...
tion), endothelial dysfunction, and activation of variou...
factors.

Microvascular Complications
Retinopathy
Diabetic retinopathy affects almost all patients with T...
60% to 80% of those with T2DM by 20 years after the...
of diabetes. It is the most common cause of blindness i...
between the ages of 20 and 74 years in the developed w...
incidence and progression of diabetic retinopathy incr...
duration of diabetes, poor glycemic control, the type o...
(T1DM more than T2DM), and the presence of hype...
smoking, dyslipidemia, nephropathy, and pregnancy...

Early interventions often are beneficial in slowing...
times reversing diabetic retinopathy, but most patient...
symptoms until the lesions are advanced. Therefor...

TABLE 66-8 SIGNS AND SYMPTOMS OF HYPOGLYCEMIA

AUTONOMIC

Sweating	Palpitations	Hunger
Pallor	Tachycardia	Nausea
Anxiety	Hypertension	Vomiting
Tremor	Irritability	Paresthesias

NEUROGLYCOPENIC

Difficulty thinking	Dizziness	Seizures
Fatigue, weakness	Visual blurring	Loss of consciousness
Somnolence	Confusion	Coma
Headache	Abnormal behavior	Death

Pathology

Hypoglycemic disorders can result when there is overproduction of hormones that lower glucose concentrations, underproduction of hormones that serve to elevate glucose levels, deficiency of substrates for endogenous glucose synthesis, or changes in cells and tissues that result in their increased consumption of glucose.

Etiologic Classification

Causes of hypoglycemia by etiologic categories are listed in Table 66-9.

Drug-Induced

The most common causes of hypoglycemia are excess insulin or insulin secretagogues (especially sulfonylureas) administered in the treatment of diabetes. Ethanol is another commonly used drug that can cause hypoglycemia. This most often occurs in the context of chronic alcoholism in an individual who is nutritionally depleted, often after binge drinking for several days or longer. Under these circumstances, hepatic glycogen stores become depleted, and the process of alcohol metabolism blocks gluconeogenesis by depriving the liver of nicotinamide adenine dinucleotide (NAD+). Commonly used pharmacologic agents that have been associated with hypoglycemia include β-blockers (especially nonselective β_2-adrenergic antagonists), ACE inhibitors, pentamidine (through toxic effects on beta cells), quinine, and quinolones.

Excess Endogenous Insulin or Insulin-like Hormones

Alimentary hypoglycemia is a disorder in which low blood glucose levels occur typically 90 to 180 minutes after meals in patients who have undergone gastric outlet surgery with resulting accelerated gastric emptying. This is distinct from the more common *dumping syndrome*, which results from rapid entry of an osmotic load into the small intestine and associated fluid shifts and autonomic responses and is not associated with hypoglycemia. "Reactive hypoglycemia" is a now outmoded term that previously was applied to adrenergic symptoms occurring 2 to 4 hours after a meal in patients who are not hypoglycemic; these individuals may experience decreased symptoms with frequent feedings and avoidance of high-carbohydrate meals.

Tumors of islet beta cells (*insulinomas*) can cause hypoglycemia by producing excess insulin in an unregulated manner. They are uncommon (1 in 250,000 patient-years), but it is important

TABLE 66-9 ETIOLOGIC CLASSIFICATION OF HYPOGLYCEMIC DISORDERS MANIFESTING IN ADULTS

DRUG-INDUCED

Antidiabetic agents (insulin, sulfonylureas, meglitinides)
Alcohol
Other pharmacologic agents (β-blockers, ACE inhibitors, pentamidine, quinine, quinolones and many others)

ALTERED GASTROINTESTINAL FUNCTION

Alimentary hypoglycemia

BETA-CELL INSULIN OVERSECRETION

Insulinoma
Non-insulinoma pancreatogenous hypoglycemia (without or with bariatric surgery)

NON–ISLET CELL NEOPLASMS

Tumor insulin-like growth factor-II secretion
Tumor glucose consumption

AUTOIMMUNE

Circulating insulin antibodies
Insulin receptor activating antibodies

ENDOCRINE DEFICIENCIES

Glucocorticoids (adrenal insufficiency), growth hormone, catecholamines, glucagon

SEVERE ILLNESS

Sepsis
Hepatic failure
Renal failure

MALNUTRITION

Anorexia nervosa

ACE, Angiotensin-converting enzyme.

to recognize them when they do occur. Insulinomas usually are small (1 to 2 cm), benign (>90%), solitary (>90%), and confined to the endocrine pancreas (99%). Some patients have an indolent course extending over many years before diagnosis, but insulinomas can produce profound hypoglycemia. There is a tendency for adrenergic symptoms to become suppressed as a consequence of repeated exposures to hypoglycemia, and neuroglycopenic symptoms may predominate, including sometimes bizarre behavioral abnormalities. Patients may eat frequently in response to the hypoglycemia and exhibit moderate weight gain.

Non-insulinoma pancreatogenous hypoglycemia is a disorder that may manifest with symptoms similar to those of insulinomas, but the pathology involves beta-cell hypertrophy and hyperplasia rather than the presence of a discrete tumor. More recently, the development of hypoglycemia with similar beta-cell hyperplasia has been described in a small number of patients, more often in females, months to years after Roux-en-Y gastric bypass surgery.

Non–islet cell neoplasms are a rare cause of hypoglycemia; they produce an insulin-like growth factor (IGF), usually a partially processed form of IGF-II designated *big IGF-II*, that can have insulin-like effects. The tumors typically are large and malignant and are most often located in the retroperitoneal space, abdomen, or thoracic cavity. Tumor types include hemangiopericytomas, hepatocellular carcinomas, lymphomas, adrenocortical carcinomas, gastrointestinal carcinoids, and mesenchymal tumors. Some large tumors cause hypoglycemia in the absence of detectable insulin-like factors.

Hormone Deficiencies

Deficiencies of insulin counter-regulatory hormones, which normally function to raise glucose levels, can result in or contribute to hypoglycemia. An example is low levels of corticosteroids caused by primary or secondary adrenocorticoid insufficiency. Deficiencies of other hormones, including catecholamines, glucagon, and growth hormone, also can cause hypoglycemia.

Severe Illness

Hypoglycemia can occur during severe illness through a number of different mechanisms in association with sepsis, hepatic insufficiency, and renal failure. Patients with severe illness appear to be particularly vulnerable to hypoglycemia when they are poorly nourished, although malnutrition alone is rarely associated with hypoglycemia.

Approach to the Diagnosis

For patients who have well-documented hypoglycemia, the diagnosis often is evident or strongly suggested by the clinical setting, history, and physical examination findings. Hypoglycemia induced by insulin or other glucose-lowering agents in diabetic patients often is immediately apparent from the medical history. Alcohol-induced hypoglycemia may be suspected in a patient with a known or suspected history of alcohol abuse and binge drinking. Identification of other candidate drugs as a cause of hypoglycemia requires a thorough medical history, and the condition can be expected to resolve if the suspect medication is stopped. The patient may have a known diagnosis of adrenal insufficiency, or this may be suggested by other clinical findings (e.g., orthostatic hypotension, increased skin pigmentation) or the development of markedly increased insulin sensitivity in a patient with T1DM. The patient may have a known tumor suggesting the possibility of a non–islet cell neoplasm as a cause of hypoglycemia. There may be a history of Roux-en-Y bypass surgery, raising the possibility of beta-cell hyperplasia. The co-occurrence of sepsis, hepatic failure, renal failure, profound malnutrition, or a known diagnosis of anorexia nervosa may suggest one of these potential underlying causes.

A number of algorithms have been developed to guide the evaluation of documented or potential hypoglycemia, including a recommended approach from an expert panel published by the Endocrine Society. If there is an opportunity to observe the patient during a symptomatic episode of presumed hypoglycemia, plasma should be obtained, if possible before treatment, for measurement of glucose, insulin, proinsulin, C-peptide, β-hydroxybutyrate, and screening for sulfonylureas and meglitinides. Hypoglycemia can be rapidly, provisionally confirmed with a test meter. After blood samples have been obtained for the tests described, glucose should be administered orally (15 to 30 g) or intravenously (25 g, or 1 ampule of 50% dextrose), and recovery of glucose levels and symptoms should be observed.

For patients with suspected or confirmed hypoglycemia developing specifically in the fasted state, it may be possible to replicate the condition by observing during several hours of daytime fasting, with or without a preceding overnight fast. The same laboratory testing panel as described earlier then can be obtained if symptoms suggestive of hypoglycemia occur. For patients who describe postprandial hypoglycemic symptoms (within 5 hours after a meal), a mixed meal (not a pure glucose load) should be provided, with blood sampling at baseline and every 30 minutes thereafter for 5 hours

For patients who do not manifest hypoglycemia with the testing procedures described despite a strong suspicion of hypoglycemia, the most frequently utilized approach is a 72-hour fast according to a protocol developed at the Mayo Clinic. Blood is obtained every 6 hours and at test termination. The test is ended at 72 hours or at an earlier time point if the plasma glucose level decreases (by glucose meter testing) with associated symptoms to 45 mg/dL (2.5 mmol/L) or lower or to less than 55 mg/dL (3 mmol/L) in a patient with prior documentation of Whipple's triad. At the end of the 72-hour test period, the patient is given 1 mg of glucagon intravenously, and blood is obtained at 10, 20, and 30 minutes, after which the patient is given a meal. The final blood sample obtained at the end of the fast (before glucagon administration) is analyzed additionally for β-hydroxybutyrate and a sulfonylurea/meglitinide panel.

For any of these test protocols, elevations of insulin, proinsulin, and C-peptide associated with hypoglycemia at the same time point are consistent with an insulinoma, beta-cell hyperplasia, the effects of an insulin secretagogue (sulfonylurea or meglitinide), or the presence of insulin antibodies. An elevation in these three hormones during a meal test in a patient who has had gastric surgery is suggestive of alimentary hypoglycemia. Plasma insulin, proinsulin, and C-peptide are not elevated in patients with hypoglycemia secondary to extrapancreatic neoplasms. This diagnosis usually can be further confirmed by evidence of a large tumor with various imaging techniques. High insulin levels, together with low proinsulin and C-peptide concentrations in the presence of hypoglycemia, is indicative of exogenous insulin administration. Factitious hypoglycemia secondary to insulin or insulin secretagogue administration is uncommon and has been observed in individuals with or without diabetes.

Treatment

The most important therapeutic step in hypoglycemia is to identify and treat the underlying causes, including drugs, alcohol, serious infection, tumors, and hypoadrenalism. The occurrence of hypoglycemia usually can be substantially improved in patients with alimentary hypoglycemia by a modified feeding regimen with frequent, small meals and avoidance of concentrated sources of rapidly digested and absorbed carbohydrate.

Non–islet cell tumor hypoglycemia is treated by tumor resection if possible. For nonresectable tumors, a debulking procedure may be effective in reducing hypoglycemia. Hypoglycemia in patients with insulinomas can be cured by resection. Persistent hypoglycemia secondary to nonresectable insulinoma can sometimes be treated effectively with diazoxide, long-acting somatostatin analogues (octreotide or lanreotide), verapamil, or phenytoin. For patients with beta-cell hyperplasia after bariatric surgery, first-line treatment includes diet modifications with more frequent, small meals and avoidance of concentrated sources of carbohydrate to decrease meal-induced insulin secretion.

For a deeper discussion of this topic, please see Chapter 229, "Diabetes Mellitus," and Chapter 230, "Hypoglycemia/Pancreatic Islet Cell Disorders," in Goldman-Cecil Medicine, 25th Edition.

SUGGESTED READINGS

American Diabetes Association clinical practice recommendations 2013, Diabetes Care 36(Suppl 1):S1–S108, 2013.

Bril V, England J, Franklin GM, et al: Evidence-based guideline: treatment of painful diabetic neuropathy. Report of the American Academy of Neurology, the American Association of Neuromuscular and Electrodiagnostic Medicine, and the American Academy of Physical Medicine and Rehabilitation, Neurology 76:1758–1765, 2011.

Coustan DR: Gestational diabetes mellitus, Clin Chem 59:1310–1321, 2013.

Cryer PE, Axelrod L, Grossman AB, et al: Evaluation and management of adult hypoglycemic disorders: an Endocrine Society clinical practice guideline, J Clin Endocrinol Metab 94:709–728, 2009.

Eckel RH, Grundy SM, Zimmet PZ: The metabolic syndrome, Lancet 365:1415–1428, 2005.

Eringsmark Regnéll S, Lernmark A: The environment and the origins of islet autoimmunity and type 1 diabetes, Diabet Med 30:155–160, 2013.

Forbes JM, Cooper ME: Mechanisms of diabetic complications, Physiol Rev 93:137–188, 2013.

Gross JL, de Azevedo MJ, Silveiro SP, et al: Diabetic nephropathy: diagnosis, prevention, and treatment, Diabetes Care 28:164–176, 2005.

Insulin pump therapy, Drug Ther Bull 50:105–108, 2012.

Inzucchi SE, Bergenstal RM, Buse JB, et al: Management of hyperglycemia in type 2 diabetes: a patient-centered approach. Position statement of the American Diabetes Association (ADA) and the European Association for the Study of Diabetes (EASD), Diabetes Care 35:1364–1379, 2012.

Kavvoura FK, Owen KR: Maturity onset diabetes of the young: clinical characteristics, diagnosis and management, Pediatr Endocrinol Rev 10:234–242, 2012.

Mauras N, Fox L, Englert K, et al: Continuous glucose monitoring in type 1 diabetes, Endocrine 43:41–50, 2013.

Nathan DM, Cleary PA, Backlund JY, et al: Intensive diabetes treatment and cardiovascular disease in patients with type 1 diabetes. Diabetes Control and Complications Trial/Epidemiology of Diabetes Interventions and Complications (DCCT/EDIC) Study Research Group, N Engl J Med 353:2643–2653, 2005.

Pickup JC: Insulin-pump therapy for type 1 diabetes mellitus, N Engl J Med 366:1616–1624, 2012.

Seaquist ER, Anderson J, Childs B, et al: Hypoglycemia and diabetes: a report of a workgroup of the American Diabetes Association and the Endocrine Society, J Clin Endocrinol Metab 98:1845–1859, 2013.

Torres JM, Cox NJ, Philipson LH: Genome wide association studies for diabetes: perspective on results and challenges, Pediatr Diabetes 14:90–96, 2013.

Obesity

Osama Hamdy

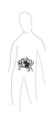

DEFINITION AND EPIDEMIOLOGY

Obesity is a disease that is usually defined as a body mass index (BMI) greater than or equal to 30 kg/m^2 (weight [kg]/(height [m])^2). A BMI of 30 to 34.9 is considered class 1 obesity, 35 to 39.9 is class 2 obesity, and 40 or higher is class 3 or severe obesity. The term "morbid obesity" previously was applied to individuals weighing at least 45 kg (100 lb) more than, or typically about 60% more than, desirable body weight; the term also has been applied to any individual with a BMI greater than or equal to 40 kg/m^2.

There is increasing recognition of limitations to defining obesity based on BMI resulting from the variable correlation between BMI and amount of body fat in different ethnic (genetic) populations or in individuals with different degrees of muscularity. Many investigators and clinicians are moving toward a definition that defines obesity as an excess of body fat sufficient to confer risk. Linking obesity to cardiometabolic risk, body fat distribution, and waist circumference is more important than measuring percentage body fat or BMI alone. People who accumulate visceral fat and clinically have higher waist circumference (metabolic obesity) are at much higher risk for cardiovascular disease and diabetes than those with the same BMI or the same percentage of body fat but a lower waist circumference. The National Cholesterol Education Program Adult Treatment Panel III (ATP III) considered a waist circumference greater than 40 inches (102 cm) in American men or 35 inches (88 cm) in American women to be among the five criteria that define the cardiometabolic syndrome. In spite of its limitations, BMI remains a simple measurement with utility in estimating a person's health risks and comparing outcomes between trials.

During the last 30 years, there has been a dramatic increase in the percentage of both adults and children in the United States who are overweight (defined as BMI of 25 to 30) or obese. According to the 2009-2010 National Health and Nutrition Examination Survey (NHANES) conducted by the Centers for Disease Control and Prevention (CDC), more than one third of U.S. adults (35.7%) were obese. This was more than double the prevalence in the 1976-1980 NHANES data (15.0%). Non-Hispanic blacks had the highest age-adjusted rates of obesity (49.5%), followed by Mexican Americans (40.4%), all Hispanics (39.1%), and non-Hispanic whites (34.3%). More recently, there appears to have been a slowing of the rate of increase or even a leveling off. Obesity prevalence varies significantly across states, from a low of 20.5% in Colorado to a high of 34.7% in Louisiana in 2012. In general, higher prevalence of adult obesity was found in the midwest (29.5%) and the south (29.4%) and lower prevalence in the northeast (25.3%) and the west (25.1%).

The percentage of children and adolescents who are overweight or obese has almost tripled since 1980. Currently, 17% of children and adolescents aged 2 to 19 years (12.5 million individuals) are obese. NHANES data from 1976-1980 and from 2009-2010 show the prevalence of obesity increasing from 5.0% to 12.1%, respectively, for children aged 2 to 5 years and from 5.0% to 18.4% for those aged 12 to 19 years. Among low-income preschool children, the prevalence of obesity increased between 1998 and 2003 from 13.0% to 15.2%, and severe obesity from 1.8% to 2.2%. These rates decreased slightly between 2003 and 2010: obesity from 15.2% to 14.9%, and severe obesity from 2.2% to 2.1%.

Overweight and obesity and their associated health problems have a significant economic impact on the U.S. health care system through direct medical expenses and indirect costs (e.g., loss of work time and productivity). Medical costs of obesity account for an estimated 10% of total U.S. medical expenditures. The estimated total annual medical costs of obesity in the United States was $147 billion in 2008, with medical costs on average $1429 higher per year for obese compared with normal-weight individuals. Approximately half of these costs were paid by Medicaid and Medicare.

PATHOLOGY OF OBESITY

Obesity develops as a consequence of genetic-environmental interactions, such that genetically prone individuals who lead a sedentary lifestyle and consume larger amounts of dietary calories are at higher risk. Children of obese parents are 80% more likely to become obese, and it is believed that this results from a combination of genetic and environmental influences.

The genetic contributions to obesity are most commonly considered to reflect the combined effects of variations in multiple genes and only rarely appear to result from a defect in a single powerful gene. Single-gene defects identified in experimental animals have been useful to demonstrate appetite and satiety mechanisms, and mutations in some of these same genes have subsequently been identified in rare human forms of genetic obesity. For example, loss-of-function mutations in the leptin gene and in the cellular receptor for leptin were first identified as a cause of obesity in laboratory mice (*ob/ob* and *db/db* mice, respectively). Leptin is a hormone that is produced in fat cells, mostly in subcutaneous fat. It is a potent satiety factor that acts in the arcuate nucleus of the hypothalamus to reduce the production of neuropeptide Y, a stimulator of food intake. After its discovery in mice, leptin gene mutations were identified as a cause of a rare form of heritable human obesity. Affected individuals develop marked obesity in childhood as a consequence of increased food intake. Leptin secretion normally follows a circadian pattern, with higher levels during evening and night hours. Loss of leptin secretion has particularly marked effects during these hours, resulting in a phenomenon known as night-eating syndrome, in which patients tend to consume large amounts of food during the night.

Other single-gene defects identified as rare causes of human obesity include loss-of-function mutations in genes encoding carboxypeptidase E, melanocortin-4 or melanocortin-3 receptors, and serotonin-2C or serotonin-1B receptors. Obesity is also a feature of many other genetic disorders in which the specific mechanisms of the obesity are less well understood. These different syndromes may have autosomal dominant, autosomal recessive, or X-linked inheritance patterns, consistent with multiple different genetic causes. Among the best known of these disorders, the Bardet-Biedl syndrome, is an autosomal recessive disorder characterized by obesity and other abnormalities, including hypogonadism in men, mental retardation, retinal dystrophy, polydactyly, and renal malformations. In Prader-Willi syndrome, loss of portions of the long arm of chromosome 15 (q11-13) is associated with obesity, poor muscle tone in infancy, defects in cognition, behavioral abnormalities (irritability), short stature, and hypogonadotropic hypogonadism.

Although known single-gene mutations account for only a small percentage of human obesity, there is evidence for widespread heritable influences in more common forms of human obesity. For example, in twin and adoptee studies, both members of identical twin pairs tend to become obese in concordance with the same weight pattern as their biologic parents, even when raised apart. Metabolic rate, spontaneous physical activity, and thermic response to food seem to be heritable to a variable extent, but the specific genes that contribute to prevalent forms of human obesity have not yet been defined. Genomic analyses in large populations have identified multiple genes or genetic regions in which polymorphisms are associated with obesity risk. These include polymorphisms in or near genes for the melanocortin-4 receptor (a protein involved in appetite suppression pathways in the hypothalamus), brain-derived neurotrophic factor (role in energy balance); the β_3-adrenergic receptor (role in visceral fat accumulation), and peroxisome proliferator-activated receptor-$\gamma 2$ (PPAR-$\gamma 2$, a transcription factor involved in adipocyte differentiation. Multiple other sites of genetic variation associated with increased obesity risk have been identified for which potential mechanistic links to obesity are not yet apparent. It is hypothesized that the heritable component of common forms of human obesity derives from the effects of variations in these and many yet unidentified genes acting both additively and synergistically.

Important environmental factors driving the recent increased prevalence of obesity include increased caloric intake (reflecting greater availability of high-calorie, low-cost foods) and decreased energy expenditure (as a consequence of decreased physical activity). Lower socioeconomic status, lower education level, cessation of smoking, and consumption of carbohydrates with a high glycemic index have been identified as specific confounders of obesity. Additional factors that may influence obesity risk include intrauterine growth and nutritional history, levels of reproductive and other hormones, and factors that may alter the feedback between energy intake and expenditure. Ultimately, an increase in total body fat results from energy intake that exceeds energy expenditure. This occurs through the operation of genetic and environmental influences, together with individual behavioral characteristics.

PATHOLOGY OF OBESITY-ASSOCIATED HEALTH RISKS

Adipose tissue is not just a passive depot for lipids. Adipocytes also function as a complex and active endocrine organ with metabolic and secretory products (hormones, prohormones, cytokines, and enzymes) that play a major role in whole-body metabolism. Relationships between obesity and both insulin resistance and endothelial dysfunction (the early stage of atherosclerosis) are mediated through the release of several hormones from adipose tissue. These hormones, designated adipocytokines or adipokines, comprise a group of pharmacologically active low- and medium-molecular-weight proteins that possess autocrine and paracrine effects and are known products of the inflammatory and immune systems. They play an important role in adipose tissue physiology and in initiating metabolic and cardiovascular abnormalities, not only in overweight and obese individuals but also in lean persons with higher visceral fat mass. Adipokines include adiponectin, leptin, tumor necrosis factor-α (TNF-α), interleukin-6 (IL-6), resistin, plasminogen activator inhibitor-1 (PAI-1), angiotensinogen, and monocyte chemoattractant protein-1 (MCP-1). An increased amount of adipose tissue or its disproportionate distribution between central and peripheral body regions is related to altered serum levels of these factors. With the exceptions of leptin and adiponectin, the adipokines are produced both from fat cells and from adipose tissue–resident macrophages in the stromal tissues surrounding fat cells. For unknown reasons, an increase in the amount of body fat is associated with increases in the number of adipose tissue macrophages and their production of cytokines.

Human adiponectin is a relatively abundant, 244-amino-acid polypeptide in plasma, accounting for 0.01% of total plasma proteins. Adiponectin gene expression in adipose tissue is associated with obesity, insulin resistance, and type 2 diabetes (T2DM). Hypoadiponectinemia is more strongly related to the degree of insulin resistance than to the degree of adiposity or glucose intolerance. Genetic polymorphisms may influence the regulation of adiponectin and lead to variations in its levels among different individuals. Several human studies have shown that high adiponectin levels protect against development of T2DM and point to the possible future use of adiponectin as an indicator of diabetes risk. Low plasma concentrations of adiponectin are observed in patients with coronary artery disease (CAD), and lower adiponectin levels have been found in diabetic patients with CAD than in those without CAD. In obesity, a 10% reduction in body weight leads to a significant increase in adiponectin (40% to 60%) in both diabetic and nondiabetic patients. Adiponectin is also involved in the modulation of inflammatory responses through attenuation of TNF-α–mediated inflammatory effects, regulation of endothelial function, and inhibition of growth factor–induced proliferation of vascular smooth muscle cells.

Leptin is a 167-amino-acid adipocyte-derived hormone that circulates in the plasma in free and bound forms. It affects energy balance by activating specific centers in the hypothalamus to

decrease food intake, increase energy expenditure, modulate glucose and fat metabolism, and alter neuroendocrine function. Leptin plasma levels increase exponentially with increased fat mass (fourfold higher in obese compared with lean individuals in one study), and this is thought to reflect resistance to leptin in obesity. Leptin therapy in lipodystrophic patients has been shown to lower blood glucose, improve insulin-stimulated hepatic and peripheral glucose metabolism, and reduce hepatic and muscle triglyceride content, suggesting that leptin acts as a signal that contributes to regulation of total body sensitivity to insulin. It has also been found that leptin is independently associated with cardiovascular mortality. Although both adiponectin and leptin are integrally related to insulin resistance, adiponectin is more strongly related to visceral abdominal fat stores, whereas leptin is more closely related to subcutaneous fat.

Adipose tissue serves as a major source of TNF-α and substantial amounts of IL-6. Levels of these two proinflammatory cytokines correlate with obesity and are strongly related to insulin resistance. Several studies have demonstrated a strong link between TNF-α and cardiovascular disease. Plasma levels of TNF-α are increased in individuals with premature cardiovascular disease independent of insulin sensitivity. Conversely, circulating levels of TNF-α decrease after weight reduction in parallel with improvements in endothelial function.

Resistin is an adipocyte-derived, cysteine-rich signaling protein that is expressed predominantly in white adipose tissue and is also detectable in serum. Resistin is thought to act at sites remote from adipose tissue, similar to other adipokines, and to contribute to insulin resistance in obesity. PAI-1 is another bioactive peptide produced by subcutaneous and visceral fat. Its circulating levels correlate better with visceral than with subcutaneous adiposity and are a strong predictor of CAD. High PAI-1 levels are associated with increased blood coagulability. Improvement in insulin sensitivity by either weight reduction or medication lowers circulating levels of PAI-1. This decrease in PAI-1 correlates with the amount of weight loss and the decline in serum triglycerides.

Visceral and subcutaneous fat differ in their production of specific adipokines, pointing to differences in endocrine function between these two adipose depots. Removal of a significant amount of only subcutaneous fat by liposuction in obese individuals with and without diabetes resulted in reduction in serum leptin but did not change the serum levels of other cytokines or any other metabolic parameters. It also did not improve insulin sensitivity or decrease the high serum insulin level observed initially in those individuals. In animal models, removal of subcutaneous fat resulted in an increase in mesenteric fat volume and increased production of TNF-α by visceral fat. Although surgical removal of visceral fat has not been attempted in humans, two studies of aging in rodent models showed that removal of visceral fat reduces the production of inflammatory adipokines and improves glucose tolerance and insulin sensitivity.

Risks Associated with Obesity

Overweight and obese individuals are at increased risk for the following health conditions:

- Cardiometabolic syndrome
- Type 2 diabetes (T2DM)
- Hypertension
- Dyslipidemia
- Coronary heart disease
- Congestive heart failure
- Atrial fibrillation
- Osteoarthritis
- Stroke
- Gall bladder disease
- Fatty liver and nonalcoholic steatohepatitis
- Sleep apnea
- Asthma
- Gastroesophageal reflux (GERD)
- Some cancers (endometrial, breast, and colon)
- Gynecologic disorders (abnormal menses, infertility, polycystic ovarian syndrome)

Weight loss of 7%-10% is associated with reduced risk for many if not all of these disorders. Recent studies have shown that significant weight reduction (15% to 25% of initial body weight) after gastric bypass surgery in class 2 and class 3 obese patients with T2DM results in transient remission of diabetes for 2 to 10 years. The relative importance of the weight loss itself and the hormonal changes associated with gastric bypass surgery to terms of diabetes remission is not yet understood.

DIAGNOSIS AND ASSESSMENT OF OBESITY

The form of obesity that characteristically occurs in men— android or abdominal obesity (apple-shaped body configuration)—is closely associated with metabolic complications such as insulin resistance, hypertension, dyslipidemia, and hyperuricemia. By contrast, the typical female or gynecoid obesity (pear-shaped body configuration), in which fat accumulates in the hips and gluteal and femoral regions, has milder metabolic complications. The waist-to-hip circumference ratio (WHR) has been used to distinguish these forms of obesity. A ratio greater than 1.0 in men or greater than 0.8 in women, indicative of visceral fat deposition and abdominal obesity, correlates with increased health risks.

Previously, the "gold standard" technique for measuring total body fat was hydrodensitometry (underwater weighing). This is based on the principle that fatty tissue is less dense than muscle. Currently, dual-energy x-ray absorptiometry (DEXA) scanning is used to accurately measure body composition, particularly fat mass and fat-free mass. It has an additional advantage of measuring regional fat distribution. DEXA is more accurate than anthropometric measures and is more cost-effective than computerized tomography (CT) or magnetic resonance imaging (MRI) scans. However, DEXA cannot distinguish between subcutaneous and visceral abdominal fat depots, nor between subcutaneous and intramuscular peripheral fat depots. Bioelectric impedance is a simpler and less expensive method for measuring total body fat, but it is greatly affected by the hydration state of the body and is less accurate overall than DEXA.

BMI is widely used as measure of obesity. It is calculated by dividing a person's body weight in kilograms by the square of the person's height in meters; alternatively, weight in pounds × 703 is divided by the square of the height in inches). A BMI between 19 and 27 has little association with cardiometabolic risk in whites. Adverse health consequences occur with a BMI of 27 or more and increase with increasing levels of BMI. Risks associated with increased BMI are more pronounced in older patients.

Waist circumference or WHR or both are often used to indirectly estimate intra-abdominal fat volume in epidemiologic studies. Although these measures show good correlation with intra-abdominal fat volume as measured by CT, they are less accurate than CT. At present, waist circumference is the easiest anthropometric measurement for routine use by health care professionals to estimate visceral adiposity and monitor changes in visceral fat volume.

The current gold standard techniques for measuring visceral fat volume are abdominal CT (at the L4-L5 vertebral level) and MRI. These methods are not widely used because of high cost and radiation exposure. In contrast to CT, MRI requires additional definition of adipose tissue by adjusting settings on the MRI scanner. Several commercial software packages are available for calculation of visceral fat volume, and it is possible to further subdivide body fat into at least three separate and measurable compartments: subcutaneous, intramuscular, and visceral fat.

Visceral fat volume determination by abdominal ultrasonography has been investigated for use in research and clinical settings. Several studies found good correlation between intra-abdominal fat volume measured by abdominal ultrasound and that measured by abdominal CT scanning. Measurements should be performed with the patient in the supine position at the end of a quiet inspiration with compression of the transducer against the abdomen. Intra-abdominal fat is quantified based on the distance between the peritoneum and the lumbar spine. Studies have shown that intra-abdominal fat measured by ultrasound has a stronger association with metabolic risk factors for CAD than does waist circumference or WHR. Recently, visceral fat has been measured using bioelectric impedance, but this technique is less accurate than CT.

⬤ TREATMENT OF OBESITY

Current guidelines for treatment of obesity are summarized in Table 67-1. The preferred intervention varies with the obesity level based on five BMI categories. The major four therapeutic options are lifestyle modification (diet and exercise), behavior modification, pharmacologic intervention, and bariatric surgery. In general, better results are obtained with a combination of different interventions rather than a single modality.

Lifestyle Modification

Key components of effective lifestyle modification most often include structured dietary interventions and individualized physical activity programs. Behavior modification strategies and patient education are also critical for achievement and maintenance of target weight loss. Evidence-based dietary guidelines should be used to design individualized patient plans in consultation with a registered dietitian or qualified health care provider. First, daily caloric intake should be reduced by a modest 250 to 500 calories. Reasonable and paced reductions can help patients continue on the recommended dietary plan for a longer time. Daily calories from carbohydrate should be reduced to approximately 40% to 45% of intake, with a total daily carbohydrate intake of no less than 130 g/day. Except in patients with renal impairment (creatinine clearance <60 mL/min) or significant microalbuminuria, protein intake should not be less than 1.2 g/kg of adjusted body weight (adjusted body weight = ideal body weight + 0.25 [current weight − ideal body weight]). This typically accounts for 20% to 30% of total calorie intake and is intended to minimize loss of lean body mass during weight reduction. The remaining 30% to 35% of calorie intake should come from fat. Trans-fats should be eliminated, and saturated fat should be reduced to less than 7% of total calorie intake. Meal plans should also include substantial soluble fiber (e.g., from fresh fruits and vegetables) and consumption of healthy carbohydrates, especially foods that are high in fiber and have a low glycemic index. Approximately 14 g of fiber per 1000 calories (20 to 35 g of fiber) per day is recommended.

Caloric intake should be adjusted downward over time until weight loss is achieved. Underlying all of these steps should be the goal of designing an individualized plan that can be maintained over the long term. Many patients find it helpful to receive a structured dietary intervention that includes specific suggestions for daily meals. Such structured diets may increase adherence and can be easier to follow than a list of general guidelines. Nutritionally complete meal replacement (e.g., in the form of shakes or bars) can be useful for some patients, especially at the start of a weight reduction program. If meal replacement is used, 100- to 200-calorie snacks (e.g., fruits and nuts) may be added at breakfast, lunch, or between meals.

Each patient should meet with an exercise physiologist to construct an individualized plan that is responsive to his or her lifestyles, capabilities, and potential cardiovascular risks. Because obese individuals frequently have difficulty exercising, this process requires careful attention. A balanced exercise plan incorporates a mix of cardiovascular, stretching, and strength exercises and should be graded to increase gradually in both duration and intensity. Patients can start with 10 to 20 minutes of daily stretching and aerobic exercise (e.g., moderate-intensity walking) with subsequent progressive increases. Any exercise

TABLE 67-1 GUIDE TO SELECTING TREATMENT BASED ON BMI CATEGORY*

TREATMENT	BMI CATEGORY				
	25-26.9	27-29.9	30-34.9	35-39.9	≧40
Diet, physical activity, behavior therapy	Yes with comorbidities	Yes with comorbidities	Yes	Yes	Yes
Pharmacotherapy		Yes with comorbidities	Yes	Yes	Yes
Weight-loss surgery			Yes with comorbidities	Yes with comorbidities	Yes with comorbidities

From National Institutes of Health (NIH), National Heart, Lung, and Blood Institute (NHLBI), North American Association for the Study of Obesity (NAASO): The practical guide to the identification, evaluation, and treatment of overweight and obesity in adults. NIH Publication No. 00-4084, Bethesda, Md., October 2000, NIH. http://www.nhlbi.nih.gov/files/docs/guidelines/prctgd_c.pdf. Accessed November 2014.

*"Yes" indicates that the treatment is indicated regardless of comorbidities.

secondary prevention of cardiovascu- by clinical trial evidence) or for primary ts with a 10-year cardiovascular risk greater d on expert opinion). Influenza vaccination ided yearly; pneumococcal immunization should ce and then repeated after age 65.

agement of Diabetes during ercurrent Illness

Diabetes often requires changes in the blood glucose management regimen during an intercurrent illness to accommodate potential decreases in nutrient intake and increases in insulin resistance secondary to disease-related release of stress hormones. Patients with T1DM require exogenous insulin administration at all times to prevent marked hyperglycemia and DKA, even if they are unable to consume nutrients during an illness (e.g., with gastroenteritis). Depending on the degree and duration of interruption of food intake, they may require a transient, partial reduction in insulin dosage as well as more frequent glucose monitoring. Alternatively, if they are consuming a normal diet, they may require a modest increase in insulin dose because of insulin resistance related to the stress of illness. T2DM patients taking oral agents who are undergoing surgical procedures or are hospitalized for serious illness often require discontinuation of the oral agents and use of insulin to control blood glucose until normal eating patterns are resumed.

For hospitalized patients, blood glucose target goals are adjusted to prevent marked hyperglycemia and at the same time protect against hypoglycemia. For noncritical illness, typical blood glucose targets include lowest levels of 90 to 100 mg/dL, premeal levels lower than 140 mg/dL, and random levels lower than 180 mg/dL. For critically ill patients, intravenous insulin infusion may be needed to allow for rapid adjustments in dosage, and the blood glucose range recommended by most expert panels is 140 to 180 mg/dL.

Gestational Diabetes

The hormonal environment of pregnancy results in insulin resistance and therefore predisposes to the development or unmasking of diabetes during pregnancy. GDM occurs in 2% to 5% of all pregnancies and is associated with consequences for both mother and fetus if untreated. For this reason, screening for GDM is routinely performed between 24 and 28 weeks of gestation in women older than 25 years of age and in younger women who fulfill one or more of the risk criteria in Table 66-6 (2a through 2d and 2g). Women who are at high risk (i.e., those who are obese, have a personal history of GDM, glycosuria, or have a first-degree relative with diabetes) should be screened earlier, at their initial obstetric or prenatal visit. A broadly accepted approach to screening is a 2-hour 75-g oral glucose tolerance test with cutoff values as specified in Table 66-2.

A detailed discussion of the approach to managing GDM and also preexisting diabetes during pregnancy is beyond the scope of this chapter. The fundamental principles include diet, exercise, and glucose-lowering oral agents or insulin as needed. Blood glucose goals are set lower than in nonpregnant individuals because of the importance of minimizing exposure of the fetus to hyperglycemia: fasting, 95 mg/dL (5.3 mmol/L) or lower;

1-hour postprandial, 140 mg/dL (7.8 mmol/L) or lower; and 2-hours postprandial, 120 mg/dL (6.7 mmol/L) or lower. HbA_{1c} levels may be useful in establishing the presence of hyperglycemia before its discovery during pregnancy, but they have limited value in managing GDM. Women with GDM should be reevaluated with a 75-g glucose tolerance test 6 to 12 weeks after delivery, at which point approximately 10% will still have overt diabetes. Up to 40% of women with GDM go on to develop diabetes in the subsequent 20 years, with this risk varying substantially depending on ethnic background and obesity. Pregnancy serves as a provocative test and not as a risk factor for the future development of diabetes.

Management of Severe Metabolic Decompensation in Diabetes

Diabetic Ketoacidosis

Diabetic ketoacidosis (DKA) develops most commonly in patients with T1DM (approximately 2.5 cases per 100 T1DM patients per year). It also can occur in those with T2DM, especially during acute illness (severe infection, medical illness, or trauma), and in a subset of *ketosis-prone* T2DM patients. DKA is present in approximately 25% of T1DM patients at diagnosis and otherwise most often develops when patients with known T1DM stop taking prescribed insulin. It is a potentially life-threatening condition that has an overall mortality rate of approximately 2.5%, with most deaths resulting from complicating or precipitating medical conditions rather than the metabolic disturbances of DKA itself.

The pathophysiology of DKA results from the combined effects of insulin deficiency and increased levels of *insulin counterregulatory (stress) hormones*. With insulin deficiency, glucose levels rise as a consequence of decreased uptake and metabolism by body tissues, the breakdown of hepatic glycogen stores (*glycogenolysis*), and net glucose production by the liver and kidney (*gluconeogenesis*). Catabolism of muscle proteins as a result of low insulin levels leads to the release of amino acids, which provide substrate that further drives gluconeogenesis. Because glucose is being synthesized endogenously, blood glucose levels rise markedly, even in the fasted state. Blood glucose levels greater than 170 mg/dL result in glycosuria. Excretion of glucose in the urine necessitates the co-excretion of large amounts of water and electrolytes (Na^+ and K^+). Patients experience polyuria but cannot compensate adequately and become progressively more fluid and electrolyte depleted. The osmotic diuresis is characterized by greater losses of water than electrolytes, and this leads to progressively increasing hyperosmolality. Because of insulin deficiency, there is decreased *lipogenesis* and accelerated *lipolysis* leading to increased levels of circulating free fatty acids, which serve as a substrate for the hepatic synthesis of ketone bodies (β-hydroxybutyrate, acetoacetate, and acetone). β-Hydroxybutyrate and acetoacetate are acids, and their rising plasma levels contribute to the development of a metabolic acidosis.

These processes can result from simple insulin deficiency, but often they are exacerbated by an underlying or precipitating illness, such as an infection. Infection results in insulin resistance secondary to increased levels of *stress hormones* (cortisol,

should be preceded by a warm-up period to minimize injuries.

Long-term lifestyle modification trials, such as the Diabetes Prevention Program, have targeted 150 minutes of exercise per week. Newer guidelines recommend 60 to 90 minutes of daily exercise, with a minimum of 150 to 175 minutes per week needed to obtain weight loss benefit. Emphasis should be placed on moderate-intensity exercise, such as walking 20-minute miles, rather than strenuous exercise. Because patients who are not used to exercising may find it difficult to incorporate physical activity into daily practice, it is also important to use a variety of exercises to maintain interest. Increasing exercise duration to 300 minutes/week was found to help in long-term maintenance of weight reduction. Frequent short bouts of exercise as brief as 10 minutes each can increase adherence to a regimen.

Behavior Modification and Patient Education

Cognitive-behavioral intervention and patient education are important components of successful weight loss programs. Whenever possible, cognitive-behavioral intervention should be conducted by an experienced psychologist. The fundamental principles of intervention typically include behavioral goal setting, stimulus control techniques, cognitive restructuring, assertive communication skills, stress management, and relapse prevention. Cognitive-behavioral support conducted in a group setting with weekly meetings is frequently successful. Patients should learn how to set *SMART* goals (*s*pecific, *m*easurable, *a*ction-oriented, *r*ealistic, *t*ime-limited). It can be helpful to emphasize real-life examples (e.g., success stories, logbook learning, recommitting to progress). The behavioral modification strategy should assist patients in identifying precipitants for deviations from a diet (e.g., timing, types of food or exercise, situations, feelings), overcoming challenges (planning ahead, delay and distraction, problem solving), managing automatic negative thinking ("detour thoughts"), coping with cravings through mindful strategic eating, preventing relapses using logbook learning, navigating social eating, and setting personal weight maintenance plans.

Pharmacologic Options

The four anti-obesity drugs currently licensed for use in the United States are orlistat, phentermine, lorcaserin, and the combination of phentermine and long-acting topiramate. Except for phentermine by itself, the three other medications are approved for long-term management of obesity.

Orlistat

Orlistat limits caloric intake through inhibition of the lipase-mediated breakdown of fat in the gastrointestinal tract. This mechanism results in an approximately 30% reduction of fat absorption and an increase in fecal fat content. In addition to weight loss, orlistat use has been associated with decreased incidence of diabetes, improved concentrations of total cholesterol and low-density lipoprotein (LDL)-cholesterol, and improved blood pressure and glycemic control in patients with diabetes. However, high-density lipoprotein (HDL)-cholesterol has been found to be slightly lowered. Most people develop side effects with variable degrees of diarrhea, flatulence, oily stools, fecal

urgency, and, rarely, fecal incontinence. There also is an increased risk of cholelithiasis. Gastrointestinal side events are usually proportional to the amount of fat intake. Supplemental fat-soluble vitamins A, D, E, and K must be taken to prevent possible deficiencies. The usual dose of orlistat is 120 mg before each meal. A 60 mg dose formulation is currently available over the counter; it is less effective but is also associated with fewer side effects.

Phentermine

Phentermine is approved for short-term treatment of obesity (up to 6 months). Because phentermine has actions similar to amphetamines, it can elevate blood pressure, increase heart rate, and stimulate the central nervous system (frequently causing insomnia), in addition to suppressing the appetite. The recommended phentermine dose is 30 mg once daily. Combining phentermine with tricyclic antidepressants or monoamine oxidase inhibitors may result in substantial increases in blood pressure and other serious reactions because of elevated serotonin levels in the blood.

Lorcaserin

Lorcaserin is a selective serotonin (5-hydroxytryptamine) receptor agonist with specificity for the 5-HT2C receptor subtype. The activation of these receptors in the hypothalamus is thought to activate production of proopiomelanocortin (POMC) and, consequently, to promote weight loss through satiety signals. Lorcaserin has 100-fold higher selectivity for 5-HT2C versus the closely related 5-HT2B receptor. Activation of the 5-HT2B receptor by the less selective agents fenfluramine and dexfenfluramine previously was linked to serious cardiac valvulopathy, but there is no evidence for this adverse effect with lorcaserin. Clinical trials showed that 47.5% of patients treated with lorcaserin lost at least 5% of their initial body weight, and 22.6% lost at least 10%, in 1 year. Lorcaserin treatment also resulted in significantly lower glycosylated hemoglobin (HbA$_{1c}$) values in patients with T2DM and improved lipid profile and decreased blood pressure in clinical studies.

Lorcaserin is approved for use as an adjunct to a reduced-calorie diet and exercise for chronic weight management in patients with initial BMI values of 30 kg/m^2 or higher and in those with BMI values of 27 kg/m^2 or higher with at least one weight-related comorbid condition (e.g., hypertension, dyslipidemia, T2DM). It is given in a dose of 10 mg twice daily. Side effects usually are mild to moderate, with the most common being headache, upper respiratory tract infection, nasopharyngitis, sinusitis, dizziness, nausea, and fatigue. The U.S. Drug Enforcement Administration has classified lorcaserin as a schedule IV drug because it has hallucinogenic properties that could lead to psychiatric complications.

Phentermine and Long-Acting Topiramate

Phentermine is an appetite suppressant and stimulant of the amphetamine and phenethylamine class (see earlier discussion for details on the use of phentermine alone for weight reduction). Topiramate is an anticonvulsant that was found to have weight loss side effects. The combination of phentermine plus low doses of topiramate has been shown to have synergistic effects on weight loss. As with lorcaserin, this combination tablet is indicated as an adjunct to a reduced-calorie diet and exercise for chronic weight management. Clinical trials showed that average weight loss after 1 year of 10.9% for patients receiving the maximum dose (phentermine/topiramate, 15 mg/92 mg) and 5.1% for those taking the recommended starting dose (3.75 mg/23 mg). The drug is taken once daily in the morning to avoid insomnia caused by the phentermine component. The initial dose of 3.75 mg/23 mg is given for 2 weeks before titration to 7.5 mg/46 mg for another 12 weeks. If a patient has not lost at least 3% of baseline body weight on the higher dosage, the drug may be discontinued or the dose may be escalated to 11.25 mg/69 mg for an additional 2 weeks before a further increase to the maximum dose of 15 mg/92 mg. If a patient has not lost at least 5% of baseline body weight after 12 weeks, the drug is discontinued gradually. Side effects include paresthesias, dry mouth, constipation, metabolic acidosis, nasopharyngitis, upper respiratory infection, and headache.

Data indicate that fetuses exposed during the first trimester to topiramate (when used alone as an anticonvulsant) have an increased risk (9.6%) of cleft lip with or without cleft palate. Therefore, the drug should not be given to women of childbearing age unless an effective method of contraception is used and a pregnancy test is conducted monthly during use. Phentermine/topiramate may increase resting heart rate up to 20 beats/minute, so the drug should be used cautiously in patients with a history of cardiac or cerebrovascular disease. Topiramate also increases the risk of suicidal thoughts or behaviors and mood disorders including depression, anxiety, and insomnia. It can also cause cognitive dysfunction, including impairment of concentration or attention, difficulty with memory, and speech or language problems, particularly word-finding difficulties. It is contraindicated in patients with closed-angle glaucoma because it increases intraocular pressure and the risk of permanent loss of vision.

Contrave is a combination of Bupropion and Naltrexone just approved by the FDA for weight loss (Medical Letter November 10, 2014).

Bariatric Surgery

At present, there are three broad categories of bariatric surgical procedures: (1) pure gastric restriction; (2) gastric restriction with some malabsorption, as represented by the Roux-en-Y gastric bypass (RYGB) procedure; and (3) gastric restriction with significant intestinal malabsorption (discussed later). The number of bariatric procedures performed in the United States increased from an estimated 13,365 in 1998 to almost 220,000 in 2008. Bariatric surgery is considered to be indicated for adults with class 3 obesity (BMI ≥40 kg/m²). In patients with less severe obesity (BMI 35 to 40 kg/m²), bariatric surgery can be considered if there are one or more high-risk comorbid conditions present, such as life-threatening cardiopulmonary disease (e.g., severe sleep apnea, obesity-related cardiomyopathy) or uncontrolled T2DM. Bariatric surgery is sometimes performed for patients with diabetes or metabolic syndrome and a BMI of 30 to 35 kg/m², although current evidence on benefit is limited. For teenagers younger than 17 years old who have attained skeletal maturity (usually by 13 years for girls and 15 years for boys), bariatric surgery has been recommended with different guidelines: BMI 35 to 40 kg/m² with at least one serious comorbid condition (e.g., T2DM, obstructive sleep apnea, pseudotumor cerebri) or BMI 50 kg/m² or higher with less serious comorbidities. Contraindications for bariatric surgery include high operative risk (e.g., congestive heart failure, unstable angina), active substance abuse, and significant psychopathology.

Different types of commonly used bariatric procedures are shown in Figure 67-1. Gastric restriction procedures induce weight loss by producing early satiety and limiting food intake. Gastric restriction by vertical banded gastroplasty (VBG) typically limits the volume of the upper gastric pouch into which the esophagus empties to 15 to 45 mL and restricts the pouch outlet to the remaining stomach to 10 to 11 ml. Currently, the laparoscopic adjustable gastric band (LAGB) has almost completely replaced the VBG procedure, because it is less invasive, adjustable, and reversible and has better outcomes.

LAGB is associated with substantially better maintenance of weight loss than lifestyle intervention alone, and it carries a very low operative mortality rate (0.1%). However, it is associated with significantly lower loss of excess weight at 5 years and 10 years and with smaller reductions in fat-free mass compared with RYGB. LAGB has been demonstrated to be safe in patients older than 55 years of age. Complications associated with the LAGB procedure include band slippage, band erosion, balloon failure, injection port malposition, band and port infections, and esophageal dilatation. Some of these problems have been decreased by use of a different method of band insertion and revision of the port connection. Overall, complication and

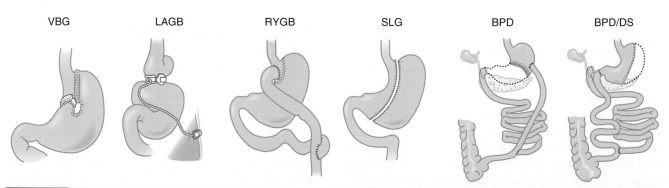

VBG   LAGB   RYGB   SLG   BPD   BPD/DS

FIGURE 67-1 Common bariatric procedures. BPD, Biliopancreatic diversion; VBG, Vertical banded gastroplasty; LAGB, laparoscopic adjustable gastric band; RYGB, Roux-en-Y gastric bypass; SLG, sleeve gastrectomy; BPD, biliopancreatic diversion; BPD/DS, BPD with duodenal switch.

mortality rates are much lower for LAGB than for RYGB. Nevertheless, RYGB is currently the most commonly performed bariatric procedure in the United States because it achieves greater weight loss.

In RYGB, the upper stomach is transected, thereby creating a very small proximal gastric pouch measuring 10 to 30 mL. The gastric pouch is anastomosed to a Roux-en-Y proximal jejunal segment, bypassing the remaining stomach, duodenum, and a small portion of jejunum. The standard Roux (alimentary) limb length is about 50 to 100 cm, and the biliopancreatic limb is 15 to 50 cm. As a result, the RYGB serves to limit food intake and induces some nutrient malabsorption.

Sleeve gastrectomy (SLG) is another restrictive surgery in which the stomach is reduced to about 25% of its original size by surgical removal of a large portion of the stomach fundus, resulting in a tube-like structure. Although the procedure permanently reduces stomach size, some dilatation of the stomach may occur later. The procedure is frequently performed by a laparoscopic technique. Because it has low operative risk, the use of sleeve gastrectomy currently is increasing more rapidly than other types of bariatric surgery. Other procedures, including biliopancreatic diversion (BPD), biliopancreatic diversion with duodenal switch (BPD/DS), and staged bariatric surgical procedures, are less commonly performed.

There is a need for more data to guide the choice of bariatric procedures for individual patients. Most procedures currently are being performed laparoscopically. This approach has the advantages of fewer wound complications, less postoperative pain, a shorter hospital stay, and more rapid postoperative recovery with comparable efficacy. However, these advantages may be offset by more frequent complications associated with techniques used for laparoscopic gastrojejunostomy creation, anastomotic strictures, and higher rates of postoperative bowel obstructions.

The Agency for Healthcare Research and Quality (AHRQ) identified a 0.19% in-hospital mortality rate for all bariatric discharges in the United States. A recent meta-analysis showed that mortality rate from bariatric surgery within 30 days was 0.08% and the mortality rate after 30 days was 0.31%. Bariatric surgery is not uniformly a "low-risk" procedure, and judicious patient selection and diligent perioperative care are mandatory. Preoperative patient selection and education as well as careful postsurgical follow-up are important for successful outcomes.

The benefits of bariatric surgery extend beyond calorie restriction and weight loss. Foregut bypass leads to improvement in the physiologic responses of gut hormones involved in glucose regulation and appetite control, including ghrelin, glucagon-like peptide-1 (GLP-1) and peptide YY[3-36] (PYY). Mechanical improvements include less weight-bearing burden on joints, improved lung compliance, and reduced fatty tissue around the neck, which can relieve obstruction to breathing and sleep apnea.

In an extensive meta-analysis of 22,000 bariatric surgeries, patients lost on average 61% of excess body weight and exhibited improvements in T2DM, hypertension, sleep apnea, and dyslipidemia. The beneficial effect of obesity surgery on T2DM is one of the most important outcomes observed, with gastric bypass and malabsorptive procedures having the greatest impact. A shorter duration of diabetes and greater weight loss are independent predictors of diabetes remission after bariatric surgery.

Improvements in fasting blood glucose levels occur before significant weight loss is achieved. Insulin-treated patients experience significant decreases in insulin requirements, and most T2DM patients are able to discontinue insulin therapy by 6 weeks after surgery. Euglycemia is maintained in some patients for up to 14 years after RYGB. Two recent randomized controlled studies compared RYGB to intensive lifestyle intervention in moderately obese patients with T2DM and found RYGB to be superior in inducing diabetes remission and reducing use of antihyperglycemic medications.

Weight loss after malabsorptive bariatric surgery usually reaches a nadir after 12 to 18 months. Over the following decade, there is weight regain of approximately 10% of body weight. Weight loss is more gradual for the restrictive LAGB procedure and may continue for several years. In purely restrictive procedures, failure to experience optimal weight loss has been associated with consumption of calorically dense liquids that can pass through the stoma without producing satiety.

PROGNOSIS

Although recent clinical data show that patients on average can maintain a 4% to 5% weight loss for 10 years with ongoing medically supervised intensive lifestyle intervention, many patients are subjected to less intensive intervention and regain their initial weight loss over months or years. Weight regain even after bariatric surgery is not uncommon and most often occurs after 2 years of peak weight loss. Loss of 10% to 20% of the initial body weight is associated with a decrease in total and resting energy expenditure, a change that retards further weight loss. Similarly, weight gain is associated with an increase in energy expenditure, which retards further weight gain. These observations suggest that the human body adopts a biologic set point or mechanism that tends to maintain body weight, and they lend support to the theory that behavior is not the sole determinant of obesity. Although long-term intensive lifestyle intervention in obese patients with T2DM resulting in approximately 5% body weight loss can significantly decrease the risks of chronic kidney disease and depression and further improve glucose control, blood pressure, physical fitness, and some lipid parameters, it has not been shown to reduce cardiovascular events or mortality. Further understanding of genetic and hormonal regulation of obesity may help researchers create more effective and long-lasting interventional tools.

For a deeper discussion on this topic, please see Chapter 220, "Obesity," in Goldman-Cecil Medicine, 25th Edition.

SUGGESTED READINGS

Aldahi W, Hamdy O: Adipokines, inflammation, and the endothelium in diabetes, Curr Diabetes Rep 3:293–298, 2003.

Angrisani L, Lorenzo M, Borrelli V: Laparoscopic adjustable gastric banding versus Roux-en-Y gastric bypass: 5-year results of a prospective randomized trial, Surg Obes Relat Dis 3:127–134, 2007.

Chang SH, Stoll CR, Song J, et al: The effectiveness and risks of bariatric surgery: an updated systematic review and meta-analysis, 2003–2012, JAMA Surg 149:275–287, 2014.

Després J-P, Moorjani S, Lupien PJ, et al: Regional distribution of body fat, plasma lipoproteins, and cardiovascular disease, Arteriosclerosis 10:497–511, 1990.

Hamdy O: The role of adipose tissue as an endocrine gland, Curr Diabetes Rep. 5:317–319, 2005.

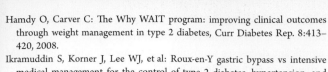

Hamdy O, Carver C: The Why WAIT program: improving clinical outcomes through weight management in type 2 diabetes, Curr Diabetes Rep. 8:413–420, 2008.

Ikramuddin S, Korner J, Lee WJ, et al: Roux-en-Y gastric bypass vs intensive medical management for the control of type 2 diabetes, hypertension, and hyperlipidemia: the Diabetes Surgery Study randomized clinical trial, JAMA 309:2240–2249, 2013.

Look AHEAD Research Group, Wing RR, Bolin P, et al: Cardiovascular effects of intensive lifestyle intervention in type 2 diabetes, N Engl J Med 369:145–154, 2013.

Maggard MA, Shugarman LR, Suttorp M, et al: Meta-analysis: surgical treatment of obesity, Ann Intern Med 142:547–559, 2005.

Schauer PR, Kashyap SR, Wolski K, et al: Bariatric surgery versus intensive medical therapy in obese patients with diabetes, N Engl J Med 366:1567–1576, 2012.

Sjostrom L, Lindroos AK, Peltonen M, et al: Swedish Obese Subjects Study Scientific Group. Lifestyle, diabetes, and cardiovascular risk factors 10 years after bariatric surgery, N Engl J Med 351:2683–2693, 2004.

Strauss RS, Bradley LJ, Brolin RE: Gastric bypass surgery in adolescents with morbid obesity, J Pediatr 138:499–504, 2001.

Malnutrition, Nutritional Assessment, and Nutritional Support in Hospitalized Adults

Thomas R. Ziegler

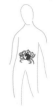

MALNUTRITION IN HOSPITALIZED PATIENTS

Numerous surveys conducted in developed countries in the 21st century continue to demonstrate the frequent rate of protein-energy malnutrition as well as depletion of specific micronutrients in patients with chronic illnesses and those requiring elective or emergent hospital admission. Hospitalized patients commonly receive inadequate amounts of calories, protein, vitamins, and minerals during their stay, and ad libitum intake of prescribed diets is typically inadequate. Studies have shown that worsening of malnutrition during hospitalization is common. This is problematic, because adequate intake of essential macronutrients (energy, carbohydrate, protein/amino acids, and fats) and micronutrients (vitamins, minerals, and electrolytes) is critical for optimal cellular and organ structure and function, muscle mass, tissue repair, immune function, ambulatory capacity, and patient recovery. Significant erosion of lean body mass (predominately derived from skeletal muscle) and deficiencies of specific vitamins and minerals are variously associated with weakness and fatigue, increased rates of infection, impaired wound healing, and delayed convalescence. This relationship is especially apparent in patients with chronic protein-energy malnutrition and body weight loss associated with illness.

Patients with acute or chronic illnesses typically have experienced several days to several months of continuous or intermittent decreased food intake due to anorexia, gastrointestinal symptoms, depression and anxiety, and other medical factors. They may also have had food intake restricted by surgical operations or diagnostic or therapeutic procedures and recovery from these. Some patients have abnormal nutrient losses due to diarrhea (e.g., with chronic malabsorptive and maldigestive disorders or infectious diarrhea), vomiting, polyuria (as in uncontrolled diabetes mellitus), wound drainage, dialysis, or other causes. Certain drugs, including corticosteroids, chemotherapeutic agents, antirejection drugs, and diuretics, are associated with skeletal muscle breakdown, gastrointestinal injury, or loss of electrolytes or water-soluble vitamins. Bedrest or markedly decreased ambulation are common in outpatient and inpatient settings and are associated with skeletal muscle wasting and impaired protein synthesis.

Catabolic and critical illnesses are associated with concomitantly increased blood concentrations of "counterregulatory" hormones derived from the adrenal glands and pancreas (e.g., cortisol, catecholamines, glucagon); release of pro-inflammatory cytokines from stimulated immune, endothelial, and epithelial cells, such as interleukins (e.g., IL-1, IL-6, IL-8) and tumor necrosis factor-α (TNF-α); and peripheral tissue resistance to anabolic hormones such as insulin and insulin-like growth factor-I (IGF-I). These hormonal and cytokine alterations increase the availability of endogenous metabolic substrates that are critical for cellular and organ function, wound healing, and host survival (e.g., glucose via glycogenolysis and gluconeogenesis, amino acids via skeletal muscle breakdown, and free fatty acids via lipolysis). This combination of decreased nutrient intake and increased tissue nutrient losses (from the actions of these hormones and cytokines), coupled with increased energy (calorie), protein, and micronutrient needs due to inflammation, infection, and cytokinemia, is responsible for the wasting and micronutrient depletion commonly observed in medical patients with acute and chronic illnesses. Common causes of protein-energy malnutrition and micronutrient depletion in medical patients are shown in Table 68-1. Obesity has become a widespread medical problem and is also a form of malnutrition; it is considered in detail in Chapter 67.

NUTRITIONAL ASSESSMENT

Serial assessment of nutritional status is a critically important component of routine medical care. The major objectives are to detect preexisting depletion of body protein, energy reserves, and micronutrients; to identify risk factors for malnutrition (see Table 68-1); and to take steps to prevent nutrient deficiencies, depletion of lean body mass, and loss of skeletal muscle. There are still no practical "gold standard" tests that can provide an index of general nutritional status. Blood concentrations of specific micronutrients (e.g., copper, zinc, thiamine, 25-hydroxyvitamin D, vitamin B_6, folate, vitamin B_{12}) and electrolytes (e.g., magnesium, potassium, phosphorus) are important to guide needs and repletion responses. Nutritional assessment involves an integration of multiple factors, including the patient's medical and surgical history, type and severity of the acute or chronic underlying illness and its anticipated

TABLE 68-1	COMMON CAUSES OF PROTEIN-ENERGY MALNUTRITION AND MICRONUTRIENT DEPLETION IN MEDICAL PATIENTS WITH ACUTE OR CHRONIC ILLNESSES

Decreased spontaneous food intake due to anorexia from chronic or acute illness, gastrointestinal symptoms (e.g., nausea, vomiting, abdominal pain), or depression and anxiety

Restricted food intake required for surgical operations or diagnostic or therapeutic procedures and gastrointestinal dysfunction after these procedures

Abnormal macronutrient and micronutrient losses from the body due to malabsorption (e.g., celiac sprue, short gut syndrome, inflammatory bowel disease, cystic fibrosis, diarrhea), maldigestion (e.g., pancreatitis), emesis, polyuria (e.g., in diabetes), wound drainage, or renal replacement therapy

Periods of increased energy expenditure (caloric needs), protein requirements, and micronutrient needs (e.g., critical illness, increased inflammation)

Catabolic effects of counterregulatory hormones (e.g., cortisol, catecholamines, glucagon), release of pro-inflammatory cytokines from stimulated immune cells and endothelial and epithelial cells such as interleukins (e.g., IL-1, IL-6, IL-8) and tumor necrosis factor-α (TNF-α), and peripheral tissue resistance to the anabolic hormones insulin and insulin-like growth factor-I (IGF-I).

Bedrest, decreased ambulation, and chemical paralysis during mechanical ventilation (skeletal muscle wasting due to impaired protein synthesis)

Administration of drugs that induce skeletal muscle breakdown, gastrointestinal injury, or loss of electrolytes and water-soluble vitamins (e.g., corticosteroids, chemotherapeutic agents, diuretics, antirejection regimens)

Socioeconomic deprivation, inadequate caregivers, ambulation difficulties in the home setting

Inadequate provision of calories, protein, and essential micronutrients (vitamins, minerals, trace elements) during hospitalization

medical and surgical course, fluid drainage sites and amounts, physical examination findings, history of body weight change (degree and temporal aspects), dietary intake pattern, use of nutritional supplements including prior administration of specialized enteral nutrition (EN) or parenteral nutrition (PN), evaluation of current organ function and fluid status, and determination of selected vitamin, mineral, and electrolyte concentrations in blood (E-Table 68-1). In the intensive care unit (ICU) setting, measured body weight typically reflects recent intravenous fluid administration and is typically much higher than recent "dry" or preoperative body weight, which is the best parameter to use.

Integration of the factors outlined in E-Table 68-1 provides important information on whether patients are likely to be adequately nourished; to have mild, moderate, or severe protein-energy malnutrition; or to have depletion or deficiency of specific vitamins, minerals, or electrolytes. Patients who have experienced an involuntary body weight loss of 5% to 10% or more of their usual body weight in the previous few weeks or months, those who weigh less than 90% of their ideal body weight (IBW), and those who have a body mass index (BMI) lower than 18.5 kg/m^2 should be carefully evaluated, because these individuals are likely to be malnourished.

Among hospitalized patients, especially those in the ICU, circulating concentrations of proteins (e.g., albumin, prealbumin) are often quite low and not useful as protein nutritional status biomarkers given their lack of specificity. Plasma concentrations of albumin and prealbumin typically fall during active inflammation or infection, in critical illness, and after traumatic injury (due to deceased synthesis by the liver and catabolism of blood proteins).They are markedly affected by non-nutritional factors,

including fluid status, capillary leak, decreased hepatic synthesis, and increased clearance from blood. Because of the long circulating half-life of albumin (18 to 21 days), concentrations in blood remain low despite adequate feeding and are slow to respond to nutritional repletion, irrespective of other confounding factors. Prealbumin has a much shorter circulating half-life (several days), and serial blood levels can be used as a general indicator of protein status in clinically stable outpatients. E-Table 68-2 illustrates physical examination findings that may be observed in associated with depletion of specific nutrients.

Energy requirements can be estimated with the use of standard equations, such as the Harris-Benedict equation, which incorporate the patient's age, gender, weight, and height to determine basal energy expenditure (BEE) (see E-Table 68-1). Physical activity and the thermic effect of macronutrient administration can be added to the BEE to arrive at the energy prescription to maintain current body weight; for most hospitalized patients and outpatients, this is estimated as 1.2 to 1.3 times the BEE, unless energy needs are decreased because the patient is sedated or on bedrest (common in the ICU). The estimated maintenance energy requirement is approximately 1.3 times BEE in ambulatory subjects. Typically, lower amounts of calories are now given in ICU patients (as discussed later). Use of data obtained from a bedside metabolic cart machine (indirect calorimeter), which measures expired breath to determine oxygen consumption and carbon dioxide production, provides accurate actual energy expenditure in most settings and can be very useful (see E-Table 68-1).

A simple and relatively accurate method to estimate energy needs is simply to use 20 to 25 kcal/day per kilogram of actual weight, dry weight, or IBW in most patients. Values for IBW are obtained from standard tables or equations. This estimation assumes that the body weight used does not reflect intravenous fluid administration or capillary leak syndromes (discussed earlier). In ICU patients, even lower caloric doses (equivalent to 15-20 kcal/kg dry weight/day) have been advocated by some, based on known complications of overfeeding (see later discussion) and limited data on clinical outcome as a function of energy dose. In clinically stable, malnourished, non-ICU patients who require nutritional repletion, higher doses of calories (up to 35 kcal/kg/day) appear to be generally well tolerated if refeeding syndrome is avoided (see later discussion). In obese subjects (defined for these calculations as patients with body weight >20% to 25% greater than ideal), an adjusted body weight value should be used for calculation of energy and protein needs, as determined by the following equation:

$$\text{Adjusted body weight} = (\text{current weight} - \text{IBW}) \times 0.25 + \text{IBW}$$

Guidelines for protein or amino acid administration are given in E-Table 68-3. Studies in nonburned ICU patients indicate that protein loads of more than 2.0 g/kg/day are not efficiently utilized for protein synthesis, and the excess may be oxidized, contributing to azotemia. In most catabolic patients requiring specialized feeding, a recommended protein dose is 1.5 g/kg/day for individuals with normal renal function. This is about twice the recommended dietary allowance (RDA) for healthy adults of 0.8 g/kg/day. The administered protein dose should be adjusted downward as a function of the degree and tempo of azotemia (in the absence of dialysis therapy) and of hyperbilirubinemia (see

E-Table 68-3). These strategies take into account the relative inability of catabolic patients to efficiently utilize exogenous nutrients and knowledge that most protein and lean tissue repletion occurs over a period of several weeks to months during posthospital convalescence. Adequate nonprotein energy is essential to allow amino acids to be effectively used for protein synthesis and not oxidized for production of energy (adenosine triphosphate, or ATP). The ratio of nonprotein calories to nitrogen used in most centers typically ranges from 75 : 1 to 125 : 1. Because nitrogen = protein/6.25, this equates to 75 to 125 nonprotein kilocalories for each 6.25 g of protein or amino acid administered.

NUTRITIONAL SUPPORT

Table 68-2 lists common clinical scenarios in which specialized oral/EN or PN support may be indicated. In these settings, consultation with a multidisciplinary nutrition support team, if available, has been shown to reduce complications and costs and to increase the appropriate use of EN and PN in both academic and community medical centers.

Oral Nutrition Support

Oral nutrition supplementation includes provision of balanced oral diets of usual foods supplemented with complete liquid (or solid) nutrient products, protein supplements (e.g., hydrolyzed whey or casein powder that can be mixed with dietary beverages), high-potency multivitamin-multimineral supplements, and/or specific micronutrients required to treat a diagnosed deficiency (e.g., zinc, copper, vitamin B_6, vitamin B_{12}, vitamin D). Special supplements designed for patients with chronic renal failure (featuring concentrated calories and low amounts of protein and electrolytes) are available, as are a variety of formulations designed for other specific disease categories (see later discussion). Several studies have shown that convalescence after stresses such as total hip replacement or gastrointestinal surgery

TABLE 68-2	SOME CLINICAL INDICATIONS FOR SPECIALIZED ORAL/ENTERAL OR PARENTERAL NUTRITION SUPPORT

Patient currently exhibits moderate to severe protein or protein-energy malnutrition or has evidence of specific deficiency of one or more essential micronutrients

Patient with involuntary body weight loss of 5-10% or more of their usual body weight in the previous few weeks or months, weighs less than 90% of ideal body weight, or has a BMI lower than 18.5 kg/m^2.

Dietary food intake in a hospital or outpatient setting likely to be <50% of needs for more than 5-10 days due to underlying illness

Patient with severe catabolic stress (e.g., ICU care, serious infection) and adequate nutrient intake unlikely for >3-5 days.

After major gastrointestinal surgery or other major operation (e.g., hip replacement, partial organ resection)

Medical illness associated with prolonged (>5-10 days) GI dysfunction (diarrhea, nausea and vomiting, GI bleeding, severe ileus, partial obstruction) and/or short bowel syndrome, chronic or severe diarrhea, or other malabsorptive disorders

Clinical settings in which adequate oral food intake may be contraindicated or otherwise significantly decreased, such as respiratory or other acute or severe organ failure, dementia, dysphagia, chemotherapy or irradiation, inflammatory bowel disease, pancreatitis, high-output enterocutaneous fistula, alcoholism, drug addiction

Chronic obstructive lung disease, chronic infection, or other chronic inflammatory or catabolic disorders with documented poor nutrient intake and/or recent weight loss

BMI, Body mass index; GI, gastrointestinal; ICU, intensive care unit; PN, parenteral nutrition.

is enhanced with the addition of one or two containers per day of complete liquid nutrient supplements. These provide calories, carbohydrate, high-quality protein, fat, and micronutrients; are lactose and gluten free; and may contain small peptides and medium-chain triglycerides to facilitate absorption of amino acid and fat, respectively. Some formulations also contain soluble fiber or prebiotics (e.g., fructo-oligosaccharides) designed to decrease diarrhea. It is probably prudent to place outpatients who exhibit or are at risk for undernutrition (see E-Tables 68-1 and 68-2) and can tolerate oral medications on a potent oral multivitamin-multimineral preparation, at least for several months.

Administration of Enteral Tube Feeding

Patients with conditions outlined in Table 68-2 may have a functional gastrointestinal tract and yet be unable to consume adequate diet orally due to medical or surgical conditions (e.g., mechanically ventilation, pancreatitis, dementia, dysphagia, trauma or burns). Although PN is commonly administered in these settings, this practice is not evidence based; academic guidelines strongly suggest that oral nutritional supplements or enteral tube feedings should be used if specialized nutrition support is indicated in patients with a functional gastrointestinal tract ("if the gut works, use it"). E-Table 68-4 shows major characteristics of common complete liquid tube feeding formulations and the types of patients for which these are typically prescribed. These products can be used for oral nutrient supplementation as tolerated. When delivered in appropriate amounts, the liquid diets provide complete nutrition for most patients, although some ICU patients and patients with malabsorption or other conditions may have special needs (see later discussion).

The feedings can be delivered by conventional nasogastric tubes into the stomach or by small-bore nasogastric or nasojejunal tubes, percutaneous gastrostomy or jejunostomy tubes, or percutaneous gastrojejunostomy tubes (in which the gastric port may be used for suction and the jejunal port for feeding). Gastric feedings can be administered by either continuous or bolus feeds, whereas small bowel feeds must employ a continuous slow infusion using an infusion pump to avoid diarrhea. Tube feedings should be initiated at a slow rate (e.g., 10 to 20 mL/hour) for 8 to 24 hours and slowly advanced to the goal rate in 8- to 24-hour increments to deliver the calculated caloric and protein needs over the next 24 to 48 hours, depending on clinical tolerance and clinical conditions. Recent guidelines emphasize placing tube-fed patients in the semirecumbent position (e.g., increase head of bed), advancing feedings cautiously (with serial evaluations for diarrhea, nausea, emesis, abdominal distention, and significant gastric residuals), and using prokinetic agents and/or postpyloric feedings if gastric feedings are not well tolerated. Recent data suggest that higher volumes of gastric residuals (e.g., >250 mL) are usually well tolerated in patients being tube fed.

Primarily based on results of animal studies, EN is associated with improved gut barrier function, decreased infectious complications, less hypermetabolism, and decreased morbidity and mortality in catabolic models, compared with PN. Salutary clinical outcomes have been shown in randomized clinical trials in patients with pancreatitis receiving EN into the jejunum, compared with PN. Based on available data, recent guidelines for ICU patients by international expert panels and academic societies suggest that enteral tube feeds should be started within 1 to 3 days after ICU admission if adequate caloric needs (e.g., >60%) cannot be achieved with oral diet and supplements alone, especially for patients with existing malnutrition. Many studies have shown that ICU patients actually receive only 60% to 75% of the amount of tube feeding ordered by physicians. This can occur because of tube feeding intolerance (e.g., high gastric residuals, emesis, diarrhea, tube dislodgement) or discontinuation of feeding for diagnostic tests or therapeutic interventions. Although supplemental PN (see later discussion) is commonly ordered in patients who are not able to achieve tube feeding rates adequate for their needs, this practice remains controversial because of the limited number of good clinical trials. Rigorous studies are now in progress to address the efficacy of this approach, motivated by data suggesting that an increase in net caloric deficit (i.e., the difference between daily calorie requirements and daily actual calories delivered, summed over time) is associated with worse clinical outcomes in medical and surgical ICU patients.

Most outpatients and hospitalized ICU and non-ICU patients tolerate standard, inexpensive enteral formulas delivered via gastric or intestinal routes that provide between 1.0 and 1.5 kcal/mL. A large variety of enteral tube feeding products is available for clinical use. The specific product chosen should be based both on clinical conditions and underlying organ function, as outlined in E-Table 68-4. Because EN products can be marketed without efficacy data from randomized, controlled clinical trials, there remains a clear need for such trials to determine optimal EN formulations for different clinical conditions.

Complications of enteral feeding include diarrhea. Diarrhea is common in hospital patients receiving tube feedings but is typically caused by factors independent of the feeding, including administration of antibiotics, sorbitol-containing or hypertonic medications (e.g., acetaminophen elixir), and infections. Diarrhea caused by tube feeding itself does occur with rapid formula administration, in patients with underlying gut mucosal disease, and in those with severe hypoalbuminemia, which causes bowel wall edema. A fiber-containing enteral formula is sometimes useful to decrease diarrhea. Other complications of tube feeding include aspiration of tube feedings into the lung; mechanical problems with nasally placed feeding tubes, including discomfort, sinusitis, pharyngeal or esophageal mucosal erosion due to local tube trauma; and, with percutaneous feeding tubes, entrance site leakage, skin breakdown, cellulitis, and pain. Metabolic complications of tube feeding include fluid imbalances, hyperglycemia, electrolyte abnormalities, azotemia, and, occasionally, refeeding syndrome (discussed later). In general, if tube feedings are deemed to be required for more than 4 to 6 weeks, a percutaneous feeding tube should be placed.

In tube-fed patients who are receiving either subcutaneous or intravenous insulin to control hyperglycemia, significant hypoglycemia due to the continued actions of insulin may occur if tube feedings are discontinued inadvertently or for diagnostic or therapeutic tests. Hospitalized patients receiving tube feedings should have their blood glucose concentration monitored on a daily basis (or several times per day as indicated) and their blood electrolytes (including magnesium, potassium, and phosphorus) and renal function monitored several times each week (or daily in the ICU setting). Other blood chemistries should be determined at least weekly. This should be accompanied by close monitoring of intake and output records (including urine, stool, and drainage outputs) and gastrointestinal tolerance. When patients are able to consume oral food, tube feeding should be decreased and then discontinued (e.g., with daily calorie counts by a registered dietitian). For patients requiring home tube feeding, it is important to consult social service professionals to ensure appropriate care and follow-up.

Administration of Parenteral Nutrition

The basic principle in considering PN therapy is that the patient must be unable to achieve adequate nutrient intake via the enteral route. PN support includes administration of standard complete nutrient mixtures that contain dextrose, L-amino acids, lipid emulsion, electrolytes, vitamins, and minerals (in addition to certain medications as indicated, such as insulin or octreotide), given via a peripheral or central vein. Administration of complete PN therapy to patients with gastrointestinal tract dysfunction has become a standard of care in most hospitals and ICUs throughout the world, although use in individual institutions varies widely. PN is life-saving in patients with intestinal failure (e.g., short bowel syndrome). Existing data indicate that PN benefits patients with preexisting moderate to severe malnutrition or critical illness by decreasing overall morbidity, and possibly mortality, compared with patients receiving inadequate EN or hydration (intravenous dextrose) therapy alone. A consensus is emerging, based on recent rigorous studies in critical illness, that PN should probably not be initiated until days 3 to 4 after ICU admission in patients who are unable to tolerate adequate EN.

Compared with PN, EN is less expensive, probably maintains intestinal mucosal structure and function to a greater extent, is safer in terms of mechanical and metabolic complications (see later discussion), and is associated with reduced rates of nosocomial infection. Therefore, the enteral route of feeding should be used and advanced whenever possible, and the amount of administered PN should be correspondingly reduced.

Generally recognized indications for PN include the following situations:

1. Patients with short bowel syndrome or other conditions causing intestinal failure (e.g., motility disorders, obstruction, severe ileus, severe inflammatory bowel disease), especially those with preexisting malnutrition.
2. Clinically stable patients in whom adequate enteral feeding (e.g., >50% of needs) is unlikely for 7 to 10 days because of an underlying illness.
3. Patients with severe catabolic stress requiring ICU care in whom adequate enteral nutrient intake is unlikely for more than 3 to 5 days.

There is no reason to withhold PN in hospitalized patients for any period of time if they exhibit preexisting moderate to severe malnutrition and are deemed to be unlikely to meet their needs by the oral or enteral route.

Generally accepted contraindications for PN include the following conditions:

1. If the GI tract is functional and access for enteral feeding is available.

2. If PN is thought to be required for 5 days or less.

3. If the patient cannot tolerate the extra intravenous fluid required for PN or has severe hyperglycemia or electrolyte abnormalities on the planned day of PN initiation

4. If the patient has an uncontrolled bloodstream infection or severe hemodynamic instability.

5. If new placement of an intravenous line solely for PN poses undue risks based on clinical judgment

6. On an individualized basis, if aggressive nutritional support is not desired by the competent patient or legally authorized representative, such as in premorbid patients or those with terminal illness.

PN can be delivered either as peripheral vein solutions or as central vein solutions through a percutaneous subclavian vein or internal jugular vein catheter for infusion into the superior vena cava (nontunneled in the hospital setting), through a subcutaneously tunneled central venous catheter (e.g., Hickman catheter) or central venous port (for chronic home PN therapy), or through a peripherally inserted central venous catheter (PICC). Although data are limited, it is clearly preferable to manage long-term central venous PN to be managed at home with the use of a tunneled central venous catheter rather than a PICC line because of the higher rate of local complications (e.g., phlebitis, catheter breakage) and possibly catheter-associated infections with PICC lines.

A comparison of typical fluid, macronutrient, and micronutrient content of peripheral and central vein PN solutions is shown in Table 68-3. Intravenous lipid emulsions (typically added to PN as a 20% soybean oil–based solution in the United States) provide both essential linoleic and α-linolenic fatty acids and energy (10 kcal/g); these are typically infused over a 24-hour period in the complete PN administration bag. The maximal recommended rate of fat emulsion infusion is approximately 1.0 g/kg/day. Most patients are well able to clear triglyceride from plasma after intravenous administration of fat emulsion. Recently, an intravenous lipid emulsion of 80% olive oil/20% soybean oil was approved for use in adult PN in the United States. It is important to monitor blood triglyceride levels at baseline and then approximately weekly and as indicated to assess clearance of intravenous fat; triglyceride levels should be maintained lower than 400 mg/dL to decrease the risk of pancreatitis or diminished pulmonary diffusion capacity in patients with severe chronic obstructive lung disease.

Central venous administration of PN allows higher concentrations of dextrose (3.4 kcal/g) and amino acids (4 kcal/g) to be delivered as hypertonic solutions; thus, lower amounts of fat emulsion are needed to reach caloric goals (see Table 68-3). Requirements for potassium, magnesium, and phosphorus are typically higher with central vein PN compared to peripheral vein PN. The higher concentrations of dextrose and amino acids allow most patients to achieve caloric and amino acid goals with only 1 to 1.5 L of PN per day. In central vein PN, initial orders typically provide 60% to 70% of non–amino acid calories as dextrose and 30% to 40% of non–amino acid calories as fat emulsion. These percentages are adjusted as indicated based on levels of blood glucose and triglyceride, respectively. Based on comprehensive data associating hyperglycemia with hospital morbidity and

TABLE 68-3	COMPOSITION OF TYPICAL PARENTERAL NUTRITION SOLUTIONS	
COMPONENT*	PERIPHERAL PN	CENTRAL PN
Volume (L/day)	2-3	1-1.5
Dextrose (%)	5	10-25
Amino acids (%)†	2.5-3.5	3-8
Lipid (%)‡	3.5-5.0	2.5-5.0
Sodium (mEq/L)	50-150	50-150
Potassium (mEq/L)	20-35	30-50
Phosphorus (mmol/L)	5-10	10-30
Magnesium (mEq/L)	8-10	10-20
Calcium (mEq/L)	2.5-5	2.5-5
Trace elements§		
Vitamins‖		

*Electrolytes in parenteral nutrition (PN) are adjusted as indicated to maintain serially measured serum levels within the normal range. The percentage of sodium and potassium salts as chloride is increased to correct metabolic alkalosis, and the percentage of salts as acetate is increased to correct metabolic acidosis. Regular insulin is added to PN as needed to achieve blood glucose goals (separate intravenous insulin infusions are commonly required with hyperglycemia in intensive care unit settings).

†Provides all essential amino acids and several nonessential amino acids. The dose of amino acids is adjusted downward or upward to goal as a function of the degree of azotemia or hyperbilirubinemia in patients with renal or hepatic failure, respectively.

‡Lipid is given as soybean oil– or olive oil/soybean oil–based fat emulsion in the United States. In Europe and other non-U.S. countries, intravenous fish oil, olive oil, medium-chain triglycerides, and combinations of these are available for use in PN. Lipid is typically mixed with dextrose and amino acids in the same PN infusion bag ("all-in-one" solution).

§Trace elements added on a daily basis to peripheral vein and central vein PN are mixtures of chromium, copper, manganese, selenium, and zinc. (These elements can also be supplemented individually.)

‖Vitamins added on a daily basis to peripheral vein and central vein PN are mixtures of vitamins A, B_1 (thiamine), B_2 (riboflavin), B_3 (niacinamide), B_6 (pyridoxine), B_{12}, C, D, and E, biotin, folate, and pantothenic acid. Vitamin K is added on an individual basis (e.g., for patients with cirrhosis). Specific vitamins can also be supplemented individually.

mortality, expert panels now recommend tight blood glucose control in ICU settings (between 80 and 130 to 150 mg/dL) and close blood glucose monitoring. Separate intravenous insulin infusions should usually be administered in the ICU when patients receiving central vein PN develop hyperglycemia.

Specific requirements for intravenous trace elements and vitamins have not been rigorously defined for patient subgroups, and in most stable patients, therapy is directed at meeting published recommended doses using standardized intravenous preparations to maintain blood levels in the normal range (see Table 68-3). Several studies have shown that a significant proportion of ICU patients have low levels of zinc, selenium, vitamin C, vitamin E, and vitamin D despite receiving specialized PN (or EN). Depletion of these essential nutrients may impair antioxidant capacity, immunity, wound healing, and other important body functions, and supplementation is recommended if serum concentrations are low. For example, zinc (and other micronutrients such as copper) should probably be increased in the PN of patients with burns, large wounds, significant gastrointestinal fluid losses, and other conditions if serum concentrations indicate low levels. Recent data suggest that thiamine depletion is not uncommon in patients receiving chronic diuretic therapy or in those with severe malabsorption.

The most common complication of peripheral vein PN is local phlebitis resulting from use of the catheter. In such cases, a small dose of hydrocortisone and heparin is typically added to the solution. Alterations in blood electrolytes can be treated with adjustment of concentrations in the peripheral PN prescription. Hypertriglyceridemia typically responds well to lowering of the total PN lipid dose. Central vein PN is associated with a much higher rate of mechanical, metabolic, and infectious complications than peripheral vein PN. Mechanical complications include those related to insertion of the central venous catheter (e.g., pneumothorax, hemothorax, malposition of the catheter, thrombosis). Infectious complications include catheter-related bloodstream infections and non–catheter-related infections. The risk for these infections appears to be increased with use of non–subclavian vein central venous access (e.g., jugular vein, femoral vein) and multiple-use catheters with non-dedicated PN infusion ports used for additional purposes such as blood drawing or medication administration. Poorly controlled blood glucose levels (>140 to 180 mg/dL) are not uncommon in patients requiring central vein PN and are associated with an increased risk of nosocomial infection. Risk factors for hyperglycemia include poorly controlled blood glucose at PN initiation; use of high dextrose concentrations (>10%) in the initial few days of PN administration or too rapid an increase in total dextrose load; insufficient exogenous insulin administration; inadequate monitoring of blood glucose responses to central vein PN administration; and administration of corticosteroids and vasopressor agents such as noreprinephrine (which stimulate gluconeogenesis and cause insulin resistance).

Recent data also suggest that inadequate or no provision of the amino acid glutamine may increase infection risk in patients requiring PN. This amino acid appears to be conditionally essential in catabolic states and serves as an important fuel for immune cells and cells of the gut mucosa. Several expert panels now recommend that glutamine be routinely added to the PN in ICU patients, but this practice remains controversial because some studies show no benefit (or even harm) in certain patient subgroups and an improvement in hospital mortality has not been documented.

Studies on nutrient utilization efficiency and metabolic complications in severely catabolic patients suggest that lower amounts of total energy and protein/amino acids should be administered than were routinely given in the past, particularly in unstable and ICU patients. High calorie, carbohydrate, amino acid, and fat loads ("hyperalimentation") are easily administered via central vein PN but can induce severe metabolic complications, including carbon dioxide overproduction, azotemia, hyperglycemia, electrolyte alterations, and hepatic steatosis and injury (E-Table 68-5). Dextrose and lipid doses in PN should be advanced over several days after initiation, with close monitoring of the blood glucose concentration, electrolytes, triglycerides, organ function tests, intake and output measurements, and the clinical course.

Refeeding syndrome with central vein PN administration is relatively common in patients at risk, including those with preexisting malnutrition, electrolyte depletion, alcoholism, or prolonged periods of intravenous hydration therapy (e.g., 5% dextrose) without nutritional support, all of which are common in hospital patients. Refeeding syndrome is mediated by administration of excessive intravenous dextrose (>150 to 250 g, for example in 1 L of PN containing 15% to 25% dextrose). This, in turn, markedly stimulates insulin release, which rapidly lowers blood concentrations of potassium, magnesium, and especially phosphorus as a result of intracellular shifts and utilization in carbohydrate metabolic pathways. Administration of high doses of carbohydrate also consumes thiamine, which is required as a cofactor for carbohydrate metabolism and can precipitate symptoms of thiamine deficiency (see E-Table 68-2), especially in patients with poor thiamine nutriture at baseline. Hyperinsulinemia also tends to cause sodium and fluid retention at the level of the kidney. Together, fluid and sodium retention, the drop in electrolytes (which can cause arrhythmias), and hypermetabolism due to excessive calorie provision can result in heart failure, especially in patients with preexisting heart disease and cardiac muscle atrophy due to prolonged protein-energy malnutrition. Prevention of refeeding syndrome requires vigilance to identify patients at risk; use of initially low PN dextrose concentrations; empiric provision of higher doses of potassium, magnesium, and phosphorus based on current blood levels and renal function; and supplemental thiamine (100 mg/day for 3 to 5 days).

If home PN is indicated, the primary physician should consult with social service professionals to identify appropriate home care companies and nutrition support professionals to assess intravenous line access, metabolic status, and the home PN order and to arrange for follow-up care and monitoring of PN. It is important not to arrange for rapid discharge of hospitalized patients newly started on PN. Obtaining appropriate venous access and monitoring of fluid and electrolyte status over a 2- to 3-day period is an important aspect of care for most patients started on PN, and it is imperative for those with severe malnutrition and those at risk for refeeding syndrome.

For a deeper discussion on this topic, please see Chapters 214, "Nutritional Assessment," and 215, "Protein-Energy Malnutrition" in Goldman-Cecil Medicine, *25th Edition.*

SUGGESTED READINGS

Casaer MP, Mesotten D, Hermans G, et al: Early versus late parenteral nutrition in critically ill adults, N Engl J Med 365:506–517, 2011.

Doig GS, Simpson F, Sweetman EA, et al, and Early PN Investigators of the ANZICS Clinical Trials Group: Early parenteral nutrition in critically ill patients with short-term relative contraindications to early enteral nutrition: a randomized controlled trial, JAMA 309:2130–2138, 2013.

Gershengorn HB, Kahn JM, Wunsch H: Temporal trends in the use of parenteral nutrition in critically ill patients, Chest 145:508–517, 2014.

Heidegger CP, Berger MM, Graf S, et al: Optimisation of energy provision with supplemental parenteral nutrition in critically ill patients: a randomised controlled clinical trial, Lancet 381:385–393, 2013.

Heighes PT, Doig GS, Sweetman EA, et al: An overview of evidence from systematic reviews evaluating early enteral nutrition in critically ill patients: more convincing evidence is needed, Anaesth Intensive Care 38:167–174, 2010.

McClave SA, Kozar R, Martindale RG, et al: Summary points and consensus recommendations from the North American Surgical Nutrition Summit, JPEN J Parenter Enteral Nutr 37(5 Suppl):99S–105S, 2013.

McClave SA, Martindale RG, Vanek VW, et al: Guidelines for the provision and assessment of nutrition support therapy in the adult critically ill patient: Society of Critical Care Medicine (SCCM) and American Society for Parenteral and Enteral Nutrition (A.S.P.E.N.), JPEN J Parenter Enteral Nutr 33:277–316, 2009.

Ziegler TR: Parenteral nutrition in the critically ill patient, N Engl J Med 361:1088–1097, 2009.

Ziegler TR: Nutrition support in critical illness: bridging the evidence gap, N Engl J Med 365:562–564, 2011.

Disorders of Lipid Metabolism

Geetha Gopalakrishnan and Robert J. Smith

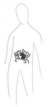

⬤ DEFINITION AND EPIDEMIOLOGY

Lipids such as free fatty acids (FFA), cholesterol, and triglycerides are hydrophobic molecules that bind proteins for transport. Nonesterified FFA travel as anions complexed to albumin. Esterified complex lipids are transported in lipoprotein particles. Lipoproteins have a hydrophobic core (cholesteryl esters and triglycerides) and an amphiphilic surface monolayer (phospholipids, unesterified cholesterol, and apolipoproteins). Ultracentrifugation separates lipoproteins into five classes based on their density (Table 69-1).

Proteins on the surface of lipoproteins (i.e., apolipoproteins) activate enzymes and receptors that guide lipid metabolism. Defects in the synthesis and catabolism of lipoproteins result in dyslipidemia. Prevalence of dyslipidemia in the United States is approximately 20% and varies with the population studied. An estimated 70% of individuals with premature coronary heart disease (CHD) have dyslipidemia. In clinical trials, treatment of dyslipidemia improved both CHD and all-cause mortality rates. Two classes of lipids, triglyceride and cholesterol, play a significant, yet modifiable, role in the pathogenesis of atherosclerosis and therefore are the focus of this chapter.

⬤ PATHOLOGY

In the intestinal lumen, dietary triglycerides and cholesterol esters are hydrolyzed by pancreatic lipase to produce glycerol, FFA, and free cholesterol. Formation of micelles enables the absorption of glycerol and FFA into the intestinal cell. The transport of free cholesterol is mediated by a cholesterol gradient that exists between the lumen and the intestinal cell. Within the cell, glycerol combines with three fatty acid chains to form triglycerides, and cholesterol is esterified to form cholesterol esters. Chylomicrons are formed from triglycerides (85% of chylomicron mass) and cholesterol esters assembled with surface lipoproteins. Chylomicrons enter into the circulation and acquire more surface apolipoproteins such as apo C-II and apo E from high-density lipoprotein (HDL) particles (Fig. 69-1). Apo C-II

activates lipoprotein lipase (LPL), which is located on the capillary endothelium. LPL hydrolyzes the core chylomicron triglycerides to release FFA, which function as an energy source. Excess fatty acids are stored in adipose tissue or utilized in hepatic lipoprotein synthesis. The triglyceride-poor chylomicron remnant is then cleared from the circulation by hepatic LDL receptors. These receptors are activated by apo E, which is located on the surface of chylomicrons.

Very-low-density lipoproteins (VLDL) are synthesized by the liver (see Fig. 69-1). FFA and cholesterol obtained from the circulation or synthesized by the liver are incorporated into VLDL particles. Any condition that increases the flux of FFA to the liver, such as poorly controlled diabetes, will increase VLDL production. The liver assembles triglycerides (55% of VLDL mass), cholesterol (20%), and surface apolipoproteins to form VLDL particles. Apo C-II, the cofactor for LPL, hydrolyzes the triglyceride core of VLDL particles to generate VLDL remnant or intermediate-density lipoprotein (IDL). The IDL, depleted of triglycerides (25%), can be cleared from the circulation by apo E–mediated LDL receptors, or it can be hydrolyzed further to form low-density lipoproteins (LDL). LDL particles are triglyceride poor (5% of LDL mass) and consist mostly of cholesterol esters (60%) and apolipoproteins. Apo B100 on the surface of LDL binds LDL receptors and facilitates LDL clearance from the circulation. Internalized LDL-cholesterol is used to synthesize hormones, produce cell membranes, and store energy.

In the liver, LDL-cholesterol is used to synthesize bile acids (see Fig. 69-1), which are secreted into the intestinal lumen along with free cholesterol. Bile acids help transport fat. Approximately 50% of the cholesterol and 97% of the bile acid entering the lumen is reabsorbed back into the circulation. The reabsorbed cholesterol regulates cholesterol and LDL receptor synthesis.

Many cells in the body, including liver parenchymal cells, synthesize cholesterol (Fig. 69-2). Acetate is converted to 3-hydroxy-3-methylglutaryl–coenzyme A (HMG-CoA). HMG-CoA reductase converts HMG-CoA to mevalonic acid, which is then

TABLE 69-1	PROPERTIES OF LIPOPROTEINS			
LIPOPROTEIN CLASS	**DENSITY (g/mL)**	**ORIGIN**	**APOLIPOPROTEINS**	**LIPID**
Chylomicrons	<0.95	Intestine	C-II, E	TG (85%), cholesterol (10%)
VLDL	<1.006	Liver	B100, C-II, E	TG (55%), cholesterol (20%)
IDL	1.006-1.019	VLDL catabolism	B100, E	TG (25%), cholesterol (35%)
LDL	1.019-1.063	IDL catabolism	B100	TG (5%), cholesterol (60%)
HDL	1.063-1.25	Liver, intestine	A-I, E	TG (5%), cholesterol (20%)

HDL, High-density lipoprotein; IDL, intermediate-density lipoprotein; LDL, low-density lipoprotein; TG, triglyceride; VLDL, very-low-density lipoprotein.

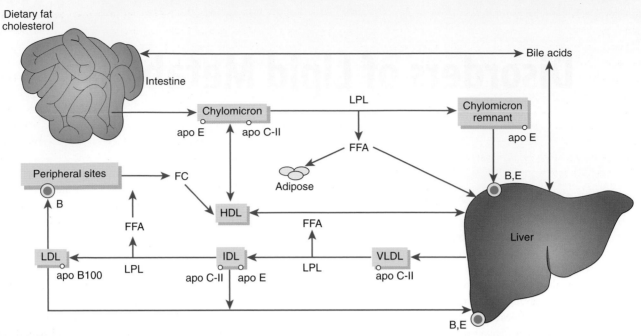

FIGURE 69-1 Normal metabolism of plasma lipoproteins (see text for details). apo, Apolipoprotein; B,E, membrane receptor for lipoproteins containing apo B and apo E (synonymous with the LDL receptor); FC, free (unesterified) cholesterol; FFA, free (unesterified) fatty acids; HDL, high-density lipoprotein; IDL, intermediate-density lipoprotein; LDL, low-density lipoprotein; LPL, lipoprotein lipase; VLDL, very-low-density lipoprotein.

LDL Cholesterol Uptake from Circulation

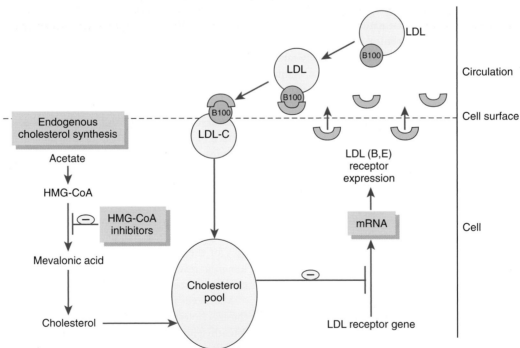

FIGURE 69-2 Regulation of low-density lipoprotein (LDL) receptor expression (see text for details). B100, Apolipoprotein B100; B,E, membrane receptor for lipoproteins containing apo B and apo E (synonymous with the LDL receptor); HMG-CoA, 3-hydroxy-3-methylglutaryl–coenzyme A; LDL-C, LDL-cholesterol; mRNA, messenger RNA.

converted to cholesterol through a series of steps. HMG-CoA reductase is the rate-limiting step in the cholesterol synthesis pathway. Drugs that inhibit this enzyme decrease cholesterol biosynthesis and cellular cholesterol pools. Internalization of LDL particles into cells is regulated by negative feedback (see Fig. 69-2). A negative cholesterol balance increases the expression of LDL receptors and subsequent uptake of cholesterol from the circulation. A positive cell cholesterol balance suppresses LDL receptor expression and decreases uptake of LDL-cholesterol into cells. Circulating LDL then enter macrophages and other tissues via scavenger receptors. Because the scavenger receptors are not regulated, these cells accumulate excess intracellular cholesterol, resulting in the formation of foam cells and atheromatous plaques.

The anti-atherogenic effect of HDL is attributed to the removal of excess cholesterol from tissue sites and other lipoproteins. HDL is synthesized in the liver and intestine (see Fig. 69-1). Excess phospholipids, cholesterol, and apolipoproteins on remnant chylomicrons, VLDL, IDL, and LDL, are transferred to HDL particles and thus increase HDL mass. Apo A-I, a surface lipoprotein on HDL particles, mobilizes cholesterol from intracellular pools and accepts cholesterol released during lipolysis of triglyceride-rich lipoproteins. It also activates lecithin-cholesterol acyltransferase (LCAT), an enzyme that esterifies cholesterol. These cholesterol esters move the hydrophilic HDL surface to the hydrophobic HDL core. Cholesterol ester transfer protein (CETP) transfers core HDL cholesterol esters to other lipoproteins such as VLDL. These lipoproteins deliver cholesterol to peripheral sites for hormone and cell membrane synthesis.

Defects in the production or removal of lipoproteins results in dyslipidemia. Both genetic and acquired conditions have been implicated in the pathogenesis of lipid disorders (Tables 69-2 and 61-3). These are discussed later in the chapter.

CLINICAL PRESENTATION

Dyslipidemia plays a significant role in the development of atherosclerosis. Increased incidence of CHD with high LDL- and low HDL-cholesterol is well documented. Excess LDL results in the formation of cholesterol plaques that deposit in arteries (atheroma), skin and tendon (xanthomas), eyelids (xanthelasma),

and iris (corneal arcus). The impact of triglycerides on vascular disease is less clear. Metabolic disorders such as diabetes and obesity are often associated with vascular disease and hypertriglyceridemia, and the atherogenic impact of other elements in these disorders is difficult to separate from the effect of hypertriglyceridemia. However, in several population-based studies, abnormal triglyceride levels correlated with increased risk for CHD. Marked hypertriglyceridemia (>1000 mg/dL) is associated with the chylomicronemia syndrome, characterized by pancreatitis and xanthomas.

DIAGNOSIS

Dyslipidemia is defined by a total cholesterol, triglyceride, or LDL level greater than the 90th percentile or an HDL level lower than the 10th percentile for the general population. Because chylomicrons are present in plasma for up to 10 hours after a meal, fasting total cholesterol, triglyceride, and lipoprotein assessments are required for diagnosis. It is advisable to confirm dyslipidemia with two separate determinations.

Total cholesterol, triglyceride, and HDL levels can be measured directly; VLDL and LDL levels usually are calculated. If the triglyceride concentration is lower than 400 mg/dL, then VLDL is calculated by dividing the triglyceride level by 5. LDL-cholesterol is estimated by subtracting VLDL and HDL from the total cholesterol. VLDL and LDL cannot be determined if triglyceride levels are greater than 400 mg/dL. In that case, the lipoprotein abnormality can be identified by inspecting the serum. When the triglyceride level exceeds 350 mg/dL, the

TABLE 69-2 GENETIC DISORDERS OF LIPID METABOLISM

DISORDER	GENETIC DEFECT	DYSLIPIDEMIA
Familial hypercholesterolemia	Mutation in the gene that encodes LDL receptor	Elevated TC and LDL
Familial defective apolipoprotein B100	Impaired binding of LDL to LDL receptor due to a defect in apo B100 protein	Elevated TC and LDL
Elevated plasma Lp(a)	Increased binding of LDL to apolipoprotein(a)	Elevated Lp(a)
Polygenic hypercholesterolemia	Increased binding of apo E4–containing lipoprotein to LDL receptor resulting in downregulation of the LDL receptor	Elevated TC and LDL
Familial combined hyperlipoproteinemia	Polygenic disorder associated with increased hepatic VLDL production, resulting in increased LDL and decreased HDL production; some individuals have a mutation in the LPL gene that affects expression and function of LPL	Elevated TC, LDL, and TG Low HDL
Familial dysbetalipoproteinemia	Lower affinity of apo E2 for LDL receptor	Elevated TG, TC, and LDL
Lipoprotein lipase deficiency	Mutation in the *LPL* gene	Elevated TG
Apolipoprotein C-II deficiency	Decrease in activation of LPL due to a deficiency of apo CII	Elevated TG
Familial hypertriglyceridemia	Overproduction of hepatic VLDL and increased catabolism of HDL	Elevated TG Low HDL

HDL, High-density lipoprotein; LDL, low-density lipoprotein; TC, total cholesterol; TG, triglyceride; VLDL, very low-density lipoprotein.

TABLE 69-3 MECHANISMS OF SECONDARY HYPERLIPIDEMIA

CLINICAL	ELEVATED LIPOPROTEIN	MECHANISM
Diabetes	Chylomicron, VLDL, LDL	Increase in VLDL production and decrease in VLDL/LDL clearance
Obesity	Chylomicron, VLDL, LDL	Increase in VLDL production and decrease in VLDL/LDL clearance
Lipodystrophy	VLDL	Increase in VLDL production
Hypothyroidism	LDL, VLDL	Decrease in LDL/LDL clearance
Estrogen	VLDL	Increase in VLDL production
Glucocorticoids	VLDL, LDL	Increase in VLDL production and conversion to LDL
Alcohol	VLDL	Increase in VLDL production
Nephrotic syndrome	VLDL, LDL	Increase in VLDL production and conversion to LDL

LDL, Low-density lipoprotein; VLDL, very-low-density lipoprotein.

serum is cloudy. After refrigeration, a white surface layer depicts excess chylomicrons, whereas a dispersed, opaque infranatant reflects a VLDL dysfunction.

Current guidelines recommend selective screening of children who have a family history of lipoprotein abnormality or premature vascular disease and adults who have an increased risk for CHD. The U.S. Preventive Services task force recommended universal screening starting at 35 years of age for men and at 45 years of age for women; there is a paucity of data supporting long-term benefits from screening of younger individuals. Either a fasting or a nonfasting total cholesterol and HDL measurement can be the initial screen. If the total cholesterol value is greater than 200 mg/dL or the HDL value is less than 40 mg/dL, then a repeat fasting lipid panel is required. If the total cholesterol value is less than 200 mg/dL and the HDL value is greater than 40 mg/dL, then retesting is recommended every 5 years. Individuals with CHD, risk factors for CHD, or CHD equivalents (i.e., symptomatic carotid artery disease, peripheral arterial disease, abdominal aortic aneurysm, or diabetes) should be screened more frequently based on risk assessment, as shown in Table 69-4. CHD risk factors include age (men >45 years, women >55 years), family history of premature CHD (affected male first-degree relative <55 years or female first-degree relative <65 years of age), smoking, hypertension, and low HDL (<40 mg/dL). HDL concentrations higher than 60 mg/dL are cardioprotective. Overall, the level of evidence to support screening is fair (level B) but increases with age, male gender, and CHD (level A).

TREATMENT

Treatment is initiated after two abnormal lipid findings. Treatment of elevated total cholesterol and LDL-cholesterol can slow the development and progression of CHD. Meta-analysis of primary and secondary prevention trials indicates that CHD mortality decreases by approximately 15% for every 10% reduction in serum cholesterol. LDL-cholesterol treatment strategies are based on risk indicators (Table 69-5). There is strong evidence that dietary modifications can reduce LDL-cholesterol and triglyceride levels (Table 69-6). However, evidence that lifestyle-induced lipid modifications improve cardiovascular outcomes is limited (level C). If target goals are not achieved, then pharmacologic therapy is considered (Table 69-7). Ample

evidence supports statin use in primary and secondary prevention of CHD (level A). Treatment effects of statin can be assessed after 1 to 2 months. Additional agents can be considered if target goals are not achieved with maximal drug dosing.

A fasting lipid panel is required to diagnose hypertriglyceridemia. Triglyceride levels higher than 200 mg/dL are classified as abnormal. Borderline triglyceride levels range from 150 to 200 mg/dL, and normal values are lower than 150 mg/dL. A diet and exercise program is recommended for all individuals with abnormal triglyceride levels (level C). However, pharmacologic treatments to reduce triglyceride levels may be considered if fasting levels are higher than 200 mg/dL, especially if the individual is at risk for CHD or pancreatitis (see Table 69-7). Fibrates, fish oil, and nicotinic acid should be considered if the triglyceride level is higher than 500 mg/dL (level C). However, for levels lower than 500 mg/dL, statins are first-line therapy (level B).

Low HDL concentrations (<40 mg/dL) can also increase the risk for CHD. In the Framingham Heart Study, every decrease in HDL of 5 mg/dL increased the risk for myocardial infarction. Both lifestyle modifications (e.g., diet low in saturated fat, exercise) and pharmacologic therapy (e.g., nicotinic acid, fibrate) can improve HDL levels. However, target goals and treatment recommendations have not been established due to a lack of evidence.

| TABLE 69-5 | THERAPEUTIC APPROACH TO REDUCE LEVELS OF LOW-DENSITY LIPOPROTEIN–CHOLESTEROL* |

RISK CATEGORY	TREATMENT GOAL: LDL (mg/dL)	LIFESTYLE CHANGES: LDL (mg/dL)	DRUG THERAPY: LDL (mg/dL)
≤One risk factor	<160	≥160	≥160-190
≥Two risk factors	<130	≥130	≥130-160
CHD or CHD risk equivalent	<100 (optional <70)	≥100	≥100-130

CHD, Coronary heart disease; HDL, high-density lipoprotein–cholesterol; LDL, low-density lipoprotein–cholesterol.

*Recommendations of the Adult Treatment Panel III, National Cholesterol Education Program (NCEP), as modified in 2004. CHD risk factors include age (men >45 yr, women >55 yr), family history of premature CHD (male first-degree relative <55 yr, female first-degree relative <65 yr), smoking, hypertension, diabetes mellitus, and HDL <40 mg/dL. Subtract a risk factor if HDL >60 mg/dL. CHD risk equivalents include symptomatic carotid artery disease, peripheral arterial disease, abdominal aortic aneurysm, and diabetes mellitus.

| TABLE 69-4 | RECOMMENDATIONS FOR SCREENING FOR DYSLIPIDEMIA* |

1. A fasting lipid profile is recommended at age 20 yr
2. Rescreen every 5 yr if
   - LDL <160 mg/dL in patients with 0-1 risk factor
   - LDL <130 mg/dL in patients with ≥2 risk factors
3. Rescreen every year if
   - LDL 130-159 mg/dL in patients with ≥2 risk factors
   - LDL <100 mg/dL in patients with CHD or CHD risk equivalent

CHD, Coronary heart disease; HDL, high-density lipoprotein–cholesterol; LDL, low-density lipoprotein–cholesterol.

*Recommendations of the Adult Treatment Panel III, National Cholesterol Education Program (NCEP), as modified in 2004. CHD risk factors include age (men >45 yr, women >55 yr), family history of premature CHD (male first-degree relative <55 yr, female first-degree relative <65 yr), smoking, hypertension, and HDL <40 mg/dL. Subtract a risk factor if HDL >60 mg/dL. CHD risk equivalents include symptomatic carotid artery disease, peripheral arterial disease, abdominal aortic aneurysm, and diabetes mellitus.

| TABLE 69-6 | RECOMMENDATIONS FOR NUTRITIONAL INTAKE* |

NUTRIENT	RECOMMENDED INTAKE
Total Fat	25-35% of total calories
Saturated	<7%
Polyunsaturated	<10%
Monounsaturated	<20%
Carbohydrates	50-60% of total calories
Protein	15% of total calories
Cholesterol	<200 mg/day
Fiber	20-30 g/day

*Recommendations of the Adult Treatment Panel III, National Cholesterol Education Program (NCEP), as modified in 2004.

TABLE 69-7 DRUGS COMMONLY USED FOR THE TREATMENT OF HYPERLIPIDEMIA

DRUG CLASS	LDL (% CHANGE)	HDL (% CHANGE)	TRIGLYCERIDES (% CHANGE)	SIDE EFFECTS
HMG-CoA inhibitors	↓ 20-60	↑ 5-10	↓ 10-30	Liver toxicity, myositis, rhabdomyolysis; enhanced warfarin effect
Cholesterol absorption inhibitors	↓ 17	No effect	↓ 7-8	Abnormal liver enzymes in combination with an HMG-CoA inhibitor, myalgia, hepatitis, rhabdomyolysis, pancreatitis, potential increase in cancer risk and cancer death
Bile acid sequestrants	↓ 15-30	Slight increase	No effect	Nausea, bloating, cramping, abnormal liver function; interferes with absorption of other drugs such as warfarin and thyroxine
Fibric acid	↓ 5-20	↑ 5-20	↓ 35-50	Nausea, cramping, myalgias, liver toxicity, enhanced warfarin effect
Nicotinic acid	↓ 10-25	↑ 15-35	↓ 25-30	Hepatotoxicity, hyperuricemia, hyperglycemia, flushing, pruritus, nausea, vomiting, diarrhea
Omega-3 fatty acids	↑ 4-49	↑ 5-9	↓ 23-45	Eructation, taste perversion, dyspepsia

HMG-CoA, Hydroxymethylglutaryl–coenzyme A reductase.

Lifestyle Modification

Lifestyle modification should be the initial step in the management of hyperlipidemia (see Table 69-6). Restricting the dietary intake of fat lowers total cholesterol by approximately 15% and LDL cholesterol by 25%. Low-fat diets that limit saturated fat content promote LDL receptor expression and increase the uptake of LDL-cholesterol from the circulation. By contrast, saturated fat downregulates hepatic LDL receptors and increases circulating LDL. Because unsaturated fats (polyunsaturated and monounsaturated) generally do not have this effect, they are the preferred form of fat intake. However, polyunsaturated fats containing fatty acids with a *trans* rather than *cis* double bond configuration (*trans*-fatty acids) increase plasma cholesterol levels similarly to saturated fat.

Limiting the intake of saturated and *trans*-unsaturated fatty acids requires appropriate calorie substitutions. Increasing carbohydrate content to achieve this goal can increase the hepatic synthesis of triglyceride. Dietary substitution with soluble fibers (e.g., oat bran) has been recommended, because these fibers have a limited effect on triglyceride levels. They also bind bile acids in the gut and thereby decrease cholesterol levels. Other polyunsaturated fats, such as omega-3 fatty acids, are cardioprotective. They are abundant in fatty fish, flaxseed oil, canola oil, and nuts. They reduce VLDL production, inhibit platelet aggregation, and decrease CHD. Even two servings per week of fatty fish such as salmon can be beneficial.

Dietary restriction of fat (<10%) is essential for the treatment of marked hypertriglyceridemia. Other factors such as carbohydrate and alcohol intake can also increase the synthesis of triglyceride. Restriction of alcohol intake to 1 or 2 servings per week and adherence to a low-fat, high-fiber diet will improve hypertriglyceridemia.

Exercise has been shown to increase LPL activity. Even a single exercise session can reduce triglycerides and increase HDL. The impact of exercise on LDL is less clear. With low- to moderate-intensity exercise regimens, clearance of VLDL particles increases LDL production. However, this effect is not seen with high-intensity exercise programs. A decrease in LDL-cholesterol occurs with high-intensity exercise, and this effect is independent of weight loss.

Pharmacotherapy

If diet and exercise modifications do not sustain a normal lipid profile, then drug therapy is appropriate (see Table 69-7). Likely benefit needs to be balanced against potential adverse effects when determining drug therapy. Many patients require two or three agents to achieve adequate control.

HMG-CoA reductase is the rate-limiting enzyme involved in cholesterol biosynthesis. Inhibition of this enzyme decreases intracellular cholesterol pools and subsequently increases uptake of LDL cholesterol from the circulation. HMG-CoA reductase inhibitors (e.g., lovastatin, pravastatin, simvastatin, fluvastatin, atorvastatin, and rosuvastatin) increase cholesterol utilization, decrease VLDL synthesis, and increase HDL synthesis. As a result, lower LDL and triglyceride levels and higher HDL levels are observed with treatment. Meta-analysis of primary and secondary CHD prevention trials found reductions in all-cause and cardiovascular mortality rates with statin therapy. These agents limit progression and may even cause regression of coronary atherosclerosis. Therefore, they represent first-line therapy in the management of abnormal LDL-cholesterol levels. Elevated liver enzymes and muscle toxicity are potential dose-related complications. Myositis can occur with statins alone, but the risk is higher when statins are used in combination with nicotinic acid or fibric acid derivatives. Some of these agents can also potentiate the effect of warfarin.

Cholesterol absorption inhibitors (e.g., ezetimibe) function by interfering with the transport of cholesterol at the intestinal brush border. They increase cholesterol utilization and decrease LDL-cholesterol levels. Despite reductions in LDL-cholesterol, improvements in cardiovascular events and mortality have not been reported with treatment. Ezetimibe may be used as a single agent or in combination with an HMG-CoA reductase inhibitor to lower LDL-cholesterol levels. In combination, this agent can increase serum transaminase levels and potentially increase the risk of cancer and cancer death.

Drugs that interfere with the absorption of cholesterol from the intestinal lumen increase cholesterol utilization and decrease circulating levels of cholesterol. Bile acid sequestrants (e.g., cholestyramine, colestipol, and colesevelam) bind bile acids in the intestinal lumen and increase fecal excretion. Subsequently, more LDL-cholesterol is used by the liver to synthesis bile acids. The decrease in cellular cholesterol pools upregulates LDL receptors and decreases the amount of LDL-cholesterol in the circulation. Mild increases in HDL-cholesterol are also seen with this agent as a result of increased intestinal HDL formation. Treatment is associated with a reduction in the incidence of CHD. Bile acid sequestrants may be used alone for mild lipid dysfunction or in combination with another lipid-lowering agent such as an HMG-CoA reductase inhibitor. Abnormal liver function and gastrointestinal symptoms (e.g., nausea, bloating, cramping) are common side effects that limit the use of bile acid sequestrants. They can also interfere with the absorption of other drugs such as warfarin and thyroxine.

Fibric acid derivatives such as gemfibrozil and fenofibrate increase FFA oxidation in muscle and liver. The reduced lipogenesis in the liver decreases VLDL and subsequent LDL production. Fibric acid derivatives also enhance LPL activity and HDL synthesis. As a result, treatment is usually associated with not only lower triglyceride and LDL levels, but also higher HDL levels. Reduced cardiovascular events have been demonstrated in a subset of individuals with high triglyceride (>200 mg/dL) and low HDL (<40 mg/dL) levels, but improvements in cardiovascular or all-cause mortality otherwise have not been confirmed with these agents. Liver toxicity and myositis are potential side effects of fibric acid derivatives, and they also interfere with the metabolism of warfarin, leading to a need for its dose adjustment.

Nicotinic acid has an antilipolytic effect and therefore decreases the influx of FFA to the liver. As a result, hepatic VLDL synthesis and LDL production are reduced. Nicotinic acid also decreases HDL catabolism. Lower triglyceride and LDL levels and higher HDL levels are observed with treatment. In addition, nicotinic acid stimulates tissue plasminogen activator and prevents thrombosis. It is the preferred agent for the reduction of lipoprotein(a) or Lp(a) (discussed later). The cardioprotective effect of nicotinic acid may be linked to its effect on Lp(a) and HDL. Side effects include hepatotoxicity, hyperuricemia, hyperglycemia, and flushing.

Omega-3 fatty acids reduce VLDL production and subsequently lower triglyceride levels (by 35%). They also modestly increase HDL (3%) and LDL (5%). The impact on lipids can occur over months to years and requires treatment doses as high as 3 to 4 g of fish oil per day. However, reductions in death due to sudden cardiac events and CHD are observed within weeks of treatment initiation. This benefit can be seen with lower treatment doses (fish oil <2 g/day) and is most likely related to the impact of omega-3 fatty acid on cardiac electrophysiology. Omega-3 fatty acids constitute 30% to 50% of fish oil supplements and 85% of prescribed pharmacologic preparations (i.e., Lovaza and Vascepa). In clinical trials, both Lovaza and Vascepa 4 g/day lowered triglyceride levels by 45%. Fish oil supplements seem to be a reasonable, cost-effective means to reduce triglyceride levels; side effects include eructation, taste perversion, and dyspepsia.

Other agents to consider are neomycin, lomitapide, and mipomersen. These agents can be considered in the management of patients with refractory LDL elevations. Neomycin complexes with bile acid and lowers LDL levels. It also inhibits production of apolipoprotein(a) in the liver and lowers Lp(a). It is recommended as adjuvant therapy for patients with familial hypercholesterolemia and Lp(a) excess. Important side effects include nephrotoxicity and ototoxicity. Lomitapide inhibits microsomal triglyceride transfer protein in the liver endecreases apo B. Significant reductions in LDL (up to 50%) are seen with treatment. Liver toxicity is a serious adverse event associated with this agent.

Mipomersen is another agent approved for use in homozygous familial hypercholesterolemia. It binds apo B messenger RNA and inhibits apo B production. Apo B is a structural component of VLDL, IDL, and LDL. Treatment reduces LDL by up to 50%. Side effects include flu-like symptoms, injection site reactions, elevations in liver enzymes, and liver toxicity. The side effect profile and expense associated with both lomitapide and mipomersen limit the use of these agents to individuals with homozygous familial hypercholesterolemia.

🔴 LIPID DISORDERS

A number of specific disorders of overproduction or impaired removal of lipoproteins result in dyslipidemia (see Tables 69-2 and 69-3). These disorders are often familial, but secondary causes also need to be considered. Comorbid conditions (diabetes, hypothyroidism), medications (estrogen, glucocorticoids, β-blockers), and lifestyle factors (diet, alcohol) can increase the production and clearance of lipoproteins. Addressing these factors can often normalize lipid levels. If abnormalities persist, evaluation of genetic factors and treatment with pharmacologic therapy may need to be considered.

Familial Hypercholesterolemia

Mutations in the gene that encodes the LDL (apo B/E) receptor result in familial hypercholesterolemia. Impairment in LDL receptor synthesis or function decreases the clearance of LDL and increases circulating LDL levels, resulting in cholesterol plaque formation. These plaques deposit in the arteries (atheroma), skin or tendons (xanthoma), eyelids (xanthelasma), and iris (corneal arcus). The homozygous form of this autosomal dominant disorder is rare. Affected individuals present early in life with elevated levels of total cholesterol (600 to 1000 mg/dL) and LDL-cholesterol (550 to 950 mg/dL). Triglyceride and HDL-cholesterol levels are normal. These patients develop CHD, aortic stenosis due to atherosclerosis of the aortic root, and tendon xanthomas (often in the Achilles tendon). If the condition remains untreated, patients with homozygous familial hypercholesterolemia typically die of myocardial infarction before 20 years of age. The heterozygous form of familial hypercholesterolemia affects 1 in every 500 individuals, with the partial receptor defect resulting in cells that display half the normal number of fully functional LDL receptors. These individuals have less strongly elevated concentrations of total cholesterol (>300 to 600 mg/dL) and LDL-cholesterol (250 to 500 mg/dL) than do those with the homozygous form. Premature CHD (before 45 years of age in men and 55 years in women) and tendon xanthomas are characteristic clinical findings.

Although familial hypercholesterolemia can be established by identifying one of the many gene mutations in the LDL receptor or by demonstrating diminished LDL receptor function, the diagnosis of familial hypercholesterolemia usually is made on the basis of clinical features. Elevated total cholesterol (>300 mg/dL) and LDL-cholesterol (>250 mg/dL) in an individual with a personal or family history of premature CHD and tendon xanthomas identifies patients at risk for familial hypercholesterolemia. Treatment requires a low-fat (<20% of total calories), low cholesterol (<100 mg/day) diet in combination with drug therapy. Usually, patients with familial hypercholesterolemia require multiple agents to lower cholesterol levels to the target range. In patients who do not tolerate the medications or who have limited receptor function, liver transplantation to provide functional receptors, ileal bypass surgery to decrease gastrointestinal absorption of bile acids, or LDL apheresis to remove excess LDL may be considered. Both lomitapide and mipomersen may also be considered as adjuvant therapy.

Familial Defective Apolipoprotein B100

In this autosomal dominant disorder, a defect in the apo B100 protein results in impaired binding of LDL particles to the LDL receptor. The disorder affects as many as 1 in 750 Caucasians with hypercholesterolemia. The clinical presentation is similar to familial hypercholesterolemia, with elevated total cholesterol and LDL-cholesterol levels associated with premature CHD and tendon xanthomas. However, the homozygous and heterozygous clinical forms of familial defective apo B100 are milder than familial hypercholesterolemia, because apo E–mediated clearance of remnant particles is still functional. Total cholesterol concentration ranges from 350 to 550 mg/dL in the homozygous and 200 to 350 mg/dL in the heterozygous disorder. DNA analysis can identify the apo B100 gene mutation and confirm the diagnosis, but genetic diagnosis is not necessary to initiate therapy. A low-cholesterol, low-fat diet in combination with a statin, bile acid resin, and/or niacin is recommended to lower cholesterol levels to target ranges.

Elevated Plasma Lipoprotein(a)

Lp(a) is a specialized form of LDL that is assembled extracellularly from apolipoprotein(a) and LDL. Lp(a), when present at elevated levels, interferes with fibrinolysis by competing with plasminogen. This leads to decreased thrombolysis and increased clot formation. Lp(a) also binds macrophages, promoting foam cell formation and atherosclerotic plaques. Screening should be considered in individuals who have a family or personal history of premature CHD without dyslipidemia and in those for whom cholesterol-lowering therapy has failed. The diagnosis can be made by documenting Lp(a) levels higher than 30 mg/dL in a patient with premature CHD. The primary goal of therapy is to lower LDL levels with agents such as statins. If LDL goals cannot be achieved, then Lp(a)-lowering therapy with niacin and neomycin may be considered.

Polygenic Hypercholesterolemia

Hypercholesterolemia in a population is mostly due to small influences of many different genes. The exact nature of these genetic defects is poorly defined, but apo E may play a role in the pathogenesis. Apo E4 on chylomicrons and VLDL remnants has a high affinity for the LDL receptor. Elevated binding of apo E4–containing lipoproteins to LDL receptors may downregulate LDL receptor synthesis and increase circulating LDL levels. Environmental factors such as diet can influence production of chylomicrons and VLDL, resulting in downregulation of the LDL receptor in conditions with high apo E4. This leads to an increased propensity for CHD, and treatment with LDL-lowering agents is recommended based on risk factors (see Table 69-7).

Familial Combined Hyperlipoproteinemia

Familial combined hyperlipoproteinemia (FCHL) is an autosomal dominant polygenic disorder that affects 1% to 2% of the population. Factors such as diet, glucose intolerance, and medications can influence the phenotypic presentation. In FCHL, the liver synthesizes excess VLDL. VLDL is hydrolyzed by LPL to produce LDL. Mutations in the *LPL* gene affecting its expression or function can decrease the efficiency of VLDL catabolism. Dysfunction of LPL is observed in one third of patients with FCHL. Diminished LPL activity increases circulating VLDL-triglyceride; furthermore, fewer VLDL remnant particles are available for HDL synthesis. Therefore, FCHL needs to be considered in all patients whose total cholesterol level is greater than 250 mg/dL, triglycerides greater than 175 mg/dL, or HDL-cholesterol less than 35 mg/dL.

There are no definitive diagnostic tests, but family screening can help confirm the diagnosis. The phenotype of FCHL is variable, with individuals displaying high LDL-cholesterol, high VLDL-triglyceride, or both based on the genetic defect and environmental factors. Patients also typically have high apo B (>120 mg/dL) and a low ratio of LDL-cholesterol to apo B100 (<1.2). They accumulate small dense LDL particles, which are thought to be atherogenic and contribute to premature CHD. Xanthomas or xanthelasmas are not a feature of this disorder. Affected individuals require a low-fat, low-cholesterol diet plus multiple lipid-lowering drugs to achieve target goals. Fibric acid derivatives, which hydrolyze the triglyceride core of VLDL particles and increase LDL production, are recommended for treatment of the hypertriglyceridemia. Patients with FCHL often additionally require a statin or niacin to lower their LDL-cholesterol level.

Familial Dysbetalipoproteinemia

Apo E on the surface of lipoprotein particles binds LDL receptors and facilitates clearance of remnant particles from the circulation. The apo E2 allele has a lower affinity for LDL receptors than apo E3 or apo E4. In individuals who are homozygous for apo E2, LPL hydrolyzes the triglyceride core and the resulting cholesterol-rich chylomicrons. VLDL and IDL remnant particles accumulate in the circulation. Expression of this phenotype usually requires a precipitating condition that increases lipoprotein production (e.g., diabetes, alcohol consumption) or decreases clearance (e.g., hypothyroidism). In addition to the more common autosomal recessive mutation of apo E described earlier, several apo E mutations have been described that result in an autosomal dominant phenotype manifesting in childhood. Premature CHD, peripheral vascular disease, and xanthomas involving the palmer crease are characteristic clinical features. Individuals with familial dysbetalipoproteinemia have elevated levels of total cholesterol (300 to 400 mg/dL) and triglycerides (300 to 400 mg/dL). Definitive diagnosis requires genetic testing to identify apo E2 homozygosity or mutation. Treatment of coexisting conditions such as diabetes and hypothyroidism can normalize lipid levels in apo E2 homozygotes. If target levels are not achieved, dietary therapy and lipid-lowering drugs such as fibric acid derivatives and HMG-CoA reductase inhibitors should also be considered.

Lipoprotein Lipase Deficiency

Mutations in the *LPL* gene resulting in deficiency of LPL synthesis or function lead to increased circulating chylomicron and VLDL particles and severe hypertriglyceridemia. Homozygous LPL deficiency is rare. It manifests in childhood with triglyceride levels higher than 1000 mg/dL. Heterozygous LPL deficiency occurs in 2% to 4% of the population and usually requires a precipitating factor, such as uncontrolled diabetes or estrogen therapy, to manifest the phenotype. These individuals have moderate hypertriglyceridemia (250 to 750 mg/dL) that can increase to levels greater than 1000 mg/dL with secondary factors. This can result in the chylomicronemia syndrome, which is characterized by marked hypertriglyceridemia (>1000 to 2000 mg/dL), pancreatitis, eruptive xanthomas, lipemia retinalis, and hepatosplenomegaly. Visual inspection demonstrates lipemic plasma. After refrigeration for 12 hours, a creamy top layer (increased chylomicrons) or turbid plasma infranatant (increased VLDL), or both, can be demonstrated. Documentation of diminished LPL activity confirms the diagnosis. A diet low in fat (<10% of total calories or 20 to 25 g/day) is the primary treatment. Secondary factors such as uncontrolled diabetes and alcohol use should be addressed, and VLDL-lowering agents (e.g., fibric acid derivatives, niacin) may be needed to prevent severe hypertriglyceridemia.

Apolipoprotein C-II Deficiency

Apo C-II is an activating cofactor for LPL. Deficiency of apo C-II is a rare autosomal recessive disorder that leads to increased chylomicrons and VLDL particles in the circulation, resulting in severe hypertriglyceridemia. Clinical manifestations are similar to those of LPL deficiency, including hypertriglyceridemia (>1000 mg/dL) and symptoms of pancreatitis, eruptive xanthomas, lipemia retinalis, and hepatosplenomegaly. Treatment recommendations include appropriate management of secondary factors such as diabetes and hypothyroidism, dietary fat restriction (<10% of calories), and drug therapy (e.g., fibric acid derivatives). For severe hypertriglyceridemia, plasma transfusion (with apo C-II) can be considered.

Familial Hypertriglyceridemia

Familial hypertriglyceridemia is an autosomal dominant disorder that is characterized by overproduction of hepatic VLDL. The exact defect or mutation is unknown. Secondary factors that increase VLDL, such as diabetes, alcohol ingestion, and estrogen therapy, appear to exacerbate this condition. Low HDL associated with familial hypertriglyceridemia is related to increased catabolism. Individuals with this condition have hypertriglyceridemia (200 to 500 mg/dL) and low HDL-cholesterol (<35 mg/dL) at presentation. This diagnosis is considered in individuals who have a family and personal history of hypertriglyceridemia, CHD, and normal LDL levels. Cloudy infranatant after overnight refrigeration of plasma identifies a disorder of VLDL metabolism. Treatment starts with management of secondary factors that may exacerbate the condition. Dietary fat restriction (<10% of calories) and drug therapy with fish oil, niacin, and fibric acid derivates should be initiated if target goals are not achieved.

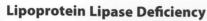 *For a deeper discussion on this topic, please see Chapter 206, "Disorders of Lipid Metabolism," in* Goldman-Cecil Medicine, *25th Edition.*

SUGGESTED READINGS

Carroll MD, Lacher DA, Sorlie PD, et al: Trends in serum lipids and lipoproteins of adults, 1960-2002, JAMA 294:1773–1781, 2005.

Expert Panel on Integrated Guidelines for Cardiovascular Health and Risk Reduction in Children and Adolescents, National Heart, Lung, and Blood Institute: Summary report, Pediatrics 128(Suppl 5):S213–S256, 2011.

Genest JJ, Martin-Munley SS, McNamara JR, et al: Familial lipoprotein disorders in patients with premature coronary artery disease, Circulation 85:2025–2033, 1992.

Gordon T, Castelli WP, Hjartland MC, et al: High density lipoprotein as a protective factor against coronary artery disease. The Farmingham Study, Am J Med 62:707–715, 1997.

Grundy SM, Cleeman JI, Merz CN, et al: Implications of recent clinical trials for the National Cholesterol Education Program (NCEP) Adult Treatment Panel III guidelines, Circulation 110:227–239, 2004.

Hokanson JE, Austin MA: Plasma triglyceride level is a risk factor for cardiovascular disease independent of high-density lipoprotein cholesterol: a meta-analysis of population-based prospective studies, J Cardiovasc Risk 3:213–224, 1996.

Jenkins DJ, Kendall CW, Marchie A, et al: Effects of a dietary portfolio of cholesterol-lowering foods vs lovastatin on serum lipids and C-reactive protein, JAMA 290:502–510, 2003.

Kumana CR, Cheung BM, Lauder IJ: Gauging the impact of statins using number needed to treat, JAMA 282:1899–1901, 1999.

National Cholesterol Education Program (NCEP) Expert Panel on Detection, Evaluation, and Treatment of High Blood Cholesterol in Adults (Adult Treatment Panel III): Third Report of the National Cholesterol Education Program (NCEP) Expert Panel on Detection, Evaluation, and Treatment of High Blood Cholesterol in Adults (Adult Treatment Panel III) final report, Circulation 106:3143–3421, 2002.

U.S. Preventive Services Task Force: Screening for lipid disorders in adults: U.S. Preventive Services Task Force recommendation statement, 2008. Available at: http://www.uspreventiveservicestaskforce.org/uspstf/uspschol.htm. Accessed August 1, 2014.

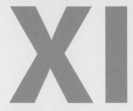

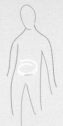

XI

Women's Health

70 Women's Health Topics
Kelly McGarry, Kimberly Babb, Laura Edmonds, Christine Duffy, Michelle Anvar, and Jennifer Jeremiah

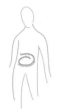

70

Women's Health Topics

Kelly McGarry, Kimberly Babb, Laura Edmonds,
Christine Duffy, Michelle Anvar, and Jennifer Jeremiah

THE SPECIALTY OF WOMEN'S HEALTH

The specialty of women's health grew out of the recognition that differences in the biology of men and women are responsible for differences in the prevalence, presentation, and management of some diseases. The focus of women's health is on conditions unique to women (e.g., pregnancy), conditions that are more common in women (e.g., breast cancer, osteoporosis, some rheumatologic diseases), and conditions that have different presentations, natural history, risk factors, and prevention or treatment strategies in women and men (e.g., heart disease, sexually transmitted infections, urinary tract infections). Specialists in this area come from all disciplines and include obstetrician-gynecologists, general internists, subspecialty internists, family medicine, radiologists, and surgeons. In this chapter, we focus on medical issues unique to women and highlight what is known about gender differences in common diseases. For more detailed discussions of specific topics, please refer to the appropriate chapters in this edition of *Cecil Essentials of Medicine* and the 25th edition of *Goldman-Cecil Medicine*.

WHAT MAKES WOMEN DIFFERENT FROM MEN?

There are substantial biologic, physiologic, and psychosocial differences between men and women. Although we have an in-depth understanding of some of the differences, others are just beginning to be elucidated, and still others remain undiscovered.

Women tend to be physically smaller than men. Women have less renal mass, and defining normal renal function takes this into account. Women typically have a 15% lower creatinine clearance rate than men with the same level of creatinine. The volume of muscle and fat varies by gender and age, which affects the metabolism of medications and estimates of kidney function. Women have smaller blood vessels than men. Until smaller intravascular catheters were created, this biologic difference made cardiac catheterizations in women technically more challenging.

Gender also influences treatment. A study of more than 700 physicians presented with several hypothetical patient scenarios found that the race and sex of a patient independently influenced how physicians managed chest pain. Women, particularly black women, were significantly less likely to be referred for catheterization than white men.

Differences in physiology affect biologic responses. For example, to increase cardiac output, women increase heart rate, whereas men increase stroke volume, in part by increasing vascular resistance. These physiologic differences may have different pathophysiologic consequences for men and women. Sympathetic tone varies by gender. Women have reduced sympathetic activity and enhanced parasympathetic activity compared with men. This may be one reason that premenopausal women tend to have lower blood pressure than age-matched men and why women may be more susceptible to orthostatic hypotension and fainting than men.

Hepatic drug clearance varies by gender, ethnicity, and race. Gender-related differences in pharmacokinetics in part determine the clinical effectiveness and potential adverse effects of drug therapy. Physiologic differences include the usually lower body weight and organ size, higher percentage of body fat, lower glomerular filtration rate, and different gastric motility in women compared with men. Molecular differences involve drug transporters and drug-metabolizing enzymes. Clinically important gender differences in pharmacodynamic processes include risk of QT prolongation, which can lead to a potentially fatal ventricular arrhythmia, torsades de pointes. A much higher percentage of women than men develop torsades after taking a variety of drugs, including certain antibiotics, antiarrhythmics, and antipsychotics. In addition to differences in drug transport and metabolism that result in different plasma and intracellular drug levels, the baseline electrocardiographic rate of corrected QT interval (QTc) is naturally longer in women than in men. Because there are gender differences in the rate of cardiac repolarization, drugs that are known to prolong the QTc interval should be carefully prescribed and monitored.

The approach to menstrual disorders is guided by an understanding of the physiology of reproduction. Estrogen levels vary substantially throughout life. With the onset of puberty, the hypothalamus begins releasing gonadotropin-releasing hormone (GnRH), leading to ovarian stimulation. The normal menstrual cycle requires precise regulation and feedback of hormones involving the hypothalamus, pituitary gland, and ovaries, with the uterus acting as an end organ for ovarian steroid effects. The menstrual cycle consists of the follicular or proliferative phase, ovulation, and the luteal or secretory phase. The physiologic changes that define the menstrual cycle, including variations in hormones, the uterine lining, and basal body temperature (taken on awakening), are graphically represented in Figure 70-1.

During the follicular phase, the hypothalamus secretes GnRH, which stimulates the pituitary to release gonadotropins, luteinizing hormone (LH), and follicle-stimulating hormone (FSH). LH and FSH then stimulate ovarian follicular development and estrogen secretion. Estrogen secretion results in proliferation of the endometrium. Eventually, one follicle with its oocyte becomes dominant, and maturation results in ovulation, which occurs soon after an LH surge. With ovulation, the oocyte leaves the dominant follicle and migrates toward the fallopian tube. The

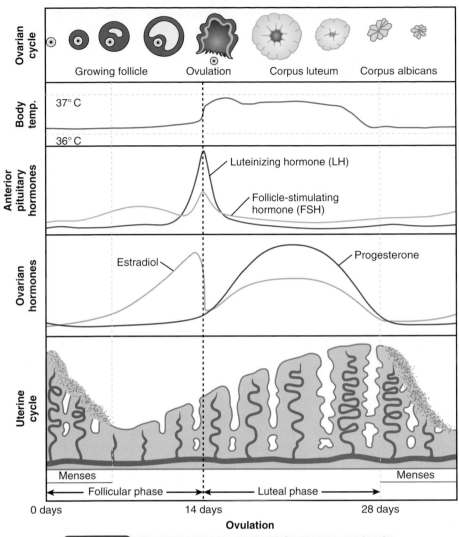

Ovarian cycle

Growing follicle   Ovulation   Corpus luteum   Corpus albicans

Body temp.

37° C

36° C

Anterior pituitary hormones

Luteinizing hormone (LH)

Follicle-stimulating hormone (FSH)

Ovarian hormones

Estradiol

Progesterone

Uterine cycle

Menses   Menses

Follicular phase   Luteal phase

0 days   14 days   28 days

Ovulation

FIGURE 70-1 The physiologic changes that define the menstrual cycle.

remaining cells in the follicle become the corpus luteum, which produces progesterone during the luteal phase. If fertilization does not occur, progesterone is secreted for about 14 days, and the follicle then involutes. This is associated with decreasing levels of estrogen and progesterone. The endometrium is shed in response to the falling estrogen and progesterone levels, and menstruation occurs.

Normal menstrual cycles usually occur monthly from adolescence until the time of menopause, which begins between the ages of 45 and 55 years. Cycle duration tends to become consistent within several years of menarche due to maturation of the hypothalamic-pituitary-ovarian hormonal axis. The median menstrual cycle length is 28 days, with a normal range between 25 and 35 days. The duration of menses typically is between 2 and 7 days. Delays in the expected onset and abnormalities of menstrual cycles often require evaluation for possible disease, including hormonal and structural disorders.

Estrogen receptors have been identified throughout the body, including reproductive organs and nonreproductive organs such as the brain, arteries, bone, smooth muscle, and urethra. Declining levels of estrogen at menopause explain some of the systemic changes that occur in postmenopausal women. The diagnostic

approach to abnormal genital bleeding and menopause is discussed later in this chapter.

Gender Differences in Societal Factors

Complex societal factors, including processes of socialization, expectations about work and home, lifestyle behaviors, and other psychosocial factors, can explain differences in the health of men and women. Research shows that women still occupy different positions in society than men. Women are less likely to be employed and more likely to have lower incomes, live in poverty, and be single parents than men. Men are more likely than women to smoke, consume alcohol, eat an unbalanced diet, and be overweight. Women are more likely than men to be physically inactive. However, both men and women of lower socioeconomic status (SES) have a higher prevalence of risky lifestyle behaviors. Women are more likely to report health problems, in part due to higher social demands and perceived obligations. Gender differences exist in perceived control and self-esteem, with women reporting lower levels of both than men, although women do report higher levels of social support.

Research has documented a relationship between health inequalities and socioeconomic inequalities in income, education, occupational status, and employment status. Women may have overall lower rates of mortality, but they paradoxically report higher levels of depression, psychiatric disorders, distress, and a variety of chronic illnesses than men. It is important to recognize the impact of these social determinants on the health of all patients and to understand that the pathways through which social position, behavior, and psychosocial forces influence health are different for men and women. Patients must be encouraged to engage in a healthy lifestyle because healthy behaviors help to prevent weight gain, high blood pressure, cardiovascular disease, diabetes, arthritis, and early mortality.

⬤ WOMEN'S HEALTH ISSUES OVER THE LIFESPAN

Issues for Adolescents

Adolescence is a period of rapid physical and emotional change, and patients may have both pediatric and adult issues. Adolescents often do not have a good understanding of health issues and are embarrassed or nervous about asking questions. Health care providers must help adolescents navigate this period of change and educate them about healthy behaviors in an open and nonjudgmental manner to create a therapeutic relationship.

Gender, Sexual Identity, and Sexual History

Adolescents often struggle with issues of gender, sexuality, and sexual behavior. They often avoid discussing these topics because of embarrassment, fear of being judged, or concerns about confidentiality. Discussing these issues in a safe, nonjudgmental manner can improve adolescents' understanding and promote healthy and responsible choices.

Individuals who identify themselves as lesbian, gay, bisexual, or transgender are at higher risk for substance abuse, intimate partner violence, and mental health issues. Asking about gender identity and sexual orientation is an important part of taking a sexual history. Many adolescents experiment, and their sexual behavior is not always a reflection of their gender identity or sexual orientation. A sexual history should include the number and gender of partners; use of contraception and barrier protection; types of sexual activities, including oral, vaginal, and anal sex; history of sexual abuse and intimate partner violence; history of coerced or forced sexual interactions; and use of alcohol or illicit substances during sex. Adolescents should be encouraged to make healthy choices regarding sexual activity, including abstaining from sex, using contraception and barrier protection, and seeking respectful partners.

Confidentiality

Adolescents often come to medical visits accompanied by a parent, and parental consent should be obtained for treatment of many medical issues. It is also important to interview all adolescents alone for part or all of the visit to discuss social and health history, because they do not feel comfortable discussing many issues in front of parents. Their history should remain confidential unless they divulge something that puts them or another individual at risk or have certain illnesses that are reportable to the department of public health. Regulations on confidentiality vary from state to state.

Adolescents often underestimate their parents' ability to understand their issues. Physicians should encourage adolescents to be open with their parents about health issues and bridge the communication divide.

Eating Disorders

Eating disorders often begin during the adolescent period. They include anorexia, bulimia, binge eating, and other disordered eating behaviors. These illnesses are characterized by distorted body image and dysfunctional behaviors that can lead to long-term physical and psychological issues. Rates of eating disorders are increasing, and white females tend to be disproportionately affected. Eating disorders often start with dieting and progressively develop into dysfunctional behaviors. Physicians who take care of adolescents should monitor weight and body mass index (BMI) and screen for alterations in body image and behaviors that suggest disordered eating. Management of eating disorders often requires a multidisciplinary approach with a primary care physician, psychologist, and nutritionist.

Sexually Transmitted Infections

Sexually transmitted infections (STIs) are common among adolescents. Human papillomavirus (HPV), *Chlamydia trachomatis*, and *Trichomonas* infections account for most cases, although gonorrhea, syphilis, herpesvirus, and human immunodeficiency virus (HIV) infections also occur.

All patients between the ages of 13 and 21 years should be screened for chlamydial and gonorrheal infections annually. Annual opt-out HIV testing is also recommended by the Centers for Disease Control and Prevention (CDC) for all patients between the ages of 13 and 64 years.

The HPV vaccine has been added to the standard pediatric immunization schedule and is recommended for girls and boys 9 to 11 years of age. If the HPV vaccine was not part of the normal schedule, it is approved for patients up to 26 years old. The vaccines have proved to be highly safe and effective, providing another means to prevent cervical cancer.

Primary Amenorrhea

Amenorrhea is defined as the lack of menses in a sexually mature female. It is categorized as primary or secondary amenorrhea. Primary amenorrhea is the lack of menarche by age 16 despite normal sexual development or the lack of menarche by age 14 in the absence of sexual development.

Primary amenorrhea is often caused by genetic or anatomic abnormalities. Breast development, presence of a uterus, and the levels of FSH and LH are important factors in determining the cause of primary amenorrhea. , Lack of a uterus despite breast development may suggest androgen insensitivity or müllerian agenesis. If the uterus exists, an outflow tract obstruction such as an imperforate hymen or a transverse vaginal septum may be identified. However, if secondary sexual characteristics are missing, measuring FSH and LH levels can help to determine the difference between hypogonadotropic hypogonadism (i.e., constitutional delay or pituitary or hypothalamic failure) and hypergonadotropic hypogonadism (i.e., premature ovarian failure or Turner syndrome).

Issues for Adult Women

Promoting Wellness and Preventive Health

Comprehensive health care for women includes gender-specific and general services and counseling to promote healthful behaviors and practices to prevent disease. Table 70-1 highlights evidence-based recommendations for preventive care specifically for women at average risk.

Screening for Cervical Cancer

Cervical cancer, the tenth leading cause of cancer death in the Unites States, occurs most often in women who have never been screened or not screened in the past 5 years. Infections with high-risk strains of HPV (16 and 18) are responsible for approximately70% of cervical cancer cases. The incidence increases with early onset of intercourse; greater number of lifetime sexual partners; co-infection with other STIs, including HIV; high parity; long-term use of oral contraceptives; and cigarette smoking. Peak incidence of HPV infection occurs among women younger than 25 years of age, but most of these infections are transient. Approximately 10% of women remain HPV positive 5 years after infection. Cervical abnormalities that do transform into cancer are thought to progress over time from less severe to more severe lesions.

The U. S. Preventive Services Task Force (USPSTF) and the American Cancer Society (ACS), American Society of Colposcopy and Cervical Pathology (ASCCP), and American Society for Clinical Pathology (ASCP) published consensus guidelines for screening average-risk women. These recommendations do not apply to women who have had cervical intraepithelial neoplasia with moderately abnormal cells (i.e., CIN 2) or higher-grade cervical lesions, cervical cancer, or in utero diethylstilbestrol (DES) exposure or to women who are immunocompromised or HIV positive (Table 70-2).

Contraception

Approximately 62% of reproductive-age women in the United States are using some form of contraception, but almost one half of pregnancies are unintended. When helping patients choose a contraceptive method, several important variables should be considered. The first is efficacy and a patient's ability to adhere to the method. The efficacy of contraceptive methods depends on appropriate use (Table 70-3). Patients' past experiences with different forms of contraception and personal preferences may help to predict how well they will comply with current regimens.

Obtaining a thorough personal and family medical history can help to determine what methods are appropriate. Certain medical issues can make a choice too risky for one patient but provide a health benefit for another. For example, oral contraceptives that increase the risk of thrombosis are contraindicated for a patient with a strong family history of venous thrombosis, but they could correct anemia in a patient with menorrhagia. The patient's sexual history and assessment of the risk for STIs play a role in contraceptive choice and education about the use of barrier methods.

Methods of Contraception

Barrier methods include the male and female condom, diaphragm, and cervical cap. The diaphragm and cervical cap need to be fitted by a medical professional, require a prescription, and need to be left in 6 to 8 hours after intercourse to be effective. The male condom, which can be purchased over the counter, has the added benefit of helping to prevent the transmission of STIs.

Combination hormonal contraceptives are the most common form of hormonal birth control. They typically contain a low dose of estrogen (≤ 35 µg) and one of several progesterones. Delivery methods include pills, patches, and intravaginal rings. Contraindications to combination hormonal contraception are related to the estrogen component and include a personal history of a thromboembolic event or known thrombogenic mutation, cerebrovascular accident (CVA), coronary artery disease (CAD), uncontrolled hypertension, migraine with aura, smoking after age 35, breast cancer, estrogen-dependent neoplasms, undiagnosed abnormal vaginal bleeding, liver tumors, and pregnancy.

Potential noncontraceptive benefits of combination oral contraceptives include regulation of menstrual flow and improvement in ovarian cyst recurrence, endometriosis, acne, polycystic ovarian syndrome, and mittelschmerz (i.e., midcycle pain). Long-term use of combination oral contraceptives has been associated with a reduced lifetime risk of endometrial and ovarian cancers. The World Health Organization (WHO) medical eligibility criteria for contraceptive use provide excellent guidance for the choice of contraceptive methods based on patients' risk factors (available at http://www.who.int/reproductivehealth/publications/family_planning/9789241563888/en/index.html [accessed August 1, 2014]). Patients should be able to take pills at approximately the same time each day.

The contraceptive patch is a form of combination hormonal contraception that is delivered transdermally. The patch is applied on a weekly basis for 3 weeks and then discontinued for 1 week. The patch delivers a higher average dose of estrogen but has lower peak doses. Another form of combination hormone delivery is the intravaginal ring. A flexible ring is inserted intravaginally for 3 weeks and then removed for 1 week when menses occur. The patch and the ring are reasonable options for patients concerned with medication compliance.

Progesterone-only contraceptives are an option for women intolerant of estrogen or at increased risk for thromboembolic events. Contraindications include active CAD, breast cancer, liver tumor, and phlebitis. They are slightly less efficacious than the combination pills, and women may experience breakthrough bleeding.

Depot medroxyprogesterone acetate (DMPA) is a progesterone-only injection administered every 12 weeks. It is a very reliable form of contraception. Major side effects include irregular bleeding (which resolves over time) and amenorrhea (50% at 1 year). Weight gain, hair changes, and acne are possible side effects. The U.S. Food and Drug Administration (FDA) issued a black box warning that DMPA may decrease bone density, especially in adolescents.

The intrauterine device (IUD) can be a great option for women who do not desire pregnancy in the next 5 to 10 years. Worldwide, it is the most widely used method of reversible

TABLE 70-1 PREVENTIVE HEALTH RECOMMENDATIONS FOR WOMEN

SCREENING	RECOMMENDATION	AGE AND INTERVAL
Alcohol	All women should be screened for alcohol misuse. Hazardous drinking defined as >7 drinks/week or >3/occasion. Drinking results in physical, social, and psychological harms, and women engaged in hazardous drinking should be provided with behavioral counseling interventions.	Beginning at age 18 and at contact with health care provider
Cardiovascular disease	All women should be assessed for their CV disease risk (hypertension, tobacco use, diabetes, family history, physical inactivity, unhealthy dietary lipids, overweight and obesity) and counseled on risk reduction strategies. The 10-yr CV risk can be calculated with risk assessment tool calculator.	At contact with health care provider
	Lipid disorders screening includes total cholesterol, HDL, LDL, and triglycerides after a 12-hr fast	Women age ≥45 and women 20-44 yr if other risk factors present; interval not clear, but every 5 yr if low risk
Cancer		
Breast cancer	Mammography	ACS suggests annually at age 40 for as long as in good health; yearly for women of any age with greater than 20% lifetime risk
		USPSTF suggests biennial screening for women age 50-74. Biennial screening before age 50 should be addressed on an individual basis. Women in poor health are unlikely to benefit from screening. Current evidence insufficient to assess the additional benefits and harms of screening in women >75 yr.
	MRI	Based on breast cancer risk calculated using NCI's breast cancer risk assessment tool
Cervical cancer	See Table 70-2	
Ovarian cancer	Routine screening is not recommended by any organization. Women at high risk (strong family history, *BRCA1* and *BRCA2* genes) may consider screening.	
Uterine cancer	Routine screening is not recommended by any organization.	Women at high risk for HNPCC can be offered screening with endometrial biopsy at age 35.
Depression	All women should be screened; multiple screening tools available. Brief intervention: (1) "Over the past 2 weeks, have you felt down, depressed, or hopeless?" (2) "Over the past 2 weeks, have you had little interest or pleasure in doing things?"	At contact with health care provider
Infectious diseases		
STIs	Counseling recommended	High-intensity behavioral counseling to prevent STIs for all sexually active adolescents and adults at increased for STIs
Chlamydia	Testing recommended	All sexually active women ages 24 and younger and older women who are at increased risk
Gonorrhea	Testing recommended	All sexually active women if they are at increased risk for infection
Hepatitis C	Testing recommended	Screen women at high risk for infection and offer one-time screening if born between 1945 and 1965
HIV	Testing recommended	Adolescents and adults ages 15-65 yr; younger adolescents and older adults who are at increased risk and all pregnant women
HPV	See Table 70-2	
Obesity	All women should be screened. Women with a BMI >30 kg/m² should be referred for behavioral interventions.	At contact with health care provider
Osteoporosis	Insufficient evidence to recommend combined calcium and vitamin D supplementation for primary prevention. Women should be counseled about daily calcium and vitamin D requirements and adequate weight-bearing and resistance exercises for prevention.	
	DEXA bone density test; fracture risk can be assessed by FRAX	All women ≥65 yr and women <65 yr whose fracture risk is equal to or greater than that of a 65-yr-old woman with no additional risk factors. Women 50-64 yrs with a 9.3% 10-yr fracture risk determined by FRAX
Stroke	Daily aspirin for prevention of stroke when potential benefit of ischemic stroke reduction outweighs potential harm of increased gastrointestinal hemorrhage	Women 55-79 yr
Thyroid disorders	USPSTF finds insufficient evidence to recommend for or against routine screening for asymptomatic women; testing recommended for symptoms.	
Tobacco use	All women should be screened and provided with smoking cessation interventions.	At contact with health care provider
Violence	Screening and counseling for interpersonal and domestic violence	At contact with health care provider

ACS, American Cancer Society; BMI, body mass index; CV, cardiovascular; DEXA, dual-energy x-ray absorptiometry; FRAX, fracture risk assessment tool; HDL, high-density lipoprotein cholesterol; HIV, human immunodeficiency virus; HNPCC, hereditary nonpolyposis colon cancer; HPV, human papillomavirus; LDL, low-density lipoprotein cholesterol; MRI, magnetic resonance imaging; NCI, National Cancer Institute; STIs, sexually transmitted infections; USPSTF, U.S. Preventive Services Task Force.

TABLE 70-2 SCREENING RECOMMENDATIONS FOR CERVICAL CANCER

AGE	USPSTF	ACS/ASCCP/ASCP	COMMENTS AND RATIONALE
<21	No screening before the age of 21 despite time of sexual activity	No screening before the age of 21 despite time of sexual activity	HPV positivity and cytologic abnormalities are likely to regress in young women.
21-29	Screening with liquid-based or conventional cytology alone every 3 yr; HPV testing should not be performed.	Screening with liquid-based or conventional cytology alone every 3 yr; HPV testing should not be performed.	HPV co-testing should not be used for women <30 yr of age because incidence of HPV is high and cytologic abnormalities are often transient, leading to unnecessary and sometimes harmful interventions
30-65	Cytology alone every 3 yr or cytology with co-testing every 5 yr	Co-testing with cytology and HPV every 5 yr (preferred method) or cytology alone every 3 yr if HPV testing in not available	
>65	No further testing if adequately screened in the past and not otherwise at increased risk for cervical cancer	No further testing if adequately screened in the past	Adequate screening defined as two negative results in the past 10 yr with one in the past 5 yr and no history of CIN2 or greater grade neoplasia. Because cancer risk decreases with age and prior normal Pap tests, overtesting may to lead to false-positive test results.
After hysterectomy	No further screening if no CIN2 or higher grade neoplasia	No further screening if no CIN2 or higher grade neoplasia	Clinicians should confirm that total hysterectomy was performed.
HPV vaccinated	Continue recommended screening	Continue recommended screening	

ACS, American Cancer Society; ASCCP, American Society of Colposcopy and Cervical Pathology; ASCP, American Society for Clinical Pathology; CIN 2, cervical intraepithelial neoplasia with moderately abnormal cells; HPV, human papillomavirus; Pap, Papanicolaou smear; USPSTF, U.S. Preventive Services Task Force.

contraception. Two types of IUDs are available in the US, and both are almost as effective as sterilization. The copper IUD can be left in 10 years, and the progesterone IUD can be left in for 5 years. The copper IUD can be associated with heavier menstrual bleeding and cramps. The progesterone IUD may initially have breakthrough bleeding, but almost one half of users become amenorrheic. Implanon is a progesterone rod that is implanted under the skin and is highly effective for 3 years. It can be placed in outpatient offices and is helpful in limiting dysmenorrhea, but it is associated with irregular menses.

Postcoital emergency contraception can be achieved with one or several hormonal options or with placement of a copper IUD. Hormonal options are available over the counter in the United States, and recommended use is up to 72 hours after intercourse. After contraception is discontinued, the time of return to fertility depends on the type of contraceptive used. The average time for return to fertility with combination hormonal contraceptives is 3 months. With DMPA, fertility can be delayed by 12 to 22 months.

Pregnancy

Preconception Counseling and Pregnancy Planning

Preconception counseling begins by obtaining a through medical history to assess potential risks to the mother and fetus. Women with a personal or family history of genetic disorders may benefit from formal genetic counseling. For the woman with no significant medical problems and no serious family medical history, education about maintaining a healthy lifestyle, nutritional supplementation, and avoidance of toxicities to the fetus are important.

In 2009, the Institute of Medicine published guidelines for weight gain during pregnancy and recommended that women planning pregnancy achieve their normal BMI before conception. Advising and assisting the overweight or obese patient in weight loss efforts before pregnancy can prevent gestational diabetes, adverse fetal outcomes, and pathologic musculoskeletal

conditions. Avoidance of tobacco, alcohol, and illicit drugs is critical because they are harmful to both mother and fetus. All women planning pregnancy or capable of becoming pregnant should be advised to take a daily multivitamin with folic acid (400 to 800 μg) to reduce the risks of neural tube defects and other congenital anomalies, including cardiovascular defects, urinary defects, and cleft lip.

Routine laboratory evaluation includes rubella titer, varicella titer (in women with a negative history of varicella), hepatitis B surface antigen, and a complete blood count (CBC), assessing for hemoglobinopathy. Women should receive HIV testing and counseling.

An important goal is to ensure that women are immune to measles, mumps, rubella, tetanus, diphtheria, poliomyelitis, and varicella. Women should receive influenza vaccine in pregnancy due to the increased risk of complications from influenza infection. Ideally, women should receive all indicated vaccinations at least 1 month before conception. Live vaccines (e.g., rubella) should not be given during pregnancy.

The patient's medications, including prescribed, over-the-counter, and herbal medications, should be reviewed to identify potential teratogens. Medications not considered absolutely necessary for the well-being of the mother or fetus should be stopped. This is not always possible or indicated for women being treated for chronic medical conditions.

Medical conditions known to increase the risk of adverse pregnancy outcomes for women and their offspring include diabetes, thyroid disease, seizure disorders, hypertension, rheumatoid arthritis, chronic renal disease, thrombophilias, asthma, and cardiovascular disease. Preconception care of these conditions can improve pregnancy outcomes. Patients usually are referred to high-risk pregnancy care for evaluation. Approximately 1% of pregnancies in the United States are complicated by pregestational diabetes. Gestational diabetes (GDM) occurs in approximately 7% of pregnancies. GDM has a high recurrence rate (30% to 80%) in subsequent pregnancies and a significantly increased

TABLE 70-3 COMPARISON OF LONG-ACTING, REVERSIBLE CONTRACEPTION METHODS

METHOD	PERCENTAGE OF WOMEN WITH AN UNINTENDED PREGNANCY DURING FIRST YEAR OF USE		PERCENTAGE OF WOMEN CONTINUING USE AT 1 YEAR[‡]
	Typical Use[*]	*Perfect Use*[†]	
No method[§]	85	85	
Spermicides[‖]	29	18	42
Withdrawal	27	4	43
Fertility awareness–based methods	25		51
Standard days method[¶]		5	
Two-day method[¶]		4	
Ovulation method[¶]		3	
Sponge			
Parous women	32	20	46
Nulliparous women	16	9	57
Diaphragm[#]	16	6	57
Condom[**]			
Female (Reality)	21	5	49
Male	15	2	53
Combined pill and progestin-only pill	8	0.3	68
Evra patch	8	0.3	68
NuvaRing	8	0.3	68
Depo-Provera	3	0.3	56
Intrauterine device (IUD)			
ParaGard (copper T)	0.8	0.6	78
Mirena (levonorgestrel intrauterine system)	0.2	0.2	80
Implanor	0.05	0.05	84
Female sterilization	0.5	0.5	100
Male sterilization	0.15	0.10	100
Emergency contraceptive pills	Use within 72 hr after unprotected intercourse reduces risk of pregnancy ≥75%.[††]		
Lactational amenorrhea method	Highly effective, temporary method of contraception[††]		

Modified from Trussell J, Wynn LL: Reducing unintended pregnancy in the United States, Contraception 77:1–5, 2008.

[*]Among typical couples who initiate use of a method (not necessarily for the first time), the percentage who experience an accidental pregnancy during the first year if they do not stop use for any other reason. Estimates of the probability of pregnancy during the first year of typical use for spermicides, withdrawal, fertility awareness–based methods, the diaphragm, the male condom, the pill, and Depo-Provera are taken from the 1995 National Survey of Family Growth (NSFG), corrected for underreporting of abortion; see the reference above for the derivation of estimates for other methods.

[†]Among couples who initiate use of a method (not necessarily for the first time) and who use it perfectly (both consistently and correctly), the percentage who experience an accidental pregnancy during the first year if they do not stop use for any other reason. Trussell and Wynn (2008) provide the derivation of the estimate for each method.

[‡]Among couples attempting to avoid pregnancy, the percentage who continue to use a method for 1year.

[§]The percentages for becoming pregnant in columns 2 and 3 are based on data from populations in which contraception is not used and from women who cease using contraception to become pregnant. Among these populations, about 89% become pregnant within 1 year. This estimate was lowered slightly (to 85%) to represent the percentage who would become pregnant within 1 year among women now relying on reversible methods of contraception if they abandoned contraception altogether.

[‖]Foams, creams, gels, vaginal suppositories, and vaginal film.

[¶]The ovulation and 2-day methods are based on evaluation of cervical mucus. The standard days method avoids intercourse on cycle days 8 to 19.

[#]With spermicidal cream or jelly.

[**]Without spermicides.

[††]The treatment schedule is one dose within 120 hr after unprotected intercourse and a second dose 12 hr after the first dose. Both doses of plan B can be taken at the same time. Plan B (one dose is one white pill) is the only dedicated product specifically marketed for emergency contraception. The U.S. Food and Drug Administration also has declared the following 22 brands of oral contraceptives to be safe and effective for emergency contraception: Ogestrel or Ovral (one dose is two white pills); Levlen or Nordetto (one dose is four light orange pills), Cryselle, Levore, Low Ogestrel, Lo/Ovral, or Quasense (one dose is four white pills), Tri Levlen or Triphasil (one dose is four yellow pills), Jolessa, Portia, Seasonale, or Trivora (one dose is four pink pills), Seasonique (one dose is four light blue-green pills), Empresse (one dose is four orange pills), Alesse, Lessira, or Levlite (one dose is five pink pills), Aviane (one dose is five orange pills), and Lutera (one dose is five white pills).

[††]To maintain effective protection against pregnancy, another method of contraception must be used as soon as menstruation resumes, the frequency or duration of breast-feedings is reduced, bottle feedings are introduced, or the baby reaches 6 months of age. The best estimates of failure rate of all types of tubal sterilization is 1.31 after 5 years and 1.85 per 100 women after 10 years; it is highest for tubal fulguration and lowest for segmental resection in the 10 years after the procedure.

risk for future development of type 2 diabetes. In women with pregestational diabetes and GDM, adequate control of diabetes reduces the risk of congenital malformations.

Thyroid disease is the second most common endocrine disease that affects reproductive-age women. Hyperthyroidism and overt hypothyroidism occur in approximately 0.2% and 2.5% of all pregnancies, respectively. Adequate treatment of thyroid illness improves pregnancy outcomes. Approximately 70% to 80% of women with rheumatoid arthritis experience remission of disease during pregnancy, although the remaining women have active or worsening disease in pregnancy. Women with systemic lupus erythematosus (SLE) often experience exacerbations in pregnancy.

SLE increases the risk of adverse fetal outcomes, including spontaneous abortion, fetal growth restriction, and preterm birth.

A few conditions confer significant mortality risks to the mother and fetus. Pulmonary hypertension (especially Eisenmenger's syndrome), congenital heart disease with hypoxia, poor functional class, and arrhythmias are associated with adverse maternal outcomes.

Medications in Pregnancy

Pregnant women should avoid the use of most medications (Table 70-4). However, the benefits of medications may outweigh the risks, particularly for women with chronic medical

TABLE 70-4	FOOD AND DRUG ADMINISTRATION CATEGORIES OF DRUG SAFETY DURING PREGNANCY
CATEGORY	**INTERPRETATION**
A	Adequate, well-controlled studies in pregnant women have not shown an increased risk to the fetus in any trimester of pregnancy.
B	Animal studies have revealed no evidence of harm to the fetus; however, there are no adequate and well-controlled studies in pregnant women. *Or* Animal studies have shown an adverse effect, but adequate and well-controlled studies in pregnant women have failed to demonstrate a risk to the fetus in any trimester.
C	Animal studies have shown an adverse effect, and there are no adequate and well-controlled studies in pregnant women. *Or* No animal studies have been conducted, and there are no adequate and well-controlled studies in pregnant women.
D	Adequate, well-controlled, or observational studies in pregnant women have demonstrated a risk to the fetus. However, the benefits of therapy may outweigh the potential risk.
X	Adequate, well-controlled or observational studies in animals or pregnant women have demonstrated positive evidence of fetal abnormalities or risks, and the use of the product is contraindicated in women who are or may become pregnant.

TABLE 70-5	CAUSES OF SECONDARY AMENORRHEA
CAUSE	**EXAMPLES**
Physiologic changes	Pregnancy, lactation, menopause
Ovarian changes	Radiation- or chemotherapy-induced ovarian failure, chromosomal abnormalities, autoimmune or idiopathic
Anovulation	Hyperandrogenism (polycystic ovary syndrome, congenital adrenal hyperplasia), hyperprolactinemia (prolactinoma, phenothiazines, narcotics, and other medications), hyperthyroidism, hypothyroidism, hypopituitarism, pituitary adenoma, Cushing's syndrome, hypothalamic hypogonadism (eating disorder, athletic triad, stress)
Medications	Hormonal, cytotoxic, others
Uterine outflow abnormalities	Surgery, Asherman's syndrome

conditions. Few medications are absolutely contraindicated in pregnancy. Decisions about continuing or stopping medications require a discussion about the risks and benefits and an informed decision on the part of the woman.

Pregnancy Complications and Risk of Future Diseases

Women with a history of gestational diabetes are at increased risk for diabetes later in life. Women whose pregnancies were complicated by a gestational hypertensive disorder, such as preeclampsia or gestational hypertension, are at increased risk for subsequent essential hypertension. Women who have a history of a child with a neural tube defect should take 4 g of folic acid daily. Women with a prior problem pregnancy may benefit from close follow-up with an obstetric provider such as a high-risk pregnancy specialist to reduce subsequent problems.

Two important conditions to recognize are postpartum depression and postpartum thyroiditis. Postpartum depression may complicate 10% to 15% of pregnancies. The symptoms are the same as those of clinical depression in a nonpregnant woman. Risk factors for postpartum depression include a history of depression before pregnancy and depression during the current pregnancy. Postpartum thyroiditis may be seen in 7% to 8% of women. Only about one third of women have the classic hyperthyroid phase followed by hypothyroidism and recovery. Another 30% exhibit only hyperthyroidism, and the remaining 40% to 50% have only hypothyroidism. Unexpected symptoms after delivery should prompt an evaluation of thyroid function.

Lesbian Health

Being lesbian is not a homogeneous experience. The racial, ethnic, and socioeconomic diversity of the United States is mirrored in the lesbian community. The Institute of Medicine released a report acknowledging that lesbian, gay, bisexual, and transgender (LGBT) individuals experience unique health care disparities and encouraged health care providers to increase cultural competence to care for these populations. Lesbians are significantly more likely than heterosexual women to experience discrimination during health care visits. Many providers do not take a sexual history or inquire about sexual orientation. Health care providers may inadvertently assume heterosexuality and communicate heterosexist attitudes, making it more difficult for patients to disclose their sexual orientation. Physicians can create a safe and welcome environment for their lesbian patients by consistently adopting gender-neutral language. For example, "Do you have a significant other?" rather than "Are you married?" It is also important that confidentiality is ensured and that staff are aware of and comfortable with lesbian patients and their families.

Between 50% and 80% of lesbians report heterosexual sexual activity (which confers the highest risk for HPV acquisition) at some point in their lives, and screening for cervical cancer should follow the same guidelines as for heterosexual women. Although many STIs occur less frequently in lesbians, screening should be considered when appropriate. Counseling about lifestyle issues and screening when appropriate are the same for lesbians as for heterosexual women.

Gynecologic Issues

Menstrual disorders are common and usually categorized as *amenorrhea* and *abnormal uterine bleeding*. Abnormalities may indicate problems related to the reproductive system or may be an early sign of an important underlying systemic illness.

Amenorrhea

Amenorrhea occurs in 5% of women each year. It is the absence of menses for at least 3 to 6 months outside of the setting of pregnancy or lactation. Women with a previously established menstrual pattern have *secondary amenorrhea* (Table 70-5). *Oligomenorrhea* occurs when menses are irregular or infrequent, with a cycle length usually greater than 35 to 40 days, and it is often associated with *chronic anovulation* or oligo-ovulation. The most common cause of secondary amenorrhea is pregnancy. Lactation causes amenorrhea for up to 6 months in a woman who is exclusively breast-feeding her infant. Prolonged amenorrhea can follow cessation of some hormonal contraceptives, especially

DMPA. Menopause should be suspected in a woman older than 45 years.

Amenorrhea and oligomenorrhea may be caused by pathologic changes at any point in the endometrial-ovarian-pituitary-hypothalamic axis. The differential diagnosis for secondary amenorrhea is broad and is categorized by the primary organ failure or dysfunction: ovarian, hypothalamic, pituitary, and uterine (in descending order of frequency).

Evaluation should begin with a history, physical examination to assess comorbidities and anatomy, and urine test for human chorionic gonadotropin (HCG). If not pregnant, further evaluation should include serum levels of TSH, prolactin, and FSH. For women who have evidence of hyperandrogenism, the serum levels of total testosterone, 17-hydroxyprogesterone, and dehydroepiandrosterone sulfate (DHEAS) should be measured. Additional testing and evaluation should be pursued based on these findings.

For women with elevated prolactin levels, normal or low FSH levels with no clear reason (e.g., weight loss, exercise, recent illness, stress) or with visual symptoms or headaches, magnetic resonance imaging (MRI) of the brain should be performed to look for pituitary abnormalities. A high serum FSH level indicates premature ovarian failure, and women should be counseled regarding management, fertility concerns, and estrogen replacement. If a woman has a normal FSH level and a history of uterine manipulation, she should have a progestin challenge to rule out outflow tract abnormalities. Women with low or normal FSH levels and a history consistent with functional hypothalamic amenorrhea due to weight loss or exercise should be counseled about healthy weight and physical activity.

Abnormal Bleeding

Abnormal bleeding can be caused by many abnormalities, including anovulation, endometrial pathology, and coagulopathies. Women with *polymenorrhea* have a cycle less than 21 days long; women with *oligomenorrhea* have an interval greater than 40 days. Women with excessive bleeding in duration or quantity have *menorrhagia. Menometrorrhagia* is excessive bleeding at irregular intervals.

Women should be asked about their bleeding, including the onset, duration, pattern, and quantity of bleeding. A classification system (Fig. 70-2) for abnormal uterine bleeding (AUB) is organized by cause (i.e., structural or nonstructural). It has eliminated the terms *menorrhagia* and *menometrorrhagia* and replaced them with *heavy menstrual bleeding* and *intermenstrual bleeding*,

respectively. In the PALM-COEIN classification, the four main structural causes for AUB are *p*olyp, *a*denomyosis, *l*eiomyoma, and *m*alignancy or hyperplasia, and the five nonstructural causes are *c*oagulopathy, *o*vulatory dysfunction, *e*ndometrial, *i*atrogenic, and *n*ot yet classified.

Evaluation of AUB assesses for evidence of ovulatory cycles by inquiring about symptoms such as breast tenderness, cramping, and fluid retention before the onset of bleeding. Absence of these symptoms suggests anovulatory bleeding and focuses the differential diagnosis on hormonal causes. Anovulatory bleeding is the result of failed ovulation and the absence of a luteal phase. The ovary secretes estrogen unopposed by progesterone and leads to continued proliferation of the endometrium. This endometrium is unstable, which results in periodic, irregular, and often heavy bleeding. Bleeding due to coagulopathy follows a typically ovulatory pattern and produces heavy, regular bleeding. A personal or family history of bleeding disorders should be sought, because a significant fraction (5% to 32%) of women with heavy menstrual bleeding have an underlying bleeding disorder.

A general physical examination seeks evidence of anemia and a systemic cause of AUB such as thyroid disease or polycystic ovary syndrome. Genitourinary examination should verify the source of bleeding and may identify a cervical polyp, which typically is associated with postcoital bleeding, or an enlarged uterus, suggesting uterine fibroids. Pregnancy must always be excluded with a urine pregnancy test; a Pap smear and cervical cultures should be obtained to assess for cervical disease or infection. Laboratory testing should include a CBC, thyroid studies, and coagulation studies. Endometrial sampling should be performed for women age 45 or older and for women younger than 45 years of age who are at risk for endometrial hyperplasia or endometrial cancer (i.e., women with obesity or a history of chronic anovulation, failed medical therapy or persistent symptoms).For women with suspected structural abnormalities, a transvaginal ultrasound study should be pursued initially.

Management of abnormal bleeding depends on the underlying pathology identified and the degree of anemia caused by the bleeding. Hemodynamically unstable women may require uterine curettage or intravenous estrogen. For hemodynamically stable women, control of bleeding is usually achieved through the use of a combination of estrogen and progestin preparations such as oral contraceptive pills. Levonorgestrel-releasing IUDs can be used for women who have contraindications to estrogen therapy or for women who require long-term therapy. Nonsteroidal anti-inflammatory drugs (NSAIDs) can be used by women who do

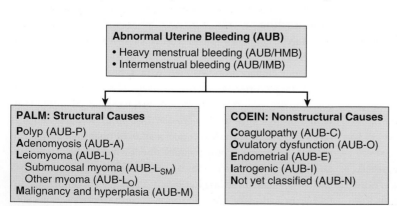

Abnormal Uterine Bleeding (AUB)
• Heavy menstrual bleeding (AUB/HMB)
• Intermenstrual bleeding (AUB/IMB)

PALM: Structural Causes
Polyp (AUB-P)
Adenomyosis (AUB-A)
Leiomyoma (AUB-L)
  Submucosal myoma (AUB-L$_{SM}$)
  Other myoma (AUB-L$_{O}$)
Malignancy and hyperplasia (AUB-M)

COEIN: Nonstructural Causes
Coagulopathy (AUB-C)
Ovulatory dysfunction (AUB-O)
Endometrial (AUB-E)
Iatrogenic (AUB-I)
Not yet classified (AUB-N)

FIGURE 70-2 The PALM-COEIN classification of abnormal uterine bleeding. (From Munro MG, Critchley HO, Broder MS, Fraser IS; FIGO Working Group on Menstrual Disorders: FIGO classification system (PALM-COEIN) for causes of abnormal uterine bleeding in nongravid women of reproductive age, Int J Gynaecol Obstet 113:3–13, 2011.)

not require contraception and who have dysmenorrhea. Surgical options, including endometrial ablation and hysterectomy, are usually reserved for women who have failed other treatments and do not desire future pregnancy.

Infertility

According to the CDC, 11% of U.S. women have trouble conceiving or carrying a pregnancy to term. Infertility is a failure to conceive after 1 year of regular intercourse without contraception. Infertility is more common with increasing age and is becoming more prevalent as women are deferring pregnancy and attempting to conceive at older ages.

Infertility may be caused by female factors or male factors. The most common female cause is an ovulatory factor (20% to 35%), which is often related to metabolic abnormalities, followed by tubal disease (20% to 25%) and uterine factors (5% to 15%). Approximately 20% to 30% of couples experience unexplained infertility. Evaluation should include a complete reproductive, medical, and gynecologic history and a physical examination to help identify metabolic or structural gynecologic abnormalities. Testing may include TSH, FSH, and prolactin levels in women with irregular menses or oligmenorrhea luteal phase serum progesterone levels or basal body temperature charting to confirm ovulation, and day 3 FSH testing in women 35 years of age or older to evaluate ovarian reserve. Further evaluation and treatment are usually performed by reproductive specialists.

Menopause

Menopause occurs when a woman has not had a menstrual cycle for 12 consecutive months or when her ovaries have been removed. The average age at menopause in western countries is 51.4 years, with a range of 40 to 58 years. Women who smoke experience an earlier menopause in a dose-dependent fashion, with an average of 1.5 years sooner than nonsmokers. Because the life expectancy of women is almost 80 years, many women spend at least one third of their lifetime in the postmenopausal period.

Although symptoms such as hot flashes and vaginal dryness may develop during menopause, the process itself is a normal part of the life cycle. This transition offers clinicians the opportunity to help women focus on important preventive health measures and define their risk for major chronic diseases, such as osteoporosis and CAD, as early as possible.

Transition from Perimenopause to Menopause

Much of our information about the menopausal transition is from the Study of Women's Health Across the Nation (SWAN). This multisite, multiethnic cohort study of women was designed to better understand the health of women during their middle years.

The transition to menopause can be erratic and prolonged over a 5- to 10-year period. It is characterized by ovarian and endocrine changes that ultimately result in the depletion of primordial oocyte stores and the cessation of ovarian estrogen production. An accelerated loss of follicles begins at about 37 years of age and is correlated with a small increase in FSH and decrease in inhibin levels. As the FSH concentration increases, the follicular phase of the cycle decreases, and one of the earliest clinical signs of the

menopausal transition is shortening of the menstrual cycle from a mean length of 30 days in the early reproductive years to 25 days in the early menopausal transition.

Later in the menopausal transition, the few remaining follicles respond poorly to FSH, and anovulation may occur. Menstrual cycles may become erratic with prolonged periods of oligomenorrhea. Ovulation may still occur, and women in this time period are advised to continue effective contraception until 12 months of amenorrhea have occurred. Ultimately, when ovarian follicles are depleted, the ovary no longer secretes estradiol but continues to secrete androgens due to continued stimulation by LH.

Perimenopausal Symptoms

Menstrual irregularities (experienced by almost 75% of women) are usually the first change noticed by women entering the menopausal transition. Although changes in the menstrual flow are expected and most women can be reassured, clinicians need to be aware of bleeding patterns that may represent underlying pathology and require evaluation (Table 70-6).

Sleep disturbances in perimenopausal women are a well-documented phenomenon. Hot flashes or sweats can disturb sleep patterns and interfere with sleep quality, resulting in fatigue, irritability, and difficulty concentrating. Vaginal dryness and dyspareunia are common symptoms that can interfere with sexual function.

Changes in mood and cognition are common complaints during the menopausal transition, but a causative link between hormonal fluctuations and mood disturbances and cognitive changes has not been established. Women who do experience significant depression at this time are more likely to have experienced depression earlier in their lives, particularly at times of hormonal change (e.g., postpartum depression, premenstrual dysphoric disorder [PMDD]). Mood issues during the perimenopausal transition should be approached in the same manner as at other ages. In addition to mood, many women in perimenopause complain of difficulties with concentration and memory. In the SWAN cohort, women had a small, transient decline in cognitive abilities during perimenopause, but anxiety and depression also had independent negative effects on cognition. Most epidemiologic studies do not demonstrate an increased risk of depression or a decline in cognitive skills during the menopausal transition.

The hot flash is the hallmark symptom of menopause. In the United States, up to 75% of women who experience a natural menopause and 90% of women who experience a surgical menopause have these vasomotor symptoms. Hot flashes may occur a few times per year or several times each day; 10% to 15% of

TABLE 70-6 ABNORMAL UTERINE BLEEDING PATTERNS IN POSTMENOPAUSAL WOMEN

Heavy menstrual bleeding (>80 mL), especially with clots
Menstrual bleeding lasting >7 days or ≥2 days longer than usual
Intervals of <21 days from the onset of one menstrual period to the onset of the next period
Spotting or bleeding between periods
Uterine bleeding after sexual intercourse

women have hot flashes that are very frequent or severe. For most women, vasomotor symptoms are self-limited, lasting on average 1 to 2 years; however, up to 25% of women may have symptoms for longer than 5 years.

The exact cause of a hot flash is not understood, although it is related to a disturbance of hypothalamic thermoregulation. Women experience a sudden onset of warmth, ranging from noticeable to markedly uncomfortable, especially over the face and upper body. This may be accompanied by significant perspiration. There are racial and ethnic differences in reported hot flashes, with African American women experiencing increased rates compared with white women and Hispanic and Asian women experiencing lower rates.

In the 1950s, it was discovered that estrogen could relieve hot flashes, and its use became widespread. In 1975, a study published in the *New England Journal of Medicine* showed that women who used estrogen for more than 7 years had a 14-fold increase in uterine cancer. Subsequent research determined that endometrial hyperplasia and cancer is reduced to essentially zero when low-dose progestin is continued for 12 to 13 days per month. Women on estrogen with an intact uterus must use progestin therapy to prevent endometrial hyperplasia and cancer.

Hormone treatment (i.e., estrogen or combined estrogen and progestin for women with an intact uterus) remains the most effective treatment of menopausal vasomotor symptoms (level A evidence). It is also FDA approved for the treatment of urogenital atrophy and the prevention of osteoporosis. In the 1990s, the results of the Heart and Estrogen/Progestin Replacement Study (HERS) found that women with preexisting heart disease had increased numbers of cardiac events when placed on estrogen.

The Women's Health Initiative (WHI) was designed to look at various hormone regimens and their effects on disease prevention, particularly cardiovascular disease, in postmenopausal women. More than 16,000 women participated in the trials, which ran for 5.6 years in the combined estrogen-progestin arm and 6.8 years in the estrogen-only arm. In the combined-therapy group, there was an increased risk for coronary heart disease (CHD) (hazard ratio [HR] = 1.29), an increased risk for stroke (HR = 1.41), an increased risk for pulmonary embolism (HR = 2.13), and increased risk for breast cancer (HR = 1.26). The combined-therapy trial was discontinued because of this excess risk.

The conclusion from the combined-therapy trial was that combination estrogen-progestin therapy should not be initiated or continued for the prevention of CHD. The estrogen-only trial did not find a significant increase in CHD or breast cancer but did show an increased risk of stroke (HR = 1.39). The conclusion was that estrogen alone should not be recommended for the prevention of chronic disease in postmenopausal women and hormone therapy should not be prescribed for disease prevention.

Postmenopausal Therapy
Hormone Therapy
Several medical societies have published guidelines for the use of postmenopausal hormone therapy, including the American College of Obstetricians and Gynecologists (ACOG) and the North American Menopause Society (NAMS). Most guidelines agree that estrogen and estrogen-progestin therapy are appropriate for the treatment of moderate to severe vasomotor symptoms and for urogenital atrophy in women who have been appropriately counseled on the risks and benefits (level B evidence). If hormone therapy is initiated, the lowest dose needed to treat the symptoms should be used and usually for a short term (i.e., 2 to 3 years and not more than 5 years). For women who have only vaginal dryness, vaginal estrogen can be used instead of oral estrogen. It may be acceptable under some circumstances, provided the woman is aware of the potential benefits and risks, to extend low-dose therapy if the benefits of treatment outweigh the risks, and a woman has failed attempts to stop (level C evidence).

Alternative Therapies
Interest in nonhormonal and "natural" alternatives in the treatment of menopausal symptoms is extremely high. As many as 75% of menopausal women have used some form of alternative or complementary treatment to relieve menopausal symptoms. Behavioral options such as dressing in layers, regular exercise, stress reduction techniques, and avoidance of known triggers are safe and may be helpful for a number of women. Some of the more common herbal remedies for menopausal symptoms include isoflavones (e.g., soy, red clover) and black cohosh. None of these therapies has consistently been shown to decrease hot flashes beyond placebo in rigorous randomized, controlled trials.

There are effective nonhormonal medication options for treatment of hot flashes, although hormone therapy is superior to these alternatives. Although paroxetine is the only other FDA-approved medical treatment for hot flashes, paroxetine and venlafaxine have been shown to decrease hot flash frequency, but they may cause sexual side effects. Gabapentin and clonidine have been shown to reduce hot flash frequency beyond placebo.

Sexual Dysfunction
According to the largest study of prevalence of female sexual dysfunction in the United States (PRESIDE study), more than 40% of women report some form of sexual problems. Women between 45 and 65 years of age are disproportionately affected, just before and after the menopausal transition. Female sexual dysfunction diagnoses in the *Diagnostic and Statistical Manual of Mental Disorders, Fourth Edition* (DSM-IV) include disorders of desire, arousal, and orgasm; dyspareunia; and vaginismus. Disorders of desire and arousal are the most common. Risk factors for dysfunction include depression and anxiety, relationship conflict, stress and fatigue, and a history of abuse. Medical and physical issues, such as pelvic floor disorders, endometriosis, and psychiatric and neurologic disease, can negatively affect sexuality.

Symptomatic vaginal atrophy occurs in up to 40% of postmenopausal women. As women age and enter menopause, the decline in estrogen levels causes thinning of the vaginal epithelium, decreased vaginal elasticity, and decreased vaginal lubrication, resulting in painful intercourse. Evaluation should include a thorough medical and sexual history and a pelvic examination, including vaginal cultures for STIs if there is pain or vaginal discharge.

Management of sexual dysfunction should be based on the underlying cause, such as evaluation of selective serotonin reuptake inhibitors (SSRIs), antihistamines, β-blockers, and antipsychotics that may affect sexual function. Nonpharmacologic therapies include counseling, lifestyle changes to decrease stress and anxiety, physical therapy for vaginismus and pelvic floor dysfunction, and lubricants and vaginal moisturizers for dyspareunia caused by vaginal dryness. For some women, vaginal lubricants and moisturizers may be sufficient and are the first-line therapy.

Pharmacologic therapy for sexual dysfunction has primarily focused on hormonal therapy. In the WHI, hormone therapy did not have a beneficial effect on sexual dysfunction, but a Cochrane review examined hormone therapy for sexual function and found a small to moderate benefit in perimenopausal or early postmenopausal women. Topical vaginal estrogen results in little systemic absorption and is very effective in relieving the symptoms of vaginal atrophy.

Genitourinary Symptoms

Urinary incontinence rates increase with age. Urinary incontinence is common after menopause, with about 25% of women affected. The cause is often multifactorial. The endothelium of the urethra and bladder becomes more fragile and less elastic with menopause. Urethral tone also decreases with age. Uterine prolapse, cystoceles, and rectoceles increase the risk of incontinence. Risk also increases as body weight increases due to increased pressure on the bladder. Urinary incontinence and its behavioral and pharmacologic treatment options are discussed in Chapter 26, "Incontinence," in *Goldman-Cecil Medicine,* 25th Edition.

🔴 MEDICAL PROBLEMS WITH UNIQUE CONSIDERATIONS FOR WOMEN

Obesity, Metabolic Syndrome, Polycystic Ovary Syndrome, and Diabetes

Rates of obesity have increased steadily in recent decades, and more than one third of U.S. adults are obese (BMI >30). Overall, obesity appears to affect men and women equally, although women of lower SES are disproportionately affected. Obesity increases the risk for many diseases, including CAD, which is the leading cause of death for men and women. In women, central obesity (waist-hip ratio >0.9) predicts the risk of CAD. The risk of many cancers (e.g., endometrial cancer) is increased for obese individuals. Obesity has specific implications for women during pregnancy. It increases the risk of numerous pregnancy-related complications, including gestational diabetes mellitus, fetal macrosomia, hypertension, shoulder dystocia, and cesarean delivery, and contributes postpartum complications such as thrombosis and infection. Obesity is also associated with irregular menses and higher rates of anovulation.

Metabolic effects related to obesity have been elucidated. The risk of cardiovascular disease related to the metabolic syndrome appears to have a stronger correlation in women. The National Cholesterol Education Program/Adult Treatment Panel III defines metabolic syndrome as the presence of three or more of five risk factors that increase the chance of developing heart disease or stroke: central obesity, elevated triglyceride levels, low levels of high-density lipoprotein (HDL) cholesterol, hypertension, and impaired fasting glucose values. Metabolic syndrome significantly increases the risk of type 2 diabetes and

cardiovascular disease, and these patients should be targeted for aggressive lifestyle modification to reduce contributory risk factors.

Polycystic ovary syndrome (PCOS) is an endocrine disorder primarily of androgen excess that affects approximately 5% to 10% of women worldwide. Reproductive and metabolic effects include anovulation, infertility, acne, hirsutism, obesity, and metabolic syndrome. Increased insulin resistance is a significant consequence of the syndrome, increasing the risk of type 2 diabetes, particularly in obese women. Women with PCOS are at increased risk for endometrial and ovarian cancers.

The risk of type 2 diabetes mellitus increases with obesity, and like obesity, the incidence of diabetes has been on the rise in the United States. More than 10% of adult Americans carry the diagnosis of diabetes, and many remain undiagnosed. Rates of diabetes are highest in black, Hispanic, and Native American groups. The increased cardiovascular disease risk conferred by diabetes is greater for women than for men, and women with diabetes have lower survival rates and quality of life after a cardiovascular event than their male counterparts. Women also have higher rates of blindness associated with diabetes. Identifying women with impaired fasting glucose values (i.e., prediabetes) can help to identify women likely to develop diabetes in the future. In addition to reviewing traditional risk factors for diabetes, a history of gestational diabetes and infant birth weight greater than 9 pounds should be considered when evaluating female patients for the risk of diabetes.

Breast Pain, Discharge, and Masses

Breast symptoms are common in practice and cause significant anxiety to patients. Although most breast complaints are about benign conditions, it is important to evaluate breast symptoms thoroughly to ensure that breast cancers are not being missed. Initial evaluation starts with obtaining a history and asking when symptoms began and how they evolved. For instance, a mass that is prominent premenstrually and then decreases in size in the follicular phase of menses is likely a benign cyst.

Breast pain is a common, nonspecific symptom that is usually benign. Localized breast pain is the only symptom in 10% to 15% of women with newly diagnosed breast cancer. Breast pain has cyclical and noncyclical patterns. Approximately two thirds of breast pain is cyclical in nature and related to the normal hormonal variations in the menstrual cycle. Noncyclical breast pain does not follow the usual menstrual pattern and is usually unilateral. Causes of noncyclical breast pain include large breasts, diet and lifestyle factors (e.g., caffeine, nicotine), inflammatory breast cancer, and various medications, including oral contraceptives, antidepressants, and antibiotics. In women older than 35 years of age, diagnostic mammography should be completed. If mammography and the physical examination are normal, reassurance can be provided. In women younger than 35 years of age, normal examination results can obviate the need for further testing.

Breast discharge is an uncommon sign of malignancy. About 5% of women with breast cancer have discharge as a symptom. Concern for malignancy is increased if the discharge occurs without provocation, is persistent, and is unilateral; if the discharge is serous, serosanguineous, or bloody; if it occurs in an older patient; or if it is associated with a mass or lump. The most common malignancy causing discharge is ductal carcinoma in situ. However, a benign intraductal papilloma is the most common cause of bloody nipple discharge.

Most bilateral discharge that occurs only with manipulation is a normal physiologic response. Galactorrhea, bilateral milk production occurring in a nonlactating woman, can be seen in many conditions, including prolactinomas, thyroid dysfunction, and chronic renal failure. It can be a response to many drugs, including antipsychotics, oral contraceptives, and marijuana.

Initial evaluation for breast discharge includes a pregnancy test, prolactin level determination, and thyroid tests. If there is concern about malignancy, a breast specialist performs cytology, immunology, and occult blood testing on the discharge and obtains mammography and ultrasound studies.

There are four categories of breast masses: abscesses, benign masses, benign tumors, and cancer. Benign masses include cysts, galactoceles, papillomas, and fibroadenomas. Cancerous masses are typically painless, dominant masses that persist. Although breast cancers have characteristically been described as hard and immobile with irregular borders, no examination finding reliably distinguishes between a benign and cancerous mass.

Persistent masses require evaluation, which may include ultrasound, mammography, and biopsy, depending on the findings from the history, physical examination, and patient's age. Women younger than 30 years of age are at lower risk for malignancy. Ultrasound is the first imaging modality indicated for young women. If the mass is a cyst, it can be aspirated if symptomatic. If the mass is solid and is not characteristic of a fibroadenoma (which can be observed or biopsied), a biopsy is indicated to rule out malignancy. In women older than 30 years of age, mammography is the first diagnostic test that should be ordered, even if the woman had a recent negative screening mammogram. Ultrasound is often done simultaneously to further evaluate the mass or an area of abnormality detected on the mammogram. Negative imaging results should not preclude further work-up of a clinically suspicious mass. Mammography misses 10% to 20% of clinically palpable breast cancers.

Pelvic Pain

Pelvic pain is characterized as acute or chronic, and both types are commonly encountered in primary care practice. Acute pelvic pain usually manifests over hours to days and may be gynecologic, gastrointestinal, or urologic in origin. Life-threatening conditions, including ruptured ectopic pregnancy and appendicitis, need to be ruled out. Gynecologic causes include complications of pregnancy, acute pelvic infection, and ovarian pathology, including cyst and torsion.

Chronic pelvic pain (CPP) is lower abdominal pain of at least 6 months' duration, and it is severe enough to cause functional impairment or require treatment. Approximately 10% of ambulatory gynecologic referrals are for CPP. The history obtained for evaluation of CPP should include characteristics of the pain; a thorough review of systems; prior medical, surgical, gynecologic, and obstetric history; and a thorough psychiatric and social history, including episodes of domestic violence as a child or an adult and periods of substance abuse.

The most common conditions associated with CPP include endometriosis, chronic pelvic inflammatory disease, interstitial cystitis, irritable bowel syndrome, pelvic floor myalgia, myofascial pain, and neuralgia. Interstitial cystitis or painful bladder syndrome is a clinical diagnosis consisting of pain, pressure, or discomfort related to the bladder and associated with lower urinary tract symptoms lasting more than 6 weeks and occurring in the absence of infection or other identifiable causes. Mental health issues, including substance abuse, somatization, depression, and physical or sexual abuse, can also cause CPP and are important to identify so that women need not undergo unnecessary testing and interventions.

Physical examination should assess for focal areas of pain, scars, hernias, or masses in the abdomen, and a pelvic examination should be performed. After the most likely diagnosis has been identified, an empirical, targeted treatment may be instituted and followed for efficacy. Further work-up should be considered if the patient does not respond or symptoms change. If empirical therapy and a thorough investigation do not yield a diagnosis, laparoscopy may be considered to identify pelvic pathology.

Depending on the underlying cause, management strategies may include heat therapy (for musculoskeletal pain), counseling and psychiatric referral, gastrointestinal referral, medications (e.g., gabapentin for neuropathic pain, NSAIDs, hormonal contraceptives), hysterectomy, and nerve transection procedures. Multidisciplinary approaches, including medications and interventions that address dietary and psychosocial factors, may be superior to medical treatment alone.

Intimate Partner Violence

Intimate partner violence (IPV) is a serious, preventable public health problem. In 2013, the USPSTF revised their guidelines to recommend that clinicians screen women of childbearing age (14 to 46 years old) for IPV and provide or refer women to intervention services when appropriate. Several screening instruments detect IPV effectively, and most experts think the benefits of detection outweigh the potential harm. Providers can choose among many tools for screening, including Hurt-Insult-Threaten-Scream (HITS), Ongoing Abuse Screen/Ongoing Violence Assessment Tool (OAS/OVAT), and Abuse Assessment Screen (AAS).

A short but effective survey may be more practical. The STaT (i.e., slapped, threatened, and thrown things) screening tool is relatively easy to implement by asking three questions: Have you ever been in a relationship in which your partner has pushed or slapped you? Have you ever been in a relationship in which your partner threatened you with violence? Have you ever been in a relationship in which your partner has thrown, broken, or punched things?

A self-administered questionnaire may be even more effective than face-to-face questioning. When screening for and discussing IPV, the provider must be nonjudgmental and compassionate and must ensure confidentiality.

Even when historical or physical examination clues are evident, IPV often remains undiagnosed by providers. Patients often conceal abusive relationships. They may blame themselves for the abuse, or they may not be emotionally ready to acknowledge the abuse. Although there are risk factors for IPV, victims are found among people of all ages, races, ethnicities, and gender and sexual identities.

Identified risk factors for IPV include younger age, female sex, lower SES, and a family history or personal history of violence.

Clues in the history include frequent emergency room visits, delay in seeking treatment, an inconsistent explanation of injuries, missed appointments, repeated abortions, late initiation of prenatal care, medication noncompliance, inappropriate affect, overly attentive or verbally abusive partner, apparent social isolation, and reluctance to undress or difficulty with examination of genitals or rectum. Common presenting complaints include somatic symptoms (e.g., chronic pain, headaches, irritable bowel symptoms), psychological symptoms (e.g., depression, anxiety, panic disorder, posttraumatic stress disorder, substance use), and gynecologic symptoms (e.g., STIs, chronic pelvic pain, unintended pregnancy). After identification, a woman may be referred to a mental health provider or social worker.

Psychiatric Issues

Fewer than one half of people who meet the diagnostic criteria for psychological disorders are identified. Patients are also reluctant to seek professional help. Only two of every five people with a mood, anxiety, or substance use disorder seek assistance within a year of onset of the disorder. Overall rates of psychiatric disorders are almost identical for men and women. However, substantial gender differences exist in the rates of common mental disorders, including depression, anxiety, and somatic complaints. In the United States, the estimated lifetime prevalence is 21% for women and 13% for men. Depression is the most common women's mental health problem, and it may have a worse prognosis for women because it is often more persistent than in men.

Advances have been made in understanding mood disturbances during specific phases of women's reproductive lives, specifically during the postpartum period, the premenstrual phase (i.e., premenstrual syndrome and PMDD), and the menopausal transition. Depression occurring at these times may represent a specific biologic response to the effects of hormonal fluctuations in the brain and may require different treatments from depression unrelated to these periods. For treating PMDD, SSRIs, oral contraceptives, alprazolam (a benzodiazepine), and GnRH agonists are effective in some women.

The disability associated with mental illness is worse for individuals with three or more comorbid disorders. Women are more likely than men to have comorbid conditions, including anxiety disorders, eating disorders, and somatization. Gender-specific risk factors for common mental disorders that disproportionately affect women include gender-based violence, low income and income inequality, low or subordinate social status, and the responsibility as caretaker of others. The high prevalence of sexual violence against women correlates with the higher prevalence of post-traumatic stress disorder (PTSD) among women than men. Somatization disorders are diagnosed almost exclusively in women. Lifetime prevalence is 0.2% to 2% if strict criteria are used. Somatoform disorders are associated with significant disability and a significantly greater number of clinic and emergency room visits than for other psychiatric diagnoses. There seem to be genetic and environmental contributions to risk.

Generalized anxiety disorder and panic disorder are about twice as prevalent among women than men, with lifetime prevalences of 5% and 3.5%, respectively. Although there is a higher prevalence of social anxiety disorder among women than men, more men may seek treatment for the disorder. Social expectations and gender roles may play a role in this difference.

More than 90% of eating disorders, anorexia nervosa, and bulimia occur in women. Approximately 0.5% to 1% of women between the ages of 15 and 30 years have anorexia, and about 1% to 3% of women have bulimia. There is a strong association between eating disorders and mood disorders, particularly depression. There are no marked gender differences in the rates of severe mental disorders such as schizophrenia and bipolar disorder, which affect less than 2% of the population.

Accessing mental health care is different for men and women. Women are more likely to seek help from and disclose mental health problems to their primary health care physician, whereas men are more likely to seek specialist mental health care and are the principal users of inpatient care. Evidence exists for possible gender bias in the treatment of psychological disorders. Physicians are more likely to diagnose depression in women than men, even when they have similar scores on standardized measures of depression or have identical symptoms at presentation. Women are more likely to be prescribed mood-altering psychotropic drugs.

Coronary Artery Disease

There are significant gender differences in the epidemiology and clinical manifestations of CAD. CAD remains the leading cause of death for men and women, but since the mid-1980s, more women than men die each year of this disease. Women with CAD tend to be diagnosed at a later age (approximately 10 years later) than men. Most CAD in women occurs postmenopausally, when estrogen levels decline. Estrogen increases levels of protective HDL cholesterol, which may affect atherosclerotic plaque progression and regression. Estrogen may also be beneficial due to its vasodilatory, antiinflammatory, and antioxidative properties.

Women with CAD are more likely than men to experience atypical symptoms, such as fatigue, abdominal pain, indigestion, nausea and vomiting, and shortness of breath. These nonclassic symptoms may partially explain why women tend to seek health care later than men. Even when women seek health care, they have a longer time to diagnosis and a longer time to medical intervention than men. Women are also more likely than men to have sudden cardiac death at presentation. They are less likely to receive proven effective therapies, such as β-blockers, aspirin, thrombolytics, and statins, and they are less often referred for invasive testing and coronary artery bypass grafting (CABG). Women are also more likely to die after a myocardial infarction and CABG compared with men.

Black and Hispanic women have a higher prevalence of cardiovascular disease risk factors than white women, including hypertension, cigarette smoking, sedentary lifestyle, hypercholesterolemia, diabetes, and obesity. Although some of these differences may be genetically based, others are likely influenced by behavioral, cultural, and psychological factors. Women of lower SES, regardless of race, have a higher prevalence of cardiovascular risk factors than women of higher SES.

Racial differences exist in the management of myocardial infarction. Black women are offered reperfusion therapy and coronary angiography at lower rates, and in-hospital mortality rates are higher compared with those of white women.

Patient factors and physician factors may contribute to the observed clinical differences in CAD between men and women. Women may delay their own care because they are caretakers.

Many women are unaware of the prevalence of CAD. In a 2006 survey, only 55% of women identified cardiovascular disease as the leading cause of death among women. Studies have shown that physicians also underestimate the magnitude of cardiovascular disease in women and that they tend to place women in lower risk categories compared with men despite equivalent risk profiles. Much of the evidence used to guide the treatment of coronary disease in women is based on trials predominantly enrolling men. Treatments and interventions found to benefit men might not provide the same benefit to women.

Osteoporosis

More than 10 million Americans have osteoporosis; 8 million are women. It is a disease that disproportionately affects women, particularly as they age. The lifetime risk of fracture of a patient with osteoporosis is as high as 40%. Most osteoporosis trials have involved mostly white women, limiting generalizability to all races and ethnicities. Racial minorities are diagnosed and treated less often.

Human Immunodeficiency Virus Infection

Since the beginning of the HIV epidemic in the 1980s, the percentage of women affected has grown considerably, with women now accounting for 25% of those living with HIV in the United States, compared with 7% when the epidemic began. African American women and Latinas are disproportionately affected. In 2010, the rate of new infections among black women was 20 times that of white women and almost 5 times that of Hispanic women (38.1 versus 1.9 and 8.0 per 100,000, respectively). Mortality rates are higher among racial minorities than among white women.

Many factors affect racial disparities. Communities in which there is a higher HIV prevalence (many African American and Latino communities) pose a greater risk of acquisition of HIV with every sexual encounter. Other factors include economic barriers, lack of insurance, stigma, and higher levels of STIs, which increase the likelihood of acquiring and transmitting HIV.

There are unique barriers to prevention of HIV in women. Women may be unaware of the partner's risk factors for HIV, such as injection drug use, multiple partners, or unprotected sex with men. Unprotected vaginal sex is a much higher risk for women than for men, and unprotected anal sex is riskier than unprotected vaginal sex. Women who have experienced sexual abuse are more likely to engage in high-risk sexual behaviors, such as exchanging sex for drugs, having multiple partners, or having sex with a partner who is physically abusive.

Although many of the clinical manifestations of HIV infection and acquired immunodeficiency syndrome (HIV/AIDS) in women are similar to those in men, significant gender-based differences exist. Women may not prioritize their own care. Women are also disproportionately affected by poverty, IPV, unstable housing, substance abuse, lack of transportation, lack of insurance, and the necessity of finding child care, all of which pose barriers to care.

Biologic differences also exist. Although women typically have lower viral loads than men despite the same level of CD4 counts,

the rates of disease progression are similar. Rates of opportunistic infections are similar for men and women. Women may have gynecologic complaints as their initial manifestation of HIV/AIDS, including *Candida* vaginitis, pelvic inflammatory disease, abnormal Papanicolaou smear results, and STIs such as herpes simplex virus, chancroid, and syphilis.

Risk for cervical abnormalities and cervical cancer is related to the degree of immunosuppression, age, and co-infection with high-risk HPV genotypes (16, 18, 52, and 58). Women with preserved CD4 counts and negative HPV test results are at relatively low risk for cervical cytologic abnormalities. Women with HIV infection are more likely to progress more rapidly to cervical cancer. The CDC recommends two cervical cytology screens at 6-month intervals in the first year after an HIV diagnosis. Those with normal results and deemed low risk (i.e., no prior abnormal Pap smear, HPV infection, or AIDS) may have the Pap smear performed annually, with more frequent examinations performed for those deemed high risk. Vulvar and perianal intraepithelial neoplasias are more common in women with HIV than HIV-seronegative women, and the lesions should be evaluated.

Antiretroviral therapy and follow-up monitoring are similar for men and women with HIV/AIDS. Women should be counseled to also use a barrier contraceptive (i.e., male or female condom), because this has proven efficacy in reducing the transmission of HIV and other STIs, although it is less effective for pregnancy prevention.

For a deeper discussion on this topic, please see Section XIX, "Women's Health," in Goldman-Cecil Medicine, *25th Edition.*

SUGGESTED READINGS

Breslau J, Kendler KS, Aguilar-Gaxiola S, et al: Lifetime prevalence and persistence of psychiatric disorders across ethnic groups in the United States, Psychol Med 1:35–45, 2005.

Committee on Practice Bulletins–Gynecology: Practice bulletin no. 128. Diagnosis of abnormal uterine bleeding in reproductive-aged women, Obstet Gynecol 120:197–206, 2012.

Department of Reproductive Health, World Health Organzation (WHO): Medical eligibility criteria for contraceptive use, ed 4, 2010. Available at http://www.who.int/reproductivehealth/publications/family_planning/9789241563888/en/. Accessed July 30, 2014.

Dunlop AL, Jack BW, Bottalico JN, et al: The clinical content of preconception care: women with chronic medical conditions, Am J Obstet Gynecol 199(Suppl B):S310–S327, 2008.

Moyer VA, U.S. Preventive Services Task Force: Screening for intimate partner violence and abuse of elderly and vulnerable adults: U.S. preventive services task force recommendation statement, Ann Intern Med 158:478–486, 2013.

Nelson H: Menopause, Lancet 371:760–770, 2008.

North American Menopause Society: The 2012 hormone therapy position statement of North American Menopause Society, Menopause 19:257–271, 2012.

Trussell J: Contraceptive technology, rev ed 19, New York, 2007, Ardent Media.

U.S. Preventive Services Task Force: Screening for family and intimate partner violence: recommendation statement. Available at http://www.uspreventiveservicestaskforce.org/3rduspstf/famviolence/famviolrs.htm. Accessed July 30, 2014

Vesco KK, Whitlock EP, Eder M, et al: Risk factors and other epidemiologic considerations for cervical cancer screening: a narrative review for the U.S. Preventive Services Task Force, Ann Intern Med 155:698–705, 2011.

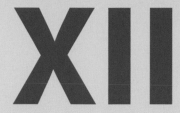

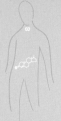
XII

Men's Health

71 Men's Health Topics
David James Osborn, Douglas F. Milam, and Joseph A. Smith, Jr.

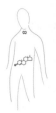

Men's Health Topics

David James Osborn, Douglas F. Milam, and Joseph A. Smith, Jr.

INTRODUCTION

This chapter addresses disorders that are unique to men because they involve the male genitalia and reproductive system. It incorporates commonly encountered and clinically important aspects of voiding, oncology, reproductive function, and endocrinology.

A. Androgen Deficiency in Adult Men

DEFINITION AND EPIDEMIOLOGY

Several clinical guidelines address the syndrome of symptomatic low testosterone levels in men. The two most referenced are from the Endocrine Society and from a collaboration of five societies, including the International Society for the Study of the Aging Male (ISSAM), International Society of Andrology (ISA), European Association of Urology (EAU), European Academy of Andrology (EAA), and American Society of Andrology (ASA). One guideline uses the term "androgen deficiency in adult men" and the other uses the term "late-onset hypogonadism" to refer to a disease process characterized by low serum testosterone levels and clinical symptoms.

The syndrome of androgen deficiency in adult men (late-onset hypogonadism) can be defined as a low level of serum testosterone (total or free) combined with three symptoms of low testosterone such as erectile dysfunction (ED), decreased libido, and lethargy or sleep disturbance. Using this general definition, the incidence of androgen deficiency ranges from 2.1% to 6% in the literature. On the other hand, the incidence of low serum testosterone (so-called low T) in men older than 40 years of age is much higher, between 17% and 38.7% in multiple studies. The clinical guidelines require only one symptom for the diagnosis of androgen deficiency, so the true incidence of androgen deficiency is probably closer to that of low T.

Over the last 10 years, there has been increased coverage of low T in the mainstream press and media. In addition, clinics specializing in testosterone replacement have proliferated. As a result, androgen use among men has increased threefold, from 0.8% in 2001 to 2.91% in 2011. This increase in the prescribing of testosterone is probably the result of both a heightened awareness about the problem and overutilization in men who have been improperly diagnosed. The diagnosis and treatment of androgen deficiency is challenging and full of potential pitfalls. Therefore, it is imperative for physicians to have a thorough understanding of this disease process, particularly in these times when information in the media and on the Internet creates an eager and motivated patient population.

PATHOPHYSIOLOGY

Normal aging sometimes results in malfunctions of the hypothalamic-pituitary-gonadal axis that lead to decreased serum testosterone levels. One of these errors is termed *primary hypogonadism* (testicular failure). In this disease process, the testicles produce an inadequate amount of testosterone (and sperm) even though there is adequate stimulation from the anterior pituitary gland in the form of elevated or normal release of luteinizing hormone (LH). Low serum testosterone also can result from failure of the pituitary gland to secrete an adequate amount of LH. When this occurs, the Leydig cells of the testicle that produce testosterone are not adequately stimulated and hence do not make a normal amount of testosterone. This form of testosterone deficiency is termed *secondary hypogonadism*. It can result from disease processes such as pituitary tumors, hemochromatosis, and obstructive sleep apnea.

Measurements of total testosterone (TT) include the concentrations of both unbound (free) and bound testosterone in the serum. Only 2% of testosterone is unbound; the other 98% is bound to proteins such as albumin or sex hormone binding globulin (SHBG). Because it is not bound to another substance, free testosterone (FT) is the more biochemically active form of testosterone. If a man has a low normal TT level but a low FT level and has clinical manifestations of this hormone deficiency, he is considered to have androgen deficiency syndrome.

Increased levels of SHBG in the serum can decrease the level of FT. The level of SHBG increases with smoking, coffee consumption, age, and disease processes such as hepatitis and hyperthyroidism. Therefore, increased levels of SHBG can contribute to androgen deficiency. Obesity decreases levels of SHBG, but it can cause androgen deficiency through the peripheral conversion of testosterone into estrogen in adipose cells. Conditions such as extreme exercise, recreational drug use, nutritional deficiency, stress, use of certain medications, and acute illness can transiently lower serum testosterone.

CLINICAL PRESENTATION

Low testosterone levels can affect a patient's general, sexual, physical, and psychological health. In Table 71-1, these symptoms are grouped according to their specific relation to androgen deficiency. Various studies have categorized and used the symptoms of androgen deficiency in different ways. For example, one clinical trial looking at the incidence of androgen deficiency defined the syndrome as the presence of 3 of 12 clinical symptoms combined with a low serum FT or TT level, whereas, in a similar trial, patients were considered to be androgen deficient if they had a low testosterone and exhibited three specific sexual symptoms. The guidelines simply state that clinicians should use the different symptoms as means to decide whether to check a patient's serum testosterone level. According to the guidelines, a patient with treatable androgen deficiency must have at least one symptom. The symptom most closely associated with androgen deficiency is decreased libido.

DIAGNOSIS

For several reasons, the diagnosis of androgen deficiency is not straightforward. By the very simplest of definitions, it requires a low serum testosterone level in conjunction with at least one clinical symptom. Most clinical guidelines suggest measuring a TT in any adult man who has symptoms associated with androgen deficiency. In general, recognizing that laboratory standards may differ, if the TT level is greater than 350 ng/dL (12.1 nmol/L), the patient does not have androgen deficiency; if the TT is lower than 200 ng/dL (6.9 nmol/L), then a symptomatic patient is considered to have androgen deficiency. If the TT level falls between those two values, FT should be assessed, and low values (typically 5 to 9 ng/dL) indicate androgen deficiency. FT tests are not recommended initially because of their greater cost. In addition, screening of asymptomatic men for low testosterone is not medically necessary.

In men with borderline testosterone levels, repeat measurement of a morning testosterone level is warranted because there is significant day-to-day variability and testosterone levels vary on a circadian rhythm. Ideally, levels should be checked within 4 hours of waking (usually between 7 and 11 A.M.), when testosterone levels are highest. It is not necessary to fast before a testosterone laboratory test; however, in a study from 2013, there

was a 25% reduction in TT levels in healthy men 60 minutes after an oral glucose tolerance test. Strength training also transiently decreases serum testosterone levels in healthy men (but typically not outside the normal range).

Testosterone levels should not be checked during acute or subacute illness. However, physicians should have a lower threshold to check the testosterone level in patients with chronic illnesses that are known to cause a symptomatically lower testosterone concentration, such as diabetes mellitus, chronic obstructive lung disease, inflammatory arthritic disease, renal disease, human immunodeficiency virus (HIV)-related disease, obesity, metabolic syndrome, and hemochromatosis. In fact, one guideline states that all patients who have a pituitary mass, HIV-associated weight loss, or a low-trauma fracture should have their testosterone level checked regardless of symptoms.

In addition, one guideline recommends checking LH levels to rule out secondary hypogonadism in all patients, whereas another recommends that LH and prolactin should be measured only in patients with TT lower than 150 ng/dL (5.2 nmol/L). In patients with disease processes (e.g., obesity, hepatitis and hyperthyroidism) that are known to alter the level of SHBG, it may be prudent to initially check FT rather than TT.

Men being considered for testosterone replacement should have their prostate-specific antigen (PSA) level measured and a digital rectal examination (DRE) performed to assess the prostate. If either is abnormal, referral to an urologist should be considered. Table 71-2 provides helpful guidelines for evaluating possible androgen deficiency.

TREATMENT

Testosterone therapy is recommended for men with androgen deficiency, and the goal of therapy should be to maintain secondary sex characteristics and improve sexual function, sense of well-being, and bone mineral density. In addition, metabolic and cardiovascular benefits are suggested by available data. Before starting treatment, clinicians should obtain baseline hematocrit and PSA levels.

There are at least nine different types of testosterone replacement formulations. In the United States, the most commonly used forms are testosterone enanthate or cypionate by intramuscular (IM) injection, transdermal testosterone patches, testosterone gels, and implantable timed-release pellets. Because of the

TABLE 71-1	SIGNS AND SYMPTOMS OF ANDROGEN DEFICIENCY
SPECIFIC SIGNS AND SYMPTOMS	**LESS SPECIFIC SIGNS AND SYMPTOMS**
Reduced sexual desire (libido) and activity	Decreased energy and self-confidence
Decreased spontaneous erections	Feeling sad, depressed mood
Breast discomfort, gynecomastia	Poor concentration and memory
Less axillary and pubic hair and less shaving	Sleep disturbance and sleepiness
Very small or shrinking testes	Mild anemia (normochromic, normocytic)
Infertility and low sperm count	Reduced muscle bulk and strength
Height loss and low bone mineral density	Increased body fat and body mass index
Hot flashes and sweats	Diminished physical or work performance

TABLE 71-2	ANDROGEN DEFICIENCY DIAGNOSIS DO'S AND DON'TS

Do check total testosterone (TT) in every symptomatic adult male >40 yr
Do confirm borderline tests with a repeat measurement
Do check in the morning
Do have a lower threshold to check testosterone in patients with certain chronic illnesses
Do consider measuring prolactin and LH level in patients with very low testosterone
Do consider checking hematocrit and PSA levels with the testosterone level to decrease blood draws
Don't check the testosterone level during acute or subacute illness
Don't start with measurement of free testosterone in most cases ($$$)
Don't monitor testosterone treatment with measurements of free testosterone ($$$)
Don't consider testosterone replacement in a patient trying to father a child

LH, Luteinizing hormone; PSA, prostate-specific antigen.

frequency of significant skin irritation with the testosterone patch, many practitioners prefer one of the other modes, usually based on patient preference. For dosage and administration of gel testosterone formulations, the clinician should refer to the package insert. For IM testosterone, a good starting dosage is 100 mg every 2 weeks. Pellet implantation is an office procedure, but adequate testosterone levels are typically maintained for 3 to 4 months.

Side Effects of Testosterone Therapy

Testosterone therapy causes decreased sperm production and usually decreased testicular volume, and it may cause acne, oily skin, and breast tenderness. In addition, testosterone can increase hematocrit and cause life-threatening erythrocytosis. If the hematocrit becomes elevated, then testosterone replacement should be suspended. Occasionally, a patient requires phlebotomy to avoid or treat dangerous erythrocytosis. Testosterone replacement is not a treatment for infertility and has in fact been investigated as method of male contraception. Patients who are interested in fathering children should not take testosterone. If necessary, human chorionic gonadotropin (HCG) may be administered for men wishing to preserve fertility.

Only oral testosterone has negative affects on the liver, so it is not necessary to monitor liver function during treatment. Testosterone therapy may worsen obstructive sleep apnea and congestive heart failure; therefore, patients in whom these conditions are untreated should not be started on testosterone therapy. Present data suggest that testosterone therapy does not worsen levels of high-density lipoproteins. Patients should be aware that testosterone therapy suppresses endogenous testosterone and sperm production. Depending on the duration of treatment, it

may take 1 to 2 months or longer after treatment discontinuation for testosterone and sperm production to return to baseline levels.

Testosterone Therapy and the Prostate

In general, testosterone therapy should be avoided in patients with a history of prostate or breast cancer. However, this is a controversial issue. Some urologists may decide that replacement is acceptable under specific circumstances because there are data to suggest that testosterone replacement may not pose an undue risk of prostate cancer recurrence or progression. In addition, there is no conclusive evidence that testosterone replacement has any effect on benign prostatic hypertrophy (BPH).

Monitoring Testosterone Treatment

TT should be measured 5 to 12 weeks after initiation of testosterone treatment. If IM testosterone is being administered every 2 weeks, morning TT levels should be checked 1 week after an injection. If a testosterone gel is used, morning TT should be checked at least 1 month after initiation of treatment. Hematocrit values should be assessed at 3 months and 6 months and then annually. If the hematocrit level is greater then 54%, the treatment should be stopped. If testosterone therapy was started to help with osteoporosis or osteopenia, a bone mineral density test should be done after 1 to 2 years. If there is an abnormality in the PSA level or it increases by 0.75 ng/mL in 1 year, referral to a urologist should be considered. If the TT level is low, the clinician should increase the dosage and reassess after 5 to 12 weeks. The goal of therapy should be a level between 400 and 600 ng/dL. Finally, therapy should be discontinued if the patient does not have clinical improvement.

B. Erectile Dysfunction

ED is defined as the inability to maintain an erection for satisfactory sexual function in the absence of premature ejaculation. Premature ejaculation is not technically a form of ED. Impotence is the most common cause of ED in the United States and is defined by an inability to attain or maintain adequate penile rigidity sufficient for intercourse. Other important, although less common, causes of ED are Peyronie's disease and trauma.

ED affects millions of American men. According to the Massachusetts Male Aging Study, 52% of men older than 40 years of age are afflicted with some form of impotence. The prevalence of impotence triples between age 40 and 70 years. By age 70 years, 15% of men experience complete ED. Age and physical health are the most important predictors of the onset of ED. Smoking is the most important lifestyle variable.

Recently, many clinics that specifically treat ED and premature ejaculation have opened across America to meet a growing need for treatment of these conditions. However, these clinics often charge money for treatments and medications that primary care physicians can provide and are covered by insurance. Therefore, it is more important than ever for primary care physicians to have a thorough understanding of this disease process.

⬤ MECHANISM OF ERECTION

Psychogenic or tactile sexual stimulation is usually the initial step in the pathway leading to penile erection. Nerve signals are carried through the pelvic plexus into the cavernous nerves of the penis. The pelvic plexus receives input from both the sympathetic and the parasympathetic nervous system. Sympathetic fibers originate in the thoracolumbar spinal cord, and parasympathetic fibers originate in the second through fourth sacral spinal cord segments (S2 through S4). Afferent somatic sensory signals are carried from the penis through the pudendal nerve to S2 through S4. This information is routed both to the brain and to spinal cord autonomic centers. Adrenergic innervation appears to play a role in the process of detumescence. High concentrations of norepinephrine have been demonstrated in the tissue of the corpora cavernosa and tributary arterioles. Afferent signals capable of initiating erection can originate within the brain, as with psychogenic stimulation, or they can result from tactile stimulation. There is no discreet center for psychogenic erections; however, the temporal lobe appears to be important.

Sexual stimulation causes the release of nitric oxide (NO) by the cavernous nerves into the neuromuscular junction

(Fig. 71-1). NO activates guanylyl cyclase, which converts guanosine triphosphate (GTP) into cyclic guanosine monophosphate (cGMP). Protein kinase G is activated by cGMP and in turn activates several proteins that decrease the intracellular concentration of calcium ions (Ca^{2+}). Decreased Ca^{2+} concentration in the smooth muscle causes muscular relaxation, cavernosal artery dilation, increased blood flow, and subsequent penile erection. The control of blood flow on the venous outflow side is less well understood.

CAUSES OF ERECTILE DYSFUNCTION

Psychogenic ED was once thought to be the most common type of ED. However, advances in understanding of the mechanics and neurophysiology of erectile function have identified other more common causes. Psychogenic ED is now thought to account for fewer than 15% of patients seen by ED specialists. The anatomic site now believed to be the most common cause of ED is the neuromuscular junction. This is the place where the cavernosal nerves meet the smooth muscle and endothelium of the deep cavernous penile arteries. The decreased release of NO by cavernosal nerves and the impaired response by smooth muscle cells that occurs at the neuromuscular junction is termed *endothelial dysfunction*. Other common causes of ED include certain endocrine disorders, vascular diseases, central and peripheral nerve disorders, and medications.

Cardiovascular Disease

In the United States, atherosclerotic vascular disease, hyperlipidemia, smoking, and hypertension are frequent causes of ED. These relationships are expected because erection is achieved by a combination of relaxation of arteriolar smooth muscle and increased venous resistance of channels penetrating the wall of the corpora cavernosa. Cardiovascular disease may decrease erectile ability by decreasing blood flow to the penile arteries, by mechanical obstruction of the vascular lumen, or, more commonly, by endothelial dysfunction. Endothelial dysfunction is the most common cause of ED. It results from interruption of the neural control mechanism of vascular smooth muscle function and leads to decreased blood flow and pressure in the corpora cavernosa.

The principal blood vessels supplying the corpora cavernosa are the cavernosal arteries, which are terminal branches of the internal pudendal artery. Diseases of large and small arteries may decrease corporal blood pressure and lead to decreased penile lengthening and rigidity. Veno-occlusive disease in the penis is also a significant cause of ED. These patients often experience normal initial rigidity, but quickly lose their erection before ejaculation occurs.

Neurogenic Erectile Dysfunction

Because the nervous system plays an integral part in the physiology of an erection, any disease process that affects the brain, the spinal cord, or the peripheral nerves can cause ED. For example, dementia, Parkinson's disease, and stroke are diseases of the brain associated with ED. Patients with spinal cord injury commonly have ED. Because of an intact reflex pathway, most patients with spinal cord injury respond to tactile sensation, but they usually require medical therapy to maintain the erection through intercourse. Iatrogenic injury to nerves during surgery (e.g., prostatectomy, rectal surgery) is also a common cause of neurogenic ED. Neurogenic ED due to decreases in penile tactile sensation can occur with increasing age.

Endocrine Disorders

Testosterone plays a permissive role in erectile function, and many endocrine disorders can directly or indirectly decrease plasma free or bound testosterone. However, androgen deficiency is an uncommon primary cause of ED because erectile ability is only partially androgen dependent. Patients with androgen deficiency typically have decreased or absent libido in addition to loss of erectile rigidity. Androgen replacement may induce return of erectile function in patients with very low or undetectable serum testosterone concentrations. More commonly, however, the impotent patient has normal or mildly decreased levels of circulating androgens. Testosterone replacement rarely restores erectile function in men with mildly decreased serum testosterone. Testosterone supplementation is never indicated for patients with normal circulating androgen levels.

The most common endocrine disorder affecting erectile ability is diabetes mellitus. In addition to causing atherosclerotic and microvascular disease, diabetes affects both the autonomic and the somatic nervous system, including loss of function of long autonomic nerves. The loss of long cholinergic neurons results in interruption of the efferent side of the erectile reflex arc. Diabetes also appears to produce dysfunction of the neuromuscular junction at the level of arterial smooth muscle in the penile corpora cavernosa. Studies have indicated markedly decreased acetylcholine and NO concentrations in the trabeculae of the corpora cavernosa in diabetic patients. These findings probably represent a combination of neural loss and

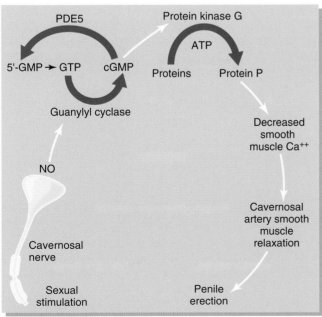

FIGURE 71-1 Sexual stimulation causes the release of nitric oxide (NO) by the cavernous nerve into the neuromuscular junction. ATP, Adenosine triphosphate; cGMP, cyclic guanosine monophosphate; GMP, guanosine monophosphate; GTP, guanosine triphosphate; PDE5, phosphodiesterase type 5.

neuromuscular junction dysfunction. Other endocrine disorders, such as hypothyroidism, hyperthyroidism, and adrenal dysfunction, can also cause ED. Because of the uncommon occurrence of thyroid and adrenal disorders in patients presenting for treatment of ED, testing of those axes is not a part of the routine work-up of ED.

Medication-Induced Erectile Dysfunction

Many commonly prescribed medications can cause or contribute to decreased erectile function. Table 71-3 lists the major classes of medications implicated in ED and suggests how commonly these medications interfere with erectile function. Changing medications may restore erectile function in some patients. However, proceeding directly to treatment of ED is usually the preferred option in all but the most straightforward cases.

Medical and Surgical Therapies

Since the introduction of sildenafil in 1998, the Process of Care Model for the evaluation and treatment of ED has been adopted. It targets the primary care provider as the initial source of care for patients with ED. Currently available therapies for ED include oral phosphodiesterase type 5 (PDE5) inhibitors, intraurethral alprostadil, intracavernous vasoactive injection therapy, vacuum constriction devices, and penile prosthesis implantation. A stepwise treatment approach starting with oral agents and progressing to more invasive therapeutic interventions should be used (Fig. 71-2). Informed patient decision making is critical to successful progression through the Process of Care pathway. Patient referral is primarily based on the need or desire for specialized diagnostic testing and management.

Oral Phosphodiesterase Type 5 Inhibitors

Current medical therapy is based on inhibition of PDE5, which degrades cGMP to inactive 5′-GMP, as shown in Figure 71-1. Sildenafil, vardenafil, avanafil, and tadalafil competitively inhibit PDE5 breakdown of cGMP. Use of a PDE5 inhibitor results in improved erectile rigidity even in patients with decreased NO or cGMP synthesis. However, not all patients respond to PDE5 inhibition. Adequate sexual stimulation and intact neural and vascular pathways are necessary to produce an adequate amount of NO and cGMP to increase deep penile artery blood flow. PDE5 inhibitors are effective in men with organic, psychogenic, neurogenic, and mixed cases of ED. The overall response rate to PDE5 inhibitors is 70%.

Unless contraindicated, PDE5 inhibition should be considered first-line therapy for most men. The combination of PDE5 inhibitors and α-adrenergic receptor blockers can result in transient hypotension. This interaction is complex and depends on the specific medication in each category. In general, it is safe to use selective α-blockers such as tamsulosin and alfluzosin with any PDE5 inhibitor. However, PDE5 inhibitors should not be used concurrently with nitrate medications because a large (>25 mm Hg) synergistic drop in blood pressure occurs in many patients. Periodic follow-up is necessary to determine therapeutic efficacy, side effects related to PDE5 inhibition, and changes in health status. Overall, 30% of men do not respond to this class of medication.

Alprostadil Intraurethral Drug Therapy

In PDE5 inhibition is not successful, an acceptable second-line medical treatment is intraurethral administration of prostaglandin E_1 (alprostadil [Muse]), which can be inserted into the urethra with the use of a pellet applicator. This method of delivery assumes substantial venous communications between the corpus spongiosum surrounding the urethra and the corpus cavernosum, and it is effective in many patients who fail oral PDE5 inhibitor medications. It is not as effective as intracavernous injection (described later). Some patients experience difficulty initiating this type of treatment, so it may be beneficial to administer the first dose in an office setting. To lubricate the urethra, patients should void before insertion of the pellet.

Up to one third of patients have normal, transient burning penile pain, and this should be discussed with the patient before treatment. Dizziness and presyncope are uncommon complications. This medication has rapid onset and minimal risk of priapism. It can be used with increased efficacy in combination with PDE5 inhibitors. Transient burning pain in the sexual partner can occur and is caused by leakage of the medication from the urethra into the vagina. This can be managed by wearing a condom.

TABLE 71-3	FREQUENCY OF DECREASED ERECTILE RIGIDITY AND EJACULATORY DYSFUNCTION BY MEDICATION CLASS	
MEDICATION CLASS	**DECREASED ERECTILE RIGIDITY**	**EJACULATORY DYSFUNCTION**
β-Adrenergic antagonists	Common	Less common
Sympatholytics	Expected	Common
α_1-Agonists	Uncommon	Uncommon
α_2-Agonists	Common	Less common
α_1-Antagonists	Uncommon	Less common*
Angiotensin-converting enzyme inhibitors	Uncommon	Uncommon
Diuretics	Less common	Uncommon
Antidepressants	Common[†]	Uncommon[‡]
Antipsychotics	Common	Common
Anticholinergics	Less common	Uncommon

*Patients are able to ejaculate, but retrograde ejaculation is seen in 5% to 30%.
[†]Uncommon with serotonin reuptake inhibitors.
[‡]Delayed or inhibited ejaculation with serotonin reuptake inhibitors.

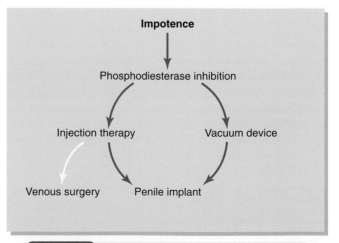

FIGURE 71-2   A logical treatment algorithm for impotence.

Intracavernosal Injection Therapy

Pharmacologic injection therapy involves the injection of vasodilator agents into the corpora cavernosa to produce erection by dilating the corporal artery smooth muscle. More than 90% of patients with ED respond to this type of therapy. Commonly used agents include alprostadil, papaverine, and phentolamine (Regitine). These medications can be used alone or in combination. As monotherapy, alprostadil is most commonly used. Of the three, only alprostadil has been evaluated in rigorous clinical trials and has specific marketing approval from the U.S. Food and Drug Administration for the treatment of ED. Phentolamine is used to potentiate the action of papaverine and can be used in combination with both alprostadil and papaverine. These vasoactive drugs can be formulated with different combinations of medications and concentrations to achieve increased efficacy and decreased side effects. *Bimix* and *trimix* are terms used to refer to a combination of two or three of these medications, respectively.

The common side effects of this type of treatment are bruising and penile pain (50%). Penile pain is more common in young patients and is usually worse with alprostadil. Therefore, a combination using lower-dose alprostadil or just papaverine and phentolamine might be beneficial in younger patients. Other, more serious risks of injection therapy include priapism and corporal scarring (Peyronie's disease). Priapism has been reported to occur in 1% to 4% of patients. Prolonged erections occur more commonly in patients with neurogenic ED, especially young men with spinal cord injury. Significant acquired penile curvature (Peyronie's disease) is seen uncommonly and usually follows several years of injection therapy. Penile curvature appears to be less common with use of alprostadil than with papaverine. The most common problem with pharmacologic injection therapy is not complications from therapy but rather the fact that 50% to 60% of patients stop using the technique within 1 year.

As with intraurethral alprostadil, initial treatment should be performed under the supervision of a physician. The medication can be injected using a self-contained medication-syringe kit or a 29-gauge (5/8-inch) insulin syringe with medication drawn from a refrigerated vial. It is advisable to start with a small test dose and slowly titrate the dosage for desired affect over several weeks. The patient should not use the medication more than once in 24 hours and should be instructed to seek medical care promptly for prolonged painful erections lasting longer than 4 hours. Typically, administration of the test dose should be carried out in the morning, and the patient should be expected to stay in close proximity to the medical office to monitor for priapism. If a patient experiences priapism after a test dose, he should seek prompt medical attention within 4 hours of injection. Priapism usually resolve without sequelae after intracavernosal injection of 0.5 to 1 mL of a 250 μg/mL solution (0.5 mg diluted in 2 mL of normal saline) of phenylephrine in a setting where blood pressure and heart rate are monitored. Formal guidelines for the treatment of priapism are available on the website of the American Urologic Association (AUA).

Vacuum Constriction Devices

Vacuum constriction devices enclose the penis in a plastic tube with an airtight seal at the penile base. Air is pumped out of the cylinder, creating a vacuum. Blood flows into the corporal bodies, leading to penile erection. A constriction band slid from the cylinder to the base of the penis maintains the erection. Simultaneous use of a vacuum device and a PDE5 inhibitor is safe and may improve outcomes. Some of the common side effects that affect patient satisfaction with these devices are coldness, numbness, and bruising of the penis.

Penile Prosthesis

A penile prosthesis, either semirigid or inflatable, is implanted in the operating room. Most patients prefer the inflatable devices because they provide a more natural erection when inflated and a flaccid penis when deflated. Although implantation of a penile prosthesis is more invasive than the other techniques, this device is the most effective long-term option for impotence treatment. Ninety percent of patients and partners are satisfied with the result.

Important interval improvements have been made in the design of implantable penile prostheses to make them more durable and resistant to infection. Improvements in the connection between tubing and corporal cylinders have cut the mechanical failure rate to less than 5% in 5 years. Components also have special coatings that either contain antibiotics or absorb antibiotics applied topically at the time of implantation. These improvements have cut the rate of postoperative infection in half.

C. Benign Prostatic Hyperplasia

BPH, a nonmalignant enlargement of the prostate gland, is a common condition in the aging male patient. It is estimated that more than 90% of all men will develop histologic evidence of BPH during the course of their lifetime; of those, at least 50% will develop lower urinary tract symptoms (LUTS) that prompt them to seek medical care. Broadly speaking, LUTS can be divided into two groups: obstructive voiding symptoms and overactive bladder symptoms (Table 71-4).

Although most patients who seek medical care for BPH do so because of the associated LUTS, these same symptoms can also result from other illnesses such as diabetes mellitus, spine disease, Parkinson's disease, multiple sclerosis, and cerebrovascular disease (Fig. 71-3). It is important to evaluate all patients for these non–BPH-related conditions to ensure optimal management. It is also important to pay close attention to medication use because a number of medications used in the elderly population can result in various urologic symptoms, including both obstructive and overactive bladder voiding symptoms.

● PATHOPHYSIOLOGY

Prostate growth and the subsequent development of BPH occur under the influence of testosterone and the more metabolically active dihydrotestosterone (DHT). Testosterone produced by the testes is converted to DHT by the action of the enzyme

5α-reductase. DHT is the major intracellular androgen and is believed to be responsible for the development and maintenance of the hyperplastic cell growth characteristics of BPH.

BPH develops predominantly in the periurethral prostatic tissue, referred to as the *transition zone* (Fig. 71-4). Tissue growth in this area leads to the phenomenon of bladder outlet obstruction (BOO), which leads to LUTS. BOO occurs as a result of two mechanisms: mechanical obstruction from increased tissue volume in the periurethral zone of the prostate and dynamic obstruction, which is caused by decreased bladder neck relaxation during voiding and increased smooth muscle tone in the bladder neck and prostate gland. Also important, but less well characterized, is the response of the bladder muscle to the increase in outlet resistance provided by those two mechanisms. As bladder outlet resistance increases, the bladder responds by increasing the force of contraction. This added work results in physical and mechanical changes in bladder function.

Early in the course of BOO, the bladder is able to compensate; however, with persistent obstruction, the patient typically develops LUTS, particularly overactive bladder symptoms such as nocturia, frequency, and urgency. These symptoms frequently drive patients to seek medical care. Later during the course of the obstructive process, the bladder wall becomes thickened and loses compliance. The subsequent loss of compliance results in a decreased functional capacity of the bladder, which exacerbates the patient's overactive bladder symptoms.

⬤ DIAGNOSIS

The initial evaluation of a patient with LUTS suggestive of BPH should include a detailed medical history that focuses on the patient's urinary symptoms as well as the past medical history, including comorbid conditions and any previous surgical procedures, general health conditions, and history of alcohol and tobacco use. The assessment of symptoms can be facilitated with the use of the AUA Symptom Index (also known as the *International Prostate Symptom Score*, or IPSS). This is a self-administered, validated questionnaire consisting of seven questions related to the symptoms of BPH and BOO. The AUA Symptom Index classifies symptoms as mild (0 to 7), moderate (8 to 19), or severe (20 to 35). Validated instruments such as the AUA Symptom Index are useful during the initial evaluation as an overall assessment of symptom severity and during follow-up visits to assess the effectiveness of any medical or surgical interventions.

A general physical examination should be performed that includes a DRE and a focused neurologic examination. Urinalysis, either by dipstick or by microscopic examination of urine sediment, is also mandatory to rule out hematuria and evidence of urinary tract infection. Glycosuria can be a significant finding, particularly if not previously identified. The initial clinical practice guidelines for the diagnosis of BPH recommended a serum creatinine measurement to assess renal function in all patients

TABLE 71-4	SYMPTOMS OF LOWER URINARY TRACT SYNDROME
OVERACTIVE BLADDER	**OBSTRUCTIVE VOIDING**
Frequency	Hesitancy
Nocturia	Slow stream
Urgency	Stop-and-start voiding
Urge incontinence	Sensation of incomplete emptying

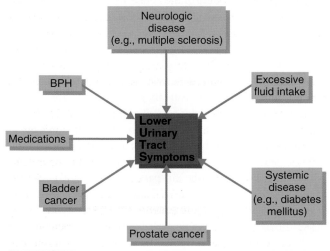

FIGURE 71-3 Causes of lower urinary tract symptoms (LUTS). BPH, Benign prostatic hyperplasia.

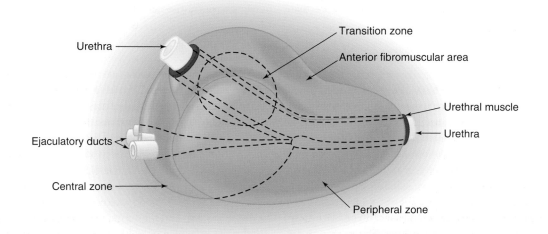

FIGURE 71-4 Zonal anatomy of the prostate gland.

with signs or symptoms suggestive of BPH. However, this recommendation came under scrutiny because of its low yield for the detection of renal insufficiency secondary to obstructive uropathy. Serum creatinine measurement is no longer a routine part of the BPH work-up. According to the same clinical practice guidelines, PSA measurement is optional during the initial evaluation. PSA can function as a surrogate for prostate volume measurement in addition to being a screening test for prostate cancer. The Medical Therapy of Prostatic Symptoms (MTOPS) study, sponsored by the National Institutes of Health, demonstrated that PSA increases linearly with prostate volume and that a PSA level greater than 4 ng/mL conveys a 9% risk of requiring surgical therapy for benign disease over a 4.5-year period.

The following additional diagnostic tests are also considered optional; however, they may be useful, particularly in patients with moderate to severe AUA symptom scores, in determining whether the patient's symptoms are compatible with obstruction from BPH. Uroflowmetry is a noninvasive method of measuring urinary flow rate. The maximal urinary flow rate, Q_{max}, is considered the most useful measurement for identifying patients with BOO. However, patients with diminished flow rates may also have impaired bladder contraction. Typical values range from 25 mL/second in a young man without BOO to 10 mL/second or slower in a man with significant BOO. Of note, patients with a flow rate of less than 15 mL/second have better outcomes after transurethral resection of the prostate (TURP, discussed later). Measurement of postvoid residual (PVR) urine may be accomplished by urethral catheterization or, preferably, by ultrasonography. Elevated PVR volumes indicate an increased risk for acute urinary retention and eventual need for surgical intervention. The MTOPS study demonstrated that 7% of men with PVR greater than 39 mL required surgical intervention over a 4.5-year period. Elevation of PVR to greater than 200 mL raises the question of functional impairment of the bladder and warrants further evaluation with urodynamic testing.

Routine evaluation of the upper urinary tracts (kidneys and ureters) with excretory urography or ultrasonography is not recommended for the average BPH patient unless there is concomitant urinary pathology (i.e., hematuria, urinary tract infection, renal insufficiency, a history of prior urologic surgery, or a history of nephrolithiasis). Likewise, transrectal ultrasonography (TRUS) is not routinely recommended unless it is used for preoperative assessment of prostate gland size while planning surgical intervention.

⬤ DIFFERENTIAL DIAGNOSIS

Many conditions can cause LUTS in the aging male. A DRE and PSA testing are helpful in distinguishing between BPH and prostate cancer. Early-stage prostate cancer is typically asymptomatic, and patients can have both conditions concurrently. Although PSA testing is not sufficiently sensitive or specific to reliably differentiate BPH from prostate cancer, it is a useful tool to stratify a patient's risk for the presence of prostate cancer.

In response to ongoing controversy about PSA screening, the AUA released a new guideline in 2013 pertaining to the early detection (screening) of prostate cancer. According to this guideline, the purpose of early detection is to decrease prostate cancer mortality. Overall, the guideline recommends against routine

prostate cancer screening (PSA and DRE) in men younger than 55 years of age. However, prostate cancer screening should be considered between the ages of 40 and 55 years in men who have higher risk of prostate cancer (i.e., family history or African American race). For men ages 55 to 69 years, the guideline recommends an individualized approach with discussion about the benefits of prostate cancer screening versus the known risks of screening and treatment. The guideline did not recommend screening in any man older than 70 years of age or in any man with less than 10 to 15 years of life expectancy.

Both the DRE and serum PSA determination have a role in the early diagnosis of prostate cancer. Prostate cancer typically arises from the peripheral portion of the prostate, which can be palpated on DRE. Induration or nodularity of the prostate on DRE should be considered suspicious for prostate cancer. PSA is a protein produced by both benign and malignant prostate cells. Serum PSA levels may be elevated in the face of prostate enlargement, inflammation, or cancer. Although an elevated PSA level is not diagnostic of prostate cancer, it can lead to a prostate biopsy to exclude cancer. Probably because of progressive enlargement in prostate size, serum PSA values increase as men age. The historical view that a PSA value lower than 4 ng/mL is "normal" has been abandoned since the recognition that PSA represents a continuum of risk based on age with no lower threshold. The comparative rate of change for PSA over time, sometimes termed *PSA velocity*, can be informative. In general, a change in PSA of more than 0.75 ng/mL is considered worrisome and may prompt a prostate biopsy.

Prostatitis is another condition that can cause LUTS. It may result from bacterial infection or from a nonbacterial inflammatory process, and the symptoms may substantially overlap those of BPH, particularly in older men. Diabetes mellitus, neurologic diseases such as Parkinson's disease or cerebrovascular disease, and other conditions of the urinary tract, such as urethral strictures, may result in LUTS in patients with BPH. Finally, many medications, particularly those with significant anticholinergic side effects, can cause symptoms mimicking those associated with BPH.

⬤ MEDICAL MANAGEMENT

Medical management is the preferred first-line treatment option for patients diagnosed with LUTS due to BPH. Most cases can be managed effectively with a minimum of side effects. The MTOPS study demonstrated that combination therapy with a long-acting α-blocker and a 5α-reductase inhibitor was more effective than single-agent therapy alone. In general, medical management is initiated for patients with moderate to severe AUA symptom scores. However, in the absence of indications for surgery (refractory urinary retention, hydronephrosis with or without renal impairment, recurrent urinary tract infections, recurrent gross hematuria, or bladder calculi), the decision to embark on any course of therapy, medical or otherwise, is principally driven by the bothersomeness of the patient's symptoms. Every patient has a different perception of his symptoms: Nocturia twice nightly may be a minor nuisance for some but may represent a significant problem for others. There is no absolute AUA symptom score or other objective measure that dictates the need for initiation of therapy for symptomatic BPH. Each patient must be evaluated individually, and the treatment course must be tailored to the patient's individual situation.

α-Adrenergic Antagonists

α-Blockers are the most commonly prescribed medications for the treatment of LUTS associated with BPH. The bladder neck and prostate are richly innervated with α-adrenergic receptors, specifically α_{1a}-receptors, which constitute about 70% to 80% of the total number of α-receptors in these areas. α_{1b}-Receptors modulate vascular smooth muscle contraction and are located in the bladder neck and prostate to a lesser degree.

Doxazosin, terazosin, tamsulosin, and extended-release alfuzosin are long-acting α-receptor antagonists. They are typically administered once daily, usually at bedtime to minimize the potential for orthostatic hypotension. These medications act through α_1-receptors and can cause vasodilation resulting in transient hypotension and lightheadedness. Blood pressure reduction is greater in patients with hypertension (average reduction, 10 to 15 mm Hg) relative to normotensive patients (average reduction, 1 to 4 mm Hg). Overall, 10% to 20% of patients experience some (often transient) side effects from these medications, including dizziness, asthenia, headaches, peripheral edema, and nasal congestion. Dose titration is recommended for doxazosin and terazosin to minimize occurrence of these adverse effects and optimize the therapeutic response. Doxazosin and terazosin require at least 4 or 5 mg, respectively, to achieve a therapeutic effect. Maximal response is usually seen within 1 to 2 weeks with doxazosin and within 3 to 6 weeks with terazosin. Overall, these drugs reduce symptom scores by 40% to 50% and improve urinary flow rates by 40% to 50% in about 60% to 65% of patients treated.

Tamsulosin is a selective α_{1a}-receptor antagonist with a long half-life. It has a significantly lower degree of nonspecific α-receptor binding compared with other α-receptor antagonists. Therefore, side effects such as postural hypotension and dizziness are less common. This drug does not appreciably affect blood pressure in hypertensive or normotensive patients. Maximal response is usually seen within 1 to 2 weeks after the initiation of therapy.

5α-Reductase Inhibitors (Finasteride and Dutasteride)

Finasteride and dutasteride block the intracellular conversion of testosterone to DHT by inhibiting the action of the enzyme 5α-reductase. This results in an approximate 18% to 25% reduction in prostate gland size over 6 to 12 months. It is most effective in reducing symptoms and preventing disease progression in patients with large prostate glands (>40 mL [Prostate measurement for clinical purposes is usually described in mL, but 1 mL= 1 g = 1 cc]), although recent evidence suggests that symptomatic improvement and stabilization of disease progression may occur in treated men with prostates as small as 30 mL. 5α-Reductase inhibition has also been shown to decrease the risk for urinary retention and subsequent surgical intervention, again predominantly in those patients with larger glands. Initial response is seen within 6 months, and maximal effect occurs 12 to 18 months after the initiation of therapy.

Finasteride and dutasteride reduce serum PSA by about 50%. This must be taken into consideration when interpreting PSA values in men taking these agents. After 6 months of therapy, the effective PSA level in a patient taking finasteride or dutasteride may be calculated by doubling the measured PSA value. Free PSA (the percentage of non–protein-bound PSA) is also reduced by about 50%. Use of finasteride or dutasteride may result in sexual dysfunction, including decreased erectile rigidity, decreased libido, and decreased ejaculate volume. ED caused by 5α-reductase inhibitor therapy is reversible and returns to baseline within 2 to 6 months after discontinuation of therapy.

Phosphodiesterase Type 5 Inhibitors

Although they are more often thought of as medications for the treatment of ED, sildenafil, vardenafil, and tadalafil have been shown to be efficacious in the treatment of the symptoms of BPH. As previously discussed, these medications work by preventing the degradation of cGMP by PDE5. This results in lower intracellular calcium levels and, consequently, smooth muscle relaxation. This process works in the vasculature of the penis as well as the smooth muscle cells of the prostate, urethra, and bladder neck. A number of randomized, double-blind, placebo-controlled trials have shown improvements in LUTS in men treated with a once-daily regimen of one of these medications. Although it has not been conclusively shown that PDE5 inhibitors are more efficacious than α-blockers, it does appear that the combination of the two medications works better than either one of them alone. The common side effects of these medications are headache, nasal stuffiness, and facial flushing.

Anticholinergic Medications

For most men, symptoms of overactive bladder make up a large component of LUTS associated with BPH. Most men with bladder outlet obstruction have symptoms of urgency, frequency, and nocturia. As in female patients, one of the best ways to treat these symptoms of overactive bladder is with daily use of anticholinergic medications such as oxybutynin, tolterodine, or solifenacin. When these medications are used in combination with an α-blocker, there can be significant improvement in LUTS in men with symptoms of overactive bladder. Except in patients with small prostates (<29 mL), it does not appear that anticholinergic monotherapy is better than combination therapy or α-blocker monotherapy. The typical side effects of this class of medications include dry mouth, constipation, nausea, and impaired cognition. The risk of urinary retention related to the use of these medications in men appears to be minimal.

● SURGICAL MANAGEMENT
Minimally Invasive Therapy

Although TURP remains the standard for surgical treatment of BPH, substantial effort has been devoted to the development of less invasive and less morbid methods of treating patients with symptomatic BPH. This has led to a number of minimally invasive therapies, primarily using different methods of generating heat within the prostate gland to cause tissue destruction. These office-based heat techniques transiently increase bladder outlet obstruction for 1 to 2 weeks due to postprocedure swelling. Maximal tissue reduction and treatment effect occur within 12 weeks.

Transurethral microwave thermotherapy (TUMT) is one of the most widely studied minimally invasive methods of treating symptomatic BPH. Catheter-mounted transducers use microwave energy (30 to 300 Hz) to heat prostatic tissue, resulting in coagulative necrosis and shrinkage of the prostate gland. The subsequent reduction in prostate transition zone volume results in an improvement in flow rates and symptom scores. Transurethral needle ablation (TUNA) uses low-level radio frequency energy to effect similar changes within the prostate gland. Other therapies currently available or in development include interstitial lasers and high-intensity focused ultrasound. All of these therapies are designed to deliver sufficient energy to the prostate to cause tissue destruction, resulting in a smaller prostate gland consequent improvement in the patient's symptoms.

The most common side effects of these treatments are temporary increases in overactive bladder symptoms, transient urinary retention, hematuria, and ejaculatory dysfunction (primarily retrograde ejaculation). Late complications such as urethral strictures and ED have been reported but are significantly less common than with traditional surgical approaches. The major benefits of these less invasive therapies are the reduction in traditional surgical morbidities (e.g., bleeding) and risks associated with general or spinal anesthesia and decreased rates of long-term complications such as incontinence, ED, bladder neck contractures, and urethral strictures. Additionally, most of these procedures can be accomplished safely on an outpatient basis, either in the office or in an ambulatory surgical setting.

Success rates for the heat-based minimally invasive therapies are intermediate between those achieved with medical management and those of traditional surgical therapy, with 65% to 75% of patients experiencing symptomatic improvement and improved flow rates. The long-term durability of these therapies appears to be good but is presently being evaluated.

Traditional Surgical Management

TURP remains the "gold standard" for the surgical management of symptomatic BPH. A TURP procedure involves removal of the transition zone of the prostate through the penis using a cutting electrocautery loop. The goals of the surgery are to reduce the transition zone prostate tissue to the level of the prostatic capsule and to create a smooth, open appearance of the prostatic urethra and bladder neck. Improvements in the conventional technique have included bipolar electrosurgical cutting, which allows saline irrigation and eliminates the chance of transient urinary retention syndrome.

Newer operating room–based therapies have evolved that produce end results similar to those of TURP. Holmium laser enucleation (HOLEP) is a surgical technique performed by specially trained urologists, generally indicated for large size prostates. Other procedures include various forms of vaporization of the transition zone tissue of the prostate. In contrast to the TURP, no pieces of prostate are removed with these procedures. The various vaporization procedures include potassium titanyl phosphate (KTP or GreenLight) laser therapy, also called photovaporization of the prostate, and bipolar plasma vaporization of the prostate (button TURP). With the exception of HOLEP, all of these procedures are useful for all but the largest prostate glands (>100 mL), which are typically best managed with open surgical enucleation. Rates of urinary incontinence, retrograde ejaculation, and urethral stricture are all higher after operating room procedures than after office-based therapies. Perioperative morbidity, including the need for blood transfusion, although substantially decreased by technical improvements, is likewise higher after TURP and similar procedures. However, standard electrosurgical resection of the prostate (TURP) is the most effective surgical treatment for symptomatic BPH short of enucleation. Success rates, as measured by improved symptom scores and increased urinary flow rates, are 80% to 90% after TURP.

Transurethral incision of the prostate (TUIP) is a more limited surgical procedure consisting of incision of the bladder neck and proximal prostatic urethra. Although it is more invasive than the heat-based therapies, success rates approach those of TURP in properly selected patients (i.e., those with prostate glands <30 mL). Morbidity after TUIP is significantly less than after TURP, but long-term durability of symptom relief is less than that seen with TURP.

Open surgical enucleation (open or simple prostatectomy) is reserved for patients with very large glands. This is an invasive surgery that typically involves a 5- to 10-cm incision in the midline of the lower abdomen and an incision in the bladder neck or the capsule of the prostate. After the incision has been made, the transition zone of the prostate (prostatic adenoma) is bluntly removed. Success rates are high, but the rate of complications is higher than with any of the other traditional surgical approaches (Table 71-5). This surgery is uncommonly performed in the United States, having been replaced by HOLEP in many centers.

⬤ CONCLUSION

The management of LUTS resulting from BPH has undergone a dramatic shift from principally a surgical approach to a medical approach. This evolution of care, coupled with the aging of the U.S. population, has resulted in a shift of care for these patients from the urologist to the primary care physician. In the absence of severe LUTS or indications for early surgical intervention, the primary care physician can now successfully manage most cases of mild to moderate BPH. If there is no response to medical therapy, the patient can be offered office-based minimally invasive surgical therapy.

TABLE 71-5 SUCCESS IN MEDICAL VERSUS SURGICAL MANAGEMENT OF BENIGN PROSTATIC HYPERPLASIA

DEGREE OF IMPROVEMENT	α_1- BLOCKERS	FINASTERIDE	TURP	TUIP	OPEN SURGERY
Symptoms (%)	48	31	82	73	79
Flow rate (%)	40-50	17	120	100	185
Mean probability (%) of achieving the stated improvements	74	67	88	80	98

TUIP, Transurethral incision of the prostate; TURP, transurethral resection of the prostate.

D. Testis Cancer

Testicular tumors are the most common solid malignancies in men aged 15 to 34 years, and the incidence of testis cancer appears to have increased over the last 25 years. The advent of platinum-based chemotherapy in the 1970s and a more recent systematic multidisciplinary approach have greatly improved the survival of patients with testicular cancer over the last 40 years. Survival now approaches 99% for low-risk disease and 80% for high-risk disease.

Cryptorchidism (undescended testicle) is a well-accepted risk factor for subsequent development of testicular cancer. Abnormalities in spermatogenesis are well documented and are thought to be a primary effect of testicular tumors; up to 15% of patients are diagnosed with testicular cancer during a work-up for male factor infertility. Also, it appears that patients with an atrophic testicle have an increased risk of testicular cancer. Testicular microlithiasis does not appear to connote an increased risk of testicular cancer, although this conclusion is somewhat controversial; patients with this incidental finding on testicular ultrasonography do not require additional surveillance beyond monthly testicular examinations. Between 2% and 3% of patients have bilateral tumors at presentation, and 5% to 10% of those with involvement of only one testicle will go on to develop cancer in the normal contralateral testicle. Despite impairments in spermatogenesis, most men with testicular cancer are capable of fathering children; discussion of fertility issues is extremely important, especially in patients who may require adjuvant therapies such as external-beam radiation and systemic chemotherapy.

The most common presenting sign or symptom of testis cancer is a firm, painless mass arising from the testis. However, patients may also have an acute scrotum at presentation as a result of tumor hemorrhage, and up to 33% of patients are treated for presumed epididymitis. Scrotal ultrasonography is diagnostic; testis cancer is usually distinguishable from benign scrotal disease because of the clear involvement of the testicular parenchyma rather than the paratesticular tissues. Signs and symptoms of advanced disease include cough, gastrointestinal symptoms (mass), back pain (retroperitoneal metastasis), neurologic symptoms (brain metastasis), lower-extremity swelling (iliac or inferior vena cava thrombus), and supraclavicular lymphadenopathy.

DIAGNOSIS AND STAGING

Initial management of the primary tumor is inguinal orchiectomy with high ligation of the spermatic cord. Histopathology distinguishes germ cell tumors (GCTs) from stromal tumors. Seminoma is the most common GCT occurring in pure form. Teratoma, yolk sac tumor, embryonal carcinoma, and choriocarcinoma are classified as nonseminomatous GCT and frequently occur as mixed GCT (more than one histologic pattern within the primary tumor). Testicular cancer is unique in that serum tumor markers (STMs) play an important role in tumor staging. STMs include HCG, α-fetoprotein (AFP), and serum lactate dehydrogenase. Elevations of serum HCG may be seen in choriocarcinomas, in embryonal carcinomas, and in 15% of seminomas. Elevated AFP can be seen in yolk sac tumors and embryonal carcinomas, and this finding excludes a diagnosis of seminoma. These STMs may be secreted either by the primary tumor or by metastatic foci (Table 71-6).

The retroperitoneal lymph nodes are the most common initial site of metastasis. Therefore, staging of the retroperitoneum with an abdominal CT scan is important in evaluating the extent of disease. However, accurate staging of the retroperitoneum remains problematic, with the literature quoting false-negative and false-positive rates of 20% to 30% with CT scanning. Common landing zones for lymph node metastasis include the precaval, interaortocaval, and preaortic lymph nodes below the renal hilum and above the aortic bifurcation. Chest radiography or thoracic CT scanning completes the clinical staging because the lungs and posterior mediastinum are the most common sites of distant metastatic disease.

TREATMENT

Histopathology, pathologic stage, and STM status are used to determine subsequent treatment after inguinal orchiectomy. All patients with elevated STMs after orchiectomy receive cisplatin-based chemotherapy, regardless of histology. Radiation therapy and retroperitoneal lymph node dissection (RPLND) have a high likelihood of failure in the face of elevated STMs.

Seminoma manifests as clinical stage I in 70% of cases, stage II in 20%, and stage III in 10%. In the past, most experts recommended radiation therapy to the retroperitoneum for patients with stage I or II disease because of the radiosensitivity of seminomas. However, patients with stage I seminoma are now more likely to undergo surveilance because of the recognition that new retroperitoneal metastases found during surveillance are sensitive to either chemotherapy or radiation. Patients with bulky stage II disease (lymph node >5 cm) and those with stage III disease should receive combination chemotherapy.

Nonseminomatous GCTs manifest more frequently at an advanced stage (stage I, in 30%, stage II in 40%, and stage III in 30%). RPLND is frequently recommended in patients with clinical stage I or low-volume stage II disease. Reasons for recommending RPLND include accurate pathologic staging of the retroperitoneum, low relapse rate (<2%) after properly performed RPLND, curative potential in the face of viable GCT, and the potential for retroperitoneal teratoma, which is resistant to chemotherapy. Side effects associated with RPLND include lymphocele, chylous ascites (0.4%), and small bowel obstruction (1% to 2%). Nerve-sparing RPLND is able to preserve antegrade ejaculation in more than 80% of patients.

TABLE 71-6 TESTIS CANCER STAGING STUDIES

Tumor markers
  AFP—elevated only with nonseminomatous tumors
  HCG—may be increased with either seminoma or nonseminomatous tumors
Abdominal CT scan—retroperitoneal nodes are most common site of regional nodal metastasis
Chest radiograph or CT scan—lung is most frequent site of distant metastasis

AFP, α-Fetoprotein; HCG, β-human chorionic gonadotropin; CT, computed tomography.

Primary chemotherapy is sometimes recommended to patients with stage I or II nonseminomatous testis cancers. Also, some men may choose surveillance alone for a stage I tumor, which implies normal serum marker status and a normal abdominal CT scan. Up to 25% may be expected to develop recurrence, usually within 2 years, and chemotherapy is used after evidence of recurrence.

Platinum-based chemotherapy is the standard for patients with advanced disease. Cure rates of 70% to 80% are achieved even in patients who have relatively bulky metastatic disease at presentation. Side effects of chemotherapy include renal dysfunction, neuropathy, Raynaud's phenomenon, hematologic toxicity, pulmonary toxicity, cardiovascular toxicity, and a 0.5% risk for secondary leukemia.

E. Male Infertility

Approximately 90% of all couples are able to conceive a child in the first year. For this reason, a male patient should not be evaluated for infertility unless he has tried to have a child for at least 1 year. Although it is difficult to localize the cause of infertility to one gender, the prevalence of male factor infertility in infertile couples is probably 25% to 50%. From a very basic perspective, male infertility is caused by problems delivering sperm, from either a decreased amount of sperm or a deficiency in the quality of the sperm. These problems can result from ED, retrograde ejaculation, ejaculatory duct obstruction, obstruction of the vas deferens, endocrine dysfunction, varicoceles, or genetic abnormalities.

● HISTORY AND PHYSICAL EXAMINATION

The evaluation of a patient with infertility should begin with a thorough history and physical examination. During the history, the clinician should include questions about how long and how frequently the couple has been trying to conceive, prior pregnancies with current or previous partners, erectile function, and use of lubricants. A detailed past medical, surgical, social, and family history is also very important.

The physical examination should commence with an overall assessment of the patient's general health. Next, the clinician should focus on examination of the genitalia. The surface of the testicle should be closely examined because studies have shown an increased incidence of testicular cancer in patients with infertility. Testicular size and consistency should also be assessed. The normal testicle has a volume of approximately 20 mL and does not feel soft or spongy. In addition, the spermatic cord should be carefully examined to confirm the presence of a vas deferens on each side. The scrotum should be examined for the presence of a varicocele, with and without performance of the Valsalva maneuver. Finally, a rectal examination should be performed to palpate for abnormalities of the prostate and seminal vesicles.

● SEMEN ANALYSIS

Semen analysis is probably the most important part of the evaluation of an infertile male patient. The patient should abstain from ejaculation for 2 to 7 days before the test, and clinical decision making should be based on at least two tests performed 7 days apart. Sperm concentration increases with days of abstinence. In a study from 2004 looking at the effect of frequency of ejaculation on sperm concentration, the concentration continued to increase after 10 days of abstinence. After the specimen has been collected by the patient, it should be delivered to the laboratory at body temperature as soon as possible. Motility significantly decreases after 2 hours.

The most important parts of the microscopic examination of the semen sample are sperm concentration, morphology, and motility. The normal sperm concentration is greater than 20 million sperm per milliliter, and a value lower than 20 million per milliliter is termed *oligospermia*. The absence of sperm is termed *azoospermia*. Depending on the laboratory, sperm morphology is usually reported as a percentage. Typically, normal morphology in more than 50% of sperm examined is considered acceptable. Morphologic studies primarily assess the size and shape of the head and tail. Motility is also expressed as a percentage and refers to the percentage of sperm that are moving in a coordinated and progressive manner. Mortality values higher than 50% are considered to be normal. Abnormal sperm motility is termed *asthenospermia*, and abnormal morphology is *teratospermia*.

Other factors checked during a semen analysis include semen volume, pH, and fructose positivity. A semen volume between 2 and 4 mL is considered normal. A volume of less than 2 mL may be a sign of ejaculatory duct obstruction (absent fluid from vas deferens and seminal vesicle) or retrograde ejaculation. Because the testicles contribute only a small portion of the fluid released during ejaculation, a vasectomy should not affect ejaculate volume. The normal range of semen pH is 7.2 to 8.0. An acidic pH may be a sign of congenital absence of the vas deferens or seminal vesicle hypoplasia. Depending on the laboratory, the fructose test result should be positive or in the normal range. Fructose is made by the seminal vesicles and provides nutrition for the sperm. Low or absent fructose may also be a sign of ejaculatory duct obstruction or seminal vesicle hypoplasia.

● OTHER DIAGNOSTIC TESTS

If a patient has an abnormal semen analysis, an endocrine evaluation should be performed. The complete initial endocrine evaluation includes measurements of LH, follicle-stimulating hormone (FSH), prolactin, and testosterone. These hormone levels should be checked in the morning (before 11 A.M.). In general, an elevated FSH is a bad prognostic sign indicating that the patient will not be found to have a correctable form of infertility. From a simplistic point of view, this is because the hypothalamic-pituitary access is trying to stimulate sperm production but the testicle is not responding. Genetic testing in the form of a chromosome analysis (karyotype and Y-linked microdeletion assessment) should be considered in patients with severe oligospermia or azoospermia to rule out disorders such as Klinefelter's syndrome and abnormalities of the Y chromosome.

As long as a normal physical examination can be performed, there is no need to do a scrotal ultrasound study on patients with infertility. If the patient has a body habitus that makes physical examination difficult, a scrotal ultrasonography may aid in the diagnosis of a clinical varicocele. In general, patients in need of further diagnostic evaluation of infertility should be referred to a specialist.

TREATMENT OF MALE INFERTILITY IN PRIMARY CARE

There are several options for the treatment of male infertility, and the choice of treatment depends on the results of the history, physical examination, and diagnostic evaluation. First, fertility is a reflection of a patient's overall general health. Decreasing the patient's stress level, improving sleep habits, and fostering a healthy diet may all have beneficial effects on fertility. There is conflicting evidence as to whether antioxidants in the form of vitamins or diet modification improve the viability of sperm. Patients can purchase antioxidant multivitamins at most supermarkets and health food stores. Because the evidence for benefit is mixed, it is important to tell the patient not to overspend on this treatment.

Other lifestyle modifications may also improve fertility. For example, avoiding hot baths and whirlpools may provide more optimal conditions for sperm production. In addition, tobacco, alcohol, and marijuana use have all been shown to negatively affect fertility in males. Certain medications also can have a negative impact on infertility. α-Blockers used to treat BPH can cause retrograde ejaculation. Exogenous testosterone replacement decreases sperm production, and at least 2 months are required for sperm production to recover once testosterone therapy is stopped.

The timing and frequency of intercourse can affect the ability to conceive. Ovulation predictor kits are readily available to patients without a prescription and may improve fertility. Because sperm can survive at least 2 days in the female genital tract, having intercourse every 2 days may maximize male sperm concentration and delivery. In addition, patients should make sure that they are not using a lubricant that has spermicidal activity.

Patients who have a palpable varicocele and oligospermia with or without defects in sperm morphology or motility may benefit from a varicocelectomy and should be referred to a urologist for further evaluation (see later discussion). The most common methods of surgical correction are varicocelectomy and gonadal vein embolization.

Patients with oligospermia and a normal or low FSH level may benefit from treatment with clomiphene citrate (Clomid). The typical dosage is 25 mg daily or 50 mg every other day for at least 2 months (it takes 64 days for new sperm to be made). Most studies of this drug have shown a significant increase in sperm production but little impact on fertility. However, it may be beneficial for selected patients with the above-mentioned laboratory values.

If a varicocele is present in an infertility patient or severe oligospermia or azoospermia does not respond to the treatments already mentioned, referral to a urologist for additional testing is warranted. Oligospermia or azoospermia with a low semen volume and a negative fructose result may suggest ejaculatory duct obstruction. If azoospermia is present with no sonographic evidence of ejaculatory duct obstruction, a testicular biopsy might be the prudent next step. If retrograde ejaculation is suspected (oligospermia, normal fructose, and low semen volume), the urologist may elect to examine a postejaculation, centrifuged urine specimen for the presence of sperm.

Once the evaluation by the urologist has been completed, he or she may recommend that the patient proceed with assisted reproductive technology (ART). The simplest form of ART is intrauterine insemination, for which patients with oligospermia and normal motility are excellent candidates. In vitro fertilization (IVF) and intracytoplasmic sperm injection (ICSI) are more costly but often successful. Even patients with azoospermia due to Klinefelter's syndrome have had frequent success (46% rate of pregnancy) with ICSI.

F. Benign Scrotal Diseases

VARICOCELE

A varicocele is classically described as an abnormal dilation of the veins of the pampiniform plexus that can be palpated as a "bag of worms" with or without having the patient performing the Valsalva maneuver while standing. When examining a patient for any scrotal pathology, it is important to have the patient stand. A clinical varicocele is one that can be palpated on physical examination. Because the occurrence of varicoceles increases with age, the prevalence in the literature is highly variable. The prevalence of a unilateral palpable left-sided varicocele is between 6.5% and 22%, and that of bilateral palpable varicoceles ranges from 10% to 20%. The prevalence of an isolated right-sided palpable varicocele is less than 1%; because of their very rare association with retroperitoneal malignancy, many clinicians perform axial imaging on patients with a unilateral right-sided varicocele. In general,

a left-sided varicocele does not have clinical significance unless it can be palpated on physical examination. A left-sided varicocele that is incidentally found during ultrasonography of the scrotum and is not palpable on examination is considered a subclinical varicocele and is typically not the source of any pathology.

Palpable and nonpalpable varicoceles are most commonly found incidentally and in most cases have no clinical significance. However, palpable varicoceles can cause ipsilateral testicular atrophy. Therefore, it is important for the clinician to compare the size of the testicles in patients who desire future fertility. If the physical examination is unclear, scrotal ultrasonography can be used to accurately measure the size of both testicles. Any patient who desires future children and has a size discrepancy greater than 20% should be monitored closely and possibly referred to a urologist. Although varicoceles are most commonly found incidentally, they may also be found during a work-up for male factor infertility, scrotal pain, or asymptomatic testicular atrophy.

The pathophysiology of varicoceles is poorly understood but involves dilation of the internal spermatic vein and transmission of increased hydrostatic pressure across dysfunctional venous valves. Stasis of blood in the venous system disturbs the counter-current heat exchange that is responsible for maintaining testicular temperature and may result in testicular parenchymal damage and impaired spermatogenesis.

Varicoceles are the most common cause of both primary infertility (patient has fathered no children) and secondary infertility (patient has fathered at least one child), accounting for 33% of cases. However, most men with palpable varicoceles are able to father children without difficulty. In a man with infertility and a palpable varicocele, semen analysis commonly reveals a low sperm count and abnormal sperm morphology and motility. After surgical correction of a varicocele in a patient with infertility, semen parameters improve in 60% to 80% and subsequent pregnancy rates range from 20% to 60%.

It is prudent to perform scrotal ultrasonography on any patient with chronic testicular pain. Varicoceles are commonly found during this evaluation, but usually only palpable (clinical) varicoceles are considered as a source of pain. If a nonpalpable varicocele is found on an ultrasound examination, the patient should not be told that it is the cause of his pain. More than 80% of men with chronic pain from a palpable varicocele have improvement in their pain after surgical correction.

Common operative techniques for treatment of a varicocele include high retroperitoneal ligation of the internal spermatic vein, microsurgical inguinal and subinguinal varicocelectomy, laparoscopic varicocelectomy, and gonadal vein embolization. The inguinal approach using microscopic magnification has the highest success and lowest complication and recurrence rates. The most common complication is hydrocele formation, whereas a rare complication is inadvertent ligation of the testicular artery resulting in testicular atrophy and loss. Surgical intervention for subclinical (nonpalpable) varicoceles is not indicated.

SPERMATOCELE (EPIDIDYMAL CYST)

Spermatoceles and epididymal cysts are dilations of the tubes that connect the testicle to the epididymis (ductuli efferentes). Although they are technically the same thing, many clinicians refer to small lesions as epididymal cysts and larger ones as spermatoceles. These cystic lesions are very common and are found in 29% of asymptomatic men on ultrasonography. After a vasectomy, 35% of men develop a new small spermatocele; therefore, distal obstruction likely contributes to their development.

On physical examination, spermatoceles are somewhat mobile, firm masses that are separate and distinguishable from the smooth border of the testicle. It may be possible to transilluminate larger lesions. They are filled with a clear fluid that usually contains abundant amounts of sperm. If the lesion cannot be transilluminated, it is advisable to perform an ultrasound study of the scrotum to distinguish a spermatocele from a solid mass. Of note, the vast majority of solid masses of the epididymis are benign. Small spermatoceles and epididymal cysts normally have no clinical significance and are typically

not the source of a patient's chronic testicular pain. They can be surgically removed if they are large or are causing discomfort for the patient.

ACUTE EPIDIDYMITIS

Acute epididymitis is a clinical syndrome that may manifest with fever, acute scrotal pain, and impressive swelling and induration of the epididymis. Pathophysiologically, epididymitis is most often caused by retrograde bacterial spread from the bladder or urethra. In men younger than 35 years of age, the most common causative agents are those organisms associated with urethritis—namely, *Neisseria gonococcus* and *Chlamydia trachomatis*. In older men, acute epididymitis is usually caused by a coliform bacteria such as *Escherichia coli* and often occurs in association with another lower urinary tract infection or bladder outlet obstruction.

The most important consideration in diagnosing acute epididymitis is differentiating this disease from acute testicular torsion. Physical examination can be nonspecific, although focal epididymal swelling and tenderness are suggestive, and the presence of white cells and bacteria in the urine is indicative of an infectious etiology. Scrotal sonography with Doppler flow can be extremely helpful in differentiating acute epididymitis from torsion in difficult cases.

Patients with acute epididymitis have significant inflammation that can also involve the testicle (epididymo-orchitis). Patients with severe epididymitis involving the testicle are often systemically ill. In most instances, initial treatment should consist of antibiotics, nonsteroidal anti-inflammatory medications, and possibly oral narcotics. In some cases, broad-spectrum antibiotics or even hospital admission may be necessary. In general, patients younger than 35 years of age should be treated with ceftriaxone and doxycycline or a single dose of azithromycin. Older patients are usually empirically treated with a fluoroquinolone or trimethoprim sulfamethoxazole for 2 to 4 weeks. Complications associated with acute epididymitis include abscess formation, testicular infarction, infertility, and chronic epididymitis or orchalgia.

HYDROCELE

A hydrocele is a serous fluid collection located between the parietal and visceral layers of the tunica vaginalis of the scrotum. Noncommunicating hydroceles usually surround the testicle and spermatic cord. Communicating hydroceles are actually indirect inguinal hernias; they contain only fluid and not bowel or fat because the opening into the peritoneal cavity is small. Communicating hydroceles can be distinguished from noncommunicating hydroceles on physical examination by gently pushing the fluid out of the scrotum and into the peritoneum. Communicating hydroceles are more commonly identified in the pediatric age group.

Patients with a noncommunicating hydrocele usually have complaints of heaviness in the scrotum, scrotal pain, or an enlarging scrotal mass. Usually the diagnosis is easily made based on the physical examination and transillumination of the scrotum. If the testis is not palpable, an ultrasound study should be performed to rule out a testicular tumor associated with a secondary or reactive hydrocele. Noncommunicating hydroceles are caused by increased secretion or decreased reabsorption of serous fluid by the tunica vaginalis. Infection, trauma, surgery, neoplastic disease, and lymphatic disease are causative in many adults, whereas the remainder of cases are idiopathic.

Treatment of symptomatic noncommunicating hydroceles is surgical. Although the recurrence rate is significantly higher with aspiration and sclerotherapy, this approach can be a good option in patients who are considered poor surgical candidates. Hydrocelectomy procedures involve either excision of the redundant tunica vaginalis or a plication of the sac without excision. After surgery, the rates of hydrocele recurrence and chronic pain are 9% and 1%, respectively.

● TESTICULAR TORSION

Testicular torsion is considered a true urologic emergency. The testicle receives its blood supply from the testicular artery (aorta), the vasal artery (inferior vesicle artery), and the cremasteric artery (inferior epigastric artery). All three vessels are transmitted to the testicle through the spermatic cord. Torsion of the spermatic cord impairs arterial inflow as well as venous outflow. If detorsion is not performed within 6 to 8 hours, testicular infarction and hemorrhagic necrosis are likely to occur. Typically, patients are younger than 21 years of age, although testicular torsion can occur later. Delay in presentation and diagnosis is more common in the adult patient population and is related to patient and physician factors.

The characteristic signs and symptoms of acute testicular torsion are the acute onset of scrotal pain, swelling, nausea, vomiting, loss of normal rugae of the scrotal skin, absent cremasteric reflex, and a high-riding, rotated, tender testicle. The diagnosis of testicular torsion remains a clinical one, however; if ultrasound equipment is readily available, all patients should have a scrotal ultrasound study before surgery. In rare cases, surgical exploration is undertaken when the index of suspicion is high but imaging is not available. Doppler ultrasonography is extremely useful in differentiating testicular torsion from other causes of acute scrotum, such as acute epididymitis, torsion of the appendix testis, and trauma.

It is possible to untwist testicular torsion by manipulating the testicle through the scrotum in the emergency room or in a physician's office. After giving the patient parenteral narcotics, the testicle can be untwisted by gently pulling down on it and, usually, rotating it laterally (like opening a book). If this is successful, the testicle will uncoil like a spring and fall into its normal position, with immediate relief of the patient's pain. Even if the procedure is successful, patients should still be taken to the operating room for bilateral orchiopexy. Of note, testicular torsion is the result of medial twisting of the testicle only 68% of the time.

Important surgical principles include surgical detorsion and assessment of testicular viability in the operating room. If the testis is determined to be viable, bilateral orchiopexy is performed using the technique of three-point fixation (sutures placed medially, laterally, and inferiorly). In the presence of infarction, orchiectomy is recommended. Orchiopexy of the contralateral testicle is always performed simultaneously. When diagnosis and surgery occur in a timely fashion, testicular salvage rates approach 70%. Delayed surgical therapy results in dropoff of the salvage rate to 40%.

SUGGESTED READINGS

Androgen Deficiency in Adult Men

Baillargeon J, Urban RJ, Ottenbacher KJ, et al: Trends in androgen prescribing in the United States, 2001 to 2011, JAMA Intern Med 173:1465–1466, 2013.

Bhasin S, Cunningham GR, Hayes FJ, et al: Testosterone therapy in men with androgen deficiency syndromes: an Endocrine Society clinical practice guideline, J Clin Endocrinol Metab 95:2536–2559, 2010.

Caronia LM, Dwyer AA, Hayden D, et al: Abrupt decrease in serum testosterone levels after an oral glucose load in men: implications for screening for hypogonadism, Clin Endocrinol (Oxf) 78:291–296, 2013.

Kvorning T, Andersen M, Brixen K, et al: Suppression of endogenous testosterone production attenuates the response to strength training: a randomized, placebo-controlled, and blinded intervention study, Am J Physiol Endocrinol Metab 291:E1325–E1332, 2006.

Meriggiola MC, Bremner WJ, Costantino A, et al: Low dose of cyproterone acetate and testosterone enanthate for contraception in men, Hum Reprod 13:1225–1229, 1998.

Morgentaler A: Testosterone therapy in men with prostate cancer: scientific and ethical considerations, J Urol 189(1 Suppl):S26–S33, 2013.

Nieschlag E, Swerdloff R, Behre HM, et al: Investigation, treatment, and monitoring of late-onset hypogonadism in males: ISA, ISSAM, and EAU recommendations, J Androl 27:135–137, 2006.

Rhoden EL, Morgentaler A: Risks of testosterone-replacement therapy and recommendations for monitoring, N Engl J Med 350:482–492, 2004.

Svartberg J, Midtby M, Bønaa KH, et al: The associations of age, lifestyle factors and chronic disease with testosterone in men: the Tromsø Study, Eur J Endocrinol 149:145–152, 2003.

Wu FCW, Tajar A, Beynon JM, et al: Identification of late-onset hypogonadism in middle-aged and elderly men, N Engl J Med 363:123–135, 2010.

Erectile Dysfunction

American Urological Association: AUA guideline on the management of erectile dysfunction: diagnosis and treatment recommendations, 2005 (website). http://www.auanet.org/education/guidelines/erectile-dysfunction.cfm. Accessed November 2014.

American Urological Association: Guideline on the management of priapism, 2003 (website). http://www.auanet.org/education/guidelines/priapism.cfm. Accessed November 2014.

Cappelleri JC, Rosen RC: The Sexual Health Inventory for Men (SHIM): a 5-year review of research and clinical experience, Int J Impotence Res 17:307–319, 2005.

Carson CC, Lue TF: Phosphodiesterase type 5 inhibitors for erectile dysfunction, Br J Urol Int 96:257–280, 2005.

Costa P, Potempa A-J: Intraurethral alprostadil for erectile dysfunction: a review of the literature, Drugs 72:2243–2254, 2012.

Feldman HA, Goldstein I, Hatzichristou DG, et al: Impotence and its medical and psychosocial correlates: results of the Massachusetts Male Aging Study, J Urol 151:54–61, 1994.

Kostis JB, Jackson G, Rosen R, et al: Sexual dysfunction and cardiac risk (the Second Princeton Consensus Conference), Am J Cardiol 96:313–321, 2005.

Montague DK, Jarow JP, Broderick GA, et al: for the Erectile Dysfunction Guideline Update Panel: The management of erectile dysfunction: an AUA update, J Urol 174:230–239, 2005.

Benign Prostatic Hyperplasia

Carter B, Albertsen P, Barry M, et al: Early detection of prostate cancer: AUA Guideline,, Linthicum, Md., 2013, American Urological Association.

D'Amico AV, Chen MH, Roehl KA, et al: Preoperative PSA velocity and the risk of death from prostate cancer after radical prostatectomy, N Engl J Med 351:125–135, 2004.

Eggener SE, Roehl KA, Catalona WJ: Predictors of subsequent prostate cancer in men with a prostate specific antigen of 2.6 to 4.0 ng/ml and an initially negative biopsy, J Urol 174:500–504, 2005.

Kaplan SA, Roehrborn CG, Rovner ES, et al: Tolterodine and tamsulosin for treatment of men with lower urinary tract symptoms and overactive bladder: a randomized controlled trial, JAMA 296:2319–2328, 2006.

Lowe FC, McConnell JD, Hudson PB, et al: for the Finasteride Study Group: Long-term 6-year experience with finasteride in patients with benign prostatic hyperplasia, Urology 61:791–796, 2003.

McConnell JD, Roehrborn CG, Bautista OM, et al: for the Medical Therapy of Prostatic Symptoms (MTOPS) Research Group: The long-term effect of doxazosin, finasteride, and combination therapy on the clinical progression of benign prostatic hyperplasia, N Engl J Med 349:2387–2398, 2003.

Roehrborn CG, Kaplan SA, Jones JS, et al: Tolterodine extended release with or without tamsulosin in men with lower urinary tract symptoms including overactive bladder symptoms: effects of prostate size, Eur Urol 55:472–479, 2009.

Wang C: Phosphodiesterase-5 inhibitors and benign prostatic hyperplasia, Curr Opin Urol 20:49–54, 2010.

Testis Cancer

Amato RJ, Ro JY, Ayala AG, et al: Risk-adapted treatment for patients with clinical stage I nonseminomatous germ cell tumors of the testis, Urology 63:144–148, 2004.

Atsu N, Eskicorapci S, Uner A, et al: A novel surveillance protocol for stage I nonseminomatous germ cell testicular tumors, Br J Urol Int 92:32–35, 2003.

Classen J, Schmidberger H, Meisner C, et al: Radiotherapy for stages IIA/B testicular seminoma: final report of a prospective multicenter clinical trial, J Clin Oncol 21:1101–1106, 2003.

DeCastro BJ, Peterson AC, Costabile RA: A 5-year follow-up study of asymptomatic men with testicular microlithiasis, J Urol 179:1420–1423, discussion 1423, 2008.

Einhorn LH, Donohue J: Cis-diamminedichloroplatinum, vinblastine, and bleomycin combination chemotherapy in disseminated testicular cancer, Ann Intern Med 87:293–298, 1977.

MacVicar GR, Pienta KJ: Testicular cancer, Curr Opin Oncol 16:253–256, 2004.

Schmoll HJ, Kollmannsberger C, Metzner B, et al: Long-term results of first-line sequential high-dose etoposide, ifosfamide, and cisplatin chemotherapy plus autologous stem cell support for patients with advanced metastatic germ cell cancer: an extended phase I/II study of the German Testicular Cancer Study Group, J Clin Oncol 21:4083–4091, 2003.

Stephenson AJ, Sheinfeld J: The role of retroperitoneal lymph node dissection in the management of testicular cancer, Urol Oncol 22:225–235, 2004.

Male Infertility

Balercia G, Regoli F, Armeni T, et al: Double-blind randomized trial on the use of L-carnitine, L-acetylcarnitine, or combined L-carnitine and L-acetylcarnitine in men with idiopathic asthenozoospermia, Fertil Steril 84:662–671, 2005.

Joesoef MR, Beral V, Aral SO, et al: Fertility and use of cigarettes, alcohol, marijuana, and cocaine, Ann Epidemiol 3:592–594, 1993.

Roth LW, Ryan AR, Meacham RB: Clomiphene citrate in the management of male infertility, Semin Reprod Med 31:245–250, 2013.

Sabanegh EJ, Agarwal A: Male infertility. In Wein AJ, Kavoussi LR, Partin AW, et al, editors: Campbell-Walsh Urology, Philadelphia, Pa., 2012, Elsevier, pp 616–647.

Schiff JD, Palermo GD, Veeck LL: Success of testicular sperm injection (corrected) and intracytoplasmic sperm injection in men with Klinefelter syndrome, J Clin Endocrinol Metab 90:6263–6267, 2005.

Benign Scrotal Diseases

Alleman WG, Gorman B, King BF, et al: Benign and malignant epididymal masses evaluated with scrotal sonography: clinical and pathologic review of 85 patients, J Ultrasound Med 27:1195–1202, 2008.

Ficarra V, Crestani A, Novara G, et al: Varicocele repair for infertility: what is the evidence? Curr Opin Urol 22:489–494, 2012.

Karmazyn B, Steinberg R, Kurareid L, et al: Clinical and radiographic criteria of the acute scrotum in children: a retrospective study in 172 boys, Pediatr Radiol 35:302–310, 2005.

Neiderberger C: Microsurgical treatment of persistent or recurrent varicocele, J Urol 173:2079–2080, 2005.

Sessions AE, Rabinowitz R, Hulbert WC, et al: Testicular torsion: direction, degree, duration and disinformation, J Urol 169:663–665, 2003.

Shridharani A, Lockwood G, Sandlow J: Varicocelectomy in the treatment of testicular pain: a review, Curr Opin Urol 22:499–506, 2012.

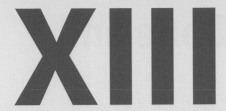

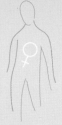

XIII

Diseases of Bone and Bone Mineral Metabolism

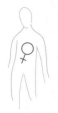

72

Normal Physiology of Bone and Mineral Homeostasis

Andrew F. Stewart

CALCIUM HOMEOSTASIS

The maintenance of normal calcium homeostasis is critical to survival for at least three reasons. First, the serum calcium concentration regulates the degree of membrane excitability in muscle and nervous tissue. Increases in serum calcium levels produce refractoriness to stimulation of neurons and muscle cells, which translates clinically into coma and muscular weakness. Conversely, reductions in serum calcium levels lead to increases in neuromuscular excitability that translate clinically into convulsions and spontaneous muscle cramps and contractions referred to as *carpopedal spasm* or *tetany*. Second, terrestrial life requires the existence of a skeleton, and calcium is the major structural cation in the skeleton. The mineral phase of the skeleton is composed of a calcium salt called *hydroxyapatite*, and reductions in bone mineral content lead to spontaneous fractures. Third, intracellular calcium has a major intracellular signaling role, and control of intracellular calcium is essential to the survival of all cells. This mechanism is used to advantage pharmacologically through the widespread clinical use of drugs that regulate intracellular calcium concentrations and calcium-channel activity for the treatment of a wide variety of human diseases. Physicians, regardless of their specialty, encounter disorders of calcium homeostasis on a regular basis.

The serum total calcium concentration is normally maintained at about 9.5 mg/dL. Of this total amount, about 4.5 mg/dL is bound to serum proteins, principally albumin, and about 0.5 mg/dL circulates as insoluble complexes such as calcium sulfate, phosphate, and citrate. The remaining 4.5 mg/dL circulates as free or unbound or ionized calcium. This free, ionized serum calcium is important clinically and physiologically. This calcium is available to be filtered at the glomerulus, to interact with cell membranes to regulate their electrical potential or excitability, and to enter and exit the skeletal hydroxyapatite crystal lattice.

It is important to maintain normal levels of ionized serum calcium, although total serum calcium is customarily measured in most clinical laboratories. In some instances, total serum calcium can change without a change in the ionized calcium level. For example, if the serum albumin level declines as a result of hepatic cirrhosis or the nephrotic syndrome, the total serum calcium also declines, but the ionized serum calcium concentration remains normal. Measuring the ionized serum calcium level directly is sometimes important.

A complex group of regulatory processes have evolved to protect the integrity of this system. When a physician encounters

patients in whom hypercalcemia, hypocalcemia, or disorders of skeletal mineralization have occurred, multiple safety control points have been breached (discussed later).

To maintain homeostatic control, the calcium ion interfaces with three important compartments, as shown in the calcium physiologic black box in Figure 72-1. Although intracellular calcium is important in intracellular signaling, it is quantitatively unimportant in overall systemic calcium homeostasis. The three critical regulatory fluxes that maintain normal serum calcium concentration are those of the intestine, kidney, and skeleton.

Calcium Fluxes into and out of Extracellular Fluid

Intestinal Calcium Absorption

The normal dietary calcium intake for an adult is about 1000 mg per day. About 300 mg of the total is absorbed (i.e., unidirectional absorption is about 30%), and this absorption occurs in the duodenum and proximal jejunum. About 150 mg of calcium per day is secreted by the liver (in bile), the pancreas (in pancreatic secretions), and the intestinal glands such that net absorption (called *fractional absorption*) of calcium is about 15% of intake.

The efficiency of calcium absorption is regulated at the level of the small intestinal epithelial cell, the enterocyte, by the active form of vitamin D, 1,25-dihydroxyvitamin D (1,25[OH]$_2$D),

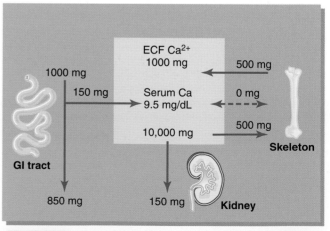

FIGURE 72-1 The calcium physiologic black box. The central box represents extracellular fluid (ECF), which contains a total of about 1000 mg of calcium. It has three regulatory interfaces with the gastrointestinal (GI) tract, skeleton, and kidney. The fluxes into and out of the ECF are measured in milligrams per day.

also called *calcitriol*. Increases in 1,25(OH)$_2$D enhance calcium absorption, and decreases in 1,25(OH)$_2$D reduce absorption of dietary calcium. Dietary calcium absorption can be increased over the short term by increasing calcium intake or increasing plasma 1,25(OH)$_2$D concentrations, or both. Pathologic increases in serum calcium (i.e., hypercalcemia) can be caused by increases in circulating 1,25(OH)$_2$D (e.g., in sarcoidosis) or by excessive calcium intake (i.e., milk-alkali syndrome). Conversely, hypocalcemia can result from a decline in 1,25(OH)$_2$D (e.g., chronic renal failure, hypoparathyroidism). If a normal individual consumes 1000 mg of calcium per day and the net absorption from the gastrointestinal (GI) tract is 150 mg per day, 850 mg of calcium will be excreted in the feces each day.

Renal Calcium Handling

The filtered load of calcium by the kidneys is about 10,000 mg per day. In terms of overall regulation of calcium homeostasis, this number is very large, making the point that the kidney is the most important moment-to-moment regulator of the serum calcium concentration. The amount also emphasizes that disorders of renal calcium handling (e.g., thiazide diuretic use, hypoparathyroidism) can be expected to produce significant abnormalities in serum calcium homeostasis.

Of the 10,000 mg filtered at the glomerulus each day, about 9000 mg (90%) is reabsorbed *proximally* by the proximal convoluted tubule, the pars recta, and the thick ascending limb of Henle loop. This 90% is absorbed in conjunction with sodium and chloride reabsorption and is not subject to regulation by parathyroid hormone (PTH). The remaining 10% (1000 mg) that arrives at the distal tubule on a daily basis is subject to regulation by PTH, which stimulates renal calcium reabsorption. The anticalciuric effect of PTH can be extremely efficient, and elevated PTH concentrations can essentially eliminate calcium excretion into the urine. This action is a potent mechanism for retaining calcium under conditions of calcium deprivation (e.g., a low-calcium diet, vitamin D deficiency, intestinal malabsorption) and can contribute to hypercalcemia under pathologic conditions, as in primary hyperparathyroidism.

About 150 mg of calcium is excreted by the kidney in the final urine on a daily basis in a healthy individual. If the kidney filters 10,000 mg of calcium each day, and if 150 mg is excreted in the final urine, 9850 mg (98.5%) is reabsorbed at proximal and distal sites. A healthy person is in zero calcium balance with respect to the outside world: intake (1000 mg/day) − output [(850 mg/day in feces) + (150 mg/day in urine)] = 0.

Skeletal Biology and Calcium Homeostasis

The skeletal compartment contains about 1.2 kg of calcium in a male adult and 1.0 kg in a female adult. Most of this calcium is in the form of crystal hydroxyapatite, a calcium phosphate salt. Although calcium contributes in an important way to the structural integrity of the skeleton, the skeleton also serves as a quantitatively large reservoir (i.e., a sink) for adding and removing calcium to and from the extracellular fluid (ECF) compartment at appropriate times.

The adult skeleton is composed of two types of bone: cortical (or lamellar) bone and trabecular (or cancellous) bone (Fig. 72-2). Cortical bone predominates in the skull and the shafts of

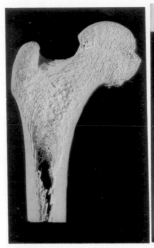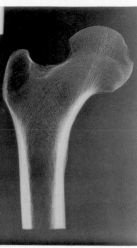

FIGURE 72-2 The structure of human bone. A human proximal femur examined using a gross pathologic specimen *(left panel)* and a radiograph of the same section *(right panel)*. Notice that two types of bone are represented. One type is cortical bone (i.e., lamellar bone), and the other is cancellous bone (i.e., trabecular bone). The proportion of trabecular and cortical bone differs by location. For example, the shaft of the femur contains mostly cortical bone, whereas the proximal end of the femoral neck and the greater trochanter contain little cortical bone and almost exclusively contain trabecular bone. This distinction is important, because most osteoporotic fractures occur at sites in which trabecular bone predominates, including the greater trochanter, the femoral neck, the vertebrae, and the distal radius. (Courtesy Webster S. S. Jee, MD, University of Utah, Salt Lake City, Utah.)

long bones, and trabecular bone predominates at other sites, such as the distal radius, the vertebral bodies, and the trochanters of the hip.

Bone is not an inert tissue, as might be imagined from visiting the dinosaur room at a natural history museum; instead, bone is a vital tissue that is continually turning over. The adult skeleton is completely remodeled every 3 to 10 years. Remodeling is perhaps best appreciated by recalling that orthopedic surgeons routinely and intentionally set fractures imperfectly, knowing that the normal processes of bone remodeling will restore the bone's original shape with the passage of time.

The cells that regulate bone turnover can be divided into those that remove old bone, those that provide new bone (Fig. 72-3) (see Chapter 74), and those that regulate these two processes. Cells that remove, or *resorb*, old bone are *osteoclasts*. These cells are large, metabolically active, multinucleated cells derived from the fusion of circulating macrophages. They deposit themselves on the surface of bone and form a *sealing zone* over the bone surface into which they secrete protons (i.e., acid), proteases (e.g., collagenase), and proteoglycan-digesting enzymes (e.g., hyaluronidase). The acid solubilizes hydroxyapatite crystals, releasing calcium, and the enzymes digest bone proteins and proteoglycans (e.g., collagen, osteocalcin, osteopontin), which constitute the nonmineral, or *osteoid*, component of bone. Osteoclasts move along the surface of trabecular bone plates and drill tunnels in cortical bone, periodically releasing the digested contents within their sealed zones into the bone marrow space and thereby creating resorption lacunae, called *Howship's lacunae*, on the trabecular bone surface. The released calcium contributes to the ECF calcium pool, and the released proteolytic products, such as

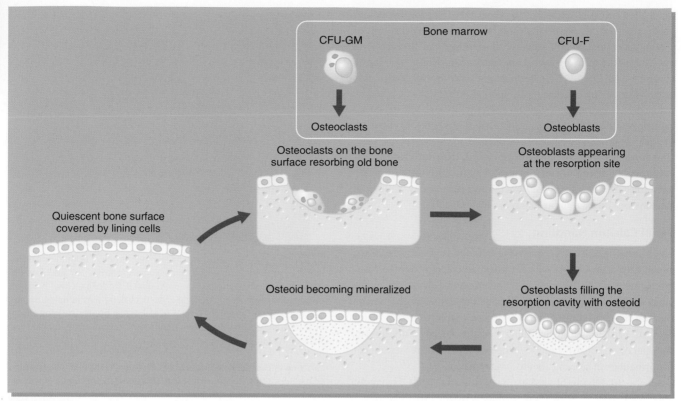

FIGURE 72-3 Cellular components of bone remodeling. Bone remodeling is a continuous process that involves the activation of osteoclast precursors in the macrophage lineage (i.e., colony-forming units of granulocyte-macrophage progenitors [CFU-GM]) that become actively resorbing osteoclasts, which tunnel into the bone surface to dig resorption lacunae. Osteoblast precursors in the fibroblast–bone marrow stromal cell lineage (CFU-F) then appear and become active at the sites of prior resorption, and they secrete new osteoid, which later mineralizes to fill the lacunae created by osteoclastic bone resorption. (From Manolagas SC, Jilka RL: Bone marrow, cytokines, and bone remodeling: emerging insights into the pathophysiology of osteoporosis, N Engl J Med 332:305–311, 1995.)

deoxypyridinoline cross-links (i.e., collagen fragments and hydroxyproline), can be used clinically as indices of bone resorption.

New bone formation is accomplished by *osteoblasts,* which are derived from marrow stromal cells or bone surface lining cells. Osteoblasts synthesize and secrete the components of the nonmineral phase of bone, called *osteoid.* The components are mostly proteins and include collagen, osteopontin, osteonectin, osteocalcin, proteoglycans, and a plethora of growth factors, including transforming growth factor-β and insulin-like growth factor-I. This complex provides the scaffolding on which the mineral crystal hydroxyapatite forms lattices.

In the past decade, attention has focused on a third, previously underappreciated bone cell type, the *osteocyte.* These cells are descendants of osteoblasts and are embedded into the mineralized phase of bone. Osteocytes physically connect with one another and to cells at the mineral surface through long dendritic processes. The dendritic processes extensively permeate the mineralized phase of bone through an elaborate canalicular network. Osteocytes serve a critical role in sensing biomechanical strain within bone, and through their cellular extensions to the cell surface, they communicate signals that attract, activate, or repress osteoclasts and osteoblasts. In this way, they determine which areas of the skeleton require new bone formation and which need to be targets of osteoclastic bone remodeling.

Through the process of bone turnover, or bone remodeling, osteoclasts continually remove old bone, and osteoblasts continually produce new osteoid that mineralizes, eventually replacing the old bone removed by osteoclasts with new bone. This process replaces old bone—and by implication, defective or damaged bone with microfractures and reduced mechanical strength—with new, mechanically strong bone, although the evidence for this action is limited. The principal therapy for osteoporosis is with the use of antiresorptives such as estrogens, estrogen-like drugs, and bisphosphonates, which dramatically reduce bone turnover while improving bone mass and bone mechanical properties.

Bone remodeling is important for systemic calcium homeostasis. Osteoclasts can be used to access calcium from the skeleton in times of need to maintain a normal serum calcium concentration. Conversely, unmineralized osteoid produced by osteoblasts can be used at appropriate times as a sink into which excess serum calcium can be deposited. Under normal circumstances, osteoclasts resorb bone at a rate such that about 500 mg of calcium is removed per day from the skeleton and delivered to the ECF compartment. At the same time, osteoblasts produce osteoid that mineralizes at a rate such that about 500 mg of calcium leaves the ECF and enters the skeleton at new sites. From the perspective of the black box shown in Figure 72-1, the skeleton is in zero calcium balance with the ECF, and the whole organism is in zero calcium balance with the external environment.

Considering the complexity of this calcium homeostatic system and the importance of maintaining tight control of serum calcium levels, an obvious need exists for systemic regulation and integration of the calcium fluxes across the GI, skeletal, and renal compartments. The two key metabolic regulatory hormones that coordinate these activities are PTH and the active form of vitamin D, 1,25(OH)₂D.

Regulatory Hormones

Parathyroid Hormone

PTH is a peptide hormone produced by the four parathyroid glands (Fig. 72-4). These glands are located behind the normal thyroid lobes, with two on the right and two on the left. Through the calcium sensor—a G protein–coupled receptor for calcium that is located on the surface of the parathyroid cell—the serum ionized calcium concentration is continuously monitored. In this exquisitely sensitive system, minor (e.g., 0.1 mg/dL) reductions in serum ionized calcium lead to PTH secretion, and minor increments in serum calcium lead to suppression of PTH secretion.

PTH is secreted as an 84-amino-acid peptide hormone that is rapidly (half-life of about 3 to 5 minutes) cleaved by the Kupffer cells in the liver into an active amino-terminal form; the carboxyl-terminal form is inactive. Continuous monitoring of the serum calcium concentration by the parathyroid glands, the immediate secretion of PTH in response to hypocalcemia, and the rapid clearance of PTH after secretion enable the parathyroid gland and PTH to regulate serum calcium with remarkable precision.

PTH targets three organs, two directly and one indirectly. The first directly targeted organ is the kidney, in which renal calcium excretion is inhibited by PTH. PTH also inhibits phosphate and bicarbonate reabsorption, which produces phosphaturia and hypophosphatemia and proximal renal tubular acidosis, respectively. The renal actions of PTH occur immediately. PTH also stimulates the production of the active form of vitamin D, 1,25(OH)₂D.

PTH also directly targets the skeleton. PTH can mobilize calcium immediately from the skeleton through activation of osteoclastic bone resorption. Over days to weeks, PTH stimulates the activity of osteoblasts to produce new bone and thereby remove calcium from the circulation. The ability to stimulate osteoclasts acutely without activating bone formation is important for the rapid delivery of calcium to the ECF.

PTH has the indirect effect of increasing intestinal calcium absorption by increasing renal synthesis of 1,25(OH)₂D. Seen in concert, PTH is secreted in response to hypocalcemia, and the actions of PTH combine to restore a low serum calcium concentration to normal by preventing renal calcium losses, by adding calcium to the ECF from the skeleton, and by indirectly stimulating (through 1,25(OH)₂D) increases in intestinal calcium absorption.

Vitamin D Metabolism

Vitamin D is two compounds: ergocalciferol (vitamin D₂) and cholecalciferol (vitamin D₃) (Fig. 72-5). Both substances are inactive precursors. One (D₃) is derived principally from skin exposed to sunlight, and the other (D₂) is derived from plant sterols. Both D₂ and D₃ are found in multivitamins and commercial dietary supplements.

Both precursors are converted constitutively by the enzyme vitamin D 25-hydroxylase (CYP2R1) in the liver to their respective 25-hydroxyvitamin D (25[OH]D) derivatives. The derivatives also are inactive precursors, but they have two types of clinical significance. First, severe liver disease such as cirrhosis prevents this essential step and leads to vitamin D–deficient syndromes collectively called *hepatic osteodystrophy*. Second, 25(OH)D is the standard clinical laboratory measure of the vitamin D status (i.e., repletion or deficiency) of patients with hypocalcemia, osteomalacia or rickets, osteoporosis and intestinal malabsorption, and other similar conditions.

25(OH)D is converted, or activated, in the renal proximal tubule by the enzyme 25-hydroxyvitamin D₃ 1α-hydroxylase (CYP27B1) to the active form of the vitamin, 1,25(OH)₂D. This substance, which is also called *calcitriol*, is regulated by PTH. Increases in PTH stimulate 1,25(OH)₂D production, and decreases in PTH diminish 1,25(OH)₂D synthesis. The primary

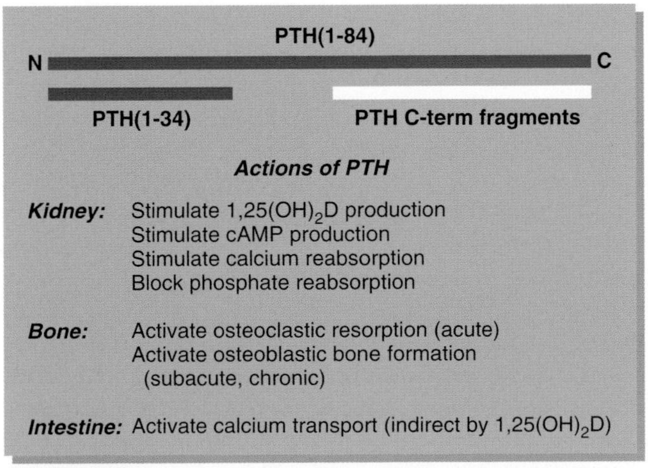

PTH(1-84)

N ————————————————————————— C

PTH(1-34)   **PTH C-term fragments**

Actions of PTH

Kidney: Stimulate 1,25(OH)₂D production
Stimulate cAMP production
Stimulate calcium reabsorption
Block phosphate reabsorption

Bone: Activate osteoclastic resorption (acute)
Activate osteoblastic bone formation
(subacute, chronic)

Intestine: Activate calcium transport (indirect by 1,25(OH)₂D)

FIGURE 72-4 Structure and actions of parathyroid hormone (PTH). PTH is secreted as an 84-amino-acid protein, which is cleaved in the liver to derivative amino-terminal and carboxyl-terminal (C-term) forms. Actions of the amino-terminally intact forms of PTH are listed. cAMP, Cyclic adenosine monophosphate; 1,25(OH)₂D, 1,25-dihydroxycholecalciferol.

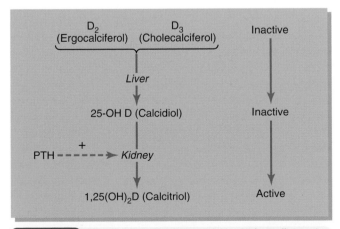

FIGURE 72-5 The vitamin D metabolic pathway. Biologically inactive vitamin D exists in two forms, D₂ and D₃, which are hydroxylated in the liver and kidney to yield the biologically active form of vitamin D: 1,25-dihydroxycholecalciferol (1,25[OH]₂D), also called *calcitriol*. PTH, Parathyroid hormone.

action of 1,25(OH)$_2$D is to regulate intestinal calcium absorption. PTH, through 1,25(OH)$_2$D, indirectly regulates calcium absorption from the diet by the intestine. The hypocalcemia of hypoparathyroidism is a result, in part, of inadequate intestinal calcium absorption. Conversely, hyperparathyroidism is associated with hypercalciuria and nephrolithiasis, both of which directly result from increases in circulating 1,25(OH)$_2$D levels. Measurement of 1,25(OH)$_2$D can be used as an index of parathyroid function and intestinal calcium absorption.

Calcitonin

Calcitonin is produced by the parafollicular or C cells of the thyroid gland in response to hypercalcemia. It was once viewed as an essential calcium-regulating hormone. Pharmacologic doses of calcitonin may reduce serum calcium levels, but little evidence exists that calcitonin has homeostatic relevance in humans.

Integration of Calcium Homeostasis

Ingestion of a greater than normal dietary calcium load (Fig. 72-6A) leads to a mild rise in the serum calcium level, followed by immediate suppression of PTH. This action immediately permits marked increases in renal calcium excretion by the distal tubule. It also immediately deceases osteoclastic activity, which prevents continued bone resorption but allows continued calcium entry from the ECF into an unmineralized osteoid sink. These two effects produce a rapid, short-term reduction in serum calcium to normal levels. However, if the high-calcium diet is maintained over the long term, these adaptations are insufficient. Continued renal calcium wasting leads to hypercalciuria (with nephrolithiasis and nephrocalcinosis), and unopposed osteoblastic bone formation leads to excessive skeletal mineralization (i.e., osteopetrosis).

Two additional responses (see Fig. 72-6B) are required to prevent the long-term adverse effects of a high-calcium diet. First, subacute or chronic suppression of PTH reduces circulating 1,25(OH)$_2$D. This reduces the efficiency of calcium absorption from the intestine, calcium entry into the ECF, and urinary calcium excretion. Second, a chronic decrement in PTH leads to a chronic decline in osteoblastic activity. No osteoid is formed, and the ability to deposit calcium into the skeletal sink is lost.

Conversely, during brief periods of dietary calcium deficiency (Fig. 72-7A), as occurs between meals, the serum calcium level declines almost imperceptibly and the PTH rises, which immediately prevents renal calcium losses from continuing. At the same time, an acute activation of osteoclasts occurs, delivering calcium into the ECF. The acute response to low calcium intake is the appropriate elimination of renal calcium losses and development of a new source of calcium entry into the ECF.

Over the longer term, the initial response is inadequate and leads to skeletal demineralization. A longer-term solution is required, and the adaptation is twofold (see Fig. 72-7B). First, a chronic low calcium intake, as may occur in a person with lactose intolerance, leads to a chronic elevation in PTH, and over a matter of days to weeks, this leads to an increase in the 1,25(OH)$_2$D level, which increases the efficiency of calcium absorption from the intestine (i.e., increase in the fractional absorption of calcium) to compensate for the reduction in dietary intake. Second, chronically elevated PTH leads to an increase in osteoblast activity and osteoid synthesis, with resultant increases in skeletal calcium deposition. In this steady-state adaptation to a low-calcium diet, PTH levels are elevated, and coupled increases in osteoclastic and osteoblastic activities take place (i.e., increased bone turnover), but net skeletal calcium losses are negligible or normal.

From an evolutionary standpoint, as life moved from a calcium-rich marine environment to a terrestrial setting in which calcium availability was unpredictable, a complex, elegant regulatory mechanism evolved that permitted survival without requiring intentional behavioral adaptations to the vagaries of calcium supply. As discussed in Chapter 73, disorders that cause hypercalcemia or hypocalcemia are always caused by abnormalities at the interfaces of the ECF with the intestine, kidney, and skeleton. The physician need only recall these homeostatic premises to dissect the pathophysiologic process with precision and treat the underlying disorder effectively.

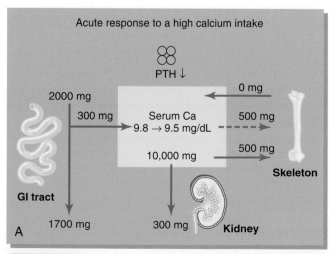

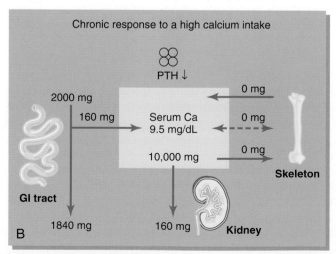

FIGURE 72-6 Responses to increases in calcium intake. **A,** The acute response. **B,** The chronic response. Details are provided in the text. GI, Gastrointestinal.

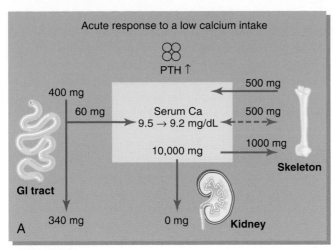
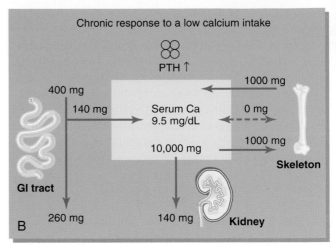

FIGURE 72-7 Responses to decreases in calcium intake. **A,** The acute response. **B,** The chronic response. Details are provided in the text. GI, Gastrointestinal; PTH, parathyroid hormone.

TABLE 72-1 THERAPEUTIC PHOSPHORUS PREPARATIONS

PREPARATION	COMPOSITION* (per mL)	pH	mOsm/ kg H₂O	PHOSPHATE (mmol/mL)	PHOSPHORUS (mg/mL)	SODIUM (mEq/mL)	POTASSIUM (mEq/mL)
ORAL							
Cow's milk (whole)	—	—	288	0.029	0.9	0.025	0.035
Neutra-Phos[†]	Na₂HPO₄, NaH₂PO₄, K₂HPO₄, KH₂PO₄	7.3	—	0.107	3.33	0.095	0.095
Phospho-Soda[†]	180 mg Na₂HPO₄ · 7H₂O + 480 mg NaH₂PO₄ · H₂O	4.8	8240	4.150	128.65	4.822	0
Acid sodium phosphate	136 mg Na₂HPO₄ · 7H₂O + 58.8 mg H₃PO₄ (NF 85%)	4.9	1740	1.018	35.54	1.015	0
Neutral sodium phosphate	145 mg Na₂HPO₄ · 7H₂O + 18.2 mg NaH₂PO₄ · H₂O	7.0	1390	0.673	20.86	1.214	0
PARENTERAL							
Neutral sodium phosphate	10.07 mg Na₂HPO₄ + 2.66 mg NaH₂PO₄ · H₂O	7.35	202	0.090	2.80	0.161	0
Neutral sodium, potassium phosphate	11.5 mg Na₂HPO₄ + 2.58 mg KH₂PO₄	7.4	223	0.100	3.10	0.162	0.019
Sodium phosphate[†]	142 mg Na₂HPO₄ + 276 mg NaH₂PO₄ · H₂O	5.7	5580	3.000	93.00	4.000	0
Potassium phosphate[†]	236 mg K₂HPO₄ + 224 mg KH₂PO₄	6.6	5840	3.003	93.11	0	4.360

From Lentz RD, Brown DM, Kjellstrand CM: Treatment of severe hypophosphatemia, Ann Intern Med 89:941-944, 1978.

H₂O, Water; K₂HPO₄, dipotassium hydrogen phosphate; KH₂PO₄, potassium dihydrogen phosphate; Na₂HPO₄, disodium hydrogen phosphate; NaH₂PO₄, sodium dihydrogen phosphate.

*Hydration states are important. For example, 268 mg Na₂HPO₄ · 7H₂O (molecular weight 268) equals 1.00 mmol, whereas 268 mg Na₂HPO₄ (molecular weight 142) equals 1.89 mmol.

†Commercial preparations: Neutra-Phos, Willen Drug Company, Baltimore, Md. (Neutra-Phos K has twice as much potassium and no sodium); Phospho-Soda, C.B. Fleet Company, Lynchburg, Va. (enema is one-third the strength of Phospho-Soda and can be used orally); sodium phosphate, Abbott Laboratories, North Chicago, Ill.; potassium phosphate, Invenex Pharmaceuticals, Grand Island, N.Y., or Abbott Laboratories. Because Neutra-Phos was not readily dissolved and its specific composition is unknown, data shown are those provided by the manufacturer.

⬤ PHOSPHATE HOMEOSTASIS

Phosphorus is an inorganic element, abbreviated as *P* in physical chemistry literature and as *Pi* in physiologic use. The biologically relevant molecule is the negatively charged, trivalent phosphate ion (PO_4). Phosphorus is the form that most clinical laboratories measure rather than the more biologically relevant phosphate ion.

Phosphate is an important physiologic buffer, and at neutral pH in blood, phosphate is apportioned between HPO_4 (divalent) and H_2PO_4 (monovalent). Physicians need to be aware that phosphorus measurements in blood are reported in milligrams per deciliter (mg/dL), whereas pharmaceutical preparations list phosphorus in millimoles (mmol). A chart converting milligrams to millimoles for some common phosphate-containing preparations is

provided in Table 72-1. These values and total doses should be reviewed for the specific phosphorus preparation being prescribed in consultation with the pharmacist and hospital formulary if necessary.

Phosphate regulates or participates in the regulation of an enormous number of biologic processes fundamental to life. They include being an integral component of the DNA double helix, shuttling oxygen from hemoglobin to cells and vice versa using 2,3-diphosphoglycerate (2,3-DPG), intracellular signaling through kinases that attach phosphate groups to other molecules, facilitating critical intracellular messenger systems such as cyclic monophosphate (cAMP) and inositol phosphates, maintaining basic intracellular redox status through the nicotinamide adenine dinucleotide phosphate (NADP-NADPH) system, and serving as the gateway to the glucose metabolic pathway through glucose 6-phosphate.

Phosphorus is primarily an intracellular ion. In addition to its critical intracellular roles, phosphate has a key extracellular role. The anion pairs with calcium in the hydroxyapatite crystal lattice that provides structural integrity to the skeleton (discussed earlier). As with calcium, phosphate is critical to skeletal strength, and disorders of phosphorus homeostasis, such as hypophosphatemic rickets, lead to pathologic skeletal fractures. The skeleton also serves as a major storage site for phosphate that is accessed in times of severe phosphate deficiency.

The broad intracellular roles for phosphate have two corollaries. First, clinically significant intracellular phosphate deficiency may exist without marked hypophosphatemia. Second, life-threatening phosphate deficiency is often unrecognized because its manifestations (i.e., reduced levels of consciousness, hypotension, respirator dependence, and muscular weakness) are non-specific but common in intensive care unit settings. Astute clinicians learn to recognize general debility as a potential sign of phosphorus deficiency. Phosphate repletion in this setting may produce dramatic results.

In contrast to regulation of the serum calcium concentration, which is very tight, the regulation of serum phosphate concentrations is relatively lax. The serum phosphorus level is maintained in a broad range between about 3.0 and 4.5 mg/dL. In contrast to extracellular calcium concentrations, extracellular phosphate concentrations are not critically important. Because phosphate is abundant in most diets, a tight systemic regulatory mechanism for serum phosphate is unnecessary.

A physiologic black box can be developed for phosphate metabolism (Fig. 72-8). The box represents the ECF, and as with calcium, it has interfaces with the GI tract, kidney, and skeleton. Because most phosphate is contained within cells, the phosphate black box has a quantitatively significant interface with the intracellular compartment.

Intestinal Phosphate Absorption

A normal diet contains about 1200 to 1600 mg of phosphorus, and about two thirds of this amount, or 800 to 1200 mg, is absorbed each day. This fixed fractional absorption of about 67% occurs in the duodenum and jejunum. In the normal world of phosphate abundance, this intake is more than ample. Under conditions of dietary phosphorus deficiency, as occurs in chronic alcoholism, intensive care units, intestinal malabsorption, or phosphate-binding antacid use, failure of adequate phosphorus absorption presents a physiologic challenge for which no physiologic remedy exists.

Skeletal Phosphate Fluxes

As with calcium, osteoclastic bone resorption and osteoblastic new bone formation (see Figs. 72-1 and 72-3) lead to skeletal phosphate exit or entry, respectively. Although the skeleton can be used as a source of phosphorus, phosphorus can be viewed as a passive passenger with calcium in the calcium regulatory process. Under pathophysiologic conditions, skeletal calcium fluxes may become important. For example, skeletal destruction in multiple myeloma or severe immobilization syndromes leads to hypercalcemia and hyperphosphatemia, which with the concomitant hypercalcemia leads to nephrocalcinosis and renal failure. Conversely, osteoblastic metastases in prostate and breast cancers and the hungry bone syndrome after parathyroidectomy lead to clinically significant hypophosphatemia.

Intracellular-Extracellular Phosphate Fluxes

Phosphate shuttles from extracellular to intracellular compartments. This issue becomes important in certain clinical settings. For example, in the setting of metabolic acidosis, phosphate leaves the intracellular compartment and may lead to hyperphosphatemia, whereas under conditions of alkalosis, serum phosphate concentrations decline, and hypophosphatemia develops as phosphate enters the intracellular compartment.

The intracellular phosphate level has important clinical implications, in part, in the settings of crush injury (i.e., rhabdomyolysis) and tumor lysis syndrome. In both conditions, large intracellular loads of phosphate are delivered into the ECF and result in hypocalcemia, seizures, nephrocalcinosis, and renal failure. Conversely, glucose shifts phosphate into cells as glucose 6-phosphate, and overzealous intravenous or oral caloric restitution in the undernourished patient can result in severe hypophosphatemia and sudden death.

Renal Phosphate Handling

The most important mechanism for maintaining a normal serum phosphorus concentration is renal phosphorus regulation. As with calcium, phosphate is filtered by the glomerulus, and 90% is reabsorbed (i.e., tubular reabsorption of filtered phosphate [TRP]). The remaining 10% is excreted (i.e., fractional excretion of phosphorus [FE_{Pi}]). The FE_{Pi} can be calculated in a spot urine sample as follows:

$$FE_{Pi} = (\text{urine Pi}\,[mg/dL]/\text{urine creatinine}\,[mg/dL])$$
$$(\text{serum creatinine}\,[mg/dL]/\text{serum phosphorus}\,[mg/dL])$$

The TRP is simple to calculate:

$$TRP = 1 - FE_{Pi}$$

The renal handling of phosphorus is best considered as a tubular maximum (Tm)–regulated process. The TmP is normally

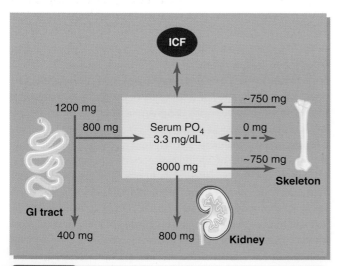

FIGURE 72-8   The phosphate physiologic black box. See Figure 72-1 for nomenclature and the text for details. GI, Gastrointestinal; ICF, intracellular fluid.

identical to a normal serum phosphorus concentration in blood, about 3.3 mg/dL. If the serum phosphate concentration rises above this level, phosphaturia occurs, and the serum phosphorus declines to 3.3 mg/dL. If the serum phosphate concentration declines below 3.3 mg/dL, filtered phosphate is entirely reabsorbed, and urinary phosphate excretion declines to zero.

The TmP can be considered as a dam in the phosphate reservoir, over which excess phosphate spills and whose level controls the concentration of serum phosphorus. The TmP is not fixed but can be moved upward or downward, depending on metabolic needs and prevailing metabolic conditions (described later).

The TRP or FE_{Pi} can be readily calculated, and the TmP can be derived from the nomogram of Bijvoet, which is shown in Figure 72-9. This process proves enormously useful in clinical practice because it is the central starting point for determining whether hypophosphatemia is principally renal or nonrenal in origin.

Parathyroid Hormone and Phosphatonins

PTH has long been appreciated to be phosphaturic; it lowers the TmP or, more accurately, inhibits proximal renal tubular phosphate reabsorption. This characteristic explains the hypophosphatemia associated with primary and secondary hyperparathyroidism and the hyperphosphatemia associated with hypoparathyroid states. Excessive PTH lowers the TmP, whereas low PTH values allow the TmP to rise to supranormal levels.

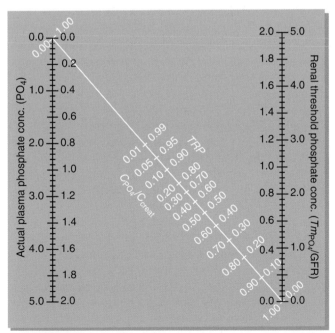

FIGURE 72-9 Nomogram shows the tubular maximum for the phosphorus glomerular filtration rate (TmP-GFR). It allows conversion of the fractional excretion of phosphorus (or its inverse, the tubular reabsorption of filtered phosphate [TRP]) into the TmP-GFR. The TRP is calculated, and a line is drawn extending from the serum phosphorus level *(left vertical line)*, through the TRP *(middle diagonal line)*, to the *right vertical line*, which represents the TmP/GFR. TmP values are provided in millimolar and milligram per deciliter units. TmP values below 1.0 mmol or 2.5 mg/dL are abnormal and indicate phosphaturia. C_{creat}, Creatinine concentration; C_{PO4}, phosphate concentration. (From Walton RJ, Bijvoet OL: Nomogram for derivation of renal threshold phosphate concentration, Lancet 2:309–310, 1975.)

The TmP level is regulated by other factors.. For example, experimental dietary phosphorus deprivation in laboratory animals and humans leads to a PTH-independent increase in the TmP, and high-phosphate feeding results in a PTH-independent decline in the TmP. For decades, investigators in this area have postulated the existence of a phosphaturic hormones called *phosphatonins*, one of which is fibroblast growth factor-23 (FGF-23). This field has progressed rapidly over the past decade, but much remains to be worked out. The main physiologic points are that a hormonal system independent of PTH also regulates renal phosphorus handling and that the kidney is the prime regulatory organ for phosphate homeostasis.

REGULATION OF SERUM MAGNESIUM

Magnesium is a divalent cation. Magnesium homeostasis parallels phosphorus homeostasis. Magnesium and phosphate are principally intracellular, with concentrations inside the cell that far exceed those outside the cell. Both substances govern key intracellular regulatory processes. In the case of magnesium, these processes include fundamental events such as DNA replication and transcription, translation of RNA, the use of adenosine triphosphate as an energy source, and regulated peptide hormone secretion.

Both substances are abundant inside all kinds of cells. Because they are well supplied in vegetarian and carnivorous diets, little evolutionary pressure exists to develop a complex regulatory network, and as with phosphate, serum magnesium concentrations are not tightly regulated. Because magnesium is principally intracellular, measurement of serum levels may provide false estimates of actual total body and intracellular magnesium status. Because magnesium is essential for fundamental processes such as gene transcription and cellular energy use, life-threatening magnesium deficiency is often unrecognized because its symptoms are frustratingly nonspecific: weakness, respirator dependence, diffuses neurologic syndromes (including seizures), and cardiovascular collapse.

Magnesium has a molecular weight of 24 (1 mole = 24 g), and because it is divalent, one equivalent is 12 g. Blood magnesium measurements are often provided in milligrams per deciliter (mg/dL) or milliequivalents per liter (mEq/L); oral magnesium supplements are expressed in milligrams per tablet or milliequivalents per vial; and urinary magnesium excretion values are given in milliequivalents or milligrams per 24 hours. Constructing a black box for magnesium is helpful (Fig. 72-10), and the magnesium values are provided in milligram and milliequivalent units.

As with phosphorus, magnesium has quantitatively important interfaces with the intestine, skeleton, intracellular supplies, and kidney. At the level of the intestine, magnesium is widely available in normal diets, and regulation is limited; the body absorbs about one third of what is ingested. In normal circumstances, dietary magnesium is abundant, absorption is ample, and magnesium deficiency does not occur. However, deficiency may occur with alcoholism, in intensive care unit settings in which adequate nutrition often is not provided, or with intestinal malabsorption.

At the level of the skeleton, magnesium is incorporated into the hydroxyapatite crystal as mineralization of osteoid occurs, and it is released by osteoclastic bone resorption (see Figs. 72-1 and 72-3). In quantitative terms, these fluxes are small.

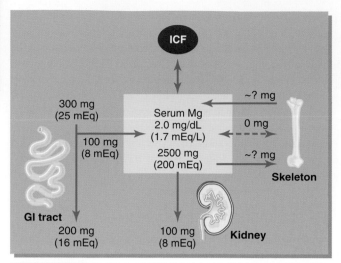

Many instances of magnesium deficiency are caused by excessive renal losses. Examples include the magnesuria that accompanies saline infusions, diuretic use, alcohol use, and secondary hyperaldosteronism states such as cirrhosis and ascites. As with calcium and phosphorus, the fractional excretion of magnesium (FE_{Mg}) can be calculated, and it should be used as an index of whether the kidney is appropriately conserving magnesium in states of hypomagnesaemia or whether renal magnesium wasting is the cause of the hypomagnesaemia. The normal FE_{Mg} is 2% to 4%. Hypomagnesemic individuals have FE_{Mg} values below 1% to 2%.

With regard to homeostatic regulation, magnesium homeostasis can best be viewed as a renal Tm-regulated process (see Renal Phosphate Handling), with the renal Tm for magnesium set at a fixed level of about 2.2 mg/dL. In this scenario, abundant dietary magnesium exists, and excessive magnesium intake is managed by spillage of excess magnesium over the Tm set at 2.2 mg/dL and into the urine. Conversely, in settings of dietary magnesium deficiency, which equate evolutionarily with caloric deficiency, short-term deficiency is prevented when serum levels fall below the renal Tm of 2.0 mg/dL. No known independent hormonal regulatory system for magnesium exists.

PROSPECTUS FOR THE FUTURE

Although it may seem that calcium, PTH, vitamin D, magnesium, and phosphorus homeostasis and skeletal biology are well understood, it should be clear that many of the physiologic details described in this chapter have been elucidated only during the past 10 to 15 years, and new regulatory proteins (e.g., fibroblast growth factor 23) and diseases continue to be identified. This area of research is dynamic, with many unanswered questions remaining.

SUGGESTED READINGS

Christov M, Juppner H: Insights form genetic disorders of phosphate homeostasis, Semin Nephrol 33:143–157, 2013.

Lentz RD, Brown DM, Kjellstrand CM: Treatment of severe hypophosphatemia, Ann Intern Med 89:941–944, 1978.

Melmed S, Polonsky KS, Larsen PR, et al, editors: Williams textbook of endocrinology, ed 12, Philadelphia, 2012, Saunders.

Rosen CJ, editor: The American Society for Bone and Mineral Research primer on metabolic bone diseases and disorders of mineral metabolism, ed 8, Washington, D.C., 2013, American Society for Bone and Mineral Research.

73

Disorders of Serum Minerals

Steven P. Hodak and Andrew F. Stewart

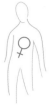

INTRODUCTION

In this chapter, we consider disorders that lead to increases or decreases in the circulating concentrations of calcium, phosphorus, and magnesium. Chapter 72 describes normal calcium, phosphorus, and magnesium metabolism.

The optimal approach to diagnosing and treating these disorders is to understand their underlying physiology and pathophysiology. Coherent diagnostic and successful therapeutic plans can then be developed. Years of experience suggest a persistent propensity to jump to the common items on the differential diagnosis list without fully considering the other options. In so doing, the correct and often easily treatable diagnosis is overlooked. For example, hypercalcemia in the setting of a pulmonary nodule may indicate the humoral hypercalcemia of malignancy, and many physicians jump to this diagnosis with its grim prognosis. However, this complex may represent hypercalcemia in a patient with treatable tuberculosis or primary hyperparathyroidism (HPT) in a person with a long-standing and inactive pulmonary scar. Complete differential diagnoses are provided in the tables that follow.

HYPERCALCEMIA

Symptoms and Signs

Hypercalcemia causes hyperpolarization of neuromuscular cell membranes and therefore refractoriness to stimulation (see Chapter 72). This condition manifests clinically as skeletal muscular weakness, smooth muscle hypoactivity with constipation and ileus, and the full spectrum of neurologic dysfunction, progressing from lassitude to mild confusion to deep coma. Hypercalcemia also leads to renal failure. It reduces the glomerular filtration rate (GFR) through afferent arteriolar vasoconstriction and activation of the calcium receptor in the distal nephron. It causes a form of nephrogenic diabetes insipidus that is associated with polydipsia and polyuria. These events lower the extracellular fluid (ECF) volume and lower the GFR.

Hypercalcemia may lead to interstitial calcium phosphate crystal deposition in the kidney (i.e., nephrocalcinosis or interstitial nephritis) and nephrolithiasis with obstructive uropathy. Hypercalcemia may also lead to shortening of the QTc interval on the electrocardiogram. Frequently, however, asymptomatic hypercalcemia is discovered on routine laboratory testing.

Whether a person develops symptoms depends on several factors. One is the degree of hypercalcemia. People with serum calcium values above 13 mg/dL usually are symptomatic. The duration of hypercalcemia is also important. A gradual increase in serum calcium, even into the severe 15- to 17-mg/dL range, may cause few symptoms if it occurs slowly enough. The overall health status and age of the person with hypercalcemia influence the severity of symptoms. For example, a child with severe immobilization-induced hypercalcemia in the 15-mg/dL range may be completely alert, whereas an elderly person with underlying Alzheimer's disease and narcotic use may become comatose with a serum calcium level of 11.5 mg/dL.

Pathophysiology

The physiologic black box described in Chapter 72 should be considered when attempting to diagnose or treat hypercalcemia. These disorders can be grouped into factitious disorders (e.g., abnormalities in serum proteins), renal disorders (e.g., thiazide diuretics, lithium use), gastrointestinal disorders (e.g., sarcoid, milk-alkali syndrome), skeletal disorders (e.g., hypercalcemia of malignancy, immobilization hypercalcemia), and combined disorders. Primary HPT is a good example of the latter, with important gastrointestinal (GI) and renal components. The diagnoses in Table 73-1 should be considered with regard to the underlying pathophysiologic mechanism and the clinical setting.

Differential Diagnosis

Malignancy-Associated Hypercalcemia

The most common cause of hypercalcemia among hospitalized patients is cancer. Hypercalcemia occurs late in the course of cancer and usually progresses rapidly, followed by death. About 50% of patients with cancer survive 30 days after the development of hypercalcemia.

Hypercalcemia usually is encountered only in patients with large tumor burdens. Conversely, small, occult cancers rarely cause hypercalcemia. The exceptions to this rule are small neuroendocrine tumors, such as islet cell tumors and bronchial carcinoids. Certain tumors are common causes of hypercalcemia, including breast, renal, squamous, and ovarian carcinomas and multiple myeloma and lymphoma. Other common cancers, such as colon, prostate, and gastric carcinomas, are not commonly associated with hypercalcemia.

Cancer may lead to hypercalcemia through several mechanisms, the most common of which is humoral hypercalcemia of malignancy (HHM). HHM accounts for about 80% of patients with malignancy-associated hypercalcemia (MAHC) and is the result of excessive secretion by tumors of parathyroid hormone–related protein (PTHrP). PTHrP mimics the actions of parathyroid hormone (PTH) on the kidney to prevent calcium excretion

TABLE 73-1   DISORDERS ASSOCIATED WITH HYPERCALCEMIA

Malignancy-associated hypercalcemia	Vitamin D and derivatives (calcitriol, dihydrotachysterol)
Humoral hypercalcemia of malignancy	Vitamin A (including retinoic acid derivatives)
Hypercalcemia caused by 1,25-dihydroxyvitamin D_3 (1,25[OH]$_2$D$_3$)–secreting lymphomas	Foscarnet
	Milk-alkali syndrome
Hypercalcemia caused by direct skeletal invasion	Immobilization plus high bone turnover
True ectopic hyperparathyroidism	Juvenile skeleton
Primary and tertiary hyperparathyroidism	Paget's disease
	Myeloma and breast cancer with bone metastases
Familial hypocalciuric hypercalcemia or familial benign hypercalcemia	Prehumoral hypercalcemia of malignancy
Granulomatous disorders	Mild primary hyperparathyroidism
Sarcoid	Secondary hyperparathyroidism (e.g., from continuous ambulatory peritoneal dialysis)
Berylliosis	
Foreign body	
Tuberculosis	Chronic and acute renal failure
Coccidioidomycosis	Recovery phase of rhabdomyolysis-induced acute renal failure
Blastomycosis	
Histoplasmosis	Chronic hemodialysis
Granulomatous leprosy	Calcitriol
Eosinophilic granuloma	Immobilization
Histiocytosis	Decreased calcium clearance
Inflammatory bowel disease	Calcium carbonate
Endocrine disorders other than hyperparathyroidism	Total parenteral nutrition (TPN)
Hyperthyroidism	Calcium-containing TPN in patients with decreased glomerular filtration rate
Pheochromocytoma	
Addisonian crisis	
Vasoactive intestinal peptide–producing tumor (VIPoma); watery diarrhea, hypokalemia, and achlorhydria (WDHA) syndrome	Chronic TPN in patients with short bowel syndrome
	Hyperproteinemia
	Volume contraction with hyperalbuminemia
Medications	Myeloma with calcium-binding immunoglobulin
Thiazides	
Aminophylline	End-stage liver disease
Lithium	Manganese intoxication
Estrogen/antiestrogen in breast cancer with bone metastases (estrogen flare)	

and on the skeleton to activate osteoclasts and induce bone resorption. PTHrP is the product of many normal cell types and, in health, is typically produced at low levels.

Tumors classically associated with the HHM mechanism are squamous carcinomas of any site (i.e., larynx, lung, cervix, and esophagus), renal carcinomas, ovarian carcinomas, and breast cancer. Hypercalcemia in HHM occurs in the absence of skeletal metastases or in the setting of a few skeletal metastases. If tumor resection or ablation is possible, hypercalcemia reverses. In addition to hypercalcemia, these patients have elevations in PTHrP concentrations and reductions in the levels of PTH, 1,25-dihydroxyvitamin D_3 (1,25[OH]$_2$D), and serum phosphorus and the tubular maximum for phosphorus (TmP) (see Chapter 72).

A second form of MAHC is caused by local tumor invasion of the skeleton, a process called *local osteolytic hypercalcemia* (LOH). LOH accounts for about 20% of patients with MAHC. In these patients, unlike those with HHM, the skeletal metastatic or primary tumor burden is large, and the offending tumor is most often a breast cancer or a hematologic neoplasm such as multiple myeloma, leukemia, or lymphoma. Local factors are secreted by tumors in the bone marrow that induce osteoclastic bone resorption. They include PTHrP, macrophage inflammatory protein 1α (MIP-1α), receptor-activating nuclear factor-κB ligand (RANKL), interleukin-6, and interleukin-1. These patients have reductions in PTH, PTHrP, and 1,25(OH)$_2$D levels, and have normal to elevated serum phosphorus values.

A third form of MAHC is secretion of 1,25(OH)$_2$D by lymphomas and dysgerminomas. This form is unusual, and the mechanism is interesting. Although direct bone involvement may occur and may contribute to hypercalcemia, the increase in 1,25(OH)$_2$D leads to intestinal calcium hyperabsorption and to systemically driven bone resorption. This condition is essentially a malignant version of the hypercalcemia that occurs in sarcoidosis (see Granulomatous Disorders).

Primary and Tertiary Hyperparathyroidism

Although MAHC is the most common cause of hypercalcemia among inpatients, primary HPT is by far the most common cause among healthy outpatients. Together, MAHC and HPT account for about 90% of cases of hypercalcemia. Most often, the hypercalcemia of HPT is mild, with serum calcium values in the range of 10.6 to 11.5 mg/dL. However, HPT occasionally produces spectacular hypercalcemia in the 20-mg/dL range. In about 85% of patients, hypercalcemia results from a single parathyroid adenoma that overproduces PTH, and in about 15% of patients, it results from multiple-gland hyperplasia. In less than 1% of patients, HPT may result from parathyroid carcinoma. For all these etiologies, the diagnosis is made by the discovery of an elevated serum PTH level in a patient with hypercalcemia. Hypophosphatemia, a reduction in the TmP, increased plasma 1,25(OH)$_2$D and serum chloride levels, and a reduction in the serum bicarbonate concentration are typical features.

Primary HPT often is asymptomatic. However, some patients develop hypercalciuria and calcium nephrolithiasis, most often as a result of calcium oxalate and, less commonly, calcium phosphate stones. Some patients with HPT, especially those with a more severe form, have a reduction in bone mineral density characterized histologically as hyperparathyroid bone disease, also called *osteitis fibrosa cystica* (see Chapter 74). Other patients may develop mild to severe renal failure as a result of the mechanisms described earlier. Each of the previously described conditions— significant osteopenia, kidney stones, reduced renal function, and a serum calcium concentration greater than 1 mg/dL above normal—is an indication for parathyroidectomy. Other patients may be monitored conservatively. In patients who refuse or are unable to undergo surgery, medical management of hypercalcemia may be attempted using bisphosphonates or the calcium receptor mimetic cinacalcet.

HPT can occur as part of one of the multiple endocrine neoplasia (MEN) syndromes. It is associated with pituitary and islet tumors (MEN 1) and with pheochromocytomas and medullary carcinoma of the thyroid (MEN 2).

Secondary HPT is an appropriate increase in circulating PTH associated with eucalcemia or hypocalcemia. It occurs in an attempt to correct hypocalcemia resulting, for example, from vitamin D deficiency or chronic renal failure

Tertiary HPT refers to HPT associated with hypercalcemia that occurs in the setting of prolonged stimulation of the parathyroid glands, such as chronic renal failure with hypocalcemia or chronic vitamin D deficiency resulting from malabsorption. Chronic parathyroid stimulation leads to parathyroid hyperplasia and sometimes adenomas, and these conditions may fail to suppress normally and cause hypercalcemia. The classic example is development of PTH-dependent hypercalcemia after successful renal transplantation.

Familial Hypocalciuric Hypercalcemia

Familial hypocalciuric hypercalcemia, also called *familial benign hypercalcemia*, is an autosomal dominant inherited disorder that results from heterozygous inactivating mutations in the calcium receptor. Parathyroid glands that bear such a defective receptor on their surface inappropriately perceive circulating calcium concentrations to be low. They therefore behave as though the patient is hypocalcemic and appropriately secrete additional PTH. This action causes the serum calcium concentration to rise, and the PTH equilibrates at a high-normal to elevated level. The hypercalcemia is usually mild, in the 11- to 12-mg/dL range, but it may be higher. Because the partially inactivated calcium receptors are expressed in the kidney, the kidney inappropriately conserves calcium, leading to hypocalciuria and contributing to hypercalcemia. Because these same calcium receptors are also expressed in the central nervous system, the hypercalcemia is not perceived, and affected individuals are therefore asymptomatic. The two names of this syndrome describe it accurately.

With the exception of the hypocalciuria and the autosomal dominant pattern of inheritance, these individuals are similar biochemically to patients with primary HPT. Because affected individuals are asymptomatic and do not develop adverse sequelae from the syndrome, its primary importance is that affected individuals be properly identified and protected from unnecessary and ineffective parathyroidectomy. Homozygous individuals, usually infants, develop severe hypercalcemia requiring urgent total parathyroidectomy.

Granulomatous Disorders

Most granulomatous disorders can lead to hypercalcemia (see Table 73-1). The prototypes are sarcoidosis, tuberculosis, and the fungal diseases listed. As with the kidney, granulomas have the ability to convert inactive 25-hydroxyvitamin D to the active metabolite, $1,25(OH)_2D$. When exposed to sunlight, ultraviolet radiation, or relatively trivial quantities of dietary vitamin D, individuals with these disorders may develop mild to severe hypercalcemia.

Hypercalcemia results from intestinal calcium hyperabsorption and $1,25(OH)_2D$-induced bone resorption; the former is the important component in most cases. Because of the hypercalcemia, PTH is suppressed, and the serum phosphorus level is elevated. The combination of hypercalcemia and hyperphosphatemia may lead to nephrocalcinosis and renal failure. Treatment focuses on correcting the underlying disorder. Measures include a low dietary calcium intake, a low vitamin D intake, limiting sun exposure, and hydration. Loop diuretics are administered to accelerate calcium clearance, and if the hypercalcemia is severe, glucocorticoids are used.

Endocrine Disorders Other Than Hyperparathyroidism

In addition to HPT, four other endocrine disorders have been associated with the development of hypercalcemia. As many as 50% of people with *hyperthyroidism* have at least mild hypercalcemia. The hypercalcemia is rarely greater than 11 mg/dL. The mechanism is thought to be an increase in osteoclast activation by thyroid hormone.

A second disorder is *pheochromocytoma*. Some of these individuals are hypercalcemic as a result of primary HPT occurring in the MEN 2 syndrome, but others become hypercalcemic as a result of PTHrP secretion by a pheochromocytoma. Hypercalcemia has also been reported in patients with hypoadrenalism and those with islet cell tumors called VIPomas.

Medications

Drugs that may cause hypercalcemia include thiazide diuretics, lithium, aminophylline, theophylline, vitamins D and A, foscarnet, and estrogens and tamoxifen in the setting of breast cancer with extensive skeletal metastases.

Milk-Alkali Syndrome

The normal intake of calcium is in the range of 600 to 1200 mg/day for most people. As reviewed in Chapter 72, absorption of calcium from the diet is tightly controlled. However, ingestion of very large quantities of calcium may overwhelm this system and lead to hypercalcemia. This condition was originally described in the 1940s in patients ingesting enormous quantities of milk, cream, and antacids. It is still encountered with some regularity in patients ingesting large quantities of calcium carbonate or other calcium-containing antacids for peptic ulcer disease. For hypercalcemia to occur, calcium intake must exceed 4 g/day, and it is often in the 10- to 20-g/day range. Severe hypercalcemia is common and may lead to renal failure.

Immobilization

Hypercalcemia due to immobilization requires two conditions: *complete immobilization* (e.g., quadriplegia) for a period of weeks, occurring on a background of *high bone turnover*, as occurs in young adults or children, HPT, Paget's disease, and malignant skeletal disease such as breast cancer with bone metastases or multiple myeloma. Immobilization activates osteoclastic bone resorption and inhibits osteoblastic activity, producing a severe uncoupling of bone resorption from formation, with rapid and enormous net losses of calcium from the skeleton into the ECF. Left untreated, the condition results in severe demineralization. The syndrome is associated with hypercalciuria, which with chronic urinary catheterization leads to urinary tract infection and severe calcium nephrolithiasis.

The most effective treatment for hypercalcemia is active weight bearing. Hydration and antiresorptive drugs such as the bisphosphonates may be used.

Chronic and Acute Renal Failure

Chronic and acute renal failure has been associated with hypercalcemia. The more common initial abnormality is hypocalcemia induced by a reduction in kidney-derived $1,25(OH)_2D$ and an increase in serum phosphate as a result of diminished glomerular filtration. However, hypercalcemia may occur in patients with chronic renal failure as a result of calcium antacid use or as a result of $1,25(OH)_2D$ or paracalcitol treatment to prevent renal osteodystrophy.

Parenteral Nutrition

Enteric and parenteral forms of nutrition have been associated with hypercalcemia. Large doses of oral calcium provided in hypercaloric enteric feeding regimens, particularly in the setting of reduced renal function, may lead to a form of the milk-alkali syndrome. More mysterious is the well-described hypercalcemic syndrome occurring in patients treated with total parenteral nutrition (TPN). These patients typically have short-bowel syndrome and are on long-term TPN. In some patients, the hypercalcemia can be traced to large amounts of calcium, vitamin D, or aluminum in the TPN solution.

Hyperproteinemia

About 50% of circulating calcium is bound to serum albumin and other proteins. Increases in serum proteins naturally lead to an artifactual increase in total, but not ionized, serum calcium concentrations. This increase is commonly observed in settings of volume depletion and dehydration. Patients with this syndrome do not display features typical of authentic hypercalcemia: reduced mental status, prolonged QTc interval on the electrocardiogram, and hypercalciuria. Treatment of the "hypercalcemia" should be avoided, because it may lead to hypocalcemic symptoms and signs such as paresthesia, tetany, and seizures.

Treatment of Hypercalcemia

A point worth emphasizing is that not everyone requires treatment for hypercalcemia. Patients with mild HPT with borderline serum calcium values and without other complications may be observed. Patients with end-stage refractory cancer with severe hypercalcemia arguably may be best served by withholding therapy. Familial hypocalciuric hypercalcemia is best left untreated.

Therapy for hypercalcemia is optimally directed at reversing the underlying pathophysiologic abnormality. Disorders associated with increased intestinal calcium absorption (e.g., sarcoid, milk-alkali syndrome, $1,25[OH]_2D_3$-secreting lymphomas) are best treated by consuming a low-calcium diet and avoiding vitamin D. Hypercalcemia in the setting of volume depletion and diminished renal function is managed by expanding the ECF volume and GFR with saline and encouraging diuresis with loop diuretics.

Medications that induce hypercalcemia should be discontinued. Disorders associated with increased osteoclastic bone resorption, such as MAHC and immobilization hypercalcemia, are best treated using inhibitors of bone resorption such as the bisphosphonates pamidronate or zoledronate. Disorders with multiple abnormalities require combinations of these measures. Resection of parathyroid tissue in patients with parathyroid disease is effective, and cinacalcet or bisphosphonates may be used if parathyroid surgery cannot be performed.

● HYPOCALCEMIA

Symptoms and Signs

Hypocalcemia leads to a reduction in the potential difference across cell membranes, producing hyperexcitability, particularly of cells of the neuromuscular class (see Chapter 72). Neuromuscular cells spontaneously fire and produce spontaneous seizures, paresthesias, and skeletal muscle contractions (i.e., carpal spasm, pedal spasm, or tetany).

Two physical signs are observed on examination: Trousseau sign, which is spontaneous contraction of the forearm muscles in response to application of a blood pressure cuff around the upper arm and inflation to above systolic pressure, and Chvostek sign, which is twitching of the facial muscles with gentle tapping of the facial nerve as it exits the parotid gland. An electrocardiographic sign is a prolonged QTc interval. Prolonged hypoparathyroidism may be associated with basal ganglia calcification, which is asymptomatic but impressive on computed tomography scans and plain x-ray films of the skull.

Pathophysiology

Hypocalcemia may result from five mechanisms: a reduction in serum binding proteins (e.g., albumin), an increase in serum phosphate with a resultant increase in the calcium-phosphate solubility product, an increase in renal calcium excretion, a reduction in intestinal calcium absorption, or a loss of calcium from the ECF into the skeleton. In practice, several of these factors are operative in several disorders. For example, in hypoparathyroidism, a reduction in intestinal calcium absorption combines with an inability to reabsorb calcium from the distal tubule to cause hypocalcemia, or in breast cancer with extensive osteoblastic metastases, increases in osteoblast activity remove calcium from the ECF, and anorexia leads to a reduction in intestinal calcium intake. This knowledge is important because effective therapy requires the underlying disorder to be appropriately managed. Giving oral vitamin D supplements to a patient with sprue may not be effective unless the underlying malabsorption is treated; parenteral vitamin D may be more effective.

Differential Diagnosis

Disorders that may lead to hypocalcemia are summarized in the following sections and Table 73-2.

Hypoparathyroidism

Hypoparathyroidism causes hypocalcemia as a result of a decrease in intestinal calcium absorption combined with reduced renal calcium reabsorption in the distal tubule. Hypoparathyroidism may be idiopathic or autoimmune, occurring in isolation or as part of the polyglandular failure syndrome in association with Graves' hyperthyroidism, Hashimoto's thyroiditis, Addison's disease, type 1 diabetes, vitiligo, mucocutaneous candidiasis, and other autoimmune disorders. Hypoparathyroidism may commonly be encountered as surgical hypoparathyroidism in patients who have undergone thyroid, parathyroid, or laryngeal surgery. Surgical and autoimmune hypoparathyroidism together account for most patients with hypoparathyroidism. Less common causes include congenital hypoparathyroidism caused by DiGeorge syndrome, isolated parathyroid failure, or genetic mutations. Rarely,

TABLE 73-2 DIFFERENTIAL DIAGNOSIS OF HYPOCALCEMIA

Hypoparathyroidism
  Surgical
  Idiopathic and autoimmune
  Infiltrative diseases
  Wilson's disease (copper)
  Hemochromatosis
  Sarcoidosis
  Metastatic (breast) cancer
  Congenital
  Isolated, sporadic
  DiGeorge syndrome
  Infant of mother with
    hyperparathyroidism
  Hereditary
  X-linked
  Parathyroid gland calcium
    receptor (Gα11 subunit)–
    activating mutations
  Parathyroid hormone (PTH)
    signal peptide mutation
  GCM2 (formerly *GCMB*)
    mutation
Pseudohypoparathyroidism
  Type Ia: multiple hormone
    resistance, Albright's hereditary
    osteodystrophy
  Type Ib: PTH resistance without
    other abnormalities
  Type Ic: specific PTH resistance,
    resulting from defect in catalytic
    subunit of PTH-receptor
    complex
  Type II: specific PTH resistance,
    postreceptor defect of adenylyl
    cyclase, undefined
Vitamin D disorders
  Absent ultraviolet exposure
  Vitamin D deficiency
  Fat malabsorption

Vitamin D–dependent rickets,
  renal 1α-hydroxylase deficiency,
  1,25-dihydroxyvitamin
  D–receptor defects
Chronic renal failure
Hepatic failure
Hypoalbuminemia
Sepsis
Hypermagnesemia and
  hypomagnesemia
Rapid bone formation
  Hungry bone syndrome after
    parathyroidectomy or
    thyroidectomy
  Osteoblastic metastases
  Vitamin D therapy of
    osteomalacia, rickets
Hyperphosphatemia
  Crush injury, rhabdomyolysis
  Renal failure
  Tumor lysis
  Excessive phosphate (PO_4)
    administration (PO, IV, PR)
Medications
  Mithramycin, plicamycin
  Bisphosphonates
  Calcitonin
  Fluoride
  Ethylenediaminetetraacetic acid
    (EDTA)
  Citrate
  Intravenous contrast
  Foscarnet
Pancreatitis
  Hypoalbuminemia
  Hypomagnesemia
  Calcium soap formation

tissue infiltrative diseases such as breast cancer, hemochromatosis (i.e., iron deposition), or sarcoidosis may destroy or replace normal parathyroid tissue.

The diagnosis is made by finding a low serum ionized calcium level in a patient with an inappropriately reduced serum PTH concentration. The phosphorus concentration usually is high normal or frankly elevated, and plasma $1,25(OH)_2D$ concentrations are reduced (see Chapter 72).

Treatment is normally directed at increasing intestinal calcium absorption through the use of large doses of calcium (up to 6-8 g of elemental calcium per day) and, when necessary, the addition of the active form of vitamin D $(1,25[OH]_2D)$, in replacement amounts of 0.25 to 1.0 µg/day. The goal is to induce sufficient intestinal calcium hyperabsorption to overwhelm the ability of the kidney to excrete it. It carries the risk of inducing significant hypercalciuria and therefore nephrocalcinosis and nephrolithiasis. Accordingly, 24-hour urinary calcium levels must be measured regularly to identify dangerously high hypercalciuria. The serum calcium concentration is maintained in the low-normal range, about 8.5 to 9.0 mg/dL. In some instances, addition of a thiazide diuretic such as hydrochlorothiazide, which stimulates renal calcium reabsorption, may be effective in preventing hypercalciuria while raising the serum calcium level.

Pseudohypoparathyroidism

Pseudohypoparathyroidism refers to a group of disorders that have in common resistance to the actions of PTH. In most cases, resistance results from different inactivating mutations in the signal-transducing protein $G_{s\alpha}$. The most common form of the syndrome, type Ia, is associated with multiple hormone resistance and a phenotype referred to as *Albright's hereditary osteodystrophy*, which includes short stature, shortened fourth and fifth metacarpals and metatarsals, obesity, mental retardation, subcutaneous calcifications, and cafe au lait spots.

Patients resemble those with hypoparathyroidism; they are hypocalcemic and have hyperphosphatemia. The diagnosis is made by the finding of an elevated circulating PTH level in a patient with hypocalcemia and hyperphosphatemia for whom other causes of hypocalcemia and secondary hypoparathyroidism have been excluded. The treatment is similar to that of hypoparathyroidism.

Vitamin D Disorders

Active vitamin D, $1,25(OH)_2D$, is required to absorb calcium from the intestine. Activation of vitamin D requires adequate amounts of vitamin D from the diet or sunlight exposure, an intact intestine through which to absorb calcium and vitamin D, an intact liver with which to convert vitamin D to 25-hydroxyvitamin D, and an intact kidney to convert 25-hydroxyvitamin D to $1,25(OH)_2D$ (see Chapter 72).

Developing hypocalcemia and osteomalacia or rickets (see Chapter 74) in settings in which one or more of the conversion steps is disrupted is common. Malabsorption syndromes, such as short-bowel syndrome and celiac sprue, lead to hypocalcemia as a result of calcium and vitamin D malabsorption. Chronic liver diseases, particularly primary biliary cirrhosis, lead to hypocalcemia and osteomalacia. Chronic renal insufficiency leads to failure to produce $1,25(OH)_2D$, with reductions in serum calcium levels and inefficient absorption of intestinal calcium.

Although Western diets are supplemented with vitamin D in milk and multivitamins, diets composed of no milk, human milk, or unsupplemented bovine milk are vitamin D deficient. Relatively trivial exposure to sunlight can provide ample vitamin D and replace dietary needs for vitamin D. However, vitamin D deficiency can occur in settings in which both sun exposure and dietary intake of vitamin D are poor (i.e., cloudy climates, excessive clothing or body covering, prolonged nursing by infants, and the standard tea and toast diet of older adults), vitamin D deficiency is the rule rather than the exception.

Certain genetic syndromes affecting vitamin D conversion can result in severe hypocalcemia. Long-term, high-dose treatment with anticonvulsants such as phenytoin or phenobarbital or their derivatives may lead to hypocalcemia and osteomalacia.

Hypoalbuminemia

Reductions in serum albumin, as occur in burn patients, the nephrotic syndrome, malnutrition, and cirrhosis, lead to reductions in serum total calcium without a reduction in the ionized total serum calcium level. Several formulas exist for correcting total serum calcium for albumin, but none is entirely accurate.

Measuring ionized calcium directly is important if the authentic ionized serum calcium concentration is needed.

Sepsis

Gram-positive and gram-negative sepsis have been associated with hypocalcemia that usually is mild. The mechanisms are poorly understood. Hypocalcemia occurring in the setting of sepsis appears to confer a particularly adverse prognosis.

Hypermagnesemia

Magnesium is a divalent cation, as is calcium, and in very high concentrations, it may mimic the actions of calcium to suppress PTH. In so doing, it leads to a functional type of hypoparathyroidism and hypocalcemia. In practice, this condition is uncommon.

Hypomagnesemia

Hypomagnesemia is one of the most common causes of hypocalcemia. It is encountered often in patients with alcoholism, malnutrition, cisplatin therapy for cancer, and intestinal malabsorption syndromes. Hypomagnesemia inhibits PTH secretion (i.e. magnesium adenosine triphosphatase is required for PTH secretion) and prevents the calcemic actions of PTH on the kidney and skeleton. Magnesium deficiency causes a functional form of hypoparathyroidism and resistance to PTH. The treatment is straightforward: magnesium replacement, which corrects the syndrome in minutes to hours. Intravenous calcium or vitamin D is ineffective.

Rapid Bone Formation

Increased rates of bone mineralization that are out of proportion to the rate of bone resorption lead to net calcium entry into the skeleton and, if these rates are large, to hypocalcemia. This state occurs in several clinical settings. One condition is the hungry bone syndrome that may follow parathyroidectomy, usually performed for HPT. Preoperatively, the rates of bone turnover (i.e., resorption and formation) are very high but are approximately coupled. Postoperatively, the rate of osteoclastic bone resorption abruptly declines with the decline in PTH, but the elevated rate of mineralization continues for days. Because of this acute postoperative imbalance, the skeleton becomes a sink for calcium, and hypocalcemia ensues.

Rapid bone formation also may occur in patients with vitamin D deficiency who have severe osteomalacia or rickets and large amounts of unmineralized osteoid. When these patients are treated with vitamin D, rapid mineralization of unmineralized osteoid occurs, the skeleton becomes a sink for calcium, and hypocalcemia ensues. Another example of this phenomenon occurs in the setting of extensive osteoblastic bone metastases, such as in prostate or breast cancer and occasionally in other malignancies.

Hyperphosphatemia

Disorders that lead to hyperphosphatemia may cause hypocalcemia as a result of exceeding the calcium-phosphate solubility product in serum. Examples of disorders that may cause the kind of severe hyperphosphatemia required include rhabdomyolysis (e.g., crush injuries), renal failure, and the tumor lysis syndrome.

Severe hyperphosphatemia may be seen after ingestion of large amounts of phosphate-containing purgatives in preparation for colonoscopy, inadvertent perforation of the rectum during the administration of phosphate enemas, and overzealous administration of intravenous phosphate. In these examples, the onset of hyperphosphatemia is relatively abrupt, and the hypocalcemia is immediate and severe. Commonly, the first sign of this sequence of events is a seizure.

Treatment involves reducing the serum phosphorus level by whatever means necessary. Giving intravenous calcium should be avoided because it is precipitated into soft tissues.

Medications

Certain medications may cause hypocalcemia, including those used to treat hypercalcemia. Fluoride compounds (e.g., anesthetic gas), chelating agents such as ethylenediaminetetraacetic acid (EDTA) and citrate (i.e., in stored blood), radiographic intravenous contrast agents, and the antiviral drug foscarnet may cause hypocalcemia.

Pancreatitis

When pancreatitis causes hypocalcemia, it is a poor prognostic sign. The classic mechanism involves the formation of calcium-free fatty acid soaps by lipases that are released from the inflamed pancreas. The free lipases then autodigest omental and retroperitoneal fat into negatively charged ions that tightly bind calcium in the ECF, causing hypocalcemia. The hypocalcemia is reversible by calcium infusion, and it self-terminates when the pancreatitis improves.

● HYPERPHOSPHATEMIA

Symptoms and Signs

Hyperphosphatemia produces no specific signs. It is usually identified incidentally on routine chemical screens or as a result of the induction of hypocalcemia.

Pathophysiology

Hyperphosphatemia develops as a result of two mechanisms. One is a large load of phosphate delivered into the ECF through the GI tract, intravenous medications, or endogenous sources such as muscle or tumor. The second mechanism is the inability to excrete phosphate, as occurs in acute or chronic renal failure. Essentially all natural foods contain phosphate, and therefore almost any diet contains substantial quantities of phosphate (see Chapter 72). Normally, phosphate is easily cleared by the healthy kidney, but this ability is lost as the GFR declines below 20 to 30 mg/dL.

Differential Diagnosis

The differential diagnoses of hyperphosphatemia are listed in the following sections and in Table 73-3.

Artifactual Occurrence

Hyperphosphatemia may occur artifactually as a result of hemolysis in blood collection tubes. One clue is that the same phenomenon occurs with potassium. The occurrence of unexplained hyperkalemia and hyperphosphatemia should trigger the

TABLE 73-3 CAUSES OF HYPERPHOSPHATEMIA	
Artifactual	Endogenous phosphate loads
Hemolysis	Tumor lysis syndrome
Increased gastrointestinal intake	Rhabdomyolysis (crush injury)
Rectal enemas	Hemolysis
Oral Phospho-Soda purgatives	Reduced renal clearance
Gastrointestinal bleeding	Chronic or acute renal failure
Intravenous phosphate loads	Hypoparathyroidism
K-Phos	Acromegaly
Blood transfusions	Tumoral calcinosis

TABLE 73-4 CAUSES OF HYPOPHOSPHATEMIA	
Inadequate phosphate (PO_4) intake	Oncogenic osteomalacia
Starvation	Fanconi's syndrome
Malabsorption	Alcoholism
PO_4-binding antacid use	Excessive skeletal mineralization
Alcoholism	Hungry bone syndrome after
Renal PO_4 losses	parathyroidectomy
Primary, secondary, or tertiary	Osteoblastic metastases
hyperparathyroidism	Healing osteomalacia, rickets
Humoral hypercalcemia of	PO_4 shift into extracellular fluid
malignancy (parathyroid	Recovery from metabolic acidosis
hormone–related protein)	Respiratory alkalosis
Diuretics, calcitonin	Starvation refeeding, intravenous
X-linked hypophosphatemic	glucose
rickets	
Autosomal dominant	
hypophosphatemic rickets	

collection of a fresh sample and immediate repeat determination of the serum phosphate level.

Increased Gastrointestinal Intake

Hyperphosphatemia may occur in patients receiving large oral phosphate loads. In a literature review, most cases of phosphate-induced hypocalcemia were caused by the administration of phosphate-containing purgatives as preparation for colonoscopy. Another underappreciated cause of this phenomenon is inadvertent perforation of the rectum during the administration of a rectal Phospho-Soda enema, with delivery of large amounts of phosphate directly into the peritoneal cavity, from which it is rapidly absorbed. Upper GI tract bleeding from ulcers of gastritis provides a large GI phosphate load and may be associated with hyperphosphatemia.

Intravenous Phosphate Loads

Large amounts of phosphate may be administered during treatment to replete potassium using potassium phosphate preparations. What appear to be trivial quantities of potassium preparation (e.g., 20 to 40 mEq of K-Phos) actually contain large amounts of phosphate and may lead to severe hyperphosphatemia and hypocalcemia (see Chapter 72). A second vehicle for delivering phosphate intravenously is transfusions of red blood cells, which ultimately hemolyze and release their copious phosphate stores.

Endogenous Phosphate Loads

Hyperphosphatemia may result from the destruction of large amounts of tissue in three situations. One is the tumor lysis syndrome, typified by a large Burkitt lymphoma responding promptly to chemotherapy with massive cell death. A second phenomenon is acute rhabdomyolysis releasing phosphate from skeletal muscle, and a third is severe hemolysis. In each case, a large phosphate load is delivered into the ECF. Combined with renal impairment common in these situations, this results in renal failure, severe hypocalcemia, seizures, and sometimes death.

Reduced Renal Clearance

Renal clearance of phosphate is the main mechanism for maintaining phosphate homeostasis. Acute and chronic disorders of the kidney lead to hyperphosphatemia. Because PTH prevents phosphate reabsorption in the proximal nephron, hypoparathyroidism is typically associated with high-normal to frankly elevated serum phosphorus values. A condition called *tumoral calcinosis*, in which the ability of the kidney to clear

phosphate is specifically defective, leads to chronic hyperphosphatemia and accumulation of calcium-phosphate salts around large joints of the appendicular skeleton. Children, particularly adolescents, have higher serum phosphate concentrations than adults.

● HYPOPHOSPHATEMIA

Symptoms and Signs

Phosphate participates in a vast array of key cellular processes, including DNA synthesis and replication, energy generation and use, oxygen uptake and delivery by erythrocytes, and maintenance of the redox state of every cell in the body (see Chapter 72). The signs of phosphate depletion are nonspecific, diffuse, and often life-threatening. These signs may include respirator dependence, congestive heart failure, coma, hypotension, and generalized weakness and malaise. Because the signs and symptoms are nonspecific, they are frequently attributed to other causes and are left untreated. They typically occur in intensive care units (ICUs). In these settings, oral nutrition is nonexistent, intravenous phosphate repletion is inadequate, and diuretics and saline infusions accelerate renal phosphate losses. Appropriate therapy can produce startling results, with patients suddenly returning from being moribund to being ambulatory, extubated, and conversant.

Chronic hypophosphatemia leads to defects in skeletal mineralization, a phenomenon called *rickets* in children or *osteomalacia* in adults. These syndromes produce weakness, bone pain, bowing of the long bones, and fractures or pseudofractures (see Chapter 74).

Differential Diagnosis

Disorders can be divided into hypophosphatemia resulting from inadequate intake, from excessive renal losses, from excessive skeletal uptake, or from shifts of phosphate from the ECF into cells (Table 73-4). From a diagnostic standpoint, measuring the TmP (see Chapter 72) is important because it provides rapid determination of which type of hypophosphatemia the patient is confronting.

Inadequate Phosphate Intake

Disorders that involve inadequate phosphate intake are associated with a high TmP. Because essentially all foods are rich in phosphate, becoming phosphate depleted based on inadequate dietary intake is difficult. However, in settings of severe caloric deprivation, inadequacies can occur. Examples include anorexia nervosa, prisoner-of-war camps, prolonged ICU care, malabsorption syndromes, and chronic alcoholism. In the first three disorders, caloric intake is scant, and little phosphate is consumed. In alcoholism, caloric intake may be high, but alcohol is devoid of phosphate. The use of phosphate-binding antacids such as aluminum hydroxide gels may lead to severe phosphate deficiency, hypophosphatemia, and osteomalacia.

Excessive Renal Phosphate Losses

Disorders involving excessive losses are associated with a low TmP. PTH is phosphaturic, and all types of HPT are associated with hypophosphatemia as long as renal function is normal. This situation is widely appreciated for primary HPT but is less well appreciated for secondary HPT, particularly in the setting of vitamin D and calcium malabsorption. A low serum phosphate level may be the first and only noticeable clue to severe vitamin D deficiency. This fact has led to the diagnosis of celiac sprue in unsuspected cases on many occasions.

PTHrP (see Malignancy-Associated Hypercalcemia) is phosphaturic, as is PTH, and patients with humoral hypercalcemia of malignancy are commonly hypophosphatemic for this reason as long as their renal function is intact. Thiazide and loop diuretics are potent phosphaturic agents, and their use without phosphate replacement therapy leads to hypophosphatemia. Ethanol is also in this category.

Certain genetic disorders may lead to severe renal phosphate wasting (see Chapter 74). These disorders include X-linked hypophosphatemia (XLH), also called *vitamin D–resistant rickets*, and autosomal dominant hypophosphatemic rickets (ADHR). Another renal phosphate-wasting syndrome is oncogenic osteomalacia, also called *tumor-induced osteomalacia* (see Chapter 74). Acquired or inherited diffuse renal proximal tubular disorders, such as Fanconi's syndrome, may lead to hypophosphatemia as a result of renal phosphate wasting.

Excessive Skeletal Mineralization

Increased bone mineralization with respect to bone resorption results in large amounts of phosphate entering the skeleton, leading to hypophosphatemia. One example is the hungry bone syndrome that occurs after parathyroidectomy (see Hypocalcemia). Other examples are osteoblastic metastases and the treatment of vitamin D–deficient rickets or osteomalacia with vitamin D.

Phosphate Shift into Extracellular Fluid

Phosphate can be shifted from serum into the intracellular compartment by a rise in ECF pH. Recovery from a metabolic acidosis (e.g., diabetic ketoacidosis) and development of a respiratory alkalosis lead to hypophosphatemia. One of the most stunning examples of this phenomenon is the shift of phosphate into cells after administration of oral carbohydrate or parenteral glucose to victims of starvation or anorexia nervosa. Insulin increases the rate of glucose uptake into cells and its subsequent phosphorylation to glucose-6-phosphate. In the setting of significantly depleted phosphate reserve, rapid consumption of oral carbohydrate or parenteral glucose may lead to profound hypophosphatemia and sudden death due to respiratory or circulatory failure. Refeeding of starvation victims should be accomplished slowly and with attention to phosphate repletion.

Treatment

Phosphorus replacement is best accomplished through the oral route and usually is given in two to four divided doses that deliver 2000 to 4000 g/day. Doses greater than 1000 to 2000 mg/day often cause diarrhea initially (phosphate is used as a purgative), but with gradual increments, larger doses may be well tolerated. Intravenous phosphate should be given only with a clear understanding of the quantities involved (see Chapter 72) and to patients for whom oral administration is not an option. Frequent monitoring of serum phosphorus, calcium, and creatinine levels is required. Intravenous dosages up to 500 to 800 mg/day may be required.

● HYPERMAGNESEMIA
Symptoms and Signs

Clinically significant hypermagnesemia is uncommon. The symptom is drowsiness, and the signs are hyporeflexia and eventual neuromuscular, respiratory, and cardiovascular collapse. It may also lead to hypocalcemia (see Hypocalcemia). Hypermagnesemia is seen in two settings: severe renal failure accompanied by the administration of magnesium-containing antacids and after the intravenous administration of large doses of magnesium sulfate for eclampsia or preeclampsia.

Differential Diagnosis

The differential diagnosis of hypermagnesemia is brief and is limited to the two disorders previously described (Table 73-5). Mild hypermagnesemia is common in patients on dialysis, but severe hypermagnesemia occurs only in the settings of renal failure accompanied by parenteral or oral magnesium salt administration, such as the use of magnesium-containing antacids or phosphate binders. Hypermagnesemia occurs commonly but in a controlled fashion in the treatment of eclampsia.

● HYPOMAGNESEMIA
Symptoms and Signs

Hypomagnesemia is common, particularly in the ICU setting, but as with hypophosphatemia, it is often overlooked or ignored. Magnesium is essential for a broad range of biologic processes,

TABLE 73-5 CAUSES OF HYPERMAGNESEMIA AND HYPOMAGNESEMIA

Hypermagnesemia	Diuretics
Renal failure accompanied by magnesium antacid use	Saline infusion
	Secondary aldosteronism
Parenteral magnesium sulfate administration for eclampsia	Cirrhosis
	Congestive heart failure
Hypomagnesemia	Osmotic diuresis, hyperglycemia
Inadequate intake	Cisplatin, aminoglycoside antibiotics, amphotericin
Starvation	Hypokalemia
Malabsorption	Hypercalcemia, hypercalciuria
Alcoholism	Proximal tubular diseases
Vomiting, nasogastric suction	Genetic defects
Excessive renal losses	

and hypomagnesemia may cause hypocalcemia, seizures, and paresthesias independent of hypocalcemia and cause a broad array of neuromuscular, cardiovascular, and respiratory symptoms.

Differential Diagnosis

Differential diagnoses are listed in the following sections and in Table 73-5.

Inadequate Intake

Inadequate intake of magnesium is common among alcoholics and the generally undernourished. It may occur as part of an intestinal malabsorption syndrome and may result from continuous vomiting or nasogastric suctioning. These situations are common in ICU settings and are often overlooked.

Excessive Renal Losses

Excessive renal losses of magnesium are common in clinical practice. Thiazide and loop diuretics cause renal magnesium losses, and saline infusion has a similar effect. Magnesium is lost by the kidney in response to aldosterone in primary hyperaldosteronism but more commonly in the secondary hyperaldosteronism associated with cirrhosis, volume depletion, congestive heart failure, and other common disorders. Osmotic diuresis, as occurs with poorly controlled diabetes mellitus, causes renal magnesium loss. Certain nephrotoxic drugs such as cisplatin, aminoglycoside antibiotics, and amphotericin induce proximal tubular injury and a severe form of renal magnesium wasting. Hypokalemia, hypercalcemia, and hypercalciuria also lead to renal magnesium excretion. Many diseases that lead to proximal tubular injury, such as

Fanconi's syndrome and interstitial nephritis, may lead to magnesium wasting.

Treatment

Magnesium can be replaced intramuscularly or intravenously. Usually, 24 to 48 mEq per 24 hours as magnesium sulfate is provided (see Chapter 72). Oral magnesium salts such as magnesium oxide are also available, but administering large doses of magnesium orally is difficult because of the cathartic effects of magnesium.

SUGGESTED READINGS

Bilezikian JP, Khan AA, Potts JT: Guidelines for the management of asymptomatic primary hyperparathyroidism: summary statement from the third international workshop, J Clin Endocrinol Metab 94:335–339, 2009.

Christov M, Juppner H: Insights from genetic disorders of phosphate homeostasis, Semin Nephrol 33:143–157, 2013.

Nakajima K, Tamai M, Okaniwa S, et al: Humoral hypercalcemia of malignancy associated with a gastric carcinoma secreting parathyroid hormone, Endocr J 60:557–562, 2013.

Nazeri AS, Reilly RF Jr: Hereditary etiologies of hypomagnesemia, Nat Clin Pract Nephrol 4:80–89, 2008.

Nesbitt MA, Hanan FM, Howles SA, et al: Mutations affecting G-protein subunit alpha-11 in hypercalcemia and hypocalcemia, N Engl J Med 368:2476–2486, 2013.

Rosen CJ, editor: The American Society for Bone and Mineral Research primer on metabolic bone diseases and disorders of mineral metabolism, ed 8, Washington, D.C., 2013, American Society for Bone and Mineral Research.

Stewart AF: Hypercalcemia associated with cancer, N Engl J Med 352:373–379, 2005.

Stewart AF: Translational implications of the parathyroid calcium receptor, N Engl J Med 351:324–326, 2004.

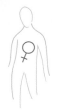

74

Metabolic Bone Diseases

Mara J. Horwitz and Andrew F. Stewart

INTRODUCTION

Metabolic bone disease is a general term used to describe a host of diffuse skeletal disorders. Many are associated with low bone mass, and some are not metabolic but have genetic, infectious, or other causes. However, metabolic bone disease remains a useful umbrella term. In its broadest sense, it includes common diseases such as osteoporosis (see Chapter 75), rare osteosclerotic disorders such as fluoride intoxication, genetic disorders, and focal skeletal diseases such as polyostotic fibrous dysplasia.

In this chapter, the focus is on the more common members of this family (Table 74-1) that may be encountered by an internist. Many additional rare metabolic bone diseases exist and, depending on the context, should be sought. Normal skeletal homeostasis and histopathology are reviewed in Chapter 72 and Figure 74-1.

Osteoclast and osteoblast activity and osteoid mineralization can be assessed by undecalcified bone biopsy of the anterior iliac crest, which is the standard for assessing bone histology. Undecalcified sections are essential because the acid-mediated decalcification performed on routine pathology specimens removes calcium and therefore cannot distinguish between mineralized mature bone and unmineralized osteoid that may be normal or pathologic. The examples shown in Figure 74-1 employ histologic sections of undecalcified bone and highlight osteoclasts, osteoblasts, and osteoid. Because tetracycline is fluorescent and incorporated into the hydroxyapatite crystals as osteoid mineralizes, administering tetracycline to patients before a bone biopsy allows assessment of the rates and efficacy of skeletal mineralization (see Fig. 74-1B and F).

DIFFERENTIAL DIAGNOSIS
Paget's Disease of Bone

Paget's disease, also called *otitis deformans*, is the second most common bone disease after osteoporosis. It affects approximately 2% of the population older than 45 years of age in the United States, but the incidence varies geographically. It is most common in those of European descent and rare in those of African or Asian descent.

In contrast to most metabolic bone diseases, which are diffuse and involve the entire skeleton, Paget's disease is a focal bone disorder. It can be *monostotic* (involving a single bone) or *polyostotic* (involving multiple bones). Paget's disease may affect any skeletal site, but it most commonly involves the pelvis, vertebrae, skull, tibia, and femur. Although Paget's disease is a chronic condition and original lesions may expand, new lesions rarely develop.

The primary cellular abnormality of Paget's disease is increased osteoclastic bone resorption, which is followed by exuberant formation of new bone that is of poor quality (see Fig. 74-1C). This marked increase in osteoblast activity accounts for the typical sclerotic lesions seen on radiographic examination (Fig. 74-2A-C), for the increased uptake of radionuclide seen on a bone scan (see Fig. 74-2D), and for increases in serum levels of alkaline phosphatase, which is the biochemical hallmark of Paget's disease.

Most patients with Paget's disease are asymptomatic, and the disorder is most often detected unexpectedly by an increased serum alkaline phosphatase level on routine testing or on a routine radiograph obtained for other reasons. At clinical presentation, patients may have bone pain, skeletal deformities, fractures, related complications such as osteoarthritis, and nerve compression syndromes (e.g., deafness, spinal stenosis). Rare complications include hypercalcemia in immobilized patients and high-output cardiac failure. Because pagetic lesions tend to be highly vascular, the skin over affected bones may be warmer than in other areas. The most dreaded complication of Paget's disease is the rare (<1%) development of osteosarcoma in a pagetic lesion.

The cause of Paget's disease is unknown but may include a viral origin and a genetic predisposition. Paget's disease is most often diagnosed using a combination of biochemical markers for bone turnover and radiologic studies. For most

TABLE 74-1	CONDITIONS, DISEASES, AND MEDICATIONS THAT CAUSE OR CONTRIBUTE TO METABOLIC BONE DISEASE
Osteoporosis (see Chapter 75)	Osteoporosis-pseudoglioma syndrome
Paget disease of bone	X-linked osteoporosis
Hyperparathyroid bone disease (i.e., osteitis fibrosa cystica)	Miscellaneous factors
Osteomalacia and rickets	Infiltrative diseases
Hypophosphatemic syndromes	Multiple myeloma
Vitamin D syndromes	Lymphoma, leukemia
Anticonvulsants	Sarcoid
Aluminum	Malignant histiocytosis
Metabolic acidosis	Mastocytosis
Renal osteodystrophy	Gaucher' disease
Genetic diseases	Hemolytic diseases (e.g., thalassemia, sickle cell anemia)
Osteogenesis imperfecta	Transplantation osteodystrophy
Hypophosphatasia	

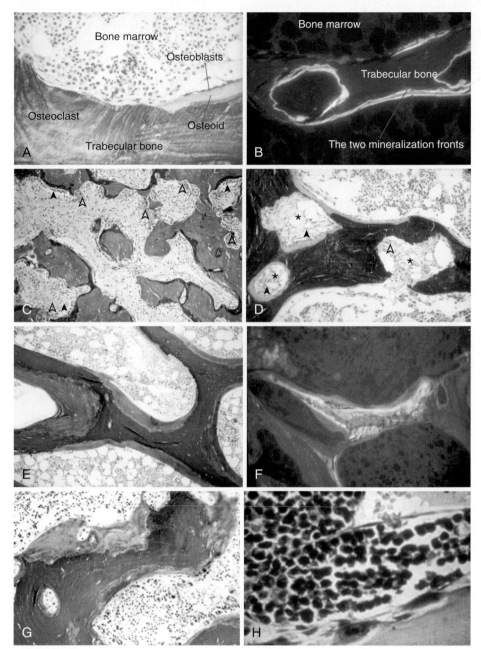

FIGURE 74-1 **A,** Normal bone histology, showing a normal bone-remodeling unit as seen in an undecalcified human anterior iliac crest biopsy. On the left, a multinucleated osteoclast has moved across the mineralized trabecular bone surface over the previous week or two, resorbing (removing) old bone. On the extreme right, the bone surface is covered by osteoid secreted by the overlying osteoblasts. In between the osteoclast- and osteoblast-covered surfaces of the trabecular bone are a large number of flat, fibroblastoid cells referred to as *lining cells*. No osteocytes are visible in this section. **B,** Tetracycline labeling of a bone biopsy from a patient with hyperparathyroid bone disease. Notice the bright yellow parallel lines on the trabecular bone surface. These lines represent the two sets of tetracycline labeling, which occurred 14 days apart. From these sets, the mineralization rate can be described in micrometers (microns) per day, the so-called *mineral apposition rate*, and it is increased dramatically in this example, as is typical of hyperparathyroid bone disease. Contrast with example **F,** which has no tetracycline labeling. **C,** Paget's disease. Enormous and abundant highly multinucleated osteoclasts *(open arrowheads)* are resorbing trabecular bone, and a comparably enormous number of osteoblasts *(closed arrowheads)* are making new but disorganized bone. The marrow space is replaced by fibrous cells. **D,** Primary hyperparathyroidism has the classic features of osteitis fibrosa cystica. Far more osteoid and osteoblasts *(closed arrowheads)* and osteoclasts *(open arrowhead)* exist than in the normal example (**A**). Three large microcysts *(asterisks)* have been created by aggressive osteoclastic bone resorption. These microcysts account for the *cystica* component of osteitis fibrosa cystica. The marrow space, particularly within the microcysts, is filled with fibroblasts, which make up the *fibrosa* component of osteitis fibrosa cystica. **E,** Osteomalacia or rickets. Notice the abundant quantities of partially and chaotically mineralized osteoid *(orange)*. These seams are the thick osteoid seams and represent osteoid that has been produced by osteoblasts but that cannot mineralize, which is the signature defect in osteomalacia and rickets. **F,** Tetracycline labeling reveals a complete absence of mineralization, diagnostic of osteomalacia or rickets. Compare with example **B. G,** Renal osteodystrophy. This photomicrograph of a biopsy from a patient on dialysis demonstrates many of the classic features of renal osteodystrophy, including evidence of aggressive osteoclastic bone resorption (i.e., numerous osteoclastic lacunae on the bone surface compared with the smooth surfaces in example **A**) and abundant, partially and chaotically mineralized areas of osteoid *(orange)*. **H,** Infiltrative bone disease as exemplified by multiple myeloma. The bone marrow is replaced by plasma cells, and two large osteoclasts in lacunae are actively resorbing the trabecular bone surface.

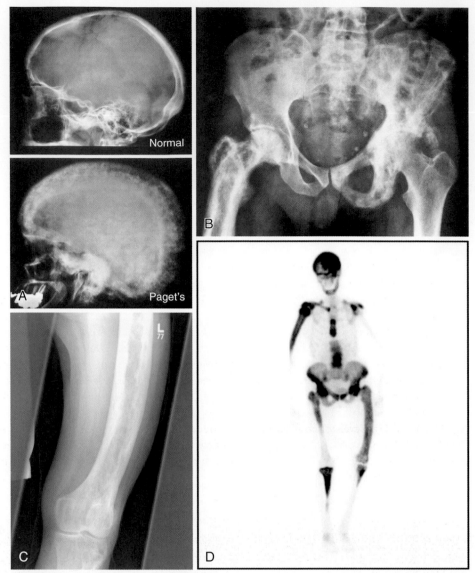

FIGURE 74-2 Typical radiologic abnormalities Paget's disease. **A,** Compare the normal skull *(top)* with the skull *(bottom)* with the classic cotton-wool appearance, an enormously expanded calvarium, and osteosclerosis of the petrous bones. **B,** Classic asymmetrical involvement of the pelvis with a mixture of lytic and blastic lesions. **C,** Bowing deformity of the femur with a markedly thickened cortex. **D,** A whole body radionuclide scan demonstrates polyostotic Paget's disease.

patients, elevated concentrations of total serum alkaline phosphatase is an adequate and sensitive indicator of disease activity. However, the serum level of bone-specific alkaline phosphatase may be a more sensitive marker than serum total alkaline phosphatase for assessing disease in patients with low levels of disease activity. A bone scan at the time of diagnosis can define the location and extent of lesions (see Fig. 74-2D). Radiographs of the affected areas confirm Paget's disease, and they are useful for evaluating complications and local disease progression (Fig. 74-2A-C).

The two major goals of therapy are to relieve symptoms and prevent complications. Indications for treatment include alleviating symptoms (e.g., bone pain, headache, neurologic complications), decreasing blood flow preoperatively to minimize bleeding during elective surgery on a pagetic site, managing hypercalcemia in an immobilized patient with severe Paget's disease, and preventing future complications of progressive local

disease, such as bowing deformities of the long bones, hearing loss as a result of temporal bone involvement, and neurologic complications resulting from foramen magnum or vertebral involvement. Treatment of Paget's disease usually involves a combination of nonpharmacologic therapy (i.e., physical therapy) and pharmacologic therapy, including antiresorptive agents and analgesics for pain management.

The mainstay of therapy is bisphosphonates, including potent aminobisphosphonates such as zoledronate, which decrease bone resorption at pagetic sites by inhibiting osteoclasts. Calcium and vitamin D supplementation is recommended for patients taking the more potent bisphosphonates to prevent hypocalcemia or secondary hyperparathyroidism.

Orthopedic surgery may be indicated when a complete fracture occurs through pagetic bone. Surgery also is indicated for realignment of a severely arthritic knee and for total joint arthroplasty in a severely affected hip or knee.

Hyperparathyroid Bone Disease

Hyperparathyroid bone disease, also called *osteitis fibrosa cystica* (OFC), results from chronically elevated concentrations of parathyroid hormone (PTH). Elevated PTH concentrations may result from primary hyperparathyroidism, in which elevated PTH levels most often result from a parathyroid adenoma or rarely from hyperplasia or carcinoma.

Secondary hyperparathyroidism is an appropriate increase in PTH levels caused by malabsorption, vitamin D deficiency, or chronic renal failure. Calcium levels are normal or subnormal.

Tertiary hyperparathyroidism refers to elevated PTH resulting from long-standing stimulation of the parathyroid glands along with hypercalcemia, as in the setting of renal failure (see Chapter 73). Chronic stimulation results in hyperplasia or adenomas.

Primary and tertiary forms of hyperparathyroidism are characterized by hypercalcemia. Patients with secondary hyperparathyroidism are eucalcemic or hypocalcemic and have elevated PTH levels.

The skeletal disease in hyperparathyroidism is typified by *high turnover,* which is characterized by coupled increases in osteoclastic bone resorption and osteoblastic synthesis of osteoid, accelerated rates of bone mineralization accompanied by microcysts in the cortex and trabeculae (the *cystica* of OFC), and increased numbers of fibroblasts and marrow stroma (the *fibrosa* of OFC) (see Fig. 74-1B and D). Levels of both serum markers of bone formation (i.e., alkaline phosphatase and osteocalcin) and markers of bone resorption (i.e., N-terminal and C-terminal telopeptides) are usually increased, reflecting the bone histology. Patients may complain of bone pain or diffuse aches and pains.

Bone density, assessed by dual-energy x-ray absorptiometry (DEXA), may be normal or low. The pathognomonic radiologic signs of severe hyperparathyroid bone disease are a salt-and-pepper appearance of the calvarium, resorption of the tufts of the terminal phalanges and distal clavicles, subperiosteal resorption of the radial aspect of the cortex of the second phalanges (Fig 74-3), and Brown tumors (i.e., collections of osteoclasts that produce gross lytic lesions) of the pelvis and long bones. These radiologic signs disappear with parathyroidectomy, and bone mass, as assessed by DEXA, typically increases rapidly and markedly after parathyroidectomy.

The treatment of hyperparathyroid bone disease involves remediation of the chronically elevated PTH concentrations by parathyroidectomy in primary or tertiary hyperparathyroidism or correction of the underlying cause of secondary hyperparathyroidism (see Chapter 73). If the hypercalcemia is mild and the bone mass is normal, no treatment may be required.

Serum calcium levels can be reduced by using a parathyroid calcium receptor mimetic. Cinacalcet is indicated for patients with chronic renal failure with secondary hyperparathyroidism, patients with parathyroid carcinoma who have failed surgical resection, and patients with severe primary hyperparathyroidism.

Moderate to severe hypocalcemia may be seen after parathyroidectomy. This condition is referred to as the *hungry bone syndrome* (see Chapter 73). Hyperparathyroid bone disease may be *pure,* occurring in patients with severe primary

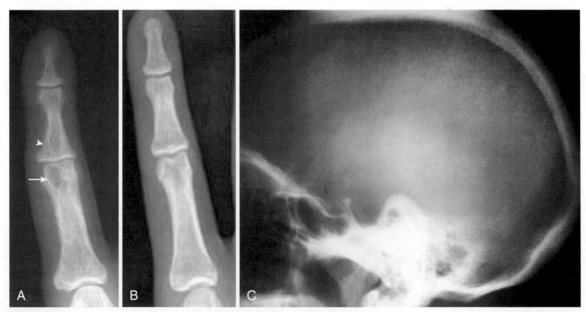

FIGURE 74-3 Skeletal radiographic changes of hyperparathyroidism. **A,** A hand film from a patient with primary hyperparathyroidism. The *arrow* indicates a typical giant cell tumor (brown tumor), which is a collection of osteoclasts that lead to macrocystic changes in bone. The *arrowhead* indicates the irregular radial surface of a phalanx resulting from subperiosteal bone resorption, which is typical of hyperparathyroidism. The brown tumor and the subperiosteal resorption refill and disappear when the offending parathyroid tumor or hyperplasia is resected. **B,** Radiograph of a normal hand for comparison. No brown tumors are seen, and the phalangeal periosteal surfaces are smooth. **C,** The classic salt-and-pepper appearance of the skull in hyperparathyroidism. The periosteal surfaces of the inner and outer cortices or tables of the calvarium are indistinct as a result of subperiosteal bone resorption. The lateral view of the calvarium is hazy and indistinct, showing micropunctations. (Courtesy J. Towers, MD, and D. Armfield, MD, University of Pittsburgh, Pittsburgh, Penn.)

hyperparathyroidism caused by a parathyroid adenoma, or it may be *mixed*, occurring in patients with vitamin D–deficient osteomalacia, immunosuppressant-induced transplant bone disease, or renal osteodystrophy.

Osteomalacia and Rickets

Although common in the United States and throughout the world, osteomalacia and rickets are often overlooked. Osteomalacia and rickets are essentially the same disorders, but by definition, rickets occurs in children with open growth plates (i.e., epiphyses), and osteomalacia occurs in adults with closed epiphyses.

The fundamental abnormality in these disorders is an inability to mineralize (i.e., form hydroxylapatite crystals) osteoid seams (see Fig. 74-1). These patients have osteoblasts and can synthesize osteoid, but it is mineralized inefficiently or not at all. This fundamental inability to mineralize osteoid results in accumulation of the characteristic thick osteoid seams seen on bone biopsy (see Fig. 74-1E and F) and a reduction in the mineral content of bone so that it is mechanically deficient. These events lead to bone pain, pseudofractures, fractures, bowing of the long bones, and other skeletal deformities (Fig. 74-4). In children with rickets, the inability to mineralize the growth plate leads to bulbous, knobby deformities of the knees, ankles, and costochondral junctions (i.e., rachitic rosary) and to dental abnormalities. The characteristic radiologic signs of osteomalacia are Looser's zones or Milkman's pseudofractures.

Mineralization disorders result from an inability to form hydroxyapatite (calcium phosphate) crystals in osteoid, the non-mineralized phase of bone. This inability may result from hypophosphatemia (common), calcium deficiency (rare), or vitamin D deficiency (common). Toxins that interfere with mineralization include aluminum, incompletely defined inhibitors of mineralization in uremic plasma, and long-term, high-dose anticonvulsants. Because calcium salts are acid soluble, chronic metabolic acidoses can result in osteomalacia or rickets. Disordered mineralization can be caused by vitamin D deficiency (e.g., malabsorption, liver disease), hypophosphatemic disorders (e.g., X-linked hypophosphatemic rickets, autosomal dominant hypophosphatemia, oncogenic osteomalacia), metabolic acidoses, drug-related disorders, and genetic conditions (e.g., vitamin D–dependent rickets types I and II, hypophosphatasia) (see Chapter 73).

The diagnosis is suggested in the setting of low bone mass, the characteristic radiologic signs described previously, hypocalcemia, elevated PTH and alkaline phosphatase levels, and unexplained bone pain or weakness. However, these are late signs, and the disorder is optimally identified and treated early. The diagnosis is supported by demonstrating reductions of plasma 25-hydroxyvitamin D or its active form, 1,25-dihydroxyvitamin D_3 ($1,25[OH]_2D_3$); hypophosphatemia; or increased alkaline phosphatase levels in an appropriate clinical setting. Hypocalciuria is typical of vitamin D deficiency. Inappropriate phosphaturia with a low tubular maximum for

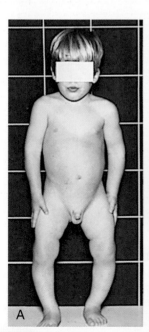
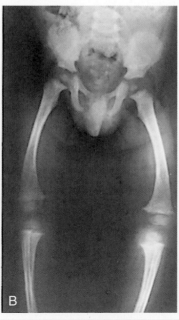
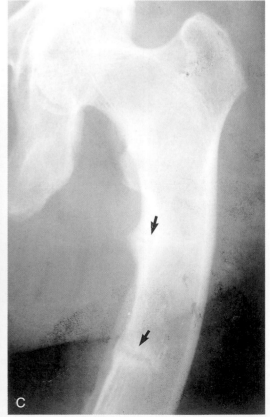

FIGURE 74-4 **A,** A typical example of rickets, with bowing of the femurs and tibias. **B,** A skeletal radiograph of a child with rickets. The weight-bearing bones of the lower extremities are bowed, and the epiphyses are open, mottled, and overgrown. **C,** Looser's zones or pseudofractures *(arrows)* are characteristic of osteomalacia or rickets. The closed epiphyses indicate the patient is an adult. This radiograph is diagnostic of osteomalacia.

phosphorus or glomerular filtration rate (see Chapter 72) typifies renal phosphate wasting disorders. The diagnosis can often be made clinically but can also be confirmed using undecalcified bone biopsy after applying oral double tetracycline labeling techniques, which are used to quantitate the degree of failure of mineralization (Fig 74-1E and F).

Treatment depends on the underlying cause and may include vitamin D formulations, calcium and phosphate supplementation, and removal of the inhibitor of mineralization when possible. These diseases are gratifying to treat because the responses are often dramatic, and patients change rapidly from being chronically ill to feeling robust and healthy.

Renal Osteodystrophy

Renal osteodystrophy is a collection of moderate to severe disorders that produce bone pain, pathologic fractures, and demineralization in the setting of end-stage renal disease or dialysis. Subclinical renal osteodystrophy is common and occurs early as a result of increased levels of phosphorous and fibroblast growth factor 23 (FGF23), which cause defects in skeletal mineralization.

Secondary hyperparathyroidism also may occur as a result of defective renal production of $1,25(OH)_2d$ combined with an increased serum phosphate concentration and calcium-phosphate precipitation into soft tissues (see Chapters 72 and 73). This circumstance evokes a marked increase in PTH secretion that causes significant increases in bone turnover, demineralization, and fracture. These patients may respond dramatically to oral or parenteral replacement of $1,25(OH)_2d$ or the calcium receptor mimetic cinacalcet, or both.

Other patients with renal osteodystrophy have adequately controlled serum levels of calcium and phosphate as a result of adequate oral calcium supplementation and phosphate binders and therefore have standard PTH levels, but they have severe osteomalacia characterized by bone pain, reduced bone mineral density on DEXA or bone biopsy, and thickened osteoid seams with a mineralization defect seen on bone biopsy (see Fig. 74-1G). These patients may respond dramatically to $1,25(OH)_2d$ replacement.

Some patients with renal osteodystrophy have combinations of secondary hyperparathyroidism and osteomalacia (see Fig. 74-1G). Others have low bone turnover or aplastic bone disease. The latter terms describe patients on dialysis who have little or no osteoblastic activity, osteoid, or osteoclastic activity—the opposite of secondary hyperparathyroidism and osteomalacia. The condition may result from previous use of inhibitors of bone turnover (e.g., aluminum intoxication); from excessive treatment with $1,25(OH)_2d$ with suppression of PTH, causing low bone turnover; or from unidentified causes.

For all bone diseases, determining the cause is essential for effective treatment. Early recognition enables treatment before bone pain and fractures occur.

Genetic Diseases

Monogenic disorders that lead to reductions in bone mass are uncommon but are seen with some frequency in practices devoted to skeletal disease. The most common of these disorders is osteogenesis imperfecta, which may be very mild or very severe and may manifest in neonates or older people, depending on the mutation involved. Patients with osteogenesis imperfecta have bone fragility and deformities, and they may have involvement of collagen-containing tissues, including the tendons, skin, and eyes.

Osteogenesis imperfecta most often results from mutations in the genes for type I collagen. In contrast, hypophosphatasia results from mutations in the tissue-nonspecific alkaline phosphatase gene (ALPL). These patients have demineralization, fracture, and bone pain, and they have little or no measurable serum alkaline phosphatase.

New monogenic causes of bone disease continue to appear. For example, the rare osteoporosis-pseudoglioma syndrome (i.e., severe autosomal dominant osteoporosis with blindness) results from inactivating mutations in the low-density lipoprotein receptor–related protein 5 gene (LRP5). Activating mutations in this gene lead to an autosomal dominant form of very high bone mass.

Infiltrative Diseases

Patients with multiple myeloma or Waldenström's macroglobulinemia classically develop skeletal demineralization, which is also true for some patients with leukemia and marrow lymphomas (see Fig 74-1H). Other disorders associated with diffuse marrow infiltration by benign or less malignant processes can lead to diffuse osteopenia, bone pain, and fracture, and they should be considered in the evaluation of unexplained osteoporosis. Examples include hemolytic anemias such as thalassemia or sickle cell disease, sarcoidosis with diffuse marrow involvement, Gaucher's disease with lipid-laden marrow giant cells, malignant mastocytosis, and diffuse histiocytosis.

Transplantation Osteodystrophy

Patients who have undergone or are undergoing organ transplantation commonly have severe osteoporosis. In some patients, this condition is caused by treatment with immunosuppressive drugs such as glucocorticoids, tacrolimus, or cyclosporine, which are potent inhibitors of bone formation and regularly lead to reductions in bone mass.

In many patients, decreased bone mineral density exists before transplantation as a result of organ failure or its treatment. For example, those with primary biliary cirrhosis also may have osteoblast failure and calcium or vitamin D deficiency. In those with end-stage lung or cardiac disease, physical inactivity and generalized malnutrition may contribute to bone demineralization. Patients with end-stage renal disease have all of the components of renal osteodystrophy. This disorder can be expected to become increasingly common as the number of organ transplantations increases.

⬤ TREATMENT

Treatment depends on the underlying disorder. If clinically indicated, primary and tertiary hyperparathyroidism are treated with surgical resection of the affected parathyroid tissue. Osteomalacia and rickets improve when the appropriate replacement drug is administered (i.e., vitamin D, calcium, or phosphate alone or in combination) or the offending agent (e.g., anticonvulsants) is removed.

Secondary hyperparathyroidism in a patient on dialysis can be treated with a combination of the active form of vitamin D ($1,25[OH]_2D_3$ [calcitriol] or analogues), calcium supplementation, phosphate binders, and cinacalcet, depending on the clinical situation. Secondary hyperparathyroidism due to vitamin D deficiency should be treated with the oral parent compound, vitamin D. Other items in Table 74-1 require attention during treatment of the underlying disorder.

These disorders are commonly amenable to treatment, and patients can have dramatic and satisfying responses to therapy. The main stumbling block is that these diagnoses may not be considered; instead, the DEXA report of osteoporosis is passively accepted without further investigation. When a patient is diagnosed with osteoporosis on the basis of a bone density study or radiograph, the physician should review the checklist in Table 74-1 and eliminate or investigate alternative disorders.

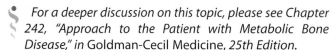
For a deeper discussion on this topic, please see Chapter 242, "Approach to the Patient with Metabolic Bone Disease," in Goldman-Cecil Medicine, *25th Edition.*

SUGGESTED READINGS

Christov M, Pereira R, Wesselig-Perry K: Bone biopsy in renal osteodystrophy: continued insights into a complex disease, Curr Opin Nephrol Hypertens 22:210–215, 2013.

Khosla S, Westendorf JJ, Oursler MJ: Building bone to reverse osteoporosis and repair fractures, J Clin Invest 118:421–428, 2008.

Lindsay R, Cosman F, Zhao H, et al: A novel tetracycline labeling strategy for longitudinal evaluation of the short term effects of anabolic therapy with a single iliac crest bone biopsy, J Bone Miner Res 21:366–373, 2006.

Moe S, Drueke T, Cunningham J, et al: Definition, evaluation and classification of renal osteodystrophy: a position statement from Kidney Disease: Improving Global Outcomes (KIDIGO), Kidney Int 69:1945–1953, 2006.

Ralston SH: Paget's disease of bone, N Engl J Med 368:644–650, 2013.

Rosen CJ, editor: Primer on the metabolic bone diseases and disorders of mineral metabolism, ed 8, Ames Iowa, 2013, J Wiley & Sons and American Society for Bone and Mineral Research.

Stewart AF: Translational implications of the parathyroid calcium receptor, N Engl J Med 351:324–326, 2004.

75

Osteoporosis

Susan L. Greenspan

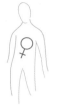

INTRODUCTION

Osteoporosis, the most common disorder of bone and mineral metabolism, affects about 50% of women and 25% of men older than 50 years. The National Institutes of Health Consensus Development Panel on Osteoporosis Prevention defines osteoporosis as a skeletal disorder characterized by compromised bone strength, predisposing a person to an increased risk of fracture. Bone strength has two main components: bone density and bone quality. Bone density reflects the peak adult bone mass and the amount of bone lost in adulthood. Bone quality is determined by bone architecture, bone geometry, bone turnover, mineralization, and damage accumulation (i.e., microfractures) (Fig. 75-1).

DEFINITION AND EPIDEMIOLOGY

In the United States, 2 million osteoporotic fractures occur each year. There are almost 300,000 hip fractures each year, which are associated with a mortality rate of more than 20% during the first year. More than 50% of patients with hip fracture are unable to return to their previous ambulatory state, and about 20% of them are placed in long-term care facilities. When defined by bone mineral densitometry, 48 million Americans have low bone mass, and 9 million have osteoporosis. Although morbidity is less with vertebral fractures, the 5-year mortality rate is similar to that for hip fractures. Only one third of radiologically diagnosed vertebral fractures receive medical attention.

PATHOLOGY AND RISK FACTORS

Peak bone mass is determined primarily by genetic factors. Men have a higher bone mass than women, and African Americans and Hispanics have a higher bone mass than whites. Other factors that contribute to the development of peak bone mass are the use of gonadal steroids, timing of puberty, calcium intake, exercise, and growth hormone.

The causes of bone loss in adults are multifactorial. The pattern of bone loss is different in women than than in men, and bone

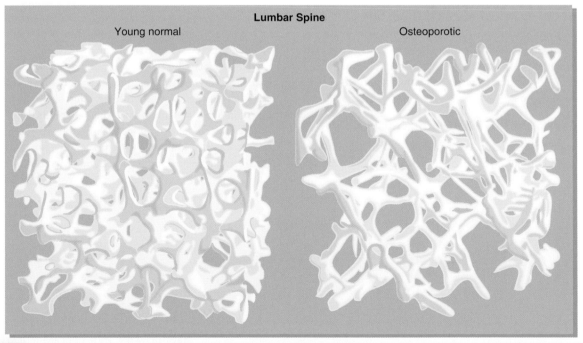

FIGURE 75-1 Three-dimensional reconstruction by microcomputed tomography of a lumbar spine sample from a young adult normal woman and from a woman with postmenopausal osteoporosis. In the osteoporotic woman, bone mass is reduced and microarchitectural bone structure is deteriorated. Whereas the platelike structure in the normal case is very isotropic, the structure in the osteoporotic case shows preferential loss of horizontal struts; the plates have become rods that are thin and farther apart, and there is a concomitant loss of trabecular connectivity. These changes lead to a reduction in bone strength that is more than would be predicted by the decrease in bone mineral density. (From Riggs BL, Khosla S, Melton LJ 3rd: Sex steroids and the construction and conservation of the adult skeleton, Endocr Rev 23:279–302, 2002; Courtesy Ralph Mueller, PhD, Swiss Federal Institute of Technology [ETH] and University of Zurich, Switzerland.)

loss is greater in sites rich in trabecular bone (e.g., spine) than cortical bone (e.g., femoral neck) (Fig. 75-2). Women lose significantly more trabecular bone than men. Estrogen deficiency during menopause contributes significantly to bone loss in women, and they may lose 1% to 5% of bone mass per year in the first few years after menopause. Women continue to lose bone mass throughout the remainder of their lives, with another acceleration of bone loss occurring after age 75 years. The mechanism of this accelerated loss in old age is not clear.

Multiple causes of secondary bone loss contribute to osteoporosis and fractures. Medications that commonly cause bone loss include glucocorticoids, antiseizure medications, excess thyroid hormone, heparin, androgen deprivation therapy, aromatase inhibitors, and depo-medroxyprogesterone. Endocrine diseases resulting in female or male hypogonadism also lead to bone loss. Hyperparathyroidism, hyperthyroidism, and hypercortisolism commonly cause bone loss, as can vitamin D deficiency. Gastrointestinal problems can contribute to decreased absorption of calcium and vitamin D (Table 75-1). Risk factors for falls (e.g., age, poor vision, previous falls, immobility, orthostatic hypotension, cognitive impairment, vitamin D insufficiency, poor balance, gait problems, weak muscles) also contribute to fractures.

● CLINICAL PRESENTATION

Unlike many other chronic diseases with multiple signs and symptoms, osteoporosis is considered a silent disease until fractures occur. Whereas 90% of hip fractures occur after a fall, two thirds of vertebral fractures are silent and occur with minimal stress, such as lifting, sneezing, and bending. An acute vertebral fracture may result in significant back pain that decreases gradually over several weeks with analgesics and physical therapy. Patients with significant vertebral osteoporosis may have height loss, kyphosis, and severe cervical lordosis, also known as a *dowager's hump*. Prolonged bisphosphonate use (>5 years) may result in an atypical femoral fracture, which may manifest as unilateral or bilateral thigh pain and result in a femoral shaft fracture with no or minimal trauma.

● DIAGNOSIS AND DIFFERENTIAL DIAGNOSIS

The diagnosis of osteoporosis is made after an acute clinical vertebral or hip fracture or on assessment of bone mineral density.

Radiography

Radiographs can reveal a vertebral compression fracture (Fig. 75-3). However, low bone mass may not be evident on radiographs until 30% of the mass has been lost. When assessing bone mass, radiographs may be read inappropriately as a result of overpenetration or underpenetration of the film. Radiographs therefore are a poor indicator of osteoporosis (with the exception of vertebral fractures), and the diagnosis is instead often based on bone mineral densitometric results.

Bone Mineral Density and Other Bone Mass Assessments

In 1994, the World Health Organization (WHO) developed a classification system for osteoporosis and low bone mass based on data from white, postmenopausal women (Table 75-2). Osteoporosis is defined as a bone mineral density less than or equal to 2.5 standard deviations (SDs) below young adult peak bone mass (T-score ≤ −2.5 SD). Low bone mass (i.e., osteopenia) is defined as a bone mass measurement between 1.0 and 2.5 SDs below adult peak bone mass (T-score between −1.0 and −2.5 SD). Normal bone mineral density is defined as assessments above 1.0 SD below adult peak bone mass (T-score ≥ −1.0 SD).

The standard for assessing bone mineral density is dual-energy x-ray absorptiometry (DEXA), which has excellent precision and accuracy. Measurements are made at the hip and spine, and in about 30% of cases, discordance is found between these measurements (Fig. 75-4). Classification should be made only if two or more vertebrae are available for analysis because of the high error rate when a single vertebra is assessed. Classification is based on the lowest value (i.e., total spine, total hip, or femoral neck).

In patients with hyperparathyroidism, in which cortical bone loss is often seen, forearm DEXA using the one-third distal radius site should also be assessed. Forearm assessments may be helpful in older patients who often have falsely elevated bone mineral density measurements at the spine as a result of atypical calcifications from degenerative joint disease, sclerosis, or aortic calcifications or in obese patients whose weight exceeds the table limit.

Bone mineral density can be measured by hip or spine quantitative computed tomography (QCT). However, less normative data are available for hip QCT, vertebral precision is inferior to

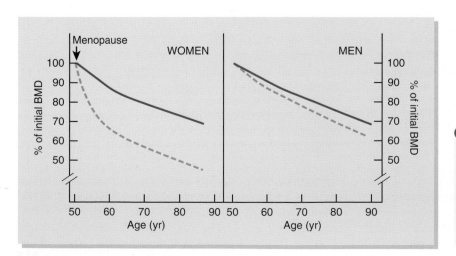

FIGURE 75-2 Patterns of age-related bone loss in women and in men. *Dashed lines* represent trabecular bone, and *solid lines* represent cortical bone. The figure is based on multiple cross-sectional and longitudinal studies using dual-energy x-ray absorptiometry. BMD, Bone mineral density. (From Khosla S, Riggs BL: Pathophysiology of age-related bone loss and osteoporosis, Endocrinol Metab Clin North Am 34:1015–1030, 2005.)

TABLE 75-1 CONDITIONS, DISEASES, AND MEDICATIONS THAT CAUSE OR CONTRIBUTE TO OSTEOPOROSIS AND FRACTURES

LIFESTYLE FACTORS

Alcohol abuse
Excessive thinness
Excess vitamin A
Falling
High salt intake
Immobilization
Inadequate physical activity
Low calcium intake
Smoking (active or passive)
Vitamin D insufficiency

GENETIC FACTORS

Cystic fibrosis
Ehlers-Danlos syndrome
Gaucher's disease
Glycogen storage diseases
Hemochromatosis
Homocystinuria
Hypophosphatasia
Idiopathic hypercalciuria
Marfan syndrome
Osteogenesis imperfecta
Parental history of hip fracture or osteoporosis
Porphyria

HYPOGONADAL STATES

Anorexia nervosa and bulimia
Athletic amenorrhea
Hyperprolactinemia
Male hypogonadism

Panhypopituitarism
Premature and primary ovarian failure
Secondary gonadal failure
Turner's syndrome, Klinefelter's syndrome

ENDOCRINE DISORDERS

Adrenal insufficiency
Cushing's syndrome
Diabetes mellitus (types 1 and 2)
Hyperparathyroidism
Thyrotoxicosis

GASTROINTESTINAL DISORDERS

Celiac disease
Gastric bypass
Gastrointestinal surgery
Inflammatory bowel disease
Malabsorption
Pancreatic disease
Primary biliary cirrhosis

HEMATOLOGIC DISORDERS

Hemophilia
Leukemia and lymphomas
Monoclonal gammopathies
Multiple myeloma
Sickle cell disease
Systemic mastocytosis
Thalassemia

RHEUMATOLOGIC AND AUTOIMMUNE DISEASES

Ankylosing spondylitis
Lupus
Rheumatoid arthritis
Other rheumatic and autoimmune diseases

CENTRAL NERVOUS SYSTEM DISORDERS

Epilepsy
Multiple sclerosis
Parkinson's disease
Spinal cord injury
Stroke

MISCELLANEOUS CONDITIONS AND DISEASES

Human immunodeficiency virus (HIV) infection/acquired immunodeficiency syndrome (AIDS)
Alcoholism
Amyloidosis
Chronic metabolic acidosis
Chronic obstructive lung disease
Congestive heart failure
Depression
End-stage renal disease
Hypercalciuria
Idiopathic scoliosis
Muscular dystrophy

Post-transplantation bone disease
Sarcoidosis
Weight loss

MEDICATIONS

Aluminum (in antacids)
Anticoagulants (heparin)
Anticonvulsants
Aromatase inhibitors
Barbiturates
Cancer chemotherapeutic drugs
Cyclosporine and tacrolimus
Depo-medroxyprogesterone (premenopausal contraception)
Glucocorticoids (≥5 mg/day of prednisone or equivalent for ≥3mo)
Gonadotropin-releasing hormone (GnRH) antagonists and agonists
Lithium
Methotrexate
Parenteral nutrition
Proton pump inhibitors
Selective serotonin reuptake inhibitors
Tamoxifen (premenopausal use)
Thiazolidinediones (e.g., Actos, Avandia)
Thyroid hormones (in excess)

Modified from National Osteoporosis Foundation: 2013 clinician's guide to Prevention and treatment of osteoporosis. Available at http://nof.org/files/nof/public/content/file/917/upload/481.pdf. Accessed August 23, 2014.

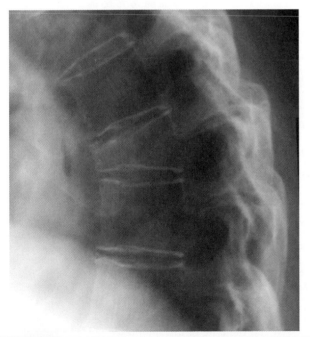

FIGURE 75-3 Lateral spine radiograph demonstrates a thoracic anterior wedge compression fracture.

TABLE 75-2 WORLD HEALTH ORGANIZATION CLASSIFICATION FOR OSTEOPOROSIS

CLASSIFICATION	CRITERIA FOR BONE MINERAL DENSITY
Normal	Above −1.0 SD of young adult peak mean value
Low bone mass (osteopenia)	Between −1.0 and −2.5 SD of young adult peak mean value
Osteoporosis	Below −2.5 SD of young adult peak mean value

SD, Standard deviation.

The National Osteoporosis Foundation (NOF) recommends obtaining a bone mineral density assessment in all women 65 years old or older and postmenopausal women younger than 65 years with a risk factor (Table 75-3). The U.S. Preventive Services Task Force (USPSTF) recommends bone density tests in all women age 65 or older and women between 60 and 64 years of age with a risk factor. The NOF recommends obtaining a bone mineral density value for men 70 years old or older; the USPSTF has not recommended screening in men. Databases are available for white, African American, Asian, and Hispanic men and women. These guidelines from the NOF and USPSTF for screening patients for osteoporosis are relatively similar for postmenopausal women but differ for older men. At the time of their review, the USPSTF did not feel there was ample evidence to determine screening guidelines for men.

The WHO developed a fracture risk assessment tool (FRAX) to predict the 10-year risk for hip or any major osteoporotic fracture for women and men between 40 and 90 years of age. The FRAX for the individual patient incorporates femoral neck

that of DEXA, and radiation doses are significantly higher than those of DEXA. Single-photon absorptiometry of the forearm and peripheral measures, such as heel ultrasound, have also been used to assess bone mass. However, the WHO classification should be used only with the central DEXA measurements.

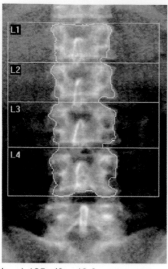

k = 1.135, d0 = 48.6
116 × 137

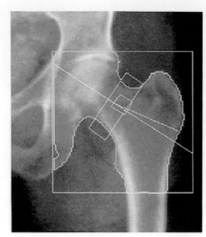

k = 1.145, d0 = 53.2
93 × 97

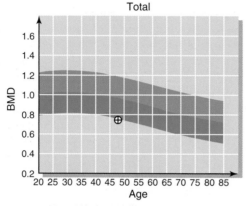

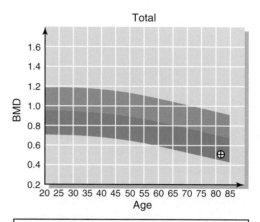

Region	Area (cm²)	BMC (g)	BMD (g/cm²)	T- Score	PR (%)	Z- Score	AM (%)
L1	12.52	8.04	0.642	−2.6	69	−2.0	74
L2	13.41	9.74	0.726	−2.7	71	−2.1	76
L3	16.21	11.96	0.738	−3.1	68	−2.5	73
L4	17.42	13.94	0.800	−2.9	72	−2.2	77
Total	59.56	43.68	0.733	−2.9	70	−2.2	75

Total BMD CV 1.0%, ACF = 1.028, BCF = 1.006, TH = 5.848
WHO Classification: Osteoporosis
Fracture Risk: High

Region	Area (cm²)	BMC (g)	BMD (g/cm²)	T- Score	PR (%)	Z- Score	AM (%)
Neck	4.68	1.89	0.404	−4.0	48	−1.6	69
Troch	10.63	4.13	0.388	−3.1	55	−1.3	75
Inter	16.59	9.90	0.597	−3.2	54	−1.3	74
Total	31.89	15.91	0.499	−3.6	53	−1.5	74
Ward's	1.19	0.32	0.268	−4.0	37	−0.9	72

Total BMD CV 1.0%, ACF = 1.028, BCF = 1.006, TH = 5.163
WHO Classification: Osteoporosis
Fracture Risk: High

FIGURE 75-4 **Left,** This patient has a lumbar spine (L1 through L4) bone mineral density (BMD) of 0.733 g/cm² *(white circle with cross on the graph)* as measured by dual-energy x-ray absorptiometry (DEXA) and a T-score of −2.9. The reference database graph displays age- and sex-matched mean BMD levels ±2 standard deviations (SDs) *(shaded areas)* derived from a normative database from the manufacturer (Hologic, Inc., Bedford, Mass.). The T-score indicates the difference in SD between the patient's BMD and that of the predicted sex-matched mean peak of a young adult; the z-value is the difference in SD between the patient's BMD and the sex-, age-, and ethnicity-matched mean BMD; and the percentage of mean is the patient's BMD as a percentage of the mean peak young adult BMD or age-matched BMD level. **Right,** This patient has a total hip BMD of 0.499 g/cm² *(white circle with cross on the graph)* as measured by DEXA, a femoral neck T-score of −4.0, and a total hip T-score of −3.6. The reference database graph displays age- and sex-matched mean BMD levels ±2 SDs *(shaded areas)* derived from the third National Health and Nutrition Examination Survey. The T-score indicates the difference in SD between the patient's BMD and the predicted sex-matched mean peak young adult BMD; the z-score is the difference in SD between the patient's BMD and the sex-, age-, and ethnicity-matched mean BMD; and the percentage of mean is the patient's BMD as a percentage of the mean peak young adult BMD or age-matched BMD level. (Bone densitometry report for the QDR-4500A bone densitometer, Bedford, Mass., Hologic, Inc.)

T-score, age, gender, height, weight, and specific risk factors, including history of adult fracture, parental hip fracture, current smoking, glucocorticoid use, rheumatoid arthritis, alcohol (≥3 drinks per day), and secondary osteoporosis. The fracture risk prediction is specific for race and country and should be used for patients not on therapy.

Bone mineral density determined by DEXA usually can be monitored after 2 years of therapy, depending on the site to be assessed and the type of therapy prescribed. For example, trabecular bone, which has greater surface area and is more metabolically active than cortical bone, is more likely to show improvements with stronger-acting antiresorptive agents. Changes in bone mass with potent antiresorptive therapy are more prominent in the spine compared with other areas. Seeing no changes in forearm bone mineral density over time is common despite good precision. Although the heel has a high percentage

TABLE 75-3 NATIONAL OSTEOPOROSIS FOUNDATION RECOMMENDATIONS FOR BONE MINERAL DENSITY TESTING

- Women age ≥65 yr and men ≥70 yr, regardless of clinical risk factors
- Younger postmenopausal women, women in the menopausal transition, and men age 50-69 yr with clinical risk factors for fracture
- Adults who have a fracture after age 50 yr
- Adults who have a condition (e.g., rheumatoid arthritis) or are taking a medication (e.g., glucocorticoids in a daily dose of ≥5 mg prednisone or equivalent for ≥3 mo) associated with low bone mass or bone loss

TABLE 75-4 NATIONAL OSTEOPOROSIS FOUNDATION GUIDELINES FOR TREATMENT

- An adult hip or vertebral fragility fracture
- Osteoporosis by DEXA T-score ≤ −2.5 SD for lumbar spine, total hip, or femoral neck after appropriate evaluation
- Low bone mass by DEXA T-scores between −1.0 and −2.5 SD at the lumbar spine or femoral neck and a WHO FRAX 10-year probability of a hip fracture ≥3% or a 10-year probability of major osteoporosis-related fractures ≥20% based on a WHO algorithm

DEXA, Dual-energy x-ray absorptiometry; FRAX, fracture risk assessment tool; SD, standard deviation; WHO, World Health Organization.

of trabecular bone, precision is poor, and monitoring should not be done at this site.

All patients with osteoporosis or low bone mass should have a work-up for secondary causes of bone loss. It should include a serum calcium level (corrected for albumin) to rule out hyperparathyroidism or malnutrition; a 25-hydroxyvitamin D level to assess for vitamin D deficiency or insufficiency; an alkaline phosphatase level to assess for Paget's disease, malignancy, cirrhosis, or vitamin D deficiency; liver and renal function tests to assess for abnormalities; a 24-hour urine calcium and creatinine assay to evaluate for hypercalciuria or malabsorption; a test for sprue in patients with anemia, malabsorption, or hypocalciuria; a thyrotropin level to rule out hyperthyroidism; and serum protein electrophoresis to rule out myeloma in older adults with anemia. Measurement of the parathyroid hormone (PTH) level often is needed to interpret the calcium and vitamin D levels. Total testosterone levels are recommended for men.

A more extensive work-up can be done in severe or unusual cases. A bone biopsy is rarely needed. Markers of bone turnover vary considerably in clinical practice, and these tests usually are reserved for research. However, they may be useful for assessing the rate of bone turnover after prolonged bisphosphonate use or a bisphosphonate holiday.

PREVENTION

General preventive measures for all patients include adequate calcium and vitamin D intake, exercise, and fall prevention techniques. The recommended daily allowance of calcium for adults, as reviewed by the Institute of Medicine, is 1200 mg. Calcium intake can be accomplished by dietary consumption, supplementation, or the combination of diet plus supplement. The supplements should be pure calcium carbonate or pure calcium citrate, taken in divided doses of about 500 to 600 mg twice daily. Calcium carbonate should be taken with meals for best absorption, whereas calcium citrate may be taken with or without food. Calcium supplements are available as tablets and in chewable and liquid forms. Foods such as orange juice, cereals, breads, and nutrition bars are calcium fortified. There is no benefit to taking more than 1200 mg per day, and excess intake may increase the risk of kidney stones and cardiovascular disease (although data are controversial).

Vitamin D is important for calcium absorption and bone mineralization. Vitamin D has nonskeletal benefits and has been associated with improvement in muscle strength and prevention of falls. Vitamin D comes from two sources: diet and photosynthesis. Because dietary sources of vitamin D are limited (e.g., fortified milk, yogurt) and patients are often advised to avoid sun exposure for prevention of skin cancer and wrinkles, many studies have documented vitamin D deficiency and insufficiency in older adults. Older patients have a reduced ability to synthesize vitamin D in the skin. Low vitamin D levels can lead to secondary hyperparathyroidism.

Vitamin D can be taken in a multivitamin, in a calcium supplement, or in pure form and is available as cholecalciferol (D_3) or ergocalciferol (D_2). Based on data from noninstitutionalized patients without osteoporosis, the daily dose recommended by the Institute of Medicine is 600 IU per day for adults up to age 70 and 800 units for those older than 70 years to achieve a level of at least 20 ng/dL (50 nmol/L). However, the NOF suggests 800 to 1000 IU per day. Elderly patients, those with malabsorption, and obese patients may need greater amounts of vitamin D. Older patients with severe vitamin D deficiency may be given 50,000 IU of vitamin D once per week for 3 months to bring serum vitamin D into the normal range. Activated vitamin D is rarely needed and should not be given on a regular basis for postmenopausal osteoporosis.

Weight-bearing exercise is important for maintaining skeletal integrity. Study results are controversial concerning different types and durations of exercise by postmenopausal women and men. However, weight-bearing or resistance training exercises usually are suggested and have been shown to improve bone mass or maintain skeletal integrity. In patients with new vertebral fractures, physical therapy is important for improving posture and increasing the strength of back muscles.

Because 90% of hip fractures and a significant number of vertebral fractures occur during a fall, preventive measures are suggested for frail older patients at risk for falling. Fall-proofing the household includes installing grab bars in the bathroom and hand rails on stairways, avoiding loose throw rugs and cords, ensuring good lighting by the bedside, and moving objects within easy reach in the kitchen. Other fall prevention measures include eliminating medications that cause dizziness or postural hypotension (if possible), assessing the need for assistive devices (e.g., canes, walkers), and ensuring appropriate footwear and good vision. The benefits of hip protectors for hip fracture reduction are disappointing and controversial, and compliance with these products is often poor.

TREATMENT AND PROGNOSIS

The NOF developed treatment guidelines that incorporate a 10-year fracture risk prediction. The NOF suggests treatment for postmenopausal women and men 50 years old or older, as shown in Table 75-4.

Patients taking glucocorticoids can fracture despite having normal bone density. The American College of Rheumatology suggests that patients starting glucocorticoids who will be treated for 3 months or longer have a bone density test and start antiresorptive therapy if indicated according to their guidelines.

Bisphosphonates

Bisphosphonates are the mainstay of osteoporosis prevention and treatment. They inhibit the cholesterol synthesis pathway in osteoclasts, causing early apoptosis and inhibiting osteoclast migration and attachment. Unlike other agents, bisphosphonates are incorporated into bone, the half-life is long, and the agent may be recycled.

In the United States, the bisphosphonates alendronate, risedronate, ibandronate, and zoledronic acid have been approved for the prevention and treatment of osteoporosis. Alendronate can increase bone mass by about 8% at the spine and 4% at the hip over 3 years. This increase has been associated with an approximately 50% reduction in spine, hip, and forearm fractures (Table 75-5). Alendronate is prescribed at 35 mg once weekly for osteoporosis prevention and 70 mg once weekly for the treatment of osteoporosis. Alendronate has been approved for use in men and patients with glucocorticoid-induced osteoporosis.

Risedronate is approved for the prevention and treatment of osteoporosis at a dose of 35 mg per week or 150 mg per month or as a delayed dose after breakfast of 35 mg per week. Large-scale, multicenter studies have shown improvements in bone mass of about 6% to 7% at the spine and 3% at the hip over 3 years. These studies revealed a 50% reduction in vertebral fractures, 40% reduction in nonvertebral fractures, and 40% reduction in hip fractures (see Table 75-5). Risedronate is approved for the treatment of osteoporosis in men and for the prevention and treatment of patients with glucocorticoid-induced osteoporosis.

Oral ibandronate is approved for the prevention and treatment of postmenopausal osteoporosis. After 3 years of treatment, ibandronate increased bone density by 6.5% at the spine and 3.4% at the hip, and it reduced new vertebral fractures by 62%. No reductions in nonvertebral or hip fractures occurred. Ibandronate is approved at an oral dose of 150 mg monthly and for treatment at an intravenous dose of 3 mg every 3 months.

Zoledronic acid is approved for the treatment of postmenopausal osteoporosis, osteoporosis in men, and steroid-induced bone loss. The 3-year pivotal trial demonstrated increases of 6.9% of bone density at the spine and 6.0% at the hip, and the drug reduced spinal fractures by 70%, nonvertebral fractures by 25%, and hip fractures by 41%. Zoledronic acid is given at a dose of 5 mg intravenously once per year for treatment and 5 mg intravenously every 24 months for prevention.

Because oral bisphosphonates are poorly absorbed, they must be taken first thing in the morning on an empty stomach with a full glass of water. Patients must wait 30 minutes (when taking alendronate and risedronate) to 60 minutes (when taking ibandronate) before eating and must not lie down. A delayed-release form of risedronate can be taken after breakfast.

Potential side effects of bisphosphonates include epigastric distress, heartburn, and esophagitis. Intravenous bisphosphonates have been associated with an influenza-like syndrome after infusion. Bisphosphonates can also cause arthralgias and myalgias. They are contraindicated in patients with renal insufficiency (i.e., estimated glomerular filtration rate of 30 to 35 mL/minute). Osteonecrosis of the jaw is a rare adverse event of abnormal bone growth in the jaw, which is more often associated with high-dose intravenous bisphosphonates in patients with cancer and poor oral hygiene. Atypical femoral shaft fractures have been reported rarely after long-term use (>5 years) of bisphosphonates. These fractures may manifest with a prodrome of unilateral or bilateral thigh pain, and fractures may occur with minimal activity. These fractures are rare after osteoporosis treatment but common in cancer patients receiving frequent high doses intravenously.

Calcitonin

Calcitonin is a 32-amino-acid peptide produced by the parafollicular cells of the thyroid gland. The pivotal clinical treatment trial did not show significant changes in bone mineral density after 3 years. However, the 200-IU dose of nasal calcitonin was associated with a 50% reduction in vertebral fractures (see

TABLE 75-5 U.S. FOOD AND DRUG ADMINISTRATION–APPROVED THERAPIES FOR PREVENTION AND TREATMENT OF OSTEOPOROSIS

AGENT	PREVENTION/ TREATMENT	DOSAGE	VERTEBRAL FRACTURE REDUCTION	HIP FRACTURE REDUCTION	WOMEN/ MEN	STEROID- INDUCED OP
Alendronate*	Yes/yes	Prev: 35 mg/wk PO Treat: 70 mg/wk PO	Yes	Yes	Yes/yes	Yes
Ibandronate*	Yes[†]/yes	150 mg/mo PO, 3 mg q3mo IV	Yes	No	Yes/no	No
Risedronate*	Yes/yes	Prev/treat: 35 mg/wk PO, 35 mg/wk PO delayed release, 150 mg/mo PO	Yes	Yes	Yes/yes	Yes
Zoledronic acid*	Yes/yes	Prev: 5 mg q2yr IV Treat: 5 mg/yr IV	Yes	Yes	Yes/yes	Yes
Calcitonin	No/yes	200 IU/day intranasal	Yes	No	Yes/no	No
Denosumab	No/yes	60 mg q6mo SC	Yes	Yes	Yes/yes	Yes
Hormone/estrogen therapy	Yes[‡]/no	Various preparations available	Yes	Yes	Yes[§]/no	No
Raloxifene	Yes/yes	60 mg/day PO	Yes	No	Yes/no	No
Teriparatide (PTH [1-34])	No/yes	20 μg/day SC	Yes	No	Yes/yes	Yes

OP, Osteoporosis; PO, oral administration; prev, prevention; PTH, parathyroid hormone; SC, subcutaneous administration; Treat, treatment.
*Alendronate, risedronate, ibandronate, and zoledronic acid are bisphosphonates.
[†]Oral only.
[‡]Short-term prevention or management.
[§]For management.

Table 75-5). No reduction in nonvertebral or hip fractures was found. The U.S. Food and Drug Administration (FDA) advisory panel is reviewing an association with cancer.

Denosumab

The receptor activator of nuclear factor-κB (RANK) and its ligand (RANKL) are mediators of osteoclast activity. Compared with placebo, denosumab, an antibody to RANKL, produced a relative increase in bone mineral density at the spine of 9.2% and hip of 6.0% over 3 years, and it reduced fractures by 68% at the spine, 40% at the hip, and 20% at nonvertebral sites. Denosumab is approved for postmenopausal women and men with osteoporosis, for men with prostate cancer on androgen deprivation therapy, and for postmenopausal women with breast cancer on aromatase inhibitors. It is given as a subcutaneous 60-mg injection every 6 months.

Estrogen Agonists-Antagonists

Estrogen agonists-antagonists were previously called selective estrogen receptor modulators (SERMs) because they have some estrogen-like and anti–estrogen-like benefits. Raloxifene is approved for the prevention and treatment of osteoporosis. The Multiple Outcomes of Raloxifene Evaluation (MORE) trial found that bone mass was increased by 4% at the spine and 2.5% at the femoral neck over 3 years. This increase was associated with a 50% reduction in vertebral fractures. No reduction in nonvertebral or hip fractures was seen (see Table 75-5). Treatment was associated with improved lipid status, as shown by decreased total and low-density lipoprotein cholesterol.

Raloxifene is not associated with endometrial hyperplasia, and patients should not have bleeding or spotting. They do not have breast tenderness or swelling. Raloxifene reduces the risk for invasive breast cancer in postmenopausal women with osteoporosis and in women at high risk for invasive breast cancer. Patients have the same small risk of deep vein thrombosis or pulmonary embolus that is found with hormone therapy. Raloxifene does not relieve postmenopausal symptoms and may exacerbate hot flashes. Studies have not found a significant impact on cardiovascular disease. Raloxifene can be given with or without food in a daily oral dose of 60 mg per day.

Hormone Therapy

Investigators of the Women's Health Initiative, a large, randomized, placebo-controlled, multicenter trial evaluating hormone therapy, reported a 36% reduction in hip and vertebral fractures after 5.2 years. In addition to improvements in bone mass, benefits include an improved lipid profile, decreased colon cancer incidence, and decreased menopausal symptoms. However, because of the potential risks of hormone therapy (i.e., cardiovascular events, breast cancer, deep vein thrombosis, pulmonary embolus, and gallbladder problems), it should be used only for prevention or management of menopausal symptoms, and other agents should be used for the treatment of osteoporosis.

Parathyroid Hormone

Recombinant human PTH (1-34), or teriparatide, is an osteoanabolic agent that increases spinal bone mineral density by 9.7%

and hip bone mineral density by 2.6% in 18 months. It is associated with a 65% reduction in vertebral fractures and a 53% reduction in nonvertebral fractures. Teriparatide is taken for up to 2 years as a subcutaneous, 20-µg daily dose for postmenopausal women and men at high risk for fracture. After therapy, patients benefit from antiresorptive therapy to prevent bone loss. Recombinant human PTH (1-84) is approved for use in Europe.

Alternative Therapies
Medical Therapies

Strontium ranelate is an approved agent for the treatment of osteoporosis in Europe, but it is not FDA approved in the United States. The mechanism of action is not fully understood, but strontium is thought to stimulate osteoblast proliferation and inhibit osteoclast formation. Inhibition of the protease cathepsin K appears to prevent bone resorption with no major impact on bone formation. Another promising osteoanabolic therapeutic target is the inhibition of sclerostin, a potent inhibitor of bone formation, with an antibody.

Combination therapy has been examined with two antiresorptive agents or an antiresorptive and osteoanabolic agent together. Overall, studies with combination therapy have suggested minor improvements in bone mass over therapy with single agents. Because studies have not shown greater fracture reduction, this type of combination therapy with two antiresorptive agents or an antiresorptive plus an osteoanabolic usually is not recommended. However, it is recommended to follow osteoanabolic therapy using teriparatide with an antiresorptive therapy such as a bisphosphonate to maintain the gain.

Vertebroplasty and Kyphoplasty

Vertebroplasty involves injection of cement (i.e., polymethylmethacrylate) into a compressed vertebra to prevent the vertebral body from further collapse. Kyphoplasty introduces a balloon into the vertebral body to expand it, followed by cement placement inside the vertebral body. This approach expands the vertebral body and may increase height. Some studies suggest a significant reduction in pain early on, but the long-term pain reduction may be similar to that of placebo. Ongoing studies are needed to determine whether differences in outcomes can be found between vertebroplasty and kyphoplasty. These procedures are recommended only for patients with significant pain from vertebral fractures and are not routinely performed in asymptomatic patients with vertebral osteoporosis.

SUGGESTED READINGS

Institute of Medicine: Dietary reference intakes for calcium and vitamin D, Washington, D.C., 2011, The National Academies Press.

Kanis JA: Diagnosis of osteoporosis and assessment of fracture risk, Lancet 359:1929–1936, 2002.

National Osteoporosis Foundation: Clinician's guide to prevention and treatment of osteoporosis, Washington, D.C., 2013, The Foundation.

Nelson HD, Helfand M: Screening for postmenopausal osteoporosis. Systematic evidence review no. 17. (Prepared by the Oregon Evidence-based Practice Center for the Agency for Healthcare Research and Quality.) Rockville, Md., 2002, Agency for Healthcare Research and Quality. Accessed at http://www.ahrq.gov/downloads/pub/prevent/pdfser/osteoser.pdf on 3 June 2010.

TABLE 77-1　CLINICAL CHARACTERISTICS OF RHEUMATOID ARTHRITIS

ARTICULAR FEATURES	EXTRA-ARTICULAR FEATURES
Morning stiffness or gelling	Rheumatoid nodules: subcutaneous, pulmonary, sclera
Symmetrical joint swelling	Lung disease
Predilection for wrists and proximal interphalangeal, metacarpophalangeal, and metatarsophalangeal joints	Vasculitis, especially skin and peripheral nerves
Erosions of bone and cartilage	Pleuropericarditis
Joint subluxation and ulnar deviation	Scleritis and episcleritis
Inflammatory joint fluid	Leg ulcers
Carpal tunnel syndrome	Felty's syndrome
Baker's cyst	

TABLE 77-2　2010 ACR/EULAR CLASSIFICATION CRITERIA FOR RHEUMATOID ARTHRITIS

For patients who have at least 1 joint with definite synovitis and for whom the synovitis is not better explained by another disease, a score of at least 6 of 10 points is needed for the classification of definite rheumatoid arthritis.

A.　Joint involvement (0-5 points)
　　1 large joint (0)
　　2-10 large joints (1)
　　1-3 small joints (with or without involvement of large joints) (2)
　　4-10 small joints (or without involvement of large joints) (3)
　　>10 joints (with involvement of at least 1 small joint) (5)
B.　Serology (0-3 points)
　　Negative RF and negative anti-CCP (0)
　　Low-positive RF or low-positive anti-CCP (2)
　　High positive RF or high positive anti-CCP (3)
C.　Acute phase reactants (0-1 points)
　　Normal CRP and normal ESR (0)
　　Abnormal CRP or abnormal ESR (1)
D.　Duration of symptoms (0-1 points)
　　<6 weeks (0)
　　≥6 weeks (1)

Aletaha D, Neogi T, Silman AJ, et al: 2010 Rheumatoid arthritis classification criteria: an American College of Rheumatology/European League Against Rheumatism collaborative initiative, Arthritis Rheum 62:2569–2581, 2010.

ACR, American College of Rheumatology; CCP, cyclic citrullinated peptide; CRP, C-reactive protein; ESR, erythrocyte sedimentation rate; EULAR, European League Against Rheumatism; RF, rheumatoid factor.

often are visible radiographically at the margins of bone and cartilage, the sites of synovial attachment. However, not all patients with RA have erosive disease. Tenosynovitis (i.e., inflammation of tendon sheaths) leads to tendon malalignment and stretching or shortening.

Common deformities are ulnar deviation at the metacarpophalangeal joints and volar subluxation at those joints and at the wrists. Flexion and extension contractures in the proximal and distal interphalangeal (PIP and DIP) joints of the fingers lead to the characteristic swan-neck deformity (i.e., flexion contracture at the DIP joint and hyperextension at the PIP joint) or boutonnière deformity (i.e., flexion contracture at the PIP and hyperextension at the DIP joint).

Synovitis at the wrists can lead to median nerve compression and carpal tunnel syndrome. Rarely, long-standing cervical spine disease may lead to C1-C2 subluxation and spinal cord compression. Rupture of synovial fluid from the knee into the calf (i.e., Baker's cyst) may mimic deep vein thrombosis or occasionally imitate cellulitis.

Extra-articular Manifestations

RA is a systemic disease with multiple extra-articular manifestations (see Table 77-1). Constitutional symptoms include fatigue, low-grade fever, weight loss, and myalgia. Extra-articular manifestations are more common in RF-positive patients with uncontrolled articular disease. On the skin, grossly palpable subcutaneous rheumatoid nodules are common along other extensor tendon surfaces, especially at the elbows, and are associated with RF positivity. Less commonly, rheumatoid nodules may occur in the lungs, pleura, pericardium, sclerae, and other sites, including the heart in rare cases. In the eyes, RA commonly is associated with keratoconjunctivitis sicca with coexistent Sjögren syndrome and less often with scleritis and episcleritis.

Lung involvement in RA usually includes interstitial lung disease and may include pleuropericarditis, producing pleural and pericardial effusions. The cardiovascular effects of RA can range from long-term inflammation leading to progressive coronary artery disease to pericarditis to a small and medium-sized vasculitis. The vasculitis of RA can produce cutaneous lesions (e.g., ulcers, skin necrosis) and mononeuritis multiplex.

RA commonly has hematologic complications and is associated with anemia of chronic disease and thrombocytosis. Patients with RA also have an increased incidence of lymphoma. Felty's syndrome (i.e., splenomegaly, leukopenia, and recurrent

pulmonary infections) is a rare complication and is often accompanied by leg ulcers and vasculitis.

DIAGNOSIS AND DIFFERENTIAL DIAGNOSIS

RA is a clinical diagnosis based on a thorough history and physical examination. Classic symptoms include morning stiffness associated with symmetrical synovitis of small joints. No single diagnostic test enables a diagnosis of RA to be made with certainty. Instead, the diagnosis depends on the accumulation of characteristic symptoms, signs, laboratory data, and radiologic findings.

Classification criteria are useful in guiding the clinical diagnosis of RA. The classification criteria have been updated to include early RA (Table 77-2) because prompt diagnosis and treatment are important to prevent disease progression, joint deformities, and disability.

The differential diagnosis for RA includes viral arthritis (e.g., parvovirus, rubella, hepatitis B and C), thyroid disorders, sarcoidosis, reactive arthritis, psoriatic arthritis, Sjögren syndrome, systemic lupus erythematosus (SLE), bacterial endocarditis, rheumatic fever, calcium pyrophosphate disease (CPPD), chronic tophaceous gout, polymyalgia rheumatic, erosive osteoarthritis, and fibromyalgia. A history and physical examination, including a thorough review of systems, help to determine the diagnosis.

RF is an antibody (typically IgM but also IgG or others) that binds to the Fc fragment of IgG. RF and IgG join to form immune complexes that are detectable in the serum of 70% to 80% of patients with RA. However, RF is not specific for RA and frequently occurs in patients with SLE, Sjögren syndrome, endocarditis, sarcoidosis, and lung and liver diseases (including hepatitis B and C infection) and in healthy individuals. In an individual patient, the titer does not correlate with disease activity, but high titers are associated with severe erosive arthritis and extra-articular disease. The finding of RF in serum alone does not establish a diagnosis of RA, but it can help to confirm the clinical impression.

Anti-CCP antibodies are a more specific marker for RA. Anti-CCP antibodies have a higher specificity (>95%) than RF, with similar sensitivity (68% to 80%). These antibodies can be detected several years before the development of clinical RA (and before RF), and they are associated with severe RA outcomes, including radiographic joint damage and a poor prognosis. Because of their higher specificity for RA, anti-CCP antibodies are useful in differentiating RA from other conditions positive for RF, including Sjögren syndrome, infection, and hepatitis.

Acute phase reactants, such as the erythrocyte sedimentation rate and C-reactive protein, are usually elevated in active inflammation but are not sensitive or specific for the diagnosis of RA. They are useful for differentiating RA from noninflammatory conditions such as osteoarthritis or fibromyalgia. Even when there is clinical evidence of joint inflammation, the values for acute phase reactants may be normal. Inflammation in RA often leads to anemia of chronic disease and thrombocytosis.

Synovial fluid analysis is usually not necessary when the diagnosis is already established, but arthrocentesis should be performed to rule out infection or crystalline arthropathy if only one joint is involved. Synovial fluid analysis is nonspecific but indicates inflammation. Radiographs, although not part of the 2010 RA classification criteria, may show characteristic periarticular osteopenia, marginal erosions, and uniform joint space narrowing in a symmetrical distribution.

For a deeper discussion of these topics, please see Chapter 257, "Laboratory Testing in Rheumatoid Arthritis," Chapter 258, "Imaging Studies in the Rheumatic Diseases," Chapter 263, "Bursitis, Tendinitis, and Other Periarticular Disorders and Sports Medicine," and Chapter 264, "Rheumatoid Arthritis," in Goldman-Cecil Medicine, 25th Edition.

⬤ TREATMENT

The ultimate goals of RA management are to reduce pain and discomfort, prevent deformities and loss of normal joint function, and maintain normal physical and social function. Although there is no cure for RA, remission can be maintained in a subset of patients. Treatment begins with effective communication between the physician and patient regarding the nature of the disease and the goals of treatment.

Nonpharmacologic therapeutic options include reduction of joint stress and physical and occupational therapy. Local rest of an inflamed joint can reduce joint stress, as can weight reduction, splinting, and the use of walking aids. Vigorous activity should be avoided during disease flares. Full range of motion of joints, however, should be maintained by a graded exercise program to prevent contractures and muscle atrophy. Physical therapy improves muscle strength and conditioning and maintains joint mobility. Occupational therapy can provide various appliances to protect joints and make daily activities easier.

Pharmacologic Approach

Studies have revealed that disease-modifying antirheumatic drug (DMARD) therapy early in the course of RA slows disease progression more effectively than delayed therapy.

Effective treatment can improve signs, symptoms, and radiographic progression, even in long-standing disease. The inflammation of RA should be controlled as completely as possible, as soon as possible, and for as long as possible. Conventional DMARDs and biologic DMARDs prevent disease progression and disability.

Symptomatic Control and Bridging Therapy

DMARDs require 1 to 6 months to work. Consequently, nonsteroidal anti-inflammatory drugs (NSAIDs), which are not disease modifying, are frequently used early in the disease process for symptomatic control. NSAIDs have significant side effects, including renal failure and increased risk of gastrointestinal bleeding, and should be used with caution in patients with multiple medical comorbidities.

Glucocorticoids remain important in the treatment of RA, especially for acute exacerbations of disease. These agents are used sparingly in low to medium doses. Although glucocorticoids are useful for brief exacerbations and decrease bone erosions, the long-term side effects of glucocorticoids can be substantial. They should be used primarily as bridging therapy for further DMARD effects. Side effects include osteoporosis, avascular necrosis of bone, obesity, hypertension, and glucose intolerance. Screening, prevention, and treatment for osteoporosis should be considered for all patients who receive long-term glucocorticoid therapy for prevention of glucocorticoid-induced osteoporosis. Intraarticular glucocorticoids are extremely effective treatment for exacerbations involving only a few joints.

For a deeper discussion of these topics, please see Chapter 243, "Osteoporosis," in Goldman-Cecil Medicine, 25th Edition.

Conventional and Biologic Disease-Modifying Antirheumatic Drugs

Many DMARDs are available for treating RA. All conventional DMARDs have a slow onset, taking 1 to 6 months to become fully effective, and they need close monitoring for toxicity.

Methotrexate is universally used as the initial DMARD in patients with moderate to severe RA because of its established efficacy and known toxicity profile (level A evidence, multiple randomized controlled trials). It can be administered once weekly by the oral or parenteral route. Known side effects include oral ulcers, nausea, hepatotoxicity, and pneumonitis.

After methotrexate failure, the subsequent choice of conventional and biologic DMARDs is not standardized and is instead based on the preferences of patients and physicians. For patients with mild RA, hydroxychloroquine or sulfasalazine, or both, may be used as first-line drugs (level B evidence). Triple therapy, the combination of methotrexate, hydroxychloroquine, and sulfasalazine, was shown in two randomized, controlled trials to be noninferior to biologic TNF-α inhibitors (level A). Tofacitinib is an oral Janus kinase inhibitor and the first kinase inhibitor of its class that reduces cytokine levels.

Biologic DMARDs are targeted, immune-based therapies that were introduced in the 1990s with the initiation of cytokine-directed TNF-α inhibitors. TNF-α inhibitors were the first of nine biologic DMARDs approved by the U.S. Food and Drug

TABLE 77-3 DISEASE-MODIFYING ANTIRHEUMATIC DRUGS

CONVENTIONAL AGENTS	TOXICITIES
Hydroxychloroquine	Retinal toxicity, requires ophthalmologic monitoring
Sulfasalazine	Nausea, bone marrow suppression
Methotrexate	Oral ulcers, nausea, bone marrow suppression, pneumonitis; contraindicated in pregnancy and coexistent lung disease
Leflunomide	Bone marrow and hepatic toxicity; cholestyramine washout if toxic; contraindicated in pregnancy
Tofacitinib (oral DMARD)	Infection rate similar to biologic DMARDs; bone marrow and hepatic toxicity, hyperlipidemia

BIOLOGIC AGENTS	MECHANISMS
Adalimumab, certolizumab, etanercept, golimumab, infliximab	Cytokine directed, anti-TNF-α
Tocilizumab	Cytokine directed, anti-IL-6
Anakinra	Cytokine directed, anti-IL-1
Abatacept	T-cell directed, inhibits costimulation
Rituximab	B-cell directed, anti-CD20

DMARDs, Disease-modifying antirheumatic drugs; IL, interleukin; TNF, tumor necrosis factor.

Administration (FDA) for the treatment of RA (Table 77-3). Five TNF-α–directed therapies are available. The TNF-α inhibitors are the most widely used biologic agents because of the rapid improvement they produce in patients resistant to methotrexate therapy. They are recommended in addition to methotrexate after methotrexate failure (level A evidence).

Most biologic DMARDs are given by intravenous or subcutaneous injection and are quite expensive. Some have an increased risk of infection, including risk of reactivation of tuberculosis. Other cytokine-directed therapies include the IL-6 receptor antagonist tocilizumab and the IL-1 receptor antagonist anakinra. Biologic DMARDs also include an inhibitor of T-cell costimulation, abatacept; and a B-cell–depleting agent, rituximab

For a deeper discussion of these topics, please see Chapter 36, "Biologic Agents," in Goldman-Cecil Medicine, 25th Edition.

Medical Care Specialized for Rheumatoid Arthritis

RA is a chronic disease that requires focused care for comorbidities. DMARDs themselves require frequent laboratory monitoring for toxicities, including bone marrow suppression, hepatotoxicity, and renal dysfunction. Opportunistic infections can occur in patients receiving biologic therapies and DMARDs. In the setting of acute infection, DMARDs and biologic therapies should be withheld. Prophylactically, all RA patients should be vaccinated for pneumococcal, influenza, and hepatitis B infection. Herpes zoster vaccine to prevent shingles should be given prior to biological agents because the vaccine is live.

RA itself is a risk factor for osteoporosis, and combined with glucocorticoid use, it can lead to severe osteoporosis and subsequent morbidity. In every RA patient, bone health should be addressed to prevent development of osteoporosis. RA is also a risk factor for cardiovascular disease due to chronic inflammation and should be aggressively monitored.

Caution should be taken preoperatively when the RA patient is being anesthetized to avoid C1-C2 subluxation and spinal cord compression. Joint replacement surgery plays an important role for patients who have had severe, destructive joint disease, particularly in the knees and hips.

PROGNOSIS

Although the underlying cause of RA is unknown, advances in cell biology, immunology, and molecular biology have led to dramatic therapeutic advancements for this disease. Conventional and biologic DMARDs improve short- and long-term outcomes. Bone erosions occur within 1 to 2 years of disease onset, and early initiation of DMARDs is essential to prevent further morbidity.

RF positivity, CCP positivity, and extra-articular features are characteristic of severe disease. The incidence of lymphoma and other malignancies is increased among patients with RA, and the overall mortality rate is increased by coexisting cardiovascular disease and infection.

Although up to 15% of patients can go into drug-free remission, long-term disability is significant. Fifty percent of patients with RA are not working after 10 years, approximately 10 times the rate in the normal population. Most patients fall between these extremes with various levels of disability. Some have a waxing and waning course over a period of years, with acute episodes of single- or multiple-joint exacerbations.

Future developments will include guidelines about when to institute biologic DMARDS, novel targeted biologic agents, and personalized approaches based on an understanding of individual disease pathogenesis.

SUGGESTED READINGS

Aletaha D, Neogi T, Silman AJ, et al: 2010 Rheumatoid arthritis classification criteria: an American College of Rheumatology/European League Against Rheumatism collaborative initiative, Arthritis Rheum 62:2569–2581, 2010.

Karlson EW, Ding B, Keenan BT, et al: Association of environmental and genetic factors and gene-environment interactions with risk of developing rheumatoid arthritis, Arthritis Care Res (Hoboken) 65:1147–1156, 2013.

McInnes IB, O'Dell JR: State-of-the-art: rheumatoid arthritis, Ann Rheum Dis 69:1898–1906, 2010.

McInnes IB, Schett G: The pathogenesis of rheumatoid arthritis, N Engl J Med 365:2205–2219, 2011.

Moreland LW, O'Dell JR, Paulus HE, et al: A randomized comparative effectiveness study of oral triple therapy versus etanercept plus methotrexate in early aggressive rheumatoid arthritis: the treatment of Early Aggressive Rheumatoid Arthritis Trial, Arthritis Rheum 64:2824–2835, 2012.

O'Dell JR, Mikuls TR, Taylor TH, et al: Therapies for active rheumatoid arthritis after methotrexate failure, N Engl J Med 369:307–318, 2013.

Saag KG, Teng GG, Patkar NM, et al: American College of Rheumatology 2008 recommendations for the use of nonbiologic and biologic disease-modifying antirheumatic drugs in rheumatoid arthritis, Arthritis Rheum 59:762–784, 2008.

Singh JA, Furst DE, Bharat A, et al: 2012 update of the 2008 American College of Rheumatology recommendations for the use of disease-modifying antirheumatic drugs and biologic agents in the treatment of rheumatoid arthritis, Arthritis Care Res (Hoboken) 64:625–639, 2012.

Spondyloarthritis

Douglas W. Lienesch

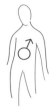

DEFINITION

Spondyloarthritis, formerly called *seronegative arthritis* or *sponydyloarthopathy*, is the name of a group of related inflammatory disorders that share certain clinical features unique among rheumatic diseases. The six types of spondyloarthritis in adults are ankylosing spondylitis, reactive arthritis, arthritis of inflammatory bowel disease (i.e., Crohn's disease and ulcerative colitis), psoriatic arthritis, and undifferentiated spondyloarthropathy. The juvenile form of spondyloarthropathy is similar to ankylosing spondylitis and usually persists into adulthood.

The cardinal clinical feature of spondyloarthritis is inflammation of the sacroiliac joints (i.e., sacroiliitis) and the spine (i.e., spondylitis). Inflammation of tendon insertion sites (i.e., enthesitis), inflammation of entire digits (i.e., dactylitis), and inflammation of one to four lower extremity joints (i.e., oligoarthritis) are typical extraspinal skeletal findings. A positive family history, eye inflammation (i.e., anterior uveitis or conjunctivitis), and the absence of rheumatoid factor and subcutaneous nodules are common.

Further classification of these disorders is based on the finding of psoriatic skin or nail changes, inflammatory bowel disease, or a history of preceding gastrointestinal or genitourinary infection. Alternatively, patients with spondyloarthritis can be classified based on the distribution pattern of joint involvement. Cases with dominant spinal disease are classified as *axial spondyloarthritis* (i.e., prototypically ankylosing spondylitis), and those without spinal disease are classified as predominately *peripheral spondyloarthritis*.

Spondyloarthritis is strongly associated with human leukocyte antigen B27 (HLA-27), a specific allele of the B locus of the HLA-encoding class I major histocompatibility complex genes. The frequency of HLA-B27 among whites is approximately 8%. However, up to 90% of white patients with ankylosing spondylitis and 80% of white patients with reactive arthritis or juvenile spondyloarthritis are HLA-B27 positive, and these percentages are even higher among patients with uveitis. The rate of HLA-B27 positivity among patients with inflammatory bowel disease or psoriasis with peripheral arthritis is not markedly increased unless they have spondylitis, in which case the frequency of HLA-B27 is 50%. The frequency of HLA-B27 varies widely among other ethnic groups and accounts for the broad variation of the prevalence of ankylosing spondylitis in different populations.

Ankylosing spondylitis is much more common among adolescent boys and young men, but this finding may reflect underdiagnosis in women, in whom disease manifestations may be milder than they are in men. Reactive arthritis is more common among men when it follows genitourinary *Chlamydia trachomatis* infection, but the sex distribution is even among patients after dysentery. Inflammatory arthritis including spondylitis affects approximately 5% to 8% of patients with psoriasis and 10% to 25% of patients with ulcerative colitis or Crohn's disease. Men and women are affected equally. The prevalence of spondyloarthritis, particularly psoriatic and reactive arthritis, is increased in populations with high human immunodeficiency virus (HIV) infection rates.

PATHOLOGY

Although the strong association of HLA-B27 with spondyloarthritis is well established, a specific role in the pathogenesis of these disorders has not been elucidated. Animal models in which rodents transgenic for HLA-B27 develop inflammatory abnormalities strikingly similar to those seen in HLA-B27–associated human diseases provide compelling indirect evidence for a pathogenic role. When raised in a germ-free environment, these animals remain disease free, suggesting a key additional environmental factor.

In addition to the strong genetic links for the risk of spondyloarthritis, important associations exist between specific bacterial agents and disease pathogenesis. Genitourinary infection with *C. trachomatis* or diarrheal illness with *Shigella, Salmonella, Campylobacter*, and *Yersinia* species can induce reactive arthritis. Several additional infectious agents are less commonly implicated. They appear to trigger an inflammatory response, possibly as a result of persistence of bacterial antigens, or cause an aberrant immunologic response to infection that results in misfolding of HLA-B27 molecules in antigen-presenting cells, generating a persistent inflammatory reaction.

No one theory of pathogenesis of spondyloarthritis explains the clinical spectrum of these disorders, and more research is clearly needed to solidify an understanding of their origin. The complex role of the immune system in the spondyloarthritis is highlighted by the observation that patients infected with HIV appear more likely to have severe disease, especially psoriatic arthritis. When HIV infection is treated with antiviral agents, the incidence of spondyloarthritis declines.

Although many of the cellular and molecular mechanisms of inflammatory joint disease have been elucidated, the pathophysiology of spondyloarthritis remains incompletely understood. Inflammation of the sacroiliac joints, spine, and entheses is a unique feature of these disorders. Pathophysiologic studies show that the inflammation originates at the interface of bone and cartilage in the sacroiliac joint and bone and fibrocartilage in the enthesis. Macrophages and CD4$^+$ and CD8$^+$ T cells are present, and the proinflammatory cytokines tumor necrosis factor-α (TNF-α) and interleukin-23 (IL-23) are abundant.

Synovial tissue becomes inflamed, and osteoclasts are activated, leading to bone resorption, reminiscent of rheumatoid arthritis joint inflammation. Unlike in rheumatoid arthritis, early bone resorption is followed by a secondary phase during which osteoblast activity predominates, leading to new bone formation in periarticular bone (i.e., hyperostosis) and around joints (i.e., osteophytosis) or vertebral bodies (i.e., syndesmophytes). Ultimately, bony fusion of joints (ankylosis) occurs. The relationship between these paradoxical phases of bone resorption and proliferation is an area of active investigation.

● CLINICAL PRESENTATION

Common Clinical Features of Spondyloarthritis

All forms of spondyloarthritis have considerable clinical overlap with one another and are most easily considered as a group of related disorders. Table 78-1 outlines the clinical features of these disorders. The cardinal clinical features common to all of them are inflammatory spine pain and an asymmetrical, predominantly lower extremity inflammatory joint or tendon disease. Inflammatory spine pain should be suspected in young patients (<40 years) who have an insidious onset of chronic low back pain or buttock pain associated with prolonged morning stiffness and relieved by exercise.

The characteristic peripheral joint disease involves one to four joints, usually in the lower extremities, and may be associated with tendon insertion inflammation (i.e., enthesitis) or sausage digits (i.e., dactylitis). Symmetrical polyarthropathy involving the upper extremities and clinically similar to rheumatoid arthritis is seen in some forms of psoriatic or inflammatory bowel disease–related spondyloarthritis. Anterior uveitis, enthesitis, dactylitis, psoriatic skin or nail changes, inflammatory bowel disease, a family history of spondyloarthritis, or a history of preceding gastrointestinal or genitourinary infection suggests spondyloarthritis. Subcutaneous nodules, rheumatoid factor, and antinuclear antibodies are usually absent.

In a given patient, the clinical features of these disorders may accumulate over a prolonged period. Some patients do not initially demonstrate the typical findings of a specific disorder. They are considered to have undifferentiated spondyloarthritis. Early disease can be subcategorized as predominately axial spondyloarthritis or predominately peripheral spondyloarthritis, depending on the site of the dominant symptoms. Many patients later have clinical findings consistent with a specific subtype of spondyloarthritis.

Inflammatory spine pain is the cardinal feature of axial disease and results from inflammation in the sacroiliac joints and spinal elements. Uncontrolled disease may lead to ankylosis (i.e., bony fusion) at sacroiliac joints and throughout the vertebral column, culminating in loss of spinal and costovertebral motion, deformity, and restrictive extrapulmonary physiology.

Enthesitis can occur in many different anatomic locations. They include spinous processes, costosternal junctions, ischial tuberosities, plantar aponeuroses, and Achilles tendons.

When peripheral arthritis of spondyloarthritis occurs, it frequently begins as an episodic, asymmetrical, oligoarticular process that often involves the lower extremities. The arthritis can progress and may become chronic and disabling. A unique feature of spondyloarthritis is the appearance of fusiform swelling of an entire finger or toe, referred to as *dactylitis* or *sausage digits.*

Anterior uveitis, or inflammation of the anterior chamber of the eye, is a common extra-articular manifestation of spondyloarthritis, especially among HLA-B27–positive patients. Acute bouts of uveitis are usually monocular, painful, and accompanied by eye redness and blurred vision. Recurrent attacks are common and can lead to blindness. Scleritis, episcleritis, and conjunctivitis are less commonly associated phenomena.

Spondyloarthritis may occasionally involve other organ systems and may cause significant morbidity and mortality. Aortitis, especially occurring in the ascending segment, can result in aortic insufficiency from aortic root dilation, aortic dissection, and cardiac conduction system abnormalities. Pulmonary fibrosis of the apical regions can occur, often in an insidious fashion. Spinal cord compression can result from atlantoaxial joint subluxation, cauda equina syndrome, or vertebral fractures. In rare cases, long-standing spondyloarthritis is associated with secondary amyloidosis.

TABLE 78-1	COMPARISON OF THE SPONDYLOARTHRITIS				
FEATURES	**ANKYLOSING SPONDYLITIS**	**POSTURETHRAL REACTIVE ARTHRITIS**	**POSTDYSENTERIC REACTIVE ARTHRITIS**	**ENTEROPATHIC ARTHRITIS**	**PSORIATIC ARTHRITIS**
Sacroiliitis	+++++	+++	++	+	++
Spondylitis	++++	+++	++	++	++
Peripheral arthritis	+	++++	++++	+++	++++
Articular course	Chronic	Acute or chronic	Acute or chronic	Acute or chronic	Chronic
HLA-B27	95%	60%	30%	20%	20%
Enthesopathy	++	++++	+++	++	++
Extra-articular manifestations	Eye, heart	Eye, GU, oral and/or GI, heart	GU, eye	GI, eye	Skin, eye
Other names	Bekhterev's arthritis, Marie-Strümpell disease	Reiter's syndrome, SARA, NGU, chlamydial arthritis	Reiter's syndrome	Crohn's disease, ulcerative colitis	

Data from Cush JJ, Lipsky PE: The spondyloarthropathies. In Goldman L, Bennett JC, editors: Cecil textbook of medicine, ed 21, Philadelphia, 2000, Saunders, pp 1499–1507.

GI, Gastrointestinal tract; GU, genitourinary tract; HLA, human leukocyte antigen; NGU, nongonococcal urethritis; SARA, sexually acquired reactive arthritis; +, relative prevalence of a specific feature.

Specific Clinical Features of Spondyloarthritis

Ankylosing Spondylitis

The cardinal clinical feature of ankylosing spondylitis is inflammatory spine pain. Over time, spine involvement ascends from the sacroiliac joints to involve all levels of the spine. Progressive loss of motion results from ankylosis of the vertebral column and apophyseal joints. Costovertebral involvement leads to decreased chest expansion and restrictive lung physiology.

Loss of mobility and secondary osteoporosis of the vertebral bodies increase the risk of traumatic spine fracture. Axial involvement of the shoulders and hips is common and associated with a worse prognosis. Peripheral oligoarthritis, enthesitis, and dactylitis are more common in females. Diagnosis requires demonstration of radiographic sacroiliitis (i.e., sacroiliac joint erosions, sclerosis, and ankylosis). Anterior uveitis is common. Aortitis, upper lobe pulmonary fibrosis, cauda equina syndrome, and amyloidosis are less common and seen in late disease.

Reactive Arthritis

Among the unique clinical features of reactive arthritis are urethritis, conjunctivitis, and certain dermatologic problems (Fig. 78-1). The urethritis may result from the chlamydial infection that triggers the disease, or it may be a sterile inflammatory discharge seen in diarrhea-associated disease. Conjunctivitis may be mild in reactive arthritis and is distinct from uveitis.

Keratoderma blennorrhagicum is a distinct papulosquamous rash usually found on the palms or soles. Circinate balanitis is a rash that may appear on the penile glans or shaft of men with reactive arthritis. Nonpitting nail thickening and oral ulcers may also occur in patients with reactive arthritis. These lesions can be confused with similar findings in patients with psoriasis and inflammatory bowel disease, respectively.

Most cases are self-limited. Chronic or relapsing arthritis and chronic spondylitis are associated with HLA-B27 and *Chlamydia* infection.

Psoriatic Arthritis

Five identifiable clinical patterns of psoriatic arthritis are recognized: distal interphalangeal joint involvement with nail pitting; asymmetrical oligoarthropathy of large and small joints; arthritis mutilans, a severe, destructive arthritis; symmetrical polyarthritis, which is identical to rheumatoid arthritis; and predominately axial disease. These patterns are not exclusive, and clinical overlap is significant.

Spondylitis or sacroiliitis may occur along with any of the other patterns. The prevalence of HLA-B27 is increased among the patients with spondylitis or sacroiliitis but not among patients with the other patterns. Psoriatic skin or nail disease predates arthritis in most cases, but both may occur concomitantly, or joint disease may precede skin involvement. Rarely, joint disease indistinguishable from psoriatic arthritis, which can occur in patients with a family history but no personal history of psoriatic skin disease.

Enteropathic Arthritis: Inflammatory Bowel Disease

Crohn's disease and ulcerative colitis (see Chapter 38) are frequently associated with inflammatory spine disease and peripheral arthritis. The peripheral arthritis is typically nonerosive, oligoarticular, and episodic, and the degree of joint involvement fluctuates with gut activity. A more chronic, symmetrical polyarthritis may occur in patients with Crohn's disease.

⬤ DIAGNOSIS AND DIFFERENTIAL DIAGNOSIS

The diagnosis of spondylarthritis remains a clinical diagnosis made by identifying typical history and physical examination phenomena, analyzing selected laboratory tests, and using musculoskeletal imaging. The diagnosis is suggested by inflammatory spine pain or chronic lower extremity asymmetric inflammatory oligoarthritis in two to four joints. In this setting, features that increase the probability of spondyloarthritis include uveitis, psoriasis, enthesitis, dactylitis, inflammatory bowel disease, family history of spondylarthropathy, elevated C-reactive protein (CRP) level, HLA-B27, preceding gastrointestinal or genitourinary infection, and sacroiliitis on radiography, computed tomography (CT), or magnetic resonance imaging MRI).

Differentiating spondyloarthritis from other inflammatory or degenerative joint or spine diseases can be challenging. Crystalline arthropathies can manifest with peripheral oligoarthritis, often in the lower extremities. However, the spine is rarely

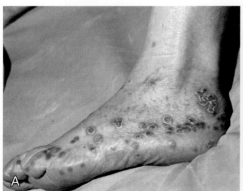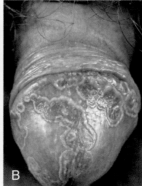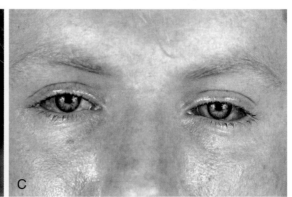

FIGURE 78-1 Reactive arthritis. **A,** Keratoderma blennorrhagicum. Red to brown papules, vesicles, and pustules with central erosion show characteristic crusting and peripheral scaling on the dorsolateral and plantar foot. **B,** Balanitis circinata. Moist, well-demarcated erosions with a slightly raised micropustular circinate border on the glans penis. **C,** Bilateral conjunctivitis associated with anterior uveitis. (From Fitzpatrick TB, Johnson RA, Wolff K, et al: Color atlas and synopsis of clinical dermatology, ed 3, New York, 1983, McGraw-Hill, pp 393, 395.)

involved, and intracellular crystals can be demonstrated in the synovial fluid. Rheumatoid arthritis and other systemic autoimmune diseases usually manifest with symmetrical polyarthritis of the upper and lower extremities associated with abnormal serologies such as rheumatoid factors, anti–cyclic citrullinated peptide (CCP) antibodies, or antinuclear antibodies. Predominately axial spondyloarthritis must be differentiated from indolent infections of the sacroiliac joints, vertebrae, or intravertebral disks; degenerative disease of the spine and disks (i.e., spondylosis); and diffuse idiopathic skeletal hyperostosis (DISH).

The radiographic features of the spondyloarthritis are highly specific and, in the correct clinical setting, greatly increase the certainty of the diagnosis. Sacroiliitis is usually the earliest radiographic sign of spine disease and results in sclerosis and erosions of the sacroiliac joints with eventual bony fusion (Fig. 78-2A). Many radiographic changes result from chronic spondylitis, including ossification of the annulus fibrosus, calcification of spinal ligaments, bony sclerosis and squaring of vertebral bodies, and ankylosis of apophyseal joints. These changes can lead to vertebral fusion and a bamboo spine appearance (see Fig. 78-2B).

Radiographic findings progress over many years of illness and may not be apparent in early disease. However, during this pre-radiographic period, MRI demonstrates bone inflammation (i.e., osteitis) and erosion at the sacroiliac joints and vertebral bodies, and CT shows bony sclerosis and joint erosions.

Bone erosions, sclerosis, and new bone formation may occur at sites of enthesitis. Erosions at bone-cartilage interface (i.e., subchondral erosions), sclerosis, and bone proliferation are hallmarks of spondyloarthritis involving peripheral joints. In severe cases such as the arthritis mutilans form of psoriatic arthritis, total or subtotal bone resorption (i.e., osteolysis) of a phalange may occur.

TREATMENT

No cure has been found for any form of spondyloarthritis, but effective treatment for many of the manifestations is available. Patient education regarding the disease is essential and allows identification of affected family members and early detection of urgent clinical features such as uveitis. Physical therapy, including a daily stretching program, postural adjustments, and strengthening, helps to maintain proper bony alignment, reduce deformities, and maximize function, particularly for those with axial disease. Selective use of orthopedic surgery may be highly effective in correcting significant spinal deformities or instability.

Nonsteroidal anti-inflammatory drugs (NSAIDs) can provide significant relief of spinal pain and stiffness, and many patients take these drugs continually for years (Centre for Evidence Based Medicine; level 1 evidence). No clear evidence indicates that systemic glucocorticoids benefit patients with spondyloarthritis, and these agents are usually avoided. Intra-articular glucocorticoid injection into the sacroiliac or other involved joints may provide temporary relief. Similarly, the role and efficacy of older immunosuppressive agents in the treatment of axial spondyloarthritis have not been established. In contrast, clinical trials have shown that the peripheral manifestations of spondylarthritis improve with sulfasalazine and methotrexate (level 2).

TNF-α blockers (i.e., infliximab, etanercept, adalimumab, and golimumab) represent a substantial breakthrough in the treatment of spondyloarthritis. The efficacy of these agents is well established, and they have rapidly become the treatment of choice for patients with axial inflammation who do not satisfactorily or fully respond to NSAIDs and physical therapy (level 1 evidence). TNF-α blockers can significantly reduce pain, improve function, and improve quality of life. They may also prevent or

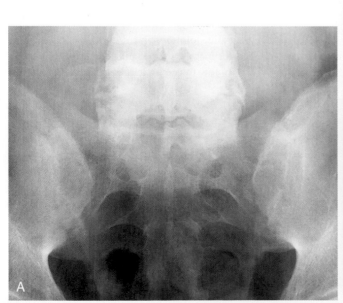
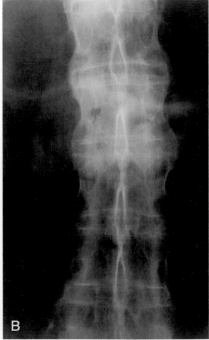

FIGURE 78-2   **A,** Bilaterally symmetrical sacroiliitis in ankylosing spondylitis. **B,** Lumbar spondylitis in ankylosing spondylitis with symmetrical, marginal bridging syndesmophytes and calcification of the spinal ligament. (From Cush JJ, Lipsky PE: The spondyloarthropathies. In Goldman L, Bennett JC, editors: Cecil textbook of medicine, ed 21, Philadelphia, 2000, Saunders, pp 1499–1507.)

slow disease progression and structural damage. The drugs are effective in psoriatic arthritis, suppress the skin and nail disease of psoriasis, and retard radiographic progression in the peripheral joints. Infliximab and adalimumab reduce gut inflammation in ulcerative colitis and Crohn's disease, with concomitant reduction in symptoms of joint and spine inflammation. Ustekinumab, an inhibitor of IL-23, has demonstrated efficacy in psoriasis and psoriatic arthritis (level 1).

Flares of uveitis require care by an ophthalmologist experienced in treating inflammatory eye diseases. Topical or intraocular glucocorticoids may suffice, but systemic therapy with glucocorticoids or immunosuppressive medications may be necessary to control the inflammation and prevent permanent visual loss. Methotrexate and TNF-α inhibitors are frequently employed (level 2 evidence).

Reactive arthritis is usually self-limited, and joint symptoms are managed with NSAIDs or intra-articular corticosteroid injections. When chronic arthritis or spondylitis develops, interventions are similar to those employed for other forms of spondyloarthritis. Evaluation and treatment of *C. trachomatis* and associated sexually transmitted diseases in patients with reactive arthritis and their sex partners are essential. Early treatment reduces the frequency of reactive arthritis. Long-term antibiotics are ineffective for gastroenteritis-associated reactive arthritis. Clinical trials of long-term antibiotics for reactive arthritis after *C. trachomatis* infection have had mixed results, and this practice requires further study before it can be adopted.

SUMMARY

Disability due to spondyloarthritis varies according to the subtype and severity of the specific syndrome. Historically, patients with spondyloarthritis usually experienced a lesser degree of disability compared with those with rheumatoid arthritis. Some patients with reactive arthritis experience self-limited disease with no long-term sequelae. Alternatively, those with more severe disease can have deformation and destruction of the axial and peripheral joints, leading to severe disability. Serious and potentially fatal extraskeletal manifestations can manifest.

With the advent of effective immunosuppressant medications such as methotrexate in psoriatic disease and biologic agents (i.e., TNF-α and IL-23 inhibitors), patients with more severe manifestations have markedly improved symptom control and quality of life.

SUGGESTED READINGS

Hreggvidsdottir H, Noordenbos T, Baeten D: Inflammatory pathways in spondyloarthritis, Mol Immunol 57:28–37, 2014.

Sieper J, Rudwaleit M, Baraliakos X, et al: The Assessment of Spondyloarthritis international Society (ASAS) handbook: a guide to assess spondyloarthritis, Ann Rheum Dis 68(Suppl lII):ii1–ii44, 2009.

Smolen JS, Braun J, Dougados M, et al: Treating spondyloarthritis, including ankylosing spondylitis and psoriatic arthritis, to target: recommendations of an international task force, Ann Rheum Dis 73:6–16, 2014.

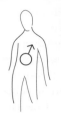

Systemic Lupus Erythematosus

Amy H. Kao and Susan Manzi

DEFINITION AND EPIDEMIOLOGY

Systemic lupus erythematosus (SLE) is the classic systemic auto-immune disease. The cause is unknown. SLE predominantly affects young women of childbearing age but can also afflict young men and older individuals of either sex.

The clinical manifestations are protean, ranging from mild symptoms of fatigue and oral ulcerations to life-threatening renal and neurologic disease. Typically, the disease fluctuates with periods of flares and clinical quiescence. However, recurrent disease flares and their treatment may ultimately lead to irreversible organ damage.

SLE is diagnosed by a thorough history, physical examination, and laboratory testing. A single diagnostic laboratory test for SLE is not available, and the diagnosis is often difficult, requiring many patient visits to numerous doctors.

Although there is no cure for SLE, patients are treated for the many chronic medical conditions associated with the disease with a variety of medications, primarily immunosuppressants. Unique consideration must be given to SLE patients regarding pregnancy, bone health, cardiovascular disease (CVD), and malignancy.

The reported incidence and prevalence of SLE vary greatly, reflecting the heterogeneity of the disease. The incidence of SLE worldwide is estimated at 1.8 to 7.6 cases per 100,000 persons per year and appears to have increased over time. Prevalence rates range from 14.6 to 149.5 cases per 100,000 persons.

During the childbearing years, the female-to-male ratio of SLE prevalence is 10:1 to 15:1. This gender discrepancy also exists but is less distinct (2:1) in young children and older patients. SLE also has a predilection for nonwhite ethnic populations, with greater prevalence rates for African Americans (three times), Afro-Caribbeans (five times), Asians (two times), and Hispanics than for whites. These patients also tend to have more severe SLE disease and worse overall prognoses than those who are white.

PATHOLOGY

Although SLE pathogenesis remains poorly understood, individuals who develop SLE likely have a genetic predisposition in the setting of immune system dysregulation, environmental triggers, and altered hormonal milieu. The genetic contribution to SLE is emphasized by the high concordance rate for mono-zygotic twins (>20%) and a lower concordance rate among other siblings (<5%). The search for genes involved in SLE pathogenesis is an active area of research. Genes coding for certain human leukocyte antigens, complement system components, immuno-

globulin receptors, and various other proteins are being considered as candidate genes for SLE.

The many immune abnormalities in SLE implicate dysregulation of the humoral and cellular immune systems in the pathogenesis of the disease. Dysregulation leads to loss of self-tolerance and autoimmune destruction of healthy tissues, hallmarked by the production of autoantibodies and immune complexes.

Various environmental triggers, including microorganisms and ultraviolet light exposure, may influence the development of SLE and lupus activity. The striking differences in SLE prevalence between genders and the effect of pregnancy on disease activity suggest a role for hormones in SLE pathogenesis.

CLINICAL PRESENTATION

Virtually any organ system may be involved in SLE. Table 79-1 outlines some of the many clinical manifestations of SLE.

Constitutional Manifestations

Fatigue, fever, lymphadenopathy, and generalized arthralgias and myalgias are common in SLE patients. The most common symptom, fatigue (>90%), can also be the most debilitating. Other reasons for fatigue, including anemia, hypothyroidism, and fibromyalgia, should be excluded when attempting to diagnose SLE.

Mucocutaneous Manifestations

Oral ulcerations may be painful or painless and are classically located on the tongue or palate. Skin manifestations of SLE are common and include the classic malar (butterfly) rash, discoid lesions (i.e., permanent scarring and disfigurement), alopecia, and photosensitivity. Subacute cutaneous SLE can manifest with a psoriasiform rash or annular lesions mimicking tinea corporis. Frequently, acne rosacea is mistaken for a malar rash. A key distinguishing feature is that erythema in lupus malar rash does not cross the nasolabial folds.

Musculoskeletal Manifestations

Arthralgias and inflammatory arthritis are common manifestations in SLE (>75%). Lupus arthritis is usually nonerosive (unlike rheumatoid arthritis), but 10% of patients have Jaccoud's arthropathy with reversible hand deformities due to inflammation and joint tendon laxity.

Cardiopulmonary Manifestations

More than 60% of SLE patients have pericarditis and pleuritis during their disease course. Subsequent pericardial or pleural effusions are typically exudative. Valvular thickening and

TABLE 79-1 CLINICAL MANIFESTATIONS OF SYSTEMIC LUPUS ERYTHEMATOSUS

CONSTITUTIONAL

Fatigue
Fever
Lymphadenopathy
Weight loss
Anorexia

MUCOCUTANEOUS

Oral, genital, nasal ulcers*
Angioedema
Alopecia
Photosensitivity*
Malar (butterfly) rash*
Discoid lesions*
Subacute cutaneous lupus
Tumid lupus
Panniculitis
Vasculitis
Chilblain
Urticaria
Periungual erythema

MUSCULOSKELETAL

Arthritis*
Arthralgias
Jaccoud's arthropathy
Avascular necrosis
Myositis

CARDIAC

Pericarditis*
Pericardial effusion
Myocarditis
Valvular thickening
Libman-Sacks endocarditis
Atherosclerotic heart disease

PULMONARY

Pleuritis*
Pleural effusion
Pneumonitis
Alveolar hemorrhage
Interstitial lung disease
Bronchiolitis obliterans
Pulmonary hypertension
Pulmonary emboli
Vasculitis
Acute reversible hypoxemic
    syndrome
Shrinking lung syndrome

RENAL

Cellular casts or glomerulonephritis*
Proteinuria or membranous
    nephropathy or nephrotic
    syndrome*

NEUROPSYCHIATRIC

Seizures*
Cerebritis/aseptic meningitis
Cerebrovascular disease
Transverse myelitis
Chorea
Headache
Cognitive impairment
Autonomic dysfunction
Cranial neuropathy
Peripheral neuropathy
Psychosis*
Anxiety
Depression
Mood disorder

HEMATOLOGIC

Leukopenia*
Lymphopenia*
Hemolytic anemia*
Nonhemolytic anemia (anemia of
    chronic disease, iron-deficiency)
Thrombocytopenia*
Antiphospholipid antibody
    syndrome

VASCULAR

Raynaud's phenomenon
Livedo reticularis
Arterial or venous thrombosis
Vasculitis (almost any location)

OCULAR

Keratoconjunctivitis sicca
Episcleritis
Scleritis
Retinal vasculitis
Arterial and venous occlusions
Optic neuritis

GASTROINTESTINAL

Hypomotility
Mesenteric vasculitis
Malabsorption
Protein-losing gastroenteropathy
    pancreatitis
Lupus enteropathy
Thrombosis of mesenteric and
    hepatic vasculature
Hepatitis
Hepatomegaly
Splenomegaly
Pancreatitis
Acalculous cholecystitis
Peritonitis

SEROLOGIC

Autoantibodies*
Hypocomplementemia
Elevated acute phase reactants

REPRODUCTIVE

Recurrent spontaneous abortions
Premature fetal delivery
Neonatal lupus

*An item in the 1997 American College of Rheumatology classification criteria for SLE.

noninfective Libman-Sacks endocarditis are frequently observed on echocardiography and autopsy studies. Myocarditis should be suspected in patients with cardiopulmonary symptoms and fever.

Renal Manifestations

Nephritis, which manifests with hematuria and proteinuria, is a major cause of morbidity and mortality for SLE patients. The International Society of Nephrology/Renal Pathology Society (ISN/RPS) revisited the 1982 World Health Organization classification of lupus nephritis (classes I through VI). ISN/RPS class IV (i.e., diffuse, proliferative) lupus nephritis is the most common form and has the worst prognosis, but it is also the most amenable to aggressive immunosuppressive therapy.

Neuropsychiatric Manifestations

Neuropsychiatric symptoms are broad, including sensorimotor neuropathy, headache, cognitive dysfunction, mood disorders, psychosis, life-threatening ischemic stroke, cerebritis, and transverse myelitis. In 2010, the European League Against Rheumatism task force recognized that "mild or moderate cognitive dysfunction is common in SLE" and recommended the "management of SLE and non–SLE-associated factors, as well as psychoeducational support to prevent further deterioration of cognitive function."

Hematologic Manifestations

Leukopenia, primarily lymphopenia, anemia, and thrombocytopenia are common in SLE. Anemia is typically results from hemolysis or chronic disease. Antiphospholipid antibodies (APAs) are detected in approximately 33% of SLE patients and are associated with recurrent thromboses, thrombocytopenia, and recurrent spontaneous miscarriages.

Vascular Manifestations

More than 40% of SLE patients have Raynaud's phenomenon. Venous clots (e.g., pulmonary emboli, deep vein thromboses) and arterial clots typically result from APAs. Leg ulcers, gangrene, thrombophlebitis, nail fold infarcts, cutaneous necrosis, and necrotizing purpura may also be seen. Small vessel vasculopathy or vasculitis can occur in any organ system and can be a life-threatening manifestation.

Ocular Manifestations

Keratoconjunctivitis sicca from secondary Sjögren's syndrome (see Chapter 85) is the most common ocular manifestation of SLE. Episcleritis, scleritis, and retinal vasculitis can occur but are less common.

For a deeper discussion of these topics, please see Chapter 266, "Systemic Lupus Erythematosus" in Goldman-Cecil Medicine, 25th Edition.

⬤ DIAGNOSIS AND DIFFERENTIAL DIAGNOSIS

SLE is a clinical diagnosis; no single test or feature is definitively diagnostic of the disease. The clinical disease of most patients evolves over time, and, in most situations, only after several years (and several different physicians' visits) are patients recognized as having SLE.

Classification

Classification criteria for SLE were established for conducting more uniform SLE research. The commonly used American College of Rheumatology classification criteria for SLE (Table 79-2) was updated in 1997. Using this system, meeting 4 of 11 criteria classifies a patient as having definite SLE.

In 2012, the Systemic Lupus International Collaborating Clinics (SLICC) further revised the classification criteria (Table 79-3) to improve clinical relevance and incorporate new knowledge into the definition of SLE immunopathogenesis. Based on the SLICC system, a patient is classified as having SLE if she has at least four of the criteria (including at least one clinical criterion and one immunologic criterion) listed in Table 79-3 or has biopsy-proven lupus nephritis (i.e., stand-alone criterion) in the setting of antinuclear antibodies (ANAs) or anti–double-stranded DNA (anti-dsDNA) antibodies. Although these classification criteria are not used for diagnostic purposes, practicing clinicians can use them along with a comprehensive examination to support the diagnosis.

Various autoantibodies are found in patients with SLE, and the prevalence of autoantibodies varies across different SLE patient cohorts and ethnic groups (Table 79-4). These autoantibodies often can be detected before the onset of SLE clinical manifestations. More than 95% of patients with SLE test positive for ANAs with titers of 1 : 160 or higher.

ANAs are evaluated by the indirect immunofluorescence antibody test, and results are reported in titers and patterns. The most common pattern in SLE is homogenous (i.e., diffuse). Antibodies to dsDNA and Smith antigen are highly specific for SLE, whereas antibodies to SSA/Ro and SSB/La antigens are also commonly found in patients with Sjögren's syndrome and rheumatoid arthritis. Certain antibodies are associated with specific clinical manifestations, particularly anti-dsDNA antibodies with lupus nephritis and anti–U1-RNP antibodies with overlapping features of systemic sclerosis or myositis. Autoantibodies alone are not diagnostic for any autoimmune disease and must be interpreted in the context of the patient's clinical presentation.

Overlap Syndrome

Some patients with clinical and laboratory features of two or more autoimmune diseases have an overlap syndrome. Mixed connective tissue disease is characterized by overlaps among SLE, scleroderma, and myositis with a high titer of anti–U1-RNP antibody levels. For patients who have multiple autoimmune manifestations but do not meet the criteria of a specific autoimmune disease, the term *undifferentiated connective tissue disease* is

TABLE 79-2	1997 AMERICAN COLLEGE OF RHEUMATOLOGY CRITERIA FOR CLASSIFICATION OF SYSTEMIC LUPUS ERYTHEMATOSUS*	
	CRITERIA	**DEFINITIONS**
1.	Malar rash	Fixed, flat or raised erythema is observed over the malar eminences, tending to spare the nasolabial folds.
2.	Discoid rash	Erythematous, raised patches develop with adherent keratotic scaling and follicular plugging; atrophic scarring may occur in older lesions.
3.	Photosensitivity	Rash occurs as a result of unusual reaction to sunlight, determined by patient history or physician observation.
4.	Oral ulcers	Oral or nasopharyngeal ulceration, usually painless, is observed by the physician.
5.	Arthritis	Nonerosive arthritis involves two or more peripheral joints, characterized by tenderness, swelling, or effusion.
6.	Serositis	a. Pleuritis: convincing history of pleuritic pain exists or rub is heard by a physician or pleural effusion is in evidence. *or* b. Pericarditis: documented by electrocardiogram or rub or evidence of pericardial effusion.
7.	Renal disorder	a. Persistent proteinuria is >0.5 g/day or scored >3+ if quantitation is not performed. *or* b. Cellular casts: may be red cell, hemoglobin, granular, tubular, or mixed.
8.	Neurologic disorder	a. Seizures: occurs in the absence of offending drugs or known metabolic derangements (e.g., uremia, ketoacidosis, or electrolyte imbalance). *or* b. Psychosis: occurs in the absence of offending drugs or known metabolic derangements (e.g., uremia, ketoacidosis, electrolyte imbalance)
9.	Hematologic disorder	a. Hemolytic anemia: develops with reticulocytosis. *or* b. Leukopenia: <4000/mm^3 is documented on two or more occasions. *or* c. Lymphopenia: <1500/mm^3 is documented on two or more occasions. *or* d. Thrombocytopenia: <100,000/mm^3 develops in the absence of offending drugs.
10.	Immunologic disorder	a. Anti–double-stranded DNA: antibody to native DNA in abnormal titer. *or* b. Anti-Smith: presence of antibody to Smith nuclear antigen. *or* c. Positive finding of antiphospholipid antibodies is based on (1) an abnormal serum level of IgG or IgM anticardiolipin antibodies, (2) a positive test result for lupus anticoagulant using a standard method, or (3) a false-positive serologic test for syphilis known to be positive for at least 6 months and confirmed by *Treponema pallidum* immobilization or fluorescent treponemal antibody absorption test.
11.	ANA	An abnormal titer of antinuclear antibody is documented by immunofluorescence or an equivalent assay at any point in time and in the absence of drugs known to be associated with drug-induced lupus syndrome.

Data from Tan EM, Cohen AS, Fries, et al: The 1982 revised criteria of the classification of systemic lupus erythematosus, Arthritis Rheum 25:1271, 1982; Hochberg MC: Updating the American College of Rheumatology revised criteria for the classification of systemic lupus erythematosus, Arthritis Rheum 40:1725, 1997.

*This classification is based on 11 criteria. For the purpose of identifying patients in clinical studies, a patient is classified as having definite SLE if any 4 or more of the 11 criteria are present (cumulative) during any interval of observation.

TABLE 79-3 SYSTEMIC LUPUS INTERNATIONAL COLLABORATING CLINICS (SLICC) CLASSIFICATION CRITERIA OF SYSTEMIC LUPUS ERYTHEMATOSUS

CLINICAL CRITERIA*	EXAMPLES
1. Acute cutaneous lupus	Bullous lupus
	Lupus malar rash (not malar discoid)
	Maculopapular lupus rash
	Photosensitive lupus rash (in the absence of dermatomyositis)
	Subacute cutaneous lupus
	Toxic epidermal necrolysis variant of SLE
2. Chronic cutaneous lupus	Classic discoid rash
	Localized (above the neck)
	Generalized (above and below the neck)
	Chilblains lupus
	Discoid lupus/lichen planus overlap
	Hypertrophic (verrucous) lupus
	Lupus erythematosus tumidus
	Lupus panniculitis (profundus)
	Mucosal lupus
3. Oral ulcers	Palate, buccal, tongue, *or* nasal ulcers (in the absence of other causes: vasculitis, Behçet's disease, infection, inflammatory bowel disease, reactive arthritis, and acidic foods)
4. Nonscarring alopecia	Diffuse thinning *or* hair fragility with visible broken hairs (in the absence of other causes: alopecia areata, drugs, iron deficiency, and androgenic alopecia)
5. Synovitis (≥2 joints)	Characterized by swelling or effusion *or* tenderness with ≥30 minutes of morning stiffness
6. Serositis	Typical pleurisy for >1 day *or* pleural effusions *or* pleural rub
	Typical pericardial pain for >1 day *or* pericardial effusion *or* pericardial rub *or* pericarditis by ECG (in the absence of other causes: infection, uremia, and Dressler's pericarditis)
7. Renal	Urine protein/creatinine (*or* 24-hr protein) ≥500 mg of protein/24 hr *or* red blood cell casts
8. Neurologic	Acute confusional state (in the absence of other causes: toxic-metabolic, uremia, and drugs)
	Mononeuritis multiplex (in the absence of other known causes: primary vasculitis)
	Myelitis
	Peripheral or cranial neuropathy (in the absence of other known causes: primary vasculitis, infection, and diabetes mellitus)
	Psychosis
	Seizure
9. Hemolytic anemia	
10. Leukopenia	<4000 cells/mm^3 detected at least once (in the absence of other known causes: Felty's syndrome, drugs, and portal hypertension)
or Lymphopenia	<1000 cells/mm^3 detected at least once (in the absence of other known causes: corticosteroids, drugs, and infection)
11. Thrombocytopenia	<100,000 cells/mm^3 detected at least once (in the absence of other known causes: drugs, portal hypertension, and thrombotic thrombocytopenic purpura)

IMMUNOLOGIC CRITERIA

1. ANAs	Above laboratory reference range
2. Anti-double stranded DNA	Above laboratory reference range, except ELISA: two times greater than laboratory reference range
3. Anti-Smith	
4. Antiphospholipid	Any of the following: lupus anticoagulant, false-positive RPR, medium- or high-titer anticardiolipin (IgA, IgG, or IgM), or anti-β_2 glycoprotein I (IgA, IgG, or IgM)
5. Low complement	Low C3
	Low C4
	Low CH50
6. Direct Coombs test	In the absence of hemolytic anemia

Modified from Petri M, Orbai AM, Alarcón GS, et al: Derivation and validation of Systemic Lupus International Collaborating Clinics classification criteria for systemic lupus erythematosus, Arthritis Rheum 64:2677–2686, 2012.

ANAs, Antinuclear antibodies; ECG, electrocardiogram; ELISA, enzyme-linked immunosorbent assay; Ig, immunoglobulin; RPR, rapid plasma reagin; SLE, systemic lupus erythematosus.

*Criteria are cumulative. A patient is classified as having SLE using lupus nephritis as a stand-alone criterion (in the setting of ANAs or anti-dsDNA antibodies) or four criteria (with at least one of the clinical criteria and one of the immunologic criteria).

TABLE 79-4 PREVALENCE OF AUTOANTIBODIES IN SYSTEMIC LUPUS ERYTHEMATOSUS

TARGET AUTOANTIGEN	POSITIVE (%)
Nuclear antigens	>95
Double-stranded DNA	30-60
Smith	10-44
Ribonucleoprotein (U1-RNP)	25-40
SSA/Ro	30-40
SSB/La	38
Phospholipids	16-60
Ribosomal P	5-10
Histone	21-90

Data from Wallace D, Hahn BH: Other clinical laboratory tests in SLE. In Dubois' lupus erythematosus and related syndromes, ed 8, Philadelphia, 2013, Saunders, pp 526–531.

used. These patients typically are early in their disease course and eventually develop a specific autoimmune disease.

TREATMENT

No cure for SLE has been identified, and treatment is aimed at educating patients, reducing inflammation, suppressing the immune system, and closely monitoring patients to identify disease manifestations as early as possible. Treatment with glucocorticoids and immunosuppressive agents has reduced the morbidity and mortality of patients with SLE, although the treatments themselves are associated with extensive toxicity. Physicians caring for SLE patients must carefully weigh the benefits of therapy against the known risks of treatment.

Patient education and prophylactic measures to prevent disease flares are crucial in the care of patients with SLE. Sunscreens (SPF ≥50) and ultraviolet radiation–protective clothing are effective in preventing photosensitivity skin rashes and systemic flares. Low-dose aspirin is frequently prescribed for patients with positive APA assays to prevent thrombotic events. Other treatments for antiphospholipid antibody syndrome (APS) are discussed later. Routine immunizations (e.g., influenza, pneumococcus) with nonlive vaccines are recommended for all patients. Psychological support is essential for patients with SLE because the disease may lead to depression and feelings of being overwhelmed.

Nonsteroidal anti-inflammatory medications may be used for mild arthralgias, but glucocorticoids remain the primary anti-inflammatory agent and one of the most effective medications for SLE. Glucocorticoids are used for almost all manifestations of SLE in regimens ranging from low, alternate-day doses to large, intravenous doses. Given the chronic nature of the disease, glucocorticoids are often used over many years, and the cumulative exposure may lead to extensive toxicity, including obesity, diabetes mellitus, accelerated atherosclerosis, osteoporosis, avascular necrosis, cataracts, and increased risk of infections. To avoid these toxicities, steroid-sparing immunomodulating or immunosuppressant agents are used.

Antimalarial medications (primarily hydroxychloroquine) are effective in SLE and are considered standard care. Antimalarials are especially beneficial for the fatigue, mild arthritis, and mucocutaneous manifestations of SLE. These medications are often used chronically and are safe to use in pregnancy. The most serious side effect is retinal toxicity, although it is uncommon. Patients taking antimalarials should have a baseline and annual ophthalmologic examination with visual field testing.

Azathioprine and methotrexate are immunosuppressive agents prescribed for SLE when glucocorticoids alone are not fully effective or to allow for a reduction in glucocorticoid dose. Toxicities of azathioprine include cytopenias, increased infection risk, and potential malignant hematologic disease. Azathioprine may be used during pregnancy for severe internal organ lupus, especially nephritis. Methotrexate is particularly effective in treating inflammatory arthritis associated with SLE. In addition to cytopenias and infections, liver function abnormalities, alopecia, nausea, and pneumonitis are potential side effects of methotrexate. Because it is teratogenic, methotrexate should be stopped 3 to 6 months before pregnancy. Azathioprine and methotrexate require regular laboratory monitoring.

Mycophenolate mofetil (MMF) is increasingly used to treat patients with internal organ involvement, particularly nephritis. Mycophenolic acid, the active metabolite of MMF, can be used in place of MMF because it may have fewer gastrointestinal side effects for some patients. Clinical trials have shown that MMF is as efficacious as intravenous cyclophosphamide for inducing remission of active lupus nephritis. MMF also has a category D rating in pregnancy, and toxicities include gastrointestinal disturbance and leukopenia.

Patients with neurologic lupus, rapidly progressive nephritis, or vasculitis of internal organs are often treated with cyclophosphamide, the most potent immunosuppressive agent used to treat SLE. Because of potential toxicities, this drug is usually reserved for the most severe manifestations of SLE. Acute toxicities of cyclophosphamide include pancytopenia, alopecia, mucositis, and hemorrhagic cystitis. Long-term use of cyclophosphamide may lead to transitional cell carcinoma, malignant hematologic disease, sterility, premature menopause, and opportunistic infections.

Great potential and optimism exist for biologic immunomodulating agents that focus on various aspects of the immune system, including B cells, interactions between B and T cells, and cytokines. The most promising agents are those that target B cells, which produce autoantibodies. Belimumab, a monoclonal antibody that inhibits B-lymphocyte stimulator, is the first therapeutic agent approved for the treatment of SLE in more than 50 years.

For a deeper discussion of these topics, please see Chapter 35, "Immunosuppressing Drugs including Corticosteroids" in Goldman-Cecil Medicine, 25th Edition.

⬤ SPECIAL ISSUES IN THE CARE OF PATIENTS WITH SLE
Pregnancy

Pregnant women with SLE have higher rates of pregnancy loss (i.e., miscarriage and stillbirths) and preterm delivery (i.e., premature rupture of membranes, preeclampsia, and intrauterine growth restriction) than their healthy counterparts. Lupus activity preceding conception, especially nephritis, hypertension, and APS, are risk factors for pregnancy complications in SLE. Pregnancy itself may place women with SLE at a greater risk of a flare, particularly if the disease was active before conception.

Neonatal lupus is a rare disorder in which maternal anti-SSA/Ro or SSB/La antibodies, or both, cross the placenta and affect the fetus. Mothers with these autoantibodies have a 2% risk of having a child with congenital heart block. These mothers are screened with fetal heart tones and fetal echocardiography beginning at 16 weeks' gestation. Treatment with a fluorinated corticosteroid (i.e., dexamethasone or betamethasone) may be beneficial, but many children with congenital heart block do not survive (30%) or have morbidities, with more than 60% requiring pacemakers.

More common manifestations of neonatal SLE are rashes, cytopenias, and hepatosplenomegaly, all of which typically resolve in 6 to 8 months after maternal antibodies are removed from the child's circulation. Mothers of children with neonatal SLE do not necessarily have SLE themselves.

With careful prenatal screening and planning, women with SLE can successfully have a healthy child. Prenatal monitoring of anti-SSA/Ro and anti-SSB/La antibodies and APAs and pre-pregnancy consultation with obstetricians caring for high-risk pregnancies are critical. Ideally, women with SLE should have clinical quiescence for 6 months before considering a planned pregnancy.

Hormone Therapy

Hormones were thought to play a role in the development of SLE because of its female predominance. Rheumatologists have historically been hesitant to prescribe estrogen therapy for fear of inducing a flare. Randomized, placebo-controlled clinical trials have helped to guide hormonal therapy in women with SLE.

A multicenter, randomized trial revealed that oral contraceptive therapy does not increase the risk of SLE flares in women with mild or stable SLE disease activity. However, this is not generalizable to all SLE women, particularly those whose disease is active or severe and those with prior thrombotic events or APAs. An effective form of birth control is necessary for young, sexually active women with SLE, especially those on teratogenic medications. Physicians must carefully discuss the risks and benefits of birth control with SLE patients.

Hormonal therapy is a controversial topic regardless of SLE status. However, it is of particular interest in SLE because some women reach menopause prematurely. In a clinical trial of hormonal therapy in SLE patients with mild or stable disease with no prior thrombotic events, APAs, or gynecologic or breast cancers, no SLE patients had severe clinical flares, but 20% did have mild to moderate flares. These findings suggest that brief (1-year) hormonal therapy may be considered for alleviating menopausal symptoms in a subset of SLE women.

Bone Health

SLE patients have higher rates of low bone mineral density, osteoporosis, and fractures than do healthy age-matched subjects. The increased risk is accounted for by traditional risk factors, such as female sex, white or Asian race, older age, and low body weight, and by SLE-associated factors. Fatigue and articular symptoms due to SLE may limit physical activity, leading to loss of bone strength.

Therapies commonly used for SLE contribute to overall loss of bone health. Corticosteroids reduce bone mass and are an independent risk factor for fractures in women with SLE. Cyclophosphamide use can lead to premature ovarian failure, another risk factor for osteoporosis. Lupus disease damage, regardless of steroid use, leads to low bone mineral density. SLE patients are advised to avoid sun exposure, which can lead to low 25-hydroxyvitamin D levels and insufficient absorption of calcium.

Because of SLE-specific risk factors for low bone mineral density, prevention of osteoporosis is extremely important (see Chapter 75). Although osteoporosis screening guidelines for SLE patients are the same as for the general population, bone density scans should be considered for patients with premature menopause and those who are or will be on chronic (>3 months) corticosteroids.

Cardiovascular Disease

As survival and therapies for SLE have improved and patients are living longer, CVD has emerged as a leading cause of morbidity and mortality. SLE patients are 5 to 10 times more likely than healthy individuals to have a coronary event. More striking, premenopausal women between 35 and 44 years of age are more than 50 times as likely as healthy women to have a myocardial infarction.

Autopsy series reveal atherosclerotic heart disease as the underlying mechanism of CVD in SLE. The cause of premature atherosclerosis in SLE is multifactorial and includes inflammatory mediators, SLE-related factors (e.g., premature menopause, corticosteroid therapy, disease activity), and traditional cardiovascular risk factors.

Although no firm cardiovascular management guidelines exist for SLE patients, the 2011 updated guidelines from the American Heart Association for prevention of CVD in women included (for the first time) autoimmune diseases (i.e., SLE and rheumatoid arthritis) in the increased-risk category. Physicians should consider premature atherosclerotic CVD and aggressively evaluate SLE patients with typical and atypical cardiac symptoms, regardless of age and sex.

Secondary Antiphospholipid Syndrome

APS is a disorder characterized by recurrent vascular thrombosis or recurrent pregnancy loss, or both, in the setting of APAs (Table 79-5). Lupus anticoagulant is part of the antiphospholipid laboratory panel and is paradoxically associated with thrombosis and recurrent pregnancy loss. The term *lupus anticoagulant* is a misnomer because the in vitro anticoagulant effect reflects the prolonged activated partial thromboplastin time (aPTT), but the term does not indicate a diagnosis of SLE or an increased risk of bleeding.

Diverse proteins binding to APAs have been recognized. APS is considered primary if it occurs in isolation and secondary if it occurs in conjunction with other autoimmune diseases. There are no major differences in severity or clinical consequences between primary and secondary APS. The reported prevalence of various APAs in SLE ranges from 16% to 55%. SLE patients with APAs have an increased risk of thromboembolism and pregnancy complications and have a higher prevalence of pulmonary hypertension, Libman-Sacks endocarditis, and neurologic complications. The term *catastrophic APS* has been coined to describe patients who exhibit multiple microthromboses, are positive for APAs, and often have a life-threatening illness resulting in multiorgan failure that can be clinically indistinguishable from sepsis or thrombotic thrombocytopenic purpura.

Treatment for APS is tailored to the patient and the clinical manifestations. For patients with vascular thrombosis, indefinite anticoagulation is usually prescribed as prophylaxis against recurrence. Warfarin is the usual drug of choice for long-term therapy, with a target of an international normalized ratio (INR) between 2 and 3. Higher INR levels (3 to 4) are not more effective and are associated with bleeding complications. Unfractionated and low-molecular-weight heparin is also an effective anticoagulant for APS and is used for patients who suffer recurrent events while on warfarin therapy or patients who are or plan to become pregnant.

Malignancy

A multicenter international cohort (SLICC) of more than 16,000 SLE patients reported an increased risk of malignancy among them compared with the general population. Most striking was a fourfold increased risk of non-Hodgkin's lymphoma. Other hematologic, vulvar, lung, and thyroid cancers were described with increased frequency, whereas breast and endometrial cancers were observed less than expected in SLE patients compared with the general population. Malignancy risk appears to be highest early in the disease course, but risk remains elevated throughout a patient's lifespan. Although lymph node

TABLE 79-5 REVISED CLASSIFICATION CRITERIA OF ANTIPHOSPHOLIPID SYNDROME

CLASSIFICATION CRITERIA*	DEFINITION
CLINICAL CRITERIA	
1. Vascular thrombosis	One or more clinical episodes of arterial, venous, or small vessel thrombosis in any tissue or organ. Thrombosis must be confirmed by objective validated criteria (i.e., unequivocal findings of appropriate imaging studies or histopathology). For histopathologic confirmation, thrombosis should be present without significant evidence of inflammation in the vessel wall.
2. Pregnancy morbidity	a. One or more unexplained deaths of a morphologically normal fetus at or beyond 10 weeks' gestation, with normal fetal morphology documented by ultrasound or by direct examination of the fetus *or*
	b. One or more premature births of a morphologically normal neonate before 34 weeks' gestation because of (i) eclampsia or severe pre-eclampsia or (ii) recognized features of placental insufficiency *or*
	c. Three or more unexplained consecutive spontaneous abortions before 10 weeks' gestation, with maternal anatomic or hormonal abnormalities and paternal and maternal chromosomal causes excluded
LABORATORY CRITERIA	
1. Lupus anticoagulant	LAC detected in plasma on two or more occasions at least 12 wk apart
2. Anticardiolipin antibody	The ACA antibody of IgG and/or IgM isotype in serum or plasma in medium or high titer (i.e., >40 GPL units, or >the 99th percentile) on two or more occasions at least 12 weeks apart, measured by a standardized ELISA
3. Anti-β_2 glycoprotein I antibody	B2GPI antibody of IgG and/or IgM isotype in serum or plasma (in titer >the 99th percentile), detected on two or more occasions at least 12 weeks apart, measured by a standardized ELISA

Modified from Miyakis S, Lockshin MD, Atsumi T, et al: International consensus statement on an update of the classification criteria for definite antiphospholipid syndrome (APS), J Thromb Haemost 4:295–306, 2006.

ACA, Anticardiolipin antibody; ELISA, enzyme-linked immunosorbent assay; B2GPI, anti-β_2 glycoprotein I antibody; Ig, immunoglobulin; LAC, lupus anticoagulant.

*Antiphospholipid antibody syndrome is diagnosed if at least one clinical criterion and one laboratory criterion are met.

enlargement is a common manifestation of SLE, physicians must consider malignancy if the lymphadenopathy does not resolve with SLE treatment, is nontender or nonmobile, or if it occurs without other lupus symptoms.

PROGNOSIS

In 1955, patients with SLE had a 5-year survival rate of only 50%. Advances in early diagnosis and treatment of lupus patients have led to the current 5- and 10-year survival rates of more than 90% and approximately 90%, respectively, in developed countries.

A bimodal pattern of mortality is seen in SLE. Early deaths (<5 years from diagnosis) are attributed to active SLE disease and infections, whereas later deaths (>5 years from diagnosis) result from chronic SLE complications and medications, atherosclerotic CVD, and infections. Data suggest that malignancy-associated morbidity and mortality are lifelong risks, but rates are the greatest early in the disease. With recent and ongoing improvements in the treatment of SLE and increasing survival rates of patients with SLE, we need to pay additional attention to comorbid conditions associated with SLE and its treatment, specifically premature atherosclerotic heart disease, malignancy, bone health, and psychosocial well-being.

SUGGESTED READINGS

Arbuckle MR, McClain MT, Rubertone MV, et al: Development of autoantibodies before the clinical onset of systemic lupus erythematosus, N Engl J Med 349:1526–1533, 2003.

Austin HA 3rd, Klippel JH, Balow JE, et al: Therapy of lupus nephritis. Controlled trial of prednisone and cytotoxics, N Engl J Med 314:614–619, 1986.

Bernatsky S, Ramsey-Goldman R, Labrecque J, et al: Cancer risk in systemic lupus: an updated international multi-center cohort study, J Autoimmun 42:130–135, 2013.

Bertsias GK, Ioannidis JPA, Aringer M, et al: EULAR recommendations for the management of systemic lupus erythematosus with neuropsychiatric manifestations: report of a task force of the EULAR standing committee for clinical affairs, Ann Rheum Dis 69:2074–2082, 2010.

Danchenko D, Satia JA, Anthony MS: Epidemiology of systemic lupus erythematosus: a comparison of worldwide disease burden, Lupus 15:308–318, 2006.

Furie R, Petri M, Zamani O, et al: A phase III, randomized, placebo-controlled study of belimumab, a monoclonal antibody that inhibits B lymphocyte stimulator, in patients with systemic lupus erythematosus, Arthritis Rheum 63:3918–3930, 2011.

Ginzler EM, Dooley MA, Aranow C, et al: Mycophenolate mofetil or intravenous cyclophosphamide for lupus nephritis, N Engl J Med 353:2219–2228, 2005.

Lee C, Ramsey-Goldman R: Bone health and systemic lupus erythematosus, Curr Rheumatol Rep 7:482–489, 2005.

Manzi S, Meilahn EN, Rairie JE, et al: Age-specific incidence rates of myocardial infarction and angina in women with systemic lupus erythematosus: comparison with the Framingham Study, Am J Epidemiol 145:408–415, 1997.

Mosca L, Benjamin EJ, Berra K, et al: Effectiveness-based guidelines for the prevention of cardiovascular disease in women—2011 update: a guideline from the American Heart Association, J Am Coll Cardiol 57:1404–1423, 2011.

Miyakis S, Lockshin MD, Atsumi T, et al: International consensus statement on an update of the classification criteria for definite antiphospholipid syndrome (APS), J Thromb Haemost 4:295–306, 2006.

Petri M, Kim MY, Kalunian KC, et al: Combined contraceptives in women with systemic lupus erythematosus, N Engl J Med 353:2550–2558, 2005.

Petri M, Orbai AM, Alarcón GS, et al: Derivation and validation of the Systemic Lupus International Collaborating Clinics classification criteria for systemic lupus erythematosus, Arthritis Rheum 64:2677–2686, 2012.

Wallace D, Hahn BH, editors: Other clinical laboratory tests in SLE. In Dubois' lupus erythematosus and related syndromes, ed 8, Philadelphia, 2013, Saunders, pp 526–531.

Systemic Sclerosis

Robyn T. Domsic

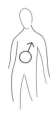

INTRODUCTION

Systemic sclerosis (SSc) is a connective tissue disease that is characterized by cutaneous and visceral fibrosis. The more common term for the disease, *scleroderma*, reflects its derivation from the Greek *scleros,* which means thick, and *derma*, which means skin.

The disorder can range from a relatively benign condition to a rapidly progressive disease leading to significant morbidity or death. Although cutaneous manifestations are the most obvious features, visceral involvement can be severe and disabling. Monitoring for potential organ complications is essential in caring for SSc patients, because early detection and treatment may minimize morbidity and mortality.

EPIDEMIOLOGY

The annual U.S. incidence of SSc is approximately 20 cases per million persons. Because patients with SSc often live for many years, the prevalence is 240 cases per million persons. Incidence and prevalence vary somewhat throughout the world, and they typically are lower in Europe and Asia. SSc more commonly affects women, with a 3 : 1 female-to-male ratio. It occurs in individuals of all ages, from childhood to the elderly, but it most frequently affects those between the ages of 40 and 60 years.

A familial pattern of inheritance is not as evident in SSc as in other connective tissue diseases. Twin studies have demonstrated only a 5% rate of concordance in monozygotic and dizygotic twins, implying that there are significant environmental contributions to its occurrence. Many patients with SSc, however, have family histories of other autoimmune diseases (e.g., thyroid disease, rheumatoid arthritis, systemic lupus erythematosus [SLE]). Genome-wide association studies have revealed a handful of genes associated with SSc that are shared with other diseases such as rheumatoid arthritis and SLE (e.g., major histocompatibility complex class I and II genes *STAT4* and *IRF5*). These findings suggest a shared genetic predisposition to autoimmune conditions.

PATHOLOGY

The pathogenesis of SSc has not been fully elucidated. There are three clearly identified components: endothelial and vascular injury with associated vasculopathy, immune system activation, and fibrosis with overproduction of collagen and other connective tissue matrix proteins (Fig. 80-1). Involvement of these systems initially became evident from autopsy studies. Vascular changes include endothelial cell injury and subintimal thickening leading to luminal narrowing with occasional vascular occlusion

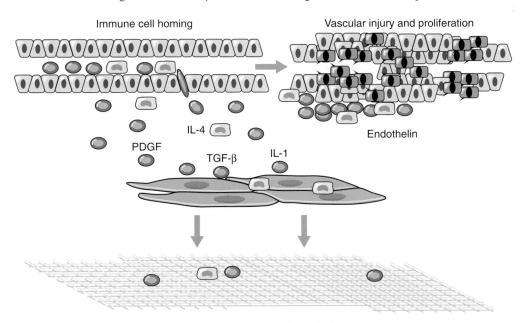

FIGURE 80-1 Pathogenetic processes in systemic sclerosis. Vascular injury leads to intimal proliferation of endothelial cells *(red)* and smooth muscle cells *(blue)*. Fibroblasts are activated to deposit increased amounts of interstitial matrix. IL, Interleukin; PDGF, platelet-derived growth factor; TGF-β, transforming growth factor-β.

and periadventitial fibrosis. Vascular changes are seen in the skin and may occur in the pulmonary, cardiac, and renal blood vessels, affecting arteries, arterioles, and capillaries. True vasculitis is conspicuously absent.

Cutaneous inflammatory infiltrates consist of activated mononuclear cells, T lymphocytes, and monocytes in the dermis, often occurring in a perivascular distribution. Dermal thickening is accompanied by excessive deposition of collagen fibrils and fibrous replacement of subcutaneous fat and secondary skin appendages such as hair follicles and sebaceous glands.

The interplay between the vascular, immunologic, and connective tissue changes is complex. Most hypotheses focus on interactions between early vascular and immunologic events leading to activation of fibroblasts, which are thought to be the effector cells in this disease. Fibroblasts are found in increased numbers in the skin and other tissues, and they develop an SSc phenotype when grown in vitro, producing an overabundance of collagen and living longer in tissue culture. Fibroblast persistence in culture suggests a perpetuated abnormality not requiring continued immune stimulation.

Other factors that may contribute to fibrosis include hypoxia and local cytokine changes. Early vascular involvement consists of an imbalance between vasodilatory and vasoconstrictive factors, endothelial cell activation with resultant leukocyte migration, smooth muscle cell proliferation, and defective vasculogenesis. Vascular activation can induce fibrosis by interleukin-mediated mechanisms.

Immune system activation is evident in several respects. First, serum levels of inflammatory markers (based on the sedimentation rate) and circulating cytokines are increased. Second, serum autoantibodies are detected in more than 95% of patients with SSc. One of nine autoantibodies is relatively specific for the disease. All of the antibodies are directed against distinct nuclear antigens. They are helpful in classifying patients, but their pathogenic role has not been elucidated. Third, there is evidence of T-cell activation, with a T_H2-predominant cytokine profile. Elevated levels of interleukins (i.e., IL-1, IL-2, IL-2R, IL-4, IL-8, IL-13, and IL-17) and interferon have been reported. The role of T_H17 cells is not understood, but studies suggest that dysregulation of these proinflammatory T cells contributes to disease pathogenesis. Fourth, there is increasing evidence of innate immune dysregulation in the setting of activated macrophages and altered expression and function of toll-like receptors.

⬤ CLINICAL PRESENTATION

Patients with SSc can have several clinical presentations, although Raynaud's phenomenon is the most common symptom. Distinctive phenotypes may manifest differently. SSc can have many internal organ manifestations, producing various clinical presentations and requiring tailored work-up protocols.

Classification by Cutaneous Features

Historically, SSc has been separated into two major clinical subsets defined by the degree and extent of skin involvement: limited cutaneous (lc) and diffuse cutaneous (dc) disease. Patients with lcSSc experience skin thickening limited to the distal extremities (i.e., below the elbows and knees). The dcSSc patients have similar distal changes in addition to involvement of

the upper arms, thighs, or trunk at some time during the disease course. Few patients (<1%) have no skin thickening but have one or more typical SSc visceral manifestation.

The term *scleroderma sine scleroderma* has been used to describe dcSSc patients whose clinical course resembles that of individuals with lcSSc. The distinct cutaneous patterns are important, because patients with dcSSc are more likely to develop internal organ complications (e.g., renal crisis, cardiac involvement) early in their illness, whereas those with lcSSc can develop internal organ involvement throughout their disease, even decades after the initial symptoms (Table 80-1). Some patients with lcSSc or dcSSC may have typical features of another connective tissue disease (most commonly polymyositis, SLE, or rheumatoid arthritis-like features), and they are considered to have *SSc in overlap*.

Serologic Classification

Serologic classification refers to SSc-associated serum autoantibodies. Patients with the same autoantibody tend to have a similar cutaneous pattern, natural history of disease, and risk of internal organ involvement.

TABLE 80-1	MANIFESTATIONS OF SYSTEMIC SCLEROSIS BY CLINICAL CLASSIFICATION	
MANIFESTATIONS	**DIFFUSE** (N = 1434)	**LIMITED** (N = 1718)
CUTANEOUS		
Puffy fingers	82%	78%
Skin induration, thickening	Widespread: trunk, face, extremities	Face, below the elbow and knee
Telangiectasias	58%	70%
Calcinosis	14%	22%
PERIPHERAL VASCULAR		
Raynaud's phenomenon	95%	97%
Digital ulcerations	42%	39%
PULMONARY		
Interstitial lung disease	37%	34%
Pulmonary arterial hypertension	5%	16%
CARDIAC		
Arrhythmias	16%	14%
Diastolic dysfunction	4%	5%
Myocarditis	6%	2%
Pericarditis	4%	3%
RENAL		
Renal crisis	18%	2%
GASTROINTESTINAL		
Esophageal hypomotility, reflux	79%	77%
Small intestine dysmotility	18%	13%
Malabsorption	11%	9%
Incontinence	2%	2%
JOINT AND MUSCULOSKELETAL		
Tendon friction rubs	53%	5%
Joint contractures	88%	38%
Myositis	10%	6%
Bland myopathy	2%	1%

Data from the University of Pittsburgh Scleroderma Databank, 1980-2012.

Serologic classification can augment the clinical classification described previously. For example, 95% of patients with anticentromere antibody have lcSSc and are at increased risk for pulmonary hypertension during the follow-up period. Individuals with anti–topoisomerase I (i.e., anti-SCL70) or anti–RNA polymerase III antibody are more likely to have dcSSc. Those with anti–RNA polymerase III antibody have an increased risk of renal crisis, and those with anti-SCL70 have a higher frequency of interstitial lung disease.

The primary internal organ risks and cutaneous associations are depicted in Figure 80-2, which illustrates the combined clinical-serologic classification of SSc. It is uncommon for patients to have more than one SSc autoantibody.

Raynaud's Phenomenon and Peripheral Vascular Involvement

Most patients with SSc experience Raynaud's phenomenon during their disease course. Raynaud's phenomenon is a triphasic vasospastic response to cold consisting of pallor (i.e., blanching) with or without cyanosis (i.e., bluish discoloration followed by reactive hyperemia (i.e., erythema) with a characteristic distinct line of demarcation on the digits separating the affected from unaffected areas.

The onset of Raynaud's phenomenon can precede the development of skin changes by years in some patients. Severe involvement may result in ischemia with loss of digital tip tissue, including digital pitting scars, ulcers, and gangrene (rare). Digital tip ulcers are more frequent in patients who are anticentromere or anti–topoisomerase I autoantibody positive. Lower extremity ulcerations in SSc patients have been increasingly reported in recent years.

Interstitial Lung Disease

Interstitial lung disease (ILD) can be one of the most serious complications of SSc and should be monitored for routinely (see Chapter 17). The initial presentation is often a nonproductive cough and a gradual onset of dyspnea on exertion over several months to years. However, the onset can be abrupt.

High-resolution chest computed tomography (CT) typically shows bibasilar fibrotic changes, which can be progressive. Pulmonary function tests reveal reduced forced vital capacity (FVC). On pathologic examination, the most frequently seen pattern is nonspecific interstitial pneumonitis. Patients with anti-SCL70 autoantibody are at the highest risk for ILD.

Pulmonary Hypertension

SSc patients can develop pulmonary hypertension of three World Health Organization (WHO) classifications (see Chapter 18). Pulmonary arterial hypertension (PAH, group 1) is the most common, with an estimated 10% to 15% of patients in cohort studies developing PAH. It occurs most commonly in those with lcSSc. The clinical presentation includes rapidly progressive dyspnea occurring over several months. Pulmonary function tests reveal a reduced diffusion capacity for carbon monoxide (D$_{LCO}$) out of proportion to any concomitant reduction in the FVC.

Less frequently, SSc patients develop pulmonary hypertension associated with ILD (group 3) or pulmonary hypertension associated with left ventricular diastolic dysfunction from myocardial fibrosis or non–SSc-associated left ventricular disorders (group 2). Screening for all types of pulmonary hypertension is performed by echocardiogram, and results should be confirmed by right heart cardiac catheterization.

Scleroderma Renal Crisis

Scleroderma renal crisis (SRC) manifests as the abrupt onset of accelerated arterial hypertension accompanied by a rise in serum creatinine levels and by microscopic hematuria and proteinuria on urinalysis. Microangiopathic hemolytic anemia and thrombocytopenia are common. Although once the major cause of mortality in SSc, SRC is now managed by aggressive blood pressure control with an angiotensin-converting enzyme (ACE) inhibitor.

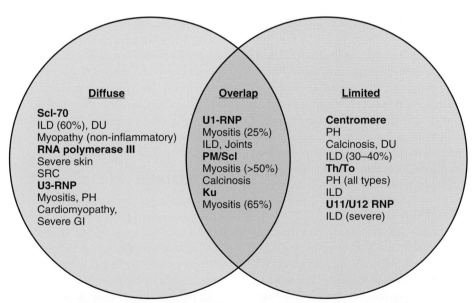

FIGURE 80-2   Clinical-serologic classification of systemic sclerosis and antibody-associated internal organ manifestations. *Bold text* indicates an antibody; clinical manifestations listed below are associated with that antibody. DU, Digital ulcers; ILD, interstitial lung disease; Ku, 70/80-kD protein (XRCC6/XRCC5); PH, pulmonary hypertension; PM, polymyositis; RNP, ribonucleoprotein; Scl, sclerosis; SRC, scleroderma renal crisis.

The typical setting for SRC is early dcSSc with a recent increase in skin thickening, palpable tendon friction rubs, and anti–RNA polymerase III antibody. During active, early dcSSc, patients should check their blood pressure once weekly and report a rise in systolic blood pressure of more than 20 mm Hg from baseline. Prednisone given at a dose of 15 mg daily or higher has been associated with the development of SRC and should be avoided in at-risk patients.

Cardiac Manifestations

Patients with SSc have three primary types of cardiac involvement: pericarditis, myocarditis, and myocardial fibrosis. The latter can lead to congestive heart failure and arrhythmias due to fibrosis of the conduction system. These complications can be asymptomatic and underrecognized in SSc patients, but pathologic changes have been found in most patients in older autopsy series. Later studies using cardiac magnetic resonance imaging (MRI) have confirmed the autopsy findings.

Diastolic dysfunction is becoming increasingly recognized as a complication of fibrosis and can be evaluated by echocardiogram during pulmonary hypertension screening. Many SSc deaths occur suddenly, possibly due to ventricular arrhythmias. It is prudent to obtain a resting electrocardiogram early in the disease course. Palpitations noticed by the patient should be addressed with a formal cardiac arrhythmia evaluation.

Gastrointestinal Tract Manifestations

At least one gastrointestinal manifestation will affect 80% or more of SSc patients, and all areas of the gastrointestinal tract may be affected. Gastrointestinal involvement is a significant cause of morbidity.

When the esophagus is affected, patients experience heartburn due to relaxation of the esophageal sphincter and distal dysphagia for solid foods due to esophageal dysmotility. Neuropathic changes and fibrosis of the muscularis of the small intestine can lead to motor dysfunction and symptoms of postprandial abdominal distention. Small intestinal hypomotility may lead to bacterial overgrowth, causing bloating and diarrhea.

When severe atony of the small intestine develops, patients occasionally develop a functional ileus or intestinal pseudoobstruction. Parenteral nutrition may be necessary for severe malabsorption with accompanying weight loss and steatorrhea. Similar to the small bowel, the colon may develop impaired motor function leading to constipation and occasionally overflow diarrhea. Wide-mouthed diverticula on the antimesenteric border of the colon can be seen. The internal anal sphincter may become fibrotic, resulting in fecal incontinence.

Musculoskeletal Manifestations

Musculoskeletal manifestations are common. Tendons can become inflamed and fibrotic, particularly in early, diffuse disease. Palpable tendon or bursal friction rubs are virtually pathognomonic of SSc and often are a harbinger of progression to dcSSc before widespread skin thickening has occurred. Finger joint flexion contractures develop frequently within the first 2 years of diffuse SSc. True arthritis with palpable synovitis should raise the question of overlap with rheumatoid arthritis.

Some patients develop a bland myopathy with nonprogressive, mild proximal muscle weakness and wasting. A few, particularly with features that overlap with other connective tissue diseases, can develop true myositis, which can result in morbidity and disability.

DIAGNOSIS AND DIFFERENTIAL DIAGNOSIS

Raynaud's disease (i.e., primary Raynaud's phenomenon) is prominent in the differential diagnosis for SSc. Features that identify Raynaud's patients who have or may later develop SSc or another connective tissue disease are abnormal nail fold capillaries (i.e., capillary dilation, megacapillaries, and avascular areas), tissue loss at the tips of the fingers, and a positive antinuclear antibody (ANA) test result. None of these features is found in Raynaud's disease.

Mixed connective tissue disease (MCTD) is also on the differential for SSc. MCTD patients have features of two or more autoimmune diseases. This most frequently includes SSc, polymyositis, and SLE. Patients are positive for anti–U1-RNP antibody, a serologic marker for MCTD. Patients with MCTD can develop any or all of the following SSc manifestations: Raynaud's phenomenon, puffy fingers, limited or diffuse skin thickening, myositis, ILD, PAH, and esophageal dysmotility.

Scleroderma mimics are sometimes difficult to distinguish from SSc (Table 80-2). They include eosinophilic fasciitis, the localized forms of scleroderma such as linear scleroderma (more frequently seen in children), and plaque or generalized morphea.

Nephrogenic systemic fibrosis is a complication of gadolinium administration for radiographic studies that occurs in the setting of renal failure. Nephrogenic systemic fibrosis manifests as symmetrical, bilateral, fibrotic, indurated papules, plaques, or subcutaneous nodules, which can be erythematosus and occur on the lower legs or hands. The lesions are often preceded by edema and may initially be misdiagnosed as cellulitis. This diagnosis should be considered in patients being evaluated for a fibrotic disorder who have renal failure, regardless of the cause of renal disease.

Scleromyxedema and scleredema are cutaneous fibrotic disorders in which excessive mucin accumulation is found on skin biopsy. Scleromyxedema can mimic dcSSc on the physical examination or can manifest with multiple, firm, nodular skin lesions (i.e., papular mucinosis). A frequent association is a monoclonal gammopathy (i.e., immunoglobulin [IgG] paraprotein). Scleredema typically involves the nape of the neck and shoulders, sparing the distal extremities. All SSc mimics lack Raynaud's phenomenon, characteristic SSc internal organ involvement, and SSc-associated serum antibodies.

TREATMENT

Because no single therapy exists for SSc, patients must be appropriately monitored for visceral involvement to allow early identification and therapy targeted at specific organ complications. Consultation with a rheumatologist is helpful in this respect, and referral of severely affected patients to a dedicated scleroderma center should be the rule.

All patients should undergo screening evaluation for ILD and pulmonary hypertension throughout the course of their disease. Current expert recommendations suggest that patients with early, diffuse disease should be monitored at least yearly for these

TABLE 80-2 SCLERODERMA MIMICS

DISORDER	DISTINGUISHING FEATURES
OTHER DISEASES	
Morphea	One or more discrete lesions; patchy or linear in distribution
Eosinophilic fasciitis	Finger flexures without sclerodactyly; characteristic groove sign when the arms are raised; puckering or dimpling of the upper arm and thigh skin; peripheral blood eosinophilia; fascia and deep subcutaneous fibrosis
Scleredema (Buschke's disease)	Prominent involvement of neck, shoulders, and upper arms; hands spared; associated with diabetes
Scleromyxedema	Association with gammopathy; skin lichenoid and thickened but not tethered; may have Raynaud's phenomenon
Graft-versus-host disease	Skin changes similar to scleroderma; vasculopathy
Nephrogenic fibrosing dermopathy	Indurated plaques or nodules on the legs or arms, sparing the face; administration of gadolinium in the setting of renal dysfunction; often preceded by edema
REACTIONS TO ENVIRONMENTAL AGENTS AND DRUGS	
Bleomycin	Skin and lung fibrosis similar to scleroderma
L-Tryptophan (1980s)	Eosinophilia-myalgia syndrome from L-tryptophan contaminant or metabolite (first described in the 1980s); fever, eosinophilia, neurologic manifestations
Organic solvents (e.g., trichloroethylene)	Clinically indistinguishable from idiopathic systemic sclerosis
Pendazocine	Localized lesions at injection sites
Toxic oil syndrome	Contaminated rapeseed oil (Spanish epidemic in 1981); similar to eosinophilia myalgia syndrome
Vinyl chloride	Vascular lesions, acro-osteolysis, sclerodactyly, no visceral disease
Gadolinium	Nephrogenic fibrosing dermopathy

complications. Patients with active dcSSc should undergo weekly monitoring of blood pressure because the abrupt appearance of hypertension suggests SRC. Early dcSSc patients should also have skin thickness scores assessed for progression or regression of cutaneous disease. For dcSSc and lcSSc, initial esophageal motility studies should be performed, and further objective studies should be ordered on the basis of symptoms.

Education of patients and family members regarding the disease and the patient's classification (i.e., early or late, diffuse or limited disease) can help to alleviate patients' anxiety. An excellent publication, *The Scleroderma Book: A Guide for Patients and Families*, is available.

Raynaud's Phenomenon

Calcium-channel blockers have been widely used for decades, and they are generally well tolerated by patients. Long-acting nifedipine is effective in more than one half of patients, and newer agents such as amlodipine are frequently prescribed (level 1B evidence). The angiotensin-receptor blocker losartan reduced the severity and frequency of Raynaud's phenomenon attacks in a placebo-controlled trial. ACE inhibitors have not proved effective in several controlled trials. Phosphodiesterase-5 (PDE-5) inhibitors have been shown to improve Raynaud phenomenon (level 1A evidence).

In patients with digital ulcerations, more aggressive therapy may be warranted. PDE-5 inhibitors have been helpful (level 1B

evidence) has been helpful. Topical nitroglycerin as a paste, gel, or patch placed at the base of the fingers may be a useful adjunct. In randomized, placebo-controlled trials, bosentan prevented the formation of new digital ulcerations in patients with SSc and Raynaud's phenomenon, although it has not been approved by th U.S. Food and Drug Administration (FDA) for this indication (level 1B evidence). Iloprost, an intravenous prostacyclin, has also been shown to reduce digital ulcerations and is frequently used in Europe, but also it is not FDA approved in the United States (level A evidence).

For patients with digital ulcers involving adjacent fingers, assessment of the ulnar and radial artery should be performed with arterial Doppler or angiography because larger arteries can become severely narrowed. Surgical interventions include sympathectomy of the digital, radial, or ulnar artery and venous bypass for ulnar or radial artery occlusion. In SSc patients with recurrent digital ulcers or other thrombotic events, evaluation for a hypercoagulable state, particularly for lupus anticoagulant, should be performed. In this circumstance, aspirin or other anticoagulants are indicated.

Cutaneous Disease

No therapeutic agent has been found to improve skin thickening in a randomized, placebo-controlled trial for patients with dcSSc. Several methodologic issues have contributed to the negative findings, including the drugs chosen, patient populations, and trial designs. In the past, considerable attention was given to methotrexate and D-penicillamine, but no convincing data support the use of either drug.

Case series with historical controls and comparisons with clinical trials have suggested a benefit for mycophenolate mofetil, although it has not been studied in a randomized setting (level B evidence).

Several reports on the benefit of autologous stem cell transplantation have been published. In an ILD study, cyclophosphamide use showed significant improvement in skin thickening in treated patients compared with placebo. Unless there is a serious internal organ complication, this potent therapy cannot be recommended because of the concern about life-threatening adverse effects, including malignancy.

Scleroderma Renal Crisis

Early diagnosis and prompt initiation of ACE inhibitors are the keys to improved survival and outcomes of SRC. ACE inhibitors should be titrated to maintain a normal blood pressure (level 3 evidence), preferably less than 125/75 mm Hg. β-Blockers are relatively contraindicated.

Even if patients with SRC become dialysis dependent initially, some may experience a slow reversal of renal vascular damage if ACE inhibitor therapy is maintained. Because up to 50% of SRC patients can spontaneously come off dialysis, transplantation evaluation should be delayed until at least 2 years after SRC onset.

Interstitial Lung Disease

Early recognition of inflammatory ILD is important if treatment is to prevent progression to distortion of lung architecture and irreversible fibrosis. A recent large, randomized, placebo-controlled trial demonstrated statistically significant but modest FVC improvement with oral cyclophosphamide at 1 year. However, after an additional year off therapy, cyclophosphamide-treated patients lost their benefit, suggesting that other treatment options are needed.

Case series with and without historical controls support the potential benefit of mycophenolate mofetil, and this drug is the subject of an ongoing randomized controlled trial. Lung transplantation can be considered for end-stage ILD.

Pulmonary Hypertension

Several agents have been approved for the treatment of PAH (see Chapter 18). Subset analyses of several placebo-controlled drug trials have shown improvement in established SSc or connective tissue disease–related PAH. They have included phosphodiesterase-5 inhibitors (e.g., sildenafil, tadalafil), endothelial receptor antagonists (e.g., bosentan, ambrisentan), and prostacyclin analogues (e.g., treprostinil, epoprostenol) (level A evidence).

Theoretically, treatment of patients with early, less severe disease should improve outcomes, but studies are only beginning to be reported. Because patients with SSc-related PAH have a worse prognosis than those with idiopathic PAH, SSc patients with PAH should be recommended to a tertiary care facility with a dedicated pulmonary hypertension clinic.

Cardiac Manifestations

Combined corticosteroids and immunosuppression can be used for myocarditis. Conventional treatment is recommended for symptomatic pericarditis (see Chapter 10), arrhythmias (see Chapter 9), and congestive heart failure (see Chapter 5).

Gastrointestinal Manifestations

Gastroesophageal reflux, which occurs in most SSc patients, can be treated with proton pump inhibitors and conservative measures, including elevation of the head of the bed and avoidance of alcohol and caffeine. If untreated, reflux esophagitis can progress to distal esophageal stricture formation.

Patients with severe esophageal, gastric, or small bowel dysmotility may improve with the use of prokinetic drugs such as metoclopramide, erythromycin, or octreotide. Rotating antibiotics may be of assistance for bacterial overgrowth. For advanced small bowel involvement with malabsorption, supplementation of iron, calcium, and fat-soluble vitamins may be required. Occasionally, total parental nutrition is necessary. Unexplained iron-deficiency anemia in SSc patients suggests the possibility of gastric antral vascular ectasias (i.e., watermelon stomach), which are treated with laser photocoagulation.

Skeletal Muscle, Joint, and Tendon Manifestations

Bland myopathy usually is nonprogressive and is treated with physical therapy. If there is evidence of myositis with elevated serum levels of muscle enzymes or abnormal electromyography or muscle biopsy, corticosteroids and immunosuppressive therapy (e.g., methotrexate, azathioprine) may be helpful.

Patients with lcSSc or dcSSc can develop contractures of the hands due to tendon involvement. Physical therapy with daily stretching exercises directed at the finger joints should be instituted as soon as possible to prevent further loss of finger motion.

For a deeper discussion of these topics, please see Chapter 267, "Systemic Sclerosis (Scleroderma)," in Goldman-Cecil Medicine, *25th Edition.*

SUGGESTED READINGS

Kowal-Bielecka O, Landewé R, Avouac J, et al: EULAR recommendations for the treatment of systemic sclerosis: a report from the EULAR scleroderma trials and research group (EUSTAR), Ann Rheum Dis 68:620–628, 2009.

Maurer B, Distler O: Emerging targeted therapies in scleroderma lung and skin fibrosis, Best Pract Res Clin Rheumatol 25:843–858, 2011.

Mayes MD: The scleroderma book: a guide for patients and families, New York, 1999, Oxford University Press.

Medsger TA: Natural history of systemic sclerosis and the assessment of disease activity, severity, functional status, and psychologic well-being, Rheum Dis Clin North Am 29:255–275, 2003.

Systemic Vasculitis

Kimberly P. Liang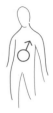

DEFINITION AND EPIDEMIOLOGY

The primary systemic vasculitides are inflammatory disorders of blood vessels that are characterized by immune-mediated injury leading to vessel necrosis, thrombosis, stenosis, or some combination of these. Vessels in any organ may be affected, but each vasculitis is characterized by different preferential vessel size or territory and tissue targeting. Although these disorders are rare, they may be organ- or life-threatening, so prompt diagnosis and treatment are necessary. The vasculitides are defined according to the 1990 American College of Rheumatology (ACR) classification criteria and the 1994 Chapel Hill Consensus Conference (CHCC) based on generally affected vessel size (small, medium, or large). Antineutrophil cytoplasmic antibody (ANCA)–associated vasculitides (AAVs) have known associations with characteristic autoantibodies. Figure 81-1 shows the major types of vasculitides. Although the ACR and CHCC definitions were not designed as diagnostic criteria, classification criteria such as these are important in clinical research study design, treatment, and prognosis. The ACR and the European League Against Rheumatism (EULAR) are currently in the process of refining diagnostic and classification criteria for primary vasculitides.

Determining the incidence and prevalence of each of the vasculitides is challenging given the rarity of the disorders, imperfect classification criteria and definitions for epidemiologic purposes, and some clinicopathologic overlaps that occur between certain types (e.g., AAVs).

Small Vessel Vasculitis

ANCA-Associated Vasculitides

Granulomatosis with polyangiitis (GPA; previously known as Wegener's granulomatosis), microscopic polyangiitis (MPA), eosinophilic granulomatosis with polyangiitis (EGPA; previously known as Churg-Strauss syndrome), and renal-limited vasculitis (RLV) affect small and medium-sized blood vessels and may be associated with ANCA. Various studies have shown AAVs to have an incidence of approximately 10 to 20 per million. The peak age at onset is 65 to 74 years, with a female-to-male ratio of 1.5 : 1. EGPA is the least common of the AAVs, with an incidence of approximately 1.0 to 3.0 per million, and it also has a weaker association with ANCA than GPA and MPA do.

Henoch-Schönlein Purpura

Henoch-Schönlein purpura (HSP) is a small vessel vasculitis that occurs most frequently in young children, with a peak age at onset of 4 to 6 years, but can also occur in adults. HSP accounts for almost half of all cases of childhood vasculitis. In children

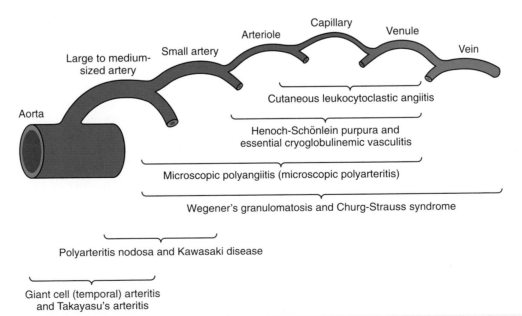

FIGURE 81-1 The vascular spectrum of the vasculitides. (From Jennette JC, Falk RJ, Andrassy K, et al.: Nomenclature of systemic vasculitides: proposal of an international consensus conference, Arthritis Rheum 37:187–192, 1994.)

younger than 17 years of age, the annual incidence of HSP is approximately 20 per 100,000. Males are more commonly affected than females (approximately 2 : 1), and HSP occurs more frequently during the winter and spring months.

Medium Vessel Vasculitis

Polyarteritis nodosa (PAN) is a medium vessel vasculitis that is characterized by arterial aneurysmal and stenotic lesions of muscular arteries, often located at segmental and branch points. In contrast to small vessel vasculitis, renal involvement in PAN is not characterized by glomerulonephritis but rather by aneurysms and stenoses of renal arteries that may result in hypertension or renal dysfunction or both. PAN may occur either as a primary vasculitis or secondary to viral infections, mainly hepatitis B or C, or human immunodeficiency virus (HIV). Determining the incidence of this vasculitis is difficult, because PAN and MPA were not differentiated until 1994.

Kawasaki disease is a medium vessel vasculitis most often seen in boys younger than 5 years of age. It is the second most common vasculitis in childhood after HSP, accounting for about 23% of all childhood vasculitis cases. In the United States, the annual incidence in children younger than 5 years old is 20 per 100,000.

Large Vessel Vasculitis

Giant cell arteritis (GCA), also known as temporal arteritis, is the most common form of vasculitis in adults. It is a large vessel vasculitis that typically affects patients of Eastern European descent, with a mean age at onset of 70 to 75 years. It affects women more commonly than men (3 : 1). About 40% of patients with GCA have the related condition, polymyalgia rheumatica (PMR), which is characterized by subacute onset of aching and stiffness in the muscles of the neck, shoulder girdle, and hip girdle. However, only 10% to 25% of patients with PMR have or will develop GCA.

Takayasu's arteritis (TAK), or "pulseless disease," is a rare large vessel vasculitis that was initially identified in young women from East Asia in the 1800s but is now described worldwide. In adults, the female-to-male ratio is about 8 : 1, with an average age at diagnosis in the mid-20s.

⬤ PATHOLOGY

For most of the systemic vasculitides, the etiology and pathogenesis of disease are largely unknown. It has been proposed that a number of diverse mechanisms contribute to the development of vascular inflammation and subsequent injury on the background of genetic susceptibility (Fig. 81-2). Proposed triggers of disease include infection and environmental exposures (e.g., chemicals, pollutants). For most vasculitides, these associations remain speculative.

Humoral and cellular immune responses, cytokine release, chemokine activation, and immune complex deposition are important in disease pathogenesis. Normal protective and repair processes in the vessel can also contribute to injury and ischemia. For example, after injury, cellular migration and proliferation occurring as part of vessel repair can result in intimal hyperplasia, and the procoagulant milieu that is protective against hemorrhage may lead to thrombosis and vessel occlusion. Impairment of blood flow in injured vessels results in tissue ischemia and

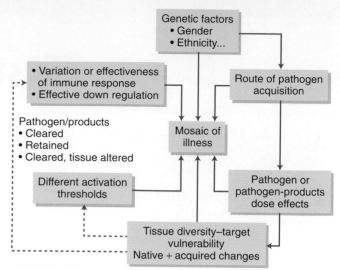

FIGURE 81-2 Factors affecting disease vulnerability and expression.

damage. The degree of blood flow impairment varies along a broad spectrum of severity and may depend on the type of vasculitis as well as the size and location of the vessels involved.

Among the AAVs, the pathology of GPA is typically characterized by necrotizing granulomatous inflammation of small blood vessels supplying the upper and lower respiratory tract. In both GPA and MPA, renal pathology shows a pauci-immune necrotizing crescentic glomerulonephritis. In EGPA, there is a strong association with allergic and atopic disorders, including allergic rhinitis, nasal polyposis, and asthma. Approximately 70% of patients with EGPA have elevated levels of immunoglobulin E (IgE) and eosinophilia of peripheral blood and tissue. Small vessel histopathology typically reveals transmural eosinophilic infiltrates with scattered plasma cells and lymphocytes and extravascular granulomas.

The pathology of HSP is characterized by a leukocytoclastic vasculitis of small vessels with IgA deposition seen on immunofluorescence. Various infectious agents, including bacteria and viruses, have been reported as triggers for HSP.

The pathology of GCA and TAK are very similar histologically. In both, large vessels demonstrate a lymphoplasmacytic inflammatory infiltrate. Giant cells and granulomas may be seen in the media, and lumen-occlusive arteritis may occur from exuberant intimal hyperplasia. Additional pathologic features include proliferation of vascular smooth muscle cells and fragmentation of the internal elastic lamina.

⬤ CLINICAL PRESENTATION AND DIAGNOSIS

Clinical manifestations of the systemic vasculitides are diverse and differ not only among disorders but also among patients. Typical clinical manifestations associated with the size of the affected vessel are detailed in Table 81-1.

Small Vessel Vasculitis

ANCA-Associated Vasculitides

GPA most commonly affects the sinuses and upper airway, the lungs, and the kidneys, although almost any organ system may be affected. Chronic refractory sinusitis, nasal crusting and ulcers,

TABLE 81-1	TYPICAL CLINICAL FEATURES* BASED ON VESSEL SIZE		
	LARGE	**MEDIUM**	**SMALL**
	Limb claudication	Cutaneous nodules	Purpura
	Asymmetrical blood pressures	Ulcers	Vesiculobullous lesions
	Absence of pulses	Livedo reticularis	Alveolar hemorrhage
	Bruits	Digital gangrene	Glomerulonephritis
	Aortic dilatation	Mononeuritis multiplex	Mononeuritis multiplex
	Aortic primary branch stenoses and/or aneurysms	Microaneurysms of mesenteric and/or renal branch arteries	Cutaneous extravascular necrotizing granulomas
			Splinter hemorrhages
			Scleritis, episcleritis, uveitis

*Constitutional symptoms in all types are fever, weight loss, malaise, anorexia, arthralgias, and myalgias.

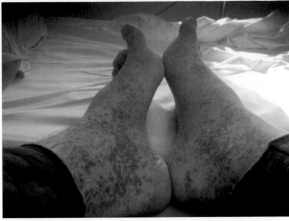

FIGURE 81-3 Palpable purpura on the lower extremities of a patient with small vessel vasculitis affecting the skin. These lesions are "palpable" because they are slightly raised (i.e., palpable even with the eyes closed), and they are typically nonblanching when palpated. (Modified from Molyneux ID, Moon T, Webb AK, Morice AH: Treatment of cystic fibrosis associated cutaneous vasculitis with chloroquine, J Cystic Fibrosis 9:439–441, 2010. Copyright 2010 European Cystic Fibrosis Society.)

epistaxis, septal perforations, and otitis media are common presenting manifestations. Chronic nasal cartilaginous inflammation and destruction may lead to the characteristic "saddle nose" deformity. Lung involvement in GPA or MPA can include pulmonary nodules (often cavitary in GPA), infiltrates, or diffuse alveolar hemorrhage due to capillaritis. Importantly, life-threatening pulmonary hemorrhage may manifest simply as progressive acute dyspnea with hypoxia or respiratory failure, and not necessarily hemoptysis. Laryngotracheal disease may manifest as hoarseness or subglottic stenosis; orbital pseudotumors can also occur from GPA, and they may cause optic nerve compression, proptosis, and/or extraocular muscle palsies.

The renal manifestations in GPA, MPA, or RLV are those of acute renal failure. Renal biopsy reveals pauci-immune necrotizing crescentic glomerulonephritis. Additional organ manifestations that may occur in either GPA or MPA include neurologic, cutaneous, musculoskeletal, cardiovascular, and constitutional signs and symptoms. Patients may have subacute symptoms (weeks to months of sinusitis, arthralgias, and fatigue) or may exhibit acute "pulmonary-renal syndrome" with rapidly progressive glomerulonephritis and life-threatening alveolar hemorrhage with respiratory failure.

In EGPA, the clinical features comprise severe asthma, eosinophilia (>1500 cells/mL), and vasculitis involving two or more organs. Additional organ involvement in EGPA may include the nervous system, kidneys, skin, heart, and gastrointestinal tract. Sinus involvement in EGPA is typically not destructive as in GPA, and pulmonary infiltrates may be fleeting.

The diagnosis of any of the AAVs is most frequently established by tissue biopsy (e.g., kidney, lung, skin, sinus, nerve). ANCA testing plays an important diagnostic role in suspected small vessel vasculitis and is helpful in differentiating between GPA and MPA. Almost 90% of patients with renal disease have positive ANCA on testing. Most GPA patients have the cytoplasmic (cANCA) antiproteinase 3 (anti-PR3) type, whereas most MPA patients have the perinuclear (pANCA) antimyeloperoxidase (anti-MPO) type. The differential diagnosis for positive ANCA testing includes drug-induced effects, infections, and other autoimmune conditions. EGPA can be distinguished from other AAVs on the basis of a prior history of adult-onset asthma or allergic rhinitis and blood or tissue eosinophilia.

The differential diagnosis for any small vessel vasculitis includes infection, disorders of coagulation, drug toxicity, atherosclerotic and embolic disease, malignancy, and secondary vasculitides associated with other autoimmune diseases.

Henoch-Schönlein Purpura

Patients with HSP have lower extremity purpura, arthritis (typically of the large joints), abdominal pain, and renal disease at presentation (Fig. 81-3). In children, arthritis and abdominal pain affect about 75% of patients; the gastrointestinal manifestations may precede the purpura by up to 2 weeks and include hematochezia. The most common renal manifestation is microscopic hematuria with or without proteinuria.

The diagnosis of HSP is most often based on clinical and laboratory evidence, although skin or renal biopsy revealing IgA deposition may be helpful in solidifying the diagnosis. By classification criteria from the EULAR, patients with HSP must have purpura or petechiae with lower limb predominance and at least one of the following: arthritis or arthralgias; abdominal pain; histopathology demonstrating IgA deposition; and renal involvement. The differential for HSP includes other causes of abdominal pain, other causes of purpura in childhood, and hypersensitivity vasculitis. Hypersensitivity vasculitis is also a small vessel vasculitis that may occur in both children and adults and may be idiopathic or triggered by infections or drug exposures. It typically manifests as an isolated cutaneous leukocytoclastic vasculitis that is self-limited with treatment of the underlying cause (e.g., treatment of infection, discontinuation of drug culprit).

Medium Vessel Vasculitis
Polyarteritis Nodosa

The most common organ systems affected in PAN are the gastrointestinal, renal, and nervous systems. Mesenteric aneurysms or stenoses resulting in gut ischemia lead to symptoms of abdominal pain or "intestinal angina" (pain after eating). Renal artery aneurysms or stenoses result in hypertension or renal dysfunction, rather than glomerulonephritis as in MPA. Neurologic involvement may manifest as mononeuritis multiplex. Orchitis may be seen, manifesting as acute testicular pain. Anemia, elevated erythrocyte sedimentation rate or C-reactive protein or both, and hypertension (if renal artery involvement is present) are common. As in all vasculitides, constitutional symptoms may also be present.

The diagnosis of PAN is made based on angiographic or biopsy findings in the appropriate clinical setting. ANCA typically are absent in PAN. A work-up for infection, including tests for hepatitis B and C and HIV, is warranted, given their known associations with PAN. The differential diagnosis includes MPA and mixed cryoglobulinemic vasculitis. The latter vasculitis shares many clinical features with PAN, including peripheral neuropathy, arthralgias, myalgias, purpura, and association with hepatitis C.

Kawasaki Disease

The clinical presentation of Kawasaki disease includes fever lasting longer than 5 days, conjunctival injection, oropharyngeal changes (strawberry tongue, mucous membrane desquamation), peripheral extremity changes (cutaneous desquamation), polymorphous rash, and cervical lymphadenopathy. Arthralgias, abdominal pain, hepatitis, aseptic meningitis, and uveitis have also been reported. Coronary artery aneurysms, one of the most serious complications of this vasculitis, appear within the first 4 weeks after onset of disease and are often detectable with echocardiography. Although areas of ectasia and small aneurysms may regress, larger aneurysms often persist and can result in coronary ischemia at any time after development, even into adulthood. Kawasaki disease is a triphasic disease, consisting of an acute febrile period lasting up to 14 days, a subacute phase of 2 to 4 weeks, and a convalescent phase that can last months to years. In the acute phase, the fever is persistent and high (>38.5° C) and is minimally responsive to antipyretics.

The differential diagnosis is wide and includes viral infections, toxin-mediated illnesses (e.g., toxic shock syndrome, scarlet fever), systemic juvenile idiopathic arthritis, hypersensitivity reactions, and drug reactions (e.g., Stevens-Johnson syndrome).

Large Vessel Vasculitis
Giant Cell Arteritis or Temporal Arteritis

At presentation, patients with GCA most commonly have new continuous headache, jaw claudication, visual disturbances (e.g., amaurosis fugax, diplopia), fatigue, and arthralgias. They are usually older than 50 years of age, have tender or thickened temporal arteries, and have an elevated erythrocyte sedimentation rate (>50 mm/hour by the Westergren method). Disease onset may be insidious or acute. Blindness due to anterior ischemic optic neuropathy occurs in 10% to 15% of patients with GCA and can occur at disease onset. Given the association between GCA and PMR, patients with PMR should be educated regarding signs and symptoms of GCA, and patients with GCA should be monitored for symptoms of PMR.

The diagnosis of GCA is often made by a biopsy of the superficial temporal artery. It is important to obtain a sufficient

length of tissue (2 to 3 cm) because the vasculitis can have "skip lesions."

Takayasu's Arteritis

The typical clinical manifestations of TAK include a systolic blood pressure difference of greater than 10 mm Hg between the arms, decreased brachial or radial artery pulses, bruits auscultated over the subclavian arteries or aorta, claudication of extremities, neck or jaw pain, headache, dizziness, hypertension, constitutional symptoms, arthralgias, and myalgias.

The diagnosis of TAK is often based on vascular imaging studies that demonstrate long, tapering stenotic lesions or aneurysmal lesions in the aorta and primary branches. The differential diagnosis includes syphilis, spondyloarthropathies, rheumatoid arthritis, inflammatory bowel disease, and connective tissue disorders. Vascular imaging studies including computed tomographic angiography and magnetic resonance angiography are typically performed for both diagnosis and disease surveillance.

⬤ TREATMENT AND PROGNOSIS
Small Vessel Vasculitis
ANCA-Associated Vasculitides

Glucocorticoids, often with other agents, are uniformly used to induce and maintain remission in AAV. They are typically initiated at a prednisone equivalent dose of 1 mg/kg/day with or without pulse methylprednisolone (1 g IV daily × 3 days), followed by a gradual taper over approximately 6 to 12 months. In addition, the standard. In addition, the standard of care in both GPA and MPA has traditionally been cyclophosphamide, either oral or intravenous, for 3 to 6 months. This has been reported to yield remission rates varying from 30% to 93% in GPA and from 75% to 89% in MPA.

Rituximab, an anti-CD20 chimeric monoclonal antibody that depletes B cells, was shown to be noninferior to cyclophosphamide in remission induction for AAV in several randomized controlled trials (RITUXVAS and RAVE trials).

Plasmapheresis, or plasma exchange therapy, is often used in combination with remission induction therapy in patients with life-threatening disease such as alveolar hemorrhage, or rapidly progressive glomerulonephritis (pulmonary-renal syndrome). The MEPEX study was a randomized controlled trial comparing plasmapheresis with high-dose methylprednisolone for severe renal vasculitis. Plasmapheresis was shown to be superior to methylprednisolone in reducing the number of patients remaining dependent on dialysis.

For limited (early) GPA, such as disease confined to the upper respiratory tract, methotrexate may be used for remission induction, rather than cyclophosphamide; this conclusion was supported by level I evidence in the NORAM trial. Trimethoprim-sulfamethoxazole was shown in two randomized controlled trials to be helpful in preventing relapses after remission induction in GPA.

Remission maintenance therapies in AAV (level I evidence) include methotrexate, azathioprine, or mycophenolate mofetil. Because there are known risks of bladder cancer, hemorrhagic cystitis, and bone marrow suppression with cumulative use of cyclophosphamide, it no longer has a role in remission maintenance in AAV.

Although AAVs were once considered diseases with considerable mortality (80% at 2 years if left untreated), the prognosis has improved significantly over the last 30 years because of improved treatments. Patient survival is now reported to be as high as 45% to 91% at 5 years. Among AAV patients with renal involvement at presentation, 20% develop end-stage renal disease within 5 years.

Henoch-Schönlein Purpura

In mild cases, the therapy for HSP is simply supportive care (i.e., hydration and analgesics). However, glucocorticoids are commonly used to hasten the resolution of symptoms; early use of glucocorticoids has been associated with improved outcomes, especially when there is severe gastrointestinal involvement. In life-threatening cases and in severe acute renal failure, additional immunosuppressive agents or plasmapheresis may be considered. The prognosis of HSP is generally good, with fewer than 1% of patients developing end-stage renal disease.

Medium Vessel Vasculitis

Polyarteritis Nodosa

Treatment of PAN includes glucocorticoids or nonsteroidal anti-inflammatory drugs (NSAIDs) or both. If disease is severe and persistent or relapsing, additional immunosuppressive agents are used, such as cyclophosphamide (especially for gastrointestinal or cardiac involvement), methotrexate, colchicine, or intravenous immunoglobulin (IVIG). In cases of PAN associated with hepatitis B or C, antiviral therapy is required not only for attaining control of the viral infection but also for treatment of the associated vasculitis itself. Corticosteroids and cyclophosphamide have improved patient outcomes, and the 1-year survival rate is now 85%. Prognosis is typically worse with more systemic complications such as renal or neurologic involvement.

Kawasaki Disease

Treatment of Kawasaki disease includes high-dose aspirin (80 to 100 mg/kg/day) for the first 48 hours, then 3 to 5 mg/kg/day. IVIG is standard therapy and has significantly decreased the incidence of coronary artery aneurysm complications in this disease. The initial IVIG dose is 2 g/kg within the first 10 days after presentation, with at least one repeat dose typically given if the first IVIG dose fails to improve the child's condition. The prognosis of Kawasaki disease, if promptly treated, is good; however, approximately 15% to 25% of patients develop coronary artery aneurysms that increase morbidity and mortality.

Large Vessel Vasculitis

Giant Cell Arteritis or Temporal Arteritis

Glucocorticoids are the cornerstone of therapy in GCA. To prevent vision loss, treatment should be instituted immediately (within 24 hours) if clinical suspicion for GCA is high or if visual disturbances are present. The initial dose of glucocorticoids is typically 1 mg/kg/day with a gradual taper. Most patients require a glucocorticoid treatment duration of 1 to 2 years, but it may be longer, especially in those with symptoms of PMR . In PMR without GCA, lower doses of glucocorticoids (10 to 20 mg/day of prednisone equivalent) are effective and provide prompt clinical response.

If patients experience relapse with glucocorticoid tapering, other immunosuppressive agents may be used. Methotrexate was shown in a meta-analysis of three randomized controlled trials to be a beneficial adjunctive agent in reducing risks of first and second relapses in GCA, with a significant decrease in the cumulative dose of glucocorticoids. Low-dose aspirin is an important adjunctive therapy in protecting against cranial ischemic events (level II evidence from two large retrospective studies). Biologic agents in GCA are still under investigation.

Takayasu's Arteritis

Glucocorticoids are also the cornerstone of therapy for TAK; they are typically initiated at a dose of 0.5 to 1 mg/kg/day. Although most patients respond to the initial dose, relapses occur in more than 50% of patients during glucocorticoid tapering. Hence, steroid-sparing agents are often used to aid in maintaining disease remission. The most commonly used steroid-sparing agents are methotrexate and azathioprine. In TAK, unlike in GCA and PMR, the tumor necrosis factor (TNF) inhibitors have shown promise in treating refractory disease. As in GCA, low-dose aspirin is believed to play a beneficial adjunctive role in preventing ischemic complications.

Revascularization interventions are often indicated in patients with TAK whose presenting symptoms include cerebrovascular disease, coronary artery disease, moderate to severe aortic regurgitation, renovascular hypertension, progressive limb claudication, or progressive aneurysm enlargement. Elective intervention should be performed when the disease is quiescent.

In both GCA and TAK, aortitis—a common manifestation of large vessel involvement—can lead to an increased risk of aortic aneurysm and subsequent dissection and rupture. In both GCA and TAK, disease flares occur in most patients, rendering them chronic, progressive and relapsing conditions.

⬤ ADDITIONAL CONSIDERATIONS IN TREATMENT

Immunosuppressive therapy is associated with an increased risk of infection. Patients receiving combination therapy with moderate- to high-dose glucocorticoid (>20 mg/day of prednisone equivalents) and another immunosuppressive agent should also receive prophylaxis for *Pneumocystis jiroveci* pneumonia (previously known as PCP). Furthermore, infections can often mimic or result in flares of systemic vasculitis. Glucocorticoid therapy should never be discontinued abruptly, even in the setting of infection, because of the risk of adrenal crisis or disease relapse or both. In most cases, other immunosuppressive agents should be discontinued if infection is suspected or diagnosed.

Glucocorticoid therapy is a common cause of bone loss (osteopenia, osteoporosis). Because significant bone loss can occur even within the first 6 months of therapy, calcium and vitamin D supplementation should be initiated, and a baseline bone density study should be obtained. Consideration should be given to additional bone protection therapies (e.g., bisphosphonates). Methotrexate and cyclophosphamide are teratogenic, and cyclophosphamide may result in premature ovarian failure. These factors must be considered when choosing therapies for women of child-bearing age. Immunosuppressive agents also can be associated with bone marrow suppression and with additional long-term risks such as malignancy.

Acknowledgments

The author wishes to acknowledge the assistance of Kathleen Maksimowicz-McKinnon, MD and Kelly Liang, MD.

> *For a deeper discussion on this topic, please see Chapter 270, "The Systemic Vasculitides," in* Goldman-Cecil Medicine, *25th Edition.*

SUGGESTED READINGS

Bloch DA, Michel BA, Hunder GG, et al: The American College of Rheumatology 1990 criteria for the classification of vasculitis: patients and methods, Arthritis Rheum 33:1068–1073, 1990.

Hoffman GS, Cid MC, Rendt-Zagar KE, et al: Infliximab for maintenance of glucocorticosteroid-induced remission of giant cell arteritis: a randomized trial, Ann Intern Med 146:621–630, 2007.

Hunder GG, Bloch DA, Michel BA, et al: The American College of Rheumatology 1990 criteria for the classification of giant cell arteritis, Arthritis Rheum 33:1122–1128, 1990.

Jennette JC, Falk RJ, Andrassy K, et al: Nomenclature of systemic vasculitides: proposal of an international consensus conference, Arthritis Rheum 37:187–192, 1994.

Jones RB, Tervaert JW, Hauser T, et al: Rituximab versus cyclophosphamide in ANCA-associated renal vasculitis, N Engl J Med 363:211–220, 2010.

Specks U, Merkel PA, Seo P, et al: Efficacy of remission-induction regimens for ANCA-associated vasculitis, N Engl J Med 369:417–427, 2013.

Stone JH, Merkel PA, Spiera R, et al: Rituximab versus cyclophosphamide for ANCA-associated vasculitis, N Engl J Med 363:221–232, 2010.

Weiss PF: Pediatric vasculitis, Pediatr Clin North Am 59:407–423, 2012.

Crystal Arthropathies

Ghaith Noaiseh

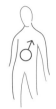

Gout

INTRODUCTION

The term *gout* refers to a heterogeneous group of diseases that result from deposition of monosodium urate (MSU) crystals in joints and soft tissue. Gout typically begins as an intermittent monoarthritis in the lower extremities; it may progress over time into a chronic, deforming and debilitating arthritis affecting almost any peripheral joint.

Gout is associated with hyperuricemia, which is defined as a serum urate level greater than 6.8 mg/dL. Above that concentration, urate can form uric acid crystals in normal physiologic conditions.

EPIDEMIOLOGY

More than 6 million adults in the United States have had gout attacks. The incidence and prevalence are markedly increasing. This is thought to be related to the aging of the population, increased use of certain medications such as diuretics, and increasing prevalence of comorbidities such as obesity, hypertension, renal disease, cardiovascular disease, and metabolic syndrome.

The incidence and prevalence are proportional to age and the degree and duration of serum urate elevation. Men are three to six times more likely to have gout than women, but the sex disparity decreases with aging, in part due to the declining levels of estrogen in postmenopausal women. Estrogen has a uricosuric effect, and this also explains why gout is uncommon in premenopausal women.

PATHOGENESIS

Pathophysiology of Hyperuricemia

Uric acid is the end product of purine metabolism in humans. Unlike many other species, humans lack the enzyme uricase, which catalyzes the conversion of uric acid into allantoin, a very soluble metabolite. Most individuals maintain uric acid levels between 4 and 6.8 mg/dL and a total body uric acid pool of approximately 1000 mg. However, accumulation of uric acid can occur and may lead to supersaturation of urate in blood. Serum uric acid levels greater than 6.8 mg/dL under normal pH and temperature may result in the precipitation of MSU crystals in joints, soft tissues, and other organs. Urate crystallization is a critical step in the progression from asymptomatic hyperuricemia to clinical gout. Unlike soluble urate molecules, MSU crystals are a potent promoter of acute inflammation.

Only about 20% of hyperuricemic patients develop gout during their lifetime. Additional factors, which are still poorly defined, are required for crystal formation.

The total body uric acid pool is closely related to the net purine accumulation, which comes from three sources: dietary purine intake, nucleic acid release from ongoing cell degradation, and de novo synthesis (endogenous purine biosynthesis). About two thirds of the daily excretion of uric acid occurs in the kidneys; the rest is eliminated by the gut. The balance between these mechanisms determines total uric acid body stores.

Hyperuricemia is caused by an imbalance between synthesis and elimination. Renal underexcretion is the cause for approximately 90% of hyperuricemia cases (Table 82-1). In the remaining 10%, hyperuricemia is caused by uric acid overproduction (>1000 mg of uric acid in a 24-hour urine collection while on a standard Western diet) or by a combination of overproduction with renal underexcretion.

Figure 82-1 summarizes the de novo biosynthesis and salvage pathways of purine metabolism. Abnormalities in the activities of key enzymes can lead to increased serum uric acid levels and development of gout. Overall, enzymatic deficiencies account for a small fraction of uric acid overproduction; most cases of uric

TABLE 82-1	CAUSES OF HYPERURICEMIA	
URATE OVERPRODUCTION	**URATE UNDEREXCRETION**
METABOLIC DISORDERS	Renal insufficiency
	Volume depletion
HGPRT deficiency (homozygous or	Metabolic acidosis (lactic acidosis
heterozygous)	and ketoacidosis)
PRPP synthetase hyperactivity	Obesity
G6PD deficiency	Ethanol
Glycogen storage diseases	Medications: low dose salicylate,
OTHERS	diuretics (thiazides, loop
	diuretics), cyclosporine,
Myeloproliferative and	tacrolimus, L-dopa, ethambutol
lymphoproliferative disorders	Familial juvenile hyperuricemic
Erythropoietic disorders (hemolytic	nephropathy
anemia, megaloblastic anemia,	Medullary cystic kidney disease
sickle cell disease, thalassemia,	Lead nephropathy
other hemoglobinopathies)	
Solid tumors	
Diffuse psoriasis	
Ethanol (particularly beer)	
Medications: cyctotoxic agents,	
nicotinic acid	
Shellfish, organ meat, red meat	
Fructose	
Obesity	

HGPRT, Hypoxanthine-guanine phosphoribosyltrasferase; PRPP, 5′-phosphoribosyl 1-pyrophosphate; G6PD, glucose-6-phosphate dehydrogenase.

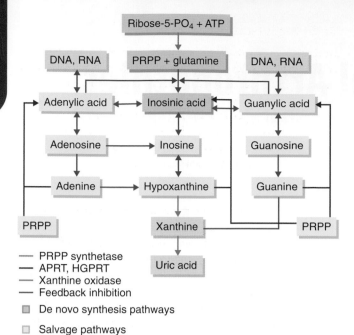

— PRPP synthetase
— APRT, HGPRT
— Xanthine oxidase
— Feedback inhibition
▢ De novo synthesis pathways
▢ Salvage pathways

FIGURE 82-1 Biochemical pathways of purine synthesis, interconversion, and degradation. APRT, Adenine phosphoribosyl transferase; ATP, adenosine triphosphate; HGPRT, hypoxanthine-guanine phosphoribosyltransferase; PRPP, 5'-phosphoribosyl 1-pyrophosphate.

acid overproduction result from increased reutilization of purine bases through salvage pathways (see Fig. 82-1). The de novo synthesis of purine is driven by the enzyme 5'-phosphoribosyl 1-pyrophosphate (PRPP) synthetase. In PRPP synthetase overactivity, overproduction of PRPP increases purine production. In salvage pathways, tissue-derived intermediate purine products (hypoxanthine, guanine, and adenine) are reutilized rather than undergoing further degradation to xanthine and uric acid. Deficiencies of hypoxanthine-guanine phosphoribosyltrasferase (HGPRT) activity result in impaired purine salvage and increased substrate for uric acid generation (Lysch-Nyhan syndrome and Kelley-Seegmiller syndrome).

Diseases associated with increased cell turnover (e.g., hemolysis, ineffective hematopoiesis, psoriasis) or with other causes of enhanced purine nucleotide breakdown (ethanol or fructose ingestion) can lead to hyperuricemia. Purine-rich foods comprise a significant portion of the daily purine load and can worsen hyperuricemia. On the other hand, consumption of low-fat dairy products is associated with reduced serum urate levels and may decrease the risk of gout.

A very small proportion of serum urate is bound to plasma proteins; therefore, urate is almost completely filtered in the glomeruli. Subsequent reabsorption and secretion occur through various organic acid transporters located on the luminal side of the proximal convoluted tubule epithelium. Only about 10% of the total filtered uric acid is excreted in the urine.

In addition to the bidirectional transport of uric acid, organic acid transporters are also responsible for eliminating other organic acids and certain medications. The function of these transporters is affected by certain medications, including thiazides, low-dose aspirin, and cyclosporine, leading to decreased uric acid excretion and hyperuricemia. Conversely, medications such as probenecid and losartan, when excreted in the tubular lumen, exert their uricosuric effect by displacing uric acid from

the transporter and increasing uric acid excretion. Certain genetic mutations affecting these transporters may lead to uric acid underexcretion. Renal insufficiency can cause hyperuricemia though decreased uric acid filtration.

Pathophysiology of Acute Gouty Attack

In some patients with prolonged hyperuricemia, tissue deposits of MSU crystals, called *microtophi*, form in the synovium and on the surface of cartilage. During an acute attack, microtophi break apart, shedding a large number of MSU crystals into the joint space and activating synovial macrophages and fibroblasts that phagocytize the crystals. This, in turn, leads to the activation of a cytosolic multiprotein complex, the NALP3 (NACHT, LRR, and PYD domains–containing protein 3) inflammasome, which generates interleukin-1β. Interleukin-1β production activates bloodstream neutrophils and endothelial cells, allowing neutrophils to cross the capillary endothelium into the joint space. Inflammation is propagated by further activation of the newly recruited neutrophils, which leads to the clinical signs of inflammation characteristic of the acute gouty attack.

MSU crystals undergo clearance by inflammatory cells that then undergo apoptosis. This, along with other mechanisms, eventually leads to resolution of the acute inflammatory process, typically after 10 to 14 days. Even after complete resolution of symptoms, a low-grade level of inflammation (intercritical inflammation) can persist in the otherwise asymptomatic joint. This inflammation may become clinically apparent in longstanding gout, and it contributes to chronic synovitis, cartilage loss, and bony erosions.

● CLINICAL FEATURES

Gout has three stages: asymptomatic hyperuricemia, acute intermittent gout, and chronic gout.

Acute Gouty Attacks

The classic picture of acute gout is rapid development of an inflammatory arthritis involving one (or occasionally two) joints. Severe pain, erythema, swelling and exquisite tenderness typically occur. The most commonly involved joints are the first metatarsophalangeal joint (podagra), followed by the joints of the ankle, midfoot, and knee. The pain intensifies over 8 to 24 hours. Acute attacks usually resolve, even without therapy, within 5 to 14 days. The clinical resolution is complete, and the patient is asymptomatic between attacks. This clinical picture can be easily confused with that of septic arthritis or cellulitis, because many patients can mount an intense systemic inflammatory response with fever, chills, and elevated inflammatory markers.

Attack-provoking factors include use of diuretics, alcohol, surgery, trauma, and consumption of foods containing high purine levels. Each of these can cause fluctuation in serum urate levels. Initiation of urate-lowering therapy can trigger attacks in the early phase by the same mechanism.

Subsequently, involvement of the upper extremities can occur, affecting the small joints of the hands, wrists, and elbows.

Chronic Gout

Transition to the chronic phase can occur if hyperuricemia is inadequately treated. This phase, called *chronic gout* (also referred to as *chronic tophaceous gout* or *chronic advanced gout*), typically develops 10 or more years after the onset of acute attacks. This phase is characterized by less severe attacks compared with the early flares and incomplete resolution of symptoms between flares as the patient continues to experience some baseline joint pain.

The characteristic lesion of chronic gout is the *tophus*, a palpable collection of MSU crystals in soft tissue or joints. It is detected in about 75% of patients who have had gout for more than 20 years. The severity and duration of hyperuricemia determine the likelihood of tophus development. Although the ears, fingers, wrist, and olecranon bursa are the typical locations, tophi can occur anywhere in the body.

DIAGNOSIS

The typical presentation of acute gouty arthritis in a characteristic joint distribution is strongly suggestive of the diagnosis, particularly if there is a history of similar attacks that completely resolved. Nevertheless, the diagnosis should be confirmed by aspiration of the involved joint. This is a critical step to rule out septic arthritis and other crystalline arthropathies such as CPPD deposition disease, which is caused by deposits of calcium pyrophosphate dihydrate (CPPD) crystals in the cartilage (see later discussion). During acute attacks, intracellular, strongly negative birefringent, needle-shaped MSU crystals are typically identified by polarized compensated microscopy. MSU crystals can also be demonstrated in tophus aspiration (Fig. 82-2A).

Bacterial infection can coexist with urate crystals in the synovial fluid; Gram stain and culture should be performed. Aspirated fluid appears cloudy, and synovial fluid analysis shows inflammatory fluid (>2000 white blood cells per microliter) with as many as 50,000 to 100,000 cells/µL or even more). Serum uric acid is not a diagnostically reliable test during acute flares because the serum urate level may be normal or even low. Laboratory testing may reveal leukocytosis and elevated inflammatory markers, both of which are nonspecific. Between attacks, MSU crystals can often be demonstrated in previously inflamed joints. This can provide support for a diagnosis of gout when the patient is asymptomatic.

Radiologic Features

During an acute attack, a plain radiograph may only show soft tissue swelling. After many years of the disease and during the chronic phase, well defined, "punched out" juxtaarticular erosions with overhanging bony edges and sclerotic margins may be seen. The joint space is preserved until late in the course of the disease. Soft tissue masses may be detected in patients with tophi. Periarticular osteopenia is absent. Ultrasound can be a promising tool in the diagnosis and management of gout.

Gout in Transplantation Patients

Hyperuricemia occurs much more frequently in transplantation patients using cyclosporine than in the normal population. Compared to patients with classic gout, these patients exhibit a significantly shorter period of asymptomatic hyperuricemia (0.5 to 4 years versus 20 to 30 years), a shorter stage of acute intermittent gout (1 to 4 years versus 10 to 15 years), and rapid development of tophi as early as 1 year after transplantation. Gouty attacks can be atypical and less severe, in part because of the concomitant use of prednisone.

DIFFERENTIAL DIAGNOSIS

Acute gouty arthropathy should be distinguished from septic arthritis and other crystal-induced arthropathies such as CPPD deposition disease. The onset of acute CPPD arthropathy is usually less abrupt, and attacks tend to last longer, up to 1 month or more. Attacks occur more often in large joints such as the knee and wrist. Forms of spondyloarthritis including reactive arthritis, psoriatic arthritis, ankylosing spondylitis, and inflammatory bowel related arthritis can also manifest with monoarticular arthritis. In these disorders, synovial fluid is inflammatory, with a leukocyte count usually in the range of 10,000 to 50,000/µL, but crystals are absent and fluid culture is negative.

In its chronic phase, gout can be confused with rheumatoid arthritis and tophi can be confused with rheumatoid nodules. Aspiration of chronically inflamed joints or a tophus can help in distinguishing the two entities.

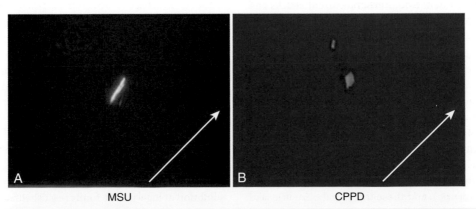

MSU   CPPD

FIGURE 82-2 Polarized microscopy image of (**A**) strongly negative birefringent monosodium urate crystals and (**B**) weakly positive calcium pyrophosphate dihydrate crystals. Arrows indicate axis of polarization. (**A**, Modified from the ACR Slide Collection on the Rheumatic Diseases. Available at http://images.rheumatology.org/. Accessed January 2015; **B**, Modified from Saadeh C, Diamond HS: Calcium pyrophosphate deposition disease. Available at: http://emedicine.medscape.com/article/330936-overview#showall. Found under "Multimedia Library." Accessed January 2015.)

TREATMENT

Management of Acute Gouty Attack

The goal of management is to quickly control the inflammation and pain. Affected joints should be rested. Application of ice to the joint is usually helpful in reducing symptoms, but it is rarely sufficient to adequately control symptoms.

Nonsteroidal anti-inflammatory drugs (NSAIDs) including ibuprofen, naproxen, indomethacin, and diclofenac are typically used, and all seem to be equally effective. Full doses of NSAIDs should be initiated immediately, and a treatment duration of 7 to 10 days may be necessary for complete resolution of symptoms. NSAIDs are inappropriate in patients with peptic ulcer disease, inflammatory bowel disease, or renal insufficiency, and they must be used with caution in patients who are at risk for cardiovascular events.

Oral colchicine can be effective if it is used early in an acute attack (i.e., within the first 24 to 48 hours). A commonly prescribed dose is 1.2 mg, followed by 0.6 mg 4 hours later for the first day, followed by dose tapering until the attack is resolved. The drug should be stopped if nausea or loose stool occurs. Use of intravenous colchicine is discouraged because of the unacceptable risk of bone marrow suppression. Intraarticular corticosteroid injection is a very effective therapy for patients with monoarticular or oligoarticular disease in whom other systemic therapies need to be avoided. Enteral or parenteral glucocorticosteroids are effective in patients with renal insufficiency, intolerance to NSAIDs or colchicine, or treatment resistance. This approach is usually reserved for polyarticular flares when intraarticular injection is not practical (i.e., too many involved joints). A common starting corticosteroid dose is prednisone, 30 to 50 mg daily.

Urate-lowering therapy (ULT) should *not* be interrupted during acute attacks. Patients with established disease should be encouraged to maintain a supply of their medication for acute attacks and to start it promptly at the onset of typical symptoms; this may shorten the duration of attacks.

Management of Intercritical and Chronic Gout

Urate-Lowering Therapy

The aim of chronic treatment is to prevent recurrent attacks and to minimize joint damage by depleting tophaceous deposits in joints and soft tissue. This is achieved by lowering the uric acid level to less than 6 mg/dL. A target serum uric acid concentration of less than 5 mg/dL should be considered in patients with chronic tophaceous gout because it can result in a faster, more effective reduction in tophus size and flare frequency. Indications for ULT in patients with gout include two or more attacks in a single year, recurrent nephrolithiasis, and presence of tophi or chronic gouty arthritis.

ULT agents are divided into three categories: those that decrease uric acid production (uricostatic), those that increase renal excretion (uricosuric), and those that metabolize uric acid (uricolytic). The optimal duration of ULT is not known, and lifelong therapy is usually recommended. ULT is typically started after resolution of an acute attack.

Uricostatic Therapy

Allopurinol and febuxostat are xanthine oxidase inhibitors that prevent urate formation. They are effective in both overproducers and undersecretors of uric acid.

Allopurinol remains the first-line and most commonly used ULT agent, particularly in patients with chronic renal insufficiency, uric acid stones, or uric acid overproduction. If renal function is normal, a starting dose of 100 mg daily is recommended because higher doses may increase the risk of allopurinol hypersensitivity, a potentially lethal complication. The risk of early flares may also be increased with higher doses. It is recommended that the allopurinol dose be titrated up by 100 mg increments every 2 to 5 weeks until the uric acid goal is reached. The maximal dose is 800 mg/day. Adverse events include rash (2%), hepatitis, vasculitis, eosinophilia, and bone-marrow suppression.

Allopurinol hypersensitivity reaction can be fatal, and the risk may be higher with concomitant use of thiazides and in patients with penicillin allergy. Fever, severe exfoliative dermatitis, eosinophilia, and hepatic and renal failure can occur. If the uric acid goal is not achieved with allopurinol titration, or if side effects occur, then febuxostat may be used.

If the target uric acid level is not achieved with monotherapy, combination therapy with a uricosuric agent and a xanthine oxidase inhibitor may be considered.

Uricosuric Therapy

In the United States, probenecid is the only available uricosuric agent. It may be used as a first-line ULT in uric acid undersecretors (<600 mg in a 24-hour urine collection), but it is ineffective in patients with renal insufficiency (glomerular filtration rate <50 mL/minute) and is contraindicated in patients with nephrolithiasis. Patients should maintain high urine volume by drinking at least 1.5 L of fluid daily.

Uricolytic Therapy

Pegloticase (pegylated recombinant uricase), administered intravenously every 2 weeks, is considered for patients whose gout is refractory to conventional ULT.

Rasburicase, another recombinant uricase, is used to prevent tumor lysis syndrome but has no role in the management of gout.

Non–Urate-Lowering Prophylactic Therapy

Anti-inflammatory prophylaxis using low-dose colchicine or NSAIDs is usually recommended in conjunction with ULT to decrease the risk of flares that often accompany initiation of ULT. Prophylactic treatment is usually continued for 6 months after the serum uric acid goal is achieved.

Lifestyle Modifications and Education

A patient newly diagnosed with gout should be evaluated for potentially modifiable risk factors and associated illnesses such as obesity, hypertension, and hyperlipidemia. Decreased consumption of high-purine foods (e.g., shellfish, liver, sweetbreads) and fructose-containing beverages, as well as reduced alcohol intake, should be recommended. Diuretics should be avoided if possible.

Treatment of Hyperuricemia in Patients Without Gout

Allopurinol and rasburicase have been used for prevention and treatment of tumor lysis syndrome associated with hyperuricemia occurring after chemotherapy. Apart from this indication, there is no evidence to support their use for the routine treatment of asymptomatic hyperuricemia.

● CALCIUM PYROPHOSPHATE DIHYDRATE DEPOSITION DISEASE

Calcium pyrophosphate dihydrate (CPPD) deposition disease is a clinically heterogeneous disorder that is characterized by the presence of intraarticular CPPD crystals. These crystals are deposited primarily in the cartilage, in the normally unmineralized pericellular matrix of hyaline and fibrocartilage. Calcification of the cartilage is promoted by alterations in the metabolism of inorganic pyrophosphate (PPi) and extracellular matrix leading to extracellular accumulation of PPi, which is necessary to the formation of CPPD crystals. Crystals are phagocytized by resident synovial macrophages, activating the intracellular NALP3 inflammasome complex and leading to recruitment and influx of neutrophils into the joint space.

CPPD deposition disease typically affects the elderly population. Up to 50% of individuals older than 85 years of age have radiographic evidence of CPPD crystal accumulation in cartilage (chondrocalcinosis), but most are asymptomatic. The most commonly involved joints are the knee menisci and the triangular fibrocartilage of the wrist.

The clinical course of CPPD deposition disease may be asymptomatic, acute, subacute, or chronic. The most common clinical manifestation, occurring in more than 50% of patients, is a peculiar type of osteoarthritis called pseudo-osteoarthritis; it is a non-inflammatory arthritis involving joints not typically affected by osteoarthritis, such as the wrist, shoulder, ankle, and metacarpophalangeal joints. Asymptomatic disease may be an incidental finding on radiographs showing chondrocalcinosis. Pseudogout is an acute monoarthritis similar in presentation to the acute gouty attack. A chronic symmetric polyarticular arthritis pattern resembling rheumatoid arthritis and a severe destructive arthropathy that mimics neuropathic arthritis on radiographs may be seen.

It is uncommon for CPPD deposition disease to affect patients younger than 50 years of age, unless the disease is familial or related to a metabolic abnormality (e.g., hyperparathyroidism). Acute pseudogout attacks may be precipitated by trauma, surgery (particularly parathyroidectomy for hyperparathyroidism), or severe medical illness. Administration of intraarticular viscosupplementation may also trigger a CPPD flare. Attacks are usually monoarticular or oligoarticular; if left untreated, they may last from a few days to a few months. Involved joints are swollen, with variable erythema and warmth. Fever, elevated erythrocyte sedimentation rate, and leukocytosis can occur.

The diagnosis is confirmed by demonstration in synovial fluid of intracellular rod- or rhomboid-shaped crystals with weak positive birefringence when examined by compensated polarized light microscopy (see Fig. 82-2B). These crystals can be difficult to detect in some patients and are frequently missed in clinical specimens.

The presence of chondrocalcinosis (radiodense deposits on radiographs) is highly suggestive of the diagnosis in the appropriate clinical context. Joint aspiration should always be performed to rule out the possibility of infection. Importantly, joint infection can cause crystal shedding, leading to a concomitant crystal-related inflammation. Synovial fluid is inflammatory (>2000 white blood cells per microliter), with an average of 24,000 cells/μL.

Therapy for CPPD deposition disease is indicated for symptomatic patients. There is no effective treatment to remove CPPD deposits from synovium or cartilage. Treatment options include intraarticular glucocorticoid injection of the affected joint or joints. NSAIDs are effective, but their potential toxicity in elderly patients may limit their utility. Severe polyarticular attacks may require short courses of systemic corticosteroids. In patients with frequent pseudogout attacks, prophylactic daily low-dose colchicine may decrease the frequency.

● APATITE-ASSOCIATED ARTHROPATHY

Abnormal accumulation of apatite (basic calcium phosphate, or BCP) may occur in hypercalcemic states and other illnesses. Unlike MSU or CPPD crystals, individual BCP crystals are not identifiable by polarized microscopy and can be seen only by electron microscopy. The most common apatite-associated condition is calcific periarthritis, which typically occurs in the shoulder.

Milwaukee shoulder is an extremely destructive BCP-associated arthropathy that occurs more commonly in elderly women. It is characterized by a large noninflammatory effusion (i.e. <2000 white blood cells per microliter) and results in destruction of the rotator cuff with subsequent marked instability and destruction of glenohumeral cartilage.

Other manifestations include acute reversible inflammatory arthropathies that resemble gout, referred to as *pseudopseudogout*, and ossifications along the anterolateral aspect of spinal vertebrae, termed *diffuse idiopathic skeletal hyperostosis* (DISH). Acute attacks of arthritis or bursitis may be self-limited. Intraarticular or periarticular injection of corticosteroids or the use of NSAIDs may shorten the duration and intensity of symptoms.

● CALCIUM OXALATE DEPOSITION DISEASE

In calcium oxalate deposition disease, or oxalosis, calcium oxalate crystals are deposited in tissue. In primary oxalosis, a hereditary metabolic disorder, this deposition leads to nephrocalcinosis, renal failure, and early mortality. Secondary oxalosis complicates long-term hemodialysis or peritoneal dialysis; crystals are deposited in bone, cartilage, synovium, and periarticular tissue. Crystal shedding into the joint space may result in inflammatory arthritis of peripheral joints. Chondrocalcinosis or soft tissue calcifications can be seen on plain radiographs. The presence of strongly birefringent bipyramidal crystals is characteristic. Treatment with NSAIDS, intraarticular corticosteroids, or colchicine usually results in moderate improvement.

Acknowledgment

The author would like to thank Dr. Douglas Lienesch, MD, for his valuable suggestions.

SUGGESTED READINGS

Choi HK: Epidemiology, pathology, and pathogenesis, chap 12. In Stone JH, Crofford LJ, White PH, editors: Primer on the rheumatic diseases, ed 13, New York, 2008, Springer.

Edwards L: Crystal deposition diseases, chap 28. In Goldman L, Schafer AI, editors: Goldman's Cecil Medicine, ed 24, Philadelphia, 2012, Saunders.

Ghosh P, Cho M, Rawat G, et al: Treatment of acute gouty arthritis in complex hospitalized patients with anakinra, Arthritis Care Res 65:1381–1384, 2013.

Harrold L: New developments in gout, Curr Opin Rheumatol 25:304–309, 2013.

Jordan KM: Up-to-date management of gout, Curr Opin Rheumatol 24:145–151, 2012.

Khanna D, Fitzgerald JD, Khanna PP, et al: 2012 American College of Rheumatology guidelines for management of gout. Part 1: systematic nonpharmacologic and pharmacologic therapeutic approaches to hyperuricemia, Arthritis Care Res 64:1431–1446, 2012.

Khanna D, Khanna PP, Fitzgerald JD, et al: 2012 American College of Rheumatology guidelines for management of gout. Part 2: therapy and anti-inflammatory prophylaxis of acute gouty arthritis, Arthritis Care Res 64:1447–1461, 2012.

Neogi T: Gout, N Engl J Med 364:443–452, 2011.

Osteoarthritis

C. Kent Kwoh

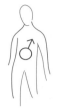

DEFINITION AND EPIDEMIOLOGY

Osteoarthritis, also known as degenerative joint disease, is the most common type of arthritis and musculoskeletal disease. It is a disease of synovial joints that encompasses the pathophysiologic changes that result from alterations in joint structure due to failed repair of joint damage and the individual's experience of illness, which is most often characterized by pain.

More than 26.9 million Americans older than 25 years have some form of osteoarthritis, and the prevalence increases with age. The radiographic prevalence varies by the joint involved. Twenty-seven percent of adults and more than 80% of those older than 65 years have evidence of hand osteoarthritis, and 37% of those older than 60 years have radiographic evidence of knee disease. The prevalence of symptomatic osteoarthritis is lower, with 7% of adults having symptomatic hand disease and 17% of those older than 45 years having symptomatic knee involvement.

Hand and knee osteoarthritis is more common among women, especially after 50 years of age, and it is more common among African Americans. Nodal osteoarthritis, involving the distal and proximal interphalangeal joints, is significantly more common in women and among female first-degree relatives.

Osteoarthritis is associated with major morbidity and is the leading cause of long-term disability in the United States. Lower extremity osteoarthritis is the most common cause of difficulty with walking or climbing stairs, preventing an estimated 100,000 elderly Americans from independently walking from their bed to the bathroom.

Osteoarthritis has a large economic impact because of direct medical costs (e.g., physician visits, laboratory tests, medications, surgery) and indirect costs (e.g., lost wages, home care). With the aging of the U.S. population, the burden of osteoarthritis is expected to increase in the coming years.

For a deeper discussion of these topics, please see Chapter 262, "Osteoarthritis," in Goldman-Cecil Medicine, 25th Edition.

PATHOLOGIC FACTORS

The causes of osteoarthritis are complex and heterogeneous, and its pathophysiology is not well understood. The cardinal feature is progressive loss of articular cartilage with associated remodeling of subchondral bone. In normal cartilage, there is continuous extracellular matrix turnover with a balance between synthesis and degradation. In osteoarthritis, there is an imbalance of these two processes, with an excess of matrix degradation that exceeds ongoing matrix synthesis. Excess degradation results from overproduction of catabolic factors such as proinflammatory cytokines and reactive oxygen species.

Osteoarthritis is best defined as joint failure, a disease process that involves the total joint, including the subchondral bone, ligaments, joint capsule, synovial membrane, periarticular muscles, and articular cartilage. After bone trauma or repetitive injury, joint failure may result from joint instability caused by muscle weakness and ligamentous laxity; nerve injury and neuronal sensitization or hyperexcitability, or both. Also contributing are low-grade systemic inflammation caused by subacute metabolic syndrome and local inflammation resulting from synovitis. Identifiable risk factors for osteoarthritis include biomechanical, metabolic, and inflammatory processes; congenital or developmental deformities of the joint that alter its shape; and genetic factors. Age, sex, and race are prominent risk factors for osteoarthritis.

Biomechanical contributors include repetitive or isolated joint trauma related to certain occupations or physical activities that involve repeated joint stress and predispose to early osteoarthritis. Altered joint shape may contribute to osteoarthritis through biomechanical factors. Obesity may contribute biomechanically or systemically through subacute or overt metabolic syndromes, both of which are associated with low-grade systemic inflammation.

Metabolic disorders such as hemochromatosis, ochronosis, Wilson's disease, and Gaucher's disease are associated with osteoarthritis. High bone mineral density is associated with hip and knee involvement. Estrogen deficiency may be a risk factor for hip or knee disease. Candidate gene studies and genome-wide scans have identified several potential genetic markers. Patients often have a family history of osteoarthritis or joint replacement.

Inflammatory joint diseases such as rheumatoid arthritis may result in cartilage degradation and biomechanical effects that lead to secondary osteoarthritis. The destruction of the joint, including articular cartilage damage, osteophyte formation, and subchondral bone remodeling, is best viewed as joint failure and the final product of a variety of etiologic factors.

The earliest finding is fibrillation of the most superficial layer of the articular cartilage. Over time, disruption of the articular surface becomes deeper, with fibrillations extending to subchondral bone, fragmentation of cartilage with release into the joint, matrix degradation, and eventually, complete loss of cartilage, leaving only exposed bone.

Early in the process, the cartilage matrix demonstrates increased water and decreased proteoglycan content, unlike the dehydration of cartilage that occurs with aging. The tidemark zone, separating the calcified cartilage from the radial zone, is invaded by capillaries. Chondrocytes initially are metabolically active and release a variety of cytokines and metalloproteinases, contributing to matrix degradation. In the later stages, this results in the penetration of fissures to the subchondral bone and the release of fibrillated cartilage into the joint space.

An imbalance between tissue inhibitors of metalloproteinases and the production of metalloproteinases may be operative in osteoarthritis. Subchondral bone remodels and increases in density. Cystlike bone cavities containing myxoid, fibrous, or cartilaginous tissue may form. Osteophytes or bony proliferations at the margin of joints at the site of the bone-cartilage interface may form at capsule insertions. Osteophytes contribute to joint motion restriction and are thought to be the result of new bone formation in response to the degeneration of articular cartilage, but the precise mechanism for their production remains unknown.

Several crystals have been identified in synovial fluid and other tissues from osteoarthritic joints, most notably calcium pyrophosphate dehydrate and hydroxyapatite. Although these crystals have potent inflammatory potential, their role in the pathogenesis of osteoarthritis remains unclear. Frequently, the crystals are asymptomatic and do not correlate with extent or severity of disease.

The diversity of risk factors predisposing to osteoarthritis suggests that many insults to the joints, including biomechanical trauma, chronic articular inflammation, and genetic and metabolic errors, can contribute to or trigger the cascade of events that results in the characteristic pathologic features described earlier. At some point, the cartilage degradative process becomes irreversible. With progressive changes in articular cartilage, joint mechanics become altered, perpetuating the degradative process.

⬤ CLINICAL PRESENTATION

Pain is the characteristic feature of osteoarthritis and the most common presenting symptom. Pain is usually worse with activity or weight bearing and better with rest. In later stages, pain may also occur at rest. Early in the disease course, pain tends to be transient, intermittent, and unpredictable. The pain may be characterized as severe, and its unpredictable nature is an extremely bothersome feature that limits activity and affects quality of life. With disease progression, pain tends to become constant but is reported to be less severe and have an aching quality. Other prominent symptoms, such as stiffness, gelling, fatigue, and sleep disturbance, often lead to functional limitation and disability.

Pain tends to localized to the specific joint involved, but it may be referred to a more distant site. The cause of pain is unclear but is likely to be heterogeneous. Pain may result from interactions among structural pathology; the motor, sensory, and autonomic innervation of the joint; and pain signal processing at the spinal and cortical levels. Specific individual and environmental factors also may be important. A subset of patients may have neuropathic pain.

Patient-specific factors may modify pain reception and pain reporting. Patients' affective status, such as depression, anxiety, and anger, may influence the level of pain reported.

Their cognitive status, including pain beliefs, expectations, and memories of past pain, and their communication skills may determine how pain is perceived and reported. Studies have shown that demographic factors such as age, sex, socioeconomic status, race or ethnicity, and cultural background may affect pain reporting.

Patients may have stiffness, particularly after prolonged inactivity, but it is not a major feature of osteoarthritis and usually lasts for less than 30 minutes. Patients do not report systemic features such as fever.

Examination of an involved joint may reveal tenderness and bony enlargement. Joint effusion and soft tissue swelling may occur with knee involvement, but they tend to be intermittent. Persistent inflammation with joint warmth, erythema, effusion, and soft tissue swelling is usually not seen. Crepitus with movement, limitation of joint motion, and joint deformity, malalignment, and joint laxity or instability may be detected on evaluation. Joint deformity as manifested by lateral subluxation is fixed and not reducible. Muscle weakness and gait abnormalities may be seen.

Several subtypes of osteoarthritis have been identified. The nodal form involves the distal interphalangeal joints (DIPs), also known as Heberden's nodes, and the proximal interphalangeal joints (PIPs), also known as Bouchard's nodes. It is most common in middle-aged women, typically those with a strong family history among first-degree relatives. Erosive, inflammatory osteoarthritis is associated with prominent destructive changes, especially in the finger joints, and it is often quite symptomatic. Generalized osteoarthritis is characterized by involvement of the DIP, PIP, and first carpal-metacarpal joints, as well as the knees, feet, and hips.

> *For a deeper discussion of these topics, please see Chapter 256, "Approach to the Patient with Rheumatic Disease," and Chapter 262, "Osteoarthritis," in* Goldman-Cecil Medicine, *25th Edition.*

⬤ DIAGNOSIS AND DIFFERENTIAL DIAGNOSIS

The diagnosis of osteoarthritis is based on the signs and symptoms previously outlined. Although there are characteristic radiographic features, they are not necessary to make the clinical diagnosis. Imaging may be used to confirm the diagnosis and exclude other diseases, but radiographs are insensitive and may not show findings early in the disease course. Despite radiographic findings of osteoarthritis, pain may have other sources, such as bursitis, tendonitis, or referred pain. For example, hip disease may manifest as knee pain.

Osteoarthritis must be distinguished from inflammatory joint diseases such as rheumatoid arthritis and the spondyloarthropathies. This is accomplished by identifying the characteristic pattern of joint involvement and the nature of the individual joint deformity. Joints commonly involved in osteoarthritis include the DIPs, PIPs, first carpal-metacarpal, cervical and lumbar spine facet joints, hips, knees, and first metatarsophalangeal joints. Involvement of the metacarpal phalangeal joints (MCPs), wrist, elbows, shoulders, and ankles is uncommon, except in the case of trauma, congenital disease, or coexisting endocrine or metabolic disease.

The characteristic radiographic features of osteoarthritis include joint space narrowing as a surrogate for cartilage loss; osteophytes and subchondral sclerosis as an indicator of new bone formation, which is characteristic of osteoarthritis; and subchondral cysts as a manifestation of myxoid or fibrous degeneration of subchondral bone. Bone attrition and subchondral bone remodeling may result in changes in bone shape. Magnetic resonance imaging (MRI) can demonstrate additional morphologic abnormalities, such as bone marrow lesions in subchondral bone, meniscal degeneration, and synovitis.

The pain and swelling of erosive hand osteoarthritis may suggest rheumatoid arthritis, although systemic inflammatory signs and other typical features of rheumatoid arthritis are absent. The prevalence of false-positive findings of rheumatoid factor and antinuclear antibody, sometimes in significant titers, is higher with increasing age. Osteoarthritis more commonly affects the distal small joints in the hands (DIPs > PIPs > MCPs and wrists), whereas rheumatoid arthritis more commonly affects proximal small joints in the hands (MCPs and wrists > PIPs > DIPs).

> *For a deeper discussion of these topics, please see Chapter 258, "Imaging Studies in the Rheumatic Diseases," Chapter 264, "Rheumatoid Arthritis," and Chapter 265, "The Spondyloarthropathies," in* Goldman-Cecil Medicine, *25th Edition.*

🔴 TREATMENT

The natural history of osteoarthritis includes periods of relative stability interspersed with rapid deterioration. Management should be individually tailored and may include a combination of nonpharmacologic, pharmacologic, and surgical approaches. The primary goal of treatment is to improve pain and function and reduce disability.

Patients should be educated regarding the objectives of treatment and the importance of lifestyle changes, exercise, pacing of activities, and other measures to unload the damaged joints. The initial focus should be on self-help and patient-driven treatments rather than on passive therapies. Patients should be encouraged to adhere to nonpharmacologic and pharmacologic therapies. Physical therapists may be helpful in providing instruction in appropriate exercises to reduce pain and preserve functional capacity. For knee and hip osteoarthritis, assistive devices such as walking aids may be useful. Graded regular aerobic, muscle-strengthening, and range-of-motion exercises are beneficial. Tai chi may also be useful.

Overweight patients should be encouraged to lose weight. A knee brace can reduce pain, improve stability, and diminish the risk of falling for patients with knee osteoarthritis and mild or moderate varus or valgus instability. Advice concerning appropriate footwear is also important. Spinal orthoses may provide benefit to patients with significant cervical or lumbar involvement. Local applications of heat, ultrasound, or transcutaneous electrical nerve stimulation (TENS) may provide short-term benefit. Acupuncture may also offer symptomatic benefit for these patients.

Pharmacologic therapy provides symptomatic relief but does not alter the course of the disease. Pharmacologic therapy should therefore be selected based on its relative efficacy and safety. The use of concomitant medications in the setting of comorbidities should be taken into account.

Acetaminophen (up to 3 g/day with caution) may be an effective initial oral analgesic for mild to moderate pain. In patients with symptomatic osteoarthritis, nonsteroidal anti-inflammatory drugs (NSAIDs) should be used at the lowest effective dose, although their long-term use should be avoided if possible. If patients are at risk for increased gastrointestinal toxicity, a cyclooxygenase-2 (COX2)–selective agent or a nonselective NSAID with co-prescription of a proton pump inhibitor or misoprostol for gastroprotection should be considered. All NSAIDs, including nonselective and COX2-selective agents, should be used with caution in patients with cardiovascular risk factors. Topical NSAIDs and capsaicin may be effective alternatives to oral analgesic or anti-inflammatory agents in knee and hand osteoarthritis and may be used as adjunctive agents, particularly in elderly patients.

Meta-analyses have shown that oral glucosamine and chondroitin sulfate have limited benefit in patients with knee osteoarthritis. If other interventions have been ineffective or are contraindicated, weak opioids and narcotic analgesics may be considered for the treatment of refractory pain. Stronger opioids should be used for the management of severe pain only in exceptional circumstances. Occasional injection of intra-articular corticosteroids (no more than once every 4 months) may provide modest short-term symptomatic benefit with minimal toxicity, especially in the knee. Patients with moderate to severe pain and effusion or other local signs of inflammation may be more responsive. Intra-articular hyaluronate appears to have little or no benefit based on current evidence.

Surgical management includes total joint replacement, which is extremely effective in relieving pain, decreasing disability, and improving function. With improvements in surgical technique and technology, the indications for total joint replacement have expanded to include younger and older age groups. Other surgical options include osteotomy and unicompartmental knee replacement. Arthroscopy is not recommended for the management of knee osteoarthritis.

🔴 PROGNOSIS

Given the obesity epidemic and the marked contact loads that increased weight places on the knee, obesity is likely the most important modifiable risk factor for the development and progression of knee osteoarthritis. One kilogram of weight loss decreases the load on the knee by 4 kg. Varus and valgus malalignments have also been identified as important risk factors for the progression of knee osteoarthritis.

> *For a deeper discussion of these topics, please see Chapter 262, "Osteoarthritis," in* Goldman-Cecil Medicine, *25th Edition.*

SUGGESTED READINGS

Blagojevic M, Jinks C, Jeffery A, et al: Risk factors for onset of osteoarthritis of the knee in older adults: a systematic review and meta-analysis, Osteoarthritis Cartilage 18:24–33, 2013.

Helmick CG, Felson DT, Kwoh CK, et al: Estimates of the prevalence of arthritis and other rheumatic conditions in the United States. Part I, Arthritis Rheum 58:15–25, 2008.

Hochberg MC, Altman RD, April KT, et al: American College of Rheumatology 2012 recommendations for the use of nonpharmacologic and pharmacologic therapies in osteoarthritis of the hand, hip, and knee, Arthritis Care Res 64:465–474, 2012.

Litwic A, Edwards MH, Dennison EM, et al: Epidemiology and burden of osteoarthritis, Br Med Bull 105:185–199, 2013.

Zhang W, Moskowitz RW, Kwoh CK, et al: OARSI recommendations for the management of hip and knee osteoarthritis, part I: critical appraisal of existing treatment guidelines and systematic review of current research evidence, Osteoarthritis Cartilage 15:981–1000, 2007.

Zhang W, Moskovitz RW, Nuki G, et al: OARSI recommendations for the management of hip and knee osteoarthritis, part II: OARSI evidence-based, expert consensus guidelines, Osteoarthritis Cartilage 16:137–162, 2008.

Nonarticular Soft Tissue Disorders

Niveditha Mohan

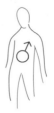

INTRODUCTION

The nonarticular soft tissue disorders account for most musculoskeletal complaints in the general population. These disorders include a large number of anatomically localized conditions (e.g., bursitis, tendinitis) and fibromyalgia syndrome, a generalized pain disorder. For most nonarticular soft tissue conditions, the etiologic factors and pathogenesis are poorly understood.

The nonarticular soft tissue syndromes can be classified according to the anatomic region involved, such as shoulder pain. After the region is defined, an attempt is made to identify the structure at fault, such as the supraspinatus tendon, bicipital tendon, or subacromial bursa. In the case of back pain, precise anatomic delineation of the structure involved (e.g., intervertebral disk, facet joint, ligament, paraspinal muscle) is frequently impossible.

EPIDEMIOLOGY

Precise data for prevalence or incidence of most nonarticular soft tissue syndromes are not available, but these conditions account for up to 30% of all outpatient visits. Fibromyalgia is considered to be the most common cause of generalized musculoskeletal pain in women between the ages of 20 and 55 years. The global mean prevalence is 2.7%.

ETIOLOGIC FACTORS AND PATHOGENESIS

The precise pathophysiology of most nonarticular soft tissue disorders remains unknown, although predisposing factors, such as overuse or repetitive activities (e.g., tennis elbow, lateral epicondylitis) or biomechanical factors (e.g., leg-length discrepancy in trochanteric bursitis), can be identified in many cases.

The term *tendinitis* implies tendon sheath inflammation, but small tendon tears, periostitis, and nerve entrapment have been proposed as potential mechanisms. Similarly, although the term *bursitis* implies bursal inflammation, demonstrable inflammation is difficult to find. In some cases (e.g., acute bursitis of the olecranon or prepatellar bursa), the mechanism is an acute inflammatory response to sodium urate crystals deposited in the soft tissue, an extra-articular manifestation of gout. The favorable response of tendinitis and bursitis to anti-inflammatory agents, including corticosteroids, supports the view that at least one component of these syndromes is the result of an inflammatory process.

In myofascial pain syndrome, the causes are even more obscure. Frequently, overuse and trauma are cited as etiologic factors, but many cases lack antedating mechanical considerations.

Investigators have examined diverse mechanisms for fibromyalgia syndrome, including studies of muscle, sleep physiologic processes, neurohormonal function, and psychological status. Although the pathophysiologic mechanisms remain unknown, an increasing body of literature points to central (central nervous system) rather than peripheral (muscle) mechanisms. Muscle tissue has been a focus of investigation for many years. Initial studies, including histologic and histochemical studies, suggested a possible metabolic myopathy; however, carefully controlled studies indicated that these abnormalities were the result of deconditioning.

Sleep studies suggested that disruption of deep sleep (stage IV) by so-called alpha-wave intrusion (i.e., normal awake electroencephalographic pattern) may play a causal role, but this finding was later observed in other disorders and more likely indicates an effect than a cause.

In some cases, musculoskeletal injury has been implicated as a trigger for fibromyalgia, but social and legal issues cloud its causative role. Several studies have suggested that subtle hypothalamic-pituitary-adrenal axis hypofunction may occur in fibromyalgia syndrome, although it remains uncertain whether these changes are constitutive or are the result of fibromyalgia. A prevailing theory of pathogenesis is dysregulation of pain pathways leading to central sensitization and marked by neurotransmitter, neurohormone, and sleep physiology irregularities.

Fibromyalgia has long been linked to psychological disturbance. Most studies have confirmed high lifetime rates of major depression, which range from 34% to 71%, associated with fibromyalgia syndrome. High lifetime rates of migraine, irritable bowel syndrome, and panic disorder have also been associated with fibromyalgia syndrome, suggesting that fibromyalgia may be part of an affective spectrum group of disorders.

CLINICAL PRESENTATION

Many of the soft tissue rheumatic syndromes involve bursae, tendons, ligaments, and muscles. Bursae are closed sacs lined with mesenchymal cells that are similar to synovial cells; the sacs are strategically located to facilitate tissue gliding. Subcutaneous bursae (e.g., olecranon, prepatellar) form after birth in response to normal external friction. Deep bursae (e.g., subacromial bursa) usually form before birth in response to movement between muscles and bones and may or may not communicate with adjacent joint cavities. Adventitious bursae (e.g., over the first metatarsal head) form in response to abnormal shearing stresses and are not uniformly found. Although most forms of bursitis involve isolated, local conditions, some may be the result of systemic conditions such as gout.

Tendinitis, bursitis, and myofascial disorders should be distinguished from articular disorders. In most cases, this can be accomplished by a careful examination of the involved structure (Table 84-1). General principles of the musculoskeletal examination are as follows:

1. Observation: If deformity or soft tissue swelling is detected, is it fusiform (i.e., surrounding the entire joint in a symmetrical fashion) or is it localized? Local rather than fusiform deformity distinguishes nonarticular disorders from articular disorders.
2. Palpation: Is tenderness localized or in a fusiform distribution? Is there an effusion? Local (not fusiform or joint line) tenderness distinguishes nonarticular disorders from articular disorders. An effusion typically indicates an articular disorder.
3. Assessing range of motion: The musculoskeletal examination includes the assessment of active range of motion (i.e., patient attempts to move the symptomatic structure) and passive range of motion (i.e., examiner moves the symptomatic structure). Articular disorders usually are characterized by equal impairment in active and passive movements as a result of the mechanical limitation of joint motion resulting from proliferation of the synovial membrane, an effusion, or derangement of intra-articular structures. Impairment of active movement characterizes nonarticular disorders to a much greater degree than passive movement.

Clinical symptoms include pain, warmth, and swelling over the site of the bursa that are worse with activity and better with rest. Bursitis can be distinguished from tendinitis by the pain during active and passive range of movement; in tendinitis, pain is elicited only during active range of movement. However, for many patients these patterns often occur simultaneously.

Muscle sprains or strains are typically diagnosed based on a history of preceding activity causing the symptom along with pain and limitation of movement when the muscle is contracted against resistance. The clinical signs and symptoms of chronic myofascial pain are more nonspecific and characterized by a distribution that is frequently nonanatomic and associated with hyperalgesia in the involved area.

Fibromyalgia syndrome is characterized by widespread pain and a host of other symptoms, including insomnia, cognitive dysfunction, depression, anxiety, recurrent headaches, dizziness, fatigue, morning stiffness, extremity dysesthesia, irritable bowel syndrome, and irritable bladder syndrome.

● DIAGNOSIS AND TREATMENT

Septic Bursitis

Superficial forms of bursitis, particularly olecranon bursitis and prepatellar and occasionally infrapatellar bursitis, are more frequently infected or involved with crystal deposition than are deep forms of bursitis, presumably due to direct extension of organisms through subcutaneous tissues. Most commonly, *Staphylococcus aureus* is isolated from infected superficial bursae. Septic bursitis should be suspected when there is cellulitis, erythema, fever, and peripheral leukocytosis.

Definitive diagnosis and exclusion of infection of subcutaneous bursae usually require aspiration of the distended bursa. The bursal fluid should be assessed for cell count, Gram stain, and culture and examined for crystals.

Nonseptic Bursitis

Nonseptic bursitis frequently appears as an overuse condition associated with sudden or unaccustomed repetitive activity of the associated extremity. The two most common types of bursitis are subacromial and trochanteric bursitis (Table 84-2).

Subacromial bursitis is the most common overall cause of shoulder pain over the lateral upper arm or deltoid muscle that is exacerbated with abduction of the arm. Subacromial bursitis is the result of compression of the inflamed rotator cuff tendon between the acromion and humeral head. Because the rotator cuff forms the floor of the subacromial bursa, bursitis in this location often results from tendinitis of the rotator cuff. Occasionally,

TABLE 84-1	DIFFERENTIATING NONARTICULAR SOFT TISSUE DISORDERS FROM ARTICULAR DISEASE		
MANIFESTATION	**NONARTICULAR SOFT TISSUE DISORDERS**	**ARTICULAR DISEASE**	
Limitation of motion	Active > passive	Active = passive	
Crepitus of articular surfaces (structural damage)	0	+/0	
Tenderness			
Synovial (fusiform pattern)	0	+	
Local	+	0	
Swelling			
Synovial (fusiform pattern)	0	+	
Local	+/0	0	

+, Present; 0, absent.

TABLE 84-2	BURSITIS SYNDROMES	
LOCATION	**SYMPTOM**	**FINDING**
Subacromial	Shoulder pain	Tender subacromial space
Olecranon	Elbow pain	Tender olecranon swelling
Iliopectineal	Groin pain	Tender inguinal region
Trochanteric	Lateral hip pain	Tender at greater trochanter
Prepatellar	Anterior knee pain	Tender swelling over patella
Infrapatellar	Anterior knee pain	Tender swelling lateral or medial to patellar tendon
Anserine	Medial knee pain	Tender medioproximal tibia (below joint line of knee)
Ischiogluteal	Buttock pain	Tender ischial spine (at gluteal fold)
Retrocalcaneal	Heel pain	Tender swelling between Achilles tendon insertion and calcaneus
Calcaneal	Heel pain	Tender central heel pad

subacromial bursitis or rotator cuff tendinitis results from osteophyte compression of the rotator cuff tendon originating from the acromioclavicular joint. The differential diagnosis includes tears of the rotator cuff, intra-articular pathologic mechanisms of the glenohumeral joint, bicipital tendinitis, cervical radiculopathy, and referred pain from the chest.

Trochanteric bursitis is the result of inflammation at the insertion of the gluteal muscles at the greater trochanter. It produces lateral thigh pain, which is often worse when the patient lies on the affected side. Women seem to be more prone to develop this condition, perhaps because of increased traction of the gluteal muscles as a result of the relatively broader female pelvis. Other potential risk factors include weight gain, local trauma, overuse activities such as jogging, and leg-length discrepancies (primarily on the side with the longer leg). These factors are thought to lead to increased tension of the gluteus maximus on the iliotibial band, producing bursal inflammation. The differential diagnosis of trochanteric bursitis includes lumbar radiculopathy (particularly of the L1 and L2 nerve roots), meralgia paresthetica (i.e., entrapment of the lateral cutaneous nerve of the thigh as it passes under the inguinal ligament), true hip joint disease, and intraabdominal pathologic processes. Other bursitis syndromes are less common and listed in Table 84-2.

Septic bursitis is treated with a combination of serial aspirations of the infected bursa and antibiotics, initially directed against *S. aureus* and then adjusted depending on the results of bursal fluid cultures. Recurrent septic bursitis may need surgical excision of the bursa. The approach to nonseptic bursitis should include rest, local heat, and unless contraindicated by peptic ulcer disease, renal disease, or advanced age, nonsteroidal anti-inflammatory drugs (NSAIDs).

The most effective approach usually is local injection of a corticosteroid. Superficial bursae with obvious swelling should be aspirated before the corticosteroid is injected. For deep bursae, such as the subacromial or trochanteric bursae, aspiration yields little or no fluid, and direct injection of a corticosteroid without attempted aspiration is reasonable. Caution is advised in attempted aspiration or injection of the iliopsoas bursa, the ischiogluteal bursa, and the gastrocnemius-semimembranosus bursa (i.e., Baker's cyst). These bursae lie close to important neural and vascular structures, and aspiration under ultrasound guidance is recommended.

Tendinitis

Most tendinitis syndromes are the result of inflammation in the tendon sheath. Overuse with microscopic tearing of the tendon is the most common risk factor for tendinitis. Tendon compression by an osteophyte may occur, such as in the rotator cuff tendon compressed by an osteophyte originating from the acromioclavicular joint.

A common form of tendinitis is lateral epicondylitis, also known as *tennis elbow* (Table 84-3). This is a common overuse syndrome among tennis players, but it can be seen in many other settings requiring repetitive extension of the forearm (e.g., painting overhead). The diagnosis is confirmed by exclusion of elbow joint pathology and the finding of local tenderness at the lateral epicondyle, which is typically exacerbated by forearm extension against resistance. Enthesopathies such as Achilles tendinitis and

TABLE 84-3 TENDINITIS SYNDROMES		
LOCATION	**SYMPTOM**	**FINDING**
Extensor pollicis brevis and abductor pollicis longus (de Quervain tenosynovitis)	Wrist pain	Pain on ulnar deviation of the wrist, with the thumb grasped by the remaining four fingers (i.e., Finkelstein test)
Flexor tendons of fingers	Triggering or locking of fingers in flexion	Tender nodule on flexor tendon on palm over metacarpal joint
Medial epicondyle	Elbow pain	Tenderness of medial epicondyle
Lateral epicondyle	Elbow pain	Tenderness of lateral epicondyle
Bicipital tendon	Shoulder pain	Tenderness along bicipital groove
Patella	Knee pain	Tenderness at insertion of patellar tendon
Achilles	Heel pain	Tender Achilles tendon
Tibialis posterior	Medial ankle pain	Tenderness under medial malleolus with resisted inversion of ankle
Peroneal	Lateral midfoot or ankle pain	Tenderness under lateral malleolus with passive inversion

peroneal and posterior tibial tendinitis may occur in the setting of an underlying seronegative arthropathy such as Reiter's disease or psoriatic arthritis. A history and clinical evaluation for these disorders should be pursued for the appropriate patient.

Therapy for tendinitis—NSAIDs, local heat, and corticosteroid injection—is similar to that for bursitis. Rest, physical therapy, occupational therapy, and occasionally ergonomic modification are useful adjuncts. The goal of corticosteroid injection in tendinitis is to infiltrate the tendon sheath rather than the tendon itself because direct injection into a tendon may result in rupture of the tendon. Corticosteroid injection of the Achilles tendon should be avoided because of the propensity of this tendon to rupture. Surgical management of tendinitis is indicated only after failure of conservative treatment. For example, chronic impingement of the supraspinatus tendon that is refractory to conservative treatment may require subacromial decompression.

Fibromyalgia Syndrome

Descriptions of fibromyalgia syndrome exist far back in the medical literature, but it remains a diagnosis of exclusion due to the lack of objective diagnostic or pathologic findings. Fibromyalgia syndrome as defined by the American College of Rheumatology (ACR) 1990 definition for use in clinical trials is a chronic, widespread pain condition with characteristic tender points on physical examination, often associated with a constellation of symptoms such as fatigue, sleep disturbance, headache, irritable bowel syndrome, and mood disorders. In 2010, the ACR developed preliminary diagnostic criteria based only on symptoms because of well-documented issues with the tender point examination (Table 84-4). These criteria do not require a tender point examination, but they provide a scale for measuring the severity of symptoms that are characteristic of fibromyalgia and show good correlation with the 1990 ACR criteria.

TABLE 84-4 2010 AMERICAN COLLEGE OF RHEUMATOLOGY FIBROMYALGIA DIAGNOSTIC CRITERIA

CRITERIA

1. Widespread pain index (WPI) ≥7, symptom severity (SS) scale score ≥5, or WPI of 3-6 and SS scale score ≥9
2. Symptoms manifest at a similar level for at least 3 months
3. Exclusion of other explanation for the pain

ASCERTAINMENT

1. WPI score
   The number of areas where the patient has had pain over the past week is assessed from 19 possible sites: left shoulder girdle, right shoulder girdle, left upper arm, right upper arm, left lower arm, right lower arm, left hip, right hip, left upper leg, right upper leg, left lower leg, right lower leg, left jaw, right jaw, chest, abdomen, upper back, lower back, and neck.
2. SS scale score
   For fatigue, waking unrefreshed, cognitive symptoms, and somatic symptoms,* the level of severity during the past week is assessed as follows: 0 = no symptoms; 1 = few symptoms; 2 = moderate number of symptoms; 3 = many symptoms.
   The SS scale score is the sum of the severity of the first three symptoms plus the severity of somatic symptoms in general. The final score is between 0 and 12.

*Somatic symptoms may include muscle pain or weakness, irritable bowel syndrome, fatigue or tiredness, cognitive or memory problems, headache, numbness or tingling, dizziness, insomnia, depression, nervousness, seizures, abdominal pain or cramps (especially upper abdomen), constipation, diarrhea, nausea, vomiting, fever, dry mouth, itching, chest pain, wheezing, Raynaud's phenomenon, hives or welts, tinnitus, hearing difficulties, heartburn, oral ulcers, loss of or change in taste, dry eyes, blurred vision, shortness of breath, loss of appetite, rash, sun sensitivity, easy bruising, hair loss, frequent or painful urination, and bladder spasms.

The clinical presentation of fibromyalgia syndrome is an insidious onset of chronic, diffuse, poorly localized musculoskeletal pain, typically accompanied by fatigue and sleep disturbance. The physical examination reveals a normal musculoskeletal system, with no deformity or synovitis. However, widespread tenderness occurs, especially at tendon insertion sites, indicating a general reduction in the pain threshold.

Approximately one third of the patients identify antecedent trauma as a precipitant for their symptoms, one third of patients describe a viral prodrome, and one third have no clear precipitant. A variety of less typical presentations has been described, including a predominantly neuropathic presentation with paresthesias (i.e., numbness and tingling) in a nondermatomal distribution, an arthralgic rather than myalgic presentation, and an axial skeletal manifestation resembling degenerative disk disease. Many patients may have undergone invasive diagnostic tests and, in some cases, inappropriate procedures such as carpal tunnel release or cervical or lumbar laminectomies.

Conditions that should be considered in the differential diagnosis of fibromyalgia syndrome include polymyalgia rheumatica (in older patients), hypothyroidism, polymyositis, and early systemic lupus erythematosus or rheumatoid arthritis. However, symptoms are exhibited for many months or years without evidence of other signs or symptoms of an underlying connective tissue disease, making other possible diagnoses unlikely.

Results of laboratory and radiographic studies are usually normal for patients with fibromyalgia syndrome. Exclusion of other conditions, such as osteoarthritis, rheumatoid arthritis, and systemic lupus erythematosus, by radiography, erythrocyte sedimentation rate, assays for rheumatoid factor or antinuclear antibody, and other tests is no longer considered necessary for the diagnosis of fibromyalgia syndrome. Fibromyalgia should be diagnosed on the basis of positive criteria.

The treatment of fibromyalgia includes reassurance that the condition is not a progressive, crippling, or life-threatening entity. A combination of treatment options, including medication and physical measures, is helpful for most patients. Medications found to be helpful in short-term, double-blind, placebo-controlled trials include amitriptyline and cyclobenzaprine. Low doses of these medications (e.g., 10 to 30 mg of amitriptyline, 10 to 30 mg of cyclobenzaprine) are moderately effective and generally well tolerated. Studies have shown that newer antidepressants of the serotonin-norepinephrine reuptake inhibitor group (e.g., duloxetine, venlafaxine, bupropion) and $\alpha_2\delta$ ligands (e.g., gabapentin, pregabalin) are also effective, particularly in combination with low doses of tricyclic antidepressants.

Patients should be encouraged to take an active role in the management of their condition. If possible, they should begin a progressive, low-level aerobic exercise program to improve muscular fitness and provide a sense of well-being. A combination approach is effective for most patients in alleviating symptoms, although a small minority of patients requires more intensive treatment strategies, such as psychiatric treatment or referral to a pain center.

SUGGESTED READINGS

Goldenberg DL, Burkhardt C, Crofford L: Management of fibromyalgia syndrome, JAMA 292:2388–2395, 2004.

Littlejohn GO: Balanced treatments for fibromyalgia, Arthritis Rheum 50:2725–2729, 2004.

Rheumatic Manifestations of Systemic Disorders; Sjögren's Syndrome

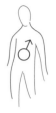

Yong Gil Hwang

INTRODUCTION

Rheumatologic manifestations may herald a variety of systemic conditions, including malignancy, endocrinopathy, and sarcoidosis (Tables 85-1 and 85-2). Musculoskeletal symptoms can precede or follow the diagnosis of these diseases. Patients may complain of joint pain, muscle weakness and pain, or reduced range of motion. Other chapters in this textbook provide detailed reviews of these systemic diseases, including rheumatologic manifestations.

RHEUMATIC SYNDROMES ASSOCIATED WITH MALIGNANCY

Paraneoplastic rheumatologic manifestations include hypertrophic osteoarthropathy (HOA), arthritis (i.e., inflammatory arthritis and carcinomatous polyarthritis), myositis, vasculitis, systemic lupus erythematosus (SLE)–like symptoms, and scleroderma. The pathophysiologic mechanisms of musculoskeletal symptoms in a patient with cancer are often unknown and remain speculative. The association is presumed if there is a close temporal relationship between the diagnosis of a malignancy and the onset of musculoskeletal symptoms or the rheumatic syndrome resolves after successful treatment of the malignancy. In many cases, however, the association may be coincidental.

Cancer may directly invade articular or periarticular structures and mimic rheumatic syndromes, as in chondrosarcoma, giant cell tumor, and osteogenic sarcoma. Musculoskeletal symptoms can occur as paraneoplastic phenomena without direct involvement by the tumor, as in dermatomyositis in patients with ovarian cancer.

The incidence of malignancy with rheumatic manifestations is unclear, but musculoskeletal symptoms occur more frequently with hematologic malignancies than with solid tumors. No single laboratory test can confirm the diagnosis of a rheumatic illness in a patient with cancer. All patients with rheumatologic syndromes should be evaluated with a thorough history, physical examination, and age-appropriate malignancy screening.

Hypertrophic Osteoarthropathy

HOA is characterized by digital clubbing, periostitis of the long bones, and arthritis. Arthritis is most prominent in large joints, and periostitis develops mostly at the distal ends of the femur,

TABLE 85-1	SYSTEMIC CONDITIONS ASSOCIATED WITH RHEUMATIC MANIFESTATIONS
MALIGNANT DISORDERS	**ENDOCRINOPATHIES**
Hypertrophic osteoarthropathy	Diabetes
Lymphoma	Hypothyroidism
Leukemia	Hyperthyroidism
Carcinoma polyarthritis	Hyperparathyroidism
HEMATOLOGIC DISORDERS	Acromegaly
	GASTROINTESTINAL DISORDERS
Hemophilia	Spondyloarthropathies
Sickle cell disease	Whipple disease
Thalassemia	Hemochromatosis
Multiple myeloma	Primary biliary cirrhosis
Amyloidosis	

TABLE 85-2	MUSCULOSKELETAL MANIFESTATIONS OF ENDOCRINE DISEASE
ENDOCRINE DISEASE	**MUSCULOSKELETAL MANIFESTATIONS**
Diabetes mellitus	Carpal tunnel syndrome
	Charcot's arthropathy
	Adhesive capsulitis
	Syndrome of limited joint mobility (cheiroarthropathy)
	Diabetic amyotrophy
	Diabetic muscle infarction
Hypothyroidism	Proximal myopathy
	Arthralgia
	Joint effusions
	Carpal tunnel syndrome
	Chondrocalcinosis
Hyperthyroidism	Myopathy
	Osteoporosis
	Thyroid acropachy
Hyperparathyroidism	Myopathy
	Arthralgia
	Erosive arthritis
	Chondrocalcinosis
Hypoparathyroidism	Muscle cramps
	Soft tissue calcifications
	Spondyloarthropathy
Acromegaly	Carpal tunnel syndrome
	Myopathy
	Raynaud's phenomenon
	Back pain
	Premature osteoarthritis
Cushing's syndrome	Myopathy
	Osteoporosis
	Avascular necrosis

tibia, and radius. The primary form of HOA (i.e., primary pachydermoperiostosis) is usually a self-limited disease of childhood. The secondary form may be generalized or localized and is mainly associated with lung cancer and suppurative lung disease.

HOA is also associated with cardiovascular disease (e.g., cyanotic congenital heart disease, infective endocarditis), hepatobiliary disorders (e.g., liver cirrhosis, primary biliary cirrhosis), and gastrointestinal disease (e.g., inflammatory bowel disease, celiac disease). Periostitis without digital clubbing can be seen in thyroid acropachy, hypervitaminosis A, fluorosis, venous stasis, hyperphosphatemia, and sarcoidosis. Isolated chronic digital clubbing, which is mainly associated with pleuropulmonary disease, does not seem to cause HOA.

The pathogenesis of HOA remains unknown, although several possible mechanisms have been proposed. HOA is usually accompanied by bone and joint pain associated with periarticular periostitis. The pain is usually exacerbated by dependency and relieved with limb elevation. Typical signs of periostitis include periosteal new bone along the distal ends of long bones, which can be seen on plain radiographs. When periostitis is not obvious on plain radiography, a bone scan is useful to demonstrate early evidence of disease. When HOA is clinically suspected, radiologic evaluation of the thorax is important because of the association between HOA and lung neoplasms.

In many cases, symptomatic management with nonsteroidal anti-inflammatory drugs or other analgesics while treating the underlying disorder provides significant relief of symptoms. In refractory cases, bisphosphonates such as pamidronate and zoledronic acid have been reported to be effective.

Rheumatoid Arthritis–Like Syndrome

Inflammatory rheumatoid arthritis–like syndrome has been associated with solid neoplasms and hematologic malignancies. Clinical characteristics associated with this paraneoplastic syndrome include acute onset or late onset, asymmetrical disease frequently involving the lower extremities, nonspecific synovitis in large joints that spares the wrists and hands without bony erosion, negative results for rheumatoid factor and cyclic citrullinated peptide antibody. However, these features are not specific and may be confused with elder-onset rheumatoid arthritis, seronegative rheumatoid arthritis, spondyloarthropathy, remitting seronegative symmetrical synovitis with pitting edema (RS3PE), or polymyalgia rheumatica (PMR).

RS3PE manifests with sudden onset of polyarthritis, pitting edema, and prominent constitutional symptoms. More than one half of RS3PE cases are associated with malignancy. Lymphoproliferative disorders such as leukemia and lymphoma may simulate various rheumatic syndromes from direct invasion of the synovium, articular tissues, or juxta-articular bone, producing synovitis or bone pain.

Lupus-Like Syndrome

Antinuclear antibodies (ANAs) can be seen in patients with solid neoplasms (e.g., gastric, cervical, and breast carcinomas, testicular seminoma), lymphomas, or myelodysplastic disorders, but the significance of these autoantibodies is not well understood. The association between SLE and occult malignancy is uncertain.

It is not necessary to search for underlying malignancy in a patient with typical manifestations of SLE. However, lupus-like autoantibodies and unexplained Coombs- positive hemolytic anemia or thrombocytopenia without clinical signs of rheumatic disease warrant further investigation for an occult neoplasm.

Raynaud's Phenomenon and Scleroderma-Like Syndrome

The sudden onset of Raynaud's phenomenon and scleroderma-like syndrome can herald an underlying tumor such as hematologic malignancies and carcinomas of the liver, ovary, testis, bladder, breast, or stomach. Scleroderma-like skin changes may also occur in patients with osteosclerotic myeloma with *p*olyneuropathy, *o*rganomegaly, *e*ndocrinopathy, *m*onoclonal gammopathy, and *s*kin abnormalities (i.e., POEMS syndrome) and in those with carcinoid tumors.

Characteristics that suggest secondary Raynaud's phenomenon include age at onset older than 50 years, symptom asymmetry, symptoms that persist year round, and rapid digital ulceration and necrosis. Secondary Raynaud's is also suggested by scleroderma-like syndromes in patients older than 50 years, rapid progression of skin sclerosis, or a poor response to therapy. The lack of Raynaud's phenomenon can be another distinguishing characteristic of paraneoplastic scleroderma-like syndrome because Raynaud's phenomenon occurs in approximately 95% of cases of systemic sclerosis.

Polymyalgia Rheumatica

Clinical symptoms and signs of PMR include shoulder and pelvic girdle pain and morning stiffness, a high erythrocyte sedimentation rate (ESR), and anemia of chronic disease. Although the association between PMR and cancer is controversial, several features are atypical for PMR and may suggest an occult malignancy: disease onset before the age of 50 years, asymmetrical or localized involvement of typical sites, an ESR less than 40 or higher than 100 mm/hr, and a poor response to low doses of glucocorticoids.

Myelodysplastic syndromes and myeloproliferative syndromes are frequently associated with PMR. Myelodysplastic syndromes also are associated with a variety of musculoskeletal symptoms and signs, including cutaneous vasculitis, monoarticular or polyarticular arthritis, lupus-like conditions, Raynaud's phenomenon, polychondritis, and pyoderma gangrenosum.

Vasculitides

Vasculitis is rarely associated with malignancy and is most commonly seen in patients with lymphoproliferative disorders and myelodysplastic syndrome. Cutaneous leukocytoclastic vasculitis is the most common manifestation of vasculitic paraneoplastic. Although clinical presentations of paraneoplastic vasculitides are indistinguishable from those of the idiopathic condition, a chronic, relapsing disease with cytopenias and poor response to conventional treatment suggest a hidden malignancy.

Inflammatory Myopathies

The association between inflammatory myopathies and malignancies has been well established.

For a deeper discussion of these topics, please see Chapter 269, "Inflammatory Myopathies," in Goldman-Cecil Medicine, 25th Edition.

Miscellaneous Conditions

Other rheumatologic syndromes that may be harbingers of neoplasia include eosinophilic fasciitis, palmar fasciitis, reflex sympathetic dystrophy, erythromelalgia, Sweet's syndrome, and osteomalacia. Up to 15% cases of Sweet's syndrome (i.e., acute neutrophilic dermatosis) are associated with malignancy, and it can manifest as an acute, self-limited polyarthritis or vasculitis. Knee pain or shoulder pain with normal physical examination findings can be a referred pain from various neoplasms.

● HEMATOLOGIC DISORDERS WITH RHEUMATIC MANIFESTATIONS

Hemophilia

Acute, painful hemophilic arthropathy of the knees, elbows, and ankles is the most common manifestation of hemophilia. Repeated episodes of hemarthrosis result in synovial proliferation and chronic inflammation, causing chronic hemophilic arthropathy.

Chronic hemophilic arthropathy is characterized by joint deformity, fibrous ankylosis, and osteophyte overgrowth. Radiography typically shows degenerative arthritis. Besides prompt administration of factor concentrate replacement, acute hemarthrosis must be treated conservatively with cold applications and joint immobilization followed by a structured physical therapy program. Aspiration (after factor replacement) is needed only if concomitant sepsis is suspected or the joint is very tense.

Sickle Cell Disease

Musculoskeletal complications of sickle cell disease include painful crises, arthropathy, dactylitis, osteonecrosis, and osteomyelitis. Sickle cell crisis is the most common musculoskeletal feature, and it can produce painful arthritis of the large joints and noninflammatory joint effusions adjacent to areas of bony crisis. Osteonecrosis of the femoral head, shoulder, and tibial plateau may result from repeated local bone ischemia or infarct.

Dactylitis manifesting as bilateral, painful, swollen hands or feet (i.e., hand-foot syndrome) may be the first manifestation of the disease in infants and young children. It usually resolves spontaneously in a few weeks. Increased risk of septic arthritis and osteomyelitis, most often due to *Salmonella* species, has been associated with hemoglobinopathies.

Multiple Myeloma

Rheumatologic manifestations of multiple myeloma include bone pain resulting from lytic bone lesions, pathologic fractures, and osteoporosis. Thoracolumbar pain in the setting of hypercalcemia, renal insufficiency, and anemia suggests the possibility of multiple myeloma. Multiple myeloma can manifest atypically and mimic specific autoimmune disorders such as Sjögren's syndrome (SS) and SLE.

Amyloidosis

Amyloidosis is a disorder of protein folding in which insoluble fibrillar proteins are deposited in the extracellular space in one or more organs, disrupting tissue structure and function. The clinical manifestations and prevalence depend on the type of amyloidosis.

Myeloma-associated amyloidosis (i.e., amyloid light-chain [AL] amyloidosis) is one of the most common forms of systemic amyloidosis. Amyloid proteins derived from monoclonal light chains can involve the synovium and the articular cartilage, producing rheumatoid arthritis–like polyarthritis. Joint stiffness is more pronounced in amyloid arthropathy, and deposition of amyloid protein at the glenohumeral joint produces enlargement of the anterior shoulder, called the *shoulder pad sign*. Other rheumatic manifestations of AL amyloidosis include muscle weakness, pseudohypertrophy of muscles, and pathologic fracture from osteolytic lesions, jaw claudication that mimics giant cell arteritis, and sicca syndrome due to exocrine gland infiltration.

The amyloid protein can be identified as apple green birefringence on Congo red staining of an abdominal fat pad aspiration or rectal mucosal biopsy specimen. The other principal systemic forms of amyloidosis are secondary amyloidosis (i.e., deposition of amyloid A [AA] protein), hereditary amyloidosis, and β_2-microglobulin–associated amyloidosis.

Endocrine Disorders

Endocrine diseases usually manifest with diffuse, poorly defined musculoskeletal symptoms and joint pain that is more often periarticular than articular. Clinical suspicion of endocrinopathy is by far the most important diagnostic step. Routine clinical laboratory tests such as ESR, ANA, rheumatoid factor, uric acid level, and an antistreptolysin O (ASO) titer are usually not helpful, and radiographs often first suggest the possibility of endocrinopathy.

Diabetes

One of the most common musculoskeletal complications of diabetes is diabetic cheiroarthropathy (i.e., diabetic hand syndrome). It is characterized by insidious development of waxy thickening of the skin of the fingers and hands and by flexion contractures of the metacarpophalangeal joints and interphalangeal joints. Patients cannot press the palms together completely without a gap with the wrists fully flexed (i.e., prayer sign). Although this syndrome is associated with the duration of diabetes and the control of blood sugar, it may develop before the onset of overt diabetes and mimic sclerodactyly.

Dupuytren contracture and stenosing flexor tenosynovitis (i.e., trigger finger) may be identified. People with diabetes are more prone to develop a carpal tunnel syndrome. Diabetic periarthritis of the shoulders (i.e., adhesive capsulitis or frozen shoulder) is more common in patients with diabetes, especially in women with a long history of diabetes. Capsulitis is characterized by staged progression of pain and restriction of shoulder motion, and bilateral involvement occurs in about one half of patients.

Patients with long-standing, poorly controlled diabetes may develop a painless, swollen, deformed joint known as a Charcot joint or neuropathic arthropathy. Tarsal, metatarsophalangeal, and tarsometatarsal joints are most commonly involved, and it can be confused with osteomyelitis on radiographs.

Diffuse idiopathic skeletal hyperostosis (DISH) is seen in up to 20% of diabetic patients, who are typically obese and older than 50 years. It is associated with neck and back stiffness rather than pain. Lateral radiographic views of the spine show four or more contiguously fused vertebrae as a result of flowing ossification of the anterior longitudinal ligament without involvement of apophyseal (facet) joints.

Diabetic amyotrophy (i.e., diabetic lumbosacral radiculoplexus neuropathy) is remarkable for acute or subacute onset of severe hip, buttock, or thigh pain followed by progressive weakness of the affected extremity. It occurs typically in older male patients who have relatively well-controlled diabetes, and there are often preceding anorexia, weight loss, and unsteady gait.

Hypothyroidism

Almost one third of patients with hypothyroidism have musculoskeletal symptoms. Arthritis of hypothyroidism can resemble early rheumatoid arthritis, affecting small joints of the hands and wrists, but it is not erosive or deforming. In contrast, myxedematous arthropathy classically involves large joints such as knees.

Many hypothyroid patients experience carpal tunnel syndrome, trigger finger, Raynaud phenomenon, and pseudogout. Acute pseudogout can be a presenting feature of hypothyroidism.

Hypothyroidism can also cause a broad spectrum of muscular diseases. Hypothyroid patients may have asymptomatic elevation of muscle enzymes, but a few patients develop proximal muscle weakness or polymyositis-like syndrome. Patients may complain of fatigue, malaise, and fibromyalgia-like generalized muscle pain. Rarely, hypothyroid myopathy manifests with muscle enlargement, stiffness, and muscle cramps (i.e., Hoffmann's syndrome).

Hyperthyroidism

Common rheumatic symptoms of hyperthyroidism include proximal myopathy, periarthritis of the shoulder, thyroid acropachy (i.e., thickened skin with periosteal new bone formation), and osteoporosis. Proximal muscle weakness is more frequently observed in elderly patients with apathetic or masked hyperthyroidism. Asking a patient to stand from a squat position can reveal the proximal muscle weakness.

Hyperparathyroidism

Musculoskeletal symptoms, often widespread and nonspecific, are common in hyperparathyroidism and can be the clinical presentation for many patients. The musculoskeletal manifestations of hyperparathyroidism include osteitis fibrosa cystica (i.e., bone pain, osteopenia, and bony cysts), subperiosteal resorption, pseudogout, rheumatoid arthritis–like disorder, diffuse osteopenia, spinal compression fracture, and proximal myopathy. Secondary hyperparathyroidism is the leading cause of renal osteodystrophy in chronic kidney disease.

Acromegaly

Acromegalic arthropathy commonly develops in the large joints and is seen in approximately 70% of the patients with acromegaly. Overgrowth of cartilage initially produces joint space widening,

but it may eventually lead to severe osteoarthritis with pain, limited range of motion, and deformity.

⬤ GASTROINTESTINAL DISEASES WITH RHEUMATIC MANIFESTATIONS

Whipple's Disease

Whipple's disease is a rare, multisystemic disease that most often affects the gastrointestinal tract. It is caused by infection with *Tropheryma whippelii*. Musculoskeletal symptoms of Whipple's disease are the most common prodrome, and they may exist for years before the diagnosis. Intermittent migratory oligoarthritis of large joints is typical, but some patients may have a florid polyarthritis. Synovial fluid is usually inflammatory with predominant mononuclear cells. Radiographs are often normal.

Hemachromatosis

Hemochromatosis is one of the most common genetic diseases among people with northern European ancestry, and it is frequently associated with osteoarthritis-like arthropathy, chondrocalcinosis, and osteoporosis. The second and third metacarpophalangeal joints of both hands are typically involved, and hooklike osteophytes on the radial side of the metacarpal are characteristic in radiographs. Chondrocalcinosis of the wrist and knee is very common in patients with hemochromatosis. Acute attacks of pseudogout can be a predominant clinical manifestation. Treatment with regular phlebotomies and iron chelation has little effect on the arthropathy.

Primary Biliary Cirrhosis

Primary biliary cirrhosis is frequently associated with other autoimmune diseases, such as limited scleroderma, rheumatoid arthritis, SS, and autoimmune thyroid disease. Vitamin D deficiency is highly prevalent among patients with primary biliary cirrhosis, and the risk of developing osteoporosis is markedly increased in women with this disease.

⬤ OTHER SYSTEMIC ILLNESSES WITH RHEUMATIC MANIFESTATIONS

Human Immunodeficiency Virus Infection

Patients with human immunodeficiency virus (HIV) disease may have osteomyelitis, osteonecrosis, reactive arthritis, or psoriatic arthritis.

Sarcoidosis

Clinical features of sarcoidosis can mimic those of many acute and chronic rheumatic diseases. Acute sarcoidosis or Löfgren's syndrome manifests with fever, erythema nodosum, hilar lymphadenopathy, and acute polyarthritis, almost invariably involving the ankles and knees. The arthritis is usually self-limited and tends to be nondeforming and nonerosive.

Chronic sarcoid arthritis is less common and usually associated with active multisystemic disease. Osseous involvement can be a focal or generalized and occurs in about 5% of patients with sarcoidosis. Bone cysts are usually asymptomatic, but they can manifest in the phalanges with sausage-like fingers or pseudoclubbing. Focal osteolytic changes can lead to pathologic fractures. Sarcoid muscle involvement is often asymptomatic, but it may manifest with proximal pain, progressive weakness, or atrophy.

SJÖGREN'S SYNDROME

Definition and Epidemiology

SS is a chronic autoimmune disorder characterized by infiltration of exocrine glands by predominantly CD4$^+$ T lymphocytes, resulting in dry eyes (i.e., keratoconjunctivitis sicca) and dry mouth (i.e., xerostomia). SS can occur as a primary disorder or can be associated with other autoimmune diseases (i.e., secondary SS) such as rheumatoid arthritis and SLE.

SS is the second most common rheumatic disease, with a community prevalence of primary SS ranging from 0.1% to 0.6% in different studies. However, many patients remain undiagnosed, and little is known about the prevalence of SS in the general population. The disease is diagnosed nine times more often in women than in men and tends to manifest in patients older than 40 years, although it may be seen among people of all ages.

Pathogenesis and Pathology

The pathogenesis of SS is not fully understood, although accumulating evidence shows that chronic immune system stimulation in genetically predisposed individuals (HLA-DR3) is important. Upregulation of type 1 interferon-regulated genes (i.e., interferon signature) and abnormal expression of B-cell activating factor (BAFF) and its receptors appear to play an important role in the development of SS.

Exocrine gland involvement is characterized by a focal lymphocytic sialadenitis and hyperplasia of salivary ductal epithelium seen on minor salivary gland biopsy. Parenchymal atrophy fibrosis or fatty infiltration, or both, are common in the elderly and should not be confused with SS.

Clinical Presentation

The clinical features of SS can be divided into exocrine gland dysfunction and extraglandular manifestations. Subjective symptoms of dry eyes and mouth are the most common problems for most affected patients. Many years can elapse before the diagnosis is established because of nonspecific initial manifestations. Patients with keratoconjunctivitis sicca complain of chronic gritty or sandy eye irritation rather than describing dryness. They may also report itching, photophobia, and the accumulation of thick mucous filaments at the inner canthus. Severe dry eyes can result in vision impairment and punctate keratopathy, which can be detected by fluorescein, lissamine green, or rose bengal staining.

Decreased saliva production can lead to dental caries, gingival recession, oral candidiasis, chronic esophagitis, weight loss due to difficulty chewing and swallowing, and nocturia. Other exocrine gland dysfunction includes recurrent nonallergic rhinitis and sinusitis, vaginal dryness with associated dyspareunia in women with SS and dry cough due to laryngeal, tracheal, and bronchial involvement. SS is a systemic disease and one third of patients with primary SS have various extraglandular features (Table 85-3).

TABLE 85-3	EXTRAGLANDULAR CLINICAL FEATURES OF SJÖGREN'S SYNDROME
SKIN AND MUCOUS MEMBRANES	**CENTRAL NERVOUS SYSTEM**
Lower extremity purpura associated with hyperglobulinemia and/or leukocytoclastic vasculitis on biopsy Photosensitive lesions indistinguishable from those of subacute cutaneous lupus erythematosus	Focal defects including multiple sclerosis, stroke Diffuse deficits including dementia, cognitive dysfunction Spinal cord involvement including transverse myelitis
PULMONARY SYSTEM	**PERIPHERAL NERVOUS SYSTEM**
Chronic bronchitis due to dryness of the tracheobronchial tree Lymphocytic interstitial pneumonitis, interstitial pulmonary fibrosis, chronic obstructive lung disease, cryptogenic organizing pneumonia, pseudolymphoma with intrapulmonary nodules	Peripheral sensorimotor neuropathy Trigeminal sensory neuropathy, optic nerve
MUSCULOSKELETAL SYSTEM	**RETICULOENDOTHELIAL SYSTEM**
Polymyositis Polyarthralgia, polyarthritis	Splenomegaly Lymphadenopathy and development of pseudolymphoma
RENAL SYSTEM	**HEPATOBILIARY SYSTEM**
Tubulointerstitial nephritis Type 1 renal tubular acidosis	Hepatomegaly Primary biliary cirrhosis
VASCULAR SYSTEM	**ENDOCRINE SYSTEM**
Raynaud's phenomenon Small vessel vasculitis, with a mononuclear perivascular infiltrate or leukocytoclastic changes on biopsy	Hypothyroidism caused by Hashimoto's thyroiditis Other autoimmune endocrinopathies

Skin

The major cutaneous manifestations of SS include dry, scaly skin, itchy annular erythema, cutaneous vasculitis, and Raynaud's phenomenon. Cutaneous vasculitis occurs in approximately 10% of patients with SS. It typically involves small and medium-sized vessels, leading to palpable purpura, urticaria, or skin ulceration. Raynaud's phenomenon can precede other features by many years, and it does not cause digital ulceration or infarcts.

Pulmonary Disease

Lung manifestations of SS include asymptomatic interstitial lung disease, pulmonary function abnormalities, and cryptogenic organizing pneumonia by lymphocytic infiltration around bronchioles. Lymph node enlargement of the lung and pulmonary lymphoproliferative disease typically is seen only in patients with primary SS.

Joints

About one half of primary SS patients are affected by joint pain, with or without evident synovitis. It usually involves the hands and knees symmetrically. Arthropathy is typically nonerosive and nondeforming. Identification of rheumatoid factor is associated with a higher prevalence of articular symptoms.

Renal Disease

Urine acidification abnormalities of the distal renal tubule leading to complete or incomplete distal renal tubular acidosis are the most common manifestation of renal involvement, but overt renal disease is less common. Glomerular diseases such as membranoproliferative glomerulonephritis and membranous nephropathy can occur in patients with SS and SLE overlap or those with cryoglobulinemia and hypocomplementemia.

Cardiovascular System

Although pericardial effusion can be seen on the echocardiogram, primary SS patients rarely have acute pericarditis. Placental transmission of maternal anti-Ro/SSA and anti-La/SSB antibodies can cause neonatal lupus and fatal fetal congenital heart block. In women with these antibodies, there is 5% risk of their first child being born with heart block. This risk rises to 15% with subsequent pregnancies. Fetal heart rate monitoring in the antenatal period is essential.

Neuromuscular Disease

Peripheral neuropathy occurs in about 10% of patients with SS and can precede sicca symptoms. Diagnosis of small fiber neuropathy may require quantitative sudomotor autonomic reflex testing or measurement of epidermal nerve density by biopsy. Cranial nerves, particularly the trigeminal and optic nerves, can be involved as a consequence of vasculitis. Although the frequency of central nervous system involvement remains controversial, focal or diffuse brain lesions and multiple sclerosis–like syndromes have been reported. Myalgia is very common, but symptomatic inflammatory myopathy is rare.

Lymphoproliferative Disease

Patients with SS are predisposed to develop lymphoma (primarily B cell in origin). Risk factors include cutaneous vasculitis, peripheral neuropathy, rheumatoid factor, cryoglobulinemia, and hypocomplementemia. Development of new masses with constitutional symptoms or persistent lymph node enlargement should raise concern for malignancy.

Gastrointestinal and Hepatobiliary Disease

Dysphagia commonly results from dryness of the pharynx and esophagus. Lymphocytic infiltration, predominantly by $CD4^+$ T cells, may cause chronic atrophic gastritis, achlorhydria, and pernicious anemia. Although liver involvement in primary SS patients is rare, histologic features show a clear association between SS and hepatic abnormalities. However, other causes of abnormal liver function test results in SS, particularly hepatitis C infection and drug toxicity, should be considered.

Diagnosis and Differential Diagnosis

Although there are no established diagnostic criteria for SS, classification criteria were developed for use in research. The American-European Consensus Group (AECG) classification is most widely accepted, and it requires demonstration of the following:

1. Signs and symptoms of inadequate tear production and decreased salivary gland function

2. Detection of autoantibodies (anti-Ro/SSA or anti-La/SSB, or both)

3. Exclusion of underlying diseases that may mimic SS, including head and neck irradiation, hepatitis C, acquired immune deficiency syndrome, preexisting lymphoma, sarcoidosis, graft-versus-host disease, and anticholinergic drug use.

A provisional classification was proposed by American College of Rheumatology and the Sjögren International Collaborative Clinical Alliance investigators (ACR-SICCA), but it has not been validated completely. The MAIN differences between the AECG and ACR-SICCA criteria are that ocular or oral dryness symptoms are not required in the latter and the ACR criteria do not distinguish between primary and secondary forms of SS.

The diagnosis of SS is made on the basis of compatible clinical and laboratory features and after the exclusion of other causes of sicca symptoms. Various tests are used to evaluate the objective glandular component of the disease. To confirm keratoconjunctivitis sicca, the Schirmer test, the rose bengal test, and tear breakup time can be used. Salivary gland scintigraphy with uptake of technetium-99m, parotid sialography, and measurement of unstimulated production of saliva (i.e., Saxon test) may provide objective evidence of xerostomia. A labial salivary gland biopsy is often essential in evaluating patients with suspected SS, particularly when the patients lack anti-Ro/SSA or anti-La/SSB antibodies. Rheumatoid factor and ANAs are commonly detected, and patients may be erroneously diagnosed with rheumatoid arthritis. Common laboratory findings include anemia, thrombocytopenia, leukopenia, raised ESR, monoclonal gammopathy, and hypergammaglobulinemia.

Other conditions can produce keratoconjunctivitis sicca symptoms, xerostomia, or lacrimal and salivary gland enlargement. The differential diagnosis of SS must consider infectious diseases such as diffuse infiltrative lymphadenopathy syndrome associated with HIV, hepatitis B and C, human T-cell lymphotropic virus infection, syphilis, and infection with mycobacteria, and it must take into account infiltrative diseases such as sarcoidosis and amyloidosis. Anticholinergic side effects from many drugs, including over-the-counter products, should be considered during assessment of dry eyes and dry mouth. Sicca symptoms may result from overlap syndromes, which may have features of SS and SLE or of SS and scleroderma.

Treatment

No cure for SS is available. Because of the diverse symptoms of SS, several medications are used to ameliorate the symptoms outlined in Table 85-4. Patients with moderate to severe involvement may require systemic medical therapy, including the use of immunosuppressive and biologic agents. There is no evidence that azathioprine, low-dose steroids, cyclosporine, infliximab, or methotrexate are useful. Hydroxychloroquine normalizes the ESR and immunoglobulin levels, but it does not increase the salivary flow rate significantly. Many clinicians use it to treat rash, fatigue, myalgia, and arthralgia. B-cell and anticytokine or antichemokine-directed therapies are active areas of research.

Prognosis

Primary and secondary forms of SS are characterized by chronic courses and different rates of progression. Systemic involvement

TABLE 85-4 TREATMENT OPTIONS FOR SJÖGREN'S SYNDROME

LOCAL TREATMENT OF EXOCRINE DYSFUNCTION

Keratoconjunctivitis Sicca

Artificial tears, preservative free
Eyeglasses and/or goggles
Punctal occlusion (plugs or electrocautery)
Topical cyclosporine drops

Xerostomia

Artificial saliva
Salivary stimulators, mechanical or electrical
Fluoride treatments and/or fastidious dental care
Sugar-free lozenges, lemon drops

Dyspareunia

Vaginal lubricants or propionic acid gels
Rigorous treatment of infection

SYSTEMIC TREATMENT OF EXOCRINE DYSFUNCTION

Pilocarpine or cevimeline
When possible, avoid or discontinue medications with anticholinergic effects

TREATMENT OF SYSTEMIC MANIFESTATIONS

Salivary gland infection: tetracycline and nonsteroidal anti-inflammatory drugs
Arthralgia: hydroxychloroquine or chloroquine
Systemic vasculitis and glomerulonephritis: glucocorticoids and/or cyclophosphamide
Leukocytoclastic vasculitis: no specific therapy
Interstitial lung disease: glucocorticoid, cyclophosphamide

of lungs, kidneys, nervous system, and skin may develop, and the risk of developing lymphoma is increased among patients with primary SS, particularly those with the previously described risk factors. The overall mortality rate for SS is not higher than that of the general population.

For a deeper discussion of these topics, please see Chapter 268, "Sjögren's Syndrome," in Goldman-Cecil Medicine, 25th Edition.

SUGGESTED READINGS

Cordner S, De Ceulaer K: Musculoskeletal manifestations of hemoglobinopathies, Curr Opin Rheumatol 15:44–47, 2003.

Garcia-Carrasco M, Ramos-Casals M, Rosas J, et al: Primary Sjögren syndrome: clinical and immunologic disease patterns in a cohort of 400 patients, Medicine (Baltimore) 81:270–280, 2002.

Hansen A, Lipsky PE, Dorner T: Immunopathogenesis of primary Sjögren's syndrome: implications for disease management and therapy, Curr Opin Rheumatol 17:558–565, 2005.

King JK, Costenbader KH: Characteristics of patients with systemic lupus erythematosus (SLE) and non-Hodgkin's lymphoma (NHL), Clin Rheumatol 26:1491–1494, 2007.

Markenson JA: Rheumatic manifestations of endocrine diseases, Curr Opin Rheumatol 22:64–71, 2010.

Ravindran V, Anoop P: Rheumatologic manifestations of benign and malignant haematological disorders, Clin Rheumatol 30:1143–1149, 2011.

Shiboski SC, Shiboski CH, Criswell L, et al: American College of Rheumatology classification criteria for Sjögren's syndrome: a data-driven, expert consensus approach in the Sjögren's International Collaborative Clinical Alliance cohort, Arthritis Care Res 64:475–487, 2012.

St Clair EW, Levesque MC, Prak ET, et al: Rituximab therapy for primary Sjögren's syndrome: an open-label clinical trial and mechanistic analysis, Arthritis Rheum 65:1097–1106, 2013.

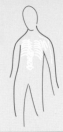

XV

Infectious Disease

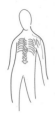

86

Host Defenses Against Infection

Bharat Ramratnam and Edward J. Wing

HOST VERSUS PATHOGEN: VICTORY, DEATH, OR COEXISTENCE

Many factors determine whether we live successfully in symbiosis with our normal microbial flora, whether we can resist exposure to outside pathogens, and whether we live or die in an environment filled with an incredibly wide spectrum of microbes. Factors include age, nutrition, underlying medical conditions (e.g., diabetes mellitus, chronic lung disease), and the nature of the exposure (e.g., microbial virulence, inoculum). The outcome is determined by our host defenses, including barriers (e.g., skin), innate immunity (e.g., phagocytes), and specific responses that include antibodies and T cell–mediated events.

The human host has developed a multilayered host defense system to counter infectious organisms, and the resulting duel between pathogen and human can lead to one of four outcomes: death of the human host, elimination of the pathogen, peaceful coexistence of both in a symbiotic relationship, or an association whose latent nature changes with time and under additional biologic pressures. For example, pneumococcal pneumonia may kill the individual, or the host's defenses may eliminate the organism. *Escherichia coli* and *Bacteroides fragilis* in the gut survive and help to protect the host in a symbiotic relationship. Most individuals exposed to *Mycobacterium tuberculosis* are asymptomatic and latently infected with an inactive nonreplicating organism. Almost one third of the world's population is latently infected, but only about 10% progress to active disease. Immunologic impairment (e.g., human immunodeficiency virus [HIV] infection) and factors such as age increase the risk of progressing from latent to active disease.

The asymptomatic nature of an infection should not automatically be equated with latency or dormancy of the pathogen. For example, chronic HIV-1 infection was incorrectly characterized as having a prolonged latent or silent stage before the host developed immunodeficiency and opportunistic infections. However, most untreated HIV-1–infected individuals harbor actively replicating virus that kill CD4⁺ T lymphocytes on a daily basis, although the aggregate effects are not appreciated until CD4⁺ T lymphocyte levels are reduced to below 200 cells/mL after 8 to 10 years of infection. Infected individuals are infectious despite their relatively asymptomatic state, and in resource-rich countries, treatment is recommended regardless of CD4⁺ T lymphocyte levels. Treatment halts viral immune destruction, reduces viral burden in genital secretions, and decreases an infected individual's risk of transmitting HIV-1.

CATEGORIES OF HOST DEFENSES AND RISKS OF INFECTION

The relative importance of the innate and adaptive defenses is best illustrated by hosts who are deficient in a particular component. For example, chemotherapy leading to the depletion of immune cells such as neutrophils renders the host more susceptible to bacterial and fungal infections. Congenital deficiency of immunoglobulins increases the risk of infections that are usually thwarted by antibody responses such as those associated with *Streptococcus pneumoniae* and *Haemophilus influenzae*. Pharmacologic inhibition of tumor necrosis factor-α (TNF-α) increases the risk of developing active tuberculosis among those with latent infection. Astute clinicians, recognizing the increased incidence of atypical infections such as those caused by *Pneumocystis jirovecii* among young men, sounded the alarm that a novel immunodeficiency syndrome had appeared that was later ascribed to HIV-1.

Host defenses to infection can be classified as nonimmunologic host defenses, innate immunity, and specific or adaptive immunity. Immune host defenses against microbial pathogens are composed of cells and molecules located in peripheral sites, such as the skin and submucosal regions, and in secondary lymphoid tissues, such as the lymph nodes, tonsils, spleen, and Peyer's patches.

For a deeper discussion of these topics, please see Chapters 45 through 50 in Section VII, "Principles of Immunology and Inflammation," in Goldman-Cecil Medicine, *25th Edition.*

Nonimmunologic Host Defenses

Nonimmunologic host defenses include epidermal and mucosal barriers that physically prevent the entry of pathogens into the body. The respiratory tract defenses depend on mucus that entraps pathogens and on ciliary action and cough that continuously clear the mucus and organisms from the lungs and upper airways. Respiratory viruses, including influenza, may inhibit ciliary action or denude the mucous membrane completely, allowing bacteria to colonize and cause infection. Stroke, medications, or other causes of reduced cough reflex may lead to poor clearance of secretions, mucus, and pathogens and cause lung infection. Smoking and industrial exposure to toxins such as silica may similarly reduce lung host defenses, such as reducing ciliary action that leads to infection. In addition to mucus and ciliary action, alveolar macrophages located in the lung parenchyma play an essential role in initial clearance and killing of pathogens.

Gastrointestinal defenses include gastric acidity, which kills many organisms, and vomiting and diarrhea, which help to clear pathogens from the gut. Bacteria vary greatly in their susceptibility to gastrointestinal host defenses. For example, as few as 10 *Shigella* organisms can cause infection, whereas 10^5 to 10^8 *Vibrio cholera* organisms are required for infection.

The urinary tract is protected physically by regular urine flow, the acidity of the urine, and antibacterial proteins. Conditions that interfere with these factors (e.g., prostatic hypertrophy, renal stones) may lead to stasis and infection. Mechanical injection of bacteria through the urethra into the bladder, as occurs in women during sexual intercourse, can lead to colonization of the bladder and infection. Injuries or devices that damage or bypass anatomic barriers frequently lead to infection. Examples include burns, intravenous catheters, intubation, urinary tract catheters, surgery, and trauma.

The normal microbiologic flora on the skin and in the respiratory and gastrointestinal tracks is an important component of host defenses. Normal florae compete with pathogens for nutrients and have antimicrobial activity of their own. Disruption of the normal flora by antibiotics allows superinfecting organisms such as *Candida* species and *Clostridium difficile* in the gut to colonize and then cause infection.

Organs that clear organisms from the bloodstream and lymph, including the liver, spleen, and lymph nodes, play an essential role after a pathogen has breached the primary anatomic barriers. Lack of a spleen increases a person's susceptibility to overwhelming sepsis caused by encapsulated bacteria including *S. pneumoniae, Neisseria meningitidis,* and *H. influenzae.* Cirrhosis of the liver allows portal vein blood to bypass the liver, increasing susceptibility to infection by gut flora.

Innate Immunity

Innate immunity refers to cells, molecules, and cellular receptors that recognize pathogens and promote inflammation nonspecifically at the site of infection. Table 86-1 compares innate and adaptive immunity. The response of innate immunity is relatively nonspecific, invariant, rapid, and without memory. Adaptive immunity is highly specific, slow during primary infection, and

TABLE 86-1	FEATURES OF THE INNATE AND ADAPTIVE IMMUNE RESPONSES	
INNATE RESPONSE	**ADAPTIVE RESPONSE**
No memory: quality and intensity of response invariant	Memory: response adapts with each exposure
Recognizes limited number of nonvarying, generic molecular patterns on or made by pathogens	Recognizes vast array of specific antigens* on or made by pathogens
Pattern recognition mediated by a limited array of receptors	Antigen recognition mediated by a vast array of antigen-specific receptors
Response immediate on first encounter	Response on first encounter takes 1-2 weeks; on second encounter, 3-7 days

From Kumar P, Clark M, editors: Kumar and Clark's clinical medicine, ed 8, London, 2012, Elsevier.

*Antigen is a molecular structure (e.g., protein, peptide, lipid, carbohydrate) that generates an immune response.

can be recalled after primary infection with a more rapid, robust response.

The molecules involved in innate and acquired immunity include cytokines, chemokines, and integrins. Cytokines are soluble proteins that have numerous functions, including promoting cellular growth and activation as well as regulating the adaptive immune response (Table 86-2). Their functions range from stimulating the production of and activating inflammatory cells, including neutrophils, macrophages, and eosinophils, to the direct antiviral action of interferons. Some activate endothelial cells and cause fever, whereas others are regulatory and downregulate the inflammatory response.

Concentration gradients of chemokines in tissue attract leukocytes to areas of inflammation. Integrins on the surface of leukocytes allow adhesion to receptors on other types of cells such as vascular endothelium. This is the first step in attracting and localizing leukocytes to areas of inflammation.

Relatively nonspecific pathogen recognition receptors on phagocytes include toll-like receptors (TLRs), which were originally described in the fruit fly, *Drosophila*; oligomerization domain–like receptors (often abbreviated as Nod-like receptors); C-type lectin-like receptors; and intracellular receptors that detect double-stranded RNA. TLRs have been studied extensively (Table 86-3). TLRs are located on several cell types, including macrophages and dendritic cells. When a pathogen is detected by its adherence to a TLR on the surface of a cell, activation of nuclear transcription factors, including nuclear factor-κB, occurs. This stimulates the production of numerous cytokines important in the inflammatory response, including interleukin-1 (IL-1), IL-6, IL-10, IL-15, TNF-α, and growth factors (see Table 86-2). These cytokines amplify the inflammatory response by activating effector cells and by stimulating the production of many other inflammatory factors, including IL-2, interferons, C-reactive protein, complement components, and growth factors.

Complement factors are soluble proteins and enzymes that are produced in the liver. Complement activation occurs through several pathways that are involved in the innate and acquired host defense system as shown in Figure 86-1. Complement activation can occur as a result of antigen-antibody immune complex binding of C1, the mannose-binding lectin pathway, or the alternative pathway, which can be activated by bacterial cell wall components.

The complement cascade results in C3 convertase, a protein that cleaves C3. Cleavage of C3 leads to the production of multiple proteins (C3a, C4a, and C5a) that stimulate histamine release from mast cells leading to vasodilatation, increased endothelial permeability, and attraction of activated neutrophils. A second cleavage product of C3, C3b, in conjunction with immunoglobulin G (IgG) stimulates phagocytosis of pathogens. Activation of C5-9 results in bacterial lysis. Patients deficient in the complement components C5-9 appear to be particularly susceptible to organisms such as *N. meningitides* and *Neisseria gonorrhoeae.* Complement activation is regulated by several regulatory proteins, such as C1 esterase inhibitor that inhibits the inappropriate activation of the classic complement activation pathway.

The inflammatory response results in the clinical signs of inflammation, including erythema, tenderness, warmth, and swelling. It can be initiated by microorganisms in tissue, tissue

TABLE 86-2   CYTOKINES

CYTOKINE	CELLULAR SOURCE	TARGETS	FUNCTION	RECEPTOR
IL-1α	Epi, fibroblasts, damaged or dying cells	Wide variety	"Dual function" cytokine involved in initiating inflammatory response and modifying gene expression	CD121a or CD121b
IL-1β	M, B	T, B, M, End, other	Leukocyte activation, increases endothelium adhesion	CD121a or CD121b
IL-2	T	TB, NK, M, oligo	T cell proliferation, regulation	CD122/CD25
IL-3	T,* Mas, Eos, NK, End	Ery, G	Proliferation and differentiation of hematopoietic precursors	CD123/CDw131
IL-4	Mas, T, M	B, T, End	Differentiation of T_H2 and B cells	CD124/CD132
IL-5	Mas, T, Eos	Eos, B	Growth differentiation of B cells and eosinophils	CD125/CDw131
IL-6	T, B, M, astrocytes, End	T, B, others	Hematopoiesis, differentiation, inflammation	CD126/CD130
IL-7	Bone marrow and thymic stroma	pB, pT	Pre/pro-B proliferation, T, upregulation of proinflammatory cytokines	CD127/CD132
IL-8	M, L, others	PMN, Bas, L	Chemoattractant	CD128
IL-9	T_H2*	T, B	Potentiates production of IgM, IgG, IgE	
IL-10	CD8⁺ T,* T_H2, (B),† M	T, B, Mas, M	Inhibits IFN-γ,TNF-β, IL-2 by T_H1 cells, DTH, stimulates T_H2	CD210
IL-11		Bone marrow stroma	Osteoclast formation	
IL-12	DC, B, T	T, NK	Potentiates IFN-γ and TNF-α production by T and NK, downregulates IL-10	CD212
IL-13	T_H2,* Mas, NK	T_H2, B, M	T_H2 modulator, downregulated IL-1, IL-6, IL-8, IL-10, IL-12	
IL-14	T	B*	Stimulates proliferation, inhibits Ig secretion	
IL-15	M, Epi	T, B*	Proliferation	
IL-16	Eos, CD8⁺ T*	CD4⁺ T*	CD4* chemoattractant	
IL-17	(T)	Epi, End, others	Osteoclastogenesis, angiogenesis	
IL-18	M	T_H1, NK	Induces IFN-γ production, enhances NK activity	
IL-32	Tn, NK, Epi	Wide variety	Proinflammatory	
TGF-β	Eos, others	Many cell types	Anti-inflammatory, promotes wound healing	
TNF-α	M,* PMN, T, B, NK	M, PMN, T, End, others	Mediator of inflammatory reactions	CD120a and CD120b
TNF-β	L	Wide variety	Mediator of inflammatory reactions	CD120a and CD120b
IFN-α	L, Epi, fibroblasts	Wide variety	Upregulates MHC class I, inhibits viral proliferation	
IFN-β	Epi, fibroblasts	Wide variety	Upregulates MHC class I, inhibits viral proliferation	
IFN-γ	CD8⁺,* (CD4⁺*), NK	T, B, M, NK, End	Antiviral, antiparasitic, inhibits proliferation, enhances MHC class I and II expression	CD119
M-CSF	L, M, G, End, Epi, others	M	Growth and differentiation of Ms	CD115
G-CSF	T,* M, End	G	Growth and differentiation of Gs	
GM-CSF	T, M, End, Mas	pG, pMye	Stimulates growth and differentiation of Gs and Mye lineage cells	CD116
MIF	M	M	Antiapoptotic activity for macrophages, promotes M survival	

From Doan T, Melvold R, Viselli S, Waltenbaugh C: Immunology, ed 2, Philadelphia, 2012, Lippincott, Williams & Wilkins.

B, B cells; Bas, basophils; CSF, colony-stimulating factor; DC, dendritic cells; DTH, delayed-type hypersensitivity; End, endothelium; Eos eosinophil; Epi, epithelium; Ery, erythrocytes; G, granulocytes; IFN, interferon; IL, interleukin; L, lymphocytes; M, macrophage; Mas, mast cells; MHC, major histocompatibility complex; MIF, macrophage migration inhibitory factor; Mye, myeloid; NK, natural killer cells; p, precursor; PMN, neutrophils; oligo, oligodendrocytes; T, T cell; TGF, transforming growth factor; T_H, helper T cell subset; TNF, tumor necrosis factor.

*Activated cells.

†Parentheses indicate that only a subset of the designated cell types produce the cytokine.

TABLE 86-3   TOLL-LIKE RECEPTORS

PRR	PAMP	PATHOGEN	PRR EXPRESSION
TLR2	Peptidoglycan	Gram-positive bacteria	mDC
TLR3	Double-stranded RNA	Viruses	mDC
TLR4	Lipopolysaccharide	Gram-negative bacteria	mDC
TLR7	Single-stranded RNA	Viruses	pDC
TLR9	Double-stranded DNA	Viruses	pDC

From Kumar P, Clark M, editors: Kumar and Clark's clinical medicine, ed 8, London, 2012, Elsevier.

mDC, Mature dendritic cell; PAMP, pathogen-associated molecular pattern; pDC, precursor dendritic cell; PRR, pattern recognition receptor; TLR, toll-like receptor.

injury, or dysfunctional adaptive immunity (e.g., autoantibodies). The response includes inflammatory molecules as previously described and tissue and migrating leukocytes. Neutrophils are central to the clinical manifestations of inflammation in tissue, and patients with neutropenia often lack the signs of inflammation at the site of serious infection.

Neutrophils are bone marrow–derived phagocytes whose production is greatly stimulated by infection through the action of macrophage-produced growth factors, including granulocyte colony-stimulating factor (G-CSF) and granulocyte-macrophage colony-stimulating factor (GM-CSF). Neutrophils circulate in blood, are attracted to sites of inflammation, and are activated

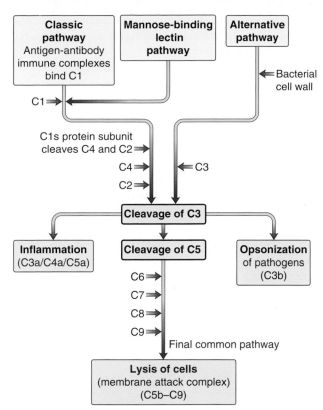

FIGURE 86-1 The complement pathway and other effector functions. (From Kumar P, Clark M, editors: Kumar and Clark's clinical medicine, ed 8, London, 2012, Elsevier.)

by chemotactic factors, including formyl peptides derived from bacteria, complement C3a and C5a, IL-8, interferon, and leukotrienes, particularly leukotriene B$_4$. Neutrophils migrate from the endovascular space into inflammatory tissue through a complicated integrin-regulated process that includes receptors on neutrophils and endothelial cells. Activated neutrophils then migrate down a chemoattractive (i.e., chemokine) gradient toward the site of inflammation.

Neutrophils are killing machines containing granules that have up to 100 different antimicrobial molecules. The contents of granules are released intracellularly into phagosomes after phagocytosis of a pathogen or released extracellularly in the vicinity of pathogens. Phagocytosis is greatly enhanced by opsonization (i.e., antibody and complement binding) of pathogens. The major microbicidal mechanism of neutrophils is the superoxide burst (i.e., production of superoxide anion catalyzed by NADPH oxidase) and then the dismutation to hydrogen peroxide. Many other granule molecules, such as cathepsins, elastases, defensins, and collagenase contribute to the killing process. Similar mechanisms exist in other phagocytes such as macrophages.

Eosinophils, which are found more in tissue than the circulation, are primarily important in host defenses against multicellular parasites such as parasitic worms. Growth and differentiation of eosinophils is promoted by IL-5. Eosinophils are activated and recruited by a variety of mediators, including complement factors and leukotrienes. Eosinophil granules contain specific cationic proteins that are toxic to parasites. Eosinophils also play key roles in the pathogenesis of allergic reactions and diseases such as asthma.

Basophils in blood and mast cells in tissue contain granules with histamine. They can be activated by complement factors and antigen-IgE binding on the surface of mast cells. Histamine is a short-acting, low-molecular-weight amine that acts through four different histamine receptors. Its actions include bronchoconstriction and bronchial smooth muscle contraction, itching, pain, vasodilation, and increased vascular permeability. Histamine also plays a role in gastric acid secretion, motion sickness, and sleep suppression. Commonly used antihistamines counter these effects.

Blood monocytes are produced in the bone marrow and circulate for several days in the blood. They then migrate into tissues, where they phagocytize pathogens and debris and kill microorganisms when activated by bacterial products such as lipopolysaccharide (LPS), interferon-γ, and other cytokines.

The properties and function of macrophages depend on the tissue. Alveolar macrophages in the lung are continuously exposed to airborne particles and pathogens, whereas microglia in the brain have a very different environment and function. Macrophages clear cellular debris after acute inflammation, and thus are the janitors of peripheral tissue. Macrophages produce a variety of cytokines important in the inflammatory process, including IL-1, TNF-α, IL-6, IL-15, and leukocyte growth factors.

Fever during inflammation and infection results from cytokines such as IL-1 and TNF-α that are released by macrophages into the circulation. These molecules increase the level of prostaglandins in the hypothalamus, which elevates the normal temperature set point. This stimulates thermoregulatory mechanisms to elevate the core body temperature.

Macrophages play a central role in granuloma formation. For example, macrophages are critical in controlling difficult-to-kill acid-fast mycobacteria such as *M. tuberculosis* or fungi by walling off viable organisms in granulomas. Macrophages also present antigen derived from microbial pathogens to T cells, helping to initiate the adaptive immune response. Cells of the myeloid lineage can control the immune response and are known as myeloid-derived suppressor cells.

Dendritic cells are derived from myeloid or lymphocytic precursors. Dendritic cells are found primarily in tissues where pathogens are likely to enter the body, such as the skin, gastrointestinal tract, spleen, and respiratory tract. These cells have branchlike cytoplasmic extensions (for which they are named), and they phagocytize pathogens in a manner similar to macrophages. They are the major antigen-presenting cells (APCs) in the body.

Natural killer (NK) cells are T lymphocytes that kill abnormal cells, including virus-infected cells and certain tumor cells. They do not require antigen sensitization for the production of perforin, a pore-forming protein with lethal effects. They are part of the first line of defense against viral infections while adaptive immunity is developing.

Adaptive Immunity

The adaptive immune response produces exquisitely specific, protective mechanisms against microbial pathogens (see Table 86-1). The specific response can be recalled rapidly by memory B and T cells years after infection if the particular pathogen is encountered again. The capacity of the adaptive immune system to protect against different pathogens is truly astounding. It has been estimated that B cells can produce 10^{14} different immunoglobulin molecules, and that T cells can have up to 10^{18} different T-cell receptors (TCRs) for specific antigens.

B Lymphocytes

Antibodies are glycoproteins produced by B cells that recognize specific structural motifs (i.e., epitopes) on microbial pathogens. In antimicrobial defense, binding of an antibody to a pathogen may inhibit the ability of the pathogen to infect a cell or the ability of a toxin to be effective (i.e., neutralization); prompt phagocytosis by phagocytic cells such as neutrophils and macrophages (i.e., opsonization); activate the complement cascade; or kill an infected cell through the process of antibody-dependent cellular cytotoxicity (ADCC).

Antibody-mediated host defense occurs mainly in the extracellular space. T cell–mediated host defenses act primarily on intracellular organisms (i.e., those that enter cells and survive intracellularly). The five major classes (i.e., isotypes) of antibodies are summarized in Table 86-4. Complement fixation is accomplished by IgM and IgG molecules, whereas opsonization is effected by IgG and IgA molecules. IgG antibodies cross the placenta, providing protective immunity to newborns for months. IgA molecules are secretory antibodies that act at mucosal surfaces and are the predominant antibody in external secretions such as mucus. IgE is responsible for allergic responses and host defenses against parasites. IgD acts as an immunomodulatory molecule with the capacity to trigger innate immune responses.

Structurally, antibodies are composed of two large heavy chains and two small light chains (Fig. 86-2). Each heavy and light chain has a constant and a variable region. Each of the five isotypes of heavy chains designates a specific antibody class (i.e., IgM, IgG, IgA, IgE, and IgD) and two types of light chains (i.e., κ and λ). The antigen-binding site of each molecule is composed of the variable region of a heavy chain and the variable region of a light chain. There are two such binding sites for each molecule. The B-cell receptor is composed of the specific immunoglobulin associated with that B cell. Unstimulated B cells express single IgM molecules on their cell surfaces. When stimulated, B cells may initially produce IgM antibodies. Later, a B cell may switch the type of immunoglobulin produced (e.g., from IgM to IgG)

and become a plasma cell producing large amounts of antibody or become a long-term memory cell. B cells do not change their antigen specificity.

The constant region of the two heavy chains comprises the Fc portion, which after immunoglobulin has bound to antigen, can then bind to Fc receptors on the cell surface of neutrophils, macrophages, and dendritic cells. This interaction binds antigen-antibody complexes to phagocytic cells and allows opsonization and phagocytosis or activation of the classic complement pathway, depending on the isotype.

Humans can generate billions of different antibodies, and this diversity results from organization of the genes that encode the variable regions of antibodies. The two major genetic strategies that allow humans to produce antibody specific to virtually any microorganism are somatic hypermutation and recombination of the variable (V), diversity (D), and joining (J) gene segments of the immunoglobulin light and heavy chains. The variable region of the heavy chain is encoded by V, D, and J genes. The variable region of the light chain is encoded by V and J genes.

There are more than 1000 different V, D, and J genes. During B-cell differentiation, somatic translocations randomly select the V, D, and J heavy chain genes and the V and J light chain genes. In this manner, an enormously diverse set of variable chains is assembled. Further genetic variation arises from somatic mutations in B cells as they encounter antigen in lymphoid tissues. B cells have specific Ig antibodies on their surface, with specificity produced by V(D)J recombinations that recognize three-dimensional structures. These molecular structures are on the surface of pathogens or are toxins produced by pathogens.

The adaptive immune cell response begins with recognition of antigen by specific B cells in lymph node follicles. IgM antibodies are produced by B cells whose Ig surface receptors have affinity for the antigen. Interaction with complementary T cells in lymph nodes may result in class switching (e.g., from IgM to IgG classes or others). The switch is called an *isotype switch* and is driven by specific cytokines, such as IL-4, IL-10, IL-5, and others produced by T cells. The isotype switch allows the host to take advantage of the different functions of different isotypes specific for the same antigen (e.g., complement fixation for IgM, opsonic activity for IgG). T-cell interaction through surface coreceptors and stimulatory soluble molecules results in B-cell division and increased

TABLE 86-4	PROPERTIES OF HUMAN IMMUNOGLOBULINS				
PROPERTY	**IgG**	**IgA**	**IgM**	**IgD**	**IgE**
H chain class	γ	α	μ	δ	ε
Molecular weight (approx.)	150,000	170,000	900,000	180,000	190,000
Complement fixation (classic)	++	0	++++	0	0
Opsonic activity (for binding)	++++	++	0	0	0
Reaginic activity	0	0	0	0	++++
Serum concentration (approx.)	1500 mg/dL	150-350 mg/dL	100-150 mg/dL	2 mg/dL	2 mg/dL
Serum half-life	23 days	6 days	5 days	3 days	2.5 days
Major functions	Recall response; opsonization; transplacental immunity	Secretory immunity	Primary response; complement fixation	Immune modulation of inflammation	Allergy; anthelmintic immunity

Ig, Immunoglobulin; +, minimal; ++++, maximal.

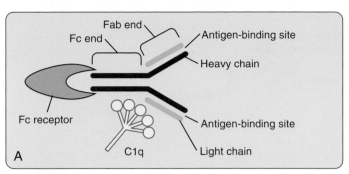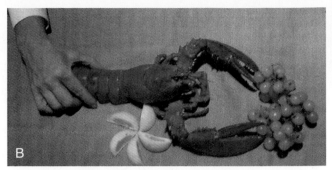

FIGURE 86-2 Structure of antibodies. Antibody molecules are composed of two heavy chains *(red lines)* and two light chains *(blue lines)* held together by disulfide bonds. The two heavy chains join to form a tail (Fc end), which can interact with receptors (FcR) on a variety of cells. The heavy and light chains contribute to the Fab end. At the 5′ or amino-terminal end, these chains form two identical antigen-binding sites, much like two lobster claws. Near the hinge region of the antibody, there is a binding site for C1q, the first component of the complement cascade. (From Birdsall H: Adaptive immunity: antibodies and immunodeficiencies. In Bennett JE, Dolin R, Blaser M, editors: Mandell, Douglas, and Bennett's principles and practice of infectious diseases, ed 8, Philadelphia, 2015, Saunders.)

antibody production. B cells may also differentiate into plasma cells that do not contain surface antibody but secrete large amounts of a single specific isotype immunoglobulin.

B cells may also undergo somatic hypermutation. In this process, cells producing antibody develop point source mutations in the immunoglobulin DNA that may increase the affinity to antigen. This may stimulate increased production of the higher-affinity antibody, thus fine tuning the B-cell response. Driven by T-cell interaction, a portion of the B cells are formed for life, and these *memory cells* have the capacity to secrete antibodies rapidly on antigen reexposure that have extremely high avidity for a particular antigen.

B cells can be activated by two routes. Some antigens can stimulate B cells to proliferate and produce antibody directly without the presence of helper CD4$^+$ T cells. They include microbial-derived molecules such as LPS, which have broad stimulatory properties. Others, such as microbial-derived repetitive motifs on polysaccharides, stimulate mature B cells more specifically. More commonly, B cells are stimulated through synergistic action with CD4$^+$ T cells. Specific antigen is bound to the surface immunoglobulin of the B cell, which triggers endocytosis, degradation of the antigen, and presentation of peptide fragments in association with MHC class II molecules on the cell surface. CD4$^+$ T cells with TCR specificity for the antigen interacts with the B cell through adhesion molecules and costimulatory activation molecules such as CD28 and CD80/86. CD4$^+$ T cells then produce cytokines such as IL-4 that drive antibody production by the B cells.

T Lymphocytes

T cells are produced in the bone marrow and then are processed and selected in the thymus. T lymphocytes have CD4 or CD8 molecules on their surface along with a TCR that has exquisite antigen specificity. During development, the TCR is produced in a process involving gene rearrangement and selection of V, D, and J clusters similar to B-cell antibody differentiation. The potential number of epitopes that T cells can respond to is greater than those that induce B cells.

As maturation takes place in the thymus, T cells whose TCRs have too high an affinity for self-molecules are eliminated. Naïve T cells, usually in regional lymph nodes or similar tissues such as

Peyer's patches in the gut, are sensitized by interaction with an APC such as the dendritic cell. The APC processes a microbial peptide antigen and then presents the antigen to the associated T cell. Presentation of antigen occurs in association with human leukocyte antigen (HLA) class II molecules for CD4$^+$ cells or HLA class I molecules for CD8$^+$ cells. CD4$^+$ cells are called helper T cells and develop into T$_H$1, T$_H$2, and T$_H$17 subsets. CD8$^+$ cells are cytotoxic T cells (Fig. 86-3).

CD4$^+$ T cells are key enhancing cells that are permissive and amplify the response of B lymphocytes, other CD4$^+$ T cells, and CD8$^+$ T cells. They also can activate cells such as phagocytes. CD4$^+$ T cells orchestrate host defenses against pathogens that are initially recognized by phagocytic cells during phagocytosis or pinocytosis. Dendritic cells, for example, incorporate external pathogens or antigens by phagocytosis or pinocytosis and then degrade them within phagosomes.

Short-chain peptide antigens, which are produced by proteolytic degradation, attach to a grove in the MHC class II molecules. The complex is then transported to the surface for presentation to naïve T lymphocytes expressing CD4 molecules on their surface. CD4$^+$ T lymphocytes with specificity for the antigen then adhere to the MHC class II/antigen complex on the surface of the APC. Accessory molecules, such as the adhesion molecule lymphocyte function–associated antigen 1(LFA-1) on T cells, which interacts with intercellular adhesion molecule 1 (ICAM-1) on the APC, are necessary to stabilize the interaction. Activating adhesion complexes such as CD28 (on T cells) and CD80/86 (on APCs) are necessary for sensitization, proliferation, and activation of T cells. Activation and proliferation is also driven by IL-2.

Activated CD4$^+$ T cells (initially called T$_H$0 cells) can be driven by IL-12 and other cytokines to become T$_H$1 cells or by IL-4 and IL-10 to become T$_H$2 cells. T$_H$17 cell differentiation is driven by transforming growth factor-β (TGF-β), IL-6, and IL-23. T$_H$1 cells mediate host defenses against intracellular pathogens such as *M. tuberculosis or Toxoplasma gondii*. They do so by producing γ-interferon that activates APCs such as macrophages that then destroy the invading intracellular pathogen. T$_H$1 cells also produce Il-12, Il-2, and TNF-α, which can enhance the immune response. They also activate cytotoxic T lymphocytes to lyse infected cells.

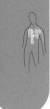

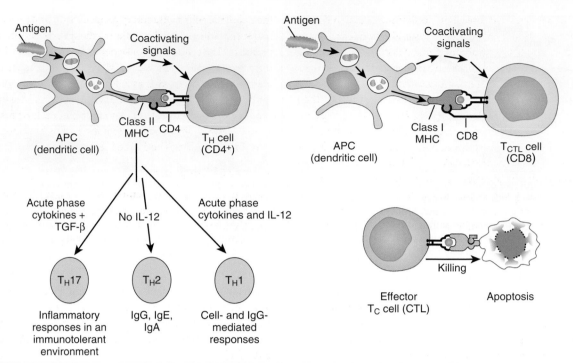

FIGURE 86-3 Overview of T-cell activation. The dendritic cell (DC) initiates the interaction with a CD4+ or CD8+ T cell through a major histocompatibility complex (MHC)–peptide interaction with the T cell receptor. The DC provides an 11-amino-acid peptide on the class II MHC, B7 coreceptor, and cytokines to activate CD4+ T cells. The CD8+ T cell is activated through the class I MHC and 8- to 9-amino-acid peptide plus the B7 coreceptor and cytokines. Presentation of antigen to CD4 T cells and cross-presentation to CD8+ T cells is shown. The cytokines produced by the DCs determine the type of helper T (T$_H$) cell. Activated CD8+ T cells can interact with and lyse target cells through T-cell receptor recognition of peptide in class I MHC molecules on target cells. APC, Antigen-presenting cell; CTL, cytotoxic T lymphocyte; Ig, immunoglobulin; TGF-β, transforming growth factor-β. (From Rosenthal KS, Tan MJ, editors: Rapid review microbiology and immunology, ed 3, Philadelphia, 2011, Mosby.)

Alternatively, CD4+ T cells can become T$_H$2 cells that drive processes such as antiparasitic activity. T$_H$2 cells stimulate B cells to produce antibodies against extracellular pathogens through the production of IL-4, and they stimulate proliferation of eosinophils for activity against parasites (e.g., worms) through the production of IL-5.

T$_H$17 cells are stimulated by IL-23 and produce IL-17, which plays an important role in amplifying the inflammatory response by attracting neutrophils to sites of infection caused by extracellular bacteria and possibly fungi. The complexity of these CD4+ T-cell subsets is still being explored.

CD8+ T cells respond to pathogens that initially enter phagocytic cells directly, such as viruses. Upon intracellular replication, viral proteins are marked for destruction by covalent binding to the protein ubiquitin. The tagged molecules are then degraded by a proteasome, which is a cytoplasmic enzyme complex. Resulting peptide chains of 6 to 24 amino acids then associate with MHC class 1 molecules in a complex intracellular process in the APC and are presented on the surface of the APC. Naïve CD8+ cells that are specific for the presented antigen adhere to the presented MHC class I/antigen complex and express IL-2 receptors. CD4+ T$_H$1 antigen-specific cells also interact with the APC, which stimulates the production of IL-2 by the CD4+ cell and increases CD80/86 expression by the APC. CD28 on the CD8+ T cell interacts with the CD80/86 on the APC to stimulate the CD8+ T cell to proliferate and differentiate into cytotoxic T lymphocytes. The cytotoxic T cells can lyse target cells expressing the appropriate MHC class I/antigen complex. Several signals,

including MHC class I/antigen recognition, IL-2 stimulation, and CD28 and CD80/86 adherence, combine to optimally initiate CD8+ cytotoxic T cells to attack virus-infected cells.

CD4+ and CD8+ T cells help to regulate the immune response. CD4+ regulatory T cells (Tregs) express CD4 and CD25 and help to regulate immune responses, particularly those related to autoimmune diseases but also some infectious diseases. CD8+ suppressor T cells inhibit some autoimmune inflammatory processes.

HOST DEFENSE RESPONSE TO PATHOGENS

Humans are constantly threatened by microbial pathogens. Organisms such as *S. pneumoniae*, group A streptococci, and respiratory viruses colonize the respiratory tract. *S. aureus*, fungi, and many other organisms live on the skin. Every type of pathogen lives in the gastrointestinal tract; some are benign, and some are dangerous.

Host defenses need to react continuously and appropriately to breaches in nonimmunologic host defenses as described earlier. For example, if a person suffers a cut on the hand, the skin barrier is breached, and pathogens may be inoculated into the subcutaneous tissues. This stimulates an immediate nonimmunologic host defense response that includes phagocytosis by cells such as macrophages, which produce cytokines such as IL-1 and TNF-α. Cytokines stimulate the expression of adhesion molecules on vascular endothelium. Neutrophils then bind to the endothelium, move into tissues, and are attracted by a chemokine gradient to the site of invasion.

A second process that breaches nonimmune host defenses results from infection by respiratory viruses. Influenza virus may damage upper and lower respiratory host defenses by destroying the respiratory epithelium, inhibiting ciliary action and mucus production. Bacterial pathogens, most commonly *S. pneumoniae,* that colonize the respiratory tract in normal hosts may then colonize and invade the lower respiratory tract, leading to pneumonia. Organisms such as *M. tuberculosis,* an intracellular pathogen, may evade upper respiratory and lower respiratory defenses and lodge in alveolar macrophages in the lung, where they can survive and multiply. Interference with alveolar macrophage function (e.g., silica exposure) may increase susceptibility to tuberculosis.

The innate immune system is critical during the early phases of infection. The response is rapid, although nonspecific, and eliminates the pathogen or holds the infection in check until the more powerful, highly specific adaptive immune system has time to respond. Phagocytes such as tissue macrophages patrol the periphery and detect pathogens through receptors such as TLRs. This activates the phagocyte, induces phagocytosis and killing, and stimulates the phagocyte to produce cytokines and chemokines that initiate the inflammatory response.

Complement may be activated through the alternative pathway and produce products to attract neutrophils, opsonize pathogens, and lyse pathogens. Vasodilation results from histamine release, and circulating neutrophils are localized to the vascular endothelium nearest the site of invasion by integrins, pass through the vascular wall, and move down a chemokine gradient to the site of infection. Opsonization helps neutrophils and other immune cells ingest and kill the pathogen. These immediate inflammatory and innate immune responses are initiated immediately and increase over hours to days. Although they are effective, these responses are temporizing measures while more specific and more effective host responses of the adaptive immune system are developing.

Immature dendritic cells in peripheral tissues are watchman for foreign molecules. Through pinocytosis and phagocytosis initiated by TLRs and other receptors, they detect pathogens; when identified, dendritic cells migrate to regional lymph nodes. There the dendritic cells mature, stop phagocytosis, and process antigen for presentation to T cells, initiating the specific adoptive immune response. The type of response depends on the type of pathogen. Intracellular pathogens such as *M. tuberculosis* stimulate a T cell–mediated response, whereas *S. pneumoniae* stimulates primarily a B-cell, antibody-mediated (humoral) response. Most infections produce components of cellular and humoral host responses in various degrees that often act in concert. For example, influenza virus induces a B-cell and T-cell response.

Humoral Response

Early in infection, complement and preexisting circulating or tissue antibodies react to pathogens directly and can initiate direct lysis, opsonization, and neutralization of pathogens. B cells may be activated by T cell–independent antigens or through interaction with CD4+ T cells and T cell–dependent antigens. B-cell populations proliferate and produce IgM antibodies initially and then with isotype switching produce other types of antibodies, including IgG and IgA. Antibodies acting in the extracellular space bind to pathogens or their products, potentially leading to neutralization, opsonization, complement fixation, and ADCC.

Cell-Mediated Response

Naïve T cells with specificity for the invading pathogen are activated, proliferate, and produce cytokines. CD4+ T cells produce cytokines that stimulate other T cells, enhance the overall inflammatory response, activate phagocytes for killing, and stimulate antibody production. Previously sensitized T cells may react rapidly with activation and proliferation on exposure to a previously recognized intracellular pathogen.

SUGGESTED READINGS

Bennett JE, Dolin R, Blaser M, editors: Mandell, Douglas, and Bennett's principles and practice of infectious diseases, ed 8, Philadelphia, 2015, Saunders.

Medzhitov R, Shevach EM, Trinchieri G, et al: Highlights of 10 years of immunology in Nature Reviews Immunology, Nat Rev Immunol 11:693–702, 2011.

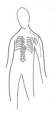

87

Laboratory Diagnosis of Infectious Diseases

Kimberle Chapin

INTRODUCTION

The ability to diagnose a greater number of infectious diseases rapidly and accurately represents a significant recent advance in medicine. Diagnosis has become readily available with point-of-care (POC) testing that is automated, molecularly based, and technologically advanced. At the same time, specimen acquisition, test selection, test performance parameters, and result interpretation have become more complex.

Up to 70% of individual patient medical diagnoses are made with the aid of a laboratory test result. Implementation of the right diagnostic technology can affect patient safety, morbidity, mortality, and health care costs. Examples of how test results can optimize patient care have been published for *Clostridium difficile* toxin molecular testing and infection control practices; algorithms for identification and treatment of sepsis to reduce morbidity and mortality; screening for colonization with methicillin-resistant *Staphylococcus aureus* (MRSA) and *S. aureus,* allowing decontamination and targeted antibiotic therapy in high-risk surgical procedures; and use of rapid molecular testing to aid in successful anti-infective intervention and stewardship programs.

This chapter highlights significant components of testing for infectious diseases and the trends in the laboratory and diagnostic technology that affect patient care. More information is available in the 2013 American Society for Microbiology (ASM) and Infectious Disease Society of America (IDSA) guideline on use of the microbiology laboratory for the diagnosis of infectious diseases. This excellent resource summarizes laboratory diagnosis of infectious diseases by basic disease categories (e.g., respiratory, genital) and contains numerous tables for rapid access of information. The document is well referenced and is updated on a regular basis; it is now available as part of the Sanford Guide–Lab Diagnosis of Infectious Diseases (http://www.sanfordguide.com/).

SPECIMEN COLLECTION AND PROCESSING

Collection of the specimen and its preservation during transportation are components of infectious disease diagnosis that are often overlooked. As part of their accreditation and inspection process, laboratories have collection procedures and criteria for rejection of specimens that are deemed inappropriate to process. These evidenced-based protocols ensure that results can reliably be used to treat patients. Examples include rejection of a sputum specimen after initial smear evaluation shows the specimen is contaminated with squamous epithelial cells and indicates normal mouth flora rather than a deep respiratory specimen. Another example is rejection of a hard stool for *C. difficile* toxin testing because it is inconsistent for a person with *C. difficile* infection, which produces watery diarrhea.

All personnel (e.g., physicians, nurses, phlebotomists) collecting specimens should be familiar with the appropriate collection devices, recommended collection techniques, and requirements for transportation to the laboratory to ensure optimal identification of the pathogen. If the practitioner requests a microbiology test not typically performed, such as for anaerobic organisms from a cerebral spinal fluid (CSF) specimen, a call should be made to the laboratory to clarify the order.

RAPID DIAGNOSTIC METHODS

Rapid or *STAT* is no longer a term foreign to direct testing for infectious diseases and the microbiology laboratory. All major areas of diagnostic testing, including direct visualization of specimens; detection of organism-specific antigens, proteins, and nucleic acids; and cell counts and biomarkers can be performed in 1 to 4 hours. Test results are often available during the time a practitioner is involved with the patient.

Table 87-1 lists the most common U.S. Food and Drug Administration (FDA)–cleared direct testing methods used in laboratories for primary specimens. Examples include Gram stain for bacteria and yeast, fluorescent calcofluor staining for fungi, *Legionella* urinary antigen for legionnaires disease, and polymerase chain reaction (PCR) for enterovirus in CSF.

Direct and *rapid* do not necessarily equate to high predictive values for a true positive or negative test result. As a result, tests commonly used in the past (e.g., bacterial antigen and India ink in CSF) are no longer routinely recommended because false-positive results are common.

DIRECT SMEAR INTERPRETATION

A direct smear interpretation can be exceedingly helpful in confirming a suspected cause (e.g., Gram stain of sputum for pneumococcal pneumonia) and can be performed usually in a few minutes to hours from receipt in the laboratory. High sensitivity and specificity, however, depend on specimens being collected appropriately (e.g., obtained before antibiotic administration) and sometimes on knowing the immune status of the patient.

Fluorescent staining with calcofluor (Fig. 87-1) and auramine have increased sensitivity for direct detection of fungal elements and acid-fast bacilli (AFB), respectively. Direct fluorescent antibody staining for parasites, viruses, or *Pneumocystis jirovecii* is specific and rapid compared with staining of histologic tissue

TABLE 87-1 FDA-CLEARED METHODS OF DIRECT TESTING FROM SPECIMENS

TEST METHODS*	DIAGNOSTIC METHOD	ANALYTE DETECTED
Smear stain preparations	Gram stain	Bacteria, yeast
	Fluorescence	DFA: *Pneumocystis jirovecii*, viruses[†]
		Auramine: mycobacteria
		Calcofluor: fungi
	Special: acid-fast (Kinyoun), partial acid-fast (PAF), India Ink[‡]	Smear use determined by laboratory and based on primary stained specimen[§]
	Wright stain	Leukocyte differentiation and count
Antigen-antibody	Latex agglutination	*Legionella* or *Streptococcus pneumoniae* urinary antigen
		Cryptococcal antigen in serum and CSF
	Lateral flow antibody/ antigen	GAS, RSV, influenza A or B
	Serology for IgG, IgM, Western blot	Multiple analytes; detection and/or confirmation of immune status and acute disease
	Biomarker	Procalcitonin,[‖] C-reactive protein
Molecular[¶]	Hybridization and signal amplification	HPV, bacterial vaginosis or vaginitis, GAS
	Amplification of RNA or DNA or both	Small bundle with ≤5 targets: sexually transmitted pathogens (GC, CT, TV)
		Multiplex amplification with ≥10 targets: blood sepsis, respiratory, gastrointestinal pathogens
		Chip array: multiple targets, HCV genotyping
	Amplification with quantification of nucleic acids	HIV, HCV, HBV

CSF, Cerebrospinal fluid; CT, *Chlamydia trachomatis*; DFA, direct fluorescent antibody; DNA, deoxyribonucleic acid; FDA, U.S. Food and Drug Administration; GAS, group A streptococci; GC, *Neisseria gonorrhoeae*; HBV, hepatitis B virus; HCV, hepatitis C virus; HIV, human immunodeficiency virus; HPV, human papillomavirus; Ig, immunoglobulin; RNA, ribonucleic acid; RSV, respiratory syncytial virus; TV, *Trichomonas vaginalis*

*One-hour, same-day testing.

[†]Because the direct fluorescent antibody (DFA) is organism specific (e.g., *P. jirovecii*, varicella zoster, herpes simplex 1 or 2, cytomegalovirus), these smears are better than histologic stains (e.g., silver stain) and Tzanck preparations (e.g., nucleated giant cells), which can yield similar appearances for many infectious causes.

[‡]Cryptococcal antigen from cerebrospinal fluid (CSF) or serum is the recommended test. India ink often yields false-positive results and is used by the laboratory for confirmation of suspected yeast in a Gram stain of CSF.

[§]For example; partial acid fast testing is performed if the Gram stain shows branching of gram-positive rods and *Nocardia* is suspected; acid fast testing is performed if the auramine-stained sample is positive.

[‖]Procalcitonin is a better marker for identification of bacterial sepsis than C-reactive protein.

[¶]Common examples of pathogens are listed for each group, but many more analytes are available.

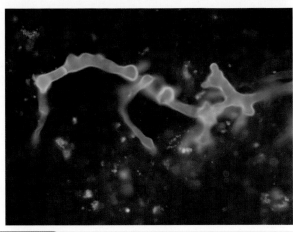

FIGURE 87-1 Calcofluor fluorescent stain depicts fungal hyphae from a wound specimen.

of these tests depend on the specimen type collected (e.g., nasopharyngeal swab is better than a throat swab for influenza A or B testing), the test analyte (e.g., group A streptococci performance is more reliable than influenza A or B), and the prevalence of disease at the time of testing.

False-positive results for rapid antigen tests are unusual, and the patient can be treated based on a positive result. In contrast, a negative test result can be quite misleading. For example, data from the novel H1N1 influenza outbreak demonstrated very poor sensitivity for rapid antigen tests (about 50%) compared with molecular tests. When a multiplex viral panel was used, other viral pathogens were identified as the cause of influenza-like illness in more than 50% of patients admitted to hospitals (Fig. 87-2). Molecular detection of influenza is recommended for hospitalized patients with influenza-like illness if a rapid antigen test result is negative. Many manufacturers have submitted amplified testing assays for influenza, seeking Clinical Laboratory Improvement Amendment (CLIA)–waived status for rapid influenza detection tests that can be performed in the laboratories of physicians' offices or urgent care centers.

Molecular Assays

Molecular identification of infectious diseases has intensified in the past 10 years. The basic categories are shown in Table 87-1.

FDA-cleared direct molecular tests include hybridization and amplification methods. The main difference between these methods is that with hybridization methods, the nucleic acid is not multiplied beyond what is already in the sample. For assays that target DNA, the sensitivity is limited because DNA exists as a single copy. For assays that target proteins or RNA, detection sensitivity is somewhat increased because these components are naturally amplified in the microbe. Familiar hybridization assays include fluorescent in situ hybridization (FISH) for targets in tissue and the protein nucleic acid (PNA) smear (Fig. 87-3). Hybridization assay systems can increase their sensitivity by pairing with signal amplification, such as for human papillomavirus (i.e., Qiagen/Digene HPV test).

In contrast, amplification assays increase the original nucleic acid copy number through a variety of processes, including PCR, transcription-mediated amplification (TMA), and isothermal loop amplification (LAMP). Real-time PCR refers to

preparations, which may take days. However, because adequate specimens are often difficult to obtain, sensitivity may be lacking with smear and culture, and alternative methods such as molecular and empirical therapy are still warranted in specific cases.

● POINT-OF-CARE OR NEAR-PATIENT TESTING

POC or near-patient testing offers rapid results, typically while the patient is still in the clinical care setting, and it allows directed treatment. However, most tests done in practitioners' offices or on-site laboratories are rapid antigen tests. The predictive values

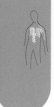

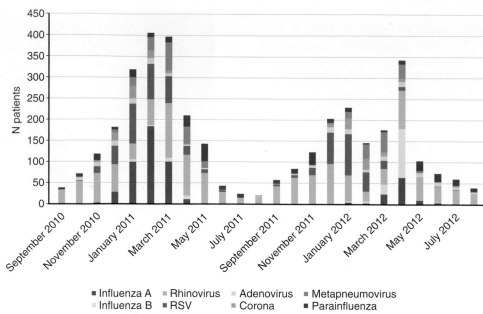

The graph represents the respiratory viruses detected from hospitalized patients who had influenza-like illness over a period of two respiratory seasons. Viral epidemiology was determined using a multiplex respiratory viral assay for 14 viral pathogens. The viral epidemiology provides helpful information for decreasing antibiotic use and discussing the likely cause of illness with patients.

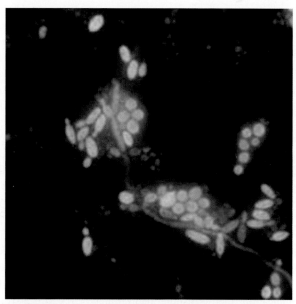

FIGURE 87-3 A protein nucleic acid (PNA) hybridization probe can be used to identify yeast from a positive blood culture. The Yeast Traffic Light PNA FISH assay identified *Candida albicans* and/or *Candida parapsilosis (green), Candida tropicalis (yellow),* and *Candida glabrata* and/or *Candida krusei (red).*

amplification and detection occurring simultaneously, enabling the analyte to be detected more quickly. Amplification assays can detect a single analyte (e.g., enterovirus from CSF) or a group of pathogens for a disease entity from a single specimen, such as sexually transmitted infections (e.g., *Chlamydia trachomatis, Neisseria gonorrhoeae,* and *Trichomonas vaginalis*).

These assays can detect numerous pathogens from a single specimen in a multiplex amplification testing format (i.e., FDA-cleared multiplex assays for 14 to 24 targets exist for respiratory or acute gastroenteritis pathogens). They also allow

quantification of the viral load for purposes of long-term treatment and assessment of clearance (i.e., human immunodeficiency virus, hepatitis B virus, and hepatitis C viral loads).

Culture

Despite advances in rapid direct and molecular diagnostics, culture is still a mainstay for infectious disease diagnosis of most specimen types, but techniques for rapid identification of cultures have been enhanced with updated technology. Blood and AFB specimens are incubated in continuously monitoring incubator cabinets that signal when a specimen is positive based on algorithmic growth curves. A positive specimen can be identified at any time of day, pulled and stained immediately after signaling positive, and tested for definitive identification and susceptibility.

Table 87-2 lists the most common identification methods used from positive broth cultures (e.g., blood) and from colony growth on a culture plate. They include several molecular hybridization methods that have become standard practice for many laboratories (see Fig. 87-3).

Although most laboratories still rely on biochemical and enzymatic phenotypic methods for identification, 16s and 18s sequencing of microbial genomes has demonstrated that the biochemical methods lack specificity. In addition, they require growth for reactions to take place, resulting in further delay of organism identification. The increased use of matrix-assisted laser desorption ionization–time of flight mass spectrometry (MALDI-TOF MS) represents a significant methodologic change. This technique relies on the protein spectral analysis of the organism for identification and takes only minutes rather than days. The technique is described in Figure 87-4.

Susceptibility testing typically requires growth of an organism in the presence of the antibiotics that are appropriate for treatment of the organism. Molecular technology has improved

TABLE 87-2 RAPID IDENTIFICATION METHODS FOR A POSITIVE CULTURE BROTH OR COLONY

METHOD*	ORGANISMS DETECTED	TIME	COST	TECHNICAL EXPERTISE
PNA fluorescent smear	Bacteria, fungi (yeast)	1-2 hr	$$	+
MALDI-TOF	Bacteria, fungi, mycobacteria	Minutes	$	+
Hybridization probes	Bacteria, dimorphic fungi, mycobacteria	1-4 hr	$$	++
Amplification†	Bacteria, viruses, mycobacteria	1-4 hr	$$$	++
16s/18s sequencing	Bacteria, fungi	1-12 hr	$$$	+++
HPLC	Mycobacteria	24 hr	$$$	+++

MALDI-TOF, Matrix-assisted laser desorption ionization–time of flight mass spectrometry; PLC, high-pressure liquid chromatography; PNA, peptide nucleic acid; $, relative cost; +, relative level of required expertise.

*Rapid methods require 2 to 24 hours. Methods presented are U.S. Food and Drug Administration cleared or have had test performance validated in the clinical laboratory. Due to required technical expertise and cost, some of these assays may not be available in the routine laboratory, and providers should inquire about availability

†Includes many different technologies, such as polymerase chain reaction (PCR), transcription-mediated amplification (TMA), and isothermal loop amplification (LAMP).

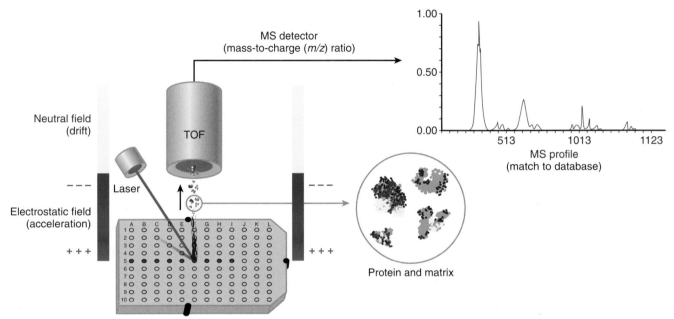

FIGURE 87-4 Matrix-assisted laser desorption–time of flight mass spectrometry (MALDI-TOF MS). Bacterial or fungal growth is selected from a culture plate and applied directly onto a MALDI slide. Samples are overlaid with a matrix and dried. Samples are then bombarded by a laser, which results in sublimation and ionization of the sample and the matrix. The ions are separated based on their mass-to-charge ratio in a tube that measures the time it takes the ions to travel. A spectral representation of these ions is generated and analyzed by software that generates a profile that is subsequently compared with a database of reference MS spectra and matched, generating identification. The process takes only minutes. Although the instrumentation is expensive, the technology is U.S. Food and Drug Administration cleared, and it yields rapid, robust, and reliable identification.

traditional screening tests for the detection of MRSA, vancomycin-resistant enterococci (VRE), carbapenem-resistant organisms, and rifampin-resistant *Mycobacterium tuberculosis*. However, the medical implications of detecting a resistance gene sequence and its expression are not fully understood.

🔴 TRENDS IN THE DIAGNOSIS OF INFECTIOUS DISEASES

Evidence-based guidelines exist for specimen work-ups in an effort to standardize reporting and interpretation of microbiologic results. They are especially useful for specimens submitted from sites potentially contaminated with normal commensal flora (e.g., urine, surface wounds, respiratory sources).

There are limitations on which microbes and how many different microbes should have full identification and susceptibility testing according to the specimen type submitted. For instance, a clean catch urine specimen is called *mixed* if three or more organisms are present in equal amounts (even if they are potential

pathogens) because the significance of any one organism cannot be determined. The specimen must be recollected. Likewise for other specimen types, listing every organism present is not considered helpful.

Other trends include limiting test ordering and the use of algorithms that may be disease or health care system based; continued efforts between microbiologists, pharmacists, and practitioners to optimize the stewardship of anti-infectives; use of multiplex testing to streamline the diagnosis of complex entities such as acute gastroenteritis; developing data on the relevance of a positive molecular result; and the increasing use of metagenomics and sequencing data to perform direct testing (e.g., blood, orthopedic specimens) and to identify infectious disease outbreaks.

SUGGESTED READINGS

Balcl C, Sungurtekin H, Gürses E, et al: Usefulness of procalcitonin for diagnosis of sepsis in the intensive care unit, Crit Care 7:85–90, 2003.

Barenfanger J, Graham DR, Kolluri L, et al: Decreased mortality associated with prompt Gram staining of blood cultures, Am J Clin Pathol 130:870–8706, 2008.

Baron EJ, Miller JM, Weinstein MP, et al: A guide to utilization of the microbiology laboratory for diagnosis of infectious diseases: 2013 recommendations by the Infectious Diseases Society of America (IDSA) and the American Society for Microbiology (ASM), Clin Infect Dis 57:e22–e121, 2013.

Buss SN, Alter R, Iwen PC, et al: Implications of culture-independent panel-based detection of Cyclospora cayetanensis [letter], J Clin Microbiol 51:3909, 2013.

Clark AE, Kaleta EJ, Arora A, et al: Matrix-assisted laser desorption ionization-time of flight mass spectrometry: a fundamental shift in the routine practice of clinical microbiology, Clin Microbiol Rev 26:547–603, 2013.

Forrest GN, Mehta S, Weekes E, et al: Impact of rapid in situ hybridization testing on coagulase-negative staphylococci positive blood cultures, J Antimicrob Chemother 58:154–158, 2006.

McCulloh R, Andrea S, Reinert S, et al: Potential utility of multiplex amplification respiratory viral panel (RVP) testing in the management of acute respiratory infection in children: a retrospective analysis, J Pediatr Infect Dis Soc 3:146–153, 2014.

McCulloh RJ, Koster M, Chapin KC: Respiratory viral testing: new frontiers in diagnostics and implications for antimicrobial stewardship, Virulence 4:1–2, 2013.

Mermel LA, Jefferson J, Blanchard K, et al: Reducing Clostridium difficile incidence, colectomies, and mortality in the hospital setting: a successful multi-disciplinary approach, Jt Comm J Qual Patient Saf 39:298–305, 2013.

Musher DM: The usefulness of sputum Gram stain and culture [letter], Arch Intern Med 165:470–471, 2005.

88

Fever and Febrile Syndromes

Ekta Gupta and Maria D. Mileno

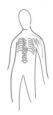

● INTRODUCTION

Fever is one of the most common problems requiring medical evaluation. Fever is an elevation in core body temperature greater than normal daily variation, which is 36.8° C ± 0.4° C (98.2° F ± 0.7° F). Documentation of true fever can be important evidence of infectious processes that warrant investigation. Although fever is characteristic of most infections, it also occurs in noninfectious conditions such as autoimmune and inflammatory diseases, malignancy, and trauma.

This chapter reviews the pathogenesis of the febrile response, the approach to the acutely ill patient with fever, and fever of unknown origin. Fever can be associated with infections, such as those from animal exposures, or with common clinical scenarios in which it may occur as the sole complaint, manifest with rash, or develop with lymphadenopathy. A word of caution about the difference between true and factitious fever is offered at the end of the chapter.

● PATHOGENESIS

Thermoregulation of core body temperature is one of the most important mechanisms in mammalian and human physiology. The hypothalamic heat-regulating set point shifts in response to infection or inflammation mediated primarily by the host's monocytes and macrophages, which are activated as they encounter exogenous bacterial substances, toxins, or the cellular products of trauma.

Monocytes and macrophages produce small proteins called *cytokines,* such as interleukin-1 (IL-1), IL-6, and tumor necrosis factor (TNF). They are collectively known as *endogenous pyrogens* because they actively increase body temperature by increasing the hypothalamic set point, which is the normal temperature for the body that is controlled by the hypothalamus. IL-1 and other endogenous pyrogens are released by macrophages at the site of infection and travel through the bloodstream to the hypothalamus, where they elevate levels of prostaglandin E_2 (PGE_2). Elevated PGE_2 levels increase the set point, and thermoregulatory mechanisms raise the body's core temperature. IL-1 also induces production of PGE_2 in peripheral tissues, which causes the nonspecific myalgias and arthralgias that often accompany fever. Prostaglandin inhibitors such as aspirin or acetaminophen block prostaglandin synthesis and reduce elevated temperatures.

Thermoregulatory control is initiated through sensory neurons in the skin, abdomen, and spinal cord. Central nervous system (CNS) thermoreceptors sense and integrate temperature information. After the hypothalamic set point is raised, the firing rates of neurons in the vasomotor center are altered, causing peripheral vasoconstriction and producing a noticeable cold sensation in the hands and feet. Blood is shunted away from the periphery to the internal organs, and this process is sufficient to raise core body temperature by 1° to 2° C.

Other signaling mechanisms have roles in thermoregulation. The adipocyte-derived hormone leptin actively controls energy homeostasis, and thermogenesis in fat tissue contributes to increasing core temperature. Thermogenesis is important in fighting infection and in responding to cold-induced heat production. Fever has direct antimicrobial effects in some infections such as neurosyphilis and salmonellosis, and elevated temperature augments humoral and cellular immune responses. IL-1 acts independently on two physiologic systems: thermoregulation and iron metabolism. IL-1 can stimulate a wide range of host defenses to conduct a synergistic response to infection.

Fever also can have deleterious effects. It may lead to disorientation and confusion in persons with underlying brain disease and in healthy older individuals. Tachycardia can increase cardiopulmonary work, precipitating congestive heart failure or myocardial infarction in persons with significant cardiopulmonary disease. Fever should be controlled with antipyretics for comfort and to avoid compromising individuals with multiple medical problems. Acetaminophen is preferred for control of fever in children because of the risk of Reye's syndrome with salicylate use.

The terms *fever*, *hyperthermia*, and *hyperpyrexia* are not synonymous. Although most patients with elevated temperature have fever (>38.3° C or 100.9° F), some conditions can increase the body temperature by overriding or bypassing the normal homeostatic mechanism and may even produce body temperatures in excess of 41° C or 105.8° F (i.e., hyperthermia), which can be rapidly fatal and does not respond to antipyretics. Rapid cooling is critical to the patient's survival in hyperthermic conditions such as heat stroke. Even in otherwise healthy individuals, heat stroke can occur after vigorous exercise and prolonged exposure to high environmental temperatures and humidity. Heat stroke is marked by temperatures greater than 40.6° C (105.1° F), altered sensorium or coma, and cessation of sweating. Treatment includes covering the patient with wet compresses followed by intravenous infusion of fluids appropriate to correct fluid and electrolyte losses.

Severe hyperthermia may be a heritable reaction to anesthetics (i.e., malignant hyperthermia) or a response to phenothiazines (i.e., neuroleptic malignant syndrome). Serotonin syndrome, which often includes fever, is classically associated with the simultaneous administration of two serotonergic agents. It can also occur after initiation of a single serotonergic drug that increases the serotonin level of individuals who are particularly sensitive to serotonin. Occasionally, persons with CNS disorders such as paraplegia and persons with severe dermatologic conditions are unable to dissipate heat and can experience hyperthermia.

Hyperpyrexia is the term for extraordinarily high fever (>41.5° C or 106.7° F), which can occur in patients with severe infections but is most commonly observed in persons with CNS hemorrhages.

● DIAGNOSTIC APPROACH TO THE ACUTELY ILL PATIENT WITH FEVER

Patterns of fever should be considered when assessing acutely ill, febrile persons. Evaluation includes determining the normal diurnal variation in body temperature, which often persists when patients have fever. Normally, body temperature peaks in the late afternoon or early evening.

Rigors (i.e., bed-shaking chills) often mark the onset of bacterial infection, typically bacteremia, although they may occur in other clinical situations, such as drug-induced fever or transfusion reactions. Wide swings in temperature may indicate an abscess. Malaria should be considered for anyone with fever who has visited or lived in malarious regions or who has relapsing fever accompanied by episodes of shaking chills and high fever separated by 1 to 3 days of normal body temperature and relative well-being. The timing of administration of anti-inflammatory drugs should be assessed because they may alter or blunt the febrile response. Most infectious diseases manifest with fever as an early finding and with subclinical and eventual clinical involvement of specific organ systems.

If fever occurs as the sole complaint or is associated with localized symptoms and signs, the diagnostic approach includes taking a thorough history, including an extensive review of systems, medical and surgical histories, and immunizations, including those from childhood. Antipyretics may be withheld to allow assessment of the fever trajectory. Elderly individuals, persons taking corticosteroids, and patients with chronic liver or renal disease may be less likely to mount a fever. All likely sources of disease, including travel, exposure to *Mycobacterium tuberculosis,* and occupational, hobby, animal, insect, and sexual contacts, should be assessed. Previous itineraries and activities, geographic risks of diseases, and the seasonality and incubation periods of possible disease exposures should be considered in returning travelers (Table 88-1).

Viral Infection

Acute febrile illnesses in young healthy adults usually are caused by viral infections, which do not require precise diagnosis because they are self-limited and seldom have therapeutic options. Upper respiratory tract symptoms of rhinorrhea, sore throat, cough, and hoarseness most often result from rhinovirus, coronavirus, parainfluenza virus, and adenoviruses. Adenovirus outbreaks occur among persons living in close quarters such as military barracks or college dormitories. Respiratory syncytial virus, human metapneumovirus, and human bocavirus infections occur in similar conditions and sometimes manifest with pneumonia.

A coronavirus causes the potentially fatal upper respiratory viral infection called *Middle East respiratory syndrome* (MERS).

TABLE 88-1	COMMON INFECTIONS IN TRAVELERS BY INCUBATION PERIOD	
DISEASE	**USUAL INCUBATION PERIOD (RANGE)**	**DISTRIBUTION**
INCUBATION <14 DAYS		
Malaria, *Plasmodium falciparum*	6-30 days	Tropics, subtropics
Dengue	4-8 days (3-14 days)	Topics, subtropics
Chikungunya	2-4 days (1-14 days)	Tropics, subtropics (Eastern Hemisphere)
Spotted fever, rickettsiae	Few days to 2-3 weeks	Causative species vary by region
Leptospirosis	7-12 days (2-26 days)	Widespread; most common in tropical areas
Enteric fever	7-18 days (3-60 days)	Especially in Indian subcontinent
Malaria, *Plasmodium vivax*	8-30 days (often >1 month to 1 year)	Widespread in tropics/subtropics
Influenza	1-3 days	Worldwide; can also be acquired en route
Acute human immunodeficiency virus (HIV) infection	10-28 days (10 days to 6 weeks)	Worldwide
Legionellosis	5-6 days (2-10 days)	Widespread
Encephalitis, arboviral (e.g., Japanese encephalitis, tick-borne encephalitis, West Nile virus)	3-14 days (1-20 days)	Specific agents vary by region
INCUBATION 14 DAYS TO 6 WEEKS		
Malaria, enteric fever, leptospirosis	See earlier incubation periods for relevant diseases	See earlier distribution for relevant diseases
Hepatitis A	28-30 days (15-50 days)	Most common in developing countries
Hepatitis E	26-42 days (2-9 weeks)	Widespread
Acute schistosomiasis (Katayama syndrome)	4-8 weeks	Most common after travel to sub-Saharan Africa
Amebic liver abscess	Weeks to months	Most common in developing countries
INCUBATION >6 WEEKS		
Malaria, amebic liver abscess, hepatitis E, hepatitis B	See earlier incubation periods for relevant diseases	See earlier distribution for relevant diseases
Tuberculosis	Primary, weeks; reactivation, years	Global distribution; rates and levels of resistance vary widely
Leishmaniasis, visceral	2-10 months (10 days to years)	Asia, Africa, South America

Modified from Centers for Disease Control and Prevention: CDC health information for international travel, 2012, New York, 2012, Oxford University Press.

It has caused pneumonia with acute respiratory distress syndrome (ARDS) and death in one half of infected individuals, and it is highly contagious.

Meningitis symptoms occur predominantly from enterovirus infections during summer months, although the symptom complex warrants urgent treatment of bacterial causes while the diagnostic process occurs. Febrile syndromes without meningitis are more common manifestations of enteroviral infections.

Arthropod-borne viruses such as California encephalitis virus; eastern, western, and Venezuelan equine encephalitis viruses; St. Louis encephalitis virus; and West Nile virus can produce self-limited febrile illnesses and encephalitis. Colorado tick fever is a biphasic illness seen after northwestern and southwestern tick exposures. It is characterized by high fevers and leukopenia. In New York State, a deer tick virus has been associated with numerous cases of fever and confusion.

Influenza causes sore throat, cough, myalgias, arthralgias, and headache in addition to fever, and it most often manifests in an epidemic pattern during winter months. It is unusual for fever to persist beyond 5 days in uncomplicated influenza. Prolonged fever in persons with diagnosed influenza warrants investigation and treatment of bacterial superinfection.

Early recognition of fever and dry cough led to the discovery and containment of the outbreak of severe acute respiratory syndrome (SARS). The epidemics of avian influenza and H1N1 pandemic strains in recent years are sobering reminders that influenza viruses have a remarkable ability to mutate, producing new immune-resistant strains on a regular basis. Preventive yearly influenza vaccination is important.

Mononucleosis syndromes of fever with detectable lymph node enlargement typify infections with Epstein-Barr virus (EBV), cytomegalovirus (CMV), primary human immunodeficiency virus (HIV), and *Toxoplasma gondii* (i.e., toxoplasmosis). Other manifestations of these infections include abnormal liver function test results, respiratory tract symptoms, and neurologic symptoms. Diagnosis of acute HIV infection, which can produce a mononucleosis-like syndrome, is an urgent issue.

Bacterial Infections

Pathogenic bacteria can infect all body parts and can cause a spectrum of localized illness warranting antibiotic therapy. For example, *Staphylococcus aureus* may cause skin abscesses or cellulitis. Highly pathogenic organisms may colonize individuals who have had contact with the health care system. Most concerning is the event of bacteria entering the bloodstream. Obtaining timely blood cultures before administering the antibiotics indicated for presumed bacterial infections in persons with common clinical syndromes can help to identify bloodstream pathogens and define the required course of treatment.

Fever may be the predominant clinical manifestation of *S. aureus* illness. This organism and the methicillin-resistant form (i.e., MRSA) frequently cause sepsis without an obvious primary site of infection. It should be considered in patients undergoing intravenous therapy or hemodialysis and in those who use intravenous drugs or who have severe chronic dermatitis. Bacteremia with staphylococci may cause hematogenous seeding of bones leading to osteomyelitis and heart valves leading to endocarditis in individuals; the bacteremia may also reflect these underlying processes. Other common causes of bacteremia and their sources include *Streptococcus pneumoniae* (i.e., pneumonia), *Escherichia coli* (i.e., urinary tract and gastrointestinal sources), streptococci (i.e., skin), and anaerobes (i.e., gastrointestinal tract).

Listeria monocytogenes bacteremia is seen predominantly in persons with depressed cell-mediated immunity. It is the most common manifestation of listeriosis in these hosts. Many with listeriosis may have meningitis and warrant lumbar puncture for cerebrospinal fluid culture.

Typhoid and paratyphoid fever (i.e., enteric fever) are common in many low-income countries. Patients may have fever alone as the primary clinical manifestation. Travelers to six countries account for 80% of U.S. cases: India, Mexico, Philippines, Pakistan, El Salvador, and Haiti. Fever with headache and an insidious onset with an unremarkable physical examination is common, although a faint and transient rash (i.e., rose spots) may appear by the second week of illness. Symptoms may include diarrhea, constipation, vague abdominal discomfort, and sometimes dry cough. Diagnosis depends on the culture of blood or stool.

Fever with Localized Symptoms and Signs

Localized bacterial infection can be apparent, as in cases of abscess, cellulitis, or otitis media, or clinically occult. It can develop as an undifferentiated febrile syndrome. Careful inspection of mucous membranes and conjunctiva may reveal petechiae, which are clues to meningococcemia or infective endocarditis. Finding heart murmurs in the setting of fever may suggest endocarditis and warrant additional blood cultures. Pulmonary signs in pneumonia include rales and evidence of consolidation, but persons with cryptococcosis, coccidioidomycosis, histoplasmosis, psittacosis, legionellosis, or pneumocystis pneumonia may show few signs.

These infections should be suspected based on exposure history and the host's immune status. It is important to assess the size of the liver, spleen, and lymph nodes, particularly in cases of viral infection. A swollen joint may indicate septic arthritis. A complete neurologic examination, including cranial nerves and testing for meningeal signs, may indicate CNS infection.

Malaria, bacterial sepsis, and bacterial infections of the lung, urinary tract, CNS, and intestines with resultant bacteremia warrant urgent initiation of empirical treatment while awaiting final identification and sensitivities. For febrile patients with features suggesting a bacterial infection, evaluation should include complete blood counts with differential and platelet counts, blood smears for those at risk for malaria or babesiosis, urinalysis, throat and blood cultures, and a chest radiograph.

Fevers with rash as a prominent feature warrant exclusion of life-threatening infectious diseases, including meningococcemia, toxic shock syndrome (TSS), and Rocky Mountain spotted fever (RMSF). Characterization of the rash can help. Clues to some of the common infections exhibiting fever as the sole feature and those causing fever with rash are provided in Tables 88-2, 88-3, and 88-4. Tables 88-5 and 88-6 list common syndromes associated with imported fevers when assessing travelers.

FEVER OF UNKNOWN ORIGIN

Most febrile conditions resolve or are readily diagnosed and treated, but some fevers can persist and remain unexplained.

TABLE 88-2   INFECTIONS EXHIBITING FEVER AS THE SOLE OR DOMINANT FEATURE

INFECTIOUS AGENT OR SOURCE	EPIDEMIOLOGIC EXPOSURE AND HISTORY	DISTINCTIVE CLINICAL AND LABORATORY FINDINGS
VIRUSES		
Rhinovirus, adenovirus, parainfluenza	None (adenovirus in epidemics)	Often URI symptoms; throat and rectal cultures; rapid viral antigen testing
Middle East respiratory syndrome (MERS)	Travel to Arabian Peninsula or contact from Middle East	Pneumonia with ARDS; viral antigen testing of sputum; PCR of normally sterile sites (CDC)
Enteroviruses (nonpolioviruses: coxsackieviruses, echovirus)	Summer, epidemic	Occasionally aseptic meningitis, rash, pleurodynia, herpangina; serologic or nucleic acid testing (PCR)
Influenza	Winter, epidemic	Headache, myalgias, arthralgias; nasopharyngeal culture, rapid viral antigen testing
EBV, CMV	Close personal contact; blood or tissue exposure; occupational or perinatal exposure	Monospot test, EBV specific antibodies; EBV PCR in immunocompromised; CMV IgM shell vial assay; CMV antigenemia assay; CMV DNA of CSF; culture and histopathology of tissues
Colorado tick fever	Southwest and northwest regions, tick exposure	Biphasic illness, leukopenia; blood, CSF cultures, serologic or PCR
Deer tick virus (Powassan virus)	New York State tick exposure	Altered mentation or encephalitis; serum and CSF IgM (CDC)
BACTERIA		
Staphylococcus aureus	IV drug users, IV catheters, hemodialysis, dermatitis	Must exclude endocarditis; blood cultures
Listeria monocytogenes	Depressed cell-mediated immunity	Meningitis may also be present; blood, CSF cultures
Salmonella typhi, Salmonella paratyphi	Food or water contaminated by carrier or patient	Headache, myalgias, diarrhea, or constipation, transient rose spots; blood, marrow, or stool cultures
Streptococci	Valvular heart disease	Low-grade fever, fatigue; blood cultures
ANIMAL EXPOSURE		
Coxiella burnetii (Q fever)	Exposure to infected livestock, parturient animals	Headache, occasionally pneumonitis, hepatitis, culture-negative endocarditis; serologic testing
Leptospira interrogans	Water contaminated by urine From dogs, cats, rodents, small mammals	Headache, myalgias, conjunctival suffusion, biphasic illness, aseptic meningitis; serologic testing

ARDS, Acute respiratory disease syndrome; CDC, Centers for Disease Control and Prevention case definition; CMV, cytomegalovirus; CSF, cerebrospinal fluid; EBV, Epstein-Barr virus; IgM, immunoglobulin M; IV, intravenous; PCR, polymerase chain reaction; URI, upper respiratory infection.

TABLE 88-3   DIFFERENTIAL DIAGNOSIS OF INFECTIOUS AGENTS PRODUCING FEVER AND RASH

MACULOPAPULAR, ERYTHEMATOUS LESIONS

Enterovirus
EBV, CMV, *Toxoplasma gondii*
Acute HIV infection
Colorado tick fever virus
Salmonella typhi
Leptospira interrogans
Measles virus
Rubella virus
Hepatitis B virus
Treponema pallidum
Parvovirus B19
Human herpesvirus 6

VESICULAR LESIONS

Varicella-zoster virus
Herpes simplex virus
Coxsackievirus A
Vibrio vulnificus

CUTANEOUS PETECHIAE

Neisseria gonorrhoeae
Neisseria meningitidis
Rickettsia rickettsii (Rocky Mountain spotted fever)
Rickettsia typhi (murine typhus)
Ehrlichia chaffeensis
Echoviruses
Streptococcus viridans (endocarditis)

DIFFUSE ERYTHRODERMA

Group A streptococci (scarlet fever, toxic shock syndrome)
Staphylococcus aureus (toxic shock syndrome)

DISTINCTIVE RASH

Ecthyma gangrenosum: *Pseudomonas aeruginosa*
Erythema migrans: Lyme disease

MUCOUS MEMBRANE LESIONS

Vesicular pharyngitis: coxsackievirus A
Palatal petechiae: rubella, EBV, scarlet fever (group A streptococci)
Erythema: toxic shock syndrome (*Staphylococcus aureus* and group A streptococci)
Oral ulceronodular lesion: *Histoplasma capsulatum*
Koplik's spots: measles virus

CMV, Cytomegalovirus; EBV, Epstein-Barr virus; HIV, human immunodeficiency virus.

TABLE 88-4 FEVER AND RASH IN VIRAL INFECTION

VIRUS	DISEASE FEATURES	INCUBATION AND EARLY SYMPTOMS
Coxsackie, ECHO virus	Maculopapular rubelliform, 1-3 mm, faint pink, begins on face, spreading to chest and extremities	Summertime No itching or lymphadenopathy
	Herpetiform vesicular stomatitis with peripheral exanthema (papules and clear vesicles on an erythematous base), including palms and soles (hand, foot, and mouth disease)	Multiple cases in household or community-wide epidemic Mostly diseases of children
Measles	Erythematous, maculopapular rash begins on upper face and spreads down to involve extremities, including palms and soles. Koplik's spots are blue-gray specks on a red base found on buccal mucosa near second molars. Atypical measles occurs in individuals who received killed vaccine and then are exposed to measles. The rash begins peripherally and is urticarial, vascular, or hemorrhagic.	Incubation period 10-14 days First, severe upper respiratory symptoms, coryza, cough, and conjunctivitis; then Koplik's spots, then rash
Rubella	Maculopapular rash beginning on face and moving down; petechiae on soft palate	Incubation 12-23 days Adenopathy; posterior auricular, posterior cervical, and suboccipital
Varicella	Generalized vesicular eruption; pruritic lesions in different stages from erythematous macules to vesicles to crusted; spread from trunk centrifugally; zoster lesions are painful and often dermatomal	Incubation 14-15 days; late winter, early spring Herpes zoster is a reactivation, occurs any season
Herpes simplex virus	Oral primary: small vesicles on pharynx, oral mucosa that ulcerates; painful and tender	Incubation 2-12 days
	Recurrent: vermilion border, one or few lesions, genital; may be asymptomatic or appear similar to oral lesions on genital mucosa	
Hepatitis B and C virus	Prodrome in one fifth; erythematous, maculopapular rash, urticaria Leukocytoclastic vasculitis occurs in hepatitis C	Arthralgias, arthritis; abnormal liver function test results; hepatitis B antigenemia
Epstein-Barr virus	Erythematous, maculopapular rash on trunk and proximal extremities Occasionally urticarial or hemorrhagic	Transiently occurs in 5-10% of patients during first week of illness
Human immunodeficiency virus	Maculopapular truncal rash may occur as early manifestation of infection	Associated fever, sore throat, and lymph node enlargement may persist for 2 or more weeks

TABLE 88-5 COMMON SYNDROMES AND DISEASES ASSOCIATED WITH FEVER IN RETURNED TRAVELERS

SORE THROAT	COUGH	ABDOMINAL PAIN	ARTHRALGIA OR MYALGIA	DIARRHEA
Bacterial pharyngitis	Amebiasis (hepatic)	Amebiasis (intestinal)	Arboviruses	Amebiasis (intestinal)
Diphtheria	Anthrax	Anthrax	Dengue	Anthrax
Infectious mononucleosis	Bacterial pneumonia	Campylobacter enteritis	Yellow fever	Campylobacter enteritis
HIV seroconversion	Filarial fever	Legionnaires disease	Babesiosis	HIV seroconversion
Lyme disease	TPE	Malaria	Bartonellosis	Legionnaires disease
Poliomyelitis	Histoplasmosis	Measles	Brucellosis	Malaria melioidosis
Psittacosis	Legionnaires' disease	Melioidosis	Erythema nodosum leprosum	Plague
Tularemia	Leishmaniasis (visceral)	Plague	Hepatitis (viral)	Relapsing fever
Viral hemorrhagic fever (Lassa)	Loeffler syndrome	Relapsing fevers	Histoplasmosis	Salmonellosis
Nonspecific viral URTI	Malaria	Salmonellosis	HIV seroconversion	Schistosomiasis (acute)
	Measles	Schistosomiasis (acute)	Legionnaires disease	Shigellosis
	Melioidosis	Shigellosis	Leptospirosis	Typhoid in children
	Plague	Typhoid fever	Lyme disease	Viral hemorrhagic fevers
	Q fever	Viral hemorrhagic fevers	Malaria	Yersiniosis
	Relapsing fever	Yersiniosis	Plague	
	Schistosomiasis (acute)		Poliomyelitis	
	Toxocariasis		Q fever	
	Trichinosis		Relapsing fevers	
	Tuberculosis		Secondary syphilis	
	Tularemia		Toxoplasmosis	
	Typhoid and paratyphoid		Trichinosis	
	Typhus		Trypanosomiasis (African)	
	Viral hemorrhagic fevers		Tularemia	
	Nonspecific viral URTIs		Typhoid and paratyphoid	
			Typhus	
			Viral hemorrhagic fevers	

From Beeching N, Fletcher T, Wijaya L: Returned travelers. In Zuckerman JN, editor: Principles and practice of travel medicine, ed 2, Boston, 2013, Wiley-Blackwell, p 271.
HIV, Human immunodeficiency virus; TPE, tropical pulmonary eosinophilia; URTI, upper respiratory tract infection.

Table 88-7 shows the most common causes of unexplained fevers.

The term *fever of unknown origin* (FUO) identifies a pattern of fever with temperatures greater than 38.3° C (101° F) on several occasions over more than 3 weeks after an initial diagnostic work-up for which the diagnosis remains uncertain. Verifying the presence or absence of fever is important; up to 35% of 347 patients admitted to the National Institutes of Health (NIH) for evaluation of prolonged fever were determined not to have significant fever or had fever of factitious origin. Cases of FUO are

TABLE 88-6   COMMON CLINICAL FINDINGS AND ASSOCIATED INFECTIONS

CLINICAL FINDINGS	INFECTIONS TO CONSIDER AFTER TROPICAL TRAVEL
Fever and rash	Dengue, chikungunya, rickettsial infections, enteric fever (skin lesions may be sparse or absent), acute HIV infection, measles, acute schistosomiasis
Fever and abdominal pain	Enteric fever, amebic liver abscess
Undifferentiated fever and normal or low white blood cell count	Dengue, malaria, rickettsial infection, enteric fever, chikungunya
Fever and hemorrhage	Viral hemorrhagic fevers (dengue and others), meningococcemia, leptospirosis, rickettsial infections
Fever and eosinophilia	Acute schistosomiasis; drug hypersensitivity reaction; fascioliasis and other parasitic infections (rare)
Fever and pulmonary infiltrates	Common bacterial and viral pathogens; legionellosis, acute schistosomiasis, Q fever, melioidosis
Fever and altered mental status	Cerebral malaria, viral or bacterial meningoencephalitis, African trypanosomiasis
Mononucleosis syndrome	Epstein-Barr virus, cytomegalovirus, toxoplasmosis, acute HIV infection
Fever persisting >2 weeks	Malaria, enteric fever, Epstein-Barr virus, cytomegalovirus, toxoplasmosis, acute HIV, acute schistosomiasis, brucellosis, tuberculosis, Q fever, visceral leishmaniasis (rare)
Fever with onset >6 wk after travel	Vivax malaria, acute hepatitis (B, C, or E), tuberculosis, amebic liver abscess

Modified from Centers for Disease Control and Prevention: CDC health information for international travel 2012, New York, 2012, Oxford University Press.

HIV, Human immunodeficiency virus.

TABLE 88-7   COMMON CAUSES OF FEVER OF UNKNOWN ORIGIN

INFECTIONS

Abscesses
Brucellosis
Catheter infections
Cytomegalovirus
Coccidioidomycosis
Histoplasmosis
Human immunodeficiency virus (HIV) infection
Infective endocarditis
Intra-abdominal, subdiaphragmatic, and pelvic disease
Liver and biliary tract disease
Lyme disease
Mycobacterium tuberculosis
Osteomyelitis
Sinusitis
Toxoplasmosis
Urinary tract infection

AUTOIMMUNE CONDITIONS

Adult Still's disease
Familial Mediterranean sarcoidosis
Rheumatoid arthritis
Systemic lupus erythematosus
Temporal arteritis

MALIGNANCY

Hepatocellular carcinoma
Leukemia
Metastatic cancers
Pancreatic cancer
Renal cell carcinoma

MISCELLANEOUS CAUSES

Deep vein thrombosis, pulmonary embolism
Hyperthyroidism
Kikuchi's disease
Periodic fever (tumor necrosis factor receptor associated)

categorized as classic FUO, health care–associated FUO, neutropenic (immune-deficient) FUO, and HIV-related FUO. Each of these FUO subtypes can have unique causes.

Classic Fever of Unknown Origin

The most common causes of classic FUO are infections, malignancies, and noninfectious inflammatory disorders; miscellaneous causes and undiagnosed cases account for the remaining categories. Historically, infections have made up the largest category, representing 25% to 50% of cases. Abscesses, endocarditis, tuberculosis, complicated urinary tract infections, and biliary tract diseases have consistently been among the most important. Abscesses account for almost one third of infectious causes, and most are intra-abdominal or pelvic in origin. Perforation of a colonic diverticulum or appendicitis can sometimes lead to large, walled-off abdominal abscesses with few localizing signs.

During the past 50 years, the improvement of imaging studies and their greater accessibility have made abdominal or pelvic abscesses and malignancies more easily detected and less likely to be the cause of prolonged, undiagnosed fever. Malignant neoplasms can induce fever directly through the production and release of pyrogenic cytokines and indirectly by undergoing spontaneous or induced necrosis or creating conditions conducive to secondary infections. Endovascular infections are usually detectable by blood cultures, although slow-growing or fastidious organisms may make detection difficult.

Infections, including tuberculosis, typhoid fever, malaria, and amebic liver abscesses, remain the most frequent causes of FUO in developing countries. The incidence of some FUOs vary in incidence according to geographic location. Classic FUO may occur as familial Mediterranean fever among Ashkenazi Jews; in Kikuchi's disease, which is an unusual form of necrotizing lymphadenitis seen primarily in Japan; and as TNF receptor–associated periodic fever (TRAPS), formerly called familial Hibernian fever, which is an inherited periodic fever syndrome described originally in Ireland.

The proportion of FUOs due to noninfectious inflammatory diseases and undiagnosed conditions has risen. Of the connective tissue diseases, juvenile rheumatoid arthritis (i.e., Still's disease), other variants of rheumatoid arthritis, and systemic lupus erythematosus predominate among younger patients. Temporal arteritis and polymyalgia rheumatica syndromes are more common among elderly patients.

Fever may be blunted or absent in up to one third of elderly individuals with serious conditions. Older people may more often have atypical clinical presentations of common infectious and noninfectious diseases. For example, elderly persons may have tuberculosis without cough or fever, infective endocarditis with fatigue and weight loss but without fever, abdominal abscesses with little abdominal tenderness found on physical examination. Leukocytosis and increased band forms are more likely to be associated with a serious infection. HIV should be considered as a possible cause of FUO in older patients, although it is not usually suspected early in the course of FUO.

Fever in returned travelers is most often caused by common infections, such as malaria and respiratory or urinary tract infections. However, fever cased by dengue, typhoid fever, or amebic liver abscess is increasingly identified, especially among international travelers returning from the tropics. Katayama fever is a febrile syndrome occurring after exposure to fresh water schistosomes in endemic areas. It may resolve spontaneously or may require treatment with antiparasitic agents to prevent sequelae that carry severe morbidity. A travel history should be obtained, and it may redirect the entire work-up.

Health Care–Associated Fever of Unknown Origin

Some FUOs are associated with health care practices, including surgical procedures, urinary and respiratory tract instrumentation, intravascular devices, drug therapy, and immobilization. Quality control measures are set up to minimize and avoid bloodstream infections and decubitus ulcers. Drug-related fever, septic thrombophlebitis, recurrent pulmonary emboli, and *Clostridium difficile* colitis must be considered in the work-up of hospitalized patients who develop fever greater than 38° C (100.4° F) for more than 3 days if it was not present on admission.

Immune Deficiency–Associated Fever of Unknown Origin

Immunosuppressed individuals have the highest incidence of FUO of any group of patients. Due to impaired immune responses, signs of inflammation other than fever are notoriously absent or diminished, producing atypical clinical manifestations and an absence of radiologic abnormalities for what otherwise would be readily diagnosed infections. In patients with impaired cell-mediated immunity, FUO often results from conditions other than pyogenic bacterial infections (e.g., fungi, CMV).

Neutropenia is a dangerous condition that can be considered a subclass of immunodeficiency. Persons with profound neutropenia are at high risk for bacterial and fungal infections. Episodes of fever are common in patients with neutropenia. Many episodes are short lived because they respond quickly to treatment or are manifestations of rapidly fatal infections.

Bacteremia and sepsis can cause rapid deterioration in neutropenic patients, and empirical, broad-spectrum antibiotics should be administered promptly without waiting for the results of cultures. However, only about 35% of prolonged episodes of febrile neutropenia respond to broad-spectrum antibiotic therapy. If fevers persist after 3 days of treatment with broad-spectrum antibiotics, diagnostic tests to explore fungal causes should be considered along with empirical antifungal treatment.

Human Immunodeficiency Virus–Related Fever of Unknown Origin

The primary phase of HIV infection is characterized by a mononucleosis-like illness in which fever is a prominent feature (see Chapter 101). After symptoms of the primary phase of HIV infection resolve, patients enter a long period of subclinical infection during which they are usually afebrile. In the later phases of

untreated HIV infection, episodes of fever become common, often signifying a superimposed illness. Many of these are potentially devastating opportunistic infections, which tend to manifest in atypical fashion because of the severe immunodeficiency. Patients with acquired immunodeficiency syndrome (AIDS) often have multiple infections simultaneously. After highly active antiretroviral therapy (HAART) has been started and the HIV viral load is effectively suppressed, the frequency of FUO in HIV-infected patients falls markedly.

Approach to the Patient with Fever of Unknown Origin

Evaluation of a patient with FUO typically includes verification that the patient has fever, consideration of the fever pattern, a comprehensive history, repeated physical examinations, appropriate laboratory investigations, key imaging studies, and invasive diagnostic procedures. The physical examination should scrutinize the patient more closely than usual because key physical abnormalities in patients with FUO are subtle and require repeated examinations to be appreciated.

Work-up of a patient with an FUO should focus on the history, physical examination, and initial laboratory data. In place of rational diagnostic thinking, there is a temptation to order multiple comprehensive laboratory and imaging studies. Rather than leading to a diagnosis, this shotgun approach may result in enormous expense, false-positive results, and unnecessary additional investigations that may obfuscate the true diagnosis.

A fundamental principle in the management of classic FUO is that therapy should be withheld, whenever possible, until the cause of the fever has been determined, so that treatment can be tailored to a specific diagnosis. The exception is in the setting of the immunocompromised host because rapid empirical treatment is most often needed.

⬤ SPECIFIC CONDITIONS AND EXPOSURES CAUSING FEVER
Fever after Animal Exposures
Q Fever

Q fever is a widespread zoonotic infection caused by the pathogen *Coxiella burnetii* that has acute and chronic manifestations. The primary source of infection is infected cattle, sheep, and goats. The organism can exist for months in soil and can become airborne. The onset of disease is typically abrupt, and high-grade fever (40° C or 104° F), fatigue, headache, and myalgias are the most common symptoms. Acute Q fever is usually a mild disease that resolves spontaneously within 2 weeks. Q fever endocarditis usually occurs in patients with previous valvular damage or immunocompromise, and it is often the predominant manifestation of chronic infection.

An immunofluorescence assay is the reference method for the serodiagnosis of Q fever. Consideration of doxycycline therapy is warranted only for patients who are symptomatic.

Leptospirosis

Leptospirosis is a zoonotic infection with protean manifestations caused by the spirochete *Leptospira interrogans*. It is distributed worldwide, but most clinical cases occur in the tropics. The organism infects rodents, cattle, swine, dogs, horses, sheep, and goats, and it is shed in the urine. Humans most often become infected after exposure to environmental sources, such as contaminated water.

Leptospirosis may manifest as a subclinical illness followed by seroconversion, a self-limited systemic infection, or a severe, potentially fatal illness accompanied by multiorgan failure. Acute illness manifests with the abrupt onset of fever, rigors, myalgias, and headache in 75% to 100% of patients. Conjunctival suffusion in a patient with a nonspecific febrile illness accompanied by lymphadenopathy, hepatomegaly, and splenomegaly points to a diagnosis of leptospirosis.

During the second phase of illness, fever is less pronounced, but headache and myalgias can be severe, and aseptic meningitis is an important manifestation. In some patients with leptospirosis, the clinical course may be complicated by jaundice (although liver failure is rare), renal failure, uveitis, hemorrhage, ARDS, myocarditis, and rhabdomyolysis (i.e., Weil's syndrome).

Because the clinical features and routine laboratory findings of leptospirosis are not specific, a high index of suspicion must be maintained. The diagnosis is usually made by serologic testing for *L. interrogans*. Symptomatic individuals warrant treatment with doxycycline.

Brucellosis

Brucellosis is a zoonotic infection caused by *Brucella melitensis*. It is transmitted to humans by contact with fluids from infected animals (i.e., sheep, cattle, goats, pigs, or other animals) or derived food products such as unpasteurized milk and cheese.

Clinical manifestations of brucellosis include fever, night sweats, malaise, anorexia, arthralgias, fatigue, weight loss, and depression. Patients may have fever and a multitude of complaints but no other objective findings. The onset of symptoms may be abrupt or insidious, developing over several days to weeks. The musculoskeletal and genitourinary systems are the most common sites of involvement. Neurobrucellosis, endocarditis, and hepatic abscesses occur in 1% to 2% of cases.

The diagnosis of brucellosis should be considered for an individual with otherwise unexplained fever and nonspecific complaints who has had a possible exposure. Ideally, the diagnosis is made by culture of the organism from blood or other sites, such as bone marrow. Serologic tests include tube agglutination and enzyme-linked immunosorbent assay (ELISA). For adults with nonfocal disease, treatment with doxycycline and rifampin is suggested.

Fever and Rash

The most concerning diseases associated with fever and rash are meningococcemia, staphylococcal TSS, and RMSF.

Bacterial Meningitis

Neisseria meningitidis is the leading cause of bacterial meningitis in children and young adults in the United States. Recent experience in New York City identified HIV patients as being at increased risk for meningococcal disease.

Manifestations of meningococcal disease can range from transient fever and bacteremia to fulminant disease, with death ensuing within hours of the onset of clinical symptoms. Acute systemic meningococcal disease may manifest as one of three syndromes: meningitis alone, meningitis with accompanying meningococcemia, and meningococcemia without clinical evidence of meningitis.

The typical initial symptoms of meningitis due to *N. meningitidis* consists of the sudden onset of fever, nausea, vomiting, headache, decreased ability to concentrate, and myalgias in an otherwise healthy patient. A petechial rash appears as discrete lesions 1 to 2 mm in diameter, most frequently occurring on the trunk and lower portions of the body. More than 50% of patients have petechiae at clinical presentation. Petechiae can coalesce into larger purpuric and ecchymotic lesions.

Staphylococcal Toxic Shock Syndrome

S. aureus strains produce exotoxins that cause three syndromes: food poisoning, caused by ingestion of *S. aureus* enterotoxin; scalded skin syndrome, caused by exfoliative toxin; and TSS, caused by toxic shock syndrome toxin 1 (TSST-1) and other enterotoxins. About one half of reported TSS cases are menstrual, associated with bacterial growth on highly absorbent tampons. Nonmenstrual TSS has been associated with surgical and postpartum wound infections, mastitis, septorhinoplasty, sinusitis, osteomyelitis, arthritis, burns, cutaneous and subcutaneous lesions (especially of the extremities, perianal area, and axillae), and respiratory infections after influenza. Some MRSA strains can produce TSST-1, and patients infected with these strains may develop TSS.

The Centers for Disease Control and Prevention (CDC) case definition for a confirmed case includes several criteria. Patients must have fever greater than 38.9° C, hypotension, diffuse erythroderma, desquamation (unless the patient dies before desquamation can occur), and involvement of at least three organ systems. Although 80% to 90% of TSS patients have *S. aureus* isolated from mucosal or wound sites, the isolation of *S. aureus* is not required for the diagnosis of staphylococcal TSS.

Rickettsial Infections

RMSF is a potentially lethal but usually curable tick-borne disease. Most cases of RMSF occur in the spring and early summer in endemic areas, particularly in the south central and southeastern states, when outdoor activity is most common. The etiologic agent, *Rickettsia rickettsii*, is a gram-negative, obligate intracellular bacterium that is usually transmitted through a tick bite. Up to one third of patients with proven RMSF do not recall a recent tick bite or recent tick contact.

In the early phases of illness, most patients have nonspecific signs and symptoms such as fever, headache, malaise, myalgias, arthralgias, and nausea with or without vomiting. Most patients with RMSF develop a rash between the third and fifth days of illness. The rash typically begins with pink, blanching macules that evolve to a deep red color and then become hemorrhagic. The lesions begin at the wrists, forearms, and ankles and then spread to the arms, thighs, trunk, and face.

The diagnosis of RMSF is based on a constellation of symptoms and signs in an appropriate epidemiologic setting (e.g., endemic area in the spring or early summer). In later illness, the diagnosis can be made by skin biopsy and confirmed serologically.

Murine typhus is a worldwide illness caused by *Rickettsia typhi* organisms that are transmitted by fleas. It produces a moderately severe illness characterized by fever, rash, and headache. Disease in the United States has been reported in Texas and Southern California.

Rickettsia africae, the cause of African tick-bite fever, occurs in travelers returning from East Africa. It produces a large eschar with a febrile syndrome similar to RMSF. Rickettsial infections respond to treatment with doxycycline and warrant rapid initiation of treatment.

Lyme Disease

Lyme disease is a tick-borne illness caused by pathogenic species of the spirochete *Borrelia burgdorferi* in the United States. Other species in Europe and Asia can cause more aggressive presentations. Localized disease includes erythema migrans in 80% of patients and nonspecific findings that resemble a viral syndrome. Erythema migrans is an expanding macule that forms an annular lesion with a clearing middle.

Early disseminated Lyme disease with acute neurologic or cardiac involvement usually occurs weeks to several months after the tick bite and may be the first manifestation of the disease. Nonspecific symptoms (e.g., headache, fatigue, arthralgias) may persist for months after treatment of Lyme disease. There is no evidence that these persistent subjective complaints represent ongoing active infection. Co-infection with *Babesia* and *Ehrlichia* is common, and these infections should be considered in persons diagnosed with Lyme disease.

Human Ehrlichiosis

The principal vector of *Ehrlichia chaffeensis*, the agent that causes human monocytic ehrlichiosis (HME), is the Lone Star tick (*Amblyomma americanum*). Patients typically have an acute illness that has an incubation period of 1 to 2 weeks. Most patients are febrile and have nonspecific symptoms such as malaise, myalgia, headache, and chills.

One feature that may distinguish HME from human granulocytic anaplasmosis (HGA), another tick-borne illness caused by *Anaplasma phagocytophilum*, is a rash (macular, maculopapular, or petechial). This rash occurs in about 30% of patients with HME but is rare in patients with HGA.

The preferred and most widely available diagnostic method for ehrlichiosis is the indirect fluorescent antibody test. The diagnosis should be considered in all patients with Lyme disease or babesiosis. Treatment with doxycycline should be initiated for all patients suspected of having ehrlichiosis or anaplasmosis.

Viral Infections Associated with Rash

The typical manifestations of viral infections associated with rash may unequivocally establish the cause of a febrile syndrome. For example, varicella-zoster virus infection manifests with distinctive lesions of chickenpox or herpes zoster (i.e., shingles). The resurgence of measles mandates the ability to recognize its rash.

Acute onset of high fever characterizes viral hemorrhagic fevers, along with bleeding complications and high mortality rates in some cases. Arthropods often transmit viral infections, including dengue, which is one of the most common causes of fever in returned travelers. The deer tick virus identified in New York State causes a syndrome of fever and confusion with or without rash.

Fever with Lymphadenopathy

Generalized and localized lymphadenopathy can be major manifestations of some infectious diseases, such as in mononucleosis syndromes, tuberculosis, HIV infection, and pyogenic infections.

Infectious mononucleosis is characterized by a triad of fever, tonsillar pharyngitis, and lymphadenopathy. EBV is a widely disseminated herpesvirus that is spread by intimate contact between susceptible persons and EBV shedders. Lymph node involvement in infectious mononucleosis is typically symmetrical and more commonly involves the posterior cervical than the anterior chains. The posterior cervical nodes are deep beneath the sternocleidomastoid muscles and must be carefully palpated. The nodes may be large and moderately tender. Lymphadenopathy may also become more generalized including enlargement of the spleen, which distinguishes infectious mononucleosis from other causes of pharyngitis.

Lymphadenopathy peaks in the first week and then gradually subsides over 2 to 3 weeks. Splenomegaly is seen in 50% of patients with infectious mononucleosis and usually begins to recede by the third week of the illness.

Patients with a clinical picture of infectious mononucleosis should have a white blood cell count with differential and a heterophile (Monospot) test. If the heterophile test result is positive, no further testing is necessary when the clinical scenario is compatible with typical infectious mononucleosis. If the heterophile test result is negative but there is still a strong clinical suspicion of EBV infection, the Monospot test can be repeated because results can be negative early in clinical illness.

If the clinical syndrome is prolonged or the patient does not have a classic EBV syndrome, immunoglobulin M (IgM) and immunoglobulin G (IgG) viral capsule antigen (VCA) and Epstein-Barr nuclear antigen (EBNA) antibodies should be measured. IgG EBNA detected within 4 weeks of symptom onset excludes acute primary EBV infection as an explanation and should prompt consideration of EBV-negative causes of mononucleosis.

Cytomegalovirus

The spectrum of human illness caused by CMV is diverse and mostly depends on the host. CMV infection in the immunocompetent host usually is asymptomatic or may manifest as a mononucleosis-like syndrome. Transmission occurs through multiple routes.

The mononucleosis syndrome associated with CMV infection has been described as typhoidal because systemic symptoms and fever predominate, and signs of enlarged cervical nodes and splenomegaly are not as commonly seen as they are in EBV infection. Diarrhea, fever, fatigue, and abdominal pain are common symptoms. Immunocompromised patients, such as those who have received transplants, may have serious, life-threatening infections such as pneumonitis, hepatitis, colitis, and retinitis. Serology provides indirect evidence of recent CMV infection based on changes in antibody titers at different time points during the clinical illness. Serologies are also helpful in determining past exposure to CMV. This information is particularly relevant for monitoring immunosuppressed hosts at risk for CMV reactivation syndromes.

Primary Human Immunodeficiency Virus Infection

Because a variety of symptoms and signs may be associated with acute, symptomatic HIV infection, all patients with mononucleosis syndromes should undergo HIV testing. Published series consistently report that the most common findings are fever, generalized lymphadenopathy, sore throat, rash, myalgia or arthralgia, and headache. The HIV plasma viral load should be assessed to detect acute infection because the ELISA result may not indicate positivity for HIV until months later.

Toxoplasmosis

Toxoplasmosis, an infection with a worldwide distribution, is caused by the intracellular protozoan parasite *T. gondii*. Humans can acquire *Toxoplasma* organisms through ingestion of contaminated meat, vertical transmission, blood transfusion, exposure to oocysts from cat feces, or organ transplantation.

Immunocompetent persons with primary infection are usually asymptomatic, but latent infection can persist for the life of the host. When symptomatic infection does occur, the most common manifestation is bilateral, symmetrical, nontender cervical adenopathy. Patients may have headache, fever, and fatigue. Symptoms usually resolve within several weeks. In AIDS patients or other immunocompromised hosts who have been previously infected, *T. gondii* infection may reactivate in the brain, causing abscesses and encephalitis.

Infections Causing Regional Lymphadenopathy

Scrofula (i.e., tuberculous cervical adenitis) develops in a subacute to chronic pattern. Low-grade fever is usually associated with a large mass of matted cervical lymph nodes. In children, *M. tuberculosis* is the etiologic agent, but in adults, *Mycobacterium avium* complex and *Mycobacterium scrofulaceum* are more commonly found. Surgical excision is the treatment of choice.

Cat-Scratch Disease

Cat-scratch disease, a condition caused by *Bartonella henselae*, is characterized by self-limited regional lymphadenopathy after a cat scratch or transmission from another vector. Other manifestations can include visceral organ, neurologic, and ocular involvement. In 85% to 90% of children, cat-scratch disease manifests as a localized cutaneous and lymph node disorder near the site of organism inoculation. In some individuals, the organisms disseminate and infect the liver, spleen, eye, bone, or CNS. Patients with localized disease usually have a self-limited illness, whereas those with disseminated disease can have life-threatening complications. *B. henselae infection* should be considered in the initial evaluation of FUO in children.

The diagnosis of cat-scratch disease is based on typical clinical findings (i.e., lymphadenopathy) associated with probable exposure to cats or fleas. Laboratory testing that supports the diagnosis includes a positive *B. henselae* antibody titer or biopsy of a lymph node with a positive Warthin-Starry stain or polymerase chain reaction (PCR) analysis of tissue.

Pyogenic Infection

S. aureus and group A streptococcal (GAS) infections can produce acute, suppurative lymphadenitis. Enlarged and tender lymph nodes usually are found in the submandibular, cervical, axillary, or inguinal areas. Patients have fever and leukocytosis. Pyoderma, pharyngitis, and periodontal infections are usually the primary sites of infection. Management includes drainage and antibiotics.

Plague

Bubonic plague is a bacterial syndrome caused by *Yersinia pestis* that usually consists of fever, headache, and a large mat of inguinal, axillary, or cervical lymph nodes. Lymph nodes suppurate and drain spontaneously. The diagnosis should be considered for acutely ill patients in the southwestern United States with possible exposure to fleas and rodents. Gram-negative coccobacilli can be seen in lymph node aspirates. The characteristic safety-pin appearance of *Y. pestis* with dark blue staining of polar bodies is seen with Wayson stain.

Sexually Transmitted Diseases

Inguinal lymphadenopathy associated with sexually transmitted diseases can be unilateral or bilateral. In primary syphilis, enlarged nodes are discrete, firm and nontender. Tender lymphadenopathies with matting are seen in lymphogranuloma venereum. The lymphadenopathy of chancroid is most often unilateral and manifests with pain and fused lymph nodes. Primary genital herpes infection also causes tender inguinal lymphadenopathy.

⬤ FACTITIOUS FEVER AND SELF-INDUCED ILLNESS

In most case series, factitious fever or self-induced illness is a relatively uncommon cause of FUO, but it may occur more often than generally appreciated. Patients with these conditions are often young women, and 50% have had training in some aspect of health care. They are often well educated, cooperative, articulate, and manipulative of family and caregivers. Patients can no longer manipulate thermometers because electronic or infrared thermometry is used, and causing factitious fever is difficult. Clues to the factitious fever diagnosis include absence of a toxic appearance despite high temperature readings, lack of tachycardia, and absent diurnal variation. Patients may appear well between episodes of fever.

Genuine fever can be induced if an individual injects or ingests pyrogenic substances such as bacterial suspensions, urine, or feces. Although intermittent polymicrobial bacteremia may suggest a diagnosis of intra-abdominal abscess, it represents self-induced infection. The discovery of needles and substances for injection in the patient's belongings may help in the diagnosis.

In most cases, a psychogenic basis for the behavior is assumed. However, one study with detailed psychological patient analyses found no evidence of major psychiatric diagnoses among individuals with self-induced or simulated illnesses. Munchausen's syndrome and Munchausen by proxy are the most extreme forms of factious fever. Patients often agree stoically to numerous highly invasive procedures to diagnose and treat themselves or their

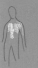

children (i.e., proxy). All of these individuals require objective but complete, tactful, and compassionate assessments and considerable psychiatric care.

SUGGESTED READINGS

Aduan RP, Fauci AS, Dale DC, et al: Prolonged fever of unknown origin (FUO): a prospective study of 347 patients, Clin Res 26:558A, 1978.

Aduan RP, Fauci AS, Dale DC, et al: Factitious fever and self-induced infection: a report of 32 cases and review of the literature, Ann Intern Med 90:230–242, 1979.

Cannon J: Perspective on fever: the basic science and conventional medicine, Complement Ther Med 21(Suppl 1):S54–S60, 2013.

Hayakawa K, Balaji R, Pranatharthi C: Fever of unknown origin: an evidence-based review, Am J Med Sci 344:307–316, 2012.

Rezai-Zadeh K, Munzberg H: Integration of sensory information via central thermoregulatory leptin targets, Physiol Behav 121:49–55, 2013.

Weber D, Cohen M, Morrell D: The acutely iii patient with fever and rash. In Mandell GL, Bennett JE, Dolin R, editors: Mandell, Douglas, and Bennett's principles and practice of infectious diseases, ed 7, Philadelphia, 2010, Churchill Livingstone, pp 791–807.

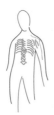

89

Bacteremia and Sepsis

Russell J. McCulloh and Steven M. Opal

DEFINITION

Sepsis is a leading cause of morbidity and death among hospitalized patients. The disease process results from a complex interplay of host immune responses and infectious microorganisms. As defined by the Surviving Sepsis Campaign, sepsis consists of proven or suspected infection combined with systemic manifestations of infection. Manifestations can include fever, altered mental status, and abnormalities in inflammation and coagulation. Severe cases can progress to multiple organ system dysfunction followed by organ failure and death.

Diagnostic criteria for sepsis are provided in Table 89-1. Severe sepsis results from sepsis-induced tissue hypoperfusion and consequent organ dysfunction. Septic shock is a combination of severe sepsis and persistent hypotension despite adequate fluid resuscitation or the need to use vasopressors to maintain a mean arterial pressure (MAP) higher than 65 mm Hg. The continuum of disease manifestations from localized infection to multiorgan failure and refractory septic shock is depicted in Figure 89-1.

Recently, a revised set of definitions was proposed. The term *sepsis* as currently used lacks specificity. Sepsis should imply a deleterious situation in which the infection-induced systemic inflammatory and coagulopathic responses have become injurious to the host. Sepsis is an infectious process characterized by tissue injury from hypoperfusion and immune dysregulation. Because sepsis always has severe ramifications for the patient, the term *sepsis* should be used instead of the current "severe sepsis." *Severe infection* should be used to describe an infection that is accompanied by systemic inflammation but without evidence of organ dysfunction remote from the site of infection (i.e., the former definition of sepsis). Whether these revised definitions can resolve the current confusion in terminology remains to be seen.

Understanding the pathophysiology of sepsis syndrome has proved helpful in differentiating and treating severe inflammatory processes that manifest with symptoms similar to sepsis, including pancreatitis, severe trauma, thermal burns, and certain toxin or environmental exposures. These processes can produce a systemic inflammatory response syndrome (SIRS), but they lack the component of infection needed to establish a diagnosis of sepsis. The remarkable clinical similarity between these severe, "sterile" inflammations and septic shock reflects their molecular profiles. Identical signaling pathways for the immune response are activated by highly conserved pathogen-associated molecular patterns (PAMPs), which are molecular motifs recognized by cells of the host's innate immune system. Damage-associated molecular patterns (DAMPs) are molecules released by injured host cells that act as endogenous danger signals to promote the inflammatory response (see Pathophysiology of Septic Shock).

EPIDEMIOLOGY

The worldwide incidence of sepsis is difficult to assess due to limited data from developing countries. In industrialized countries, reported rates of sepsis range from 22 to 300 cases per 100,000 people. Sepsis may account for up to 6% of adult deaths. In the United States, more than 750,000 cases of sepsis and 200,000 sepsis-related deaths occur annually. The risk of mortality depends on the severity of illness and multiple host factors (discussed later). Overall, estimates of death from sepsis range

TABLE 89-1 DIAGNOSTIC CRITERIA FOR SEPSIS*

GENERAL VARIABLES

Fever (>38.3° C)
Hypothermia (core temperature <36° C)
Heart rate>90 beats/min or more than 2 SD above the normal value for age
Tachypnea
Altered mental status
Significant edema or positive fluid balance (>20 mL/kg over 24 hr)
Hyperglycemia (plasma glucose >140 mg/dL or 7.7 mmol/L) in the absence
  of diabetes

INFLAMMATORY VARIABLES

Leukocytosis (WBC count >12,000 mm^3)
Leukopenia (WBC count <4000 mm^3)
Normal WBC count with more than 10% immature forms
Plasma C-reactive protein >2 SD above the normal value
Plasma procalcitonin >2 SD above the normal value

HEMODYNAMIC VARIABLES

Arterial hypotension (SBP <90 mm Hg, MAP <70 mm Hg, or an SBP
  decrease [40 mm Hg in adults or <2 SD below normal for age])

ORGAN DYSFUNCTION VARIABLES

Arterial hypoxemia (Pao$_2$/FIO$_2$ <300)
Acute oliguria (urine output <0.5 mL/kg/hr for at least 2 hr despite
  adequate fluid resuscitation)
Creatinine increase (0.5 mg/dL or 44.2 μmol/L)
Coagulation abnormalities (INR >1.5 or aPTT >60 sec)
Ileus (absent bowel sounds)
Thrombocytopenia (platelet count <100,000/mm^3)
Hyperbilirubinemia (plasma total bilirubin, 4 mg/dL or 70 μmol/L)

TISSUE PERFUSION VARIABLES

Hyperlactatemia (1 mmol/L)
Decreased capillary refill or mottling

From Dellinger RP, Levy MM, Rhodes A, et al: Surviving Sepsis Campaign: international guidelines for management of severe sepsis and septic shock, 2012, Intensive Care Med 39:165–228, 2013.
  aPTT, Activated partial thromboplastin time; FIO$_2$, fraction of inspired oxygen; INR, international normalized ratio; MAP, mean arterial pressure; Pao$_2$, partial pressure of oxygen; SBP, systolic blood pressure; SD standard deviations; WBC, white blood cell.
  *The criteria include documented or suspected infection and some of the variables listed.

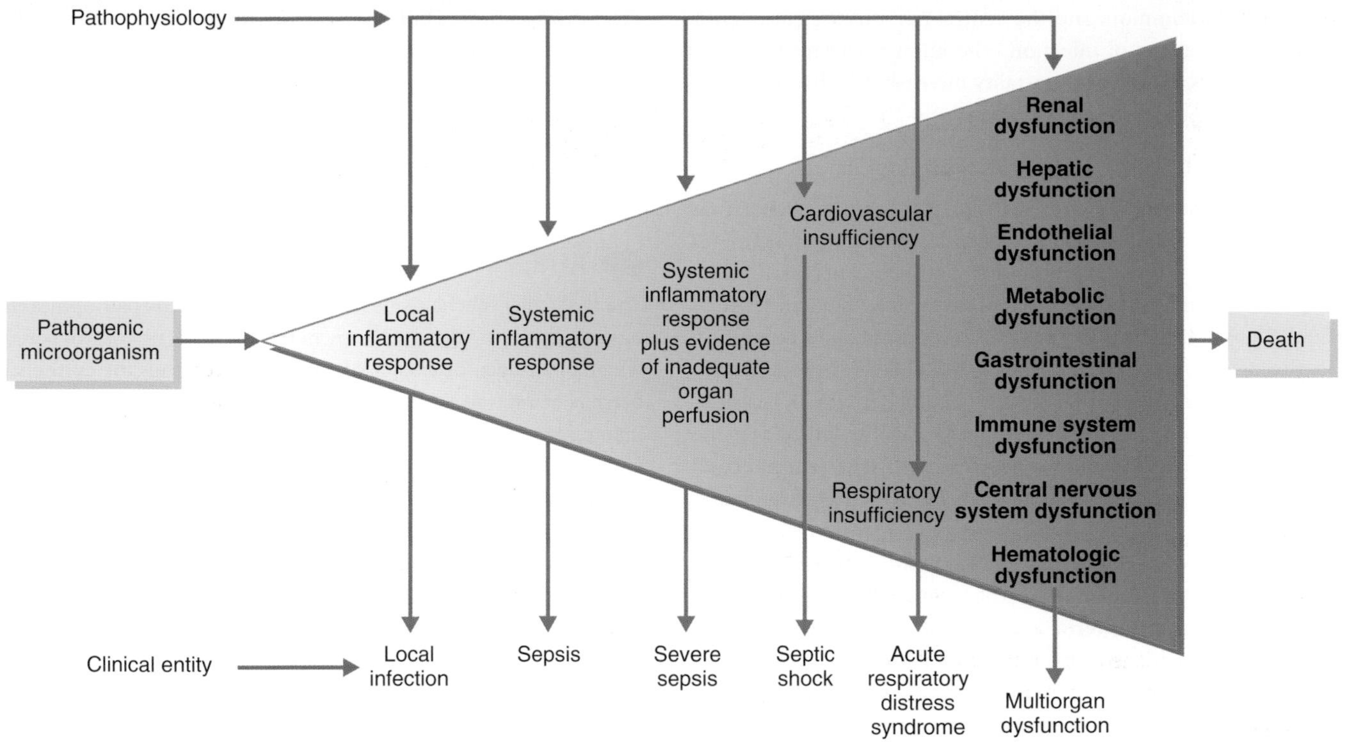

Pathophysiology →

Pathogenic microorganism →

Local inflammatory response

Systemic inflammatory response

Systemic inflammatory response plus evidence of inadequate organ perfusion

Cardiovascular insufficiency

Respiratory insufficiency

Renal dysfunction

Hepatic dysfunction

Endothelial dysfunction

Metabolic dysfunction

Gastrointestinal dysfunction

Immune system dysfunction

Central nervous system dysfunction

Hematologic dysfunction

→ Death

Clinical entity →

Local infection

Sepsis

Severe sepsis

Septic shock

Acute respiratory distress syndrome

Multiorgan dysfunction

FIGURE 89-1 The spectrum of illness and nomenclature for sepsis pathophysiology.

TABLE 89-2 MICROORGANISMS COMMONLY IDENTIFIED IN SEPTIC PATIENTS BASED ON HOST FACTORS

HOST FACTOR	ORGANISMS TO CONSIDER
Asplenia	Encapsulated organisms, particularly *Streptococcus pneumoniae*, *Haemophilus influenzae*, *Neisseria meningitidis*, *Capnocytophaga canimorsus*
Cirrhosis	*Vibrio*, *Salmonella*, and *Yersinia* species; encapsulated organisms, other gram-negative rods
Alcohol abuse	*Klebsiella* species, *S. pneumoniae*
Diabetes	Mucormycosis, *Pseudomonas* species, *Escherichia coli*, group B streptococci
Neutropenia	Enteric gram-negative rods, *Pseudomonas*, *Aspergillus*, *Candida*, *Mucor* species, *Staphylococcus aureus*, streptococcal species
T-cell dysfunction	*Listeria*, *Salmonella*, and *Mycobacterium* species, herpesviruses (including herpes simplex, cytomegalovirus, varicella-zoster virus)
Acquired immunodeficiency syndrome	*Salmonella* species, *S. aureus*, *Mycobacterium avium* complex, *S. pneumoniae*, group B streptococci

from 20% of mild to moderate cases to more than 60% of patients with septic shock.

The financial impact of sepsis cases is immense. Each episode of sepsis costs approximately $50,000 in health care expenditures, for a total of more than $17 billion dollars annually in the United States alone.

Bacterial infections are the most common cause of sepsis. Bloodstream infections due to bacteria account for the largest proportion of hospitalizations. The rates are highest for premature infants, the advanced elderly (especially those older than 85 years of age), and patients with intravenous catheters, implanted devices, or severe medical morbidities such as severe burns or hematologic malignancies.

Pathogens most commonly identified in bloodstream infections include staphylococci (e.g., *Staphylococcus aureus*), group A streptococci, *Escherichia coli*, *Klebsiella* species, *Enterobacter* species, and *Pseudomonas aeruginosa*. Immunocompromised patients and patients with long-term intravascular catheters are at increased risk for fungal bloodstream infections from *Candida*

species, and some species may be resistant to commonly used antifungal medications. Given the broad variety of potential pathogens, clinicians face the dual challenges of an accurate and timely diagnosis and choice of appropriate empirical therapy.

Several epidemiologic factors can guide the clinician in cases of sepsis when a source has not been identified. Table 89-2 lists microorganisms that are associated with certain host factors that predispose a patient to infection and sepsis. Host factors associated with worse outcomes include extremes of age, use of immunomodulating or immunosuppressing medications, and concomitant chronic medical conditions.

Several diagnostic and treatment factors are associated with severity of illness and clinical outcome. Delay in effective antimicrobial therapy correlates with worse outcomes. Infection with multidrug-resistant organisms may cause a delay in effective therapy, and for some organisms, particularly gram-negative enteric rods, the delay may be independently related to worse outcomes. Certain organisms (e.g., *P. aeruginosa*) are more virulent. The primary infection site also is important; respiratory sites are the most common, and the central nervous system often is the most lethal site of infection. The number of organ systems involved plays a role, with mortality increasing as the number of dysfunctional organ systems increase.

PATHOLOGY AND IMMUNOPATHOGENESIS

The pathologic findings of fatal septic shock are often rather bland on gross examination and even histologic examination of tissue samples. The most common finding is increased tissue edema in the interstitial spaces and excess lung fluid and pleural fluid. Signs of hyaline membrane formation and fibrin deposition in the alveoli are common and indicate the fibroproliferative stage of acute respiratory distress syndrome (ARDS). Occasionally, punctate or macroscopic evidence can be detected in the adrenal tissues, as can diffuse petechiae in tissues and mucosal surfaces that indicate disseminated intravascular coagulation (DIC).

The kidneys usually appear normal, and necrosis of kidney tissues is distinctly uncommon. The term *acute tubular necrosis* is a misnomer, and the term *acute kidney injury* (AKI) is more appropriate for describing the functional and usually reversible loss of kidney function found in septic shock without accompanying evidence of glomerular or tubular necrosis.

An important finding at autopsy is identification of the infectious focus that caused septic shock. The focal infection that precipitated sepsis is readily identifiable in most deceased patients despite days to weeks of seemingly appropriate antimicrobial therapy directed against the pathogens. If careful histochemical studies are performed shortly after a patient succumbs to sepsis,

excessive apoptosis (but not necrosis) of immune effector cells is identifiable in lung, spleen, lymph nodes, and hepatic tissues. Electron microscopy of tissues after death from sepsis often reveals loss of tight junctions along epithelial and endothelial surfaces. Electron microscopy also demonstrates diffuse mitochondrial swelling and degradation and clearance of intracellular organelles (i.e., autophagy).

PATHOPHYSIOLOGY OF SEPTIC SHOCK

The molecular mechanisms that underlie the basic pathophysiology of septic shock have been determined. Sepsis is triggered when a pathogen or cluster of pathogens breaches the epithelial barriers at a tissue site, evades clearance by humoral and cellular innate immune defenses, and causes an invasive infection. On entry into the host tissues, microbial pathogens are first sensed by myeloid cells of the innate immune system by pattern recognition receptors (e.g., toll-like receptors [TLRs]) on the cell surface and in endosomal compartments. TLRs detect highly conserved molecular motifs of microbes. Examples include lipopolysaccharide (LPS), the endotoxin produced by gram-negative bacteria; bacterial lipopeptides from gram-positive bacteria; β-glucans of the cell wall of fungi; viral RNA genomes and proteins; bacterial flagella; and DAMPs released from injured host cells, including intracellular structures such as histone proteins, mitochondrial DNA, and high-mobility group box 1 (Fig. 89-2).

TLRs and related intracellular pattern recognition receptors, including the inflammasome elements, retinoic acid–inducible gene 1 (*RIG1*)–like helicases, and cytoplasmic microbial TLR4, alert the host to infection. TLR4 is the long sought-after LPS

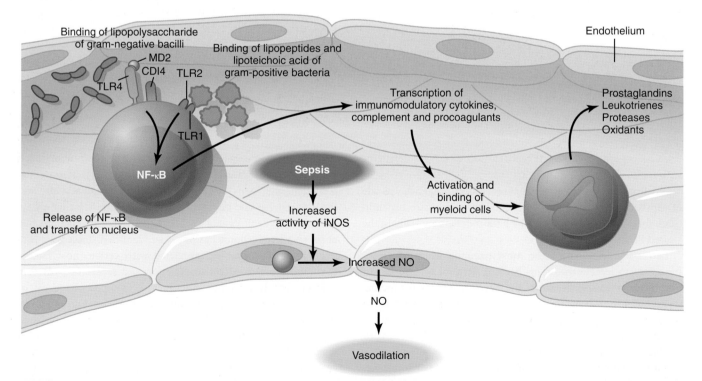

FIGURE 89-2 Immunopathogenesis of sepsis. Early recognition of bloodstream infection begins with sensing by pattern recognition receptors: toll-like receptor 4 (TLR4); cluster determinant 14 (CD14); myeloid differentiation factor 2 (MD2) for gram-negative bacterial lipopolysaccharide and TLR2 for lipoteichoic acid and other elements from gram-positive bacteria. Engagement of the TLRs by their ligands signals transcription of the acute phase response genes by the nuclear factor-κ light-chain enhancer of activated B cells (NF-κB, which is a monocyte). Septic shock is initiated by systemic release of an array of vasoactive mediators, including nitric oxide (NO) produced by cytokine-inducible NO synthase (iNOS).

receptor of the human innate immune system. LPS is released from the cell membrane of gram-negative bacteria on their destruction. LPS is first bound to a carrier protein, LPS-binding protein, and the LPS monomer is then delivered to a membrane-associated, multiligand, pattern recognition receptor, CD14. LPS monomers are then passed to a soluble protein (i.e., myeloid differentiation factor 2 [MD2]) and bind to the ectodomain of TLR4. After this LPS/MD2/TLR4 complex is completed and dimerized, intracellular signaling alerts the host to the invasive infectious challenge. The pathway induces a series of phosphorylation events of adaptor proteins and signaling molecules that terminate in the activation and translocation of transcriptional activating factors such as nuclear factor-κB (NF-κB) into the nucleus. The transcription factors bind to promoter sites of the acute phase protein network, resulting in an acute outpouring of inflammatory, host defense, and coagulation components.

Other TLRs, such as TLR5 (i.e., bacterial flagella) and the TLR2/TLR1 and TLR2/TLR6 heterodimers (i.e., bacterial lipopeptides, lipoteichoic acid, and other elements of bacteria and fungi), are expressed on the cell surface of immune effector cells that recognize different molecular patterns. Nucleic acid recognition–specific TLRs reside in endosomal vacuoles, where they detect microbial DNA (TLR9), single-stranded RNA (TLR7 and TLR8), and double-stranded RNA (TLR3).

An array of complement elements, cytokines, chemokines, prostanoids (e.g., prostaglandins), vasoactive peptides, platelet-activating factor, and proteases are generated, resulting in activation of neutrophils, monocytes, macrophages, dendritic cells, lymphocytes, and endothelial cells in a combined effort to wall off the infectious process, clear the pathogens, and begin the process of tissue repair. This defense system efficiently clears pathogens from the host after local injury and the inevitable minor breaches of the epithelial barriers by microorganisms that occur over a lifetime.

If the inflammatory process is unchecked and accompanied by large numbers of pathogens or even a few highly virulent organisms (e.g., plague, tularemia, anthrax, hemorrhagic fever viruses) to which the host has no preexisting immunity, a generalized, inflammatory, and injurious process known as *sepsis* evolves over a short time, and it can be deleterious or lethal to the host. The same inflammatory response that can be lifesaving in localized infection can become life-threatening if it becomes sustained and generalized.

Endothelial membranes throughout the body are activated and become proadherent and procoagulant surfaces that promote neutrophil and platelet adherence. Neutrophils release proteases, cytokines, reactive oxygen radicals, and vasoactive prostanoids that damage endothelial cells and their function. Cytokine-inducible nitric oxide synthase is upregulated, resulting in massive generation of nitric oxide (NO). NO is a potent vasodilator, and in combination with other vasoactive peptides and phospholipid mediators, it promotes diffuse opening of capillary beds and increased permeability, with loss of intravascular fluids into the interstitial spaces. Reactive oxygen species combine with NO to generate highly injurious reactive nitrogen intermediates (e.g., peroxynitrite) that damage mitochondrial function and induce apoptosis. Systemic hypotension rapidly develops, and septic shock ensues. Immediate action by the clinician is mandatory to correct the hemodynamic status and resolve the underlying infection.

CLINICAL PRESENTATION

Despite the vast improvements in understanding the pathophysiologic basis of sepsis, clinical diagnosis remains limited to the medical history, symptomatic assessment, and nonspecific laboratory and hemodynamic criteria. Compounding the problem is the need for prompt institution of appropriate antimicrobial therapy, making early recognition of sepsis critically important. Patients with general findings as outlined in Table 89-1 should undergo thorough and prompt evaluation for a possible infectious cause, including bacterial cultures of blood and (when indicated) other body fluids. Localizing signs and symptoms should prompt a thorough physical examination and directed imaging to identify a nidus of infection. Defects of natural defensive barriers, such as transcutaneous devices or intravascular catheters, should be assessed for infection and removed if suspected to be the origin of the septic process.

Many patients have fever or chills, but older patients and those on immunomodulating medications may not mount a fever. Hypothermia portends a worse prognosis or more severe illness. Tachypnea may be an indicator of respiratory compensation for underlying metabolic acidosis or the early signs and symptoms of ARDS.

Mental status changes can result from metabolic derangements caused by sepsis, hypoglycemia, the underlying infectious process, or concomitant hypotension. This symptom can be difficult to identify in the elderly patient with dementia, and caution should be exercised in the evaluation and treatment of the otherwise stable elderly patient with possible mental status changes.

Skin findings (e.g., cellulitis, abscess) can provide clues to the cause of sepsis and may indicate the state of peripheral systemic perfusion. Several microorganisms can cause specific skin manifestations in systemic infection. *S. aureus* and streptococci can cause diffuse erythroderma, bullous lesions, or generalized desquamation. Bacteremia caused by several gram-negative organisms, including *P. aeruginosa* and enteric organisms, can result in ecthyma gangrenosum, particularly in immunocompromised patients. These lesions are round and 1 to 15 cm in diameter, and they have a central area of necrosis and peripheral erythema. Infection with *Neisseria meningitidis* can result initially in lower extremity petechiae progressing to diffuse purpura, which likely portends septic shock and a high risk of death. A similar clinical presentation can be observed in other unusual infectious diseases, such as overwhelming pneumococcal sepsis in the asplenic host or disseminated neisserial infections in patients with late complement deficiencies.

Hemodynamic instability, particularly hypotension with or without accompanying oliguria, is commonly associated with sepsis. Instability can result from poor cardiac output, intravascular fluid depletion, or low systemic vascular resistance. Hypotension can initially respond to intravenous fluid resuscitation, but in cases of severe sepsis and septic shock, it may require additional support with vasopressors. Intensive cardiac monitoring may be necessary to gauge the relative need for intravenous fluids or vasopressors after initial fluid resuscitation measures are attempted.

Patients in septic shock can be tachycardic and hypotensive. They may have relatively warm extremities (i.e., warm shock or distributive shock), or they may be peripherally vasoconstricted, with mottled and cool extremities (i.e., cold shock). Warm shock is the predominant finding in most adult patients at the onset of septic shock, with evidence of diffuse vasodilation, bounding pulses, and a compensatory high cardiac output despite evidence of diminished myocardial performance. Increased cardiac output is accomplished primarily by increased heart rate in an attempt to maintain blood pressure and perfuse vital organs. If shock is not promptly corrected, myocardial dysfunction ensues and cold shock evolves over the next several hours. Older patients with limited cardiac reserves tolerate shock poorly and are more likely to develop cold shock. Evidence of septic shock at presentation that is refractory to early resuscitation portends a poor prognosis, with mortality rates exceeding 70%.

Besides hypotension, oliguria can represent developing AKI. It can arise from a combination of the disease process, infecting organism, and medications. Inflammatory cytokines, microbial toxins, systemic hypotension, and iatrogenic renal injury from medications can result in AKI. Other causes of renal injury include interstitial injury from infection or medications and immune complex–mediated injury, as seen in cases of endocarditis.

Besides tachypnea, pulmonary symptoms seen in septic patients include marked hypoxia due to interstitial edema, inflammation, or hemodynamic instability. ARDS is defined as an arterial partial pressure of oxygen less than 50 mm Hg despite fractional inspired oxygen of greater than 50%, together with diffuse alveolar infiltrates and a pulmonary capillary wedge pressure of less than 18 mm Hg. ARDS occurs in up to 40% of septic patients. The diffuse pulmonary inflammation in ARDS results in increased pulmonary vascular permeability, which complicates fluid resuscitation efforts because excessive fluid can exacerbate pulmonary edema and hypoxia. Altered mental status and sepsis-related myopathy also result in airway compromise and weak respiratory effort, necessitating invasive ventilatory support.

Patients with sepsis can have marked hematologic changes. They may have neutrophilic leukocytosis, which is often accompanied by increased immature cell counts, or they can be markedly leukopenic (particularly lymphopenic), often in cases of severe septic shock. Transient neutropenia is often seen in the early phase of septic shock and results from activation and adherence of neutrophils along endothelial surfaces in the microcirculation. This is rapidly followed by prolonged neutrophilia as sepsis-induced inflammatory cytokines stimulate bone marrow synthesis of new white blood cells.

Thrombocytopenia and coagulopathy can occur, and patients have petechiae or purpura at presentation. Severe derangements in coagulation can produce DIC, which can lead to thrombin deposition throughout the microcirculation. Excessive activation and degradation of clotting factors can deplete coagulation factors, resulting in diffuse hemorrhage. Excessive mucosal bleeding around airway tubes and prolonged bleeding from venipuncture sites presage internal bleeding events. Massive gastrointestinal hemorrhage can occur, which can cause or exacerbate hypotension and shock.

Derangements in glucose homeostasis can be seen at presentation. This can take the form of hyperglycemia in diabetics receiving glucose-containing fluids or acute metabolic derangement due to infection. Hypoglycemia is more common in patients with underlying liver disease. Increased anaerobic metabolism due to poor tissue oxygenation and coupled with mitochondrial dysfunction and impaired hepatic clearance of lactic acid may result in increased serum lactate levels and metabolic acidosis.

DIAGNOSIS

Accurate diagnosis of sepsis relies on the history, physical examination, and general laboratory investigation. Diagnostic criteria for sepsis in adults based on the Surviving Sepsis Campaign guidelines are listed in Table 89-1.

Accurate and timely identification of the underlying infectious cause is essential. For patients able to provide a history, an assessment of medical comorbidities, potential exposures, prior infections, and immune system abnormalities may help to guide empirical antimicrobial therapy and the laboratory investigation, particularly microbial cultures. Two sets of blood cultures drawn from a fresh venipuncture and from existing indwelling intravascular lines (before initiation of empirical antimicrobial therapy if possible) help to identify the causative organism in many cases. Symptomatic assessment and physical examination should suggest a location of focal infection that can help to guide radiologic studies and interventions to drain pus.

Beyond microbial cultures, several other laboratory studies can help to define the severity of illness and provide baseline data for monitoring the response to therapy. Basic laboratory testing, including a complete blood count with differential, chemistries, and creatinine and aminotransferase levels, can help to identify significant organ dysfunction. Oxygen saturation by pulse oximetry should be measured promptly to identify gas exchange capacity and the need for ventilatory support. Coagulation studies should be obtained, particularly for patients with evidence of DIC and those who are thrombocytopenic. For patients with altered mental status or marked respiratory difficulty, arterial blood gas sampling can help define the underlying derangement and physiologic compensation and can indirectly gauge the severity of illness.

Levels of inflammatory markers, including C-reactive protein and procalcitonin, usually are elevated. An elevated procalcitonin level can help to establish the diagnosis of severe sepsis and provide some prognostic data and a measure of response to therapy. In cases of sepsis due to pneumonia, serial measurement of procalcitonin can help to guide the duration of antibiotic therapy.

Other testing should be directed toward identifying the potential cause. Patients with severe diarrhea should undergo testing for antibiotic-associated *Clostridium difficile* infection. Imaging studies should focus on identifying infectious sources and facilitate drainage of fluid collections or abscesses. Computed tomography may be of use in such circumstances, although for the critically ill patient who is not stable for transport, bedside radiographic studies, especially ultrasound, should be considered.

Multiple tests of physiologic function and advanced microbiologic diagnostic tests are increasingly used in clinical practice. They include polymerase chain reaction (PCR)–based assays for identifying bacteria and viruses and various assays of inflammatory cytokines and other biomarkers alone and in combination as potential diagnostic and prognostic aids.

TREATMENT

Septic shock is a medical emergency. Immediate attempts to reestablish physiologic hemodynamics, vital organ support, and oxygen delivery to tissues should accompany early diagnosis and treatment of infection. Patients should be transferred to the intensive care unit as soon as possible to receive optimal monitoring, hemodynamic support, and expert supportive care.

Early recognition, prompt resuscitation, and early institution of appropriate antimicrobial agents are the most important determinants of a successful outcome. If appropriate, draining infectious foci (i.e., source control) should be done as soon as possible. Key elements of the 2012 Surviving Sepsis Champaign guidelines are summarized in Table 89-3.

An essential element in the treatment of sepsis is early administration of antibiotics active against the causative pathogen. Treatment is best given within 1 hour of the onset of septic shock, and an empirical, broad-spectrum antimicrobial regimen is usually employed until the results of cultures of blood and the site of infection become available. A suggested initial treatment regimen is provided in Table 89-4. Failing to treat the causative pathogen until its identity and susceptibility profile become available days later is associated with adverse outcomes. After the pathogen is identified, de-escalation to the simplest monotherapy to which it is susceptible is important.

PROGNOSIS

Despite advances in clinical practice and treatment, sepsis mortality rates remain high, ranging from 20% to 30% among relatively healthy adults to more than 80% among the elderly, immunocompromised, and those with significant chronic medical comorbidities. Patients may experience significant weakness, wasting, and debilitation due to severe catabolism, poor

TABLE 89-3 RECOMMENDED INITIAL MANAGEMENT OF SEPSIS IN ADULTS

- Start resuscitation immediately in patients with hypotension or serum lactate level >4 mmol/L.
- Obtain appropriate cultures before starting antibiotics if doing so does not significantly delay therapy.
- Evaluate for a focus of infection amenable to source control (e.g., abscess drainage).
- Remove intravascular catheters if potentially infected.
- Begin broad-spectrum antibiotics within the first hour of severe sepsis and septic shock. Initial antibiotic regimen is based on likely source of sepsis, likely pathogens, and local antibiotic susceptibility patterns of common pathogens.
- Begin fluid resuscitation using crystalloids as the first choice. If colloids are used, avoid starches and consider albumin in selected patients who have hypoalbuminemia or require large-volume fluid resuscitation.
- Give fluid challenge of up to 30 mL/kg of crystalloids over 15-30 min in septic patients with suspected volume depletion; larger volumes of fluids may be needed in some patients. The goals for resuscitation should be a central venous pressure of 8-12 mm Hg, a mean arterial pressure (MAP) ≥65 mm Hg, and a superior vena cava oxygen saturation ≥70% or mixed venous oxygen saturation ≥65%.
- Maintain targeted MAP of ≥65 mm Hg; if fluids are not effective in reestablishing adequate blood pressure, begin vasopressors. After hemodynamic parameters are stabilized, limit fluid therapy to prevent pulmonary fluid accumulation and exacerbation of hypoxemia.
- Use norepinephrine, centrally administered, as the vasopressor of choice. Epinephrine is the second choice, followed by vasopressin as salvage therapy. Dobutamine may be useful if an inotrope is needed. Avoid dopamine except for special situations (i.e., low risk of tachyarrhythmia and persistent bradycardia).
- Give red blood cells when the hemoglobin concentration decreases to <7 g/dL; target hemoglobin level is 7-9 g/dL.
- Target a tidal volume of 6 mL/kg in patients with acute respiratory distress syndrome.
- Give low-molecular-weight heparin or unfractionated heparin for deep vein thrombosis prophylaxis; use graduated pressure stockings or intermittent compression devices if heparin therapy is contraindicated.
- Provide stress ulcer prophylaxis using histamine H_2-blockers or a proton pump inhibitor.
- Provide expert supportive care; provide low-dose nutrition for the first week; consider stress-dose steroids if refractory septic shock occurs; maintain blood glucose in the 110-180 mg/dL range.

Data from Dellinger RP, Levy MM, et al: Surviving Sepsis Campaign: international guidelines for the management of severe sepsis and septic shock, 2012, Crit Care Med 41:580–637, 2013.

TABLE 89-4 INITIAL ANTIBIOTIC RECOMMENDATIONS FOR ADULT PATIENTS WITH SEPSIS

INDICATION	RECOMMENDED DOSAGES*
Empirical coverage (source unknown)	Vancomycin 15 mg/kg q12h plus piperacillin-tazobactam[†] 3.375 g IV q6h or imipenem 0.5 g IV q6h or meropenem 1.0 g IV q8h with or without an aminoglycoside (e.g., tobramycin 5 mg/kg IV q24).[‡]
Community-acquired pneumonia (CAP)	Ceftriaxone 1 g IV q24h plus azithromycin 500 mg IV q24h or a fluoroquinolone (e.g., moxifloxacin 400 mg IV q24h or levofloxacin 750 mg IV q24h).[§]
Community-acquired urosepsis	Piperacillin-tazobactam 3.375 g IV q6h or ciprofloxacin 400 mg. IV q12h
Meningitis	Vancomycin 15 mg/kg IV q6h plus ceftriaxone 2 g IV q12h plus dexamethasone 0.15 mg/kg IV q6h × 2-4 days, preferably before antibiotics; add ampicillin 2 g IV q4h if *Listeria* is suspected.
Nosocomial pneumonia	Vancomycin 15 mg/kg q12h plus piperacillin-tazobactam 4.5 g IV q6h or imipenem 0.5 g IV q6h or meropenem 1 g IV q8h or cefepime 2 g IV q8h plus an aminoglycoside (e.g., amikacin 15 mg/kg IV q24h or tobramycin 5-7 mg/kg IV q24h) or levofloxacin 750 mg IV q24h. Some authorities substitute linezolid 600 mg IV q12h for vancomycin if MRSA is a significant concern or known to be the cause.
Neutropenia	Cefepime 2 g IV q8h; add vancomycin 15 mg/kg IV q12h if a central line is present and infection is a concern. Add antifungal coverage with caspofungin 70 mg IV × 1, then 50 mg IV q24h if fever persists ≥5 days. For suspected or proven invasive aspergillosis, voriconazole 6 mg/kg IV q12h × 2, then 4 mg/kg IV q12h should be used.
Cellulitis and skin infections	Vancomycin 15 mg/kg IV q12h. Add piperacillin-tazobactam 3.375 g IV q6h in diabetics and immunocompromised patients. If necrotizing fasciitis is suspected, add clindamycin 900 mg. IV; surgical débridement is crucial.

IV, Intravenous; MRSA, methicillin-resistant *Staphylococcus aureus*.
*Assumes normal renal function; dose adjustments are required with impaired creatinine clearance.
[†]Substitute aztreonam 2 g IV q8h if patient is allergic to penicillin.
[‡]Monitor drug levels of aminoglycosides (i.e., peak and trough).
[§]Substitute Cefepime or a carbapenem and azithromycin ± an aminoglycoside if the patient has severe CAP or health care–associated pneumonia.

nutrition, and prolonged hospitalization. Prolonged rehabilitation in a skilled facility after the initial hospitalization and additional home-based therapy may be required. Patients may have permanent disabilities, including impaired renal function or persistent debilitation from procedures required to treat the underlying infection.

SUGGESTED READINGS

Angus DC, Linde-Zwirble WT, Lidicker J, et al: Epidemiology of severe sepsis in the United States: analysis of incidence, outcome, and associated costs of care, Crit Care Med 29:1303–1310, 2001.

Angus D, van der Poll T: Severe sepsis and septic shock, N Engl J Med 369:840–851, 2013.

Black G: Gyroscope: a survival of sepsis, West Conshohocken, Pa., 2011, Infinity Publishing.

Dellinger RP, Levy MM, Rhodes A, et al: Surviving Sepsis Campaign: international guidelines for management of severe sepsis and septic shock, 2012, Intensive Care Med 39:165–228, 2013.

Hotchkiss RS, Coopersmith CM, McDunn JE, et al: The sepsis seesaw: tilting toward immunosuppression, Nat Med 15:496–497, 2009.

Melamed A, Sorvillo FJ: The burden of sepsis-associated mortality in the United States from 1999 to 2005: an analysis of multiple-cause-of-death data, Crit Care 13:R28, 2009.

Vincent JL, Opal SM, Marshall JC, et al: Sepsis definitions: time for a change, Lancet 381:774–775, 2013.

90

Infections of the Central Nervous System

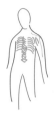

Allan R. Tunkel, Marjorie A. Janvier, and Avindra Nath

● INTRODUCTION

Infections of the central nervous system (CNS) are associated with significant morbidity and mortality. This chapter focuses on meningitis, encephalitis, and brain abscesses in the parenchyma and parameningeal areas.

● MENINGITIS AND ENCEPHALITIS

Contact with offending infectious agents such as viruses, bacteria, fungi, protozoa, and helminths can cause inflammation of the meninges covering the brain and spinal cord (i.e., meningitis) or lead to inflammation of the brain parenchyma (i.e., encephalitis). These infectious agents can penetrate the CNS by direct seeding or hematogenous spread and cause a constellation of symptoms. The clinician must rapidly initiate a diagnostic evaluation and begin appropriate management.

Meningitis

Definition

Meningitis is defined as inflammation of the leptomeninges that cover the brain and spinal cord. It is identified by an abnormal increase in the number of white blood cells in cerebrospinal fluid (CSF). Inflammation can be caused by many infectious agents (i.e., bacteria, viruses, fungi, and parasites) and also can occur as a result of noninfectious conditions, including tumors or cysts, medications (e.g., nonsteroidal anti-inflammatory drugs, antimicrobial agents), systemic illnesses (e.g., systemic lupus erythematosus, Behçet's disease, sarcoidosis), or neurologic procedures (e.g., neurosurgery, spinal anesthesia, intrathecal injections).

The clinical presentation can be acute, subacute, or chronic based on the virulence of the organism. Acute meningitis is a syndrome characterized by the onset of symptoms within hours to several days, whereas chronic meningitis characterized by clinical and CSF findings that remain abnormal for at least 4 weeks. Acute meningitis is most often caused by bacteria and viruses, whereas chronic meningitis is most often caused by spirochetes, mycobacteria, and fungi.

Epidemiology and Etiology

Bacterial Meningitis

In the United States, the epidemiology of bacterial meningitis has changed significantly over the past several decades with the introduction of conjugate vaccines against *Haemophilus influenzae* and *Streptococcus pneumoniae*. A surveillance study found that about 4000 cases of bacterial meningitis and 500 deaths occurred annually between 2003 and 2007. The leading causes of bacterial meningitis were *S. pneumoniae* (58% of cases), *Streptococcus agalactiae* (18% of cases), *Neisseria meningitidis* (14% of cases), *H. influenzae* (7% of cases), and *Listeria monocytogenes* (3% of cases).

Specific etiologic agents may be more likely based on the patient's age and various risk factors (Table 90-1). In one study of 352 episodes of community-acquired pneumococcal meningitis, 70% of cases were associated with an underlying disorder. Conditions associated with pneumococcal meningitis include splenectomy or asplenic states, multiple myeloma, hypogammaglobulinemia, alcoholism, malnutrition, chronic liver or kidney disease, and diabetes mellitus. Patients often have contiguous or distant foci of infection such as pneumonia, otitis media, mastoiditis, sinusitis, endocarditis, and head trauma with a CSF leak.

The group B streptococcus (i.e., *S. agalactiae*) is a common etiologic agent of meningitis in neonates, with 52% of cases occurring during the first year of life. Risk factors for *S. agalactiae* meningitis in adults include age older than 60 years, pregnancy or the postpartum state, diabetes mellitus, and other chronic diseases and immunosuppressed states.

N. meningitidis usually causes meningitis in children and adults. Most cases in the United States are caused by serogroups B, C, and Y; serogroups A and W135 usually cause disease outside of the United States. Because of *N. meningitidis* in the upper

TABLE 90-1	COMMON BACTERIAL PATHOGENS AND FACTORS PREDISPOSING TO MENINGITIS
PREDISPOSING FACTOR	**BACTERIAL PATHOGENS**
Age	
<1 mo	*Streptococcus agalactiae, Escherichia coli, Listeria monocytogenes*
1-23 mo	*S. agalactiae, E. coli, Haemophilus influenzae, Streptococcus pneumoniae, Neisseria meningitidis*
2-50 yr	*S. pneumoniae, N. meningitidis*
>50 yr	*S. pneumoniae, N. meningitidis, L. monocytogenes,* aerobic gram-negative bacilli
Immunocompromised state	*S. pneumoniae, N. meningitidis, L. monocytogenes,* aerobic gram-negative bacilli (including *Pseudomonas aeruginosa*)
Basilar skull fracture	*S. pneumoniae, H. influenzae,* group A β-hemolytic streptococci
Head trauma; post neurosurgery	*Staphylococcus aureus,* coagulase-negative staphylococci (especially *Staphylococcus epidermidis*), aerobic gram-negative bacilli (including *P. aeruginosa*)

From Tunkel AR, van de Beek D, Scheld WM: Acute meningitis. In Bennett JE, Dolin R, Blaser M, editors: Mandell, Douglas, and Bennett's principles and practice of infectious diseases, ed 8, Philadelphia, 2015, Saunders.

respiratory tract, outbreaks of meningitis due to *N. meningitidis* may occur in persons living in close quarters, such as among household members, in daycare, in college dormitories, and among the incarcerated. One outbreak of serogroup C disease was reported in New York City among men who have sex with men, and outbreaks caused by serogroup B were reported on the campuses of Princeton University and University of California, Santa Barbara. Patients with deficiencies in the terminal complement components (C5-C8 and perhaps C9) and properdin are at increased risk for meningococcal infections.

The incidence of meningitis due to *H. influenzae* has declined more than 90% with the widespread use of routine vaccination with the *H. influenzae* type b conjugate vaccine. Isolation of this microorganism in older children and adults suggests certain underlying conditions, such as sinusitis, otitis media, epiglottitis, pneumonia, diabetes mellitus, alcoholism, splenectomy or asplenic states, head trauma with CSF leak, and immune deficiency.

Meningitis caused by *L. monocytogenes* is most common in neonates, adults older than 50 years, alcoholics, immunosuppressed adults, and in patients with chronic conditions such as diabetes mellitus and renal disease. Given the likely gastrointestinal portal of entry for this microorganism, outbreaks of listerial infection have been associated with ingestion of contaminated coleslaw, raw vegetables, milk, and cheese. Sporadic cases have been linked to contaminated turkey franks, alfalfa tablets, cantaloupe, diced celery, hog's head cheese, and processed meats.

Gram-negative meningitis is rare; it usually affects debilitated persons and those with a breach in the meninges as a result of trauma or neurosurgical procedures. *Staphylococcus aureus* meningitis is usually found in the early period after neurosurgery or trauma, in those with CSF shunts, or in patients with underlying conditions such as diabetes mellitus, alcoholism, chronic kidney disease requiring hemodialysis, injection-drug use, and malignancies. *Staphylococcus epidermidis* is the most common cause of meningitis in patients with CSF shunts.

Viral Meningitis

Enteroviruses are the leading identifiable cause of the *aseptic meningitis syndrome*, a term used to define any meningitis (particularly with lymphocytic pleocytosis) for which a cause is not apparent after initial evaluation, routine CSF stains, and cultures. The Centers for Disease Control and Prevention (CDC) estimate that 10 to 15 million symptomatic enteroviral infections occur annually in the United States; of these, 30,000 to 75,000 are meningitis cases.

Many other viruses can cause the aseptic meningitis syndrome, including mumps virus (in unimmunized populations), human immunodeficiency virus (HIV), several arboviruses (e.g., St. Louis encephalitis virus, the California encephalitis group of viruses, Colorado tick fever virus, West Nile virus), and herpesviruses. The syndrome of herpes simplex virus (HSV) meningitis is most commonly associated with primary genital infection. The DNA of HSV has been detected in the CSF of patients with the syndrome of recurrent benign lymphocytic meningitis (previously known as Mollaret's meningitis), with almost all cases caused by herpes simplex virus type 2 (HSV-2).

Spirochetal Meningitis

The most common spirochetes associated with meningitis are *Treponema pallidum* (the etiologic agent of syphilis) and *Borrelia burgdorferi* (the etiologic agent of Lyme disease). The incidence of syphilitic meningitis is greatest in the first 2 years after initial infection, occurring in 0.3% to 2.4% of untreated cases. The overall incidence of neurosyphilis has increased, with many cases reported in patients with HIV infection. The nervous system is involved in at least 10% to 20% of patients with Lyme disease while erythema migrans is apparent or 1 to 6 months later.

Tuberculous Meningitis

Tuberculous meningitis accounts for approximately 15% of cases of extrapulmonary tuberculosis in the United States. CNS disease is much more common in less developed areas of the world. Factors associated with reactivation of latent foci and progression to the syndrome of late generalized tuberculosis include advanced age, immunosuppressive drug therapy, gastrectomy, pregnancy, and chronic medical conditions. The epidemiology of tuberculosis has been influenced by the advent of HIV infection, in which extrapulmonary disease (including CNS disease) occurs in more than 70% of cases.

Fungal Meningitis

The incidence of fungal meningitis has increased dramatically in recent years because of the increased numbers of immunosuppressed patients. *Cryptococcus neoformans* is the most common fungal cause of clinically recognized meningitis, occurring most commonly in persons who are immunosuppressed or have chronic medical conditions. HIV-infected patients are in the highest-risk group. Cases have also been documented in apparently healthy individuals.

Coccidioides immitis is a thermal dimorphic fungus that is endemic in the semiarid regions of the Americas and desert areas of the southwestern United States (e.g., California, Arizona, New Mexico, Texas), where about one third of the population is infected. Less than 1% of patients develop disseminated infection, and one third to one half of those have meningeal involvement.

Other fungi less commonly cause CNS infection. *Histoplasma capsulatum* is endemic to fertile river valleys, principally the Mississippi and Ohio River basins. *Candida* meningitis is uncommon.

Clinical Presentation

Acute Meningitis

Adult patients with acute meningitis typically seek medical attention within hours to days of illness. Patients with bacterial meningitis classically exhibit fever, headache, meningismus, and signs of cerebral dysfunction (i.e., confusion, delirium, or a declining level of consciousness ranging from lethargy to coma). All signs may not be seen in a given patient. The meningismus may be subtle, marked, or accompanied by Kernig's sign or Brudzinski's sign, although the sensitivity of these signs is only 5% in adults. Cranial nerve palsies (especially involving cranial nerves III, IV, VI, and VII) and focal cerebral signs are seen in 10% to 20% of cases. Seizures occur in about 30% of patients. Older adult patients with bacterial meningitis, especially those with underlying conditions (e.g., diabetes mellitus, cardiopulmonary disease), may have disease that manifests insidiously with lethargy or obtundation, no fever, and various signs of meningeal inflammation. Older adult patients may have an antecedent or concurrent bronchitis, pneumonia, or paranasal sinusitis.

Viral meningitis is typically a self-limited illness. The clinical manifestations of enteroviral meningitis depend on the host's age and immune status. In adolescents and adults, more than one half of the patients have nuchal rigidity. Adults usually have headache, which often is severe and frontal. Photophobia is also common in older patients. Nonspecific symptoms and signs include vomiting, anorexia, rash, diarrhea, cough, upper respiratory findings (especially pharyngitis), and myalgias. Other clues to the diagnosis of enteroviral disease are the time of year (more prevalent in summer and autumn months) and known epidemic disease in the community. The duration of illness of enteroviral meningitis is usually less than 1 week, and many patients report improvement after lumbar puncture, presumably from the reduction in intracranial pressure.

Meningitis associated with HSV-2 infections is usually characterized by stiff neck, headache, and fever. Patients with recurrent benign lymphocytic meningitis characteristically develop a few to 10 episodes of meningitis lasting 2 to 5 days, followed by spontaneous recovery. These patients have acute onset of headache, fever, photophobia, and meningism; about 50% of patients have transient neurologic manifestations, including seizures, hallucinations, diplopia, cranial nerve palsies, or altered consciousness.

Subacute or Chronic Meningitis

Subacute or chronic meningitis caused by spirochetes, mycobacteria, or fungi in the adult patient can linger for weeks to years before clinical presentation. The patient may initially have no overt symptoms, suffer from low-grade headaches and fever, or experience gradual mental status and other neurologic changes.

Syphilitic meningitis usually manifests in a manner similar to that of other forms of aseptic meningitis. Patients complain of headache, nausea, and vomiting. Other findings include stiff neck (60%), fever, seizures, cranial nerve palsies, and less commonly, other focal neurologic abnormalities.

Meningitis is the most important neurologic abnormality of acute disseminated Lyme disease, usually following erythema migrans by 2 to 10 weeks. Patients with Lyme meningitis have headache as the single most common symptom. Other findings include photophobia, nausea, vomiting, and stiff neck. About one half of patients with Lyme meningitis have mild cerebral symptoms consisting most commonly of somnolence, emotional lability, depression, impaired memory and concentration, and behavioral symptoms. Approximately 50% of patients also have cranial neuropathies, with facial nerve palsy occurring in 80% to 90% of cases.

In the usual patient with tuberculous meningitis, an insidious prodrome characterized by malaise, lassitude, low-grade fever, intermittent headache, and changing personality ensues. Within 2 to 3 weeks, the meningitic phase manifests as protracted headache, meningismus, vomiting, and confusion. In some adults, the initial prodromal stage may take the form of a slowly progressive dementia, whereas others may have a rapidly progressive meningitis syndrome indistinguishable from pyogenic bacterial meningitis. Fever is an inconstant finding on physical examination (50% to 98% of cases). Meningismus and signs of meningeal irritation are not uniform findings (absent in 25% to 80% of children and adults). Focal neurologic signs frequently consist of unilateral or, less commonly, bilateral cranial nerve palsies; cranial nerve VI is most commonly affected.

The time course of fungal meningitis depends on the clinical setting. Cases may manifest acutely, subacutely, or chronically; some of the fungal meningitides may cause symptoms that persist for years in the absence of antifungal treatment. In contrast, the same organisms can produce severe symptoms and signs within a few days and without clinical signs of meningeal irritation in the immunocompromised patient. In patients without acquired immunodeficiency syndrome (AIDS), cryptococcal meningitis typically manifests as a subacute process after days to weeks of symptoms. Headache is the most frequent complaint. Fever, meningismus, and personality changes also may occur; confusion, irritability, and other personality changes reflecting meningoencephalitis occur in about one half of patients. Ocular abnormalities occur in about 40% of patients and include papilledema and cranial nerve palsies.

In AIDS patients, manifestation of cryptococcal meningitis can be subtle, with minimal or no symptoms. AIDS patients may have only headache and lethargy. Although fever is common, meningeal signs occur in a minority of these patients.

Patients with meningeal coccidioidomycosis usually complain of headache, low-grade fever, weight loss, and mental status changes. About one half of patients develop disorientation, lethargy, confusion, or memory loss. Meningeal signs are uncommon. The presenting symptoms of *Histoplasma* meningitis are nonspecific. Symptoms usually include headache and fever. Only about one half of patients have focal neurologic mental status symptoms. Candidal meningitis also manifests with nonspecific findings.

Diagnosis

Clinically suspected meningitis is diagnosed by analysis of CSF obtained by lumbar puncture (Table 90-2). Table 90-3 illustrates general findings for patients with meningitis based on cause, and the following sections detail specific methods for establishing an etiologic diagnosis.

Bacterial Meningitis

Gram stain examination of CSF permits rapid, accurate identification of the causative microorganism in 60% to 90% of patients with bacterial meningitis, and it has a specificity of nearly 100%. CSF culture is the gold standard in diagnosis and is positive in 80% to 90% of patients with community-acquired bacterial meningitis if CSF is obtained before the start of antimicrobial therapy. The probability of identifying the organism decreases for patients who have received prior antimicrobial therapy. It has been suggested that CSF sterilization may occur more rapidly after initiation of parenteral antimicrobial therapy than previously suggested, with complete sterilization of CSF containing meningococcus within 2 hours and the beginning of sterilization of pneumococcus by 4 hours into therapy.

Several rapid diagnostic tests have been developed to aid in the etiologic diagnosis of bacterial meningitis. Latex agglutination techniques detect the antigens of *H. influenzae* type b, *S. pneumoniae*, *N. meningitidis*, *E. coli* K1, and the group B streptococci. However, because bacterial antigen testing does not appear to modify the decision to administer antimicrobial therapy and false-positive results have been reported, routine use of this modality for rapid determination of the bacterial cause of meningitis is not recommended. It can be considered for patients who have been pretreated with antimicrobial therapy and when CSF Gram stain and culture results are negative.

Nucleic acid amplification tests, such as polymerase chain reaction (PCR), have been used to amplify DNA from patients with meningitis caused by several meningeal pathogens. The test characteristics for broad-based bacterial PCR demonstrated a sensitivity of 100%, a specificity of 98.2%, a positive predictive value of 98.2%, and a negative predictive value of 100%.

Differentiation of Bacterial from Viral Meningitis

In patients without a positive CSF Gram stain or culture, the diagnosis of acute bacterial meningitis is often difficult to establish or reject. A combination of clinical features, with or without test results, has been assessed to develop models in an attempt to accurately predict the likelihood of bacterial meningitis compared with other potential causes (most often viruses). In a published meta-analysis of bacterial meningitis score validation studies in which 5312 patients were identified from eight studies, 4896 (92%) had sufficient clinical data to calculate the bacterial meningitis score, which identified children with CSF pleocytosis who were at very low risk for bacterial meningitis. Low-risk features were a negative CSF Gram stain, a CSF absolute neutrophil count less than 1000 cells/mm^3, a CSF protein level less than 80 mg/dL, and a peripheral absolute neutrophil count less than 10,000 cells/mm^3. Despite the positive results of this meta-analysis and other studies, clinical judgment should continue to be used in decisions about the need for administration of empirical therapy in patients with suspected bacterial meningitis.

Several proteins have been examined for their usefulness in the diagnosis of acute bacterial meningitis. C-reactive protein (CRP) detected in serum or CSF and serum procalcitonin concentrations have been elevated in patients with acute bacterial meningitis and may be useful in discriminating between bacterial and viral meningitis. In patients with meningitis in whom the CSF Gram stain result is negative and analysis of other parameters is inconclusive, serum concentrations of CRP or procalcitonin that are normal or below the limit of detection have a high negative predictive value in the diagnosis of bacterial meningitis.

PCR is the most promising alternative to viral culture for the diagnosis of enteroviral meningitis. Enteroviral reverse transcription PCR (RT-PCR) has been tested in clinical settings by numerous investigators and found to be more sensitive than culture for the detection of the enterovirus; the sensitivity has ranged from 86% to 100% and specificity from 92% to 100% for the diagnosis of enteroviral meningitis. For patients with HSV-2 meningitis, PCR appears promising for the diagnosis. In patients

---

TABLE 90-2 CEREBROSPINAL FLUID TESTS FOR PATIENTS WITH SUSPECTED CENTRAL NERVOUS SYSTEM INFECTION

ROUTINE TESTS

WBC count with differential
RBC count*
Glucose concentration[†]
Protein concentration
Gram stain
Bacterial culture

SELECTED TESTS BASED ON CLINICAL SUSPICION

Viral culture[‡]
Smears and culture for acid-fast bacilli
Venereal Disease Research Laboratory (VDRL) test
India ink preparation
Cryptococcal polysaccharide antigen
Fungal culture
Antibody tests (IgM or IgG, or both)[§]
Nucleic acid amplification tests (e.g., PCR)[||]
Cytology[¶]
Flow cytometry

From Tunkel AR: Approach to the patient with central nervous system infection. In Bennett JE, Dolin R, Blaser M, editors: Mandell, Douglas, and Bennett's principles and practice of infectious diseases, ed 8, Philadelphia, 2015, Saunders.

CSF, Cerebrospinal fluid; IgG, immunoglobulin G; IgM, immunoglobulin M; PCR, polymerase chain reaction; RBCs, red blood cells; WBCs, white blood cells.

*Check in the first and last tubes; in patients with a traumatic tap, there should be a decrease in the number of RBCs with continued flow of CSF. The following formula can be used for determining whether the numbers of CSF red blood cells and white blood cells are consistent with a traumatic tap (all units are number of cells/cubic mm):

Adjusted WBCs in CSF

$$= \text{Actual WBCs in CSF} - \frac{\text{WBCs in blood} \times \text{RBCs in CSF}}{\text{RBCs in blood}}$$

[†]Compare with serum glucose concentration measured just before lumbar puncture.
[‡]Yield of viral culture may be low.
[§]May be useful for specific causes of meningitis and encephalitis.
[||]Most useful for specific viral causes of encephalitis and causes of chronic meningitis.
[¶]In patients with suspected malignancy.

TABLE 90-3 CEREBROSPINAL FLUID FINDINGS FOR PATIENTS WITH INFECTIOUS CAUSES OF MENINGITIS

CAUSE OF MENINGITIS	WHITE BLOOD CELL COUNT (cells/mm³)	PRIMARY CELL TYPE	GLUCOSE (mg/dL)	PROTEIN (mg/dL)
Viral	50-1000	Mononuclear*	>45	<200
Bacterial	1000-5000[†]	Neutrophilic[‡]	<40[§]	100-500
Tuberculous	50-300	Mononuclear[||]	<45	50-300
Cryptococcal	20-500[¶]	Mononuclear	<40	>45

From Tunkel AR: Approach to the patient with central nervous system infection. In Bennett JE, Dolin R, Blaser M, editors: Mandell, Douglas, and Bennett's principles and practice of infectious diseases, ed 8, Philadelphia, 2015, Saunders.

*May be neutrophilic early in presentation.
[†]May range from <100 to >10,000 neutrophils/mm³.
[‡]About 10% of patients have a cerebrospinal fluid (CSF) lymphocyte predominance.
[§]Should always be compared with a simultaneous serum glucose level; ratio of CSF to serum glucose is ≤0.4 in most cases.
[||]A therapeutic paradox may exist in which a mononuclear predominance becomes neutrophilic during antituberculosis therapy.
[¶]More than 75% of patients with acquired immunodeficiency syndrome have <20 cells/mm³.

with recurrent benign lymphocytic meningitis, detection of HSV-2 has been strongly associated with typical cases in patients without symptoms or signs of genital infection.

Spirochetal Meningitis

For the diagnosis of CNS involvement in patients with syphilis, no single routine laboratory test is definitive. The specificity of the CSF Venereal Disease Research Laboratory (VDRL) test for the diagnosis of neurosyphilis is high, but the sensitivity is low (reactive tests in only 30% to 70% of patients). A reactive CSF VDRL test result in the absence of blood contamination is sufficient to diagnose neurosyphilis; a nonreactive result does not exclude the diagnosis. The diagnosis of neurosyphilis is based on elevated CSF concentrations of white blood cells or protein, or both, in the appropriate clinical and serologic setting.

The best currently available laboratory test for the diagnosis of Lyme disease is demonstration of specific serum antibody to *B. burgdorferi*, and this positive test result for a patient with a compatible neurologic abnormality is strong evidence for the diagnosis. However, these tests are not standardized, and marked variations are seen between laboratories.

Tuberculous Meningitis

The identification of tuberculous organisms in CSF by specific stains is difficult because of the small population of organisms. In many series, less than 25% of specimens were smear positive and less than 50% were culture positive. The technique of PCR for detecting fragments of mycobacterial DNA in CSF specimens appears to be a promising tool. The Gen-Probe technique is based on amplification of ribosomal RNA derived from *Mycobacterium tuberculosis* using a labeled DNA probe. A 5-year retrospective study of the performance of this test found a sensitivity and specificity of 94% and 99%, respectively, for patients with positive CSF cultures.

Fungal Meningitis

Conclusive proof that a fungal organism is causing the meningitis rests on identification of the fungus in CSF, although CSF cultures are not always positive in cases of fungal meningitis. The yield of CSF culture in cryptococcal meningitis is excellent for non-AIDS and AIDS patients. For patients with cryptococcal meningitis, CSF India ink examination remains a rapid, effective test that is positive in 50% to 75% of cases; the yield increases up to 88% among patients with AIDS. In contrast, only 25% to 50% of patients with other fungal meningitis have positive CSF cultures.

Because cultures may be negative or require long periods before yielding positive results for patients with fungal meningitis, adjunctive studies (particularly serologic tests) may be helpful for the diagnosis. The latex agglutination test for cryptococcal polysaccharide antigen is sensitive and specific for the diagnosis of cryptococcal meningitis. Cryptococcal polysaccharide antigen also can be found in the serum and CSF, usually in severely immunosuppressed patients such as those with AIDS. Serologic antibody tests (i.e., coccidioidal and histoplasmal antigens) and antigen urine tests (i.e., histoplasmal antigen) may be useful in other cases of fungal meningitis.

Treatment

Initial Treatment of the Patient with Acute Meningitis

Acute bacterial meningitis is a life-threatening illness, and early detection, work-up, and antimicrobial therapy are imperative to reduce morbidity and mortality. The initial management of a patient with presumed bacterial meningitis includes performance of a lumbar puncture to determine whether the CSF formula is consistent with that diagnosis (Fig. 90-1). If meningitis is purulent, institution of antimicrobial therapy should be based on the results of Gram staining (Table 90-4). However, if no etiologic agent can be identified by this means or performance of the lumbar puncture is delayed, institution of empirical antimicrobial therapy after obtaining blood cultures should be based on the patient's age and underlying disease status (Table 90-5).

It is reasonable to proceed with the lumbar puncture without computed tomography (CT) of the head if the patient does not meet any of the following criteria: new-onset seizures, an immunocompromised state, signs that are suspicious for space-occupying lesions (i.e., papilledema or focal neurologic signs, not including cranial nerve palsy), or moderate to severe impairment of consciousness. Patients at risk should undergo CT of the head before lumbar puncture to rule out brain shift (i.e., result of an intracranial mass lesion or generalized brain edema) because of

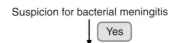

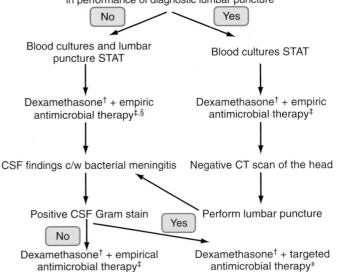

FIGURE 90-1 Management algorithm for adults with suspected bacterial meningitis. *Palsy of cranial nerve VI or VII is not an indication to delay lumbar puncture. †See text for recommendations for use of adjunctive dexamethasone in patients with bacterial meningitis. ‡See Table 90-5. §Dexamethasone and antimicrobial therapy should be administered immediately after CSF is obtained. ‖See Table 90-4. CNS, Central nervous system; CT, computed tomography; c/w, consistent with; STAT, intervention should be done emergently. (From Tunkel AR, Hartman BJ, Kaplan, SL, et al: Practice guidelines for the management of bacterial meningitis, Clin Infect Dis 39:1267–1284, 2004.)

TABLE 90-4	Recommended Antimicrobial Therapy for Acute Bacterial Meningitis
Microorganism*	**Antimicrobial Therapy**
Haemophilus influenzae type b	Third-generation cephalosporin[†]
Neisseria meningitidis	Third-generation cephalosporin[†]
Streptococcus pneumoniae	Vancomycin plus a third-generation cephalosporin[†,‡]
Listeria monocytogenes	Ampicillin or penicillin G[§]
Streptococcus agalactiae	Ampicillin or penicillin G[§]

Modified from Tunkel AR, Hartman BJ, Kaplan, SL, et al: Practice guidelines for the management of bacterial meningitis, Clin Infect Dis 39:1267–1284, 2004.
   *Pathogen presumptively identified by positive Gram stain.
   [†]Cefotaxime or ceftriaxone.
   [‡]Some experts would add rifampin if dexamethasone is also given.
   [§]Addition of an aminoglycoside should be considered.

TABLE 90-5	EMPIRICAL THERAPY FOR PURULENT MENINGITIS
PREDISPOSING FACTOR	**ANTIMICROBIAL THERAPY**
Age	
<1 mo	Ampicillin plus cefotaxime or ampicillin plus an aminoglycoside
1-23 mo	Vancomycin plus a third-generation cephalosporin*[†]
2-50 yr	Vancomycin plus a third-generation cephalosporin*[†‡]
>50 yr	Vancomycin plus ampicillin plus a third-generation cephalosporin*
Immunocompromised state	Vancomycin plus ampicillin plus cefepime or meropenem
Basilar skull fracture	Vancomycin plus a third-generation cephalosporin*
Head trauma; after neurosurgery	Vancomycin plus ceftazidime, cefepime, or meropenem

Modified from Tunkel AR, Hartman BJ, Kaplan, SL, et al: Practice guidelines for the management of bacterial meningitis, Clin Infect Dis 39:1267–1284, 2004.
   *Cefotaxime or ceftriaxone.
   [†]Some experts add rifampin if dexamethasone is also given.
   [‡]Add ampicillin if meningitis caused by *Listeria monocytogenes* is suspected.

TABLE 90-6	ANTIMICROBIAL THERAPY FOR PATIENTS WITH MENINGITIS
MICROORGANISM	**THERAPY OF CHOICE**
BACTERIA	
Haemophilus influenzae	
β-Lactamase negative	Ampicillin
β-Lactamase positive	Ceftriaxone or cefotaxime
Neisseria meningitidis	
Penicillin MIC <0.1 µg/mL	Penicillin G or ampicillin
Penicillin MIC 0.1-1.0 µg/mL	Ceftriaxone or cefotaxime
Streptococcus pneumoniae	
Penicillin MIC ≤0.06 µg/mL	Penicillin G or ampicillin
Penicillin MIC ≥0.12 µg/mL	
Ceftriaxone or cefotaxime MIC <1.0 µg/mL	Ceftriaxone or cefotaxime
Ceftriaxone or cefotaxime MIC ≥1.0 µg/mL	Vancomycin* plus ceftriaxone or cefotaxime
Enterobacteriaceae[†]	Ceftriaxone or cefotaxime
Pseudomonas aeruginosa	Ceftazidime[†] or cefepime[†]
Acinetobacter baumannii[†]	Meropenem
Listeria monocytogenes	Ampicillin or penicillin G[‡]
Streptococcus agalactiae	Ampicillin or penicillin G[‡]
Staphylococcus aureus	
Methicillin-sensitive	Nafcillin or oxacillin
Methicillin-resistant	Vancomycin*
Staphylococcus epidermidis	Vancomycin*
SPIROCHETES	
Treponema pallidum	Penicillin G
Borrelia burgdorferi	Ceftriaxone or cefotaxime
MYCOBACTERIA	
Mycobacterium tuberculosis	Isoniazid + rifampin + pyrazinamide + ethambutol
FUNGI	
Cryptococcus neoformans	Amphotericin B preparation[§] + flucytosine
Coccidioides immitis	Fluconazole
Histoplasma capsulatum	Liposomal amphotericin B
Candida species	Amphotericin B preparation[§] ± flucytosine

MIC, Minimum inhibitory concentration.
   *Addition of rifampin may be considered; see text for indications.
   [†]The choice of a specific antimicrobial agent must be guided by in vitro susceptibility testing.
   [‡]Addition of an aminoglycoside should be considered.
   [§]Amphotericin B deoxycholate, liposomal amphotericin B, or amphotericin B lipid complex.

the potential risk of herniation if a lumbar puncture is performed. In this setting, emergency empirical antimicrobial therapy, and adjunctive dexamethasone therapy (if indicated), after obtaining blood cultures should be initiated before sending the patient to the CT scanner.

Specific Antimicrobial Therapy for Meningitis

After the infecting meningeal pathogen is isolated and susceptibility testing results are known, antimicrobial therapy can be modified for optimal treatment of patients with bacterial meningitis (Table 90-6). Recommended dosages of antimicrobial agents for adults with infections of the CNS are shown in Table 90-7.

One pathogen requires special discussion. Specific therapy for pneumococcal meningitis depends on the in vitro susceptibility of the organism to penicillin and the third-generation cephalosporins. Results of surveillance studies in the United States show that the prevalence of penicillin-resistant *S. pneumoniae* ranges from 25% to more than 50%; rates are as high as 60% in some parts of Latin America and as high as 80% in some countries in Asia. Penicillin can never be recommended as empirical therapy in patients with suspected pneumococcal meningitis. As an empirical regimen, the combination of vancomycin plus a third-generation cephalosporin (i.e., cefotaxime or ceftriaxone) is

recommended. After susceptibility studies of the isolated pneumococcus are performed, antimicrobial therapy can be modified for optimal treatment (see Table 90-7).

Viral meningitis is usually a benign self-limited illness. Recovery of patients with HSV-2 meningitis is usually complete without neurologic sequelae, and it is not clear whether antiviral treatment alters the course of mild meningitis.

The preferred antimicrobial regimen for the treatment of CNS syphilis is intravenous aqueous crystalline penicillin G at a dosage of 18 to 24 million units daily in divided doses every 4 hours or by continuous infusion for 10 to 14 days. Alternatively, procaine penicillin (2.4 million units intramuscularly daily) plus probenecid (500 mg orally four times daily), both for 10 to 14 days, can be used.

Parenteral antimicrobial therapy is usually needed to treat the neurologic manifestations of Lyme disease, including meningitis. The current recommendation is to treat most patients with Lyme meningitis with intravenous ceftriaxone at a dosage of 2 g daily

TABLE 90-7	RECOMMENDED DOSAGES OF ANTIMICROBIAL AGENTS FOR MENINGITIS IN ADULTS WITH NORMAL RENAL AND HEPATIC FUNCTION	
ANTIMICROBIAL AGENT	**TOTAL DAILY DOSE***	**DOSING INTERVAL (hr)**
Amikacin[†]	15 mg/kg	8
Amphotericin B deoxycholate	0.7-1.0 mg/kg	24
Ampicillin	12 g	4
Cefepime	6 g	8
Cefotaxime	8-12 g	4-6
Ceftazidime	6 g	8
Ceftriaxone	4 g	12-24
Ethambutol[§]	15 mg/kg	24
Fluconazole	400-800 mg[‡]	24
Flucytosine[§,‖]	100 mg/kg	6
Gentamicin[†]	5 mg/kg	8
Isoniazid[§,¶]	300 mg	24
Liposomal amphotericin B	3-4 mg/kg	24
Meropenem	6 g	8
Nafcillin	9-12 g	4
Oxacillin	9-12 g	4
Penicillin G	24 million units	4
Pyrazinamide[§]	15-30 mg/kg	24
Rifampin[§]	600 mg	24
Tobramycin[†]	5 mg/kg	8
Sulfamethoxazole-trimethoprim	10-20 mg/kg[**]	6-12
Vancomycin[††]	30-60 mg/kg	8-12

*Unless indicated, therapy is administered intravenously.
[†]Need to monitor peak and trough serum concentrations.
[‡]Dose of 800-1200 mg is recommended for patients with coccidioidal meningitis.
[§]Oral administration.
[‖]Maintain serum concentrations of 50-100 µg/mL.
[¶]Initiate therapy at a dose of 10 mg/kg.
[**]Dosage based on trimethoprim component.
[††]Maintain serum trough concentrations of 15-20 µg/mL.

for 14 days (range, 10 to 28 days); no evidence supports treatment durations longer than 4 weeks.

In patients with tuberculous meningitis, the most important principle of therapy is early initiation on the basis of strong clinical suspicion; it should not be delayed until proof of infection has been obtained. The American Thoracic Society, in conjunction with the CDC and the Infectious Diseases Society of America, recommends 2 months of isoniazid, rifampin, ethambutol, and pyrazinamide, followed by 7 to 10 months of isoniazid and rifampin for patients with drug-sensitive tuberculous meningitis. Therapy for tuberculous meningitis may need to be individualized, with longer durations of therapy used for patients with more severe illness or HIV.

Therapy for cryptococcal meningitis in patients with AIDS is usually an amphotericin B preparation (i.e., amphotericin B deoxycholate, liposomal amphotericin B, or amphotericin B lipid complex) plus flucytosine for 2 weeks, followed by consolidation therapy with fluconazole for 8 weeks. For non-AIDS patients with cryptococcal meningitis, the optimal use of fluconazole is less clear. In a retrospective review of HIV-1–negative patients with CNS cryptococcosis, the patients were more likely to receive an induction regimen containing amphotericin B and subsequent therapy with fluconazole. Most experts recommend high-dose fluconazole (800 to 1200 mg daily) as first-line therapy for coccidioidal meningitis.

The current recommendation is to treat *Histoplasma* meningitis with liposomal amphotericin B over 4 to 6 weeks, followed by itraconazole for at least 1 year. Amphotericin B, alone or in combination with flucytosine, also is the treatment of choice for *Candida* meningitis.

Adjunctive Therapy

For adult patients with bacterial meningitis, adjunctive dexamethasone should be administered to those with suspected or proven pneumococcal meningitis. This recommendation is based on a prospective, randomized, double-blind trial enrolling 301 adults with bacterial meningitis. Adjunctive dexamethasone was associated with a reduction in the proportion of patients who had unfavorable outcomes (15% vs. 25%, $P = .03$) and in the proportion of patients who died (7% vs. 15%, $P = .04$). The benefits were most striking for the subgroup of patients with pneumococcal meningitis and those with moderate to severe disease as assessed by the admission Glasgow Coma Scale.

Dexamethasone is administered at a dosage of 10 mg intravenously every 6 hours (with the first dose given concomitant with or just before the first dose of an antimicrobial agent for maximal attenuation of the subarachnoid space inflammatory response) for 4 days. Adjunctive dexamethasone should not be used in patients who have already received antimicrobial therapy or the meningitis is found not to be caused by *S. pneumoniae*. Despite the positive benefits of adjunctive dexamethasone for adults with bacterial meningitis described previously, the routine use of adjunctive dexamethasone for patients with bacterial meningitis in the developing world has been controversial.

Tuberculous meningitis is associated with persistent morbidity and mortality despite the availability of effective antituberculous chemotherapy. Use of adjunctive corticosteroids has abrogated the signs and symptoms of disease, and early treatment with adjunctive dexamethasone should be used in all patients with tuberculous meningitis.

Patients with cryptococcal meningitis may have increased intracranial pressure or hydrocephalus, or both. Therapeutic modalities for these complications include shunting of CSF and frequent, high-volume lumbar punctures.

Encephalitis

Definition

Encephalitis is inflammation of the brain parenchyma that is associated with neurologic dysfunction. In the absence of pathologic evidence of brain inflammation, an inflammatory response in the CSF or parenchymal abnormalities on neuroimaging are often used as surrogate markers of brain inflammation; however, encephalitis can occur without significant CSF pleocytosis or demonstrable neuroimaging abnormalities. Encephalitis and meningitis share many features. Both syndromes can manifest with fever, headache, and altered mental status, although the encephalitis patient suffers from more severe alterations in mental status.

There is also clinical overlap between encephalitis and encephalopathy. Patients with encephalopathy, however, exhibit confusion early in the course of their illness that can quickly progress to obtundation. Causes of encephalopathy include metabolic disturbances, hypoxia, ischemia, intoxications, organ dysfunction, paraneoplastic syndromes, and systemic infections.

Epidemiology and Etiology

Encephalitis causes significant morbidity and mortality, and it is a significant burden on the health care system. The hospital admission rate in one study was 7.3 per 100,000 people. The case-fatality rate among patients with encephalitis varies from 3.8% to 7.4% and is significantly higher among patients also infected with HIV. There is significant morbidity among survivors of encephalitis, with resultant loss of productivity and the need for prolonged rehabilitation or skilled nursing care.

Infectious causes of encephalitis are diverse and include viruses (most common), bacteria, fungi, and parasites. Clues in the patient's history that aid identification include seasonal variation, geographic location, prevalence of disease in the local community, travel history, recreational activities, occupational exposures, insect contact, animal contact, vaccination history, and immune status of the patient.

The most commonly identified viral causes in the United States are herpes simplex virus type 1 (HSV-1), West Nile virus, and the enteroviruses, followed by other herpesviruses (e.g., varicella-zoster virus). Other agents may be highly endemic regionally (e.g., La Crosse virus in the Midwest) or internationally (e.g., rabies virus, Japanese encephalitis virus). Bacterial agents, including *Ehrlichia* species and *Rickettsia rickettsii*, are potentially treatable causes of encephalitis, and prompt administration of appropriate antimicrobial therapy may be lifesaving.

Perhaps the most challenging aspect of encephalitis is that no pathogen is identified in 50% to 70% of cases. Up to 10% of patients have a noninfectious cause.

Clinical Presentation

Because encephalitis is infrequently confirmed by pathologic means, the signs and symptoms of neurologic dysfunction are used as surrogate markers, and they are often nonspecific. The clinical signs and symptoms of encephalitis are determined by the specific area of the brain involved and by the severity of the infection. Some organisms show neurotropism for particular anatomic sites. HSV-1 infection almost universally involves the temporal lobe, and the clinical presentation typically includes temporal lobe seizures. With this comes an associated change in personality, decreasing consciousness, focal neurologic findings (including dysphagia), paresthesias and weakness, and focal seizures. Sudden onset of fever and headache can also accompany these mental status changes.

Diffuse brain involvement is frequently seen with arboviral infections, and it is associated with global impairment in neurologic function and coma. Fever and headache frequently precede the onset of altered mental status, which can range from mild confusion to obtundation. Other neurologic manifestations may include behavioral changes (e.g., psychosis), focal paresis or paralysis, cranial nerve palsies, and movement disorders (e.g., chorea). About 80% of patients infected with West Nile virus are asymptomatic, and about 20% have only fever. Symptomatic patients may have fever, headache, myalgia, and flaccid paralysis. A maculopapular rash is seen in 50% of patients.

Evidence of inflammation or infection at sites distant from the CNS may be useful in making a microbiologic diagnosis for patients with encephalitis and myelitis. For instance, rickettsial diseases, varicella-zoster virus, and West Nile virus often have associated skin manifestations. Stomatitis and ulcerative lesions in the mouth or an exanthem in a peripheral distribution can suggest enterovirus infection. Patients with tuberculous and fungal meningoencephalitis may have suggestive pulmonary findings.

A syndrome frequently misclassified as encephalomyelitis based on the similar clinical presentation is postinflammatory encephalomyelitis. The most widely cited example is acute disseminated encephalomyelitis (ADEM), which is seen primarily in children and adolescents. ADEM is characterized by poorly defined white matter lesions on magnetic resonance imaging (MRI) that enhance after gadolinium administration. Postinflammatory encephalomyelitis is likely mediated by an immunologic response to an antecedent antigenic stimulus such as infection or immunization. Viral infections associated with ADEM include measles, mumps, rubella, varicella-zoster, Epstein-Barr, cytomegalovirus, herpes simplex, hepatitis A, and coxsackievirus. Immunizations temporally associated with ADEM include vaccines for Japanese encephalitis, yellow fever, measles, influenza, smallpox, anthrax, and rabies, but a direct causal association with these vaccines is difficult to establish. ADEM usually begins between 2 days and 4 weeks after the antigenic stimulus, and patients develop rapid onset of encephalopathy, with or without meningeal signs. The neurologic features depend on the location of the lesions.

Another important disorder to consider is anti–*N*-methyl-D-aspartate receptor (NMDAR) encephalitis, which is the most common cause of autoimmune encephalitis after ADEM. The disorder is seen in patients of all ages but occurs mostly in young adults and children with or without teratomas. Patients usually have an acute behavioral change, psychosis, and catatonia that evolves to include seizures, memory deficit, dyskinesias, speech problems, and autonomic and breathing dysregulation. Symptoms are more often neurologic in children and psychiatric in adults, but in most cases, symptoms progress to a similar syndrome.

Diagnosis

The initial laboratory testing of an individual should include a complete blood count, tests of renal and hepatic function, and coagulation studies. A low white blood cell count, low platelet count, and elevated liver transaminase levels may suggest *Ehrlichia* or *Anaplasma* infection. A baseline chest radiograph should be obtained because a focal infiltrate can suggest particular pathogens (e.g., fungal or mycobacterial infections).

Neuroimaging studies are important to perform for all patients with encephalitis; MRI is more sensitive at detecting abnormalities than CT, and it is the preferred study. Diffusion-weighted MRI is superior to conventional MRI for the detection of early signal abnormalities in viral encephalitis caused by HSV, enterovirus 71, and West Nile virus. In patients with HSV encephalitis, there may be significant edema and hemorrhage in the temporal lobes. Patients with flavivirus (e.g., West Nile virus, Japanese encephalitis virus) encephalitis may display characteristic patterns of mixed-intensity or hypodense lesions on T1-weighted images of the thalamus, basal ganglia, and midbrain. In patients with ADEM, MRI usually reveals multiple focal or confluent areas of signal abnormality in the subcortical white matter and, sometimes, in subcortical gray matter on T2-weighted and fluid attenuation inversion recovery (FLAIR) sequences; the lesions are usually enhancing and display similar stages of evolution.

Electroencephalography is rarely specific for a given pathogen in patients with encephalitis, but results can be helpful in identifying the degree of cerebral dysfunction by detecting subclinical seizure activity, and it may provide information about the specific area of the brain involved. Many patients with HSV encephalitis demonstrate a temporal lobe focus with periodic lateralizing epileptiform discharges (PLEDs).

Lumbar puncture with CSF analysis (i.e., cell count and differential, glucose and protein levels) and a measurement of the opening pressure should be performed unless there is a specific contraindication. Most patients with viral encephalitis have a mononuclear cell pleocytosis with cell counts ranging from 10 to 1000/mm^3. Early in the disease process, CSF pleocytosis may be absent, or there may be an elevation in neutrophils. The CSF protein concentration is typically elevated, but usually less than 100 to 200 mg/dL, whereas the CSF glucose concentration is typically normal. CSF viral cultures are usually not recommended.

Brain biopsy has largely been replaced by CSF molecular tests. For certain types of infections, however, brain biopsy may be diagnostic. In rabies infections, for example, Negri bodies are a distinctive histopathologic feature. Intranuclear eosinophilic amorphous bodies surrounded by a halo may be seen in diseases such as HSV encephalitis.

Testing for specific agents includes laboratory methods such as antigen detection, culture, serology, and molecular diagnostics. HSV encephalitis is a treatable and relatively common cause of encephalitis, and an HSV PCR should be performed on the CSF of all patients with a clinical diagnosis of encephalitis. False-negative PCR test results can occur within the first 72 hours after onset, and if HSV encephalitis is strongly suspected (e.g., in a patient with temporal lobe involvement), a repeat HSV PCR on a second sample of CSF within 3 to 7 days is recommended. Enterovirus and varicella PCR should be done on CSF because they are also common causes of encephalitis; however, detection of antibodies to varicella-zoster virus in the CSF appears to have greater sensitivity than detection of viral DNA.

Testing for other agents should be individualized with consideration of the patient's exposures, travel, season of the year, and clinical and laboratory characteristics. Many infections require acute and convalescent (i.e., paired) serum samples to determine a diagnosis. A serum specimen collected during the acute phase of the illness should be stored and tested in parallel when the convalescent serum sample is drawn. Immunoglobulin M (IgM) and immunoglobulin G (IgG) capture enzyme-linked immunosorbent assays (ELISAs) have become useful and widely available for the diagnosis of arboviral encephalitis. Detection of intrathecal IgM antibody is a specific and sensitive method for the diagnosis of West Nile virus infection. There is substantial cross-reactivity among the flaviviruses (e.g., West Nile virus, St. Louis encephalitis virus, Japanese encephalitis virus); plaque-reduction neutralization assays may be helpful in distinguishing which flavivirus is involved in the event of elevated titers.

Serologic testing for *Rickettsia*, *Ehrlichia*, and *Anaplasma* species should be performed for all encephalitis patients during the appropriate season and with travel to or residence in endemic areas, especially because these are treatable causes. Empirical therapy should not be withheld from patients with a compatible clinical presentation because antibodies are not always detectable early in the course of illness.

Identification of NMDAR antibodies confirms the diagnosis of anti-NMDAR encephalitis and should lead to the search for a tumor. The tumor is almost always an ovarian teratoma.

Treatment

One of the most important first steps in managing encephalitis is to consider treatable causes. Specific antiviral therapy is usually limited to infections caused by herpesviruses (especially HSV-1 and varicella-zoster virus) and HIV. Acyclovir (10 mg/kg intravenously every 8 hours in adults with normal renal function) should be administered to patients with encephalitis. Empirical therapy for acute bacterial meningitis should be initiated when clinical and laboratory testing is compatible with bacterial infection. If rickettsial or ehrlichial infections are suspected, empirical doxycycline should be administered. The management of West Nile virus infection is supportive care.

In patients with suspected postinfectious encephalomyelitis (i.e., ADEM), high-dose intravenous corticosteroids (1 g of methylprednisolone intravenously daily for at least 3 to 5 days) are usually recommended, followed by an oral taper for 3 to 6 weeks. For patients diagnosed with anti-NMDAR encephalitis, treatments have included corticosteroids, intravenous immunoglobulins, and plasmapheresis. If a tumor is detected, removal is important because it accelerates improvement and decreases relapses.

BRAIN ABSCESS

CNS infections can manifest as abscesses in the parenchyma or as parameningeal infections. Prion infections produce clinical signs confined to the brain and spinal cord.

Definition

A *brain abscess* is a focal collection of infected material in the brain parenchyma that results in a necrotic center surrounded by inflammatory cells.

Pathology and Pathophysiology

Brain abscesses produce symptoms and findings similar to those of other space-occupying lesions (e.g., brain tumors), but they often progress more rapidly and affect meningeal structures more frequently than tumors. They originate or extend from extracerebral locations. Examples include blood-borne metastases from unknown sources, lungs, or heart (i.e., endocarditis); direct extensions from parameningeal sites of infection (i.e., otitis, cranial osteomyelitis, facial infections, and sinusitis); and infections from sites of recent or remote head trauma or neurosurgical procedures.

The infection is often polymicrobial. Commonly isolated pathogens are aerobic and microaerobic streptococci and gram-negative anaerobes such as *Bacteroides* and *Prevotella*. Less common are gram-negative aerobes and *Staphylococcus*.

Actinomyces, Nocardia, and *Candida* are found even less often. In immunosuppressed individuals, *Cryptococcus* (i.e., microabscesses) and *Toxoplasma* are common causes of abscesses. Surgical specimens are culture positive for 70% of antibiotic-treated patients and 95% of patients undergoing surgery before antibiotic administration.

Clinical Presentation

The classic clinical picture is composed of elements reflecting the infectious nature of the lesion (e.g., fever), those related to focal brain involvement, and those due to an increasing intracranial mass effect. Elements of one or two categories are often absent in a given case, particularly early in the disease course. For example, almost one half of patients may not have a fever or leukocytosis. Recent onset of a headache is the most common symptom, which may increase in severity associated with focal signs related to the location of the abscess (e.g., hemiparesis, aphasia), followed by obtundation and coma. Seizures precede the diagnosis in 30% of cases. *Toxoplasma* abscesses are often associated with movement disorders due to their propensity for the basal ganglia. The period of evolution may be as brief as hours or as long as days to weeks with more indolent organisms.

Diagnosis

CSF examination should be avoided; it is seldom diagnostic, and results can be normal. Lumbar puncture in the setting of a mass lesion carries the risk of transtentorial herniation. Because the brain abscess is seeded from a peripheral site of infection, a search for other sites of infection can help to identify the causative organisms and determine adequate treatment.

MRI with intravenous gadolinium provides better soft tissue contrast than CT and is particularly useful for detecting multiple abscesses and posterior fossa abscesses or for demonstrating cerebritis, the extent of a mass effect, associated venous thrombosis, and the response to therapy. In the early cerebritis stage, CT results may be normal, but the MRI FLAIR sequence is very sensitive for visualization of brain edema. On T1-weighted images, the area of cerebritis is seen initially as a low-signal-intensity, ill-defined area. T1-weighted images in the later stages of infection show the formation of a rim of slightly higher signal intensity and central necrosis. Contrast administration typically shows ring enhancement with central necrosis. This area of central necrosis appears bright on diffusion-weighted images and dark on apparent diffusion coefficient (ADC) images (Fig. 90-2). MRI of tumors shows the opposite features. Differentiating a brain abscess from tumor is important for the stereotactic approach to ring-enhancing lesions before biopsy or surgical excision. An abscess should be drained centrally, whereas a tumor should be biopsied along its rim.

Nocardia brain abscesses are often mutilobulated. *Listeria* brain abscesses are often located in the brain stem.

Treatment

A suspected brain abscess requires urgent intervention. Unless the surgical procedure poses a substantial risk, aspiration of the lesion is needed for microbial diagnosis. If treatment of cerebral edema is necessary, high-dose intravenous dexamethasone (16 to 24 mg/day in four divided doses) may be used for short periods until surgical intervention is possible. Corticosteroids may retard formation of a capsule around the brain abscess and the immune response to infection.

Seizures should be controlled because the tonic phase of a generalized seizure may increase intracranial pressure. In a patient with a large abscess, seizures may trigger a brain herniation. Seizure prophylaxis should be initiated in all patients with

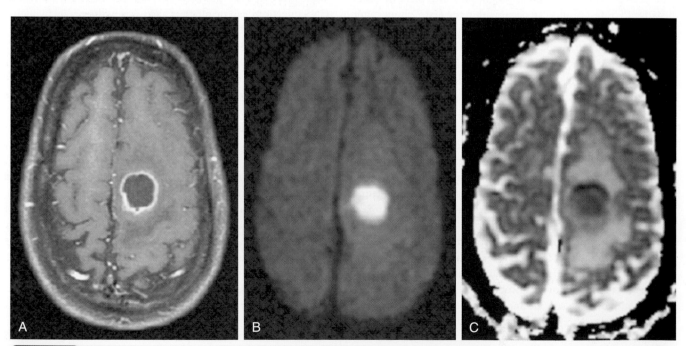

FIGURE 90-2 Magnetic resonance imaging features of a brain abscess. **A,** Contrast-enhanced scan shows a ring-enhancing lesion in the left frontal lobe. **B,** The diffusion-weighted image shows restricted diffusion in the cavity due to viscous pus and cellular material. **C,** Corresponding apparent diffusion coefficient map shows dark, viscous material in the cavity and surrounding edema.

cortical or temporal lobe abscesses. Anticonvulsants that can be administered intravenously are the drugs of choice.

Successful antibiotic management of brain abscess is based on knowledge of proven or suspected pathogens and antibiotic properties, such as CNS drug penetration capabilities and the spectrum of activity. Empirical antibiotic therapy without surgical intervention may be used if the primary source of infection outside of the CNS is identified, in patients with cerebritis without capsule formation, or in those with multiple, small abscesses or abscesses in basal ganglia or brain stem. If the organism is unknown, empirical therapy may include vancomycin, metronidazole, and a third-generation cephalosporin. In brain stem abscesses, the possibility of *Listeria* infection should be considered, and treatment should include intravenous ampicillin. In HIV-infected patients with multiple ring-enhancing lesions, empirical therapy for toxoplasmosis should be initiated even if the patient is seronegative for *Toxoplasma*.

Patients undergoing empirical therapy should be followed with repeated CT or MRI. Those who fail to respond should undergo surgical intervention. An important aspect of the management strategy is eradication of the predisposing condition or cause of the brain abscess, such as an oral, ear, cardiac, or pulmonary infection.

⬤ PARAMENINGEAL INFECTIONS
Definition

Parameningeal infections include those infections that produce suppuration in potential spaces covering the brain and spinal cord (i.e., epidural abscess and subdural empyema) and those that produce occlusion of the contiguous venous sinuses and cerebral veins (i.e., cerebral venous sinus thrombosis).

Subdural Empyema
Definition

Subdural empyema refers to infection in the space separating the dura and arachnoid.

Pathology and Pathophysiology

Two thirds of subdural empyemas result from frontal or ethmoid sinus infections, 20% from inner ear infections, and the remainder from trauma or neurosurgical procedures. The empyema is caused by direct or indirect extension from infected paranasal sinuses through a retrograde thrombophlebitis. Unilateral empyema is most common because the falx prevents passage across the midline, but bilateral or multiple empyemas can occur. Cortical venous thrombosis or brain abscess develops in about one fourth of patients. In some patients, the subdural empyema may be associated with an epidural abscess or meningitis. These infections occur more often in children than in adults.

Clinical Presentation

Initial symptoms are caused by chronic otitis or sinusitis with superimposed lateralized headache, fever, and obtundation. Vomiting, meningeal signs, and focal neurologic abnormalities (i.e., hemiparesis or seizures) follow. If untreated, obtundation

progresses, and the septic mass and swollen underlying brain produce venous thrombosis or death from herniation.

The major differential diagnosis is meningitis. Nuchal rigidity and obtundation occur in meningitis and subdural empyema, but papilledema and lateralizing deficits are more common in empyema.

Diagnosis

Lumbar puncture should be avoided in patients with subdural empyema to prevent cerebral herniation. Contrast-enhanced CT or MRI can be diagnostic of empyema, showing an extra-axial, crescent-shaped mass with an enhancing rim lying just below the inner table of the skull over the cerebral convexities or in the interhemispheric fissures. On MRI, subdural empyemas have decreased signal intensity on T1-weighted imaging and increased signal intensity on T2-weighted scans. Similar to brain abscess, subdural empyema has high signal intensity on diffusion-weighted images and low signal intensity on ADC maps.

Treatment

Treatment requires prompt surgical drainage of the empyema cavity and high-dose intravenous antibiotics directed at organisms found at the time of craniotomy.

⬤ MALIGNANT EXTERNAL OTITIS

Chapter 91 discusses infections of the head and neck.

⬤ SPINAL EPIDURAL ABSCESS
Definition and Epidemiology

A *spinal epidural abscess* is an infection in the epidural space between the dura and the bones of the spine around the spinal cord. It can cause paralysis and death. The incidence is 0.5 to 1.0 cases per 10,000 hospital admissions in the United States, and the frequency is increased among injection drug users.

Pathology and Pathophysiology

Infections of the epidural space originate from contiguous spread or through hematogenous routes from a distant source. Cutaneous infection, particularly in the back, is the most common remote source, especially among injection drug users. Abdominal, respiratory tract, and urinary sources are also common. As the use of epidural catheters has increased for pain management, epidural abscess and hematoma have been increasingly reported.

The anatomy of the epidural space dictates the location of the abscess. Because the size of the intravertebral canal remains relatively constant but the circumference of the spinal cord changes, abscess formation is maximal in the thoracic and lumbar regions and minimal at the cervical spine enlargement. Due to the loose connections between the dura and the bones of the spine, the abscess can extend to multiple levels, causing severe and extensive neurologic manifestations.

Causative organisms can be identified by culture or Gram stain from pus obtained at exploration (90% of patients), blood cultures (60% to 90%), or CSF (20%). *S. aureus* is most common, followed by streptococci and gram-negative organisms. Tuberculous abscesses may occur in as many as 25% of patients in high-risk populations. In a recent epidemic, iatrogenic infection occurred with rare fungi after epidural injections of corticosteroids that were contaminated with a plant pathogen, *Exserohilum rostratum*, that rarely infects humans.

Clinical Presentation

The classic triad of fever, spinal pain, and neurologic deficits may not be identified in all patients, leading to a delay in diagnosis. Patients are usually febrile and have acute or subacute neck or back pain. An important physical finding is focal tenderness over the affected spinous processes. Stiff neck and headache are common. The pain can be mistaken for sciatica, a visceral abdominal process, chest wall pain, or cervical disk disease. If it goes unrecognized at this stage, the symptoms can evolve over a few hours to a few days to weakness, loss of lower extremity reflexes, and paralysis distal to the spinal level of the infection. In this clinical setting, spinal epidural abscess should be assumed, systemic antibiotics begun, and urgent neuroradiologic imaging pursued.

Diagnosis

The diagnosis is made by CT or MRI (Fig. 90-3). The differential diagnosis includes transverse myelitis, intervertebral disk herniation, epidural hemorrhage, and metastatic tumor. These conditions can usually be detected by MRI. Epidural abscess is often accompanied by diskitis or osteomyelitis of the vertebral bodies.

Treatment

Unless culture and sensitivities dictate otherwise, a penicillinase-resistant penicillin should be started empirically as antistaphylococcal treatment for presumed bacterial infection. If methicillin resistance is suspected, vancomycin should be used. Considering the severity of the disease, additional gram-negative coverage with a third-generation cephalosporin or a quinolone may be needed.

Surgical decompression was previously considered mandatory, but early diagnosis by MRI may allow for effective medical therapy if started before the occurrence of neurologic complications. These patients should be monitored closely, and if signs of neurologic deterioration emerge, surgical intervention may be necessary.

⬤ SINUS THROMBOSIS

Septic Cavernous Sinus Thrombosis

Septic cavernous sinus thrombosis usually results from spread of infection from facial structures through facial veins or from the sphenoid or ethmoid sinuses. Symptoms include headache or lateralized facial pain, followed in a few days to weeks by fever and involvement of the orbit (i.e., proptosis and chemosis due to obstruction of the ophthalmic vein). Paralysis of oculomotor nerves follows rapidly. In some instances, sensory dysfunction occurs in the first and second divisions of the trigeminal nerve along with a decrease in the corneal reflex. Further involvement of the contiguous orbital contents follows, with mild papilledema and decreased visual acuity that sometimes progresses to blindness.

Extension to the opposite cavernous sinus or to other intracranial sinuses with cerebral infarction or increased intracranial pressure due to impaired venous drainage can result in stupor, coma, and death. The CSF is abnormal if there is accompanying meningitis or parameningeal infection. The most common causative organism is *S. aureus*, followed by streptococci and pneumococci; anaerobic infection may occur.

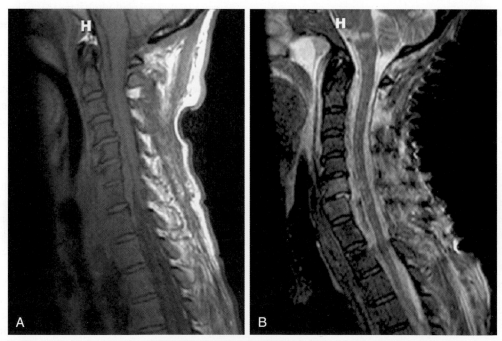

FIGURE 90-3 Magnetic resonance imaging shows an epidural abscess due to *Staphylococcus* in the cervical spine of a patient with human immunodeficiency virus infection. **A,** Noncontrast T1-weighted image shows an extensive lesion in the epidural space that extends from C2 to C7. Notice straightening of the cervical spine. **B,** After a laminectomy from C2 to T1 and fusion, the short tau inversion recovery (STIR) image shows fluid collection in the epidural space as a high-signal-intensity lesion. Normal curvature of the spine is seen.

Diagnosis of cavernous sinus thrombosis is usually made by MRI with a venogram. Radiologic evaluation includes imaging of the sphenoidal and ethmoidal sinuses, which may require drainage if infected. Empirical antimicrobial therapy should include an antistaphylococcal agent. An empirical combination therapy with parenteral metronidazole, vancomycin, and ceftriaxone can achieve reasonable CSF and brain penetration and is likely to be active against *S. aureus* and the usual sinus pathogens. Parenteral nafcillin can be added for identified or suspected methicillin-sensitive *S. aureus*.

Lateral Sinus Thrombosis

Septic thrombosis of the lateral sinus results from acute or chronic infections of the middle ear. The infection spreads through emissary veins that connect the mastoid with the lateral venous sinus. It may spread to involve the sigmoid sinus. The symptoms include ear pain followed over several weeks by fever, headache, nausea, vomiting, and vertigo. Mastoid swelling may be seen. Sixth cranial nerve palsies and papilledema can occur, but other focal neurologic signs are rare.

The diagnosis can be established by magnetic resonance angiography. Treatment includes an empirical regimen of broad-spectrum intravenous antibiotics to cover staphylococci and anaerobes (i.e., nafcillin or oxacillin with penicillin or metronidazole), but surgical drainage (i.e., mastoidectomy) may be required.

Septic Sagittal Sinus Thrombosis

Septic sagittal sinus thrombosis is uncommon and occurs as a consequence of purulent meningitis, infections of the ethmoidal or maxillary sinuses spreading through venous channels, infected compound skull fractures, or neurosurgical wound infections (rare). Symptoms include manifestations of elevated intracranial pressure (i.e., headache, nausea, and vomiting) that evolve rapidly to stupor and coma. Diagnosis and treatment is similar to the lateral venous sinus thrombosis described earlier.

⬤ NEUROLOGIC COMPLICATIONS OF INFECTIVE ENDOCARDITIS
Epidemiology

Neurologic complications occur in one third of patients with bacterial endocarditis, and they triple the mortality rate of the disease. Most complications are related to valvular vegetations. Cerebral (but not systemic) emboli from mitral valve endocarditis are increasingly common. Most emboli, regardless of the bacterial cause of the infection, occur before or early in the course of treatment. By 2 weeks of therapy, the risk of embolization decreases dramatically. Mycotic aneurysms in the brain complicate endocarditis in 2% to 10% of patients and are more common in acute than subacute disease.

Pathophysiology and Clinical Manifestations

Cerebral emboli are distributed in the brain in proportion to cerebral blood flow. Most emboli lodge in the branches of the middle cerebral artery peripherally, with resultant hemiparesis. Focal seizures may result. Multiple microabscesses, however, can result in a diffuse encephalopathy similar to that seen in sepsis.

Mycotic aneurysms occur most commonly in the middle cerebral artery, with the aneurysms located distally in the vessel. This differentiates them from congenital berry aneurysms.

Clinical Manifestations

Patients often develop strokes, impaired consciousness, meningitis, focal seizures, and new-onset severe headaches. Strokes may manifest as ischemic lesions or hemorrhagic lesions in the brain parenchyma or subarachnoid space. Patients may have other signs of systemic microembolisms or retinal lesions, splinter hemorrhages in the nail bed, or microscopic hematuria.

Diagnosis

The diagnosis of neurologic involvement from endocarditis is best made with CT or MRI. MRI findings in endocarditis include ischemic lesions, hemorrhagic lesions, subarachnoid hemorrhage, brain abscess, mycotic aneurysm, and cerebral microbleeds. The CSF is abnormal in 70% of patients and simulates purulent meningitis (i.e., polymorphonuclear predominance, elevated protein level, and low glucose level) or a parameningeal infection (i.e., lymphocytic predominance, modest protein elevation, and normal glucose level). Multiple blood cultures may be needed to identify the organisms.

Multidetector CT angiography may be necessary to diagnose aneurysms. Small brain abscesses may complicate the course of endocarditis, but macroscopic abscesses are rare, with most occurring in the setting of acute rather than subacute endocarditis. Multiple microabscesses may escape detection on CT and are not amenable to surgical drainage.

Treatment

Antibiotic treatment of the primary disease is indicated. Stroke is usually treated conservatively. There are no controlled trials for the management of unruptured mycotic aneurysms. The aneurysms may decrease in size with antibiotic therapy, but the risk of rupture is high, and most clinicians advocate surgical management with clipping of the aneurysm or endovascular coiling. However, endovascular coiling may not prevent hemorrhage associated with rupture of a new aneurysm. Patients with infective endocarditis who do not respond to conservative medical therapy can have prompt valve replacement despite intracerebral hemorrhage.

⬤ PRION DISEASES
Etiology

Several human diseases have been attributed to a unique infectious protein, the prion. The infectious form of the prion protein is rich in β-sheets, detergent insoluble, multimeric, and resistant to proteinase K treatment.

Prion illnesses (i.e., transmissible spongiform encephalopathies) can be classified as sporadic, hereditary, or acquired. The most common form is sporadic Creutzfeldt-Jakob disease (sCJD). Familial forms include Gerstmann-Sträussler-Scheinker syndrome and familial fatal insomnia.

Acquired forms are caused by the transmission of an abnormal prion protein (PrP) from human to human or from cattle to humans. Accidental transmission of CJD between humans appears to have occurred with cadaveric dura mater grafting, corneal transplantation, receipt of human growth hormone or pituitary gonadotropin, contaminated electroencephalogram electrodes, and contaminated surgical instruments. This form of CJD has been called iatrogenic CJD (iCJD).

The appearance of variant CJD (vCJD) in Great Britain, which was associated with the outbreak of bovine spongiform encephalopathy and the contamination of beef, greatly increased interest in this group of illnesses. Kuru is another transmissible spongiform encephalopathy that was spread in New Guinea by cannibalism, a practice that ceased in the 1950s. The disease is now almost extinct.

Sporadic Creutzfeldt-Jakob Disease

Epidemiology

Illness from sCJD is seen worldwide, with an incidence of 0.5 to 1.0 cases per 1 million people in the general population per year.

Clinical Manifestations

CJD is frequently diagnosed incorrectly initially. Prodromal symptoms include altered sleep patterns and appetite, weight loss, changes in sexual drive, and impaired memory and concentration. Disorientation, hallucinations, depression, and emotional lability are early signs, followed by a rapidly progressive dementia associated with myoclonus (about 90% of patients). Myoclonus is usually provoked by tactile, auditory, or visual startle stimuli. CJD has an abrupt onset in 10% to 15% of patients.

Other distinctive features include seizures, autonomic dysfunction, and lower motor neuron disease, suggesting amyotrophic lateral sclerosis. Cerebellar ataxia occurs in one third of patients.

Pathology

The pathologic hallmarks of CJD are spongiform or vacuolar changes in the brain without cellular inflammatory infiltrates. The pathogenic isoform of the prion protein can be demonstrated in brain tissue by immunocytochemical staining and by Western blot analysis. The fundamental process involved in human prion propagation is intercellular induction of protein misfolding and seeded aggregation of misfolded prion protein.

Diagnosis

The clinical tetrad supporting the diagnosis of CJD consists of a subacute progressive dementia, myoclonus, typical periodic complexes on electroencephalography, and normal CSF. FLAIR MRI sequences shows extensive curvilinear hyperintensity along the neocortex, called *cortical ribboning*, which affects frontal, parietal, and temporal lobes (in decreasing order of frequency). Routine CSF study is usually normal. A CSF test for the protein 14-3-3, which is released into spinal fluid when brain cells die, in the appropriate clinical context is highly specific and sensitive for CJD.

Treatment

No effective therapy exits. The disease is inexorably progressive. The median time to death from onset is 5 months, and 90% of patients with sporadic CJD die within 1 year.

Although the illness is not communicable in the conventional sense, a risk exists in handling material contaminated with the prion protein. Gloves should be worn when handling blood, CSF, and other body fluids. Instruments must be disinfected and sterilized appropriately.

For a deeper discussion of these topics, please see Chapter 412, "Meningitis: Bacterial, Viral, and Other"; Chapter 413, "Brain Abscess and Parameningeal Infections"; Chapter 414, "Acute Viral Encephalitis"; and Chapter 415, "Prion Diseases," in Goldman-Cecil Medicine, *25th Edition.*

SUGGESTED READINGS

Brouwer MC, Thwaites GE, Tunkel AR, et al: Dilemmas in the diagnosis of acute community-acquired bacterial meningitis, Lancet 380:1684–1692, 2012.

Carfrae MJ, Kesser BW: Malignant otitis externa, Otolaryngol Clin North Am 41:537–549, 2008.

Colby DW, Prusiner SB: Prions, Cold Spring Harb Perspect Biol 3:a006833, 2011.

Connor DE Jr, Chittiboina P, Caldito G, et al: Comparison of operative and nonoperative management of spinal epidural abscess: a retrospective review of clinical and laboratory predictors of neurological outcome, J Neurosurg Spine 19:119–127, 2013.

Glaser CS, Honarmand S, Anderson LJ, et al: Beyond viruses: clinical profiles and etiologies associated with encephalitis, Clin Infect Dis 43:1565–1577, 2006.

Solomon T, Michael BD, Smith PE, et al: Management of suspected viral encephalitis in adults—Association of British Neurologists and British Infection Association National Guidelines, J Infect 64:347–373, 2012.

Thigpen MC, Whitney CG, Messonnier NE, et al: Bacterial meningitis in the United States, 1998-2007, N Engl J Med 364:2016–2025, 2011.

Titulaer MJ, McCracken L, Gabilondo I, et al: Treatment and prognostic factors for long-term outcome in patients with anti-NMDA receptor encephalitis: an observational cohort study, Lancet Neurol 12:157–165, 2013.

Tunkel AR, Glaser CA, Block KC, et al: The management of encephalitis: clinical practice guidelines by the Infectious Diseases Society of America, Clin Infect Dis 47:303–327, 2008.

Tunkel AR, Hartman BJ, Kaplan SL, et al: Practice guidelines for the management of bacterial meningitis, Clin Infect Dis 39:1267–1284, 2004.

van de Beek D, Brouwer MC, Thwaites GE, et al: Advances in treatment of bacterial meningitis, Lancet 380:1693–1702, 2012.

van de Beek D, Drake JM, Tunkel AR: Nosocomial bacterial meningitis, N Engl J Med 362:146–154, 2010.

Venkatesan A, Tunkel AR, Bloch KC, et al: Case definitions, diagnostic algorithms, and priorities in encephalitis; consensus statement of the International Encephalitis Consortium, Clin Infect Dis 57:1114–1128, 2013.

Weisfelt M, van de Beek D, Spanjaard L, et al: Clinical features, complications, and outcome in adults with pneumococcal meningitis: a prospective case series, Lancet Neurol 5:123–129, 2006.

Infections of the Head and Neck

Edward J. Wing

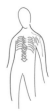

COMMON COLD

Definition and Epidemiology

The common cold is a syndrome of sore throat, rhinorrhea, and nasal congestion caused by viruses. Adults average two or three colds per year, and children have five to seven colds each year. The common cold accounts for 110 million visits to health care providers, an estimated 20 million lost work days, and at least $3 billion in expenses for medications. Viruses are transmitted most efficiently by direct contact, but aerosol transmission also occurs.

Pathogenesis and Microbiology

The pathogenesis varies with the pathogen. For example, rhinovirus has no histological effect on the mucosal epithelium, whereas influenza virus destroys it. The syndrome is caused by many viruses including rhinovirus (30% to 40%), influenza virus, parainfluenza virus, adenovirus, coronavirus, respiratory syncytial virus, enteroviruses and metapneumovirus. No organism can be identified in 25% to 30% of cases.

Clinical Presentation

Symptoms include an initial sore throat that develops into rhinorrhea, nasal congestion, sneezing, and cough after several days. Patients may also complain of fever, malaise, and hoarseness. The presence of myalgias may indicate influenza virus, whereas conjunctivitis may indicate adenovirus or enteroviruses. Symptoms peak from 3 to 6 days and last from 7 to 10 days, but viral shedding can occur 2 to 3 weeks after infection.

Laryngitis frequently accompanies the common cold. Patients complain of hoarseness, voice breaks or aphonia. Laryngitis typically lasts 3 days and is self limited. Unusual causes of laryngitis include group A streptococci, *Hemophilus influenzae*, *Corynebacterium diphtheriae*, *Mycobacterium tuberculosis*, and fungi.

Croup is a subglottic viral infection manifesting in children typically under 3 years of age. Patients present with a characteristic rough and stridulous cough and stridor on breathing. Diagnosis is clinical and treatment symptomatic.

Treatment

Treatment of the common cold is symptomatic; treatments include decongestants for nasal congestion, nonsteroidal anti-inflammatory drugs (NSAIDs) for fever and myalgia, lozenges for sore throat, and dextromethorphan for cough. Zinc and Echinacea have not been shown to be effective. There is also no convincing evidence supporting preventative measures. Viral laryngitis and croup are treated symptomatically; there is no evidence that antibiotics help.

For a deeper discussion of these topics, please see Chapter 361, "The Common Cold," in Goldman-Cecil Medicine, 25th Edition.

ACUTE BACTERIAL SINUSITIS

This section focuses on acute community-acquired bacterial sinusitis.

Definition and Epidemiology

Bacterial sinusitis is inflammation and bacterial infection of the paranasal sinuses. Bacterial sinusitis follows the common cold in 0.5% to 2.0% of cases in adults and in 6% to 13% of cases in children. Sinusitis accounts for 23 million health care visits each year and 20 million antibiotic prescriptions per year.

Pathogenesis

Sinusitis occurs when the sinus ostias narrow from inflammation, mucosal cilia become dysfunctional and disrupted, and mucus becomes viscous. The sinuses, which are normally sterile, become colonized with nasal bacteria and infection results. The major organisms identified by sinus puncture are *Streptococcus pneumoniae* and *H. influenzae* (Table 91-1); 30% to 40% of cultures are negative. Fungi cause a rare syndrome of rhinocerebral mucormycosis in diabetics.

Clinical Presentation

The symptoms and signs of acute bacterial sinusitis have a large overlap with the common cold. Table 91-2 shows the sensitivity and specificity of symptoms and signs in sinusitis. Nasal discharge/obstruction, facial pain, and maxillary toothache are suggestive. Physical findings of nasal discharge, facial pain, and pain on palpation of the sinuses are nonspecific and variable. Most important is that symptoms of the common cold peak between days 3 and 6 and resolve by day 10. Sinus infection occurs characteristically after 10 days of infection. There are three patterns of acute bacterial sinusitis: symptoms persisting for more than 10 days; severe symptoms, including fever and purulent nasal discharge over 3 to 4 days; and common cold symptoms that improve and then suddenly worsen.

Diagnosis

The diagnosis of acute bacterial sinusitis is most often made on clinical grounds as noted previously. Imaging can be helpful in situations in which the diagnosis is unclear or there are complications. Unfortunately, the common cold can also result in positive findings. Computed tomography (CT) is the procedure of choice if indicated.

TABLE 91-1   BACTERIAL CAUSE OF ACUTE SINUSITIS

| | ADULTS (*n* = 339) | | CHILDREN (*n* = 30) | |
ORGANISM	Number of Isolates	% of Isolates	Number of Isolates	% of Isolates
Streptococcus pneumoniae	92	41	17	41
Haemophilus influenza	79	35	11	27
Anaerobes	16	7		
Streptococcal species	16	7	3	7
Moraxella catarrhalis	8	4	9	22
Staphylococcus aureus	7	3		
Other	8	4	1	2

Mandell GL, Bennett JE, Dolin R, editors: Mandell, Douglas, and Bennett's principles and practice of infectious diseases, ed 7, Philadelphia, 2009, Churchill Livingstone.

TABLE 91-2   DAGNOSTIC SIGNS AND SYMPTOMS OF SINUSITIS

SYMPTOM OR SIGN	SENSITIVITY (%)	SPECIFICITY (%)	LIKELIHOOD RATIO
Maxillary toothache	18	93	2.5
No improvement with decongestants	41	80	2.1
Cough	70	44	1.3
Sore throat	52	56	1.2
Headache	68	30	1.0
Purulent secretion	51	76	2.1
Abnormal transillumination	73	54	1.6
Sinus tenderness	48	65	1.4
Fever	16	83	0.9

From Williams JW Jr, Simel DL, Roberts L, Samsa GP: Clinical evaluation for sinusitis: making the diagnosis by history and physical examination, Ann Intern Med 117:705–710, 1992.

Treatment

Acute bacterial sinusitis resolves spontaneously within 2 weeks without antibiotic therapy. Antibiotic therapy hastens the resolution of symptoms and is recommended by guidelines from the major national organizations of internists, pediatricians, allergists, and otolaryngologists. Careful review of randomized controlled trials as reported in the Cochrane Database Systemic Reviews, however, concludes that the risks of antibiotics outweigh the benefits in routine cases in adults. The antibiotics of choice are amoxicillin or amoxicillin and clavulinic acid given for 10 days. Macrolides, sulfamethoxazole-trimethoprim, and doxycycline may be less effective because common bacteria are developing resistance. Patients should respond within 48 to 72 hours. Intranasal saline irrigation has been shown to give symptomatic relief. Intranasal steroids may help individuals with underlying allergic rhinitis. There are no convincing data supporting use of antihistamines or α-adrenergic agonists. Surgery may be indicated for people with unresponsive sinusitis or those with intracranial or orbital complications.

Complications that are unusual include intracranial pathology such as subdural empyema, epidural abscess, brain abscess, meningitis and venous sinus thrombosis. Extracranial complications include orbital cellulitis, orbital abscess and subperiosteal abscess (Fig. 91-1). Immediate surgical intervention is indicated for orbital or intracranial abscesses. Refer to the Infectious Diseases Society of America guidelines for upper/respiratory tract infections for treat details.

⬤ PHARYNGITIS, STOMATITIS, LARYNGITIS, AND EPIGLOTITIS

Pharyngitis

Definition and Epidemiology

Pharyngitis or sore throat is mucous membrane inflammation localized to the posterior pharynx and contiguous membranes. Stomatitis, laryngitis, and epiglottitis are similar processes in the indicated locations. These infections are extremely common. In the acute care setting in the United States, for example, pharyngitis accounts for 7 million pediatric and 6 million adult visits each year. Peak incidence is typically in the winter months.

Etiology

Viruses cause 70% to 90% of cases of pharyngitis with rhinovirus being the most common. Adenovirus, which typically occurs in the late winter, is common in children less than 5 years of age and in young adults. Enteroviruses cause syndromes of herpangina (e.g., coxsackie group A); hand, foot, and mouth disease (e.g., coxsackie A16 and enterovirus 71); and nonspecific illnesses (e.g., group B coxsackie and echovirus). Herpes simplex virus causes pharyngitis and stomatitis in children and college students. Many other viruses cause pharyngitis, including Epstein-Barr virus, influenza virus, parainfluenza virus, and cytomegalovirus.

Group A streptococci (GAS) accounts for 10% to 30% of cases in children and 5% to 0% of cases in adults. In winter months up to 50% of cases may be due to GAS. Other bacterial causes, including group C and G streptococci and *Fusobacterium necrophorum*, are much less common. Noninfectious causes of pharyngitis include Beçhet's syndrome, Kawasaki disease, and aphthous stomatitis.

Clinical Presentation

The main job of clinicians is to distinguish GAS from viral pharyngitis. Typically, GAS presents with sudden onset of pain on swallowing, tender cervical lymph nodes and fever without cough and coryza. Viral etiologies may be accompanied by cough, coryza, and conjunctivitis (typically adenovirus). Scarlet fever consisting of a fine maculopapular rash like "sand paper" that desquamates and a strawberry tongue (prominent lingual papillae) indicates GAS. However, even experienced clinicians can distinguish viral from bacterial causes of pharyngitis only 50% of the time.

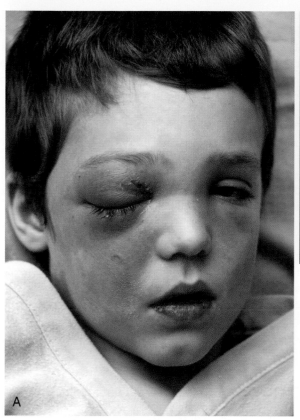

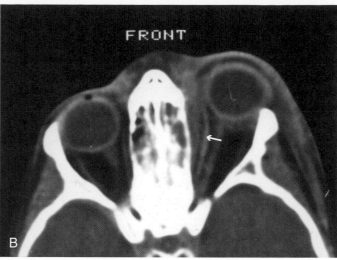

FIGURE 91-1 **A,** A child has an orbital abscess as a complication of ethmoid sinusitis. Notice the marked edema and proptosis. **B,** Computed tomography scan of the orbit shows a subperiosteal abscess *(arrow)*. (**A,** Courtesy Gary Williams, MD; **B,** From DeMuri GP, Wald ER: Sinusitis. In Bennett JE, Dolin R, Blaser M, editors: Mandell, Douglas, and Bennett's principles and practice of infectious diseases, ed 8, Philadelphia, 2015, Saunders.)

Complications include peritonsillar abscess or Quinsy that occur in adolescents and young adults. Patients appear ill and may have a muffled or "hot potato" voice and foul-smelling breath. The uvula may be displaced and there may be trismus and drooling. Less common complications include contiguous neck space infections. *F. necrophorum* can cause a rare syndrome called postangina septicemia or Lemierre's syndrome, which manifests with severe sore throat and fever. The lateral pharyngeal space becomes infected with resulting septic thrombophlebitis of the internal jugular vein. The mortality rate can be as high as 50%. Treatment is intravenous penicillin and drainage of any abscess. Table 91-3 lists the danger signs in patients with sore throat.

Diagnosis

Identifying GAS infection is important because treatment can prevent poststreptococcal complications including acute rheumatic fever, scarlet fever and peritonsillar abscess (i.e., quinsy). Rapid antigen detection tests for GAS are specific but only 66% to 90% sensitive. The diagnostic standard is a culture of a careful swab of the tonsils and pharynx. If clinical and epidemiological data suggest GAS, a rapid antigen detection test should be performed. If positive, the patient should be treated. If negative in children and adolescents, a culture should be done and if the culture is positive treatment is indicated. In adults, culture is not always necessary because the rate of complications is low and the incidence of a rheumatic fever is exceptionally low. Otherwise, symptomatic therapy is indicated.

Treatment

Treatment of viral pharyngitis is symptomatic; treatment of GAS pharyngitis is oral penicillin or amoxicillin for 10 days. For patients with a penicillin allergy, first generation cephalosporins

TABLE 91-3 SEVEN DANGER SIGNS IN PATIENTS WITH SORE THROAT

1. Persistence of symptoms longer than 1 week without improvement
2. Respiratory difficulty, particularly stridor
3. Difficulty in handling secretions
4. Difficulty in swallowing
5. Severe pain in the absence of erythema
6. A palpable mass
7. Blood, even small amounts, in the pharynx or ear

(non–life-threatening allergy), clindamycin or clarithromycin for 10 days, or azithromycin for 5 days are reasonable alternatives.

Oral Cavity Infections

Stomatitis

Many viruses can cause stomatitis (see Pharyngitis). In particular, herpes simplex virus causes stomatitis and is characterized by vesicles and moderate pain. Treatment of primary infection is with oral acyclovir or valcyclovir. Other viruses such as enteroviruses can also cause stomatitis.

Periodontal Infections

Periodontal infections include gingivitis, periodontitis (i.e., the major cause of tooth loss in adults), and periodontal abscess. Acute necrotizing ulcerative gingivitis or Vincent's angina is characterized by acute pain of the gingiva, a pseudomembrane, and halitosis. Débridement and antibiotics are indicated.

Neck Space Infections

Neck space infections usually result from dental caries. Dental infections can lead to neck space infections involving the lateral

pharyngeal space, the retropharyngeal space, and the submandibular and sublingual space (e.g., Ludwig's angina). These infections are medical emergencies and need to be dealt with surgically as well as with antibiotic treatment. Ludwig's angina is characterized by swelling in the submandibular space, an elevated tongue, and difficulty eating (Fig. 91-2). Treatment consists of surgical decompression and drainage and intravenous antibiotics. Table 91-4 lists neck space infections requiring drainage and decompression.

Aphthous Ulcers

Aphthous ulcers are shallow ulcerations typically lasting for several days to weeks located on the anterior structures of the mouth. The cause is unknown. Treatment is symptomatic except for individuals with extensive persistent disease in whom steroids or thalidomide may be indicated

Thrush

Thrush refers to superficial *Candida albicans* infection of the tongue, hard and soft palate, and pharynx, which results in a sore

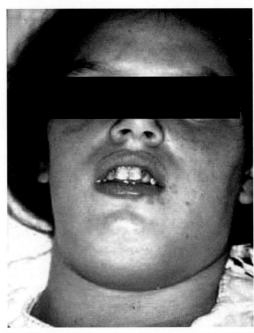

FIGURE 91-2 Early appearance of a patient with Ludwig's angina, who has a brawny, boardlike swelling in the submandibular spaces. (From Megran DW, Scheifele DW, Chow AW: Odontogenic infections, Pediatr Infect Dis 3:262, 1984.)

TABLE 91-4 PARAPHARYNGEAL SOFT TISSUE SPACE INFECTIONS AND INDICATIONS FOR SURGICAL DRAINAGE

INFECTION	INDICATIONS FOR SURGERY
Peritonsillar abscess (quinsy)	Abscess or respiratory compromise
Lateral pharyngeal space abscess	Abscess
Jugular vein septic thrombophlebitis	Febrile after 5-6 days of medical therapy
Retropharyngeal abscess	Abscess or respiratory compromise
Ludwig's angina	Abscess or respiratory compromise

mouth and oropharyngeal pain on swallowing. On inspection there are creamy white plaques on the tongue, hard and soft palates, and the pharynx. Patients who are immunocompromised secondary to corticosteroid treatment or underlying conditions such as HIV are susceptible. Treatment is typically topical antifungal agents or oral fluconazole for 5 to 7 days.

Bacterial Epiglottitis

Acute bacterial epiglottitis caused by *H. influenzae* was previously an uncommon but life-threatening illness of children under the age of 5. With widespread use of the *H. influenzae* vaccine in children, the incidence has decreased by 99% in children. More often, the disease occurs in adults in whom a variety of bacteria are responsible, including *S. pneumoniae, Staphylococcus aureus,* β-hemolytic streptococci, and *Klebsiella pneumoniae.* Patients typically present with fever and toxicity, drooling, dysphagia, and holding the head extended. Speaking is painful and the laryngeal tracheal area is very tender. Examination may reveal a cherry red visible epiglottitis. Coordinated care, if necessary in the OR, is critical to maintain the airway. Broad-spectrum antibiotics are indicated. Steroids are commonly used but data are lacking to support their use.

● ACUTE BACTERIAL OTITIS EXTERNA AND MEDIA
Acute Bacterial Otitis Externa

Acute localized otitis externa is a superficial infection of the outer portion of the ear canal usually related to furunculosis caused by *S. aureus.* It can be treated with oral anti-staphylococcal antibiotics. Acute diffuse otitis externa (i.e., swimmer's ear) begins with itching and progresses to moderate/severe pain on manipulation of the pinna or tragus. The canal is erythematous and swollen. The usual organism is *Pseudomonas aeruginosa.* Treatment consists of acetic acid and alcohol lavage with or without topical antibiotics such as ciprofloxacin or neomycin plus polymyxin.

Malignant otitis externa is a rare infection usually found in elderly diabetic patients that progresses over weeks to months. It is characterized by deep seated pain, otorrhea and granulation tissue on the posterior inferior wall of the external canal. CT scan is the initial imaging modality of choice. The infection can progress to skull-based osteomyelitis and meningitis and has a significant mortality. Treatment is surgical débridement and antipseudomonal systemic therapy.

Acute Bacterial Otitis Media
Definition and Epidemiology

Acute bacterial otitis media is an acute bacterial infection of the middle ear. Almost all children have at least one episode of otitis media in the first 10 years of life, making it the most common bacterial infection seen in children. It accounts for one fourth of all office visits and is the second most common reason for surgical procedures in children (the most common is circumcision). It appears that about one third of children are prone to infection and have multiple episodes, another third have intermediate susceptibility, whereas another third will be relatively resistant.

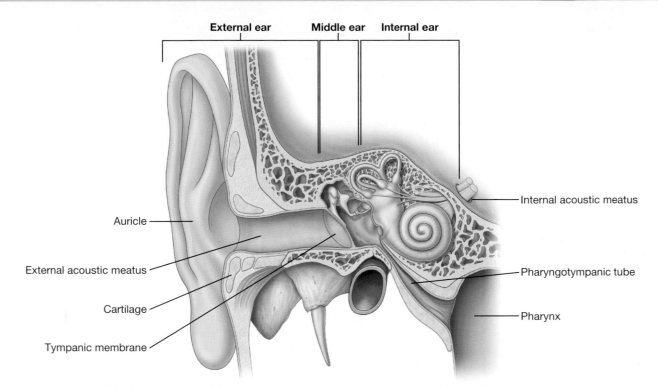

FIGURE 91-3 Eustachian tube. (From Drake RL: Gray's basic anatomy, Philadelphia, 2012, Elsevier, pp 413–592.)

Pathogenesis

While the disease in adults mimics that in children, children are more susceptible because their Eustachian tubes are shorter and more horizontal (Fig. 91-3). Disease typically results from Eustachian tube blockage and dysfunction that occurs during viral infection. Bacteria colonize the middle ear and cannot be eliminated. The most common causative bacteria are *S. pneumoniae,* nontypable *H. influenzae,* and *Moraxella catarrhalis.*

Clinical Presentation

Acute bacterial otitis media presents with ear pain in over two thirds of patients. The diagnosis can be difficult in young children because the history may be absent or inaccurate. Physical diagnosis typically shows middle ear effusion and an abnormal tympanic membrane that is red and bulging or retracted. Movement of the membrane is limited on application of positive or negative pressure. Perforation, drainage, fever and decreased hearing may occur. Patients may also have vertigo, tinnitus, and nystagmus. The course of otitis media is usually self-limited with most cases resolves within one week.

Treatment

Treatment has been controversial because for most patients otitis media is a self-limited disease. Studies suffer from the difficulty in making an accurate diagnosis and lack of placebo controls. Overuse of antibiotics has resulted in the development of resistant organisms in the United States, complicating treatment of respiratory infections. Antibiotics shorten the course of the disease and may prevent complications such as mastoiditis, facial palsy, brain abscess, epidural abscess and cholesteatoma, although convincing data are lacking because the incidence of these complications has decreased in all patient populations.

Guidelines recommend the use of antibiotics in otitis media, particularly for patients at high risk, for patients in whom there is complicated disease, or when pain relief is important. The failure rate with antibiotics is less. The concerns about antibiotic resistance, however, have made withholding antibiotics and closely observing the patient a reasonable option. A Cochrane review of antibiotics for sore throat, acute otitis media, bronchitis, and the common cold concluded that antibiotics could be delayed if clinicians felt it safe. If symptoms worsen or persist over 48 to 72 hours, then antibiotics should be initiated.

S. pneumoniae, H. influenzae, and *M. catarrhalis* have each shown significant resistance to penicillin in resistant years. Despite these increased rates, amoxicillin or amoxicillin/clavulinic acid continue to be the drugs of choice. Alternative choices include cephalosporins or macrolide antibiotics. If there is no improvement after three days, switching antibiotics should be considered.

Serous otitis media refers to fluid in the ear in the absence of signs or symptoms of infection. This is usually self-limited and resolves in 2 to 4 weeks. Persistent fluid for greater than 3 months associated with hearing loss, however, is an indication for tube placement.

SUGGESTED READINGS

Carfrae MJ, Kesser BM: Malignant otitis externa, Otolaryngol Clin North Am 41:537–549, 2008.

Lemiengre MB, van Driel ML, Merenstein D, et al: Antibiotics for clinically diagnosed acute rhinosinusitis in adults, Cochrane Database Syst Rev 10:CD006089, 2012.

Shulman ST, Bisno AL, Clegg HW, et al: Clinical practice guideline for the diagnosis and management of group A streptococcal pharyngitis: 2012 update by the Infectious Diseases Society of America, Clin Infect Dis 55:1279–1282, 2012.

Spurling GK, Del Mar CB, Dooley L, et al: Delayed antibiotics for respiratory infections, Cochrane Database Syst Rev (4):CD004417, 2013.

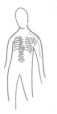

92

Infections of the Lower Respiratory Tract

John R. Lonks

DEFINITION AND EPIDEMIOLOGY

Pneumonia, which is inflammation of the lung parenchyma, is usually caused by an acute infection. When the disease onset occurs outside of the hospital, it is referred to as *community-acquired* pneumonia. It ranges in severity from a mild, self-limited disease to one that is fatal. Community-acquired pneumonia is common, and most patients with pneumonia are treated in the outpatient setting.

Pneumonia is one of the most common reasons for hospitalization among all age groups and accounts for approximately 1 million hospitalizations per year. Each year, approximately 50,000 people in the United States die of influenza and pneumonia. Influenza or pneumonia is the leading cause of death due to infection and the ninth most common cause of death overall.

Numerous microorganisms cause pneumonia, including bacteria, viruses, mycobacteria, and fungi. These agents range from microorganisms that are part of the normal flora to exogenous microorganisms that are inhaled. Noninfectious diseases can mimic pneumonia. The incidence of pneumonia is lowest during early adulthood and increases with each decade of life (Fig. 92-1).

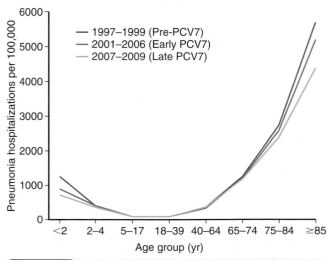

FIGURE 92-1 Rate of hospitalization for pneumonia by age group. PCV7, 7-valent pneumococcal conjugate vaccine. (From Griffin MR, Zhu Y, Moore MR, et al: U.S. hospitalizations for pneumonia after a decade of pneumococcal vaccination, N Engl J Med 369:155–163, 2013.)

PATHOLOGY

Bacterial pneumonia usually causes lobar pneumonia, which is consolidation of an entire lobe or a large portion of a lobe, or bronchopneumonia, which is patchy consolidation of the lung. Pneumococcal lobar pneumonia has four stages of the inflammatory response: consolidation, red hepatization, gray hepatization, and resolution. The initial congestion is characterized by fluid, with some neutrophils and bacteria, filling the alveoli. Red hepatization is characterized by red blood cells along with numerous neutrophils and fibrin filling the alveoli. With gray hepatization, there is breakdown of red blood cells and persistence of fibrin and neutrophils. The consolidated exudate within the alveolar spaces then undergoes resolution.

Pathophysiology

The lower respiratory tract is virtually sterile. Normal host defenses that protect against pneumonia include mucus production and cilia; in combination, they form the mucociliary escalator.

Impairment of host defenses leads to increased risk of pneumonia. Loss or suppression of the cough reflex due to stroke and other neurologic diseases, drugs, and alcohol increases the risk of developing pneumonia, as do aging and associated medical illnesses.

Environmental factors such as smoking and respiratory irritants impair ciliary function and increase the risk of developing pneumonia. Mechanical obstruction of an airway by a tumor or foreign body leads to decreased clearance of microorganisms and may produce postobstructive pneumonia. In addition to mechanical clearance, innate host defenses such as phagocytes and antibodies are essential after microorganisms reach the alveoli. Alveolar macrophages and other components of innate immunity are the first line of defense. Subsequently, opsonizing antibodies and neutrophils play an essential role. Impairment of these host defenses (e.g., alveolar macrophages by silica exposure, neutrophils by chemotherapy, antibodies by hypogammaglobulinemia) increases susceptibility to pneumonia. Those infected with human immunodeficiency virus (HIV) are at increased risk for pneumococcal pneumonia.

The two main mechanisms of entry of microorganism into the lung are microaspiration of organisms that colonize the upper respiratory tract and inhalation of airborne particles that contain a pathogenic microorganism. When a sufficient inoculum enters the lung and normal host defenses are not able to clear the inoculum; bacterial replication leads to a lower respiratory tract infection.

Transmission of Respiratory Pathogens

Some pathogens are transmitted from person to person by droplet transmission. Droplets are created when a person coughs, sneezes, or talks. Transmission can occur during medical procedures such as suctioning, endotracheal intubation, cardiopulmonary resuscitation, or cough-producing procedures. The greatest distance of transmission is unresolved. Historically, a distance of 3 feet or less was assumed for person-to-person droplet transmission. Some data suggest that transmission may occur from as far away as 6 feet. Respiratory droplets have also been defined by their size, usually greater than 5 μm in diameter.

Crowding, as occurs in prisons, barracks, and shelters, is associated with increased spread. Pathogens that are transmitted by the droplet route include *Streptococcus pneumoniae*, *Mycoplasma pneumoniae*, and influenza virus.

Infectious agents such as *Mycobacterium tuberculosis*, fungi, and anthrax spores are airborne. Microorganisms transmitted in this fashion can be spread over long distances (>6 feet) by air currents and normal airflow. The size of the droplet nuclei particles that are transmitted by the airborne route are usually 5 μm or less in diameter.

Etiologic Agents

Many bacteria and viruses cause pneumonia. *S. pneumoniae* (i.e., pneumococcus) is the most common, and the classic description of pneumonia is based on disease caused by pneumococci. Most cases of pneumococcal pneumonia occur between December and April. Pneumococci transiently colonize the upper respiratory tract. Microaspiration leads to entry into the lower respiratory tract. If aspirated in sufficient quantity so that normal host defenses do not clear the bacteria, the patient develops pneumonia. Pneumococci have a polysaccharide capsule that prevents phagocytosis. Antibodies against the polysaccharide capsule, which are acquired from prior exposure or vaccination, opsonize pneumococci, enabling phagocytosis.

Other bacteria that can colonize the oropharynx and cause pneumonia when aspirated include *Haemophilus influenzae*, less commonly *Staphylococcus aureus*, and rarely *Streptococcus pyogenes* (i.e., group A β-hemolytic streptococcal infection). Similarly, *Moraxella catarrhalis* in patients with chronic obstructive pulmonary disease and in the elderly and *Klebsiella pneumoniae* in alcoholics colonize the oropharynx and cause pneumonia. Most cases of community-acquired pneumonia are monomicrobial.

Patients with pneumococcal pneumonia can develop infections at other sites, including empyema, pericarditis, meningitis, endocarditis, and septic arthritis. Approximately one of five patients with pneumococcal pneumonia has bacteremia.

M. pneumoniae usually causes milder disease. Its peak incidence is during the first 2 decades of life. Patients usually do not require hospitalization, but some develop severe disease.

Chlamydophila pneumoniae (formerly called *Chlamydia pneumoniae*) is a common cause of community-acquired pneumonia. It usually causes a milder disease and is seen more commonly among patients treated in the outpatient setting.

Legionella, an environmental organism, can cause pneumonia. *Legionella pneumophila* is the most common species of pneumonia, but *Legionella micdadei* and *Legionella bozemanii* can also cause pneumonia. Most cases are sporadic. Outbreaks have occurred from contaminated point sources such as cooling towers and air conditioning units. Transmission usually occurs through inhalation of aerosol particles; microaspiration of water containing *Legionella* has also occurred.

Infrequently, *S. aureus* causes bacterial pneumonia, sometimes as a complication of influenza infection. Community-acquired methicillin-resistant strains (MRSA) have caused secondary bacterial pneumonias.

Viruses, particularly influenza viruses, cause a minority of pneumonias in adults. Patients with influenza are at risk for secondary bacterial pneumonia, most commonly due to *S. pneumoniae*, *H. influenzae*, or *S. aureus*. Respiratory syncytial virus (RSV), a pathogen that usually infects children, has been found more frequently as a cause of pneumonia among the elderly. Adenovirus rarely causes pneumonia in young adults. During 2003, the severe acute respiratory syndrome (SARS) virus emerged in Guangdong Province in southern China, and after initial international spread, it was contained. In 2012, the Middle East respiratory syndrome coronavirus (MERS-CoV) emerged as a cause of severe pneumonia. Most cases occurred in the Middle East.

Viruses such as the influenza viruses predispose patients to secondary bacterial pneumonia. Influenza infection may damage the respiratory epithelium, and resulting dysfunctional innate immune responses enhance susceptibility to secondary bacterial infection.

Fungi that cause pneumonia are not part of the normal flora. Certain dimorphic fungi (e.g., *Histoplasma capsulatum*, *Blastomyces dermatitidis*, and *Coccidioides immitis*) that reside in the soil cause pneumonia when they are inhaled. Dimorphic fungi form hyphae at ambient temperatures and yeasts at body temperature. The hyphal form is the transmissible form of the fungus. The yeast form is not transmissible from person to person.

These fungi are limited to certain geographic areas: *H. capsulatum* in the Mississippi, Missouri, and Ohio River valleys; *B. dermatitidis* in Southern states bordering the Mississippi and Ohio River basins and Midwestern states bordering the great lakes; and *C. immitis* in the Southwestern United States. *H. capsulatum*, *B. dermatitidis*, and *C. immitis* cause disease in the normal host. *Aspergillus*, a mold, is ubiquitous in the environment; it rarely causes disease in the immunocompetent host. Patients who are immunocompromised or have abnormal airways are at risk for infection with *Aspergillus* but rarely with other molds such as *Zygomycetes* species (Mucorales order), which do have a predisposition for infecting patients with diabetes mellitus.

M. tuberculosis is not part of the normal flora. It is transmitted by small aerosol particles (<5 μm) that are inhaled directly into the alveolus. *M. tuberculosis* is a slow-growing organism that usually causes chronic symptoms; however, it rarely can manifest acutely. Patients with HIV infection, those treated with biologic agents such as tumor necrosis factor (TNF) inhibitors, and the very young and old are particularly susceptible.

The normal flora of an acutely ill hospitalized patient is different from that of a healthy outpatient. Hospitalized patients are more frequently colonized with *S. aureus,* including methicillin-resistant strains, and gram-negative bacilli, including *Pseudomonas aeruginosa.* When a hospitalized patient aspirates his or her oropharyngeal flora, it may contain one of these organisms. Microorganisms that almost never cause pneumonia include *Candida* species and enterococci.

For a deeper discussion of these topics, please see Chapter 9, "Overview of Pneumonia," in Goldman-Cecil Medicine, 25th Edition.

CLINICAL PRESENTATION

Patients with pneumonia usually have an acute onset of fever, chills, cough, sputum production, dyspnea, and sometimes pleuritic chest pain. Patients may produce blood-tinged sputum that appears rust colored, a classic sign of pneumonia due to *S. pneumoniae.* Extrapulmonary signs and symptoms may include nausea, vomiting, diarrhea, abdominal pain, headache, confusion, arthralgia, myalgias, and change in mental status. Signs and symptoms can be blunted or absent in the elderly. Rales or rhonchi may be heard on auscultation of the chest. A leukocytosis with a left shift (i.e., increased band forms), pulmonary signs and symptoms, and a new infiltrate seen on the chest radiograph are used to diagnose pneumonia.

DIAGNOSIS AND DIFFERENTIAL DIAGNOSIS

When pneumonia is suspected, the next step is to determine the etiologic diagnosis. Unfortunately, there is no single diagnostic test with a high sensitivity and high specificity. The sputum Gram stain provides useful diagnostic information. Although epithelial cells from the upper respiratory tract and oropharyngeal flora may contaminate an expectorated sputum sample, careful examination of the sputum Gram stain can reveal an area of the specimen that originated from the lower respiratory tract and contains neutrophils, and examination for bacteria in that area can be helpful. However, some patients do not produce sputum, and prior antibiotic use can alter sputum results.

S. pneumoniae is a gram-positive coccus that forms pairs and chains; the cocci are sometimes pointed at one end (i.e., lancet shaped). *H. influenzae* is a pleomorphic gram-negative rod. *S. aureus* is a gram-positive coccus that forms "grape-like" clusters. *M. catarrhalis* is gram-negative diplococcus. These distinct morphologic features allow a presumptive diagnosis of a specific etiologic agent when seen on a Gram stain of sputum (Fig. 92-2).

Mycoplasma, Legionella, Mycobacterium, and *Chlamydophila* species are not seen on the sputum Gram stain. *Mycobacteria* are seen with special acid-fast staining.

Culture of sputum can reveal the etiologic diagnosis, and results should be correlated with findings from the sputum Gram stain. However, pneumococci are fastidious. A study of patients with bacteremic pneumococcal pneumonia found that only 55% of sputum cultures grew pneumococci. *Mycoplasma* species, *Legionella* species, *Mycobacterium* species, and *C. pneumoniae* do not grow on routine agar. Special culture media are required for certain bacteria, such as Löwenstein-Jensen medium for

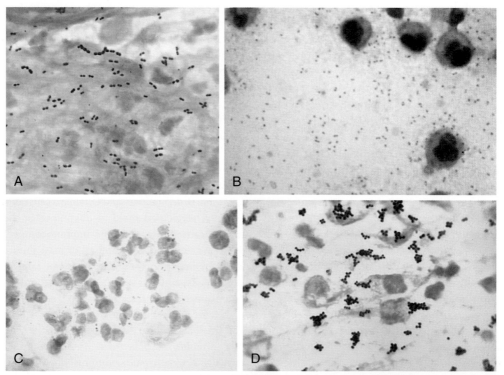

FIGURE 92-2 Sputum Gram stain. **A,** *Streptococcus pneumoniae.* **B,** *Haemophilus influenzae.* **C,** *Moraxella catarrhalis.* **D,** *Staphylococcus aureus.* PCV7, 7-Valent pneumococcal conjugate vaccine. (**A,** From Murray PR: Medical microbiology, ed 7, Philadelphia, 2013, Elsevier; **B,** From de la Maza LM, Pezzlo MT, Shigei JT, Peterson EM: Color atlas of medical bacteriology, Washington, D.C. 2004, ASM Press; **C,** From Ferri F: Ferri's color atlas and text of clinical medicine, Philadelphia, 2009, Elsevier; **D,** From Donowitz GR: Acute pneumonia. In Mandell GL, Bennett JE, Dolin R, editors: Mandell, Douglas, and Bennett's principles and practice of infectious diseases, ed 8, Philadelphia, 2015, Churchill Livingstone.)

Mycobacteria and buffered charcoal yeast extract (BCYE) for *Legionella*.

Blood cultures can be helpful. However, the ratio of bacteremic to nonbacteremic pneumococcal pneumonia is approximately 1 : 4. A positive blood culture is very helpful because the etiologic agent is definitely identified and susceptibility data are available to determine appropriate therapy.

Other diagnostic studies used to identify the causative organism include *Legionella* urinary antigen, *Histoplasma* urinary antigen, polymerase chain reaction (PCR) for respiratory viruses, and serologic testing for *Mycoplasma* and *C. immitis*.

Chest radiography of patients with pneumococcal pneumonia can show a consolidative lobar infiltrate or a bronchopneumonic (patchy) pattern; less commonly, it causes an interstitial pattern. A definitive etiologic diagnosis cannot be made based on the chest radiographic appearance.

Not all patients with a new pulmonary infiltrate have pneumonia. Congestive heart failure is commonly confused with pneumonia. Noninfectious causes of pulmonary infiltrates and fever include pulmonary infarction, granulomatosis with polyangiitis (i.e., Wegener's granulomatosis), drug reactions, tumor, cryptogenic organizing pneumonia, hypersensitivity pneumonitis, collagen vascular disease, and acute respiratory distress syndrome (ARDS).

TREATMENT

The definitive treatment for pneumonia is to eradicate the infecting microorganism. Antibiotics are used to kill bacteria and decrease or stop the spread of infection in the lungs. Normal host responses are needed to repair the inflammatory damage in the lungs.

Penicillin therapy has reduced the mortality rate of bacteremic pneumococcal pneumonia from 84% to 17%. However, antibiotics have little to no effect on the mortality rate during the first 5 days of illness.

After the etiologic agent has been identified, the appropriate antibiotic can be given (Table 92-1). If a specific etiologic diagnosis is not made, empirical treatment with one of many antimicrobial agents is recommended. Guidelines are available at http://www.idsociety.org/IDSA_Practice_Guidelines (accessed November 1, 2014).

The decision to admit a patient with pneumonia is based on clinical prediction rules. The pneumonia severity index (PSI) stratifies patients into one of five risk groups. Those in a low-risk group are treated as outpatients, whereas those in a higher-risk group are admitted to the hospital for treatment. The CURB-65 score (*c*onfusion, *u*rea, *r*espiratory rate, *b*lood pressure, and *age* ≥65 years) developed by Lim and colleagues is easier to calculate but has not been as rigorously validated as the PSI. Psychosocial and other factors that affect the decision to admit a patient are not included in the PSI or CURB-65.

> For a deeper discussion of these topics, please see Chapter 9, "Overview of Pneumonia," in Goldman-Cecil Medicine, 25th Edition.

PROGNOSIS AND PREVENTION

Patients with bacteremic pneumococcal pneumonia have a higher mortality rate (21%) compared with those who have nonbacteremic pneumococcal pneumonia (13%). Among patients with bacteremic pneumococcal pneumonia, the mortality rate increases with advancing age (Fig. 92-3), number of lobes involved (i.e., one lobe, 12%; two lobes, 24%; and three lobes, 63%), and white blood cell (WBC) count (i.e., leukopenia, 35%; normal peripheral WBC count, 24%; and leukocytosis, 14%). Mortality rates are different for each capsular type of pneumococcus. For example the mortality rate for patients infected with capsular type I is 3%, compared with 22% for patients infected with capsular type III. Patients who survive usually recover without sequelae.

The influenza vaccine protects against not only influenza but also bacterial pneumonia, because patients who do not have influenza are not at risk for secondary bacterial pneumonia. The 13-valent pneumococcal conjugate vaccine followed 6 to 12 months later by the 23-valent pneumococcal polysaccharide vaccine is recommended for those 65 years of age and older who have not been previously vaccinated. Adults less than 65 years with certain immunocompromising conditions or

TABLE 92-1	TREATMENT OF PNEUMONIA BY SPECIFIC ETIOLOGIC AGENT	
ETIOLOGIC AGENT	**PREFERRED ANTIMICROBIAL**	**ALTERNATIVE ANTIMICROBIAL**
Streptococcus pneumoniae	Penicillin	Cephalosporin, moxifloxacin, levofloxacin
Haemophilus influenzae	Cefuroxime, ceftriaxone	
Mycoplasma pneumoniae	Macrolide	Moxifloxacin, levofloxacin
Legionella species	Macrolide or quinolone	
Methicillin-susceptible *Staphylococcus aureus*	Nafcillin	Cephalosporin
Methicillin-resistant *Staphylococcus aureus*	Vancomycin (intravenous)	Sulfamethoxazole-trimethoprim (oral) or doxycycline
Moraxella catarrhalis	Amoxicillin/clavulanate, cefuroxime, ceftriaxone, sulfamethoxazole-trimethoprim	

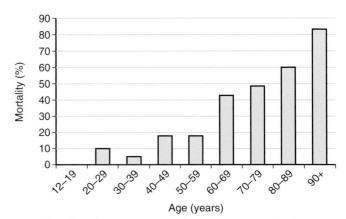

FIGURE 92-3 Mortality rates for bacteremic pneumococcal pneumonia by age group. (Data from Austrian R, Gold J: Pneumococcal bacteremia with especial reference to bacteremic pneumococcal pneumonia, Ann Intern Med 60:759–776, 1964.)

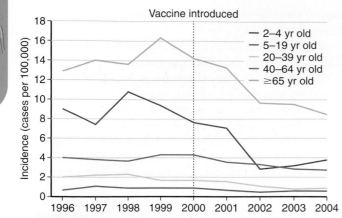

FIGURE 92-4 Incidence of penicillin-resistant pneumococcal infection from before and after the introduction of the pneumococcal conjugate vaccine for different age groups. (From Kyaw MH, Lynfield R, Schaffner W, Schaffner W, et al: Effect of introduction of the pneumococcal conjugate vaccine on drug-resistant Streptococcus pneumoniae, N Engl J Med 354:1455–1463, 2006.)

(Fig. 92-4). Use of the pediatric conjugate vaccine has reduced the number of adult hospital admissions for pneumonia (see Fig. 92-1). It also has decreased antibiotic resistance because the capsular types of pneumococci that are more likely to be antibiotic resistant are included in the vaccine.

specific underling medical conditions that put them at a higher risk of pneumococcal infections should also be vaccinated. The conjugate pneumococcal vaccine has reduced invasive pneumococcal disease in children, and decreased carriage in children has reduced transmission and subsequent disease in adults

SUGGESTED READINGS

Austrian R, Gold J: Pneumococcal bacteremia with especial reference to bacteremic pneumococcal pneumonia, Ann Intern Med 60:759–776, 1964.

Fine M, Auble T, Yealy D: A prediction rule to identify low-risk patients with community acquired pneumonia, N Engl J Med 336:243–250, 1997.

Griffin M, Zhu Y, Moore M: U.S. hospitalizations for pneumonia after a decade of pneumococcal vaccination, N Engl J Med 369:155–163, 2013.

Kyaw M, Lynfield R, Schaffner W, et al: Effect of introduction of the pneumococcal conjugate vaccine on drug-resistant *Streptococcus* pneumonia, N Engl J Med 354:1455–63, 2006.

Lim WS, Van der Eerden MM, Laing R: Defining community acquired pneumonia severity on presentation to hospital: an international derivation and validation study, Thorax 58:377–382, 2003.

Mandell L, Wunderink R, Anzueto A: Infectious Diseases Society of America/American Thoracic Society consensus guidelines on the management of community-acquired pneumonia in adults, Clin Infect Dis 44:S27–S72, 2007.

Tomczyk S, Bennett NM, Stoecker C, et al: Use of 13-valent pneumococcal conjugate vaccine and 23-valent pneumococcal polysaccharide vaccine among adults aged ≥65 years: recommendations of the Advisory Committee on Immunization Practices (ACIP), MMWR Morb Mortal Wkly Rep 63(37): 822–825, 2014.

93

Infections of the Heart and Blood Vessels

Cheston B. Cunha and Eleftherios Mylonakis

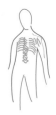

INFECTIVE ENDOCARDITIS

Definition

Infective endocarditis (IE) is an infection of the endocardium of one or more cardiac valves or, less commonly, the mural endocardium. The pathologic lesion of IE is the vegetation (infected platelet and fibrin thrombus). The pathologic findings of IE were first described in 1646 by Lazare Rivière, a French physician at the University of Montpellier. At autopsy, Rivière described "small round outgrowths resembling the lungs in texture, the largest of which was about the size of a hazelnut, which blocked the aortic valve." The term *endocarditis* was first used in 1835 by the French physician Jean-Baptiste Bouillaud, but it was not until the 1880s that Sir William Osler was able to synthesize many of the prior clinical, pathologic, and microbiologic findings into a unified description of the disease.

Over the past 6 decades, the epidemiology, risk factors, and treatment of endocarditis have changed significantly. In the preantibiotic era, IE was uniformly fatal. Since the advent of antibiotics and valve replacement surgery, IE can be effectively treated and mortality can be significantly reduced, provided the diagnosis is made early. Despite progress, new challenges continue to arise in diagnosis and treatment. As more patients undergo intravascular manipulation, have intracardiac or intravascular devices placed, and harbor more resistant organisms, effective therapy for IE remains a challenge.

Traditionally, IE has been classified, based on the acuteness of onset, as subacute bacterial endocarditis (SBE) or acute bacterial endocarditis (ABE). This classification reflects the virulence of the causative agent: *Staphylococcus aureus* is a common cause of ABE, whereas low-virulence organisms such as viridans streptococci are more likely to be the cause of SBE. IE may also be subdivided according to the nature of the involved valve, as native valve endocarditis (NVE) or prosthetic valve endocarditis (PVE), or by the number of valves involved (multivalvular IE). Some hosts, particularly intravenous drug abusers, are predisposed to IE. IE from invasive procedures is classified as health care–associated IE or nosocomial IE. Endocarditis may be further divided according to the causative organism. These categories are often combined (e.g., *S. aureus* tricuspid valve nosocomial ABE).

Epidemiology

SBE is most common in older adults, and over the last 50 years, the average age of patients diagnosed with IE has gradually increased. More than one half of all cases of IE occur in patients older than 50 years of age. Rheumatic heart disease has decreased in the modern era and is now a less common predisposing factor.

Recent estimates are that the overall annual incidence of IE in the United States is 12.7 cases per 100,000 persons, a significant increase from prior years. The age-adjusted hospital admission rate has increased by 2.4% annually, mirroring this increase in incidence. SBE usually involves the mitral valve or, less commonly, the aortic valve. IE of the pulmonic valve is relatively rare, and right-sided ABE occurs primarily in intravenous drug abusers. Individuals with congenital heart disease may be predisposed to IE, depending on the lesion.

Pathogenesis

Normal cardiac endothelium is relatively resistant to bacterial invasion. If the cardiac endothelium is damaged, an uninfected platelet and fibrin thrombus may form. This nonbacterial thrombotic endocarditis may become infected due to bacteremia, forming a vegetation. Endothelial damage may result from degenerative valvular disease, rheumatic heart disease, congenital heart disease, or intracardiac instrumentation or devices.

Predisposing Cardiac Factors

Approximately 15% of patients diagnosed with NVE have underlying congenital heart disease. Of these diseases, tetralogy of Fallot has the highest IE potential. Other lesions that predispose to IE include ventricular septal defect, bicuspid valves, and coarctation of the aorta. Significant mitral valve regurgitation is the most important predisposing factor for IE, with mitral valve prolapse accounting for 20% of NVE cases. Degenerative valvular disease predisposes to SBE in the elderly, and the mitral valve is most frequently involved. Aortic valve IE is rare in hypertrophic cardiomyopathy or asymmetric septal hypertrophy.

Noncardiac Predisposing Factors

Central venous catheters and intracardiac devices can cause endocardial injury, predisposing to IE. The most frequent nosocomial IE pathogens are *S. aureus*, coagulase-negative staphylococci, group D enterococci, and aerobic gram-negative bacilli. Infections with these organisms usually occur less than 1 month after the procedure. Nosocomial IE may affect normal or abnormal valves. Because ABE pathogens are more virulent, nosocomial IE is associated with a high mortality rate.

Low-virulence and noninvasive organisms (e.g., viridans streptococci) are the most common SBE pathogens. The SBE potential of viridans streptococci is directly related to the thickness of the capsule, which permits adherence to damaged cardiac valves. Viridans streptococci are normal inhabitants of the mouth and gastrointestinal tract. Invasive dental procedures frequently cause transient bacteremias that may result in SBE on damaged but not normal cardiac valves. Transient bacteremias of viridans streptococci may form a vegetation in the sterile platelet and fibrin thrombus covering an area of damaged endothelium. The gastrointestinal or genitourinary tract is the usual source of bacteremia in cases of native valve SBE due to group D enterococci.

Diagnosis

Clinical Features

The cardinal clinical features of IE are fever (90% of cases) and heart murmur (85%). In the antibiotic era, fever may not be present if the patient has been taking antibiotics for another reason. SBE often manifests with sweats, malaise, and anorexia. The course of SBE tends to be more indolent and may be accompanied by back pain, joint pains (>50% of patients), or embolic stroke. As SBE progresses, circulating immune complexes may deposit in the kidney, causing interstitial nephritis, glomerulonephritis, and even renal failure. Osler's nodes (painful, subcutaneous nodules on the distal pads of the fingers or toes), Janeway's lesions (hemorrhagic, nonpainful macules on the palms and soles) and Roth's spots (retinal hemorrhages with small central clearing) are classic findings related to microemboli and SBE immune-mediated vasculitis.

Patients with ABE tend to have a more fulminant course because of the greater virulence of the pathogen. The fever of ABE is usually high (>102° F) and is often accompanied by rigors. If there is mechanical dysfunction of the valve, symptoms of congestive heart failure will predominate. Often, a presenting feature of right-sided ABE is septic pulmonary emboli with pleuritic chest pain. The clinical findings of SBE and ABE are presented in Table 93-1.

Clinically, PVE may be considered as early (<2 months after implantation of the valve) or late (>2 months). Early PVE is caused by virulent pathogens (e.g., S. aureus) that infect the prosthetic valve before endothelialization is complete. Endothelialization of a mechanical valve is partially protective against transient bacteremias in late PVE. Over time, bioprosthetic valves have the same IE potential as mechanical ones.

An otherwise unexplained high-grade or continuous bacteremia and murmur should suggest IE. An acute versus subacute presentation correlates with the virulence of the IE pathogen. If blood cultures are negative, a diagnosis of infectious culture-negative endocarditis (CNE) should be considered if a murmur, vegetation, and peripheral manifestations of IE are present. The clinical diagnosis of IE relies on a combination of clinical, laboratory, and echocardiographic findings. Epidemiologic clues to the potential IE pathogens are outlined in Table 93-2. The most important finding in IE is the demonstration of continuous bacteremia, usually by multiple positive blood cultures. Table 93-3 contains the modified Duke criteria that are frequently used to predict the likelihood that a patient has IE.

TABLE 93-1 CLINICAL FINDINGS FOR SUBACUTE BACTERIAL ENDOCARDITIS (SBE) AND ACUTE BACTERIAL ENDOCARDITIS (ABE)

SYMPTOMS AND FINDINGS*	ABE	SBE
Anorexia	−	+
Weight loss	−	±
Myalgias or arthralgias	+	±
Fatigue	−	+
Dyspnea	+	−
Pleuritic chest pain†	+	−
Low back pain	+	+
Headache	+	±
Mental status changes	+	±
Acute confusion	+	−
Cerebrovascular accident	−	+
Sudden unilateral blindness	−	+
Left upper quadrant pain	Splenic abscess	Splenic infarct
Fever	>102° F‡	<102° F
New or changing heart murmur	±	−
Splenomegaly	−	+
Petechiae	+	+
Osler's nodes	−	+
Janeway's lesions	+	−
Splinter hemorrhages	±	+
Roth's spots	−	+
Congestive heart failure (LVF)	+	−

Modified from Cunha BA, Gill MV, Lazar JM: Acute infective endocarditis: diagnostic and therapeutic approach, Infect Dis Clin North Am 10:811–834, 1996.

LVF, Left ventricular fibrillation; +, present; −, absent; ±, present or absent.
*Otherwise unexplained.
†With septic pulmonary emboli from tricuspid valve ABE.
‡Fever may be <102° F in intravenous drug abusers with ABE.

Early PVE pathogens such as S. aureus and Pseudomonas aeruginosa are typically highly virulent and invasive. Late PVE more closely resembles SBE, is caused by less virulent pathogens, and has a more indolent course. The most common etiologic agents are coagulase-negative staphylococci, but viridans streptococci also cause late PVE. Nosocomial IE results from invasive intravascular or intracardiac procedures that damage the endothelium or the valves; it can also be caused by direct extension of infection, such as from ABE associated with a pacemaker wire. The organisms causing nosocomial IE originate from the skin (e.g., S. aureus, coagulase-negative staphylococci), from gastrointestinal or genitourinary procedures (e.g., group D enterococci), or from central venous catheters, ports, or hemodialysis catheters (e.g., Candida spp, aerobic gram-negative bacilli). IE related to total parenteral nutrition (TPN) is most often caused by Candida spp; other TPN-associated fungemias cause IE less frequently. In intravenous drug abusers, tricuspid valve ABE is usually caused by S. aureus or P. aeruginosa (depending on the geography and drug-related materials).

Infectious CNE is caused by organisms that are difficult to culture, such as Legionella spp, Brucella spp, Tropheryma whipplei, and Coxiella burnetii (which produces Q fever). Legionnaires' disease may cause NVE or PVE. CNE due to Brucella spp can be a difficult diagnosis, but an antecedent history of contact with livestock or consumption of unpasteurized dairy products should suggest the diagnosis, and echocardiography often reveals large

TABLE 93-2 CLUES TO THE LIKELY PATHOGEN IN INFECTIVE ENDOCARDITIS

EPIDEMIOLOGIC FEATURES	PATHOGENS
Intravenous drug abuse	*Staphylococcus aureus*
	Pseudomonas aeruginosa
	β-Hemolytic streptococci
	Aerobic GNB
	Polymicrobial
	Fungi
Indwelling cardiovascular device	*S. aureus*
	CoNS
	Aerobic GNB
	Corynebacterium spp
Genitourinary disorders, infection, manipulation	*Enterococcus* spp
	Group B streptococci (*Streptococcus agalacti, Listeria monocytogenes*)
	Aerobic GNB
Chronic skin disorders	*S. aureus*
	β-Hemolytic streptococci
Poor dentition, dental procedures	Viridans streptococci
	Nutritionally variant streptococci (*Abiotrophia* spp, *Granulicatella* spp)
	Gemella spp
	HACEK organisms†
Alcoholic cirrhosis	*Streptococcus pneumoniae*
	Bartonella spp
	L. monocytogenes
	β-Hemolytic streptococci
Burns	*S. aureus*
	Aerobic GNB
	P. aeruginosa
	Fungi
Diabetes mellitus	*S. aureus*
	β-Hemolytic streptococci
	S. pneumoniae
Early PVE	*S. aureus*
	Aerobic GNB
	Fungi
	Corynebacterium spp
Late PVE	CoNS
	S. aureus
	Viridans streptococci
	Enterococcus spp
	Corynebacterium spp
	Legionella spp
Dog or cat exposure	*Bartonella* spp
	Pasteurella spp
	Capnocytophaga spp
Contact with contaminated milk or infected farm animals	*Brucella* spp
	Coxiella burnetii (Q fever)
	Erysipelothrix rhusiopathiae
Homelessness	*Bartonella* spp.
Human immunodeficiency virus infection	*S. pneumoniae*
	Salmonella spp
	S. aureus
Pneumonia and meningitis*	*S. pneumoniae*
Solid organ transplants	*S. aureus*
	Aspergillus fumigatus
	Enterococcus spp
	Candida spp
Gastrointestinal lesions	*Streptococcus bovis*
	Enterococcus spp

Modified from Baddour LM, Wilson WR, Bayer AS, et al: Infective endocarditis: diagnosis, antimicrobial therapy, and management of complications: a statement for healthcare professionals from the Committee on Rheumatic Fever, Endocarditis, and Kawasaki Disease, Council on Cardiovascular Disease in the Young, and the Councils on Clinical Cardiology, Stroke, and Cardiovascular Surgery and Anesthesia, American Heart Association; endorsed by the Infectious Diseases Society of America, Circulation 111:e394–e433, 2005.

CoNS, Coagulase-negative staphylococci; GNB, gram-negative bacilli; PVE, prosthetic valve endocarditis.

*With alcoholic cirrhosis.

†HACEK organisms: *Haemophilus* spp, *Aggregatibacter actinomycetemcomitans, Cardiobacterium hominis, Eikenella corrodens*, and *Kingella kingae*.

TABLE 93-3 MODIFIED DUKE CRITERIA FOR DIAGNOSIS OF INFECTIVE ENDOCARDITIS

DIAGNOSTIC CRITERIA

Definite IE (any of the following):
  Positive findings for IE in the pathology or microbiology of the vegetation
  Two major criteria
  One major and three minor criteria
  Five minor criteria
Possible IE (any of the following):
  One major and one minor criteria
  Three minor criteria
Not IE (any of the following):
  Definite alternative diagnosis or resolution with <4 days of antibiotic therapy
  Does not meet the criteria of possible IE

MAJOR CRITERIA

Positive blood cultures for IE (any of the following):
  Typical microorganism for IE from two separate blood cultures:
  • Viridans streptococci, *Streptococcus gallolyticus* (formerly *Streptococcus bovis* biotype I), or the nutritional variant strains (*Granulicatella* spp and *Abiotrophia defectiva*)
  • HACEK group: *Haemophilus* spp, *Aggregatibacter actinomycetemcomitans*), *Cardiobacterium hominis, Eikenella corrodens*, and *Kingella kingae*
  • *Staphylococcus aureus*
  Community-acquired enterococci, in the absence of a primary focus
Persistently positive blood culture, defined as recovery of a microorganism consistent with IE from any of the following:
  Blood cultures drawn more than 12 hr apart
  All of three or a majority of four or more separate blood cultures, with first and last drawn at least 1 hr apart
  *Single positive blood culture for *Coxiella burnetii* or antiphase I IgG antibody titer >1 : 800
Evidence of endocardial involvement
Positive echocardiogram for IE:
  *TEE is recommended in patients with prosthetic valves rated at least "possible IE" by clinical criteria, or with complicated IE (paravalvular abscess); TTE as first test in other patients
  Definition of positive echocardiogram (any of the following):
  • Oscillating intracardiac mass, on valve or supporting structures, or in the path of regurgitant jets, or on implanted material, in the absence of an alternative anatomic explanation
  • Abscess
  • New partial dehiscence of prosthetic valve
New valvular regurgitation (increase in or change in preexisting murmur is not sufficient)

MINOR CRITERIA (*Echocardiographic minor criteria have been eliminated)

Predisposition: predisposing heart condition or intravenous drug use
Fever: 38.0° C (100.4° F)
Vascular phenomena: major arterial emboli, septic pulmonary infarcts, mycotic aneurysm, intracranial hemorrhage, conjunctival hemorrhages, Janeway's lesions
Immunologic phenomena: glomerulonephritis, Osler's nodes, Roth's spots, rheumatoid factor
Microbiologic evidence: positive blood culture but not meeting major criterion (excluding single positive cultures for coagulase-negative staphylococci and organisms that do not cause endocarditis) or serologic evidence of active infection with organism consistent with IE

Modified from Li JS, Sexton DJ, Mick N, et al: Proposed modifications to the Duke criteria for the diagnosis of infective endocarditis, Clin Infect Dis 30:633–638, 2000.

IE, Infective endocarditis; IgG, immunoglobulin G; TEE, transesophageal echocardiography; TTE, transthoracic echocardiography.

*Represents a change from the previously published Duke criteria.

TABLE 93-4 NONPECIFIC LABORATORY TESTS FOR INFECTIVE ENDOCARDITIS	
LABORATORY FINDINGS	**PERCENTAGE**
Anemia	70-90
Leukocytosis	20-30
Elevated ESR	90-100
C-reactive protein (CRP)	100
Histiocytes in blood smear	25
Positive rheumatoid factor (RF)	50
Circulating immune complexes	65-100
Microscopic hematuria	30-50

Data from Brusch JL: Clinical manifestations of endocarditis. In Brusch JL, editor: Infective endocarditis, New York, 2007, Informa Healthcare, pp 143–166.

ESR, Erythrocyte sedimentation rate.

TABLE 93-5 DIAGNOSTIC APPROACH TO CULTURE-NEGATIVE ENDOCARDITIS

VALVULAR BIOPSY UNAVAILABLE

1. Q fever and *Bartonella* serology: If negative, then use lysis-centrifugation system for blood cultures and inform microbiology laboratory of concern for fastidious organisms to allow use of special media and culture techniques: thioglycolate-, pyridoxal hydrochloride–, or L-cystine–enriched media for *Abiotrophia*; buffered charcoal yeast extract (BCYE) agar for *Legionella*; prolonged incubation for HACEK organisms*
2. Rheumatoid factor (RF), antinuclear antibodies (ANA)
3. PCR for *Bartonella* spp and *Tropheryma whipplei*
4. Nested PCR for fungi, tissue for *Cryptococcus neoformans* capsular antigen and urine for *Histoplasma capsulatum* antigen: If negative, then obtain serum serology studies for *Mycoplasma pneumoniae, Legionella pneumophila, Brucella melitensis,* and *Bartonella* spp by Western blot

VALVULAR BIOPSY AVAILABLE

1. Broad-range PCR for bacteria (16S rRNA) and fungi (18S rRNA)
2. Histologic examination with direct staining for *Chlamydia* spp, *Coxiella burnetii, Legionella* spp, fungi, and *T. whipplei*
3. Primer extension enrichment reaction (PEER) or autoimmunohistochemistry (AIHC)

Modified from Fournier PE, Thuny F, Richet H, et al: Comprehensive diagnostic strategy for blood culture-negative endocarditis: a prospective study of 819 new cases, Clin Infect Dis 51:131–140, 2010; and Mylonakis E, Calderwood SB: Infective endocarditis in adults, N Engl J Med 345:1320, 2001.

PCR, Polymerase chain reaction; rRNA, ribosomal RNA.

*HACEK organisms: *Haemophilus* spp, *Aggregatibacter actinomycetemcomitans, Cardiobacterium hominis, Eikenella corrodens,* and *Kingella kingae.*

vegetations. A difficult infectious CNE diagnosis is Q fever. Q fever SBE may be suggested by a history of animal contact. Clinical findings of Q fever are often present, but the diagnosis can be missed because Q fever vegetations are not easily visualized.

Laboratory Findings

With IE, many nonspecific laboratory abnormalities may occur (Table 93-4); when placed in the appropriate context, these can be a significant aid to diagnosis.

Echocardiography is an important element in diagnosis and management; it should be performed for all patients with suspected IE. In those with a low likelihood of having IE or small body habitus, a transthoracic echocardiogram (TTE) may be sufficient. Although TTE is often sufficient to screen for NVE, the "gold standard" remains transesophageal echocardiogram (TEE), which is more sensitive at detecting smaller vegetations, paravalvular abscess, and PVE. If the TTE or TEE demonstrates a vegetation but blood cultures remain negative, the diagnosis of infectious CNE should be considered. A tiered diagnostic approach to such cases is presented in Table 93-5.

Diagnosis of *Legionella*-related IE is based on an antecedent pneumonia and elevated titers of urinary antigen. *Brucella*-related IE is confirmed by titers or by polymerase chain reaction or both. A clue to Q fever CNE is enhanced valve uptake on positron-emission tomography (PET) or computed tomography (CT), and such a result should prompt testing for Q fever. With the advent of sophisticated microbiologic testing, HACEK organisms (*Haemophilus* spp, *Aggregatibacter actinomycetemcomitans* [formerly called *Actinobacillus actinomycetcomitans*], *Cardiobacterium hominis, Eikenella corrodens,* and *Kingella kingae*) grow relatively rapidly and no longer manifest as CNE.

Radiologic testing in IE is primarily focused on identifying complications of IE. Although echocardiography is still the preferred method for detecting vegetations, improvements in multislice CT scans have allowed chest CT to detect vegetations and valvular abnormalities in addition to the septic emboli seen in right-sided IE. Magnetic resonance imaging (MRI) of the spine is useful in patients with IE who report back pain; it is the preferred method to detect the presence of vertebral osteomyelitis caused by IE. Mental status changes should prompt CT or MRI imaging of the head to assess xor septic emboli to the brain. Although it is less invasive than TEE, cardiac MRI often lacks the special resolution to detect smaller vegetations; however, it may

be helpful in identifying aortic root pseudoaneurysms, sinus of Valsalva aneurysms, and embolic vascular lesions.

Differential Diagnosis and Mimics

The diagnosis of SBE is based an otherwise unexplained high-grade or continuous bacteremia caused by a known endocarditis pathogen plus a cardiac vegetation. Depending on the duration before presentation (usually 1 to 3 months), IE may be accompanied by peripheral manifestations such as Osler's nodes, Janeway's lesions, splinter hemorrhages, or conjunctival hemorrhages. Splenomegaly or embolic phenomena may also accompany SBE. However, peripheral manifestations that are seen in SBE may also be present in other disorders. Before ascribing peripheral manifestations to SBE, physicians need to rule out other systemic disorders and confirm the diagnosis of SBE.

Clinically, the disorders most likely to mimic SBE are Libman-Sacks endocarditis (associated with systemic lupus erythematosus [SLE]), marantic endocarditis (caused by a malignancy, usually lymphoma, lung cancer, or pancreatic cancer), and atrial myxoma. Myocarditis of any etiology may mimic SBE with fever, murmur, and peripheral embolic phenomena. Cardiomegaly, which is usually present with myocarditis, is typically absent with SBE. Leukopenia and thrombocytopenia may be clues to viral myocarditis, and either finding argues against a diagnosis of SBE. Cardiac echocardiography shows myocarditis but no vegetations, and bacteremia is not present.

SLE, particularly between flares, may mimic SBE with low-grade fevers, murmur, peripheral manifestations, and splenomegaly. Laboratory findings in SLE include the anemia of chronic disease and a mildly to moderately elevated erythrocyte sedimentation rate (ESR). Even if Libman-Sacks vegetations are present, SBE is rare in SLE. A lupus flare may resemble ABE with high fevers (>102° F), tender fingertips (mimicking Osler's nodes), and funduscopic findings of cotton-wool spots or Roth's spots. Conjunctival and splinter hemorrhages are rare in SLE but common in SBE. Microscopic hematuria is the usual renal manifestation of SBE (i.e., focal glomerulonephritis), but full-blown nephritis with proteinuria and hematuria are typical of SLE renal involvement. Although clinical findings of SLE and SBE may overlap, SBE is ruled out by the absence of high-grade or continuous bacteremia.

Atrial myxomas may mimic SBE with fever, murmurs, and embolic phenomena (e.g., splinter hemorrhages). Highly elevated ESR levels are common with atrial myxomas, but biologically false-positive results on Venereal Disease Research Laboratory (VDRL) testing, elevated rheumatoid factors, and renal involvement are not seen. On TTE or TEE, atrial myxomas appear as masses or vegetations on the atrial surface rather than on a valve as in IE. SBE is ruled out by the absence of bacteremia.

Besides clinical mimics of SBE, there are also echocardiographic mimics, including papillary fibromas, thrombi, calcified valves, myxomatous degeneration, and marantic endocarditis. These disorders are usually unaccompanied by fever or bacteremia. The term *marantic endocarditis* refers to uninfected vegetations with a murmur and negative blood cultures that occur secondary to malignancy. Patients with marantic endocarditis are afebrile unless fever is caused by the underlying malignancy (e.g., lymphoma). The patient with marantic endocarditis due to lymphoma may have fever, splenomegaly, and other manifestations of SBE. Negative blood cultures effectively rule out IE. Infectious CNE (e.g., Q fever) may show little or no visible vegetations. Infectious CNE should be considered if fever, murmur, and vegetation are present along with peripheral manifestations of IE.

Treatment

Effective treatment of IE depends on the antibiotic susceptibility of the pathogen, the penetration of the antibiotic into the vegetation, and the appropriate duration of antibiotic therapy. Antibiotics selected for IE preferably should be bactericidal. In IE, the organisms are deeply embedded in the vegetation, and prolonged therapy is necessary for penetration and sterilization of the vegetation. Early in IE therapy, blood cultures rapidly become negative, but treatment is continued because infection in the vegetation has not been eradicated. Multiplication of bacteria, which is required for bactericidal activity of antibiotics, is reduced within vegetations and is one reason for the requirement for prolonged antibiotics. It is important to note that in cases of *Staphylococcus aureus* endocarditis, blood cultures may not clear rapidly and may remain positive for days despite appropriate antibiotic therapy. Penetration into the vegetation is critical; for example, viridans streptococci are highly susceptible to β-lactam antibiotics but require a prolonged course of antimicrobial therapy to eradicate the pathogens in the vegetation.

Whereas some cases of uncomplicated IE may be treated with 2 weeks of antimicrobial therapy, the usual duration of monotherapy or combination therapy is 4 to 6 weeks, depending on the pathogen. Effective antimicrobial therapy does not eliminate supportive or embolic complications of endocarditis. Therapeutic failure is usually related to valvular destruction, a complication that may require valve replacement. Suppurative intracardiac or extracardiac complications usually require drainage for cure of

TABLE 93-6	PRINCIPLES OF THERAPY FOR INFECTIVE ENDOCARDITIS

1. Antibiotic selection initially is made empirically on the basis of physical examination and clinical history.
2. Bactericidal antibiotics are prescribed.
3. The MIC and MBC are measured to insure adequate dosing of the agent.
4. Intermittent dosing provides superior penetration into the thrombus compared with continuous infusion; penetration is directly related to peak serum level.
5. The patient should be treated in a health care facility for the first 1-2 wk.
6. The usual duration of therapy is 4-6 wk.
7. A 4-wk course is appropriate for an uncomplicated case of NVE (a shorter course of 2 wk may be appropriate in some cases); a 6-wk course is required for the treatment of PVE and those infections with large vegetations (i.e., infection by HACEK organisms*).

Modified from Brusch JL: Diagnosis of infective endocarditis. In Brusch JL, editor: Infective endocarditis, New York, 2007, Informa Healthcare, pp 241–254.
MBC, Minimal bactericidal concentration; MIC, minimal inhibitory concentration.
*HACEK organisms: *Haemophilus* spp, *Actinobacillus actinomycetcomitans*, *Cardiobacterium hominis*, *Eikenella corrodens*, and *Kingella kingae*.

IE. The overarching principles of IE therapy are presented in Table 93-6, and Table 93-7 provides an outline of specific antibiotic regimens that may be used to treat IE.

Complications of endocarditis may be intracardiac or extracardiac, and they may also be classified by damage mechanism (i.e., immunologic versus infectious). The infectious intracardiac complications of IE include purulent pericarditis and paravalvular abscess; they manifest clinically with persistent fever or persistent bacteremia despite appropriate antibiotic therapy. Complications may be septic or immunologic; for example, splenic involvement may be immunologic (splenic infarct) or septic (splenic abscess). Embolic events are related to vegetation size. Bland central nervous system emboli (e.g., aseptic meningitis) may complicate SBE, whereas septic emboli (e.g., acute bacterial meningitis) may complicate ABE. Particularly with ABE, there may be valvular perforation or destruction resulting in acute congestive heart failure. It is often these complications that dictate whether and when surgery will occur. The indications for surgical intervention are shown in Table 93-8. As a general principle, paravalvular abscess or intractable congestive heart failure requires urgent surgical intervention. Persistent vegetations or embolic disease that occurs after 1 week of appropriate antibiotic therapy should also prompt surgical consideration.

Prognosis

The prognosis of all forms of IE depends directly on any complications related to the infection. Consequently, early diagnosis and initiation of appropriate antibiotic therapy is the key to limiting mortality. Recent studies have supported the role of early surgical intervention, when appropriate, as a significant aid to decreasing morbidity and mortality, specifically in relation to having fewer embolic events. If treated in a timely fashion and with appropriate antibiotics, the cure rate for viridans streptococci and S. bovis is estimated to be 98% in NVE and up to 88% in PVE. Right-sided endocarditis in intravenous drug abusers is usually caused by S. aureus and typically has a cure rate of 90% in NVE and 75% to 80% in PVE. However, among non–intravenous drug abusers, cure rates in IE involving *S. aureus* are far lower: 60% to 70% in NVE and 50% in PVE. When gram-negative bacilli or fungal organisms are the causative agent,

TABLE 93-7 ANTIMICROBIAL TREATMENT OF INFECTIVE ENDOCARDITIS

CAUSATIVE ORGANISM	NATIVE VALVE		PROSTHETIC VALVE	
	ANTIBIOTIC THERAPY	COMMENTS	ANTIBIOTIC THERAPY	COMMENTS
Penicillin-susceptible viridans streptococci, *Streptococcus bovis*, and other streptococci with MIC of penicillin ≤0.1 µg/mL	Penicillin G or ceftriaxone for 4 wk*	A 2-wk regimen of penicillin G or ceftriaxone combined with gentamicin may be considered in patients with right-sided NVE without evidence of embolic disease (excluding pulmonary emboli) or other complications.	Penicillin G for 6 wk and gentamicin for 2 wk*	Shorter duration of treatment with an aminoglycoside (2 wk) is usually appropriate for PVE due to penicillin-susceptible viridans streptococci, *S. bovis*, or other streptococci with MIC of penicillin ≤0.1 µg/mL.
Relatively penicillin-resistant streptococci (MIC of penicillin >0.1 to 0.5 µg/mL)	Penicillin G for 4 wk and gentamicin for 2 wk*		Penicillin G for 6 wk and gentamicin for 4 wk*	
Streptococcus species with MIC of penicillin >0.5 µg/mL, *Enterococcus* species, or *Abiotrophia* species	Penicillin G or ampicillin and gentamicin for 4-6 wk*	6 wk of therapy is recommended for patients with symptoms lasting >3 mo, myocardial abscess, or selected other complications.	Penicillin G or ampicillin and gentamicin for 6 wk*	A recent study by Fernando-Hidalgo et al. showed that the combination of ampicillin and ceftriaxone is as effective as the combination of ampicillin and gentamicin for treating *Enterococcus faecalis* IE.
Methicillin-susceptible staphylococci	Nafcillin or oxacillin for 4-6 wk, with or without addition of gentamicin for the first 3-5 days of therapy[†]	In the few patients infected with a penicillin-susceptible staphylococcus, penicillin G may be substituted for nafcillin or oxacillin.	Nafcillin or oxacillin with rifampin for 6 wk and gentamicin for 2 wk[†]	It may be prudent to delay initiation of rifampin for 1 or 2 days, until therapy with two other effective antistaphylococcal drugs has been initiated.
Methicillin-resistant staphylococci	Vancomycin, with or without addition of gentamicin, for the first 3-5 days of therapy		Vancomycin with rifampin for 6 wk and gentamicin for 2 wk	If the staphylococcus is resistant to gentamicin, an alternative third agent should be chosen on the basis of in vitro susceptibility testing.
Right-sided staphylococcal NVE in selected patients	Nafcillin or oxacillin with gentamicin for 2 wk	This 2-wk regimen has been studied for infections caused by an oxacillin- and aminoglycoside-susceptible isolate. Exclusions to short-course therapy include any cardiac or extracardiac complications associated with IE, persistence of fever for ≥7 days, and infection with HIV. Patients with vegetations >1-2 cm should probably be excluded from short-course therapy.		
HACEK organisms[‡]	Ceftriaxone for 4 wk	Ampicillin and gentamicin for 4 wk is an alternative regimen, but some isolates may produce β-lactamase, thereby reducing the efficacy of this regimen.	Ceftriaxone for 6 wk	Ampicillin and gentamicin for 6 wk is an alternative regimen, but some isolates may produce β-lactamase, thereby reducing the efficacy of this regimen.

Modified from Mylonakis E, Calderwood SB: Infective endocarditis in adults, N Engl J Med 345:1318–1330, 2001.

HIV, Human immunodeficiency virus; IE, infective endocarditis; NVE, native valve endocarditis; PVE, prosthetic valve endocarditis.

*Vancomycin therapy is indicated for patients with confirmed immediate hypersensitivity reactions to β-lactam antibiotics.

[†]For patients who have IE due to methicillin-susceptible staphylococci and are allergic to penicillin, a first-generation cephalosporin or vancomycin may be substituted for nafcillin or oxacillin. Cephalosporins should be avoided in patients with confirmed immediate-type hypersensitivity reactions to β-lactam antibiotics.

[‡]HACEK organisms: *Haemophilus* spp, *Actinobacillus actinomycetcomitans*, *Cardiobacterium hominis*, *Eikenella corrodens*, and *Kingella kingae*.

cure rates are significantly lower (40% to 60%). Increased age, diabetes, aortic valve involvement, and developing complications of IE including congestive heart failure and emboli to the central nervous system are all highly predictive of increased mortality and morbidity.

Infective Endocarditis Prophylaxis

The most recent American Heart Association guidelines state that not all patients require antibiotic prophylaxis and that prophylaxis should be considered only for a specific subset of patients. Antibiotic prophylaxis is indicated for patients with prosthetic heart valves, cardiac transplant recipients with valvular disease, patients with a history of IE, and patients with certain forms of congenital heart disease. Among patients with congenital heart disease, only those with unrepaired or partially repaired lesions and those with prosthetic material should receive prophylactic antibiotics (grade IIa recommendation).

Typically, antibiotic regimens used for prophylaxis against IE prior to invasive procedures above the waist are directed against viridans streptococci. For invasive dental procedures, the recommended prophylactic agent is amoxicillin, 2 g PO as a single dose 30 to 60 minutes before the procedure. In patients with penicillin allergy, clindamycin or a macrolide may be substituted.

● ENDARTERITIS AND SUPPURATIVE PHLEBITIS

The term *infectious endarteritis* refers to an intravascular infection of the arteries that affects coarctation of the aorta, aortic

TABLE 93-8 ECHOCARDIOGRAPHIC INDICATIONS FOR SURGICAL INTERVENTION IN INFECTIVE ENDOCARDITIS

VEGETATION

Persistent vegetation after systemic embolization

Anterior mitral valve leaflet vegetation (particularly if ≥1 embolic events occur during the first 2 wk of antimicrobial therapy)*

Increase in vegetation size despite appropriate antimicrobial therapy*[†]

VALVULAR DYSFUNCTION

Acute aortic or mitral insufficiency with signs of ventricular failure[†]

Heart failure unresponsive to medical therapy[†]

Valve perforation or rupture[†]

Large abscess or extension of abscess despite appropriate antimicrobial therapy[†]

PARAVALVULAR EXTENSION

Valvular dehiscence, rupture, or fistula[†]

New heart block[†]

Large abscess or extension of abscess despite appropriate antimicrobial therapy[†]

Modified from Baddour LM, Wilson WR, Bayer AS, et al: Infective Endocarditis: diagnosis, antimicrobial therapy, and management of complications: a statement for healthcare professionals from the Committee on Rheumatic Fever, Endocarditis, and Kawasaki Disease, Council on Cardiovascular Disease in the Young, and the Councils on Clinical Cardiology, Stroke, and Cardiovascular Surgery and Anesthesia, American Heart Association; endorsed by the Infectious Diseases Society of America, Circulation 111:e394–e433, 2005.

*Surgery may be required because of risk of embolization.

[†]Surgery may be required because of failure of medical therapy or heart failure.

valve shunts, or a patent ductus arteriosus, analogous to IE at other sites. As with IE, continuous or high-grade bacteremia in the absence of an intracardiac vegetation should suggest the diagnosis. Imaging studies (e.g., PET scans) delineate the extent of arterial involvement. Treatment is the same as for IE.

The term *suppurative thrombophlebitis* refers to an intravenous infection that is characterized by an intravenular abscess; it is a complication of the use of central venous catheters. Patients have phlebitis with high fevers (>102° F, compared with <102° F in uncomplicated phlebitis with fevers) and bacteremia due to a skin organism (e.g., *S. aureus*). Treatment consists of a combination of antibiotic therapy and resection of the involved venous segment.

 ## CENTRAL VENOUS CATHETER–RELATED BLOODSTREAM INFECTIONS

Central venous catheter–related bloodstream infections are relatively common, with an annual incidence of approximately 200,000 in the United States. Central venous catheter infection should be suspected if the patient develops fevers, chills, or hypotension without another obvious source of infection. The likelihood of infection increases with the length of time the catheter is in place. In addition to the clinical signs, blood cultures, drawn from the periphery as well as the line, should demonstrate growth of the causative organism. If the culture drawn from the catheter shows growth of bacteria at least 2 hours earlier than the peripheral blood cultures do, infection associated with the central line, rather than bacteremia in the setting of a catheter, should be strongly suspected.

Treatment of catheter-related infections varies depending on what action will be taken with the catheter (i.e., removal,

exchange, or salvage). In any case, empirical antibiotic therapy should be initiated against the most likely pathogens. Empirical therapy should cover *S. aureus* and nosocomial gram-negative bacilli. Therapy may then be modified based on the results of blood cultures or catheter tip culture. If a catheter-related bloodstream infection is suspected, immediate removal of the catheter should occur if the infection has led to septic shock or IE. The line also should be removed if blood cultures remain positive for the causative organism for 72 hours longer, or if evidence of septic thrombophlebitis develops.

Salvage therapy may be considered in hemodynamically stable patients except when the infection is caused by *S. aureus, P. aeruginosa, Bacillus* spp, *Micrococcus* spp, *Propionibacterium acnes* or other propionibacteria, fungi, or mycobacteria. Salvage therapy relies on concurrent use of systemic antimicrobial agents and antibiotic or ethanol locks.

Guidewire exchange should be reserved for cases in which there is a high risk for complications if the original catheter were to be removed. Guidewire exchange has a lower chance of eliminating the infection than does removal of the catheter.

For a deeper discussion of these topics, please see Chapter 76, "Infective Endocarditis," in Goldman-Cecil Medicine, 25th Edition.

SUGGESTED READINGS

Baddour LM, Cha YM, Wilson WR: Clinical practice: infections of cardiovascular implantable electronic devices, N Engl J Med 367:842–849, 2012.

Bor DH, Woolhandler S, Nardin R, et al: Infective endocarditis in the U.S., 1998–2009: a nationwide study, PLoS ONE 8(e60033):2013.

Brouqt P, Raoult D: Endocarditis due to rare and fastidious bacteria, Clin Microbiol Rev 14:177–207, 2001.

Fournier PE, Thuny F, Richet H, et al: Comprehensive diagnostic strategy for blood culture-negative endocarditis: a prospective study of 819 new cases, Clin Infect Dis 51:131–140, 2010.

Fernández-Hidalgo N, Almirante B, Gavaldà J, et al: Ampicillin plus ceftriaxone is as effective as ampicillin plus gentamicin for treating *Enterococcus faecalis* infective endocarditis, Clin Infect Dis 56:1261–1268, 2013.

Garcia-Cabera E, Fernandez-Hidalgo N, Almirante B, et al: Neurological complications of infective endocarditis: risk factors, outcome, and impact of cardiac surgery: a multicenter observational study, Circulation 127:2272–2284, 2013.

Kang DH, Kim YJ, Kim SH, et al: Early surgery versus conventional treatment for infective endocarditis, N Engl J Med 366:2466–2473, 2012.

Kiefer T, Park L, Tribouilloy C, et al: Association between valvular surgery and mortality among patients with infective endocarditis complicated by heart failure, JAMA 306:2239–2247, 2011.

Li JS, Sexton DJ, Mick N, et al: Proposed modifications to the Duke criteria for the diagnosis of infective endocarditis, Clin Infect Dis 30:633–638, 2000.

Mermel LA, Allon M, Bouza E, et al: Clinical practice guidelines for the diagnosis and management of intravascular catheter-related infection: 2009 Update by the Infectious Disease Society of America, Clin Infect Dis 49:1–45, 2009.

Mylonakis E, Calderwood SB: Infective endocarditis in adults, N Engl J Med 345:1318–1330, 2001.

Wilson W, Taubert KA, Gewitz M, et al: Prevention of infective endocarditis: guidelines from the American Heart Association: a guideline from the American Heart Association Rheumatic Fever, Endocarditis, and Kawasaki Disease Committee, Council on Cardiovascular Disease in the Young, and the Council on Clinical Cardiology, Council on Cardiovascular Surgery and Anesthesia, and the Quality of Care and Outcomes Research Interdisciplinary Working Group, Circulation 116:1736–1754, 2007.

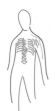

94

Skin and Soft Tissue Infections

Sajeev Handa

DEFINITION

Skin and soft tissue infections (SSTIs) comprise infections of skin, subcutaneous tissue, fascia, and the muscle by a multitude of organisms.

EPIDEMIOLOGY

SSTIs are among the most common infections found in all age groups, although the exact incidence is unknown. Several factors predispose to development of SSTIs:

- Epidermal breaks caused by trauma, surgical wounds, human or animal bites, or dry and irritated skin with concomitant tinea infection
- Immunosuppressed states caused by malnutrition, diabetes mellitus, or acquired immunodeficiency syndrome (AIDS)
- Chronic venous or lymphatic insufficiency

PATHOLOGY

Infectious Mechanisms

Microbes penetrate the integument after entering through a cut, bite, or hair follicle. Components of the host's defense system, including oxygen radicals, complement, immunoglobulins, macrophages, lymphocytes, and granulocytes, are recruited to the site of invasion through a vast plexus of dermal capillaries.

Bacteria contain proteins whose N-terminal amino acid sequence begins with an N-formyl-methionine group that is chemoattractive to phagocytes, including macrophages and granulocytes. Other microbial cell wall components, such as the zymosan of yeast, endotoxins of gram-negative bacteria, and the peptidoglycans of gram-positive bacteria, activate the alternative complement pathways, producing serum-derived chemotactic factors. Efflux of phagocytes occurs from the capillary through endothelial cell interstices and follows the gradient of chemotactic factors derived from bacteria and serum to the site of active infection.

Activated endothelial cells also produce chemotactic cytokines such as interleukin-8 (IL-8). Activated granulocytes synthesize leukotriene B_4 from arachidonic acid, a potent chemoattractant for leukocytes. Production of proinflammatory cytokines such as IL-1, IL-6, and tumor necrosis factor augments immune function, inducing fever, priming neutrophils, and increasing antibody production and synthesis of acute phase reactants such as C-reactive protein.

Cytokine-driven stimulation of endothelial cells generates nitric oxide and prostaglandins, both of which cause vasodilatation. The net physiologic effect is greater blood flow to the tissue, causing acute inflammation. As described by Celsus (30 BC-38 AD), acute inflammation is characterized by rubor (i.e., redness), calor (i.e., increased heat), tumor (i.e., swelling), dolor (i.e., pain), and, as added by Virchow in the 19th century, function laesa (i.e., loss of function). Chapter 86 discusses host defenses against infection in more depth.

Pathologic Manifestations

Impetigo is characterized by thick, crusted lesions with rounded or irregular margins that typically occur on the face. Most cases are caused by *Staphylococcus aureus*, including methicillin-resistant *S. aureus* (MRSA), or by group A streptococci (e.g., *Streptococcus pyogenes*). Certain strains of streptococci causing impetigo have been implicated in the development of poststreptococcal glomerulonephritis.

Folliculitis is a superficial bacterial infection of the hair follicles. Purulent material is found in the epidermis. It manifests as clusters of multiple, small, raised, pruritic, erythematous lesions that are typically less than 5 mm in diameter.

Furuncles (i.e., boils) are infections of the hair follicle. Purulent material extends through the dermis into the subcutaneous tissue, where small abscesses may form. A carbuncle is coalescence of several inflamed follicles into a single inflammatory mass. Purulent drainage exudes from multiple follicles.

Cellulitis is superficial inflammation of the skin and underlying tissues. It is characterized by erythema, warmth, and tenderness of the involved area (Fig. 94-1). Erysipelas is a variant of cellulitis that is predominantly caused by toxin-producing *S. pyogenes*. It manifests as a superficial, spreading, warm, erythematous (fiery red) lesion distinguished by its indurated and elevated margin. Lymphatic involvement and vesicle formation are common. Groups B, C, and D streptococci may also be implicated (Fig. 94-2).

Necrotizing fasciitis is a progressive and rapidly spreading inflammatory reaction deep in the fascia that is associated with secondary necrosis of the subcutaneous tissues. Thrombosis of the dermal vessels is responsible for tissue necrosis. Necrotizing fasciitis may be polymicrobial (type I), involving aerobic microbes (e.g., streptococci, staphylococci, gram-negative bacilli) and anaerobes (e.g., *Peptostreptococcus*, *Bacteroides*, *Clostridium* species), or it may be monomicrobial (type II) and caused by *S. pyogenes* (Fig. 94-3). When involving the scrotum and perineal area, it is known as *Fournier's gangrene*.

Pyomyositis is a less serious infection involving the musculature that results from direct inoculation of bacteria. For example,

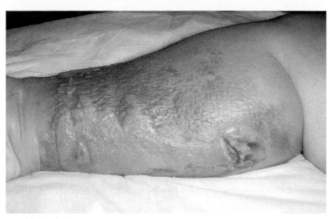

FIGURE 94-1 Ill-defined erythema and edema with bullae formation is characteristic of lower extremity cellulitis. (From Pride HB: Cellulitis and erysipelas. In Zaoutis LB, Chiang VW, editors: Comprehensive pediatric hospital medicine, Philadelphia, 2007, Mosby, Fig. 156-1.)

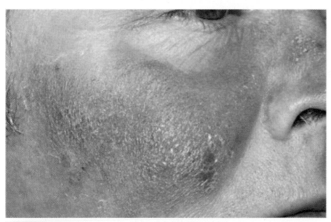

FIGURE 94-2 Sharply defined erythema and edema is characteristic of erysipelas. (From Pride HB: Cellulitis and erysipelas. In Zaoutis LB, Chiang VW, editors: Comprehensive pediatric hospital medicine, Philadelphia, 2007, Mosby, Fig. 156-2.)

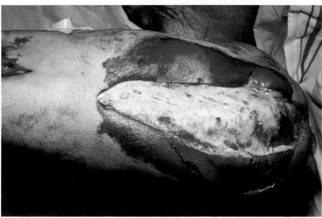

FIGURE 94-3 Spontaneous necrotizing fasciitis due to *Clostridium septicum*. The patient developed sudden onset of severe pain in the forearm. Swelling rapidly ensued, and he sought medical treatment. Crepitus was found on physical examination, and gas in the soft tissue was verified with routine radiographs. Immediate surgical débridement revealed necrotizing fasciitis but sparing of the muscle. Notice the purple-violaceous appearance of the skin. (From Stevens DL, Aldape MJ, Bryant AE. Necrotizing fasciitis, gas gangrene, myositis and myonecrosis. In Cohen J, Powderly WG, Opal SM, editors: Infectious diseases, ed 3, London, 2010, Mosby, Fig. 10-11.)

infection can result from injection drug use or from secondary seeding by *S. aureus* or group A β-hemolytic streptococci from an incidental bacteremia or a hematoma caused by nonpenetrating trauma.

Ecthyma is an ulcerative pyoderma of the skin that extends into the dermis (unlike impetigo). It is caused by group A streptococci and *Pseudomonas* species.

ETIOLOGY AND CLINICAL PRESENTATION
Causative Organisms

A multitude of organisms can cause SSTIs. However, three are most common: *S. pyogenes, S. aureus,* and *Streptococcus agalactiae.*

S. pyogenes (i.e., group A β-hemolytic streptococci) is a gram-positive coccus that may cause erysipelas, streptococcal cellulitis, necrotizing fasciitis, myositis, myonecrosis, and streptococcal toxic shock syndrome. Streptococcal cellulitis arises from infection of wounds, burns, or surgical incisions and may progress to involve large areas. Injection drug users and individuals with impaired lymphatic drainage are at high risk. Systemic manifestations include fever, chills, malaise with or without associated lymphangitis, and bacteremia. In contrast to erysipelas, the affected area is not raised, and the demarcation between involved skin and uninvolved skin is indistinct. The lesions tend to be more pink than fiery red.

Streptococcal toxic shock syndrome manifests with hypotension and is associated with acute kidney injury, elevated aminotransferases, rash or soft tissue necrosis, and coagulopathy. It may be complicated by the acute respiratory distress syndrome. Isolation of the organism from a sterile site provides a definite diagnosis.

S. aureus is a gram-positive coccus that is found in the anterior nares of up to 30% of healthy people. It is responsible for a variety of invasive and suppurative infections. Localized SSTIs include furuncles, carbuncles, bullous and nonbullous impetigo, mastitis, ecthyma, cellulitis, and wound and foreign body infections. Bacteremia may be complicated by septicemia, endocarditis, pericarditis, pneumonia, empyema, osteomyelitis, and abscesses of the soft tissue, muscle, and viscera.

Staphylococcal toxic shock syndrome is typically associated with tampon use but may occur after childbirth or surgery and can be associated with cutaneous lesions. It manifests with the acute onset of fever, erythroderma, hypotension, and multisystem involvement (e.g., acute kidney injury, elevated levels of aminotransferases, coagulopathy, nausea, vomiting, diarrhea).

Community-associated MRSA is the most common identifiable cause of SSTIs in the emergency department. Isolates contain genes encoding for multiple toxins, including cytotoxins that result in leukocyte destruction and tissue necrosis.

S. agalactiae (a group B streptococcus) is a gram-positive diplococcus. It may account for up to one third of SSTIs among adults. Cellulitis, foot ulcers, and infection of decubitus ulcers are common manifestations. Cellulitis has been associated with foreign bodies such as breast or penile implants. Less commonly, polymyositis, blistering dactylitis, and necrotizing fasciitis may occur.

Other Organisms

Aeromonas hydrophila, Aeromonas veronii, and *Aeromonas schubertii* are gram-negative rods found in salt and fresh water. They may cause mild to severe wound infections after injury, producing cellulitis, myonecrosis, and rhabdomyolysis. Necrotizing fasciitis has been reported with *A. veronii* and *A. schubertii* infections. *Aeromonas* wound infections have also been reported as a result of the medicinal use of leeches.

Arcanobacterium haemolyticum is a gram-positive, weakly acid-fast bacillus. It has been isolated from soft tissue infections, including chronic ulcers, cellulitis, and paronychia.

Bacillus anthracis is a gram-positive bacillus that forms spores. Transdermal inoculation of the spores from even incidental trauma can result in cutaneous anthrax. It manifests initially as a small, pruritic papule that becomes surrounded by painless, non-purulent vesicles that easily rupture, leaving a black eschar at the base of the ulceration. Uncomplicated disease heals without scar formation in 1 to 3 weeks. Serious cutaneous disease is marked by extensive edema, worsening inflammation, and toxemia (Fig. 94-4).

Bartonella henselae is a gram-negative bacillus that causes cat-scratch disease. Between 3 and 10 days after a bite or scratch from a cat or other vector, a tender, erythematous papule appears. Lymphadenopathy ipsilateral to the site of inoculation occurs 1 to 3 weeks later, and the patient typically experiences constitutional symptoms. The lymphadenopathy may take months to resolve.

Capnocytophaga canimorsus is a thin, gram-negative bacillus with tapered ends. It is strongly associated with dog (primarily) and cat bites and scratches. Asplenic patients are at particular risk for sepsis due to this organism.

Clostridium perfringens is an anaerobic, large, gram-positive rod. It can cause cellulitis or life-threatening necrotizing infections of skin, muscle, and other soft tissues. The latter is characterized by rapidly progressive tissue destruction, gas in tissues, shock, and death. Conditions such as trauma or illicit drug injection produce anaerobic tissue conditions that favor the organism. The condition can also develop in patients with bowel carcinoma or neutropenia. Gram stain of tissue or exudate reveals large, gram-positive rods and no inflammatory cells.

Edwardsiella tarda is a gram-negative rod found in fresh water environments. It is associated with wound infections, abscesses, and bacteremia. The mortality rate is high among patients with liver disease and iron overload.

Eikenella corrodens is a gram-negative bacillus that is part of the normal human oral flora. It is an important pathogen in human bite wounds, closed-fist injuries, and infections seen in chronic finger or nail biters. Severe soft tissue infection may occur, leading to septic arthritis and osteomyelitis.

Erysipelothrix rhusiopathiae is a gram-positive rod, but it may appear as gram-negative because of rapid decolorization. Its major reservoir is in domestic swine, and infection occurs by direct cutaneous contact through a cut or abrasion. Disease is characterized as erysipeloid (i.e., subacute cellulitis with vesiculation), as a diffuse cutaneous eruption with systemic symptoms, or as bacteremia that is often associated with endocarditis.

Francisella tularensis is a gram-negative coccobacillus found in rabbits, hares, hamsters, and rodents. Ulceroglandular tularemia occurs 3 to 5 days after humans are inoculated cutaneously during contact with any of these species. A papule is formed initially, followed by ulceration with enlargement of the regional lymph nodes. Vesicles may be seen. If left untreated, the ulcer remains for weeks before healing, leaving a residual scar. Suppuration of the affected lymph nodes is the most common complication, occurring despite appropriate treatment (Fig. 94-5). *B. anthracis* and *F. tularensis* have been used as agents in bioterrorism.

Cryptococcus neoformans, Candida albicans, Histoplasma capsulatum, Blastomyces dermatitidis, Coccidioides immitis, and opportunistic fungi can have skin manifestations. Opportunistic fungi, including *Aspergillus* species, fungi in the order Mucorales, and *Fusarium* species, can infect the skin of immunocompromised patients. Skin manifestations of fungal infections include papules, nodules, circumscribed erythematous lesions, ulcers, verrucous lesions, and eschars.

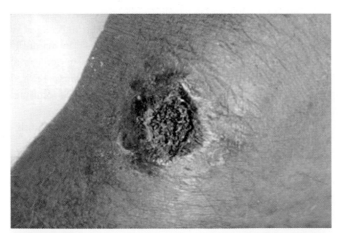

FIGURE 94-4 Cutaneous anthrax lesion on the skin of the forearm caused by the bacterium *Bacillus anthracis.* (From Centers for Disease Control and Prevention: Public health image library. Available at http://phil.cdc.gov/Phil/home.asp. Accessed October 31, 2014.)

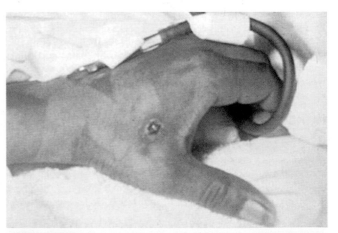

FIGURE 94-5 Tularemic ulcer with eschar formation after percutaneous inoculation of *Francisella tularensis.* (From Beard CB, Dennis DT: Tularemia. In Cohen J, Powderly WG, Opal SM, editors: Infectious diseases, ed 3, London, 2010, Mosby.)

Exposure to herpes simplex virus types 1 and 2 (HSV-1 and HSV-2) at abraded skin sites allows entry into the epidermis and dermis. Infection typically occurs from sexual contact, but it occasionally occurs at extraoral or extragenital sites, such as the hands of health care workers, producing a painful erythema primarily at the junction of the nail bed and skin (i.e., whitlow). This progresses to a vesicopustular lesion that can mimic a bacterial infection (i.e., paronychia). Sexually transmitted diseases are discussed in Chapter 100.

Mycobacterium marinum is an atypical, acid-fast bacillus; it is the most common atypical mycobacterium that causes infection in humans. After inoculation of a skin abrasion or puncture wound in salt or fresh water (nonchlorinated), lesions appear as papules on an extremity. Lesions progress to shallow ulcers and form scars. Typically, lesions are solitary, but they may take on the appearance of ascending, sporotrichoid-like, nodular lymphangitis that may involve the local joint or tendons.

Mycobacterium leprae is a slow-growing, acid-fast bacillus that cannot be grown in vitro. It is the cause of leprosy (Hansen's disease). It is primarily transmitted by the airborne route and causes chronic disfiguring skin lesions and nerve damage.

> *For a deeper discussion of this topic, please see Chapter 326, "Leprosy (Hansen's Disease)" in* Goldman-Cecil Medicine, *25th Edition.*

Pasteurella multocida is a gram-negative coccobacillus that may occur at the site of a scratch or bite from a dog or cat. Cellulitis results within 24 hours of the injury, producing swelling, erythema, tenderness, serous or purulent discharge with or without regional lymphadenopathy, chills, and fever.

Pseudomonas aeruginosa is a gram-negative rod and primarily a nosocomial pathogen. In the community, serogroup 0:11 may cause folliculitis related to the use of hot tubs, whirlpools, and swimming pools. Typically, the eruption occurs 48 hours after exposure and consists of tender, pruritic papules, papulopustules, or nodules. It is an important pathogen in burn wound infections, which may progress to sepsis.

Sporothrix schenckii is a dimorphic fungus ubiquitous primarily in the tropical parts of North and South America. Cutaneous inoculation from thorny plants (e.g., rose bushes) is followed by development of a painless papule that enlarges slowly to become a nodular lesion with a violaceous hue or ulceration. Secondary lesions may form along the lymphatic drainage distribution.

Primary varicella-zoster virus (VZV) infection occurs by the respiratory route but may occur through contact with infected lesions. Viremia results in crops of papules that primarily occur on the trunk and progress to vesicles and then to pustules, followed by crusting. Zoster or shingles represents reactivation of the latent virus in the sensory neurons of the dorsal root ganglion, resulting in pain that proceeds to a rash in the distribution of the affected dermatome in a few days. The appearance of papules and vesicles in a unilateral dermatomal distribution confirms the diagnosis. Ramsay Hunt syndrome occurs when the VZV infection involves the geniculate ganglia and causes a painful eruption in the ear canal and tympanic membrane that is associated with ipsilateral seventh cranial nerve palsy. Vesicles that appear on the tip of the nose (i.e., Hutchinson's sign) may be preceded by development of ophthalmic zoster and involvement of the cornea.

Immunosuppressed individuals are at higher risk for disseminated disease.

Vibrio vulnificus is a gram-negative bacillus that is spread by contamination of a superficial wound with warm seawater. It can cause rapidly developing and intense cellulitis, necrotizing vasculitis, and ulcer formation. Aggressive soft tissue infection may occur with necrosis, fever, sepsis, and bullae formation. Ingestion of raw oysters, particularly by immunocompromised (e.g., liver cirrhosis, iron overload) patients may be followed 1 to 3 days later by septicemia associated with necrotizing cutaneous lesions.

Table 94-1 provides a classification for the spectrum of skin involvement by bacteria and fungi.

DIAGNOSIS

A thorough medical history is critical; it should assess the specific risk factors, such as travel history, animal contacts, marine exposures, occupational and avocational hazards (e.g., farming, gardening), and immune status. If an animal bite has occurred, the timing of the bite, circumstances of injury, and health status of the animal should be determined. Human bites are classified as self-inflicted, occlusal (i.e., intentional), or closed-fist injuries.

In addition to wound assessment, evaluation for other transmissible pathogens, including human immunodeficiency virus (HIV), HSV, *Treponema pallidum* (the etiologic agent of syphilis), and hepatitis B and C viruses, should be pursued. A thorough clinical examination should follow. Initial antimicrobial management, if indicated, is directed by the history and physical examination findings.

Evaluation of hospitalized patients should include a complete blood count and a basic metabolic panel. The C-reactive protein level may be useful as a marker for inflammation and guidance for treatment. The creatine phosphokinase concentration may be helpful, but it is not specific for cases of compartment syndrome and necrotizing fasciitis involving the musculature. Cultures are not indicated for uncomplicated common forms of SSTIs managed in the outpatient setting. The benefit of blood cultures for cellulitis in hospitalized patients is uncertain because the yield is low. Cultures are indicated for patients who require incision and drainage because of the risk of deep structure and underlying tissue involvement.

The most sensitive and specific test for the diagnosis of HSV and VZV cutaneous lesions is nucleic acid amplification. A sample is scraped from the base of an active dermal lesion with a swab. Direct fluorescent antibody testing is less sensitive. Incision and drainage of these lesions is contraindicated.

Special Diagnostic Considerations
Animal Bites

Blood cultures, tissue biopsy, and aspirates for culture of aerobic or anaerobic organisms are preferred methods in cases of animal bites.

Human Bites

Wounds swabs may produce misleading information in cases of human bites. A Gram stain should be performed to assess

TABLE 94-1 CLASSIFICATION OF BACTERIAL AND MYCOTIC INFECTIONS OF THE SKIN

DISEASE OR DISORDER	MICROORGANISMS
PRIMARY PYODERMAS	
Impetigo	*Staphylococcus aureus*, group A streptococci
Folliculitis	*S. aureus*, *Candida* spp, *Pseudomonas aeruginosa* (diffuse folliculitis)
Furuncles and carbuncles	*S. aureus*
Paronychia	*S. aureus*, group A streptococci, *Candida*, *P. aeruginosa*
Ecthyma	Group A streptococci, *Pseudomonas* spp.
Erysipelas	Group A streptococci
Chancriform lesions	*Treponema pallidum*, *Haemophilus ducreyi*, *Sporothrix*, *Bacillus anthracis*, *Francisella tularensis*, *Mycobacterium ulcerans*, *Mycobacterium marinum*
Membranous ulcers	*Corynebacterium diphtheriae*
Cellulitis	Group A or other streptococci, *S. aureus*; rarely, various other organisms
INFECTIOUS GANGRENE AND GANGRENOUS CELLULITIS	
Streptococcal gangrene and necrotizing fasciitis	Group A streptococci, mixed infections with Enterobacteriaceae and anaerobes
Progressive bacterial synergistic gangrene	Anaerobic streptococci plus a second organism (*S. aureus*, *Proteus* spp.)
Gangrenous balanitis and perineal phlegmon	Group A streptococci, mixed infections with enteric bacteria (*Escherichia coli*, *Klebsiella* spp.), anaerobes
Gas gangrene, crepitant cellulitis	*Clostridium perfringens* and other clostridial species; *Bacteroides* spp., peptostreptococci, *Klebsiella* spp., *E. coli*
Gangrenous cellulitis in immunosuppressed patients	*Pseudomonas*, *Aspergillus* spp., agents of mucormycosis
PREEXISTING SKIN LESIONS WITH SECONDARY BACTERIAL INFECTIONS	
Burns	*P. aeruginosa*, *Enterobacter* spp., various other gram-negative bacilli, various streptococci, *S. aureus*, *Candida* spp., *Aspergillus* spp.
Eczematous dermatitis and exfoliative erythrodermas	*S. aureus*, group A streptococci
Chronic ulcers (varicose, decubitus)	*S. aureus*, streptococci, coliform bacteria, *P. aeruginosa*, peptostreptococci, enterococci, *Bacteroides* spp., *C. perfringens*
Dermatophytosis	*S. aureus*, group A streptococci
Traumatic lesions (abrasions, animal bites, insect bites)	*Pasturella multocida*, *C. diphtheriae*, *S. aureus*, group A streptococci
Vesicular or bullous eruptions (varicella, pemphigus)	*S. aureus*, group A streptococci
Acne conglobata	*Propionibacterium acnes*
Hidradenitis suppurativa	*S. aureus*, *Proteus* spp. and other coliforms, streptococci, peptostreptococci, *P. aeruginosa*, *Bacteroides* spp.
Intertrigo	*S. aureus*, coliforms, *Candida* spp.
Pilonidal and sebaceous cysts	Peptostreptococci, *Bacteroides* sp., coliforms, *S. aureus*
Pyoderma gangrenosa	*S. aureus*, peptostreptococci, *Proteus* spp. and other coliforms, *P. aeruginosa*
CUTANEOUS INVOLVEMENT IN SYSTEMIC INFECTIONS	
Bacteremias	*S. aureus*, group A streptococci (and other groups such as D), *Neisseria meningitidis*, *Neisseria gonorrhoeae*, *P. aeruginosa*, *Salmonella typhi*, *Haemophilus influenzae*
Infective endocarditis	Viridans streptococci, *S. aureus*, group D streptococci, and others
Fungemias	*Candida* spp., *Cryptococcus* spp., *Blastomyces dermatitidis*, *Fusarium*
Listeriosis	*Listeria monocytogenes*
Leptospirosis (Weil's disease and pretibial fever)	*Leptospira interrogans* serotypes
Rat-bite fever	*Streptobacillus moniliformis*, *Spirillum minus*
Melioidosis	*Burkholderia pseudomallei*
Glanders	*Burkholderia mallei*
Carrión's disease (verruga peruana)	*Bartonella bacilliformis*
SCARLET FEVER SYNDROMES	
Scarlet fever	Group A streptococci, rarely *S. aureus*
Scalded skin syndrome	*S. aureus* (phage group II)
Toxic shock syndrome	Group A streptococci, *S. aureus* (pyrogenic toxin–producing strains)
PARAINFECTIOUS AND POSTINFECTIOUS NONSUPPURATIVE COMPLICATIONS	
Purpura fulminans (manifestation of disseminated intravascular coagulation)	Group A streptococci, *N. meningitidis*, *S. aureus*, pneumococcus
Erythema nodosum	Group A streptococci, *Mycobacterium tuberculosis*, *Mycobacterium leprae*, *Coccidioides immitis*, *Leptospira autumnalis*, *Yersinia enterocolitica*, *Legionella pneumophila*
Erythema multiforme–like lesions (rarely), guttate psoriasis	Group A streptococci
OTHER LESIONS	
Erythrasma	*Corynebacterium minutissimum*
Nodular lesions	*Candida*, *Sporothrix*, *S. aureus* (botryomycosis), *M. marinum*, *Leishmania brasiliensis*; leprosy due to *M. leprae* can cause popular lesions, nodular, and ulcerative lesions
Hyperplastic (pseudoepitheliomatous) and proliferative lesions (e.g., mycetomas)	*Nocardia* spp., *Pseudallescheria boydii*, *Blastomyces dermatitidis*, *Paracoccidioides brasiliensis*, *Phialophora*, *Cladosporium*
Vascular papules/nodules (bacillary angiomatosis, epithelioid angiomatosis)	*Bartonella henselae*, *Bartonella quintana*
Annular erythema (erythema chronicum migrans)	*Borrelia burgdorferi*

Modified from Mandell GL, Bennett JE, Dolin R, editors: Mandell, Douglas, and Bennett's principles and practice of infectious diseases, ed 7, Philadelphia, 2009, Churchill Livingstone.

organisms, neutrophils (i.e., inflammation), and squamous epithelial cells (i.e., superficial contamination). If feasible, tissue biopsy or aspiration of the infected site can provide specimens for aerobic and anaerobic culture.

Traumatic Wounds

The optimal time to acquire specimens for cultures is immediately after débridement of the wound site. Analysis of initial cultures should focus on common pathogens, and additional testing should be reserved for uncommon or rare infections associated with unusual circumstances, such as *Vibrio* species after salt water exposure. Tissue biopsy and special stains may be required in certain situations, such as suspected infection with *M. marinum*.

Burn Wounds

Before sampling, the burn area must be clean and devoid of topical antimicrobial agents. Surface swabs or tissue biopsies are recommended for obtaining culture samples, and histopathologic examination can monitor for the presence and extent of infection. Quantitative evaluation of swab or culture specimens is recommended twice weekly to monitor colonization. Evidence of systemic infection related to the wound should prompt blood cultures.

Diabetic Foot Infections

Superficial swab cultures of ulcerations can be misleading and should be avoided. If surgical débridement is performed, deep tissue specimens should be sent to the microbiology laboratory for evaluation.

Radiographs should be obtained if bone involvement is suspected, and they may also be useful in demonstrating soft tissue gas before crepitus is detected (Fig. 94-6). Magnetic resonance imaging is the most sensitive modality. Chapter 87 discusses the laboratory diagnosis of infectious diseases in more detail.

Differential Diagnosis

Many noninfectious conditions can mimic SSTIs:

- Brown recluse spider bite
- Contact dermatitis
- Gout
- Psoriatic arthritis with distal dactylitis
- Reiter's syndrome

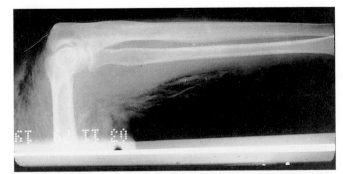

FIGURE 94-6 Radiograph of patient with clostridial myonecrosis shows gas in the tissues. (Courtesy J.W. Tomford, MD.)

- Relapsing polychondritis
- Ruptured Baker's cyst
- Mixed cryoglobulinemia due to immune complex disease from chronic hepatitis C or B infection (may have an erythematous rash)
- Pyoderma gangrenosum
- Sweet's syndrome (acute febrile neutrophilic dermatosis)
- Venous stasis

TREATMENT
Pharmacologic and Supportive Care

Mild cases of cellulitis may be managed on an outpatient basis with dicloxacillin, amoxicillin, or cephalexin. Clindamycin or levofloxacin may be used in patients allergic to penicillin. Severe cellulitis should be managed with parenteral cefazolin, nafcillin, or oxacillin. Clindamycin or vancomycin may be used in patients with allergies to penicillin. Concomitant tinea infection should be treated with a topical antifungal agent such as clotrimazole or terbinafine.

Mild cases of community-acquired MRSA may be managed with clindamycin, trimethoprim-sulfamethoxazole, or tetracycline if antibiotics are indicated. The latter two agents do not, however, provide adequate streptococcal coverage. Severe cases requiring parenteral antibiotics require vancomycin, daptomycin, telavancin, ceftaroline, clindamycin, or linezolid. A β-lactam antibiotic may be considered for hospitalized patients with nonpurulent cellulitis, with modification to MRSA-active treatment if is there is no clinical response. Cellulitis associated with an abscess requires surgical drainage.

In addition to supportive care, urgent surgical consultation should be obtained in the event that crepitus, bullae, rapidly evolving cellulitis, or pain disproportional to physical examination findings suggests necrotizing fasciitis. Initial parenteral therapy with vancomycin, daptomycin, linezolid with piperacillin-tazobactam, cefepime plus metronidazole, or a carbapenem is appropriate. Type II necrotizing fasciitis due to *S. pyogenes* or clostridial myonecrosis should prompt combined therapy with parenteral penicillin and clindamycin. The use of intravenous immune globulin in cases of necrotizing fasciitis remains controversial.

Compartment syndrome requires emergent surgical decompression to prevent muscle necrosis and irreversible neuronal damage. Cellulitis or wound infections attributed to *A. hemolyticum* may be treated with clindamycin, erythromycin, vancomycin, or tetracycline. HSV and VZV infections are susceptible to acyclovir, famciclovir, or valacyclovir if treatment is indicated.

Special Treatment Considerations
Animal Bites

Mild cases of animal bites may be treated with amoxicillin-clavulanate. For patients with a penicillin allergy, a fluoroquinolone plus clindamycin or sulfamethoxazole-trimethoprim plus metronidazole are alternatives that may be used in oral or parenteral forms. Inpatient parenteral agents including ampicillin-sulbactam or piperacillin-tazobactam may be used for patients who are not allergic to penicillin.

Tularemia is treated with gentamicin, tobramycin, streptomycin, doxycycline, or ciprofloxacin. Azithromycin is the drug of choice for cat-scratch disease. For individuals at risk for *E. rhusiopathiae* infection, the treatment of choice is penicillin or ampicillin or use of a third-generation cephalosporin or fluoroquinolone in penicillin-allergic patients.

Animal handlers with cutaneous anthrax infection require treatment with ciprofloxacin or levofloxacin. Cases of suspected bioterrorism must be reported immediately.

Marine Lacerations and Punctures

The treatment regimen for marine lacerations and punctures should include doxycycline and ceftazidime or a fluoroquinolone. Treatment of fresh water injuries should include a third- or fourth-generation cephalosporin (i.e., ceftazidime or cefepime) or a fluoroquinolone. If *M. marinum* is suspected, treatment with clarithromycin, minocycline, doxycycline, sulfamethoxazole-trimethoprim, or rifampin plus ethambutol is appropriate.

Human Bites

Patients who have human bite wounds without evidence of infection should receive prophylactic treatment with amoxicillin-clavulanate for 3 to 5 days. Closed-fist injuries require radiographic evaluation and consultation with a hand surgeon for possible wound exploration. Parenteral treatment with ampicillin-sulbactam or moxifloxacin is recommended.

Burn Wounds

Systemic therapy with antibiotics and antifungals are reserved for burn patients demonstrating signs of sepsis or septic shock. Infection due to mucormycoses requires liposomal amphotericin B.

Diabetic Foot Infections

Simple infections such as cellulitis are most often caused by group A streptococci or *S. aureus* and should be managed accordingly. If ulcers do not have purulence or inflammation, antimicrobials are not indicated. Severe limb-threatening infections require surgical evaluation and broad-spectrum antibiotic coverage because infection tends to include aerobic and anaerobic organisms. Empirical therapy directed at *P. aeruginosa* is not usually necessary unless the patient has other risk factors. MRSA-active treatment is recommended for patients with a history of MRSA, when the local prevalence of MRSA is high in the community, or if the infection is severe. All wounds require adequate wound irrigation and débridement.

⬤ PROGNOSIS

Full recovery is expected for patients with simple SSTIs provided they receive appropriate treatment. For those who develop complications such as necrotizing fasciitis, the estimated mortality rate is between 30% and 70%. The prognosis is guarded for patients with multiple comorbidities and those who are immunosuppressed.

SUGGESTED READINGS

Baddour L: Skin abscesses, furuncles and carbuncles, UpToDate. Available at http://www.uptodate.com/contents/skin-abscesses. Accessed October 31, 2014.

Baron EJ, Miller JM, Weinstein MP, et al: A guide to utilization of the microbiology laboratory for diagnosis of infectious diseases: 2013 recommendations by the Infectious Diseases Society of America (IDSA) and the American Society of Microbiology (ASM). Available at http://www.idsociety.org/uploadedFiles/IDSA/Guidelines-Patient_Care/PDF_Library/Laboratory%20Diagnosis%20of%20Infectious%20Diseases%20Guideline.pdf

Cohen J, Powderly WG, Opal SM, editors: Infectious diseases, ed 3, London, 2010, Mosby.

Golstein EJ: Bite wounds and infectious, Clin Infect Dis 14:633–640, 1992.

Herchline T: Cellulitis treatment and management. Available at http://emedicine.medscape.com/article/214222-overview. Accessed October 31, 2014.

Lipsky BA, Berendt AR, Cornia PB, et al: 2012 Infectious Diseases Society of America clinical practice guideline for the diagnosis and treatment of diabetic foot infections, Clin Infect Dis 54:132–173, 2012.

Liu C, Bayer A, Cosgrove SE, et al: Clinical practice guidelines by the Infectious Diseases Society of America for the treatment if methicillin-resistant *Staphylococcus aureus* infectious in adults and children, Clin Infect Dis 52:e18–e55, 2011.

Stevens DL, Bisno AL, Chambers HF, et al: Practice guidelines for the diagnosis and management of skin and soft-tissue infections, Clin Infect Dis 41:1373–1406, 2005.

95

Intraabdominal Infections

Edward J. Wing

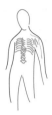

INTRODUCTION

Intraabdominal infections are serious conditions that usually result from perforation or obstruction of abdominal organs. These infections often require surgical intervention to drain abscesses, repair perforations, and relieve obstructions. The cause is typically polymicrobial infection, including aerobic and anaerobic bacteria that require broad antibiotic coverage. Guidelines for diagnosis and therapy have been developed by the Surgical Infection Society and the Infectious Diseases Society of America (Tables 95-1, 95-2, and 95-3). This chapter focuses on the most common intraabdominal infections found in adults.

APPENDICITIS

Definition and Epidemiology

Appendicitis is an acute inflammation of the appendix that is usually caused by an obstruction of the lumen by an appendicolith. Appendicitis is the most common cause of emergency surgery worldwide. In the United States in 2007, appendicitis accounted for 295,000 hospital discharges and $7.4 billion in hospital costs. The lifetime risk is 7% to 12%, with a slight preponderance among men.

Pathology

The normal appendix is 5 to 10 cm long and typically lies anterior to the cecum. Locations that affect the clinical manifestations include retrocecal, pelvic, and retroileal variants. Obstruction of the proximal appendix is typically caused by an appendicolith;

less common causes are tumors, mesenteric lymphadenitis, parasites, and seeds. Obstruction leads to swelling, compromise of the blood supply, and inflammation with a resulting neutrophilic infiltrate of the appendicular wall. Gangrene of the wall and rupture eventually occurs.

TABLE 95-2 REGIMENS USED FOR INITIAL EMPIRICAL TREATMENT OF BILIARY INFECTION IN ADULTS

INFECTION	REGIMEN
Community-acquired acute cholecystitis of mild to moderate severity	Cefazolin, cefuroxime, or ceftriaxone
Community-acquired acute cholecystitis of severe physiologic disturbance, advanced age, or immunocompromised status	Imipenem-cilastatin, meropenem, doripenem, piperacillin-tazobactam, ciprofloxacin, levofloxacin, or cefepime, each in combination with metronidazole*
Acute cholangitis after bilioenteric anastomosis of any severity	Imipenem-cilastatin, meropenem, doripenem, piperacillin-tazobactam, ciprofloxacin, levofloxacin, or cefepime, each in combination with metronidazole*
Health care–associated biliary infection of any severity	Imipenem-cilastatin, meropenem, doripenem, piperacillin-tazobactam, ciprofloxacin, levofloxacin, or cefepime, each in combination with metronidazole, vancomycin added to each regimen*

From Solomkin JS, Mazuski JE, Gradley JS, et al: Diagnosis and management of complicated intraabdominal infection in adults and children: guidelines by the Surgical Infection Society and the Infectious Diseases Society of America, Surg Infect 11:79–109, 2010.
*Because of increasing resistance of *Escherichia coli* to fluoroquinolones, local population susceptibility profiles and, if available, isolate susceptibility should be reviewed.

TABLE 95-1 AGENTS AND REGIMENS FOR THE INITIAL EMPIRICAL TREATMENT OF EXTRABILIARY COMPLICATED INTRAABDOMINAL INFECTION

REGIMEN	COMMUNITY-ACQUIRED INFECTION IN CHILDREN	COMMUNITY-ACQUIRED INFECTION IN ADULTS	
		Mild to Moderate Severity*	High Risk or Severity†
Single agent	Ertapenem, meropenem, imipenem-cilastatin, ticarcillin-clavulanate, and piperacillin-tazobactam	Cefoxitin, ertapenem moxifloxacin, tigecycline, and ticarcillin-clavulanic acid	Imipenem-cilastatin, meropenem, doripenem, and piperacillin-tazobactam
Combination	Ceftriaxone, cefotaxime, cefepime, or ceftazidime, each in combination with metronidazole; gentamicin or tobramycin, each in combination with metronidazole or clindamycin and with or without ampicillin	Cefazolin, cefuroxime, ceftriaxone, cefotaxime, ciprofloxacin, or levofloxacin, each in combination with metronidazole†	Cefepime, ceftazidime, ciprofloxacin, or levofloxacin, each in combination with metronidazole*

From Solomkin JS, Mazuski JE, Gradley JS, et al: Diagnosis and management of complicated intraabdominal infection in adults and children: guidelines by the Surgical Infection Society and the Infectious Diseases Society of America, Surg Infect 11:79–109, 2010, Table 2.
*Includes perforated or abscessed appendicitis and other infections of mild to moderate severity.
†Includes severe physiologic disturbance, advanced age, and immunocompromised states.
‡Because of increasing resistance of *Escherichia coli* to fluoroquinolones, local population susceptibility profiles and, if available, isolate susceptibility should be reviewed.

TABLE 95-3	INTRAVENOUS ANTIBIOTICS FOR EMPIRICAL TREATMENT OF COMPLICATED INTRAABDOMINAL INFECTION
ANTIBIOTIC	**ADULT DOSAGE***
β-LACTAM/β-LACTAMASE INHIBITOR COMBINATION	
Piperacillin-tazobactam	3.375 g q6h[†]
Ticarcillin-clavulanic acid	3.1 g q6h; FDA labeling indicates 200 mg/kg/day in divided doses q6h for moderate infection and 300 mg/kg/day in divided doses q4h for severe infection
CARBAPENEMS	
Doripenem	500 mg q8h
Ertapenem	1 g q24h
Imipenem-cilastatin	500 mg q6h or 1 g q8h
Meropenem	1 g q8h
CEPHALOSPORINS	
Cefazolin	1-2 g q8h
Cefepime	2 g q8-12h
Cefotaxime	1-2 g q6-8h
Cefoxitin	2 g q6h
Ceftazidime	2 g q8h
Ceftriaxone	1-2 g q12-24h
Cefuroxime	1.5 g q8h
Tigecycline	100-mg initial dose, then 50 mg q12h
FLUOROQUINOLONES	
Ciprofloxacin	400 mg q12h
Levofloxacin	750 mg q24h
Moxifloxacin	400 mg q24h
Metronidazole	500 mg q8-12h or 1500 mg q24h
AMINOGLYCOSIDES	
Gentamicin or tobramycin	5-7 mg/kg[‡] q24h[§]
Amikacin	15-20 mg /kg[‡] q24h[§]
Aztreonam	1-2 g q6-8h
Vancomycin	15-20 mg/kg[∥] q8-12h[§]

From Solomkin JS, Mazuski JE, Gradley JS, et al: Diagnosis and management of complicated intraabdominal infection in adults and children: guidelines by the Surgical Infection Society and the Infectious Diseases Society of America, Surg Infect 11:79–109, 2010.

FDA, U.S. Food and Drug Administration.

*Dosages are based on normal renal and hepatic function.

[†]For *Pseudomonas aeruginosa* infection, dosage may be increased to 3.375 g q4h or 4.5 g q6h.

[‡]Initial dosage regimens for aminoglycosides should be based on adjusted body weight.

[§]Monitoring of serum drug concentration should be considered for dosage individualization.

[∥]Initial dosage regimens for vancomycin should be based on total body weight.

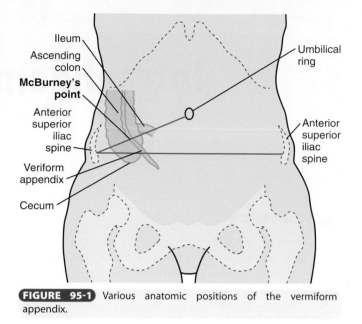

FIGURE 95-1 Various anatomic positions of the vermiform appendix.

umbilicus (Fig. 95-1). Seventy-five percent of patients vomit once or twice.

Evidence of peritoneal irritation includes rebound and guarding. Patients are typically supine and do not want to move. Pain may also be elicited by flexion and internal rotation of the right hip (i.e., obturator sign) or passive extension of the right hip (i.e., psoas sign). Palpation of the left lower quadrant pain may produce right lower quadrant pain (i.e., Rovsing's sign).

Patients usually have little fever or tachycardia. Determining whether a patient has a ruptured appendix, which occurs in 25% of cases, can be difficult. If the clinical presentation is delayed 4 to 5 days and rupture has occurred, there may be fever, tachycardia, and a palpable mass.

Variations in the presentation include initial right lower quadrant pain, back and flank pain (i.e., retrocecal appendix), suprapubic pain (i.e., pelvic appendix), and left lower quadrant pain (i.e., long appendix). The elderly may have no periumbilical or right lower quadrant pain. Children may not be able to give an accurate history, and in pregnant women, the appendix may be pushed upward by the expanding uterus. At 8 months' gestation, the pregnant woman's pain may be in the right upper quadrant.

Diagnosis

The diagnosis of acute appendicitis is important but can be difficult. A careful meta-analysis reported that the history, physical examination, and inflammatory markers are singly unreliable predictors of the diagnosis, but when combined, they are accurate. A careful history and physical examination should be obtained. Pain migrating from the umbilical area to the right lower quadrant should be sought in the history. Signs of peritoneal irritation, including rebound, percussion tenderness, guarding, and rigidity, should be determined. The total white blood cell count, number of neutrophils, percentage of bands, and level of C-reactive protein should be measured.

The Alvarado system was developed to aid in the diagnosis of appendicitis (Table 95-4). Using the mnemonic MANTRELS, it

The bacteriology of acute appendicitis, including rupture, is polymicrobial, with gut aerobes (*Escherichia coli* is most common) and anaerobes (*Bacteroides fragilis* is most common). Typically, 10 to 14 different organisms can be isolated. This picture is similar to other intraabdominal infections such as diverticulitis.

Clinical Presentation

Classically, acute appendicitis begins with anorexia followed by periumbilical pain. The pain is steady, moderately severe, and sometimes cramping. After 4 to 6 hours, the pain migrates to the right lower quadrant, where the site of maximal tenderness is located at McBurney's point. This point is 0.5 to 2 inches inside the right anterior spinous process of the ilium on a line to the scores the impact of eight factors: *m*igration, *a*norexia, *n*ausea and vomiting, *t*enderness in the right lower quadrant, *r*ebound of pain, *e*levation of temperature, *l*eukocytosis, and *s*hift to the left. A patient with a score of 5 or 6 is usually observed, but an individual with a score of 7 or greater should undergo surgery.

Two prospective trials demonstrated the accuracy of helical computed tomography (CT) with contrast for the diagnosis of acute appendicitis. The initial CT findings of appendicitis are enlargement of the appendix, usually to an appendiceal diameter of more than 6 mm (Fig. 95-2). The wall is thickened and enhances with contrast. Later findings include inflammation,

thickening of the cecal wall, and pericecal fat stranding. An appendicolith is a helpful sign. If perforation has occurred, extensive inflammatory changes are seen, which may include an abscess cavity. Although there has been controversy about whether CT scans are necessary or more accurate than clinical assessment in every case, the current standard of care in emergency departments includes a CT scan. Use of CT has reduced the rate of finding normal appendices at surgery from between 11% and 15% to between 3% and 5%.

Diagnostic ultrasound is accurate if carefully performed and can be particularly useful in small children and pregnant women. Because of its accuracy and lack of ionizing radiation, magnetic resonance imaging (MRI) has become the scanning modality of choice in many centers for children, pregnant women, and other patients. Nonetheless, CT scanning is rapid and more likely available, and it is therefore the procedure of choice for most patients.

The differential diagnosis for acute appendicitis is long. It includes urinary tract infection and stones; gynecologic problems such as a ruptured ovarian cyst, ectopic pregnancy, and pelvic inflammatory disease; and bowel pathology, including diverticulitis and Crohn's disease.

Treatment

Laparoscopic (75% of procedures) or open appendectomy is the treatment of choice for emergent cases. If rupture is identified, antibiotics and drainage are indicated. Pretreatment antibiotics in all cases prevent wound infection and intraabdominal infections as indicated by a Cochran review. Antibiotics to cover *E. coli*

TABLE 95-4	ALVARADO OR MANTRELS* SYSTEM FOR DIAGNOSING ACUTE APPENDICITIS	
FEATURES SCORED	**VARIABLE**	**VALUE**
Symptoms	Migration	1
	Anorexia	1
	Nausea-vomiting	2
Signs	Tenderness in right lower quadrant	2
	Rebound of pain	1
	Elevation of temperature (≥37.3° C)	1
Laboratory values	Leukocytosis (white blood cell count >10.000/µL)	2
	Shift to the left (>75% neutrophils)	1
Total score		10

From Wray CJ, Kao LS, Millas SG, et al: Acute appendicitis: controversies in diagnosis and management, *Curr Probl Surg* 50:54–86, 2013.

*MANTRELS mnemonic: *M*igration, *a*norexia, *n*ausea and vomiting, *t*enderness in right lower quadrant, *r*ebound of pain, *e*levation of temperature, *l*eukocytosis, *s*hift to the left.

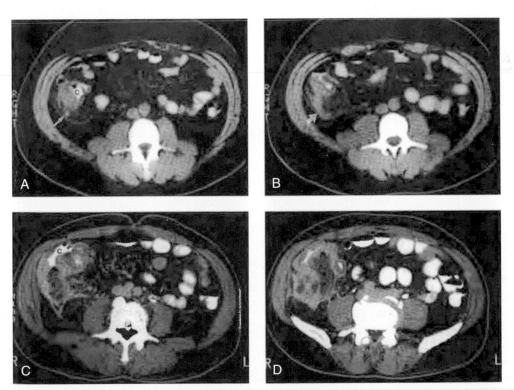

FIGURE 95-2 Computed tomography (CT) of acute appendicitis. **A,** CT scan of uncomplicated appendicitis shows an appendicolith *(arrow)*. **B,** CT scan shows a dilated appendix *(arrow)* and surrounding inflammation in the pericolic fat. **C** and **D,** Two views at different levels of perforated appendicitis with abscess formation. C, Cecum. (From Novelline RA, editor: *Squire's fundamentals of radiology*, ed 6, Cambridge, Mass., 1964, Harvard University Press, Figures 13.43 and 13.44.)

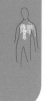

and *B. fragilis* are recommended by the guidelines from the Surgical Infection Society and Infectious Diseases Society of America (see Tables 95-1 and 95-3). The recommendations also apply to other intraabdominal infections, such as diverticulitis. Antibiotics should be stopped after surgery in simple cases. If rupture has occurred, it is usually safe to stop antibiotics after 5 to 7 days.

Some studies over the past decade have advocated antibiotics alone for the treatment of acute appendicitis. Although provocative and potentially a future direction for care, the lack of a sufficient number of controlled trials, the difficulty of confirming the diagnosis in trials, and the high recurrence and complication rates make this approach unsuitable for general application.

Prognosis

The mortality rate in the United States is extremely low for uncomplicated cases. Rupture, however, results in an overall 1% mortality rate and a 5% rate in elderly patients. Wound infection occurs in 1% to 20%. The rate of fetal loss in pregnant women with appendicitis is 1.5%, but the rate is 20% to 35% in cases of rupture.

⬤ DIVERTICULITIS
Definition and Epidemiology

Diverticulitis is inflammation and infection resulting from perforation of diverticula of the bowel wall, usually in the sigmoid colon. Diverticulitis is diagnosed in more than 2 million patients each year and accounted for 219,000 hospital discharges in 2009 in the United States. It is also the most common cause of sigmoid colon resection.

Diverticula occur in less than 10% of people younger than 40 years and in 50% to 80% of those older than 80 years. Between 10% and 25% of individuals with diverticulosis develop diverticulitis. Rates of diverticulosis in rural Africa and Asia are less than 1%. Diet is thought to be a critical risk factor. Supporting this hypothesis was a study measuring diverticulosis in Japanese populations in Japan (1% prevalence) and individuals of Japanese heritage living in the United States (52% prevalence).

Pathology

Diverticula are herniations of the mucosa and muscularis through the colonic wall between the taeniae coli where the main blood vessels penetrate the wall. Diverticulitis results from macroscopic or microscopic perforations, resulting in inflammation, local infection, and in severe cases, free air and diffuse peritonitis (Fig. 95-3).

Clinical Presentation and Diagnosis

Noninflamed diverticula cause no symptoms. Patients with uncomplicated diverticulitis have left lower quadrant pain often accompanied by nausea and fever. CT, which is the diagnostic test of choice, may show pericolic soft tissue stranding, colonic wall thickening, and a phlegmon. Between 10% and 20% of patients have severe pain, tenderness, fever, and leukocytosis, and they require hospital admission for intravenous antibiotics. The differential diagnosis for diverticulitis includes urinary tract infection, gastroenteritis, inflammatory bowel disease, perforated colonic cancer, appendicitis, and bowel obstruction.

Complicated diverticulitis occurs when the perforation is not contained. Patients may have severe abdominal pain, free air, guarding, rigidity, and multisystem failure. Complications include abscess seen in pericolic, retroperitoneal, or pelvic areas on CT; purulent or feculent peritonitis; and colovesical, colovaginal, or coloenteric fistulas (5% occurrence). Percutaneous drainage of abscesses or surgery, including sigmoid resection, is usually indicated in these situations.

Treatment and Prognosis

Uncomplicated diverticulitis can be treated on an outpatient basis with oral antibiotics, and more severe cases are treated with intravenous antibiotics for 7 to 10 days on an inpatient basis (see Tables 95-1 and 95-3). Although data from a Cochrane review and a controlled trial conducted in Sweden suggest that not all patients need to be treated with antibiotics, the standard of care in the United States is to treat with antibiotics. The most important organisms to cover in this polymicrobial infection are *E. coli* and *B. fragilis*. Complicated diverticulitis requires point source control (i.e., drainage or bowel resection), intravenous antibiotics to cover bowel flora, and systemic resuscitation. Fistulas require surgical resection and repair.

Colonoscopy should be done 6 to 8 weeks after an episode of diverticulitis to rule out colonic cancer. The recurrence rate of diverticulitis is approximately 20%. A high-fiber diet, weight loss, and exercise are recommended to prevent recurrence. Sigmoid resection may be considered after the second recurrence, depending on age, medical condition, and the frequency and severity of episodes. If the sigmoid colon is removed, more than 95% of patients have no further episodes.

⬤ CHOLECYSTITIS AND CHOLANGITIS
Definition and Epidemiology

Gallstones occur in 11% to 36% of the population. Approximately 20% of patients with gallstones develop temporary obstruction of the cystic duct at some time. This results in biliary colic (i.e., episodes of right upper quadrant pain) lasting 1 to 5 hours. Cholecystitis occurs when the cystic duct is obstructed for longer periods. Intraluminal pressure increases, compromising blood and lymphatic flow, and it may result in acute inflammation and infection.

Among patients with gallstones, 6% to 12% have stones in the common duct or choledocholithiasis. Cholangitis results from obstruction of the common duct, usually by common duct stones, leading to inflammation and often to severe infection.

Clinical Presentation

Patients with biliary pain have various sites of maximal pain and radiation of pain (Fig. 95-4). Classic signs of acute cholecystitis include unremitting right upper quadrant pain that is more severe than biliary colic, fever, anorexia, nausea, and vomiting. Murphy's sign (i.e., inspiratory arrest with deep palpation of the right upper quadrant) is positive. Accuracy is increased by assessing the gallbladder with ultrasound and eliciting pain with the probe (i.e., sonographic Murphy's sign).

Elderly patients and patients with diabetes may have more subtle clinical presentations. A mild leukocytosis may be

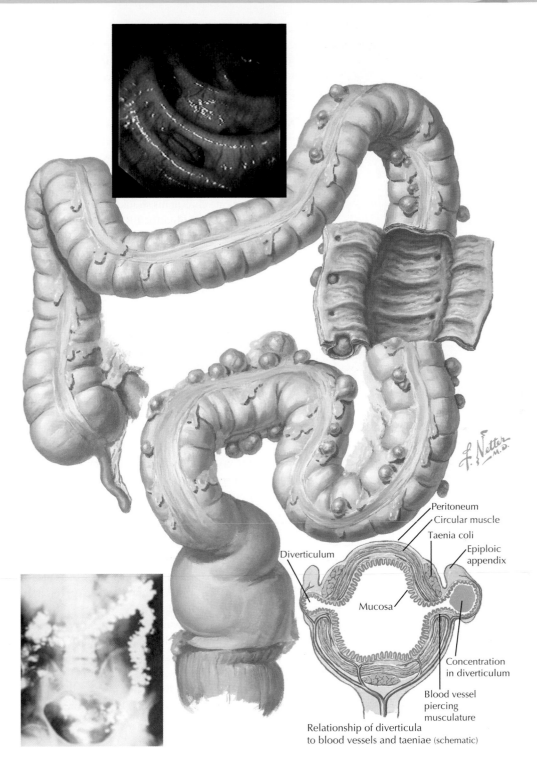

FIGURE 95-3   Diverticulosis. (From the Netter Collection of Medical Illustrations. Available at www.netterimages.com. Accessed October 31, 2014.)

identified. Bacterial contamination of the gallbladder occurs in 15% to 30%. If obstruction continues, gangrenous cholecystitis, necrosis of the gallbladder wall and abscess or empyema may occur. Perforation, which rarely occurs, is usually limited to the subhepatic space. Infection by gas-forming organisms may result in emphysematous cholecystitis.

Acute cholangitis with common duct obstruction can cause mild and self-limited disease to fulminant, life threatening infection. Two thirds of patients have Charcot's triad (i.e., right upper quadrant pain, fever, and jaundice). Fever is often accompanied by rigors. The addition of hypotension and mental status changes results in Reynolds pentad (i.e., jaundice, fever, abdominal pain, shock, and altered mental status), a sign of severe disease. Leukocytosis and elevated alkaline phosphatase and bilirubin levels are typical. Bile cultures usually show bowel organisms, and blood cultures are positive in 30% to 40% of cases.

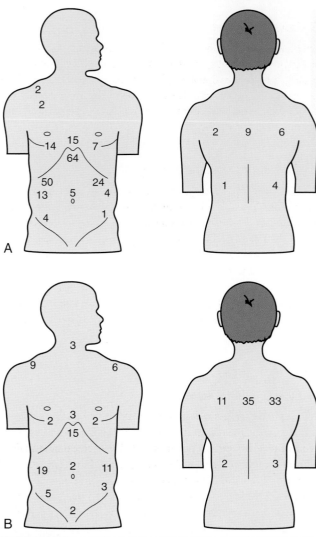

FIGURE 95-4 **A,** Sites of the most severe pain during an episode of biliary pain in 107 patients with gallstones (% values add up to >100% because of multiple responses). The subxiphoid and right subcostal areas were the most common sites; note that the left subcostal region was not an unusual site of pain. **B,** Sites of pain radiation (%) during an episode of biliary pain in the same group of patients. (Modified from Burnicardi FC, Andersen DK, Billiar TR, et al: Schwartz's principles of surgery, ed 9, New York, 2009, McGraw-Hill.)

For a deeper discussion of these topics, please see Chapter 155, "Diseases of the Gallbladder and Bile Ducts," in Goldman-Cecil Medicine, 25th Edition.

Diagnosis

Ultrasonography is 95% sensitive and specific for the diagnosis. In cholecystitis, ultrasound shows a thickened gallbladder wall and pericholecystic fluid. In cholangitis, ultrasound shows a dilated common duct, but obstructing gallstones are difficult to identify. Endoscopic retrograde cholangiopancreatography (ERCP) is required for a definitive diagnosis of cholangitis. The differential diagnosis includes peptic ulcer disease with or without perforation, pancreatitis, appendicitis, hepatitis, myocardial infarction, and pneumonia.

Treatment

Biliary colic is usually self-limited. Acute cholecystitis usually requires intervention to relieve obstruction of the cystic duct, but it may remit spontaneously. Laparoscopic cholecystectomy is indicated emergently if there is gangrene or perforation; otherwise, surgery should be done within 1 to 3 days. Antibiotics are routinely given to cover bowel flora. Ceftriaxone can be given for mild to moderate disease, whereas broader coverage such as imipenem-cilastatin or piperacillin-tazobactam should be given for more severe disease (see Tables 95-1, 95-2, and 95-3).

Acute cholangitis should be treated initially with fluid resuscitation and antibiotics. ERCP is indicated for diagnosis and relief of obstruction. Emergency decompression of the biliary tract by ERCP or surgery may be indicated for severely ill patients.

● INFECTIONS OF SOLID ORGANS
Hepatic Abscess

Liver abscess is usually caused by bacteria or *Entamoeba histolytica*. Both are rare. The incidence of bacterial abscess is 10 to 20 cases per million people per year, and the incidence of amebic abscess is 1 case per million per year in the United States. Worldwide, however, 10% of people are infected with gastrointestinal *E. histolytica*, and liver abscess is the most common extraintestinal manifestation.

The biliary tract is the most common source of infection for bacterial hepatic abscess. Other sources include direct extension (e.g., perforated appendicitis), portal vein (e.g., abdominal infection), hepatic artery (e.g., bacterial line infection), and trauma. In 20% to 40% of cases, no cause is found. The bacteriology of hepatic abscess reflects the source, with polymicrobial bowel flora being the most common. Hematogenous sources are usually staphylococcal or streptococcal species. Less common organisms include *Klebsiella pneumoniae*, which is identified particularly in case series from Asia, and *Candida* species found in immunocompromised patients.

Liver abscess usually manifests with fever for days to weeks. Right upper quadrant abdominal pain and tenderness are found in one half of patients and jaundice in one fourth. Peripheral blood leukocyte counts are elevated in three fourths, and two thirds have an obstructive liver profile with an elevated alkaline phosphatase level. Table 95-5 illustrates the differences between amebic and bacterial liver abscesses.

Patients with amebic liver abscess tend to be younger men with more right upper quadrant pain and a more acute course than those with bacterial hepatic abscess. There often is a history of travel or residence in a highly endemic geographic area.

Ultrasound is the preferred initial diagnostic test because it is rapid and can help to identify biliary sources. CT is more specific and can identify other causes of liver abscess, such as extension from an intraabdominal abscess. The right lobe is most commonly infected, and 50% of cases are multifocal.

Drainage of liver abscesses is essential. Percutaneous aspiration of the abscess is therapeutic and diagnostic. Repeated aspirations or catheter placement may be necessary. Antibiotics are directed by the likely source and by results of Gram stain and culture. Blood cultures are positive in 50% of cases and may be

TABLE 95-5	AMEBIC AND PYOGENIC LIVER ABSCESSES	
FEATURE	**AMEBIC LIVER ABSCESS**	**PYOGENIC LIVER ABSCESS**
EPIDEMIOLOGY		
Male-to-female ratio	5-18	1.0-2.4
Age (yr)	30-40	50-60
Duration (days)	<14 (≈75% of cases)	5-26
Mortality (%)	10-25	0-5
SYMPTOMS AND SIGNS*		
Fever	80	80
Weight loss	40	30
Abdominal pain	80	55
Diarrhea	15-35	10-20
Cough	10	5-10
Jaundice	10-15	10-25
Right upper quadrant tenderness	75	25-55
LABORATORY TESTS*		
Leukocytosis	80	75
Elevated alkaline phosphatase	80	65
Solitary lesion	70	70

From Sifri CD, Madoff LC: Infections of the liver and biliary system. In Mandell GL, Bennett JE, Dolin R, editors: Mandell, Douglas, and Bennett's principles and practice of infectious diseases, ed 7, Philadelphia, 2009, Churchill Livingstone.
   *Approximate percentage of cases.

the only positive culture. Therapy is usually given for 4 to 6 weeks. Rupture or sepsis syndrome occurs rarely. Surgery may be necessary if there is a lack of response, rupture, or complex multilocular abscesses.

The serologic analysis for *E. histolytica* is 95% sensitive but cannot distinguish gastrointestinal disease from hepatic abscess. Treatment for amebic infection is oral metronidazole for 7 to 10 days.

Pancreatic Infection

Although most episodes of pancreatitis are self-limited, infected necrotizing pancreatitis has a mortality rate approaching 30%. Acute pancreatitis is characterized by upper abdominal pain that often radiates to the back and is accompanied by nausea and vomiting. The serum amylase concentration is greater than three times the normal value, and CT shows typical inflammation in the pancreas. Eighty percent of acute pancreatitis cases are mild, whereas 20% of cases are moderate to severe.

Patients with infected necrotizing pancreatitis typically develop fever, leukocytosis, and increased abdominal pain several weeks after the onset of pancreatitis. The standard of care includes antibiotics to cover cultured microorganisms (typically enteric bacteria or *Staphylococcus aureus*), and surgical débridement is delayed for 4 to 6 weeks if possible. Because early surgical intervention may increase the mortality rate, delayed débridement is recommended.

Pancreatic abscess usually occurs 2 to 6 weeks after an episode of acute pancreatitis. Treatment is percutaneous drainage plus antibiotics. Distinguishing pancreatic necrosis from necrosis plus infection and pseudocyst from abscess can be difficult.

For a deeper discussion of these topics, please see Chapter 144, "Pancreatitis," in Goldman-Cecil Medicine, *25th Edition.*

Splenic Abscess

Splenic abscess usually results from a hematogenous source, particularly endocarditis; consequently, the infecting bacteria are usually streptococcal and staphylococcal species. Patients have left upper quadrant pain, fever, an enlarged spleen, and an elevated white blood cell count. Ultrasound is diagnostic, and splenectomy is curative. Percutaneous aspiration plus antibiotics can also be effective.

Extravisceral Abscesses

Extravisceral abscesses typically occur from perforation of the bowel, resulting from inflammation or iatrogenic sources such as endoscopy and surgery. Other causes include peritonitis, ruptured solid organ abscess, and penetrating trauma. The clinical presentation varies widely with the location and cause. CT is the most useful imaging modality. Point source control, usually with percutaneous aspiration or surgical drainage, is essential for treatment. Antibiotic coverage is secondary and should be directed at the cause as identified by location, Gram stain, and culture.

● PERITONITIS

Primary Peritonitis

Primary or spontaneous bacterial peritonitis usually occurs in patients with cirrhosis and ascites or in children with nephrotic syndrome. The source is not apparent. The bacteriologic analysis reflects aerobic bowel flora, including *E. coli*, *K. pneumoniae*, and gram-positive organisms. Anaerobes are uncommon.

Clinical presentation includes fever, abdominal pain, ascites, and deteriorating liver function test results. Diagnosis is likely if aspirated ascitic fluid has greater than 250 neutrophils/μL. A diagnosis of primary peritonitis is made if a secondary source is ruled out. Culture and Gram stain may be negative. Patients usually respond after 48 to 72 hours of antibiotics. Patients with cirrhosis and ascites who have had one episode of spontaneous peritonitis are at risk for further episodes and are candidates for antibiotic prophylaxis. A meta-analysis of 13 trials concluded that prophylaxis resulted in decreased morbidity and mortality.

Secondary Peritonitis

Secondary peritonitis usually results from perforation of bowel and contamination by mixed enteric organisms. Other sources include rupture of the urinary tract or gynecologic organs. Bacteriology usually identifies polymicrobial infection with aerobes and anaerobes, reflecting the mucosal surface of the source. The peripheral blood leukocyte count is usually elevated.

Patients are usually febrile and have signs of peritoneal irritation: abdominal wall tenderness, rebound, and rigidity. Tenderness may be maximal over the origin of the peritonitis (e.g., ruptured viscus). Because movement causes pain, patients keep their knees bent and have quiet respirations.

Ultrasound and CT may reveal the origin of peritonitis. Aspiration of ascitic fluid usually reveals the causative organisms. Antibiotic therapy to cover the suspected or identified organisms should be begun immediately. It usually includes coverage of bacteria causing intraabdominal infection as discussed previously.

Surgical approach is aimed at controlling the source (e.g., perforated appendix), débridement, and drainage of abscesses.

Peritonitis during Peritoneal Dialysis

Rates of peritonitis during long-term peritoneal dialysis average less than 1 case in 24 months, but a few patients have higher rates. Bacteria usually represent skin flora, with *Staphylococcus epidermidis*, *S. aureus*, and streptococcal species predominating. Most patients have abdominal pain and tenderness but no fever. Neutrophil counts greater than 100 cells/μL and bacteria in a cloudy dialysate confirm the diagnosis.

Treatment can usually be accomplished intraperitoneally on an outpatient basis. Several antibiotic regimens have proved effective. Removal of the peritoneal catheter may be necessary (10% to 20% of cases) if there is a catheter tunnel infection, an unusual organism such as a fungus, or persistent infection.

Tuberculous Peritonitis

Primary tuberculous peritonitis often has a gradual onset. Symptoms include fever, abdominal pain, and weight loss. Pulmonary tuberculosis often exists. Signs may include tender, "doughy" masses or ascites. Symptoms and signs may be subtle.

Peritoneal fluid is exudative and contains 500 to 2000 cells/μL, mostly lymphocytes. Culture of peritoneal fluid is positive in only 25% of cases. The diagnosis is made by biopsy of nodules seen on the peritoneum during laparoscopy. Treatment consists of standard antituberculous therapy.

SUGGESTED READINGS

Alvarado A: A practical score for the early diagnosis of acute appendicitis, Ann Emerg Med 15:557–564, 1986.

Attasaranya S, Fogel EL, Lehman GA: Choledocholithiasis, ascending cholangitis and gallstone pancreatitis, Med Clin North Am 92:925–960, 2008.

Chabok A, Pahlman L, Hjern F, et al: Randomized clinical trial of antibiotics in acute uncomplicated diverticulitis, Br J Surg 99:532–539, 2012.

Fagenholz PJ, Demoya MA: Acute inflammatory surgical disease, Surg Clin North Am 94:1–30, 2014.

Shabanzadeh DM, Wille-Jorgensen P: Antibiotics for uncomplicated diverticulitis, Cochrane Database Syst Rev (11):CD009092, 2012.

Soares-Weber K, Brezis M, Tur-Kaspa R, et al: Antibiotic prophylaxis of bacterial infections in cirrhotic inpatients: a meta-analysis of randomized controlled trials, J Gastroenterol 38:193–200, 2003.

Solomkin JS, Mazuski JE, Gradley JS, et al: Diagnosis and management of complicated intra-abdominal infection in adults and children: guidelines by the Surgical Infection Society and the Infectious Diseases Society of America, Surg Infect 11:79–109, 2010.

Wilkins T, Embry K, George R: Diagnosis and management of acute diverticulitis, Am Fam Physician 87:612–620, 2013.

Wray CJ, Kao LS, Millas SG, et al: Acute appendicitis: controversies in diagnosis and management, Curr Probl Surg 50:54–86, 2013.

96

Infectious Diarrhea

Awewura Kwara

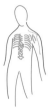

DEFINITION AND EPIDEMIOLOGY

Acute diarrhea is defined as an increase in frequency of bowel movements, to three or more times daily with at least 200 g of stool per day, lasting less than 14 days. In clinical practice, three or more loose stools per day is considered to represent diarrhea. *Infectious diarrhea* is diarrhea that has an infectious etiology and is often associated with symptoms and signs of enteric involvement, such as nausea, vomiting, abdominal cramps, passage of bloody stool (dysentery), or systemic symptoms. When diarrhea lasts longer than 14 days, it is considered to be *persistent diarrhea*. The term *chronic diarrhea* refers to illness that last longer than 1 month. Organisms responsible for infectious diarrhea include bacteria, viruses, and parasites.

Globally, there are an estimated 1.7 billion cases of diarrhea annually, with acute infectious diarrhea causing more than 2 million deaths per year. Infectious diarrhea is the second leading cause of death in children younger than 5 years of age, killing an estimated 760,000 such children every year. In the United States, an estimated 211 to 375 million episodes of acute diarrhea occur annually, with more than 900,000 hospitalizations and about 6000 deaths. Foodborne illnesses alone account for about 76 million cases and 5000 deaths in the US each year.

PATHOLOGY

Diarrhea is an alteration of movement of ions and water that leads to an increase in water content, volume, or frequency of stools. Under normal conditions, up to 9 L of fluid is passed through the adult gastrointestinal tract daily. Almost 98% of this fluid is absorbed, and only 100 to 200 mL is excreted in stools. Enteric pathogens or microbial toxins that are ingested can overcome host defenses and alter this balance toward a net secretion, leading to diarrhea. A large number of microorganisms are normally ingested with every meal. Host defense mechanisms against enteric pathogens include low gastric pH, rapid transit of bacteria through the proximal small intestine, cellular immune responses, and antibody production. In addition, large numbers of normal bacterial flora inhabit the intestines and prevent colonization by enteric pathogens.

Alteration of the normal defense mechanisms can put individuals at risk for infectious diarrhea. Individuals with gastric resection or achlorhydric states have increased frequency of infection due to *Salmonella*, *Giardia lamblia*, and helminths, whereas some organisms, such as *Shigella* or rotavirus, survive the extreme acidity of the gastric environment. Some viral, bacterial, and parasitic infections are more common in patients with impaired cellular or humoral immunity. More than 99% of the normal colonic flora is made up of anaerobic bacteria; they produce fatty acids and cause acidic pH, which is important for resistance to colonization. Alteration of the bacterial flora due to broad-spectrum antibiotic therapy predisposes some individuals to the development of *Clostridium difficile* infection.

The virulence factors employed by enteric pathogens include inoculum size, adherence factors, toxin production, and invasion. Organisms such as *Shigella*, enterohemorrhagic *Escherichia coli* (EHEC), *G. lamblia*, and *Entamoeba histolytica* need as few as 10 to 100 organisms to produce infection, whereas *Vibrio cholerae* needs 10^5 to 10^8 organisms to cause disease. Many pathogens, including *V. cholerae* and enterotoxigenic *E. coli* (ETEC), must adhere to the gastrointestinal tract to establish infection. They produce virulence factors that allow the organisms to attach to the brush border of the intestinal epithelium. Several enteric pathogens produce disease through the production of toxins. These include enterotoxins that cause secretory diarrhea, cytotoxins that cause cell destruction and inflammatory diarrhea, and neurotoxins that act on the nervous system. Other bacteria cause disease by invasion and destruction of mucosal epithelial cells.

Enterotoxin-Induced Secretory Diarrhea

Ingested enterotoxin-producing bacteria colonize the small bowel and multiply to large numbers. The bacteria then produce enterotoxin, which binds to the mucosa and causes watery diarrhea through hypersecretion of isotonic fluid that overwhelms the absorptive capacity of the colon. *V. cholerae* produces the cholera toxin, a heterodimeric protein composed of one A and five B subunits. The enterotoxin binds to the intestinal mucosa and activates adenylate cyclase to produce cyclic adenosine monophosphate (cAMP), which causes increased chloride secretion and decreased sodium absorption, leading to hypersecretion of fluid. ETEC, which causes traveler's diarrhea, produces both a heat-labile enterotoxin that acts by the same mechanism as the cholera toxin and a heat-stable enterotoxin that causes secretory diarrhea through activation of guanylate cyclase to produce cyclic guanosine monophosphate (cGMP).

Cytotoxin-Induced Diarrhea

In contrast to enterotoxins, cytotoxins elaborated by enteric pathogens destroy mucosal epithelial cells, causing bloody diarrhea with inflammatory cells (dysentery). *Shigella dysenteriae* produces the shiga toxin, which causes dysenteric diarrhea in patients with shigellosis. Other toxin-producing bacteria include *Vibrio parahaemolyticus*, *C. difficile*, and shiga toxin–producing strains of *E. coli* (STEC) that cause hemorrhagic colitis and hemolytic-uremic syndrome (HUS).

Invasive Diarrhea

Some bacteria cause dysentery through direct invasion and destruction of intestinal mucosa rather than through production of a cytotoxin. *Shigella* and enteroinvasive *E. coli* invade and multiply in epithelial cells and spread to adjacent cells. Diarrhea is often accompanied by fever, abdominal cramps, and small amounts of bloody mucoid stools. Other bacteria, such as *Salmonella typhi* and *Yersinia enterocolitica*, penetrate the mucosa before disseminating into the bloodstream to cause a systemic illness.

Bacterial Food Poisoning

Bacterial food poisoning is caused by ingestion of preformed toxins in food; this results in a toxic illness rather than an enteric infection. The toxins may include cytotoxins, enterotoxins, and neurotoxins. Pathogens that produce bacterial food poisoning include *Staphylococcus aureus, Clostridium perfringens,* and *Bacillus cereus*. These organisms grow in food and produce toxins that are ingested directly in the food. Symptoms occur soon after food ingestion, with incubation periods of 1 to 16 hours and high attack rates. The illness is rarely associated with fever, and symptoms usually resolve within 12 to 24 hours after onset.

The staphylococcal and *B. cereus* toxins act on the nervous system to cause vomiting. *S. aureus* causes vomiting and diarrhea within 2 to 7 hours after ingestion of improperly cooked or stored food containing its heat-stable enterotoxin. *C. perfringens* produces secretory and cytotoxin-induced watery diarrhea within 8 to 14 hours after ingestion of contaminated vegetables, meat, or poultry. *B. cereus* often contaminates fried rice, vegetables, or sprouts; it produces one of two toxins which cause disease resembling that of *S. aureus* or *C. perfringens* infection within 1 to 6 hours after ingestion. Ingestion of the bacteria with subsequent

in vivo toxin production often results in disease with a longer incubation period (8 to 16 hours).

● SPECIFIC PATHOGENS

The epidemiologic and clinical features of common enteric pathogens and the recommended methods for diagnosis and treatment are summarized in Tables 96-1 and 96-2.

Shigella

Diarrhea due to *Shigella* occurs after ingestion of fecally contaminated food or water. The main species include *S. dysenteriae, Shigella flexneri, Shigella boydii,* and *Shigella sonnei*. Ingestion of as few as 10 to 100 microorganisms can lead to infection because the bacteria are relatively resistant to gastric acid. Person-to-person transmission is common, and the attack rate is highest among infants and young children in child care centers. The incubation period is 6 to 72 hours. Illness may initially manifest as noninflammatory, watery diarrhea caused by enterotoxin production or multiplication of bacteria in the small intestines. Invasion of the colonic epithelium and mucosa often manifests as dysentery. Complications of shigellosis include HUS, which is associated with *S. dysenteriae* type 1, and Reiter's chronic arthritis syndrome, which is associated with *S. flexneri* infection.

Salmonella

Salmonella typhi causes typhoid fever, but not diarrhea. Nontyphoidal salmonellosis results from ingestion of contaminated meat, dairy, or poultry products or from direct contact with animals such as birds, pet turtles, snakes, and other reptiles. An oral inoculum of 10^5 to 10^8 organisms is needed but smaller inocula can cause disease in patients with impaired gastric acidity or compromised immunity. The organisms invade the distal

TABLE 96-1	EPIDEMIOLOGIC AND CLINICAL CHARACTERISTICS OF COMMON ENTERIC PATHOGENS	
ORGANISM	**EPIDEMIOLOGIC FEATURES**	**COMMON CLINICAL FEATURES**
Campylobacter jejuni	Consumption of undercooked poultry, travel to tropical and semitropical regions	Acute watery diarrhea, fever, abdominal pain, fecal evidence of inflammation (positive fecal leukocytes, lactoferrin, or occult blood)
Vibrio cholerae	Inadequately cooked seafood, travel to endemic regions	Acute dehydrating watery diarrhea; fever is usually absent
Clostridium difficile	Antibiotic use, recent hospitalization, elderly patients with coexisting conditions	Diarrhea with fever, fecal evidence of inflammation, marked leukocytosis
Enterotoxigenic *Escherichia coli*	Travel to tropical and semitropical regions	Watery diarrhea, abdominal cramps, nausea and vomiting; leukocytes absent in stools
Nontyphoidal *Salmonella*	Foodborne outbreaks, exposure to animals	Acute watery diarrhea, fever, abdominal pain, evidence of inflammation
Shigella	Person-to-person transmission, daycare center contact	Severe diarrhea with fever, abdominal pain, bloody diarrhea, fecal evidence of inflammation
Shiga toxin–producing *E. coli*	Foodborne outbreaks, undercooked hamburgers, raw seed sprouts, water and wading pool exposure	Abdominal pain, bloody stools, absence of fever, fecal evidence of inflammation
Noncholeraic *Vibrio*	Ingestion of shellfish and undercooked seafood	Watery diarrhea, abdominal cramps, nausea; fever and vomiting are less frequent
Yersinia enterocolitica	Contaminated food or water, inadequately cooked meats, unpasteurized milk	Acute watery diarrhea, fever, abdominal pain, bloody diarrhea
Norovirus	Winter outbreaks in congregate settings, outbreaks on cruise ships	Watery diarrhea, nausea, vomiting, abdominal pain
Cyclospora	Foodborne outbreaks, travel to tropical and subtropical regions (especially Nepal)	Persistent noninflammatory diarrhea
Cryptosporidium	Waterborne outbreaks, travel to tropical and subtropical regions	Persistent noninflammatory diarrhea
Entamoeba histolytica	Travel to tropical regions, recent immigration from endemic regions	Bloody diarrhea, extraintestinal involvement (liver abscess)
Giardia lamblia	Waterborne outbreaks, travel to mountainous areas of North America, Russia	Abdominal pain, persistent watery diarrhea, flatulence, steatorrhea, nausea and vomiting

TABLE 96-2 DIAGNOSIS AND RECOMMENDED ANTIMICROBIAL TREATMENT FOR DIARRHEA WITH SPECIFIC PATHOGENS IN ADULTS

ORGANISM	DIAGNOSIS	RECOMMENDATIONS
Campylobacter jejuni	Routine stool culture	Erythromycin 250 mg qid or azithromycin 500 mg daily for 7 days
Vibrio cholerae O1	Stool culture in special salt-containing media (TCBS), test isolate for O1 serotype	Doxycycline 300 mg single dose, or single dose of fluoroquinolone, or tetracycline 500 mg qid for 3 days, or TMP-SMZ 160/800 mg bid for 3 days
Clostridium difficile	Stool test for *C. difficile* toxin A or B by EIA, or PCR for the B toxin gene	Stop implicated antibiotic. For mild to moderate illness, metronidazole 500 mg tid for 10 days; for severe illness, vancomycin 125 mg qid for 10-14 days
Enterotoxigenic *Escherichia coli*	Stool culture for *E. coli*, with assay for enterotoxin	Fluoroquinolone orally for 3 days (e.g., ciprofloxacin 500 mg bid, levofloxacin 500 mg daily, norfloxacin 400 mg bid). If susceptible, TMP-SMZ 160/800 mg bid for 3 days
Nontyphoidal *Salmonella*	Routine stool culture	Antimicrobials not recommended. If extraintestinal involvement or immunocompromise is present, TMP-SMZ (if susceptible) or quinolone as above, or ceftriaxone 100 mg/kg/day in one or two divided doses for 7 to 14 days, or longer if endovascular infection or relapsing
Shigella	Routine stool culture	Fluoroquinolone for 3 days (e.g., ciprofloxacin 500 mg bid, levofloxacin 500 mg daily, norfloxacin 400 mg bid). If susceptible, TMP-SMZ 160/800 mg bid for 3 days
Shiga toxin–producing *E. coli*	Stool culture with sorbitol-MacConkey agar, followed by serotyping for O157, then H7, with EIA for shiga toxins	Antibiotics and antimotility drugs should be avoided
Noncholeraic *Vibrio*	Stool culture in special salt-containing media (TCBS)	Fluoroquinolone orally for 3-5 days (ciprofloxacin 500 mg bid, levofloxacin 500 mg daily, norfloxacin 400 mg bid)
Yersinia enterocolitica	Stool culture on MacConkey media incubated at 25° to 28° C	Antibiotics usually not required. For severe infection or bacteremia, treat with TMP-SMZ or fluoroquinolone or doxycycline plus aminoglycoside
Cyclospora	Stool trichrome or acid-fast stain for parasites	TMP-SMZ 160/800 mg bid for 7-10 days
Cryptosporidium	Stool trichrome or acid-fast stain for parasites, EIA for *Cryptosporidium* species	Self-limited in immunocompetent persons. If severe or if patient is immunocompromised, consider paromomycin 500 mg tid for 7 days
Isospora	Stool trichrome or acid-fast stain for parasites	TMP-SMZ 160/800 mg bid for 7-10 days
Entamoeba histolytica	Stool examination for ova and parasites, EIA for *E. histolytica*	Metronidazole 750 mg tid for 5-10 days, plus iodoquinol 650 mg tid for 20 days or paromomycin 500 mg tid for 7 days
Giardia	Stool examination for ova and parasites, EIA for *Giardia* species	Metronidazole 500 to 750 mg tid for 7-10 days

bid, Twice a day; EIA, enzyme immunoassay; PCR, polymerase chain reaction; qid, four times a day; tid, three times a day; TCBS, thiosulfate-citrate-bile salts-sucrose agar; TMP-SMZ, trimethoprim-sulfamethoxazole.

ileum and cause diarrhea with fever, nausea, or vomiting. Diarrhea usually resolves in 2 to 3 days. Complications include bacteremia and metastatic seeding of atherosclerotic plaques and prostheses. Antimicrobial treatment does not shorten the duration of diarrhea and may prolong intestinal carriage in stools; therefore, antibiotics are indicated only for cases of severe disease or extraintestinal involvement.

Campylobacter jejuni

Disease caused by *Campylobacter jejuni* usually results from ingestion of undercooked poultry or direct contact with animals. The infective dose is 10^4 to 10^6 organisms, with an incubation period of 1 to 5 days. Acute watery diarrhea is the most common presentation; less frequently, systemic symptoms including fever may occur. Prodromal symptoms such as fever, myalgia, headache, and malaise may precede diarrhea. Complications include reactive arthritis, especially associated with the human leukocyte antigen B27 (HLA-B27), and Guillain-Barré syndrome, which can occur 2 to 3 weeks after diarrhea has resolved. Antibiotic therapy shortens the carriage state.

Vibrio

V. cholerae can be divided by the O-antigen of lipopolysaccharide into more than 150 strains. The toxigenic strains *V. cholerae* O1 and O139 produce cholera toxin and are associated with clinical illness. The infectious oral inoculum is about 10^5 to 10^8 organisms, with an incubation period of 6 hours to 5 days. Classic cholera starts with vomiting, abdominal pain, and diarrhea. Diarrhea progresses to voluminous watery stools which have been described as "rice water" because they are clear with flecks of mucus. Massive diarrhea can lead to dehydration and shock within a few hours. The illness may be fulminant, with death occurring 3 to 4 hours after onset. Fever and bacteremia are rare. In endemic areas, the diagnosis is usually made on clinical grounds.

The characteristics of noncholeraic *Vibrio* species are covered in Tables 96-1 and 96-2.

Diarrhea-Causing *Escherichia coli*

There are several types of diarrheagenic *E. coli*, each with a different pathogenesis leading to diarrhea. In addition to ETEC and STEC, these include enteropathogenic, enteroinvasive, enteroaggregative, and diffusely adherent *E. coli*. ETEC is the most common cause of traveler's diarrhea. It results in an enterotoxin-mediated watery diarrhea with abdominal cramps and vomiting. Enteropathogenic *E. coli* has been associated with epidemic diarrhea in neonates.

EHEC or STEC is acquired by eating contaminated food or water. The oral inoculum is 10 to 100 organisms, with an incubation period of 3 to 4 days. Most disease in the United States is caused by *E. coli* O157:H7, an enterohemorrhagic strain. It is classically associated with bloody diarrhea, abdominal pain, and fecal leukocytes. Systemic complications include HUS in children and thrombotic thrombocypenia purpura in adults.

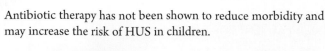

Antibiotic therapy has not been shown to reduce morbidity and may increase the risk of HUS in children.

Clostridium difficile

C. difficile is the main cause of nosocomial diarrhea among adults in the United States. Virtually all antibiotics have been implicated in the development of *C. difficile* infection, but the most common agents are clindamycin, cephalosporins, fluoroquinolones, and penicillins. Spores occur in the environment and are resistant to alcohol-based handwashing solutions. The spores of toxigenic *C. difficile* are ingested, survive gastric acidity, geminate, and colonize the lower intestinal tract, where they elaborate two exotoxins, toxin A (an enterotoxin) and toxin B (a cytotoxin). The toxins disrupt cell and tight junctions, leading to fluid leakage. The cellular toxicity results in formation of a pseudomembrane.

The epidemic strain referred to as the North American pulsed-field gel electrophoresis type 1 (NAP1) strain is associated with a severe course, higher mortality, and increased risk of relapse. Three bacterial factors have been implicated in outbreaks of *C. difficile* infection caused by the NAP1 strain, including increased production of toxins A and B, fluoroquinolone resistance, and production of a binary toxin. Patients often have abdominal pain and watery diarrhea but may also have bloody stools. Markers of severe infection include pseudomembranous colitis, acute renal failure, marked leukocytosis, hypotension, and toxic megacolon. The indigenous intestinal microbiota is important for colonization resistance and for recovery from antibiotic-associated *C. difficile* colitis.

Yersinia enterocolitica

Y. enterocolitica is a zoonosis caused by ingestion of contaminated food or water or undercooked meats. Oral inoculation requires 10^9 organisms for infection, with an incubation period of 3 to 7 days. The illness may mimic acute appendicitis and may be complicated by ileal perforation, mesenteric adenitis, or terminal ileitis. Postinfectious reactive polyarthritis and Reiter's syndrome may occur.

Viral Causes of Diarrhea

Viruses tend to cause diarrhea by adhering to the intestinal mucosa and disrupting the absorptive and secretory processes without causing inflammation. They may invade intestinal villous epithelial cells and cause sloughing of villi. Rotavirus was the most common cause of severe diarrhea in children in the past, but the incidence has fallen dramatically with widespread use of the rotovirus vaccine. Norovirus is highly contagious and is a very common cause of foodborne gastroenteritis in adults and children in the United States. It has been the cause of epidemic diarrhea on cruise ships. There is neither a vaccine nor specific treatment. Other viruses that cause diarrhea are adenoviruses, sapoviruses, and astroviruses. The incubation period is usually longer than 14 hours, and vomiting may be a prominent feature of diarrheal disease caused by viral agents.

Protozoan Causes of Diarrhea

Important parasitic causes of diarrhea include *G. lamblia*, *Cryptosporidium parvum*, and *E. histolytica*. Contaminated water sources tend to be the cause of outbreaks. *G. lamblia* multiplies in the small intestine and attaches to or invades, but does not destroy, mucosa cells. Ingestion of a few organisms can lead to disease. *C. parvum*, *Isospora belli*, and *Cyclospora cayetanesis* occasionally cause self-limited diarrhea in immunocompetent individuals but may cause severe disease in patients with advanced acquired immunodeficiency syndrome (AIDS). *E. histolytica* causes a syndrome ranging from mild diarrhea to fulminant amebic colitis and extraintestinal amebic abscesses.

Traveler's Diarrhea

Traveler's diarrhea affects 10% to 40% of travelers from industrialized countries who visit tropical and semitropical developing countries. The causative agent is identified in about one half of cases, and 80% of those identified are bacterial pathogens, most often ETEC or enteroaggregative *E. coli*. Other bacterial causes include *Shigella*, *Salmonella*, *Campylobacter*, *Aeromonas*, noncholeraic *Vibrio*, and *Plesiomonas*. The viral etiologies include rotavirus and norovirus; parasitic causes are rare. Patients with traveler's diarrhea should be treated empirically with antibiotics without stool examination.

● CLINICAL PRESENTATION

The epidemiologic and clinical characteristics are important to identify the potential etiologic agent and to guide management (see Table 96-1). The initial evaluation should consider the severity of illness, signs of dehydration, and intestinal inflammation indicated by the fever, abdominal pain, blood in stools (dysentery), or tenesmus. Important epidemiologic clues in the history include age, travel history, ingestion of undercooked or raw food and meat, antibiotic use, sexual activity, daycare attendance, and outbreaks involving others with similar exposure (see Table 96-1). Fever (temperature 38.5° C or 101.3° F or higher) is associated with invasive pathogens that cause intestinal inflammation. The examination should determine the severity of dehydration and need for rehydration as well as the likely cause. Signs of dehydration or hypovolemia include lax skin turgor and tenting, dry mucus membranes, decreased urination, tachycardia, and hypotension.

● DIAGNOSIS AND DIFFERENTIAL DIAGNOSIS

The approach to diagnosis and management of infectious diarrhea is shown in Figure 96-1. Examination of stools for erythrocytes and white blood cells (leukocytes) using methylene blue staining or the lactoferrin test can help differentiate diarrhea caused by invasive pathogens from that caused by noninvasive pathogens. Most cases of diarrheal illnesses are self-limited, and almost half resolve within 1 day. Therefore, microbiologic investigation is usually not necessary for patients who are seen within 24 hours of the onset of illness unless certain conditions are present.

The indications for stool culture include severe diarrhea (six or more stools per day), diarrhea lasting longer than 1 week, fever, dysentery, hospitalization, inflammatory diarrhea, and multiple cases in a suspected outbreak. Routine stool culture will identify *Shigella*, *Salmonella*, *Campylobacter*, and *Aeromonas*. If the patient has bloody diarrhea or HUS, stool culture for *E. coli* O157 and tests for shiga-like toxin should be performed. Enzyme immunoassay for *C. difficile* toxins A and B or polymerase chain reaction

ASK ABOUT:

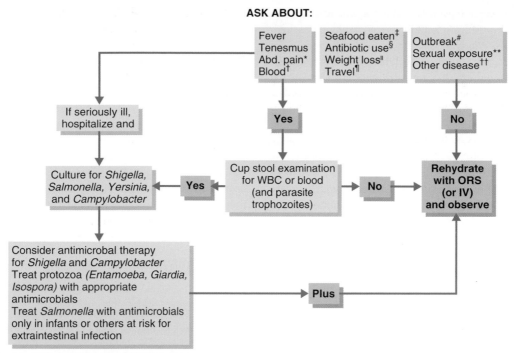

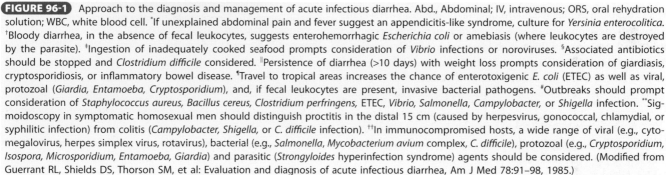

FIGURE 96-1 Approach to the diagnosis and management of acute infectious diarrhea. Abd., Abdominal; IV, intravenous; ORS, oral rehydration solution; WBC, white blood cell. *If unexplained abdominal pain and fever suggest an appendicitis-like syndrome, culture for *Yersinia enterocolitica*. †Bloody diarrhea, in the absence of fecal leukocytes, suggests enterohemorrhagic *Escherichia coli* or amebiasis (where leukocytes are destroyed by the parasite). ‡Ingestion of inadequately cooked seafood prompts consideration of *Vibrio* infections or noroviruses. §Associated antibiotics should be stopped and *Clostridium difficile* considered. ‖Persistence of diarrhea (>10 days) with weight loss prompts consideration of giardiasis, cryptosporidiosis, or inflammatory bowel disease. ¶Travel to tropical areas increases the chance of enterotoxigenic *E. coli* (ETEC) as well as viral, protozoal (*Giardia, Entamoeba, Cryptosporidium*), and, if fecal leukocytes are present, invasive bacterial pathogens. #Outbreaks should prompt consideration of *Staphylococcus aureus, Bacillus cereus, Clostridium perfringens*, ETEC, *Vibrio, Salmonella, Campylobacter*, or *Shigella* infection. **Sigmoidoscopy in symptomatic homosexual men should distinguish proctitis in the distal 15 cm (caused by herpesvirus, gonococcal, chlamydial, or syphilitic infection) from colitis (*Campylobacter, Shigella*, or *C. difficile* infection). ††In immunocompromised hosts, a wide range of viral (e.g., cytomegalovirus, herpes simplex virus, rotavirus), bacterial (e.g., *Salmonella, Mycobacterium avium* complex, *C. difficile*), protozoal (e.g., *Cryptosporidium, Isospora, Microsporidium, Entamoeba, Giardia*) and parasitic (*Strongyloides* hyperinfection syndrome) agents should be considered. (Modified from Guerrant RL, Shields DS, Thorson SM, et al: Evaluation and diagnosis of acute infectious diarrhea, Am J Med 78:91–98, 1985.)

for toxin B should be obtained if there is a history of recent antibiotic use, hospitalization, or age greater than 65 years with coexisting conditions, immunosuppression, or neutropenia. Consider protozoa, and check stools for ova and parasites (e.g., trophozoites) and/or for *Giardia* antigen test if diarrhea duration is greater than 7 days. If a patient has AIDS, stools should be checked for *Cryptosporidium*, *Microsporidium*, and *Mycobacterium avium* complex.

TREATMENT

Initial therapy should include fluid and electrolyte repletion with or without antimicrobial therapy. Oral rehydration is often adequate unless the patient is comatose or severely dehydrated. Nutritional support with continued feeding improves outcomes in children. In children, the BRAT diet (bananas, rice, applesauce, and toast) with avoidance of milk products is often recommended, but supporting evidence is limited.

Oral Fluid Therapy

In most patients with diarrhea, fluid repletion can be achieved with oral rehydration therapy using isotonic fluids containing glucose and electrolytes. An effective solution can be prepared by the addition of 2 tablespoons of sugar, one fourth of a teaspoon

of salt (NaCl), and one fourth of a teaspoon of baking soda ($NaHCO_3$) to 1 L of boiled drinking water. In the United States, fluids containing sodium in the range of 45 to 75 mEq/L (such as Pedialyte or Rehydrolyte solutions) are recommended. Fluid should be administered in large quantities until there is clinical evidence that fluid balance is restored, and then as maintenance therapy. Oral rehydration therapy can be life-saving for patients in developing countries with severe diarrhea.

Intravenous Fluid Therapy

Massive fluid loss due to diarrhea should be rapidly replaced by the administration of intravenous fluids. Lactated Ringer's solution is the fluid of choice because the composition is similar to electrolyte loss during diarrhea. The rate of fluid administration and maintenance should be guided by clinical signs including vital signs, appearance of the mucosa, neck veins, and skin turgor.

Antimicrobial Therapy

Most cases of infectious diarrhea do not require antimicrobial therapy. However, antibiotics may decrease the volume of diarrhea (e.g., in cholera) or the duration and severity of the illness. Antibiotics are effective in the treatment of shigellosis, traveler's diarrhea, *Campylobacter* infection, and *C. difficile* infection. In uncomplicated salmonellosis, antibiotics may prolong the shedding of salmonella. The choice and dose of antimicrobials for specific pathogens are described in Table 96-2. For traveler's diarrhea in adults, empiric therapy with ciprofloxacin 500 mg twice a day, or trimethoprim-sulfamethoxazole (TMP-SMZ) 160/800 mg twice a day, for 3 to 5 days is adequate. For antibiotic-associated *C. difficile* colitis, broad-spectrum antibiotics should be discontinued, if possible. The first-line therapy is metronidazole 500 mg three times a day orally for 10 to 14 days. For severely ill patients, oral vancomycin 125 mg four times a day for 10 to 14 days should be initiated. Persistently recurrent *C. difficile* disease has been treated successfully with replacement of bowel flora.

Symptomatic Therapy

Antidiarrheal agents such as loperamide and bismuth subsalicylate can be used in some instances for symptomatic relief. Loperamide inhibits intestinal peristalsis and has some antisecretory properties. When used with or without antibiotics in cases of traveler's diarrhea, it may reduce the duration of diarrhea by about 1 day. Antimotility agents should be avoided in patients with bloody or suspected inflammatory diarrhea. The use of these agents has been implicated in prolonging the duration of fever in shigellosis, development of toxic megacolon in *C. difficile* colitis, and development of HUS in children with STEC infection. Bismuth subsalicylate can alleviate stool output in children as well as the symptoms of abdominal pain, diarrhea, and nausea in patients with traveler's diarrhea.

PROGNOSIS

The prognosis is generally good but is variable depending on the etiology and the severity of illness. Most patients recover completely within 3 to 5 days. However, serious complications including death, can occur. Serious disease and death is usually seen in individuals who become severely dehydrated, infants, elderly patients, and those with underlying medical conditions or immunosuppression (e.g., AIDS). Untreated severe dehydration may lead to shock, renal failure, and death. Postinfectious reactive polyarthritis and Reiter's syndrome can complicate cases due to *Yersinia*, *Campylobacter*, *Shigella*, and Guillain-Barré syndrome may occur after diarrhea caused by *Campylobacter*.

SUGGESTED READINGS

Dupont HL: The Practice Parameters Committee of the America College of Gastroenterology: Guidelines on acute infectious diarrhea in adults, Am J Gastroenterol 92:1962–1975, 1997.

Dupont HL: Bacterial diarrhea, N Engl J Med 361:1560–1569, 2009.

Guerrant RL, Van Gilder T, Steiner TS, et al: Practice guidelines for the management of infectious diarrhea, Clin Infect Dis 32:331–351, 2001.

Kelly CP, Lamont JT: *Clostridium difficile*—more difficult than ever, N Engl J Med 359:1932–1936, 2008.

Thielman NM, Guerrant RL: Acute infectious diarrhea, N Engl J Med 350:38–47, 2004.

97

Infections Involving Bones and Joints

Jerome Larkin

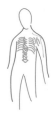

DEFINITION

The term *osteomyelitis* refers to infection of any component of the bony skeleton, whereas *septic arthritis* refers to infection of native or prosthetic joints. Associated structures such as tendons, ligaments, and bursae can also become infected, especially if they involve prosthetic or biografted material. Osteomyelitis and septic arthritis can each occur as a result of seeding during an episode of bacteremia, as a consequence of vascular insufficiency, as a complication of trauma, or by extension from a contiguous focus of infection in an adjacent tissue or structure.

In the case of hematogenous infection, the bacteremia itself may be relatively transient and of little clinical consequence. Hematogenous osteomyelitis is common in children but accounts for only about 20% of osteomyelitis in adults. The vertebrae and pelvis are the most commonly involved sites.

Peripheral vascular disease leading to tissue hypoxia, often related to diabetes, hypertension, hyperlipidemia, or smoking, is the biggest risk factor for the development of osteomyelitis in adults older than 50 years of age. There is often antecedent soft tissue infection or destruction as a result of vascular insufficiency and neuropathy. It is most common in the lower extremities, particularly in the feet, and often occurs in diabetics.

Trauma, especially when it involves open fracture, with its attendant disruption of the bony architecture and vascular supply, is a major risk factor for development of osteomyelitis and septic arthritis. This is particularly true when an open fracture (such as from a fall or a motor vehicle accident), is heavily contaminated with soil or other environmental materials. Such fractures often require internal fixation (i.e., placement of rods, screws, or other metal devices) to stabilize the bone. The presence of such internal fixation devices provides a nidus for bacteria and other microorganisms, including fungi, to elude the immune system and incubate. Chronic osteomyelitis is a possible complication of such injuries and is often a result of multiple or unusual organisms. It may occur despite aggressive débridement and prophylactic antibiotic treatment at the time of injury and can arise months or even years afterward. Individuals who experience prolonged periods of immobility (e.g., paraplegia) are also at risk for osteomyelitis. Infection typically involves the pelvis, sacrum, and lower spine, corresponding to areas of unrelieved pressure and resulting pressure sores.

Osteomyelitis may be thought of as being acute or chronic. The former is typically hematogenous and associated with signs of inflammation in the overlying soft tissue, with onset occurring over the course of days to 1 week. Radiographs are usually normal at presentation. Chronic osteomyelitis is typically more indolent, with onset over the course of months. It is more likely to show bony destruction on plain radiographs at the time of presentation and is often associated with a draining sinus tract. Sequestra (areas of dead bone) and involucra (new bone formed around sequestra) may also be seen on radiographs. Whereas with acute osteomyelitis, a 6-week course of antibiotics may effect a cure, chronic osteomyelitis more typically requires surgical intervention and a prolonged (≥3 months) course of antibiotic therapy.

PATHOPHYSIOLOGY

Characteristics of the vascular supply of the bone and properties of the most common pathogen, *Staphylococcus aureus*, may combine to lead to infection. Although bone is generally resistant to infection, the vasculature of the metaphysis contains capillary loops composed of a single layer of discontinuous endothelial cells, which may allow bacteria to enter the extracellular matrix. Additionally, these capillary beds appear to lack functionally active phagocytes. *S. aureus* is able to elaborate proteins expressed on its surface that promote adherence to tissues of the extracellular matrix. When engulfed by osteoblasts, *S. aureus* can survive for prolonged periods in an almost sporelike state, leading to potential recurrences of infection. Finally, many bacteria can elaborate biofilms that allow them to elude clearance by the immune system. Prosthetic material, such as that used in joint replacements and other grafts, can serve as a platform for the formation of such biofilms.

In the case of septic arthritis, there is usually some underlying joint abnormality (e.g., rheumatoid arthritis), although this abnormality may be as mundane as osteoarthritis. It is hypothesized that relatively trivial injuries, which may even go unnoticed or unremembered by the patient, can cause minor bleeding into the joint, providing a hospitable environment for bacteria to incubate.

CLINICAL PRESENTATION AND DIAGNOSIS

Patients with osteomyelitis often have pain at the site of infection. The overlying soft tissue may have signs of inflammation or tissue destruction; the latter is often seen in diabetics with soft tissue ulceration. Historically, the diagnosis of osteomyelitis relied on the presence of lucency on plain radiographs of the affected area. The diagnosis could be confirmed histologically by bone biopsy with culture to identify the pathogenic organism. Currently, the diagnosis is typically based on magnetic resonance imaging (MRI) with gadolinium, which demonstrates marrow edema with or without bony destruction. Alternatively, the diagnosis may be made by three-phase bone scanning or computed tomography. These modalities may be especially helpful for patients with renal insufficiency who cannot undergo gadolinium-enhanced studies due to the risk of nephrogenic systemic fibrosis. An elevated C-reactive protein (CRP) level or erythrocyte sedimentation rate (ESR) supports the diagnosis.

Microbiologic diagnosis of osteomyelitis is made by positive blood cultures or by bone biopsy and culture. Culture of cutaneous ulcers is typically not helpful because the results usually demonstrate multiple colonizing organisms and do not correlate with organisms isolated on bone culture. An exception is the isolation of *S. aureus* or *Salmonella* from a draining fistula or, on occasion, *Pseudomonas* from an ulcer. In the former case, the bacterium can be presumed to be the pathogen; in the latter, a decision would have to be made to include coverage of *Pseudomonas* spp in an empirical antibiotic regimen. If cultures of bone obtained by bone aspirate under radiographic guidance are negative, either the procedure should be repeated or an open biopsy with culture should be performed.

Septic arthritis almost always manifests with the cardinal features of inflammation (i.e., erythema, swelling, warmth, and pain) when it involves the extremities. Fever is frequently present, and there is often an associated bacteremia. Septic arthritis of the spine, pelvis, or hip may require imaging, usually MRI, because these sites are difficult to assess by examination alone. Persistent back, pelvic, or hip pain that is otherwise unexplained should prompt radiographic evaluation even in the absence of fever.

The diagnosis of septic arthritis ultimately relies on joint aspiration. Such procedures should occur before the administration of antibiotics. Fluid should be sent for cell count with differential, crystal analysis, Gram stain, aerobic and anaerobic culture, and fungal and acid-fast stains and cultures. Positive stains or cultures are taken as evidence of infection in most cases in which an appropriate clinical syndrome is also present. White blood cell (WBC) counts higher than 50,000 cells/μL are suggestive of infection. In cases that are difficult to diagnosis and in instances in which antibiotics were given before aspiration, it may be appropriate to have cultures held for up to 14 days. Specialized culture techniques for fastidious organisms such as anaerobes and nutritionally deficient streptococci may be required. Ultimately, tagged WBC scans may help to clarify the presence or absence of septic arthritis in difficult cases. Evolving molecular technologies such as polymerase chain reaction (PCR) and 16S ribosomal sequencing may offer alternative and more rapid and precise diagnosis in the future.

Most cases of osteomyelitis and septic arthritis are caused by *Staphylococcus* spp, *Streptococcus* spp, and aerobic gram-negative bacilli, although almost any pathogenic microorganism can cause such an infection in the appropriate circumstance. Infecting *Staphylococcus* spp include both *S. aureus* and coagulase-negative staphylococci. The latter are often implicated in prosthetic joint infections and infections associated with orthopedic hardware. *Streptococcus* spp that cause bone and joint infections include groups A, B, C, G, and F, as well as *Abiotrophia* and *Gemella* (formerly termed "nutritionally deficient streptococci").

Gram-negative organisms account for as many as 30% of hematogenous infections. They are seen more commonly in the elderly as a result of urinary tract infection with associated bacteremia. Isolated species include *Escherichia coli*, *Haemophilus influenzae*, and *Haemophilus parainfluenzae*. Infections with *Serratia marcescens* and *Pseudomonas* spp are associated with exposure to water and are usually nosocomial or related to intravenous drug use.

Fungi such as *Candida*, *Aspergillus*, and *Zygomycetes* may cause bone and joint infections particularly in immune-compromised patients, diabetics, and those who have suffered trauma. *Nocardia* and other acid-fast organisms may be seen after trauma or in association with prosthetic joints, and several attempts at débridement may be needed before the organism can be isolated. *Propionibacterium acnes* is often isolated from shoulder infections, especially those involving prosthetic joints. The variety of potential pathogens underscores the need to obtain appropriate specimens for culture before administration of antibiotics.

Infection with *Borrelia burgdorferi*, the causative agent of Lyme disease, can lead to a multifocal or monoarticular septic arthritis. Fluid analysis is consistent with bacterial septic arthritis but is negative for typical organisms on culture. Associated findings of erythema migrans, diffuse myalgias and arthralgias, cranial nerve palsies, fever, and aseptic meningitis may also be present. PCR analysis of joint fluid has a reported sensitivity between 30% and 75%. Diagnosis relies on serology and associated findings in patients who reside in endemic areas. Later-stage disease may manifest with a less inflammatory-appearing effusion, often without any other symptoms. Treatment is with doxycycline or ceftriaxone, depending on the stage of disease.

Neisseria gonorrhoeae can cause a solitary or multifocal septic arthritis often associated with tenosynovitis and skin lesions. It is usually seen in sexually active younger adults. Culture of the joint fluid may be negative, but testing of specimens from the pharynx, urethra, or rectum is usually positive by nucleic acid amplification. The treatment of choice is ceftriaxone.

DIFFERENTIAL DIAGNOSIS

The differential diagnosis of both osteomyelitis and septic arthritis includes noninfectious inflammatory disorders such as gout, pseudogout, rheumatoid arthritis, inflammatory bowel disease, and other inflammatory and autoimmune disorders. Occasionally, neoplasms such as sarcomas or metastatic lesions may manifest similarly to osteomyelitis. Infection with several viruses such as rubella, parvovirus B19, and hepatitis B virus can manifest with arthritis.

Chronic recurrent multifocal osteomyelitis is a noninfectious inflammatory lesion of bone that is thought to be autoimmune in nature and is characterized by findings on MRI similar to those of osteomyelitis. It is culture-negative and unresponsive to antibiotics. The diagnosis is one of exclusion and often is made only after several attempts at diagnosing and treating presumed bacterial osteomyelitis. Although it is typically seen in children, it can also occur in adults.

TREATMENT

Treatment of osteomyelitis involves débridement of appropriate infected or necrotic tissue and the administration of antibiotics. It is critically important to remove all necrotic or devitalized tissue. If not removed, such tissue may serve as a nidus of chronic or recurrent infection. In this regard, it is often necessary to remove any fixating hardware, plastic device, bone graft, or other donor tissue if the infection has been present for longer than 1 month or is recurrent. Cadaveric donor tissue infections often are caused by atypical organisms such as *Clostridium* spp. Historically, sequestra developed in sites of chronically infected bone. These are produced by the action of the immune system and histologically are characterized by granulomatous tissue that serves to isolate the infection. Although this reaction is effective in containing the infection, it represents a risk for recurrence as well as an area of bone weakening. Any sequestra that are discovered should be surgically excised.

Infection that occurs in the immediate postoperative period (i.e., within 1 month after placement of hardware and grafts) and appears to involve only the soft tissue may be treated with débridement and antibiotics alone with a reasonable chance of success. Occasionally, infected hardware must be left in place to stabilize the bone while a fracture is healing. In such cases, it may be necessary to continue antibiotic treatment until the hardware can be removed. Infected spine hardware, which must remain in place, may necessitate prolonged antibiotic treatment, at times even indefinitely. The addition of rifampin for susceptible staphylococcal infections with retained hardware improves the overall cure rates.

Septic arthritis requires either repeated aspiration or serial débridement of the joint until active purulence has resolved. This is indicated by decreasing cell counts and sterilization of joint fluid cultures. Prosthetic joint infection typically requires removal of the infected prosthesis and placement of an antibiotic spacer for 4 to 6 weeks while antibiotics are administered. This is followed by placement of a new prosthesis after all signs and symptoms of infection have resolved. Selected infections with coagulase-negative *Staphylococcus* and *Streptococcus* spp may be treated with débridement, joint retention, and a course of antibiotics lasting 6 weeks or longer. Consideration should then be given to chronic suppressive antibiotic therapy, assuming that an appropriate agent is available.

Antibiotic treatment should be with agents that are active against the infecting organism, depending on culture and susceptibility data. β-lactams are the preferred agents in most cases. Therapy with quinolones for Enterobacteriaceae and, in combination with rifampin, for *Staphylococcus* spp may be considered. These drugs have the advantage of high oral bioavailability that results in tissue levels that approach or are equal to those achieved when they are given intravenously. Care should be taken regarding drug interactions with rifampin as well as the risks of *Clostridium difficile* colitis and Achilles tendon rupture with quinolones. In the face of negative cultures, empirical therapy with an agent that is active against typical pathogens, including methicillin-resistant *S. aureus* (MRSA), is reasonable. Caution should be exercised in the use of daptomycin because there have been failures in the treatment of bone infections with this drug. Vancomycin remains the standard agent for empirical therapy to cover resistant staphylococci (e.g., MRSA). Prior administration of antibiotics may lead to negative cultures even in cases of unequivocal infection. In this situation, empirical therapy should be based on the activity of the agents previously administered as well as the potential pathogens based on exposure history.

In all cases, the clinical response to treatment of the infection should inform subsequent decision making regarding the need for additional débridement or changes in antibiotic therapy. Monitoring of inflammatory markers such as CRP or ESR is helpful in determining the adequacy of response to treatment. In particular, if these markers are elevated at the start of treatment, they should fall to normal or near-normal levels by the time the treatment is finished. Signs and symptoms of inflammation at the site of infection should have also resolved by the cessation of treatment. There have been few randomized controlled trials comparing different durations of antimicrobial therapy. In general, acute osteomyelitis should be treated for 4 to 6 weeks. It is reasonable to continue treatment if the patient has improved but has failed to resolve elevated inflammatory markers or local signs of inflammation. Such patients should be closely monitored and evaluated for the need for additional débridement or other measures aimed at diagnosis and source control. Chronic osteomyelitis may require 12 or more weeks of therapy, and treatment is usually individualized based on the clinical situation.

Patients undergoing therapy should also be monitored weekly for toxicity to antibiotics. Assessment of renal and hepatic function, complete blood counts, and drug levels are typically monitored, depending on the specific agent used. In the case of aminoglycosides, renal function and peak and trough levels of antibiotics should be measured twice weekly. Adjunctive therapies such as bone grafting, revascularization procedures, and the placement of muscle flaps to cover and protect exposed bone may be used in the appropriate clinical situation.

Native joint septic arthritis may be treated with a 4-week course of antibiotics; prosthetic joint infections are typically treated for 6 weeks or longer. Monitoring for toxicity and response to treatment is similar to that for osteomyelitis.

⬤ PROGNOSIS

The prognosis for most cases of osteomyelitis or septic arthritis is excellent, assuming adequate diagnosis, débridement, and antimicrobial therapy. The most common complication is residual pain and/or decreased function of the affected bone or joint. However, these effects are relatively rare and relatively minor. An exception is prosthetic joint infections: 25% to 50% of patients experience some loss of function as a result of the infection. Recurrence rates for chronic osteomyelitis, especially in diabetics, may be as high as 30%. In more complex cases, such as open contaminated fractures or infected hardware that require retention, complications including non-union, prosthesis failure, and chronic osteomyelitis may occur. Ultimately, infections that cannot be controlled may lead to the need for amputation and its attendant loss of function and mobility. Occasionally, bone or joint infections can disseminate to other joints or to the bloodstream, resulting in life-threatening sepsis. Such cases usually involve infection with *S. aureus* and fortunately remain the exception.

For a deeper discussion on this topic, please see Chapter 272, "Infections of Bursae, Joints, and Bones," in Goldman-Cecil Medicine, 25th Edition.

SUGGESTED READINGS

Lew DP, Waldvogel FA: Osteomyelitis, Lancet 364:369–379, 2004.

Osmon DR, Berbari EF, Berendt AR, et al: Diagnosis and management of prosthetic joint infection: clinical practice guidelines by the Infectious Diseases Society of America. Executive summary, Clin Infect Dis 56:1–25, 2013.

Ross JJ: Septic arthritis, Infect Dis Clin North Am 19:799–817, 2005.

Shuford JA, Steckelberg JM: Role of oral antimicrobial therapy in the management of osteomyelitis, Curr Opin Infect Dis 16:515–519, 2003.

Spielberg B, Lipsky BA: Systemic antibiotic therapy for chronic osteomyelitis in adults, Clin Infect Dis 54:393–497, 2012.

Stengel D, Bauwens K, Sehouli J, et al: Systematic review and meta-analysis of antibiotic therapy for bone and joint infections, Lancet Infect Dis 1:175–188, 2001.

Tice AD, Hoaglund PA, Shoultz DA: Outcomes of osteomyelitis among patients treated with outpatient parenteral antimicrobial therapy, Am J Med 114:723–728, 2003.

Waldvogel FA, Medoff G, Swartz MN: Osteomyelitis: a review of clinical features, therapeutic consideration and unusual aspects, N Engl J Med 282:316–322, 1970.

98

Urinary Tract Infections

Joao Tavares and Steven M. Opal

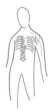

DEFINITION AND DIAGNOSIS

The term *urinary tract infection* (UTI) refers to significant bacteriuria in a patient with symptoms or signs attributable to the urinary tract and no alternative diagnosis. UTI includes asymptomatic bacteriuria, urethritis, cystitis, pyelonephritis, catheter-associated UTI, prostatitis, and urosepsis. This chapter focuses primarily on the two major forms of UTI, cystitis and pyelonephritis.

A practical classification divides these infections into uncomplicated and complicated UTI. Uncomplicated UTIs are episodes of cystitis and mild pyelonephritis occurring in healthy, premenopausal, sexually active, nonpregnant women with no history suggestive of abnormalities in the urinary tract. All other episodes of UTI are deemed to be potentially complicated and deserving of further evaluation.

The presence of dysuria, increased frequency of urination, suprapubic tenderness, and hematuria associated with bacteriuria or pyuria on urinalysis is unequivocally consistent with the diagnosis of cystitis. Back or flank pain, nausea, vomiting, and the presence of fever or rigors suggest infection of the upper urinary tract, although it is not easy to distinguish cystitis from pyelonephritis on clinical grounds alone. The diagnosis of UTI gets more difficult when patients cannot ascribe symptoms to the urinary tract (e.g., patients with paraplegia or neurogenic bladder, confused elderly or sedated patients) or when they have atypical symptoms, such as changes in mental status, agitation, or hypotension. Sometimes patients have urinary symptoms without bacteriuria (the pyuria-dysuria or "urethral syndrome" commonly caused by *Chlamydia trachomatis* or other difficult-to-culture genitourinary pathogens).

Bacteriuria is the hallmark of UTI. In women, *asymptomatic bacteriuria* is defined as two consecutive voided midstream urine specimens with isolation of the same bacterial strain at levels of at least 10^5 colony-forming units (CFU) per milliliter from patients without genitourinary symptoms. In men, a single clean-catch, midstream voided urine specimen with one bacterial species at a concentration greater than 10^5 CFU/mL defines asymptomatic bacteriuria. The diagnosis of asymptomatic bacteriuria is also established in both women and men from a single catheterized urine specimen (not an indwelling catheter) with one bacterial species isolated at concentrations greater than 10^2 CFU/mL.

To increase the sensitivity of the tests, *significant bacteriuria* is defined as greater than 10^2 CFU/mL of urine in a woman with symptoms of uncomplicated cystitis and pyuria (≥ 5 white blood cells per milliliter of urine per high-power field). Among women with symptoms of uncomplicated pyelonephritis and men with UTI, significant bacteriuria is defined as greater than 10^4 CFU/mL plus pyuria. In patients with complicated UTI, a concentration of 10^5 CFU/mL or higher is required for the definition of significant bacteriuria independently of pyuria.

In order for these definitions to be valid, the urine must remain in the bladder for at least 2 hours, and after urine collection the sample should be incubated immediately. If urine is not incubated immediately, it can be refrigerated for up to 8 hours before proper incubation.

The presence of asymptomatic bacteriuria is not equivalent to UTI except for pregnant women, neutropenic patients, and individuals with anatomic or functional defects in the urinary tract. The presence of white blood cell casts indicates pyelonephritis, and this finding suggests a complicated UTI with obstructive lesions of the kidney or collecting system (e.g., papillary necrosis). It is difficult to define asymptomatic bacteriuria in the patient who has undergone renal transplantation, and bacteriuria in such patients often indicates the need to treat for UTI.

LABORATORY FINDINGS

Young, sexually active women with typical symptoms of UTI have a high pretest probability for UTI. Therefore, no laboratory test is indicated. In this population, pretreatment urine analysis and culture are indicated only if the diagnosis is not straightforward or if an antibiotic-resistant organism is suspected. Urine analysis and culture are indicated in all cases of suspected complicated UTI. Blood cultures are mandatory for patients with suspected pyelonephritis. Imaging studies are indicated if kidney stones, malignancy, obstructive uropathy, and urologic malformations are suspected.

EPIDEMIOLOGY

At the extremes of age, men are more prone to UTI than women. In young boys, urethral malformation is commonly the cause, and in older men, UTI is usually caused by bladder neck obstruction secondary to prostatic hypertrophy. Homosexual men are at increased risk for acquiring UTIs. Teenage girls and sexually active women have more UTIs than their male counterparts. A higher than expected incidence of UTI among young girls might suggest sexual abuse. Sexually active women have the highest rate of UTI. Postmenopausal women have increased prevalence of UTI due to estrogen deficiency and age-related pelvic relaxation with poor bladder emptying.

The most common etiologic agent in patients with uncomplicated UTI is *Escherichia coli* (90% of cases), followed by *Staphylococcus saprophyticus*. Other agents include *Klebsiella* spp, *Enterococcus faecalis, Enterococcus faecium, Proteus* spp, *Providencia stuartii*, and *Morganella morganii*. In patients with complicated UTI, *E. coli* is still the most frequent uropathogen, but at a lower rate than in uncomplicated UTI. Other causative organisms are *Pseudomonas aeruginosa, Acinetobacter baumannii, Enterobacter* spp, *Serratia marcescens, Stenotrophomonas maltophilia, Enterococcus* spp, and *Candida* spp.

Anaerobic agents are infrequent causes of UTI; when present, they represent fistulae between the digestive tract and the urinary tract. *Staphylococcus aureus* UTI most often represents bacteremia with bacteriuria resulting from clearance of bloodstream bacteria by the kidney. Whereas 1% of individuals with a UTI get pyelonephritis, 20% to 40% of pregnant women with a UTI develop pyelonephritis, and 30% of patients with pyelonephritis have bacteremia. In diabetic and transplanted patients with UTI, the incidence of bacteremia is higher.

PATHOGENESIS

There are at least three routes by which bacteria can enter the bladder or kidney: ascending, hematogenous, and lymphatic. Lymphatic spread is the least common route. The hematogenous route is important for gram-positive organisms such as *S. aureus* or *Candida* spp but unimportant for gram-negative bacilli. The ascending route is the most important for enteric bacteria, and this mechanism is supported by higher frequency of UTI in women, given the shorter length of the female urethra, and in individuals with an indwelling Foley catheter.

Before reaching the urinary bladder or kidney, the microorganism must colonize the external part of the urinary tract.

Probably the most important aspect in the establishment of UTI is the interaction between host factors (e.g., secretor phenotype, P1 blood group, uroplakin I and II) and bacterial virulence factors (the adhesins, P fimbriae, and type I fimbriae [pili]). The urinary bladder is normally covered by a glycosaminoglycan surface that prevents binding of bacteria that transiently enter the bladder. P-fimbriated uropathogenic *E. coli* bind to alpha 1-4 linked, galactose-galactose disaccharide moieties found on uroepithelial cells, and these gal-gal glycolipids are also expressed on the P1 blood group. People with P1 blood group are overrepresented among individuals with either recurrent UTI and pyelonephritis. Also, people who lack P1 blood group are less prone to complicated UTI.

Studies have shown that P-fimbriated *E. coli* is present in 60% to 100% of isolates from patients with UTI. Ascending UTI infection can be inhibited experimentally by epithelial cell surface receptor analogues. Type I fimbriae bind to glycoprotein uroplakin I and II. *E. coli* expressing type I fimbriae are responsible for most cases of cystitis.

Once *E. coli* is attached to uroepithelial cells, both mechanical and biochemical factors facilitate the development of full-blown UTI. The local trauma and mechanical massage of the urethra during sexual intercourse help deliver bacteria into the bladder and, if vesicoureteral reflux or another ureteral anatomic defect is present, into the kidney. Foley catheter placement also helps to propel bacteria into the bladder, and all patients with a long-term indwelling catheter in place will eventually develop UTI. All uropathogenic organisms have the ability to multiply in the urine.

From the standpoint of the host, other factors associated with the development of UTI are a new sex partner (within 1 year), use of diaphragms and spermicides, family history of UTI in a first-degree relative, and lower expression of CXCR1, an

	CYSTITIS			PYELONEPHRITIS		
ANTIMICROBIAL AGENT	**USEFUL THERAPEUTICALLY**	**DOSE AND DURATION**	**COMMENTS**	**USEFUL THERAPEUTICALLY**	**DOSE AND DURATION**	**COMMENTS**
Nitrofurantoin monohydrate macrocrystals	*Yes, first line	100 mg bid for 5 days	Cheap, well tolerated SE: N, H Low impact on microbiome	No	NA	Reduced renal tissue penetration
Trimethoprim-sulfamethoxazole	*Yes, first line	160/800 mg bid for 3 days	If resistance is known to be <20% SE: rash, urticaria, N, V	Yes	160/800 mg bid for 14 days	*If organism susceptibility is known †If not, give an initial LA IV agent
Fosfomycin trometamol	*Yes, first line	3 g single-dose sachet	May be less efficient SE: N, D, H	No	NA	Active against MRSA ESBL, VRE
Fluoroquinolones (ciprofloxacin levofloxacin)	†Yes, second line	3-day regimen 250 mg bid 250 mg qd	High collateral damage SE: N, V, D, H, tendinitis	*Yes, first line	Dose varies; 7-14 days	If resistance is known to be <10%
β-Lactams	†Yes, second line	Dose varies by agent; 5-7 days	Less effective, increased side effects SE: N, V, D, rash, urticaria	†Yes Use cautiously Less efficient	Dose varies; 10-14 day regimen	†Give an initial LA IV agent

TABLE 98-1 THERAPY FOR UNCOMPLICATED URINARY TRACT INFECTIONS

Data from Gupta K, Hooton TM, Naber KG, et al: International clinical practice guidelines for the treatment of acute uncomplicated cystitis and pyelonephritis in women: a 2010 update by the Infectious Diseases Society of America and the European Society for Microbiology and Infectious Diseases—executive summary, Clin Infect Dis 52:561–564, 2011.

D, Diarrhea; ESBL, extended-spectrum β-lactamase; H, headache; IV, intravenous; LA, long acting; N, nausea; NA, not applicable; MSRA, methicillin-resistant *Staphylococcus aureus*; SE, side effects; V, vomiting; VRE, vancomycin-resistant enterococci.
*AI level of evidence from current guidelines.
†AIII level of evidence from current guidelines.
‡BI level of evidence from current guidelines.

interleukin 8 receptor. Pathogenic factors associated with the development of UTI are flagellae, diverse adhesins, siderophores, toxins, polysaccharide coating, and the ability to cause a deleterious inflammatory response.

Patient behaviors that are not associated with UTI include precoital or postcoital voiding patterns, daily beverage consumption, frequency of urination, delayed voiding habits, wiping patterns, tampon use, douching, use of hot tubs, and type of underwear.

TREATMENT

The goal of treatment in uncomplicated UTI is to decrease symptoms and prevent complications. Treatment should be guided by two important principles: the prevalence of resistant genitourinary pathogens in the community and collateral damage to ecologic microbiota (i.e., the risk of propagation of resistant organisms). First-line agents for uncomplicated UTI are nitrofurantoin, trimethoprim-sulfamethoxazole (TMP-SMX), and fosfomycin trometamol; alternative agents are the fluoroquinolones (except moxifloxacin) and the β-lactams (Table 98-1).

Treatment of complicated UTI should be based on culture results and the other comorbidities that are present. Recurrent UTI in sexually active women can be prevented with postcoital TMP-SMX 40/200 mg single dose (if the patient has more than two UTIs per year related to coitus) or with daily, every other day, or weekly antibiotic. If the patient has a UTI unrelated to coitus or there are fewer than two UTIs per year related to coitus, the prevention of the UTI recurrence can be achieved with patient-initiated therapy. Daily topical application of intravaginal estriol can be helpful in postmenopausal women. After completion of the treatment, urine culture is indicated for pregnant women and on an individualized basis for other patients with complicated UTI.

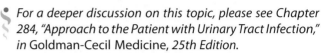

For a deeper discussion on this topic, please see Chapter 284, "Approach to the Patient with Urinary Tract Infection," in Goldman-Cecil Medicine, *25th Edition.*

SUGGESTED READINGS

Gupta K, Hooton TM, Naber KG, et al: International clinical practice guidelines for the treatment of acute uncomplicated cystitis and pyelonephritis in women: a 2010 update by the Infectious Diseases Society of America and the European Society for Microbiology and Infectious Diseases—executive summary, Clin Infect Dis 52:561–564, 2011.

Gupta K, Trautner B: In the clinic: urinary tract infection [review], Ann Intern Med 156:ITC3-1–ITC3-15, quiz ITC-13–ITC-16, 2012.

Hooton TM: Clinical practice: uncomplicated urinary tract infection [review], N Engl J Med 366:1028–1037, 2012.

Hooton TM, Bradley SF, Cardenas DD, et al: Diagnosis, prevention, and treatment of catheter-associated urinary tract infection in adults: 2009 International Clinical Practice Guidelines from the Infectious Diseases Society of America, Clin Infect Dis 50:625–663, 2010.

Nicolle LE, Bradley S, Colgan R, et al: Infectious Diseases Society of America guidelines for the diagnosis and treatment of asymptomatic bacteriuria in adults, Clin Infect Dis 40:643–654, 2005.

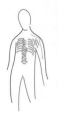

99

Health Care–Associated Infections

Steven "Shaefer" Spires and Thomas R. Talbot

INTRODUCTION

A health care–associated infection (HAI) is an infection that did not exist or was not incubating at the time of admission to the health care facility. Infections with an onset of more than 48 hours after admission and within 7 to 30 days after facility discharge are defined as HAIs. These infections can occur in all types of health care settings, including acute care units, long-term care facilities, rehabilitation facilities, outpatient dialysis clinics, and outpatient surgical centers.

HAIs cause a substantial degree of morbidity and mortality. A 2011 survey conducted by the Centers for Disease Control and Prevention (CDC) Emerging Infection Program reported an acute care hospital HAI prevalence of 6.8%. Extrapolating from acute care admission data (about 35 million admissions per year), approximately 2 million acute care HAIs occur annually in the United States. Beyond the extensive morbidity and mortality they cause, HAIs are costly, calculated as $13,973 per infection in one review. These costs are likely to be underestimated because of incomplete estimation of the outpatient costs of parenteral antibiotics, skilled nursing care, physical rehabilitation, and lost work days.

As of January 2011, the Centers for Medicare and Medicaid Services (CMS) required public reporting of certain facility-specific HAI outcomes as part of value-based purchasing. As of January 2013, the following acute care–related HAIs are required for reporting by CDC's National Healthcare Safety Network (NHSN): catheter-associated urinary tract infections (CAUTIs) and central line–associated bloodstream infections (CLABSIs) in intensive care units (ICUs), colon and abdominal hysterectomy surgical site infections (SSIs), hospital-onset *Clostridium difficile* infections (CDIs), and hospital-onset methicillin-resistant *Staphylococcus aureus* (MRSA) bacteremias. The importance of preventing HAIs has never been more apparent.

The major types of HAIs include the infections reported to CMS, hospital-acquired pneumonia (HAP) or ventilator-associated pneumonia (VAP), and multidrug-resistant organisms (MDROs). MDROs are pathogens with resistance to various important antibiotics (e.g., MRSA, vancomycin-resistant *Enterococcus* (VRE), antibiotic-resistant gram-negative bacilli). This chapter reviews the major classes of HAIs, with a focus on prevention, diagnosis, and treatment.

HEALTH CARE EPIDEMIOLOGY AND INFECTION PREVENTION

In the age of increasing MDROs, shortage of new antibiotics, and public reporting of HAIs, the importance of efforts to prevent HAIs is growing. The fields of health care epidemiology and infection prevention focus on the practices of tracking HAIs in a systematic fashion (i.e., surveillance) to implement evidence-based HAI prevention practices.

Although HAIs were once thought to be the cost of being critically ill and receiving care in a hospital, several key events occurred during the past decade that shifted that perception. In 2006, Pronovost and colleagues implemented a "simple and inexpensive intervention" in 103 ICUs in the state of Michigan while participating in the Michigan Health and Hospital Association Keystone ICU project. This landmark study showed a reduction in the median rate of CLABSIs from 2.7 per 1000 catheter days to zero. These results shifted the discussion from merely controlling HAIs to preventing them. Other major events have included recognition and effectiveness of using bundles of evidence-based practices to reduce HAIs; recognition of the HAI burden in nonacute, non-ICU settings; and importance of quality improvement science in reducing HAIs.

The prevention of HAIs has become increasingly possible, and various types of prevention interventions can reduce the HAI burden dramatically. In 2010, Wenzel and Edmund described these interventions as horizontal and vertical strategies (Table 99-1). Horizontal infection prevention strategies are broad practices (e.g., hand hygiene, isolation precautions) aimed at preventing many or all types of HAIs, regardless of the specific pathogen, procedure, or device. Vertical HAI prevention strategies are directed at specific types of HAIs or target a specific organism. Vertical strategies include using procedural checklists or standardized bundles and MRSA decolonization.

CATHETER-ASSOCIATED URINARY TRACT INFECTIONS

In a survey performed by the CDC in 2011, CAUTIs were the second most common device-associated infection. The incidence of CAUTIs in 2011 ranged from 0 to 4.2 per 1000 catheter days, compared with the 2006-2007 period, when rates were between 3.4 and 7.7 per 1000 catheter days. The estimated additional cost of a CAUTI was $589 to $758 per infection in 1998 dollars, and

TABLE 99-1	STRATEGIES FOR PREVENTING HEALTH CARE–ASSOCIATED INFECTIONS

HORIZONTAL STRATEGIES (TO PREVENT ALL OR MANY TYPES OF HAI)

1. Standard precautions
   - Hand hygiene
   - Use of appropriate PPE
   - Respiratory hygiene and cough etiquette
   - Appropriate environmental cleaning and waste disposal
2. Chlorhexidine bathing in ICUs*
3. Isolation precautions appropriate for pathogen
4. Steps to prevent needlestick injuries
5. MDRO decolonization
6. Education of health care workers on IC/IP protocols

VERTICAL STRATEGIES (SPECIFIC TO HAI TYPE)

CAUTI

Urinary catheter placed only for appropriate indications:
 Urinary retention or obstruction
 Need for accurate UOP measurement in critical illness
 Incontinence and perineal or sacral wounds
 Comfort care use for terminal illness
Consider alternatives:
 Condom catheters
 Intermittent catheterization
Proper insertion and maintenance:
 Maintain aseptic technique
 Properly secure catheter to patient
 Maintain closed drainage system
 Maintain unobstructed flow
Urinary catheter premeditated stop order or RN-initiated discontinuation policy
Anti-infective catheters if infection rates remain high

VAP

Use noninvasive ventilation when able
On intubation:
 Semirecumbent position (30-45 degrees) unless contraindicated
 Hypopharyngeal suctioning
 Avoid gastric overdistention
 Use cuffed ET tube
 Oral care (with chlorhexidine oral rinse), tooth brushing
 Keep ventilatory circuit closed unless changing for soiling or malfunctioning
 Daily targeted sedation management
 Spontaneous breathing trial if screening finds applicable
Use weaning protocols to minimize duration of ventilation

CLABSI

Use checklist for device insertion:
 Bundle supplies
 All present use at least face mask, then proceduralist uses sterile gown and gloves, mask, and head cap
 Avoid femoral line placement if possible
 Skin antisepsis with alcohol and >0.5% chlorhexidine
 Use of chlorhexidine-impregnated dressing or sponge at insertion site
 Empower personnel to stop nonemergent insertion if improper technique is followed
Maintenance:
 Access as infrequently as feasible
 Scrub the access hub or port with antiseptic
Daily audits for assessment of device need and potential discontinuation

SSI

Preoperative strategies:
 Nonirritative hair removal with clippers (not razors)
 Eradicate remote infection
 Decolonization of *Staphylococcus aureus* if carrier
 Smoking cessation
 Glucose control, hemoglobin A_{1c} <7% if possible
 Avoid immunosuppressive medication in perioperative period
 Identify and address malnutrition
Intraoperative strategies:
 In OR: proper ventilation, minimize traffic, proper attire, and surgical scrub
 Proper skin preparation (chlorhexidine plus alcohol or povidone plus alcohol) and draping
 Antimicrobial prophylaxis; proper timing, dosing, and intraoperative redosing
 Maintain normothermia
 Glucose control
 Tissue oxygenation, preoperative and postoperative supplementation

CDI

Prevention of acquisition:
 Antimicrobial stewardship
Prevention of transmission:
 Contact precautions (e.g., empirical placement for those suspected of CDI before confirmation of diagnosis)
 Hand hygiene with soap and water before leaving the patient's room
 Continue contact precautions until discharge
Appropriate environmental cleaning with bleach-containing agents

CAUTI, Catheter-associated urinary tract infection; CDI, *Clostridium difficile* infection; CLABSI, central line–associated bloodstream infection; ET, endotracheal; HAI, health care–associated infection; IC/IP, infection control or prevention; ICU, intensive care unit; MDRO, multidrug-resistant organism; OR, operating room; PPE, personal protective equipment; RN, registered nurse; SSI, surgical site infection; UOP, urine output; VAP, ventilator-associated pneumonia.

*Current data are not strong for prevention of CAUTI, VAP, and CDI by this method.

the total annual cost associated with CAUTIs in U.S. hospitals in 2007 was estimated between $390 and $450 million.

CAUTI complications include cystitis, pyelonephritis, and in up to 4%, bacteremia. Although urinary catheter–associated bacteremias are rare, they are an underappreciated cause of health care–associated bacteremias and have been estimated to cost an additional $3744 per episode. Most of the epidemiologic data on CAUTIs are from ICU patients. However, some studies describe rates of CAUTI among the non-ICU population that are similar to rates among ICU patients when calculated in catheter days, and in some instances, the absolute number of infections is higher outside of the ICU.

Most health care–associated urinary tract infections are catheter associated. A catheterized patient's daily risk of developing bacteruria is about 3% to 10%. Indwelling urinary catheters disrupt several mechanisms of the natural defense against infection, including urine flow, length of the urethra, and micturition to prevent attachment of potential pathogens to the uroepithelium. Tamm-Horsfall proteins, the most abundant soluble proteins in the urine, play a significant role by binding uropathogenic bacteria, facilitating wash out, and lowering the threshold for activating local innate immunity. These soluble proteins are prevented from entering the lower urinary tract by the catheters.

An indwelling catheter allows colonization, attachment, and biofilm formation by certain microorganisms. Most of the organisms causing CAUTIs arrive by ascending the urethra from the meatus and perineum. The most common uropathogens identified in CAUTIs are *Escherichia coli*, *Candida* species, *Klebsiella* species, *Pseudomonas aeruginosa*, and *Enterococcus* species (Fig. 99-1).

Common symptoms of a urinary tract infection (e.g., dysuria, urinary frequency) may not be useful in diagnosing a patient with an indwelling catheter. However, the most common clinical manifestations of a CAUTI are fever (≥38°C) and bacteruria. Other signs and symptoms of a CAUTI can include rigors,

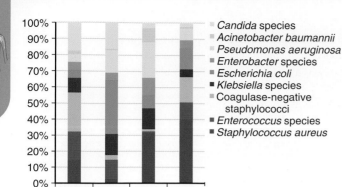

FIGURE 99-1 Causative pathogens by specific type of health care–associated infection as reported to the Centers for Disease Control and Prevention National Healthcare Safety Network. CAUTI, Catheter-associated urinary tract infections; CLABSI, central line–associated bloodstream infections; SSI, surgical site infections; VAP, ventilator-associated pneumonia. (Modified from Sievert DM, Ricks P, Edwards JR, et al: Antimicrobial-resistant pathogens associated with healthcare-associated infection: summary of data reported to the National Health-care Safety Network at the Centers for Disease Control and Prevention, 2009-2010, Infect Control Hosp Epidemiol 34:1–14, 2013.)

altered mental status, pelvic or suprapubic pain, costovertebral angle tenderness, and acute onset of hematuria without another underlying cause. One of these signs or symptoms plus a positive urine culture with a known uropathogen ($>10^5$ colony-forming units) strongly suggests a CAUTI. Pyuria (>5 leukocytes/mL of urine) is not always a reliable indicator for infection in patients with indwelling catheters; pyuria and asymptomatic bacteriuria are not necessarily indications for treatment. Risk factors for CAUTI acquisition include duration of catheterization, underlying fatal illness, age older than 50 years, having a nonsurgical underlying illness, and nonadherence to proper catheter care (E-Table 99-1).

The most effective method of preventing CAUTIs is to avoid placing urinary catheters unless absolutely necessary and to restrict catheter use to institutionally accepted indications. Proper insertion and care of urinary catheters are paramount (see Table 99-1). Maintenance of unobstructed flow with the collection bag below the bladder, use of a closed catheter system (even when sampling urine), and discontinuation of the catheter as soon as appropriate are key elements for preventing a CAUTI. Nurse-directed discontinuation protocols in which frontline personnel have defined parameters for removing catheters without requiring a provider's order are increasingly used to eliminate unnecessary catheters. The routine use of antimicrobial-coated catheters is not recommended except when infection rates remain elevated despite proper adherence to all other prevention strategies.

Treatment of asymptomatic bacteriuria usually is not recommended. Treatment of CAUTI is based on current Infectious Disease Society of America (IDSA) guidelines, and the choice of antimicrobial regimen should be based on the local antibiogram and identified syndrome (e.g., pyelonephritis). Before treatment, urine culture and sensitivity results are used to evaluate a resistant organism and tailor an empirical antimicrobial regimen.

Most clinicians prefer to replace or discontinue the catheter after a urinary tract infection is diagnosed. Guidelines recommend replacement if it has been in place for more than 2 weeks.

PNEUMONIA TYPE	DEFINITION
TABLE 99-2	**DEFINITIONS OF TYPES OF NOSOCOMIAL PNEUMONIA**
Health care–associated pneumonia (HCAP)	Pneumonia in any patient who was hospitalized in an acute care hospital for 2+ days within 90 days of infection; resided in an NH or LTCF; received recent IV antibiotic therapy, chemotherapy, or wound care within the past 30 days of the current infection; or attended a hospital or hemodialysis clinic
Hospital-acquired pneumonia (HAP)	Pneumonia that occurs at least 48 hours after admission and that was not incubating at the time of admission
Ventilator-associated pneumonia (VAP)	Pneumonia that arises 48-72 hours after endotracheal intubation

Data from American Thoracic Society, Infectious Diseases Society of America: Guidelines for the management of adults with hospital-acquired, ventilator-associated, and healthcare-associated pneumonia, Am J Respir Crit Care Med 171:388–416, 2005.
IV, Intravenous; LTCF, long-term care facility; NH, nursing home.

There is good evidence based on review by expert committees (grade A-III evidence) that duration of treatment can be 7 days if symptoms quickly resolve or 10 to 14 days if resolution is delayed. There is moderate evidence based on expert committees' opinions (grade B-III) that a 5-day course of levofloxacin can be considered if patients are not severely ill and the organism is sensitive to the drug. In nonpregnant women younger than 65 years of age, a 3-day course of antibiotic therapy can be considered after the urinary catheter has been removed (grade B-II).

HOSPITAL-ACQUIRED PNEUMONIA

HAP has become the most common HAI. Most HAPs occur in the ICU, and more than 90% are VAPs. Health care–associated pneumonia (HCAP) is considered along with HAP because of the etiologic similarities. Other definitions are given in Table 99-2.

The incidence of HAP or VAP is difficult to determine due to the various definitions that have been used for surveillance and the subjective nature of these diagnoses. Some studies have estimated that the incidence of VAP ranges from 2 to 16 cases per 1000 ventilator days. VAP is associated with increased length of hospital stay (10 days in one study), costs (approximately $40,000), and mortality (attributable mortality rate of 13%, highest among surgical patients).

Risk factors for VAP include conditions that lead to increased aspiration or impairment of host defenses and bacterial colonization of the respiratory and upper gastrointestinal tracts (see E-Table 99-1). In a ventilated patient, the body's natural mechanical defense mechanisms (e.g., ciliated epithelium, mucus, cough) are interrupted, leading to colonization of the lower airways by potentially pathogenic organisms. The most significant source of these organisms tends to be the patient's own oropharynx and upper gastric contents.

The most commonly implicated respiratory pathogens are *S. aureus* and *P. aeruginosa,* followed by several Enterobacteriaceae species and *Acinetobacter baumannii* (see Fig. 99-1). Colonization with MDROs correlates with increasing duration of hospitalization. Guidelines argue that late (>4 days after admission) compared with early HAP may be the most useful factor when determining empirical antimicrobial therapy. Although bacteria play the largest role in HAP, fungi and viruses also must be considered in immunosuppressed patients.

TABLE 99-3 MODIFIED CLINICAL PULMONARY INFECTION SCORE (CPIS)

CLINICAL CRITERIA	INFORMATION	POINTS*
Temperature (°C)	≥36.5 and ≤38.4	0
	≥38.5 and ≤38.9	1
	≤36 or ≥39	2
Leukocyte count (per µL)	≥4,000 and ≤11,000	0
	<4,000 or >11,000	1
	<4,000 or >11,000 + ≥500 bands	2
Tracheal secretions	Absent/rare	0
	Abundant/nonpurulent	1
	Abundant + purulent	2
PaO_2/FIO_2 (mm Hg)	>240 or ARDS	0
	≤240 and no evidence of ARDS	2
Chest radiographic findings	No infiltrate	0
	Diffuse or patchy infiltrate	1
	Localized infiltrate	2
Microbiology†	Negative	0
	Positive	2

Data from Fartoukh M, Maitre B, Honore S, et al: Diagnosing pneumonia during mechanical ventilation: the clinical pulmonary infection score revisited, Am J Respir Crit Care Med 168:173–179, 2003.

ARDS, Acute respiratory distress syndrome.

*With the use of these clinical criteria, a clinical pulmonary infection score of 6 or greater has an 85% sensitivity for detecting pulmonary infection.

†Gram stain results of directed or blind, protected endotracheal aspirate.

One definition of HAP or VAP includes clinical, radiographic, and microbiologic criteria. The Clinical Pulmonary Infection Score (CPIS) system is useful in determining when antimicrobial therapy is necessary (Table 99-3). A score of 6 or greater has 85% sensitivity in diagnosing a pulmonary infection. Signs and symptoms indicating an infection include fever (≥38°C), peripheral leukocytosis, purulent sputum, and worsening respiratory status. A tracheal aspirate for Gram stain and culture provides the last piece of diagnostic information. When several of these signs and symptoms exist in the absence of a pulmonary infiltrate, alternative diagnoses should be considered, including ventilator-associated tracheobronchitis.

Duration of hospitalization is a significant factor to consider when initiating empirical therapy because of the increasing likelihood of MDRO colonization with prolonged length of stay. In early HAP (≤4 days), more community-acquired organisms may be targeted, except when the patient has certain qualifiers for HCAP (see Table 99-2) or is known to be colonized with resistant organisms. However, in late HAP (including VAP and HCAP), the IDSA guidelines recommend adding empirical coverage for resistant gram-positive organisms (including MRSA) and for multidrug-resistant Enterobacteriaceae (level II evidence according to the American Thoracic Society [ATS]/IDSA guidelines for HAP). Dual coverage for multidrug-resistant *P. aeruginosa* should also be considered. An example of an empirical regimen for late-onset HAP is vancomycin or linezolid plus an antipseudomonal β-lactam/β-lactamase inhibitor, carbapenem, or cephalosporin.

INFECTIONS ASSOCIATED WITH VASCULAR CATHETERS

The NHSN collects data on CLABSIs, and public reporting is required for CLABSIs in ICUs. In 2011, the incidence of CLABSIs ranged from 0 to 3.7 cases per 1000 catheter days, compared with 1 to 5.6 cases per 1000 catheter days in 2006

through 2007. Although CLABSIs have the lowest prevalence among HAIs, the cost per episode and morbidity rate remain high. The estimated additional cost of an infection related to an intravenous catheter is $4000 to $56,000 per episode. The attributable increase in length of stay has been between 6.5 and 22 days, and the attributable mortality rate is about 10% among hospitalized patients.

The most common pathogens that cause primary CLABSIs are flora arising at the percutaneous insertion site or from contamination of the catheter hub. Hematogenous seeding from a gastrointestinal or other endovascular source occurs but is less likely. The most common pathogens that cause CLABSIs are coagulase-negative staphylococci, *Candida* species, *S. aureus*, and *Enterococcus* species (see Fig. 99-1). The risk factors for CLABSI are provided in E-Table 99-1. The rising proportion of infections caused by *Enterococcus* species and *Candida* species since the 2006-2007 period suggests that skin colonization is being adequately addressed by the adoption of evidence-based prevention strategies and that an increasing fraction of CLABSIs are caused by secondary hematogenous seeding. Patients who are more severely ill, are neutropenic, have burns, or are on total parenteral nutrition are also at increased risk for candidemia. Other types of catheter-related infections include phlebitis, exit site infection, and pocket and tunnel infection.

Many CLABSIs are preventable through the use of evidence-based prevention practices for line insertion and maintenance. Strategies include appropriate decolonization of the skin before insertion with chlorhexidine plus alcohol, use of maximal sterile barriers (i.e., proceduralist wears sterile gloves and gown, cap, and mask, and a large barrier drape is placed over the patient), hand hygiene, and sterile technique (see Table 99-1). Appropriate maintenance of the central line mandates scrubbing the hub with antiseptic and discontinuing the catheter as soon as it is not needed.

For a patient with a fever or systemic symptoms who has a central venous catheter, a bloodstream infection should be suspected. The diagnostic evaluation should begin with paired peripheral and catheter blood samples for culture before initiation of antimicrobial therapy. In a suspected case of bloodstream infection, the exudate at the exit site should be cultured.

The type of device (e.g., peripheral vs. central, short term vs. long term), associated infectious complications, and the implicated organism all play a role in treatment. For CLABSIs associated with short-term, nontunneled catheters and no complicating factors (e.g., suppurative thrombophlebitis, endocarditis, intravascular hardware), it may be appropriate to treat for 7 to 14 days after removal of the catheter. However, for long-term catheters, salvage may be attempted with systemic plus antibiotic lock therapy (level B-II evidence, indicating a moderate amount of evidence from well-designed clinical trials or cohort or case series). Salvage of catheters associated with *S. aureus* bacteremia and fungemia have largely been unsuccessful, and it is not recommended. In the setting of an endovascular complication, removal of the catheter is strongly recommended, and systemic antibiotic therapy should be prolonged (i.e., 4 to 6 weeks) (level B-II). In many cases, septic thrombophlebitis may require surgical attention. Tunnel and pocket infections may also require débridement, but after the catheter is removed, 7 to 14 days of antimicrobial therapy should be sufficient.

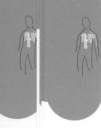

Treatment

Despite the classic staging of syphilis as primary, secondary, latent, or tertiary, the disease is best thought of in terms of early infection (<1 year) or late infection (≥1 year) when considering treatment. *T. pallidum* remains sensitive to penicillin. Individuals with early syphilis can be treated with a single intramuscular injection of benzathine penicillin G (Bicillin), which achieves high and prolonged serum concentrations. Individuals with late syphilis or disease of unknown duration should be treated with three weekly injections of intramuscular benzathine penicillin G (Table 100-3). This cures most patients.

Although penicillin remains the drug of choice, doxycycline may also be used in individuals who have severe allergies to penicillin. However, every effort should be made to use penicillin because of the sensitivity of the organism. For pregnant women who are allergic to penicillin, penicillin desensitization should occur in collaboration with a pharmacist and an allergist specialist. As a result of treatment, individuals may experience a febrile reaction (i.e., Jarisch-Herxheimer reaction). Symptoms are caused by killing of the spirochetes and should not be confused with an allergic reaction.

The co-epidemic of syphilis and HIV has led to an increase in individuals with manifestations of neurosyphilis. In cases of syphilis with neurologic symptoms, a lumbar puncture is warranted to rule out neurologic involvement. Any pleocytosis or increase in protein concentration warrants treatment for neurosyphilis. A cerebrospinal fluid (CSF) sample should be sent for VDRL testing, but the test lacks sensitivity (50%), and a negative test result does not rule out neurosyphilis. Usually, HIV-negative individuals with syphilis without neurologic symptoms should not undergo a lumbar puncture. Many HIV-infected individuals with syphilis, however, have asymptomatic neurosyphilis. The clinical implications of this are unclear, but these individuals may fail intramuscular therapy at a high rate. Some experts recommend CSF examination in all HIV-infected individuals with a CD4⁺ count lower than 350 cells/μL or a nontreponemal titer greater than 1 : 32. These criteria capture almost everyone with asymptomatic neurosyphilis.

Individuals with neurosyphilis should be treated with intravenous penicillin G for 10 to 14 days. In tertiary disease with manifestations of neurologic disease, treatment with intravenous penicillin halts disease progression but does not reverse existing structural damage. Ocular disease or other similar neurologic manifestations should be treated as neurosyphilis. Nontreponemal titers should be followed to ensure an appropriate response. Repeat treatment may be necessary in a small number of cases.

Prognosis

Although penicillin is the treatment of choice for syphilis, it has not been validated in clinical trials but is based on a long history of clinical use. However, a significant number of individuals with syphilis do not respond with the recommended decline in nontreponemal titer. Individuals who do not respond should be retreated.

For a deeper discussion of these topics, please see Chapter 319, "Syphilis," in Goldman-Cecil Medicine, *25th Edition.*

Herpes Simplex Virus

Definition and Epidemiology

Herpes simplex virus types 1 and 2 (HSV-1/2) cause a wide variety of clinical disease. HSV-1 is usually the cause of herpes labialis (i.e., cold sores), and HSV-2 is the cause of genital herpes, although there may be overlap. After infection occurs, HSV-1/2 enters a latent state and may later reactivate to cause disease in a subset of individuals.

The overall prevalence of HSV-1 and HSV-2 in the population is approximately 60% and 20%, respectively. However, the incidence of HSV-1 infection approaches 90% to 100% among middle-aged adults. Seroprevalence of HSV-2 is associated with a patient's sexual activity, including number of partners and history of other STIs, and with age, gender (women ae at higher risk than men), and race or ethnicity. More than 50 million people in the United States are infected with genital HSV-1/2, and most are asymptomatic. CDC guidelines do not recommend routine screening for HSV-1/2 in people without symptoms. There is no evidence that screening for HSV-1/2 reduces its spread or has an impact on the disease. HSV-1/2 is not a reportable disease in the United States.

Pathology

HSV-1 and HSV-2 are two of eight double-stranded DNA human herpesviruses. Others are varicella-zoster virus (VZV), cytomegalovirus (CMV), Epstein-Barr virus (EBV), and human herpesviruses 6, 7, and 8. Infection with one type of HSV does not prevent or increase the chances of infection with other types. After initial infection, HSV-1/2 enters a latent state within neuronal cells of sensory or autonomic peripheral ganglia. Reactivation can occur at any time and is mediated in part by immune factors. HSV-1 most commonly infects the trigeminal ganglia and HSV-2 the sacral nerve root ganglia (S2-S5).

Clinical Presentation

Transmission of HSV-1/2 is through skin-to-skin contact, including sexual contact at mucosal surfaces, including the oropharynx,

TABLE 100-3	SYPHILIS TREATMENT	
CLINICAL CATEGORY	**REGIMEN OF CHOICE**	**ALTERNATIVE***
Early syphilis (<1 year)	Benzathine penicillin, 2.4 million units IM, given once	Penicillin desensitization Doxycycline, 100 mg PO bid for 14 days Tetracycline, 500 mg PO qid for 14 days Azithromycin 2 g PO qd
Late syphilis (≥1 year) or unknown duration	Benzathine penicillin, 2.4 million units IM, given once each week for 3 wk	Penicillin desensitization Doxycycline, 100 mg PO bid for 28 days Tetracycline, 500 mg PO qid for 28 days
Neurosyphilis	Penicillin G, 4 million units IV q4h or 24 million units by continuous infusion qd for 10-14 days	Penicillin desensitization Ceftriaxone 2 g qd IM or IV for 10-14 days

*If patient has a penicillin allergy.

vagina, rectum, cervix, and conjunctivae. Importantly, transmission may occur in the absence of symptoms.

The stages of HSV-1/2 infection include primary, latent, and recurrent. Primary infection of genital HSV-1/2 may include fever, headache, other systemic symptoms, and the classic local symptoms of painful genital vesicles or ulcers (multiple) and lymphadenopathy. Oral infections of HSV-1 may include gingivostomatitis and pharyngitis. Symptoms may vary from none to serious and require hospitalization. HSV-1/2 then enters a latent state. Reactivation occurs in a subset of individuals with symptoms less severe than those of primary infection. Some individuals have no reactivation, and others have more than three reactivations per year.

Complications of HSV-1/2 infection include meningitis and proctitis. Recurrent episodes of meningitis (i.e., Mollaret's meningitis) may be caused by HSV-1/2. Other manifestations of HSV-1/2 include herpetic whitlow (e.g., infection of a finger of a health care worker), herpes gladiatorum (e.g., HSV-1/2 skin infections in athletes such as wrestlers), and ocular disease (e.g., keratitis, acute retinal necrosis). HSV-1/2 infection may rarely be associated with erythema multiforme, hepatitis, and encephalitis.

Diagnosis and Differential Diagnosis

The diagnosis of HSV-1/2 is typically made clinically. If possible, lesions should be tested for HSV-1/2 using viral culture (50% sensitivity), PCR, or direct fluorescent antibody (DFA) testing. Alternatively, serology testing for immunoglobulin M (IgM) and immunoglobulin G (IgG) antibodies is available. This test should be reserved for individuals with suspected primary infection or to document chronic infection, and it should usually not be used for screening purposes.

Treatment

Recommended regimens for primary HSV-1/2 infection include acyclovir (400 mg orally three times per day for 7 to 10 days or 200 mg orally five times per day for 7 to 10 days), famciclovir (250 mg orally three times each day for 7 to 10 days), or valacyclovir (1 g orally twice each day for 7 to 10 days). Treatment can also be used for reactivation disease: acyclovir (400 mg orally three times each day for 5 days, 800 mg orally twice each day for 5 days, or 800 mg orally three times each day for 2 days), famciclovir (125 mg orally twice each day for 5 days or 1000 mg orally twice each day for 1 day or 500 mg once followed by 250 mg twice each day for 2 days), or valacyclovir (500 mg twice each day for 3 days or 1 g orally once each day for 5 days).

Individuals with frequent recurrences may be candidates for suppressive therapy. Severe disease should be treated with intravenous acyclovir (5 to 10 mg/kg intravenously every 8 hours). Duration and transition to oral medication should be based on clinical improvement but is usually 7 to 10 days. The safety of systemic acyclovir, valacyclovir, and famciclovir therapy in pregnant women is not established.

Prognosis

Although HSV-1/2 infection cannot be cured, most people are asymptomatic, and suppressive therapy is available. Individuals with HSV-1/2 infection should be educated regarding the disease, including transmission and available treatments. They should be encouraged to discuss their status with sexual partners, including the possibility that transmission may occur in the absence of symptoms. Individuals should abstain from sex during an outbreak.

Chancroid

Chancroid is a rare cause of genital ulceration in the United States. The infection is caused by the gram-negative rod *Haemophilus ducreyi* and is endemic in parts of Africa and the Caribbean. Classic symptoms include a single or multiple, painful, nonindurated genital ulcers and inguinal lymphadenopathy. Growth of the organism in cultures requires hemin-containing media, and it may appear as a school of fish on Gram stain. PCR may be available in certain areas.

Testing for HSV-1/2 and syphilis should always be performed. Recommended treatment regimens include azithromycin (1 g orally once), ceftriaxone (250 mg intramuscularly once), or ciprofloxacin (500 mg orally twice each day for 3 days). Ciprofloxacin is contraindicated in pregnant and lactating women.

Granuloma Inguinale

Granuloma inguinale is also known as donovanosis. It is caused by the gram-negative bacterium *Klebsiella granulomatis*. The disease is rare in the United States (24 cases in 2010) but endemic in regions of Africa, India, Oceania, and the Caribbean. Clinical manifestations include painless, ulcerative genital lesions with erythema. Classic Donovan bodies may be observed on histopathology.

The recommended treatment regimen is doxycycline (100 mg orally twice each day for at least 3 weeks). Alternative regimens include azithromycin, ciprofloxacin, and sulfamethoxazole-trimethoprim. Azithromycin may be useful for treating granuloma inguinale during pregnancy. Doxycycline and ciprofloxacin are contraindicated in pregnant women.

Other Causes of Genital Ulcers

Other causes of genital ulcers should be considered when the results of routine testing are negative. Noninfectious causes include trauma, Behçet's disease, malignancy, and drug-mediated disease

⬤ OTHER SEXUALLY TRANSMITTED INFECTIONS
Genital Warts

Human papillomavirus (HPV) is responsible for a spectrum of cutaneous and mucosal disease, ranging from genital warts to invasive cancer. HPV has been linked to cervical, anal, and oropharyngeal cancer. There are more than 100 types of HPV. Sexually transmitted HPV infection is responsible for genital warts and anogenital carcinoma. More than 80% of sexually active adults acquire HPV infection in their lifetime. Genital warts tend to be benign and asymptomatic, and 90% are caused by HPV types 6 and 11. The HPV types most often linked to anogenital carcinoma are 16 and 18; HPV-16 is the most common.

Warts are usually described as flat and papular in the genital regions. Diagnosis of genital warts is usually made by clinical examination. If unclear, a biopsy may be performed. Treatment

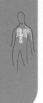

of genital warts may include podofilox (0.5% solution or gel), imiquimod (5% cream), sinecatechins (15% ointment), cryotherapy, podophyllin resin (10% t0 25% concentration), trichloroacetic acid (TCA), and surgical excision.

HPV vaccination is available with Gardasil (quadrivalent vaccine) and Cervarix (bivalent vaccine). The main objective of vaccination is to prevent cervical and other cancers. The vaccines are also effective in preventing genital warts. The vaccines are most effective before sexual debut. Guidelines suggest vaccination of males and females between the ages of 11 to 26 years. Vaccines may be administered to individuals as young as 9 years old. The guidelines state there is insufficient evidence to vaccinate individuals older than 26 years.

Pubic Lice

Pubic lice (i.e., *Pediculosis pubis*) may spread from the genitalia to other areas of the body. The most common symptom is pruritus. Small macules and localized lymphadenopathy may occur. Diagnosis of this STI is made by light microscopy of the organism.

Treatment includes permethrin (1% cream applied to affected areas, rinsed off in 10 minutes) or pyrethrins (similar application). Alternative medications include malathion (0.5% lotion) or ivermectin. Clothing, bed sheets, and other linens should be thoroughly washed.

Scabies

Scabies is caused by the skin mite *Sarcoptes scabiei*. Transmission occurs by skin contact, and among adults, it is usually sexual. Clinical presentation usually includes pruritus and small erythematous papules that are classically present on the wrists, forearms, fingers, and genital areas.

Diagnosis is usually based on clinical presentation and examination of skin scrapings. Recommended treatment regimens include permethrin (5% cream applied from the neck down and washed off after 8 to 14 hours) or ivermectin.

SUGGESTED READINGS

Centers for Disease Control and Prevention: Sexually transmitted diseases surveillance 2012, Atlanta, 2013, U.S. Department of Health and Human Services.

Cook RL, Hutchison SL, Østergaard L, et al: Systematic review: noninvasive testing for *Chlamydia trachomatis* and *Neisseria gonorrhoeae*, Ann Intern Med 142:914–925, 2005.

Geisler WM, Lensing SY, Press CG, et al: Spontaneous resolution of genital *Chlamydia trachomatis* infection in women and protection from reinfection, J Infect Dis 207:1850–1856, 2013.

Jensen JS: *Mycoplasma genitalium*: the aetiological agent of urethritis and other sexually transmitted diseases, J Eur Acad Dermatol Venereol 18:1–11, 2004.

Platt R, Rice PA, McCormack WM: Risk of acquiring gonorrhea and prevalence of abnormal adnexal findings among women recently exposed to gonorrhea, JAMA 250:3205–3209, 1983.

Rockwell DH, Yobs AR, Moore MB Jr: The Tuskegee study of untreated syphilis: the 30th year of observation, Arch Intern Med 114:792–798, 1964.

Schroeter AL, Lucas JB, Price EV, et al: Treatment for early syphilis and reactivity of serologic tests, JAMA 221:471–476, 1972.

Vall-Mayans M, Caballero E, Sanz B: The emergence of lymphogranuloma venereum in Europe, Lancet 374:356, 2009.

Workowski KA, Berman S, et al, for the Centers for Disease Control and Prevention (CDC): Sexually transmitted diseases treatment guidelines, 2010, MMWR Recomm Rep 59:1–110, 2010.

Human Immunodeficiency Virus Infection and Acquired Immunodeficiency Syndrome

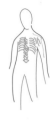

Brian T. Montague, Aadia I. Rana, Edward J. Wing, and Timothy P. Flanigan

DEFINITION AND EPIDEMIOLOGY

The human immunodeficiency virus (HIV) is a retrovirus from the lentivirus family. The first descriptions of the disease came in 1982, when HIV-associated wasting occurring in large numbers of young adults in a Ugandan fishing community was described as "slim disease." In the United States in the same year, the designation acquired immunodeficiency syndrome, or AIDS, was applied to a syndrome identified in previously healthy men who had sex with men (MSM). It was characterized by serious infections with unusual opportunistic pathogens, such as pneumonia from *Pneumocystis carinii* (now called *Pneumocystis jirovecii*) or development of the formerly rare tumor, Kaposi's sarcoma. Such infections had previously been found only among patients with severe cellular immunodeficiency, and studies confirmed profound immunodeficiency in these individuals. When similar opportunistic infections (OIs) were subsequently observed in injection drug users and in men with hemophilia along with their female sexual partners, it became clear that this syndrome was caused by an agent transmitted either through sexual contact or through infusion of blood or blood products.

The HIV virus was identified in 1983, and its role as the causative agent of AIDS was confirmed in 1984. By 1993, AIDS had become the leading cause of death among American adults aged 25 to 44 years, a trend that was dramatically reversed by the introduction of effective combination antiretroviral therapy (ART) at the end of 1995. By the end of 2006, approximately 1.1 million persons in the United States were living with HIV and AIDS, and an estimated 56,300 persons are estimated to have become infected that year. More than 20% of people living with HIV remain unaware of their status; they are at risk for serious health complications and for transmitting the virus to others.

TRANSMISSION

Although it was initially observed most frequently among homosexual men and intravenous drug users in the United States, heterosexual intercourse has been the dominant mode of HIV transmission throughout most of the world. The virus is present in semen and cervicovaginal secretions of infected individuals and can be transmitted by either partner during vaginal or anal intercourse. The concurrent presence of other sexually transmitted diseases, especially those associated with genital ulcerations, strongly facilitates sexual transmission of HIV.

Vertical transmission of HIV from an infected mother to her child may occur in utero, during labor, or through breastfeeding. In the absence of antiretroviral treatment (ART), HIV infects 25% to 30% of infants born to HIV-infected mothers. The rate of vertical transmission can be reduced to less than 2% by prenatal and perinatal treatment of the mother and postnatal treatment of the infant with effective antiretroviral drugs.

Before the nationwide implementation of a blood screening test in late 1985, infection by means of transfused blood or blood products accounted for almost 3% of AIDS cases in the United States. Since 1985, all blood products in North America have been screened for HIV antigens and antibodies to HIV. The risk of transfusion-acquired HIV infection in North America and western Europe is now exceedingly small, but not absent.

HIV infection may occur after accidental parenteral exposures among health care workers. After injury by an HIV-contaminated hollow needle, the risk of infection is approximately 0.3%. Observational data suggest that this risk can be reduced at least 10-fold by prompt postexposure prophylaxis.

For a deeper discussion of these topics, please see Chapter 387, "Prevention of Human Immunodeficiency Virus Infection," in Goldman-Cecil Medicine, *25th Edition.*

EPIDEMIOLOGY

HIV is a reportable condition in the United States. Individual states and the Centers for Disease Control and Prevention (CDC) together monitor incident cases of HIV, the number of persons known to be living with HIV, and the incidence of AIDS diagnosis. The CDC has established clear surveillance criteria for the diagnosis of AIDS, which include having a CD4+ T-helper lymphocyte count (CD4 count) lower than 200 cells/mm^3, having been diagnosed with any of a large number of OIs indicative of defects in cellular or humoral immunity, and having certain neoplasms or other conditions associated with severe immunodeficiency. With ART, the clinical significance of an AIDS diagnosis is more limited, although tracking the number of AIDS cases remains important epidemiologically as a marker of late diagnosis and limitations in access to care.

Since the early 1980s, HIV infection has become a worldwide pandemic. HIV continues to spread throughout all continents. Since the late 1990s, exceptionally rapid transmission has occurred throughout India, Southeast Asia, Southern Africa, the former Soviet Union, and some parts of Eastern Europe. Because of latency between HIV infection and the development of AIDS-associated illnesses, the clinically recognized epidemic of AIDS has lagged 6 to 8 years behind the spread of the virus into new populations. Worldwide, 1.7 million deaths were attributed to HIV in 2011, and an estimated 34 million people were living with HIV, including 3.3 million children. In 2011, an estimated 2.5 million people were newly infected with HIV—a 24% decrease from the 3.1 million estimated in 2001. In 2009, there were an estimated 370,000 new infections in children and between 42,000 and 60,000 maternal deaths. Persons from sub-Saharan Africa accounted for 70% of all new HIV infections globally. Morbidity and mortality from HIV and associated infections in many resource-poor communities has been high. As access to ART in low- and middle-income countries improves, morbidity and mortality from HIV should fall, leading to an increase in the prevalence of those living with HIV.

In the United States, HIV infection has increased rapidly among women in the last decade; in several rural areas of the Southeast, women accounted for more than one half of new cases in 2005. Over the last several years, there has also been a resurgence of HIV infection among young MSM. A disproportionate number of North American men and women infected by HIV are African American or Hispanic. Transmission by injection drug use has been a major factor in this imbalance, given that it has occurred most commonly in impoverished inner-city areas, where intravenous drug abuse is most prevalent. Since 2003, transmission by injection drug use has significantly declined in the United States, whereas heterosexual transmission has continued to increase. Recent studies in the United States have shown clearly that even when treatment is readily available, the fraction of persons who are retained in care and achieve virologic suppression remains as low as 25% (Fig. 101-1). There are increasing calls for coordinated interventions directed toward identifying persons with HIV, linking them to care, promoting retention, and supporting sustained adherence to antiviral therapy. This is termed the Seek, Test, Treat, and Retain (STTR) strategy for HIV control.

For a deeper discussion of these topics, please see Chapter 384, "Epidemiology of Human Immunodeficiency Virus Infection and Acquired Immunodeficiency Syndrome," in Goldman-Cecil Medicine, 25th Edition.

PATHOLOGY

The core of HIV contains two single-stranded copies of the viral RNA genome, together with the virus-encoded enzymes reverse transcriptase, protease, and integrase (Fig. 101-2). Surrounding the structural (p24 and p18) proteins is a lipid bilayer derived from the host cell, through which protrude the transmembrane (gp41) and surface (gp120) envelope glycoproteins. The HIV envelope glycoproteins have a high affinity for the CD4 molecule on the surface of T-helper lymphocytes and other cells of monocyte-macrophage lineage. After HIV binds to CD4, the envelope undergoes a conformational change that facilitates

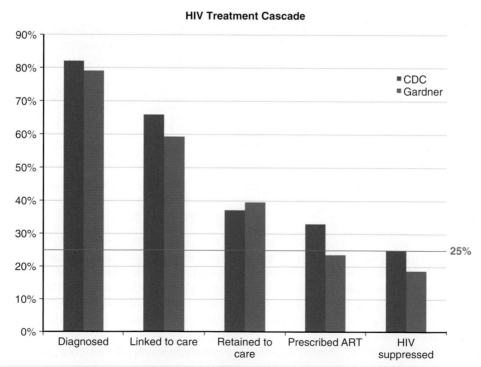

FIGURE 101-1 The HIV treatment cascade. Estimates show the progressive loss to follow-up as one moves from diagnosis to linkage to care, retention, and achievement of virologic suppression with antiretroviral therapy. (Data from HIV in the United States: the Stages of Care. CDC Fact Sheet, 2012. Available at http://www.cdc.gov/hiv/pdf/research_mmp_StagesofCare.pdf. Accessed November 3, 2014; and from Gardner EM, McLees MP, Steiner JF, et al: The spectrum of engagement in HIV care and its relevance to test-and-treat strategies for prevention of HIV infection, Clin Infect Dis 52:793-800, 2011.)

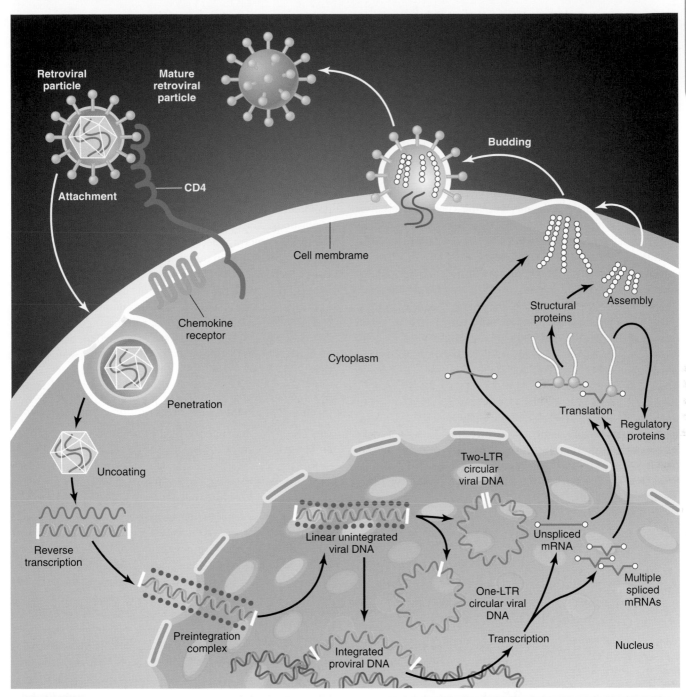

FIGURE 101-2 HIV viral replication. Key steps in the pathway targeted by antiretroviral therapy include membrane binding and fusion, reverse transcription, integration of proviral DNA, and protein synthesis. LTR, Long terminal repeat; mRNA, messenger RNA. (Modified from Furtado MR, Callaway DS, Phair JP, et al: Persistence of HIV-1 transcription in patients receiving potent antiretroviral therapy, N Engl J Med 340:1614–1622, 1999.)

binding to another cellular coreceptor (the most important of these are the chemokine receptors CCR5 and CXCR4). This second binding event promotes a major conformational change that causes approximation of the viral and cellular membranes; fusion of these membranes is mediated by insertion of the newly exposed fusion domain of the envelope gp41 into the host cell membrane.

As a result of these processes, the HIV nucleoprotein complex enters the cytoplasm, where the RNA viral genome undergoes reverse transcription by the virally encoded reverse transcriptase. The resulting double-stranded viral DNA enters the nucleus, where proper localization of the viral preintegration complex is mediated by host proteins, and integration of the DNA provirus into the host chromosome is catalyzed by the retroviral integrase. Latently infected resting memory CD4 lymphocytes serve as reservoirs of persistent infection for the life of the infected patient even with effective ART (see later discussion). However, the bulk of viral replication takes place in activated T cells, which are both more susceptible to HIV infection and more capable of supporting productive HIV replication.

When a CD4 lymphocyte is activated, expression of HIV messenger RNA (mRNA) is enhanced. Core proteins, viral enzymes, and envelope proteins are encoded by the *gag, pol,* and *env* genes of HIV, respectively. Recent data indicate that more than 100 host proteins, in addition to the viral proteins, may be important for viral replication. Viral particles are assembled at the cell membrane, each containing two copies of unspliced mRNA within the core as the viral genome, and virions then are released from the cell by budding. Productive viral replication is lytic to infected T cells. A number of other host cells, including macrophages and certain dendritic cells, are also infected by HIV, but viral replication does not appear to be lytic to these cells.

Following acute infection, high-level viral multiplication occurs in mucosal lymphoid tissues of the gut and in other lymphatic sites, and plasma HIV RNA levels (i.e., the plasma viral load [PVL]) often exceed 1 million copies per milliliter during the second to fourth weeks after infection. Almost all instances of acute HIV infection are caused by R5 tropic viruses, viruses that use the chemokine receptor CCR5 for cellular entry. During subsequent weeks, the PVL decreases, often rapidly. This decrease in viremia results largely from a partially effective immune response. After 6 to 12 months, the PVL typically stabilizes at a level denoted the viral *set point*, and it may remain at approximately that level for several years (Fig. 101-3). The set point, assessed as the PVL at 6 to 12 months after infection, is a significant predictor of the subsequent rate of progression of HIV disease but accounts for only half of the population variability in disease progression rates.

After recovery from the acute retroviral syndrome, the patient may feel entirely well for several years, but even in the asymptomatic infected individual, more than 100 billion new virions may be produced daily. Rapid production and turnover of circulating CD4 cells also occurs throughout the course of HIV infection,

and a progressive decline in circulating CD4 cells occurs in most individuals. As disease progresses, a more dramatic CD4 cell decline is observed, following a sharp rise in the PVL (see Fig. 101-3). Cell lysis associated with HIV replication accounts only partially for this progressive loss of CD4 cells. During the years of clinical latency, virions are present in large numbers in the follicular dendritic processes of the germinal centers of the lymph nodes, which undergo both hyperplasia and progressive fibrosis. As HIV disease progresses over several years, the lymphatic tissue atrophies and plasma viremia intensifies. In later-stage HIV disease, there is often persistent high-level viremia.

The decline in the number of CD4 cells is accompanied by profound functional impairment of the remaining lymphocyte populations. Anergy may develop early in HIV infection and eventually occurs in almost all persons with AIDS. T-helper lymphocyte proliferation in response to antigenic stimuli is dramatically impaired, T-cell cytotoxic responses are diminished, and natural killer cell activity against virus-infected cells is greatly impaired. Decrease in function as well as number of CD4 cells is central to the immune dysfunction, and this impairment partly underlies the failure of B-lymphocyte function, as measured by impaired capacity to synthesize antibody in response to new antigens.

For a deeper discussion of these topics, please see Chapter 385, "Immunopathogenesis of Human Immunodeficiency Virus Infection," in Goldman-Cecil Medicine, *25th Edition.*

CLINICAL PRESENTATION

Acute HIV Infection and the Acute Retroviral Syndrome

Up to 50% of HIV-infected persons report a mononucleosis-like syndrome (*acute retroviral syndrome*) occurring 2 to 6 weeks after initial infection. The symptoms may include fever, sore throat, lymph node enlargement, rash, arthralgias, and headache, and they usually persist for several days to 3 weeks (Table 101-1). The rash is typically maculopapular and short-lived and usually affects the trunk or face. Ten percent of infected individuals experience an acute, self-limited aseptic meningitis, which on lumbar puncture is characterized by cerebrospinal fluid (CSF) pleocytosis with detectable HIV in the CSF. The acute retroviral syndrome is often sufficiently severe that the patient seeks medical attention. It is critical to maintain a high index of suspicion for acute HIV retroviral syndrome because a very high plasma HIV RNA level during this period indicates a high likelihood of HIV transmission to sexual or needle-sharing partners, or from mother to infant.

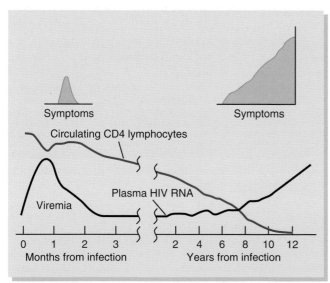

FIGURE 101-3 Natural history of HIV without antiretroviral therapy. Following acute infection, an initial burst of viral replication causes an immediate drop in the CD4 count. Partially effective cell-mediated immunity suppresses viral replication to a nadir level and allows for a rise in the CD4 count to a plateau that is less than a normal CD4 count. Left without treatment, the CD4 count declines somewhat proportionally to the nadir viral level until the patient begins to experience significant immune deficiency. At that time, the viral count may rise and the patient typically becomes symptomatic. Though this usually occurs within 8 to 10 years, considerable variability exists, with some patients progressing to AIDS within a few years and others without a significant decline in CD4 count after 20 years.

TABLE 101-1	SIGNS AND SYMPTOMS ASSOCIATED WITH HIV ACUTE RETROVIRAL SYNDROME	
SIGN OR SYMPTOM		**FREQUENCY (%)**
Fever		98
Lymph node enlargement		75
Sore throat		70
Myalgia or arthralgia		60
Rash		50
Headache		35

Spectrum of Disease Associated with HIV

Untreated HIV infection usually results in a slow, nonlinear progression to severe immunodeficiency. However, the progression of disease varies greatly among individuals. Within 10 years after infection, approximately 50% of untreated individuals will develop AIDS, 30% will have milder symptoms, and fewer than 20% will be entirely asymptomatic (see Fig. 101-3). Children and adolescents progress to AIDS at a slower rate than older persons; fewer than 30%, in the absence of ART, will develop AIDS within 10 years after HIV infection. The rate of progression of immunodeficiency is not influenced by the route of HIV transmission and, in the long term, does not appear to differ by gender, although typically women with HIV infection tend to experience more rapid disease progression with lower levels of HIV in plasma.

First Impacts of HIV

Clinically recognized lymph node enlargement occurs in 35% to 40% of asymptomatic HIV-infected persons but is not significantly associated with either rate of progression of immunodeficiency or subsequent development of lymphoma. During early HIV infection, thrombocytopenia, probably caused by autoimmune platelet destruction, is common. Most HIV-infected individuals remain asymptomatic until their CD4 count falls to less than 200 cells/mm^3, a fact that contributes to the late diagnosis of disease. In parts of the world where tuberculosis is hyperendemic, persons with HIV with CD4 counts greater than 200 cells/mm^3 are at high risk for development of tuberculosis.

Early Immunodeficiency

Patients with moderate immunodeficiency (CD4 counts between 200 and 500 cells/mm^3) exhibit diminished antibody response to protein and polysaccharide antigens, as well as decreased cell-mediated immune function. These functional impairments are manifested clinically by a threefold to fourfold increase in the incidence of bacteremic pneumonias caused by common pulmonary pathogens (especially *Streptococcus pneumoniae* and *Haemophilus influenzae*) and by a marked increase in incidence of active pulmonary tuberculosis in endemic areas (Table 101-2).

Mucocutaneous lesions may be the first manifestations of immune dysfunction. These include reactivation of varicellazoster (shingles), recurrent genital herpes simplex virus (HSV) infections, oral or vaginal candidiasis, and oral hairy leukoplakia (see later discussion). The earliest clinical manifestation of HIV infection in women may be frequent recurrence of *Candida* vaginitis in the absence of predisposing factors. Recurrent large, painful genital, perianal, or perineal ulcers caused by HSV type 2, are more frequent in women than in men. HIV-infected women show an increased prevalence of high-grade squamous intraepithelial lesions on Papanicolaou (Pap) smear. Both men and women may show similarly increased rates of dysplasia or neoplasia on rectal Pap smear.

Opportunistic Infections

With advanced immunodeficiency, indicated by CD4 counts lower than 200 cells/mm, patients are at high risk for development of OIs (see Table 101-2). Before the availability of effective

TABLE 101-2 PROGRESSIVE COMPLICATIONS OF HIV INFECTION BY CD4 COUNT

CD4 COUNT (CELLS/MM^3)	OPPORTUNISTIC INFECTION OR NEOPLASM
>500	Herpes zoster
	Tuberculosis
200-500	Oral hairy leukoplakia
	Candida pharyngitis (thrush)
	Kaposi's sarcoma, mucocutaneous
	Bacterial pneumonia, recurrent
	Cervical or anal neoplasia
100-200	*Pneumocystis jirovecii* pneumonia
	Histoplasmosis capsulatum infection, disseminated
	Kaposi's sarcoma, visceral
	Progressive multifocal leukoencephalopathy
	Lymphoma, non-Hodgkin's
<100	*Candida* esophagitis
	Cytomegalovirus retinitis
	Mycobacterium avium-intercellulare
	Toxoplasma gondii encephalitis
	Cryptosporidium parvum enteritis
	Cryptococcus neoformans meningitis
	Herpes simplex virus, chronic, ulcerative
	Cytomegalovirus esophagitis or colitis
	Primary central nervous system lymphoma

antiretroviral drugs and use of prophylactic antibiotics, 60% of HIV-infected North American men developed *Pneumocystis* pneumonia (PCP). Incidence of *Toxoplasma* encephalitis before the availability of ART in the United States was estimated to be as high as 3.9 per 100 patient-years. CD4 counts lower than 50 cells/mm^3 indicate profound immunosuppression and, in the absence of effective ART, are associated with a high mortality rate within the subsequent 12 to 24 months.

Cytomegalovirus (CMV) retinitis, which can lead rapidly to blindness, and disseminated *Mycobacterium avium-intracellulare* (MAI) infection occur frequently in the absence of therapy. They respond adequately to specific therapy only if it is accompanied by effective control of viral replication.

DIAGNOSIS AND DIFFERENTIAL DIAGNOSIS

Identification of persons with HIV and support of linkage to effective care are critical public health priorities. Recent studies have demonstrated reduced transmission of HIV associated with ART. Despite the acknowledged priority of early diagnosis, the median CD4 count at diagnosis has remained fairly constant in the range of 175 cells/mm^3, indicating persistent delays in testing and treatment.

The CDC and the U.S. Preventive Services Task Force recommend that all persons between the ages of 13 and 64 years be tested for HIV once, with repeat testing and testing outside of this age group based on assessed risk for infection and reinfection. All pregnant women should routinely be offered HIV testing. The CDC, to meet this goal, further recommends that HIV testing be considered a part of routine medical care, without any requirement for written consent or formal pretest and posttest counseling. Pretest discussion is important to ensure that patients appreciate that they are being tested and that treatment is available if they are found to be HIV positive.

Standard testing for HIV infection begins with detection of antibodies to HIV in serum or in oral fluid. Positive antibody tests are confirmed by assessing for the presence of at least two viral proteins through Western blot assays. These techniques are highly sensitive in detecting HIV antibody, but individuals who have been infected recently may be antibody negative. During a window period, typically 1 to 2 weeks, infected persons have detectable HIV RNA and core p24 antigen in their plasma. If the initial enzyme-linked immunosorbent assay (ELISA) result is negative in a person recently exposed to HIV, repeat ELISA at 6 weeks and 3 months are indicated. In a person who is at high risk for HIV exposure, an indeterminate Western blot reaction pattern often represents early seroconversion; in such cases, a positive plasma HIV RNA concentration (i.e., >10,000 copies/mL) indicates acute HIV infection.

Rapid point-of-care testing methods play an important role in HIV testing in many clinical and community settings. These rapid test kits can provide results within 30 minutes, but they require confirmation by antibody-based tests. Fourth-generation assays for HIV have recently been developed; they combine tests for antibodies and viral proteins in a single assay.

⬤ TREATMENT

Initial Counseling and Ambulatory Evaluation

Once HIV infection is recognized, the physician should discuss, in an unhurried manner, the clinical course and treatment of HIV infection and the use of immunologic and virologic studies (e.g., CD4 counts, PVL assays) to guide therapy. The physician should then emphasize that, with effective currently available ART, HIV disease progression can be prevented indefinitely. Stigma related to HIV remains an important concern and a key barrier to engagement in care. Addressing this as part of post-test counseling and intake to care is key to retention in care for persons newly diagnosed.

Prevention of further transmission through unprotected sex or sharing of needles must be discussed at the first visit and periodically thereafter. It is important to emphasize that these high-risk activities place not only the other person but also the patient at risk because they may lead to transmission of new and potentially drug-resistant HIV strains to the patient.

The initial evaluation should include both an HIV-oriented review of systems and a complete physical examination. In particular, the skin must be examined for HIV-associated rashes and Kaposi's sarcoma. Examination of the oral cavity may reveal thrush, gingivitis, hairy leukoplakia, superficial ulcers caused by HSV, aphthous ulcers, or lesions characteristic of Kaposi's sarcoma. In persons with very advanced disease, the optic fundi may have hemorrhagic lesions characteristic of CMV retinitis. Lymph node enlargement, hepatomegaly, splenomegaly, and any genital lesions should all be carefully noted. Neurologic examination for both peripheral neuropathy and decreased global cognition deserves close attention.

Laboratory Monitoring

The CD4 count and the PVL should be measured at the first visit, and the patient should be shown the results. Graphic illustrations of the interaction between PVL and CD4 can be useful to increase patient understanding. HIV genotyping to assess for drug resistance should also be performed (see later discussion).

The PVL is a key measure of treatment adherence and is repeated at intervals, initially every 3 to 4 months. For patients with suppressed virus who are stable on ART, current guidelines allow for PVL monitoring at 6-month intervals. For those who are not taking or have only recently started ART and have a CD4 count lower than 200 cells/mm^3, CD4 monitoring is typically repeated every 3 to 4 months along with the PVL monitoring. Once a patient is stable on treatment, with suppressed virus (<200 copies) and CD4 counts higher than 200 cells/mL, the value of CD4 monitoring is less clear, and guidelines allow for extending the monitoring interval to yearly.

Screening for Associated Infections
Tuberculosis

Purified protein derivative (PPD) testing should be performed early in the course of HIV infection. Induration of 5 mm or more should be considered positive. Any patient with a positive PPD test result should be evaluated for the presence of active tuberculosis; if no active disease is present, the patient should receive 9 months of prophylaxis with isoniazid or combination drug therapy for a shorter period (see Chapter 92). If active tuberculosis is identified, multidrug therapy should be initiated after careful consideration of possible interactions with antiretroviral medications.

Sexually Transmitted Diseases

Serologic testing for syphilis should be followed by prompt treatment if the patient is confirmed to be positive. Syphilis infections are common within many populations highly impacted by HIV, and co-infection with syphilis increases the risk of transmission of HIV to others. Regular screening is recommended.

Hepatitis

Liver disease is an important cause of morbidity and mortality for persons with HIV. Screening for hepatitis A, B, and C at baseline is recommended, and those not immune to hepatitis A or B should receive immunization. Hepatitis C is highly prevalent among persons who acquired HIV from injection drug use, and increasing numbers of cases of sexual transmission of hepatitis C among MSM with HIV are being described. Given the lack of an effective vaccine for hepatitis C, regular screening is recommended for persons with ongoing risk of exposure.

Other Infections

Screening for antibodies to *Toxoplasma gondii* should be considered for persons with low CD4 counts who are potentially in need of prophylaxis. Persons from endemic areas may be screened for histoplasmosis and coccidiomycosis and considered for prophylaxis if positive.

Immunization

Antibody responses to polysaccharides are better among patients with higher CD4 counts. The optimal timing of immunization is uncertain. For persons with low CD4 counts, most physicians provide initial immunization and reimmunization for certain vaccines after immune reconstitution occurs. Live vaccines should be avoided in persons with CD4 counts lower than 200 cells/mm^3.

Pneumococcus

All persons with HIV should receive a dose of PCV14 (Prevnar13), followed by a dose of PPV23 (Pneumovax) at least 8 weeks later. If previously vaccinated with PPV23, the patients should receive PCV13 at least 1 year after PPV23. Patients should have a CD4 cell count greater than or equal to 200/microliter. A second PPV23 dose is recommended 5 years after the first PPV23.

Influenza Virus

Persons with HIV have excess morbidity and mortality associated with influenza and its complications. They should receive seasonal influenza vaccination yearly.

Herpes Zoster

Reactivation of herpes zoster viral infection, resulting in shingles, is a significant cause of morbidity among persons with HIV disease. Because the singles vaccine is a live attenuated vaccine, additional studies were conducted to assess the safety of this vaccine in persons with HIV. Although there were no reports of excess risk in these trials, final review is still pending, and the vaccine does not carry an indication from the U.S. Food and Drug Administration (FDA) for use in persons with HIV.

Human Papillomavirus

The CDC recommends use of the human papillomavirus (HPV) vaccine in boys or girls at age 11 or 12 regardless of HIV status, in MSM, and in persons with immune compromise, including those with HIV, up to the age of 26 if not previously vaccinated.

Hepatitis A and B Viruses

Persons with HIV should be assessed by serology for prior exposure to hepatitis A and B. Those found to be susceptible to infection should receive immunization.

Other Health Screening

Cervical Cancer

HIV-infected women should have two Pap smears 6 months apart; if the they are both normal, Pap smears should be repeated once a year. Persons with cellular atypia on a Pap smear should be referred for colposcopy.

Rectal Cancer

HPV is associated with risk of cervical cancer in women and rectal cancer in both men and women. Although some advocate for regular screening, clear guidelines have not yet been developed for rectal cancer.

⬤ ANTIRETROVIRAL THERAPY

The goal of ART is to ensure that HIV-infected persons can lead symptom-free, productive lives. Currently available therapy makes achieving this goal possible in almost all individuals with early, asymptomatic HIV infection who have not acquired major resistance mutations as a result of earlier, suboptimal ART. The current recommendations in the United States are that therapy should be offered to all persons infected with HIV. In much of the world, thresholds for treatment based on CD4 count are still in effect, reflecting in part the allocation of limited resources to those who are likely to experience the most immediate benefits.

Antiretroviral Drug Regimens

Evidence-based guidelines for ART have been developed by the U.S. Department of Health and Human Services. The most commonly used antiretroviral agents are presented in Table 101-3. The current preferred and alternative regimens for first-line treatment are summarized in Table 101-4. With rare exceptions, all recommended regimens consist of at least three fully active drugs. Increasingly, coformulation of medications has allowed the combination of multiple drugs to be taken in single tablets. Three single-tablet daily regimens are currently approved for the treatment of HIV, and more are in development. The reduced pill burden can significantly improve adherence to treatment and minimize the risk of treatment failure. The World Health Organization publishes guidelines for HIV treatment programs in resource-limited settings. They delineate first- and second-line therapies selected based on efficacy, cost, and availability.

Clinical trials assessing the benefits of early treatment have demonstrated the many health impacts of HIV that occur even before the onset of demonstrable immune deficiency. Persons who undergo structured treatment interruptions and delay treatment until their CD4 count drops to less than 500 cells/mm^3 experience higher rates of cardiovascular disease, kidney disease, liver disease, and neurocognitive disorders. Although the risk increases with declining CD4 count and worsening immune function, early effects can in some cases be demonstrated before the onset of marked immunodeficiency. The demonstrated benefit of initiating ART before the CD4 count drops to less than 500 cells/mm^3 was primarily attributable to these noninfectious complications of HIV disease.

TABLE 101-3	MOST FREQUENTLY USED ANTIRETROVIRAL MEDICATIONS BY CLASS	
DRUG CLASS		**MEDICATION**
Nucleoside/nucleotide reverse transcriptase inhibitors (NRTIs)		Tenofovir
		Abacavir
		Lamivudine
		Emtricitabine
		Zidovudine
		Didanosine*
		Stavudine*
Non-nucleoside reverse transcriptase inhibitors (NNRTIs)		Efavirenz
		Nevirapine
		Etravirine
		Rilpivirine
Protease inhibitors†		Atazanavir
		Darunavir
		Fosamprenavir
		Lopinavir
		Saquinavir
Integrase inhibitors		Raltegravir
		Elvitegravir
		Dolutegravir
CCR5 inhibitor		Maraviroc
Fusion inhibitor		Fuseon

*Infrequently used due to toxicity.
†Most protease inhibitors require a second medication to boost the levels of the drug by inhibiting drug metabolism. Ritonavir at a dose of 100 mg daily is most commonly used. Cobicistat was recently approved for use as part of a fixed-dose combination, and its potential for expansion is currently being studied.

TABLE 101-4 PREFERRED AND ALTERNATIVE REGIMENS FOR FIRST-LINE ANTIRETROVIRAL THERAPY ACCORDING TO DHHS GUIDELINES

PILL BURDEN	COMBINATION*	LIMITATIONS†
PREFERRED REGIMENS		
Single pill	Atripla (tenofovir, emtricitabine, efavirenz)	CrCl >50, teratogenicity
2 pills once daily	Truvada (tenofovir, emtricitabine) + dolutegravir	CrCl >50
3 pills once daily	Truvada (tenofovir, emtricitabine) + atazanavir + ritonavir	CrCl >50, cirrhosis Child Pugh class A
3 pills once daily	Truvada (tenofovir, emtricitabine) + darunavir + ritonavir	CrCl >50, cirrhosis Child Pugh class A
BID regimen: 1 pill daily, 1 pill twice daily	Truvada (tenofovir, emtricitabine) + raltegravir	CrCl >50
ALTERNATIVE REGIMENS		
Single pill	Complera (tenofovir, emtricitabine, rilpivirine)	CrCl >50,† PPI contraindicated
Single pill	Stribild (tenofovir, emtricitabine, elvitegravir, cobicistat)	CrCl >70,† cirrhosis Child Pugh class A
Single pill	Triumeq (abacavir lamivudine dolutegravir)	HLAB5701 negative, CrCl >50
3 pills once daily	Epzicom (abacavir, lamivudine) + atazanavir + ritonavir	HLA-B5701 negative,† CrCl >50,† cirrhosis Child Pugh score <5
3 pills once daily	Epzicom (abacavir, lamivudine) + rilpivirine	HLA-B5701 negative, CrCl >50,† PPI contraindicated, cirrhosis Child Pugh score <5
BID regimen: 1 pill daily, 1 pill twice daily	Truvada (tenofovir, emtricitabine) OR Epzicom (abacavir, lamivudine) + etravirine	CrCl >50,† HLA-B5701 negative (abacavir), cirrhosis Child Pugh score <5 (abacavir)
4 pills once daily	Truvada (tenofovir, emtricitabine) OR Epzicom (abacavir, lamivudine) + fosamprenavir + ritonavir	CrCl >50,† HLA-B5701 negative (abacavir), cirrhosis Child Pugh score <5 (abacavir)
5 pills once daily	Truvada (tenofovir, emtricitabine) OR Epzicom (abacavir, lamivudine) + lopinavir/ritonavir	CrCl >50,† HLA-B5701 negative (abacavir), cirrhosis Child Pugh score <5 (abacavir)

CrCl, Creatinine clearance (measured in mL/min/17.3 m²); DHHS, U.S. Department of Health and Human Services; HLA, human leukocyte antigen; PPI, proton pump inhibitors.

*New antiretroviral medications as well as new formulations of medications are approved frequently. For the most up-to-date listing of preferred and alternative regimens, refer to the DHHS Guidelines for the Use of Antiretroviral Medications (see Recommended Readings).

†Tenofovir, lamivudine, and emtricitabine all require dose adjustment when the CrCl drops to <50, preventing the use of fixed-dose combinations.

‡HLA-B5701 is a genetic marker indicating risk for a hypersensitivity reaction to abacavir. Screening is indicated before the medication is started, and abacavir should not be used if the marker is present.

As persons with HIV live longer on ART, more typical diseases associated with aging become the focus of care. It can be challenging to distinguish what additive effects HIV may have to the risks associated with these conditions, particularly if comorbid substance use, smoking, and other risk factors are highly prevalent. As HIV is controlled with treatment, recognizing these risks and focusing on providing the best quality primary care will be critical to helping ensure that patients with HIV live full and healthy lives.

Baseline Resistance Testing and Development of Drug Resistance

Inconsistent intake of ART can lead to the development of HIV strains resistant to antiviral medications. At least 16% of new infections (one in six) contain mutations affecting susceptibility to one or more antiretroviral medications. For this reason, measurement of baseline resistance is recommended before ART is initiated. Close monitoring of persons with inconsistent adherence is critical. Some resistance mutations, particularly M184V, which confers resistance to lamivudine and emtricitabine, have been observed to develop with as little as a few weeks of inconsistent treatment.

When to Change Therapy

When an effective antiretroviral regimen is initiated in an asymptomatic patient with no previous ART, the PVL should decrease sharply, usually by 10-fold in 4 weeks and to an undetectable level (<50 copies/mL) within 16 to 24 weeks. If reduction of this magnitude is not achieved, the physician should assess with the patient whether adherence has been adequate. If adherence has been nearly complete (>95%), the physician and patient should consider retesting for resistance mutations and changing to another effective regimen. Minority viral subpopulations carrying resistance mutations can rapidly overtake the sensitive virus once the selective pressure exerted by the medications. These subpopulations may become detectable only while on treatment.

If a given regimen achieves a reduction of PVL below detectable limits and continuing adherence is achieved, the patient can anticipate effective viral suppression for many years and perhaps indefinitely. Small elevations in PVL on a single determination are usually not significant. One may consult the International AIDS Society—USA resistance guidelines, which are regularly updated (www.iasusa.org/guidelines/index.html). If an antiretroviral drug must be stopped for any reason, it is important to stop temporarily all antiretroviral drugs. Alternatively, a completely new effective regimen may be initiated to sustain complete virologic suppression.

Prophylaxis against Opportunistic Infections

During the first 15 years of the HIV pandemic, the most effective medical interventions for HIV infection were prophylactic measures against OIs. The greatest success was in preventing PCP in individuals with CD4 counts lower than 200 cells/mm³; routine use of prophylaxis resulted in a greater than fourfold decrease (from 60% to <15%) in the frequency of PCP as the initial OI in North American men with HIV infection.

Specific antimicrobial prophylaxis (Table 101-5) is also effective for prevention of *T. gondii* encephalitis in patients with anti-*Toxoplasma* antibodies and CD4 counts lower than 100 cells/mm³ and for prevention of active tuberculosis in patients with positive tuberculin skin test results at any CD4 level. Prophylaxis against disseminated MAI infection is recommended at lower CD4 counts (<50 cells/mm³). Prophylaxis against CMV retinitis

TABLE 101-5 RECOMMENDATIONS FOR PRIMARY AND SECONDARY PROPHYLAXIS FOR PERSONS WITH HIV INFECTION

PATHOGEN	CD4 THRESHOLD (CELLS/MM³)	ADDITIONAL INDICATION	PREFERRED	ALTERNATE
PRIMARY PROPHYLAXIS				
Pneumocystis jirovecii	<200		TMP-SMX SS or DS tablet daily	Dapsone, atovaquone
Toxoplasmosis	<100	Anti-*Toxoplasma* IgG detectable	TMP-SMX SS or DS tablet daily	Pyrimethamine-dapsone and pyrimethamine-sulfadoxine
Mycobacterium avium-intercellulare	<50		Azithromycin 1200 mg weekly	Clarithryomicin 500 mg bid
SECONDARY PROPHYLAXIS				
Mycobacterium tuberculosis	Any	History of exposure to TB confirmed by PPD test or IGRA	Isoniazid depending on sensitivities	Rifampin, isoniazid+rifapentene
Cryptococcosis	<200	History of cryptococcal meningitis or cryptococcal antigen positive	Fluconazole	NA
Coccidomycosis	<150	Antihistoplasma IgG detectable or history of coccidiomycosis	Fluconazole or itraconazole	NA
Histoplasmosis	<150	Anticoccidomyces IgG detectable	Itraconazole	NA
Cytomegalovirus (CMV)	<50	Ocular or extraocular findings consistent with CMV infection	Ganciclovir 3 g/day	NA

DS, Double-strength; IgG, immunoglobulin G; IGRA, interferon-γ release assay; NA, not applicable; PPD, purified protein derivative; SS, single-strength; TB, tuberculosis; TMP-SMX, trimethoprim-sulfamethoxazole.

is moderately effective in patients with CD4 counts lower than 50 cells/mm³, but prompt initiation of effective ART with early treatment of active disease is the currently preferred strategy. Prophylaxis is very effective against recurrent HSV type 2 infection (with acyclovir, famciclovir, or valacyclovir) and against recurrent *Candida* esophagitis (with fluconazole) but should generally be reserved for those patients with recurrent symptomatic disease. Persons from areas where histoplasmosis or coccidiomycosis is endemic should be considered for primary prophylaxis (with fluconazole) if they have detectable antibodies and their CD4 count is lower than 150 cells/mm³. No guidelines exist for cryptococcal antigen screening.

After the CD4 count rises on ART, withdrawal of prophylaxis against specific OIs is reasonable. After initiation of effective ART and two consecutive CD4 counts at least 3 months apart that exceed 100 cells/mm³, prophylaxis against CMV and MAI may be withdrawn safely; likewise, if the two consecutive counts exceed 200 cells/mm³, prophylaxis against PCP and *T. gondii* may be withdrawn.

For a deeper discussion of these topics, please see Chapter 389, "Prophylaxis and Management of Complications of HIV/AIDS: Infectious, Neoplastic, and Metabolic," in Goldman-Cecil Medicine, 25th Edition.

MANAGEMENT OF SPECIFIC CLINICAL MANIFESTATIONS OF HIV INFECTION

Clinical manifestations of HIV include not only OIs associated with immunodeficiency but also HIV-associated malignancies and other noninfectious complications of HIV. The manifestations of HIV vary significantly in time of onset (see Table 101-2). Before the onset of infectious complications, some HIV-associated cancers such as non-Hodgkin's lymphoma and HPV-associated carcinomas can develop. Infectious complications such tuberculosis can manifest at any CD4 count and occur with increased frequency in association with HIV. Infectious complications that occur with higher CD4 counts respond to routine

therapy for the specific infection (e.g., appropriate β-lactam antibiotic for pneumococcal pneumonia, standard multidrug therapy for pulmonary tuberculosis), whereas OIs occurring with CD4 counts lower than 200 cells/mm³ require chronic suppressive therapy after treatment of the acute infection (e.g., PCP pneumonia, CMV retinitis, *Cryptococcus neoformans* meningitis).

For a deeper discussion of these topics, please see Chapter 389, "Prophylaxis and Management of Complications of HIV/AIDS: Infectious, Neoplastic, and Metabolic," in Goldman-Cecil Medicine, 25th Edition.

Initial Assessment of HIV-Associated Illnesses

Assessment of a patient's immunologic status is key in the evaluation of persons with HIV when there is a new presenting illness or complaint. If the patient is on ART and has had a recent CD4 assessment, that count is the best indicator of their status. Persons without recent CD4 testing should be presumed to be immunocompromised unless there is clear information to suggest the contrary. If there has been a treatment interruption, the CD4 count should return to its prior nadir after about 12 months of interruption. During an acute illness, the absolute CD4 count may decline; therefore, a measured CD4 count during an acute illness can underestimate an individual's true immune function.

Constitutional Symptoms

Nonspecific symptoms may be the initial clinical manifestations of severe immunodeficiency. Patients may develop unexplained fever, night sweats, anorexia, weight loss, or diarrhea. These symptoms may last for weeks or months before the development of identifiable OIs in patients who do not receive effective ART. Most persistent fevers occurring late in the course of HIV infection reflect a definable OI. The most common cause of unexplained fever and anemia in patients with CD4 counts lower than 50 cells/mm³ is disseminated MAI infection. This may be diagnosed by bone marrow biopsy, but blood cultures in

Mycobacterium-selective media are usually positive. Treatment usually results in resolution of fever and weight gain. Aggressive non-Hodgkin's lymphoma may cause unexplained fever and weight loss, a rapidly enlarging spleen, or asymmetrical lymph node enlargement.

Wasting and Changes in Body Morphology

Cachexia may be prominent in advanced HIV disease. In some instances, the wasting is caused by an intercurrent infectious process. Heightened production of tumor necrosis factor may contribute to fever, cachexia, and hypertriglyceridemia in advanced HIV disease. If orthostatic hypotension occurs, especially if it is associated with hyperkalemia, the possibility of adrenal insufficiency, which rarely can result from CMV adrenalitis, should be investigated. Most patients with AIDS-associated cachexia gain weight and achieve a sense of well-being after initiation of effective ART. If the cachexia is refractory, weight gain may be enhanced by administration of recombinant growth hormone, nonmethylated androgens, or megestrol, but definitive indications for these therapies have not been established.

Older antiviral agents, particularly nucleoside/nucleotide reverse transcriptase inhibitors (e.g., didanosine, stavudine) and the early protease inhibitors, were associated with alterations in fat distribution known as lipodystrophy and lipoatrophy. Patients with long-term exposure to these medications may develop a loss of fat in the face and on the extremities. At the same time, they develop prominent central obesity including a buffalo hump and marked abdominal obesity. These changes typically persist even after the medication is discontinued and are associated with increased risk of cardiovascular disease.

Cutaneous Disease

Cutaneous infections ultimately occur in most patients with untreated HIV infection. Persons with HIV experience both higher rates of more typical skin infections (e.g., folliculitis, cellulitis) and OIs such as disseminated herpes zoster or HSV, bacillary angiomatosis, and fungal infections. Most of these diseases respond to specific therapy. Noninfectious skin manifestations include exacerbation of underlying psoriasis, seborrhea dermatitis, and eosinophilic folliculitis. Skin lesions can equally be associated with some disseminated infectious complications or malignancies. If a patient has unexplained constitutional symptoms, a thorough skin examination may provide important findings to support a diagnosis.

For a deeper discussion of these topics, please see Chapter 392, "Skin Manifestations in Patients with Human Immunodeficiency Virus Infection," in Goldman-Cecil Medicine, 25th Edition.

Oral Disease

Oral *Candida* stomatitis (thrush) is often the earliest recognized OI. Early thrush may be entirely asymptomatic; as the infection becomes more extensive, it causes pain on eating. The characteristic cheesy white exudate on the mucous membranes can easily be scraped off, and the underlying mucosa may be normal or inflamed.

Xerostomia is common among patients with HIV and is often underappreciated. It can be a significant contributor to poor dentition and gingivitis, which can contribute to other adverse health consequences for the patient.

Severe gingivitis can be a significant problem in patients with AIDS, leading to local and systemic infection as well as loss of teeth.

Oral ulcers may be caused by HSV, but often they represent aphthous lesions of uncertain cause. Small oral aphthous ulcers may respond to topical corticosteroids, whereas large oral or esophageal ulcers require oral administration of thalidomide or corticosteroids. It is important to obtain cultures for HSV and CMV to exclude a viral origin before initiating corticosteroid or thalidomide therapy. Thalidomide should not be used in women of childbearing age because of its teratogenic effect.

Oral hairy leukoplakia is a white, lichenified, plaque-like lesion most commonly seen on the lateral surfaces of the tongue that is probably caused by Epstein-Barr virus (EBV). It is painless, may remit and relapse spontaneously, and almost always responds to effective ART.

Kaposi's sarcoma has a predilection for the oral cavity and skin. Oral lesions may be purple, red, or blue and may be raised or flat. Usually painless, these lesions cause symptoms when they enlarge, bleed, or ulcerate (see later discussion).

Esophageal Disease

Symptomatic esophageal disease seldom occurs with CD4 counts greater than 100 cells/mm^3. Pain on swallowing and substernal burning are common and most often indicate *Candida* esophagitis, particularly when oral thrush is present. Diagnostic esophagoscopy with biopsy, cytology, and culture should be performed if symptoms do not rapidly respond (within 3 to 5 days) to antifungal therapy.

If esophagoscopy shows ulcerative lesions, they are usually caused by CMV (50%), aphthae (45%), or HSV (5%). Because each of these lesions is responsive to appropriate therapy, definitive etiologic diagnosis is essential. CMV esophageal ulcers respond well to intravenous ganciclovir or foscarnet therapy for 2 to 3 weeks or until resolution is confirmed endoscopically. Esophageal ulcerations caused by HSV usually respond well to intravenous acyclovir.

For a deeper discussion of these topics, please see Chapter 390, "Gastrointestinal Manifestations of HIV and AIDS," in Goldman-Cecil Medicine, 25th Edition.

Pulmonary Diseases

Pulmonary infections are common in persons living with HIV and range from nonspecific interstitial pneumonitis to life-threatening pneumonias (Table 101-6). HIV-infected persons have a threefold to fourfold increased risk of bacterial pneumonia, usually caused by encapsulated bacteria, including *S. pneumoniae* and *H. influenzae*. The increased risk begins with modest degrees of immunodeficiency (CD4 counts of 200 to 500 cells/mm^3). The onset is often abrupt, and the response to prompt initiation of therapy is usually good; however, delay in appropriate antimicrobial therapy may result in a fulminant downhill course. For those with CD4 counts greater than 200 cells/mm^3,

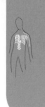

TABLE 101-6 PULMONARY COMPLICATIONS OF HIV INFECTION: DIFFERENTIAL DIAGNOSIS AND TREATMENT

CONDITION	CHARACTERISTICS	CHEST RADIOGRAPH	DIAGNOSIS	TREATMENT
Pneumocystis jirovecii pneumonia	Subacute onset, dry cough, dyspnea	Interstitial infiltrate most common	BAL or induced sputum for organism by stain	TMP-SMX, pentamidine or atovaquone or primaquine + clindamycin
Bacterial (*Pneumococcus*, *Haemophilus* most common)	Acute onset, productive cough, fever, chest pain	Lobar or localized infiltrate	Sputum Gram stain and culture, blood culture	Cefuroxime or alternative antibiotics
Tuberculosis	Chronic cough, weight loss, fever	Localized infiltrate, lymphadenopathy	Sputum acid-fast stain and mycobacterial culture	Isoniazid, rifampin, pyrazinamide, ethambutol
Kaposi's sarcoma	Asymptomatic or mild cough	Pulmonary nodules, pleural effusion	Open lung biopsy	Chemotherapy

BAL, Bronchoalveolar lavage; TMP-SMX, trimethoprim-sulfamethoxole.

therapy should follow existing guidelines for empirical treatment of pneumonia (see Chapter 92). Pursuit of diagnostic studies that can support a definitive diagnosis is important, particularly if the patient's CD4 count is near 200 cells/mm^3 or the features or clinical course of pneumonia are atypical.

As with acute bacterial pneumonia, active pulmonary tuberculosis may develop at a time when the CD4 count remains well above 200 cells/mm^3 (see Table 101-6). Chest radiographs in HIV-infected patients may show features of primary tuberculosis, including hilar adenopathy, lower or middle lobe infiltrates, miliary pattern, or pleural effusions, as well as classic patterns of reactivation. Extrapulmonary *Mycobacterium tuberculosis* infection also occurs with increased frequency in patients with advanced immunodeficiency. Both pulmonary and extrapulmonary tuberculosis respond promptly to the use of four antituberculosis drugs.

Pneumonia caused by PCP remains a common life-threatening infection in persons with AIDS. Patients frequently report a gradual onset of nonproductive cough, fever, and shortness of breath with exertion; a productive cough suggests another process. A substernal "catch" with inspiration is common and is suggestive of PCP. In contrast to the acute onset of PCP in other immunocompromised patients, AIDS patients with PCP may have pulmonary symptoms for weeks before consulting a physician. Arterial hypoxemia is typical and rapidly worsens with slight exertion. Oxygen desaturation with exercise, as measured by pulse oximetry, can suggest the diagnosis. The chest radiograph often shows a subtle interstitial pattern but may be entirely normal. The presence of pleural effusions suggests a cause other than PCP.

If PCP is suspected clinically, therapy should be started immediately; treatment for several days does not interfere with the ability to make a specific diagnosis. Confirmation of PCP is essential; delay in establishing a correct diagnosis of another treatable condition may be lethal. An induced sputum sample can sometimes confirm the diagnosis, but most patients require bronchoalveolar lavage, which is adequate to diagnose PCP in more than 95% of patients. Treatment with high-dose trimethoprim-sulfamethoxazole (TMP-SMX) for 3 weeks is effective therapy (see Table 101-6). Patients with PCP and arterial hypoxemia (oxygen tension 75 mm H$_2$O on breathing of room air) benefit from the administration of corticosteroids (40 mg of prednisone twice daily), with tapering of the drug over a 3-week period.

For a deeper discussion of these topics, please see Chapter 391, "Pulmonary Manifestations of Human Immunodeficiency Virus and Acquired Immunodeficiency Syndrome," in Goldman-Cecil Medicine, 25th Edition.

Disseminated histoplasmosis and coccidioidomycosis occur with much greater frequency in persons with HIV infection. Either fungal infection can cause nodular infiltrates or a miliary pattern on chest radiography. Histoplasmosis usually involves bone marrow as well as skin, and examination of the bone marrow often shows the organism. Standard treatment of disseminated mycoses in AIDS patients is high-dose liposomal amphotericin. Because relapse is common, oral azole therapy (fluconazole for coccidioidomycosis, itraconazole for histoplasmosis) must be continued even after resolution of signs and symptoms. For patients treated for histoplasmosis, secondary prophylaxis may be discontinued after 1 year of therapy, provided that the CD4 count is at least 150 cells/mm^3, blood cultures are negative, and the HIV serum *Histoplasma* antigen titers are low. Patients treated for systemic, meningeal, or diffuse pulmonary coccidioidomycosis have a greater risk of relapse and probably should continue suppressive therapy indefinitely.

For a deeper discussion of these topics, please see Chapter 332, "Histoplasmosis," and Chapter 333, "Coccidioidomycosis," in Goldman-Cecil Medicine, 25th Edition.

Cardiovascular Disease

As the population with HIV ages, cardiovascular disease is becoming an increasingly important cause of morbidity and mortality. Persons with HIV experience higher rates of cardiovascular disease. Even with suppressive ART, some increased risk remains, likely attributable in part to risk factors such as persistent residual immunologic activation, high rates of tobacco use, hyperlipidemia, metabolic syndrome, diabetes, or chronic kidney disease.

Pericarditis and Pericardial Effusions

Pericardial effusions are a well recognized complication of HIV disease and may be result from infections or malignancy (see Chapter 10). In many cases, no specific cause is identified and effusions resolve without specific treatment. In places where tuberculosis is endemic, constrictive pericarditis secondary to tuberculosis is an important consideration. In addition, pericarditis and effusions secondary to acute infections and both non-Hodgkin's lymphoma and Kaposi's sarcoma may occur.

Congestive Heart Failure

In addition to ischemic cardiomyopathy, persons with HIV may develop congestive heart failure due to an HIV-associated dilated cardiomyopathy and infectious myocarditis.

Gastrointestinal Diseases

HIV affects the gastrointestinal tract early in infection, with profound depletion of memory CD4 T cells in gut-associated lymphoid tissue within the first few weeks of infection. However, symptomatic disease of the gut is unusual in the early stage of infection.

With advanced immunodeficiency (CD4 count <50 cells/mm^3), gastrointestinal disease manifesting as dysphagia, diarrhea, or colitis is common. Each process may contribute to inadequate nutrition, compounding the weight loss associated with advanced HIV disease. Nausea and vomiting are often related to medications. If symptoms of nausea and vomiting do not respond to empirical therapy with histamine-2 (H$_2$) antagonists or antiemetics, more extensive gastrointestinal evaluation is indicated.

For a deeper discussion of these topics, please see Chapter 390, "Gastrointestinal Manifestations of HIV and AIDS," in Goldman-Cecil Medicine, 25th Edition.

Diarrhea

Diarrhea occurs, at least intermittently, in many persons with advanced immunodeficiency and may be caused by a variety of microorganisms (Table 101-7) as well as by certain antiretroviral and other medications. In many instances, no clear cause is found. Stool specimens should be cultured for the common bacterial pathogens. *Salmonella, Campylobacter,* and *Yersinia* species are frequent causes; the diarrhea usually responds to standard antimicrobial therapy. Patients may also have recurrent episodes of diarrhea associated with *Clostridium difficile* toxin; this probably reflects the frequent use of broad-spectrum antibiotics.

In cases of persistent diarrhea, a fresh stool specimen should be examined for parasites, using a modified acid-fast stain for *Cryptosporidium parvum,* microsporidia, and *Isospora belli,* the most common enteric protozoal infections in AIDS patients. Microsporidial infection may require biopsy with electron microscopy for diagnosis. Although cryptosporidiosis can be self-limited, massive diarrhea (up to 10 L/day) may occur.

Isosporiasis responds to oral TMP-SMX, and several microsporidial species respond to albendazole. Symptoms of both cryptosporidiosis and isosporiasis resolve with effective ART.

If stool diagnostic studies are negative and diarrhea persists, patients should undergo endoscopy (see Chapter 34). Biopsy of the duodenum or small bowel may show histologic evidence of cryptosporidial, microsporidial, MAI, or CMV infection. Biopsy of the colon may be indicate HSV proctitis, CMV colitis, or MAI infection. For patients with refractory diarrhea, symptomatic treatment may improve the quality of life.

Hepatitis

Abnormalities on liver function testing are common in HIV disease and often are nonspecific. Elevations of serum alanine aminotransferase and aspartate aminotransferase often represent chronic active hepatitis B or C but may reflect hepatic inflammation caused by medications, including TMP-SMX and antiretroviral agents. Alcohol use is highly prevalent among persons with HIV and may contribute, as can use of other drugs such as MDMA ("ecstasy").

Marked elevations in serum alkaline phosphatase levels may reflect infiltrative disease of the liver (e.g., MAI, CMV, tuberculosis, tumor) but also may occur in patients with acalculous cholecystitis, cryptosporidiosis, or AIDS-associated sclerosing cholangitis. Syphilitic hepatitis has been well described and may be characterized by a more pronounced elevation in alkaline phosphatase.

Viral hepatitis, particularly hepatitis C, is an important cause of morbidity and mortality among persons with HIV. More than 80% of persons with HIV who have a history of injection drug use are co-infected with hepatitis C, and the risk of progression to end-stage liver disease is greater for those with HIV hepatitis C co-infection. Occult hepatitis infections (antibody negative but with detectable RNA or DNA) have been described for both hepatitis B and hepatitis C, particularly in the context of advanced immunodeficiency. The response to hepatitis C therapy has historically been significantly worse for those co-infected with HIV, but this may be less true with the new generation of direct-acting agents for treatment of hepatitis C.

Genital Diseases

Primary and secondary syphilis remains a concern among persons with HIV, particularly MSM. Early neurologic

TABLE 101-7 AIDS-ASSOCIATED DIARRHEA: DIFFERENTIAL DIAGNOSIS AND TREATMENT

CAUSE	CHARACTERISTICS	DIAGNOSIS	TREATMENT
Cryptosporidium parvum	Variable from high-frequency to large-volume diarrhea	Acid-fast stain of stool	Nitazoxanide ART
Clostridium difficile	Abdominal pain, fever common	*C. difficile* toxin in stool or endoscopy	Metronidazole or vancomycin
Cytomegalovirus	Small bowel movements with blood or mucus (colitis)	Colonoscopy and biopsy	Ganciclovir
Mycobacterium avium-intracellulare	Abdominal pain, fever, retroperitoneal lymphadenopathy	Blood culture or endoscopy with biopsy	Multidrug regimen including clarithromycin, ethambutol
Salmonella or *Campylobacter*	Sometimes with blood or mucus in bowel movements (colitis)	Stool culture	Fluoroquinolone (check sensitivities)
Microsporidia	Watery diarrhea	Calcofluor white or trichrome staining of stool; electron microscopy of biopsy material	Albendazole, ART
Isospora belli	Watery diarrhea	Acid-fast stain of stool	TMP-SMX

ART, Antiretroviral therapy; TMP-SMX, trimethoprim-sulfamethoxazole.

involvement has been well described, and a thorough history and examination to exclude neurologic complications is important in the evaluation of incident cases. Treatment regimens for persons with HIV, based on stage of presentation, are the same as for those without HIV. However, persons with HIV take longer to achieve a full reduction in rapid plasma reagin (RPR) titer and may continue to have low-level demonstrable RPR titers even after successful treatment.

Recurrent genital ulcers are most often caused by HSV. Viral culture or specific immunofluorescence of ulcer scrapings confirms the diagnosis.

Candida species, most often *Candida albicans*, can cause an irritating vulvovaginitis in women with HIV infection as well as in healthy HIV-seronegative women. A potassium hydroxide preparation of the cheesy white exudate reveals budding yeast or pseudohyphae.

Bacterial vaginosis and trichomoniasis are common, and although both typically respond to specific treatment (e.g., metronidazole), bacterial vaginosis often recurs.

For more information on sexually transmitted diseases, see Chapter 100.

Nervous System Diseases

Nervous system complications ultimately occur in most persons with untreated HIV infection. They range from mild cognitive disturbances or peripheral neuropathy to severe dementia and life-threatening central nervous system (CNS) infections. As with other lentiviruses, HIV enters microglial cells of the CNS early in the course of infection. Both direct neuronal destruction and effects of viral proteins on neuronal cell function may contribute to nervous system disease in AIDS.

Cognitive Dysfunction

Intellectual impairment rarely occurs early in HIV infection, but subtle changes (e.g., decreased learning accuracy and learning speed) may be present in patients with only moderate immunodeficiency. AIDS dementia complex (ADC) often begins insidiously and usually progresses over months to years. ADC is characterized by poor concentration, diminished memory, slowing of thought processes, motor dysfunction, and occasionally behavioral abnormalities characterized by social withdrawal and apathy. Symptoms of clinical depression overlap with many of the characteristics of early ADC and must be considered carefully in differential diagnosis and therapy.

Computed tomography (CT) of the head in ADC reveals only atrophy, with enlarged sulci and ventricles, but these findings do not reliably predict cognitive deficits. The CSF is most often normal on examination. Motor abnormalities may include a progressive gait ataxia. As the disease progresses, patients may develop focal neurologic complications characterized by spastic weakness of the lower extremities and incontinence secondary to vacuolar myelopathy.

Focal Lesions of the Central Nervous System

A large variety of neurologic problems can complicate the later stages of HIV infection. A neuroanatomic classification of these manifestations is presented in Table 101-8. Some of the more frequent or treatable problems are discussed here and in the next section.

Several opportunistic complications of HIV infection produce focal CNS lesions. Patients with focal neurologic signs, seizures of new onset, or recent onset of rapidly progressive cognitive impairment should undergo magnetic resonance imaging (MRI) or CT of the brain. Toxoplasmosis, CNS lymphoma, and progressive multifocal leukoencephalopathy (PML) are the most common causes of CNS focal lesions in this setting (Table 101-9).

In the absence of ART, *T. gondii* encephalitis occurs in up to one third of HIV-infected patients who have serologic evidence of *T. gondii* infection, but is rare in individuals who have no such antibodies. Patients often have progressive headache and focal neurologic abnormalities, usually associated with fever. CT with contrast usually shows multiple ring-enhancing lesions. MRI is a more sensitive technique and often shows multiple small lesions

TABLE 101-8 NEUROANATOMIC CLASSIFICATION OF NEUROLOGIC COMPLICATIONS OF HIV INFECTION

CATEGORY	CONDITION
Meningitis and headache	Aseptic meningitis
	Cryptococcal meningitis
	Tuberculous meningitis
	Neurosyphilis
Diffuse brain diseases	
With preservation of consciousness	AIDS dementia complex
	Neurosyphilis
With decreased arousal	*Toxoplasma* encephalitis
	Cytomegalovirus encephalitis
Focal brain diseases	Tuberculous brain abscess
	Primary central nervous system lymphoma
	Progressive multifocal leukoencephalopathy
	Cerebral toxoplasmosis
	Neurosyphilis
Myelopathies	Subacute or chronic progressive vacuolar myelopathy
	Cytomegalovirus myelopathy
Peripheral neuropathies	Predominantly sensory polyneuropathy
	Toxic neuropathies
	Autonomic neuropathy
	Cytomegalovirus polyradiculopathy
Myopathies	Noninflammatory myopathy
	Zidovudine myopathy

TABLE 101-9 NEUROLOGIC COMPLICATIONS OF HIV INFECTION

	CLINICAL ONSET			NEURORADIOLOGIC FEATURES		
CONDITION	*Time*	*Alertness*	*Fever*	*Number of Lesions*	*Characteristics of Lesions*	*Location of Lesions*
Cerebral toxoplasmosis	Days	Reduced	Common	Usually multiple	Spherical, ring enhancing	Basal ganglia, cortex
Primary CNS lymphoma	Days to weeks	Variable	Absent	One or few	Irregular, weakly ring enhancing	Periventricular
PML	Weeks to months	Variable	Absent	Often multiple	Multiple lesions visible on MRI	White matter

MRI, Magnetic resonance imaging; PML, progressive multifocal lymphoma.

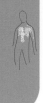

not apparent on CT. Management includes initiation of empirical therapy with pyrimethamine, sulfadiazine, and folinic acid. Brain biopsy should be reserved for patients with neurologic deterioration, those with no serum antibodies to *T. gondii* who have neuroimaging findings atypical for toxoplasmosis, those with discordant results between PCR of the CSF for EBV and thallium-enhanced single-photon emission computed tomography (SPECT) scans, and those whose lesions do not respond after 10 to 14 days of antiprotozoal treatment. After the initial response, patients must remain on chronic suppressive therapy until a sustained rise in CD4 count (>200 cells/mm^3) is achieved with effective ART.

Primary CNS lymphoma complicates advanced HIV infection in 3% to 6% of cases and is almost invariably associated with detectable EBV DNA in the CSF. Lesions may be single or multiple and are often weakly ring enhancing. Irradiation often provides remission, which may be sustained as immune function is restored by effective ART.

PML is a demyelinating disease caused by a papovavirus (JC virus). Presenting signs and symptoms may include progressive dementia, visual impairment, seizures, and hemiparesis. MRI usually shows multiple lesions predominantly involving the white matter. These lesions are usually less visible on CT than on MRI and are not ring enhancing, helping to distinguish PML from other mass lesions of the CNS. There is no effective specific treatment for PML; the disease often, but not always, regresses in response to effective ART.

For a deeper discussion of these topics, please see Chapter 394, "Neurologic Complications of Human Immunodeficiency Virus Infection," in Goldman-Cecil Medicine, *25th Edition.*

Central Nervous System Diseases without Prominent Focal Signs

Evaluation of the HIV-infected patient with fever and headache is difficult because of the often subtle manifestations of serious CNS lesions in immunocompromised patients. Management of bacterial meningitis is the same as for non-immunocompromised patients. Meningeal diseases in HIV-infected patients often fall into the broad categories of aseptic meningitis, chronic meningitis, and meningoencephalitis.

For a deeper discussion of these topics, please see Chapter 394, "Neurologic Complications of Human Immunodeficiency Virus Infection," in Goldman-Cecil Medicine, *25th Edition.*

Aseptic Meningitis

Patients with aseptic meningitis, which can be a manifestation of the acute retroviral syndrome, complain most often of headache. Their sensorium is generally intact, and findings on neurologic examination are normal. In the individual with established HIV infection, aseptic meningitis may result from several potentially treatable causes.

Chronic Meningitis

Patients with chronic meningitis characteristically have headache, fever, difficulty in concentrating, or changes in sensorium.

CSF examination shows low glucose concentration, elevated protein level, and mild to modest lymphocytic pleocytosis.

Cryptococcal meningitis is the most common type. The presence of cryptococcal antigen in serum or CSF or a positive CSF India ink preparation establishes the diagnosis. Treatment with amphotericin B for at least 2 weeks, followed by high-dose fluconazole, is usually effective. Serial lumbar punctures, with removal of CSF to decrease intracranial pressure, may be necessary in the early management of cryptococcal meningitis.

M. tuberculosis can cause subacute or chronic meningitis in the HIV-infected patient. Antituberculosis therapy should be considered in the setting of chronic meningitis if the cryptococcal antigen test is negative.

Coccidioides immitis or *Histoplasma capsulatum* may cause subacute or chronic meningitis in patients who reside in, or have a history of travel to, endemic regions (i.e., the U.S. southwestern deserts and the Ohio and Mississippi River drainage areas, respectively).

Neurosyphilis in patients with HIV is more common and may manifest earlier after infection. Patients may experience headaches and dizziness in the early phases, which can be followed by personality change, ischemic strokes, ataxia, seizures, and paralysis.

Meningoencephalitis

Patients with meningoencephalitis manifest alterations in sensorium varying from mild lethargy to coma. Patients are usually febrile, and neurologic examination often shows evidence of diffuse CNS involvement. CT or MRI may show only nonspecific abnormalities, whereas electroencephalography often is consistent with diffuse disease of the brain.

CMV encephalitis is rare and difficult to diagnose; it occurs only in the setting of CD4 counts lower than 50 cells/mm^3. Patients may demonstrate confusion, cranial nerve abnormalities, or long tract signs. CSF findings may resemble those of bacterial meningitis, with a modest polymorphonuclear leukocyte pleocytosis and depressed CSF glucose levels. CT scanning or MRI may reveal periventricular abnormalities. Many patients have associated CMV retinitis. PCR detection of CMV DNA in CSF appears to be a sensitive and specific method for diagnosis of CMV encephalitis and polyradiculopathy (persistent back pain and weakness of the lower extremities).

Meningoencephalitis caused by HSV is unusual in HIV infection.

HIV-Associated Malignancies

The incidence of AIDS-associated malignancies has declined significantly since the advent of effective ART. Among HIV-infected MSM, the frequency of Kaposi's sarcoma fell from 40% at the outset of the epidemic to less than 15% in 1999. Human herpesvirus 8 is the causative agent. In many instances, lesions resolve after institution of effective ART. Systemic chemotherapy can cause remission in many patients with symptomatic visceral disease. Kaposi's sarcoma remains common in many parts of the developing world.

Non-Hodgkin's lymphomas (largely B cell, with small noncleaved or immunoblastic histology) occur 150 to 250 times more often in HIV-infected persons than in the general population. Up to 40% of AIDS-related systemic lymphomas, and almost all of those in a primary CNS location, are related to EBV. Extranodal presentation of these tumors is the rule, and there is a high frequency of gastrointestinal or intracranial presentation. Chemotherapy for systemic disease or radiation therapy for CNS disease usually provides a clinical response, which may be maintained if it is accompanied by effective ART.

Other malignancies, including Hodgkin's disease, have an increased incidence in patients with untreated HIV infection. Now that more treated persons are surviving , an increasing incidence of a variety of non-AIDS–defining malignancies is being observed. Among these, increased rates of anal cancer, non–small cell lung cancer, Hodgkin's disease, and liver cancer (related to hepatitis viruses) have been associated with HIV.

For a deeper discussion of these topics, please see Chapter 394, "Neurologic Complications of Human Immunodeficiency Virus Infection," in Goldman-Cecil Medicine, 25th Edition.

Renal Disorders

Renal insufficiency in patients with HIV may be a consequence of nephrotoxic drug administration, long-term use of certain antiviral agents (particularly tenofovir), substance use (e.g., heroin), or HIV-associated nephropathy (HIVAN). HIVAN typically improves with ART. In some cases, renal biopsy is indicated to establish a diagnosis, particularly if rapid decline in glomerular function is observed. In the United States, HIVAN is seen almost exclusively in African Americans and usually manifests as heavy proteinuria and progressive renal insufficiency. Without treatment, most patients develop end-stage renal disease within several months. Treatment is primarily with combination antiretroviral drugs.

Musculoskeletal and Rheumatologic Disorders

Musculoskeletal complaints are common among patients with HIV, and distinguishing acute complications of HIV from more indolent degenerative joint disease or recurrent muscle strain is important. Septic arthritis is a particular concern in persons who use injection drugs or have hemophilia.

Reiter's syndrome has been associated with HIV, and patients with HIV may experience a more severe or more prolonged course. Flares related to immune reconstitution have been described; they frequently respond quickly to doxycycline.

Declining CD4 counts in persons with psoriasis is associated with flares of both cutaneous disease and psoriatic arthritis. Standard therapy for both can now be supplemented if necessary with disease-modifying antirheumatic drugs.

Both lupus and rheumatoid arthritis, when present, may be relatively quiescent in persons with low CD4 counts. When treatment for HIV is initiated and the CD4 count rises, these persons may experience flares of their underlying connective tissue disease.

Avascular necrosis of the hip has been well described in persons with HIV, including those on ART. MRI may be necessary to confirm the diagnosis, and surgery is the mainstay of treatment.

Muscle weakness, if localized, may be indicative of myelopathy-neuropathy. If weakness is proximal or is associated with myalgia and tenderness, myopathy should be suspected. ART is the primary treatment for HIV-associated myopathy. Myopathy may rarely be caused by zidovudine toxicity.

Immune Reconstitution Inflammatory Syndrome

Persons with low CD4 counts at the start of treatment who experience a rapid rise in CD4 count on treatment may be at risk for development of what is termed the immune reconstitution inflammatory syndrome (IRIS). The syndrome results from the development of a pronounced immune response to a previously tolerated antigen, usually an infection. The specific symptoms depend on the pathogen or antigen and the involved area of the body. Entities commonly associated with IRIS include *M. tuberculosis* and other mycobacteria, *Pneumocystis* pneumonia, cryptococcal infections, herpesviruses, and hepatitis B or C virus. Treatment is supportive, although in severe cases, for example IRIS associated with meningitis or inflammation of the lungs leading to respiratory compromise, corticosteroids may be used to reduce inflammation and alleviate the symptoms.

For a deeper discussion of these topics, please see Chapter 395, "Immune Reconstitution Inflammatory Syndrome in HIV/AIDS," in Goldman-Cecil Medicine, 25th Edition.

PREVENTION OF HUMAN IMMUNODEFICIENCY VIRUS INFECTION

Three approaches—behavioral modification, treatment of sexually transmitted diseases, and ART—have had a major impact on HIV transmission. All of these activities are supported by expanded testing and improved linkage to care.

In several communities at increased risk for HIV (e.g., homosexually active men in the United States and western Europe, young adults in Uganda and Thailand), adoption of safer sexual practices, specifically the use of condoms during sexual activity, has been associated with a decrease in incidence of HIV infection. Sustaining these behavioral changes over long periods is challenging and requires behavioral reinforcement. Several recent controlled trials have demonstrated that male circumcision can decrease the risk of acquiring HIV infection by more than half.

Increasingly, ART is becoming a key goal of prevention programs. Antiretroviral treatment of HIV-infected pregnant women and their infants in the peripartum period has decreased maternal-child transmission from 25% to less than 5% in North America. If a pregnant woman maintains viral suppression during pregnancy and during breast-feeding, the risk of transmission to her infant is less than 1%.

Prophylactic use of ART has been shown to be effective for postexposure prophylaxis after occupational exposures to HIV and after unprotected sexual exposures. Recently, studies have shown the benefit of preexposure prophylaxis in preventing transmission of HIV among high-risk MSM, and the fixed-dose combination of tenofovir and emtricitabine has received an FDA indication for this use. The most compelling reinforcement of the importance of ART for prevention was a large multisite clinical trial of discordant couples that demonstrated a reduction of almost 100% in transmission to partners.

The development of an effective vaccine is the target of active research. Early clinical trials of vaccine candidates are ongoing but to date have demonstrated, at most, limited protection. Induction of brisk T-cell responses to HIV antigens has neither protected against HIV acquisition nor decreased the magnitude of HIV replication among vaccinated subjects. A legitimate goal for vaccines, the induction of antibody responses that can broadly inhibit or neutralize the infectivity of diverse HIV strains, has so far eluded vaccine developers.

For a deeper discussion of these topics, please see Chapter 387, "Prevention of Human Immunodeficiency Virus Infection," in Goldman-Cecil Medicine, 25th Edition.

PROGNOSIS

With ART, survival in many cohorts approaching that of age-matched controls. Because of the high rates of co-infection with viral hepatitis in many populations, liver disease remains a significant cause of morbidity and mortality, accounting for a significant portion of the early mortality still associated with HIV. In endemic areas, tuberculosis is a similar cause of early mortality among persons with HIV infection. Even with effective ART, persons with HIV still experience some excess risk of cardiovascular disease as well some non–AIDS-defining malignancies such as non-Hodgkin's lymphoma. The key message for persons living with HIV is that if they stay in care and maintain adherence to ART, they can expect to live a relatively normal life.

SUGGESTED READINGS

Aberg JA, et al: Primary care guidelines for the management of persons infected with HIV: 2013 update by the HIV Medicine Assocation of the Infectious Diseases Society of America, Clin Infect Dis 58:1–10, 2014.

Castel AD, Magnus M, Greenberg AE: Pre-exposure prophylaxis for human immunodeficiency virus, Infect Dis Clin North Am 28(4):563–583, 2014.

Center for Disease Control and Prevention, Project Workgroup: Recommendations for HIV prevention with adults and adolescents with HIV in the United States, 2014. Available at: http://stacks.cdc.gov/view/cdc/26062. Accessed December 2014.

Cohen MS, Chen YQ, McCauley M, et al: Prevention of HIV-1 infection with early antiretroviral therapy, N Engl J Med 365(6):493–505, 2011.

Gardner EM, McLees MP, Steiner JF, et al: The spectrum of engagement in HIV care and its relevance to test-and-treat strategies for prevention of HIV infection, Clin Infect Dis 52:793–800, 2011.

International Antiviral Society–USA: Practice Guidelines, Topics in Antiviral Medicine, Available at: https://www.iasusa.org/guidelines. Accessed December 2014.

Panel on Antiretroviral Guidelines for Adults and Adolescents: Guidelines for the use of antiretroviral agents in HIV-1-infected adults and adolescents, Department of Health and Human Services, Available at: http://aidsinfo.nih.gov/contentfiles/lvguidelines/AdultandAdolescentGL.pdf. Accessed December 2014.

Rajasuriar R, Wright E, Lewin SR: Impact of antiretroviral therapy (ART) timing on chronic immune activation/inflammation and end-organ damage, Curr Opin HIV AIDS 10:35–42, 2015.

Smith CJ, Ryom L, Weber R, et al: Trends in underlying causes of death in people with HIV from 1999 to 2011 (D:A:D): a multicohort collaboration, Lancet 384:241–248, 2014.

World Health Organization: Global health observatory (GHO), HIV/AIDS, Available at: http://www.who.int/gho/hiv/en/. Accessed December 2014.

102

Infections in the Immunocompromised Host

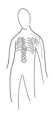

Staci A. Fischer

● INTRODUCTION

With the development of increasingly complex and potent treatments for autoimmune, malignant, and chronic end-organ diseases, the spectrum of opportunistic infections continues to grow. Infections are the primary complication of many conditions causing immune deficiency, from congenital syndromes manifesting early in life to malignancy occurring in the elderly (Table 102-1). Success in challenging fields such as transplantation depends on preventing, quickly diagnosing, and effectively treating infections.

● DEFINITION AND EPIDEMIOLOGY

The approach to the immunocompromised patient with possible infection should begin with an assessment of the arms of the immune system affected by the patient's underlying diseases and treatments.

Neutropenia

Neutropenia is a combined absolute neutrophil and band count of less than 500 cells/mm^3. It is common after chemotherapy and may be prolonged in patients with hematologic malignancies and after hematopoietic stem cell transplantation (HSCT) (see Table 102-1). In these settings, patients may develop infections from their own microbial flora or from ubiquitous environmental organisms (Table 102-2). Because some chemotherapy agents cause mucositis and other breaches of protective barriers, bacterial infections predominate in this setting, most commonly as oral mucosal, skin, soft tissue, and sinopulmonary infections. Intravenous catheter-related infections and translocation of bacteria from the gastrointestinal tract may also occur. Because *Pseudomonas* species are associated with the highest mortality rate in this setting, empirical therapy for fever in the neutropenic patient should always include antibacterial therapy to cover this organism.

Neutropenic patients are at risk for invasive fungal infection, particularly in the setting of prolonged neutropenia. *Candida* species infections are common. Sinopulmonary infections caused by *Aspergillus* and the molds of the Mucorales order are associated with considerable morbidity and mortality.

Nonchemotherapy drugs may also cause neutropenia, with a less predictable risk of infection. Responsible agents include β-lactam antibiotics, carbapenems, amphotericin B, antipsychotics, antiepileptics (e.g., carbamazepine, valproic acid, phenytoin), hydralazine, sulfonamides, and nonsteroidal anti-inflammatory agents.

The risk of infection in patients with neutropenia is inversely related to their absolute neutrophil count (i.e., neutrophils plus bands); the lower the neutrophil count and the more prolonged the period of neutropenia, the higher the risk of infection. Because chemotherapeutic agents attack native cells with rapid turnover rates, mucosae in the oropharyngeal and gastrointestinal tracts are frequently interrupted, allowing commensal and colonizing bacteria (e.g., viridans streptococci, *Escherichia coli*, *Klebsiella, Enterococcus, Pseudomonas*), viruses (most commonly herpes simplex virus), and fungi (especially *Candida*) to escape and replicate. In patients on prophylactic antimicrobials while neutropenic, resistant organisms can break through, resulting in bloodstream infections and sepsis with multidrug-resistant organisms.

Cell-Mediated Immunity Defects

Cell-mediated immunity defects may result from infection with certain viruses (notably human immunodeficiency virus [HIV], hepatitis C virus, and cytomegalovirus [CMV]) or from immunosuppressive agents routinely used in solid organ transplantation and in the prophylaxis and treatment of graft-versus-host disease (GVHD) in allogeneic HSCT recipients (see Table 102-1). Cell-mediated immunity defects complicate T-cell lymphoma and primary immunosuppressive conditions such as common variable immune deficiency disease (CVID). CVID, the most common primary immunodeficiency, manifests with recurrent bacterial infections (notably pneumonia and bronchitis), usually between the ages of 20 and 50 years. Patients with T-cell dysfunction or deficiency are at risk for opportunistic infections such as *Listeria monocytogenes*, CMV, *Pneumocystis jirovecii*, and invasive fungal infections (see Table 102-2).

L. monocytogenes is the most common cause of bacterial meningitis in transplant recipients. CMV causes latent infection in T cells, and the seropositive patient with late-stage HIV infection or a transplant may reactivate CMV, causing viremia or focal infection of the gastrointestinal tract, liver, lungs, or retina. Seronegative recipients of seropositive organs are at high risk for developing donor-transmitted CMV infection, which can result in long-term allograft dysfunction in addition to symptomatic infection.

P. jirovecii, a fungal pathogen, causes hypoxemia and interstitial pulmonary infiltrates in those with advanced HIV infection or T-cell dysfunction from transplantation or GVHD. Reactivation, acquisition, or donor-derived transmission of endemic fungal infections, including *Blastomyces, Coccidioides*, and *Histoplasma*, can occur. Environmental fungi, including *Aspergillus*, Mucorales

TABLE 102-1 CONDITIONS CAUSING IMMUNE DEFICIENCY

NEUTROPHILS AND PHAGOCYTES

Neutropenia
- Congenital syndromes
- Drug-related neutropenia (e.g., chemotherapy, antimicrobial agents, antipsychotics, anticonvulsants)
- Autoimmune neutropenia
- Cyclic neutropenia
- Myelodysplastic syndrome
- Fanconi's anemia
- Aplastic anemia
- Myeloproliferative disorders (e.g., acute myeloid leukemia)

Neutrophil dysfunction
- Chédiak-Higashi syndrome
- Hyperimmunoglobulin E syndrome (Job's syndrome)
- Chronic granulomatous disease
- Leukocyte adhesion deficiency
- Immunosuppressive medications (e.g., mycophenolate, azathioprine)
- Warts, hypogammaglobulinemia, infections, and myelokathexis (WHIM)
- Viral infections (e.g., human immunodeficiency virus, human herpesvirus 6)

CELL-MEDIATED IMMUNITY

Immunosuppressive agents for transplantation
- Cyclosporine, tacrolimus, sirolimus
- Daclizumab, basiliximab
- Mycophenolate, azathioprine
- Antilymphocyte therapies (e.g., Thymoglobulin, alemtuzumab)

Corticosteroids

Cytotoxic drugs (e.g., cyclophosphamide)

Fludarabine

Anti–tumor necrosis factor-α agents (e.g., adalimumab, etanercept, infliximab, certolizumab, golimumab)

Graft-versus-host disease (GVHD)

DiGeorge syndrome (i.e., thymic hypoplasia)

Severe combined immunodeficiency (SCID)

Ataxia-telangiectasia

Wiskott-Aldrich syndrome

End-stage renal disease

Malnutrition

Human immunodeficiency virus (HIV) infection

T-cell lymphoma

Idiopathic CD4+ lymphopenia

HUMORAL IMMUNITY

Common variable immune deficiency (CVID)

Splenectomy, splenic aplasia (e.g., sickle cell disease)

Nephrotic syndrome

Protein-losing enteropathy

Multiple myeloma

B-cell lymphoma

Chronic lymphocytic leukemia

Waldenstrom's macroglobulinemia

Severe combined immune deficiency

Ataxia-telangiectasia

Wiskott-Aldrich syndrome

Hyperimmunoglobulin M syndrome

Selective IgA deficiency

X-linked agammaglobulinemia

Immunosuppressive therapies (e.g., cyclophosphamide, azathioprine, mycophenolate)

Medications (e.g., rituximab, azathioprine, sulfasalazine, gold, cyclosporine, carbamazepine, valproic acid, phenytoin, alemtuzumab, chloroquine)

Hypogammaglobulinemia complicating solid organ and hematopoietic stem cell transplantation

COMPLEMENT DEFICIENCY

C2 deficiency

Mannose-binding lectin deficiency

C3 deficiency

Factor H deficiency

Factor I deficiency

Terminal pathway (C5-C9) deficiency

TABLE 102-2 ORGANISMS ASSOCIATED WITH IMMUNE DYSFUNCTION

NEUTROPHILS AND PHAGOCYTES

Staphylococcus auereus
Pseudomonas aeruginosa
Enterobacteriaceae
Streptococcus mitis, viridans streptococci
Aspergillus species
Candida species
Mucorales order fungi (cause mucormycosis)
Fusarium species
Herpes simplex virus (HSV)

Cryptococcus neoformans
Aspergillus species
Candida species
Pneumocystis jirovecii
Strongyloides stercoralis
Cryptosporidium species
Toxoplasma gondii
Leishmania species

HUMORAL IMMUNITY

Mycoplasma species
Streptococcus pneumoniae
Haemophilus influenzae
Campylobacter jejuni
Ureaplasma urealyticum
Chlamydia pneumoniae
Salmonella species
Giardia lamblia
Echovirus
Varicella-zoster virus

CELL-MEDIATED IMMUNITY

Herpesviruses (HSV, varicella-zoster virus, Epstein-Barr virus, human herpesviruses 6 and 8)
JC virus
BK virus (especially in kidney transplants)
Human papilloma virus (HPV)
Respiratory viruses (e.g., influenza, metapneumovirus, parainfluenza, respiratory syncytial virus)
Listeria monocytogenes
Nocardia species
Salmonella species
Mycobacterium species (*M. avium complex* in human immunodeficiency virus infection)

COMPLEMENT DEFICIENCY

Recurrent sinopulmonary infections
Streptococcus pneumoniae
Haemophilus influenzae
Neisseria gonorrhoeae
Neisseria meningitidis

order fungi (which cause mucormycosis) and other molds, may be inhaled, causing sinopulmonary infections in neutropenic hosts. Infection may be complicated by dissemination to sites such as the skin and brain.

Bacterial infection with organisms such as *Nocardia* and *Legionella* and parasitic or protozoal infections such as *Strongyloides stercoralis* and *Babesia* are common in patients with cell-mediated immune defects.

Humoral Immunity

Humoral immunity is critical to control infection by encapsulated bacteria such as *Neisseria meningitidis*, *Streptococcus pneumoniae*, and *Haemophilus influenzae*. Patients with hypogammaglobulinemia, protein-losing conditions such as enteropathy or nephrotic syndrome, splenectomy, or chronic lymphocytic leukemia have significant defects in humoral immunity, predisposing them to infection with these organisms (see Table 102-1). Transplant recipients on immunosuppressive therapy for many years may develop hypogammaglobulinemia, predisposing them to similar infections. The use of agents such as rituximab, a monoclonal antibody against CD20, in malignancy and transplantation may result in significant B-cell defects and infection with encapsulated bacteria.

Complement Deficiency

Patients deficient in complement factors have a higher risk of autoimmune disease and can develop recurrent infections. Sinopulmonary infections, particularly from *S. pneumoniae* and *H. influenzae*, are common. Patients with deficiencies of terminal pathway components (C5 to C9) develop recurrent infections with *N. meningitidis* and *Neisseria gonorrhoeae*.

Although this chapter focuses on systemic immune deficiencies, it is important to consider local processes that increase the risk of focal infections in certain hosts. For example, the cystic fibrosis or chronic obstructive pulmonary disease patient with multiple bouts of pneumonia may develop localized bronchiectasis, in which normal mucociliary clearance mechanisms are inadequate to control and prevent infection. These areas are prone to recurrent bacterial infections, particularly with *Pseudomonas*. Similarly, the patient with lymphedema of a limb lacks the benefit of lymphatic drainage of early infections and is predisposed to recurrent cellulitis of the affected extremity.

PATHOLOGY

Infections in the immunocompromised host are often caused by organisms of low virulence that are able to cause infection due to impaired or absent normal defense mechanisms. Diagnosis of infection may be hampered by the small number of organisms required to cause disease and by the lack of inflammation associated with immunosuppressive conditions and therapies.

CLINICAL PRESENTATION

The clinical presentation of immunocompromised hosts with infection may be different from that seen in the immunocompetent patient. In the transplant population, typical signs and symptoms of infection such as fever, erythema, and leukocytosis may be absent as a result of the effect of immunosuppressive medications. Infections that are normally limited in scope may become disseminated in the immunocompromised host. For example, pyelonephritis involving the renal allograft may be complicated by bacteremia and acute kidney injury, both of which are uncommon in normal hosts.

Assessing the immunocompromised host with possible infection involves performing a detailed physical examination, including close inspection of the oral and periodontal tissues, perianal area, and skin. Even minor changes (e.g., faint erythematous rash, gum line erythema) may point to the source of a fever. Symptoms and signs of infection such as fever may not exist. On review of systems, subtle findings such as chills and sweats may be the only sign of an opportunistic infection. A classic finding is perianal or rectal pain without swelling or erythema, indicating a perirectal abscess in neutropenic patients. Laboratory clues to infection such as leukocytosis in the patient with systemic bacterial infection or eosinophilia in the patient with disseminated *Strongyloides* infection may be absent as a result of immunosuppressive therapy.

In many cases, the initial presentation of congenital or acquired immune deficiency states is the development of unusual or recurrent infections, and recognition of the immune defects associated with the infections can guide the diagnostic work-up. For example, the nonimmunosuppressed patient with *P. jirovecii* infection should undergo investigation for T-cell immune defects, most importantly HIV infection. The patient with recurrent *N. meningitidis* infections should be tested for possible late component complement deficiencies. Details on the manifestations of infection with the pathogens listed in Table 102-2 are found elsewhere in this textbook.

DIAGNOSIS AND DIFFERENTIAL DIAGNOSIS

Diagnosis of infection in the immunocompromised host can be more difficult than in the normal host, and the differential diagnosis of infections can be quite broad. Because defects in humoral and cell-mediated immunity may limit the ability to develop antibody responses to infection, serologic tests have poor sensitivity for these patients. Cultures—including standard bacterial cultures and those facilitating growth of acid-fast bacilli and fungi—are often critical to making a diagnosis of infection. Because some of the pathogens causing infection in these settings are commensals or colonizers, interpretation of a positive culture result may be difficult. For example, the growth of *Candida* species in bronchoscopy specimens most likely reflects upper airway and pharyngeal colonization.

Sensitive assays to detect the DNA or RNA of opportunistic viruses—most commonly through quantitative polymerase chain reaction (PCR)—have become crucial diagnostic tests for infections such as CMV, human herpesvirus 6 (HHV-6), and BK virus, and they may help to guide the duration of antiviral therapy. Biologic markers of fungal infection such as serum galactomannan and β-D-glucan assays may suggest a diagnosis of invasive infection with molds such as *Aspergillus*.

In many cases, the diagnosis of infection may be elusive, requiring biopsy and histopathologic examination of involved tissues to determine the underlying pathogen. This process combined with tissue cultures may be needed to make a definitive diagnosis of infection in the immunocompromised host, and it can help differentiate colonization from infection with a particular organism. Biopsy of skin lesions, bone marrow, or liver may provide a diagnosis when cultures and other standard tests are unrevealing.

In neutropenic patients with fever, the procalcitonin level may be elevated in the setting of bacteremia, but it is normal in patients with fungal infections. 18-Fluorodeoxyglucose positron-emission tomography/computed tomography can help localize infection in the immunocompromised patient, in whom the sensitivity of nuclear medicine studies with indium-111, technetium-99m, or gallium may be limited.

TREATMENT AND PREVENTION OF INFECTIONS

Treatment of infections in the immunocompromised host requires rapid diagnosis and, when possible, improvement of the underlying immune disorder to help reconstitute natural immune function. In many cases, treatment must be broad spectrum and empirical while awaiting results of diagnostic testing. Delay of therapy for these patients is associated with a higher risk of dissemination and death. Details on the specific treatment recommendations for individual pathogens are found elsewhere in this textbook.

Neutropenia

For patients with neutropenic fever, empirical therapy should always include coverage for *Pseudomonas aeruginosa* because it is associated with a high mortality rate. Empirical therapy should also be guided by the individual patient's antimicrobial administration history, prior infections, colonization status (e.g., methicillin-resistant S. aureus [MRSA], vancomycin-resistant

Enterococcus [VRE]), and local susceptibility data. Broad-spectrum agents such as piperacillin-tazobactam and cefepime may be used. Carbapenems may be indicated in the patient with recent hospitalization, recent broad-spectrum antibacterial administration, or with a history of infection with extended-spectrum β-lactamase–producing Enterobacteriaceae. After a pathogen is identified in cultures and susceptibility data are available, antimicrobial therapy should be narrowed.

If a neutropenic patient remains febrile for 3 to 5 days without an identified locus or pathogen of infection, empirical glycopeptide therapy (e.g., vancomycin to cover *S. aureus,* particularly in the setting of an indwelling central catheter) and antifungal therapy are recommended to cover staphylococci and *Aspergillus* and other fungi common in this setting. Although amphotericin B products have been a mainstay of therapy for many years, voriconazole is the preferred agent to treat suspected aspergillosis because of its better efficacy in the neutropenic host.

Reconstitution of immune function in the patient with neutrophil deficiency or dysfunction can help prevent or treat infection. Administration of granulocyte colony-stimulating factor (G-CSF) (i.e., filgrastim or pegfilgrastim) with chemotherapy for solid tumors can prevent and treat absolute neutropenia and therefore reduce the risk of infection. For patients with drug-induced neutropenia, similar benefit can be attained. G-CSF usually is contraindicated in patients with myeloid malignancies and myelodysplasia due to the potential for stimulation of growth of dysplastic or malignant cells.

Several measures can help decrease the risk of infection in patients with neutropenia, including prevention of exposure to potential pathogens and antimicrobial prophylaxis. Periodontal care with oral rinses with sterile water or saline four to six times per day and gentle teeth brushing may help prevent periodontal infection and streptococcal bacteremia. Daily chlorhexidine bathing may decrease colonization with multidrug-resistant organisms that can be acquired while hospitalized. Ingestion of a low-microbial diet (e.g., no raw fruits or vegetables) and avoidance of dried or fresh flowers and potted plants may decrease exposure to fungi, including *Aspergillus.*

Housing in high-efficiency particulate air (HEPA)–filtered rooms with positive air pressure and adequate ventilation is the standard of care in HSCT units to decrease the risk of exposure to airborne pathogens. For patients at home, avoiding construction areas (including home renovation projects) while neutropenic may decrease the risk of invasive fungal infection. Patients visiting medical offices or hospitals should wear a mask, including when ambulating in the hallways or being transported for testing. Strict handwashing and hand hygiene are paramount to preventing infection. Avoidance of rectal thermometers, suppositories, enemas, and tampons while neutropenic has been recommended to prevent infection. Patients with well water should use filters to decrease the risk of *Cryptosporidium* infection. Minimization of mucositis with newer chemotherapeutic agents can help decrease the risk of infection in patients with malignancy.

Solid data support the use of quinolones (e.g., ciprofloxacin, levofloxacin) as prophylaxis for serious infection in patients with anticipated neutropenia for 7 or more days. Penicillin is often added to prevent infection with viridans streptococci in patients on a mucositis-inducing chemotherapy regimen. Antifungal prophylaxis with voriconazole or posaconazole decreases the incidence of invasive fungal infections in patients undergoing HSCT and those with hematologic malignancies undergoing induction chemotherapy. Certain cancer patients, including those with acute lymphoblastic leukemia or those on high-dose corticosteroids, methotrexate, fludarabine, bleomycin, l-asparaginase, or cytarabine, have sufficient T-cell dysfunction to warrant prophylaxis against *P. jirovecii* (discussed later). Herpes simplex virus (HSV) prophylaxis with acyclovir is indicated for those with a history of symptomatic HSV infection or seropositivity.

Humoral Immunity Defects

Patients with hypogammaglobulinemia and CVID are at risk for infection with encapsulated organisms such as *S. pneumoniae.* Replacement of immunoglobulin G (IgG) with intravenous immune globulin (IVIG) at a dose of 400 to 600 mg/kg monthly can help prevent infections in these patients. Immunization may not be protective against *S, pneumoniae, H. influenzae,* or *N. meningitidis* due to poor seroconversion rates.

Hematopoietic Stem Cell Transplantation

Infection risk after HSCT depends on the source of stem cells, the type of conditioning chemotherapy regimen administered, and the risk and degree of GVHD (Fig. 102-1). Myeloablative regimens (including chemotherapy and total body irradiation) often result in severe mucositis, putting patients at risk for the infections detailed previously. Although the risk of infection in autologous transplants is relatively low due to earlier engraftment, recipients of matched unrelated donor allogeneic

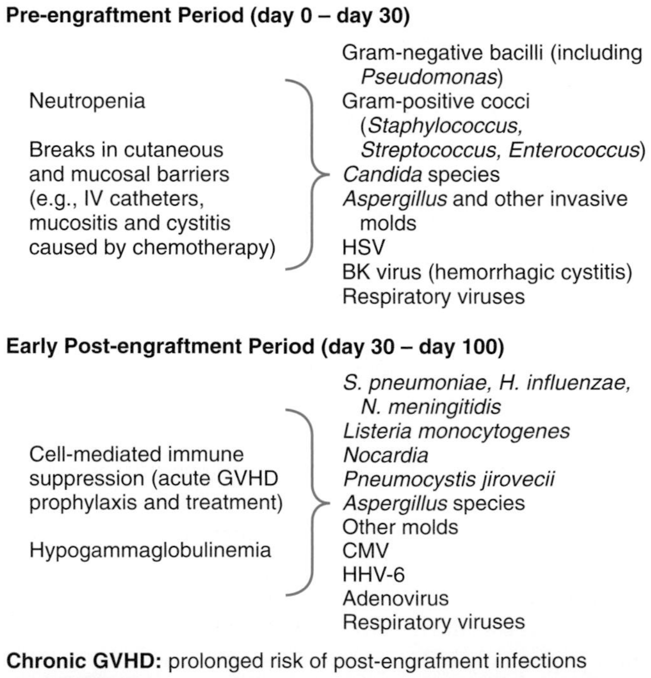

Pre-engraftment Period (day 0 – day 30)

Neutropenia

Breaks in cutaneous and mucosal barriers (e.g., IV catheters, mucositis and cystitis caused by chemotherapy)

Gram-negative bacilli (including *Pseudomonas*)
Gram-positive cocci (*Staphylococcus, Streptococcus, Enterococcus*)
Candida species
Aspergillus and other invasive molds
HSV
BK virus (hemorrhagic cystitis)
Respiratory viruses

Early Post-engraftment Period (day 30 – day 100)

Cell-mediated immune suppression (acute GVHD prophylaxis and treatment)

Hypogammaglobulinemia

S. pneumoniae, H. influenzae, N. meningitidis
Listeria monocytogenes
Nocardia
Pneumocystis jirovecii
Aspergillus species
Other molds
CMV
HHV-6
Adenovirus
Respiratory viruses

Chronic GVHD: prolonged risk of post-engrafment infections

FIGURE 102-1 Timing of infection after hematopoietic stem cell transplantation. CMV, Cytomegalovirus; GVHD, graft-versus-host disease; HHV, human herpesvirus; HSV, herpes simplex virus; IV, intravenous.

transplants are at significant and prolonged risk for opportunistic infections due to the high rate of GVHD associated with these allografts, resulting in prolonged T-cell–mediated immunosuppression and delayed immune reconstitution. Umbilical cord blood transplants are associated with prolonged neutropenia as a result of the small volume of cells available for transplantation, placing patients at risk for infection. The risk of GVHD, however, is lower with the use of umbilical cord cells.

Immediately after HSCT, stem cell recipients are neutropenic. During this pre-engraftment period, pathogens characteristic of prolonged neutropenia can cause infection. Prophylaxis with voriconazole or posaconazole, levofloxacin or ciprofloxacin, acyclovir, and penicillin is common to prevent infections during this vulnerable period.

After engraftment, the risk of GVHD is high for many allogeneic transplant recipients, resulting in administration of corticosteroids, methotrexate, cyclosporine, tacrolimus, sirolimus, or mycophenolate for prophylaxis. After GVHD develops, high-dose corticosteroids usually are given. In refractory cases, additional T-cell–active immunosuppressive agents, including antithymocyte globulin, tacrolimus, sirolimus, cyclophosphamide, and alemtuzumab, may be required. Patients on these agents are at risk for infections from CMV, *Nocardia*, HHV-6, *P. jirovecii*, adenovirus, invasive molds, and other opportunists. In some cases, patients require chronic immunosuppressive therapy to control GVHD, putting them at risk for infection indefinitely and requiring long-term antibiotic prophylaxis. If GVHD is successfully prevented, immunosuppressive therapy is discontinued after 6 to 12 months.

In uncomplicated HSCT cases without GVHD, functional humoral immunity takes 1 to 2 years to return to normal, and patients are at risk for encapsulated organisms despite being successfully engrafted. Standard immunizations are re-administered 1 to 2 years after transplantation because pretransplantation antibodies are often lost.

Human Immunodeficiency Virus Infection

Chapter 101 provides a detailed discussion of treatment and prophylaxis of infections occurring in HIV-infected patients.

Solid Organ Transplantation

Organ transplant recipients are at lifelong risk of infection, although the pathogens involved change over time (Fig. 102-2). In the first month after transplantation, patients develop infections related to the surgical procedures and hospitalization. Urinary tract infection in the renal transplant recipient, pneumonia in the lung transplant recipient, and sternal wound infection in the heart transplant recipient tend to manifest in the first 4 weeks postoperatively. Common nosocomial infections such as catheter-related bloodstream infection and *Clostridium difficile* may also occur. Anastomotic leaks in pancreas and liver transplant recipients may cause polymicrobial intra-abdominal abscesses.

Patients with incubating infection at the time of transplantation and induction immunosuppression can develop disseminated infection with viral or bacterial pathogens, which is associated with a high mortality rate. Careful evaluation of the recipient at the time of hospital admission for transplantation is

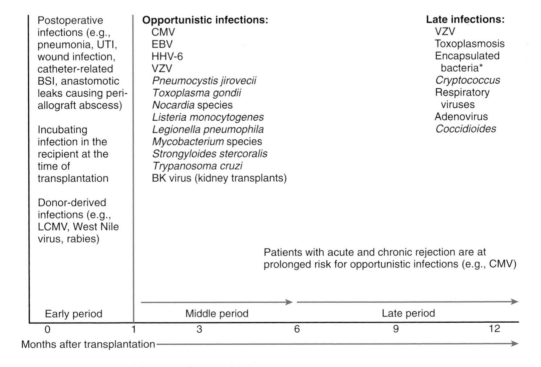

FIGURE 102-2 Timing of infections after solid organ transplantation. BSI, Bloodstream infection; CMV, cytomegalovirus; COPD, chronic obstructive pulmonary disease; EBV Epstein-Barr virus; HCV, hepatitis C virus; HHV-6, human herpesvirus 6; HIV, human immunodeficiency virus; LCMV, lymphocytic choriomeningitis virus; UTI, urinary tract infection; VZV, varicella-zoster virus.

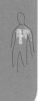

essential for positive early outcomes. Rarely, donor-transmitted infections can occur, including viral pathogens such as rabies virus, West Nile virus, lymphocytic choriomeningitis virus (LCMV), HIV, and hepatitis B and C viruses. Organ banks and transplantation centers continue to work to improve the sensitivity and specificity of donor testing paradigms to prevent transmission of infection.

The most common time for opportunistic infections such as CMV, *Listeria*, *Legionella*, and invasive fungal infections such as *Aspergillus* is 1 to 6 months after transplantation. Later infection may be seen in those receiving lymphocyte-depleting induction agents (e.g., thymoglobulin, alemtuzumab) to prevent acute rejection at the time of transplantation or in those with episodes of acute rejection.

Because CMV causes symptomatic infection and is associated with chronic allograft dysfunction, prophylaxis or preemptive treatment of infection with valganciclovir is used. Seronegative recipients of a CMV-seropositive organ are at highest risk for infection. Lung transplant recipients, who are at significant risk for *Aspergillus* infection in the first 6 months after transplantation, receive prophylactic voriconazole to prevent invasive fungal infection. Lung recipients are at lifelong risk for respiratory viral infections. Lung transplant recipients may also receive azithromycin to improve the prognosis for bronchiolitis obliterans syndrome, the most common manifestation of chronic allograft dysfunction.

Heart transplant recipients are at particular risk for reactivation of donor-transmitted infection with *Toxoplasma gondii*, which can cause early myocarditis or late cerebral disease. Serologic (IgG) screening of the donor and recipient, with sulfamethoxazole-trimethoprim prophylaxis used in seropositive recipients or seronegative recipients of a seropositive heart, is the standard of care in cardiac transplantation centers.

P. jirovecii can cause infection in solid organ transplant recipients, which usually occurs 6 to 12 months after transplantation. Pneumonitis similar to that seen in patients with HIV is the most common manifestation, although extrapulmonary infection (particularly in the liver and spleen) can be seen in transplant recipients. Prophylaxis with sulfamethoxazole-trimethoprim (or atovaquone in sulfa-allergic patients) is indicated for 12 months after transplantation. If high-dose corticosteroids or antilymphocyte therapy is required for treatment of acute rejection, prophylaxis should be restarted.

Almost all liver transplant recipients with underlying active hepatitis B or C have reactivation of the infection. Treatment of hepatitis B with lamivudine or other antiviral agents is often successful in suppressing infection when started at the time of transplantation. Although more difficult, post-transplantation treatment of symptomatic hepatitis C with interferon, ribavirin, and protease inhibitors may prolong hepatic function. Newer direct acting agents are being studied in the post-transplant setting.

In patients with no episodes of acute rejection, the risk of opportunistic infections often declines with time. Late infections (≥12 months after transplantation) may still occur, with varicella-zoster virus (VZV), HSV (particularly encephalitis) *Cryptococcus neoformans*, JC virus (i.e., progressive multifocal leukoencephalopathy), and community-acquired infections such as influenza

and *S. pneumoniae* most commonly reported. Patients with hypogammaglobulinemia complicating long-term immunosuppressive therapy may benefit from IVIG to help prevent infections.

Although not always possible, especially with lifesaving heart, lung, or liver transplants, reduction of immunosuppression in the organ transplant recipient with invasive fungal infection, viral infection, or bacterial sepsis may assist in recovery. Reinstitution of immunosuppressive therapy may be indicated as infection resolves.

A significant challenge in treating infections in the patient with a solid organ transplant or GVHD complicating HSCT is the cytochrome P-450 metabolism of antimicrobial agents such as the azoles, macrolides, rifampin, echinocandins, nucleoside reverse transcriptase inhibitors (NRTIs), protease inhibitors, and non-nucleoside reverse transcriptase inhibitors (NNRTIs). Careful monitoring of levels of calcineurin inhibitors (e.g., cyclosporine, tacrolimus) is indicated for patients on these and other agents that can induce or inhibit P-450 metabolism.

Although the immunocompromised patient may not seroconvert from vaccinations such as the annual influenza vaccine, immunization of household contacts and health care workers can prevent exposure and therefore infection of the most vulnerable hosts. Immunocompromised patients should avoid live virus vaccines (e.g., measles/mumps/rubella, varicella, yellow fever) that can be associated with disseminated infection. Specialized protocols exist for immunization of immunocompromised children.

 PROGNOSIS

The prognosis of infections in immunocompromised hosts relies on accurate and rapid diagnosis and early institution of appropriate antimicrobial therapy. Use of cidal therapies (versus static agents) is recommended. Manipulation of the immune response to infection through G-CSF administration (in neutropenic patients), administration of IVIG (in hypogammaglobulinemic patients), or decreasing immunosuppressive therapy (in kidney or pancreas transplant recipients) may improve survival.

The prognosis for infections in these settings is worse for older patients, those requiring intensive care unit (ICU) admission, and those in whom rapid immune reconstitution is not possible. Tumor lysis syndrome, acute respiratory failure, and sepsis increase mortality. Patients with underlying acute leukemia and those with other comorbidities, including cardiovascular disease, renal failure, liver disease, or lung disease have a significantly worse prognosis, particularly in the setting of invasive fungal infection. The attributable mortality rate for invasive aspergillosis is 20% to 50% when patients require ICU admission (Fig. 102-3).

CONCLUSIONS

Care of the immunocompromised host with infection requires meticulous monitoring of symptoms, detection of often subtle physical findings, and an understanding of the arms of the immune system involved in a particular patient's illness. With successes in treatment of malignancies and end-organ disease, the breadth of infections causing infection in these hosts continues to widen.

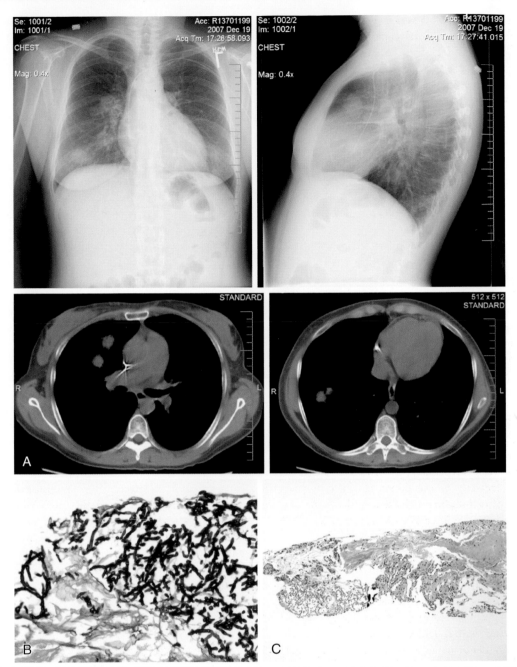

FIGURE 102-3 Invasive pulmonary aspergillosis in a kidney transplant recipient with myelodysplasia. At presentation, the patient was afebrile and had dyspnea on exertion without cough. **A,** Anteroposterior and lateral chest radiographs *(top)* and computed tomography scans *(bottom)* of the chest. **B,** Transbronchial lung biopsy demonstrates hyphae in tissue (hematoxylin and eosin stain, ×100). **C,** Silver stain of biopsy tissue demonstrates acute-angle branching hyphae. Cultures grew *Aspergillus fumigatus*.

SUGGESTED READINGS

Bennett CL, Djulbegovic B, Norris LB, et al: Colony-stimulating factors for febrile neutropenia during cancer therapy, N Engl J Med 368:1131–1139, 2013.

Blumberg EA, Danziger-Isakov L, Kumar D, et al: Infectious disease guidelines, ed 3, Am J Transplant 13:1–371, 2013.

Bow EJ, Bacteriol D: Infection in neutropenic patients with cancer, Crit Care Clin 29:411–441, 2013.

Boysen AK, Jensen BR, Poulsen LO, et al: Procalcitonin as a marker of infection in febrile neutropenia: a systematic review, Mod Chemother 2:8–14, 2013.

Buckley RH: Primary cellular immunodeficiencies, J Allergy Clin Immunol 109:747–757, 2002.

Choi SW, Levine JE, Ferrara JL: Pathogenesis and management of graft-versus-host-disease, Immunol Allergy Clin North Am 30:75–191, 2009.

Copelan EA: Hematopoietic stem-cell transplantation, N Engl J Med 354:1813–1826, 2006.

Fischer SA: Emerging viruses in transplantation: there is more to infection after transplant than CMV and EBV, Transplantation 86:1327–1339, 2008.

Flowers CR, Seidenfeld J, Bow EJ, et al: Antimicrobial prophylaxis and outpatient management of fever and neutropenia in adults treated for malignancy: American Society of Clinical Oncology clinical practice guideline, J Clin Oncol 31:794–810, 2013.

Freifeld AG, Bow EJ, Sepkowitz KA, et al: Executive summary: clinical practice guideline for the use of antimicrobial agents in neutropenic patients with

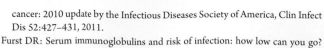

cancer: 2010 update by the Infectious Diseases Society of America, Clin Infect Dis 52:427–431, 2011.

Furst DR: Serum immunoglobulins and risk of infection: how low can you go? Semin Arthritis Rheum 39:18–29, 2008.

Green M, Michaels MG: Epstein-Barr virus infection and posttransplant lymphoproliferative disorder, Am J Transplant 13:41–54, 2013.

Kotton CN: CMV: prevention, diagnosis and therapy, Am J Transplant 13:24–40, 2013.

Paul M, Yahav D, Bivas A, et al: Anti-pseudomonal beta-lactams for the initial, empirical, treatment of febrile neutropenia: comparison of beta-lactams [review], Cochrane Database Syst Rev 11:1–117, 2010.

Steinberg JP, Robichaux C, Tejedor SC, et al: Distribution of pathogens in central line-associated bloodstream infections among patients with and without neutropenia following chemotherapy: evidence for a proposed modification to the current surveillance definition, Infect Control Hosp Epidemiol 34:171–175, 2013.

Tam JS, Routes JM: Common variable immunodeficiency, Am J Rhinol Allergy 27:260–265, 2013.

Thom KA, Kleinberg M, Roghmann MC: Infection prevention in the cancer center, Clin Infect Dis 57:579–585, 2013.

Tomblyn M, Chiller T, Einsele H, et al: Guidelines for preventing infectious complications among hematopoietic cell transplantation recipients: a global perspective, Biol Blood Marrow Transplant 15:1143–1238, 2009.

103

Infectious Diseases of Travelers: Protozoal and Helminthic Infections

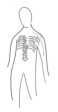

Rebecca Reece, Aadia I. Rana, and Erna Milunka Kojic

INTRODUCTION

Medical advice for overseas travelers, recommended protective measures, and the diagnosis and treatment of common parasitic diseases endemic in the United States and abroad are reviewed in this chapter.

PREPARATION OF TRAVELERS

More than 27 million Americans travel internationally every year, and more than 60% of them travel to developing regions of the world. Increases in international travel are associated with exposures to infectious diseases worldwide and bring the issues of prevention and management of health problems in travelers into the office of every physician. The risk of becoming ill while traveling internationally depends on the destination and duration of the trip, the underlying health and age of the traveler, and activities undertaken while abroad. Major issues to be addressed before traveling include required and recommended immunizations, malaria prophylaxis, and traveler's diarrhea, as well as measures to prevent tick and mosquito bites. Information about health risks in specific geographic areas, updated weekly, can be obtained from the Centers for Disease Control and Prevention (CDC) through its publications or website (www.cdc.gov/travel/destinations/list).

Immunizations

All international travelers should ensure they are up-to-date on routine vaccinations. Only yellow fever vaccination may be required by law for international travel, but other immunizations are often strongly recommended, depending on the destination, type, and duration of travel. Before immunization, a thorough history should be obtained to determine the safety of immunizations and any allergies to eggs or chick embryo cells. Pregnant women and individuals who are immunocompromised by human immunodeficiency virus (HIV), malignancy, or chemotherapy pose specific and important concerns requiring review before receiving vaccinations.

Hepatitis A

In the United States, the most frequently identified risk for hepatitis A infection is travel. The risk varies with living conditions, length of stay, and incidence of hepatitis A in the area visited. In some areas, the disease affects an estimated 1 of every 500 to 1000 travelers on a 2- to 3-week trip. Therefore, hepatitis A vaccination is recommended for all susceptible persons traveling to or working in countries with intermediate or high endemicity of infection. Hepatitis A vaccine should be given at least 2 weeks before departure but remains effective if given up until the time of travel. A single dose provides protection for 1 to 2 years; a booster 6 to 18 months later is required for long-lasting immunity (at least 20 years and possibly lifelong).

Influenza

Although influenza is not necessarily considered a travel-related illness, the influenza vaccine should be considered in the panel of vaccines offered to the traveler. Influenza seasons can occur at different times of the year in different parts of the world. If a patient cannot be immunized, a course of the antiviral medication oseltamivir can be provided to take at the first sign of a flu-like illness.

Japanese Encephalitis

Japanese encephalitis (JE) virus is closely related to the West Nile and Saint Louis encephalitis viruses and is transmitted to humans through the bite of an infected mosquito. JE virus is the most common vaccine-preventable cause of encephalitis in Asia. It occurs throughout most of Asia and parts of the western Pacific. The overall incidence of JE among people from non-endemic countries traveling to Asia is estimated to be less than 1 case per 1 million travelers. However, expatriates and travelers who stay for prolonged periods in rural areas with active JE virus transmission are likely to be at similar risk as the susceptible resident population (i.e., 5 to 50 cases per 100,000 children per year). Even during brief trips, travelers might be at increased risk if they have extensive outdoor or nighttime exposure in rural areas during periods of active transmission. Short-term (<1 month) travelers whose visits are restricted to major urban areas are at minimal risk for JE. A new inactivated JE vaccine, a two-dose series given 28 days apart, was approved in 2009 for use in people 17 years of age and older; pediatric clinical trials are being conducted to enable its licensure for use in children.

Measles

In the United States, most measles cases result from international travel, and measles remains a common disease in many parts of the world. Currently, measles vaccination is recommended at 15 months of age, with a second vaccination after age 5. Individuals born after 1956 who have no physician-documented record of immunization or who have received a booster after early childhood should have a one-time booster before travel.

Meningococcal Meningitis

Vaccination for meningococcal disease is recommended to persons who travel to or reside in countries in which the bacterium *Neisseria meningitidis* is hyperendemic or epidemic, particularly if they will be in close contact with the local population. Vaccination is recommended for travelers to Saudi Arabia during the Hajj, along the meningitis belt of sub-Saharan Africa, and in other locations for which travel advisories have been issued (information available on the CDC website). The meningococcal conjugate vaccine (MCV4) is preferred for people age 9 months through 55 years, and the meningococcal polysaccharide vaccine (MPSV4) is the recommended vaccine for persons older than 55.

Polio

Polio remains endemic in some regions of Asia and Africa. Before traveling to areas where poliomyelitis cases are still occurring, travelers should ensure that they have completed the recommended age-appropriate polio vaccine series and have received a booster dose with the inactivated polio vaccine as an adult.

Typhoid

International travelers are at greatest risk for contracting typhoid in the Indian subcontinent, Central America, western South America, and sub-Saharan Africa. Vaccination is recommended for travel to endemic areas where exposure to contaminated food and water is likely. Both a live oral vaccine (four enteric-coated capsules given over 7 days) and an injectable vaccine (single-dose) are available; they are essentially equivalent in effectiveness, which ranges from 50% to 70%.

Yellow Fever

The yellow fever vaccine is a live, attenuated virus vaccine that is recommended for persons traveling to areas in South America and Africa where yellow fever is endemic. Vaccination is protective for at least 10 years and must be given at designated vaccination centers. Severe adverse events are rare and include yellow fever vaccine–associated viscerotropic and neurologic disease, both of which are more common in elderly persons and in those with thymus disease. Because the adverse events occur more commonly in people older than 60 years of age, a careful assessment of risks and benefits for these travelers should be made before vaccination.

Other Vaccines

Some individuals live for prolonged periods in developing countries or are at special risk for contracting certain highly contagious diseases. Consideration should be given to immunization against hepatitis B, plague, and rabies. Tetanus vaccinations should be up to date: for travel, a tetanus booster within the previous 5 years is recommended. The cholera vaccine is not available in the United States. Worldwide, two oral cholera vaccines are available, but vaccination offers limited protection. Therefore, the vaccine is not recommended for travelers, but standard cholera prevention and control measures are emphasized.

Malaria Prophylaxis

Malaria infection is associated with significant morbidity and mortality, particularly if the causative agent is *Plasmodium falciparum*. The need for, as well as the type of, malaria prophylaxis depends on known resistance patterns and the exact itinerary within a given country because the risk of transmission is regional. In general, travelers to areas where chloroquine-sensitive *P. falciparum* strains are exclusively found (i.e., parts of Central America, the Caribbean, North Africa, and the Middle East) should take chloroquine phosphate (300-mg base or 500-mg salt) weekly, starting 1 week before travel to malarious areas and continuing during the trip and for 4 weeks after leaving the area.

Travelers to Southeast Asia, sub-Saharan Africa, South America, and South Asia, where chloroquine-resistant *P. falciparum* is common may take mefloquine (Lariam), atovaquone-proguanil (Malarone), or doxycycline. Mefloquine may be associated with neurologic side effects (dizziness, tinnitus, and vivid dreams) and, rarely, with significant neuropsychiatric side effects. A U.S. Food and Drug Administration (FDA) black box warning issued in 2013 indicated that the neurologic side effects can occur at any time and persist indefinitely; this has lent some caution to the prescription of mefloquine. Mefloquine is also not completely effective in Myanmar, rural Thailand, or some parts of East Africa, where resistance is a growing problem. Atovaquone-proguanil and doxycycline are effective in Southeast Asia and may be used in other areas of chloroquine resistance. Atovaquone-proguanil is well tolerated but must be taken every day. Daily doxycycline can be associated with photosensitivity, esophagitis, and, occasionally, vaginal candidiasis.

Where it is approved, primaquine can be used for primary prophylaxis in areas with higher rates of *Plasmodium vivax* or *Plasmodium ovale* infection. It has the advantage of both preventing acute infection from all malaria parasites and preventing the later recurrent infections of *P. vivax* and *P. ovale*. It cannot be used in individuals with glucose-6-phosphate dehydrogenase (G6PD) deficiency. Emphasis must also be given to the use of mosquito bite prevention measures, including netting, screens, permethrin for clothing, and insect repellents.

Traveler's Diarrhea

Each year between 20% and 50% of international travelers develop diarrhea. Bacterial infections such as enterotoxigenic *Escherichia coli* are most common, but other causes include parasites and viruses. The average duration of an episode of traveler's diarrhea is 3 to 6 days, but about 10% of episodes last longer than 1 week. The diarrhea may be accompanied by abdominal cramping, nausea, headache, low-grade fever, vomiting, or bloating. Travelers with fever greater than 101°F (38°C), bloody stools, or both should see a physician at once (see Chapter 96).

Diarrheal illness can be avoided by taking precautions with regard to food and beverages. All water and ice should be presumed to be unsafe. Salads are often contaminated by protozoal cysts; along with street vendor foods, they are the most dangerous foods encountered by most travelers. Food should be well cooked, and unpasteurized dairy products should be avoided.

Prophylactic antibiotics are not generally recommended. Diphenoxylate (Lomotil) and loperamide (Imodium) may provide symptomatic relief of mild diarrhea. First-line treatment includes fluoroquinolones, taken orally for 3 days. In some countries, such as Thailand and Nepal, fluoroquinolone resistance, especially among *Campylobacter* species, has been on the rise; azithromycin is an alternative in these situations.

Special Problems

Pregnant Women

Although travel is rarely contraindicated during a normal pregnancy, complicated pregnancies require special consideration and may warrant a recommendation that travel be delayed. The risk of obstetric complications is highest during the first and third trimesters.

Most live-virus vaccines are contraindicated during pregnancy. Yellow fever vaccine, for which pregnancy is considered a precaution by the Advisory Committee on Immunization Practices (ACIP), should be avoided if possible. If travel is unavoidable and the risks for yellow fever virus exposure are believed to outweigh the risks of vaccination, a pregnant woman should be vaccinated. Pregnant women should avoid or delay travel to malaria-endemic areas because no prophylactic measures provide complete protection. If travel is unavoidable, pregnant women should take utmost precautions to avoid mosquito bites; for chemoprophylaxis, chloroquine and mefloquine are the drugs of choice for destinations with chloroquine-sensitive and chloroquine-resistant malaria, respectively.

Acquired Immunodeficiency Syndrome

Many countries bar entry to persons with acquired immunodeficiency syndrome (AIDS). Several countries require serologic testing for the human immunodeficiency virus (HIV) from all travelers applying for visa lasting longer than 3 months; official documentation is required well in advance of travel. Patients with HIV infection need special preparation before travel to developing countries because of their increased susceptibility to certain illnesses (e.g., pneumococcal infection, tuberculosis). Issues of HIV infection and other sexually transmitted diseases should be discussed, especially with young, sexually active adults.

The Returning Traveler

The most common medical problems encountered by travelers after their return home are diarrhea, fever, respiratory illnesses, and skin lesions. A detailed history should focus on the traveler's exact itinerary, including dates of travel, exposure history (e.g., food indiscretions, drinking-water sources, freshwater contact, sexual activity, animal contact, insect bites), style of travel (urban versus rural), immunization history, and use of antimalarial chemoprophylaxis.

Diarrhea

Traveler's diarrhea is an acute condition that usually resolves within 2 weeks. If the traveler's diarrhea is not responsive to empiric antibiotic treatment, a work-up should be performed to evaluate for *Giardia lamblia* (see later discussion). Three stool specimens for ova and parasites and a stool culture are indicated (E-Fig. 103-1). If *Giardia* tests are negative, an empirical trial of metronidazole for treatment of a possible infection with *Giardia* or other protozoan (e.g., amebiasis) should be considered. Noninfectious causes such as temporary lactose intolerance, irritable bowel syndrome, and, less commonly, inflammatory bowel disease should also be in the differential diagnosis.

Fever

Malaria should be the first diagnosis considered in a febrile traveler who has returned from a malarious area. *P. falciparum* malaria can be fatal if it is not diagnosed and treated promptly. Detection of the *Plasmodium* species on Giemsa-stained blood smears by light microscopy is the standard tool for diagnosis of malaria. Rapid diagnostic tests for detection of malaria parasite antigens are becoming increasingly important tools in resource-limited endemic settings because of their accuracy and ease of use.

Travelers with chloroquine-sensitive *P. falciparum* malaria should be treated with chloroquine. Reasonable agents for uncomplicated malaria caused by chloroquine-resistant *P. falciparum* include atovaquone-proguanil, artemisinin derivative combinations (if available), and mefloquine- or quinine-based regimens. Quinine- and mefloquine-based regimens are more frequently associated with adverse effects, and mefloquine should not be used to treat *P. falciparum* malaria acquired in the Thai-Myanmar-Cambodia area because of high resistance rates.

Severe malaria is defined as acute malaria with major signs of organ dysfunction or a high level of parasitemia (>5%) or both. It should be treated with intravenous quinidine for 7 days with close monitoring of the QTc interval. In many parts of the world, intravenous artesunate is used, but it may be associated with high rates of relapse.

Other important causes of fever after travel include viral hepatitis (hepatitis A and E), typhoid fever, bacterial enteritis, arboviral infections (e.g., dengue, chicungunya), rickettsial infections, and, in rare instances, leptospirosis, acute HIV infection, and amebic liver abscess.

Skin Diseases

Sunburn, insect bites, skin ulcers, and cutaneous larva migrans are the most common skin conditions affecting travelers after their return home. Persistent skin ulcers should prompt a work-up for cutaneous leishmaniasis, mycobacterial infection, or fungal infection. Careful, complete inspection of the skin is important in detecting the rickettsial eschar in a febrile patient or the central breathing hole in a "boil" caused by myiasis.

PROTOZOAL INFECTIONS

Protozoal infections, though endemic to certain regions, can be encountered all around the world, partly because of the increase in travel and migration (Table 103-1). They cause a tremendous burden of disease in the tropics and subtropics as well as more

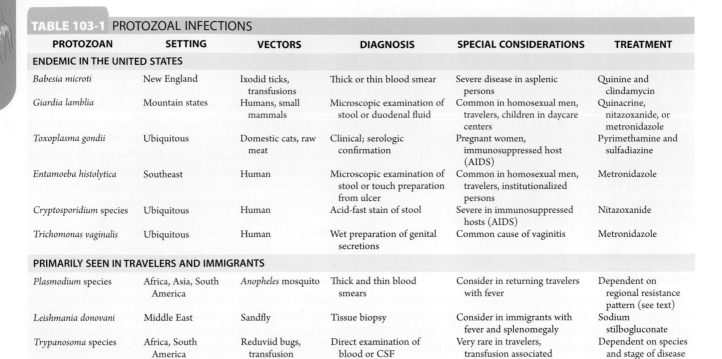

TABLE 103-1 PROTOZOAL INFECTIONS

PROTOZOAN	SETTING	VECTORS	DIAGNOSIS	SPECIAL CONSIDERATIONS	TREATMENT
ENDEMIC IN THE UNITED STATES					
Babesia microti	New England	Ixodid ticks, transfusions	Thick or thin blood smear	Severe disease in asplenic persons	Quinine and clindamycin
Giardia lamblia	Mountain states	Humans, small mammals	Microscopic examination of stool or duodenal fluid	Common in homosexual men, travelers, children in daycare centers	Quinacrine, nitazoxanide, or metronidazole
Toxoplasma gondii	Ubiquitous	Domestic cats, raw meat	Clinical; serologic confirmation	Pregnant women, immunosuppressed host (AIDS)	Pyrimethamine and sulfadiazine
Entamoeba histolytica	Southeast	Human	Microscopic examination of stool or touch preparation from ulcer	Common in homosexual men, travelers, institutionalized persons	Metronidazole
Cryptosporidium species	Ubiquitous	Human	Acid-fast stain of stool	Severe in immunosuppressed hosts (AIDS)	Nitazoxanide
Trichomonas vaginalis	Ubiquitous	Human	Wet preparation of genital secretions	Common cause of vaginitis	Metronidazole
PRIMARILY SEEN IN TRAVELERS AND IMMIGRANTS					
Plasmodium species	Africa, Asia, South America	*Anopheles* mosquito	Thick and thin blood smears	Consider in returning travelers with fever	Dependent on regional resistance pattern (see text)
Leishmania donovani	Middle East	Sandfly	Tissue biopsy	Consider in immigrants with fever and splenomegaly	Sodium stilbogluconate
Trypanosoma species	Africa, South America	Reduviid bugs, transfusion	Direct examination of blood or CSF	Very rare in travelers, transfusion associated	Dependent on species and stage of disease

AIDS, Acquired immunodeficiency syndrome; CSF, cerebrospinal fluid.

temperate climates. Immunosuppression associated with various conditions, particularly HIV infection, leads to more severe manifestations. Of all protozoal diseases, malaria causes the most deaths globally, approximately 1 million people each year.

Protozoal Infections in the United States

Giardiasis

Giardiasis is a common cause of nonbloody diarrhea in returning travelers. *G. lamblia* and *Giardia intestinalis* are found worldwide, including in the United States. However, giardiasis is most commonly diagnosed in travelers returning from Latin America, Southeast Asia, or the Middle East. Transmission is by the fecal-oral route in the setting of contaminated food or water or public swimming areas, or by person-to-person contact in certain risk populations such as men who have sex with men. It is usually a self-limited diarrheal illness that lasts 2 to 4 weeks but may persist longer. Rarely, individuals have associated fevers, nausea, or vomiting. The diagnosis is made by microscopic examination of stool for cysts or trophozoites or by an antigen detection test. Treatment options include metronidazole, tinidazole, or nitazoxanide.

Amebiasis

Amebiasis is another diarrheal illness that occurs in travelers. Like *Giardia*, *Entamoeba histolytica* is found worldwide, and transmission is by the fecal-oral route. However, most infected individuals (80%) are asymptomatic. The presentation in those acutely infected includes bloody or watery diarrhea with abdominal cramping lasting up to 4 weeks. In immunocompromised individuals, a severe invasive infection can occur with risk of necrotizing colitis or bowel perforation. Extraintestinal amebiasis can occur as well, particularly liver abscesses. The diagnosis can be made by microscopic examination of stool for ova and

parasites or by antigen detection tests of stool or serum. Treatment is with metronidazole or tinidazole in symptomatic individuals, followed by paromomycin or iodoquinol.

Protozoal Infections Common in Travelers and Immigrants

Leishmaniasis

Leishmaniasis is transmitted by the sandfly and can manifest with cutaneous, mucocutaneous, or visceral involvement. The skin finding is a persistent ulcer with raised edges in a traveler returning from the Middle East (Old World: *Leishmania major*, *Leishmania tropica*) or Latin America (New World: *Leishmania braziliensis*, *Leishmania peruviana*, others). Diagnosis is by tissue biopsy. Visceral leishmaniasis can have hepatic, splenic, or bone marrow involvement and is more commonly identified in immigrants from Asia (*Leishmania donovani*) or South America (*Leishmania chagasi*). Diagnosis is by tissue biopsy or culture of the involved organ.

Treatment varies based on severity of presentation and resistance characteristics. Most cutaneous lesions are self-limited, but treatment options include sodium stibogluconate (Pentostam) or paromomycin. For visceral involvement, treatment includes sodium stibogluconate, amphotericin B, or a combination of these two agents.

African Trypanosomiasis

African trypanosomiasis, or African sleeping sickness, is a protozoal infection caused by *Trypanosoma rhodesiense* (East Africa) or *Trypanosoma gambiense* (Central and West Africa), which is transmitted by the tsetse fly. Presenting symptoms include fever, headache, and central nervous system involvement. The disease is rarely reported in travelers returning from sub-Saharan Africa

TABLE 103-2 HELMINTHIC INFECTIONS

HELMINTH	SETTING	VECTORS	DIAGNOSIS	TREATMENT
ENDEMIC IN THE UNITED STATES				
Pinworm (enterobiasis)	Ubiquitous	Human	Direct examination for ova	Mebendazole, albendazole
Ascaris lumbricoides	Southeast	Human	Stool examination for ova	Mebendazole, albendazole
Trichuris trichiura	Southeast	Human	Stool examination for ova	Mebendazole, albendazole
Hookworm	Southeast	Human	Stool examination for ova	Mebendazole, albendazole
COMMON IN TRAVELERS AND IMMIGRANTS				
Strongyloides stercoralis	Developing world	Human	Stool examination for larvae	Thiabendazole, ivermectin
Schistosoma species	Developing world	Snails	Stool or urine examination for ova	Praziquantel
Wuchereria and *Brugia* species	Asia, some parts of Africa	Mosquitoes	Nocturnal blood examination	Ivermectin
Onchocerca volvulus	Africa, South and Central America	Black flies	Biopsy	Ivermectin
Loa loa	Africa	Tabanid flies	Blood examination, clinical setting	Diethylcarbamazine or ivermectin
Clonorchis sinensis	Asia	Undercooked fish and snails	Stool examination for ova, radiology	Praziquantel
Echinococcus species	Worldwide	Canines and livestock	Radiology, serology, biopsy	Surgery, supportive therapy
Taenia solium (cysticercosis)	Developing world	Humans, pigs	Radiology, serology	Surgery, albendazole
T. solium, Taenia saginata, Diphyllobothrium latum (tapeworms)	Worldwide	Pigs, bovine, fish	Stool examination for ova or proglottids	Praziquantel

but should be considered in immigrants from these areas. Frequently, the patient remembers a chancre at the site of the insect bite (E-Fig. 103-2). The diagnosis is made by microscopic examination of blood, lymph, or cerebrospinal fluid for the parasite (E-Figs. 103-3 and 103-4). Treatment varies by species and is highly toxic. Consultation with an expert in infectious disease or tropical medicine is recommended.

American Trypanosomiasis

American trypanosomiasis, or Chagas' disease, is caused by *Trypanosoma cruzi* and is endemic in Central and South America. Transmitted by contact with feces of reduviid bugs (kissing bugs) (E-Fig. 103-5), it can also be acquired through blood transfusion or organ transplantation from an infected individual. The risk to travelers is extremely low but increases with prolonged stays in poor-quality housing. The presentation has an acute phase of 3 months followed by a chronic infection for life. The classic acute presentation involves swelling and erythema of the eyelid and ocular tissue at the entry site of infection, known as the Romana sign. However, most individuals are asymptomatic throughout the infection and are identified only at the time of blood donation. Between 20% and 30% of individuals develop manifestations of chronic infection decades later that can include cardiomegaly and heart failure, megaesophagus, or megacolon.

Diagnosis in the acute phase is by microscopic examination of peripheral blood (E-Fig. 103-6). In the chronic phase, various serologic analyses are available to aid in diagnosis. Treatment is recommended early because it may prevent chronic manifestations. In the United States, antitrypansomal drugs are available through the CDC in consultation with an expert in the field. For most chronic manifestations, however, treatment is supportive.

⬤ HELMINTHIC INFECTIONS

Infestation by nematodes, or roundworms, is the most common parasitic infection in the world. The intestinal nematodes *Ascaris* and *Trichuris* are the two most prevalent types. Other important helminths include *Strongyloides, Enterobius*, schistosomes, and tapeworms (see later discussion). Although most helminths are found worldwide, they disproportionately affect the developing world and pose potential risk to travelers to those areas (Table 103-2).

Helminthic Infections Common in the United States

Pinworm

Enterobiasis is common in the United States and worldwide. Children are predominantly infected, and transmission is by the fecal-oral route. The clinical presentation is perianal pruritus. Diagnosis is made by the tape test, in which transparent tape is applied to the perianal skin overnight and then examined microscopically for ova on the tape. Treatment is with mebendazole.

Roundworm

Ascaris lumbricoides is found worldwide, including in the United States, but mostly affects people in the developing world. Although affected individuals are usually asymptomatic, some develop pulmonary infiltrates during the migration phase of the worm or obstruction of the biliary, pancreatic, or intestinal tract. These manifestations usually occur in the setting of high worm burden. Diagnosis is by stool examination for ova and parasites (E-Fig. 103-7). Treatment is with mebendazole.

Whipworm

Trichuris trichiura are called whipworms because of their characteristic shape in the adult form. Like *Ascaris*, this is an intestinal nematode that infects mostly children. It is usually asymptomatic except in the setting of heavy worm burden, which can lead to rectal prolapse and bloody diarrhea among children in the developing world. Diagnosis is made by stool examination for ova and parasites or by endoscopy revealing colitis and the presence of adult worms. The treatment of choice is mebendazole.

Hookworm

Ancylostoma duodenale and *Necator americanus* (hookworms) are similar to roundworms in their worldwide distribution and are common among immigrants from Asia and sub-Saharan Africa. Infection occurs through direct penetration of the skin by the larvae, which travel through the lymphatics and the bloodstream to the lungs and are then swallowed. Infected individuals may be asymptomatic, or they may develop pruritic dermatitis at the site of entry. As with the roundworm, pulmonary infiltrates can occur during the migration phase; this is known as Loeffler's syndrome. Chronic iron deficiency anemia associated with heavy hookworm infection can be severe and debilitating. Eosinophilia is common. The diagnosis is made by stool examination for ova and parasites (E-Fig. 103-8). The treatment is mebendazole.

Helminth Infections Common in Travelers and Immigrants

Strongyloidosis

Strongyloides stercoralis is a helminthic parasite that is found worldwide, although more commonly in the tropics. Infection occurs from contact with contaminated soil; the larva penetrates the skin, migrates to the lungs, and is then swallowed by the individual. The infection is usually asymptomatic, but infection can persist into the chronic phase decades later. Those with symptoms usually have gastrointestinal complaints of bloating, diarrhea, and abdominal pain. Eosinophilia is a common finding in these individuals. In immunocompromised individuals, a hyperinfection syndrome with dissemination of the organism can occur. Hyperinfection syndrome has a higher mortality rate and occurs usually in immigrants who become immunosuppressed as a result of chemotherapy, use of steroids, or illness. Diagnosis is made by stool examination (approximately 30% to 50% sensitivity) (E-Fig. 103-9) or by serology but does not distinguish between chronic and acute disease. Treatment is with ivermectin for 2 days; in the setting of hyperinfection, a longer course is required.

Schistosomiasis

Schistosomiasis is found throughout the tropics and the developing world. Also known as blood flukes, schistosomes use freshwater mollusks as their intermediate host and penetrate the skin of individuals, leading to infection. The three major species are: *Schistosoma mansoni* (Africa, Middle East, South America), *Schistosoma haematobium* (Africa, Middle East), and *Schistosoma japonicum* (China, Philippines, and Southeast Asia). Acute infection can manifest with dermatitis, although most cases are asymptomatic. Chronic infection develops from the immune response to egg deposition. *S. haematobium* can lead to urinary obstruction or hematuria, whereas *S. mansoni* and *S. japonicum* can lead to hepatosplenomegaly, hepatic fibrosis, obstruction of portal blood flow, and varices. *S. japonicum* can infect the central nervous system causing ring enhancing lesions and seizures. Diagnosis is by examination of stool or urine for schistosome eggs in individuals from endemic areas, who have a high egg burden; among travelers, in whom the egg burden is usually low, serology is used for diagnosis The treatment of choice is praziquantel.

Lymphatic Filariasis (Elephantiasis)

Wuchereria bancrofti and *Brugia malayi* are found throughout the tropics; they are lymph-dwelling filariae that cause elephantiasis. The presentation can vary from acute lymphadenitis, to asymptomatic microfilaremia, filarial fevers, or tropical pulmonary eosinophilia. Lymphadentitis can involve both upper and lower extremities with both of these filarial species, but scrotal involvement only occurs with *W. bancrofti*. The diagnosis is made by examination of a peripheral blood smear for microfilariae obtained between 10 PM and 4 AM because these organisms are nocturnally periodic.

Diethylcarbamazine is used for lymphatic filariasis to eradicate the microfilariae and the adult worms. However, the management of chronic lymphatic obstruction remains a challenge because it is not fully reversible and requires supportive therapy.

Loa loa (Eyeworm)

Loiasis is caused by the eyeworm (*Loa loa*) and is found in West and Central Africa. Presentation can vary and may include pruritus, subcutaneous swellings, joint manifestations, or neurologic symptoms. In the rarest presentation, the adult worm can be seen in the anterior chamber of the individual's eye. Diagnosis is confirmed by the presence of microfilariae in blood samples or isolation of the adult worm. Treatment is as for lymphatic filariasis, with diethylcarbamazine.

River Blindness

Onchocerca volvulus infection mostly occurs in regions of West and Central Africa but also in South and Central America. Pruritic dermatitis is the most common presentation; but involvement of the eye is the most serious presentation. Ocular involvement occurs in endemic areas in individuals with heavy worm burden. The complications can begin with conjunctivitis and photophobia. Corneal involvement with the microfilariae causes an inflammatory reaction leading to sclerosing keratitis and blindness. River blindness is the most common cause of blindness in Africa. The diagnosis is made by examination of skin snips for microfilariae. Ivermectin is the drug of choice; an initial single dose is followed by a repeat dose at 3 or 6 months to suppress any further microfilariae.

Clonorchiasis

Clonorchis sinensis is the Chinese liver fluke. This is an important infection to consider in Asian immigrants who have symptoms consistent with biliary tract disease, including right upper quadrant pain, anorexia, and weight loss. Though the disease is uncommon, untreated infections can lead to cholangiocarcinoma. Treatment is curative with praziquantel in 85% of cases.

Cysticercosis

Cysticercosis is caused by the pork tapeworm, *Taenia solium*. Individuals report new-onset seizures or headaches. Head computed tomographic (CT) scans show ring-enhancing lesions. The diagnosis is usually based on the history and imaging findings, and confirmation can be made by immunoblot assay. Treatment depends on the site of infection and symptoms. It may include antiparasitic treatment, antiseizure medications, and surgical removal. The antiparasitic drug of choice is praziquantel or albendazole. Expert consultation before treatment is recommended because of the risk of increasing focal cerebral edema and seizure activity.

Intestinal Tapeworms

Tapeworms that commonly infect humans include *Taenia solium* (from raw pork), *Taenia saginata* (raw beef), and *Diphyllobothrium latum* (raw fish). Most infections are asymptomatic except in the case of invasive disease with *T. solium,* as discussed earlier (see Cysticercosis). Praziquantel is the treatment of choice for all three tapeworms.

Echinococcus

The tapeworm *Echinococcus granulosus* causes hydatid disease with production of a cystic liver mass. This occurs in immigrants from sheep-raising parts of the world such as South America, Central Asia, and the Middle East. The characteristic appearance of the cyst includes a calcified wall with a dependent hydatid on CT scans. This appearance and the supporting history help to make the diagnosis; the serologic testing available can be falsely negative. Treatment is surgical removal of the cyst without rupture or spillage of the contents. Albendazole is usually given before surgical removal.

Less common is *Echinococcus multilocularis,* which causes alveolar cyst disease. This more aggressive infection leads to liver lesions as well as brain and lung involvement. Treatment includes resection of liver lesions in combination with antiparasitic therapy with mebendazole or albendazole. However, these agents are not parasitocidal, so the mortality rate remains high. Other potential therapies, such as amphotericin B and nitazoxanide, are being explored.

SUGGESTED READINGS

Arguin P: Approach to the patient before and after travel. In Goldman L, Schafer A, editors: Cecil Textbook of Medicine, ed 24, Philadelphia, 2012, Saunders, pp 1800–1803.

Centers for Disease Control and Prevention: CDC Health Information for International Travel 2014, New York, 2014, Oxford University Press.

Jeronimo S, de Queiroz Sousa A, Pearson R: Leishmaniasis. In Guerrant RL, Walker DH, Weller PF, editors: Tropical Infectious Diseases: Principles, Pathogens, and Practices, ed 3, Philadelphia, 2011, Saunders, pp 696–706.

Kirchoff L: Trypanosoma species (American trypanosomiasis, Chagas' disease): biology of trypanosomes. In Mandell GL, Bennett JE, Dolin R, editors: Principles and Practice of Infectious Diseases, ed 7, Philadelphia, 2010, Churchill Livingstone, pp 3481–3488.

Leder K, Torresi J, Libman M, et al: GeoSentinel surveillance of illness in returned travelers, 2007-2011, Ann Intern Med 158:456–468, 2013.

U.S. Department of Commerce, Office of Travel and Tourism Industries: Profile of U.S. resident travelers visiting overseas destinations: 2011 Outbound. Available at: http://travel.trade.gov/outreachpages/download_data_table/2011_Outbound_Profile.pdf. Accessed November 3, 2014.

XVI

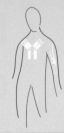

Neurologic Disease

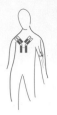

104

Neurologic Evaluation of the Patient

Frederick J. Marshall

INTRODUCTION

To arrive at an accurate neurologic diagnosis, the clinician generates and tests hypotheses about the location and the mechanism of injury to the nervous system. Hypotheses are refined as the clinician progresses from the interview to the physical examination to the laboratory assessment of the patient. The focus is first placed on entities that are common, serious, and treatable. Typical clinical presentations of patients with common diseases account for 80% of cases, unusual presentations of patients with common diseases account for 15%, typical presentations of patients with rare diseases account for 5%, and unusual presentations of patients with rare diseases account for less than 1%.

TAKING A NEUROLOGIC HISTORY

The clinician must determine the location, quality, and timing of symptoms. He or she must ask the patient to report the progression of symptoms rather than a litany of diagnostic procedures and specialty evaluations. Establishing when the patient last felt normal is important. Ambiguous descriptors such as *dizzy* should be rejected in favor of evocative descriptors such as *light-headed* (which may implicate cardiovascular insufficiency) or *off balance* (which may implicate cerebellar or posterior column dysfunction).

Family members and other witnesses should corroborate historical information when appropriate. Historical information should include the medical and surgical histories; current medications; allergies; family history; review of systems; and social history, including the patient's level of education, work history, possible toxin exposures, substance use, sexual history, current life circumstance, and overall function.

Clues to localization are sought during the interview. For example, pain is usually caused by a lesion of the peripheral nervous system, whereas aphasia (i.e., disordered language processing) indicates an abnormality of the central nervous system. Because sensory and motor functions are anatomically relatively distant in the cerebral cortex but progressively closer together as fibers converge in the brain stem, spinal cord, roots, and peripheral nerves, the coexistence of sensory loss and motor dysfunction in a limb implies a large lesion at the level of the cortex or a smaller lesion lower down in the neuraxis. Small lesions in areas of high traffic such as the spinal cord or brain stem can result in widespread neurologic dysfunction, whereas small lesions elsewhere may be asymptomatic.

Table 104-1 lists the potential localizing values of common neurologic symptoms to help address the issue of lesion localization. Tables 104-2 and 104-3 list symptoms that are commonly associated with lesions at specific locations in the nervous system. Some symptoms can result from a lesion at any of several levels of the nervous system. For example, double vision can result from a focal lesion in the brain stem, peripheral nerves (cranial nerve III, IV, or VI), neuromuscular junction, or extraocular muscles; or it can be nonfocal and result from an increase in intracranial pressure. Associated symptoms (or their lack) may lead the interviewer to reject certain hypotheses that at first seemed most likely. Table 104-4 lists the most important types of neuropathologic conditions and provides examples of diseases in each category.

Some neuroanatomic locations point to a specific diagnosis or a limited number of diagnoses. For example, disease of the neuromuscular junction is usually caused by an autoimmune process such as myasthenia gravis (common) or Eaton-Lambert myasthenic syndrome (uncommon). The exceptions—botulism and congenital myasthenic disorders—are rare. Alternatively, some areas of the nervous system (e.g., the cerebral hemispheres) are vulnerable to practically any of the categories of disease outlined in Table 104-4.

The pace and temporal order of symptoms are important. Degenerative diseases usually progress gradually, whereas vascular diseases (e.g., stroke, aneurysmal subarachnoid hemorrhage) progress rapidly. Certain symptoms such as double vision almost invariably develop abruptly, even if the underlying disorder has been developing gradually over days to weeks.

TABLE 104-1	POTENTIAL LOCALIZING VALUE OF COMMON NEUROLOGIC SYMPTOMS
POTENTIAL LOCALIZING VALUE	**SIGN OR SYMPTOM**
High	Focal weakness, sensory loss, or pain
	Focal visual loss
	Language disturbance
	Neglect or anosognosia
Medium	Vertigo
	Dysarthria
	Clumsiness
Low	Fatigue
	Headache
	Insomnia
	Dizziness
	Anxiety, confusion, or psychosis

TABLE 104-2 SYMPTOM LOCALIZATION IN THE CENTRAL NERVOUS SYSTEM

SIGN OR SYMPTOM	LOCATION
CEREBRAL HEMISPHERES	
Unilateral weakness or sensory complaints	Contralateral cerebral hemisphere
Language dysfunction	Left hemisphere (frontal and temporal)
Spatial disorientation	Right hemisphere (parietal and occipital)
Anosognosia (lack of insight into deficit)	Right hemisphere (parietal)
Hemivisual loss	Contralateral hemisphere (occipital, temporal, and parietal)
Flattening of affect or social disinhibition	Bihemispheric (frontal and limbic)
Alteration of consciousness	Bihemispheric (diffuse)
Alteration of memory	Bihemispheric (hippocampus, fornix, amygdala, and mammillary bodies)
CEREBELLUM	
Limb clumsiness	Ipsilateral cerebellar hemisphere
Unsteadiness of gait or posture	Midline cerebellar structures
BASAL GANGLIA	
Slowness of voluntary movement	Substantia nigra and striatum
Involuntary movement	Striatum, thalamus, and subthalamus
BRAIN STEM	
Contralateral weakness or sensory complaints in the body with ipsilateral weakness or sensory complaints in the face	Midbrain, pons, and medulla
Double vision	Midbrain and pons
Vertigo	Pons and medulla
Alteration of consciousness	Midbrain, pons, medulla (reticular formation)
SPINAL CORD	
Weakness and spasticity (ipsilateral) and anesthesia (contralateral) below a specified level	Corticospinal and spinothalamic tracts
Unsteadiness of gait	Posterior columns
Bilateral (can be asymmetrical) weakness and sensory complaints in multiple contiguous radicular distributions	Central cord

TABLE 104-3 SYMPTOM LOCALIZATION IN THE MOTOR UNIT*

SIGN OR SYMPTOM	LOCATION
ANTERIOR HORN CELL	
Weakness and wasting with muscle twitching (fasciculation) but no sensory complaints	Anterior horn of spinal cord (diffuse or segmental)
SPINAL ROOT	
Weakness and sensory loss confined to a known radicular distribution (pain, a common feature, may spread)	Cervical, thoracic, lumbar, and sacral
PLEXUS	
Pain, weakness, and sensory loss in a limb; not limited to a single radicular or peripheral nerve distribution	Brachial and lumbosacral (may also be caused by polyradiculopathy)
NERVE	
Pain, distal weakness, and/or sensory changes confined to a single peripheral nerve distribution	Peripheral nerves (mononeuropathy)
Pain, distal weakness, and/or sensory changes affecting both sides symmetrically (usually starting in feet)	Peripheral nerves (polyneuropathy)
Pain, distal weakness, and/or sensory changes affecting scattered single peripheral nerve distributions	Peripheral nerves (mononeuropathy multiplex)
Unilateral special sensory loss	Cranial nerves I, II, V, VII, VIII, and IX
Unilateral facial weakness involving entire one half of face	Cranial nerve VII (ipsilateral)
NEUROMUSCULAR JUNCTION	
Progressive weakness with repeated use of a muscle; no sensory complaints	Ocular, pharyngeal, and skeletal
MUSCLE	
Proximal weakness; no sensory complaints	Diffuse and various patterns

*Anterior horn cell and the peripheral nervous system.

TABLE 104-4 CATEGORIES OF NEUROLOGIC DISEASE

DISEASE CATEGORY	EXAMPLE	DISEASE CATEGORY	EXAMPLE
GENETIC		**DEGENERATIVE**	
Autosomal dominant	Huntington's disease	Central	Parkinson's disease
Autosomal recessive	Friedreich's ataxia	Central and peripheral	Amyotrophic lateral sclerosis
X-linked recessive	Duchenne muscular dystrophy	**AUTOIMMUNE**	
Mitochondrial	Progressive external ophthalmoplegia	Central demyelinating	Multiple sclerosis
Sporadic	Down syndrome	Peripheral demyelinating	Guillain-Barré syndrome
NEOPLASTIC		Neuromuscular junction	Myasthenia gravis
Intrinsic	Glioblastoma	**TOXIC AND METABOLIC**	
Extrinsic	Metastatic melanoma	Endogenous	Uremic encephalopathy
Paraneoplastic	Cerebellar degeneration	Exogenous	Alcoholic neuropathy
VASCULAR		**OTHER STRUCTURAL**	
Stroke	Thrombotic, embolic, lacunar, hemorrhagic	Trauma	Spinal cord injury
Structural	Arteriovenous malformation	Hydrodynamic	Normal pressure hydrocephalus
Inflammatory	Cranial arteritis	Psychogenic	Hysterical paraparesis
INFECTIOUS			
Bacterial	Meningococcal meningitis		
Viral	Herpes encephalitis		
Protozoal	Toxoplasmosis		
Fungal	Cryptococcal meningitis		
Helminthic	Cysticercosis		
Prion	Creutzfeldt-Jakob disease		

NEUROLOGIC EXAMINATION

Performance of the main elements of a general screening neurologic examination is imperative (Table 104-5), but the examination should be tailored to confirm or disprove the clinical hypotheses generated from the patient's history. Unexpected signs must be explained, often with a return to the history for further clarification.

The examination is approached as if only one of two possible injuries has occurred—the final common pathway to a structure is disrupted, or the input to that pathway is disrupted (Fig. 104-1). In the case of the motor system, the *final common pathway* is the motor unit and includes the anterior horn cells giving rise to axons in a nerve, the nerve itself, the neuromuscular junction, and the muscle. Injury to any of these structures results in dysfunction of the muscle. Conversely, if these structures are intact, observing the muscle function may be possible under the right circumstances. If all modes of engaging the final common pathway fail to elicit a response, the clinician can conclude that the lesion is located somewhere within the final common pathway.

For example, a man with paralysis of facial movement on one side that is caused by a lesion of cranial nerve VII cannot smile voluntarily, close his eye, or wrinkle his forehead on the affected side. Spontaneous laughter or smiling as an automatic response to a joke also fails to move the paretic side. If the problem is central, however, facial movement with involuntary (spontaneous) smiling may be preserved or increased. This observation is common in patients with facial weakness caused by a stroke.

Central input to a final common pathway in the nervous system is usually tonically inhibitory. Damage to this input typically results in overactivity of the involved muscle group. Signs of damage to central inhibitory systems include spasticity and hyperreflexia (i.e., motor cortex, subcortical white matter,

---

TABLE 104-5 ELEMENTS OF A GENERAL SCREENING NEUROLOGIC EXAMINATION

SYSTEMIC PHYSICAL EXAMINATION

Head (trauma, dysmorphism, and bruits)
Neck (tone, bruits, and thyromegaly)
Cardiovascular (heart rate, rhythm, and murmurs; peripheral pulses and jugular venous distention)
Pulmonary (breathing pattern, cough and cyanosis)
Abdomen (hepatosplenomegaly)
Back and extremities (skeletal abnormalities, peripheral edema, and straight-leg raising)
Skin (neurocutaneous stigmata and hepatic stigmata)

MENTAL STATUS

Level of consciousness (awake, drowsy, and comatose)
Attention (coherent stream of thought, serial 7s)
Orientation (temporal and spatial)
Memory (short and long term)
Language (naming, repetition, comprehension, fluency, reading, and writing)
Visuospatial skills (clock drawing and figure copying)
Judgment, insight, thought content (psychotic)
Mood (depressed, manic, and anxious)

CRANIAL NERVES

Olfactory (smell in each nostril)
Optic (afferent pupillary function, funduscopic examination, visual acuity, visual fields, and structural eye findings)
Oculomotor, trochlear, and abducens (smooth pursuit and saccadic eye movements, nystagmus, efferent pupillary function, and eyelid opening)
Trigeminal (jaw jerk, facial sensation, afferent corneal reflex, and muscles of mastication)
Facial (efferent corneal reflex, facial expression, eyelid closure, nasolabial folds, and power and bulk)
Vestibulocochlear (nystagmus, speech discrimination, Weber test, and Rinne test)
Glossopharyngeal and vagus (afferent and efferent gag reflex and uvula position)
Spinal accessory (power and bulk of sternocleidomastoid and trapezii muscles)
Hypoglossal (position, bulk, and fasciculations of tongue)

MOTOR EXAMINATION

Pronator drift (subtle corticospinal lesion)
Tone and bulk of muscles (basal ganglia lesion yields rigidity, cerebellar lesion yields hypotonia, corticospinal lesion yields spasticity, nonspecific bihemispheric disease yields paratonia, hypertrophy indicates dystonia, pseudohypertrophy indicates muscle disease, and atrophy indicates lower motor neuron disease)
Adventitious movements (tremor, tic, dystonia, and chorea indicate disease of the basal ganglia; asterixis and myoclonus may indicate toxic metabolic process)
Power of major muscle groups (scale 0-5)

Upper extremities: deltoids, biceps, triceps, wrist extension and flexion, finger extension and flexion, and interossei
Lower extremities: hip flexion, extension, abduction, and adduction; knee extension and flexion; ankle dorsiflexion, plantar flexion, inversion, and eversion; toe extension and flexion

SENSORY EXAMINATION

Light touch (posterior columns)
Pinprick (spinothalamic tract)
Temperature (spinothalamic tract)
Joint position sense (posterior columns)
Vibration (posterior columns)
Graphesthesia (cortical sensory)
Double simultaneous stimulation (cortical sensory)
Two-point discrimination (posterior columns and cortical sensory)

REFLEX EXAMINATION

Standard reflexes (grades 0-4)
Biceps
Triceps
Brachioradialis
Knee jerk
Ankle jerk
Pathologic reflexes
Babinski's sign (if present)
Myerson's sign (if present)
Snout (if present)
Jaw jerk (if brisk)
Palmomental (if present)
Hoffmann sign (if brisk)

COORDINATION AND GAIT

Finger-nose-finger (action tremor suggesting cerebellar disease)
Rapid alternating movements (dysdiadochokinesia suggesting cerebellar disease)
Fine motor movements (slowness and small amplitude suggesting basal ganglia or corticospinal tract abnormalities)
Heel-to-shin (ataxia suggesting cerebellar disease)
Arising from chair with arms folded across chest (inability in advanced basal ganglia, cerebellar, corticospinal, or muscle disease)
Walking naturally (look for decreased arm swing, spasticity, broad base, festination, waddle, footdrop, start hesitation, and dystonia)
Tandem gait (look for ataxia)
Walking with feet everted or inverted (look for latent dystonia)
Hopping on each foot separately (look for latent dystonia)
Stand with feet together and eyes open, eyes closed (sensory ataxia and cerebellar disease)
Response to retropulsive stress (loss of postural righting mechanisms)

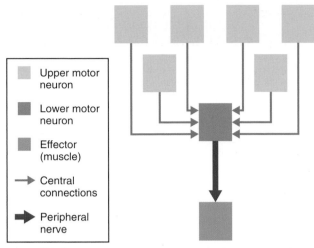

FIGURE 104-1 The nervous system can be conceptually reduced to a series of higher-order inputs that converge on final common pathways. For example, upper motor neurons converge on lower motor neurons, whose axons form the final common pathway to an effector muscle.

Legend in figure:
- Upper motor neuron
- Lower motor neuron
- Effector (muscle)
- → Central connections
- ➤ Peripheral nerve

TABLE 104-6	INDICATIONS FOR LUMBAR PUNCTURE

URGENT (DO NOT WAIT FOR BRAIN IMAGING)

Acute central nervous system infection in the absence of focal neurologic signs

LESS URGENT (WAIT FOR BRAIN IMAGING)

Vasculitis, subarachnoid hemorrhage, or cryptic process
Increased intracranial pressure in the absence of mass lesion on magnetic resonance imaging or computed tomography
Intrathecal therapy for fungal or carcinomatous meningitis
Symptomatic treatment for headache from idiopathic intracranial hypertension or subarachnoid hemorrhage

or corticospinal pathways in the brain stem and spinal cord); dystonia, rigidity, tremor, and tic (i.e., basal ganglia or extrapyramidal systems); and ataxia and dysmetria (i.e., cerebellum). An exception is hypotonia, which is caused by cerebellar disease.

⬤ TECHNOLOGIC ASSESSMENT

Laboratory investigations and special testing should be used to confirm a clinical suggestion and to finalize the diagnosis. Testing should be selectively performed because of expense, risk, and discomfort to the patient. Frequently helpful tests are discussed in subsequent sections. Diagnostic tests should never be ordered without a specific differential diagnosis firmly in mind. Many neurodiagnostic tests disclose incidental abnormalities unrelated to a patient's symptomatic disease process.

Lumbar Puncture

Investigation of the cerebrospinal fluid (CSF) is indicated in a small number of specific circumstances, usually meningitis and encephalitis (Table 104-6). When taken, a CSF specimen should be routinely sent for laboratory testing to determine cell and differential counts, protein and glucose levels, and bacterial cultures. The CSF should also be examined for its color and clarity. Cloudy or discolored CSF should be centrifuged and examined for xanthochromia in comparison with water. Additional, special studies may be obtained as appropriate, including Gram stain; fungal, viral, and tuberculous cultures; cryptococcal and other antigens; tests for syphilis; Lyme titers; malignant cytologic patterns; paraneoplastic and other specific protein antibodies; and oligoclonal bands. Polymerase chain reaction for specific viruses may also be appropriate. Assessment of specific CSF proteins such as tau, phosphorylated tau, and amyloid-β in patients at risk for dementia is considered more useful in research than clinical settings. The 14-3-3 protein may be found in patients with rapid-onset dementia.

Recording the opening and closing pressures is important. Tissue infection in the region of the puncture site is an absolute contraindication to lumbar puncture. Relative contraindications include known or probable intracranial or spinal mass lesion, increased intracranial pressure as a result of mass lesions, coagulopathy caused by thrombocytopenia (usually correctable), anticoagulant therapy, and bleeding disorders.

Rare but severe complications of lumbar puncture include transtentorial or foramen magnum herniation, spinal epidural hematoma, spinal abscess, herniated or infected disk, meningitis, and adverse reaction to a local anesthetic agent. More common and relatively benign complications include headache and backache.

Tissue Biopsies

In selected specialty centers, a diagnostic biopsy is performed on various tissues, including brain, peripheral nerve (see Chapter 121), muscle (see Chapter 121), and skin. Occasionally, biopsy provides the only means of arriving at a definitive diagnosis.

Electrophysiologic Studies

Electrophysiologic studies include electroencephalography, electromyography, nerve conduction studies, and evoked potentials. These studies are helpful in situations in which the patient cannot be examined or interviewed adequately.

Electroencephalography is most often used to investigate seizures (see Chapter 118). It can document encephalopathy, in which case the background electrical activity of the brain is slowed, and it is also used in the evaluation of brain death.

Electromyography is useful in the differential diagnosis of muscle disease, neuromuscular junction disease, peripheral nerve disease, and anterior horn cell disease (see Chapter 121). Nerve conduction studies (see Chapters 122 and 123) may show decreased amplitude (characteristic of axonal neuropathy) or decreased velocity (characteristic of demyelinating neuropathy).

Visual-evoked potential studies are commonly used in the evaluation of possible multiple sclerosis (see Chapter 120). Asymmetrical slowing of the cortical response to visual pattern stimulation suggests demyelination in the optic nerve or central optic pathways. Brain stem auditory-evoked potential studies are useful in the diagnosis of diseases affecting cranial nerve VIII or its central projections. Lesions at the cerebellopontine angle and the brain stem cause abnormal delay in conduction. Brain stem auditory-evoked potentials are helpful in the diagnosis of deafness in infants. Somatosensory-evoked potentials are used to identify a slowing of central sensory conduction that results from demyelinating disease, compression, or metabolic derangements.

TABLE 104-7 MAGNETIC RESONANCE IMAGING VERSUS COMPUTED TOMOGRAPHY

MAGNETIC RESONANCE IMAGING (MRI)

Resolution 1-2 mm (higher with newer 3-Tesla magnets)
Gadolinium contrast relatively safe, except in severe renal insufficiency
Unaffected by bone; multiple planes of imaging available; functional (physiologic) imaging capacity

COMPUTED TOMOGRAPHY

Resolution >5 mm
Iodine contrast associated with anaphylaxis and rash
Faster acquisition than MRI
Metallic objects such as pacemaker or aneurysm clip preclude MRI
Acute hemorrhage well visualized
Better tolerated by patients who are severely ill or claustrophobic

TABLE 104-8 NEUROLOGIC CONDITIONS FOR WHICH GENETIC TESTS ARE AVAILABLE

- Neuromuscular diseases: nerve (Charcot-Marie-Tooth disease); muscle (myotonic dystrophy, Duchenne-Becker muscular dystrophy); anterior horn cell (spinal muscular atrophy, familial amyotrophic lateral sclerosis)
- Movement disorders: spinocerebellar ataxia, multiple types; Friedreich's ataxia; dystonia (*DYT1* mutation); Huntington's disease
- Mental retardation (fragile X syndrome)
- Mitochondrial diseases: *mitochondrial encephalomyelopathy, lactic acidosis, and strokelike symptoms* (MELAS syndrome); *myoclonus epilepsy with ragged red fibers* (MERRF syndrome).

They are also used to evaluate spinal cord–mediated sensory abnormalities.

Imaging Studies

Magnetic resonance imaging (MRI) and computed tomography (CT) are high-resolution imaging techniques that provide extraordinary diagnostic precision for central nervous system lesions. Most neurologic diseases, however, can have normal CT and MRI findings. Moreover, many abnormal findings on CT and MRI bear no relation to the diagnosis responsible for the patient's symptoms.

Table 104-7 compares CT with MRI. MRI is used for most purposes, although CT has the advantage of wider accessibility, greater speed of acquisition, and better tolerability by the patient. CT detects acute hemorrhage and is preferred for emergencies. MRI provides more detail and simultaneously obtains images in the horizontal, vertical, and coronal planes. Contrast media for CT or MRI are useful in the diagnosis of tumors, abscesses, and other processes that derange the blood-brain barrier. MRI can be used for functional imaging and spectroscopy; both techniques have great promise for the evaluation of cognitive and metabolic disorders, epilepsy, multiple sclerosis, and many other conditions.

MR- and CT-angiography allow noninvasive visualization of the major vessels of the head and neck. Conventional angiography with an intra-arterial injection of contrast agent is used for evaluation of many intracranial vascular abnormalities, including small aneurysms and arteriovenous malformations, and inflammation of small blood vessels.

Noninvasive ultrasonography of the carotid and vertebral arteries can define stenotic vessels. It has been supplemented by transcranial Doppler technology, which allows characterization of blood flow in intracranial arteries.

Single-photon emission CT (SPECT) is useful for the evaluation of intracranial blood flow. The development of iodine-123 ioflupane injection (DaTscan) makes it possible to visualize the dopamine transporter to follow cell loss in patients with Parkinson's disease.

Positron-emission tomography (PET) is a functional imaging technology that can demonstrate specific metabolic derange-

ments. It is useful for evaluating local abnormalities of glucose and oxygen metabolism. PET is of particular value in defining the site of origin of focal seizures. Customized ligands may be used to identify specific pathologic processes. Examples include florbetapir F-18 (Amyvid), a U.S. Food and Drug (FDA)–approved agent for estimating β-amyloid neurotic plaque density in Alzheimer's disease, and fluorodopa F18, which is under FDA review for diagnostic use in Parkinson's disease.

Genetic and Molecular Testing

There are more neurologic diseases than diseases of all other systems combined. Discoveries have revolutionized the diagnostic approach to many of these diseases, and new genetic tests are discovered every year. Table 104-8 outlines the tests that are commercially available.

Genetic testing for a disorder requires the clinician to perform a thoughtful and caring evaluation of the patient, usually with input from and evaluation of the patient's family. Important ethical issues surround the use of genetic tests, including the ability to ensure privacy, to ensure adequate psychological and social support for patients who may be given devastating news, and to address adequately the appropriateness of prenatal screening or presymptomatic testing when no treatment is available.

PROSPECTUS FOR THE FUTURE

Novel imaging techniques and molecular diagnostic studies are beginning to shed light on the pathogenesis of neurologic conditions that have been identifiable only by clinical phenomenology. Studies of previously untreatable neurodegenerative disorders are now targeting presymptomatic individuals in the hope that earlier intervention can modify disease outcomes. Despite these and foreseeable future advances, the clinical aspects of neurologic disease remain fundamentally important in understanding the impact of disease on patients and their families.

SUGGESTED READINGS

Biller J, editor: Practical neurology, ed 4, Philadelphia, 2012, Lippincott Williams & Wilkins.
Griggs RC, Jozefowicz R, Aminoff MJ: Approach to the patient with neurologic disease. In Goldman L, Schafer AI, editors: Goldman's Cecil medicine, ed 24, Philadelphia, 2012, pp 2228–2235.

105

Disorders of Consciousness

Mohamad Chmayssani and Paul M. Vespa

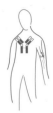

INTRODUCTION

Coma is a sleeplike state in that the patient is unresponsive and the eyes remain closed even with vigorous stimulation. A poorly responsive state in which the eyes are open, or an agitated and confused state, or delirium is not coma but may represent early stages of the same disease processes and should be investigated in the same manner.

Consciousness requires that the brainstem reticular activating system and its cortical projections be intact and functioning. The reticular formation begins in the midpons and ascends through the dorsal midbrain to synapse in the thalamus; it then innervates higher centers through thalamocortical connections. Knowledge of this anatomic substrate provides the short list of regions to be investigated in the search for a structural cause of coma: Brainstem or bihemispheric dysfunction satisfies these anatomic requirements, whereas structural lesions elsewhere are not the cause of the patient's unconsciousness. In addition to structural lesions, meningeal inflammation, metabolic encephalopathy, and seizures diffusely affect the brain and complete the differential diagnosis for the patient in coma.

PATHOPHYSIOLOGIC FACTORS

Meningeal irritation caused by infection or blood in the subarachnoid space is an essential early consideration in coma evaluation because its cause requires immediate attention (especially with purulent meningitis) and may not be diagnosed by computed tomography (CT).

Hemispheric mass lesions result in coma either by expanding across the midline laterally to compromise both cerebral hemispheres or by impinging on the brainstem to compress the rostral reticular formation. These processes—*lateral herniation* (lateral movement of the brain) and *transtentorial herniation* (vertical movement of the brain)—most commonly occur together. At the bedside, clinical signs of an expanding hemispheric mass evolve in a level-by-level, rostral-caudal manner (Fig. 105-1). Hemispheric lesions of adequate size to produce coma are readily seen on CT.

Brainstem mass lesions produce coma by directly affecting the reticular formation. Because the pathways for lateral eye movements—the pontine gaze center, medial longitudinal fasciculus, and oculomotor (third nerve) nucleus—traverse the

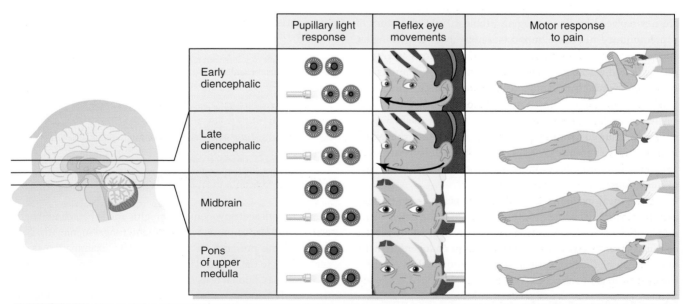

FIGURE 105-1 The evolution of neurologic signs in coma from a hemispheric mass lesion as the brain becomes functionally impaired in a rostral-caudal manner. The terms *early diencephalic* and *late diencephalic* refer to levels of dysfunction just above and just below the thalamus, respectively. (From Aminoff MJ, Greenberg DA, Simon RP: Clinical neurology, Stamford, Conn., 1996, Appleton and Lange.)

TABLE 105-1	MULTIFOCAL DISORDERS INDICATING METABOLIC COMA
Disseminated intravascular coagulopathy	Thrombotic thrombocytopenic purpura
Sepsis	Fat emboli
Pancreatitis	Hypertensive encephalopathy
Vasculitis	Diffuse micrometastases

reticular activating system, impairment of reflex eye movements is often the critical element of diagnosis of a brainstem lesion. A comatose patient without impaired reflex lateral eye movements does not have a mass lesion compromising brainstem structures in the posterior fossa. CT is not able to show some lesions in this region. Posterior fossa lesions may block the flow of cerebrospinal fluid from the lateral ventricles, resulting in the dangerous situation of *noncommunicating hydrocephalus.*

Metabolic abnormalities are caused by deficiency states (e.g., thiamine, glucose), by derangements of metabolism (e.g., hyponatremia), or by the presence of *exogenous toxins* (e.g., drugs) or *endogenous toxins* (e.g., organ system failure). Metabolic abnormalities result in diffuse dysfunction of the nervous system; therefore, with rare exceptions, they produce no localized signs such as hemiparesis or unilateral papillary dilation. The diagnosis of *metabolic encephalopathy* means that the examiner has found no focal anatomic features on examination or neuroimaging studies to explain coma but that a specific metabolic cause has not been established. Drugs have a predilection for affecting the reticular formation in the brainstem and for producing paralysis of reflex eye movement on examination. *Multifocal structural disorders* may simulate metabolic coma (Table 105-1).

In the late stages of status epilepticus, motor movements may be subtle even though *seizure activity* is continuing throughout the brain (nonconvulsive status epilepticus). Once seizures stop, the so-called *postictal state* can also cause unexplained coma.

DIAGNOSTIC APPROACH

The history and examination are essential in the diagnosis and are not replaced by brain imaging (Table 105-2). A history of a premonitory headache supports a diagnosis of meningitis, encephalitis, or intracerebral or subarachnoid hemorrhage. A preceding period of intoxication, confusion, or delirium points to a diffuse process such as meningitis or endogenous or exogenous toxins. The sudden apoplectic onset of coma is particularly suggestive of ischemic or hemorrhagic stroke affecting the brainstem or of subarachnoid hemorrhage or intracerebral hemorrhage with intraventricular rupture. Lateralized symptoms of hemiparesis or aphasia before coma occur in patients with hemispheric masses or infarctions.

The physical examination is critical, quickly accomplished, and diagnostic. The issues are three: (1) Does the patient have meningitis? (2) Are signs of a mass lesion present? and (3) Is this condition a diffuse syndrome of exogenous or endogenous metabolic etiology? Emergency management should then be instituted accordingly (Table 105-3).

Identification of Meningitis

Signs of meningeal irritation are not invariably present and have differing sensitivities depending on the cause: They are extremely

TABLE 105-2	CAUSES OF COMA WITH NORMAL COMPUTED TOMOGRAPHY SCAN
Meningeal disorders	Endogenous toxins, deficiencies, derangements
Subarachnoid hemorrhage (uncommon)	Hypoxia and ischemia
Bacterial meningitis	Hypoglycemia
Encephalitis	Hypercalcemia
Subdural empyema	
	Osmolar causes
Exogenous toxins	Hyperglycemia
Sedative drugs and barbiturates	Hyponatremia
Anesthetics and γ-hydroxybutyrate*	Hypernatremia
Alcohols	Organ system failure
Stimulants	Hepatic encephalopathy
Phencyclidine[†]	Uremic encephalopathy
Cocaine and amphetamine[‡]	Pulmonary insufficiency (carbon dioxide narcosis)
Psychotropic drugs	
Cyclic antidepressants	Seizures
Phenothiazines	Prolonged postictal state
Lithium	Spike-wave stupor
Anticonvulsants	Hypothermia or hyperthermia
Opioids	
Clonidine[§]	Brainstem ischemia
Penicillins	Basilar artery stroke
Salicylates	
Anticholinergics	Pituitary apoplexy
Carbon monoxide, cyanide, and methemoglobinemia	Conversion or malingering

*General anesthetic, similar to γ-aminobutyric acid; used as a recreational drug and body building aid. It has a rapid onset and rapid recovery, often with myoclonic jerking and confusion. It causes deep coma lasting 2 to 3 hours (Glasgow Coma Scale score = 3) with maintenance of vital signs.
[†]Coma associated with cholinergic signs: lacrimation, salivation, bronchorrhea, and hyperthermia.
[‡]Coma after seizures or status epilepticus (i.e., a prolonged postictal state).
[§]An antihypertensive agent that is active through the opiate receptor system; overdose is frequent when used to treat narcotic withdrawal.

TABLE 105-3	EMERGENCY MANAGEMENT

1. Ensure airway adequacy.
2. Support ventilation and circulation.
3. Obtain blood for glucose, electrolytes, hepatic and renal function, prothrombin and partial thromboplastin times, complete blood count, and drug screen.
4. Administer 100 mg of thiamine intravenously (IV).
5. Administer 25 g of dextrose IV (typically 50 mL of 50% dextrose) to treat possible hypoglycemic coma.*
6. Treat opiate overdose with naloxone (0.4-2 mg IV repeated every 2-3 minutes as needed).
7. The specific benzodiazepine antagonist flumazenil (0.2 mg IV every 1 min, x1-5 doses; max is 1 mg) should be given for reversal of benzodiazepine-induced coma or conscious sedation.[†]

*The glucose level is poorly correlated with the level of consciousness in hypoglycemia; stupor, coma, and confusion are reported with blood glucose concentrations ranging from 2 to 60 mg/dL.
[†]Not recommended in coma of unknown origin because seizures may be precipitated in patients with polydrug overdoses that include benzodiazepines with tricyclic antidepressants or cocaine.

common with acute pyogenic meningitis and subarachnoid hemorrhage and less common with indolent, fungal meningitis. Nevertheless, the presence of these signs on examination is the central clue to the diagnosis. Missing these signs results in time-consuming additional tests such as brain imaging and the potential loss of a narrow window of opportunity for directed therapy.

Passive neck flexion should be carried out (Fig. 105-2) in all comatose patients unless a history of head trauma exists. When the neck is passively flexed by attempting to bring the chin within

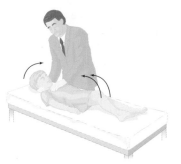

FIGURE 105-2 Elicitation of Brudzinski's sign of meningeal irritation, as seen in infectious meningitis or subarachnoid hemorrhage. (From Aminoff MJ, Greenberg DA, Simon RP: Clinical neurology, Stamford, Conn., 1996, Appleton and Lange.)

a few fingerbreadths of the chest, patients with irritated meninges reflexively flex one or both knees. This sign, called *Brudzinski's reflex*, is usually asymmetrical and not dramatic, but any evidence of knee flexion during passive neck flexion mandates that the cerebrospinal fluid be examined.

Is CT required before lumbar puncture in this setting? In the absence of lateralized signs (e.g., hemiparesis) supporting a superimposed mass lesion, a spinal puncture should be performed immediately. Although rare cases of herniation after lumbar puncture have been reported in children with bacterial meningitis, the urgency of diagnosis and treatment at the point of coma is paramount. The time required for CT may result in a fatal therapeutic delay. An alternative approach involves obtaining blood cultures and immediately initiating antibiotic therapy with subsequent lumbar puncture. With this approach, the cerebrospinal fluid cell count, glucose determination, and protein content are unchanged, and Gram stain and culture often remain positive despite a short period of antibiotic treatment. Bacterial antigens in the cerebrospinal fluid or blood can also be detected.

Separation of Structural from Metabolic Causes of Coma

The goal of this differential diagnosis is achieved by neurologic examination. Because the evaluation and potential treatments for structural and metabolic coma are widely divergent and the disease processes in both categories are often rapidly progressive, initiating prompt medical and surgical evaluation may be lifesaving. Identification of a structural versus a metabolic cause is accomplished by focusing on three features of the neurologic examination: the *motor response* to a painful stimulus, *pupillary function*, and *reflex eye movements*.

Motor Response

Asymmetrical or reflex function of the motor system provides the clearest indication of a mass lesion. Elicitation of a *motor response* requires that a painful stimulus be applied, to which the patient will react. The patient's arms should be placed in a semiflexed posture, and a painful stimulus should be applied to the head or trunk. Strong pressure on the supraorbital ridge or pinching of the skin on the anterior chest or inner arm is the most useful method; finger nail bed pressure is also used, but it makes the interpretation of upper limb movement difficult.

The neurologic examination of a patient with an expanding hemispheric mass lesion is shown in Figure 105-1. Hemispheric masses in their *early diencephalic* stage (i.e., compromising the brain above the thalamus), produce appropriate movement of one upper extremity—that is, movement toward the painful stimulus. The attenuated contralateral arm movement reflects a hemiparesis. This lateralized motor response in a comatose patient establishes the working diagnosis of a hemispheric mass. As the mass expands to involve the thalamus (*late diencephalic* stage), the response to pain becomes reflex arm flexion associated with extension and internal rotation of the legs (*decorticate posturing*); asymmetry of the response in the upper extremities is seen. With further brain compromise at the midbrain level, the reflex posturing in the arms changes such that both arms and legs respond by extension (*decerebrate posturing*); at that level, the asymmetry tends to be lost. At this point, the pupils become midposition in size, and the light reflex is lost, first unilaterally and then bilaterally. With further progression to the level of the pons, the most frequent finding is no response to painful stimulation, although spinal-mediated movements of leg flexion may occur.

The classic postures illustrated in Figure 105-1, and particularly their asymmetry, strongly support the presence of a mass lesion. However, these motor movements, especially early in coma, are most frequently seen as fragments of the fully developed, asymmetrical flexion or extension of the arms (illustrated as decorticate and decerebrate postures in Figure 105-1). A small amount of asymmetrical flexion or extension of the arms in response to a painful stimulus carries the same implications as the full-blown postures of decortication or decerebration.

Metabolic lesions do not compromise the brain in a progressive, level-by-level manner as do hemispheric masses, and they rarely produce the asymmetrical motor signs typical of masses. Reflex posturing may be seen, but it lacks the asymmetry of decortication seen with a hemispheric mass, and it is not associated with the loss of pupillary reactivity at the stage of decerebration.

Pupillary Reactivity

In metabolic coma, one feature is central to the examination: Pupillary reactivity is present. This reactivity is seen both early in metabolic coma, when an appropriate motor response to pain may be retained, and late in coma, when no motor responses can be elicited. The pupillary reaction in metabolic coma is lost only when coma is so deep that the patient requires ventilatory and blood pressure support.

Reflex Eye Movements

The presence of inducible lateral eye movements reflects the integrity of the pons and midbrain. These reflex eye movements (see Fig. 105-1) are brought about with the use of passive head rotation to stimulate the semicircular canal input to the vestibular system (so-called *doll's eyes maneuver*) or by inhibiting the function of one semicircular canal by infusing ice water against the tympanic membrane (caloric testing).

In metabolic coma, reflex eye movements may be lost or retained. Lack of inducible eye movements with the doll's eyes maneuver, in the setting of preserved pupillary reactivity, is virtually diagnostic of drug toxicity. With metabolic coma of non–drug-induced origin, such as organ system failure, electrolyte disorders, or osmolar disorders, reflex eye movements are preserved.

Brainstem mass lesions are most commonly caused by hemorrhage or infarction. Reflex lateral eye movements, the pathways for which traverse the pons and midbrain, are particularly affected, and the reflex postures of decortication and decerebration typical of brainstem injury are common. Lesions restricted to the midbrain (e.g., embolization from the heart to the top of the basilar artery) cause sluggish pupillary reflexes or their absence, with or without impaired medial eye movements; both are controlled by the third cranial nerve. With lesions restricted to the pons (e.g., intrapontine hypertensive hemorrhage), pupils are reactive but very small (pinpoint or pontine pupils), reflecting focal impairment of sympathetic innervations; pinpoint pupils are rare. Ocular bobbing (spontaneous symmetrical or asymmetrical rhythmic vertical ocular oscillations) is most often a manifestation of a pontine lesion.

Seizures occurring in a patient with acute brain injury (such as that resulting from encephalitis, hypertensive encephalopathy, hyponatremia, hypernatremia, hypoglycemia, or hyperglycemia) or chronic brain injury (such as dementia or mental retardation) often result in prolonged postictal coma. The examination shows reactive pupils and inducible eye movements (in the absence of overtreatment with anticonvulsants), and often up-going toes or focal signs are often observed (Todd's paresis).

Nonconvulsive status epilepticus should be considered as a diagnosis even if there are no obvious seizure movements. Nonconvulsive seizures can cause coma and also can complicate other etiologies of coma, including infectious and metabolic disorders. Nonconvulsive seizures should be suspected in patients with (1) a seemingly prolonged "postictal state" after generalized convulsive seizures or prolonged alteration of alertness after an operative procedure or neurologic insult; (2) acute onset of impaired consciousness or fluctuating mentation interspersed with episodes of normal awareness; (3) altered mental status or consciousness associated with facial myoclonus or nystagmoid eye movements; or (4) episodic blank staring, aphasia, automatisms e.g., lip-smacking, fumbling with fingers), or acute-onset aphasia without an acute structural lesion. The diagnosis is made by electroencephalography (EEG) (see Chapter 118). EEG provides information about brain electrical activity even when brain function is depressed and cannot be evaluated otherwise, as in comatose patients. EEG is essential to detect electrical seizures and document their duration as well as the response to therapy and to improve coma prognostication.

Current evidence suggests that the presence of nonconvulsive seizures or periodic discharges, delay to diagnosis, and duration of nonconvulsive status in patients with or without acute brain injury are independent predictors of worse outcome.

● PROGNOSIS IN COMA

Therapeutic hypothermia has been demonstrated to improve neurologic outcomes in patients who have return of spontaneous circulation but remain comatose after cardiac arrest. Historically, prognostication after cardiac arrest was solely based on neurologic examination. Although this still holds true for the most part,

there has been extensive work using additional means besides the physical examination to better predict prognosis. Pupillary, corneal, and motor responses are the best clinical indicators of prognosis that can be assessed at bedside. Such responses give some indication of the functionality of the brainstem, which is the most resilient portion of central nervous system. Any signs of damage to the brainstem is strong evidence of cortical injury (Fig 105-3).

Current guidelines endorse the utility of EEG for predicting poor outcome in comatose survivors of cardiac arrest not treated with hypothermia. The early onset of generalized myoclonic status is an ominous sign. Serum biomarkers have been used in evaluating prognosis among comatose patients after cardiac arrest. Neuron-specific enolase (NSE) is the most promising biomarker and has been extensively studied. NSE levels of >30 ng/mL or higher have been found to predict persistent coma. Similarly, somatosensory evoked potentials (SSEPs), as electrophysiologic markers, are most helpful for predicting which patients will remain in a persistent coma. In particular, the bilateral absence of the N20 cortical response (a negative peak at 20 ms) to median nerve stimulation after 24 hours predicts a grave outcome. Despite tremendous potential, the role of neuroimaging as a prognostic tool after hypoxic-ischemic injury from cardiac arrest has yet to be clearly defined. Severe reductions in the apparent diffusion coefficient (ADC), as well as bilateral

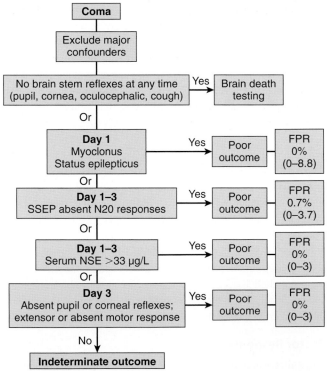

FIGURE 105-3 Decision algorithm for use in prognostication of comatose survivors after cardiopulmonary resuscitation (CPR). The numbers in parentheses show the exact 95% confidence intervals. FPR, False-positive rate; N20, a negative peak at 20 ms on SSEP; NSE, neuron-specific enolase; SSEP, somatosensory evoked potential. (Data from Wijdicks EFM, Hijdra A, Young GB, et al: Practice parameter: prediction of outcome in comatose survivors after CPR [an evidence-based review]: report of the Quality Standards Subcommittee of the American Academy of Neurology, Neurology 67:203–210, 2006.)

hippocampal hyperintensities on magnetic resonance imaging (MRI), suggests severe global damage and extensive ischemic injury and is highly indicative of poor outcome.

The use of therapeutic hypothermia quite likely influences the clinical examination and ancillary test findings. There is a scarcity of data about the utility of physical examination, EEG, and evoked potentials in predicting outcomes among cardiac arrest patients with induced hypothermia. It is well accepted that one should consider observation for longer than 72 hours before prognosticating outcome in patients treated with hypothermia.

COMA-LIKE STATES

Patients with *locked-in syndrome* have a lesion (usually a hemorrhage or an infarct) that transects the brainstem at a point below the reticular formation (thereby sparing consciousness) but above the ventilatory nuclei of the medulla (thereby maintaining cardiopulmonary function) (Table 105-4). Such patients are awake, with eye opening and sleep-wake cycles, but the descending pathways through the brainstem that are necessary for volitional vocalization or limb movement have been transected. Voluntary eye movement, especially vertically, is preserved, and patients can open and close their eyes or produce appropriate numbers of blinking movements in answer to questions. The EEG is usually normal, reflecting normal cortical function.

Psychogenic unresponsiveness is a diagnosis of exclusion. The neurologic examination shows reactive pupils and no reflex posturing in response to pain. Eye movements during the doll's eyes maneuver show volitional override rather than the smooth, uninhibited reflex lateral eye movements of coma. Ice water caloric testing either arouses the patient because of the discomfort produced or induces cortically mediated nystagmus rather than the tonic deviation typical of coma. The slow, conjugate roving eye movements of metabolic coma cannot be imitated and therefore rule out psychogenic unresponsiveness. Likewise, the slow, often asymmetrical, and incomplete eye closure seen after passive eye opening in a comatose patient cannot be feigned and also rules out psychogenic coma. In contrast, conscious patients usually exhibit some voluntary muscle tone in the eyelids during passive eye opening. The EEG in psychogenic unresponsiveness is that of normal wakefulness, with reactive posterior rhythms on eye opening and eye closing. In patients with catatonic stupor, lorazepam administration may produce awakening.

The vegetative state (VS), now also called *unresponsive wakefulness syndrome*, is exhibited by patients with eye opening and sleep-wake cycles. The reticular activating system of the brainstem is intact to produce wakefulness, but the connections to the cortical mantle are interrupted, precluding awareness.

A VS is termed *persistent* after 3 months if the brain injury was medical or after 12 months if the brain injury was traumatic. The determination as to when *persistent* equals *permanent* cannot be stated absolutely. Prediction early in VS of which patients will remain persistently vegetative is particularly difficult in cases of trauma. Lesions of the corpus callosum and dorsolateral brainstem seen on MRI 6 to 8 weeks after trauma correlated with persistence of VS at 1 year. A combined analysis of morphologic MRI studies and post-traumatic brainstem spectroscopy can be a predictor of persistent vegetative states (PVS) and minimally conscious states (MVS). In rare cases, patients show late improvement, but they do not return to normal. Bilateral absence of SSEPs in the first week predicts death or VS.

Patients in a PVS open their eyes diurnally and in response to loud sounds; blinking occurs with bright lights. Pupils react, and eye movements occur both spontaneously and with the doll's eyes maneuver. Yawning, chewing, swallowing, and, uncommonly, guttural vocalizations and lacrimation may be preserved. Spontaneous roving eye movements (very slow, with constant velocity) are particularly characteristic and distressing to the patient's visitors because the patient appears to be looking about the room. The brainstem origin of the eye movements is documented by their being readily redirected by the oculocephalic (doll's eyes) reflex. The limbs may move, but motor responses are only primitive; pain usually produces decorticate or decerebrate postures or fragments of these movements.

MCS is a newly described entity in which patients do not meet criteria for PVS. Both patients in PVS and those in MCS demonstrate severe alteration in consciousness. In contrast to PVS, subjects with MCS exhibit evidence of limited interaction with the environment by visually tracking, following simple commands, answering yes or no (not necessarily reliably), or having intelligible verbalization or restricted purposeful behavior. It is estimated that the rate of misdiagnosis between the VS and MCS is about 40%.

Novel applications of functional neuroimaging in patients with disorders of consciousness may aid in differential diagnosis, prognostic assessment, and identification of pathophysiologic mechanisms. In one study, authors prospectively evaluated cortical activation in response to a familiar voice in seven patients in VS and four subjects in MCS. All four of the MCS patients and only two of the VS patients showed activation that extended beyond the primary auditory cortex to hierarchically higher-order associative temporal areas. Over the course of 3 months, these two VS patients improved clinically to MCS.

Brain death characterizes the *irreversible cessation* of brain function. Therefore, death of the organism can be determined based on death of the brain. Although local laws may dictate some details, the standard definition permits a diagnosis of brain death based on documentation of irreversible cessation of all brain function, including function of the brainstem (Table 105-5). Documentation of *irreversibility* requires that the cause of the coma is known, that the cause is adequate to explain the clinical

TABLE 105-4	LOCKED-IN SYNDROME	
Clinical features	**Recovery possible**
Eye opening	Onset over 1-12 wk (vascular)* *or*
Reactive pupils	Onset over 4-6 mo (nonvascular)*
Volitional vertical eye movements in response to command	
Muteness	**Prognosis favorable**
Quadriparesis	Normal CT scan*
Sleep-wake cycles	Early recovery of lateral eye movements*
Causes	
Pontine vascular lesions (common)	
Head injury, brainstem tumor, pontine myelinolysis (rare)	

CT, Computed tomography.
*Implications for care.

TABLE 105-5 CRITERIA FOR CESSATION OF BRAIN FUNCTION*

ANATOMIC REGION TESTED	CONFIRMATORY SIGN
Hemispheres	Unresponsive and unreceptive to sensory stimuli including pain[†]
Midbrain	Unreactive pupils[‡]
Pons	Absent reflex eye movements[§]
Medulla	Apnea[‖]

CO_2, Carbon dioxide; PCO_2, partial pressure of carbon dioxide.

*Sequential testing is necessary for a clinical diagnosis of brain death; it should be done at least every 6 hours in all cases and at least every 24 hours in the setting of anoxic-ischemic brain injury.

[†]The patient does not rouse, groan, grimace, or withdraw limbs. Purely spinal reflexes (deep tendon reflexes, plantar flexion reflex, plantar withdrawal, and tonic neck reflexes) may be maintained.

[‡]Most easily assessed by the bright light of an ophthalmoscope viewed through its magnifying lens when focused on the iris. Unreactive pupils may be either midposition, as they will be in death, or dilated, as they often are in the setting of a dopamine infusion.

[§]No eye movement toward the side of irrigation of the tympanic membrane with 50 mL of ice water. The oculocephalic response (doll's eyes maneuver) is always absent in the setting of absent oculovestibular testing.

[‖]No ventilatory movements in the setting of maximum CO_2 stimulation (≥60 mm Hg); with apnea, PCO_2 passively rises 2 to 3 mm Hg/min). Disconnect the ventilator from the endotracheal tube and insert a cannula with 6 L of oxygen per minute.

TABLE 105-6 EXCLUSIONARY CRITERIA FOR BRAIN DEATH

Seizures	Hypothermia (<32.2° C)
Decorticate or decerebrate posturing	Neuromuscular blockade
Sedative drugs	Shock

TABLE 105-7 CONFIRMATORY TESTS FOR BRAIN DEATH

EEG isoelectricity	Deep coma from sedative drugs or hypothermia (temperature <20° C) can produce EEG flattening.
Nuclear medicine	The most common radionuclide modality for brain imaging uses the tracer HMPAO. Absence of isotope uptake ("hollow skull phenomenon") indicates no brain perfusion and supports the diagnosis of brain death.
Transcranial Doppler	Findings of small systolic peaks without diastolic flow or a reverberating flow pattern suggest high vascular resistance and support the diagnosis of brain death. No cerebral blood flow is the most definitive confirmatory test.
CT angiography	Nonopacification of the cortical segments of MCAs and ICVs appears to be highly sensitive for confirming brain death, with a specificity of 100%. Lack of opacification of the ICVs is the most sensitive sign.

CT, Computed tomographic; EEG, electroencephalogram; HMPAO, ^{99m}Tc-labeled hexamethylpropyleneamineoxime; ICV, internal cerebral vein; MCA, middle cerebral artery.

findings of brain death, and that exclusionary criteria are absent (Table 105-6). Confirmatory tests are sometimes used but are not required for diagnosis (Table 105-7). Brain death results in asystole, usually within days (mean, 4 days), even if ventilatory support is continued. Recovery after appropriate documentation of brain death has never been reported. Removal of the ventilator results in terminal rhythms (most often complete heart block without ventricular response), junctional rhythms, or ventricular tachycardia. Purely spinal motor movements may occur in the moments of terminal apnea (or during apnea testing in the absence of passive administration of oxygen); these may include arching of the back, neck turning, stiffening of the legs, and upper extremity flexion.

SUGGESTED READINGS

Bernard SA, Gray TW, Buist MD, et al: Treatment of comatose survivors of out-of-hospital cardiac arrest with induced hypothermia, N Engl J Med 346:557–563, 2002.

Bernat JL: Chronic disorders of consciousness, Lancet 367:1181–1192, 2006.

Fins JJ, Master MG, Gerber LM, et al: The minimally conscious state: a diagnosis in search of an epidemiology, Arch Neurol 64:1400–1405, 2007.

Greer DM, Scripko PD, Wu O, et al: Hippocampal magnetic resonance imaging abnormalities in cardiac arrest are associated with poor outcome, J Stroke Cerebrovasc Dis 22:899–905, 2013.

Laureys S, Celesia GG, Cohadon F, et al: Unresponsive wakefulness syndrome: a new name for the vegetative state or apallic syndrome, BMC Med 8:68, 2010.

Laureys S, Schiff ND: Coma and consciousness: paradigms (re)framed by neuroimaging, Neuroimage 61(2):478–491, 2012.

Meaney PA, Bobrow BJ, Mancini ME: Cardiopulmonary resuscitation quality: improving cardiac resuscitation outcomes both inside and outside the hospital–a consensus statement From the American Heart Association, Circulation 124:417–435, 2013.

Peberdy MA, Callaway CW, Neumar RW, et al: Cardiac arrest care: 2010 American Heart Association guidelines for cardiopulmonary resuscitation and emergency cardiovascular care, Circulation 122(18 Suppl 3):S768–S786, 2010. [Errata in Circulation 123:e237, 2011, and Circulation 124:e403, 2011.].

Plum F, Posner JB: The diagnosis of stupor and coma. Contemporary Neurology Series, vol 71, ed 4, New York, 2007, Oxford University Press.

Rodriguez RA, Nair S, Bussiere M, et al: Long-lasting functional disabilities in patients who recover from coma after cardiac operations, Ann Thorac Surg 95:884–891, 2013.

Wijdicks EFM: The diagnosis of brain death, N Engl J Med 344:1215–1221, 2001.

Wijdicks EFM, Hijdra A, Young GB, et al: Practice parameter: prediction of outcome in comatose survivors after cardiopulmonary resuscitation (an evidence-based review), Neurology 67:203–210, 2006.

Wu O, Soresenen AG, Benner T, et al: Comatose patients with cardiac arrest: predicting clinical outcome with diffusion-weighted MR imaging, Radiology 252:173–181, 2009.

Young GB: Neurologic prognosis after cardiac arrest, N Engl J Med 361:605–611, 2009.

Zandbergen EGJ, Hijdra A, Koelman JH, et al: Prediction of poor outcome within the first 3 days of postanoxic coma, Neurology 66:62–68, 2006.

106

Disorders of Sleep

Selim R. Benbadis

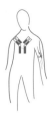

INTRODUCTION

Sleep disorders can be classified in various ways. The international classification uses an axial system to define three categories: dyssomnias, parasomnias, and sleep disorders associated with mental or neurologic diseases. From a practical point of view, sleep disorders are better classified by their clinical presentation, which is the approach taken here. This chapter focuses on primary sleep disorders rather than sleep disturbances that result from self-evident medical or psychiatric diseases.

DISORDERS OF EXCESSIVE DAYTIME SLEEPINESS

History

A careful sleep history is the starting point. It often uncovers likely causes of excessive daytime sleepiness (EDS), such as medications, systemic illnesses, sleep deprivation, or circadian rhythm disturbances. Most of the causes of EDS (e.g., insufficient sleep time, lifestyle, circadian rhythm disorders) do not require a specialized sleep evaluation. The history can elicit symptoms that suggest specific causes such as sleep-disordered breathing (i.e., sleep apnea) or narcolepsy.

To subjectively quantify EDS, various scales have been developed. The most useful in clinical practice is the Epworth Sleepiness Scale (ESS), which is an extension of the history. The ESS consists of a brief questionnaire on the likelihood of dozing off in eight situations. This yields a score between 0 and 24 (Table 106-1). Although there is no strict cutoff, scores above 10 or 11 indicate sufficiently severe EDS to warrant investigation. In addition to being disabling for the individual, EDS is a public health concern because it impairs performance and may cause motor vehicle and industrial accidents in a way comparable to alcohol intoxication.

Examination

The examination of patients with EDS should include a general neurologic examination. If sleep-disordered breathing is suspected, the upper airway should also be examined.

Sleep Studies

Polysomnography (PSG) is an all-night sleep study that measures multiple parameters such as sleep staging, respiration, leg movements, and electrocardiographic patterns. Portable or home adaptations of formal laboratory PSG are increasingly used.

The multiple sleep latency test (MSLT) and the maintenance of wakefulness test (MWT) are used to measure and quantify EDS. They consist of a series of daytime naps during which sleep latency (i.e., latency to stage N1) is measured and sleep stages are determined. The MSLT is better standardized than the MWT. Normal sleep latency is greater than 12 minutes; latency of less than 5 minutes is evidence for severe sleepiness.

SLEEP-DISORDERED BREATHING

Definition and Epidemiology

Sleep-disordered breathing encompasses a spectrum of conditions typified by the most common: obstructive sleep apnea (OSA). The spectrum of obstructive disease extends from primary, isolated, or trivial snoring to upper airway resistance syndrome (i.e., compensated OSA) to OSA of mild, moderate, or severe degree. The degree is determined by PSG.

OSA has a prevalence of about 2% to 4%. It affects more men than women, and the incidence increases with age. Central sleep apnea is much less well defined. It has the same definitions but has no evidence of obstruction.

Pathophysiology

The pathophysiology of OSA is recurrent upper airway closure or collapse with resulting oxygen desaturation leading to arousals. Obstruction typically occurs at the level of the nasopharynx

TABLE 106-1 EPWORTH SLEEPINESS SCALE
How likely are you to doze off or fall asleep in the following situations in contrast to just feeling tired? The situations refer to your usual way of life. Even if you have not done some of these things recently, try to work out how they would have affected you. Use the following scale to choose the most appropriate number for each situation.

0 = would never doze
1 = slight chance of dozing
2 = moderate chance of dozing
3 = high chance of dozing

What is your chance of dozing in the following situations?

Sitting and reading	_____
Watching TV	_____
Sitting and inactive in a public place (theater or meeting)	_____
As a passenger in a car for an hour without a break	_____
Lying down to rest in the afternoon when possible	_____
Sitting and talking to someone	_____
Sitting quietly after lunch (without alcohol)	_____
In a car while stopped for a few minutes in traffic	_____
Total	_____

Modified from Johns MW: A new method for measuring daytime sleepiness: the Epworth Sleepiness Scale, Sleep 14:540–545, 1991.

or oropharynx. The sleep fragmentation caused by arousal is responsible for sleep deprivation and EDS.

Clinical Manifestation

OSA typically manifests with a combination of EDS and snoring in a patient who is overweight. Other symptoms include apneic pauses or "choking" witnessed by the bed partner, and less specific symptoms such as morning headaches, depression, impaired cognition, and sexual dysfunction. On examination, the body mass index (>10 kg/m^2) and neck circumference (>17 inches for men or 16 inches for women) predict OSA. If the patient is not obese, abnormalities of the craniofacial anatomy or upper airways (e.g., retromicrognathia, macroglossia, tonsillar hypertrophy) should be sought.

Diagnosis and Differential Diagnosis

Other causes of EDS should be considered, but in a typical case of OSA, the diagnosis is usually obvious and easily confirmed by overnight PSG. Apneas are defined as cessation (90% reduction) of airflow, whereas hypopneas are 30% to 90% reductions of airflow; both last 10 seconds or longer. These events are called *obstructive* if they occur with respiratory effort and *central* if they occur with no respiratory effort. The apnea-hypopnea index (AHI) is the total number of apneas plus hypopneas per hour, and an AHI score greater than 5 is considered abnormal. An AHI score of 5 to 10 is mild, 10 to 15 is moderate, and more than 15 is severe.

Respiratory effort–related arousals are episodes of decreased airflow with increased effort and crescendo snoring that result in arousals, and they define upper airways resistance syndrome. They represent a compensated degree of OSA. The PSG quantifies the severity in terms of event frequency (i.e., AHI), oxygen desaturation, sleep disturbances (i.e., arousals and fragmentation), and arrhythmias. With some limitations, diagnostic PSG can be performed at home with portable systems if OSA is the likely cause and there are no signs of underlying neurologic disease.

Treatment and Prognosis

Depending on severity, treatment modalities include weight loss, positional measures to prevent sleeping supine, oral appliances for mild disease, and positive airway pressure (PAP) modalities and surgery for moderate to severe disease. For patients with moderate to severe OSA, the initial treatment is PAP; its main limitation is patient compliance. Maximizing the patient's comfort with nasal pillows, humidification, and attention to mask fit is important. PAP requires a titration study to determine the type continuous positive airway pressure (CPAP) (e.g., auto-CPAP, bilevel PAP) and pressure settings appropriate for each patient. When PAP modalities do not work, stimulants and wake-promoting agents can be used as adjuncts to help EDS.

Central sleep apnea is often associated with other cardiopulmonary abnormalities such as heart failure. It is also treated with CPAP initially, but it often requires specialized pulmonary care.

It is important to treat OSA because it has many complications. They include hypertension, coronary artery disease, stroke, diabetes mellitus, depression, and cognitive impairment.

NARCOLEPSY

Definition and Epidemiology

Narcolepsy affects at least 2 in 1000 individuals. Narcolepsy includes a tetrad of excessive sleepiness, cataplexy, sleep paralysis, and hypnagogic hallucinations. The full tetrad occurs in approximately 1 of 5000 people.

Pathophysiology

Narcolepsy is a disorder of rapid eye movement (REM) sleep regulation caused by disordered hypocretin neurotransmission, likely resulting from an autoimmune loss of hypocretin neurons in the lateral hypothalamus. It has a major genetic component, as evidenced by strong human leukocyte antigen (HLA) associations such as HLA-DQB1*0602 in black and white populations and HLA-DR2 in Japanese populations. The daytime symptoms of narcolepsy are accompanied by the intrusion of REM sleep into wakefulness.

Clinical Presentation

The mean age of onset of narcolepsy is in the mid-20s, but two peaks occur around 15 and 35 years of age. EDS is severe and almost constant, and the urge to sleep can be sudden and irresistible (i.e., sleep attacks).

Of the three accessory symptoms, cataplexy is the most specific and helpful for diagnosis. Cataplexy without narcolepsy is exceptional. Narcolepsy without cataplexy is more difficult to identify, and overlaps occur with idiopathic hypersomnia. Cataplexy is characterized by brief (seconds to a few minutes) loss of muscle tone (i.e., intrusion of REM atonia) triggered by emotions, most commonly laughter but also elation, surprise, and fear. If severe, the patient may fall. With milder attacks, a head nod or slurred speech can occur.

Hypnagogic hallucinations that are vivid and dreamlike and that occur at sleep onset are more specific for narcolepsy than hypnopompic (i.e., sleep offset) hallucinations. Sleep paralysis is the often frightening experience of inability to move while aware, usually on awakening. In addition to the tetrad, patients frequently have episodes of automatic behaviors with no recall, which can resemble complex partial seizures. Nocturnal sleep is often fragmented by frequent arousals, vivid dreams, or leg movements.

Diagnosis and Differential Diagnosis

Other causes of EDS, especially the more common OSA, should be sought. A PSG should be obtained the night before the MSLT. The PSG can exclude OSA as a cause of EDS, and an MSLT with a sleep latency of less than 8 minutes and two sleep-onset episodes of REM confirms the diagnosis. Alternatively, a CSF hypocretin level less than 110 pg/mL can confirm the diagnosis. HLA typing is more useful to exclude narcolepsy than to diagnose it because it is sensitive but not specific.

Treatment and Prognosis

Stimulants (e.g., amphetamines, methylphenidate) are still used for the treatment of EDS, but newer wake-promoting agents are more widely used. They include modafinil (100 to 400 mg twice daily) and the longer-acting, once-daily armodafinil (150 to

250 mg per day). Sodium oxybate (3 to 9 g each day) is also used to treat EDS, cataplexy, and disrupted nocturnal sleep. It is potent but short acting; it is typically administered at bedtime and again a few hours later. Sodium oxybate and modafinil may be synergistic in treating EDS. For cataplexy, antidepressants can be used (Table 106-2).

Prognosis is usually good with adequate treatment. However, narcolepsy, when severe, can remain disabling and require accommodations such as scheduled naps.

IDIOPATHIC HYPERSOMNIA

Definition and Epidemiology

Idiopathic hypersomnia is a poorly characterized syndrome with no known pathologic substrate. It is therefore a diagnosis of elimination. It is much less common than narcolepsy.

Clinical Manifestation

Patients have lifelong EDS with non-REM (long and unrefreshing) naps, and none of the REM-type accessory symptoms of narcolepsy. By definition, there must be no other cause of EDS. Patients also wake up unrefreshed (i.e., sleep inertia) from nocturnal sleep and long daytime naps, and they can have prolonged states of fogginess (i.e., sleep drunkenness).

Diagnosis and Differential Diagnosis

Other causes of EDS must be excluded, and the PSG should be normal with no sleep-disordered breathing and no sleep fragmentation such as seen in narcolepsy. MSLT confirm sleep latency of less than 8 minutes but without sleep-onset REM.

Treatment and Prognosis

Treatment includes the same stimulants and wake-promoting agents as used for narcolepsy. The response is typically less satisfactory. The response to treatment is varies, and accommodation in the workplace is usually necessary.

KLEINE-LEVIN SYNDROME

Kleine-Levin syndrome is a rare, recurrent or cyclic hypersomnia with a prevalence of 1 case per 1 million people. Its cause is unknown. Its onset is usually in the second decade, with episodes of hypersomnia lasting days to weeks and with associated hyperphagia, hypersexuality, confusion, and hallucinations. Episodes tend to recur every few months and at least once each year. Other symptomatic causes of EDS must be excluded.

Stimulants and wake-promoting agents and lithium are used for treatment. With time, episodes tend to become less severe, less prolonged, and less frequent.

PERIODIC LIMB MOVEMENT DISORDER

Definition and Epidemiology

Periodic limb movement disorder (PLMD) is characterized by repetitive movements (usually of the legs) that occur during sleep. This can be purely a PSG finding, but it is often associated with restless legs syndrome (RLS).

Pathophysiology

PLMD is caused by decreased dopamine neurotransmission.

Clinical Manifestations

Leg movements may be reported by the bed partner, and the patient may report EDS, insomnia, or symptoms of RLS (i.e., urge to move legs or walk due to unpleasant "creepy-crawly" sensations at rest). Most patients with RLS have PLMD, but the reverse is not true.

Diagnosis and Differential Diagnosis

RLS is diagnosed by the history. PLMD is diagnosed by PSG. Once established, the search for a cause of secondary PLMD should investigate the same causes as RLS: polyneuropathy, spinal cord disease, pregnancy, iron-deficiency anemia (i.e., ferritin levels), B_{12} deficiency, uremia, medications, primary sleep disorders, narcolepsy, or OSA.

Treatment and Prognosis

Similar to RLS, pramipexole or ropinirole is used at lower doses than for treating Parkinson's disease (Table 106-3). Prognosis is usually good with treatment.

For a deeper discussion of these topics, please see Chapter 410, "Other Movement Disorders," in Goldman-Cecil Medicine, *25th Edition.*

INSOMNIA

Definition and Epidemiology

Insomnia is defined as difficulty initiating or maintaining sleep. Severe, chronic insomnia can have major health consequences, including depression, anxiety, drug or alcohol use, and overall higher mortality rates.

Insomnia is the most common sleep complaint in the general population. Up to one third of the population report at least occasional difficulties sleeping. Chronic insomnia (>1 month) affects about 10% of the population.

Pathophysiology

Insomnia can be caused by pain, medical conditions (e.g., chronic obstructive pulmonary disease), psychiatric conditions, and

TABLE 106-2 AGENTS PROMOTING WAKEFULNESS

DRUG	DOSE RANGE (MG)
Amphetamine (Dexedrine, Desoxyn, Adderall, Adderall XR)	5-60
Methylphenidate (Ritalin, Metadate, Methylin, Concerta)	10-60
Modafinil (Provigil)	200-400
Armodafinil	150-250

TABLE 106-3 TREATMENTS FOR RESTLESS LEGS SYNDROME

DRUG	DOSE RANGE (MG)
Levodopa or carbidopa (Sinemet)	50-200
Ropinirole (Requip)	0.25-4.0
Pramipexole (Mirapex)	0.125-0.5

medications. Acute or short-term insomnia is caused by identifiable factors and can become a chronic, persistent problem. Chronic insomnia results from predisposing (genetic), precipitating (environmental), and perpetuating (behaviors) factors. With the exception of rare conditions such as the prion disease, fatal familial insomnia, insomnia alone is almost never the symptom of a neurologic disease.

Clinical Manifestations

Insomnia may manifest as the inability to fall asleep (i.e., onset insomnia) or to stay asleep (i.e., maintenance insomnia). In addition to nighttime symptoms, the diagnosis demands daytime symptoms considered to be the consequence of insomnia (e.g., fatigue, EDS, poor concentration, altered mood, headache).

Adjustment insomnia is an acute reaction to some type of stress. When the trigger combines with a propensity for poor or fragile sleep, the condition can become chronic (>1 month) and lead to maladaptive behaviors and a conditioned arousal associated with sleep. This is known as *psychophysiologic insomnia,* and it is by far the most common insomnia syndrome. A vicious cycle is created by poor sleep habits that worsen the insomnia. Because of its chronicity, it is typically associated with poor sleep habits, multiple treatment trials, and anxiety about sleep. If there was no trigger at onset, there may be a lifelong history of poor sleep (i.e., idiopathic insomnia) with the same end result of psychophysiologic insomnia.

Paradoxical insomnia and *sleep-state misperception* are terms applied to patients who claim to not sleep. However, when studied objectively, they have normal sleep amounts and architecture.

Diagnosis and Differential Diagnosis

The diagnosis is based on the history, which should include a sleep diary. Identifiable medical, psychiatric, or drug-related disease and other sleep disorders (e.g., OSA) require exclusion. Sleep studies (PSG and MSLT) are occasionally helpful.

Treatment and Prognosis

Nondrug treatments include common sense sleep hygiene recommendations (e.g., avoiding caffeine, exercising late in the day) (Table 106-4) and behavior modifications to avoid the conditioned arousal responses associated with sleep (e.g., using the

---

TABLE 106-4   SLEEP HYGIENE

1. Maintain a regular schedule each day.
2. Wake at the same time each morning.
3. Exposure to natural light entrains the circadian rhythm.
4. Exercise in the morning or early afternoon; avoid vigorous exercise in the evening.
5. Avoid napping during the day, especially after 3 PM.
6. Avoid stimulants such as caffeine and nicotine and avoid alcohol close to bedtime.
7. Avoid large meals close to bedtime.
8. Maintain regular and relaxing routines at bedtime.
9. Maintain a comfortable sleep environment.
10. Reserve the bed for sleep; avoid other activities (e.g., TV, radio, reading).
11. Sleep only when sleepy.
12. Try to resolve worries (or list for future thought) before sleeping.
13. Get out of bed if not sleeping in 20 minutes.

---

bedroom only for sleep and sex). Other strategies include cognitive behavior therapy specifically for insomnia (CBT-I), relaxation techniques, biofeedback, and behavioral changes such as sleep restriction therapy and stimulus control therapy.

The principles of the pharmacologic treatment of insomnia include using the lowest effective dose, intermittent (not daily) use, using the appropriate (i.e., short or intermediate half-life) drug based on the type of insomnia (i.e., onset or maintenance), and limiting the duration of treatment. Treatment should be tapered to avoid rebound. Medications should be used only in combination with nondrug (i.e., behavioral) treatments. Behavioral treatment has been effective.

Over-the-counter sleep aids (usually antihistamines) are typically safe, but use is limited by anticholinergic and hangover effects. Melatonin may promote sleep and be used for circadian rhythm disorders, including jet lag. The selective melatonin agonist ramelteon is helpful for sleep-onset insomnia. Other treatments are listed in Table 106-1.

Prognosis is usually good with the combination of drug and nondrug treatments. Behavior modification may be limited by the willingness of patients to participate.

● PARASOMNIAS

Parasomnias are undesirable phenomena that occur in sleep or during transition to or from sleep. They usually consist of complex and seemingly purposeful behaviors, sometimes dramatic, of which the patient is not aware. They are often classified by the sleep stage in which they arise.

Slow-Wave Sleep Parasomnias

Definition and Epidemiology

Slow-wave sleep parasomnias include disorders of arousals, including sleep talking, night terrors (i.e., pavor nocturnus), sleep walking (i.e., somnambulism), nocturnal wandering, and confusional arousals (i.e., sleep drunkenness), with considerable overlap among these entities.

Pathophysiology and Clinical Manifestations

Characterized by partial arousals and intermediate states between wakefulness and sleep, slow-wave sleep parasomnias tend to begin in childhood. A family history of similar symptoms is common.

Episodes are often triggered by precipitants such as fever, intercurrent illness, sleep deprivation, or alcohol. They tend to occur in the first third of the night, when delta sleep predominates. They are characterized by typical slow-wave sleep arousals. Patients appear confused, may have slurred speech, and take several minutes to regain orientation. Slow-wave sleep has a higher threshold for arousal.

Sleep talking usually consists of fragments of barely intelligible sentences. Sleep walking and nocturnal wandering typically include ambulation. Night terrors (i.e., sleep terrors or pavor nocturnus) are dramatic, with an abrupt arousal, a scream, and autonomic hyperactivity (e.g., mydriasis, diaphoresis, flushing, piloerection, tachycardia). The child appears terrified and is inconsolable. Episodes last a few minutes and are not recalled the next morning.

Diagnosis and Differential Diagnosis

The main differential diagnosis is nocturnal seizure, which occasionally requires epilepsy monitoring (video electroencephalogram) if the episodes are frequent. For episodic symptoms, the use of home video (by cell phone) is more reliable than description by witnesses. Nocturnal seizures tend to be more stereotyped than parasomnias, and they often include tonic or clonic motor activity.

Treatment and Prognosis

Reassurance and measures to avoid injuries usually are sufficient. For episodes with injurious behaviors, low-dose benzodiazepines (clonazepam, 0.5 to 1 mg) are often effective. Prognosis is good, and most patients do not require treatment.

Rapid Eye Movement Behavior Disorder

Definition and Epidemiology

REM behavior disorder (RBD) is a disorder of REM sleep regulation in which there is a dissociation of REM features with loss of the muscle atonia, leading to patients acting out their dreams. RBD typically affects patients after the age of 50 (usually older) and the male-to-female ratio is 10 : 1.

Pathophysiology

REM inhibition is lost due to bilateral degeneration of REM atonic neurons in the pons. RBD occurs with α-synucleinopathies (i.e., Parkinson's disease, multiple system atrophy, and dementia with Lewy bodies), and RBD typically heralds these neurodegenerative diseases, sometimes by 10 to 15 years.

Clinical Manifestations

Typically, the episodes are reported by the bed partner and consist of high-amplitude, flailing, injurious behaviors during sleep. When awakened, the patient typically recalls the dream. As is typical of REM arousals, the patient is alert and coherent immediately (unlike slow-wave sleep arousal). Medications, especially psychotropics, can exacerbate RBD.

Diagnosis and Differential Diagnosis

The diagnosis can usually be made by the history alone, and PSG is not needed. When performed, PSG shows a lack of REM atonia or increased phasic and tonic REM. Like slow-wave parasomnias, the main differential diagnosis is nocturnal seizure, and this occasionally requires epilepsy monitoring. Home video (cell phones) recordings can be useful.

Treatment and Prognosis

Low-dose clonazepam (0.5 to 2 mg) is usually effective. Symptoms initially respond to treatment, but a neurodegenerative disease is likely to become evident.

For a deeper discussion of these topics, please see Chapter 100, "Obstructive Sleep Apnea," and Chapter 405, "Disorders of Sleep," in Goldman-Cecil Medicine, *25th Edition.*

SUGGESTED READINGS

Buysse DJ: Insomnia, JAMA 309:706–716, 2013.

Ebisawa T: Analysis of the molecular pathophysiology of sleep disorders relevant to a disturbed biological clock, Mol Genet Genomics 288:185–193, 2013.

Faraut B, Boudjeltia KZ, Vanhamme L, et al: Immune, inflammatory and cardiovascular consequences of sleep restriction and recovery, Sleep Med Rev 16:137–149, 2012.

Mignot EJ: A practical guide to the therapy of narcolepsy and hypersomnia syndromes, Neurother 9:739–752, 2012.

Ohayon MM: From wakefulness to excessive sleepiness: what we know and still need to know, Sleep Med Rev 12:129–141, 2008.

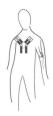

107

Cortical Syndromes

Sinéad M. Murphy and Timothy J. Counihan

ANATOMY

The paired cerebral hemispheres are connected by a large band of white matter fibers, the *corpus callosum*. Each hemisphere consists of four anatomically and functionally distinct regions: the frontal, temporal, parietal, and occipital lobes (Fig. 107-1). The two cerebral hemispheres supplement each other functionally in a variety of behavioral and sensorimotor tasks; however, certain functions, particularly language, manual dexterity, and visuospatial perception, are strongly lateralized to one hemisphere. Language function is lateralized to the left hemisphere in 95% of the population; although 15% of people are left-handed, the right hemisphere is dominant for language in only between 10% and 27% depending on the degree of left-handedness. Visuospatial functions are largely subserved by the right (nondominant) hemisphere. The Rolandic fissure separates the motor cortex (precentral gyrus) from the sensory cortex (postcentral gyrus). In these regions, cortical representations of the different parts of the body are arranged as the motor (frontal lobe) and sensory (parietal lobe) homunculi (Fig. 107-2).

CLINICAL ASSESSMENT

Symptoms and signs caused by cortical lesions may be less consistent than deficits caused by lesions of the spinal cord or more peripheral nerves, and patients may be unaware of the extent of their deficit. This makes a collateral history and careful examination (including cognitive assessment) important. In addition, there is substantial individual variability among patients. The rate of onset of symptoms and the tempo of progression influence the extent of the clinical deficit. The homuncular arrangement of cortical motor and sensory representation may allow for more precise localization of a lesion. For instance, motor or sensory signs confined to the lower extremities may suggest a parasagittal lesion, whereas signs involving the face and upper limb may originate in laterally placed cortical lesions.

REGIONAL SYNDROMES

Table 107-1 summarizes some of the eponymous syndromes and clinical features associated with damage to individual lobes.

Aphasia

Aphasia or *dysphasia* refers to a loss or impairment of language function as a result of damage to the specific language centers of the dominant hemisphere. It is distinct from dysarthria, which is a disturbance in the articulation of speech. The principal types of aphasia are summarized in Table 107-2.

Writing is almost invariably affected in patients with disturbances of language (Fig. 107-3). An exception to this occurs in the syndrome of *alexia without agraphia,* which results from a lesion in the dominant occipital lobe and splenium of corpus callosum (usually caused by infarction in the territory of the posterior cerebral artery). The patient's language center is "disconnected" from the contralateral (unaffected) visual cortex. Such patients can write a sentence but are unable to read what they have written.

Clinical assessment for aphasia requires testing of fluency, comprehension, repetition, naming, reading, calculation, and writing. *Anomia* (difficulty in recalling the names of objects) in isolation has little localizing value.

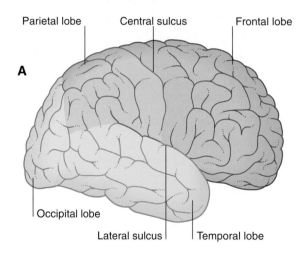

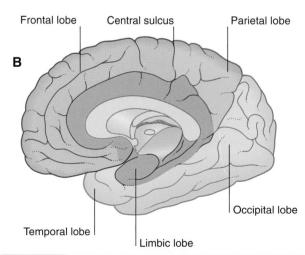

FIGURE 107-1 Lateral (**A**) and medial (**B**) views of the cerebral hemispheres. (From FitzGerald MJT, editor: Clinical neuroanatomy and neuroscience, ed 6, Philadelphia, 2011, Saunders, Fig. 2-1.)

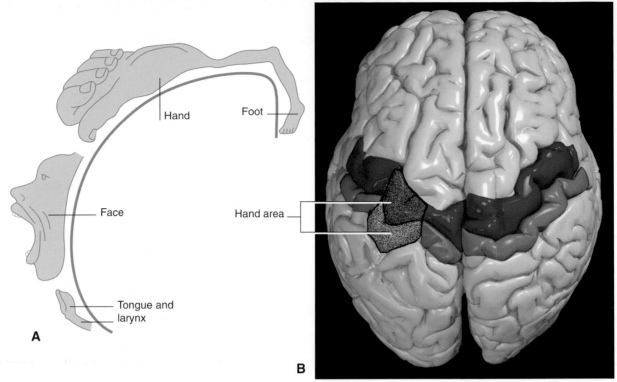

FIGURE 107-2 **A**, Homuncular arrangement shows the correlations with the primary motor cortex lying anterior to the central sulcus and the somatosensory cortex posteriorly (**B**). (Modified from Kretschmann HJ, Weinrich W: Neurofunctional systems: 3D reconstructions with correlated neuroimaging: text and CD-ROM, New York, 1998, Thieme.)

TABLE 107-1 CORTICAL SYMPTOMS AND SIGNS

DOMINANT HEMISPHERE	NONDOMINANT HEMISPHERE	EITHER HEMISPHERE
FRONTAL LOBE		
Broca's aphasia	Motor dysprosody	Contralateral spastic weakness
Transcortical motor aphasia		Forced eye deviation
Pure agraphia		Executive dysfunction, poor sequencing
		Akinetic mutism, urinary incontinence (bilateral lesions)
		Disinhibition, emotional lability, abulia
		Frontal lobe release signs (pout, grasp, snout, rooting, palmomental)
		Alien hand
PARIETAL LOBE		
Wernicke aphasia	Contralateral sensory neglect	Contralateral sensory loss
Transcortical sensory aphasia	Constructional apraxia	
Apraxia	Anosagnosia	
Gerstmann's syndrome (acalculia, finger agnosia, right-left disorientation, agraphia)	Dressing apraxia	
Conduction aphasia		
TEMPORAL LOBE		
Anomic or sensory aphasia	Impaired recognition of facial emotional expressions	Contralateral superior quadrantanopia
Verbal amnesia	Visuospatial amnesia	Amnesia
Transcortical sensory aphasia	Sensory dysprosody/amusia	Klüver-Bucy syndrome (oral-exploratory behavior, passivity, hypersexuality) bilateral lesions
Pure word deafness		Auditory hallucinations
		Complex visual hallucinations
		Olfactory hallucinations
		Visual/experiential delusions
OCCIPITAL LOBE		
Alexia without agraphia		Anton's syndrome (visual agnosia, denial of blindness)
		Contralateral homonymous hemianopia
		Visual hallucinations
		Optic apraxia, absent optokinetic nystagmus, palinopsia
		Balint's syndrome (simultanagnosia, optic ataxia, oculomotor apraxia); bilateral lesions, usually occipitoparietal

TABLE 107-2 PRINCIPAL TYPES OF APHASIA

TYPE	LESION SITE	FLUENCY	COMPREHENSION	REPETITION	NAMING	OTHER SIGNS
Broca's (expressive)	Inferior frontal lobe	↓	Good	↓	↓	Contralateral weakness
Wernicke's (receptive)	Posterior superior temporal lobe	Good	↓	↓	↓	Homonymous hemianopia
Transcortical motor	Inferior frontal gyrus	↓	Good	Good	May be normal	May be contralateral weakness
Transcortical sensory	Middle temporal gyrus, thalamus	Good	↓	Good	Usually normal	May be normal
Conduction	Supramarginal gyrus	Good	Good	↓	↓	None
Global	Frontal lobe (large)	↓	↓	↓	↓	Hemiplegia

↓, Reduced.

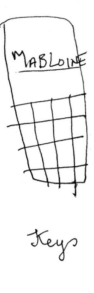

FIGURE 107-3 Neologisms written by a patient with aphasia who was attempting to name cell phone, keys, camera, watch, pen, bag, and boots.

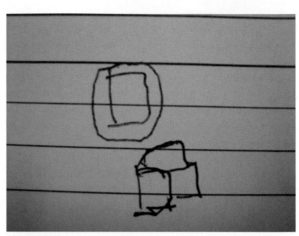

FIGURE 107-4 Attempts to draw a cube by a patient with a neurodegenerative disorder demonstrate constructional apraxia.

Broca's aphasia is characterized by a severe disruption in the fluency of speech, with profound impairments of expression in both speech and writing. Comprehension may be mildly affected. The language disturbance is almost invariably accompanied by contralateral face and arm weakness as a result of the proximity of the motor homunculus to Broca's speech area.

Wernicke's aphasia is characterized by an inability to comprehend spoken or written language. Affected patients speak fluently, but the content is meaningless; they may use words that are close in meaning to the intended word (semantic paraphasias) or words that sound like the intended word (literal paraphasias). Patients may be misdiagnosed as having a psychiatric disorder because they lack an associated hemiparesis.

Conduction aphasia is characterized by normal comprehension and fluent speech but an inability to repeat. The responsible lesion lies in the arcuate fasciculus connecting Broca's and Wernicke's areas. *Global aphasia* results from large lesions of the frontal lobe; all aspects of language are affected. Lesions of the language areas of the nondominant hemisphere result in *dysprosody*. For instance, patients with lesions in the inferior frontal lobe of the nondominant hemisphere, analogous to Broca's area, speak with a monotonous voice, losing the natural cadence of speech.

In *dysarthria*, the language function is intact (which can be confirmed by having the patient write a sentence), but patients have difficulty articulating. Dysarthria can result from a lesion anywhere along the path from the cerebral cortex to the bulbar muscles.

Agnosia and Apraxia

Agnosia is the inability to recognize a specific sensory stimulus despite preserved sensory function. For instance, visual agnosia is the inability to recognize a visual stimulus despite normal visual acuity. Other agnosia syndromes include the inability to recognize sounds (auditory agnosia), color (color agnosia), or familiar faces (prosopagnosia). Usually, the responsible lesions are located in the occipitotemporal region.

Apraxia refers to an inability to perform learned motor tasks despite sufficient sensorimotor function to physically execute the movement; it is a disorder of motor planning (Fig. 107-4). The responsible lesions are usually in the dominant inferior parietal lobe. A simple test of apraxia is to ask the patient to perform a pantomime (e.g., combing his or her hair, blowing out a candle).

Lesions of the nondominant parietal lobe often result in *hemispatial neglect*: the patient does not attend to stimuli in the contralateral (usually the left) visual field or on the contralateral side of the body. In a milder form of neglect, called *extinction,* patients can attend to stimuli contralateral to the side of the brain with the lesion (and the lesion is usually on the right side), but when presented with bilateral stimuli simultaneously, they respond only on the ipsilateral (right) side. *Anosognosia,* or the lack of awareness of one's deficit, frequently accompanies hemispatial neglect. In severe cases, patients may even deny that the affected limb belongs to them.

⬤ PROSPECTUS FOR THE FUTURE

There have been many advances in neuroimaging technology that allow neuroscientists to study not only the structural and functional anatomy of a particular brain structure but also its metabolic activity. Functional magnetic resonance imaging (fMRI) permits mapping of the metabolic anatomy of subcortical gray and white matter structures, such as the basal ganglia, and their roles in conditions such as dystonia. These modalities allow one to study white matter tracts (tractography) in great detail, using a technique called diffusion tensor imaging.

Similarly, modern MRI technology is now able to discriminate brain tissue that is infarcted from tissue that is ischemic (and therefore potentially still viable) in the setting of acute stroke. Positron emission tomography (PET) and single-photon emission computed tomography (SPECT) are nuclear medicine imaging techniques that are increasingly used in the diagnosis of neurodegenerative disorders. It is likely that these techniques will become increasingly available in the acute hospital setting.

SUGGESTED READINGS

Brazis PW, Masdeu JC, Biller J: Localization in clinical neurology, ed 6, Philadelphia, 2011, Lippincott Williams & Wilkins.

Carota A, Calabrese P: The achromatic "philosophical zombie," a syndrome of cerebral achromatopsia with color anopsognosia, Case Rep Neurol 5:98–103, 2013.

Goldenberg G: Apraxia in left handers, Brain 136:2592–2601, 2013.

Knopman DS: Regional cerebral dysfunction: higher mental functions, chapter 408. In Goldman's Cecil Medicine, ed 24, Philadelphia, 2012, Saunders.

Mesulam MM: Primary progsressive aphasia and the language network, Neurology 81:456–462, 2013.

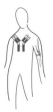

108 Dementia and Memory Disturbances

Frederick J. Marshall

MAJOR DEMENTIA SYNDROMES

Dementia is progressive loss of intellectual function coupled with loss of meaningful function in daily life. Memory loss is the central feature, and specific dementia syndromes characteristically cause particular forms of memory impairment. Dementia syndromes also produce specific abnormalities of cognition in language, spatial processing, praxis (i.e., learned motor behavior), and executive function (i.e., ability to plan and sequence events). *Cortical dementia* and *subcortical dementia*, although older terms, remain helpful for subdividing the dementias (Table 108-1).

Table 108-2 provides the differential diagnosis of neurodegenerative causes of dementia, and Table 108-3 outlines other causes of dementia. Neurodegeneration is the most common underlying cause of dementia and is seen in Alzheimer's disease (AD), frontotemporal dementia, and diffuse Lewy body disease.

Most causes of dementias are currently untreatable. Potentially correctable causes account for less than 5% of dementia cases. Structural processes or infections must be considered, along with metabolic and nutritional diseases. Every patient with dementia should have tests of serum electrolytes and vitamin B_{12} and assessments of liver, renal, and thyroid function. Serologic studies for syphilis and Lyme exposure should be done if risk factors are identified. Chronic infections (see Chapter 90) and normal-pressure hydrocephalus should be considered. Brain imaging should be performed.

Neuropsychological testing characterizes the pattern of cognitive and memory impairments and is helpful in the differential diagnosis. The Montreal Cognitive Assessment (MoCA) (Table 108-4) is a standard test that can be used as a bedside or office screening tool for identifying patients with dementia. This examination is superior to the Mini-Mental Status Examination (MMSE) in that it is sensitive to abnormalities in a wider array of cognitive domains, including visual-spatial or executive

TABLE 108-2 ETIOLOGIC DIAGNOSIS OF NEURODEGENERATIVE DEMENTIA IN ADULTS

Alzheimer's disease*
Parkinson's disease*
Diffuse Lewy body disease*
Progressive supranuclear palsy
Corticobasal ganglionic degeneration
Striatonigral degeneration
Olivopontocerebellar degeneration
Huntington's disease
Frontotemporal dementias
Pick's disease
Frontotemporal dementia without characteristic neuropathology
Frontotemporal dementia with motor neuron disease
Hallervorden-Spatz disease

*Denotes conditions for which symptomatic treatment is available.

TABLE 108-3 OTHER CAUSES OF PROGRESSIVE DEMENTIA IN ADULTS

STRUCTURAL DISEASE OR TRAUMA	INFECTIOUS DISEASE
Normal-pressure hydrocephalus* Neoplasms* Dementia pugilistica (multiple concussions in boxers)	Human immunodeficiency virus type 1* Tertiary syphilis* Creutzfeldt-Jakob disease Progressive multifocal leukoencephalopathy
VASCULAR DISEASE	Whipple's disease*
Vascular dementia† Vasculitis*	Chronic meningitis* Cryptococcal meningitis* Others
HEREDOMETABOLIC DISEASE	**METABOLIC OR NUTRITIONAL DISEASE**
Wilson's disease* Neuronal ceroid lipofuscinosis (Kufs' disease) Other late-onset lysosomal storage diseases	Vitamin B_{12} deficiency* Thyroid hormone deficiency or excess* Thiamine deficiency* (Korsakoff's syndrome) Alcoholism†
DEMYELINATING OR DYSMYELINATING DISEASE	**PSYCHIATRIC DISEASE**
Multiple sclerosis† Metachromatic leukodystrophy	Pseudodementia from depression*

*Denotes conditions for which preventive or corrective treatment is available.
†Denotes conditions for which symptomatic treatment is available.

TABLE 108-1 DISTINGUISHING CHARACTERISTICS OF CORTICAL AND SUBCORTICAL DEMENTIAS

CORTICAL DEMENTIA

Symptoms: major changes in memory, language deficits, perceptual deficits, praxis disturbances
Affected brain regions: temporal cortex (medial), parietal cortex, and frontal lobe cortex
Examples: Alzheimer's disease, diffuse Lewy body disease, vascular dementia, frontotemporal dementias

SUBCORTICAL DEMENTIA

Symptoms: behavioral changes, impaired affect and mood, motor slowing, executive dysfunction, less severe changes in memory
Affected brain regions: thalamus, striatum, midbrain, striatofrontal projections
Examples: Parkinson's disease, progressive supranuclear palsy, normal-pressure hydrocephalus, Huntington's disease, Creutzfeldt-Jakob disease, chronic meningitis

function, naming, attention, fluency; abstract reasoning, short-term memory encoding and retrieval, and orientation.

In addition to the MoCA, patients with dementia should have tests of praxis (e.g., show how you would comb your hair; show how you would blow out a match) and neglect (e.g., testing of double-simultaneous extinction to visual, tactile, and auditory stimuli). Depending on the results of these screening procedures, more detailed neuropsychological studies can be pursued.

Alzheimer's Disease

AD accounts for approximately 70% of dementia cases among older adults. Almost 5.3 million persons in the United States are affected, and this number may approach 18 million by 2050 as the population ages. AD places enormous burdens on the patient, family, and society. The annual direct and indirect expenditures are estimated to exceed $150 billion. The disease occurs in 32% to 47% of persons older than 80 years of age. Incidence at age 65 is one in 200 people per year. Incidence at age 80 is one case per 10 people per year. More than 50% of caregivers develop depression or major medical illness.

AD has many causes, but none is fully defined. All causes produce similar clinical and pathologic findings. The disease is characterized by the progressive loss of cortical neurons and the formation of amyloid plaques and intraneuronal neurofibrillary tangles. β-Amyloid (Aβ) is the major component of the plaques, and hyperphosphorylated tau protein is the major constituent of the neurofibrillary tangles. The process starts in the hippocampus and entorhinal cortex and spreads to involve diffuse areas of association cortex in the temporal, parietal, and frontal lobes. The relative deficiency of cortical acetylcholine (resulting from the loss of neurons in the nucleus basalis) provides the rationale for symptomatic treatment of the disease with centrally acting acetylcholinesterase inhibitors.

Pathogenesis

AD is often categorized as a young-onset, hereditary or familial form, which is rare and for which three specific genetic abnormalities have been determined, or as a common, sporadic form that typically occurs in persons older than 65 years of age (Table 108-5).

The autosomal dominant, early-onset forms of AD have in common abnormalities of Aβ production and processing, which have provided clues to the molecular pathogenesis of sporadic AD. Abnormal processing of amyloid precursor protein into the amyloidogenic peptide Aβ (1-42) is thought to be important in the pathogenesis of AD. It is thought to provoke downstream abnormalities of tau protein processing, with hyperphosphorylation of tau yielding intraneuronal tangles.

The apolipoprotein E (Apo E) gene *(APOE)* was found to be a susceptibility locus for sporadic AD in late-onset familial AD pedigrees. The gene is polymorphic (ε2, ε3, ε4), and first-degree relatives of AD patients, who inherit both ε4 alleles, have a more than 60% lifetime risk of developing AD. Apo E-ε4 interacts selectively with Aβ and with tau protein, but how Apo E-ε4 increases the risk of AD remains unknown.

Clinical Features

AD begins gradually and affects memory, orientation, language, visuospatial processing, praxis, judgment, and insight. Depression is common early in AD, and psychosis with agitation and behavioral disinhibition often occur in advanced stages. Patients become dependent on others for all activities of daily living. The rate of progression of AD is varies but usually takes 5 to 15 years to progress from presentation to advanced illness.

Diagnostic criteria are outlined in Table 108-6. Although a definitive diagnosis of AD requires biopsy (rarely done) or autopsy confirmation, these diagnostic criteria establish the diagnosis with more than 85% specificity in moderately demented patients. The positron emission tomography (PET) ligand

TABLE 108-4 ELEMENTS OF THE MONTREAL COGNITIVE ASSESSMENT

COGNITIVE DOMAIN	ITEMS	SCORE
Visual-spatial or executive	Complete a trail-making task, copy a cube, draw a clock	5
Naming	Name three depicted animals	3
Attention	Recall 5 digits forward, 3 digits backward, maintain letter vigilance, subtract 7s serially	6
Language	Repeat two phrases, generate a list of words starting with a specific letter	3
Abstraction	Identify the similarity between nouns (train/bicycle; watch/ruler)	2
Delayed recall	Recall five words rehearsed twice previously (face, velvet, church, daisy, red)	5
Orientation	Identify the date, month, year, day, place, and city	6
Total possible score		30

From Nasreddine ZS, Phillips NA, Bedirian V, et al: The Montreal Cognitive Assessment, MoCA: a brief screening tool for mild cognitive impairment, J Am Geriatr Soc 53:695–699, 2005.

TABLE 108-5 FAMILIAL VERSUS SPORADIC ALZHEIMER'S DISEASE

CHROMOSOME AND GENE	AGE AT ONSET (YR)	% OF ALL FAD CASES	% OF ALL SAD CASES
FAMILIAL ALZHEIMER'S DISEASE*			
Chromosome 1, *PSEN2* (presenilin 2)	40-80	5-10	<0.5
Chromosome 14, *PSEN1* (presenilin 1)	30-60	70	<1
Chromosome 21, *APP* (amyloid-β precursor protein)	35-65	5	<0.5
SPORADIC ALZHEIMER'S DISEASE†			
No single determinant gene‡	Usually >60	—	98

*Familial Alzheimer's disease (FAD) has early onset and is autosomal dominant.
†Sporadic Alzheimer's disease (SAD) has late onset and may be polygenetic and/or environmental.
‡Apolipoprotein E-ε4 allele on chromosome 19 increases the risk compared with the ε2 or ε3 allele.

TABLE 108-6   DIAGNOSTIC CRITERIA FOR PROBABLE ALZHEIMER'S DISEASE

Progressive functional decline and dementia established by clinical examination and mental status testing and confirmed by neuropsychological assessment

Insidious onset

Clear-cut history of worsening cognition by report or observation

Initial and most prominent cognitive deficits evident on history and examination in one of the following categories:

    Amnestic presentation (plus at least one other domain)

    Nonamnestic presentations (plus deficits in other domains): language, visuospatial, executive dysfunction

No evidence of vascular dementia, dementia with Lewy bodies, frontotemporal dementias, or other concurrent active neurologic or non-neurologic medical comorbidity or use of medication that could have a substantial effect on cognition

florbetapir F 18 (Amyvid), which binds to amyloid plaques, has been approved by the U.S. Food and Drug Administration (FDA) for use in the clinical diagnosis of AD. It can be positive in patients without clinical signs of dementia. Similarly, cerebrospinal fluid (CSF) assays for Aβ, tau, and phosphorylated tau protein loads have been commercialized as aids to diagnosis, but they are not universally used due to the invasive nature of the testing and the relatively good accuracy of the clinical diagnosis.

PET and CSF assays are in widespread use for stratification of subjects in emerging large-scale, prospective, randomized studies of individuals at risk for preclinical disease. Changes in brain morphometry are identifiable on structural imaging many years before onset of clinical symptoms.

Treatment

Although their benefits are modest, the cholinesterase-inhibiting drugs donepezil (Aricept), rivastigmine (Exelon), and galantamine (Razadyne) represent important advances. These drugs may be given in once-daily formulations. Rivastigmine is also available as a transdermal patch.

In clinical trials, cholinesterase inhibitors benefited less than 50% of patients. They have not been shown to prevent AD in patients with mild cognitive impairment (MCI), a condition in which the memory or another domain of cognition is impaired in the absence of meaningful dysfunction in daily life. Approximately 12% of patients with MCI go on to develop AD per year, with roughly two thirds of patients with MCI developing clinical AD within 5 years of symptom onset.

Gingko biloba has no role in the treatment or prevention of AD. The glutamate antagonist memantine (Namenda) has been shown to prolong daily function in patients with moderate to advanced AD.

Treatment strategies in clinical trials over the past decade have included decreasing Aβ peptide production by blocking α-secretase or β-secretase or upregulating cleavage of the amyloid precursor protein at the α-secretase site. Studies of active and passive immunization have been designed to lower brain Aβ levels. However, these approaches have failed to deliver on the promise of AD disease modification, necessitating a wide-reaching reassessment of current theories of disease pathogenesis.

There is an emerging concept of preclinical AD, with many biomarkers showing changes years before clinical manifestations.

Several large, prospective, interventional studies targeting this population are getting underway or are planned on the inference that intervening later in the disease process (when symptoms of dementia have manifested) may be too late. Novel molecular and immunologic approaches continue to hold promise for disease-modifying treatments in the future.

Nursing services provide oversight of hygiene, nutrition, and medication compliance. Antipsychotics, antidepressants, and anxiolytics are useful for patients with behavioral disturbances, which are the most common cause of nursing home placement. Patients and families can be referred to a local Alzheimer's Association chapter for further information on available community support.

Prevention

There is no high or even moderate level of evidence that any intervention decreases the risk of AD. There is a low level of evidence that a Mediterranean diet, folic acid, HMG-CoA reductase inhibitors (i.e., statins), higher levels of education, light alcohol intake, cognitively engaging activities, and physical activity (particularly at high levels) may decrease the risk of AD.

There is a moderate level of scientific evidence that conjugated equine estrogen with methyl-progesterone increases the risk of AD. There is a low level of scientific evidence that some nonsteroidal anti-inflammatory drugs, depressive disorder, diabetes mellitus, hyperlipidemia in midlife, current tobacco use, traumatic brain injury, pesticide exposure, and relative social isolation increase the risk of AD.

Diffuse Lewy Body Disease

Lewy bodies are pathologic inclusions that are the hallmark of Parkinson's disease when they are restricted to the brain stem (see Chapter 114). Patients with diffuse Lewy body disease have clinical parkinsonism (i.e., slow movement, rigidity, and balance problems) combined with early and prominent dementia. Pathologically, Lewy bodies are found in the brain stem, limbic system, and cortex. Visual hallucinations and cognitive fluctuations are common, and patients are unusually sensitive to the adverse effects of neuroleptic medication.

Diffuse Lewy body disease may represent the second most common cause of dementia after AD. However, the common concurrence of the pathologic features of diffuse Lewy body disease with the classic neuritic plaques and neurofibrillary tangles of AD complicates the identification of the cause of dementia in a given patient.

Vascular Dementia

Approximately 10% to 20% of older patients with dementia have radiographic evidence of focal stroke on magnetic resonance imaging (MRI) or computed tomography (CT), combined with focal signs on the neurologic examination. When the dementia syndrome begins with a stroke and progression of the illness is stepwise (suggesting recurrent vascular events), the diagnosis of vascular dementia is likely.

Patients typically develop early incontinence, gait disturbances, and flattening of affect. A subcortical dementing process attributed to small vessel disease in the periventricular white matter has been referred to as *Binswanger's disease*, but it may be a radiographic finding rather than a true disease. Appropriate treatment of risk factors for vascular disease—blood pressure control, smoking cessation, diet modification, and anticoagulation (in select settings such as atrial fibrillation)—is mandatory and may be of benefit.

Frontotemporal Dementias

Patients with the behavioral variant of frontotemporal dementia (FTD) are frequently socially disinhibited, but they may also be lethargic and lack motivation and spontaneity. Patients with the progressive nonfluent aphasia variant of FTD have loss of speech fluency with poor articulation and syntactic errors but relative preservation of comprehension. Those with the semantic dementia variant of FTD remain fluent with normal phonation but have progressive difficulty with naming and word comprehension. Memory and spatial skills and praxis are relatively preserved early on in all of these forms, whereas executive function, emotional regulation, and conduct are relatively impaired.

There are several frontotemporal lobar degenerations (FTLDs), including Pick's disease (now referred to as FTLD-tau). In some families, a mutation in the microtubule-associated protein tau gene *(MAPT)* on chromosome 17 causes tau-positive frontotemporal dementia with parkinsonism (FTDP-17). Transactive response DNA-binding protein (TDP-43) pathology accounts for 40% of FTD with or without motor neuron disease. Although mutations in the fused in sarcoma gene *(FUS)* had previously been identified as a cause of familial amyotrophic lateral sclerosis (ALS), some also give rise to 5% to 10% of clinically diagnosed FTD (typically the behavioral variant). Hexanucleotide repeat expansions in *C9orf72* cause neurodegeneration in FTD and ALS. RNA processing is abnormal in both conditions.

As in AD, all forms of FTD progress for years. No intervention slows the inevitable decline of these patients. Approximately 50% of patients have a family history of the disease.

Parkinson's Disease

Almost 50% of patients with Parkinson's disease (see Chapter 114) become demented by the time they reach the age of 85 years. The dementia of Parkinson's disease affects executive function out of proportion to its impact on language and visuospatial processing. Thought processes appear to slow down (i.e., bradyphrenia), analogous to the slowing of movement (i.e., bradykinesia).

Because dementia occurs relatively late in the progression of Parkinson's disease, most patients are taking drugs to improve their movement disorder by enhancing dopaminergic neurotransmission. These drugs can induce psychosis. Dose reductions should be attempted before the diagnosis of underlying dementia is made for these patients. Acetylcholinesterase inhibition has been helpful for patients with dementia caused by Parkinson's disease, and the FDA has specifically approved rivastigmine for this indication.

Normal-Pressure Hydrocephalus

The triad of dementia (typically subcortical), gait instability, and urinary incontinence suggests the possibility of normal-pressure hydrocephalus. These patients appear to walk with their feet stuck to the floor, without lifting up the knees and with a broad base. Symptoms evolve over the course of weeks to months, and

brain imaging reveals ventricular enlargement out of proportion to the degree of cortical atrophy.

Numerous diagnostic tests have been described, including radionuclide cisternography and MRI flow studies. The most important test remains the clinical response to removal of large volumes of CSF through serial lumbar punctures or the temporary placement of a lumbar drain, followed by examination of the patient's gait and cognitive function. Neurosurgical placement of a permanent ventriculoperitoneal shunt may correct the problem. Patients likely to benefit from shunt placement have a clear response to the removal of 30 to 40 mL of spinal fluid, with improved gait and alertness within minutes to hours of the procedure. The cause of normal-pressure hydrocephalus is a derangement of the CSF hydrodynamics. Shunt placement is most likely to be effective if normal-pressure hydrocephalus occurs after severe head trauma or subarachnoid hemorrhage.

Prion Infection, Chronic Meningitis, and Dementia Related to Acquired Immunodeficiency Syndrome

Creutzfeldt-Jakob disease (CJD) is a subacute, dementing, transmissible illness with typical onset between 40 and 75 years of age and an incidence of one case per 1 million people (see Chapter 90). The disease causes spongiform degeneration and gliosis in widespread areas of the cortex. Clinical variants of the disorder are differentiated by the relative predominance of cerebellar symptoms, extrapyramidal hyperkinesias, or visual agnosia and cortical blindness (i.e., Heidenhain variant).

Ninety percent of patients with CJD have myoclonus, compared with 10% of patients with AD. Patients with all forms of the disease share a relentlessly progressive dementia and disruption of personality over weeks to months. The electroencephalogram shows characteristic abnormalities, including diffuse slowing and periodic sharp waves or spikes.

The transmissible agent, a prion protein, is invulnerable to routine modes of antisepsis. CSF can be tested for the 14-3-3 protein, although this test is not as sensitive or specific for CJD as once hoped (see Chapter 90). Diffusion-weighted MRI images show characteristic cortical ribbon changes.

Certain infectious agents can cause the subacute or chronic development of subcortical dementia. These chronic meningitides are discussed in Chapter 90.

Human immunodeficiency virus accesses the central nervous system through monocytes and the microglial system and causes associated neuronal cell loss, vacuolization, and lymphocytic infiltration. The dementia associated with this infection is characterized by bradyphrenia and bradykinesia. Patients have executive dysfunction, impaired memory, poor concentration, and apathy. Treatment of the underlying viral infection with protease inhibitors and reverse transcriptase inhibitors may slow the progression of the dementia (see Chapter 90).

⬤ OTHER MEMORY DISTURBANCES
Structure of Memory

Memory function is divided into introspective processes (i.e., declarative, explicit, aware memories) and processes that are not accessible to introspection (i.e., nondeclarative, implicit, procedural memories). Short-term memory (e.g., words on a list) is a form of declarative memory. Other forms include the conscious recall of episodes from personal experience (i.e., episodic memory), and factual knowledge (i.e., semantic memory) that can be consciously recalled and stated (i.e., declared). Declarative memory involves consciously *knowing that* .... Patients with amnesia resulting from lesions of the medial temporal lobes or midline diencephalic structures have deficits of declarative memory.

Nondeclarative memory encompasses several distinct and neuroanatomically less clearly localized functions related to the performance of specific learned motor, cognitive, or perceptual tasks. Nondeclarative (procedural) memories involve unconsciously *knowing how* .... Deficits in nondeclarative memory may involve various areas of association neocortex, depending on the nature of the task (e.g., parietal-temporal-occipital junction cortex for visual perceptual tasks, frontal association cortex for motor tasks). Patients with amnesia resulting from lesions of the medial temporal lobes tend to perform normally on tests of nondeclarative memory.

Anterograde amnesia is the inability to learn new information. It commonly occurs after brain injury or in association with dementia. The inability to recollect prior information is retrograde amnesia. Both types of amnesia usually occur together in brain injury syndromes, although the extent of one type or the other may vary. The degree of anterograde amnesia after head injury correlates with the severity of the injury.

Isolated Disorders of Memory Function

Memory can be impaired in relative isolation as a consequence of head injury, thiamine deficiency (i.e., Korsakoff's syndrome), benign forgetfulness of aging, transient global amnesia, or psychogenic disease.

Head injury typically results in retrograde amnesia in excess of anterograde amnesia, with both forms stretching out over time from the discrete event. As time passes, these disrupted memories gradually return, although rarely to the point at which the events immediately surrounding the trauma are recalled.

Korsakoff's syndrome is characterized by the near-total inability to establish new memory. Patients often confabulate responses when they are asked to convey the details of their current circumstance or to relay the content of a recently presented story. Deficiency of thiamine and other nutritional deficiencies in the context of chronic alcoholism are the most common underlying causes. Thiamine is a necessary cofactor in the metabolism of glucose, and thiamine must be replenished at the same time glucose is administered whenever a comatose patient is seen in the emergency department.

Aging is associated with mild loss of memory, exhibited by difficulty in recalling names and by forgetfulness for dates. Population-based assessments of neuropsychological function have demonstrated that poor performance on delayed-recall tasks is the most sensitive indicator of cognitive change with advancing age. Verbal fluency, in contrast, remains intact with advancing age, and vocabulary may increase with time, even into old age.

Transient global amnesia is a dramatic memory disturbance that affects older patients (>50 years). Patients usually have only one episode; occasionally, episodes recur over the course of several years. Patients have complete temporal and spatial disorientation; orientation for person is preserved. Near-total retrograde and anterograde amnesia persists for various periods, typically 6 to 12 hours. Patients are often anxious and may repeat the same question over and over again. Transient global amnesia may be confused with psychogenic amnesia, fugue state, or partial complex status epilepticus. Transient global amnesia is thought to reflect underlying vascular insufficiency to the hippocampus or midline thalamic projections.

Unlike patients with organic memory disturbances, patients with psychogenic amnesia typically have inconsistent loss of recent and remote memory, relatively more loss of emotionally charged memory (rather than relatively less loss of such memory in organic disease), and an apparent indifference to their own plight; they ask few questions. Most characteristically, patients with psychogenic amnesia tend to express disorientation to person (asking, *Who am I?*), a phenomenon seldom seen in organic memory disturbance.

Patients with severe depression may exhibit pseudodementia. Vegetative signs, including changes in appetite, weight, and sleep pattern, are common, whereas signs of cortical impairment, such as aphasia, agnosia, and apraxia, are rare. Memory and bradyphrenia improve with antidepressant therapy. Depression often coexists with other causes of dementia, such as AD, Parkinson's disease, and vascular dementia.

For a deeper discussion on this topic, please see Chapter 402, "Alzheimer's Disease and Other Dementias," in Goldman-Cecil Medicine, *25th Edition.*

SUGGESTED READINGS

Bateman RJ, Xiong C, Benzinger TLS, et al: Clinical and biomarker changes in dominantly inherited Alzheimer's disease, N Engl J Med 367:795–804, 2012.

Carrillo MC, Brashear HR, Logovinsky V, et al: Can we prevent Alzheimer's disease? Secondary "prevention" trials in Alzheimer's disease, Alzheimers Dement 9:123–131, 2013.

Castellani RJ, Perry G: Pathogenesis and disease-modifying therapy in Alzheimer's disease: the flat line of progress, Arch Med Res 43:694–698, 2012.

Iqbal K, Flory M, Soininen H: Clinical symptoms and symptom signatures of Alzheimer's disease subgroups, J Alzheimers Dis 37:475–481, 2013.

Ling SC, Polymenidou M, Cleveland DW: Converging mechanisms in ALS and FTD: disrupted RNA and protein homeostasis, Neuron 79:416–438, 2013.

McKhann GM, Knopman DS, Chertkow H, et al: The diagnosis of dementia due to Alzheimer's disease: recommendations from the National Institute on Aging and the Alzheimer's Association workgroup, Alzheimers Dement 7:263–269, 2011.

Perry DC, Miller BL: Frontotemporal dementia, Semin Neurol 33:336–341, 2013.

109

Major Disorders of Mood, Thoughts, and Behavior

Jeffrey M. Lyness

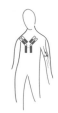

CLASSIFICATION OF MENTAL DISORDERS

Mental (psychiatric) disorders are alterations in thoughts, feelings, or behaviors that produce substantive subjective distress or affect the patient's functional status. Many mental disorders are caused by the direct effects of drugs, systemic disease, or neurologic disease on brain physiology. They may be broadly considered as secondary psychiatric disorders, as opposed to the primary or idiopathic psychiatric disorders. The distinguishing feature of neurocognitive disorders is impairment in intellectual functions such as level of consciousness, orientation, attention, or memory; however, these disorders also often include disruption of mood, thoughts, and behaviors similar to that seen in other psychiatric syndromes. Neurocognitive disorders are the focus of Chapters 105 and 108.

The noncognitive secondary syndromes by definition cause psychiatric phenomena similar to their idiopathic counterparts. During the evaluation of any patient with new or worsened psychiatric symptoms, it is essential to conduct a thorough evaluation for other medical causes, including a careful history and physical examination (with a screening neurologic examination) that often are supplemented by laboratory evaluations. Table 109-1 outlines important causes of psychiatric syndromes. Although some conditions are likely to produce certain psychiatric syndromes, many manifest as any of several psychiatric syndromes. Conversely, a psychiatric syndrome may be caused by any of a wide range of conditions.

Because the cause of primary psychiatric disorders is unknown, approaches to classification depend on reliable empirical observations of phenomena clustered into recognizable syndromes. Table 109-2 shows the most important psychiatric syndromes

and the disorders in which they may manifest. Table 109-3 shows the major idiopathic disorders, excluding addictive disorders (see Chapter 126). Many psychiatric disorders manifest with multiple syndromes. For example, major depression with psychotic features manifests with a depressive syndrome and a psychotic syndrome. In evaluating a patient with new or worsened psychiatric symptoms, the clinician must construct a differential diagnosis based on syndromes alongside the differential diagnosis based on potential secondary causes.

DEPRESSIVE AND BIPOLAR DISORDERS

Depressive and bipolar disorders are characterized by idiopathic episodes of depression alone (i.e., unipolar) or mania and depression (i.e., bipolar). The core symptoms of depressive episodes include emotional symptoms (e.g., dysphoria, irritability, anhedonia, loss of interests), ideational symptoms (e.g., thoughts with hopeless, worthless, guilty, or suicidal themes), and neurovegetative symptoms and signs (e.g., anergia; psychomotor slowing or agitation; decreased concentration; altered sleep, appetite, and weight).

Major depressive disorder is defined by episodes of a least five symptoms, including depressed mood, anhedonia, or loss of interests, that occur almost every day for at least 2 consecutive weeks, sufficient to cause significant distress and affect functional status. Other prominent symptoms may include associated anxiety, somatic worry, or new somatic symptoms, and in the most severe cases, psychotic symptoms, including nihilistic or self-deprecatory (i.e., mood-congruent) delusions.

Major depression is common, with a 12-month prevalence of approximately 7% and a lifetime prevalence of up to 10% among men and 20% to 25% in women. New depressive episodes have an annual incidence of approximately 3%. First onset may occur at any age but is most common in the third through fifth decades of life. Whereas most episodes of major depression fully remit spontaneously or with treatment, the lifetime risk of recurrence is at least 50% to 70%, and up to 20% of patients may experience chronic symptoms over many years. Major depression is a leading correlate of disability worldwide, is an important determinant of death by suicide, and is associated with increased risk of death from comorbid physical illnesses. Persistent depressive disorder (i.e., dysthymia) is a condition defined by chronic depressive symptoms, often of insufficient severity to meet criteria for major depression.

Depressive disorders are heterogeneous, with many potential pathogenic mechanisms. Genetic factors, such as polymorphisms

TABLE 109-1	IMPORTANT CAUSES OF PSYCHIATRIC SYNDROMES
CENTRAL NERVOUS SYSTEM CONDITIONS	**SYSTEMIC DISEASES**
Tumor	Cardiovascular diseases
Toxins	Pulmonary diseases
Vascular disorders	Cancer
Seizure	Infection
Infection	Nutritional disorders
Genetic disorders	Endocrine disorders
Congenital malformation	Metabolic disorders
Demyelinating conditions	**DRUGS**
Degenerative conditions	Drug intoxication
Hydrocephalus	Drug withdrawal

TABLE 109-2   IMPORTANT PSYCHIATRIC SYNDROMES

SYNDROME	MAIN SYMPTOMS AND SIGNS	DISORDERS
Neurocognitive	Impairment in intellectual functions (e.g., level of consciousness, orientation, attention, memory, language, praxis, visuospatial, executive functions)	Neurocognitive disorders Intellectual disability (if onset in childhood)
Mood	Depressive: lowered mood, anhedonia, negativistic thoughts, neurovegetative symptoms	Neurocognitive disorders Mood disorders (bipolar or depressive) (primary or secondary)
	Manic: elevated or irritable mood; grandiosity; goal-directed hyperactivity with increased energy; pressured speech; decreased sleep need	Psychotic disorders (schizoaffective disorder)
Anxiety	All include anxious mood and associated physiologic signs and symptoms (e.g., palpitations, tremors, diaphoresis)	Neurocognitive disorders Mood disorders (bipolar or depressive) (primary or secondary)
	May include various types of dysfunctional thoughts (e.g., catastrophic fears, obsessions, flashbacks) and behaviors (e.g., compulsions, avoidance behaviors)	Psychotic disorders (primary or secondary) Anxiety disorders (primary or secondary)
Psychotic	Impairments in reality testing: hallucinations, thought process derailments	Neurocognitive disorders Mood disorders (bipolar or depressive) (primary or secondary) Psychotic disorders
Somatic symptom syndromes	Somatic symptoms with associated distressing thoughts, feelings, or behaviors	Mood disorders (bipolar or depressive) (primary or secondary) Anxiety disorders (primary or secondary) Obsessive-compulsive and related disorders Trauma-related disorders Somatic symptom disorders
Personality pathology	Dysfunctional enduring patterns of emotional regulation, thought patterns, interpersonal behaviors, impulse regulation	Neurocognitive disorders Personality change due to another medical condition Personality disorders

Data from American Psychiatric Association: Diagnostic and statistical manual of mental disorders, ed 5, Washington, D.C., 2013, American Psychiatric Association.

of the serotonin transporter protein, affect vulnerability to depressive episodes in the face of psychosocial stressors. Depression is polygenic and multifactorial, with genetic factors accounting for about 40% of the risk. Alterations in the functioning of brain serotonergic and noradrenergic systems and of the hypothalamic-pituitary-adrenal axis are found in depression. Neuroimaging studies show smaller hippocampal volumes and altered metabolic activity in several regions, including the anterior cingulate cortex. However, the information in these studies is not sufficient for making the clinical diagnosis, which depends on identification of the clinical syndrome. Dysfunctional, negativistic patterns of thinking, impaired social relationships, and stressful life events also contribute to depression.

Mild to moderate forms of major depression respond to focused psychotherapies or antidepressant medications (level A evidence) (Table 109-4). More severe forms of depression do not respond to psychosocial interventions alone. Severe or refractory depression may be treated safely and effectively with electroconvulsive therapy (level A). Other evidence-based somatic therapies include light therapy (for depression with a seasonal component) and vagal nerve stimulation (levels B and C). Data suggest that the dissociative anesthetic ketamine, an N-methyl-D-aspartate (NMDA) receptor antagonist, may rapidly improve patients with treatment-resistant depression, although the general clinical applicability of ketamine remains to be determined.

Bipolar disorder (i.e., bipolar I) is characterized by recurrent episodes of mania, usually with episodes of major depression. Manic episodes include elevated (euphoric) or irritable mood, goal-directed hyperactivity (often for pleasurable activities with poor judgment leading to substantial adverse consequences such as sexual, spending, or gambling sprees), pressured speech, increased energy level with a decreased need for sleep, and distractibility.

Compared with unipolar depression, bipolar disorder has a lower 12-month prevalence (approximately 0.6%) and a younger average age of onset (typically late teens to 20s). Unlike unipolar depression, bipolar disorder is slightly more common among males. Most patients return to baseline functioning between acute mood episodes, but some have a deteriorating course, and others have frequent debilitating episodes (i.e., rapid cycling of four episodes per year).

Genetic factors play a greater role in the pathogenesis of bipolar disorder than in major depressive disorder, accounting for approximately 50% of the risk and representing a greater than 50-fold increase over the population base rate. Bipolar disorder is polygenic and has been linked in individual families to different loci. The pathogenesis is unclear but likely involves dysregulation of frontostriatal systems. Structural neuroimaging studies show increased ventricular-to-brain ratios, suggesting parenchymal atrophy. Psychosocial stressors often play a role in precipitating episodes of mania and depression.

The mainstay of treatment for bipolar disorder is mood stabilizer medications (e.g., lithium, anticonvulsants such as valproic acid and carbamazepine) for acute episodes and maintenance therapy (level A evidence). The anticonvulsant lamotrigine may be particularly useful for bipolar depression. Antipsychotic medications are useful for acute manic episodes and may have a role in maintenance therapy. Benzodiazepines may be used to treat acute agitation and aggression while waiting for more definitive antimanic therapies to take effect. Antidepressants have long been used for depressive episodes, although they may precipitate manic episodes.

Electroconvulsive therapy is effective for refractory mania (level B evidence) and depression (level A). Psychosocial treatments alone do not effectively treat mania and may be less effective for bipolar depression, but psychoeducation and support to

TABLE 109-3 MAJOR IDIOPATHIC (PRIMARY) DISORDERS OF MOOD, THOUGHTS, AND BEHAVIOR

MOOD DISORDERS	PERSONALITY DISORDERS
Depressive (Unipolar)	**Cluster A: Odd Eccentric**
Major depressive disorder Persistent depressive disorder (dysthymia)	Schizoid personality disorder (detachment from social relationships, restricted emotional expression)
Bipolar	Schizotypal personality disorder (social and emotional deficits, cognitive or perceptual distortions, eccentric behavior)
Bipolar disorder Cyclothymic disorder Bipolar II disorder (bipolar disorder not otherwise specified)	Paranoid personality disorder (pervasive distrust and suspiciousness)
ANXIETY DISORDERS	**Cluster B: Dramatic or Emotional**
Panic disorder (without or with agoraphobia) Generalized anxiety disorder Social phobia Specific phobia	Borderline personality disorder (instability of interpersonal relationships, self-image, and affects, and impulsivity)
OTHER CONDITIONS WITH ANXIETY AS A PROMINENT FEATURE	Narcissistic personality disorder (grandiosity, need for admiration, lack of empathy)
Obsessive-compulsive disorder Acute stress disorder, posttraumatic stress disorder	Antisocial personality disorder (disregard for and violation of the rights of others) Histrionic personality disorder
PSYCHOTIC DISORDERS	**Cluster C: Anxious or Fearful**
Schizophrenia Schizophreniform disorder Brief psychotic disorder Schizoaffective disorder Delusional disorder	Avoidant personality disorder (social inhibition, feelings of inadequacy, hypersensitivity to criticism)
SOMATIC SYMPTOM DISORDERS	Dependent personality disorder (pervasive and excessive need to be taken care of, leading to submissive and clinging behavior and fears of separation)
Somatic symptom disorder Illness anxiety disorder Conversion (functional neurologic symptom) disorder Psychological factors affecting physical condition Factitious disorder (i.e., Munchausen's syndrome)	Obsessive-compulsive personality disorder (preoccupation with orderliness, perfectionism, and mental and interpersonal control, at the expense of flexibility, openness, and efficiency)

Data from American Psychiatric Association: Diagnostic and statistical manual of mental disorders, ed 5, Washington, D.C., 2013, American Psychiatric Association.

TABLE 109-4 PSYCHOTHERAPIES FOR DEPRESSION AND ANTIDEPRESSANT MEDICATIONS

NAME	APPROACH OR MECHANISM OF ACTION
PSYCHOTHERAPY	
Cognitive psychotherapy	Identify and correct negativistic patterns of thinking
Interpersonal psychotherapy	Identify and work through role transitions or interpersonal losses, conflicts, or deficits
Problem-solving therapy	Identify and prioritize situational problems; plan and implement strategies to deal with top-priority problems
COMMONLY USED ANTIDEPRESSANTS	
Selective serotonin reuptake inhibitors (SSRIs) Citalopram and escitalopram Fluoxetine Paroxetine Sertraline	Inhibit presynaptic reuptake of serotonin
Serotonin and norepinephrine reuptake inhibitors (SNRIs) Duloxetine Venlafaxine and desvenlafaxine	Inhibit presynaptic reuptake of serotonin and norepinephrine
Tricyclic antidepressants (TCAs) Amitriptyline Desipramine Doxepin Imipramine Nortriptyline	Inhibit presynaptic reuptake of serotonin and norepinephrine (in various proportions depending on the specific TCA)
Monoamine oxidase inhibitors (MAOIs) Isocarboxazide Phenelzine Selegiline Tranylcypromine	Inhibit monoamine oxidase, the enzyme that catalyzes oxidative metabolism of monoamine neurotransmitters Selective MAO-B inhibitor
Other drugs Bupropion	Unknown, although it is weak inhibitor of presynaptic reuptake of norepinephrine and dopamine
Mirtazapine	Serotonin (5-hydroxytryptamine [5-HT]) antagonist at α_2 and 5-HT2 receptors
Trazodone	Inhibits presynaptic reuptake of serotonin; antagonist at 5-HT2 and 5-HT3 receptors
Vilazodone	Inhibits presynaptic reuptake of serotonin; agonist at 5-HT1A receptors

manage psychosocial stressors and encourage medication compliance improve longer-term outcomes.

A spectrum of less severe bipolar disorders includes conditions marked by episodes of hypomania (i.e., low-level manic symptoms without psychosis or significant impairment in functioning). They include bipolar II disorder, characterized by episodes of hypomania and major depression, and cyclothymic disorder, characterized by hypomania and low-level depression not meeting criteria for major depression. Because patients with bipolar II disorder are most likely to seek care during depressive episodes, it is important to inquire about a history of manic symptoms to avoid precipitating mania with the use of antidepressant medications. The pathogeneses of these less severe mood disorders is unclear.

● DISORDERS WITH ANXIETY AS A PROMINENT FEATURE

The idiopathic anxiety disorders manifest with troublesome thoughts and somatic symptoms (Table 109-5) along with the emotional sensation of anxiety. A panic attack is a transient episode of crescendo anxiety, catastrophic thoughts (e.g., fears of dying, going insane, losing self-control), and somatic symptoms. If panic attacks or other clinically significant anxiety symptoms occur only in predictable response to environmental stimuli, the anxiety disorder is known as a *phobia*, which may further be classified as agoraphobia (i.e., anxiety about being in places from which escape may be difficult or embarrassing such as being alone, in crowds, in tunnels, or on bridges), social phobia (i.e., anxiety in interpersonal situations); and specific phobia (i.e., anxiety provoked by other situations or objects such as blood, animals, or heights). Panic disorder manifests with recurrent panic attacks, some of which are unexpected and unpredictable, along with anticipatory anxiety (i.e., fear of having another attack) and avoidance behaviors (i.e., avoiding situations that

TABLE 109-5   COMMON SOMATIC SYMPTOMS OF ANXIETY

CARDIORESPIRATORY	GENITOURINARY
Palpitations	Urinary frequency or urgency
Chest pain	**NEUROLOGIC OR AUTONOMIC**
Dyspnea or sensation of being smothered	Diaphoresis
GASTROINTESTINAL	Warm flushes
	Dizziness or presyncope
Sensation of choking	Paresthesia
Dyspepsia	Tremor
Nausea	Headache
Diarrhea	
Abdominal bloating or pain	

may provoke a panic attack or in which having an attack is perceived to be embarrassing or dangerous).

Other disorders may not cause discrete panic attacks. Obsessive-compulsive disorder is characterized by recurrent obsessions (i.e., thoughts, impulses, or mental images that are anxiety-producing, perceived as intrusive and inappropriate, and resistant to attempts to suppress or neutralize them) and compulsions (i.e., repetitive behaviors or mental acts performed in response to obsessions or other rigid rules). Recognizing its distinct pathogenesis involving striatofrontal function and central serotonergic systems, it has been classified separately from the anxiety disorders.

Individuals exposed to severely stressful events (typically involving the actual or threatened loss of life or limb) may experience any of a wide variety of psychiatric sequelae. If the sequelae include symptoms of intrusion (e.g., intrusive memories, dreams, flashbacks, intense distressing responses to reminders of the trauma), avoidance of distressing memories or external reminders, negative cognitions and mood (e.g., amnesia for aspects of the event, negativistic thoughts about oneself in general or self-blame for the event, diminished interests or activities, feelings of detachment), and alterations in arousal and reactivity, the disorder is called *acute stress disorder* (duration up to 1 month) or *posttraumatic stress disorder* (duration is more than 1 month). Enduring anxiety symptoms that are not captured by these diagnoses or by diagnoses of cognitive, mood, or psychotic disorders may be diagnosed as *generalized anxiety disorder*.

These disorders are common, with point prevalence of 1% to 2% each for panic disorder and obsessive-compulsive disorder and up to 10% for phobias. Although there are fewer data on long-term outcome than for mood disorders, many of these disorders tend to have a chronic waxing and waning course. Most of these disorders have a first onset in the teens, 20s, and 30s, although new-onset anxiety is common in later life. The cause is rarely a primary anxiety disorder (see Table 109-2).

The pathogeneses of most anxiety disorders may be understood as inappropriate activation of the stress response system involving a variety of neuroendocrine and autonomic outputs and coordinated by the central nucleus of the amygdala and other brain structures. The amygdala receives excitatory glutamatergic inputs from cortical sensory areas and the thalamus and has outputs to the major monoaminergic centers (e.g., noradrenergic neurons of the locus coeruleus, dopaminergic neurons of the ventral tegmental area, and serotonergic neurons of the raphe nuclei), which project to the many brain regions subserving the symptoms of anxiety.

The identification and correction of dysfunctional patterns of thinking (i.e., cognitive therapy) and the extinction of pathologic behaviors and positive reinforcement of more functional behaviors (i.e., behavior therapy) are evidence-based psychotherapies useful in most anxiety disorders (level A evidence). They are the sole therapies for specific phobias and may be the sole or primary therapy for most other anxiety disorders or combined with pharmacotherapy.

Antidepressant, anxiolytic, and other drug therapies are used in treatment. Increasingly, antidepressant medications have replaced anxiolytics as the mainstay of pharmacotherapy for panic disorder, posttraumatic stress disorder, generalized social phobia, and generalized anxiety disorder. For obsessive-compulsive disorder, only antidepressant agents with pronounced activity on the serotonergic system (i.e., clomipramine and selective serotonin reuptake inhibitors [SSRIs]; see Table 109-4) are efficacious.

PSYCHOTIC DISORDERS

Psychosis is a loss of reality testing, manifested as hallucinations (i.e., false sensory perceptions), delusions (i.e., fixed false beliefs), and thought process derailments. Schizophrenia is the prototypic psychotic disorder; it includes acute episodes of psychosis (i.e., positive symptoms) and often declining overall functioning over time related to the negative symptoms such as affective flattening, abulia, apathy, and social withdrawal.

The lifetime prevalence of schizophrenia is slightly less than 1%, and its chronic, debilitating course takes a considerable toll on patients, families, and society. Peak onset is in late adolescence to young adulthood, with slightly younger ages for males than females. The annual incidence is approximately 15 cases per 100,000 people, but with marked variability across study samples and populations. The condition is slightly more common in males than females.

The pathogenesis of schizophrenia remains unknown, but it is clearly multifactorial. Genetic factors account for up to 50% of the risk, with multiple loci implicated. Studies of postmortem brains indicate a nongliotic neuropathologic process with subtle disruptions of cortical cytoarchitecture. It is likely that psychosocial factors and neurodevelopment interact with a nonlocalizable brain lesion present at birth or acquired early in life. Dopaminergic mesocortical and mesolimbic pathways are important in the production of psychotic symptoms.

Antipsychotic medications, often with adjunctive benzodiazepines, are used to treat acute psychotic episodes. Although maintenance antipsychotic medications help reduce the severity and frequency of acute psychotic episodes (level A evidence), comprehensive psychosocial rehabilitation programs are required to help patients manage interpersonal and other stressors and to improve overall clinical outcomes. Adjunctive cognitive-behavioral therapy also may improve outcomes for some patients (level A). Second-generation (atypical) antipsychotic medications have replaced first-generation antipsychotics in common U.S. practice because of their lower rates of extrapyramidal side effects, including tardive dyskinesia. However, second-generation drugs contribute to an increase in obesity and metabolic syndrome.

Schizoaffective disorder is a chronic, recurrent disorder with a prevalence slightly lower than that of schizophrenia. It is characterized by episodes of nonmood psychosis and mood episodes (i.e., manic or depressed) with psychotic features. Its diagnosis therefore cannot be based on the patient's clinical findings at any one point in time but requires knowledge of the overall course. The outcomes of schizoaffective disorder are heterogeneous but on average are intermediate between schizophrenia and mood disorders. Treatment is symptomatic, using antipsychotic, mood stabilizing, and antidepressant medications to target specific psychotic and mood symptoms.

Delusional disorder is characterized by delusions in the absence of thought process disorder, prominent hallucinations, or the negative symptoms of schizophrenia. The delusions may be potentially plausible (i.e., not bizarre). Delusional disorder has a lifetime prevalence of approximately 0.2%. It often is only partially responsive to antipsychotic medications, but patients' functioning may be largely unimpaired if they are able with the aid of antipsychotics and psychotherapy to avoid acting on their delusions. The pathogeneses of the nonschizophrenic primary psychotic disorders remain largely unknown.

● SOMATIC SYMPTOM DISORDER AND RELATED DISORDERS

Formerly called *somatoform disorders*, these conditions include somatic symptoms and associated thoughts, feelings, or behaviors that are distressing and disabling. Prominent types include somatic symptom disorder (i.e., excessive thoughts, feelings, or behaviors associated with one or more somatic symptoms), illness anxiety disorder (i.e., illness preoccupation and health-related behaviors disproportionate to somatic symptoms), conversion (i.e., functional neurologic symptom) disorder (i.e., neurologic somatoform symptoms incompatible with recognized neurologic or general medical conditions), and psychological factors affecting physical conditions. Factitious disorder (i.e., Munchausen's syndrome) is a mental disorder in which patients consciously produce stigmata of disease (e.g., simulated or artificially induced fever or hypoglycemia) for the unconscious gain of assuming the sick role.

Although identifiable physical disease is insufficient to fully explain the patient's presentation, in all these conditions other than factitious disorder, the patient's distress and dysfunction are *not* consciously produced and are just as distressing to patients as would be similar symptoms produced by other medical conditions. Malingering is the conscious feigning of illness for conscious gain and therefore is not a mental disorder.

● PERSONALITY DISORDERS

Personality is defined as the repertoire of enduring patterns of inner mental experience and behavior, including affect and impulse regulation, defense and coping mechanisms, and interpersonal relatedness. Personality traits must be distinguished from time-limited states. For example, a patient who exhibits dependent features solely while acutely depressed does not have a dependent personality.

A personality disorder is diagnosed when personality traits lead to pervasive (if variable) subjective distress or dysfunction in a broad range of situations. The major personality disorders are listed in Table 109-3. Personality and personality disorders are

the result of complex interactions among genetic, environmental, and developmental factors. Approaches to patients with personality disorders depend on the specific type, but in most clinical circumstances other than long-term psychotherapy, the realistic goal is not to alter fundamental personality structure but to help the patient maximize use of personality strengths (e.g., optimal defense mechanisms) while minimizing the harmful effects of emotional dysregulation, unhelpful defenses, and destructive behaviors.

Although not the mainstay of most treatments for personality disorders, pharmacotherapy can be useful in selected patients (e.g., antipsychotics to target escalating paranoia in paranoid personality disorder, mood stabilizers or antidepressants to target emotional dysregulation in borderline personality disorder). Patients with personality disorders are also prone to mood, anxiety, eating, addictive, and other treatable psychiatric disorders.

● PROSPECTUS FOR THE FUTURE

Advances in neuroscience will lead to better pharmacologic or other somatic therapies. One example, deep brain stimulation, is being studied for severe refractory mood and anxiety disorders. In the future, regimens tailored for each individual may be based on genomic or proteomic profiles. These same advances may help identify patients for whom evidence-based psychotherapies or other psychosocial interventions are most likely to be effective. Identification of more specific and powerful risk markers may lead to the development of preventive interventions for at-risk individuals or groups. The current U.S. health care system, however, provides barriers that often prevent implementation of mental health treatments, although this may change in light of recent incentives to improve the health of populations.

SUGGESTED READINGS

American Psychiatric Association: Diagnostic and statistical manual of mental disorders, ed 5, Arlington, VA, 2013, American Psychiatric Association.

Anderson IM, Haddad PM, Scott J: Bipolar disorder, BMJ 345:e8508, 2012.

Bateman AW: Treating borderline personality disorder in clinical practice, Am J Psychiatry 169:560–563, 2012.

Gask L, Evans M, Kessler D: Clinical review: personality disorder, BMJ 347:f5276, 2013.

Geddes JR, Miklowitz DJ: Treatment of bipolar disorder, Lancet 381:1672–1682, 2013.

Kupfer DJ, Frank E, Phillips ML: Major depressive disorder: new clinical, neurobiological, and treatment perspectives, Lancet 379:1045–1055, 2012.

Leucht S, Tardy M, Komossa K, et al: Antipsychotic drugs versus placebo for relapse prevention in schizophrenia: a systematic review and meta-analysis, Lancet 379:2063–2071, 2012.

Leucht S, Cipriani A, Spineli L, et al: Comparative efficacy and tolerability of 15 antipsychotic drugs in schizophrenia: a multiple-treatments meta-analysis, Lancet 382:951–962, 2013.

Murrough JW, Iosifescu DV, Chang LC, et al: Antidepressant efficacy of ketamine in treatment-resistant major depression: a two-site randomized controlled trial, Am J Psychiatry 170:1134–1142, 2013.

Rector NA, Beck AT: Cognitive behavioral therapy for schizophrenia: an empirical review, J Nerv Ment Dis 200:832–839, 2012.

Tol WA, Barbui C, van Ommeren M: Management of acute stress, PTSD, and bereavement: WHO recommendations, JAMA 310:477–478, 2013.

Wetherell JL, Petkus AJ, White KS, et al: Antidepressant medication augmented with cognitive-behavioral therapy for generalized anxiety disorder in older adults, Am J Psychiatry 170:782–789, 2013.

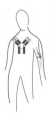

110

Autonomic Nervous System Disorders

William P. Cheshire, Jr.

DEFINITION AND EPIDEMIOLOGY

The autonomic nervous system reaches throughout the body and governs all visceral activity. Its central network and peripheral sympathetic and parasympathetic divisions integrate complex organ functions, maintain internal homeostasis in response to environmental change, modulate the flight-or-fight physiologic response to stress, and enable circulation, digestion, and procreation.

Benign dysautonomias are common. Neurally mediated syncope and situational reflex syncope in response to emotional distress, carotid sinus stimulation, micturition, defecation, coughing, straining, or other factors occur in about 20% of people during a lifetime and account for 1% to 3% of all emergency room visits. Hyperhidrosis of the palms and soles affects about 1% of the population. Anhidrosis can contribute to increased mortality rates during severe heat stress.

One of the most disabling manifestations of autonomic failure is orthostatic hypotension, the prevalence of which increases with age, physical inactivity, and in diseases that impair sympathetic adrenergic nerves. Orthostatic hypotension affects about 5% to 20% of the elderly.

Diabetes mellitus is the most common cause of autonomic neuropathy in industrialized nations. About 30% of diabetics develop autonomic neuropathy, and symptomatic orthostatic hypotension occurs in 5% of patients. Other features of autonomic neuropathy include constipation in 40% to 60% of diabetics, gastroparesis in 20% to 40%, bladder dysfunction in 30% to 80%, and erectile impotence in more than 30% of men.

> For a deeper discussion of these topics, please see Chapter 25, "Common Clinical Sequelae of Aging," and Chapter 229, "Diabetes Mellitus," in Goldman-Cecil Medicine, 25th Edition.

PATHOLOGY

Many brain, spinal cord, peripheral nerve, and systemic disorders that impair autonomic nerves can cause autonomic dysfunction or failure. They include a wide range of degenerative, traumatic, cerebrovascular, autoimmune, genetic, metabolic, toxic, and pharmacologic conditions.

Small-caliber peripheral autonomic nerves are unmyelinated or thinly myelinated, and small-fiber peripheral neuropathies that cause distal sensory loss may also involve sympathetic or parasympathetic nerves. Diabetic autonomic neuropathy results from microvascular damage to autonomic nerves. Several hereditary, infectious, metabolic, toxic, and drug-induced sensory and autonomic neuropathies are recognized causes.

Accumulation of abnormal proteins distinguishes some of the degenerative dysautonomias. Oligodendroglial cytoplasmic inclusions composed of aggregates of misfolded α-synuclein are pathognomonic of multiple system atrophy. Abnormally folded sympathetic neuronal accumulation of α-synuclein occurs in Lewy body disorders such as Parkinson's disease. Peripheral autonomic nerve deposition of β-pleated sheet amyloid protein causes a severe autonomic neuropathy, which is frequently seen in primary amyloidosis, immunoglobulin light chain–associated disease, and hereditary amyloidosis, although rarely in reactive amyloidosis.

Other dysautonomias have an autoimmune basis. Autonomic instability has long been recognized in Guillain-Barré syndrome, which is an acute inflammatory, demyelinating polyradiculoneuropathy associated with antiganglioside antibodies (e.g., anti-GM_1, anti-GM_3). The list of autoimmune autonomic neuropathies includes acute autonomic ganglionopathy; patients with acute pandysautonomia have antibodies against the nicotinic acetylcholine receptor in autonomic ganglia, which is sometimes associated with lung cancer or thymoma. Additional paraneoplastic autonomic neuropathies include those associated with antineuronal nuclear antibody type 1 (i.e., ANNA-1 or anti-Hu) and antibodies against collapsing response mediator proteins (i.e., CRMP-5 or anti-CV2). Lambert-Eaton myasthenic syndrome is associated with antibodies to voltage-gated calcium channels. Antibodies to voltage-gated potassium channels cause autoimmune neuromyotonia and dysautonomia with hyperhidrosis and orthostatic intolerance.

Pharmacologic agents frequently alter autonomic function. Diuretics, sympatholytic drugs, α-adrenoreceptor blockers, and vasodilators can cause or contribute to orthostatic hypotension. Anticholinergics and carbonic anhydrase inhibitors decrease sweating, whereas opioids and selective serotonin reuptake inhibitors increase sweating. Opioids slow intestinal transit. Anticholinergics, tricyclic antidepressants, and antihistamines may cause urinary retention.

Functional dysautonomias are medical conditions in which autonomic function is impaired in the absence of a known structural neurologic deficit. Some psychological disorders may manifest with autonomic symptoms because emotional and autonomic centers are closely linked in the limbic system.

For a deeper discussion of these topics, please see Chapter 420, "Peripheral Neuropathies," Chapter 188, "Amyloidosis," and Chapter 47, "Mechanisms of Immune-Mediated Tissue Injury," in Goldman-Cecil Medicine, 25th Edition.

CLINICAL PRESENTATION

Clinical manifestations of autonomic disorders vary according to which nerves are involved and how severely. Autonomic signs and symptoms may be benign or serious, paroxysmal or continuous, or localized or generalized, and they may represent hypofunction or hyperfunction.

Afferent autonomic lesions that separate central autonomic nuclei from incoming information needed to gauge an appropriate response may cause excessive or erratic autonomic outflow. An example of afferent dysautonomia is the volatile hypertension in carotid arterial baroreceptor failure after irradiation to treat laryngeal carcinoma. Spinal cord injuries above the level of sympathetic outflow at T5 can cause autonomic dysreflexia, a condition of paroxysmal sympathetic surges with hypertension, diaphoresis, flushing, and headache. Catastrophic brain disorders such as subarachnoid hemorrhage, trauma, or hydrocephalus may also cause autonomic storms if hypothalamic circuits are released from cortical inhibition.

More common are efferent autonomic lesions, which cause failure of outflow to neuroeffector junctions, resulting in inadequate excitatory or inhibitory autonomic responses. An example of efferent dysautonomias is autonomic peripheral neuropathy, which may accompany distal sensory loss and decreased Achilles tendon jerks.

Adrenergic failure impairs the cardiac and peripheral vascular response needed to maintain blood pressure during orthostatic stress. Typical symptoms of adrenergic failure include lightheadedness or fatigue on standing that is relieved by sitting.

Vagal failure impairs cardiac parasympathetic tone that may protect against arrhythmogenic sympathetic activity. Patients have a fixed heart rate that does not vary with respiration.

Sudomotor failure with extensive anhidrosis may coexist with tonic pupils and areflexia (i.e., Ross syndrome), and it can increase the risk of heat exhaustion or heat stroke. A dramatic example of regional sudomotor failure is harlequin syndrome, in which hemifacial cutaneous sympathetic denervation divides the pale and dry denervated half of the face from the intact half that flushes red in response to heat stress. Horner's syndrome (i.e., unilateral ptosis, miosis, and anhidrosis) may be identified.

The clinical hallmark of generalized autonomic failure is severe orthostatic hypotension without pulse acceleration. In at least one half of patients, it is accompanied by supine and nocturnal hypertension, a reversal of the normal diurnal decrease in blood pressure during sleep. In addition to vagal and sudomotor failure, patients with generalized autonomic failure may have constipation, gastroparesis, bladder dysfunction, male erectile dysfunction, dry mouth, or dry eyes. Some have postprandial hypotension, in which a large meal high in carbohydrate content causes a reduction in blood pressure.

One of the most severe autonomic disorders is multiple system atrophy, which is a sporadic, progressive, ultimately fatal neurodegenerative disorder in which autonomic failure occurs in combination with parkinsonism or cerebellar ataxia. Bladder hypotonia with overflow incontinence and nocturnal respiratory stridor may occur. The parkinsonian phenotype (i.e., Shy-Drager syndrome) tends to respond poorly to levodopa. Orthostatic hypotension is also common in Lewy body disorders such as Parkinson's disease. Pure autonomic failure consists of widespread autonomic failure without other neurologic features.

In contrast to autonomic failure, neurally mediated syncope occurs in patients with a functioning autonomic nervous system in which there is a reversal of normal autonomic outflow. Prodromal features typically include pallor, sweating, nausea, abdominal discomfort, mydriasis, increased respiratory rate, and cognitive slowing, which may progress to transient loss of consciousness if the patient continues in an upright posture. Withdrawal of peripheral sympathetic vasomotor tone (i.e., vasodepressor syncope) or an increase in parasympathetic tone (i.e., vasovagal syncope) causes a fall in blood pressure, heart rate, and cerebral perfusion.

Orthostatic intolerance refers to a heterogeneous group of conditions in which patients have difficulty sustaining the autonomic outflow needed to maintain blood pressure during the gravitational stress of prolonged standing. Some patients experience a gradual decline in blood pressure, but others experience an abnormal increase in heart rate without a drop in blood pressure.

For a deeper discussion of these topics, please see Chapter 62, "Approach to the Patient with Suspected Arrhythmia," Chapter 67, "Arterial Hypertension," Chapter 136, "Disorders of Gastrointestinal Motility," and Chapter 409, "Parkinsonism," in Goldman-Cecil Medicine, 25th Edition.

DIAGNOSIS AND DIFFERENTIAL DIAGNOSIS

A careful history and discerning physical examination are essential for reaching a diagnosis. The astute clinician inquires about the time course of symptoms and the circumstances that provoke or modify them. How long have they been present? Are they stable, improving, or worsening? Do they occur consistently or episodically? Orthostatic disorders are typically worse in the early morning, in heat, and after physical exercise or a large meal. How well the patient tolerates standing in line or taking a warm shower are helpful clues to identifying orthostatic intolerance.

Physical signs of autonomic dysfunction may include pupillary asymmetry or sluggishness, ptosis, or mucosal dryness. An acutely distended bladder may be suspected by percussion. Asymmetrical sweating may be visible or palpable.

The most important part of the examination, but one that is frequently omitted, is measurement of orthostatic blood pressure (Fig. 110-1). Blood pressure and heart rate should be assessed when the patient is resting supine and again after standing for 1 to 3 minutes or longer. Correlation with symptoms is key. Patients with orthostatic hypotension may appear less alert, or they may shift weight from one leg to the other to improve venous return, lower the head to bring the cerebral circulation closer to the level

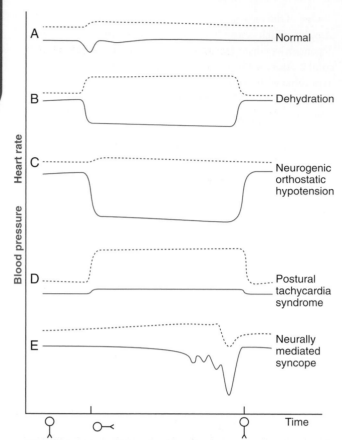

FIGURE 110-1 Orthostatic blood pressure profiles. **A,** The normal response to standing or head-up tilt is no change or a small decrease in blood pressure that recovers within one-half minute and a small increase in heart rate. **B,** Dehydration causing intravascular hypovolemia may cause a fall in blood pressure accompanied by reflex tachycardia. **C,** Neurogenic orthostatic hypotension may cause a more profound drop in blood pressure. Hypotension occurs immediately and is sustained without recovery during standing and often without adequate compensatory tachycardia. **D,** Postural tachycardia syndrome and other forms of orthostatic intolerance are characterized by an abnormal increase in heart rate without orthostatic hypotension. **E,** Neurally mediated syncope develops after standing for some time, may be preceded by oscillations in blood pressure, and may be accompanied by bradycardia with loss of consciousness in about 7 seconds if cerebral perfusion is not restored.

of the heart, or exhibit lower extremity rubor if cutaneous vasomotor function is impaired.

Orthostatic hypotension is a reduction in systolic blood pressure of at least 20 mm Hg or a reduction in diastolic blood pressure of at least 10 mm Hg, with or without symptoms, within 1 to 3 minutes of assuming an erect posture. Neurogenic orthostatic hypotension is typically sustained with continued standing and lacks the reflex tachycardia that may be seen if hypotension is caused by blood loss, dehydration, or excessive venous pooling.

Orthostatic intolerance is a sustained increase in postural heart rate of more than 30 beats per minute in adults (40 in adolescents). In postural tachycardia syndrome, the standing heart rate consistently exceeds 120 beats per minute.

Laboratory testing of autonomic responses under controlled conditions is useful to determine the presence, severity, and distribution of autonomic failure. Clinical autonomic testing typically evaluates beat-to-beat blood pressure and heart rate responses to the Valsalva maneuver, upright tilt, and periodic deep breathing, along with quantitative assessment of sweating responses. Ambulatory blood pressure testing is useful for the assessment of episodic or postprandial hypotension, nocturnal hypertension, and the volatile hypertension of autonomic storms.

⬤ TREATMENT

Treatment options for orthostatic hypotension are outlined in Table 110-1. The goal is to enable the patient to stand long enough to engage in daily activities without symptoms. Medication is not always needed and can potentially exacerbate recumbent hypertension. Orthostatic intolerance was shown in a randomized controlled trial to improve after endurance exercise training (level A evidence).

Generalized hyperhidrosis may be reduced by oral anticholinergic agents such as 1 to 2 mg of glycopyrrolate taken one to three times daily (level B evidence). Topical glycopyrrolate reduces regional gustatory sweating (level A). Subdermal botulinum toxin injections are helpful for some forms of focal hyperhidrosis (level A), and palmar hyperhidrosis may respond to tap water iontophoresis (level B) or, in severe cases, to endoscopic thoracic sympathotomy (level A).

For a deeper discussion of these topics, please see Chapter 418, "Autonomic Disorders and Their Management," in Goldman-Cecil Medicine, 25th Edition.

⬤ PROGNOSIS

Orthostatic intolerance and neurally mediated syncope are frequently benign, manageable, and improve or recover with time. Autonomic failure, in contrast, can signify a more serious prognosis, depending on the nature and extent of its pathophysiology. Persistent or severe orthostatic hypotension carries a worse prognosis.

Diabetic cardiovascular autonomic neuropathy doubles the risk for silent myocardial ischemia and overall mortality. Amyloid autonomic neuropathy is especially grave, with a median survival of less than 1 year if the patient has orthostatic hypotension. Pure autonomic failure may remain stable for many years, although some patients with this phenotype eventually develop signs of multiple system atrophy, which denotes a life expectancy of 7 to 9 years after diagnosis.

Regular physical exercise can reverse the autonomic deconditioning that comes from inactivity. In the elderly, it may compensate for some age-associated decline in autonomic function (level B evidence).

For a deeper discussion of these topics, please see Chapter 418, "Autonomic Disorders and Their Management," in Goldman-Cecil Medicine, 25th Edition.

TABLE 110-1 TREATMENT OF ORTHOSTATIC HYPOTENSION

INTERVENTION	RATIONALE	DOSAGE	EVIDENCE LEVEL
CONSERVATIVE			
Avoid prolonged bed rest and increase time spent upright	Reverses physiologic deconditioning		B
Liberalize fluid intake	Expand plasma volume	2-2.5 L/day	B
Increase sodium intake	Expand plasma volume	Salt 10-20 g/day	A
Compressive leg garments and abdominal binder	Reduce venous pooling	15-20 mm Hg	B
Physical counter-maneuvers	Tensing limb muscles augments venous return	Isometric contractions for 30 sec	A
Water bolus treatment	Sympathetic reflex increases blood pressure for 1-2 hr	16 oz. plain water	A
Elevate heads of bed 4 inches	Decrease nocturnal natriuresis and nocturnal hypertension		C
Avoid large meals high in carbohydrate content	If patient is subject to postprandial hypotension		B
PHARMACOLOGIC			
Discontinue or decrease dose of blood pressure–lowering drugs			A
Midodrine	α-Adrenergic agonist, constricts capacitance vessels	5-10 mg tid	A
Fludrocortisone	Retains sodium and sensitizes peripheral vascular α-adrenergic receptors	0.1-0.4 mg/day	B
Pyridostigmine	Stimulates sympathetic ganglionic transmission	30-60 mg bid or tid	B

SUGGESTED READINGS

Benarroch EE: Postural tachycardia syndrome: a heterogeneous and multifactorial disorder, Mayo Clin Proc 87:1214–1225, 2012.

Feldstein C, Weder AB: Orthostatic hypotension: a common, serious and under-recognized problem in hospitalized patients, J Am Soc Hypertens 6:27–39, 2013.

Figueroa JJ, Basford JR, Low PA: Preventing and treating orthostatic hypotension: as easy as A, B, C, Cleve Clin J Med 77:298–306, 2010.

Freeman R, Wieling W, Axelrod FB, et al: Consensus statement on the definition of orthostatic hypotension, neurally mediated syncope and the postural tachycardia syndrome, Auton Neurosci 161:46–48, 2011.

Guzman JC, Armaganijan LV, Morillo CA: Treatment of neurally mediated reflex syncope, Cardiol Clin 31:123–129, 2013.

Karayannis G, Giamouzis G, Cokkinos DV, et al: Diabetic cardiovascular autonomic neuropathy: clinical implications, Expert Rev Cardiovasc Ther 10:747–765, 2012.

Koike H, Watanabe H, Sobue G: The spectrum of immune-mediated autonomic neuropathies: insights from the clinicopathological features, J Neurol Neurosurg Psychiatry 84:98–106, 2013.

Logan IC, Witham MD: Efficacy of treatments for orthostatic hypotension: a systematic review, Age Ageing 41:587–594, 2012.

Pop-Busui R, Cleary PA, Braffett BH, et al: Association between cardiovascular autonomic neuropathy and left ventricular dysfunction: DCCT/EDIC study (Diabetes Control and Complications Trial/Epidemiology of Diabetes Interventions and Complications), J Am Coll Cardiol 61:447–454, 2013.

Singer W, Sletten DM, Opfer-Gehrking TL, et al: Postural tachycardia in children and adolescents: what is abnormal? J Pediatr 160:222–226, 2012.

Spallone V, Ziegler D, Freeman R, et al: Cardiovascular autonomic neuropathy in diabetes: clinical impact, assessment, diagnosis, and management, Diabetes Metab Res Rev 27:639–653, 2011.

Stewart JM: Common syndromes of orthostatic intolerance, Pediatrics 131:968–980, 2013.

Wenning GK, Geser F, Krismer F, et al: The natural history of multiple system atrophy: a prospective European cohort study, Lancet Neurol 12:264–274, 2013.

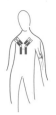

111

Headache, Neck and Back Pain, and Cranial Neuralgias

Timothy J. Counihan

HEADACHE

Definition and Epidemiology

Headache is caused by irritation of pain-sensitive intracranial structures, including the dural sinuses; the intracranial portions of the trigeminal, glossopharyngeal, vagus, and upper cervical nerves; the large arteries; and the venous sinuses. Many structures are insensitive to pain, including the brain parenchyma, the ependymal lining of the ventricles, and the choroid plexuses. The insensitivity of the brain parenchyma to pain accounts for the common clinical observation of patients who, despite having large intracerebral lesions (such as a hematoma or a brain tumor), complain of little or no headache. The term "cervicogenic" headache is sometimes used to indicate that the source of headache (usually occipital in location) arises from an abnormality in the cervical spine.

Classification of Headache

Headache is generally classified into primary, secondary, and cranial neuralgia syndromes (Table 111-1; Table 111-2; Table 111-3). It is essential that the clinician make every effort to make an accurate clinical diagnosis of the presenting headache syndrome; Table 111-4 provides some key questions in the assessment of the patient with headache.

Migraine

Definition

Migraine is a common episodic neurologic disorder characterized by disabling headache preceded in one third of patients by various combinations of neurologic, gastrointestinal, and autonomic phenomena (termed the "aura"). The diagnosis is based on the headache's characteristics and associated symptoms. Results of the physical examination as well as the laboratory studies are usually normal.

TABLE 111-1 PRIMARY HEADACHE SYNDROMES

Migraine	Other primary headache syndromes
Tension-type headache	• Primary stabbing headache
Trigeminal autonomic cephalgias	• Exertional/Sex headache
• Cluster	• Primary thunderclap headache
• Paroxysmal Hemicrania	• Hemicrania continua
• SUNCT	

SUNCT, Sudden-onset Unilateral Neuralgiform (Headache with) Conjunctival Tearing.

TABLE 111-2 SECONDARY HEADACHE SYNDROMES

Post-traumatic	**Disordered Homeostasis**
Vascular	• Hypoxia or hypercapnia (e.g., obstructive sleep apnea)
• Subarachnoid hemorrhage	• Dialysis-associated headache
• Vasculitis	• Hypoglycemia
• Arterial Dissection (carotid or vertebral)	**Medication**
Non-Vascular	• Side effects (e.g. dipyridamole,nitrates, cyclosporine)
• Idiopathic Intracranial Hypertension (Pseudotumor cerebri)	• Withdrawal
• Low CSF pressure (e.g. post lumbar puncture or CSF leak)	**Syndrome of Transient Headache and Neurological Deficits with CSF Lymphocytosis (HANDL)**
• Tumor	
• Chiari malformation	
Infection	**Cervicogenic**
• Meningitis	
• Abscess	
• Sinusitis	

CSF, Cerebrospinal fluid.

TABLE 111-3 COMMON CRANIAL NEURALGIAS AND RELATED DISORDERS

Trigeminal neuralgia
Glossopharyngeal neuralgia
Occipital neuralgia
Other cranial branch neuralgias (e.g., superior orbital neuralgia)
Central facial pain syndromes (e.g., cold-stimulus headache)

TABLE 111-4 KEY QUESTIONS IN THE ASSESSMENT OF HEADACHE

1. For how long have you been having headaches?
2. What were they like when they first began? Were they intermittent, daily persistent, or progressive from the beginning?
3. What is the length of time from the start of the headache until its peak intensity?
4. Are there any warning symptoms (e.g., aura)?
5. Does the headache interfere significantly with normal activity (e.g., work, school)?
6. What aggravates the headache (e.g., light, noise, odors)?
7. What do you do for relief from the headache (e.g., rest, move around, take medication)?
8. What time of day are the headaches most likely to occur? Do they regularly awaken you from sleep?
9. Are you aware of any specific triggers (e.g., foods, stress, lack of sleep, menstrual cycle)?
10. Does anyone else in the family have headaches?

TABLE 111-5 CLASSIFICATION OF MIGRAINE	
Migraine without aura	Migraine variants
Migraine with aura	• Hemiplegic migraine
	• Migraine with basilar aura
	• Vestibular Migraine
	• Retinal Migraine

The prevalence of migraine is up to 18% in women and 6% in men. It is estimated that 28 million Americans have disabling migraine headaches. All varieties of migraine may begin at any age from early childhood on, although peak ages at onset are adolescence and early adulthood.

Several subtypes of migraine are described (Table 111-5). The two most common are migraine without aura and migraine with aura; migraine without aura accounts for 70% of patients. Migraine auras are focal neurologic symptoms that precede, accompany, or, rarely, follow an attack. The aura usually develops over 5 to 20 minutes, lasts less than 60 minutes, and can involve visual, sensorimotor, language, or brainstem disturbances. The most common aura is typified by positive visual phenomena (such as scintillating scotomata) that often precede the headache. The differential diagnosis of an aura includes a focal epileptic seizure arising from the visual cortex of the occipital lobe, or a transient ischemic attack (TIA). In the latter, there is no evolution of symptoms, and the symptoms themselves are typically "negative" (such as a hemianopia) rather than the "positive" visual phenomenon of phosphenes that is characteristic of the migrainous aura. The pain of migraine is often pulsating, unilateral, and frontotemporal in distribution and usually accompanied by anorexia, nausea, and, occasionally, vomiting. In characteristic attacks, patients are markedly intolerant of light (photophobia) and seek rest in a dark room. There may also be intolerance to sound (phonophobia) and occasionally to odors (osmophobia). The diagnosis of migraine requires the presence of at least one of these features, particularly in the absence of gastrointestinal symptoms. The presence of these symptoms results in a syndrome that is invariably disabling for the patient, to the extent that for the duration of the attack he or she is unable to function normally. In children, migraine is often associated with episodic abdominal pain, motion sickness, vertigo, and sleep disturbances. Onset of typical migraine late in life (older than age 50) is rare, although recurrence of migraine that had been in remission is not uncommon. Recurrent migraine headache associated with transient hemiparesis or hemiplegia occurs rarely as a clearly genetically determined (Mendelian) disease (*familial hemiplegic migraine*).

Migraine with basilar aura is unusual and occurs primarily in childhood. Severe episodic headache is preceded, or accompanied by, signs of bilateral occipital lobe, brainstem, or cerebellar dysfunction (e.g., diplopia, bilateral visual field abnormalities, ataxia, dysarthria, bilateral sensory disturbances, other cranial nerve signs, and occasionally coma). *Vestibular migraine* is characterized by symptoms of vertigo with or without the other typical migraine symptoms.

Complications of Migraine

Status Migrainosus refers to a severe migraine lasting greater than 72 hours. *Migrainous infarction* is a rare complication of migraine

with aura. The term *migralepsy* has been suggested for patients in whom an aura triggers a seizure.

Pathophysiology of Migraine

A migraine attack is the end result of the interaction of a number of factors of varying importance in different individuals. These factors include a genetic predisposition, a susceptibility of the central nervous system to certain stimuli, hormonal factors, and a sequence of neurovascular events. A positive family history is reported in 65% to 91% of cases. Three distinct ion channel gene mutations have been identified in patients with familial hemiplegic migraine (FHM), including a mutation in the P/Q type calcium channel on chromosome 19 (FHM 1) and a gene encoding a Na/K- ion pump on chromosome 1 (FHM 2). These findings lend support to the theory that migraine may be a true channelopathy in which mutations of diverse channels result in a common phenotype. The etiology of migraine in the majority of patients remains unknown.

The migrainous aura is likely caused by a "cortical spreading depression," corresponding to a wave of neuronal depolarization spreading over the cortex from posterior to anterior. One of the key structures in the mechanism of pain in migraine is the trigeminal vascular system. Stimulation of the trigeminal nucleus caudalis can activate serotonin receptors and nerve endings on small dural arteries and result in a state of neurogenic inflammation. It is postulated that these processes, in turn, stimulate perivascular nerve endings, with resultant orthodromic stimulation of trigeminal nerve and pain referred to its territory. Furthermore, positron emission tomographic (PET) studies have demonstrated activation of brainstem neuromodulatory structures, including the periaqueductal grey matter, locus coeruleus, and raphe nuclei during a migraine attack.

Treatment of Migraine

The goals of treatment are (1) making an accurate and confident diagnosis of migraine to reassure the patient that there is no more sinister cause for the headache; (2) relieving acute attacks; and (3) preventing pain and associated symptoms of recurrent headaches. The first step is to inform the patient that he or she has a migraine. The benign nature of the disorder and the patient's central role in the treatment plan should be emphasized. It is important that the patient keep a headache diary, which serves to help identify covert headache triggers, assists in monitoring headache frequency and response to treatment, and actively involves the patient in the management of the condition. A sustained pain-free therapeutic response should aim to have the patient pain-free at two hours with no recurrence and no need for subsequent rescue medication.

Acute Migraine Attack

Acute attacks are best alleviated using a stratified, rather than stepped care approach, using single agents or varying combinations of drugs as well as with behavioral modification therapy. Many attacks of migraine respond to simple analgesics, such as acetaminophen, aspirin, or nonsteroidal anti-inflammatory agents (NSAIDs). Opioid drugs and butalbital should not be used in the routine management of patients with migraine. Overuse of analgesics is particularly frequent in headache patients; therefore, one of the most important aspects of therapy is the monitoring of amounts of analgesic used. In patients who are nauseated, it is often helpful to prescribe an anti-emetic agent early in an attack. Phenothiazine drugs have antiemetic, prokinetic, and sedative properties, but they can produce involuntary movements as an acute adverse effect (acute dystonic reaction) or with prolonged use (tardive dyskinesias).

A number of *migraine-specific* serotonin agonist drugs have become available. These agents, commonly referred to as "triptans," are useful in the acute treatment of migraine, having a rapid onset of action. The increasing availability of non-oral (parenteral, inhaled, and transdermal) preparations has largely circumvented the problem of emesis and gastroparesis in migraine patients resulting in greater efficacy. For instance, sumatriptan, available as a subcutaneous preparation, results in a headache response rate of close to 70% (Fig. 111-1). Although triptans are highly effective in alleviating migraine, patients must be carefully instructed in their appropriate use. Moreover, a response to these medications does not confirm a diagnosis of migraine.

Treating Acute Migraine in the Emergency Room

Migraine is one of the most common reasons for emergency room visits and presents some treatment challenges; typically migraine is more difficult to treat once it is fully established. It is essential to confirm that the diagnosis is accurate, even in patients with an established history of migraine. Patients will usually be aware that the headache will have started as their typical migraine, although it may be more severe than usual. In patients who state that the new headache is different to their usual headache, consideration should be given to exclude a more sinister cause.

Thereafter the core principles of treatment include reassurance that the headache can be treated effectively, hydration, pain control, and relief of accompanying symptoms such as nausea and photophobia. The majority of patients presenting with acute migraine as an emergency will have already tried some form of abortive therapy, and they are likely to be dehydrated. In this setting parenteral therapy with an NSAID, a triptan, and an anti-emetic is often effective (Fig. 111-1)

Migraine Prevention

Several agents have a strong evidence base for efficacy in the prevention of migraine (Table 111-6). The use of these agents should be restricted to patients who have frequent attacks (usually more than four per month) and who are willing to take daily medication. With any of the medications, an adequate trial period should be given, using adequate doses, before it is declared ineffective. Combination therapy is occasionally required but is not routinely prescribed. For a preventative drug to be considered successful, it should reduce the headache frequency rate by at least 50%. Other medications commonly used for migraine prevention include gabapentin, cyproheptadine, methysergide, and clonidine, but these have limited evidence to support their use as first line therapy. Magnesium supplementation, the plant extract feverfew, butterbur, and high-dose riboflavin (vitamin B_2) have been effective in some patients.

Future of Migraine Treatment

The most significant recent advance in acute migraine treatment relates to calcitonin gene-related peptide (CGRP) receptor antagonists. Stimulation of trigeminal ganglia neurons results in

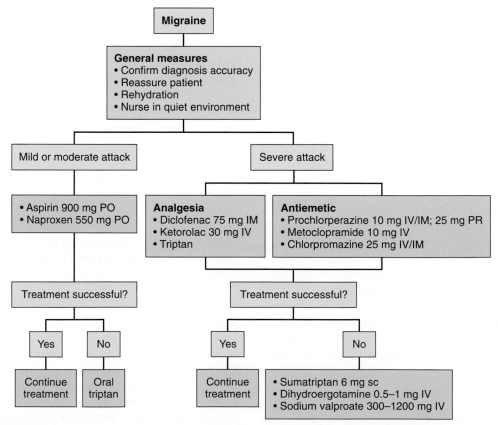

FIGURE 111-1   Algorithm for the treatment of migraine. DHE, Dihydroergotamine; IM, intramuscular; IV, intravenous; NS, normal saline; NSAIDs, nonsteroidal anti-inflammatory drugs; SC, subcutaneous.

TABLE 111-6 PREVENTIVE THERAPIES FOR MIGRAINE

DRUG CLASS	AGENT	DOSE RANGE	EVIDENCE LEVEL	ADVERSE EFFECTS
β-adrenoceptor blockers	Propranolol	80-240 mg	A	Contraindicated in asthma, syncope
	Metoprolol	50-150 mg	A	
	Timolol	10-20 mg	A	
Antiepileptic drugs	Divalproex sodium	200-1500 mg	A	Weight gain, thrombocytopenia, tremor
	Topiramate	25-150 mg	A	Renal calculi, weight loss, amnesia,
	Gabapentin	300-1800 mg	U	glaucoma, dysequilibrium
Antidepressants	Amitriptyline	10-150 mg	B	Somnolence
	Nortriptyline	25-100 mg	N/A	Insomnia, hypertension
	Venlafaxine	37.5-150 mg	B	
Calcium channel blockers	Verapamil	180-480 mg	U	Constipation, hypotension, edema
	Flunarizine*	5-10 mg	N/A	Weight gain, depression
Other	Onabotulinum toxin A	Variable	N/A	Discomfort, ecchymosis

Level of Evidence A, Medication with established efficacy; Level B, medication probably effective; Level U, inadequate data to support use; N/A, not considered in recent evidence review.
*Not available in the US.

release of CGRP; telcagepant, a CGRP receptor antagonist has been found to have similar efficacy to oral triptan therapy. Greater insights into the genetic basis for migraine has enhanced our understanding of ion channel dysfunction in this disorder, and are likely to lead to new therapeutic targets.

Cluster Headache

Clinical Features

Cluster headache is the prototypic trigeminal autonomic cephalgia, entirely distinct from migraine, although there may be some clinical overlap. It is uncommon, occurring in less than 10% of all patients with headache. Unlike migraine, it is much more common in men than in women, and the mean age at onset is later in life. Also, unlike migraine, cluster headache rarely begins in childhood, and there is less often a family history. The pain in cluster headache is of extreme intensity, is strictly unilateral, and is associated with congestion of the nasal mucosa and injection of the conjunctiva on the side of the pain. Increased sweating of the ipsilateral side of the forehead and face may occur. There may be associated ocular signs of Horner syndrome: miosis, ptosis, and the additional feature of eyelid edema. Attacks often awaken patients, usually 2 to 3 hours after the onset of sleep ("alarm-clock headache"). In contrast to migraineurs, the pain is not relieved by resting in a dark, quiet area; on the contrary, patients sometimes seek activity that can distract them. The duration of headache is usually around 1 hour, although it may recur several times in a day, paroxysmally (in *clusters*) for several weeks.

These periods of frequent headaches are separated by headache-free periods of varying duration, often several months or years. Attacks have a striking tendency to be precipitated by even small amounts of alcohol. There are rare variants of cluster headache: a "chronic variety" in which remissions are brief (less than 14 days); *"chronic paroxysmal hemicrania,"* in which attacks are shorter and strikingly more prevalent in women; and *"hemicrania continua,"* in which there is continuous, moderately severe, unilateral headache. The cause of all these syndromes is unknown, although the distribution of the pain suggests dysfunction of the trigeminal nerve.

Treatment

Therapy for cluster headache may be abortive for acute headache or prophylactic to prevent headache. Acute headache may respond to oxygen by mask (7 to 10 L/min for 15 minutes), which is effective within several minutes in 70% of patients. Sumatriptan and dihydroergotamine are also effective. Preventive medications include lithium, divalproex sodium, verapamil, methysergide, and corticosteroids. Paroxysmal hemicrania and related syndromes are often strikingly responsive to indomethacin.

Tension-Type Headache

In contrast to migraine, tension-type headache is featureless. The pain is usually not throbbing, but rather steady and often described as a "pressure feeling" or a "viselike" sensation. It is usually not unilateral and may be frontal, occipital, or generalized. There is frequently pain in the neck area, unlike in migraine. Pain commonly lasts for long periods of time (days) and does not rapidly appear and disappear in attacks. There is no "aura." Photophobia and phonophobia are not prominent. Although tension-type headache may be related by the patient to occur or be exacerbated at times of particular emotional stress, the pathophysiology may relate to sustained craniocervical muscle contraction; hence, a more useful term for this syndrome is *muscle-contraction headache.*

A careful evaluation should be made of the patient's psychosocial milieu and the presence of anxiety or depression. The tricyclic antidepressant drugs in low doses have proven the most useful for prevention of tension-type headache. Although the best documented is amitriptyline, newer agents with fewer side effects may be equally effective. Nonpharmacologic therapies such as relaxation therapy, massage, physiotherapy, or acupuncture may be useful in refractory cases. Intramuscular botulinum toxin injections have been used both in migraine and tension-type headache, but are of established benefit only in patients with chronic migraine.

Other Defined Primary Headache Syndromes

Other acute short-lasting headache syndromes need to be differentiated from migraine, cluster, or tension headache. These include primary "thunderclap" headache, *primary stabbing headache, primary exertional headache,* and coital headache. The latter may be indistinguishable from the headache of intracranial aneurysm rupture and requires computed tomography (CT) and lumbar puncture to exclude subarachnoid hemorrhage (SAH). All of these headache syndromes are more common in migraineurs. Two additional rare, short-lasting headache syndromes deserve mention: short-lasting unilateral neuralgiform headache with conjunctival tearing (SUNCT); and *hypnic* headache. The latter refers to multiple episodes of very brief headache that awaken the patient (typically an older woman) from sleep. The syndrome of SUNCT causes multiple very brief (seconds to minutes) episodes of cluster-like headache and autonomic disturbance.

Chronic daily headache is defined arbitrarily as headache lasting for more than 4 hours on more than 15 days in the month for more than 3 months. In clinical practice this means that the patient has a headache more often than not. In these cases it is important to establish whether the headache syndrome began as an episodic disorder (as in migraine or tension-type headache) or whether it consists of new daily persistent headaches.

New Daily Persistent Headache
New daily persistent headache needs to be distinguished from tension-type or migraine headaches that have transformed into chronic daily headache, and necessitates investigation to exclude a secondary cause.

Headache may be a manifestation of underlying structural brain disease (Table 111-2). Headache can be seen in all forms of cerebrovascular disease, including infarction, intracerebral hemorrhage, and SAH, although headache is rarely prominent in cerebral infarction. In contrast, the headache in SAH is usually extremely severe and often described by the patient as "the worst headache of my life." Nuchal rigidity, third nerve palsy (usually involving the pupil), and retinal, preretinal, or subconjunctival hemorrhages may be found. CT of the head usually shows subarachnoid, intraventricular, or other intracranial blood.

Certain symptoms raise suspicion for a structural brain lesion (Table 111-7).

The patient with headache and fever presents a common diagnostic problem in the emergency department. Neck stiffness is a common symptom. Meningismus is confirmed by eliciting Brudzinski and Kernig signs. Vomiting occurs in about 50% of patients. Suspicion for meningitis should prompt immediate investigation, including a lumbar puncture. If the patient shows focal signs, papilledema, or profound alteration in level of consciousness, CT of the head before lumbar puncture is required to rule out focal disease such as an abscess or subdural empyema. These lesions, however, are rare.

Acute Sinusitis
Head and face pain is the most prominent feature of sinusitis. Malaise and low-grade fever are usually present. The pain is dull, aching, and nonpulsatile; is exacerbated by movement, coughing, or straining; and is improved with nasal decongestants. The pain is most pronounced on awakening or after any prolonged recumbency, and is diminished with maintenance of an upright posture.

The location of the pain depends on the sinus involved. Maxillary sinusitis provokes ipsilateral malar, ear, and dental pain with significant overlying facial tenderness. Frontal sinusitis produces frontal headache that may radiate behind the eyes and to the vertex of the skull. Tenderness to frontal palpation may be present with point tenderness on the undersurface of the medial aspect of the superior orbital rim. In ethmoidal sinusitis, the pain is between or behind the eyes with radiation to the temporal area. The eyes and orbit are often tender to palpation, and, in fact, eye movements themselves may accentuate the pain. Sphenoidal sinusitis causes pain in the orbit and at the vertex of the skull and occasionally in the frontal or occipital regions. Given that the trigeminal nerve mediates pain perception from the sinuses, many patients who complain of "sinus headaches" are probably suffering from the trigeminovascular disturbance of migraine, rather than sinusitis. Chronic sinusitis is seldom a cause of headache.

Brain Tumors
Posterior fossa tumors (particularly of the cerebellum) frequently produce headache, especially if hydrocephalus occurs because cerebrospinal fluid (CSF) flow is partially obstructed. Supratentorial tumors, however, are less likely to cause headache and are more frequently heralded by altered mental status, focal deficits, or seizures. Although increased intracranial pressure is often associated with headache, it is usually not the primary mechanism because uniform pressure elevations do not usually produce distortions of pain-sensitive structures.

Idiopathic Intracranial Hypertension
Idiopathic intracranial hypertension (IIH), also called *benign intracranial hypertension,* is defined as a syndrome of elevated intracranial pressure without evidence of focal lesions, hydrocephalus, or frank brain edema. It usually occurs between the ages of 15 and 45 years and is more frequent in obese women. The disorder is characterized by headache with features of raised intracranial pressure. The headache is usually insidious in onset, is typically generalized, is relatively mild in severity, and is often worse in the morning or after exertion (e.g., straining or coughing).

At times, patients have visual disturbances, such as restricted peripheral visual fields, enlarged blind spots, visual blurring (*obscurations*), or diplopia secondary to abducens nerve palsies. Funduscopic examination shows papilledema, which is often more impressive than the clinical picture. IIH is usually a benign and self-limited disorder, but it may lead to visual loss, including blindness.

The condition has been associated with drugs—vitamin A intoxication, nalidixic acid, danazol (Danocrine), and isotretinoin (Accutane)—as well as corticosteroid withdrawal and systemic disorders such as hypoparathyroidism and lupus.

CT scans are usually normal but can show small ventricles and an "empty sella" in some cases. CSF opening pressure is elevated, usually in the range of 250 to 450 mm of water, with the pressure fluctuating markedly when monitoring occurs over a prolonged period. Some cases of IIH are caused by cerebral venous sinus

TABLE 111-7	DIFFERENTIAL DIAGNOSIS OF ACUTE HEADACHE—MAJOR CAUSES
Migraine	Acute hydrocephalus
Cluster headache	Meningitis or encephalitis
Stroke	Giant cell arteritis (often chronic)
• Subarachnoid hemorrhage	Tumor (usually chronic)
• Intracerebral hemorrhage	Trauma
• Cerebral infarction	
• Arterial dissection (carotid or vertebral)	

occlusion. These cases can occur in hypercoagulable states, including peripartum, in association with the combined oral contraceptive pill, and in association with antiphospholipid antibody syndrome. After secondary causes of IIH have been eliminated, the patient should have dietary counseling for weight loss. Carbonic anhydrase inhibitors (acetazolamide) and corticosteroids have proved useful in headache control. As a second-line agent, furosemide also acts to lower CSF production. Serial lumbar punctures are understandably unpopular with patients even though transient headache relief is obtained. CSF shunting procedures (ventriculoperitoneal shunt) are occasionally necessary. For patients with progressive visual loss, optic nerve sheath fenestration preserves or restores vision in 80% to 90% of cases and provides headache relief in a majority.

Idiopathic Intracranial Hypotension

Also known as *low pressure headache*, idiopathic intracranial hypotension is commonly encountered as a sequela of lumbar puncture, resulting from leakage of CSF through the dural sac. Low pressure headaches may also occur spontaneously as a result of rupture of subarachnoid cysts. The headache is initially characteristically positional, being severe on standing but relieved rapidly on lying down. Occasionally the headache is associated with focal or "false localizing" signs, especially abducens nerve palsies.

Post-Traumatic Headache

Headache following trauma has no specific quality and is associated with irritability, concentration impairment, insomnia, memory disturbance, and light-headedness. Anxiety and depression are present to variable degrees. Multiple treatment options are available, and amitriptyline and nonsteroidal anti-inflammatory agents are useful. Occasionally, muscle relaxants and anxiolytics are beneficial. Training is occasionally associated with the onset of typical migraine.

Giant Cell Arteritis

Headache occurs in 60% of patients with giant cell arteritis, a granulomatous vasculitis of medium and large arteries. Over 95% of patients are 50 years of age or older. Malaise, fever, weight loss, and jaw claudication occur early, in addition to headache. Polymyalgia rheumatica, a syndrome of painful stiffness of the neck, shoulders, and pelvis, is found in half the patients (Chapter 131). Visual impairment secondary to ischemic optic neuritis may occur. The headache is usually described as aching and is exacerbated at night and after exposure to cold. The superficial temporal artery is frequently swollen, tender, and may be pulseless. The erythrocyte sedimentation rate is usually elevated; the mean is 100 mm/hr. Anemia is frequently present. Temporal artery biopsy usually confirms the diagnosis, but, because the arteritis is segmental, large or multiple sections may be required. Prednisone therapy is often dramatically effective and must be given promptly to preserve vision on the affected side.

Evaluation of the patient with acute headache

It is important to distinguish benign from ominous causes of headache. A detailed history (the quality, location, duration, and time course of the headache) helps in determination of which patients have a symptomatic structural intracranial lesion (Table 111-7; Table 111-8; Table 111-4)). Pain intensity is not of much diagnostic value, except for the patient who complains of the acute onset of the worst headache of his or her life). The quality of pain ("throbbing," "pressure," "jabbing") and the location may also be helpful, especially if the pain is of extracranial origin, such as temporal in temporal arteritis. Posterior fossa lesions cause occipitocervical pain, occasionally associated with unilateral retro-orbital pain. In general, multifocal pain usually implies a benign cause. It is most important to clarify the acuity of onset of the headache; patients who describe the onset of pain as "like being hit on the head with a bat" should be suspected of having the sentinel headache of subarachnoid headache. Equally important is to establish the time course of the headache. Is this paroxysmal, nonprogressive headache (typical of migraine or tension-type headache)? Or is the headache daily persistent (such as in temporal arteritis) or progressive (suggesting the presence of a structural brain lesion)? Patients should be asked about any known triggers for the headache, such as menses, particular foods, caffeine, alcohol, or stress. Positional headache (headache that is maximal in the upright position and disappears rapidly on lying down) is characteristic of intracranial hypotension (low pressure headache). Diurnal variation in headache severity may give a clue to cause; morning headache or headache that awakens a patient from sleep may indicate raised intracranial pressure or sleep apnea as a cause. The presence of associated symptoms such as visual disturbances, nausea, or vomiting should be noted. The history should include inquiries about medications, especially use of analgesics and over-the-counter remedies. Information regarding the patient's past medical history as well as family history should also be taken into consideration. In the majority of patients with headache, the physical and neurologic examination findings are normal, although special attention may be directed toward examination of the eyes for papilledema, as well as the temporal arteries for a palpable nonpulsatile artery. Assessment of the patient with acute nontraumatic headache in the emergency room can be challenging; it is essential to establish how the headache evolved. Acute-onset severe headache should prompt investigation to exclude SAH, intracranial hemorrhage, acute obstructive hydrocephalus, and meningitis (Table 111-7). Appropriate initial investigations should include brain imaging with CT or magnetic resonance imaging (MRI). Patients with suspected meningitis without focal neurologic signs or impaired consciousness should not have their lumbar puncture delayed unnecessarily before imaging. All patients should have standard

TABLE 111-8	CLINICAL FEATURES OF HEADACHES SUGGESTING A STRUCTURAL BRAIN LESION	
SYMPTOMS	**SIGNS**
Worst of the patient's life	Nuchal rigidity
Progressive	Fever
Onset >50 years of age	Papilledema
Worse in early morning—awakens patient	Pathologic reflexes or reflex asymmetry
Marked exacerbation with straining	Altered state of consciousness
Focal neurologic dysfunction	

blood tests, including blood cultures if bacterial meningitis is suspected.

A wide variety of systemic diseases have headache as a prominent symptom; some of the more prevalent disorders are summarized in Table 111-2.

CRANIAL NEURALGIAS

Neuralgias are differentiated from other head pains by the brevity of the attacks (usually 1 to 2 seconds or less) and by the distribution of the pain (Table 111-3).

Trigeminal Neuralgia

In trigeminal neuralgia (tic douloureux), stabbing, spasmodic pain occurs unilaterally in one of the divisions of the trigeminal nerve. It lasts seconds, but it may occur many times a day for weeks at a time. It is characteristically induced by even the lightest touch to particular areas of the face, such as the lips or gums. Trigeminal neuralgia is the most frequent neuralgia of the elderly and is thought to be caused by compression of the trigeminal nerve root in the pons by an aberrant arterial loop. A small minority of cases are caused by multiple sclerosis, cerebellopontine angle tumors, aneurysms, or arteriovenous malformations, although in these cases (unlike "true" trigeminal neuralgia) there are usually objective signs of neurologic deficit, such as areas of diminished sensation. In these cases of "symptomatic" neuralgia, the pain is often atypical. MRI is indicated in patients who have sensory loss, those who are under 40, and those with bilateral or atypical symptoms. Trigeminal neuralgia may be life threatening when it interferes with eating. Neuralgic pain is often responsive to treatment with standard doses of an anticonvulsant such as phenytoin, carbamazepine, gabapentin, pregabalin, and, occasionally, baclofen. Antidepressant drugs such as amitriptyline and, more recently, duloxetine may also be useful in this setting. Combination therapy, including an antidepressant, anticonvulsant, and opiate analgesic has been shown to have synergistic effects.

If medical treatments are unsuccessful, surgical treatment may be indicated: microvascular decompression or radiofrequency lesioning of the sensory portion of the trigeminal nerve.

Glossopharyngeal Neuralgia

Glossopharyngeal neuralgia is less common than trigeminal neuralgia. Brief paroxysms of severe, stabbing, unilateral pain radiate from the throat to the ear or vice versa and are frequently initiated by stimulation of specific "trigger zones" (e.g., tonsillar fossa or pharyngeal wall). Swallowing often provokes an attack; yawning, talking, and coughing are other potential triggers. Microvascular decompression is necessary if medical treatment is ineffective.

Postherpetic Neuralgia

Herpes zoster produces head pain by cranial nerve involvement in one third of cases. In some cases a persistent intense burning pain follows the initial acute illness. The discomfort may subside after several weeks or persist (particularly in the elderly) for months or years. The pain is localized over the distribution of the affected nerve and associated with exquisite tenderness to even the lightest touch. The first division of the trigeminal nerve is the most frequent cranial nerve involved (ophthalmic herpes) and is occasionally associated with keratoconjunctivitis. When the seventh nerve is affected ("geniculate herpes"), the pain involves the external auditory meatus and pinna. Occasionally, concomitant facial paralysis may occur (Ramsay Hunt syndrome).

Occipital Neuralgia

Occipital neuralgia is a syndrome that includes occipital pain starting at the base of the skull and often provoked by neck extension. Physical examination shows tenderness in the region of the occipital nerves and altered sensation in the C2 dermatome. Treatment includes the use of a soft collar, muscle relaxants, physical therapy, and local injections of analgesics and anti-inflammatory agents. The term *cervicogenic headache* is often used to describe headache associated with myofascial trigger points in the neck. Importantly, cervical spondylosis (discussed below) is not usually typically associated with headache.

CERVICAL SPONDYLOSIS

Cervical spondylosis is a degenerative disorder of the cervical intervertebral disks leading to osteophyte formation and hypertrophy of adjacent facet joints and ligaments. In contrast to the lumbar spine, herniation of cervical intervertebral disks (nucleus pulposus) accounts for only 20% to 25% of cervical root irritation. Cervical spondylosis one of the most common pathologies seen in office practice and is present radiographically in over 90% of the population older than 60 years of age. For unknown reasons, the degree of anatomic abnormality is not directly correlated with the clinical signs and symptoms. Clinical disease may represent a combination of normal, age-related, degenerative changes in the cervical spine and a congenital or developmental stenosis of the cervical canal; the process may be aggravated by trauma. Cervical spinal myelopathy results from a combination of degenerative disc disease, spondylosis aggravated by biomechanical instability, as well as stiffening and buckling of the ligamentum flavum. It may manifest as a painful stiff neck, with or without symptoms or signs of cervical root irritation or spinal cord compression. Patients with root irritation (cervical radiculopathy) complain of pain and paresthesias radiating down the arm roughly in the dermatomal distribution of the affected nerve root. More typically, the pain radiates in a myotomal pattern, whereas numbness and paresthesias follow a dermatomal distribution. Discrete sensory loss is uncommon and less prominent than symptoms (Table 111-9). For relief, patients often adopt a position with the arm elevated and flexed behind the head. Pain is exacerbated by turning the head, ear down, to the side of the pain (Spurling maneuver). Objective neurologic findings may be limited to reflex asymmetry because weakness may be obscured by pain. Patients who have some degree of spinal cord compression demonstrate gait and bladder disturbances and evidence of spasticity on examination of the lower extremities. These patients require investigation with MRI. Plain radiographs of the cervical spine add little information except in patients with rheumatoid arthritis in whom basilar invagination or atlantoaxial subluxation is suspected.

Cervical spondylosis is so common in the general population that it may be present coincidentally in a patient with another disease of the spinal cord. Among other diseases that may mimic cervical spondylosis are multiple sclerosis, amyotrophic lateral

TABLE 111-9 COMMON CERVICAL ROOT SYNDROMES

DISK SPACE	ROOT AFFECTED	MUSCLES AFFECTED	DISTRIBUTION OF PAIN	DISTRIBUTION OF SENSORY SYMPTOMS	REFLEX AFFECTED
C4-5	C5	Deltoid, biceps	Medial scapula; shoulder	Shoulder	Biceps
C5-6	C6	Wrist extensors	Lateral forearm	Thumb; index finger	Triceps
C6-7	C7	Triceps	Medial scapula	Middle finger	Brachioradialis
C7-T1	C8	Hand intrinsics	Medial forearm	Fourth and fifth fingers	Finger flexion

sclerosis, and, less commonly, subacute combined system disease (vitamin B_{12} deficiency). Conservative treatment includes the use of anti-inflammatory medication, cervical immobilization, and physical therapy for isometric strengthening of neck muscles once pain has subsided. Surgery should be considered if there is progression of the neurologic deficit, especially the emergence of signs of cervical cord compression. There is some evidence to suggest that cervical spondylosis is an active degenerative disease rather than simply the process. Furthermore, early studies with the glutamate antagonist riluzole suggest a potential role in reducing disease progression.

ACUTE LOW BACK PAIN

Low back pain without sciatica (radiating radicular pain) is common, with a reported point prevalence of up to 33%. Acute low back pain lasting several weeks is usually self-limiting, with a low risk for serious permanent disability. Risk factors for prolonged disability include psychological distress, compensation conflict over work-related injury, and other coexistent pain syndromes. The evaluation of patients with acute low back pain should focus on distinguishing pain of mechanical origin from neurogenic pain caused by nerve root irritation. The same pathologic changes that affect the cervical spine may also affect the lumbar spine. Because the spinal cord ends at the level of the first lumbar vertebra, lumbar canal stenosis from intervertebral disk disease and degenerative spondylosis will affect the roots of the cauda equina. The most common levels for lumbar degenerative disk disease are at L4 to L5 and L5 to S1, resulting in the common complaint of sciatica caused by irritation of the lower lumbar roots. Pain tends to improve with sitting or lying down, in contrast to the pain from spinal or vertebral tumors, which is aggravated by prolonged recumbency. Examination shows loss of the normal lumbar lordosis, paraspinal muscle spasm, and exacerbation of pain with straight leg rising, owing to stretching of the lower lumbar roots. About 10% of disk herniations occurs lateral to the spinal canal, in which case the more rostral root is compressed. Percussion of the spine may elicit focal tenderness of one of the vertebrae, suggesting bony infiltration by infection or tumor.

Spinal stenosis of the lumbar region may manifest as "neurogenic claudication," which is usually described as unilateral or bilateral buttock pain that is worse on standing or walking and relieved by rest or flexion at the waist. Patients may have pain that is worse when walking downhill, in contrast to patients with vascular claudication, whose pain is maximal when walking up an incline.

MRI in many patients with isolated low back pain shows nonspecific findings; MRI assessment early in the course of an episode of low back pain does not improve clinical outcome. MRI should be limited to patients with back pain who have associated neurologic symptoms or signs, especially new onset disturbances of bladder or bowel continence or perineal sensory symptoms suggestive of a *cauda equina syndrome*. Patients with risk factors for malignancy, infection, or osteoporosis, as well as those with pain maximal at rest (or nocturnal pain) require imaging. Patients with primary and metastatic tumor can present with acute back pain (Chapter 119). Moreover, developmental anomalies are often associated with pain (Chapter 115).

Treatment strategies for lumbar pain are similar to those for cervical pain, with surgery reserved for patients with neurologic signs and clear pathologic processes seen on imaging studies. Most cases of acute low back pain, even with rupture of an intervertebral disk, can be treated conservatively with a short period of rest, muscle relaxants, and analgesics. Prolonged bed rest is recommended only for patients in severe pain. Patient education regarding proper posture and appropriate back exercises is helpful, as is a formal physical therapy program. Chiropractic manipulation should not be performed for patients who have evidence of neurologic injury or spine instability.

For a deeper discussion on this topic, please see Chapter 398, "Headaches and Other Head Pain," in Goldman-Cecil Medicine, 25th Edition.

SUGGESTED READINGS

Bronfort G, Evans R, Anderson AV, et al: Spinal manipulation, medication, or home exercise with advice for acute and subacute neck pain: a randomized trial, Ann Intern Med 156:1–10, 2012.

Cherkin DC, Sherman KJ, Kahn J, et al: A comparison of the effects of 2 types of massage and usual care on chronic low back pain: a randomized, controlled trial, Ann Intern Med 155:1–9, 2011.

El Barzouhi A, Vleggeert-Lankamp CL, Lycklama à Nijeholt GJ, et al: Magnetic Resonance Imaging in follow up assessment of sciatica, N Engl J Med 368:999–1007, 2013.

Fehlings MG, Tetreault LA, Wilson JR, et al: Cervical Spondylitic Myelopathy. Current State of the art and future directions, Spine 38:S1–S8, 2013.

Gelfand AA, Goadsby PJ: A neurologist's guide to acute migraine treatment in the emergency room, Neurohospitalist 2:51–59, 2012.

Headache Classification Subcommittee of the International Headache Society: The International Classification of Headache Disorders: 3rd edition, Cephalalgia 33:629–808, 2013. Available at: http://ihs.classification.org/en/.

Rana MV: Managing and treating headache of cervicogenic origin, Med Clin North Am 97:267–280, 2013.

Rizzoli PB: Acute and preventive treatment of migraine, Continuum 18:764–782, 2012.

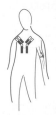

112

Disorders of Vision and Hearing

Eavan McGovern and Timothy J. Counihan

● DISORDERS OF VISION AND EYE MOVEMENTS

Examination of the Visual System

Acuity

The clinical examination of visual function should begin with testing visual acuity. Patients who wear corrective lenses should wear them during testing, and testing should be performed using a Snellen chart at a distance of 20 feet (Fig. 112-1). The smallest line the patient can read is documented as the visual acuity; for instance, acuity of 20/40 refers to letters that the patient sees maximally at 20 feet, which a normal individual can see at 40 feet. When errors of refraction are responsible for decreased visual acuity, vision may be improved by having the patient look through a pinhole. Corrected vision in one eye of less than 20/40 suggests damage to the lens (cataract) or retina or a disorder of the anterior visual (prechiasmal) pathway. Color vision in each eye should also be tested using Ishihara color plates; even when visual acuity is normal, patients with lesions of the optic nerve may complain that colors appear "washed out" in the affected eye.

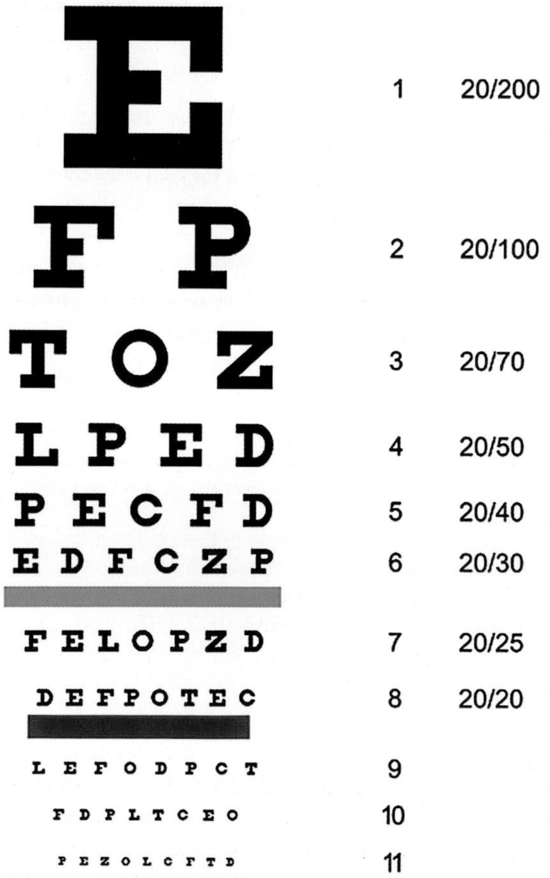

Visual Fields

Thorough examination of the visual fields can often localize lesions interrupting the afferent (sensory) visual system (Fig. 112-2). Visual fields in all four quadrants should be tested by comparing the patient's field with that of the examiner (confrontation). The examiner's head should be level with that of the patient's, and a white pin used to map peripheral visual fields and a red pin to assess for the presence of a scotoma. Asking the patient to count the number of the examiner's extended fingers is more sensitive than presenting moving objects in detecting visual field deficits. The field should be tested first unilaterally and then bilaterally because uncovering a defect (particularly in the left hemifield) with bilateral testing only (extinction) suggests a lesion in the contralateral parietal lobe.

Partial or complete visual loss in one eye only implies damage to the retina or optic nerve anterior to the optic chiasm, whereas a visual field abnormality involving both eyes implies a defect at or posterior to the optic chiasm. *Scotomas* are areas of partial or complete visual loss and may be central or peripheral. Central scotomas result from damage to the macula. A scotoma affecting one half of a visual field is known as a *hemianopia*. Field defects are said to be *homonymous* if the same part of the visual field is affected in both eyes; a homonymous hemianopia implies a postchiasmal lesion. A homonymous defect may be *congruous* (the visual defect is identical in each hemifield) or *incongruous* (the visual defect is not identical in each hemifield).

Quadrantanopias are smaller defects in the visual field and may be superior (which suggests a temporal lobe lesion) or inferior (which suggests a parietal lobe lesion). Bitemporal hemianopia implies a lesion at the chiasm, such as a pituitary tumor. An altitudinal hemianopia occurs with vascular damage to the retina. Scintillating scotomas are hallucinations of flashing lights. If they are monocular, they may be caused by retinal detachment; binocular scintillations suggest occipital oligemia (as in migraine) or seizure. Any suspicious findings on bedside confrontation testing warrant formal visual field testing using perimetry (Fig. 112-3).

Pupils

Examination of the pupils should begin with observation of papillary size and shape at rest. Pupil constriction is mediated by the parasympathetic system of the oculomotor (third cranial) nerve,

E	1	20/200
F P	2	20/100
T O Z	3	20/70
L P E D	4	20/50
P E C F D	5	20/40
E D F C Z P	6	20/30
F E L O P Z D	7	20/25
D E F P O T E C	8	20/20
L E F O D P C T	9	
F D P L T C E O	10	
P E Z O L C F T D	11	

FIGURE 112-1 Snellen Chart.

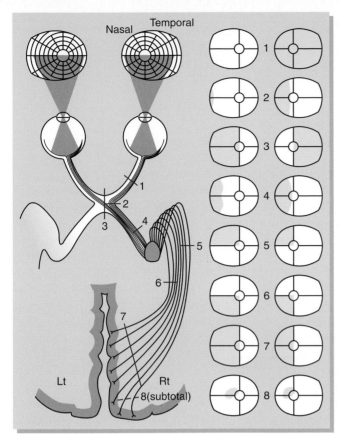

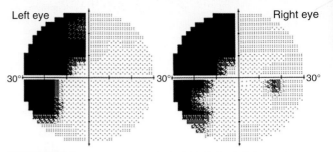

FIGURE 112-3 Humphrey visual fields demonstrating an incongruent homonymous hemianopia.

FIGURE 112-2 Visual fields that accompany damage to the visual pathways. *1*, Optic nerve: unilateral amaurosis. *2*, Lateral optic chiasm: grossly incongruous, incomplete (contralateral) homonymous hemianopia. *3*, Central optic chiasm: bitemporal hemianopia. *4*, Optic tract: incongruous, incomplete homonymous hemianopia. *5*, Temporal (Meyer) loop of optic radiation: congruous partial or complete (contralateral) homonymous superior quadrantanopia. *6*, Parietal (superior) projection of the optic radiation: congruous partial or complete homonymous inferior quadrantanopia. *7*, Complete parieto-occipital interruption of optic radiation: complete congruous homonymous hemianopia with psychophysical shift of foveal point often sparing central vision, giving "macular sparing." *8*, Incomplete damage to visual cortex: congruous homonymous scotomas, usually encroaching at least acutely on central vision. (From Baloh RW: Neuro-ophthalmology. In Goldman L, Bennett JC, editors: Cecil textbook of medicine, ed 21, Philadelphia, 1998, WB Saunders, p 2236).

whereas dilation is mediated by the sympathetic system. If the balance of these systems is disrupted, *anisocoria* (unequal pupil size) results. The pupils should be examined in both dim and bright light. If the anisocoria increases going from dim to bright light, a lesion of the parasympathetic system is likely. *Physiologic anisocoria* is characterized by pupillary asymmetry that is unchanged irrespective of the ambient light intensity; this occurs in approximately 20% of the population.

Both the direct and consensual light responses should be noted for each eye; in the latter, when the light is shone in one eye, both pupils should constrict. This is best tested using the "swinging light test," in which the light is moved quickly from one eye to the other. When light is shone into one eye, both eyes should constrict simultaneously. If there is dilation of one pupil as the light is moved to it from the other side, an abnormality of the optic nerve in that eye should be

suspected. This abnormality is referred to as an *afferent pupillary defect*. The accommodative pupillary response is tested by asking the patient to look first in the distance and then at the examiner's finger, held 12 inches away. The pupils should constrict symmetrically and rapidly. *Argyll-Robertson pupils* are small, irregular pupils that constrict to near vision (accommodation reflex) but not in response to light. They are associated with neurosyphilis, diabetes, and other disorders. This so-called *light-near dissociation* may also occur in rostral dorsal midbrain lesions, in which there may be associated abnormalities of vertical gaze, eyelid retraction, and convergence retraction nystagmus (Parinaud Syndrome). This uncommon constellation of clinical findings is frequently noted in patients with lesions of the pineal gland.

The presence of ptosis should be noted. A large, unreactive pupil with ptosis indicates a lesion of the oculomotor nerve *(third cranial nerve palsy)* interrupting the parasympathetic nerve supply to the pupil. The associated paralysis of the medial and inferior rectus and inferior oblique muscles (see later discussion) results in distortion of the eye (inferolaterally, *"down and out"*) and a subjective complaint of diplopia by the patient. Common causes of a third nerve palsy include compression by an aneurysm of the posterior communicating artery by transtentorial herniation, or from ischemia, usually in the setting of diabetes or vasculitis. A third nerve palsy caused by ischemia often spares the pupil but results in complete paralysis of the oculomotor and eyelid levator muscles. Acute painful third nerve palsy should be treated as an emergency, with the need to investigate for an intracranial aneurysm.

A small, poorly reactive pupil with associated ptosis is known as *Horner syndrome* and results from damage to the sympathetic fibers to the pupil, which may occur anywhere along their course from the hypothalamus, brainstem, and ascending sympathetic chain from the superior cervical ganglion to the orbit. There may be associated unilateral anhidrosis resulting from damage to sympathetic fibers. Horner syndrome may be the first sign of an apical lung tumor (Pancoast) or may occur in diseases affecting the carotid artery.

Tonic (Adie) pupils constrict slowly and incompletely in response to light. This is usually an incidental finding on examination but may be associated with areflexia (Holmes-Adie syndrome). Reaction to accommodation is preserved, and it has been suggested that the disorder is a result of parasympathetic denervation. *Hippus* refers to pupillary unrest with synchronous oscillation of the pupil size; it is considered a normal

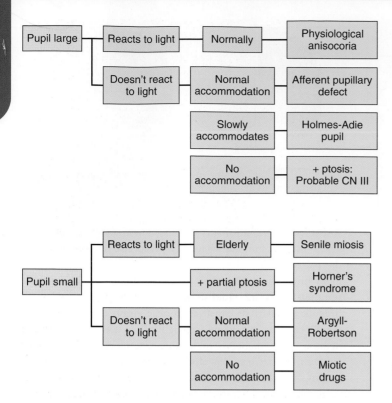

FIGURE 112-4 Algorithm for the approach to unequal pupils (anisocoria).

phenomenon. Figure 112-4 summarizes common pupillary abnormalities and their associated features.

Eye Movements

The history helps in evaluating the patient with diplopia. Is the diplopia primarily horizontal or vertical, or is it greater looking to the right or to the left? Double vision that varies during the day suggests myasthenia gravis. Is the diplopia maximal with near or distant vision? Greater difficulty with near vision suggests impairment of the medial rectus, oculomotor nerve, or convergence system, whereas abducens nerve weakness results in horizontal diplopia when objects are viewed at a distance. Diplopia that worsens on going down stairs may suggest a fourth nerve lesion. Monocular diplopia is usually caused by diseases of the retina or lens and is corrected by having the patient look through a pinhole, unless the cause is psychogenic.

The examination should begin by determining the position of the head and eyes with the eyes in primary gaze. There are four components to oculomotor function:

1. Pursuit eye movements: Smooth pursuit eye movements allow fixation on a moving object. Ask the patient to follow a moving target such as a pin in all directions of gaze.
2. Saccadic eye movements: These movements allow rapid switching of gaze from one target to another. Both horizontal and vertical saccadic movements should be checked.
3. Vestibulo-ocular reflex: This reflex enables fixation on an object even if the head is moving. It is assessed by using the *Doll's Eye Maneuver*.
4. Convergence Response: This tests the ability of the eyes to track an object as it is brought close to the limit of accommodation. Ask the patient to look into the distance and then at your finger held close to their eyes.

Both smooth pursuit and (voluntary) saccadic eye movements in horizontal and vertical directions are checked to determine whether the movements are conjugate or disconjugate. Disconjugate eye movements suggest a disorder of the brainstem (at the level of the ocular motor nuclei or their connections), the peripheral nerves (cranial nerves III, IV, or VI), individual eye muscles (ocular myopathy), or the neuromuscular junction (myasthenia gravis or botulism). A large deficit in the range of eye movements may provide sufficient diagnostic information. However, in many cases, although the patient complains of diplopia, no clear misalignment is visible on testing eye movements. The corneal reflection test may help identify misalignment in these cases. The patient is instructed to look at a light shining directly at the eyes. If the eyes are normally aligned, the light reflection will be about 1 mm nasal to the center of the cornea. If one eye is deviated medially, the reflection will be displaced outward; the reflection will be displaced inward if the eye is deviated outward.

The abducens (sixth cranial) nerve supplies the lateral rectus muscle. The trochlear (fourth cranial) nerve subserves the superior oblique muscle, which intorts the eye as well as depresses the eye in adduction (such as when a patient tries to look downstairs). All other muscles are supplied by the oculomotor nerve (Fig. 112-5). Abnormalities of the cranial nerves in the brainstem are usually accompanied by other signs, such as weakness, ataxia, or dysarthria. The abducens nerve has a long ascending course through the posterior fossa, where it is prone to compression at multiple sites and as a result of raised intracranial pressure; hence, a sixth nerve palsy may be a false localizing sign. Conjugate eye movement is regulated by supranuclear pathways from the cerebral hemisphere to the medial longitudinal fasciculus in the brainstem. A lesion in the cerebral hemisphere resulting from hemorrhage, infarction, or tumor disrupts conjugate gaze to the contralateral side, so that the eyes "look away" from the

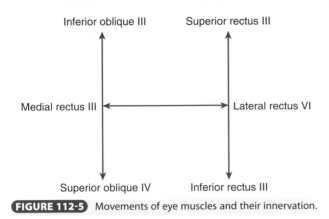

FIGURE 112-5 Movements of eye muscles and their innervation.

Inferior oblique III

Superior rectus III

Medial rectus III ⟷ Lateral rectus VI

Superior oblique IV

Inferior rectus III

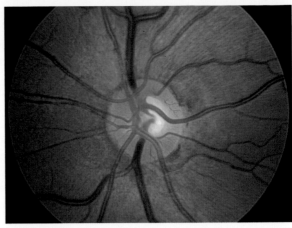

FIGURE 112-6 A normal optic disk on fundoscopic examination.

TABLE 112-1	MAJOR CAUSES OF ACUTE OPHTHALMOPLEGIA	
CONDITION	DIAGNOSTIC FEATURES
BILATERAL	
Botulism	Contaminated food; high-altitude cooking; pupils involved
Myasthenia gravis	Fluctuating degree of paralysis; responds to edrophonium chloride (Tensilon) IV
Wernicke encephalopathy	Nutritional deficiency; responds to thiamine IV
Acute cranial polyneuropathy	
Brainstem stroke	Antecedent respiratory infection; elevated CSF protein level
	Other brainstem signs
UNILATERAL	
P Comm aneurysm	Third cranial nerve, pupil involved
Diabetic-idiopathic	Third or sixth cranial nerve, pupil spared
Myasthenia gravis	As above
Brainstem stroke	As above

CSF, Cerebrospinal fluid; IV, intravenous; P Comm, posterior communicating artery.

hemiplegia. Lesions of the brainstem cause conjugate paralysis to the ipsilateral side (eyes looking toward the side of the hemiplegia). Lesions of the medial longitudinal fasciculus, which connects the nuclei of the oculomotor and abducens nerves, lead to *internuclear ophthalmoplegia*. In this case, horizontal gaze results in failure of adduction in one eye and nystagmus in the abducting eye. The lesion is on the side of failed adduction; bilateral lesions are frequently seen in multiple sclerosis. Table 112-1 lists the major causes of acute opthalmoplegia.

Funduscopy

The retina should be carefully examined in each patient by direct ophthalmoscopy, which provides a magnified view of the fundus without the necessity for dilation of the pupil (Fig. 112-6).

Monocular Visual Loss

Loss of vision in one eye may be caused by lesions of the cornea, lens, vitreous, retina, or optic nerve. Careful funduscopic examination will usually reveal ocular and retinal lesions, but acute lesions of the optic nerve (optic neuritis) may not be associated with abnormalities of the optic nerve head. *Optic neuritis* is characterized by inflammation of the optic nerve accompanied by

non-homonymous visual defects. The term *papillitis* refers to ophthalmoscopically observable changes in the optic nerve; *retrobulbar neuritis* refers to this condition without observable changes in the funduscopic examination findings ("the doctor sees nothing and the patient sees nothing").

The patient with optic neuritis complains of difficulty with vision in the affected eye. Loss of vision may be insidious and recognized only when the unaffected eye is accidentally occluded. Patients often complain of periorbital pain on eye movement on presentation. The evolution of visual loss is highly variable, progressing over a period ranging from less than a day to several weeks, although most patients will have reached their maximal visual deficit in 3 to 7 days. Patients may describe their vision as blurred or dim, and colors may appear less bright than usual or "gray." Red desaturation may occur with optic neuritis and may be detected using Ishihara color plates. At the time the patient is first examined, visual acuity may range from almost 20/20 to the extreme of total blindness. Examination of the visual field shows defects within the central 25 degrees, with central and paracentral scotomas being the most common types. An afferent pupillary defect is frequently present. The funduscopic examination is abnormal in only about one half of the cases. The disc may appear hyperemic with blurred margins, and hemorrhages, when present, are few and found only on the disc or in the area immediately surrounding the disc. Optic neuritis should be treated acutely with high-dose intravenous corticosteroids because this is proven to shorten time to recovery. The most common cause of optic neuritis is multiple sclerosis. Bilateral optic neuritis is much less common and may coincide with longitudinally extensive transverse myelitis, known as *neuromyelitis optica* (NMO) or *Devic disease*. The recent discovery of antibodies directed toward aquaporin 4 (a water channel present on astrocytes and vascular endothelial cells), associated with NMO, has identified this as a separate disease entity, with a different treatment regimen emerging for it. The NMO antibody is the first sensitive and specific biomarker associated with a central demyelinating disorder.

The optic nerve may be compressed by tumors that originate in the nerve itself or in the region of the optic chiasm. Pathologic processes that appear acutely as optic disc edema frequently result in a secondary optic atrophy, including papilledema, optic neuritis, and ischemic optic neuropathy. Glaucoma is responsible for more cases of optic atrophy in the adult population than any other cause. In young patients with inherited optic atrophy, Leber hereditary optic neuropathy is often the cause; it is usually bilateral. *Foster-Kennedy* syndrome is optic atrophy in one eye with papilledema in the other eye, secondary to a tumor compressing the atrophied optic nerve and causing raised intracranial pressure to produce papilledema in the opposite eye.

Ischemic optic neuropathy occurs in two forms. The *atherosclerotic* variety occurs mostly between the ages of 50 and 70 years, and no evidence of systemic disease is present. The *arteritic* form is usually a manifestation of giant cell arteritis; there may be systemic manifestations of the disease, including headache, scalp tenderness, and generalized myalgias. Laboratory evaluation shows anemia and elevated erythrocyte sedimentation rate in almost every case. Patients with arteritis should be treated with high doses of corticosteroids to prevent permanent loss of vision.

Acute transient monocular blindness is usually the result of embolization to the central retinal artery from an atheromatous plaque in the carotid artery (*amaurosis fugax*). Any complaint of transient visual loss constitutes an emergency, and steps must be taken to prevent permanent loss of vision by making a prompt diagnosis and initiating appropriate therapy. Examples of sight-saving procedures include corticosteroid therapy for cranial arteritis, reduction of intraocular pressure for acute glaucoma, and carotid surgery, anticoagulation, or antiplatelet therapy for embolic cerebrovascular disease.

Binocular Visual Loss

Gradual bilateral visual loss caused by optic nerve lesions is rare. Causes include Leber hereditary optic neuropathy and a toxic nutritional–deficiency state. Acute transient bilateral visual loss (visual obscuration) may be a symptom of raised intracranial pressure caused by a brain tumor or idiopathic intracranial hypertension (IIH); papilledema is often severe. IIH, formerly known as *pseudotumor cerebri,* requires prompt investigation and treatment to prevent potential bilateral visual failure. It is often associated with a high body mass index (BMI) and is more common in young females. Vitamin A and tetracycline ingestion have been associated with the condition. Unilateral or bilateral lateral rectus palsy may be present. It is one of the few situations in which, after imaging, performance of a lumbar puncture is safe in the setting of marked bilateral papilledema. Cerebral venous sinus thrombosis may mimic IIH and should be screened for with neuroimaging.

Bilateral damage to the optic radiations or visual cortex results in cortical blindness. The pupillary light reflex is normal, as are the funduscopic examination findings, and the patient may occasionally be unaware that he or she is blind (*Anton syndrome*). Patients are often misdiagnosed as having a conversion reaction. Transient cortical blindness occurs most often in basilar artery insufficiency but is also seen in hypertensive encephalopathy. Positive visual phenomena (e.g., phosphenes, scintillating scotomas) are characteristic of migrainous aura and probably reflect oligemia to the occipital lobes from vasoconstriction. Arteriovenous malformations, tumors, and seizures may produce similar symptoms and should be distinguished from migraine with aura by a careful history and examination as well as by imaging in appropriate cases.

Visual hallucinations are visual sensations independent of external light stimulation; they may be either simple or complex, may be localized or generalized, and may occur in patients with a clear or clouded sensorium. Visual illusions are alterations of a perceived external stimulus in which some features are distorted. The simplest visual phenomena consist of flashes of light (photopsias), blue lights (phosphenes), or scintillating zigzag lines, which last a fraction of a second and recur frequently or which appear to be in constant motion. These can arise from dysfunction within the optic pathways at any point from the eye to the cortex. Glaucoma, incipient retinal detachment, retinal ischemia, or macular degeneration can cause simple visual hallucinations based on dysfunction in the eye. Lesions of the occipital lobe are often associated with simple hallucinations; classic migraine is by far the most common condition of this type. Complex visual hallucinations such as seeing objects as people, animals, landscapes, or various indescribable scenes occur most frequently with temporal lobe lesions or parieto-occipital association areas. Visual hallucinations of epileptogenic origin are typically stereotyped.

⬤ HEARING AND ITS IMPAIRMENTS

Symptoms of Auditory Dysfunction

The main symptoms of lesions within the auditory system are hearing loss and tinnitus. Hearing loss can be classified as conductive, sensorineural, mixed, or central, based on the anatomic site of pathology (Figs. 112-7 and 112-8). Tinnitus can be either subjective or objective. Conductive hearing loss results from lesions involving the external or middle ear. Patients with a conductive hearing loss can hear speech in a noisy background as well as in a quiet background, because they can understand loud speech as well as anyone. The ear often feels full, as if it is blocked. The Weber test localizes to the deaf ear, if the deafness is unilateral.

Sensorineural hearing loss usually results from lesions of the cochlea or the auditory division of the vestibulocochlear (eighth cranial) nerve. Patients with sensorineural hearing loss often have difficulty hearing speech that is mixed with background noise and may be annoyed by loud speech. They usually hear low tones better than high-frequency ones. Distortion of sounds is common with sensorineural hearing loss. Central (retrocochlear) hearing disorders are rare and result from bilateral lesions of the central auditory pathways, including the cochlear and dorsal olivary nuclear complexes, inferior colliculi, medial geniculate bodies, and auditory cortex in the temporal lobes. Damage to both auditory cortices may result in pure word deafness, in which patients are selectively unable to discriminate language but may be able to hear nonverbal sounds.

Tinnitus is the perception of a noise or ringing in the ear that is usually audible only to the patient (subjective), although, rarely, an examiner can hear the sound as well. The latter, so-called *objective tinnitus,* can be heard when the examining physician places a stethoscope against the patient's external auditory canal. Tinnitus that is pulsatory and synchronous with the heartbeat suggests a vascular abnormality within the head or neck (see Fig. 120-7). Aneurysms, arteriovenous malformations, and vascular tumors can produce this type of tinnitus.

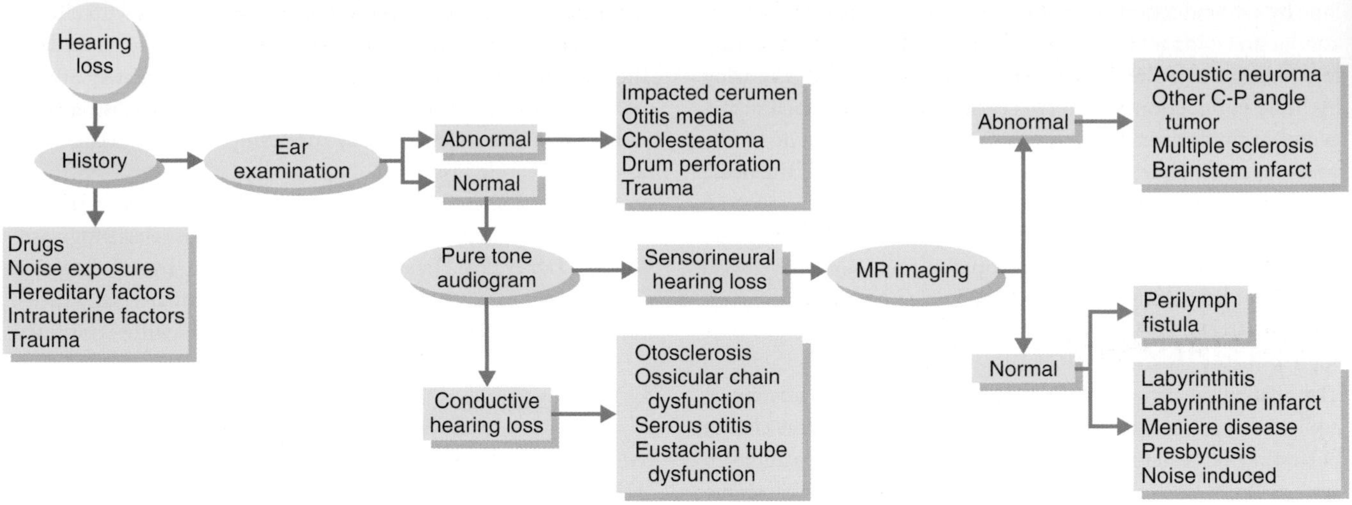

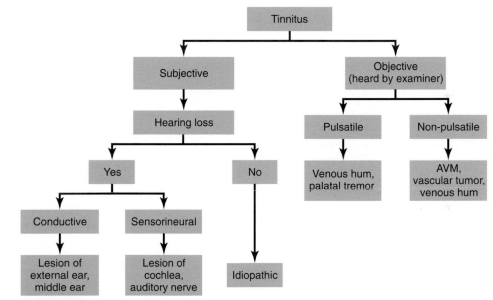

FIGURE 112-7 Evaluation of deafness (unilateral and bilateral). C-P, Cerebellopontine; MR, magnetic resonance. (Modified from Baloh RW: Hearing and equilibrium. In Goldman L, Bennett JC, editors: Cecil textbook of medicine, ed 21, Philadelphia, 1998, WB Saunders, p 2250).

FIGURE 112-8 Algorithm for the approach to the patient with tinnitus. AVM, Arteriovenous malformation.

Subjective tinnitus, heard only by the patient, can result from lesions involving the external ear canal, tympanic membrane, ossicles, cochlea, auditory nerve, brainstem, and cortex. The character of the tinnitus does not usually aid in determining the site of the disturbance. For this, one must rely on associated symptoms and signs. When tinnitus results from a lesion of the external or middle ear, it is usually accompanied by a conductive hearing loss. The patient may complain that his or her voice sounds hollow and that other sounds are muffled. Because the masking effect of ambient noise is lost, the patient may be disturbed by normal muscular sounds such as chewing, tight closure of the eyes, or clenching of the jaws. The characteristic tinnitus associated with Meniere's syndrome is low pitched and continuous, although fluctuating in intensity. Often the tinnitus becomes very loud immediately preceding an acute attack of vertigo and then may disappear after the attack. Tinnitus resulting from lesions within the central nervous system is usually not associated with hearing loss but is nearly always associated with other neurologic symptoms and signs. High-dose salicylates frequently result in tinnitus.

Examination of the Auditory System

A quick test for hearing loss in the speech range is to observe the response to spoken commands at different intensities (whisper, conversation, and shouting). The examiner must be careful to prevent the patient from reading his or her lip movement. A high-frequency stimulus such as a watch tick should also be used because sensorineural disorders often involve only the higher frequencies. Tuning fork tests permit a rough assessment of the hearing level for pure tones of known frequency. The Rinne test compares the patient's hearing by air conduction with that by bone conduction. A 512-cps tuning fork is first held against the mastoid process until the sound fades. It is then placed 1 inch from the ear. Normal subjects can hear the fork about twice as long by air conduction as by bone conduction. If hearing by bone conduction is longer than by air conduction, a conductive hearing loss is suggested. The Weber test compares the patient's hearing by bone conduction in the two ears. The fork is placed at the center of the forehead, and the patient is asked where he or she hears the tone. Normal subjects hear it in the center of the head, patients with unilateral conductive loss hear it on the affected side, and patients with unilateral sensorineural loss hear it on the side opposite the loss. Otoscopic examination may reveal impacted cerumen as a cause of conductive hearing loss.

Causes of Hearing Loss

The bilateral hearing loss commonly associated with advancing age is called *presbycusis*. Presbycusis is not a distinct disease entity but rather represents multiple effects of aging on the auditory system. Presbycusis may include conductive and central dysfunction, although the most consistent effect of aging is on the sensory cells and neurons of the cochlea; as a result, higher tones are lost early.

Otosclerosis is a disease of the bony labyrinth that usually manifests itself by immobilizing the stapes and thereby producing a conductive hearing loss. Seventy percent of patients with clinical otosclerosis notice hearing loss between the ages of 11 and 30. There is a family history of otosclerosis in approximately 50% of cases. *Stapedectomy*, a procedure in which the stapes is replaced with a prosthesis, is effective in correcting the conductive component of hearing loss.

A lesion of the cerebellopontine angle, such as a vestibular schwannoma, often causes unilateral hearing loss that progresses slowly (Table 112-2); symptoms are caused by compression of the nerve in the narrow confines of the canal (Fig. 112-9). The most common symptoms associated with vestibular

TABLE 112-2	CAUSE OF ACUTE UNILATERAL SENSORINEURAL DEAFNESS	
COCHLEAR		**RETROCOCHLEAR**
Idiopathic (85%)		Demyelination
Trauma		Vestibular schwannoma (usually
Meniere's disease		gradual onset)
Lyme's disease		Stroke
Syphilis		
Autoimmune disease		

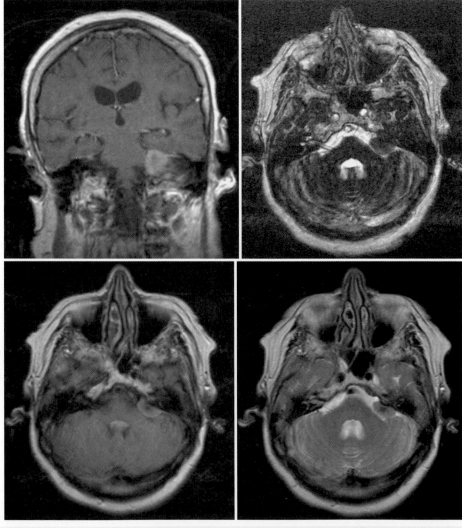

FIGURE 112-9 Magnetic resonance imaging scan of the brain showing coronal and axial views of a tumor of the left cerebellopontine angle, consistent with a schwannoma.

schwannomas are slowly progressive hearing loss and tinnitus from compression of the cochlear nerve. Vertigo occurs in fewer than 20% of patients, but approximately 50% complain of imbalance or disequilibrium. Next to the auditory nerve, the cranial nerves most commonly involved by compression are the seventh (facial weakness) and fifth (sensory loss). Loss of the corneal reflex on the affected side is often the first clinical sign. Treatment in most cases is surgical removal.

Meniere's syndrome (endolymphatic hydrops) is characterized by fluctuating hearing loss and tinnitus, episodic vertigo, and a sensation of fullness or pressure in the ear. Typically the patient develops a sensation of fullness and pressure, along with decreased hearing and tinnitus in one ear. Vertigo rapidly follows, reaching a maximum intensity within minutes and then slowly subsiding over the next several hours. The patient is usually left with a sense of unsteadiness and dizziness for days after the acute vertiginous episode. In the early stages the hearing loss is completely reversible, but in later stages a residual hearing loss remains. Up to 50% of patients with idiopathic Meniere's syndrome frequently have a positive family history, suggesting genetic predisposing factors. The key to the diagnosis of Meniere's syndrome is to document fluctuating hearing levels in a patient with the characteristic clinical history. Medical therapy for endolymphatic hydrops includes dietary sodium restriction and oral diuretics.

Acute unilateral deafness usually results from damage to the cochlea and may be caused by viral or bacterial labyrinthitis or vascular occlusion in the territory of the anterior inferior cerebellar artery. Perilymphatic fistulas may also cause abrupt unilateral deafness, usually in association with tinnitus and vertigo.

Drugs that cause acute irreversible bilateral hearing loss include aminoglycosides, cisplatin, and furosemide. Salicylates may cause reversible hearing loss and tinnitus.

Treatment of Hearing Loss

The best treatment is prevention, particularly by the appropriate use of earplugs for those working in a noisy environment. Hearing aids help patients with conductive hearing loss, and developments with cochlear implants may help patients with sensorineural hearing loss.

Prospectus for the Future

Optical coherence tomography (OCT) is an emerging technology in the assessment of retinal layer thickness. This technology has been used in multiple sclerosis research. It has been used to correlate retinal layer thickness with severity of multiple sclerosis. This may have important implications for future research in this field.

For a deeper discussion on this topic, please see Chapter 423, "Diseases of the Visual System," and Chapter 424, "Neuro-Opthalmology," in Goldman-Cecil Medicine, *25th Edition.*

SUGGESTED READINGS

Drori T, Chapman J: Diagnosis and classification of neuromyelitis optica (Devic's syndrome), Autoimmune Rev 13:531–533, 2014.
Toosy AT, Mason DF, Miller DH: Optic neuritis, Lancet Neurol 13:83–99, 2014.

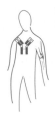

113

Dizziness and Vertigo

Kevin A. Kerber

DEFINITION/EPIDEMIOLOGY

Dizziness is a common term that is used by patients and providers to group a variety of different symptoms including a spinning sensation, lightheadedness, disorientation, or imbalance. Other more vague symptoms are also often labeled as "dizziness." Vertigo is the term used for a false sense of movement, typically spinning. The problem with defining the type of dizziness is that patients are often inconsistent when describing dizziness. In addition, the type of dizziness generally does not adequately discriminate among disorders. Approximately 30% of the general population reports having had some type of bothersome dizziness.

PATHOLOGY

Pathology that causes dizziness can stem from many systems of the body. Understanding the vestibular system and common peripheral vestibular disorders is of central importance in the evaluation of patients with dizziness. This is because the dilemma is often discriminating a benign peripheral vestibular disorder from a focal brain lesion. The vestibular system is a common source of confusion. Many clinicians assume a "peripheral" cause in the absence of motor, sensory, or language deficits, but this approach is flawed. A more effective approach is to aim to "rule in" a *specific* peripheral vestibular disorder. The three common peripheral vestibular disorders all have highly characteristic history and examination features, thus enabling this approach. When a specific peripheral vestibular disorder does not fit, then one must consider other potential etiologies.

BASIC VESTIBULAR SYSTEM CONCEPTS

The peripheral vestibular system maintains a balanced tonic input to the brain. The input represents the circuitry that links the inner ear to eye movements, the vestibulo-ocular reflex (VOR). A normal functioning VOR is important for balance and maintaining clear vision when moving. Vertigo ensues when an imbalance is caused by a lesion (e.g., vestibular neuritis) or aberrant stimulation (e.g., benign paroxysmal positional vertigo). A characteristic sign of vestibular system imbalance is nystagmus: rhythmic slow and fast movements of the eyes in opposite directions. The location of pathology determines the pattern of nystagmus (Table 113-1). Dysfunction at the semicircular canal level leads to nystagmus in the plane of the affected canal. Therefore problems in the vertical canals (i.e., posterior and anterior canals) lead to vertical and torsional nystagmus, whereas problems in the horizontal canal lead to horizontal nystagmus. At the vestibular nerve level a mixed horizontal-torsional nystagmus is generated because input from all the semicircular canals converge at this level and the signals from the vertical canals mostly cancel each other out. The pathways and thus the patterns of eye movements become less predictable with lesions of the central vestibular pathways, although some general rules apply. Pure vertical (downbeat or upbeat) spontaneous nystagmus, bidirectional gaze-evoked nystagmus (look left, beats left; look right, beats right) (Video 113-1), and persistent downbeating positional nystagmus are signs of central dysfunction (see Table 113-1).

Another characteristic sign of vestibular disturbance is a positive head-thrust test (Video 113-2). A person with an intact VOR will maintain gaze on a stationary, straight-ahead target after a brief, small-amplitude, high-acceleration movement of the head to one side. A person with vestibular impairment on one side loses this reflex on the ipsilateral side and therefore, after the quick head movement, will need to make a re-fixation voluntary eye movement (i.e., a "saccade") back to the target because the eyes moved with the head. This so-called "catch-up" or "corrective" saccade is easily appreciated at the bedside and indicates vestibular deafferentation.

TABLE 113-1	COMMON TYPES AND PATTERNS OF NYSTAGMUS		
TYPES	**PATTERNS**	**LOCALIZATION**	**PRINCIPAL CAUSES**
Spontaneous	Unidirectional horizontal ≫ torsional	Vestibular nerve, or less commonly the brainstem	Vestibular neuritis, or less commonly stroke
	Downbeat, upbeat, or pure torsional	Brain	Stroke
Gaze-evoked	Unidirectional	Vestibular nerve	Vestibular neuritis (recovery pattern)
	Bidirectional	Brain	Stroke, cerebellar syndrome, medication side effect*
Positional	Burst of upbeat torsional with DH	Posterior SCC	BPPV
	Horizontal with supine positional testing	Horizontal SCC or less commonly the brainstem	BPPV, brainstem lesion
	Persistent downbeat	Brain	Chiari malformation, cerebellar degeneration

BPPV, Benign paroxysmal positional vertigo; DH, Dix-Hallpike positional test; SCC, semicircular canal; ≫, greater than.
*Most common with antiepileptic drugs.

CLINICAL PRESENTATION

Patients usually present with acute constant dizziness, recurrent spontaneous attacks, or recurrent positional attacks. Less commonly, patients present with chronic constant dizziness. The physical examination is a critical part of the assessment. If the general examination is unrevealing, then the focus should shift to the ocular motor examination because vestibular disorders have highly characteristic findings, particularly regarding the presence and pattern of nystagmus (see Table 113-1). Hearing should be tested one ear at a time with either tuning forks or finger rub.m

DIFFERENTIAL DIAGNOSIS

The differential diagnosis can generally be categorized as follows: a peripheral vestibular disorder, a central nervous system disorder, a general medical disorder (e.g., anemia, metabolic derangement, anxiety disorder), or a chronic otherwise undefined disorder. There are three common peripheral vestibular disorders: vestibular neuritis, Meniere's disease, and benign paroxysmal positional vertigo (BPPV). An understanding of these three disorders is important because each one is the primary consideration for the cause of one of the three common dizziness presentation categories (Table 113-2). In addition, these disorders are the prototypes for most pathology that involves the peripheral vestibular system.

Vestibular neuritis manifests with the abrupt onset of severe vertigo, nausea, and imbalance without other neurologic symptoms. The disorder is caused by a viral disturbance of the vestibular nerve, analogous to Bell's palsy. On examination, the acute peripheral vestibular pattern of nystagmus is seen (see Table 113-2; Video 113-3). A positive head-thrust test in the direction of the affected ear (but in the direction opposite the fast phase of nystagmus) further supports vestibular nerve localization. If the nystagmus changes direction with gaze (i.e., look left, beat left; then look right, beat right), then vestibular neuritis is not the diagnosis because these findings localize to the central nervous system. Small strokes of the cerebellum or brainstem can closely mimic vestibular neuritis.

Meniere's disease is characterized by recurrent episodes of vertigo, nausea, and imbalance typically lasting hours; prominent auditory features must be present to make the diagnosis. Early in the course, auditory symptoms fluctuate along with vertigo attacks, but later they become a fixed symptom. The auditory symptoms are nearly always unilateral at the onset and consist of hearing loss, roaring tinnitus, or severe fullness in one ear. If attacks are brief (i.e., minutes rather than hours), then transient ischemic attacks should be considered. The dizziness of migraine can also closely mimic Meniere's disease.

Patients with BPPV report very brief episodes (<1 minute) of vertigo triggered by head movement; most often tilting the head back to look up, getting in or out of bed, or rolling over in bed. Dizziness from any cause may worsen after certain movements, but the dizziness of BPPV is *triggered* by certain movements. The most common form of BPPV occurs when otoliths enter the posterior canal. Posterior canal BPPV is identified at the bedside using the Dix-Hallpike test (Fig. 113-1). In response to the Dix-Hallpike test, otoliths move in the canal and lead to a burst of upbeat-torsional nystagmus lasting about 20 to 30 seconds (Video 113-4). BPPV is less commonly caused by otoliths in the horizontal canal and very rarely the anterior canal. When the otoliths are in one of these other canals, the pattern of nystagmus is different from that of posterior canal BPPV, as are the repositioning maneuvers used to treat BPPV. Positional vertigo and nystagmus are common in patients with migraine. If a persistent downbeating nystagmus is seen during the Dix-Hallpike test, then a central nervous system cause (e.g., Chiari malformation, cerebellar tumor, or cerebellar degeneration) should be considered.

If the patient reports imbalance as the principal symptom and has a gait disorder, then the following causes should be considered: stroke (if the onset was acute), a musculoskeletal disorder, peripheral neuropathy, bilateral vestibulopathy (frequently attributable to ototoxicity, particularly from gentamicin), or a neurodegenerative disorder involving the cerebellum.

If a specific peripheral vestibular disorder is not identified and the neurologic examination is normal, then general medical causes should be considered. The list of medications should be

TABLE 113-2	COMMON CATEGORIES OF DIZZINESS PRESENTATIONS		
	ACUTE CONSTANT DIZZINESS	**RECURRENT SPONTANEOUS ATTACKS**	**RECURRENT POSITIONAL ATTACKS**
Primary consideration	Vestibular neuritis	Meniere's disease	BPPV
Key features	Constant vertigo, unidirectional horizontal nystagmus,* positive head-thrust test†	Vertigo lasting hours, unilateral auditory symptoms	Positionally triggered, brief (<1 min) attacks Upbeat-torsional burst of nystagmus in DH position, cured by Epley maneuver‡
Red flags	Other CNS features, other patterns of nystagmus, imbalance as the principal symptom, chest pain, cardiovascular risk factors	Other CNS features, CNS patterns of nystagmus, imbalance as the principal symptom, attacks lasting only minutes, chest pain, cardiovascular risk factors, recent onset, crescendo pattern	Other CNS features, CNS patterns of nystagmus
Other considerations	Stroke, myocardial infarction, metabolic disturbances, demyelinating attack	TIA, cardiac arrhythmia, migraine, panic attacks	Horizontal or anterior canal BPPV, migraine, Chiari malformation, posterior fossa tumor, orthostatic hypotension

BPPV, Benign paroxysmal positional vertigo; CNS, central nervous system; DH, Dix-Hallpike; TIA, transient ischemic attack.

*This nystagmus never changes direction. Gaze in the direction of the fast phase will increase the velocity of the nystagmus, whereas gaze in the opposite direction will decrease the velocity of the nystagmus.

†The head-thrust test will be positive in the direction of the affected ear, which is opposite the direction of the fast phase of nystagmus.

‡These features apply to BPPV stemming from the posterior canal.

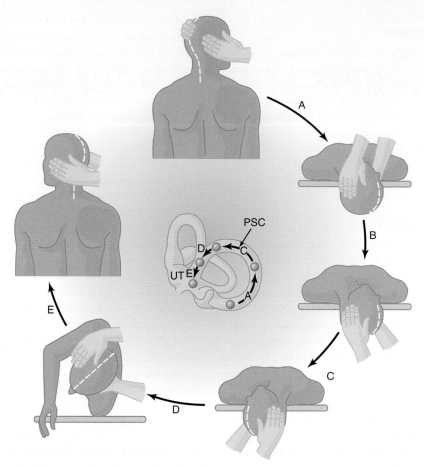

FIGURE 113-1 Repositioning treatment for benign paroxysmal positional vertigo designed to move endolymphatic debris out of the posterior semicircular canal (PSC) of the right ear and into the utricle (UT). The patient is seated, and the patient's head is turned 45 degrees to the right **(A).** The head is then lowered rapidly to below the horizontal **(B).** The examiner shifts hand positions **(C),** and the patient's head is rotated rapidly 90 degrees in the opposite direction, so it now points 45 degrees to the left, where it remains for 30 seconds **(D).** The patient then rolls onto the left side without turning the head in relation to the body and maintains this position for another 30 seconds **(E)** before sitting up. The treatment is repeated until nystagmus is abolished. The procedure is reversed for treating the left ear. (Modified from Foster CA, Baloh RW: Episodic vertigo. In Rakel RE, editor: Conn's Current Therapy, Philadelphia, 1995, WB Saunders.)

carefully scrutinized because dizziness is a common medication side effect. Dizziness can be a prominent symptom of anxiety and panic disorders. Vestibular migraine should be on the differential diagnosis of any dizziness presentation. When none of these seem to fit, the examination findings are normal, and the symptom has been present for more than several months, then the patient likely has chronic dizziness—typically considered a benign hypersensitivity disorder.

TREATMENT

Vestibular rehabilitation is the treatment of choice for patients with vestibular neuritis. If Meniere's disease is diagnosed, then a low-salt diet or a diuretic may alleviate the frequency of episodes. However, neither of these treatments is of established efficacy. Ablative surgical procedures are appropriate in refractory Meniere's disease. The treatment of BPPV involving the posterior canal is the highly effective and guideline-supported repositioning maneuver described by Epley (see Fig. 113-1). Patients with chronic dizziness may benefit from lifestyle modifications (e.g., exercise, optimizing sleep and diet, and stress management).

Migraine prophylactic agents are reasonable to initiate, but their effectiveness for dizziness has not been established. Acute symptoms can be effectively managed with an antihistamine, a benzodiazepine, or an antiemetic. However, these are not appropriate long-term treatment regimens.

PROGNOSIS

The prognosis in patients with dizziness is generally favorable. The main goals are to identify the patients at significant probability of having a dangerous disorder, to relieve the acute symptoms, and to take appropriate steps to reduce the likelihood of recurrent events.

SUGGESTED READINGS

Baloh RW, Kerber KA, Honrubia V: Clinical Neurophysiology of the Vestibular System, ed 4, New York, 2011, Oxford University Press.

Fife TD, Iverson DJ, Lempert T, et al: Practice parameter: Therapies for benign paroxysmal positional vertigo (an evidence-based review): Report of the Quality Standards Subcommittee of the American Academy of Neurology, Neurology 70:2067–2074, 2008. (Accompanying video clips are accessible at www.aan.com/go/practice/guidelines.)

114

Disorders of the Motor System

Kevin M. Biglan

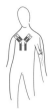

INTRODUCTION

The motor system is broadly divided into the pyramidal and extrapyramidal systems. The pyramidal system is a single neuron system, which originates in the primary motor cortex of the frontal lobes and, with white matter projections, coalesces to form the internal capsule; it then traverses the brainstem (as the cerebral peduncles in the midbrain, the basis pontis in the pons and the pyramids in the medulla where the majority of neurons decussate to form the corticospinal tracts), and ultimately synapses on the lower motor neurons in the anterior horn of the spinal cord (Fig. 114-1). The extrapyramidal system consists primarily of the basal ganglia and the cerebellum, and provides coordinating and integrating information to the pyramidal tract system under the influence of various afferent feedback loops. The components and pathways of the basal ganglia (Fig. 114-2) and cerebellum (Fig. 114-3) influence and modulate voluntary motor activity of the motor cortex.

Disorders of the motor system affect the components of the pyramidal and extrapyramidal systems. The approach to the patient with motor dysfunction depends on the ability to accurately localize the neuroanatomical region affected through a careful history and focused examination.

SYMPTOMS AND SIGNS OF MOTOR SYSTEM DISORDERS

Table 114-1 summarizes the neuroanatomic localization of diseases and the associated symptoms and signs characteristic of dysfunction at those levels. While "weakness" is a frequent complaint, it does little to help with the localization of the problem because it can occur with any disorder of the motor system and does not always reflect weakness on examination. In addition, weakness of insidious onset may be completely overlooked by the patient. Some patients may complain of feeling numb, or that the limb is asleep, uncoordinated, or fatigued. Symptoms referable to impaired balance and gait are common. Patients with distal weakness may complain of impairment in fine motor tasks, buttoning buttons, opening jars/doors, handwriting, stumbling, or tripping with walking. Proximal weakness of the upper extremities will result in difficulty performing tasks over their heads, including washing their hair or applying makeup. Proximal weakness of the lower extremities is often manifested as difficulty with stairs or getting up from sitting. Bulbar weakness with dysarthria and dysphagia may be referable to a variety of diseases of the motor system and can often provide important clues to the differential diagnosis. Involuntary movements may reflect diseases of the basal ganglia but, similar to weakness, may not be appreciable to

the patient; therefore, information from a secondary observer is beneficial. Complaints of diffuse motor incoordination including deficits in speech, fine motor coordination, and gait imbalance suggest cerebellar dysfunction.

SIGNS OF CENTRAL MOTOR SYSTEM DYSFUNCTION

Central nervous system diseases affecting the motor system are divided into abnormalities of pyramidal tract (upper motor neuron), basal ganglia, and cerebellum. Each presents with distinct clinical signs; however, overlapping syndromes may occur, which suggests more diffuse disease processes.

Upper motor lesions affecting the motor cortex and the subcortical white matter prior to the medullary decussation are associated with contralateral weakness, whereas lesions of the medulla and corticospinal tracts in the spinal cord post-decussation cause ipsilateral weakness. Both are associated with upper motor neuron signs. Lesions of the spinal cord may cause mixed upper motor neuron dysfunction below the lesion and lower motor neuron dysfunction at the level of the lesion due to involvement of descending corticospinal tracts and peripheral motor neurons originating in the anterior horn. Dysfunction of upper motor neurons traditionally causes distal greater than proximal weakness, increased muscle tone with spasticity, increased muscle stretch reflexes with clonus, and pathologic reflexes (Babinski's sign). There is little or no muscle atrophy. Acute lesions of the spinal cord can initially cause a flaccid paralysis with areflexia that eventually evolves into a typical upper motor neuron syndrome.

The basal ganglia are important for the planning, initiation, and execution of movements. They facilitate desired movements while inhibiting unwanted movements through pathways that ultimately interact with primary motor cortex. Disorders of basal ganglia function often cause movement disorders characterized by heterogeneous and mixed impairments in voluntary movement not associated with muscle weakness, and often involuntary movements. Disorders of tone are common and variable. Speech and posture are often affected. Patients may have involuntary movements when awake but, with rare exceptions, the involuntary movements are abolished during sleep. Gait dysfunction with postural instability may be seen.

The cerebellum constantly monitors afferent input from muscles, joints, and motor cortex and integrates planned movements to fine tune motor control through efferent projections that regulate motor cortex activity. Disorders causing cerebellar signs may result from direct impairment of cerebellar function or impairment in afferent and efferent pathways of the cerebellum. Cerebellar disorders result in signs that reflect difficulty with

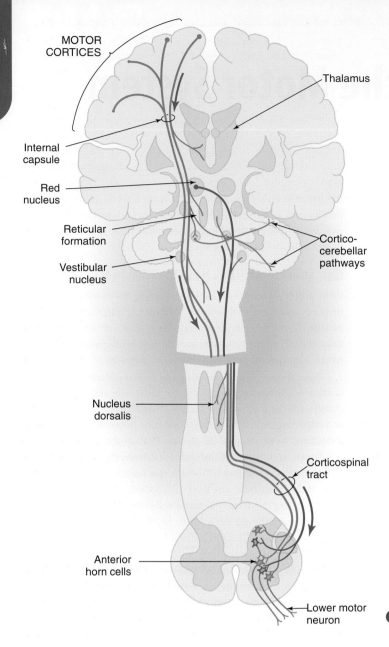

MOTOR CORTICES

Thalamus

Internal capsule

Red nucleus

Reticular formation

Vestibular nucleus

Cortico-cerebellar pathways

Nucleus dorsalis

Corticospinal tract

Anterior horn cells

Lower motor neuron

FIGURE 114-1 Normal human voluntary motor system.

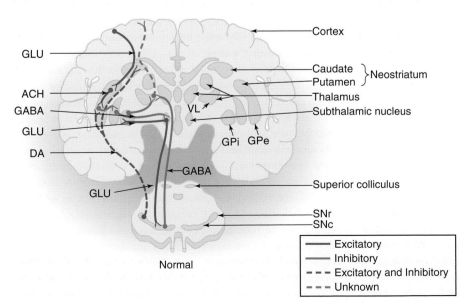

Cortex

GLU

ACH

GABA

GLU

DA

GABA

GLU

Caudate ⎫ Neostriatum
Putamen ⎭

Thalamus

VL

Subthalamic nucleus

GPi   GPe

Superior colliculus

SNr
SNc

Normal

—— Excitatory
—— Inhibitory
--- Excitatory and Inhibitory
- - - Unknown

FIGURE 114-2 Anatomy of the basal ganglia and their connections. The feedback loop proceeds from cerebral prefrontal areas to the basal ganglia and eventually back from the basal ganglia to the thalamus to the motor cortex. This ultimately regulates the descending corticospinal motor system. ACH, Acetylcholine; DA, dopamine; GABA, γ-aminobutyric acid; GLU, glutamate; GP, globus pallidum (e, external; i, internal); SN, substantia nigra (c, compacta; r, reticulate); VL, ventrolateral. (From Jankovic J: The extrapyramidal disorders: Introduction. In Goldman L, Bennett JC, editors: Cecil Textbook of Medicine, ed 21, Philadelphia, 2000, Saunders, p 2078).

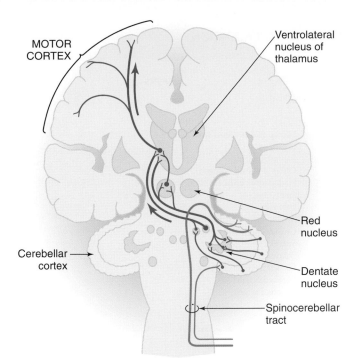

MOTOR
CORTEX

Ventrolateral
nucleus of
thalamus

Cerebellar
cortex

Red
nucleus

Dentate
nucleus

Spinocerebellar
tract

FIGURE 114-3 Corticocerebellar loop. The major cerebellar input is from the spinocerebellar tract. Outflow is to the motor cortex via the mesencephalon and thalamus.

monitoring and regulating motor actions. Eye movement abnormalities include square wave jerks on ocular fixation, jerky slow pursuit movements, hypo- and hyper-metric point-to-point saccades, and nystagmus. The characteristic speech pattern, a scanning dysarthria, displays an abnormal modulation of speech volume and velocity. Speech prosody is also affected. Voluntary movements are irregular and uncoordinated with irregularities in amplitude, velocity, and rhythm. With sustained posture a tremor may develop and increase in amplitude with prolonged sustention. On directed movements there is an irregular placement of the limb (i.e. dysmetria) with voluntary movements, such as finger to nose or heel to shin testing. An intention tremor (increasing amplitude of tremor as one approaches target) is characteristic of cerebellar dysfunction. Patients have difficulty regulating muscle contractions with an increase in rebound when the examiner pushes against a limb and the patient is asked to keep the limb still, or a reduced ability to check a movement when resistance to muscle contraction is suddenly removed.

SIGNS OF PERIPHERAL MOTOR SYSTEM DYSFUNCTION

Disorders affecting the peripheral motor system reflect disease of the motor unit: the anterior horn cell, peripheral nerve, neuromuscular junction, and muscles. All may be associated with weakness, muscle atrophy, hypotonia, hyporeflexia, fasciculations, and fibrillations. Anterior horn cell diseases cause a pure motor disorder with profound atrophy and prominent fasciculations. Paradoxically, the most common cause of anterior horn cell disease, amyotrophic lateral sclerosis, is associated with both upper and lower motor neuron syndrome: individuals have weakness, muscle wasting with spasticity, and increased muscle stretch reflexes. The motor neuron exits the spinal cord via a nerve root,

in the limb multiple roots combine to form a plexus, and then individual peripheral nerves innervate specific muscles. Lesions of nerve roots, plexus, and peripheral nerves are often associated with both weakness and sensory symptoms in the regions innervated by the specific roots, plexus, or nerves. Muscle stretch reflexes are reduced or absent. The distribution of weakness, sensory, and reflex findings assists in accurate localization. Peripheral nerve disorders may affect single nerves, such as median nerve in carpal tunnel syndrome, or multiple nerves, such as polyneuropathy in diabetes. In the former setting combined motor and sensory findings are the rule, whereas in the latter, occasional pure motor neuropathies occur. Polyneuropathy is usually associated with a distal gradient of both motor and sensory abnormalities that can be slowly or rapidly ascending depending on the underlying etiology.

Neuromuscular junction disorders are characterized by fluctuating weakness and fatigability. Tone and reflexes are usually unaffected with the exception of Lambert-Eaton Syndrome, in which muscle stretch reflexes are reduced or absent. Muscle mass and sensation are preserved. On examination, an individual may demonstrate fatigable weakness with strength recovery after rest. Bulbar symptoms and signs may be prominent with a nasal speech pattern, various abnormalities of eye movements, ptosis, and neck weakness.

Disorders of the muscle classically result in proximal greater than distal limb weakness with some exceptions, such as inclusion body myositis and myotonic dystrophy, in which distal weakness predominates. Muscle diseases, especially toxic or inflammatory conditions, may be associated with myalgia and tenderness to muscle palpation. Muscle stretch reflexes are normal to slightly reduced. Sensation is preserved.

DIFFERENTIAL DIAGNOSIS OF PYRAMIDAL TRACT DISORDERS

Any disease affecting the nervous system can cause pyramidal tract dysfunction. Structural lesions due to stroke, tumor, infection, trauma, inflammatory and demyelinating diseases can cause pyramidal tract dysfunction with variable presentations depending on the underlying disease process and the variable involvement of non-motor systems. These disorders are discussed elsewhere.

Hereditary spastic paraplegia (HSP) is a rare and heterogeneous group of inherited disorders that causes progressive pyramidal tract dysfunction manifest clinically by spastic paraparesis.

DIFFERENTIAL DIAGNOSIS OF PERIPHERAL MOTOR SYSTEM DISORDERS

Similar to pyramidal tract dysfunction, lesions resulting from direct tumor involvement, infection, trauma, and inflammatory and demyelinating processes may all affect the peripheral motor system. In addition, specific inherited and acquired degenerative disorders may affect the peripheral motor system (Chapters 121, 122, and 123).

MOVEMENT DISORDERS

Movement disorders are a heterogeneous group of disorders associated with basal ganglia dysfunction. Movement disorders refer to the involuntary or abnormal movement, known as the

TABLE 114-1 SYMPTOMS AND SIGNS APPROACH TO NEUROANATOMIC LOCALIZATION OF MOTOR SYSTEM DYSFUNCTION

NEUROANATOMIC LOCALIZATION	SYMPTOMS	SIGNS
CENTRAL NERVOUS SYSTEM		
PYRAMIDAL TRACT		
Cortical	Weakness Cortical symptoms (e.g. aphasia)	Hemiparesis or focal weakness Spasticity Babinski's sign Other cortical findings
Subcortical	Isolated weakness/clumsiness	Hemiparesis of face and body Spasticity Babinski's sign Absence of cortical findings
Brainstem	Weakness Bulbar symptoms Somnolence	Crossed facial and body paresis Spasticity Babinski's sign Cranial nerve findings (e.g. INO) Cerebellar signs Impaired arousal
Spinal Cord	Weakness Sensory loss, paresthesia/dysesthesia Gait imbalance and falls Back pain Bowel and bladder dysfunction	Paraparesis > hemiparesis Sensory level Absence of bulbar signs Babinski's sign Hoffman's sign
BASAL GANGLIA	Changes in gait, gait imbalance, and falls Changes in voice Impairment in voluntary motor actions Involuntary movements Behavioral changes	Tone abnormalities (rigidity) Postural abnormalities Postural instability Gait disorders Akinesia/hypokinesia Tremor Chorea/ballism/athetosis Dystonia Tics
CEREBELLAR	Gait imbalance and falls Slurred speech Tremor with intentional tasks Incoordination	Oculomotor abnormalities Hypotonia Gait ataxia Titubation Scanning dysarthria Dysmetria Intention tremor Past pointing Dysdiadokinesis Excessive rebound Impaired check
PERIPHERAL NERVOUS SYSTEM		
ROOTS (RADICULAR)	Pain radiating into limb/trunk Localized sensory loss, parasthesias, dysesthesias Localized weakness	Combined motor and sensory deficits in a radicular distribution Reduced MSR in region subserved by root(s) Muscle atrophy
PLEXUS	Localized sensory loss, parasthesias, dysesthesias in a single limb Localized weakness in a single limb Bowel and bladder symptoms in lumbosacral plexus	Combined motor and sensory deficits involving multiple roots and subserving multiple nerves Reduced MSR in region subserved by multiple roots Muscle atrophy
PERIPHERAL NERVE	Polyneuropathy Distal/bilateral sensory loss, parasthesias, dysesthesias Distal/ascending and bilateral weakness Mononeuropathy Localized pain and sensory symptoms	Distal predominant weakness Stocking-glove sensory loss Reduced MSR Hypotonia Muscle atrophy
NEUROMUSCULAR JUNCTION	Fluctuating weakness Worsening weakness over the course of the day or with physical activity Diplopia Slurred speech Absence of sensory symptoms	Bulbar weakness Normal MSR Normal muscle bulk Fatigable weakness Normal sensory exam
MUSCLE	Proximal greater than distal weakness Myalgias Absence of sensory symptoms	Proximal weakness Normal muscle tone and bulk Normal to reduced MSR

INO, Intranuclear ophthalmoplegia; MSR, muscle stretch reflexes.

movement phenomenon, or may be used to describe a syndromic disorder in which involuntary or abnormalities of movement are cardinal features of the disease. In contrast to most seizures, the involuntary movements occur when the patient is conscious, but are absent during sleep.

Movement disorders can be classified as either hyperkinetic or hypokinetic. Hyperkinetic phenomena include tremor, chorea, dystonia, tics, myoclonus, and other involuntary movements. Hypokinetic disorders encompass the Parkinsonian disorders characterized by a paucity of spontaneous movement (akinesia) and low amplitude slow movements (bradykinesia). While this classification strategy is a valuable means for approaching the patient with abnormal movements, many movement disorders include both hyperkinetic and hypokinetic phenomena. Idiopathic Parkinson's disease is the prototypical hypokinetic movement disorder, but it is associated with the hyperkinetic phenomenon of tremor in over 60% of patients. Similarly, Huntington disease, a traditionally hyperkinetic disorder, is associated with bradykinetic voluntary movements.

Parkinsonism

Parkinsonism is the most common of the extrapyramidal disorders and is characterized by akinesia, rigidity, tremor, and postural instability. Parkinsonism is caused by a wide variety of degenerative disorders, medication and toxins, and systemic diseases. Table 114-2 summarizes the differential diagnosis of Parkinsonism.

Idiopathic Parkinson's Disease

Idiopathic Parkinson's disease (PD) accounts for most individuals with Parkinsonism and is the second most common adult onset neurodegenerative disease after Alzheimer's disease. The average age of onset is around 60 years with an increasing prevalence associated with aging and a slight male preponderance. The motor symptoms of PD result from the selective loss of dopaminergic neurons in the substantia nigra-pars compacta that project to the striatum. The pathological hallmark of PD is the presence of eosinophilic cytoplasmic neuronal inclusions known as Lewy bodies containing α-synuclein.

Clinically, PD is characterized by its motor phenomenon with asymmetric rigidity, bradykinesia, rest tremor, and postural instability. However, PD is also characterized by secondary, nonmotor manifestations (facial hypomimia, hypophonia, dysphagia, micrographia, and flexed posture), autonomic dysfunction (orthostatic hypotension, constipation, hyperactive bladder, and impaired temperature regulation), behavioral symptoms (depression, anxiety, psychosis), cognitive impairment and dementia, sleep disorders (impaired sleep architecture, restless legs syndrome, REM sleep behavior disorder), and sensory phenomena.

Until recently the diagnosis of PD was made based on the findings of an adult onset disorder of unilateral onset, persistent asymmetry of motor findings, and responsiveness of motor features to levodopa therapy. In addition, a number of "red flags" on history or examination might suggest an atypical or secondary cause of Parkinsonism (Table 114-3). However, Dopamine Transporter (DAT) SPECT imaging has recently been approved to assist in distinguishing PD from PD mimics, notably drug-induced Parkinsonism and essential tremor with parkinsonian features. The dopamine transporter is responsible for re-uptake of dopamine into presynaptic terminals and is, therefore, an indirect measure of nigro-striatal neuronal density. In PD, nigrostriatal neurons are lost asymmetrically; on dopamine transporter imaging, this is characterized by asymmetric reduction in dopamine transporter signal in the striatum. Unfortunately, this imaging method does not distinguish atypical Parkinsonism from PD.

A number of monogenic causes of Parkinsonism have been identified. Mutations in α-synuclein (SNCA), leucine-rich repeat kinase 2 (LRRK2), vacuolar protein sorting 35 (VPS35), and eukaryotic translation initiation factor 4-γ (EIF4G1) are associated with autosomal dominant Parkinsonism. Autosomal dominant causes account for less than 2% of all adult onset Parkinson's disease cases with higher frequencies in certain populations due to founder effects. Autosomal recessive monogenic causes include parkin, PTEN-induced kinase 1 (PINK1), and Parkinson protein 7 (DJ-1) and are relatively common in familial cases with onset before the age of 45. An improved understanding of these genetic causes suggests an important role of impairment in lysosomal pathways and protein degradation in PD pathogenesis.

PD is a slowly progressive disorder associated with accumulating disability. No treatments have been proven to slow progression; however, ongoing efforts continue to identify putative

TABLE 114-2   DIFFERENTIAL DIAGNOSIS OF PARKINSONISM

DEGENERATIVE/ INHERITED CAUSES	Idiopathic Parkinson's disease
	Multiple system atrophy
	Progressive supranuclear palsy
	Dementia with Lewy body
	Corticobasal degeneration
	Frontotemporal dementia with Parkinsonism
	Huntington's disease
	Wilson's disease
	Dopa-responsive dystonia
	Pantothenate kinase–associated neurodegeneration
SECONDARY CAUSES	Dopamine receptor blocking medications (e.g. antipsychotics, metoclopramide, prochlorperazine)
	Presynaptic dopamine depleting medications (tetrabenazine)
	Cerebrovascular disease
	Toxins (MPTP, manganese, carbon monoxide)

MPTP, 1-methyl-4-phenyl-1,2,3,6-tetrahydropyridine.

TABLE 114-3   "RED FLAGS" IN THE DIAGNOSIS OF PARKINSON'S DISEASE

CLINICAL OR HISTORICAL "RED FLAG"	SUGGESTED DIAGNOSIS
Early postural instability and falls	PSP, MSA, CBD, DLB, Vascular
Early dysphagia	PSP, CBD
Early or spontaneous hallucinations	DLB
Early dementia or dementia predating PD	DLB
Early or severe dysautonomia	MSA
Pyramidal tract and/or Cerebellar signs	MSA
Antipsychotic exposure	Tardive or drug-induced
Acute onset and/or non-progressive	Vascular

CBD, Corticobasal degeneration; DLB, dementia with Lewy body; MSA, multiple system atrophy; PSP, progressive supranuclear palsy.

Table 114-4 MEDICATIONS FOR PARKINSON'S DISEASE

ANTICHOLINERGIC AGENTS

Trihexyphenidyl (Artane)
Benztropine (Cogentin)

DOPAMINE PRECURSORS (COMBINED WITH PERIPHERAL AROMATIC AMINO ACID DECARBOXYLASE INHIBITORS)

Carbidopa-levodopa (Sinemet, Sinemet-CR, Parcopa) (regular, controlled-release, and orally disintegrating)
Benserazide-levodopa (Madopar) (marketed in Europe)

DOPAMINE AGONISTS

Apomorphine (Apokyn) (injectable short acting), bromocriptine (Parlodel)
Pramipexole (Mirapex)
Rotigotine (Neupro) (transdermal patch)
Ropinirole (Requip, Requip XR)

MONOAMINE OXIDASE TYPE B (MAO-B) INHIBITORS

Selegiline (deprenyl) (Carbex, Eldepryl, Zelapar)
Rasagiline (Azilect)

CATECHOL *O*-METHYLTRANSFERASE (COMT) INHIBITORS

Tolcapone (Tasmar)
Entacapone (Comtan)

CATECHOL *O*-METHYLTRANSFERASE (COMT) INHIBITORS COMBINED WITH CARBIDOPA-LEVODOPA

Entacapone-carbidopa-levodopa (Stalevo)

disease modifying therapies. Treatments of the motor symptoms can reduce disability and improve function (Table 114-4). The mainstay of treatment is levodopa, the precursor to dopamine, given with a dopa-decarboxylase inhibitor to maximize CNS penetration of levodopa and minimize systemic side effects. Other symptomatic treatments stimulate dopamine receptors in the brain or inhibit the breakdown of levodopa and dopamine (Table 114-4). This approach to symptom management is effective early in the course of the disease; however, as the disease continues to progress, it may be complicated by the development of motor fluctuations, drug-induced dyskinesias, and psychosis.

Atypical Parkinsonism

Atypical Parkinsonism or "Parkinson plus" disorders refer to a heterogeneous group of inherited and sporadic neurodegenerative disorders characterized by Parkinsonism and a reduced or absent response to dopaminergic therapy. The most common are multiple system atrophy (MSA), progressive supranuclear palsy (PSP), dementia with Lewy bodies (DLB), and corticobasal degeneration (CBD).

MSA is a sporadic neurodegenerative disorder characterized clinically by the variable combination of Parkinsonism, autonomic dysfunction, cerebellar dysfunction, and extrapyramidal motor signs. The term MSA was coined to encompass three previously distinct clinical entities: striatonigral degeneration with prominent parkinsonism, olivopontocerebellar atrophy with prominent cerebellar dysfunction, and Shy-Drager syndrome with prominent autonomic dysfunction, particularly profound orthostatic hypotension. The identification of a shared neuropathological correlate of neuronal inclusions consisting of α-synuclein bolstered the shared nomenclature of these disorders. Currently, the preferred classification refers to either MSA-parkinsonism type or MSA-cerebellar type depending on the predominant clinical symptoms and signs. An MSA-autonomic type is proposed for those with an overwhelmingly autonomic presentation. Although relatively rare, MSA is among the most frequently encountered of the atypical Parkinsonisms with an overall incidence of 0.6/100,000 and an increasing incidence with age. It is universally fatal with a mean survival of 7 to 9 years, though longer disease duration is sometimes seen. Treatment is challenging and largely symptomatic. Some patients may be partially responsive to dopaminergic therapy and levodopa is recommended for individuals with prominent parkinsonism. Autonomic manifestations can be managed with symptomatic treatments to address orthostatic hypotension, constipation, and bladder symptoms (see Chapter 110).

Progressive supranuclear palsy is a relentlessly progressive disorder characterized by early gait instability and falls, prominent and early dysphagia, early speech difficulties progressing to a non-fluent aphasia, dementia, and supranuclear gaze palsy; death occurs on average 5 years after diagnosis. Supranuclear gaze palsy, in its fully realized form, is characterized by vertical greater than horizontal gaze palsy with preserved oculocephalic reflexes. Early, the gaze palsy may manifest by the presence of square wave jerks, difficulty initiating saccades, and loss of the fast phase on optokinetic nystagmus testing. Patients have a wide-eyed stare and lid lag may be present. Opposed to the flexed posture and asymmetry of PD, individuals with progressive supranuclear palsy have extensor trunk posturing and greater axial rigidity with relatively appendicular symmetry. Up to 20% of patients may have a modest response to levodopa therapy.

Dementia with Lewy bodies is the second most common degenerative cause of dementia after Alzheimer's disease. It is characterized clinically by Parkinsonism, dementia preceding or within 1 year of the motor symptoms, propensity for psychosis, early falls, and fluctuations in cognition and arousal. Motorically, it may be indistinguishable from Parkinson's disease. Patients have a high risk for psychosis associated with dopaminergic therapy and antipsychotics may cause worsening of Parkinsonism and even death making management of these patients challenging.

Corticobasal degeneration is a rare and heterogenous disorder. The characteristic Parkinsonian disorder presents with marked asymmetric Parkinsonism, focal limb dystonia, cortical sensory findings, alien limb phenomenon, and myoclonus. However, it may present with primary cortical cognitive symptoms and have features of progressive supranuclear palsy. It is a relentlessly progressive and fatal illness. Treatment is symptomatic.

Secondary Parkinsonism

There are many causes of secondary Parkinsonism, including medications, toxins, and cerebrovascular disease. Medications associated with Parkinsonism include any medication that reduces dopaminergic tone in the brain, either through direct blockade of post-synaptic dopamine receptors (e.g. antipsychotics) or through depletion of pre-synaptic dopamine stores (e.g. tetrabenazine). Metoclopramide, a medication commonly used to treat gastroparesis, is a frequent cause because its dopamine blocking effects may be overlooked. Drug-induced Parkinsonism can be indistinguishable from Parkinson's disease and is frequently asymmetric. Treatment consists of withholding the offending agent, recognizing that it may take months for the symptoms to resolve. Even then, patients exposed to dopamine blocking agents may develop a tardive Parkinsonism (i.e., a drug-induced Parkinsonism that persists even after the offending agent is removed). DAT SPECT imaging can be useful in distinguishing drug-induced or tardive Parkinsonism from Parkinson's Disease.

Cerebrovascular disease is a common cause of secondary Parkinsonism. Tremor is uncommon in vascular Parkinsonism; lower extremity bradykinesia and gait difficulties dominate the clinical picture. Patients may have a history of clinical strokes with acute deteriorations followed by plateaus; however, many patients have vascular risk factors and a history of gradual decline.

Tremor

Tremor is a rhythmic, oscillatory movement of a body part. Tremor is classified by its distribution (e.g., voice, limb) and whether it is present at rest, with sustained posture (sustention), or with action. Action tremor can further be classified as an intention tremor, in which the tremor worsens as one approaches target. Intention tremor is characteristic of cerebellar disease. Tremor has multiple etiologies, including medications, alcohol and drug withdrawal, systemic disease (e.g. hyperthyroidism), structural brain lesions, or as a component of a neurodegenerative disease.

Essential tremor is among the most common movement disorders and the most common cause of tremor. Essential tremor has a worldwide prevalence of 2% to 4% with increasing incidence with aging. Clinically it is characterized by postural tremor of the upper extremities. An intention tremor develops with disease progression and may be disabling. Involvement of the head and voice are common. Mild Parkinsonian features (e.g., tremor at rest, rigidity with activation) may develop and can make distinguishing incipient Parkinson's disease challenging. The condition is often familial with an autosomal dominant pattern of inheritance and tends to improve with alcohol ingestion. Propranolol and primidone are of similar benefit (Table 114-5).

Chorea

Chorea is characterized by brief, irregular, random, non-rhythmic movements that flow from one body part to another. It is often associated with athetosis and ballism. These conditions lie on a spectrum of choreic phenomenon with ballism characterized by proximal large amplitude flinging movements on one end, chorea in the middle with lower amplitude random flowing movements and athetosis characterized by slower distal writhing movements on the other. Chorea is often associated with a variety of secondary clinical features detailed in Table 114-6.

There are many etiologies of choreic disorders reflecting a wide variety of processes affecting the basal ganglia and specifically the striatum. Generally, chorea either represents the primary manifestation of an inherited disorder or is acquired secondary to basal ganglia insults due to various comorbid medical conditions, medications or toxins, or structural abnormalities. Table 114-7 summarizes the differential diagnosis of chorea categorized by genetic and acquired causes.

Huntington's Disease

Huntington's disease (HD) is an autosomal dominant, progressively disabling, and fatal neurodegenerative disease; it is and the most common cause of inherited adult onset chorea. The causative mutation is an expansion of an unstable cytosine-adenine-guanine (CAG) trinucleotide repeat of the IT-15 gene on the short arm of chromosome 4.

HD may emerge at any age, with the peak incidence between 35 and 40 years of age with death occurring 10 to 20 years after onset. Age of onset and rate of progression of the disease are inversely associated with CAG repeat length with the longest repeats associated with juvenile onset disease and a more rapid disease progression.

HD is characterized clinically by the triad of an extrapyramidal movement disorder, progressive cognitive decline (dementia), and an array of behavioral disturbances. Chorea is the prototypical motor manifestation of HD occurring in 90% of patients. Cognitive impairment is invariable in HD and typically progresses from selective deficits in psychomotor, executive, and visuospatial abilities to more global impairment with higher cortical functions usually spared. Psychiatric illness has been recognized as an important feature of HD since George Huntington reported on the "tendency to insanity and suicide."

The juvenile variant of HD, in which age of onset occurs before 20, typically has an akinetic-rigid phenotype and paternal inheritance and only rarely chorea. Paternal inheritance of the HD gene is the rule for onset before the age of 10 and paternal inheritance predominates (about 3 : 1 paternal : maternal) for onset before the age of 20.

TABLE 114-5	TREATMENT OPTIONS FOR ESSENTIAL TREMOR
FIRST LINE	Propranolol
	Primidone
SECOND LINE	Topirimate
	Zonisamide
	Benzodiazepines
	Other beta-blockers
	Gabapentin/Pregabalin
MEDICATION FAILURE	Botulinum toxin injections
	Deep brain stimulation

TABLE 114-6	SECONDARY FEATURES ASSOCIATED WITH CHOREA
ATHETOSIS	Slow, writhing movements of distal limbs
BALLISM	Rapid, flinging movements of proximal limbs
PARAKINESIS	Incorporation of an involuntary movement into a voluntary movement (e.g. crossing and uncrossing of legs, adjusting glasses)
MOTOR IMPERSISTENCE	Inability to maintain tongue protrusion, "milk maid's grip"
PARTIALLY SUPPRESSIBLE	Brief ability to voluntary reduce the severity of movements
DEEP TENDON REFLEX CHANGES	"hung up" or "pendular" reflexes
GAIT DISORDERS	Irregular or dance like gait

TABLE 114-7 DIFFERENTIAL DIAGNOSIS OF CHOREA

GENETIC DISORDERS	Autosomal dominant	Huntington's disease
		Spinocerebellar ataxia (SCA 17 >1-3)
		DRPLA
		Neuroferritinopathy
		Benign hereditary chorea
	Autosomal recessive	Neuroacanthocytosis
		Wilson's disease
		Ataxia (Friedreich's, ataxia-telangiectasia, ataxia with oculomotor apraxia)
		Disorders associated with brain iron accumulation (PKAN)
	X-linked	McLeod's syndrome
		Lesch-Nyan's syndrome
ACQUIRED/SPORADIC	Medications	Direct side effects
		Tardive dyskinesia
	Immune mediated	Sydenham's chorea
		Systemic lupus erythematosus
		Anti-phospholipid antibody syndrome
		Vasculitis
		Paraneoplastic (*CRMP5* gene, anti-Hu)
	Infectious	HIV/AIDS
		Variant CJD
		Neurosyphilis
	Endocrine	Hyperthyroidism
		Chorea gravidarum
	Metabolic	Hyperglycemia
		Electrolyte disturbances
		Acquired hepatocerebral degeneration
	Vascular	Basal ganglia infarcts/hemorrhage
	Miscellaneous	Polycythemia vera
		Post-cardiac bypass pump
		Multiple sclerosis
		Sporadic neurodegenerative disorders

CJD, Creutzfeld-Jakob disease; DRPLA, dentatorubropallidoluysian atrophy; PKAN, pantothenate-kinase-associated neurodegeneration; SCA, spinocerebellar ataxia.

The neuropathology of HD is characterized by selective neuronal vulnerability, particularly involving the caudate and putamen of the corpus striatum. Microscopically, the pathological hallmark of the disease is the preferential loss of medium-sized spiny neurons projecting from the striatum to the external pallidum. While HD is associated with a variety of motoric phenotypes, it remains the prototypical choreiform disorder and the most common cause of inherited adult onset chorea. In addition, HD represents one of the most important genetic disorders of adulthood. HD was the first disease recognized to arise from a trinucleotide expansion and serves as a model for the experimental therapeutics of adult-onset neurodegenerative diseases.

Huntington's Disease Phenocopies

Approximately 10% of individuals with an autosomal dominant HD-like disorder will not carry the causative mutation for HD. Among these "phenocopies," only a small minority will have an identifiable genetic mutation. The most common genetic causes in the Caucasian population include spinocerebellar ataxia (SCA) 17, Friedreich's ataxia, HD-like 2, and familial prion disease (HD-like 1). Alternative diagnoses include dentatorubropallidoluysian atrophy (DRPLA), SCA 1-3, and neuroferritinopathy. A benign form of an autosomal dominant chorea, benign familial chorea, without significant behavioral or cognitive impairment can occur.

Wilson's Disease

Wilson's disease is a rare, autosomal recessive disorder of impaired copper metabolism with copper accumulation and neurological and hepatic dysfunction. It causes heterogenous movement disorder including chorea, dystonia, Parkinsonism, and tremor; dystonia and tremor tend to predominate. Onset with movement disorder occurs in about 50% of individuals, the others presenting with liver disease. The mean age of onset is 20; it rarely occurs after the age of 40. Untreated it is invariably fatal; early treatment is associated with better clinical outcomes; therefore, a high level of suspicion should be maintained. Diagnosis is confirmed by the presence of Kayser-Fleischer corneal rings in the setting of increased urinary copper excretion or elevated copper on liver biopsy. Although ceruloplasmin is usually low in symptomatic patients, it is not definitive, and confirmatory testing with ophthalmologic screen, 24-hour urinary copper or liver biopsy is necessary. Treatment consists of drugs that facilitate copper excretion, such as zinc, trientine, tetrathiomolybdate, penicillamine (the latter falling from favor because of its toxicities).

Sydenham's Chorea

Sydenham's chorea is one of the most common causes of childhood onset chorea and is an immune complication of group A streptococcal infection. It presents acutely months after the streptococcal infection, is frequently asymmetric, and may cause behavioral symptoms in addition to chorea. Other features of rheumatic fever may also be present and echocardiography should be performed on any child with suspected Sydenham's. Treatment of the underlying infection, management of complications of rheumatic fever, and supportive care are generally sufficient with the majority of patients having resolution of symptoms by 1 year. A history of Sydenham's may predispose a female patient to adult onset chorea during pregnancy (chorea gravidarum) or in response to estrogen treatment.

Medications and Tardive Dyskinesia

Numerous medications have been associated with chorea. The most common direct cause of drug-induced chorea is levodopa-induced dyskinesias in individuals with Parkinson's disease. Tardive dyskinesia is a late complication of treatment with dopamine receptor blocking agents, usually neuroleptic antipsychotics, and may have chorea as a prominent feature. Advancing age, female gender, and use of high potency antipsychotics are associated with an increased risk for this complication. While removal of the offending agent is critical to prevent worsening, symptoms persist in approximately two thirds of patients and treatment can be challenging.

Dystonia

Dystonia is a heterogenous class of movement disorders characterized by sustained muscle contractions that lead to twisting movements, abnormal postures, and repetitive movements. The classification of dystonia is challenging, having undergone numerous revisions over time, and is based on age of onset, distribution (focal versus generalized), association with neurological signs other than dystonia, and cause, if known. Mutations in at least 23 different genes are associated with dystonia. In general, the specific mutation does not reliably predict the phenotype. Childhood onset dystonia often has an underlying genetic cause, tends to generalize, and has a more severe course; while adult onset focal dystonia of the neck (e.g. cervical dystonia) tends to be non-progressive without a defined genetic cause.

Adult onset focal dystonias are by far the most common dystonias encountered clinically. Cervical dystonia is the most common dystonia, followed by focal dystonias involving the face and jaw muscles (blepharospasm, oromandibular dystonia or the combination); laryngeal and limb dystonias are rare. Adult onset limb dystonias are usually task-specific; dystonic contraction only occurs during specific voluntary actions (e.g., writer's cramp, musician's dystonia). This task specificity may be lost over time and occur even at rest. Focal adult onset limb dystonia that is not task specific can be the earliest manifestation of Parkinsonism and Parkinson's disease.

A mutation in the *TOR1A* gene is the most common cause of early onset generalized dystonia. DYT1 is an autosomal dominant disorder with reduced penetrance (30%). Onset is usually during childhood (10 to 15 years of age) with focal limb dystonia with action that rapidly generalizes often sparing the craniocervical muscles. It accounts for less than 50% of childhood onset dystonia in non-Jews and approximately 80% in children of Ashkenazi Jewish descent.

Dopa-responsive dystonia is a rare but important cause of childhood onset dystonia. It is inherited in autosomal dominant fashion with reduced penetrance (30%) with females more commonly affected than males. It is characterized by lower extremity dystonia, Parkinsonism, and diurnal variability with the symptoms worsening as the day progresses and improving with sleep. As the name suggests, it is exquisitely sensitive to levodopa therapy. The condition is often misdiagnosed and untreated; therefore, patients with childhood onset dystonia should have a trial of levodopa.

Myoclonus dystonia syndrome is an autosomal dominant disorder with alcohol responsive myoclonic jerks and dystonia. Dystonia is often focal with cervical dystonia and writer's cramp predominating. Onset is usually prior to the age of 20 years and psychiatric symptoms are common.

Rapid-onset dystonia Parkinsonism is a rare autosomal dominant condition with reduced penetrance that presents over hours or weeks with craniofacial and limb dystonia, dysarthria, bradykinesia, and postural instability. After initial progression the disorder stabilizes. The rapid onset and triggers, including emotional trauma or physical exertion, often result in it being misdiagnosed as a somatoform disorder.

Treatment of dystonia consists of a combination of oral medications and focused botulinum toxin injections. Oral medications include anticholinergics, benzodiazepines, and muscle relaxants. Deep brain stimulation has shown recent benefit in treating dystonia resulting from multiple causes.

Tics and Tourette's Syndrome

Tics are rapid, stereotyped, non-rhythmic movements or vocalizations. They can mimic many normal motor activities and movement disorders and occur on a background of otherwise normal activity and motor function. The key differentiating characteristics of tics are that they are associated with an irresistible urge or sensation that is temporarily relieved with performance of the tic. Tics are voluntarily suppressible but suppressing them results in increasing urge and rebound exacerbation of tics. Tics of childhood are extremely common and if transient, require no treatment.

Tourette's syndrome (TS) is a tic disorder, beginning in childhood with both motor and vocal tics persisting for more than one year. Approximately 50% of individuals with TS will also have features of obsessive compulsive disorder and/or attention deficit disorder. These other features are often more disabling than the tics themselves. In the majority of individuals there is partial or complete resolution of symptoms by adulthood. Treatment of tics and associated comorbidities should be reserved only for functionally disabling symptoms. A combination of behavioral approaches (comprehensive behavioral intervention for tics), oral medications, and botulinum toxin injections can be effective at minimizing the impact of symptoms. Extreme cases with persistence in adulthood may respond to deep brain stimulation.

● CEREBELLAR ATAXIAS

The ataxias are a heterogeneous group of conditions reflecting impaired cerebellar function or impairment in cerebellar afferent and efferent pathways. Structural lesions due to abnormalities of brain development, stroke, tumor, infection, trauma, and inflammatory and demyelinating diseases can frequently affect cerebellar function and result in cerebellar symptoms and signs. Table 114-8 summarizes the differential diagnosis of the ataxic disorders divided by genetic and acquired causes.

Inherited/Genetic Ataxias

Progressive ataxia in coordination and gait disturbance are the cardinal features of the inherited ataxias. Autosomal dominant spinocerebellar ataxias (SCA) may present with a pure cerebellar syndrome or be associated with other extrapyramidal, pyramidal,

TABLE 114-8 DIFFERENTIAL DIAGNOSIS OF CEREBELLAR ATAXIA

GENETIC DISORDERS	Autosomal dominant	Spinocerebellar Ataxias
		Episodic ataxia
		DRPLA
	Autosomal recessive	Friedreich's ataxia
		Ataxia-telangiectasia
		Ataxia with oculomotor apraxia
		Ataxia with vitamin E deficiency
	X-linked	Fragile X-associated tremor/ataxia syndrome
	Mitochondrial	Polymerase gamma (POLG)
ACQUIRED/ SPORADIC	Medications/Toxins	Alcohol
		Phenytoin
		Fluorouracil
		Heavy metals
		Carbon monoxide
	Developmental	Chiari malformations
		Dandy-Walker malformations
		Pontocerebellar hypoplasia
	Immune mediated	Paraneoplastic (anti-Hu/Yo/Ri)
		Pediatric post-viral
		Behçet's disease
	Infectious	HIV/AIDS
		PML
		CJD
		Lyme disease
	Metabolic	Thiamine deficiency (Wernicke's encephalopathy)
		vitamin E/B12 deficiency
		Thyroid disease
	Vascular	Cerebellar stroke/hemorrhage
	Neoplastic	Primary and metastatic tumors
		Paraneoplastic (anti-Hu/Yo/Ri)
	Miscellaneous	MSA-cerebellar
		Multiple sclerosis

CJD, Cruetzfeldt-Jakob disease; DRPLA, dentatorubropallidoluysian atrophy; MSA, multiple system atrophy; PML, progressive multifocal leukoencephalopathy.

cognitive, or behavioral features. They are usually adult onset with variable genetic mutations, including trinucleotide repeats, mutations in noncoding regions, and point mutations. Genetic testing is available for many of the common spinocerebellar ataxias and new mutations are being identified in a rapid and ongoing basis. Currently there are no treatments to address disease progression and symptomatic treatment is limited.

The fragile X mental retardation (FMR1) gene contains a CCG trinucleotide repeat expansion of greater than 200 in the fully penetrant mutation associated with mental retardation in boys. Recently a pre-mutation associated with repeats of 55-200 in the FMR1 gene has been found to be the cause of the adult onset neurodegenerative disorder, fragile X–associated tremor/ataxia syndrome (FXTAS). Clinically, affected males have a progressive cerebellar tremor and ataxia. Fragile X–associated tremor/ataxia syndrome has been under-recognized and may be the most common genetic cause of late onset ataxia. Treatment is largely symptomatic and the disease results in progressive disability.

Autosomal recessive ataxias are rare conditions with onset in childhood. Friedreich's ataxia (FA) is the most common and best characterized of these disorders. It results from an unstable GAA expansion on chromosome 9. Clinically it is characterized by childhood onset gait ataxia and clumsiness. The ataxia reflects a combination of spinocerebellar degeneration and peripheral sensory loss. Frank weakness secondary to pyramidal tract dysfunction is a late complication. Non-neurological manifestations include cardiomyopathy, diabetes mellitus, and skeletal deformities, which add to the morbidity and mortality of the disease. Since identification of the mutation, late onset forms of the disease with less systemic involvement and milder symptoms have been identified. Therefore, Friedreich's ataxia should be considered in the differential of adult onset sporadic ataxias.

Ataxia with vitamin E deficiency is a childhood onset ataxia with a Friedreich's ataxia phenotype. Treatment with high dose vitamin E may slow the progression of neurological symptoms. Ataxia with vitamin E deficiency should be considered in any child with signs and symptoms of Friedreich's ataxia that do not carry the Friedreich's ataxia mutation.

Sporadic/Acquired Ataxias

Insidious onset of cerebellar ataxia without a family history can be a diagnostic challenge. Alcohol abuse, toxins, multiple system atrophy, and mitochondrial disorders are diagnostic considerations.

Acute or subacute onset ataxia is most often associated with cerebrovascular disease, demyelinating illness, or direct or indirect effects of cancer. Paraneoplastic cerebellar degeneration is one of the more common paraneoplastic syndromes usually associated with gynecological, breast, lung cancer, or lymphoma. A variety of anti-neuronal antibodies have been implicated; however, anti-Hu/Yo/Ri are most frequently seen. The cerebellar syndrome often predates the identification of the cancer. Treatment of the underlying cancer and plasma exchange are sometimes beneficial.

Vitamin B12 and vitamin E deficiency secondary to malabsorption can present with ataxic gait as a result of posterior column sensory deficits. In the appropriate clinical situation, Wernicke's encephalopathy due to thiamine deficiency needs to be considered as an acute cause of gait ataxia.

SUGGESTED READINGS

Aarsland D, Påhlhagen S, Ballard CG, et al: Depression in Parkinson disease—epidemiology, mechanisms and management, Nat Rev Neurol 8(1):35–47, 2011.

Abdo WF, van de Warrenburg BP, Burn DJ, et al: The clinical approach to movement disorders, Nat Rev Neurol 6:29–37, 2010.

Albanese A, Bhatia K, Bressman SB, et al: Phenomenology and Classification of Dystonia: A Consensus Update, Mov Disord 28:863–873, 2013.

Anheim M, Tranchant C, Koenig M: The autosomal recessive cerebellar ataxias, N Engl J Med 366:636–646, 2012.

Armstrong MJ, Miyasaki JM: Evidence-based guideline: pharmacologic treatment of chorea in Huntington disease: Report of the Guideline Development Subcommittee of the American Academy of Neurology, Neurology 79:597–603, 2012.

Barker RA, Barrett J, Mason SL, et al: Fetal dopaminergic transplantation trials and the future of neural grafting in Parkinson's disease, Lancet Neurol 12(1):84–91, 2013.

Beato R, Maia DP, Teixeira AL Jr, et al: Executive functioning in adult patients with Sydenham's chorea, Mov Disord 25:853–857, 2010.

Berardelli A, Wenning GK, Antonini A, et al: EFNS/MDS-ES/ENS recommendations for the diagnosis of Parkinson's disease, Eur J Neurol 20(1):16–34, 2013.

Charlesworth G, Bhatia KP, Wood NW: The genetics of dystonia: new twists in an old tale, Brain 136(Pt 7):2017–2037, 2013.

Finsterer J, Löscher W, Quasthoff S, et al: Hereditary spastic paraplegias with autosomal dominant, recessive, X-linked, or maternal trait of inheritance, J Neurol Sci 318(1–2):1–18, 2012.

Fox SH, Katzenschlager R, Lim SY, et al: The Movement Disorder Society Evidence-Based Medicine Review Update: Treatments for the motor symptoms of Parkinson's disease, Mov Disord 26(Suppl 3):S2–S41, 2011.

Garcia-Borreguero D, Ferini-Strambi L, Kohnen R, et al: European guidelines on management of restless legs syndrome: report of a joint task force by the European Federation of Neurological Societies, the European Neurological Society and the European Sleep Research Society, Eur J Neurol 19(11):1385–1396, 2012.

Hauser RA, Cantillon M, Pourcher E, et al: Preladenant in patients with Parkinson's disease and motor fluctuations: a phase 2, double-blind, randomised trial, Lancet Neurol 10:221–229, 2011.

Jellinger KA: Neuropathology of sporadic Parkinson's disease: evaluation and changes of concepts, Mov Disord 27(1):8–30, 2012.

Jinnah HA, Berardelli A, Comella C, et al: The focal dystonias: Current views and challenges for future research, Mov Disord 28(7):926–943, 2013.

Kehagia AA, Barker RA, Robbins TW: Cognitive impairment in Parkinson's disease: the dual syndrome hypothesis, Neurodegener Dis 11(2):79–92, 2013.

Kieburtz K, Wunderle KB: Parkinson's disease: evidence for environmental risk factors, Mov Disord 28(1):8–13, 2013.

Killoran A, Biglan KM, Jankovic J, et al: Characterization of the Huntington intermediate CAG repeat expansion phenotype in PHAROS, Neurology 80(22):2022–2027, 2013.

Knight T, Steeves T, Day L, et al: Prevalence of tic disorders: a systematic review and meta-analysis, Pediatr Neurol 47(2):77–90, 2012.

Kordower JH, Bjorklund A: Trophic factor gene therapy for Parkinson's disease, Mov Disord 28(1):96–109, 2013.

Lee JM, Ramos EM, Lee JH, et al: CAG repeat expansion in Huntington disease determines age at onset in a fully dominant fashion, Neurology 78:690–695, 2012.

Lipsman N, Schwartz ML, Huang Y, et al: MR-guided focused ultrasound thalamotomy for essential tremor: a proof-of-concept study, Lancet Neurol 12(5):462–468, 2013.

Okun MS: Deep-brain stimulation for Parkinson's disease, N Engl J Med 367(16):1529–1538, 2012.

Olanow CW, Schapira AH: Therapeutic prospects for Parkinson disease, Ann Neurol 74(3):337–347, 2013.

Parkinson MH, Boesch S, Nachbauer W, et al: Clinical features of Friedreich's ataxia: classical and atypical phenotypes, J Neurochem 126(Suppl 1):103–117, 2013.

Phukan J, Albanese A, Gasser T, et al: Primary dystonia and dystonia-plus syndromes: clinical characteristics, diagnosis, and pathogenesis, Lancet Neurol 10(12):1074–1085, 2011.

Pringsheim T, Wiltshire K, Day L, et al: The incidence and prevalence of Huntington's disease: a systematic review and meta-analysis, Mov Disord 27(9):1083–1091, 2012.

Sailer A, Houlden H: Recent advances in the genetics of cerebellar ataxias, Curr Neurol Neurosci Rep 12(3):227–236, 2012.

Scahill L, Woods DW, Himle MB, et al: Current controversies on the role of behavior therapy in Tourette syndrome, Mov Disord 28:1179–1183, 2013.

Seibyl J, Russell D, Jennings D, et al: Neuroimaging over the course of Parkinson's disease: from early detection of the at-risk patient to improving pharmacotherapy of later-stage disease, Semin Nucl Med 42:406–414, 2012.

Seppi K, Weintraub D, Coelho M, et al: The Movement Disorder Society Evidence-Based Medicine Review Update: Treatments for the non-motor symptoms of Parkinson's disease, Mov Disord 26(Suppl 3):S42–S80, 2011.

Tabrizi SJ, Scahill RI, Owen G, et al: Predictors of phenotypic progression and disease onset in premanifest and early-stage Huntington's disease in the TRACK-HD study: analysis of 36-month observational data, Lancet Neurol 12(7):637–649, 2013.

Trinh J, Farrer M: Advances in the genetics of Parkinson disease, Nat Rev Neurol 9(8):445–454, 2013.

Vidailhet M, Jutras MF, Grabli D, et al: Deep brain stimulation for dystonia, J Neurol Neurosurg Psychiatry 84(9):1029–1042, 2013.

Visanji NP, Brooks PL, Hazrati L-N, et al: he prion hypothesis in Parkinson's disease: Braak to the future, Acta Neuropathol Commun 1:2, 2013.

Zesiewicz TA, Shaw JD, Allison KG, et al: Update on treatment of essential tremor, Curr Treat Options Neurol 15:410–423, 2013.

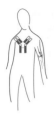

115

Congenital, Developmental, and Neurocutaneous Disorders

Maxwell H. Sims and Jennifer M. Kwon

This chapter describes some of the most important congenital nervous system malformations and neurodevelopmental disorders. Advances in imaging and molecular genetic diagnostic technology have improved our understanding of these disorders. Neuroimaging facilitates diagnosis and informs early management of malformations of the brain and spinal cord. The remarkable advances in genetic sequencing and microarray technology are improving our understanding of the etiology and pathogenesis of neurodevelopmental disorders due to single genes, like Fragile X syndrome, Rett syndrome, tuberous sclerosis, and neurofibromatosis, as well as the genetically heterogeneous disorders autism and ADHD.

CONGENITAL MALFORMATIONS

Malformations of the central nervous system develop during fetal life. Table 115-1 summarizes the timeline of early neural and cortical development and the defects that may occur during these stages. Malformations developing early in embryogenesis can be more severe than those arising later, after the basic structures of the nervous system are in place.

Brain Malformations

Disorders of Ventral Induction

Definition/Epidemiology

Ventral induction is the early stage of brain development where brain vesicles and the face begin to form. Malformations that arise during this time include holoprosencephaly (HPE), agenesis of the corpus callosum (ACC), and septo-optic dysplasia

(SOD). In clinical practice, ACC is the most commonly seen, with an estimated prevalence in the general population of greater than 0.5%, higher in those with developmental disabilities. The estimated prevalence of HPE is 1/10,000, and SOD is even rarer, occurring in 3/100,000.

Pathology

During ventral induction, the prosencephalon forms and undergoes cleavage and midline formation. Abnormal prosencephalon cleavage leads to HPE, a spectrum of abnormalities ranging from alobar HPE (cortex with a single ventricle) to semi-lobar and lobar HPE (cerebral hemispheres are mostly separated except for the frontal lobes) (Figure 115-1). In all cases, there is some fusion between the two cerebral hemispheres, often accompanied by facial anomalies. ACC and SOD represent more discrete abnormalities localized to specific midline structures and occur later in prosencephalic development.

Clinical Presentation

Children with HPE, ACC, and SOD have varying degrees of developmental disability and other congenital anomalies. In HPE, especially, the close timing of this defect with facial development may lead to midline anomalies like cleft lip, hypotelorism, or cyclopia. Children with SOD will have vision problems and optic nerve hypoplasia on examination; they can also have pituitary dysfunction. The clinical presentations range from severe—where individuals develop multiple complications related to their severe neurologic impairments—to nearly normal, as in the case of ACC associated with no other defects.

TABLE 115-1 STAGES OF PRENATAL NEURAL DEVELOPMENT (SIMPLIFIED)

	STAGE	STRUCTURES FORMING	POST-CONCEPTUAL AGE	ANOMALIES SEEN*
NEURAL TUBE, BRAIN VESICLE DEVELOPMENT (KANEKAR)	Dorsal induction	Neural tube closure	18-26 days (3-5 weeks)	Anencephaly, spina bifida, myelomeningocele, Chiari 2 malformation
	Ventral induction (ref Kanekar)	Brain vesicle and face development	5-10 weeks	Holoprosencephaly agenesis of the corpus callosum, septo-optic dysplasia
CORTICAL DEVELOPMENT (REF BARKOVICH, OSBORNE)	Proliferation	Development of neuroblasts and glioblasts	2-4 months (neuroblasts)	Microcephaly, megalencephaly
	Migration	Formation of 6 cortical layers	Peak occurrence at 2-4 months, though occurs from 8 weeks to 8 months	Lissencephaly, periventricular heterotopias
	Post-migrational organization	Cortex formed		Polymicrogyria, schizencephaly

*NB: Some anomalies (such as microcephaly, polymicrogyria) can arise from different stages. So even though it may seem intuitive to think of microcephaly as a disorder of neuronal proliferation, there are some forms of microcephaly that develop well after migration.

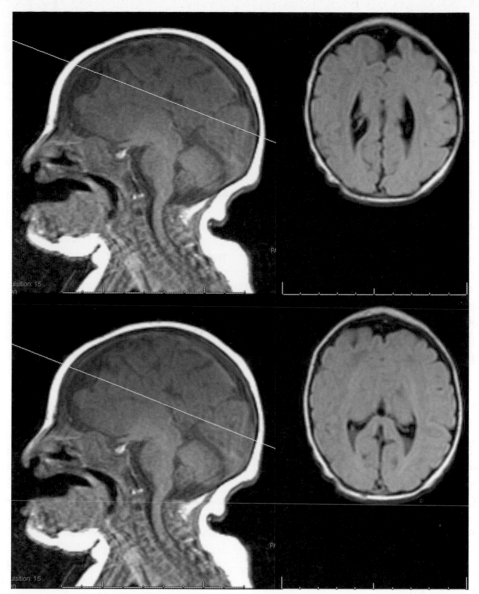

FIGURE 115-1 Semilobar HPE. MRI (sagittal T1 image taken at midline paired with and the axial FLAIR image whose location is indicated by the scout line) of 13 day old with hypotelorism and microcephaly. There is presence of partial fusion of the frontal lobes with lack of interhemispheric fissure/falx and septum pellucidum. The body and genu of corpus callosum is likewise poorly formed. There is appropriate separation of the thalami.

Diagnosis/Differential

Neuroimaging is the primary method of diagnosing HPE, ACC, and SOD. MRI allows for specific anatomic diagnoses and for delineating the full extent of brain malformations. Ophthalmology examination can also detect hypoplastic optic nerves. HPE, ACC, and SOD are associated with a number of genetic syndromes, including trisomies and familial disorders.

Treatment

Surgical treatment can improve associated craniofacial anomalies (e.g., cleft lip) and hormone replacement is needed for pituitary dysfunction (seen in SOD). These patients can present with a wide range of medical problems related to their underlying disabilities, including the development of joint contractures, hip dislocations, impaired swallowing, and respiratory insufficiency.

Prognosis

Survival has improved for these children thanks to aggressive treatment and management of associated medical problems. Long-term outcome depends on the degree of neurologic impairment and associated medical comorbidities.

Disorders of Neuronal Migration and Organization

Definition/Epidemiology

These disorders, including lissencephaly, schizencephaly, polymicrogyria and pachygyria, are caused by disrupted migration of neuronal progenitor cells, resulting in the abnormal appearance of cortical sulci and gyri. The more severe forms of lissencephaly occur in approximately 1/100,000 births. Other migrational disorders have a more variable presentation and, while their true incidence is unknown, they are more common than lissencephaly.

Pathology

Neuronal migration is a complex, highly-regulated process integral to formation of normal cortical architecture that occurs throughout gestation but peaks from 2 to 4 months. In the case of lissencephaly and pachygyria, the brain appearance is smoother because there are fewer convolutions of the cortical surface. In polymicrogyria syndromes, the brain is more irregular in appearance due to an increased number of abnormally small gyri. In schizencephaly, clefts form from the surface of the brain to the lateral ventricle; the clefts are often lined by polymicrogyri.

Clinical Presentation

Lissencephaly has a severe presentation with marked motor disability and seizures. Polymicrogyria and schizencephaly, depending on the extent and location, often result in less severe developmental disabilities. All neuronal migration disorders are associated with high risk of seizures.

Diagnosis/Differential

Neuroimaging is the primary method of diagnosing the neuronal migration disorders. Further diagnostic evaluation is often done because these disorders are heterogeneous in etiology and may be associated with other genetic syndromes or environmental factors, such as teratogens or intrauterine infections. Single gene mutations are responsible for many malformation syndromes and identification of these genes can aid in counseling and prognosis.

Treatment

The most common medical issue in this population is intractable epilepsy which is treated with medications and possibly by surgical resection of the abnormal epileptogenic cortex. In the case of severe neurologic impairment, a number of medical complications can arise: orthopedic complications from immobility and spasticity; failure to thrive and aspiration from poor oromotor coordination; vulnerability to pulmonary infections; and complications due to respiratory insufficiency.

Prognosis

Long-term outcome depends on the degree of neurologic impairment and, to a lesser extent, the etiology of the migration disorder. Genetic evaluation is useful for prognostic counseling and management.

Chiari Malformation, Type 1 (CMI)

Definition/Epidemiology

Chiari malformation, type 1 (CMI) is cerebellar tonsillar ectopia with displacement of the cerebellar tonsils more than 5 mm below the foramen magnum, usually accompanied by deformity of tonsils and evidence of altered CSF flow (indicated by loss of peritonsillar CSF space or impaired CSF flow dynamics.) It is common, likely occurring in 0.5 % of the population.

Pathology

The cerebellar tonsils are inferiorly displaced, elongated, and compressed by the foramen magnum. This displacement can cause increased intracranial pressure and change CSF flow dynamics, leading to development of syringomyelia.

Clinical Presentation

In CM1 cases with severe displacement, there may be lower cranial neuropathies, disordered sleep, headaches, and vertigo, among other symptoms. If there is an associated syringomyelia, this may also result in symptoms (see discussion of syringomyelia.) Rarely, patients may experience difficulty with balance and gait.

Diagnosis/Differential

MRI is most useful for making the diagnosis. CSF flow studies may be helpful to establish clinical significance of the Chiari malformation. Since any cause of increased intracranial pressure can lead to tonsillar herniation, it is important to exclude idiopathic intracranial hypertension and CNS mass lesions.

Treatment

Surgical decompression by removing suboccipital bone and posterior C1 vertebrae may be necessary when the symptoms are severe and when syringomyelia is present, symptomatic, and worsening. Otherwise, conservative management is sufficient.

Prognosis

CM1 is generally not disabling. Surgical decompression is generally effective and prognosis is good.

Spinal Cord Malformations

Spina Bifida

Definition/Epidemiology

Failure to completely close the neural tube during the 24th to 26th days post conception can result from defects anywhere along the neuroaxis. These abnormalities are termed neural tube defects (NTDs), the most common of which occur caudally, and are collectively termed spina bifida. Spina bifida occurs in about 1 in 2800 births in the United States. The prevalence of NTDs varies by geography and is influenced by genetic and environmental factors. Use of folic acid at the time of conception and during pregnancy can significantly reduce NTD rates.

Pathology

The neural plate folds and seals itself to form the neural tube in a process, called neurulation, from gestation day 18 to 28. The central portion of the neural tube closes first, then the cranial and caudal portions. Abnormal caudal closure can be associated with overlying bony and skin defects, leading to "open" NTDs, such as myelomeningocele (MMC). The severe neuropathology seen in MMC may not be due only to the lack of caudal tube closure, but also to exposure of neural tube contents to amniotic fluid, trauma, and the leakage of CSF leading to downward herniation of the cerebellum. In cases of "closed" spina bifida where the abnormal caudal cord tissue is covered by fat or skin, neurologic function is less impaired.

Clinical Presentation

The more severe and disabling the defect, the earlier it will present. A large MMC is clinically obvious at birth. MMC can be diagnosed prenatally as well. MMC causes severe distal spinal cord dysfunction, including paralysis and sensory loss in the legs, and loss of bladder control. Nearly all children with MMC have an associated Chiari malformation, "type II" (CM2, also called an Arnold-Chiari malformation). CM2 is characterized by displacement of the cerebellum and lower brainstem through the foramen magnum, usually causing obstructive hydrocephalus. Spina bifida does not have to be associated with an open defect. In cases of closed NTD, patients may present with leg spasticity, foot deformities, and bladder abnormalities, and the overlying skin may show nevi, lipomas, abnormal dimples, or hairy tufts.

Diagnosis/Differential

MRI is the method of choice for evaluation of NTDs. In the case of a child with an open caudal defect, the imaging should look for other associated nervous system abnormalities, such as CM2 and hydrocephalus. Closed NTDs are definitively diagnosed by MRI, but patients may present with symptoms later. Other disorders that can present with gait abnormalities and deformities include spastic diplegia, vitamin B12 deficiency, multiple sclerosis, and other conditions presenting with spastic paraparesis.

Treatment

Treatment is surgical repair of the MMC with subsequent shunting of the hydrocephalus. Bladder dysfunction may necessitate intermittent catheterization and treatment of urinary tract infections and genitourinary reflux. A recent clinical trial indicated that fetal surgery before 26 weeks gestation to repair the MMC defect resulted in better neurologic outcomes, possibly by preventing the spinal cord injury and CSF leakage that can occur during the third trimester with an open defect.

Prognosis

Infants with open NTDs such as MMC have a much more severe presentation and course than those born with closed defects. Fetal surgery at qualified centers may improve MMC outcome.

Syringomyelia

Definition/Epidemiology

Syringomyelia or syrinx is a cystic cavitation of the central portion of the spinal cord. The estimated prevalence of 8/100,000 is likely an underestimate.

Pathology

The central canal cysts are most commonly located in the cervical spine and consist of CSF-filled space lined by glial cells, in contrast to hydromyelia, where the dilated central canal is lined with ependymal cells. The syrinx can be septated and irregular, and it may develop in association with Chiari malformations (CM1 and CM2), trauma, tumor, or a tethered cord.

Clinical

The classic presentation is a dissociated sensory loss (pain and temperature loss with preservation of light touch and proprioception) in the neck, arms, or legs. A cervical lesion produces a cape-like dissociated sensory loss of the arms and shoulder, along with atrophy of the hands and arms with increased tone and hyperreflexia in the legs. Extension into the medulla (syringobulbia) may cause lower cranial neuropathies.

Diagnosis/Differential

Diagnosis is confirmed by MRI, which will also differentiate the cysts from neoplasms, infections, and other spinal cord lesions.

Treatment

If the syrinx is associated with CM1 or CM2, then posterior fossa decompression or shunting of the hydrocephalus may improve the symptoms. Direct evacuation or shunting of the syrinx itself is less frequently done and not of established benefit.

Prognosis

Syringomyelia can be slowly progressive but spontaneous resolution has been seen. Therefore, conservative treatment has been advocated, especially in children.

DEVELOPMENTAL DISORDERS

Autism Spectrum Disorder

Definition/Epidemiology

Autism spectrum disorder (ASD) is characterized by 1) impaired social communication and interactions and 2) restricted and repetitive behaviors. The prevalence of ASD is 1/88 and is four times higher in boys than girls.

Pathology

The marked social impairments that characterize ASD are not associated with specific pathology or physical findings.

Clinical Presentation

ASD presents in early childhood with lack of interest or inclination to relate to others. Young children with autism may be physically healthy with good motor skills, but they are hard to engage, do not reliably respond to their name being called, and are slow to develop social and communicative gestures such pointing and waving.

Diagnosis/Differential

The lack of a clear biologic marker or simple clinical test means that the diagnosis of ASD relies on careful evaluation of the child by experienced examiners. (See Table 115-2 for DSM-V criteria for ASD). ASD may be difficult to diagnosis or distinguish from other forms of mental retardation and psychiatric disorders. ASD should be distinguished from acquired encephalopathies (e.g., epilepsy or encephalitis).

Treatment

The mainstay of treatment is prompt initiation of appropriate behavioral and early enrichment services. The treatments for ASD are aimed at improving social interactions and communication; not surprisingly, there is no set treatment that works for all. Rather, treatment of this disorder often requires coordination of medical, educational, and community services.

Prognosis

Patients with ASD respond to appropriate treatments over time, but these may be highly resource intensive. Some children with ASD, especially those who have normal verbal and intellectual skills and a higher level of adaptive functioning, may develop skills for independent living and work.

Attention Deficit/Hyperactivity Disorder (ADHD)

Definition/Epidemiology

ADHD is a common neurodevelopmental disorder occurring in about 5% of children and 2.5% of adults, worldwide. ADHD is marked by inappropriate inattention, impulsivity, and hyperactivity that, in turn, cause impaired functioning, as compared to typical same-age peers.

Pathology

Despite extensive neuroimaging studies, there are no consistent pathologic brain findings or neurotransmitter abnormalities in ADHD. ADHD appears to be highly heritable. The behaviors of ADHD likely are a common phenotype caused by multiple etiologies.

Clinical Presentation

ADHD presents before age 12 years with developmentally inappropriate inattention, hyperactivity, and impulsivity resulting in significant impairment in at least two different settings (e.g., home, school, work, with friends), by multiple observers, and the disruptive symptoms should have persisted for at least 6 months. Table 115-3 lists the symptoms of inattention and hyperactivity/impulsivity that fulfill diagnostic criteria for ADHD.

Diagnosis/Differential

ADHD is a primary disorder of attention and should be distinguished from attentional deficits that are secondary to other disorders. Causes of secondary inattention include learning disability, hearing impairment, and psychiatric disorders. ADHD can also coexist with autism spectrum disorders. Table 115-3 outlines the criteria used for diagnosis of ADHD.

Treatment

Stimulant medications such as methylphenidate and amphetamines are the primary class of medication used in ADHD. Other nonstimulant medications such as atomoxetine and guanfacine are also used. All children with ADHD benefit from behavioral interventions designed to help children re-focus and stay on task.

TABLE 115-2	DSM-5 CRITERIA FOR AUTISM SPECTRUM DISORDER
REQUIRED DOMAIN	**CRITERIA**
Deficits in social communication/ interaction (must have all three criteria)	Problems reciprocating social or emotional interaction, including difficulty establishing or maintaining back-and-forth conversations and interactions, inability to initiate an interaction, and problems with shared attention or sharing of emotions and interests with others.
	Severe problems maintaining relationships—ranges from lack of interest in other people to difficulties in pretend play and engaging in age-appropriate social activities, and problems adjusting to different social expectations.
	Nonverbal communication problems such as abnormal eye contact, posture, facial expressions, tone of voice and gestures, as well as an inability to understand these.
Restricted and Repetitive Behavior (at least 2 criteria must be met)	Stereotyped or repetitive speech, motor movements or use of objects.
	Excessive adherence to routines, ritualized patters of verbal or nonverbal behavior, or excessive resistance to change.
	Highly restricted interests that are abnormal in intensity or focus.
	Hyper or hypo reactivity to sensory input or unusual interest in sensory aspects of the environment.
Symptoms must be present in early childhood, but may not become fully manifest until social demands exceed capacities.	
Symptoms need to be *functionally impairing* and not better described by another DSM-5 diagnosis.	

TABLE 115-3	DSM-5 CRITERIA FOR ADHD

Inattention: 6 or more symptoms in inattention for children up to age 16, or 5 or more symptoms in those 17 years or older; symptoms present for at least 6 months.

- Often fails to give close attention to details or makes careless mistakes in schoolwork, at work, or with other activities.
- Often has trouble holding attention on tasks or play activities.
- Often does not seem to listen when spoken to directly.
- Often does not follow through on instructions and fails to finish schoolwork, chores, or duties in the workplace (e.g., loses focus, side-tracked).
- Often has trouble organizing tasks and activities.
- Often avoids, dislikes, or is reluctant to do tasks that require mental effort over a long period of time (such as schoolwork or homework).
- Often loses things necessary for tasks and activities (e.g. school materials, pencils, books, tools, wallets, keys, paperwork, eyeglasses, mobile telephones).
- Is often easily distracted
- Is often forgetful in daily activities.

Hyperactivity and Impulsivity: 6 or more symptoms of hyperactivity-impulsivity inattention for children up to age 16, or 5 or more symptoms in those 17 years or older; symptoms present for at least 6 months.

- Often fidgets with or taps hands or feet, or squirms in seat.
- Often leaves seat in situations when remaining seated is expected.
- Often runs about or climbs in situations where it is not appropriate (adolescents or adults may be limited to feeling restless).
- Often unable to play or take part in leisure activities quietly.
- Is often "on the go" acting as if "driven by a motor."
- Often talks excessively.
- Often blurts out an answer before a question has been completed.
- Often has trouble waiting his/her turn.
- Often interrupts or intrudes on others (e.g., butts into conversations or games)

In addition, the following conditions must be met:
- Several inattentive or hyperactive-impulsive symptoms were present before age 12 years.
- Several symptoms are present in two or more settings, (e.g., at home, school or work; with friends or relatives; in other activities).
- There is clear evidence that the symptoms interfere with, or reduce the quality of, social, school, or work functioning.
- The symptoms do not happen only during the course of schizophrenia or another psychotic disorder. The symptoms are not better explained by another mental disorder (e.g. Mood Disorder, Anxiety Disorder, Dissociative Disorder, or a Personality Disorder).

Prognosis

ADHD generally responds to treatment, but there are often residual school difficulties. Improvement depends on age at diagnosis, associated intelligence, and the effectiveness of clinical follow-up.

Rett Syndrome

Definition/Epidemiology

Rett Syndrome is an X-linked dominant disorder caused by a mutation of the methyl-cytosine binding protein (MECP2), a transcriptional repressor. The prevalence in girls is 1/10,000. In boys, MECP2 mutations are lethal or result in severe encephalopathy.

Pathology

Girls with Rett syndrome have a characteristic constellation of behaviors, but there are no specific pathologic hallmarks. Microcephaly is typically seen, with reduced frontotemporal brain volume. The loss of MECP2 function prevents the protein from regulating gene expression during critical developmental periods in infancy.

Clinical Presentation

Patients with Rett syndrome develop normally during their first year then lose communication skills with deceleration of head growth. A classic feature is loss of hand function and stereotypic hand wringing. Seizures are common.

Diagnosis/Differential

Diagnosis is confirmed by mutational testing of the MECP2 gene. Other conditions that can cause a similar presentation include Angelman syndrome, mitochondrial disorders, and neuronal ceroid lipofuscinosis.

Treatment

Girls usually required ongoing medical management of seizures, along with therapy for their gross and fine motor delays. They receive long-term enrichment and support for their intellectual disability.

Prognosis

While girls survive into adulthood, most will not acquire speech or functional skills; they will remain dependent for their care.

Fragile X Syndrome (FX)

Definition/Epidemiology

X-linked disorder caused by expanded CGG triplet repeats (>200 CGG repeats) in the first exon of the fragile X mental retardation gene *(FMR1)*. Considered an X-linked recessive disorder, females can be symptomatic though they may have milder intellectual disability compared with male. FX is the most common genetic cause of mental retardation, affecting 1/4000 males and 1/8000 females.

Pathology

Boys with FX have a characteristic constellation of behaviors and clinical findings on examination, but there are no specific pathologic hallmarks.

Clinical Presentation

Children with FX syndrome present with mild-to-moderate social anxiety, shyness, distractibility, hyperactivity, stereotypic movements, and intellectual disability. They are generally diagnosed before school age. Children have a distinctive appearance: relative macrocephaly with a long narrow face, and prominent ears, pubertal macro-orchidism, soft skin, and joint laxity. Individuals with 55 to 200 CGG repeats (the "pre-mutation" range) develop ataxia and tremor and cognitive dysfunction (Fragile X associated tremor/ataxia syndrome, FXTAS) in adulthood, at a median age of onset of 60 years.

Diagnosis/Differential

Diagnosis is confirmed by testing for increased repeats in the FMR gene. Other etiologies of intellectual disability and autism can be mistaken for FX. Adults with FXTAS are often diagnosed with a variety of other conditions which may present similarly (e.g., parkinsonism, other ataxia syndromes, tremor).

Treatment

Treatment focuses on appropriate behavioral and educational services. In older individuals with movement disorders, the treatment is supportive.

Prognosis

Patients with FX respond to training and education over time, but their intellectual disability may make it difficult for them to live independently. FXTAS tends to cause, gradual, progressive neurologic deterioration over many years.

⬤ NEUROCUTANEOUS DISORDERS

Neurocutaneous disorders are congenital, often hereditary disorders characterized by pathognomonic cutaneous and central nervous system lesions that uniquely distinguish each disease. The most important of these syndromes are neurofibromatosis 1 and 2, tuberous sclerosis complex, and Sturge-Weber syndrome. One disorder, von Hippel-Lindau disease, is often included with the neurocutaneous syndromes though skin findings are generally absent. Many neurocutaneous disorders are associated with abnormal, non-cancerous growth of tissues often in a disorganized manner. There is considerable variability in the spectrum of clinical manifestations.

Neurofibromatosis 1 (NF1)

Definition/Epidemiology

Autosomal dominant disorder caused by mutation of the gene, *NF1*, that encodes the protein, neurofibromin. NF1 is characterized by altered skin pigmentation, tumors, and abnormalities of bones, connective tissue, and brain. This is a relatively common disorder occurring in 1/3500 individuals.

Pathology

Neurofibromin is a tumor suppressor gene, and loss of function can lead to dysregulated cell growth and differentiation, accounting for the variety of tumors—cutaneous neurofibromas, plexiform neurofibromas, and gliomas—that can occur in NF1.

Malignant tumors can also occur, likely due to malignant transformation.

Clinical Presentation

Patients can present with NF1 in a variety of ways. All NF1 patients can be identified by clinical criteria before 20 years of age, but those with mild symptoms may not realize they have the disorder. Diagnosis is based on clinical criteria, having two or more of the following: (1) six or more café-au-lait macules larger than 5 mm in prepubertal patients or more than 15 mm in postpubertal individuals (Fig. 115-2), (2) two or more neurofibromas of any type or one plexiform neurofibroma, (3) axillary or inguinal freckling, (4) sphenoid bone dysplasia, (5) optic nerve glioma, (6) iris Lisch nodules, and (7) a family history of NF1. Other comorbid conditions frequently seen are learning disabilities, macrocephaly, and epilepsy. Important complications of NF1 include scoliosis, gastrointestinal neurofibromas, pheochromocytomas, and renal artery stenosis.

Diagnosis/Differential

The diagnostic criteria outlined above are highly sensitive and specific. Neuroimaging and DNA testing can be useful as well. There are many other disorders that present with hyperpigmented skin macules. Schwannomatosis and neurofibromatosis type 2 (see Neurofibromatosis type 2) may also be mistaken for NF1.

Treatment

Most individuals with NF1 do not require specific treatment though ongoing periodic surveillance is recommended. Many identified tumors can be followed without surgery. Painful subcutaneous neurofibromas can be excised, though they may recur. Genetic counseling should be provided to all patients and families.

Prognosis

There is as much variability in disease course as there is in clinical presentation. Even within families, some individuals

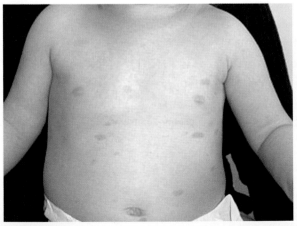

FIGURE 115-2   Multiple café-au-lait spots in a child with neurofibromatosis type 1. (From Shah KN: The diagnostic and clinical significant of café-au-lait macules, Pediatr Clin N Am 57:1131-1153, 2010, Fig. 3.)

may have only skin findings with no symptoms, while others have more complications including malignant transformation of plexiform neurofibromas. While it is an autosomal dominant condition, about half of the cases are sporadic due to new mutations.

Neurofibromatosis 2 (NF2)

Definition/Epidemiology

Neurofibromatosis type 2 (NF2) is an autosomal-dominant adult onset disease characterized by bilateral vestibular schwannomas and brain tumors. It is caused by mutations in the gene, *NF2*, whose protein product is merlin (schwannomin). It affects approximately 1/30,000 individuals.

Pathology

Despite the name, the primary tumor types seen in NF2 are schwannoma and meningioma. Merlin behaves as a tumor suppressor gene.

Clinical Presentation

The diagnosis is generally made when bilateral VIII nerve tumors are identified (often by MRI). The diagnosis can be made based on other clinical criteria (some combination of family history of NF2; presence of characteristic tumors—meningioma, schwannoma, neurofibroma, or posterior subcapsular lenticular opacities.) Symptoms of NF2 begin in the second to fourth decades usually with onset of hearing loss. Skin lesions are present in a minority of patients with NF2.

Diagnosis/Differential

NF2 is frequently misdiagnosed as NF1, especially if there are café-au-lait spots. Patients with NF2 may be misdiagnosed as having isolated meningioma or unilateral vestibular schwannoma if other findings are not sought. Schwannomatosis can be distinguished by the absence of vestibular schwannomas.

Treatment

Eventual removal of the schwannomas and other tumors is usually indicated, though later in life when the tumors are larger and causing significant symptoms. There may be post-surgical complications and tumors may recur.

Prognosis

The vestibular tumors, leading to deafness and vestibular symptoms contribute greatly to the morbidity of this condition. Mortality is related to tumor growth.

Tuberous Sclerosis Complex (TSC)

Definition/Epidemiology

Tuberous Sclerois Complex (TSC) is an autosomal dominant disorder of early cellular differentiation, proliferation, and migration, which results in hamartomatous lesions involving multiple organs at different stages. Sporadic cases are frequent because of spontaneous mutations. The incidence is 1/6000. Two genes, *TSC1* and *TSC2*, are known to cause TSC and account for approximately 85% of cases. TSC1 for approximately 30% and TSC2 69% of confirmed cases.

Pathology

The gene product for *TSC1* is hamartin and for *TSC2*, tuberin. Both gene products interact with the mammalian target of rapamycin (mTOR), which is essential in cell growth, proliferation, and angiogenesis. Hamartin and tuberin join to form a combined tumor suppressor complex (TSC1:TSC2 complex) that acts to inhibit mTOR signaling. Mutations that impair function of the TSC1:TSC2 complex lead to unregulated growth and proliferation.

Clinical Presentation

Like NF1, TSC has variable presentation depending on the location and extent of lesions. The organs most affected include the brain (cortical tubers, subependymal giant cell astrocytomas [SEGAs]), heart (cardiac rhabdomyomas), skin (facial angiofibromas, hypomelanotic skin macules or "ash leaf spot," shagreen patches, and subungual fibromas), kidney (renal angiomyolipoma), eye (retinal hamartoma), and lung (pulmonary lymphangioleiomyomatosis). Seizures, most commonly infantile spasms, are the usual early clinical presentation.

Diagnosis/Differential

The spectrum of tumors seen in TSC patients can also be seen in isolation. Biopsy may be needed to distinguish facial angiofibromas from acne and other skin lesions.

Treatment

Treatment is directed toward the epilepsy, especially for infantile spasms. A surgical approach may be necessary for intractable epilepsy. SEGAs are slow growing tumors that may enlarge and cause obstruction, especially during adolescence and early adulthood. Surgical treatment of SEGAs causing hydrocephalus can be effective but associated with significant morbidity. Everolimus is a pharmacologic mTOR inhibitor that is effective at reducing the size and growth of SEGAs and is useful for delaying the need for surgery or in those cases where surgery is not an option. Renal angiomyolipomas are prone to hemorrhage and may need to be resected, and pulmonary lymphangioleiomyomatosis may cause life-threatening complications. These renal and pulmonary tumors may also respond to the mTOR inhibitors, everolimus and sirolimus. Cognitive disability may require special education.

Prognosis

The variability in outcome depends on the extent and type of presenting symptoms. Refractory seizures, developmental delays, and CNS lesions have poor prognoses. The development of renal angiolipomas, especially multiple tumors, is also associated with poorer outcome.

Sturge-Weber Syndrome (SWS)
Definition/Epidemiology

SWS is variably characterized by an upper facial vascular nevus (port-wine stain), leptomeningeal angiomatos (cerebral venous malformation), and glaucoma with ocular capillary malformations. The disorder occurs sporadically in less than 1 in 20,000 births.

Pathology

The port-wine stain represent a collection of congested capillaries of subepidermal tissue. If there is an associated leptomeningeal vessel abnormality, it tends to be ipsilateral to the port-wine stain. The leptomeningeal vascular malformation makes the underlying brain susceptible to injury, possibly from venous stasis and abnormal perfusion. Cortical injury can lead to increased susceptibility to seizures, which in turn can increase the metabolic demands of already poorly perfused tissue.

Clinical Presentation

Clinical features include focal epilepsy, cognitive impairment, and, less frequently, hemiparesis, hemianopia, and glaucoma.

Diagnosis/Differential

The diagnosis is usually made by observing a port-wine stain in the cranial nerve V1 distribution with neuroimaging confirmation of the intracranial abnormality. Magnetic resonance imaging is a more reliable tool for diagnosis because calcifications on computed tomographic scans are classic but unnecessary for the diagnosis. However, 80% of people with a facial port-wine stain have no associated brain involvement. SWS should be distinguished from other disorders involving abnormal intracranial vessels and intractable seizures and neurologic dysfunction. These include moyamoya disease, other vascular malformations, and tuberous sclerosis.

Treatment

Aspirin (3-5 mg/kg/day) may reduce the frequency of stroke-like events. Aggressive treatment of seizures is indicated as well. If antiepileptic drugs do not control seizures, surgical excision of epileptogenic areas may be indicated. Laser treatment of the port-wine stain is of cosmetic benefit. Patients require regular ophthalmologist visits to screen for and surgically treat glaucoma.

Prognosis

Prognosis depends on the degree of underlying intellectual and developmental disability and control of seizures.

Von Hippel-Lindau Disease (Central Nervous System Angiomatosis)
Definition/Epidemiology

Von Hippel–Lindau (VHL) disease is an autosomal-dominant disorder caused by a defective tumor suppressor gene, *VHL*, associated with a variety of vascular tumors in multiple organs, including cerebellar and retinal hemangioblastomas and renal cell carcinomas. Incidence is 1/36,000.

Pathology

VHL is a tumor suppressor gene and increases susceptibility to various vascular tumors.

Clinical Presentation

VHL disease is variably associated with retinal angiomas, brain and spinal cord hemangioblastomas, renal cell carcinomas, pheochromocytomas, angiomas of the liver and kidney, and cysts of the pancreas, kidney, liver, and epididymis. Symptoms typically begin during the third or fourth decade. Retinal inflammation with exudates, hemorrhage, and retinal detachment may antedate cerebellar symptoms (headache, vertigo, and vomiting) or signs (incoordination, dysmetria, and ataxia).

Diagnosis/Differential

The diagnosis of VHL disease is suspected in individuals with characteristic lesions such as hemangioblastomas, multiple renal cysts and renal cell carcinoma, pheochromocytoma, and endolymphatic sac tumors. Clinical diagnostic criteria have been established. Molecular genetic testing of *VHL* detects mutations in 90% to 100% of those meeting clinical criteria.

Treatment

Early evaluation and repeated imaging studies are indicated once the diagnosis has been made, and genetically at-risk relatives should also be evaluated. Retinal detachments and tumors are treated by laser therapy. Surveillance for brain tumors, renal cell carcinomas, pheochromocytomas, and epididymal tumors is instituted and appropriated medical and surgical interventions are provided.

Prognosis

Survival depends on management of tumors. Aggressive surveillance has increased survival (where the median had been less than 50 years).

For a deeper discussion on this topic, please see Chapter 417, "Congenital, Developmental, and Neurocutaneous Disorders," in Goldman-Cecil Medicine, 25th Edition.

SUGGESTED READINGS

Adzick NS, Thom EA, Spong CY, et al: A randomized trial of prenatal versus postnatal repair of myelomeningocele, N Engl J Med 364:993–1004, 2011.

Barkovich AJ, Guerrini R, Kuzniecky RI, et al: A developmental and genetic classification for malformations of cortical development: update 2012, Brain 135:1348–1369, 2012.

Cuddapah VA, Pillai RB, Shekar KV, et al: Methyl-CpG-binding protein 2 (MECP2) mutation type is associated with disease severity in Rett syndrome, J Med Genet 51:152–158, 2014.

Grzadzinski R, Huerta M, Lord C: DSM-5 and autism spectrum disorders (ASDs): an opportunity for identifying ASD subtypes, Mol Autism 4:12–17, 2013.

Gutmann DH, Parada LF, Silva AJ, et al: Neurofibromatosis type 1: modeling CNS dysfunction, J Neurosci 32:14087–14093, 2012.

Hagerman RJ, Berry-Kravis E, Kaufmann WE, et al: Advances in the treatment of Fragile X syndrome, Pediatrics 123:378–390, 2009.

Kanekar S, Kaneda H, Shively A: Malformations of dorsal induction, Semin Ultrasound CT MR 32:189–199, 2011.

Kanekar S, Shively A, Kaneda H: Malformations of ventral induction, Semin Ultrasound CT MR 32:200–210, 2011.

Lo W, Marchuk DA, Ball KL, et al: Updates and future horizons on the understanding, diagnosis, and treatment of Sturge-Weber syndrome brain involvement, Dev Med Child Neurol 54:214–223, 2012.

Nigg JT: Attention-deficit/hyperactivity disorder and adverse health outcomes, Clin Psychol Rev 33:215–228, 2013.

Richard S, Gardie B, Couvé S, et al: Von Hippel-Lindau: how a rare disease illuminates cancer biology, Semin Cancer Biol 23:26–37, 2013.

Vaz SS, Chodirker B, Prasad C, et al: Risk factors for nonsyndromic holoprosencephaly: a Manitoba case-control study, Am J Med Genet A 158A:751–758, 2012.

Volpe P, Campobasso G, De Robertis V, et al: Disorders of prosencephalic development, Prenat Diagn 29:340–354, 2009.

Volkow ND, Swanson JM: Adult attention deficit – hyperactivity disorder, NEJM 369:1935–1944, 2013.

Wallingford JB, Niswander LA, Shaw GM, et al: The continuing challenge of understanding, preventing, and treating neural tube defects, Science 339:1047–1054, 2013.

116

Cerebrovascular Disease

Mitchell S.V. Elkind

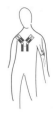

INTRODUCTION

Stroke is a major public health problem throughout the world due to its high prevalence and mortality, and its association with significant disability even among survivors. Stroke is the fourth leading cause of death in the United States, and a leading cause of death in other countries, particularly in Asia. It is the leading cause of serious disability, and results in enormous costs measured in both health care dollars and lost productivity. Major strides have been made in understanding the epidemiology, etiology, and pathogenesis of cerebrovascular disease, which have led to new approaches to diagnosis and treatment.

DEFINITION AND EPIDEMIOLOGY

The term *cerebrovascular disease* encompasses a host of disorders that share pathology localized to the vessels of the brain and spinal cord, including ischemic stroke, transient ischemic attack (TIA), intracerebral hemorrhage (ICH), subarachnoid hemorrhage (SAH), cerebral venous and sinus thrombosis, and disorders of the vessels themselves unassociated with cerebral injury (Table 116-1). Strokes may also be classified as either ischemic (i.e., due to lack of blood flow) or hemorrhagic. With widespread use of sensitive brain imaging, such as diffusion-weighted MRI (DWI), cerebral injury from ischemia can be seen among patients whose symptoms last only a few minutes. A definition from an expert panel in 2013 defines an *ischemic stroke* as "an episode of neurological dysfunction caused by focal cerebral, spinal, or retinal infarction." A *stroke due to ICH* was defined as "rapidly developing clinical signs of neurologic dysfunction due to a focal collection of blood within the brain parenchyma or ventricular system which is not due to trauma." Importantly, the pathology, and not the duration of the symptoms, is considered paramount.

Ischemic strokes may be further classified into etiologic subgroups, based on the mechanism of the ischemia and the type and localization of the vascular lesion. Cardioembolism as the source occurs in 15% to 30% of cases, large vessel atherosclerotic infarction varies from 14% to 40%, and small-vessel lacunar infarcts account for 15% to 30%. Stroke from other determined causes, such as arteritis or dissection, account for less than 5% of cases. In 30% to 40% of ischemic infarcts the cause cannot be determined. Intracranial hemorrhage may also be subdivided into subtypes, based on the site and vascular origin of the blood: subarachnoid, when the bleeding originates in the subarachnoid spaces surrounding the brain; and intracerebral, when the hemorrhage is into the brain parenchyma. Other forms of intracranial bleeding, such as subdural hemorrhage and epidural hemorrhage, are generally associated with trauma and not usually manifestations of stroke.

A further complicating issue is that advanced imaging techniques permit the detection of abnormalities consistent with infarction or microhemorrhage that are unassociated with any clinical symptoms. Therefore, current definitions distinguish between "stroke," which involves clinical symptoms, and "cerebral infarction," which need not be associated with symptoms of cerebral injury. However, these so-called "silent infarcts" are not so silent; they are associated with cognitive decline, dementia, gait disorders, functional disability, and an increased risk of clinical strokes. Because these subclinical infarcts are approximately five times more common than clinically evident strokes, including them (and microbleeds) within the rubric of *cerebrovascular disease* substantially increases the recognized burden of cerebrovascular disease.

In the United States, there are 6.4 million stroke survivors (prevalence of 3%), and there are approximately 600,000 new (incident) and 200,000 recurrent strokes per year. Of these

---

TABLE 116-1 COMMON FORMS OF CEREBROVASCULAR DISEASE

Ischemic cerebrovascular disease
  Symptomatic
  • Ischemic stroke
    • Cerebral infarction
    • Spinal cord infarction
    • Retinal infarction
  • Transient ischemic attack
  • Transient monocular blindness (*amaurosis fugax*)
  Asymptomatic
  • Cerebral infarction/spinal cord infarction/retinal infarction

Hemorrhagic cerebrovascular disease
  • Intracerebral hemorrhage
  • Subarachnoid hemorrhage
  • Intraventricular hemorrhage
  • Subdural hemorrhage
  • Epidural hemorrhage
  • Cerebral microbleeds

Other forms of cerebrovascular disease
  • Cerebral vein thrombosis
  • Dural sinus thrombosis

Disorders of cerebral autoregulation
  • Posterior reversible encephalopathy syndrome
  • Hypertensive encephalopathy
  • Reversible cerebral vasoconstriction syndrome

Vascular abnormalities
  • Aneurysms
  • Arteriovenous malformations
  • Cavernous malformations
  • Fibromuscular dysplasia

strokes, about 87% are ischemic infarctions, 10% primary hemorrhages, and 3% SAHs. Among adults age 35 to 44, the incidence of stroke is 30 to 120/100,000 per year, and for those age 65 to 74, the incidence is 670 to 970/100,000 per year. Stroke incidence rates are approximately twice as high for African Americans as for whites. In northern Manhattan, Caribbean Hispanics had an incidence rate intermediate between that of whites and blacks. Temporal trends in stroke incidence suggest that stroke incidence rates have been declining since 1950; however, disparities in stroke incidence and mortality have increased.

Stroke incidence increases with age, but strokes do occur in young adults and children, and may be missed if the diagnosis is not considered. Although stroke incidence rates are higher for men than women at most ages, among young adults the rates are similar or higher among women, probably related to pregnancy, hormonal contraception, and other hormone-related differences. At older ages, incidence rates among women are again greater, and because women tend to live longer than men, overall about 60,000 more women than men have a stroke each year.

⬤ MODIFIABLE RISK FACTORS

Well-established modifiable stroke risk factors include hypertension, cardiac disease (particularly atrial fibrillation), diabetes, hyperlipidemia, cigarette use, physical inactivity, alcohol abuse, asymptomatic carotid stenosis, and a history of TIAs (Table 116-2).

Hypertension is the most powerful modifiable stroke risk factor and is associated with both ischemic and hemorrhagic

TABLE 116-2   STROKE RISK FACTORS

NON-MODIFIABLE RISK FACTORS	Age
	Sex
	Race/ethnicity
	Family history
	Genetic disorders
WELL-ESTABLISHED MODIFIABLE RISK FACTORS	Hypertension/blood pressure
	Diabetes mellitus/hyperglycemia
	Cardiac disorders
	Atrial fibrillation
	Valvular heart disease
	Recent myocardial infarction
	Cardiomyopathy/heart failure
	Bacterial endocarditis
	Hyperlipidemia
	Cigarette smoking
	Carotid stenosis
	TIAs
	Physical inactivity
	Hypercoagulable states (e.g., antiphospolipid antibody syndrome, cancer-associated)
	Alcohol abuse
	Substance abuse (e.g., cocaine, IV drug abuse)
OTHER POTENTIAL RISK FACTORS	Migraine
	Sleep apnea
	Cardiac disorders
	Paroxymsal supraventricular tachycardia
	Patent foramen ovale/atrial septal aneurysm
	Aortic atheroma
	Infections (e.g. varicella zoster virus, influenza)
	Inflammation
	Others

strokes. Risk of stroke decreases with lower systolic and diastolic blood pressures, and this graded decrement in risk persists down to levels as low as 115/75. There is no clearly defined threshold level below which stroke risk levels off.

Cardiac disease is associated with an increased risk of ischemic stroke. Atrial fibrillation accounts for up to 24% of cerebral infarction in the elderly. Atrial fibrillation (AF) is the most important cardiac cause of embolic stroke, but other cardiac diseases, including valvular heart disease, myocardial infarction (MI), coronary artery disease (CAD), congestive heart failure (CHF), and electrocardiographic evidence of left-ventricular hypertrophy are also associated with stroke risk. Recent evidence also suggests that other atrial abnormalities, such as paroxysmal supraventricular tachycardia, may also increase risk of stroke, even in the absence of atrial fibrillation. Other possible sources of cardiac emboli include patent foramen ovale, aortic arch atherosclerotic disease, atrial septal aneurysms, and valvular strands.

Hyperlipidemia is a stroke risk factor, though its relationship to stroke is more complicated than for heart disease, primarily because of the many types of stroke. Lipid abnormalities, such as elevations in low density lipoprotein (LDL) and decreased levels of high density lipoprotein, are strongly associated with atherosclerotic stroke.

The role of alcohol as a stroke risk factor depends on stroke subtype and quantity consumed. Alcohol consumption has been shown to be a risk factor for both ICH and SAH in a linear fashion, whereas a J-shaped relationship exists between alcohol and ischemic stroke, such that modest consumption (up to two drinks daily in men, and one daily in women) is protective against stroke and heavy consumption (five or more drinks per day) increases risk.

Asymptomatic carotid artery disease, particularly with 75% or greater stenosis, is associated with increased stroke risk (approximately 2% per year). The risk of stroke also depends, however, on the rate of progression of the stenosis, collateral circulation, and the stability of the atherosclerotic plaque.

TIAs are a strong predictor of subsequent stroke. The first several days after a TIA have the greatest stroke risk, with recent series demonstrating a 5% risk at 2 days and 10% risk at 90 days. Patients with transient monocular blindness (*amaurosis fugax*) have a better outcome than those with hemispheric ischemic attacks. The stroke risk after TIA depends on the underlying cause of the ischemia, including the presence and severity of underlying atherosclerotic disease or atrial fibrillation. Age, hypertension, the presence of diabetes, clinical syndromes, including aphasia and hemiparesis, and duration of at least 10 minutes predict patients at higher risk of stroke. Patients with TIA with evidence of infarction on MRI are also at higher risk. Other potential stroke risk factors include migraine, oral contraceptive use, drug abuse, sleep apnea, infection, and inflammation.

⬤ PATHOLOGY

Understanding the pathology of cerebrovascular disease requires an appreciation of the vascular anatomy of the brain, the vascular pathologies that can affect brain vessels, and the response of brain tissue to ischemia and hemorrhage.

Clinical Implications of Vascular Anatomy

The brain is perfused by four major vessels, the paired carotid and vertebral arteries. These originate extracranially as branches off the aorta and great vessels and course through the neck and base of the skull to reach the intracranial cavity (Fig. 116-1). The carotid and its branches constitute the anterior circulation, and the vertebral arteries and its branches the posterior circulation. Anterior and posterior circulations communicate with one another through the posterior communicating arteries. The left and right sides of the anterior circulation communicate with each other through the anterior communicating artery. The major vessels at the base of the brain and these communicating vessels constitute the Circle of Willis, the anastomotic network that allows for collateral blood flow when individual vessels are stenotic or occluded. Because variants in the circle of Willis are common, collateral flow may not be sufficient in many cases of blockage, and the risk of ischemic stroke, therefore, depends on a patient's individual anatomy.

The right common carotid artery usually begins as a branch from the innominate artery, whereas the left common carotid artery originates directly from the aortic arch. The common carotid arteries bifurcate into the internal and external carotid arteries, usually at the level of the fourth cervical vertebrae. The

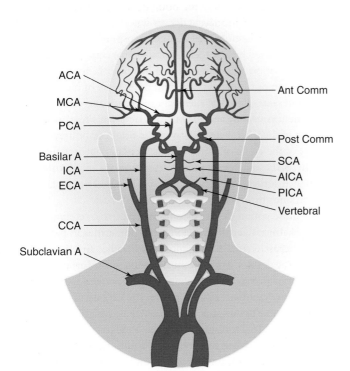

FIGURE 116-1 Coronal view of the extracranial and intracranial arterial supply to the brain. Vessels forming the circle of Willis are highlighted. A, Artery; ACA, anterior cerebral artery; AICA, anterior inferior cerebellar artery; Ant Comm, anterior communicating artery; CCA, common carotid artery; ECA, external carotid artery; ICA, internal carotid artery; MCA, middle cerebral artery; PCA, posterior cerebral artery; PICA, posterior inferior cerebellar artery; Post Comm, posterior communicating artery; SCA, superior cerebellar artery. (Modified from Lord R: Surgery of occlusive cerebrovascular disease, St. Louis, 1986, Mosby.)

internal carotid arteries have no branches in the neck and face, and enter the cranium through the carotid canal. There are four main segments of each internal carotid artery: cervical, petrous, cavernous, and supraclinoid. The siphon is the term used to describe the hairloop turn made by the cavernous and supraclinoid segments, and it is at this level that the ophthalmic artery originates, providing the first major branch of the internal carotid artery and supplying blood flow to the optic nerve and retina. Thus, internal carotid artery disease commonly causes ocular ischemia, leading to a transient ischemic attack (*amaurosis fugax*) or infarction of the optic nerve or retina, a warning sign of impending cerebral stroke. The internal carotid arteries then give off the superior hypophyseal, posterior communicating, and anterior choroidal arteries, before terminating intracranially by dividing into the middle and anterior cerebral arteries. In addition to the eye, the paired carotid systems supply approximately 80% of the hemispheric blood flow, including the frontal, parietal, and anterior temporal lobes. In up to 15% of individuals, the posterior cerebral artery (PCA) also arises directly from the internal carotid artery (the so-called fetal origin PCA), so that the entire hemisphere including the occipital lobe is supplied by the internal carotid artery. The anterior choroidal artery supplies a number of structures in addition to the choroid plexus, including the inferior portion of the posterior limb of the internal capsule, the hippocampus, and portions of the globus pallidus, posterior putamen, lateral geniculate, amygdala, and ventrolateral thalamus.

The middle cerebral artery (MCA) is the largest branch of the internal carotid artery. Its first portion, or stem, is often referred to as the M1 segment, and this usually bifurcates into superior and inferior divisions or, less often, trifurcates into three major divisions (upper, middle, and lower). The MCA stem gives rise to the medial and lateral lenticulostriates, which supply the extreme capsule, claustrum, putamen, most of the globus pallidus, part of the head and the entire body of the caudate, as well as the superior portions of the anterior and posterior limbs of the internal capsule. The divisions of the MCA supply almost the entire lateral cortical surface of the brain, including the insula, operculum, and frontal, parietal, temporal, and occipital cortices.

The anterior cerebral artery (ACA) also has a proximal, or A1, segment, which ends at the junction with the anterior communicating artery. The ipsilateral ACA then continues as the distal, or A2, segment. An important branch is the recurrent artery of Heubner, which supplies the head of the caudate nucleus, and several cortical branches supply the medial and orbital surfaces of the frontal lobe.

The vertebral arteries generally originate from the subclavian arteries, course through the transverse foramina of the cervical vertebrae, pierce the dura, and enter the cranial cavity through the foramen magnum. The two vertebral arteries join to form the basilar artery at the level of the pontomedullary junction. Anterior and posterior spinal arteries and the posterior inferior cerebellar artery (PICA), which supplies the inferior surface of the cerebellum, arise from the distal segments of the vertebrals. The lateral medulla is supplied by the multiple, perforating branches of PICA or the direct penetrating branches of the vertebral artery. Occlusion of the distal vertebral artery may, therefore, cause infarction of the lateral medulla (Wallenberg syndrome), characterized by vertigo, imbalance, Horner syndrome, dysphagia, and sensory loss.

After originating as the union of the right and left vertebral arteries, the basilar artery travels up the ventral pons. Paramedian and circumferential penetrating arteries exit the basilar to dive into the pontine parenchyma. Proximally, the basilar gives off the paired anterior inferior cerebellar arteries (AICA), and more distally the superior cerebellar arteries (SCA); these perfuse the ventrolateral aspect of the cerebellar cortex. An internal auditory (labyrinthine) artery arises either directly from the basilar or from the anterior cerebellar artery to supply the cochlea, labyrinth, and part of the facial nerve. Ischemia in the basilar territory may, therefore, cause hearing loss and vertigo, sometimes as an isolated symptom.

The basilar artery terminates in the right and left posterior cerebral arteries (PCAs). A series of penetrators arise from the posterior communicating and posterior cerebral arteries to supply the hypothalamus, dorsolateral midbrain, lateral geniculate, and thalamus. The posterior cerebral artery supplies the inferior temporal lobe, and the medial and inferior surfaces of the occipital lobe. In some patients a single large penetrating vessel at the midline of the terminal basilar artery may supply medial aspects of both thalami (the artery of Percheron); emboli occluding this vessel may, therefore, cause bilateral thalamic infarcts, with a decrease in alertness and vertical gaze abnormalities, without significant motor deficit.

The brain's anastomotic network includes not only the connections through the Circle of Willis, but also intercommunicating systems extracranially and more distal connections intracranially through meningeal anastomoses that cover the cortical and cerebellar surfaces (pial-pial collaterals). These networks all protect the brain from ischemia by providing alternate routes to circumvent obstructions in the main arteries.

Venous anatomy is more variable than arterial. Superficial veins drain into the transverse, superior sagittal, and cavernous sinuses. The deep venous drainage is via the great vein of Galen, which drains into the straight sinus, and in turn drains into the torcula along with the sagittal sinus. Blood drains from the torcula to the transverse sinus, then to the sigmoid sinus, and thereafter the jugular vein. Anterior venous drainage is via the cavernous sinus, which communicates with the contralateral cavernous sinus, the transverse sinus via the superior petrosal sinus, and the inferior petrosal sinus, which drains directly into the jugular bulb.

Vascular Pathogenesis

There are multiple mechanisms leading to brain ischemia. Hemodynamic infarction occurs as a result of reduced perfusion, usually in the setting of arterial stenosis due to atherosclerosis. In some cases, stenosis may be due to arterial dissection, vasculitis, fibromuscular dysplasia, or other arteriopathies. Embolism occurs when a thrombus originating from a more proximal source (e.g., arterial or cardiac) travels through the arteries and occludes a cerebral artery. Paradoxical embolism occurs when a thrombus crosses from the venous circulation to the left side of the heart through a patent foramen ovale or, less commonly, an intrapulmonary arteriovenous shunt. Other particles that may embolize include neoplasm, fat, air, or other foreign substances.

Air emboli can follow injuries or procedures involving the lungs, the dural sinuses, or jugular veins. Fat embolism usually results from a bone fracture. Septic emboli arise from bacterial endocarditis.

Intracranial hemorrhage results from the rupture of a vessel anywhere within the cranial cavity. Intracranial hemorrhages may be classified by location (e.g., extradural, subdural, subarachnoid, intracerebral, intraventricular), by the nature of the ruptured vessel (e.g., arterial, capillary, venous), or by cause (e.g., primary, secondary). Trauma is often involved in the generation of extradural hematoma from laceration of the middle meningeal artery or vein, and subdural hematomas from traumatic rupture of veins that traverse the subdural space.

Intracerebral hemorrhage is characterized by bleeding into the substance of the brain, usually originating from a small penetrating artery. Hypertension has been implicated as the cause of weakening in the walls of arterioles and the formation of microaneurysms (i.e., Charcot-Bouchard aneurysms). The most common sites for hypertensive arterial hemorrhage are the putamen, pons, cerebellum, and thalamus. Blood under arterial pressures destroys or displaces brain tissue. Amyloid angiopathy, due to the vascular deposition of β-amyloid protein similar to that seen in Alzheimer disease has been implicated as an important cause of lobar hemorrhage in elderly patients. Other causes of hemorrhage include arteriovenous malformations, aneurysms, moyamoya disease, bleeding disorders or anticoagulation, trauma, tumors, cavernous angiomas, and illicit drug abuse.

Subarachnoid hemorrhage occurs when blood is localized to the surrounding membranes and cerebrospinal fluid. It is most frequently caused by leakage of blood from a cerebral aneurysm. The combination of congenital and acquired factors leads to a degeneration of the arterial wall and the release of blood, under arterial pressures, into the subarachnoid space and cerebrospinal fluid. Aneurysms may be distributed at different sites throughout the base of the brain, particularly at the origin or bifurcations of arteries of the circle of Willis. Other secondary causes that may lead to SAH include trauma, arteriovenous malformations, bleeding disorders or anticoagulation, amyloid angiopathy, or cerebral sinus thrombosis.

The most common intrinsic disorder of the cerebral blood vessels is atherosclerosis, which shares similarities in pathology with atherosclerosis throughout the body. Arteriosclerotic plaques may develop at any point along the carotid artery and the vertebrobasilar system, but the most common sites are the bifurcation of the common carotid artery, the origins of the MCAs and ACAs, and the origins of the vertebral from the subclavian arteries (Fig. 116-2). In the past it was thought that intracranial atherosclerotic disease required significant stenosis (>50%) to cause symptoms. However, recent pathological and radiological studies provide evidence that substenotic lesions can also cause strokes due to plaque rupture and acute thrombosis, as is the case elsewhere in the body.

Small-vessel disease refers to the occlusion of a penetrant branch of a larger artery, usually due to microatheroma or to lipohyalinosis, a degenerative disorder of the vessel characterized by deposition of fatty and proteinaceous material. Hematological disorders and coagulopathies, including leukemia, Waldenstrom macroglobulinemia, polycythemia, primary and secondary

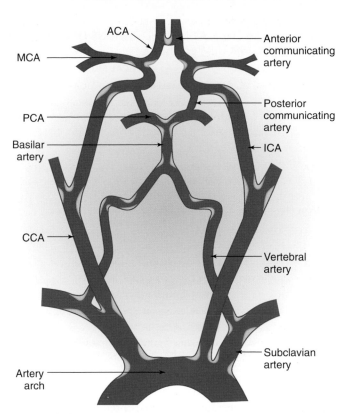

FIGURE 116-2 Sites of predilection for atheromatous plaque. ACA, Anterior cerebral artery; CCA, common carotid artery; ICA, internal carotid artery; MCA, middle cerebral artery; PCA, posterior cerebral artery. (From Caplan LR: Stroke: a clinical approach, ed 2, Boston, 1993 Butterworth-Heinemann.)

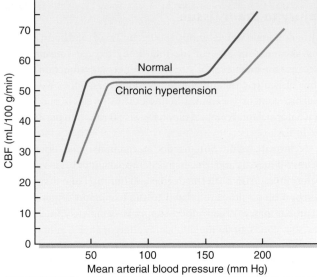

FIGURE 116-3 Autoregulatory cerebral blood flow (CBF) response to changes in mean arterial pressure in normotensive and chronically hypertensive persons. Note the shift of the curve toward higher mean pressures with chronic hypertension. (From Pulsinelli WA: Cerebrovascular diseases-principles. In Goldman L, Bennett JC, editors: Cecil textbook of medicine, ed 21, Philadelphia, 2000, Saunders, p 2097.)

antiphospholipid antibody syndrome, and genetic defects of the coagulation cascade, may also lead to occlusive thrombi and emboli.

The cerebral circulation differs from the systemic circulation. The brain is protected by the anastomoses described above. In addition, *cerebral autoregulation* maintains a constant cerebral perfusion pressure over a range of systemic blood pressures (Fig. 116-3). Cerebral arterioles have a well-developed muscular coat that allows constriction in response to increased blood pressure, and dilation with hypotension. The arterioles are also exquisitely sensitive to changes in peripheral arterial concentrations of carbon dioxide ($PaCO_2$) and oxygen (PaO_2). When the partial pressure of CO_2 decreases, such as after hyperventilation, the arterioles constrict and blood flow is reduced. In healthy individuals, cerebral autoregulation maintains a constant cerebral blood flow over mean arterial pressures of 60 to 140 mm Hg. In patients with chronic hypertension, the autoregulatory curve is shifted to the right, so that even minor reductions in blood pressure levels may not be tolerated. At blood pressures above these limits, moreover, as in severe hypertension, autoregulatory capacity may be overwhelmed, leading to breakthrough edema and hemorrhage. In the setting of infarction or hemorrhage, cerebral autoregulation is also impaired, resulting in cerebral dependence on systemic blood pressure to maintain adequate perfusion. Thus, decreasing the blood pressure in the setting of acute ischemia is hazardous.

Specific disorders may originate from autoregulatory dysfunction: posterior reversible encephalopathy syndrome (PRES) and the reversible cerebral vasoconstriction syndrome (RCVS). In posterior reversible encephalopathy syndrome, there is loss of autoregulatory control with leakage of fluid across the blood-brain barrier, primarily in the posterior regions of the brain. Patients present with elevated blood pressures, headaches, seizures, and loss of visual function. Reversible cerebral vasoconstriction syndrome, a recently recognized syndrome, remains incompletely characterized, and shares features with posterior reversible encephalopathy syndrome. The two disorders overlap in 10% or more of cases. Patients with reversible cerebral vasoconstriction syndrome are typically young women who present with acute, severe headache, have minimal or no neurological deficits, and may have evidence of non-aneurysmal, superficial SAH as well as vasospasm of the cerebral arteries. Sympathetic innervation of the vessels is also less in the posterior circulation than anteriorly, leading to a reduced ability of the posterior circulation to adapt to changes in blood pressure, and may contribute to the propensity for edema to form in the occipital lobes during hypertensive crises.

In addition, focal cerebral activity, such as occurs when activating brain regions responsible for moving a limb, is accompanied by accelerated metabolism in the appropriate region, and is accommodated by slight increases in local blood flow and oxygen delivery. Exploitation of this increased local energy demand and delivery is what allows imaging of functional brain activity using MRI, which can detect subtle changes in regional cerebral blood flow.

Intracerebral capillaries also lack adventitia, with astrocytes serving as the vascular component of the neurovascular unit. Tight junctions at the capillary level play an important role in the blood-brain barrier, which limits permeability between the vascular compartment and the brain tissue.

Injury to Brain Tissue

The adult brain weighs about 1500 g, or 2% of total body weight, but accounts for 20% of the total body oxygen consumption. Because the brain cannot store much energy, dysfunction results after only a few minutes of deprivation when either oxygen or glucose content is reduced below critical levels. In the resting state, normal total cerebral blood flow is 50 mL/min per 100 g of brain tissue.

Neuronal dysfunction occurs at cerebral blood flow levels below 50 mg/dL, and irreversible neuronal injury begins at levels below 30 mg/dL. Both the degree and duration of reductions in cerebral blood flow are related to the likelihood of permanent neuronal injury. When blood supply is completely interrupted for 30 seconds, brain metabolism is altered; after 1 minute, neuronal function may cease. After 5 minutes, anoxia initiates a chain of events that may result in cerebral infarction; however, if oxygenated blood flow is restored quickly enough, the damage may be reversible, as with a TIA.

Research into the cellular basis of cerebral ischemia has led to the concept of the "ischemic cascade." As perfusion of the brain decreases, a chain of events at the neuronal level begins with failure of the membrane sodium/potassium (Na/K) pump, the depolarization of the neuronal membrane, the release of excitatory neurotransmitters such as glutamate and glycine that hyperstimulate their receptors, and the opening of calcium channels. Calcium enters the neuron through various voltage-sensitive and receptor-mediated channels (e.g., the N-methyl-d-aspartate receptor). The influx of calcium is at the root of further neuronal injury, with damage to organelles and further destabilization of neuronal metabolism and normal function resulting. These events may lead to delayed neuronal death, even after restoration of blood flow, and are a target of experimental neuroprotective strategies.

Recent research has distinguished between the "core" infarct and an "ischemic penumbra," or shadow. The core represents a central region of necrosis, or tissue that dies very quickly after blood flow ceases. The penumbra represents the surrounding region of brain tissue, in which neurons are dysfunctional but potentially salvageable. Recanalization of occluded vessels with blood flow into infarcted tissue, particularly when delayed, results in "reperfusion injury." Increased use of MRI has shown that petechial hemorrhagic infarction is very common, occurring in the majority of strokes, even when not suspected clinically.

⬤ CLINICAL PRESENTATION

The signs and symptoms of strokes are varied, and depend on the type of stroke, the region of the nervous system affected by the lack of flow or hemorrhage, and the patient's handedness (Table 116-3). In general, embolic ischemic strokes are characterized by the sudden onset of a neurological deficit, generally painless. Thrombotic strokes may have a stuttering or progressive course due to fluctuating hypoperfusion and gradual occlusion. Arterial dissections, as well as hemorrhages, are more often associated with headaches than ischemic stroke. Hemorrhagic strokes and large hemispheric infarcts can lead to decrease in consciousness due to increased intracranial pressure.

TABLE 116-3	CLINICAL MANIFESTATIONS OF ISCHEMIC STROKE
OCCLUDED VESSEL	**CLINICAL SIGNS**
ICA	Ipsilateral blindness (variable) MCA syndrome
MCA	Contralateral hemiparesis, hemisensory loss (face or arm more than leg) Aphasia (dominant) or anosognosia (nondominant) Homonymous hemianopsia (variable)
ACA	Contralateral hemiparesis, hemisensory loss (leg more than arm) Abulia (especially if bilateral)
VA or PICA	Ipsilateral facial sensory loss, hemiataxia, nystagmus, Horner syndrome Contralateral loss of temperature or pain sensation Dysphagia
SCA	Gait ataxia, nausea, vertigo, dysarthria
BA	Quadriparesis, dysarthria, dysphagia, diplopia, somnolence, amnesia
PCA	Contralateral homonymous hemianopsia, amnesia, sensory loss

ACA, Anterior cerebral artery; BA, basilar artery; ICA, internal carotid artery; MCA, middle cerebral artery; PCA, posterior cerebral artery; PICA, posterior inferior cerebellar artery; SCA, superior cerebellar artery; VA, vertebral artery.

Most emboli occur in the territory of the MCAs. Lesions of the dominant (almost always left) hemisphere are characterized by variable combinations of right hemiparesis, right hemisensory loss, right visual loss, impaired gaze to the right side of space, and language disturbance. When the superior division of the middle cerebral artery is affected, the language impairment is predominantly motor: the patient either cannot speak or produces sparse, agrammatic speech, despite an ability to fully comprehend spoken and written material. When the inferior division is affected, the patient may produce fluent, prosodic, but nonsensical speech and be unable to follow instructions. Larger infarcts of the dominant hemisphere produce a total loss of language function, leaving the patient mute and uncomprehending.

Lesions of the non-dominant (right) hemisphere produce deficits of the left side of the body. Language is preserved but the patient may demonstrate impaired attention, particularly to the left side of space and fail to appreciate the presence of people or objects to their left, and may even fail to recognize the left side of their own body (asomatagnosia). This neglect phenomenon may extend even to an awareness of any deficit of functioning on their part, and they may be unaware there is a problem (anosagnosia). These patients may be found at home, lying on the floor paralyzed yet unaware that anything is the matter; their unawareness can delay their presentation to the hospital for treatment and similarly limit their participation in rehabilitation. Lesions in the right hemisphere may also cause dysprosody, the non-dominant equivalent of aphasia, which is characterized by a lack of the emotional and gestural components of speech, despite preservation of its semantic content; many of these patients have a flat affect or appear to be depressed.

Infarcts in the territory of the anterior cerebral arteries often cause weakness limited to the legs, due to location of the representation of the legs in the medial part of the hemispheres. They may have incontinence, lack initiative (abulia), and have gaze palsies. In some cases their deficits may be more extensive and mimic those of middle cerebral artery infarctions. Posterior cerebral artery infarcts lead to visual loss, often without any motor deficit. With involvement of the medial temporal lobes supplied by the PCAs, there may also be behavioral disturbances, including delirium and amnesia.

Brainstem infarcts cause specific syndromes due to the affected neural pathways and nuclei. Midbrain infarcts often produce vertical gaze deficits and impaired consciousness if the reticular activating system is involved.

Many cerebral infarctions do not cause weakness, such as fluent (or Wernicke's) aphasia, cortical visual loss, and Wallenberg syndrome. Because the inferior division of the MCA supplies the lateral temporal lobe and parietal lobes, including Wernicke's area, occlusion of that vessel may cause a prosodic, fluent speech with multiple paraphasic errors and poor comprehension, while sparing the motor strip in the frontal lobe. Emboli traveling up the basilar artery may cause significant infarction in the territory of both posterior cerebral arteries, causing complete blindness, sometimes without awareness of the deficit on the part of the patient, due to infarction of both occipital lobes (the "top of the basilar syndrome"). Behavioral abnormalities, memory loss, and eye movement abnormalities may also occur, due to the involvement of the medial temporal lobe structures and the midbrain eye movement centers. Small emboli to branches of the superior division of the MCA may cause focal weakness of the hand, particularly fine finger movements, simulating a peripheral compression neuropathy.

In patients presenting with dizziness, it is particularly difficult to distinguish stroke from vestibular neuronitis or Ménière's disease (see Chapter 113). The presence of a normal head-thrust test, skew deviation, or direction-changing nystagmus are all signs of stroke, rather than a peripheral cause. Patients should be followed until they can walk without imbalance; patients with nausea and vomiting due to cerebellar infarction may develop fatal brainstem compression due to swelling.

The signs and symptoms of *subarachnoid hemorrhage* differ from other stroke types due to the absence of focal deficits. Instead, patients present with abrupt onset of severe headache (i.e., "the worst headache of my life"), vomiting, altered consciousness, and sometimes coma, typically without localizing signs.

Thrombosis of cerebral veins or the larger draining dural sinuses present with a combination of headache due to elevated intracranial pressure, seizures, and focal deficits due to hemorrhage. Rarely the syndrome of *thunderclap headache*, or sudden severe headache without any focal signs similar to that occurring in SAH, may be due to venous thrombosis. Occlusion of the cerebral venous sinuses may occur in association with a hyperviscosity or hypercoagulable state, including pregnancy or hormonal contraceptive use. Imaging findings include bilateral hemorrhagic infarctions in a parasagittal distribution and extensive white matter edema. Contrast-enhanced CT may demonstrate the *empty delta* sign, indicating a filling defect in the sagittal sinus. Magnetic resonance venography (MRV) and T1 weighted MRI images confirm the presence of thrombus; cerebral angiography is seldom needed to confirm the diagnosis.

● DIAGNOSIS AND DIFFERENTIAL DIAGNOSIS

The benefit of thrombolytic therapy within 3 hours of onset of acute ischemic stroke requires urgent differentiation of ischemic stroke from hemorrhage and other causes of sudden neurological symptoms. Headache, vomiting, seizures, and coma, are more common in hemorrhagic stroke, though these are never reliable enough to preclude imaging. The distinction is straightforward in most cases once a head CT is performed. The hyperdense signal of blood in the parenchyma on CT almost invariably distinguishes hemorrhage from ischemia. In exceptional cases the typical hyperdensity of ICH is absent owing to severe anemia or to its subacute state, during which blood may be indistinguishable from brain tissue. Certain imaging findings on initial CT further support a presumed diagnosis of infarction, such as a hyperdense vessel sign indicative of thrombus in the vessel, or loss of the gray-white junction and sulci in the cortex, and loss of the demarcation of the insular cortex and deep gray nuclei, both of which are early indicators of ischemia and edema (Fig. 116-4). CT angiography often identifies the site of vascular occlusion.

Imaging in the setting of suspected acute ischemia does not definitively diagnose ischemia, but rather excludes hemorrhage; if clinical symptoms are consistent with cerebral ischemia, then thrombolytic treatment is indicated. Primary stroke centers must perform and interpret CT scans within 30 minutes of the arrival of a patient with suspected stroke. MRI can also effectively exclude acute hemorrhage, and diffusion-weighted imaging sequences are more sensitive to the earliest changes of ischemia (Fig. 116-5), but the speed and availability of CT make it the initial imaging modality of choice at most centers. MRI scanning may then be used to provide additional information. Specific MRI sequences have greater sensitivity to blood than CT, and many identify hemorrhagic infarction missed by CT.

Clinical features at stroke onset may suggest a subtype of cerebral infarction but require confirmatory laboratory data. Cerebral embolism is suggested by sudden onset and a syndrome of circumscribed focal signs attributable to cerebral surface infarction, such as pure aphasia or pure hemianopia. Unless the source of embolization is obvious on hospital admission, blood cultures, electrocardiographic monitoring, and echocardiography are indicated.

A diagnosis of atherosclerotic infarction is suggested if there were previous TIAs, particularly when the symptoms are stereotypical. Doppler ultrasonography or MRA can usually identify the stenosis. In equivocal cases, CT angiography or conventional angiography may be needed. Small penetrating vessel infarcts, *lacunar infarcts*, usually spare cortical functions, such as language and cognition, but cause loss of elementary neurologic function, such as strength, sensation, and coordination. Up to 25% of patients with lacunar infarcts have large-vessel disease or a cardioembolic source, so it is important to carry out a complete etiologic evaluation in all stroke patients.

Up to 50% of patients with transient deficits lasting less than 24 hours have evidence of infarction on imaging, and the risk of stroke and other vascular events is as high after TIA as after completed stroke. In the acute setting, when decisions about thrombolysis must be made, it is virtually impossible to know which

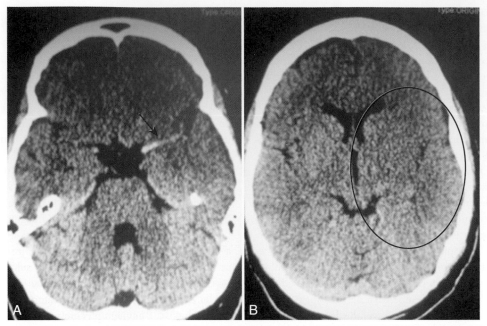

FIGURE 116-4 Early signs of infarction on computed tomography of the brain. **A,** Hyperdense middle cerebral artery sign *(red arrow),* and **B,** hypoattenuation of the left caudate and lentiform nuclei, loss of the insular ribbon, and sulcal effacement *(outlined in red).*

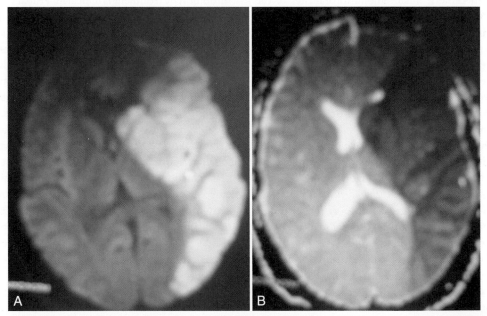

FIGURE 116-5 Magnetic resonance imaging scan of the brain of the same patient shown in Figure 116-4. **A,** Diffusion-weighted image shows bright signal in the left middle cerebral artery territory. **B,** Apparent diffusion coefficient shows dark signal in the same area, confirming acute infarction.

patients with ischemia will have symptoms resolve without infarction (thus, having a TIA) and which will have a completed infarction. Patients with either stroke or TIA need immediate attention to secondary prevention strategies. In terms of choosing treatments, the important issue is to identify the cause of the cerebral ischemia, rather than its duration. Entities other than cerebral ischemia can masquerade as strokes and TIAs. Among patients diagnosed with stroke in emergency departments, 20% or more have a stroke *mimic,* including seizure, migraine, systemic

infection, brain tumor, and toxic-metabolic encephalopathy. Other sources of misdiagnosis are listed in Table 116-4.

In patients with a prior of history cerebral infarct or hemorrhage, new *metabolic derangements,* including infections, may precipitate a recrudescence of the original stroke syndrome. Hypoglycemia, hyponatremia, urinary tract infection, pneumonia, and starting initiation of a psychotropic medication can each precipitate this phenomenon. The patient returns to normal over hours to days when the new insult is treated or reversed. Such

TABLE 116-4 STROKE MIMICS AND DIFFERENTIAL DIAGNOSIS

COMMON MIMICS

Metabolic encephalopathy (hypoglycemia, hyponatremia, etc.)
Systemic infection
Seizure
Migraine
Brain tumors

OTHER MIMICS

Transient focal neurological symptoms associated with amyloid angiopathy
Positional vertigo
Cardiac events
Syncope
Trauma (especially acceleration-deceleration without evidence of external injury)
Subdural hematoma
Herpes simplex virus encephalitis
Transient global amnesia
Dementia
Demyelinating disease
Cervical spine disease/radiculopathy/fracture
Myasthenia gravis
Parkinsonism
Hypertensive encephalopathy
Conversion disorder
Intoxication/substance abuse

metabolic and infectious causes of neurologic deterioration must be excluded in patients with a history of earlier brain injury before diagnosing a new stroke. Focal signs may also occur with metabolic disturbances in patients without a prior history of stroke.

External signs of injury are usually present in brain *trauma*, but they need not be present after acceleration-deceleration injury, such as from a motor vehicle accident. The most frequent sites of brain contusions are the frontal and temporal poles, which are not typical locations for strokes.

Seizures may occasionally complicate acute stroke, but they may also mimic stroke. Unlike stroke, seizures are often characterized by obtundation, an amnestic state, clonic activity, incontinence, or tongue biting. The postictal deficit, often called a *Todd's paralysis*, resembles stroke and weakness or language and other cortical deficits may occur. The deficits after seizure usually resolve within hours after the seizure, but occasionally persist for up to a week, making the distinction from stroke difficult. Seizures may also develop months or years after an infarct or hemorrhage, and the postictal state in these patients may recapitulate the initial stroke syndrome.

Migraine with persistent aura often mimics stroke or TIA. Aura alone, without headache (i.e., acephalgic migraine), is sometimes experienced by those who previously suffered from migraine with aura. Migraine aura typically produces a visual disturbance that marches across the vision of both eyes as an advancing, enlarging blind spot that takes 20 to 30 minutes to resolve. Subsequent unilateral, pounding headache suggests the diagnosis, but may not occur. Less often, migrainous auras take the form of sensory symptoms. The speed of the march is generally slower than the rapid spread of symptoms in stroke.

As many as 10% of *brain tumors* present with acute transient symptoms reflecting intratumoral hemorrhage or focal seizures. Seizures often precede focal signs. CT scan usually demonstrates an enhancing mass even when symptoms are mild.

TABLE 116-5 EVIDENCE-BASED PRIMARY PREVENTION OF ISCHEMIC STROKE

RISK FACTOR	TREATMENT
Hypertension	Anti-hypertensives
Myocardial infarction	HMG-CoA reductase inhibitors
Hyperlipidemia	HMG-CoA reductase inhibitors
Atrial fibrillation	Anticoagulation (warfarin, other agents)
Diabetes mellitus/vascular disease	ACE inhibitor
Diabetes mellitus type II, obesity	Metformin
Aymptomatic carotid stenosis (60-99%)	Carotid endarterectomy
High vascular risk populations	Antiplatelet therapy

⬤ TREATMENT

Stroke prevention and treatment are directed toward: (1) preventing the first stroke (primary prevention); (2) limiting damage from the stroke; (3) optimizing functional recovery following stroke; and (4) avoiding recurrence (secondary prevention). Specific measures for treatment and prevention depend on the patient's risk factors and stroke mechanism. The diagnostic evaluation of the stroke patient dictates optimal therapy.

Primary Prevention of Stroke

Randomized trials have demonstrated that specific interventions prevent first stroke among patients with specific risk factors (Table 116-5). Treatment of hypertension, for example, is associated with up to a 45% reduction in the risk of stroke (Level A). Among patients with atrial fibrillation, the use of warfarin is associated with a 60% to 70% relative reduction in risk of stroke, though younger patients without any accompanying heart disease, hypertension, or diabetes may be managed with antiplatelet agents alone (Level A). Hydroxymethylglutaryl-coenzyme A (HMG-CoA) reductase inhibitors, or statins, have been shown in some primary prevention studies, and in studies of patients with heart disease, to reduce the risk of a first stroke as well as that of heart disease (Level A). The effects on stroke risk are more modest than the effects on heart disease, possibly reflecting the greater heterogeneity among causes of stroke compared to heart disease. For patients with asymptomatic carotid stenosis of at least 60%, carotid endarterectomy reduces the risk of stroke, though the effect is much more modest than in symptomatic patients, and the number of patients needed to treat to prevent one stroke is greater. Because many of the large randomized trials of endarterectomy for asymptomatic patients were conducted in the era before the current recommended use of statins and antiplatelet agents, it is no longer clear that surgery is superior to medical therapy. New trials are addressing medical versus surgical treatment.

Antiplatelet therapy is not of established benefit for prevention of a first stroke. In a large primary prevention study, for example, aspirin use was associated with an increased risk of both ischemic and hemorrhagic stroke, despite reducing the risk of ischemic heart disease. However, other studies have shown that aspirin reduces the risk of ischemic stroke among women over the age of 45 (Level B).

Observational studies provide evidence that certain behaviors prevent stroke. Smoking cessation leads to a reduction by 5 years in stroke risk to levels similar to non-smokers. Consumption of alcohol in moderation, up to 2 drinks daily for men and one daily for women is associated with a lower level of stroke risk than in those who do not drink. Physical activity, weight loss when appropriate, and management of diabetes are recommended.

Acute Treatment of Ischemic Stroke

For patients with ischemic stroke evaluated within 3 hours of symptom onset with no evidence of hemorrhage on a brain CT or MRI, recombinant tissue plasminogen activator (rt-PA), a thrombolytic agent, improves functional outcomes at 3 months compared to placebo. Among the 624 ischemic stroke patients treated within 3 hours in the original landmark study, the proportion of patients achieving normal or near-normal neurological and functional status by 3 months was significantly higher among those receiving rt-PA, though there was no definite benefit at 24 hours. The proportion of patients who achieved independence in their performance of activities of daily living was increased from 38% to 50%, an absolute benefit of 12%. The absence of an immediate (24-hour) benefit, coupled with the finding of a benefit at 3 months, is consistent with the hypothesis that thrombolytic treatment works to reduce the size of the infarct penumbra by reperfusing tissue before permanent infarction of the entire territory occurs, despite some irreversible injury to a core component.

Patients treated with rt-PA had a tenfold increase in incidence of hemorrhagic conversion of the infarction (from 0.6% in placebo-treated patients to 6.0% in rt-PA–treated patients). Overall, the rates of neurological deterioration and mortality within the first day after stroke were similar between the groups. Rt-PA was approved for patient use by the FDA in 1996, and it is now considered standard of care for ischemic stroke patients presenting within 3 hours (Level A). Specific guidelines for eligibility and exclusion must be met when using rt-PA to reduce the risk of complications (Table 116-6).

Because of the potential to reduce cerebral perfusion below the limits permitted by autoregulation in the setting of acute brain injury, current guidelines recommend that blood pressure not be reduced acutely after ischemic stroke, and systolic blood pressure levels as high as 220 mm Hg are allowed. Before and following thrombolytic treatment, however, systolic blood pressure should be kept below 180 mm Hg to reduce the risk of hemorrhagic conversion. In addition, antiplatelet and anticoagulant medications must be withheld for 24 hours after rt-PA.

Subsequent meta-analyses and individual trials have demonstrated that the benefit of thrombolytic therapy decreases as the time interval between symptom onset (the presumed beginning of ischemia) and treatment increases, but that the therapeutic time window may persist as long as 4.5 hours after stroke. Advanced imaging techniques, such as diffusion-weighted (DWI) and perfusion-weighted images (PWI), that can distinguish irreversibly injured versus underperfused or "at risk" tissue have been investigated as a means to identify ischemically viable tissue that may respond to revascularization. Recent trial results, however, have not confirmed their value, at least using the imaging parameters under study.

TABLE 116-6	ELIGIBILITY AND EXCLUSION CRITERIA FOR TREATMENT OF ACUTE ISCHEMIC STROKE WITH INTRAVENOUS RT-PA

ELIGIBILITY

Age ≥18 years
Diagnosis of ischemic stroke causing measurable neurological deficit
Well-documented onset of symptoms <4.5 hours before beginning treatment

MAJOR EXCLUSION CRITERIA

Stroke or head trauma within the preceding 3 months
Major surgery within the preceding 2 weeks
History of intracerebral hemorrhage
Systolic blood pressure >185 mm Hg
Diastolic blood pressure >110 mm Hg
Rapidly improving or minor neurological symptoms and signs
Symptoms suggestive of subarachnoid hemorrhage
Gastrointestinal or urinary tract bleeding within 3 weeks
Arterial puncture at a noncompressible site within 1 week
Platelet count <100,000/mm^3
INR >1.7

RELATIVE EXCLUSION CRITERIA (MUST WEIGH RISKS AND BENEFITS)

Seizure at stroke onset
Myocardial infarction within 6 weeks
Infective endocarditis
Hemorrhagic eye disorder
Blood glucose <30 mg/dL (2.7 mmol/L)
Blood glucose >400 mg/dL (21.6 mmol/L)
Patients requiring very aggressive therapy for blood pressure reduction

Interventional techniques to revascularize occluded vessels has promise in the management of patients with ischemic stroke. For patients with MCA occlusions presenting up to 6 hours after symptom onset, there is evidence that intra-arterial thrombolytic agents delivered via catheter into the face of the occluding thrombus can improve functional outcomes, despite an increase in risk of hemorrhage similar to that seen with intravenous rt-PA (Level B). More recently, the FDA has approved the use of mechanical devices specifically engineered to facilitate clot extraction and dissolution in the setting of ischemic stroke. These devices are promising in that they are associated with higher recanalization rates of occluded vessels than occurs spontaneously, but they have not yet been demonstrated to lead to better clinical outcomes than standard treatment with intravenous rt-PA in randomized trials. There is evidence, however, that earlier treatment (within 2 hours) may lead to better outcomes, and further studies are ongoing to test whether other devices used quickly enough will improve clinical outcomes.

Treatment with heparin and various heparinoids for acute stroke are not of benefit and are not recommended in acute stroke. In some patients with massive hemispheric strokes, surgical decompression (hemicraniectomy) can be lifesaving with acceptable functional outcomes, particularly for younger patients (Level A).

Since stroke is characterized by a cascade of events that can cause further neuronal injury for hours or days after stroke, experimental animal stroke studies have tested strategies that might limit this injury (i.e., neuroprotection), including drugs targeting N-Methyl-D-Aspartate (NMDA)-receptors, glycine receptors, calcium channels, adhesion molecules, free radicals, albumin, inflammation, and membrane constituents. However, none of these have been of benefit in human clinical trials.

Treatment of Intracerebral Hemorrhage

Treatment of ICH is primarily supportive. Many patients require management in the intensive care setting to manage elevated blood pressure and secondary complications, such as respiratory failure, aspiration, and hemodynamic instability in severely neurologically compromised patients. In many cases, patients also require management of intracranial pressure using osmotic agents, such as mannitol or hypertonic saline, or therapeutic hyperventilation. In some patients, surgical evacuation of hematomas may be lifesaving, although trials have thus far failed to show that most ICH patients benefit from surgical decompression. Among more than 1000 participants randomized in a large international study, there was no evidence of benefit of surgical over medical therapy, apart from a potential benefit in the subgroup of patients with small superficial hemorrhages. Most hemorrhages that occur deep within the hemispheres probably cause the majority of their damage immediately after the ictal hemorrhage, so that evacuation does not save tissue and may introduce further damage.

One of the major recent insights into the pathogenesis of cerebral injury associated with ICH has been the recognition that a large proportion of hemorrhages continue to expand during the early hours after onset. As a result, there has been increased interest in the use of prothrombotic agents to reduce this expansion and to limit secondary cerebral injury. Though preliminary studies on the potential benefits of infusing factor VII as a prothrombogenic agent showed promise, subsequent and more definitive studies did not confirm a benefit in the majority of patients, although it remains possible that subgroups of patients, including those with warfarin-associated hemorrhage, may benefit.

For cerebellar hemorrhages, surgical decompression may be lifesaving, and it is essential to recognize the signs and symptoms of incipient brainstem compression and herniation (i.e., headache, vertigo, nausea, vomiting, and truncal ataxia without focal weakness, declining sensorium, and gaze-palsy). Neuroimaging studies that support the need for surgical decompression include hematoma greater than 3 cm, fourth ventricular shift, cisternal obliteration, and ventricular enlargement. Lumbar puncture is contraindicated with ICH, particularly with cerebellar hemorrhages because life-threatening tonsillar herniation and midbrain compression may occur. Great caution must be taken in these patients subjected to ventriculostomy for the purposes of reducing intracranial pressure because upward cerebellar herniation may occur.

The management of aneurysmal SAH is complicated. Recurrent bleeding risks and mortality are high; therefore, definitive therapy is elimination of the ruptured aneurysm. This may be accomplished surgically or with interventional embolization techniques, such as with coils deposited in the aneurysm. Even after securing the aneurysmal site of bleeding, however, several other complications may ensue, including vasospasm, cerebral infarction, cerebral edema, seizures, ventricular dilatation, the syndrome of inappropriate ADH secretion (SIADH), and cardiac failure. Antifibrinolytic agents, such as epsilon-amino-caproic acid, used to preserve the thrombus around an aneurysm, and thereby preventing rebleeding, have been unsuccessful.

Transcranial Doppler screening may be used daily to detect early changes of vasospasm; continuous EEG monitoring and multimodality monitoring of vital signs are other emerging ways to detect cerebral dysfunction while still reversible. Vasospasm may be minimized with the calcium channel antagonist, nimodipine, which crosses the blood-brain barrier; use of nimodipine has become standard of care in SAH patients for up to 3 weeks after hemorrhage. Hydration, hyperosmolar therapy, hypertensive therapy, and angioplasty of vascular spasm may also be used to reduce risk of infarction. Hydrocephalus may require ventricular shunting.

Rehabilitation and Recovery

A team approach to stroke rehabilitation, starting with a stroke recovery unit with experienced physiatrists and physical therapists, has proven beneficial for the optimum recovery of patients. A specialized stroke unit is particularly helpful in avoiding complications such as infections, contractures, decubiti, and in maximizing independence for patients. Speech and occupational therapists help patients improve their swallowing, communication, and daily living skills.

Constraint-induced therapy is a specific type of physical therapy that involves having a hemiparetic patient wear a large mitt to prevent use of the unaffected limb for several hours daily, forcing the patient to use the affected limb for most tasks. In a randomized trial, constraint-induced therapy with intensive task-directed therapy was associated with functional improvement compared to standard physical therapy (Level B). Further studies are still needed to determine whether the use of constraints or the intensive nature of the therapy itself is responsible for the improvements in function since it is both intensive and expensive.

Depression is a frequent accompaniment of stroke, reflecting both the physical disability and altered brain chemistry. Depression may respond to selective serotonin-reuptake inhibitors (SSRIs) and tricyclic antidepressants. Escitalopram administered prophylactically to stroke patients was effective in preventing the development of depression, though other studies have not confirmed this (Level B). There is also evidence from other trials that SSRI treatment facilitates functional recovery after stroke.

Secondary Stroke Prevention

The optimal secondary prevention strategy for an individual patient depends on the stroke mechanism. For stroke or TIA caused by carotid stenosis of 70% or more of the vessel diameter, carotid endarterectomy (CEA) by a skilled surgeon with an acceptable complication rate (<5%) is preferable to medical therapy in good surgical candidates (Level A). For patients at high risk of surgical complications, including those over age 80, those with cardiac or pulmonary disease, or those with radiation-induced arteriopathy, stenting reduces the risks of cardiac complications (Level B). Trials that tested whether carotid angioplasty and stenting are more effective or safer than carotid endarterectomy in patients at low surgical risk have not demonstrated any benefit over open surgery (Level A). Among patients with symptomatic intracranial stenosis (lesions not amenable to surgery), a recent randomized trial demonstrated that best medical therapy, including aggressive risk factor control, was associated with a lower recurrence risk (Level B).

Anticoagulation is indicated in patients with definite cardio-embolic sources of stroke, such as mechanical valves or atrial fibrillation. In embolic strokes caused by atrial fibrillation, anticoagulation with warfarin was superior to aspirin, with a relative risk reduction of about 68% (Level A). Recommended options for secondary prevention among patients with atrial fibrillation now include warfarin with an INR between 2.0 and 3.0, or use of one of the newer antithrombotic agents, such as dabigatran, riva-roxaban, edoxaban, or apixaban (Level A). For patients who cannot tolerate anticoagulants because of a risk of ICH or bleeding elsewhere, newer treatment modalities, including interventions to exclude the left atrial appendage from the circulation using devices or cinching procedures, show promise in early trials, though they are not yet approved (Level B).

Other causes of cardiogenic emboli require different treatments. Infected prosthetic valves need replacement if emboli persist on antibiotics, or if patients develop heart failure. Emboli from myxomatous tumors of the atria frequently require surgical removal of tumor. The need for anticoagulation among patients with less well-established sources of emboli, such as paradoxical embolism through a patent foramen ovale or aortic arch embolization, is unproven, and current guidelines do not support its use in this setting (Level A). Closure of patent foramen ovale using umbrella-like devices may reduce the risk of recurrent stroke in selected patients (younger patients without other stroke risk factors), though recent trials have not proven this effect; further trials in highly selected patients are ongoing.

All patients with ischemic stroke without a definite indication for anticoagulation, and in whom no contraindication is present, should receive long-term antiplatelet therapy, which reduces the risk of recurrence by 20% to 25% (Level A). Agents currently approved for this purpose include aspirin, dipyridamole, and clopidogrel, a thienopyridine derivative ADP receptor inhibitor. Head-to-head trials have failed to demonstrate a benefit of one of these agents over another; the combination of aspirin and dipyridamole was more effective than either agent alone, but long-term treatment with the combination of aspirin and clopidogrel was no more effective than aspirin alone and increased the risk of significant bleeding. A more recent trial in China suggested that there may be benefit to the combination of aspirin and clopido-grel when used for the short term after stroke or TIA, and a similar study is ongoing in the United States. Aspirin doses as low as 30 mg daily appear effective and have fewer side effects, such as gastrointestinal bleeding, than higher doses. The FDA recommends doses between 50 and 325 mg daily for stroke prevention.

Clinical trials provide evidence for increased use of anti-hypertensive agents in patients with stroke and TIA. There are theoretical concerns about lowering blood pressure in patients with existing cerebrovascular disease due to the possibility that in patients with arterial disease of cerebral vessels and reduced autoregulation, a reduction in blood pressure could worsen perfusion and precipitate clinical events or affect cognition. Randomized trials like PROGRESS provide evidence, however, that blood pressure reduction among patients with cerebrovascular disease reduces risks of recurrent stroke by 28% independently

of a history of hypertension (Level A). Guidelines currently focus on the use of blood pressure agents to achieve recommended target blood pressure levels, rather than on specific agents, which should be individualized depending on a patient's comorbidities.

Trials using HMG-CoA reductase inhibitors, or statins, among cardiac and other vascular disease high-risk patients have demonstrated benefits in stroke risk reduction. The Stroke Prevention by Aggressive Reduction in Cholesterol Levels (SPARCL) trial provides more direct evidence of the benefit of statin therapy in secondary prevention of stroke among patients presenting with stroke or TIA (Level A). SPARCL randomized patients with recent stroke or TIA to atorvastatin 80 mg daily or placebo. Over 5 years, atorvastatin reduced the risk of the primary outcome, recurrent stroke, from 13.1% to 11.2%, an absolute risk reduction of about 2%.

Among those with diabetes, diet and exercise, oral hypoglycemic drugs, and insulin are recommended to obtain glycemic control. While glycemic control reduces risks of microvascular complications, the benefit in reducing macrovascular complications is less certain. In one trial, tight glycemic control of a prospective cohort of newly diagnosed diabetics was not found to significantly reduce stroke risk. Ongoing trials are addressing the use of newer agents in secondary stroke prevention among those with insulin resistance.

Behavioral risk factors are difficult to control, but are important. Smoking is addictive, and cessation may necessitate psychologic counseling and medical aids, such as nicotine patches or varenicline. Physical activity should be encouraged, as a sedentary lifestyle is associated with elevations in blood pressure and stroke risk. Alcohol consumption in excess of 2 drinks daily should be discouraged, though there is evidence that moderate alcohol consumption may have protective effects against stroke risk. It should be noted, however, that there is only Level B evidence that control of these risk factors reduces recurrent stroke risk.

PROGNOSIS

The immediate period after an ischemic stroke carries the greatest risk of death, with fatality rates ranging from 8% to 20% in the first 30 days. Age and stroke severity are the most important predictors of prognosis. Case fatality rates are worse for hemorrhagic strokes, ranging from 30% to 80% for intracerebral hemorrhage and 20% to 50% for subarachnoid hemorrhage.

Stroke survivors continue to have a three to fivefold increased risk of death, compared with the age-matched general population. Annual aggregate estimates of death have been 5% for minor stroke and 8% for major stroke. Survival is influenced by age, hypertension, cardiac disease, and diabetes. Patients with lacunar infarcts appear to have a better long-term survival than do those with the other infarct subtypes.

Recurrent stroke is frequent. The immediate period after a stroke carries the greatest risk for early recurrence; rates range from 3% to 10% during the first 30 days. Thirty-day recurrence risks vary by infarct subtypes; the greatest rates are in patients with atherosclerotic infarction and the lowest rates in patients with lacunes. After the early phase, the risk of stroke recurrence continues to threaten the quality of life of a stroke survivor.

Long-term stroke recurrence rates range in different studies from 4% to 14% per year, with aggregate annual estimates of 6% for minor stroke and 9% for major stroke. These rates have been decreasing with the advent of the improved protection strategies outlined above. Recurrent stroke contributes to the burden of dementia and functional decline after stroke. Importantly, cardiac events are also increased in stroke survivors, and pose a major threat of death.

For a deeper discussion on this topic, please see Chapters 64, "Cardiac Arrhythmias with Supraventricular Origin," and 70, "Atherosclerosis, Thrombosis, and Vascular Biology," in Goldman-Cecil Medicine, *25th Edition.*

SUGGESTED READINGS

Amarenco P, Bogousslavsky J, Callahan A 3rd, et al: The Stroke Prevention by Aggressive Reduction in Cholesterol Levels (SPARCL) Investigators. High-Dose Atorvastatin after Stroke or Transient Ischemic Attack, N Engl J Med 355:549–559, 2006.

Broderick JP, Palesch YY, Demchuk AM, et al: Endovascular therapy after intravenous t-PA versus t-PA alone for stroke, N Engl J Med 368:893–903, 2013.

Carroll JD, Saver JL, Thaler DE, et al: Closure of patent foramen ovale versus medical therapy after cryptogenic stroke, N Engl J Med 368:1092–1100, 2013.

Furie KL, Kasner SE, Adams RJ, et al: Guidelines for the prevention of stroke in patients with stroke or transient ischemic attack: a guideline for healthcare professionals from the American Heart Association/American Stroke Association, Stroke 42:227–276, 2011.

Giugliano RP, Ruff CT, Braunwald E, et al: Edoxaban versus warfarin in patients with atrial fibrillation, N Engl J Med 369:2093–2104, 2013.

Goldstein LB, Bushnell CD, Adams RJ, et al: Guidelines for the primary prevention of stroke: a guideline for healthcare professionals from the American Heart Association/American Stroke Association, Stroke 42:517–584, 2011.

Howard G, Lackland DT, Kleindorfer DO, et al: Racial differences in the impact of elevated systolic blood pressure on stroke risk, JAMA Intern Med 173:46–51, 2013.

Jauch EC, Saver JL, Adams HP, et al: Guidelines for the early management of patients with acute ischemic stroke: A Guideline for Healthcare Professionals From the American Heart Association/American Stroke Association, Stroke 44:870–947, 2013.

Kamel H, Elkind MSV, Bhave PD, et al: Paroxysmal Supraventricular Tachycardia and the Risk of Ischemic Stroke, Stroke 44:1550–1554, 2013.

Kidwell CS, Jahan R, Gornbein J, et al: A trial of imaging selection and endovascular treatment for ischemic stroke, N Engl J Med 368:914–923, 2013.

Lackland DT, Elkind MSV, D'Agostino R, et al: Inclusion of stroke in cardiovascular risk prediction instruments: a statement for healthcare professionals from the American Heart Association/American Stroke Association, Stroke 43:1998–2027, 2012.

Mayer SA, Brun NC, Begtrup K, et al: Efficacy and safety of recombinant activated factor VII for acute intracerebral hemorrhage, N Engl J Med 358:2127–2137, 2008.

Meier B, Kalesan B, Mattle HP, et al: Percutaneous closure of patent foramen ovale in cryptogenic embolism, N Engl J Med 368:1083–1091, 2013.

Mendelow AD, Gregson BA, Fernandes HM, et al: Early surgery versus initial conservative treatment in patients with spontaneous supratentorial intracerebral haematomas in the International Surgical Trial in Intracerebral Haemorrhage (STICH): a randomised trial, Lancet 365:387–397, 2005.

Robinson RG, Jorge RE, Moser DJ, et al: Escitalopram and problem-solving therapy for prevention of poststroke depression: a randomized controlled trial, JAMA 299:2391–2400, 2008.

Rothwell PM, Eliasziw M, Gutnikov SA, et al: Analysis of pooled data from the randomised controlled trials of endarterectomy for symptomatic carotid stenosis, Lancet 361:107–116, 2003.

Rutten-Jacobs LC, Arntz RM, Maaijwee NA, et al: Long-term mortality after stroke among adults aged 18 to 50 years, JAMA 309:1136–1144, 2013.

Saver JL, Fonarow GC, Smith EE, et al: Time to treatment with intravenous tissue plasminogen activator and outcome from acute ischemic stroke, JAMA 309:2480–2488, 2013.

Singhal AB, Biller J, Elkind MS, et al: Recognition and management of stroke in young adults and adolescents, Neurology 81:1089–1097, 2013.

SPS3 Study Group, Benavente OR, Coffey CS, et al: Blood-pressure targets in patients with recent lacunar stroke: the SPS3 randomised trial, Lancet 382(9891):507–515, 2013.

Wang Y, Wang Y, Zhao X, et al: Clopidogrel with aspirin in acute minor stroke or transient ischemic attack, N Engl J Med 369:11–19, 2013.

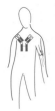

117

Traumatic Brain Injury and Spinal Cord Injury

Geoffrey S.F. Ling

Traumatic brain injury (TBI) and traumatic spinal cord injury (TSCI) are leading causes of traumatic death and disability. Over 8 million patients suffer TBI each year; the vast majority (over 80%) are mild TBI or concussion. Approximately 52,000 patients in the U.S. die from severe TBI as a direct consequence. An additional 11,000 patients are severely disabled by TSCI. The vast majority are due to falls, motor vehicle accidents, sports-related occurrences, and assaults. Among the almost 5.5 million TBI and TSCI survivors, most require prolonged rehabilitation.

TYPES OF INJURY

Certain lesions require neurosurgical intervention while others do not. TBI conditions for which emergency neurosurgery are needed are penetrating wounds, intracerebral hemorrhage with mass effect, including subdural and epidural blood, and bony injury, such as displaced fracture and vertebral subluxation. However, focal, hypoxic-anoxic, diffuse axonal and diffuse microvascular injuries typically do not require surgery.

MANAGEMENT

Tramatic Brain Injury (TBI)

Patients with mild or moderate TBI typically recover quickly and fully. It is critical to first remove the TBI victim from play or work to prevent further injury. Diagnosis of mild TBI or concussion begins simply with identifying affected patients. This is often difficult because these patients suffer transient alteration of consciousness with only a minority completely losing consciousness. Most have memory impairment. As a result, patients are typically unaware that they are injured. Thus, it is important that colleagues, coaches, athletic trainers, parents, and other observers have a heightened suspicion when a potential head injury event occurs. If so, then a sideline point-of-injury screening tool should be administered, such as a standardized assessment of concussion (SAC) or sports concussion assessment tool version 3 (SCAT3). SAC is a neuropsychological battery that tests orientation, immediate memory, concentration, and memory recall. An abnormal score is less than 25. If abnormal, the patient is at high risk for having suffered a concussion and thus should be brought to medical attention for further evaluation, diagnosis and treatment.

In the early stage of management, it is important that a neurologist or medical practitioner skilled in managing TBI perform a detailed history, physical, and neurologic examination, especially assessment of cognitive function. In the history, the practitioner should determine the duration of altered sensorium, amnesia or loss of consciousness a patient may have suffered. The American Academy of Neurology Guidelines uses a grading scale for concussion that is based primarily on the length of these intervals (Table 117-1). Longer periods of abnormal sensorium are associated with higher grades. Higher grades necessitate longer periods of convalescence. Other clinical guides that may be used include the Cantu Grading System and the Colorado Medical Society Guidelines.

The decision to obtain neuroimaging is based on the index of suspicion of intracranial hemorrhage or skull fracture. Both CT and MRI are inadequate in ruling out mild TBI, which is a clinical diagnosis. If a patient has lost consciousness, persistent altered mentation, abnormal GCS score, focal neurologic deficit, or is clinically deteriorating, then neuroimaging should be obtained.

In general, patients with mild TBI do not require major medical intervention; almost all do well after adequate convalescence. It is essential that patients have adequate time for recovery; they should not return to play or work until fully recovered. A second head injury before full recovery may be catastrophic, the second impact syndrome (SIS), which leads to worse clinical outcome, including death.

The patient must be allowed to rest with minimal cognitive burden. There are no specific medications to foster recovery. Treatment is focused on ameliorating symptoms according to published evidence-based guidelines, such as VA/DoD Clinical Practice Guidelines for the Management of Concussion/mild TBI. In general, headache, the most common complaint, can be treated with acetaminophen or a nonsteroidal anti-inflammatory agent. Triptans can be considered if there are features of migraine. Dizziness can be treated with physical therapy. Meclizine should be reserved only for symptoms that are severe enough to impair activities of daily function. Insomnia can be treated with proper sleep hygiene. A sedative can be used acutely and should be

TABLE 117-1	GLASGOW COMA SCORE (GCS)	
BEST EYE RESPONSE	**BEST VERBAL RESPONSE**	**BEST MOTOR RESPONSE**
1 = No eye opening	1 = No verbal response	1 = No motor response
2 = Eye opening to pain	2 = Incomprehensible sounds	2 = Extension to pain
3 = Eye opening to verbal command	3 = Inappropriate words	3 = Flexion to pain
4 = Eyes open spontaneously	4 = Confused	4 = Withdrawal from pain
	5 = Orientated	5 = Localizing pain
		6 = Obeys commands

GCS, Eye Response + Verbal Response + Motor Response.

limited to non-benzodiazepine agents such as zolpidem. Visual and auditory symptoms should be evaluated by appropriate medical specialists.

The patient is able to return to play or work after at least 24 hours of recovery and when cleared to do so by a neurologist or clinical practitioner experienced in the management of concussion. In many states statutes specify these requirements. In general, the patient is able to return to play when symptoms no longer require treatment. At this point, many practitioners will subject the patient to provocative testing such as performing exertion (e.g., running) followed by cognitive testing. If this does not cause symptoms to recur and the patient performs well cognitively, then he or she is allowed to return to full activity.

For moderate to severe TBI the initial care goals are the "ABCs" of airway, breathing, and circulation. Next is "D" for disability (neurologic). Every patient should undergo a detailed neurologic examination to ascertain the level of neurologic disability. An initial Glasgow Coma Score (GCS) should be assigned to each patient. The GCS (Table 117-2) categorizes patients with TBI and provides a quantifiable measure of impairment.

Patients with severe TBI are those who present with GCS scores of eight or less. To optimize outcome, medical management should adhere to currently accepted clinical guidelines such as the Brain Trauma Foundation "Clinical Guidelines for Severe TBI." An important early intervention is airway protection, usually by endotracheal intubation. If elevated intracranial pressure (ICP) is suspected, elevate the patient's head to 30° and keep it midline, ideally with a rigid neck collar (at least until the cervical spine can be evaluated for stability). Mannitol should be given intravenously at a dose of 0.5-1.0 gm/kg. Hyperventilation may also be used with a goal of pCO_2 34-36 mm Hg. ICP should be kept less than 20 mm Hg with the cerebral perfusion pressure (CPP) greater than 60 mm Hg. A head CT without contrast should be done as soon as possible to identify lesions that will require surgery and to determine the extent of injury.

If ICP remains poorly controlled, one can consider administering an intravenous bolus of 23% hypertonic saline (50 mL) followed by continuous infusion of 2% or 3% hypertonic saline (75-125 mL/hr) through a central venous catheter. If these interventions are unsuccessful, pharmacological coma or surgical decompression should be considered. Pharmacological coma can be induced with pentobarbital. This is given as a loading dose of 5 mg/kg intravenously, followed by an infusion of 1-3 mg/kg/hr. Alternatively, propofol can be used, which is administered as a loading dose of 2mg/kg intravenously, followed by an infusion up to 200 µg/min. Continuous EEG monitoring is helpful as the limit of drug-induced coma is achieving ICP control or cerebral electrical burst-suppression. Persistently elevated ICP after all these efforts is ominous. Consideration should be given to frontal or temporal lobe decompression and hemicraniectomy.

To meet CPP goals, patients must first be adequately hydrated. The goal of TBI fluid management is to increase the osmolar gradient between systemic vasculature and brain. For this purpose, hyperosmolar intravenous solutions are used, such as normal saline. Other options are hypertonic saline (e.g., 3% sodium solutions). If meeting CPP goals is difficult with intravenous fluids alone, vasoactive pharmacologic agents such as norepinephrine and phenylephrine can be administered. These two agents are preferred because they are considered to have the least effect on cerebral vasomotor tone. Barbiturates and propofol are myocardial depressants, therefore aggressive cardiovascular management will probably be necessary when pharmacological coma is induced.

Agitation can be treated with lorazepam or haloperidol. If inadequate, then infusions of midazolam or propofol may be used. Pain should be controlled: acetaminophen and nonsteroidal anti-inflammatory agents are adequate for mild discomfort; however, for moderate to severe pain, narcotic analgesics such as fentanyl or morphine should be used. A benefit of opioids is that they can be reversed by naloxone to allow reassessment of neurologic status.

Hypoxia, seizures, and fever must be avoided. Maintaining pO_2 at approximately 100 mm Hg is sufficient. Phenytoin is administered for the first 7 days after injury because it will reduce early onset seizures. After 7 days it should be stopped. It can be restarted if seizures recur. Fever should be reduced with antipyretics such as acetaminophen, using a cooling blanket if needed. Other important management considerations include prevention of gastric stress ulcer, deep vein thrombosis (DVT), and decubitus ulcers. Feeding should be instituted as soon as practical to maintain nutrition.

After the initial few hours, efforts should be made to reduce hyperventilation, which is indicated only for initial emergency management. After 12 hours, metabolic compensation negates the ameliorative effects of respiratory alkalosis caused by the hypocapnic state induced by hyperventilation.

Repeated neurologic examination and continuous ICP and CPP measurement are indicated. Generally, the peak period of cerebral edema is from 48 to 96 hours after TBI. Thereafter, the edema resolves spontaneously and clinical improvement should follow.

TABLE 117-2 AMERICAN ACADEMY OF NEUROLOGY CONCUSSION MANAGEMENT

GRADE 1 (MILD)	GRADE 2 (MODERATE)	GRADE 3 (SEVERE)
Remove from duty/work/play	Remove from duty for the rest of the day	Take to emergency department
Examine immediately and at 5-minute intervals	Examine frequently for signs of CNS deterioration	Neurologic evaluation, including appropriate neuroimaging
May return to duty/work/play if clear within 15 minutes	Physician's neuro exam ASAP (within 24 hours)	Consider hospital admission
	Return to duty/work/play after 1 full asymptomatic week (after being cleared by physician)	

GRADE OF CONCUSSION	RETURN TO PLAY/WORK
Grade 1 (first)	15 minutes
Grade 1 (second injury)	1 week
Grade 2 (first)	1 week
Grade 2 (second injury)	2 weeks
Grade 3 (first) (brief LOC)	1 week
Grade 3 (first) (long LOC)	2 weeks
Grade 3 (second injury)	1 month
Grade 3 (third injury)	Consult a neurologist

A complication of TBI is post-concussive syndrome (PCS). Diagnosis can be made using the Post-Concussion Symptom Scale (PCSS) and Graded Symptom Checklist (GSC). The most common symptoms of PCS are headache, difficulty concentrating, appetite changes, sleep abnormalities, and irritability. PCS has a variable presentation and duration depending on the patient and the severity of TBI. In general, PCS lasts for a few weeks post-injury. However, uncommonly, it can persist beyond a year or more. Treatment is symptomatic. For headache, nonsteroidal anti-inflammatory agents, migraine drugs, and biofeedback can be effective. For cognitive dysfunction, neuropsychological testing may be helpful in determining appropriate intervention, which may include cognitive behavior therapy.

Traumatic Spinal Cord Injury (TSCI)

The emergency management of traumatic injury to the spinal cord has greatly improved with adherence to the American Association of Neurological Surgeons "Guidelines for the Management of Cervical Spine and Spinal Cord Injuries." Therapy begins with the "ABC" of airway, breathing, and circulation. A secure airway is absolutely vital. For patients suffering from high cervical lesions, spontaneous ventilation will be lost. Lesions below C5 may also impair ventilatory capability. If the airway or ventilatory efforts are compromised, emergency intubation is required. For a patient in whom cervical spine trauma has not been assessed, the preferred method is nasotracheal intubation using fiberoptic guidance. Other approaches are nasotracheal (blind) or orotracheal intubation, provided that cervical spine alignment is maintained by traction.

Maintaining an intravascular volume is essential in TSCI. Hypotension may be due to either neurogenic shock or hypovolemia. For neurogenic shock, vasopressive pharmacologic agents, such as phenylephrine, may be needed. If tachycardia is present, then hypovolemia is the more likely etiology and fluid resuscitation with normal saline is the appropriate initial management.

After addressing the "ABC's," a neurologic history and examination should be obtained. An accompanying TBI needs be considered. Up to 50% of TSCI patients have an associated TBI. Neuroimaging is often indicated, but not all patients need radiographic study. A normal neurologic assessment obviates the need for imaging studies; however, a complaint of burning hands or of pain over the spine, numbness, tingling, or weakness indicates possible spinal cord injury. The time of injury should be recorded as accurately as possible. A detailed neurologic examination is needed to identify the level of the injury, the completeness of any deficits, and to document the degree of neurologic dysfunction at the earliest time possible. The level of the injury is the lowest spinal cord segment with intact motor and sensory function. The prognosis for neurologic improvement is better if the lesion is incomplete than complete. Following the acute injury, serial examinations must be made frequently.

If spinal cord injury is suspected, the patient should be immediately and appropriately immobilized with a rigid collar or back board, or both. Radiologic evaluation should begin with plain x-rays of the bony spine. Abnormalities on x-rays should lead to further neuroimaging. Bony vertebrae should be examined with CT and the spinal cord with MRI. Intervertebral and paravertebral soft tissue are best studied with MRI. A chest x-ray should also be obtained in order to visualize the lower cervical and thoracic vertebrae. Presence of a pleural effusion in the setting of a possible thoracic spine injury suggests a hemothorax.

If the C-spine x-rays are normal but the patient complains of neck pain, then ligamentous injury may be present. Ligamentous injury is evaluated by flexion-extension C-spine x-rays. However, in the acute period, pain may prevent an adequate study. These patients should be kept in a rigid cervical collar for a few days until the pain and neck muscle spasm resolves. At that time, imaging may be performed. If abnormal, the patient will need surgical evaluation.

The use of methylprednisolone for TSCI is no longer advocated.

Spinal Cord Syndromes

There are three main spinal cord syndromes: Anterior cord, Brown-Sequard, and Central cord. Anterior cord syndrome is associated with deficits referable to bilateral anterior and lateral spinal cord columns. There is loss of touch sensation, pain, temperature, and motor function below the level of the lesion. The posterior column functions of proprioception and vibratory sensation remain intact. In Brown-Sequard syndrome, the deficits are due to injury to a lateral half of the cord. There is functional loss of ipsilateral motor, touch, proprioception and vibration, and contralateral pain and temperature. Central cord results in a "man in a barrel" syndrome: motor paralysis of both upper extremities with sparing of the lower extremities. Weakness is greater proximally than distally. Pain and temperature sensations are generally reduced, but proprioception and vibration are spared.

Spinal Shock

Spinal shock may occur after acute injury causing a temporary loss of spinal reflexes below the level of injury. Neurologic examination will reveal loss of muscle stretch reflexes, bulbocavernosus reflex, and the anal wink. In high cervical injuries, the lower reflexes (bulbocavernosus and anal wink) may be preserved. There may also be the "Schiff-Sherrington" phenomenon, in which reflexes are affected above the level of injury. Additionally, there may be loss of autonomic reflexes leading to neurogenic shock and ileus and urinary retention.

Acute and Subacute Management

In the intensive care unit, the patient will need continued treatment. Once methylprednisolone therapy has completed, there is no need for further steroid use. TSCI patients require close cardiovascular and respiratory monitoring. Other issues are genitourinary, bowel, infectious disease, nutrition, skin, and prophylaxis against ulcers and deep vein thrombosis formation.

Patients suffering from spinal cord injury are at risk for neurogenic shock and dysautonomia with resulting peripheral vasodilation and hypotension. Lesions at T3 or above compromise sympathetic tone with hypotension accompanied by bradycardia: the classic neurogenic shock triad of bradycardia, hypotension, and peripheral vasodilation.

Dysautonomia is treated by ensuring adequate circulating volume. The goal is to fluid resuscitate to a euvolemic state. Blood can be used if the patient is anemic (i.e., hematocrit less than 30%). If blood is not required, then either colloid (e.g., albumin solutions) or crystalloid (e.g., normal saline) may be used. Central venous pressure (CVP) should be maintained at 4-6 mm Hg. Hypervolemia should be avoided because it will exacerbate peripheral edema. Once an adequate circulating volume has been achieved, vasopressive agents can be used, (e.g., phenylephrine, norepinephine, or dopamine). The mean arterial pressure (MAP) should be 85 mm Hg or greater. Symptomatic bradycardia can be treated with atropine.

Patients with TSCI are at risk for ventilatory compromise. Patients whose injuries are at C5 or higher typically require mechanical ventilation with an appropriate tidal volume (6-10 mL/kg), FiO$_2$ and mandatory machine driven rate. The FiO$_2$ inspired oxygen concentration should give a pO$_2$ between 80-100 mm Hg. The rate should be set to give a pCO$_2$ of 40 mm Hg. Positive end-expiratory pressure (PEEP) should also be used to minimize atelectasis. If the patient does not show signs of ventilatory recovery within 2 weeks of intubation, a tracheostomy should be considered. Lesions below C5 may also be associated with inadequate spontaneous ventilation. Mid-cervical lesions may be associated with intact but compromised diaphragm function. If suspected, a "sniff" test under fluoroscopy can be performed to determine if both hemidiaphragms are functioning properly. If not, intubation/tracheostomy with volume-controlled ventilation may be needed. If intact, then pressure support (PS) ventilation sufficient to maintain an appropriate tidal volume with oxygenation and PEEP should be set as described above.

Patients with cervical lesions at C6 and below, including the thoracic cord, do not require mechanical ventilation. However, their ventilatory effort may be inadequate because the thoracic cord innervates intercostal muscles, which are accessory muscles of respiration. Such patients have decreased cough and inability to increase ventilation when needed, leading to atelectasis and inability to clear secretions, which can cause pneumonia. Such patients need assistance with clearing their airway: chest percussion, suctioning, and encouragement in coughing.

Thromboembolic disease is a leading cause of morbidity and mortality in patients with TSCI: up to 80% will develop DVT without prophylaxis. All patients with TSCI should receive both anticoagulation and have mechanical compression devices applied to their legs. Sequential compression devices (SCD) or compression stockings should be placed as soon as possible. When hemostasis is assured, low molecular weight heparin (LMWH) should be initiated. Unfractionated heparin may also be used in conjunction with SCD but LMWH is preferred. An inferior vena cava filter may be placed in those patients in whom anticoagulation therapy is contraindicated, but it should not be the primary means of preventing DVT.

Mid-low thoracic spinal cord injury can lead to ileus. A nasogastric tube should be placed to decompress the stomach. Parental nutrition should be started as soon as possible. Enteral feeding should be delayed until gastrointestinal motility returns, usually between 2 to 3 weeks. Pharmacologic agents that promote motility are metoclopromide, erythromycin, and cisapride. Gastric ulcer should be prevented with medication: H2 receptor antagonists, proton pump inhibitors, antacids, or sucralfate. Pancreatitis and trauma-related bowel perforation occur: loss of abdominal muscle tone and visceral sensation may mask usual clinical findings of pain, guarding, or rigidity.

Bladder tone may be lost due to spinal shock. A Foley catheter should be placed and maintained for a minimum of 5 to 7 days to drain the bladder and to evaluate circulatory volume and renal status. Once spinal shock resolves, autonomic dysreflexia may occur from bladder distention: skin flushing and hypertension. Clinical examination by palpation and percussion will reveal a distended bladder, which can be treated with intermittent catheterization or bladder training. Phenoxybenzamine may be helpful in this condition.

Nutrition should be given. Until enteral feeding can begin, parenteral nutrition should be used. A caloric level of 80% of the Harris-Benedict prediction should be used for quadriplegic patients. The full Harris-Benedict predicted amount should be used for patients with thoracic spine injuries and below. Skin care is essential to prevent decubitus ulcers. Mechanical kinetic beds, regular log rolling (every 2 hours), and padded orthocics are all useful in minimize this complication.

Orthotics, physical therapy, and occupational therapy (for cervical cord injury) are useful. Therapy should begin as soon as the spine is stabilized with the goal of minimizing contractures and beginning the rehabilitation. Once therapy begins, energy expenditure will increase requiring additional nutrition. If intermittent compression devices need to be removed during therapy, heparin dose may need to be increased.

⬤ PROGNOSIS

Tramatic Brain Injury (TBI)

The most useful prognostic indicator following TBI is the neurologic examination at presentation. Clearly, the better the neurologic examination, the higher the likelihood of improved recovery. The initial GCS score is a very reliable prognostic indicator. The lower the initial GCS score, the less likely a patient will have meaningful neurologic or functional recovery.

Tramatic Spinal Cord Injury (TSCI)

For TSCI, the completeness of the injury is the most useful prognosticator. The American Spine Injury Association Impairment Scale grades spinal cord injury on the basis of completeness (Table 117-3). A grade "A" or complete motor and sensory deficit below the lesion is the most ominous prognosis. If such a lesion persists longer than 24 hours, there is little reasonable likelihood of meaningful recovery. On the other hand, partial injuries, even severe, have substantial probability of recovery.

⬤ FUTURE

TBI and TSCI are serious neurologic conditions with significant implications on society. Prevention remains the most effective way of reducing the incidences of these diseases. Introduction of practice guidelines have contributed to improved outcome from TBI and TSCI. Sadly, morbidity remains a serious problem. Medical management is largely confined to supportive efforts primarily directed towards minimizing secondary injury, optimizing perfusion and oxygenation, and preventing nonneurologic morbidity. Surgical intervention helps restore structural stability, minimize further injury, and reduce the lesion. However

TABLE 117-3   AMERICAN SPINAL INJURY ASSOCIATION IMPAIRMENT SCALE

GRADE	INJURY TYPE	DEFINITION
A	Complete	No motor or sensory function below the lesion
B	Incomplete	Sensory but no motor function
C	Incomplete	Some motor strength (<3)
D	Incomplete	Motor strength >3
E	None	Sensory & motor normal

neither reverses neuronal death nor fully prevents secondary injury processes. There are ongoing significant medical research efforts to improve our understanding of the pathogenesis of these diseases and find ways to mitigate them. As new pharmacologic, medical, and surgical approaches are introduced, there will be increasing opportunities to restore these patients.

For a deeper discussion on this topic, please see Chapter 399, "Traumatic Brain Injury and Spinal Cord Injury," in Goldman-Cecil Medicine, 25th Edition.

SUGGESTED READING

Centers for Disease Control (CDC): State laws governing return to play following traumatic brain injury. Available at www.cdc.gov/concussion/policies.html.

Consensus Statement on TBI. American Academy of Neurology, Neurology 48:581–585, 1997.

Cushman JG, Agarwal N, Fabian TC, et al: EAST practice management guidelines work group: practice management guidelines for the management of mild traumatic brain injury: the EAST practice management guidelines work group, J Trauma 51:1016–1026, 2001.

Giza CC, Kutcher JS, Ashwal S, et al: Summary of evidence-based guideline update: Evaluation and management of concussion in sports: Report of the Guideline Development Subcommittee of the American Academy of Neurology, Neurology 80:2250–2257, 2013.

The Brain Trauma Foundation, The Amer Assn Neurol Surg and The Congress of Neurosurgery: Guidelines for the management of severe traumatic brain injury, J Neurotrauma 24:S1–106, 2007.

VA/DoD clinical practice guidelines for the management of concussion/mild TBI, J Rehabil Res Dev 46:CP1–68, 2009.

Walters BC, Hadley MN, Hurlbert RJ, et al: Guidelines for the management of acute cervical spine and spinal cord injuries: 2013 update, Neurosurgery 60(Suppl 1):82–91, 2013.

118

Epilepsy

Michel J. Berg

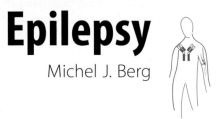

DEFINITION/EPIDEMIOLOGY

Epileptic seizures are defined as a transient occurrence of signs and/or symptoms due to abnormal excessive or synchronous neuronal activity in the brain. Seizures are a common sign of brain dysfunction. A wide variety of symptoms can occur depending on the brain networks involved including involuntary movements, abnormal sensations and behaviors, and impaired consciousness.

Seizures often occur during the course of medical or neurological illnesses in which brain function is temporarily deranged (symptomatic seizures) (Table 118-1). The most common secondary causes of seizures are metabolic derangements (such as hypoglycemia or hyponatremia), intoxications (alcohol, cocaine), acute head trauma, and hypoxic-ischemic conditions (cardiac arrest, syncope, embolic stroke). Symptomatic seizures are usually self-limited and recurrent seizures do not occur after the underlying disorder is corrected. Thus, symptomatic seizures do not constitute epilepsy.

Epilepsy is a chronic disease of the brain characterized by an enduring predisposition to generate epileptic seizures. The diagnosis of epilepsy requires the occurrence of at least one epileptic seizure, but typically is not applied unless there are at least two unprovoked seizures occurring more than 24 hours apart or one unprovoked seizure and a high probability of further seizures

TABLE 118-1 CAUSES OF SYMPTOMATIC SEIZURES*

ACUTE ELECTROLYTE DISORDERS

Acute hyponatremia (<120 mEq/L)
Acute hypernatremia (>155 mEq/L)
Hyperosmolality (>310 mOsm/L)
Hypocalcemia (<7 mg/dL)
Hypoglycemia (<30 mg/dL)

DRUGS

Quinolone antibiotics, isoniazid, penicillins (in renal insufficiency)
Theophylline, aminophylline, ephedrine, phenylpropanolamine, terbutaline
Tramadol, lidocaine, meperidine (in renal insufficiency)
Tricyclic antidepressants
Cyclosporine
Cocaine (crack), phencyclidine, amphetamines; alcohol withdrawal

CENTRAL NERVOUS SYSTEM DISEASE

Hypertensive encephalopathy, eclampsia
Hepatic and uremic encephalopathy
Sickle cell disease, thrombotic thrombocytopenic purpura
Systemic lupus erythematosus
Meningitis, encephalitis, brain abscess
Acute head trauma, stroke, brain tumor

*The metabolic derangements and drugs listed in Table 118-1 also lower the seizure threshold in people with epilepsy.

based on additional data such as an epileptiform EEG. The phrase *seizure disorder* is synonymous with the word, epilepsy. Individuals with epilepsy have increased seizure susceptibility (lowered seizure threshold). Genetic factors and prior brain injury (from a multitude of causes) are the major contributors to this susceptibility. The diagnosis of epilepsy encompasses the neurobiological, cognitive, psychological, and social consequences of this condition.

There are many different *epilepsy syndromes* (the epilepsies) with the three major categories being focal epilepsy, idiopathic (genetic) generalized epilepsy, and symptomatic generalized epilepsy (discussed later). Classification of the epilepsy syndrome depends on a number of factors, including the seizure type, etiology, genetic mutations, neuroimaging, and response to therapy.

The care of people with seizures suffers from imprecise terminology usage. The word "epilepsy" is a noun, as in, "a person with epilepsy." The word "epileptic" is an adjective, as in, "an epileptic seizure." An individual with epilepsy should not be labeled as an "epileptic." That is, from the psychosocial perspective, people with epilepsy are more than just an enduring predisposition to seizures and their consequences. Epilepsy is thought of as a disorder, but, to emphasize the impact of the recurrent seizures, epilepsy should be considered a disease. Epileptic seizures, also referred to as electrical seizures, are distinct from nonepileptic (or nonelectrical) seizures, which have a psychological basis and are best referred to as psychogenic nonepileptic attacks (less appropriately termed pseudoseizures; see later). Most seizures in someone with epilepsy occur in an unpredictable fashion. It is this unpredictable timing that results in the major negative impact of epilepsy on quality of life. If functionally impairing seizures occur during waking hours *(diurnal seizures)* then activity restrictions are required, including restriction from driving, operating heavy machinery, climbing heights, and unobserved swimming or bathing (showering with a good drain should be advised). These activity restrictions lead to loss of independence. The psychological impact of having intermittent involuntary loss of body control and the dependency imposed by the activity restrictions are major contributors to the increased incidence of comorbid depression in people with epilepsy (up to 50%).

In many people with epilepsy there are more seizures during sleep due to increased synchronization of neuronal activity. Seizures that occur exclusively in sleep constitute *nocturnal epilepsy*. In women with epilepsy (WWE), seizures sometimes occur more often during the week around menses or at ovulation (*catamenial epilepsy*). Sleep deprivation, alcohol consumption, infectious illnesses, certain medications, and severe emotional stressors can further lower the seizure threshold and are associated with more seizures in people with epilepsy (Table 118-1).

Seizures can occur at any time. Ten percent of the population in developed countries has a seizure at some time during their life. In contrast, 0.7% to 1% has current epilepsy (prevalence) and 3% to 4% has epilepsy at some time during their life (lifetime prevalence). In the United States, there are approximately 125,000 new cases of epilepsy diagnosed each year (incidence). The incidence and prevalence are biphasic, with epilepsy being more common in childhood (primarily because of perinatal injury, infections, and genetic factors) and in old age (because of stroke, tumors, and dementia) (Fig. 118-1). In developing countries the frequency of epilepsy is higher because of factors such as increased brain infections with organisms such as cysticercosis.

PATHOLOGY

Prior to the 1990s, the underlying cause was not determined in most people with epilepsy. The advent of MRI and, more recently, genetic analysis has substantially improved our ability to identify the cause of many types of epilepsy. About 70% of adults and 40% of children with new-onset epilepsy have partial (focal) seizures implying a cerebral injury or lesion. The most common lesions are hippocampal sclerosis, neuronal and glial tumors, vascular malformations, neuronal migration disorders (e.g., cortical dysplasia), hamartomas, encephalitis, autoimmunity, cerebral trauma, embolic stroke, and hemorrhage. Hippocampal sclerosis

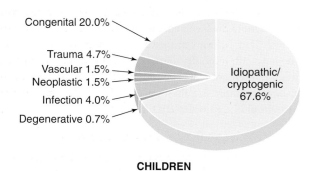

Congenital 20.0%
Trauma 4.7%
Vascular 1.5%
Neoplastic 1.5%
Infection 4.0%
Degenerative 0.7%
Idiopathic/cryptogenic 67.6%

CHILDREN

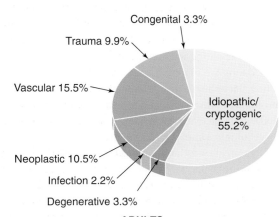

Congenital 3.3%
Trauma 9.9%
Vascular 15.5%
Neoplastic 10.5%
Infection 2.2%
Degenerative 3.3%
Idiopathic/cryptogenic 55.2%

ADULTS

FIGURE 118-1 Etiology of epilepsy, according to age, in all newly diagnosed cases in Rochester, Minnesota, 1935–1984. (Modified from Hauser WA, Annegers JF, Kurland LT: Incidence of epilepsy and unprovoked seizures in Rochester, Minnesota: 1935–1984, Epilepsia 34:453–468, 1993.)

(sometimes referred to as mesial temporal sclerosis) is particularly common and can occur in isolation or secondary to another epileptogenic lesion (dual pathology). It consists of loss of pyramidal cells and gliosis in several hippocampal subfields. Hippocampal sclerosis is associated with temporal lobe epilepsy and short-term memory dysfunction. Not all patients with cerebral lesions develop epilepsy; how or why a particular lesion becomes epileptogenic is poorly understood.

Hereditary influences have long been associated with epilepsy. During the past several decades, a number of gene mutations have been associated with specific epilepsy syndromes, both focal and generalized. Many of the mutations occur in ion channels, which, not surprisingly, lead to neuronal dysfunction and epilepsy. Two important phenotypic examples of channelopathies are genetic (generalized) epilepsy with febrile seizures plus (GEFS+) and Dravet syndrome (also known as severe myoclonic epilepsy of infancy). GEFS+ is typically associated with a partial loss of function mutation in the voltage-gated sodium channel gene, *SCN1A*, whereas a complete loss of function mutation in the same gene results in Dravet syndrome. Less commonly, mutations in other ion channel genes can lead to the same phenotypic expressions. GEFS+ can begin at any age, although is usually evident in childhood, with various seizure types in different affected family members; some may have febrile seizures after age 6 years (febrile seizures plus), whereas others may have myoclonic, absence, or partial seizures. In contrast, Dravet syndrome typically presents at 6 to 8 months of age with prolonged hemiclonic seizures associated with an intercurrent fever. Adults with Dravet syndrome are typically mentally retarded with spasticity or ataxia, gait dysfunction, and occasion nocturnal clonic seizures as well as other seizure types. Recognition of Dravet syndrome is important because certain antiepileptic drugs (AEDs) can cause permanent clinical deterioration (e.g., lamotrigine, phenytoin), whereas others are particularly beneficial (e.g., topiramate, levetiracetam, valproate, benzodiazepines).

CLINICAL PRESENTATION

Classification and Clinical Manifestations

Seizures are classified by their clinical symptoms and signs. The manifestations of a seizure depend on whether its onset includes most or only a part of the cerebral cortex, on the functions of the involved cortical areas, and on the subsequent pattern of spread within the brain. Seizures are of two broad types: those with onset limited to a specific region of cerebral cortex (*partial or focal seizures*) and those with onset that involves the cerebral cortex diffusely (*generalized seizures*). Seizures are dynamic with an evolving electrical discharge. Thus, highly focal (*simple partial*) seizures can progress into more widespread (*complex partial*) seizures and partial seizures can evolve into secondarily generalized tonic-clonic seizures.

In an individual, seizures are typically stereotyped, although a person can have more than one seizure type and a specific seizure type can have varying intensities. The behaviors that occur during the seizure are termed the *seizure semiology*. The seizure itself is referred to as the ictus and the period of time during which the seizure occurs is termed the *ictal phase*. The time after the seizure, until the patient is fully recovered, is the *postictal phase* and the time between seizures (which can be seconds to years) is the *interictal phase*.

The *epilepsy syndromes* can be divided into three major categories: *focal epilepsy, idiopathic (primary) generalized epilepsy,* and *symptomatic generalized epilepsy.* This classification is based on the widely used scheme of the International League against Epilepsy. This scheme is undergoing revision. In the future, the epilepsies may be classified as genetic, structural/metabolic, and unknown cause. The current classification of the epilepsy syndromes closely follows the classification of the seizures. In the following paragraphs, the specific seizure types are described followed by a description of the attendant epilepsy syndromes.

Partial Seizures (Seizure Types)

In *partial seizures* (also known as localization-related or focal seizures) a localized region of the brain has abnormal neurons that intermittently fire hypersynchronously, recruiting the surrounding, otherwise normal neurons, generating a seizure. If the abnormal neuronal firing is confined, there may be no clinical manifestation and the event, which can only be detected with EEG, is termed a *subclinical* or *electrical seizure.*

Simple Partial Seizures

If the electrical discharge involves a clinically functional small area, a *simple partial seizure (SPS)* occurs and manifests as a symptom without impairment of consciousness. The symptom may be a sensation, autonomic function (e.g., nausea or another epigastric sensation), abnormal thought (e.g., fear, dèjá vu), or involuntary movement. An SPS is commonly called an *aura* and can serve as a warning that a more intense seizure is about to occur. Auras occur in about 60% of patients with focal epilepsy.

During an SPS the patient can interact normally with their environment except for limitations imposed by the seizure itself on specific functions. Thus, SPSs are divided into *SPS without impairment*, which do not interfere with function (e.g., just an internal sensation) and *SPS with impairment*, which can interfere with function (e.g., a jerking limb that would disrupt the ability to drive safely).

The motor signs of a seizure can be *clonic* (rhythmic jerking) or *tonic* (stiffening) movements of a discrete body part. An SPS restricted to the precentral (Rolandic) gyrus that spreads to involve adjacent areas of the primary motor cortex, is expressed as clonic movements that progress in an orderly sequence (*Jacksonian march*) that reflects the motor cortex homunculus topographic organization (e.g., mouth to hand to arm to leg).

Complex Partial Seizures

A *complex partial seizure (CPS)* is a focal-onset seizure with impairment of consciousness. The degree of consciousness impairment ranges from minimal to complete unresponsiveness. The patient's eyes are almost always open during the ictus indicating an awake state (albeit impaired). The eyes may close after the seizure ends and the patient typically experiences some degree of postictal confusion, fatigue, and sometimes headache (with the head pain often ipsilateral to the seizure focus due to the increased metabolic demand). An CPS typically lasts 1 to 3 minutes with a postictal state of a few minutes to hours. The specific signs and symptoms that occur during a partial

TABLE 118-2	LOCALIZATION OF SEIZURES BY SYMPTOMS AND ICTAL MANIFESTATIONS
LOCUS	**MANIFESTATION**
TEMPORAL LOBE	
Uncus/amygdala	Foul odor
Middle/inferior temporal gyrus	Visual changes: micropsia, macropsia
Parahippocampal-hippocampal area	Déjà vu; jamais vu
Amygdala-septal area	Fear, pleasure, anger, dreamy sensation
Auditory association cortex	Voices, music
Insular, anterior temporal cortex	Lip smacking, drooling, abdominal symptoms, cardiac arrhythmia
FRONTAL LOBE	
Motor cortex	Contralateral clonic movements of face, fingers, hand, foot
Premotor cortex	Contralateral arm extension, hypermotor behaviors
Language areas	Speech arrest, aphasia
Lateral cortex	Contralateral eye deviation
Bifrontal	Absence-like seizure
Parietal lobe cortex	Sensory symptoms
Occipital lobe cortex	Visual hallucinations (often in color), teichopsias, metamorphopsias

seizure characteristically reflect the location of seizure onset (Table 118-2). The location of the focus is important because it can predict the nature of the pathology and directs diagnostic testing. Both medical and surgical treatment is determined, in part, by focus location.

Psychomotor, temporal lobe, and *limbic seizures* are terms that have been used in the past to describe a variety of ictal behaviors now classified as CPSs, but they are not synonymous. Not all complex partial seizures arise from the temporal lobe, nor do all involve the limbic system. Similarly, certain temporal lobe and limbic phenomena may not be associated with the alteration in awareness that is required to term it a CPS.

Secondarily Generalized Convulsive Seizures

A focal-onset seizure that spreads throughout the brain results in a *secondarily generalized seizure.* Typically there is a tonic phase that consists of extensor posturing lasting 20 to 60 seconds followed by progressively longer periods of inhibition manifesting as a clonic phase that lasts up to another minute: hence the descriptive name *generalized tonic-clonic (GTC)* seizure. The terms convulsion, GTC, grand-mal, and major-motor seizure are often used interchangeably, although GTC is a specific phenomenological description of the behavior. In some patients, a few clonic jerks precede the tonic-clonic sequence; in others, only a tonic or clonic phase is present.

As a partial seizure transitions into a secondarily generalized convulsion the arm contralateral to the seizure focus may extend first, while the ipsilateral arm is flexed at the elbow. This is termed the *figure-4 sign* and is useful for lateralizing the seizure focus. A loud *tonic-cry* may occur at the onset of a convulsion as air is forcibly expelled through tightly contracted vocal cords. The eyes are open and commonly described to roll upward. During a convulsion, breathing stops and cyanosis may develop. Foaming at the mouth may be present. Oral trauma, especially biting the tongue, is typical. Urinary incontinence is common. Fecal incontinence is rare. First aid involves turning the patient onto a side as the seizure ends to allow the saliva to drool out the mouth, decreasing the likelihood of aspiration. Witnesses commonly describe a GTC as lasting 5 to 10 minutes or longer; however, the GTC phase rarely lasts longer than 2 minutes. The postictal phase is marked by transient deep stupor, followed in 15 to 30 minutes by a lethargic, confused state, sometimes with automatic behaviors. As recovery progresses, many patients complain of headache, muscle soreness, mental dulling, lack of energy, or mood changes lasting for hours to days. Convulsions result in a number of striking, but transient, physiologic changes, including hypoxemia, lactic acidosis, elevated catecholamine levels, and increased serum concentrations of creatine kinase, prolactin, corticotropin, and cortisol. Complications include oral trauma, vertebral compression fractures, shoulder dislocation, aspiration pneumonia, and, very rarely, sudden death, which may be related to acute pulmonary edema, cardiac arrhythmia, or suffocation. Sudden Unexplained Death in Epilepsy (SUDEP) has garnered increased attention during the past decade, but remains poorly understood.

Partial seizures of all intensities may be followed by a transient neurological abnormality reflecting postictal depression of the epileptogenic cortical area. Thus, focal weakness may follow a partial motor seizure or numbness a sensory seizure. These reversible neurological deficits are referred to as *Todd's paralysis* and last minutes to hours, rarely more than 48 hours. Examination of a patient immediately after a seizure may show transient focal abnormalities that indicate the site or at least the side of seizure origin.

Focal Epilepsy (Epilepsy Syndrome)

Focal (localization-related, partial) *epilepsy* is characterized by recurrent partial seizures. It is divided into two main groups, idiopathic and symptomatic.

Idiopathic Focal Epilepsy

The idiopathic focal epilepsies are thought to be due to subtle genetic developmental anomalies that manifest in childhood and remit during puberty. There are several syndromes including occipital, frontal, and the most common type, *benign epilepsy with central midtemporal spikes* (BECTS), which is also known as *benign Rolandic epilepsy* (BRE). BECTS represents about 15% of all pediatric epilepsies. In BECTS, seizures usually begin between the ages of 3 and 12 years in an otherwise normal child. The seizures consist of brief simple partial hemifacial motor or sensory events. There is typically twitching of one side of the face, speech arrest, drooling, and paresthesias of the face, gums, tongue, or inner cheeks. These signs may be so minor that they escape notice, although the affected child often points to his face and goes to a parent and holds on until it is over; the child then quickly resumes normal activity. Seizures may progress to include hemiclonic movements or hemitonic posturing. Secondarily generalized tonic-clonic seizures occasionally occur, usually during sleep. The parents may report only the convulsions; the focal signature can be missed unless the child is carefully questioned. The EEG reveals distinctive, stereotyped epileptiform discharges over the central and midtemporal regions that are dramatically activated by sleep with a normal underlying background.

Prognosis for BECTS is invariably good, as it is for most of the other benign focal epilepsy syndromes; the seizures disappear and the EEG normalizes by mid to late adolescence. Outcome is not affected by treatment, but AEDs prevent recurrent attacks.

Symptomatic Focal Epilepsy

The symptomatic focal epilepsies are the most common type of epilepsy and are classified based on the cerebral lobe involved during the initial phase of the seizure. Temporal lobe epilepsy is the most frequent, followed by frontal, with rarer cases of parietal and occipital. Although sometimes not identified in life, all cases of symptomatic focal epilepsy have an underlying focal abnormality in the cerebral cortex such as a scar, malformation, growth, or abnormal gene expression. An individual patient with symptomatic focal epilepsy usually has a single focus. However, the focus can involve a large, multilobar circuit. Some patients have multiple foci, each with different seizure manifestations.

Temporal lobe epilepsy (TLE) is the most common epilepsy syndrome of adults, accounting for at least 40% of epilepsy cases. Habitual seizures typically begin in childhood or adolescence although onset in adulthood occurs. There may be a history of childhood febrile seizures. Most patients have complex partial seizures, some of which secondarily generalize. *Medial temporal lobe seizures* involve the hippocampal and amygdalar areas. A rising epigastric sensation or vague cephalic sensation is the most common aura symptom. Less frequently, the classical symptom of a foul smell, déjà vu, or other odd thinking occurs. Olfactory auras are referred to as *uncinate seizures* because of their origin in or near the uncus of the medial temporal lobe. In *lateral (neocortical) temporal lobe seizures* language impairment (dominant hemisphere), recurring vocalizations (nondominant hemisphere), eye blinking, or formed visual or auditory hallucinations can occur. As a temporal lobe seizure spreads to involve the dominant temporal lobe or bilateral temporal lobe structures, including the limbic system, the seizure becomes complex. A blank stare is often described by witnesses. Automatic motor behaviors, termed *automatisms,* are common in seizures that involve the limbic system (usually in the temporal lobe). Automatisms include oro-alimentary signs (e.g., lip-smacking, repetitive swallowing) and repetitive hand movements (manual automatisms).

Frontal lobe epilepsy (FLE) can be difficult to diagnose because the scalp EEG may be normal or not reveal a classic epileptic discharge, even during seizures. Depending on the area involved there are at least four different *premotor* frontal lobe seizure semiological patterns. *Supplementary motor* seizures (superior frontal gyri, posterior aspect) consist of contralateral versive posturing of the head and arms such that a fencing posture is assumed; the contralateral arm is extended, the head is turned strongly to that side, and the ipsilateral arm is flexed and held either up above the head or across the chest. *Lateral frontal* seizures manifest as contralateral head and eye deviation. *Hypermotor* seizures (frontal, poorly localized) can be dramatic and consist of wild asynchronous movements and are often confused with psychogenic nonepileptic attacks; thus, they are sometimes termed *pseudo-pseudoseizures*. Almost all hypermotor seizures last less than 40 seconds and typically occur 1 to 5 times a night during sleep and less often during waking. Obscene verbal expletives are commonly uttered loudly during hypermotor seizures.

Frontal absence seizures are rare and are due to diffuse, bisynchronous frontal epileptic activity. These consist of staring and mimic typical or atypical absence seizures (see later). Seizures arising in the posterior frontal lobe motor cortex (precentral gyrus) are classically clonic with a Jacksonian march.

Parietal and occipital lobe epilepsy involve sensory structures and at least initially, have only subjective symptoms. *Parietal lobe seizures* consist of somatosensory sensations or higher cognitive function disruption. The somatosensory sensations can have a Jacksonian march with sensory symptoms progressing along the sensory homunculus. *Occipital lobe seizures* involve unformed or poorly formed visual hallucinations that are often in color (in contrast to the visual aura of migraine, which is black, gray, and white). Forced eye deviation can occur with occipital seizures. Occipital seizures can have a prolonged discharge lasting tens of minutes that is subclinical or minimally clinical before propagating. Parietal and occipital seizures do not become complex until propagating to the temporal lobes or limbic system. *Reflex seizures* are precipitated by a specific stimulus, such as touch, a musical tune, a particular movement, reading, flashing lights, or certain complex visual images. With the exception of the photosensitive response in juvenile myoclonic epilepsy (see later) which is relatively common, reflex seizures are rare and classified as a type of parietal or occipital lobe epilepsy because these regions mediate sensory functions.

Posttraumatic epilepsy is a type of symptomatic focal epilepsy distinguished by its etiology. The likelihood of developing posttraumatic epilepsy relates directly to the severity of the head injury. The relative risk for developing epilepsy after a penetrating wound to the brain (e.g., bullet or shrapnel) is up to six hundred times that in the general population. Severe closed head injuries result in epilepsy in 20% of patients. Severe closed head injuries are defined by the presence of an intracranial hemorrhage (subdural, epidural, subarachnoid, or cerebral contusion), unconsciousness or amnesia lasting more than 24 hours, or persistent abnormalities on neurological examination, such as hemiparesis

or aphasia. Although the majority of the patients with a severe head injury develop seizures within 1 to 2 years, new-onset epilepsy may appear after 20 years or longer. Mild closed head injuries (uncomplicated brief loss of consciousness, no skull fracture, absence of focal neurological signs, and no contusion or hematoma) may minimally increase the risk of seizures. Posttraumatic epilepsy is always focal or multifocal, although only convulsions may be clinically evident, especially with multifocal injury. Several early seizures within a week of a head injury do not necessarily predict that future epilepsy will be present.

Primary Generalized Seizures (Seizure Types)

Primary generalized seizures begin diffusely and involve both cerebral hemispheres simultaneously from the outset. Primary generalized seizures should be distinguished from partial seizures because in some cases they have similar clinical features, yet respond to different treatments.

Absence seizures (historically termed petit mal) occur mainly in children and are characterized by sudden, momentary lapses in awareness with staring. Sometimes rhythmic blinking occurs with a slight loss of neck tone. Most absence seizures last less than 10 seconds. If the absence lasts longer than 20 seconds, automatisms are usually present, making differentiation from partial seizures based on clinical observation difficult. The EEG has a characteristic pattern of generalized 3 per second spike and slow waves (Fig. 118-2) during an absence seizure. Behavior and awareness return to normal immediately after the seizure ends, although brief confusion may be present if the surroundings changed during the seizure. There is no postictal period and usually no recollection that a seizure occurred.

Myoclonic seizures manifest as rapid, recurrent, brief muscle jerks that can occur unilaterally or bilaterally, synchronously or asynchronously, without loss of consciousness. To be a seizure, the myoclonus must have a corresponding discharge on EEG. Other types of myoclonus, such as benign nocturnal (hypnic) jerks, or subcortical and spinal myoclonus related to lesions,

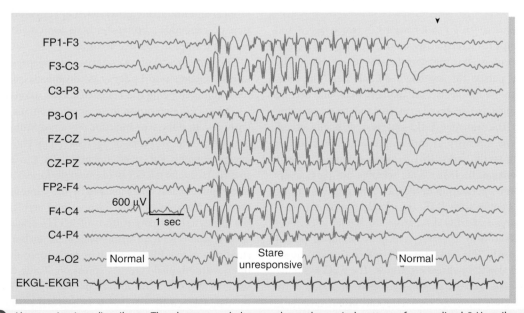

FIGURE 118-2 Absence (petit mal) epilepsy. The electroencephalogram shows the typical pattern of generalized 3-Hz spike-wave complexes associated with a clinical absence seizure.

which do not have an EEG correlate, are not considered epileptic seizures. The jerks of myoclonic seizures range from small movements of the face or hands to massive bilateral spasms that simultaneously affect the head, limbs, and trunk. Repeated myoclonic seizures may crescendo and evolve into a generalized tonic-clonic seizure. Although myoclonic seizures can occur at any time, clusters shortly after awakening are typical.

Primary generalized tonic-clonic seizures may begin with a few myoclonic jerks or abruptly with a tonic phase lasting 20 to 60 seconds and then a clonic phase of similar duration followed by a postictal state. Although there are usually no focal features, sometimes head turning occurs; this movement does not suggest a specific localization. If the onset is missed, it is often not possible to distinguish a primary generalized convulsion from a secondarily generalized one due to focal epilepsy.

Idiopathic Generalized Epilepsy (Epilepsy Syndrome)

The idiopathic (primary) generalized epilepsies (IGEs) are likely polygenic resulting from a combination of mutations and polymorphisms in genes involved in thalamocortical circuitry. Different members of the same family often have dissimilar phenotypes. However, only rare IGE genes have been identified. A person with IGE has a 10% chance of passing the condition to a child. Most people with IGE have normal intelligence.

Childhood absence epilepsy (CAE; pyknolepsy, petit mal epilepsy) is the most common type of childhood epilepsy. It begins between 3 to 12 years of age with a peak at 7 years. Children with CAE have frequent absences (often hundreds per day) and are sometimes initially thought to have attention problems or to be daydreamers. Parents tend to report more absences at meal times, but that is due to closer observation; the absences are present throughout the day. One half of children with CAE have occasional GTC seizures. CAE is self-limited and seizures and the EEG abnormalities resolve by young adulthood. The absence seizures of CAE are typically provoked by hyperventilation, a useful procedure in the office setting and during an EEG.

Juvenile myoclonic epilepsy (JME) begins between age 8 and 20 years old. It is characterized by clusters of myoclonic seizures in the morning, starting shortly after awakening. The clusters typically persist for several to 30 minutes. The jerks are predominantly in the arms and last less than one second each. Consciousness is preserved. An affected teenager often fails to mention the morning jerks unless specifically asked. Sometimes there is a history of throwing breakfast utensils or toothbrushes due to the jerks. JME is often diagnosed after a morning GTC seizure. In JME, GTC seizures are particularly common after sleep deprivation or alcohol consumption during the prior night. People with JME are usually photic sensitive. That is, the seizures and EEG discharges are activated by flickering lights between 5 to 20 Hz (*photic-paroxysmal* or *photic-convulsive* response). This is a type of reflex seizure. Some people with JME also have absence seizures. The EEG is similar to that seen in CAE, but the generalized spike and slow wave discharges are slightly faster (3 to 4 Hz) and often have polyspike components. In contrast to CAE, the seizures in JME persist into adulthood and can be lifelong, although they lessen with age.

Less common IGE phenotypes include *juvenile absence epilepsy (JAE)* and *generalized tonic-clonic seizures alone (GTCA)*. In JAE the predominant seizure type is absence with onset in the teenage years and, like JME, persists into adulthood. In GTCA the predominant seizure type is a convulsion, sometimes with a predilection for the morning. Less frequent absences or myoclonic seizures can occur in GTCA. Although onset of IGE is typically during childhood or teenage years, rare cases occur with onset in all ages of adulthood and are called a*dult absence epilepsy (AAE)*.

Symptomatic Generalized Seizures (Seizure Types)

Symptomatic generalized seizures involve rapidly synchronized abnormal brain activity across the corpus callosum or involving midbrain structures occurring in brains with diffuse or multifocal dysfunction usually from early life.

Drop seizures can be either or both tonic and atonic. "Drop" implies that if the patient is upright they fall with no protective reflexes. Patients with drop seizures often suffer head injuries and should wear a helmet except when they are directly attended by a care provider, in a secure chair, or lying down. During a *tonic seizure*, the arms abruptly thrust forward at a 90 degree angle to the body and the entire body stiffens. Classically the fall is backwards. During an *atonic seizure*, tone is abruptly lost in the postural muscles and the patient falls forward.

Atypical absence seizures manifest as staring or mental slowing associated with a slow generalized spike and slow wave discharge (2.5 Hz or less) on the EEG. They may last minutes or even hours. Fluctuating levels of awareness and gradual onset and offset is described with atypical absences.

Symptomatic Generalized Epilepsies (Epilepsy Syndrome)

Symptomatic generalized epilepsies occur in people with multifocal or diffuse brain dysfunction from early in life. There is usually an associated encephalopathy with some degree of developmental delay. In addition to all of the seizure types that occur in focal and idiopathic generalized epilepsy, people with symptomatic generalized epilepsies have tonic and atonic drop seizures and atypical absence seizures.

There are several unrelated types of epilepsy under the Symptomatic Generalized Epilepsy syndrome classification, with the most common being the *Lennox-Gastaut syndrome (LGS)*.

The *LGS* is a common form of symptomatic generalized epilepsy due to diffuse or multifocal brain dysfunction. LGS presents from 2 to 10 years of age. Sixty percent have preexisting encephalopathy and developmental delay and 20% had infantile spasms (see later). LGS is responsible for 5% to 10% of childhood epilepsy. It is characterized by the combination of tonic or atonic seizures, myoclonic seizures, and atypical absences with the characteristic EEG pattern of 2.5 Hz or slower generalized spike and slow waves. During sleep there are bursts of diffuse fast rhythms on the EEG consistent with tonic or atonic seizures often with minimal clinical expression. Tonic-clonic and partial seizures also occur. Almost all people with LGS have developmental delay with associated behavioral disorders. LGS is a chronic condition requiring supervision; many ultimately live in group homes. If drop seizures are present, and the patient is ambulatory, a helmet should be prescribed for protection.

Infantile Spasms are often a precursor of the LGS, although not formally classified as symptomatic generalized epilepsy. By definition, infantile spasms begin during the first year of life. They affect approximately 1 in 5000 children. The epileptic spasms manifest as flexor or extensor tonus, myoclonus, or a mixed pattern. The spasms last 1 to 20 seconds each and occur in clusters for up to 20 minutes. *West Syndrome* is the combination of epileptic spasms, hypsarrhythmia (a chaotic, disorganized epileptiform EEG pattern), and mental retardation. It is common for the term infantile spasms to be used synonymously with West syndrome. Infantile spasms have a poor prognosis with over 90% developing mental retardation and most progressing to symptomatic generalized epilepsy; a small percent of cryptogenic cases recover. There are many causes of infantile spasms including perinatal insults, cerebral malformations, CNS infections, tuberous sclerosis, and inborn errors of metabolism.

Other Seizure Conditions

Febrile seizures affect between 3% and 5% of children younger than the age of 6 years. About 30% of children have more than one episode; the likelihood of recurrence is greater if the first seizure occurs before 1 year of age or there is a family history of febrile seizures. There are a number of genes that, when mutated, predispose to febrile seizures. Although most affected children have no long-term consequences, febrile seizures increase the risk of developing epilepsy later in life. This risk is low for most children (2% to 3%), but is 10% to 15% in those who had prolonged or focal febrile seizures (*complicated febrile seizures*), a family history of nonfebrile seizures, or neurological abnormalities before the first febrile seizure.

⬤ DIAGNOSIS

Accurate diagnosis is the cornerstone of epilepsy treatment. The diagnostic evaluation has three objectives: to determine that the events are epileptic seizures, to identify a specific underlying cause, and to establish if the seizures are symptomatic and isolated or if epilepsy is present and, if so, to determine the specific epilepsy syndrome.

History and Examination

The patient's and witnesses' descriptions of the events are central to diagnosis. Extra attention should be given to exploring details of the behavior during the seizure. The setting of the seizure can suggest acute causes such as drug withdrawal, central nervous system infection, trauma, or stroke. Recent-onset seizures in an adult suggest a new intracranial lesion. A remote history of seizures suggests epilepsy. Any focal feature before, during, or after the seizure suggests a structural brain lesion requiring appropriate investigation. The pattern of the seizures and the patient's age are often important clues to the seizure and epilepsy type.

The physical examination is normal in most patients with epilepsy. Examination should seek overt or subtle focal neurological signs: slight unilateral lower facial paresis, clumsy fine finger movements, or mild hyperreflexia. These can be present in focal epilepsy with a contralateral seizure focus. Careful skin examination is indicated to detect features of neurocutaneous syndromes such as a facial port-wine stain involving the upper eyelid in Sturge-Weber syndrome, hypopigmented macules (ash-leaf spots), shagreen patch, facial angiofibromas in tuberous sclerosis, and café-au-lait spots and axillary freckling in neurofibromatosis. Asymmetry in the size of the hands, feet, or face signifies a long-standing abnormality of the cerebral hemisphere contralateral to the smaller side. Absence seizures can be triggered in untreated children with hyperventilation for 2 to 3 minutes.

Laboratory Tests—EEG

Electroencephalography (EEG) is the most helpful diagnostic test for seizures and epilepsy. EEG findings help establish the diagnosis, classify the seizures correctly, identify the epilepsy syndrome, and make therapeutic decisions. In combination with suitable clinical findings, *epileptiform* EEG discharges, termed *spikes* or *sharp waves*, strongly support a diagnosis of epilepsy. In patients with recurrent seizures, focal epileptiform discharges are consistent with focal epilepsy, whereas generalized epileptiform activity usually indicates a generalized form of epilepsy. However, most EEGs are obtained between seizures, and interictal abnormalities alone cannot prove or disprove a diagnosis of epilepsy. Up to 50% of patients with epilepsy show epileptiform abnormalities on their initial EEG. The chance of capturing epileptiform activity is enhanced by sleep deprivation the night before the test so that the patient sleeps during a portion of the EEG recording. Serial EEGs increase the yield of positive tracings. A small proportion of patients with epilepsy have normal interictal EEGs despite all efforts to record an abnormality.

The interpretation of the interictal EEG is confounded by two factors. Epileptiform discharges occur in about 2% of normal people; many of these may be asymptomatic markers of a genetic trait, especially in children. Also, the interpretation of the EEG is subjective. Normal benign variant waveforms and artifacts can be misinterpreted as epileptiform activity and erroneously considered to be evidence of seizure susceptibility.

Epilepsy can be definitively established by recording a characteristic ictal discharge during a representative clinical attack. This is uncommon during routine EEG recordings, but can be accomplished with *inpatient video–EEG long-term monitoring* performed at many epilepsy centers throughout the world. Inpatient video-EEG monitoring is indicated in people who have ongoing seizures despite being treated with appropriate antiseizure medications. About one third of patients admitted for long-term monitoring are found to not have epilepsy; these patients have psychogenic nonepileptic attacks. In the 25 to 30% of people with focal epilepsy who continue to have disabling seizures despite trials with multiple AEDs, inpatient video-EEG monitoring to define the seizure focus is a critical test for determining candidacy for resective epilepsy surgery.

Laboratory Tests—Neuroimaging

Brain MRI complements EEG findings by identifying structural pathology that is causally related to the development of epilepsy. MRI is the best test to detect epileptogenic cerebral lesions including hippocampal sclerosis, neuronal migration disorders, tumors, focal atrophy, arteriovenous malformations, and cavernous malformations. It is important to obtain a complete imaging study that includes T1-weighted, T2-weighted, and inversion-recovery sequences in coronal and axial planes with and without contrast. Imaging in the coronal plane perpendicular to the long axis of the hippocampus has improved detection of hippocampal atrophy and hippocampal high T2 signal; findings that correlate with the pathological finding of hippocampal sclerosis and an epileptogenic temporal lobe. Additional sequences that should be routine include T2-weighted gradient-echo (GRE), to detect hemosiderin indicating old hemorrhage associated with vascular malformations or trauma, and diffusion-weighted images (DWI) for cytotoxic edema sometimes present with acute cerebral injury from prolonged seizures.

An MRI should be obtained in all patients suspected of having epilepsy except those with definite benign epilepsy with centrotemporal spikes (BECTS) or definite idiopathic generalized epilepsy (e.g., CAE and JME). CT scan with contrast is an alternate study for those who cannot have MRI, but is not as good at detecting small lesions. Any patient with seizures and abnormal neurological findings or focal slow-wave abnormalities on EEG should have neuroimaging. Repeat neuroimaging should be considered if there is an unexplained change in seizure pattern to evaluate for a new lesion.

Positron emission tomography (PET) and single-photon emission computed tomography (SPECT) use physiologically active, radio-labeled tracers to image the brain's metabolic activity (PET) or blood flow (SPECT). SPECT is most useful when an ictal and interictal study are combined to identify an extratemporal seizure focus. Abnormalities on PET or SPECT can be present when brain structure on MRI is normal.

Other Tests

Routine blood tests rarely offer diagnostic assistance in otherwise healthy patients with epilepsy. Serum electrolytes, liver function tests, and complete blood count are useful with acute new onset seizures and as baseline studies before antiepileptic drug therapy is started. Adolescents and young adults with unexplained seizures should be screened for substance abuse (especially cocaine) with blood or urine studies. Genetic testing should be considered in specific cases with suspected phenotypes, especially if a positive genetic test would alter therapy, such as in SCN1A associated epilepsies (e.g., Dravet syndrome). Lumbar puncture is indicated only if there is a suspicion of meningitis, encephalitis, or a CNS glucose transporter abnormality. Repeated generalized seizures and status epilepticus can increase cerebrospinal fluid protein content slightly and produce a mild pleocytosis for 24 to 48 hours; cerebrospinal fluid pleocytosis should be attributed to seizures only in retrospect after excluding an intracranial inflammatory process. An electrocardiogram (ECG) should be obtained in any young person with a first generalized seizure if there is a family history of arrhythmia, sudden unexplained death, or episodic unconsciousness. An ECG should also be obtained in any patient with a personal history of cardiac arrhythmia or valvular disease.

DIFFERENTIAL DIAGNOSIS

Not every paroxysmal event is a seizure, and misidentification of other conditions leads to ineffective, unnecessary, and potentially harmful treatment. Misdiagnosis accounts for patients who have not responded to antiepileptic drug treatment. The conditions confused with epilepsy depend on the age of the patient and the nature and circumstances of the attacks (Table 118-3).

TABLE 118-3 NONEPILEPTIC EPISODIC DISORDERS THAT MAY RESEMBLE SEIZURES
Movement disorders: subcortical myoclonus, paroxysmal choreoathetosis, episodic ataxias, hyperekplexia (startle disease)
Migraine: confusional, vertebrobasilar, visual auras
Syncope
Behavioral and psychiatric: psychogenic nonepileptic attacks (pseudoseizures), hyperventilation syndrome, panic/anxiety disorder, dissociative states
Cataplexy (usually associated with narcolepsy)
Transient ischemic attack
Alcoholic blackouts
Hypoglycemia

Nonepileptic paroxysmal disorders that are confused with epileptic seizures have sudden, discrete abnormal behaviors, variable responsiveness, changes in muscle tone, and various postures or movements.

Psychogenic nonepileptic attacks (PNEA), such as pseudoseizures and psychogenic nonelectrical seizures, frequently cause intractable "epilepsy" in adults. PNEA are due to the unconscious mind converting emotional conflicts or stressors into a physical state, mimicking a seizure. Some patients with psychogenic seizures also have epilepsy. Definitive diagnosis requires video-EEG documentation, although a history of atypical and nonstereotyped attacks, emotional or psychological precipitants, psychiatric illness, lack of response to antiepileptic drugs, and repeatedly normal interictal EEGs suggest psychogenic attacks. About 80% of patients with PNEA have been the victims of physical or sexual abuse. PNEA are more common in females.

Panic attacks (anxiety attacks) with hyperventilation can superficially resemble partial seizures with affective, autonomic, or special sensory symptoms. Hyperventilation typically causes perioral and finger tingling. Prolonged hyperventilation results in muscle twitching or spasms (tetany); affected patients may faint.

Syncope (see Chapter 9) refers to the symptom complex that occurs when there is a transient global reduction in cerebral perfusion associated with cardiovascular dysfunction. Loss of consciousness lasts only a few seconds, uncommonly a minute or more, and recovery is usually rapid. If the cerebral ischemia is sufficiently severe, the syncopal episode may include tonic posturing of the trunk or clonic jerks of the arms and legs and incontinence (*convulsive syncope*).

Some forms of *migraine* can be mistaken for seizures, especially if the headache is atypical or mild. The visual aura, present in some migraineurs, is typically black, gray, and white; a colored aura almost always indicates an epileptic seizure. Basilar artery migraine, usually in children and young adults, can include lethargy, mood changes, confusion, disorientation, vertigo, bilateral visual disturbances, and loss of consciousness.

TREATMENT

If the cause of symptomatic seizures is corrected, AEDs are usually not necessary. Adults with a single, unprovoked seizure and normal clinical and laboratory findings frequently do not have subsequent seizures; AEDs are usually not indicated if only one seizure has occurred. However, patients with focal neurological findings on clinical, radiological, or EEG examinations are more likely to have repeated seizures. In individual patients, social considerations may dictate treatment after a single seizure.

Medication Therapy

If seizures are recurrent, the goal of treatment is complete seizure freedom. In the United States, as of 2013, there were 25 AEDs in standard use to treat epilepsy with several other medications sometimes used as adjuncts. There is no perfect AED; all have potential toxic side effects and idiosyncratic reactions. For over one half of people with epilepsy the appropriate AED for their type of seizures can be completely effective and well tolerated. However, for about one quarter of people with epilepsy, no AED or combination of AEDs is completely effective. Once the seizure type and epilepsy syndrome is determined, an initial and, if needed, subsequent AED, should be chosen based on both its anticipated efficacy and toxicity profile. All AEDs can cause sedation, cognitive dysfunction, and incoordination in some patients, especially at high levels. Various rare, sometimes life threatening, reactions can occur with all of the AEDs. Commonly encountered situations are:

Idiopathic generalized epilepsy (CAE, JME, others)

- In all idiopathic generalized epilepsies, valproate or lamotrigine are the first line agents and result in complete seizure control in 85% to 90% of patients.
  - Valproate tends to cause weight gain and has been associated with the development of polycystic ovary syndrome, particularly in adolescent females. It results in hair loss in about 5%. It has an increased risk of teratogenicity.
  - Lamotrigine has a small but significant risk of a severe rash (e.g., toxic epidermal necrolysis, Stevens Johnson syndrome) for about the first 2 months after starting. A slow dose escalation substantially lowers this risk. Lamotrigine's metabolism is substantially inhibited by valproate, so in combination, lower doses of lamotrigine are required. Occasionally lamotrigine worsens myoclonus, but it is effective in most cases of JME.
- Second line options include clobazam, topiramate, levetiracetam, and zonisamide.
- In childhood absence epilepsy with exclusively absence seizures, ethosuximide should be the first choice. If any convulsions have occurred, valproate or lamotrigine should be used.
- If there is a history of more than 5 minutes of crescendo absences or myoclonus (often described as a "foggy" state) culminating in a convulsion, then oral benzodiazepines (lorazepam or diazepam) can abort the cluster and prevent a convulsion.
- Absences and myoclonus can be exacerbated by carbamazepine, oxcarbazepine, and GABAergic compounds including gabapentin, pregabalin, and tiagabine. These AEDs should be avoided in idiopathic generalized epilepsy.

Focal Epilepsy

- Almost all of the AEDs (except ethosuximide) can be effective in focal epilepsy. The choice of the first AED should be guided by side effect concerns and pharmacokinetics.
- Phenytoin is the most commonly used AED in focal epilepsy in developed countries. It is typically loaded in the emergency room after the initial seizures and subsequently continued.

However, phenytoin has substantial short- and long-term toxicity and its levels are difficult to regulate due to saturation kinetics and multiple drug interactions. Its toxicities include hirsuitism, coarsening of features, and gingival hyperplasia, especially in children and adolescents. Long-term toxicities include osteomalacia, peripheral neuropathy, and cerebellar degeneration with permanent incoordination. Peak level toxicities include nystagmus, gait instability, ataxia and, if the level rises above 50, acute cerebellar degeneration and cardiac arrhythmias.

- Carbamazepine, oxcarbazepine, topiramate, levetiracetam, lamotrigine, and zonisamide are currently used as first line therapy for partial seizures. Carbamazepine and oxcarbazepine can cause hyponatremia. Topiramate can lead to weight loss (often desired), but also has undesirable cognitive side effects and predisposes to renal stones. Levetiracetam can cause severe mood changes and marked sedation, but is usually well tolerated. Lamotrigine needs to be titrated slowly due to the rash risk. Zonisamide, which also predisposes to renal stones, has a long half-life (48 to 72 hours) so is a good option for intermittently noncompliant patients.
- Patients of Asian ancestry should be tested for the HLA-B*1502 allele and patients of Northern European ancestry tested for the HLA-A*3101 allele prior to initiating treatment with carbamazepine, oxcarbazepine, and eslicarbazepine. Patients with these alleles are at increased risk of Stevens Johnson syndrome and toxic epidermal necrolysis when exposed to these drugs.
- Adjunctive treatment for partial seizures includes clobazam, valproate, pregabalin, lacosamide, gabapentin, perampanel, and primidone. The proportion of gabapentin absorbed decreases with increasing dose, which limits its effectiveness. For most, pregabalin is a better choice. Primidone is rapidly converted to phenobarbital by some people, limiting its use.
- Phenobarbital is the most widely used AED in the world due to its low cost. However, it causes sedation and cognitive impairment, and it should be avoided except in difficult to control epilepsy. The exception is neonatal seizures where it is the most commonly accepted AED.

Symptomatic generalized epilepsy (LGS, others)

- All AEDs have a role in the treatment of symptomatic generalized epilepsy, but seizure freedom is rarely achieved. At a minimum, control of the more severe seizures, including drop seizures and convulsions should be the target of therapy. Polytherapy is usually required.
- Valproate is commonly the initial medication instituted.
- Added efficacy can occur with clobazam, lamotrigine, topiramate, levetiracetam, rufinamide, and zonisamide.
- Felbamate may be effective, but its use should be limited to epileptologists due to the significant risk of fatal aplastic anemia and liver failure.
- The vagus nerve stimulator (see later) has a specific role in reducing the severity of seizures in this condition.
- Dravet syndrome and possibly the related syndrome of GEFS+ respond best to topiramate, levetiracetam, and benzodiazepines. Some drugs, including lamotrigine and phenytoin, worsen Dravet syndrome.

Dosing of AEDs must be done with care. Only a few of the AEDs are safe to load or start at a full therapeutic dose. Most should be started with a gradual dose escalation. Management guidelines are: (1) The type of seizures and epilepsy should be defined and the preferred medication should be given in usual doses and then increased until seizure control is complete or side effects occur (Table 118-4); (2) If seizures persist at toxic levels, or if major side effects occur, another agent should be tried; (3) Do not stop one agent until another has been added. Otherwise, status epilepticus may occur; (4) If seizures persist after two agents have been given to toxic levels, consider referral to a specialized epilepsy center for complex combination therapy and video-EEG long-term monitoring; (5) Toxic levels of some AEDs (e.g., phenytoin and carbamazepine) can cause seizures; (6) Extended release and longer acting AEDs are preferred for most patients; (7) Patients should be counseled to adhere to the medication regimen. Pill boxes should be encouraged. Medication noncompliance is a leading cause of poor seizure control.

Epilepsy Surgery

In most patients, epilepsy is controlled with medication. When seizures cannot be controlled by adequate trials of two appropriate single agents or by the combination of two agents, the epilepsy is termed *medically intractable* (or *refractory*), a situation encountered in approximately 25% of patients with symptomatic focal epilepsy. Such patients are at risk for the consequences of seizures: inability to drive; stigmatization by schools, employers, and families; and threats to personal educational and occupational goals. In appropriately selected cases, epilepsy surgery can abolish seizures with restoration of normal neurological function. The accurate localization of a small, safely resectable seizure focus requires intensive investigation at a specialized center.

Dietary Therapy

The *ketogenic diet* is a very high fat diet with restricted carbohydrates and protein carefully designed to cause a ketotic state mimicking starvation, but supplying adequate nutrition. It is mainly used in developmentally delayed children with severe symptomatic generalized epilepsy. The ketogenic diet can be effective in this most refractory form of epilepsy, resulting in seizure-freedom in 15% to 20%. However, the diet is hard to maintain and requires a dedicated, cooperative caregiver and a specially trained dietician.

The *modified Atkins diet* (MAD) and *low glycemic-index diet* are scaled-down versions of the ketogenic diet with mainly carbohydrate restriction. These diets are more palatable than the ketogenic diet and can be tolerated by adults. The slight ketosis achieved sometimes results in a dramatic seizure reduction in any form of epilepsy.

Neurostimulators

The *vagus nerve stimulator* is an implanted device similar in appearance to a cardiac pacemaker. The stimulating electrode is placed on the left vagus nerve in the neck and programmed to stimulate the nerve for 30 seconds every 3 to 5 minutes. Swiping a magnet over the device gives an extra stimulation that can sometimes abort a seizure. In up to two thirds of patients, partial seizures are reduced by 50% or more and seizure intensity decreases.

Another strategy in medically refractory focal epilepsy is the *responsive neurostimulator*. Chronically implanted electrodes at the seizure foci are used to rapidly detect seizure onset and abort the seizure within a few seconds by delivering an electrical stimulation directly to the seizure focus. *Deep brain stimulation* to the bilateral anterior nuclei of the thalami may also improve seizure control.

Status Epilepticus

Status epilepticus can occur with partial or generalized epilepsy and is defined as prolonged or rapidly recurring seizures without full intervening recovery. *Acute repetitive seizures* are defined as a cluster of seizures over minutes to hours with intervening recovery.

Convulsive status epilepticus (Grand mal, major-motor) is a medical emergency. Continuous generalized epileptic activity can damage the brain permanently. The most frequent cause is abrupt withdrawal of AEDs (e.g., noncompliance) in a person with known epilepsy. Other precipitants include withdrawal of alcohol or drugs in a habitual user, cerebral infection, trauma, hemorrhage, and brain tumor.

TABLE 118-4   FREQUENTLY PRESCRIBED ANTIEPILEPTIC DRUGS

NONPROPRIETARY AED NAME	ADULT TOTAL DOSE PER DAY	DOSE FREQUENCY (IN HOURS)	"THERAPEUTIC" CONCENTRATIONS
Carbamazepine	800-1600 mg	6-8 (12 for sustained release)	6-12 µg/mL
Ethosuximide	750-1500 mg	8-12	40-100 µg/mL
Gabapentin	900-3600 mg	6-8	Uncertain
Lacosamide	200-600 mg	12	Uncertain
Lamotrigine*	100-800 mg	12	2-15 µg/mL
Levetiracetam	500-3000 mg	12	15-45µg/mL
Clobazam	20-60 mg	12	Uncertain
Oxcarbazepine	600-2400 mg	8-12	15-45µg/mL
Phenobarbital	60-240 mg	24	15-40 µg/mL
Phenytoin	200-600 mg	24	10-20 µg/mL
Pregabalin	100-600 mg	8-12	Uncertain
Topiramate	50-600 mg	12	2-20 µg/mL
Valproate	500-6000 mg	8 (12-24 for sustained release)	50-120 µg/mL
Zonisamide	100-600 mg	24	Uncertain

*Slow initial dose titration mandatory for lamotrigine and often indicated for other agents.

Complex partial status epilepticus manifests as a sustained state of confusion often associated with motor and autonomic automatisms. Some attacks produce bizarre behavior or stupor. Patients may resist assistance due to their abnormal state, which can last for hours or even days. The EEG usually shows nearly continuous discharging activity predominating in one or both temporal regions.

Absence status epilepticus (petit mal status) resembles complex partial status and consists of a confused state with some automatic behaviors. The EEG is characteristic with continuous runs of generalized 3 to 4 Hz spike and slow wave activity. The condition occurs in children or young adults with known absence epilepsy. Rarely, absence status occurs as the first manifestation of epilepsy in adults with no history of seizures. *Atypical absence status* with fluctuating confusion lasting for hours or longer occurs in patients with symptomatic generalized epilepsy (e.g., Lennox-Gastaut syndrome) and is accompanied by a generalized spike and slow wave pattern of 2.5 Hz or slower on the EEG.

Partial motor status, also known as *epilepsy partialis continua*, ranges from highly focal, clonic movements of the face or hand to jerks that involve most of the limb or half the body. The clonus frequency can vary from one every three seconds to three per second. It is relatively uncommon. Its causes include stroke, trauma, neoplasms, encephalitis, and hyperglycemia; sometimes the cause never becomes clear. Epilepsy partialis continua often resist all efforts at treatment and neurosurgical removal of the causative lesion is sometimes required.

Physicians infrequently witness seizures; most of the time they learn about the semiology during the history. Merely observing a patient in the midst of a seizure does not indicate that the patient should be treated for status epilepticus. However, once status epilepticus is diagnosed, treatment is urgent. The longer status epilepticus lasts, the more difficult it is to terminate and the more likely it is to cause brain damage. Aggressive therapy is mandatory for convulsive status epilepticus (Table 118-5). If initial therapy is not rapidly effective, anesthetic agents requiring intubation and ventilation should be used within an hour of onset. Complex partial status can also result in permanent neuronal injury and should similarly be treated aggressively, although therapeutic decisions are often made to try to stop complex partial status with agents that do not cause respiratory depression to avoid intubation. Absence status is unlikely to result in permanent sequelae and usually responds promptly to benzodiazepine treatment. Investigation of the cause of the status epilepticus should be undertaken during the treatment and continued after the seizures stop. Severe hyperglycemia can produce refractory partial motor and complex partial status; seizures stop once hyperglycemia is corrected.

Postanoxic status myoclonus is accompanied by generalized polyspike epileptiform discharges on the EEG but is usually unresponsive to treatment for status epilepticus. It typically indicates an irreversible condition with a poor prognosis.

⬤ GENETIC COUNSELING AND PREGNANCY
Heredity

Patients with epilepsy should be advised about the hereditary risks to their offspring, although in most people with epilepsy it does not influence their decision about having children. The

TABLE 118-5 TREATMENT OF CONVULSIVE STATUS EPILEPTICUS

TIME (MIN)	STEPS
0-5 (ABCs)	Give O$_2$; ensure adequate ventilation Monitor: vital signs, ECG, oximetry Establish intravenous access; obtain blood samples for glucose level, complete blood cell count, electrolytes, Ca, Mg, toxins, and AED levels
6-9 (glucose) (benzodiazepine)	Give glucose if blood glucose level is low or unavailable. In adults give 100 mg thiamine as well. Intravenously administer 1-2 mg of lorazepam or midazolam or 5-10 mg of diazepam as initial therapy. Alternatively use rectal diazepam gel 0.2 mg/kg.
10-20	If the initial dose of benzodiazepine is not effective, then continue to intravenously administer either lorazepam 1-2 mg every 5 minutes up to a maximum of 0.1 mg/kg or diazepam 5-10 mg every 5 minutes up to a maximum of 30 mg in patients over 12 years old. If diazepam or midazolam is used and the status epilepticus stops, phenytoin (or another AED) should be administered promptly to prevent recurrence of seizures as diazepam and midazolam's duration of action against seizures can be less than 30 minutes.
21-40 (phenytoin)	If status epilepticus persists, administer 20 mg/kg of fosphenytoin* intravenously no faster than 3 mg/kg/min up to 150 mg/min in adults. (Alternatively use phenytoin at maximum 1mg/kg/min up to 50 mg/min in adults in a proximal IV.) Monitor carefully for hypotension, arrhythmia, local extravasation.
>40 (phenobarbital) (intubate)	If the seizures do not stop after fosphenytoin/phenytoin, give 20 mg/kg of phenobarbital intravenously at maximum 100 mg/min. When phenobarbital is given after a benzodiazepine, ventilatory assistance is usually required.
(general anesthesia)	If status epilepticus persists, give general anesthesia (e.g., propofol, midazolam, or lorazepam drip) to induce a burst suppression pattern (EEG monitoring, if available, should be instituted). Vasopressors or supplemental IV fluids are often necessary.
(alternatives)	Alternative/additional treatments include IV valproate (30 mg/kg) load, levetiracetam, and lacosamide.

ABCs, Airway, breathing, and circulation; AED, antiepileptic drug.
*Always dosed in phenytoin-equivalents (PE).

idiopathic epilepsies have complex inheritance with about 10% of children of an affected parent developing seizures. There are over 200 Mendelian-inherited syndromes with epilepsy, all rare.

Teratogenicity

Children of mothers taking antiseizure medications have a birth defect rate of 6% to 9%, which is two to three times that of the general population. Convulsions, however, pose a substantial risk to the mother and fetus. Thus, AEDs should not be stopped during pregnancy. Two AEDs, valproate and carbamazepine, have been incriminated in neural tube closure defects. Since the neural tube closes by 28 days of fetal development, this defect develops before the mother is aware she is pregnant. Phenytoin, phenobarbital, and primidone have been associated with a spectrum of neurodevelopmental abnormalities. All five of these older AEDs are classified as pregnancy category D by the FDA and should be avoided if possible. Large registries suggest that the newer AEDs have less teratogenicity, but the data are incomplete. Use of two or more AEDs (polytherapy) increases the teratogenic risk. Pregnancies in women with epilepsy should be planned. During the year prior to conception, an attempt should be made to minimize the teratogenic potential of the AEDs by changing to a newer AED, to monotherapy from polytherapy, or tapering off the AEDs, if there are reasons to believe that seizures will not recur (see later). The lowest effective dose of the AEDs should be used, but this must be balanced with the risk of a breakthrough seizure. Folic acid deficiency is a well-established factor in neural tube closure defects in the general population. There is little evidence that additional folic acid in a well-nourished woman with epilepsy decreases the AED effects on neural tube closure. However, it is common practice to place women with epilepsy of childbearing age on supplemental folic acid (1 mg) as prophylaxis against a neural tube closure defect. Once pregnancy is planned or recognized, the dose of folic acid is commonly increased to 4 mg per day.

Management during and after Pregnancy

Women with epilepsy have a 1.5- to 3-fold increased rate of complications of pregnancy, including bleeding, toxemia, abruptio placentae, and premature labor. They should be managed as high risk pregnancies. High-quality (focused or type 2) ultrasound, maternal serum alpha-fetoprotein level (elevated in neural tube closure defects), and amniocentesis for chromosomal analysis are used to identify fetal malformations.

During pregnancy AED concentrations decrease due to increased hepatic and renal clearance and increased plasma volume. The free fraction of highly protein-bound AEDs (e.g., phenytoin and valproate) typically increases due to decreased albumin concentration and increased competition for binding sites by sex steroids. Thus, it is essential to monitor drug levels (free levels for highly protein-bound AEDs) prior to conception and at regular intervals throughout pregnancy. Hepatic induction of glucuronidation can dramatically reduce lamotrigine levels, sometimes requiring doubling or tripling of the lamotrigine dose to maintain prepregnancy levels. Lamotrigine levels should be measured at least every month throughout pregnancy. Similarly, oxcarbazepine levels fall by about one third beginning in the first trimester and, thus, the dose should be increased and the level checked at least each trimester.

Emesis, a common problem during early pregnancy, can result in missed and partial doses of AEDs. The expectant mother should have specific instructions to retake a full or partial dose of her AEDs if vomiting occurs after medications are taken. After the child is born, the dose of AEDs should be tapered to the pre-pregnancy amount within days to weeks. The AED levels can be checked 1 to 2 weeks after completing the taper to confirm they are at the patient's baseline. In general, breastfeeding is not contraindicated in women taking antiepileptic drugs.

During the postpartum period the mother with epilepsy may be at increased risk of seizures, especially if her seizures are activated by lack of sleep. To decrease this risk, a support person should perform at least one of the nighttime feedings. Patients whose seizure semiology would put the infant at risk (e.g., dropping or excessively clutching the baby) require childcare modification or supervision.

PSYCHOSOCIAL CONCERNS

Ongoing epileptic seizures often have major emotional consequences for the patient and family. Comorbid depression is present in up to 50% of patients with refractory epilepsy and 20% of patients with controlled epilepsy. Anxiety disorders are also common. Both are often unrecognized and untreated. In people with epilepsy, quality of life impairment is better correlated with depression than seizure frequency. The unpredictable nature of seizures and the necessary activity restrictions cause dependence, decreased self-worth, embarrassment, underemployment, and helplessness. Reduced libido and hyposexuality are common in patients with epilepsy and are often unrecognized.

Family dynamics are often disrupted by the presence of epilepsy. Both families and patients often fear seizures (seizure phobia). Family members may think their loved one is dying when they have a convulsion, especially for the first time. Patients with epilepsy are helped most by complete seizure control, but reassurance and optimistic social guidance can aid immeasurably. Once seizure control is achieved, affected persons should be encouraged to live a near normal life, using common sense as a guide. Although activity restrictions may eventually be lifted, patients with past epilepsy (with the exception of CAE and benign epilepsy with centro-temporal spikes, which completely remit) should be advised to avoid head contact sports, high alpine climbing, scuba diving, and professions requiring work at heights, large amounts of driving, or weapon use.

All states grant automobile driver's licenses to patients with epilepsy provided that no seizures have occurred for specified periods (typically six months to one year). Life and health insurance policies can generally be obtained. Epilepsy foundations and local social service organizations can assist patients with case coordination, including social and vocational considerations.

PROGNOSIS

Sixty to 70% of people with epilepsy achieve a 5-year remission of seizures within 10 years of diagnosis. About half of these patients are eventually seizure-free without AEDs. Factors favoring remission include an idiopathic form of epilepsy, a normal neurological examination, and onset in early to middle childhood (excluding neonatal seizures). Approximately thirty percent of patients continue to have seizures and never achieve a permanent remission with medications. In the United States, the prevalence of intractable epilepsy is 1 to 2 per 1000 population. Such patients should be evaluated at an epilepsy center. Injuries due to seizures are common. Advising patients not to cook, or to use back burners or microwave ovens, can prevent some serious burns. A helmet is advisable for those with drop seizures.

Sudden unexplained death in epilepsy (SUDEP) occurs in 1 per 1000 patients per year taking all forms of epilepsy together. In the most refractory epilepsies, the SUDEP rate is greater than 1 per 200 patients per year. SUDEP may be due to excessive autonomic nervous system sympathetic tone during an unwitnessed seizure with resultant cardiac arrhythmia or pulmonary edema. Suffocation can occur after an unwitnessed convulsion if the patient ends up face down in a pillow. Accidental deaths related to seizures (e.g., motor vehicle collisions) further increase the death rate.

Aspiration with convulsions is common, but can be prevented by turning the head to one side as the convulsion ends.

DISCONTINUING ANTIEPILEPTIC DRUGS

Many patients with epilepsy become seizure-free on medication for an extended period of time. Some patients can discontinue antiepileptic drugs without a relapse. Successful drug withdrawal is most likely if initial seizure control was readily achieved using monotherapy, there were relatively few seizures before remission, and the EEG and neurological examination are normal just before the AEDs are tapered off. A seizure-free interval of at least 2 years is important to reduce the likelihood of relapse; some advocate that seizure-freedom should be present for at least 5 years unless the epilepsy syndrome is known to remit (e.g., CAE or BECTS). Conversely, risk of relapse is high if seizure control was difficult to establish and required polytherapy, if there were frequent convulsions before control was achieved, a focal abnormality is present on neurological examination, or if the EEG demonstrates focal disturbances of background activity or epileptiform activity at the time AED withdrawal is considered.

For a deeper discussion of this topic, please see Chapter 403, "The Epilepsies," in Goldman-Cecil Medicine, *25th Edition.*

SUGGESTED READINGS

Berg AT, Scheffer IE: New concepts in classification of the epilepsies: Entering the 21st century, Epilepsia 52:1058–1062, 2011.

Christensen J, Grønborg TK, Sørensen MJ, et al: Prenatal valproate exposure and risk of autism spectrum disorders and childhood autism, JAMA 309(16):1696–1703, 2013.

Fazel S, Wolf A, Langstrom N, et al: Premature mortality in epilepsy and the role of psychiatric comorbidity: a total population study, Lancet 382:1646–1654, 2013.

French JA, Pedley TA: Clinical Practice. Initial Management of Epilepsy, N Engl J Med 359:166–176, 2008.

Krumholz A, Wiebe S, Gronseth G, et al: Practice Parameter: Evaluating an apparent unprovoked first seizure in adults (in evidence-based review): report of the Quality Standards Subcommittee of the American Academy of Neurology and the American Epilepsy Society, Neurology 69:1996–2007, 2007.

Kumada T, Miyajima T, Hiejima I, et al: Modified Atkins Diet and Low Glycemic Index Treatment for Medication-Resistant Epilepsy: Current Trends in Ketogenic Diet, J Neurol Neurophysiol S2:007, 2013.

Manjunath R, Paradis PE, Parisé H, et al: Burden of uncontrolled epilepsy in patients requiring an emergency room visit or hospitalization, Neurology 79(18):1908–1916, 2012.

Petit-Pedrol M, Armangue T, Peng X, et al: Encephalitis with refractory seizures, status epilepticus, and antibodies to the GABAA receptor: a case series, characterization of the antigen, and analysis of the effects of antibodies, Lancet Neurol 13:276–286, 2014.

119

Central Nervous System Tumors

Bryan J. Bonder and Lisa R. Rogers

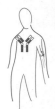

DEFINITION/EPIDEMIOLOGY

Central nervous system (CNS) tumors are of two types, primary or metastatic. Primary tumors arise from a variety of cell types within the parenchyma of the brain or spinal cord or the meninges adjacent to the brain or spinal cord. Metastatic tumors result from spread of systemic cancer to the brain, spinal cord, or meninges. This chapter considers both primary and metastatic brain tumors.

The incidence of primary malignant and nonmalignant brain tumors in the United States is 14.8/100,000. Approximately 20,500 individuals were diagnosed with primary malignant brain tumors in 2007 in the United States. High-grade gliomas and meningiomas are the most common types of adult primary brain tumors. The incidence of primary brain tumors is low in young adults but increases with advancing age and reaches a plateau between the ages of 65 and 79 years. There is a recent rise in the incidence of primary brain tumors among elderly patients, but part of this increase is due to improved detection methods. Meningiomas are the most common benign intracranial tumor and account for up to one third of benign brain tumors. The incidence of primary CNS lymphoma (PCNSL) is increasing in all age groups, accounted for only in part by CNS lymphoma associated with the acquired immunodeficiency syndrome (AIDS). Population-based studies suggest an incidence rate of 10/100,000 population with brain metastasis, but brain metastatic tumors are more common than primary CNS tumors. Because incidence rates are based on tumor registries and many patients with brain metastasis do not undergo surgery, they are underrepresented in these statistics.

Primary brain tumors are the second most common cancers in children. Medulloblastomas are the most common malignant pediatric brain tumor. In the United States, between 350 and 500 new cases of pediatric and adult medulloblastomas are diagnosed each year, and the majority of these are pediatric.

The cause of most CNS tumors is unknown. Aside from exposure to ionizing radiation, no environmental agents are known to be causative. Hereditary syndromes that are associated with an increased risk of CNS tumors include neurofibromatosis 1 and 2, tuberous sclerosis, von Hippel-Lindau disease, Li-Fraumeni syndrome, and Turcot's syndrome, but account for less than 1% of primary CNS tumors. Although the chromosomal abnormalities associated with many of these syndromes is known, the specific mechanisms leading to CNS neoplasia have not been defined.

PATHOLOGY

The World Health Organization classification defines brain tumors based on the cell of origin and includes a grading system, which is of use in predicting the biological behavior of the tumor. Most adult primary brain tumors are of neuroepithelial origin and result from neoplastic transformation of astrocytes, oligodendrocytes, or ependymocytes. Astrocytomas are the most common primary brain tumor in adults. Meningiomas derive from arachnoidal cap cells in the meningeal covering of the brain. Common locations of meningioma are the cerebral convexity, falx and parasagittal area, olfactory groove, sphenoid wing, and posterior fossa. They are comprised of heterogeneous histopathology patterns and careful neuropathological assessment is needed for accurate grading.

PCNSL is a rare form of non-Hodgkin lymphoma, typically of B cell origin. It presents within the white matter of the cerebral hemispheres, often in a periventricular location, and is often multiple, especially in AIDS patients. Brain metastasis develops when tumor cells gain access to the systemic circulation and embolize to the brain. Metastases occur most commonly from solid tumors arising in the breast, lung, colon, and skin (melanoma). Lung cancer, both non-small and small cell type, is the most common tumor overall to metastasize to the brain and constitutes up to 50% of cases of brain metastasis. In women, breast cancer is the most common source of brain metastasis. Malignant melanoma is a much less common systemic cancer but carries a high risk of brain metastasis; up to 50% of stage IV melanoma patients develop brain metastasis. Colon and renal cell carcinoma are also common underlying tumors. Other solid tumors are less frequent. Medulloblastomas are of primitive neuro-ectodermal origin and are highly cellular. Homer Wright rosettes can be found in up to 40% of cases. Medulloblastomas are grade IV tumors as they are invasive and rapidly growing, with a tendency to disseminate through the CSF.

CLINICAL PRESENTATION

Symptoms and signs caused by brain tumors typically result from compression or invasion of adjacent neural tissue by the tumor or from vasogenic edema resulting from disruption of the blood-brain barrier caused by vessel compression or invasion from tumor or from "leaky" blood vessels present within tumors. Neoangiogenesis associated with tumor growth typically results in embryonic vessels that lack a normal blood-brain barrier. Because of the uncompromising rigidity of the cranial vault, both histologically benign and malignant tumors may cause symptoms even when they are small. Symptoms caused by low-grade primary brain tumors tend to be slowly progressive whereas those in mid-grade and high-grade histology are acute or subacute (over weeks to months). The exception is the clinical presentation of a low-grade glioma with seizure. Metastatic tumors often present in a subacute fashion but may present acutely when hemorrhage into the tumor occurs. Hemorrhage into metastatic brain tumors is most common with renal cell, melanoma, lung, and choriocarcinomas.

The clinical symptoms and signs depend on the location of tumor. In most pediatric patients with brain tumor, tumors arise in the posterior fossa and result in diplopia, ataxia, dysphagia, or nausea/vomiting. Most of adult brain tumors arise in the cerebral hemispheres and present with symptoms and signs related or supratentorial structure involved: unilateral limb weakness, aphasia, and memory loss are common. Tumors in either location may present with generalized symptoms arising from increased intracranial pressure or meningeal irritation. Headache occurs in up to two thirds of patients as a presenting sign. There are no characteristics unique to this headache, but useful clinical clues include a new or different headache pattern, a progressively worsening headache, and one that occurs at night or on awakening. The pain may localize to the side of the tumor in patients with supratentorial tumors, whereas patients with infratentorial tumors frequently describe pain in the retro-orbital, retroauricular, or occipital region. Other generalized symptoms include changes in mood or personality, a decrease in appetite, and nausea. Projectile vomiting, common in children with posterior fossa tumors, is rare in adults. Meningiomas generally grow slowly; they may also be found incidentally during the evaluation of unrelated neurologic symptoms. Seizures are a frequent presenting sign of low-grade gliomas. Seizures may develop over the course of the illness in a high percentage of other patients with glioma, often in association with tumor progression.

⬤ DIAGNOSIS/DIFFERENTIAL

All patients suspected of having a brain tumor should undergo a contrast-enhanced magnetic resonance imaging (MRI) brain scan. If MRI is not available or is contraindicated because of a pacemaker or other condition, brain computed tomography (CT) should be obtained. Brain MRI is preferred because it is more useful in imaging the temporal and posterior fossae and it is more sensitive in detecting the extent of parenchymal involvement by tumor of any type. In addition, advanced sequences such as diffusion, perfusion, and spectroscopy add to the diagnostic accuracy of imaging. Vasogenic edema resulting from leakage of intravascular fluid through a disrupted blood-brain barrier can accompany any type of brain tumor and is easily visible on MRI.

High-grade gliomas typically appear as irregularly shaped contrast-enhancing masses surrounded by edema. Central necrosis is characteristic of glioblastoma (Fig. 119-1). Anaplastic gliomas appear similar, except for less frequent tumor necrosis. Although there are exceptions, most low-grade gliomas do not enhance after intravenous contrast injection (Fig. 119-2). Meningiomas typically demonstrate smooth and homogeneous enhancement originating from the extra-axial space and may also compress adjacent brain. PCNSLs typically present as multiple contrast-enhancing lesions within the white matter but in rare

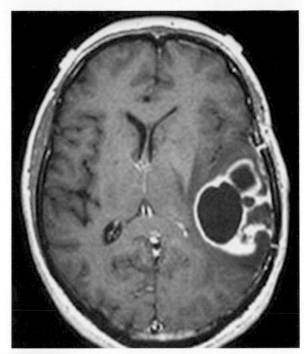

FIGURE 119-1 Contrast-enhanced T1-weighted MRI demonstrates irregular contrast enhancement with central necrosis in the left temporal lobe. There is adjacent vasogenic edema and mass effect on midline structures.

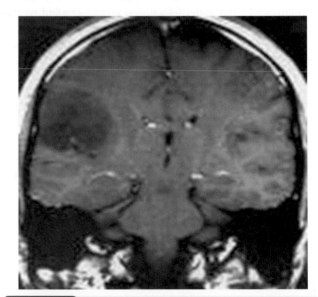

FIGURE 119-2 Coronal T-weighted MRI following contrast injection in a low-grade astrocytoma shows low attenuation and no contrast enhancement, typical of a low-grade glioma.

instances do not show contrast enhancement. Brain metastases are often located at the grey-white junction of the brain and demonstrate homogeneous enhancement or peripheral enhancement surrounding a necrotic center. When single, a brain metastasis cannot be accurately distinguished from other neoplasm or nonneoplastic entities. Medulloblastomas are usually large by the time they are identified and demonstrate homogeneous enhancement within or superior to the floor of the fourth

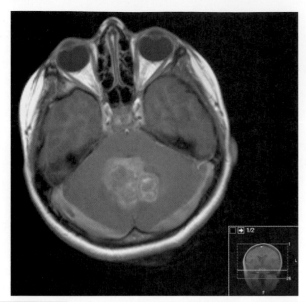

FIGURE 119-3 Contrast-enhanced T1-weighted MRI shows a large enhancing tumor in the midline of the cerebellum with compression of the fourth ventricle.

ventricle location (Fig. 119-3). They are often accompanied by hydrocephalus. The desmoplastic variant of medulloblastomas can be located lateral to the fourth ventricle.

The differential diagnosis of contrast-enhancing lesions includes brain abscess, but infection is a consideration only in rare clinical situations. Diffusion-weighted magnetic resonance images can be useful in distinguishing tumor from infection. Low-grade gliomas can be misdiagnosed as cerebral infarction, especially on brain CT. Periventricular enhancement in PCNSL can sometimes be confused with active multiple sclerosis lesions or with brain metastasis. Dural pathologies such as sarcoidosis, meningeal infection, or dural metastasis can mimic a meningioma. Posterior fossa ependymomas in children can mimic medulloblastomas.

Biopsy or resection is the preferred method to establish the histology and grade of primary brain tumors. Exceptions include PCNSL in which malignant cells are identified in the CSF or by vitreous biopsy to establish the diagnosis, and brainstem gliomas in which the MRI appearance is characteristic and biopsy is considered dangerous.

TREATMENT

Maximal surgical resection is the goal for patients with benign and malignant primary brain tumors with the exception of PCNSL in which clinical deterioration can result from resection, and biopsy alone is recommended for diagnosis. Surgical resection provides tissue for analysis and often relieves neurological symptoms; maximal surgical resection improves outcome. Surgical resection is also indicated in patients with a single brain metastasis and who have limited systemic disease with a prognosis of at least 3 months. Small patient series also indicate that resection of up to three brain metastases can be beneficial in extending overall survival and improving quality of life. More than three metastases are typically treated with radiation therapy without surgery.

Standard therapy for newly diagnosed glioblastoma is maximal resection and external beam radiation of 60Gy over 6 weeks in combination with daily temozolomide followed by temozolomide for 6 months. In a prospective randomized trial of newly diagnosed glioblastoma patients, the median survival with radiation and temozolomide was 14.6 months versus 12.1 months with radiation alone. In addition, the 2-year survival rate was superior with the combined regimen (26.5%) versus radiation alone (10.4%). O-6-methylguanine DNA methyltransferase (MGMT) is a DNA repair gene that reduces the efficacy of temozolomide and other DNA-damaging treatments for cancer. Methylation of the MGMT promoter in tumor tissue silences this gene and results in improved survival in glioblastoma. Determination of the promoter status of MGMT is often obtained as a part of clinical research trials but is rarely used in clinical practice.

The introduction of "targeted agents" that are designed to deactivate oncogenic pathways is a major advance in cancer treatment, including glioblastoma. Bevacizumab, a monoclonal antibody to vascular endothelial growth factor, is associated with a high response rate (6 month progression-free survival of 46%) in recurrent glioblastoma, although the effect on overall survival is not significant. Molecular markers in glioblastoma that are predictive and prognostic of outcome have not yet been identified. There is some evidence that tissues harboring IDH1 mutations are correlated with a superior outcome compared with wild type IDH1. The discovery of molecular "drivers" may lead to identification of targets for therapy.

Anaplastic gliomas are treated by maximal surgical resection, followed by external beam radiation. Despite the overall better prognosis for anaplastic gliomas, chemotherapy is frequently recommended but of uncertain benefit. One anaplastic glioma exquisitely sensitive to chemotherapy is the AO with codeletions of 1p and 19q. Small clinical trials have evaluated the benefit of chemotherapy alone in these patients. Deferring radiation until the time of tumor progression may reduce the CNS toxicity associated with brain radiation.

The long-term progression-free survival and overall survival of low-grade glioma patients is better than those with glioblastoma or anaplastic glioma, but malignant transformation occurs in up to 50% of such patients and close monitoring is required. Patients with low-grade gliomas should be treated initially with surgical resection. Postsurgical management of low-grade gliomas remains controversial, specifically whether radiation should be administered at diagnosis or delayed until the time of progression. The only prospective clinical trial to compare early versus delayed radiation therapy demonstrated that early radiation does not improve survival but does delay the time to tumor progression. In general, radiation therapy is deferred for patients younger than 40 years of age who have undergone complete resection. An ongoing cooperative group trial seeks to determine if temozolomide chemotherapy added to radiation offers a survival advantage over radiation alone.

Maximal surgical resection is important in patients with meningioma to reduce the risk of relapse. When complete removal is not possible, radiation therapy should be considered, depending upon the location of the tumor and regardless of grade. Radiation therapy is recommended regardless of the extent of resection for malignant meningioma. Chemotherapy for this disease has been disappointing.

Symptoms and imaging abnormalities associated with PCNSL often improve with the administration of corticosteroids because of the cytotoxic effects of steroids on lymphoma cells. However, administration of steroids before brain biopsy reduces the yield of tissue biopsy. Surgical biopsy, but not resection, is the recommended method for diagnosis. The treatment for this tumor is currently evolving as new treatments emerge. Methotrexate chemotherapy is the most effective treatment. Combining high-dose methotrexate with standard-dose brain radiation carries a risk of neurotoxicity, especially in elderly patients, but reduced-dose whole brain radiation following methotrexate chemotherapy is currently under study.

Standard therapy for patients with a single brain metastasis is complete resection if the tumor is in a noneloquent part of the brain and if the extent of systemic disease predicts a survival of at least 4 to 6 months. In addition, some patients with limited systemic cancer show a survival benefit with resection of up to three metastatic tumors. Resection is typically followed by whole brain radiation or stereotactic surgery to the tumor margin. If the patient does not receive whole brain radiation, close observation with periodic MRI scans is indicated to assess for recurrence at the original site or at other sites in the brain. For patients presenting with more than three metastases, whole brain radiation as indicated. A meta-analysis of the addition of stereotactic radiosurgery and whole brain radiation did not identify a survival benefit when compared with whole brain radiation therapy alone, except for patients with a single brain metastasis (6.5 versus 4.9 months). A variety of systemic chemotherapies show therapeutic efficacy in newly diagnosed and recurrent brain metastasis, depending upon the sensitivity of the brain metastasis to the agent, rather than to delivery of the drug to the lesion.

The extent of resection is prognostic in medulloblastomas. Staging evaluations for the extent of disease include postoperative MRI of the brain and spine and lumbar CSF sampling. Prospective randomized trials and single-arm trials suggest that adjuvant chemotherapy administered during and after craniospinal radiation improves the progression-free survival and overall survival in both average and poor risk groups. The therapy for children younger than 3 years of age excludes craniospinal radiation therapy because of the long-term deleterious effects and includes surgery and chemotherapy alone. Distinct subgroups of medulloblastomas have been identified, and profiling of these subgroups reveals distinct genomic events, several of which represent actionable targets for therapy.

Vasogenic edema associated with parenchymal and meningeal tumor causes neurological symptoms and signs, and it can be life-threatening. Treatment with corticosteroids often reduces edema and improves neurologic function. Dexamethasone is the preferred steroid because of its long half-life. Patients with symptoms related to vasogenic edema often improve within 48 hours of dexamethasone administration. Doses used for treatment of tumor-related edema are typically 4-24 mg/day given in divided doses (2 to 4 times daily). Because steroids can be associated with a variety of adverse effects, the lowest dose and duration of administration should be sought. In patients with severe neurologic signs related to brain edema, an intravenous bolus of 10 to 20 mg dexamethasone should be considered. If the neurologic signs are life-threatening, including signs of brain herniation, mannitol and dexamethasone should be administered and urgent neurosurgical consultation obtained. Seizures should be aggressively managed with antiepileptic drugs. Nonenzyme inducing antiepileptic drugs are generally favored because of a better safety profile than enzyme-inducing drugs and because of the lack of interaction with other medications prescribed to treat the tumor, including steroids and chemotherapy. Prophylactic antiepileptic drugs are generally not recommended for patients with a primary or metastatic brain tumor when there is no history of seizure.

PROGNOSIS

The histology of high-grade glioma, performance status, and age are important predictors of prognosis. Glioblastoma has the worst prognosis, with a median survival of just over 1 year even with aggressive therapy. Good prognosis patients can live more than 2 years. Data from the nationwide Surveillance, Epidemiology, and End Results registry identified an overall median survival of 15 months and 42 months for patients with anaplastic astrocytomas and anaplastic oligodendrogliomas, respectively. This analysis did not include the status of 1p19q chromosomal loss, and the more favorable survival of patients with codeletions was not demonstrated. Low-grade gliomas have a median survival of approximately 5 years, but there is individual variation depending on age, size of tumor, and extent of resection.

Recurrence rates in meningioma depend upon grade and vary from greater than 25% in grade 1 to greater than 90% in grade 3. Risk factors for recurrence include incomplete resection, tumor grade, young age, specific subtypes, brain infiltration, and high proliferative rate.

Five-year survival rates in meningioma are approximately 69% overall but vary significantly with tumor grade. Survival in PCNSL ranges from 1 to several years, depending on patient age and treatment modality. Performance status, age, status of the extracranial tumor, and number of brain metastases are factors that predict prognosis in patients with brain metastasis. The median survival ranges from 3 to 6 months in patients with multiple metastases treated with whole brain radiation therapy. Patients with a single metastasis with limited extracranial disease who undergo surgical resection and whole brain radiation therapy have significantly improved survival (40 weeks) as compared with those who undergo whole brain radiation therapy alone (15 weeks). Importantly, the improved survival is accompanied by a longer period of functional independence. The 5-year progression-free survival in medulloblastomas is 70% to 85%. However, more than one third of patients experience recurrence, and there is no standard therapy at the time of recurrence. Median survival after recurrence is usually less than 1 year. For children less than 3 years of age at diagnosis, 5-year progression-free survival ranges between 30% and 70%, depending on the extent of dissemination at diagnosis.

SUGGESTED READINGS

American Cancer Society: www.cancer.org. Accessed October 22, 2013.
Backer-Grøndahl T, Moen BH, Torp SH: The histopathological spectrum of human meningiomas, Int J Clin Exp Pathol 5:231–242, 2012.

Barnholtz-Sloan JS, Yu C, Sloan AE, et al: A nomogram for individualized estimation of survival among patients with brain metastasis, Neuro-Oncol 14:910–918, 2012.

CBTRUS: Primary brain and central nervous system tumors diagnosed in the United States in 2004–2007, Central Brain Tumor Registry of the United States Statistical Report 2011.

De Braganca KC, Packer RJ: Treatment options for medulloblastoma and CNS primitive neuroectodermal tumor (PNET), Curr Treat Options Neurol 15:593–606, 2013.

Nuño M, Birch K, Mukherjee D, et al: Survival and prognostic factors in anaplastic gliomas, Neurosurgery 73:458–465, 2013.

Patil CG, Pricola K, Sarmiento JM, et al: Whole brain radiation therapy (WBRT) alone versus WBRT and radiosurgery for the treatment of brain metastases, Cochrane Database Syst Rev (9):CD006121, 2012.

Rutkowski S, von Hoff K, Emser A, et al: Survival and prognostic factors of early childhood medulloblastoma: an international meta-analysis, J Clin Oncol 28:4961–4968, 2010.

Taylor M, Northcott P, Korshunov A, et al: Molecular subgroups of medulloblastoma: the current consensus, Acta Neuropathol 123:465–472, 2012.

van den Bent MJ, Brandes AA, Taphoorn MJ, et al: Adjuvant procarbazine, lomustine, and vincristine chemotherapy in newly diagnosed anaplastic oligodendroglioma: long-term follow-up of EORTC brain tumor group study 26951, J Clin Oncol 31:344–350, 2013.

Wang Z, Bao Z, Yan W, et al: Isocitrate dehydrogenase 1 (IDH1) mutation-specific microRNA signature predicts favorable prognosis in glioblastoma patients with IDH1 wild type, J Exp Clin Cancer Res 32:59, 2013.

120

Demyelinating and Inflammatory Disorders

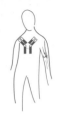

Anne Haney Cross

INTRODUCTION

In demyelinating CNS disorders, previously normal myelin is lost due to an acquired, typically inflammatory disease. The prototypic CNS demyelinating disorder is multiple sclerosis (MS). Other disorders of this type include neuromyelitis optica (NMO), acute disseminated encephalomyelitis (ADEM), acute transverse myelitis (TM), and optic neuritis (ON).

MULTIPLE SCLEROSIS
Definition/Epidemiology

According to the National Multiple Sclerosis Society, MS affects over 2 million people worldwide. It is a presumed autoimmune disorder, although the exact etiology is still not fully understood. MS begins as a relapsing remitting disease in greater than 80% of patients and ultimately becomes progressive in greater than 50% of untreated patients. Patients with progressive MS accumulate neurologic disability, with or without discrete relapses. MS is more common in females, with the current female to male ratio in North America and in Europe estimated at 2-4 : 1. An exception is primary progressive MS (see Clinical Presentation), where the female to male ratio is 1 : 1.

MS is most common in persons of northern European ancestry. Recent genome-wide association studies indicate that many genes affect the risk of MS, although most confer only a small risk of disease (odds ratios less than 1.5). Alleles within the HLA-DR region (DRB1*15:01 > DRB1*13:03 > DRB1*03:01) are the most well-established and confer the greatest risk with odds ratios between 1.5 and 4 for most populations of northern European ancestry.

Environmental factors can also confer risk for MS. Modifiable factors include low vitamin D blood level, high body mass index during adolescence/young adulthood, and smoking cigarettes. Seropositivity to the Epstein Barr virus increases the risk of MS; a symptomatic case of infectious mononucleosis confers greater risk than seropositivity alone. Though relatively high at 1/1000 to 1/500, the incidence of MS appears relatively stable in North America, the United Kingdom, and Europe. Incidence of MS may be increasing in several regions where MS was not previously prevalent, such as Iran, Turkey, Sicily, and South Africa. These reports of increasing incidence may reflect a real increase or just improved recognition and diagnosis.

Pathology

Classically, MS causes demyelinating CNS white matter lesions with relative sparing of axons. The most common pathology of active lesions in white matter is perivascular mononuclear cell infiltration (monocyte/macrophages, lymphocytes), with a variable presence of antibody and activated complement. Acutely active white matter lesions display blood-brain barrier breakdown, which is manifest on MRI by gadolinium enhancement. Despite its categorization as a "white matter disease," gray matter is frequently damaged in MS. Gray matter lesions have been under-recognized because they are difficult to see by MRI, and are often not appreciated pathologically without special stains. Such gray matter lesions may occur in the white matter tracts within deep gray structures such as the thalamus or be within gray matter itself, such as in the cerebral cortex. Cortical gray matter lesions can be subpial, extend into cortex from underlying white matter (leukocortical), or be wholly within the cortex. Cortical lesions are characterized by activated microglia and relatively fewer infiltrating lymphocytes and macrophages when compared with white matter MS lesions. Ectopic lymphoid tissue containing B cells, a finding associated with chronic inflammation, has also been observed in meninges of progressive MS subjects.

Clinical Presentation

MS may manifest with a variety of symptoms and signs. Common presentations include: optic neuritis, diplopia (often caused by internuclear ophthalmoplegia due to a propensity of MS to affect the medial longitudinal fasciculus), TM, brainstem syndromes, sensory disturbances, and weakness. Less frequent presentations include seizures, cognitive problems, bladder control problems, and pain. Clinically isolated syndrome (CIS) refers to a single attack that is likely due to CNS demyelination. CIS may be acute or subacute in onset, and may involve a single or more than one CNS region. CIS presentations may look identical to MS attacks, but a formal diagnosis of MS cannot be made until the occurrence of separation of lesions in time. Ultimately, most CIS patients do develop MS. In one study, over 85% of CIS patients with even one silent abnormality on brain or spinal cord magnetic resonance imaging (MRI) eventually developed clinically definite MS. On the other hand, only about 20% of those without any other MRI abnormalities developed clinically definite MS.

Three main clinical subtypes of MS are defined based on clinical course: relapsing remitting, secondary progressive, and primary progressive. Relapsing remitting MS is characterized by clinical stability between individual attacks from which the patient may or may not fully recover. Secondary progressive MS patients have gradual neurologic deterioration and may also have superimposed attacks. Secondary progressive MS develops following an initial relapsing-remitting course in a substantial proportion of relapsing remitting patients, although this proportion may be declining with the advent of disease-modifying therapies. About 10% of MS patients have primary progressive MS, which is characterized by gradual downhill progression from onset without any clinical attacks. It has been proposed to discontinue the uncommon fourth clinical designation, progressive relapsing MS, in favor of *primary progressive MS with activity*.

Diagnosis

The diagnosis of MS requires dissemination of CNS disease in time and in space. No other disease should provide a better explanation. MRI, spinal fluid analyses, evoked potentials (EPs) and ocular coherence tomography (OCT) are tools that may aid in the diagnosis. The McDonald criteria (Table 120-1) allow new MRI lesions to be used to define disease in time after an initial first attack (clinically isolated syndrome). These criteria have made diagnosis easier, without losing significant specificity.

MRI

Classic features seen on brain and spinal cord MRI greatly aid in the certainty of diagnosis. MS lesions are characterized by increased intensity on T2-weighted (T2w) and T2-FLAIR (fluid attenuated inversion recovery) images (Fig. 120-1A). Lesions are usually ovoid, and often localize to the periventricular or subcortical regions, the corpus callosum, the brainstem, and the cervical spinal cord. Periventricular lesions are typically at right angles to the lateral ventricles and bear the moniker "Dawson's fingers." On sagittal images, lesions in the corpus callosum are usually flame-shaped (Fig 120-1C). On T1w images, MS lesions may be isointense or hypointense. T1w hypointensity in a chronic inactive lesion denotes underlying tissue damage, including axonal loss (Fig.120-1D). Enhancement of lesions following administration of gadolinium containing contrast agents indicates blood-brain barrier breakdown, and that a lesion is active (Fig. 120-1B). Enhancing lesions are also often T1w hypointense, but the hypointensity resolves more than 50% of the time. A ring pattern of enhancement is common. Most enhancing MS lesions display no edema or mass effect, but occasional "tumefactive" MS lesions have significant edema on MRI and may require biopsy for diagnosis.

Spinal Fluid Analysis

Evidence of increased intrathecal immunoglobulin synthesis is present in more than 90% of MS patients. Elevated concentrations of CSF IgG and IgM, CSF-restricted oligoclonal bands of immunoglobulin (Fig. 120-2), and a high intrathecal IgG synthesis rate are seen. The IgG index, which is derived from the ratio of CSF to serum IgG and takes BBB integrity into account, is elevated. A mild lymphocytic pleocytosis is frequently seen in CSF during MS relapses.

TABLE 120-1 THE 2010 REVISED MCDONALD CRITERIA

CLINICAL PRESENTATION	LESIONS	ADDITIONAL DATA NEEDED FOR MS DIAGNOSIS*
≥2 attacks	Objective clinical evidence of ≥2 lesions or objective clinical evidence of 1 lesion and reasonable historical evidence of a prior attack	None
≥2 attacks	Objective clinical evidence of 1 lesion	DIS demonstrated by >1 T2w lesion in at least 2 of 4 MS-typical regions of CNS, or 2nd clinical attack at alternate site in CNS
1 attack	Objective clinical evidence of ≥2 lesions	DIT demonstrated by simultaneous presence of asymptomatic gad+ lesion and non-enhancing lesions or a new T2w and/or gad+ lesion on follow-up MRI after a baseline scan, or 2nd clinical attack
1 attack	Objective clinical evidence of 1 lesion (CIS)	For DIS, ≥1 T2w lesion in at least 2 of 4 MS-typical regions of CNS; For DIT, as above; or await a 2nd clinical attack implicating different CNS region
Gradual neurologic progression suggestive of MS (PPMS)	1 year or more of disease progression plus 2 of 3 of following criteria: evidence for DIS in the brain based on ≥1 T2w lesions characteristic of MS, evidence of DIS in the spinal cord ≥2 T2w cord lesions positive CSF (elevated IgG index or oligoclonal bands not present in serum)	

(Modified from Polman CH, Reingold SC, Banwell B, et al: Diagnostic criteria for multiple sclerosis: 2010 revisions to the McDonald criteria, Ann Neurol 69(2): 292–302, 2011, Table 4.)

DIS, Dissemination in space; DIT, dissemination in time.

*These criteria were developed using CIS presentations and are therefore most applicable in patients who present with a typical CIS suggestive of CNS inflammatory demyelinating disease. Alternative diagnoses that might better explain the disorder must be considered and reasonably excluded.

Evoked Potentials

Evoked potentials (EPs) detected by surface electrode recording have in the past been useful in detecting subclinical demyelination in the brainstem (auditory EPs), spinal cord (somatosensory EPs), and optic nerves (visual EPs). The advent of high resolution MRI has made these tests less useful.

Optical Coherence Tomography

Optical coherence tomography (OCT) is a safe and rapid means to image the retina and detect evidence of prior optic neuritis. OCT uses safe infrared light to provide images of the retinal layers, including the retinal nerve fiber layer (RNFL) which contains axons that form the optic nerve. The RNFL is thinner than normal in those with remote optic neuritis. Also, RNFL thickness correlates with neurodegenerative aspects of MS, such as brain atrophy.

Differential Diagnosis

The diagnosis of MS requires the exclusion of diseases that might better explain the clinical scenario. The differential diagnosis of MS is broad (Table 120-2). Some diseases that can mimic MS

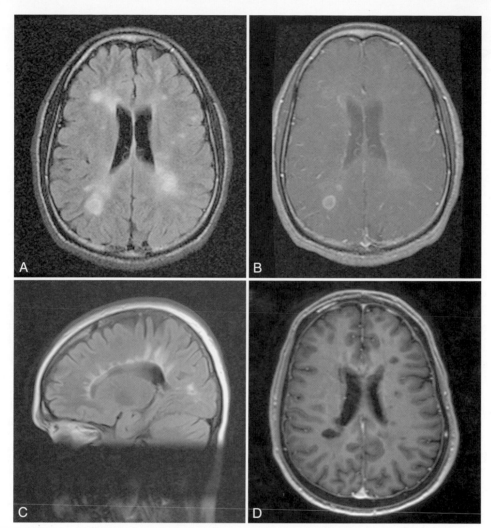

FIGURE 120-1 **A,** Axial fluid-attenuated inversion recovery (FLAIR) image of the brain from a patient with MS revealing classical periventricular and deep white matter high-signal intensity lesions. **B,** Axial T1-weighted image following gadolinium contrast administration in the same patient as **A**. Enhancing lesions after gadolinium contrast administration, indicating loss of integrity of the blood-brain barrier that is seen with active MS lesions. One enhancing lesion in the right parietal region is ring enhancing. **C,** Sagittal FLAIR image of the brain of an MS patient demonstrating classical flame-shaped pericallosal lesions radiating outward from the ventricle. **D,** Axial T1-weighted image showing areas of T1 low signal intensity ("black holes").

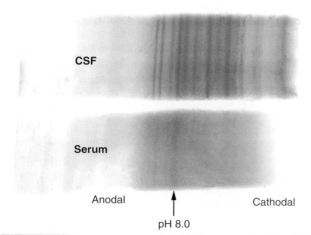

Anodal ↑ Cathodal
pH 8.0

FIGURE 120-2 Isoelectric focusing gel of cerebrospinal fluid (CSF) and serum of a patient with multiple sclerosis. The CSF *(upper lane)* shows oligoclonal bands cathodal to the pH 8.0, which are not seen in the serum *(lower lane)*.

CSF

Serum

have relapses and others display progressive courses. "Red flags" that are atypical for MS, such as non-CNS symptoms (arthritis, rash, pulmonary, or GI symptoms), bilateral hearing loss, peripheral neuropathy, or atypical time of onset (early childhood or after age 50) should lead the clinician to question the diagnosis of MS.

For a deeper discussion of these topics, please see Chapter 411, "Multiple Sclerosis and Demyelinating Conditions of the Central Nervous System," in Goldman-Cecil Medicine, *25th Edition.*

Treatment

MS treatment can be divided into three categories: treatment of symptoms (e.g. spasticity, fatigue, or depression), treatment of acute relapses, and disease-modifying therapies. This discussion will be largely limited to the latter two categories. Table 120-3 lists some major symptoms and their therapies in MS.

TABLE 120-2   DIFFERENTIAL DIAGNOSIS OF DEMYELINATING DISEASES

DISEASE CATEGORY*	EXAMPLES OF DISORDERS[†]
Immune-mediated /autoimmune	Multiple sclerosis, neuromyelitis optica (NMO), acute demyelinating encephalomyelitis (ADEM), idiopathic optic neuritis, CRION, idiopathic transverse myelitis, Behçet's disease
Infectious	Progressive multifocal leukoencephalopathy (PML), HTLV-I, HIV, CNS abscess, Lyme disease, Whipple disease, neurosyphilis
Metabolic	Vitamin B12, vitamin E or copper deficiency, central pontine and extrapontine myelinolysis
Neurodegenerative	spinocerebellar ataxias, spine disease (e.g. compressive cervical spondylopathy)
Rheumatologic	Sarcoidosis, systemic lupus erythematosus, antiphospholipid antibody syndrome, Sjögren syndrome
Genetic Disorders	Adrenomyeloleukodystrophy/adrenomyeloneuropathy, hereditary spastic paraparesis, CADASIL, Leber's optic neuropathy, Perlizeus-Merzbacher, Wilson's disease
Neoplastic/Paraneoplastic	CNS Lymphoma, meningeal carcinomatosis, paraneoplastic CRMP-5 IgG, anti-Amphiphysin-1 Abs
Vascular	CNS vasculitis (e.g., giant cell arteritis, primary CNS vasculitis, etc.), spinal dural fistula, Susac syndrome
Iatrogenic	TNF inhibitors, CNS irradiation

*Several of the disorders listed could be placed in more than one category.
[†]This list is not comprehensive.

TABLE 120-3   SELECTED MS SYMPTOMS AND THEIR MANAGEMENT

SYMPTOM/SIGN	TREATMENT(S)
Stiffness/cramps/spasms/spasticity	baclofen, tizanidine (evidence level A)
Fatigue	Amantadine, modafinil, armodafinil, amphetamines
Depression	Selective serotonin reuptake inhibitors, cognitive behavior therapy
Pain/paresthesias/trigeminal neuralgia	gabapentin, carbamazepine, oxcarbazepine, pregabalin, amitriptyline
Gait impairment	Fampridine SR (Evidence level A)
Nystagmus, with visual impairment	Gabapentin
Dizziness/Vertigo	Meclizine, dimenhydrinate, benzodiazepines
Urinary urgency/incontinence/ neurogenic bladder	Oxybutynin, tolterodine, other anticholinergics, BOTOX injection
Impotence/erectile dysfunction	Sildenafil, tadalafil, testosterone supplementation if low
Tonic spasms	Phenytoin, carbamazepine

Relapses that alter function or cause pain are typically treated with corticosteroids. Severe relapses are usually managed with intravenous methylprednisolone at 500-1000 mg daily for 3 to 5 doses, followed by a short oral corticosteroid taper (usually prednisone). Oral corticosteroid tapering courses may be used for mild relapses. Blood pressure, serum electrolytes and glucose, and patient mood should be monitored during corticosteroid therapy. Based on the multi-center Optic Neuritis Treatment Trial (ONTT), this regimen will lead to more rapid recovery from the attack, but is unlikely to alter the degree of eventual recovery (evidence level A).

For severe relapses that do not respond to high-dose IV corticosteroids, a small randomized study showed that plasma exchange can be effective. Plasma exchange was followed by rapid functional improvement in over 40%, with early initiation of plasma exchange treatment the single factor most associated with significant improvement (level A). Subjects in this trial likely included patients with neuromyelitis optica (NMO) and acute disseminated encephalomyelitis (ADEM), in addition to MS.

Relapsing remitting MS (RRMS) is one of only a handful of chronic neurologic disorders with effective disease modifying therapies. The beta-interferons (BIFNs) and glatiramer acetate (GA) are FDA-approved for relapsing remitting MS (level A).

The BIFNs and GA all reduced annualized relapse rate by about 30% in early pivotal studies. Most have also been shown to delay progression to definite MS in patients with clinically isolated syndrome who are at high risk for developing MS.

As of 2015, twelve different DMTs with seven different mechanisms of action are available for MS (Table 120-4). The approved agents have distinct and variable risk profiles. As there are currently no biomarkers that direct the choice of disease modifying therapies for an individual patient, selection of the disease modifying therapy for an individual is based on disease course and severity, patient comorbidities, and individual preferences.

Five BIFNs are approved for use in relapsing remitting MS and clinically isolated syndrome in the United States. They differ in dosage, side effects, and incidence of neutralizing antibody induction. Three BIFNs are identical to endogenous human BIFN-1a (poly ethyleneglycol has been covalently attached to one of the three for longer duration of effect); the other two are BIFN-1b, which differs by one amino acid. BIFNs are immunomodulators, though their exact mechanism of action in MS is not fully established. BIFN therapy is associated with increased circulating soluble VCAM-1, which could produce an effect similar to that of the monoclonal antibody natalizumab. Patients taking BIFNs require monitoring of hepatic transaminases and CBC; elevation of transaminases is uncommon, but may require dose adjustment or discontinuation. Common side effects include a "flu-like" feeling for several hours after a dose, which is usually improved by nonsteroidal anti-inflammatory medications or acetaminophen. BIFNs are given by injection and, as with any injectable drug, skin infection can occur. BIFNs are rated Pregnancy Category C; the BIFNs should be discontinued before conception.

Glatiramer acetate is given as a daily 20 mg subcutaneous injection, or 40 mg SQ three times per week. The drug is a random polymer of four amino acids that are abundant within myelin basic protein, a major protein in CNS myelin. It is considered immunomodulatory not immunosuppressive, although its mechanism of action is not fully understood. Glatiramer acetate has no known drug interactions, and laboratory monitoring is not needed. Side effects include injection site reactions and an uncommon transient tachycardia reaction that occurs soon after an injection. Lipoatrophy at injection sites may develop with prolonged use. Glatiramer acetate is pregnancy category B, and is

TABLE 120-4 DISEASE MODIFYING MEDICATIONS FOR MS

DRUG (BRAND NAME), DOSING	APPROVED	MS INDICATION	MECHANISM OF ACTION
Interferon beta 1b (Betaseron, Extavia), 250ug SQ qod	1993, 2009	RRMS, CIS	Inhibits "pro-inflammatory" cytokines, such as interferon (IFN)-gamma, tumor necrosis factor alpha, and lymphotoxin. Increases IL-10. Adhesion molecule and class II MHC induction reduced.
Interferon beta 1a (Avonex) 30ug IM weekly	1996	RRMS, CIS	
Interferon beta 1a (Rebif) 22 or 44ug SQ 3x /wk.	2002	RRMS	
Interferon beta 1a (Plegridy) 125ug SQ every 14 days	2014	Relapsing forms of MS	
Glatiramer acetate (Copaxone) 20mg SQ daily, or 40mg SQ 3x/wk	1996 2014	RRMS, CIS	Alters T cell cytokine profile toward that of Th2 immunomodulatory cells.
Mitoxantrone (Novantrone) 12mg/m^2 IV q 3 months	2000	Worsening RRMS, relapsing SPMS PRMS	Anthracenedione chemotherapeutic agent
Natalizumab (Tysabri) 300mg IV q 4 weeks	2004/2006	Relapsing MS*	Monoclonal antibody targeting the alpha-4-integrins, part of the VLA-4 adhesion molecule.
Fingolimod (Gilenya) 0.5mg po daily	2010	Relapsing MS, approved for treatment naïve patients	Down-modulates sphingosine-1-phosphate receptors, lymphocytes unable to migrate out of lymphoid tissue. May have direct effects in CNS
Teriflunomide (Aubagio) 7mg or 14mg po daily	2012	Relapsing MS, approved for treatment naïve patient	Inhibits dihydroorotate dehydrogenase, thus inhibiting proliferation of activated lymphocytes
Dimethyl fumarate (Tecfidera) 240mg po BID	2013	Relapsing MS, approved for treatment naïve patients	Activates nuclear factor erythroid 2-related factor 2 (Nrf2) pathway which enhances response to oxidative stress
Alemtuzumab (Lemtrada) IV infusion, SQ in development	2014	Relapsing forms of MS	Monoclonal antibody that lyses cells expressing CD52

considered the safest MS disease modifying therapy to use in women who may become pregnant.

Mitoxantrone is an anthracenedione chemotherapeutic agent that is FDA approved for secondary progressive MS, progressive relapsing MS, or worsening relapsing-remitting MS. It is administered by IV infusion every 3 months and has a lifetime dose limit due to dose-related cardiotoxicity. In a prospective randomized 2-year study enrolling worsening relapsing-remitting or secondary progressive MS patients, those that received mitoxantrone had longer time to first treated relapse and improved level of disability compared with those randomized to placebo (level A). Beneficial effects were still measurable 12 months after treatment discontinuation. In addition to dose-limiting cardiotoxicity, mitoxantrone is associated with leukemia in approximately 1% of MS patients. Because of these risks and with the advent of more targeted medications, mitoxantrone is not commonly used in the United States.

Natalizumab is a humanized monoclonal antibody targeting the α-4-integrins, part of the VLA-4 adhesion-related heterodimer. The dose is 300 mg given intravenously every 4 weeks. A 2-year phase 3 trial of natalizumab showed 68% reduction in annualized relapse rate, 42% reduction in sustained disability, and over 90% reduction in gadolinium-enhancing lesions compared with placebo (level A). Natalizumab was temporarily removed from the market in 2005 due to an association with progressive multifocal leukoencephalopathy, a severe viral disorder caused by the JC virus. Because of its association with progressive multifocal leukoencephalopathy, this drug is generally recommended in cases of an inadequate response or intolerance of an alternate MS therapy. Patients receiving it must take part in a risk-mitigation program and can only be infused at certified infusion centers. Natalizumab is pregnancy category C.

Fingolimod was the first oral disease modifying therapy to be approved for relapse rate reduction in MS. This once daily 0.5 mg capsule reduces annualized relapse rate by about 50% and disability progression by about 25% versus placebo (level A). Fingolimod has several risks, including macular edema, pulmonary dysfunction, bradycardia, and herpetic infections.

It is contraindicated in some settings, such as recent myocardial infarction or uncontrolled heart failure, and with certain medications (such as class IA and class III anti-arrhythmic drugs). Medical monitoring for potential bradycardia for at least 6 hours is necessary for the first dose. Fingolimod is pregnancy category C.

Teriflunomide is a once daily oral tablet of 7 mg/day or 14 mg/day. Two phase 3 studies in relapsing patients with relapsing forms of MS found that the 14 mg/day dose significantly reduced annualized relapse rate by over 30% and disability progression by around 30% (level A). The 7 mg dose had a lesser beneficial effect. Thus, the 14 mg daily dose is favored by many clinicians. Teriflunomide can cause hepatotoxicity, and it is contraindicated in pregnancy (pregnancy category X). If necessary, teriflunomide can be rapidly eliminated from the body using cholestyramine, otherwise it persists for long periods. Teriflunomide is closely related to the drug leflunomide, approved for rheumatoid arthritis in 1998.

Dimethyl fumarate is a capsule taken orally twice daily. In phase 3 trials, it reduced MS relapse rates by 44 to 53% and also improved MRI outcomes (level A). The white blood cell count may drop and should be monitored. As of late 2014, one fatal case of PML in a person taking the medication and with persistent low lymphocyte counts has occurred. Adverse effects include flushing, gastrointestinal side effects, and rash. Dimethyl fumarate is pregnancy category C.

Alemtuzumab is a monoclonal antibody targeting cells expressing CD52, which includes T and B lymphocytes, monocytes, and other mononuclear white blood cells. In the CARE-MS I and II studies in RRMS patients, alemtuzumab was compared not to placebo, but instead to 44 μg BIFN-1a given subcutaneously three times per week. Patients treated with alemtuzumab had lower annualized relapse rate (by 49% and 53.8%) and disability progression (by 28% and 42%). Alemtuzumab leads to a profound drop in the white blood cell count, which may last for months or even years. In trials, secondary autoimmune diseases developed in a sizeable proportion of alemtuzumab-treated subjects, with autoimmune thyroid disease being most common.

Prognosis

MS is highly variable. It is occasionally "benign" in which case the disease has little impact on quality of life. It can also be severe with considerable disability or early death. Most patients fall in between these extremes. Poor prognostic indicators at onset of MS include primary progressive course, male gender, frequent attacks, prominent motor or cerebellar findings, and high initial MRI lesion burden. Expected lifespan of people with MS is reduced overall by 7 to 14 years. Suicide rate is 1.7 to 7.5 times that of the general population. Albeit controversial, the use of disease modifying therapies (BIFNs and GA) likely improves not only relapse rate but long-term disability and even mortality. In one non-randomized study, early initiation of disease modifying therapies within a year of symptom onset was associated with better long-term outcomes.

● NEUROMYELITIS OPTICA (DEVIC'S DISEASE)

Definition/Epidemiology

Neuromyelitis optica (NMO), also called Devic's Disease, is an inflammatory CNS disorder causing both demyelination and necrosis. NMO can be monophasic, but is more often characterized by attacks of optic neuritis and longitudinally extensive TM that are not necessarily concurrent. NMO was once believed to be a subtype of MS, but now is known to be a different disorder associated in most cases with autoantibodies to the aquaporin 4 (AQP4) water channels, which are strongly expressed by astrocytes. Histopathological changes in NMO are mostly in the spinal cord and optic nerve; the brain is less involved. AQP4 is expressed outside of the CNS in the kidney, stomach, and other tissues, but curiously no pathology has been recognized in the non-CNS organs expressing AQP4.

NMO is much less common than MS, with estimates by the Guthy-Jackson Charitable Foundation of 4,000 patients in the United States, and a half million worldwide. It is even more female-preponderant than MS, with female to male ratio estimated from 4 : 1 to 8 : 1. Children and adults both develop NMO. Unlike MS, NMO is *not* associated with HLA-DRB1*15:01, and it affects those of Asian, African, and Hispanic ancestry disproportionately.

Clinical Presentation

NMO presents clinically as an acute attack of optic neuritis and/or TM; it often takes a relapsing course. Gradually progressive NMO has not been described (helping to distinguish it from progressive MS). Other autoimmune diseases often occur together with NMO including Sjögren's syndrome, systemic lupus erythematosis, Hashimoto's disease, and myasthenia gravis.

Diagnosis/Differential

In 2004, researchers first reported the presence of a serum IgG autoantibody to cerebral vessels in NMO; this was later found to target aquaporin 4. NMO-IgG/ AQP4-IgG is highly specific (>90%) and relatively sensitive (~75%) for NMO. Fulfilling two out of three of the following criteria is reported to be 99% sensitive and 90% specific for NMO in the setting of optic neuritis and TM: (1) longitudinally extensive spinal cord lesion, which is greater than or equal to 3 segments in length (Figure 120-3); (2) NMO-IgG positivity; and (3) brain MRI not typical or diagnostic for MS. NMO-IgG seropositive patients with isolated optic neuritis or longitudinally extensive TM are currently described as having "NMO spectrum disorder."

For a deeper discussion of these topics, please see Chapter 411, "Multiple Sclerosis and Demyelinating Conditions of the Central Nervous System," in Goldman-Cecil Medicine, *25th Edition.*

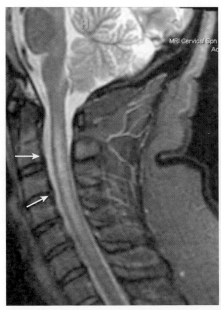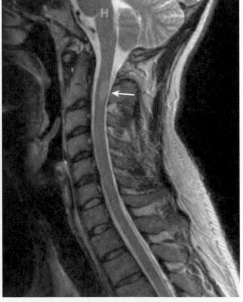

FIGURE 120-3 **A,** Sagittal T2w image of the upper spinal cord in a 37-year-old female with NMO. She developed quadriparesis over several days, and was AQP4-IgG seropositive. Two years later she had right eye optic neuritis, which left her with visual acuity of only 20/200. The spinal cord lesion *(arrows)* had mild mass effect and was contiguous over 6 vertebral segments. **B,** Sagittal T2w image of the upper spinal cord in a 24-year-old male with MS shows a lesion *(arrow)* in the posterior cord at C2. This patient had moderate vibration loss in the legs but was otherwise asymptomatic.

Pathology

NMO lesions affect both white and gray matter and are located mainly in the spinal cord and optic nerves. In the brain, they are most common in the hypothalamus and around the fourth ventricle. NMO lesions center on blood vessels, where IgG, IgM, and complement activation products are seen. The vessels are abnormally thickened and hyalinized. Active NMO lesions show infiltration by mononuclear cells (lymphocytes, monocytes), neutrophils, and eosinophils. Older lesions display demyelination, axon loss, and death of oligodendroglia and neurons. In vitro and animal studies indicate that AQP4-IgG itself is pathogenic, causing complement- and antibody-mediated damage.

Treatment

Acute relapses are treated with high-dose corticosteroids. If these are not effective, plasma exchange is usually tried.

Because NMO is a rare disease, large multi-center randomized, controlled trials of disease modifying therapies are lacking. Several short case series have pointed toward possible efficacy of azathioprine plus prednisone, rituximab, and mycophenolate mofetil for prevention of future attacks (level C). Eculizumab, a monoclonal antibody that inhibits the complement cascade, was used in a small open-label trial in AQP4-IgG positive NMO patients. Over one year, 85% had no relapses and no patient progressed in disability (level B). Of note, beta-interferons are not effective for NMO and may actually increase the rate of attacks.

Prognosis

The necrotic nature of NMO results in worse outcomes than MS. Seropositive NMO patients tend to have more frequent and severe relapses than AQP4-IgG negative patients. Death can be a consequence and is often due to respiratory failure. The death rate in a retrospective study covering 1950-1997 was over 30%. Less than 10% mortality was reported in a more recent retrospective study of Caucasian NMO patients.

● ACUTE DISSEMINATED ENCEPHALOMYELITIS

Acute disseminated encephalomyelitis (ADEM) is an acute, inflammatory, presumed immune-mediated disorder of the CNS that is encountered primarily in children but may occur in adults. An antecedent viral infection, or occasionally a vaccination, is common. ADEM presents with multifocal neurologic symptoms and signs. These can include encephalopathy, which may manifest as reduced level of consciousness (even coma), or as behavioral changes (e.g. confusion or irritability). Fever is common. Seizures, optic neuritis, and spinal cord involvement can all occur. Males and females are about equally affected. ADEM is usually monophasic, although relapsing ADEM has been described. On MRI, both white and gray matter CNS regions are affected. Gray matter involvement can include the basal ganglia, a region not typically affected in MS. The periventricular white matter region is often spared, unlike MS. When present, enhancement with gadolinium occurs in all lesions simultaneously. CSF often shows pleocytosis and an elevated protein, but no infection. Findings typical of MS, such as oligoclonal bands, are not usual. No randomized prospective treatment trials for acute disseminated encephalomyelitis are reported. Intravenous methylprednisolone followed by a prednisone taper is typically administered,

and the response is usually good (level D). Over 80% of cases recover well. As ADEM is only rarely recurrent, long-term immunomodulatory/immunosuppressive therapy is not indicated. A rare hemorrhagic form of ADEM (Weston Hurst syndrome) is more severe and can lead to death or severe disability.

● ACUTE TRANSVERSE MYELITIS

Transverse myelitis (TM) is an inflammatory spinal cord syndrome presenting with abrupt or subacute onset of motor and/or sensory loss below a specific spinal level. Control of bladder and bowel is often affected, as is autonomic function below the level. Back pain and paresthesias may be prominent. Many cases of acute TM are idiopathic, but treatable causes must be ruled out. An urgent MRI with and without gadolinium should be obtained to look for compressive etiologies needing immediate treatment. After a compressive etiology has been ruled out, a lumbar puncture to assess CSF for cell count, glucose, and protein, and cultures and PCRs for infectious causes should be done. The usual tests for MS should be performed, and CSF should be analyzed for evidence of neoplastic etiology. Serum AQP4-IgG, paraneoplastic panels and chest CT should be considered. CSF may also be tested for NMO-IgG, angiotensin converting enzyme, and paraneoplastic antibodies when no etiology is forthcoming.

Acute TM can be the presenting episode for MS (where the TM is generally incomplete and asymmetric) or NMO (where the TM affects ≥3 spinal cord segments). Acute TM can also be caused by spinal cord infarction due to occlusion of the anterior spinal artery. Infections by viruses can cause acute or subacute TM. The most common viruses associated with acute TM are varicella zoster, herpes virus type 2, and cytomegalovirus. The retroviruses HTLV-I and HIV can each cause a myelopathy that is usually subacute. West Nile virus can cause a myelopathy that resembles poliomyelitis, with flaccid paralysis due to infection and death of anterior horn cells. Subacute TM may be caused by vitamin B12 or copper deficiency, or infiltrating or compressive syndromes such as tumors or abscesses. Nitrous oxide anesthesia can precipitate an acute onset myelopathy in the case of borderline vitamin B12 deficiency. Rheumatologic disorders such as Sjögren's disease, systemic lupus erythematosus, and Behçet's disease can all cause TM. Paraneoplastic syndromes associated with anti-CRMP-5 and anti-amphiphysin can cause a tract-specific myelopathy. The history and physical examination should be performed with these disorders in mind.

Treatment is determined by the most likely etiology. Idiopathic TM is treated much like TM in MS or NMO, with intravenous methylprednisolone at 500 mg to 1000 mg/day, usually followed by a short oral prednisone taper (evidence level D). When response to intravenous methylprednisolone is suboptimal, plasma exchange should be considered.

● IDIOPATHIC ACUTE OPTIC NEURITIS

Inflammatory demyelinating optic neuritis can occur as part of MS or NMO, or as an idiopathic entity. Classically, optic neuritis presents over hours with loss of vision together with pain exacerbated by eye movement. Vision loss may range from subclinical to frank blindness. Color vision and contrast sensitivity are disproportionately affected. On examination, a relative afferent pupillary defect is seen in unilateral optic neuritis. Acute demyelinating optic neuritis is often retrobulbar without papillitis. On MRI, the optic nerve can be swollen and enhance after gadolinium contrast. After recovery from the acute episode, the optic disk may appear pale, and the relative afferent pupillary defect may persist. Transient worsening of vision when the body temperature rises due to exercise or fever (Uhthoff's phenomenon) may occur following recovery. The differential diagnosis includes other causes of acute monocular or binocular vision loss, such as Leber's hereditary optic neuropathy, giant cell arteritis, and acute non-arteritic anterior ischemic optic neuropathy.

The Optic Neuritis Treatment Trial studied patients with acute optic neuritis (either idiopathic or due to MS) who were randomized to one of three treatments, intravenous methylprednisolone versus oral prednisone taper versus oral placebo. Visual acuity initially recovered faster in the intravenous methylprednisolone group, but by 6 months later there was no difference among the three groups (level A). Recovery of vision was good. Patients from this trial were examined 10 years later and acuity in the affected eyes was 20/20 or better in 74% and less than 20/200 in only 3%. However, recurrence of optic neuritis was common, and had occurred in either eye in 35% of the patients. Recurrences were more frequent in those who had MS than those with idiopathic optic neuritis ($P < .001$).

● CHRONIC RELAPSING INFLAMMATORY OPTIC NEUROPATHY

First described in 2003, chronic relapsing inflammatory optic neuropathy (CRION) is an inflammatory optic neuropathy characterized by acute relapses, but often with more severe visual loss than idiopathic optic neuritis or optic neuritis associated with MS. Patients with CRION can have onset at any age and the entity has been described worldwide. Prevalence rates and epidemiology are still unclear. As in other types of optic neuritis, eye pain at onset is frequent. Return of pain can herald a relapse. Uveitis is present in a small percentage of cases. Five diagnostic

criteria for CRION have been suggested: (1) optic neuritis with at least one relapse, (2) objective visual loss, (3) AQP4-IgG seronegative, (4) contrast enhancement on MRI of acutely inflamed optic nerve, and (5) response to immunosuppressive treatment and relapse on withdrawal. Other diseases that might present similarly, such as sarcoidosis and giant cell arteritis, should be ruled out. Treatment for acute CRION is similar to that for other causes of optic neuritis, using intravenous methylprednisolone followed by oral corticosteroids. Relapses are common upon corticosteroid discontinuation. Successful long-term treatment with "steroid sparing" agents such as methotrexate, azathioprine, or mycophenolate mofetil has been reported. The underlying pathology is not yet known, but the disease appears inflammatory based on clinical presentation, imaging, and specific medication response. Eventual visual outcomes are often poor. One report indicated that visual acuity was less than 20/200 in one third of CRION patients.

SUGGESTED READINGS

Kim SH, Huh SY, Lee SJ: A 5-Year Follow-up of Rituximab Treatment in Patients with Neuromyelitis Optica Spectrum Disorder, JAMA Neurol 70:1110–1117, 2013.

Klaver R, De Vries HE, Schenk GJ, et al: Grey matter damage in multiple sclerosis: a pathology perspective, Prion 7:66–75, 2013.

Langer-Gould A, Brara SM, Beaber BE, et al: Incidence of multiple sclerosis in multiple racial and ethnic groups, Neurology 80:1734–1739, 2013.

Petzold A, Plant GT: Chronic relapsing inflammatory optic neuropathy: a systematic review of 122 cases reported, J Neurol 261:17–26, 2014.

Polman CH, Reingold SC, Banwell B, et al: Diagnostic criteria for multiple sclerosis: 2010 revisions to the McDonald criteria, Ann Neurol 69(2):292–302, 2011.

West TW, Hess C, Cree BA: Acute transverse myelitis: demyelinating, inflammatory, and infectious myelopathies, Semin Neurol 32(2):97–113, 2012.

Wootla B, Watzlawik JO, Denic A, et al: The road to remyelination in demyelinating diseases: current status and prospects for clinical treatment, Expert Rev Clin Immunol 9(6):535–549, 2013.

121

Neuromuscular Diseases: Disorders of the Motor Neuron and Plexus and Peripheral Nerve Disease

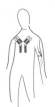

Carlayne E. Jackson

INTRODUCTION

Neuromuscular diseases are classified into four groups, according to which portion of the motor unit is involved (Table 121-1). Motor neuron and peripheral nerve diseases are considered in this chapter; myopathies are considered in Chapter 122, and neuromuscular junction diseases are considered in Chapter 123. The symptoms and signs of the neuromuscular diseases are at times indistinguishable. However, some useful general rules apply to assist with localization based on the distribution of weakness, presence or absence of sensory symptoms, reflex abnormalities, and specific associated clinical features (Table 121-2).

Electromyography and Nerve Conduction Studies

Electromyography (EMG) and nerve conduction studies can also be useful diagnostic tools in localizing the lesion in a patient with a suspected neuromuscular disease. The measurement of electrical activity arising from muscle fibers is performed by inserting a needle electrode percutaneously into a muscle. Normal muscle is electrically silent at rest. Spontaneous activity during complete relaxation occurs in myotonic disorders, in inflammatory myopathies, and in denervated muscles. Spontaneous activity of a single muscle fiber is called a *fibrillation,* and such activity of part of or an entire motor unit is called a *fasciculation.* In myotonia, repeated muscle depolarization and contraction occur despite voluntary relaxation. Abnormalities in motor unit potentials occur during the course of denervation; with the development of reinnervation, the remaining motor units increase in amplitude and become longer in duration and polyphasic (E-Fig. 121-1). Conversely, in muscle diseases such as the muscular dystrophies and other diseases that destroy scattered fibers within a motor unit, the motor unit action potentials are of lower amplitude and shorter duration and are polyphasic. A reduced recruitment (interference) pattern from maximum voluntary effort occurs in denervation. Conversely, in patients with primary muscle disease, submaximal voluntary effort produces a full recruitment pattern despite marked weakness.

Nerve conduction is studied by stimulating a peripheral nerve (e.g., the ulnar) with surface electrodes placed over the nerve. The resulting action potential is recorded by electrodes placed over the nerve more proximally in the case of large sensory nerve fibers and over the muscle distally in the case of motor nerve fibers in a mixed motor sensory nerve. For sensory nerves, the sensory nerve action potential (SNAP) is quantitated, and for motor nerves, the compound muscle action potential (CMAP) is quantitated.

TABLE 121-1	CLASSIFICATION OF NEUROMUSCULAR DISEASES	
SITE OF INVOLVEMENT	**TYPICAL EXAMPLES**
ANTERIOR HORN CELL	
Without upper motor neuron involvement	Spinal muscular atrophy Progressive muscular atrophy Bulbospinal muscular atrophy Poliomyelitis West Nile virus
With upper motor neuron involvement	Amyotrophic lateral sclerosis Primary lateral sclerosis
PERIPHERAL NERVE	
Mononeuropathy	Carpal tunnel syndrome Ulnar palsy Meralgia paresthetica
Multiple mononeuropathies	Mononeuritis multiplex (e.g., polyarteritis nodosa), leprosy, sarcoidosis, amyloidosis
Polyneuropathies	Diabetic neuropathy Charcot-Marie-Tooth disease Guillain-Barré syndrome
NEUROMUSCULAR JUNCTION	
	Myasthenia gravis Lambert-Eaton syndrome
MUSCLE	
	Duchenne muscular dystrophy Dermatomyositis

TABLE 121-2 CLINICAL FEATURES OF THE NEUROMUSCULAR DISEASES

CLINICAL FEATURE	ANTERIOR HORN CELL	PERIPHERAL NERVE	NEUROMUSCULAR JUNCTION	MUSCLE
DISTRIBUTION OF WEAKNESS	Asymmetrical limb or bulbar	Symmetrical, usually distal	Extraocular, bulbar, proximal limb	Symmetrical, proximal limb
ATROPHY	Marked and early	Mild, distal	None (or very late)	Slight early; marked later
SENSORY INVOLVEMENT	None	Dysesthesias, loss of sensation	None	None
REFLEXES	Variable (depending on degree of upper motor neuron involvement)	Decreased out of proportion to weakness	Normal in myasthenia gravis, depressed in Lambert-Eaton syndrome	Decreased in proportion to weakness
CHARACTERISTIC FEATURES	Fasciculations, cramps	Combined sensory and motor abnormalities	Fatigability	Usually painless

⬤ DISEASES OF THE MOTOR NEURON (ANTERIOR HORN CELL)

Amyotrophic Lateral Sclerosis

Definition and Epidemiology

The most common *acquired* motor neuron disease, amyotrophic lateral sclerosis (ALS), is a progressive, typically fatal disorder. The incidence is approximately 2 per 100,000 population, and there is a slight male predominance. The peak age of onset is in the sixth decade, although the disease can occur at any time throughout adulthood. Epidemiologic studies have incriminated risk factors for ALS including exposure to insecticides, smoking, participation in varsity athletics, and military service in the Gulf War. The cause of ALS is largely unknown, with 95% of cases considered "sporadic," and 5% related to an autosomal dominant disease (familial ALS [FALS]). FALS is an adult-onset disease that is clinically and pathologically indistinguishable from sporadic ALS. FALS is caused by mutations in many genes, including the C9orf72, SOD1, TARDBP, FUS, ANG, ALS2, SETX, and VAPB genes. Mutations in C9orf72 can also cause sporadic ALS. (E-Table 121-1).

Pathology

ALS results from degeneration of the cortical motor neurons originating in layer five of the motor cortex and descending via the pyramidal tract (resulting in upper motor neuron signs and symptoms) and from degeneration of the anterior horn cells in the spinal cord and their brainstem homologues innervating bulbar muscles (resulting in lower motor neuron signs and symptoms) (Table 121-3).

Clinical Presentation

Clinical symptoms relating to the upper motor neuron degeneration include loss of dexterity, slowed movements, muscle weakness, stiffness, and emotional lability. Signs on neurologic examination that confirm an upper motor neuron lesion include pathologic hyperreflexia, spasticity, and extensor plantar responses (Babinski's sign). Lower motor neuron signs and symptoms caused by anterior horn cell degeneration include weakness, muscle atrophy, fasciculation, and cramps. Fasciculations in the absence of associated muscle atrophy or weakness are usually benign and may be aggravated by sleep deprivation, stress, and excessive caffeine ingestion. Muscle weakness in patients with ALS usually begins distally and asymmetrically and may manifest as a monoparesis, hemiparesis, paraparesis,

TABLE 121-3 SYMPTOMS AND SIGNS ASSOCIATED WITH AMYOTROPHIC LATERAL SCLEROSIS

SYMPTOMS	SIGNS
UPPER MOTOR NEURON DEGENERATION	
Loss of dexterity	Pathologic hyperreflexia
Slowed movements	Babinski's sign
Weakness	Hoffman's sign
Stiffness	Jaw jerk
Pseudobulbar affect	Spasticity
LOWER MOTOR NEURON DEGENERATION	
Weakness	Muscle atrophy
Fasciculations	Fibrillation potentials on electromyography
Cramps	Neurogenic atrophy on muscle biopsy

or quadriparesis. It may also be limited initially to the bulbar region, resulting in difficulty with swallowing, speech, and movements of the face and tongue. For unclear reasons, ocular motility is spared until the very late stages of the illness. Bowel and bladder function and sensation remain spared throughout the course of the disease. Degeneration of the corticobulbar projections innervating the brainstem can lead to pseudobular affect causing difficulty controlling laughter and/or tearfulness. Up to 50% of patients with ALS may also have a component of frontotemporal dementia characterized by executive dysfunction, poor insight, personality changes (disinhibition, impulsivity, and apathy), abnormal eating habits, poor hygiene, and language dysfunction.

Diagnosis and Differential Diagnosis

The diagnosis of ALS remains one of "exclusion," in which other potential causes must be ruled out through a variety of neuroimaging, laboratory, and electrodiagnostic investigations (E-Table 121-2). For example, compression of the cervical spinal cord or cervicomedullary junction from tumors or cervical spondylosis can produce weakness, atrophy, and fasciculations in the upper extremities and spasticity in the lower extremities, closely resembling ALS.

Treatment

Specialized multidisciplinary clinic referral should be considered for patients with ALS to optimize health care delivery (Level B) and prolong survival (Level B). The only current U.S. Food and Drug Administration (FDA)–approved therapy for ALS is riluzole 50 mg twice per day, which in clinical trials prolonged

TABLE 121-4	SYMPTOM MANAGEMENT FOR MOTOR NEURON DISEASES	
RESPIRATORY INSUFFICIENCY		**SPASTICITY**
Noninvasive positive pressure ventilation Cough-assist devices		Baclofen 10-20 mg qid Dantrium 25-100 mg qid
DYSARTHRIA		**PSEUDOBULBAR AFFECT**
Augmentative speech device		Serotonin reuptake inhibitors Amitriptyline 25-75 mg qhs Dextromethorphan/Quinidine 20/10 mg bid
DYSPHAGIA		
Percutaneous endoscopic gastrostomy placement Suction machine		**WEAKNESS**
SIALORRHEA		Ankle foot orthosis Wheelchair Elevated toilet seat
Amitriptyline 25-75 mg qhs Glycopyrrolate 1-2 mg q8h Botulinum toxin		

TABLE 121-5	CLINICAL SPECTRUM OF MOTOR NEURON DISEASES*	
UPPER AND LOWER MOTOR NEURON INVOLVEMENT		**LOWER MOTOR NEURON INVOLVEMENT**
Sporadic amyotrophic lateral sclerosis *Familial amyotrophic lateral sclerosis*		Motor neuronopathy related to malignancy or paraproteinemia Poliomyelitis West Nile virus Postpolio syndrome *Hexosaminidase deficiency* Progressive muscular atrophy *Spinal muscular atrophy* Type I: Infantile onset (Werdnig-Hoffmann disease) Type II: Late infantile onset Type III: Juvenile onset (Kugelberg-Welander disease)
UPPER MOTOR NEURON INVOLVEMENT		
Primary lateral sclerosis *Familial spastic paraparesis*		

*Italicized disorders are hereditary.

survival by 2 to 3 months (Level A). The mechanism of this effect is not known with certainty; however, riluzole may reduce excitotoxicity by diminishing presynaptic glutamate release. Initiation of noninvasive positive pressure ventilation (NPPV) on a spontaneous timed mode has also been shown to prolong survival up to 20 months, slow the rate of forced vital capacity (FVC) decline (Level B), and improve quality of life (Level C). NPPV should be initiated when the forced vital capacity (FVC) is less than 50%, the maximal inspiratory pressure is less than 60 cm, or when patients report symptoms that suggest nocturnal hypoventilation (e.g., daytime fatigue, frequent arousals, supine dyspnea, morning headaches). A cough-assist device can be used to assist with clearing upper airway secretions and has been shown to minimize the risk of pneumonia in clinical trials (Level C). A percutaneous gastrostomy (PEG) tube should be considered for prolonging survival and stabilizing body weight (Level B) in patients with impaired oral food intake. Symptomatic therapy for spasticity, pseudobulbar affect, muscle cramping, and sialorrhea is also essential in maintaining patient dignity and quality of life (Table 121-4). Augmentative speech devices can assist patients with communication and computer access.

Prognosis

Mean survival from onset of symptoms is 2 to 5 years, with 10% of patients surviving beyond 10 years. The majority of deaths are related to respiratory muscle failure and aspiration pneumonia.

Other Acquired Motor Neuron Diseases

Other motor neuron diseases involve only particular subsets of motor neurons (Table 121-5). Progressive muscular atrophy (PMA) is a pure lower motor neuron disease that accounts for 8% to 10% of patients with motor neuron disease. Weakness is typically distal and asymmetrical, and bulbar involvement is rare. Patients with PMA generally have a better prognosis than those with ALS, with a survival of 3 to 14 years. Primary lateral sclerosis (PLS) is a pure upper motor neuron syndrome in which patients demonstrate either a slowly progressive spastic paralysis or dysarthria. This is a rare disorder, accounting for 2% of all motor neuron cases. Survival is generally years to decades.

Spinal Muscular Atrophy

Spinal muscular atrophy (SMA) is a hereditary form of motor neuron disease in which only the lower motor neuron is affected. The SMAs may begin in utero, in infancy, in childhood, or in adult life and represent the first class of neurologic disorders in which a developmental defect in neuronal apoptosis most likely produces the disease. Two genes are involved in SMA types 1 to 3: the neuronal apoptosis inhibitor protein (NAIP) and survival motor neuron (SMN) genes.

Bulbospinal muscular atrophy (BSMA) or Kennedy's disease is an X-linked recessive disorder in which the mean age at onset is 30 years; the range is from 15 to 60 years. BSMA is a trinucleotide repeat disorder with a CAG expansion encoding for a polyglutamine tract in the first exon of the androgen receptor gene, on chromosome Xq11-12. The mechanism by which disruption of the androgen receptor gene alters the function of bulbar and spinal motor neurons is not known. An inverse correlation exists between the number of CAG repeats and the age of onset of the disease. Affected individuals exhibit chin fasciculations, midline furrowing and atrophy of the tongue, and proximal weakness. Dysphagia and dysarthria are common, and up to 90% of patients demonstrate gynecomastia and infertility. Two findings distinguishing this disorder from ALS are the absence of upper motor neuron signs and in some patients the presence of a subtle sensory neuropathy.

● DISORDERS OF THE BRACHIAL AND LUMBOSACRAL PLEXUS

The roots within the cervical, lumbar, and sacral regions organize into the cervical, lumbar, and sacral plexuses before giving rise to individual peripheral nerves. Diseases of these plexuses (plexopathies) tend to be *focal* in symptoms and signs, whereas many diseases of the peripheral nerves and muscles are *generalized*.

Brachial Plexopathy

The brachial plexus is constituted by mixed nerve roots from C5 to T1 that fuse into upper, middle, and lower trunks above the level of the clavicle and redistribute into lateral, posterior, and medial cords below that landmark (E-Fig. 121-2). Symptoms include weakness, pain, and sensory loss in the shoulders or arms.

Upper trunk lesions may be due to trauma and idiopathic brachial plexitis (see later discussion). Lower trunk lesions may result from malignant tumor invasion, thoracic outlet syndrome, or as a complication of sternotomy. If the entire plexus is involved, radiation injury, trauma, and late metastatic disease are the most common causes.

Acute Autoimmune Brachial Neuritis

Acute autoimmune brachial neuritis is characterized by the abrupt onset of severe pain, usually over the lateral shoulder, but at times extending into the neck or entire arm. The acute pain generally subsides after a few days to a week; by this time, weakness of the proximal arm becomes apparent. The serratus anterior, deltoid, and supraspinatus are the most commonly affected muscles, but other muscles of the shoulder girdle may also be affected. In rare cases, most of the patient's arm and even the ipsilateral diaphragm are involved. Sensory loss is usually slight and generally involves the axillary nerve distribution. Weakness lasts weeks to months and be accompanied by severe atrophy of the shoulder girdle. No therapy has been shown to alter or shorten the clinical course, although steroids and analgesics may reduce pain. Most patients recover within several months to 3 years. The disorder frequently follows an upper respiratory infection or an immunization, but in many instances no antecedent illness occurs. It is bilateral in one third of cases but is always asymmetrical; it may recur in 5% of patients. Recurrent brachial plexopathies that are painless may be related to an autosomal dominant disorder, hereditary neuropathy with liability to pressure palsies (HNPP), caused by a deletion, or point mutation of PMP-22 protein (chromosome 17p).

Lumbosacral Plexopathy

The lumbosacral plexus is formed from the ventral rami of spinal nerves T12 to S4. These divide within the plexus into ventral and dorsal branches that form the femoral, sciatic, and obturator nerves. The plexus is located within the substance of the psoas major muscle. Clinical features include proximal pain and weakness in anterior thigh muscles (femoral) or posterior thigh muscles and the buttocks. Bowel and bladder dysfunction may also occur. Diabetes, malignant invasion, radiation therapy, infection (herpes zoster), psoas abscess, trauma, and retroperitoneal hemorrhage are common causes. An autoimmune form is much less frequent than brachial neuritis.

● DISORDERS OF THE PERIPHERAL NERVES
Definition and Epidemiology

Peripheral neuropathy refers to a large group of disorders that can produce focal (mononeuropathy or multiple mononeuropathies) or generalized nerve dysfunction (polyneuropathies) (Table 121-6). Peripheral neuropathies are prevalent neurologic conditions, affecting 2% to 8% of adults, with the incidence increasing with age. They range in severity from mild sensory abnormalities, found in up to 70% of patients with long-standing diabetes, to fulminant, life-threatening paralytic disorders such as Guillain-Barré syndrome (GBS).

Mononeuropathies are disorders in which only a single peripheral nerve is affected. The most common cause is nerve

TABLE 121-6	CLASSIFICATION AND CAUSES OF PERIPHERAL NEUROPATHY
TYPE OF NEUROPATHY	**EXAMPLES**
MONONEUROPATHIES	
Compressive	Carpal tunnel syndrome, ulnar palsy
Hereditary	Hereditary neuropathy with predisposition to pressure palsies
Inflammatory	Bell's palsy
Multiple mononeuropathies	Vasculitis (mononeuritis multiplex), diabetes, leprosy, sarcoidosis, amyloidosis
POLYNEUROPATHIES	
Hereditary	Charcot-Marie-Tooth disease
Endocrine	Diabetes, hypothyroidism
Metabolic	Uremia, liver failure
Infections	Leprosy, diphtheria, human immunodeficiency virus, Lyme disease
Immune mediated	Guillain-Barré syndrome, chronic inflammatory demyelinating polyneuropathy
Toxic	Lead, arsenic, alcohol, drug induced
Paraneoplastic	Lung cancer

entrapment such as median nerve compression resulting in carpal tunnel syndrome or peroneal nerve injury causing footdrop (Table 121-7). When more than one peripheral nerve is involved, the term *mononeuropathy multiplex* or *multiple mononeuropathies* is often used. Multiple mononeuropathies are most commonly seen in diabetes mellitus and vasculitis but also occur in leprosy, vasculitis, sarcoidosis, hereditary neuropathy with predisposition to pressure palsies, and amyloidosis.

Polyneuropathies are a group of disorders affecting the motor, sensory, and autonomic nerves. These disorders may predominantly affect the nerve axon (axonal neuropathies), myelin sheath (demyelinating neuropathies), or the small- to medium-sized blood vessels supplying the nerves (vasculitic neuropathies). The clinical features of the polyneuropathies reflect the pathology of the underlying process.

Pathology

In the symmetrical *axonal* polyneuropathies, the underlying pathology is usually a slowly evolving type of axonal degeneration that involves the ends of long nerve fibers first and preferentially. With time, the degenerative process involves more proximal regions of long fibers, and shorter fibers are affected. This pattern of distal axonal degeneration or *dying back* of nerve fibers results from a wide variety of metabolic, toxic, and endocrinologic causes.

In the *demyelinating* polyneuropathies, the underlying pathology involves the myelin sheath.

Demyelination of a peripheral nerve at even a single site can block conduction, resulting in a functional deficit identical to that seen after axonal degeneration. In contrast to repair by regeneration, however, repair by remyelination can be rapid. Autoimmune attack on the myelin sheath occurs in the inflammatory demyelinating neuropathies (GBS and chronic inflammatory demyelinating polyneuropathy [CIDP]) and some neuropathies associated with paraproteinemias (see later discussion). Inherited disorders of myelin such as Charcot-Marie-Tooth (CMT) disease comprise the other major category of demyelinating neuropathies. Other causes include toxic, mechanical, and

TABLE 121-7 COMMON MONONEUROPATHIES

	PRECIPITATING FACTORS	MOTOR SIGNS AND SYMPTOMS	SENSORY SIGNS AND SYMPTOMS	TREATMENT
MEDIAN NERVE				
Entrapment at the wrist (carpal tunnel syndrome)	Repetitive wrist flexion or sleep	Weakness in thenar muscle; inability to make a circle with the thumb and index fingers	Numbness, tingling, and/or pain in thumb, index finger, middle finger, and medial half of ring finger. Tinel and Phalen signs	Neutral wrist splint, carpal tunnel injections or surgery
ULNAR NERVE				
Entrapment at the elbow	External compression in condylar groove, fracture of humerus	Weakness or atrophy of the interossei and thumb adductor	Sensory loss in the little finger and contiguous half of the ring finger	Elbow pads; ulnar nerve transposition or decompression of cubital tunnel
RADIAL NERVE				
Entrapment at the spiral groove	Prolonged sleeping on arm after drinking excessive amounts of alcohol: "Saturday night palsy"	Wrist drop with sparing of elbow extension; weakness of finger and thumb extensors	Sensory loss on dorsum of hand	Spontaneous recovery; wrist splint
FEMORAL NERVE				
	Abdominal hysterectomy, hematoma, prolonged lithotomy position, diabetes	Weakness and atrophy of quadriceps	Sensory loss in anterior thigh and medial calf	Physical therapy
LATERAL FEMORAL CUTANEOUS NERVE				
Meralgia paresthetica	Obesity, pregnancy, diabetes, constrictive belts	None	Sensory loss, pain, or tingling over anterolateral thigh	Weight loss; spontaneous recovery
PERONEAL NERVE				
Entrapment at the fibular head	Habitual leg crossing, knee casts, prolonged squatting, profound weight loss	Weakness of ankle dorsiflexors or evertors and toe extensors	Sensory loss in anterolateral leg and dorsum of foot	Ankle-foot orthosis; remove source of compression
SCIATIC NERVE				
	Injection injury, fracture or dislocation of hip	Weakness of hamstrings, ankle plantar flexors or dorsiflexors	Sensory loss in buttock, lateral calf and foot	Ankle-foot orthosis; physical therapy
TIBIAL NERVE				
Entrapment in tarsal tunnel	External compression from tight shoes, trauma, tenosynovitis	None	Sensory loss and tingling in sole of foot	Tarsal tunnel injection, eliminate source of compression, medial arch support

physical injuries to nerves. Although these examples have nearly pure demyelination, many neuropathies have both axonal degeneration and demyelination. This mixed pathologic abnormality reflects the mutual interdependency of the axons and the myelin-forming Schwann cells. Vasculitic neuropathies occur as a result of disease of the small- or medium-sized blood vessels that leads to ischemia and infarction of isolated peripheral nerves. The term *mononeuritis multiplex* is also used to describe this clinical situation, in which there is multifocal involvement of individual nerves.

Clinical Presentation

The clinical picture of an *axonal* polyneuropathy includes early loss of muscle stretch reflexes at the ankle and weakness that initially involves the intrinsic muscles of the feet, the extensors of the toes, and the dorsiflexors at the ankle. The motor signs are usually mild in contrast to the sensory abnormalities, which may include numbness, tingling, and burning sensations (dysesthesias). The sensory symptoms usually begin symmetrically in the toes and feet and then ascend proximally to the legs in a "stocking" distribution. When the sensory abnormalities reach the level of the knees, the symptoms begin in the hands, in a "glove"

distribution. Truncal and abdominal dysesthesias may develop once the sensory abnormalities ascend to the level of the elbows.

The prominent clinical feature of an acquired *demyelinating* polyneuropathy is weakness that affects not only the distal muscles, but also the proximal and facial muscles. Unlike in an axonal neuropathy, sensory loss is rarely the presenting symptom. Patients generally have diffuse hyporeflexia or areflexia.

Vasculitic neuropathies typically present with acute or subacute asymmetrical, predominantly distal weakness and sensory loss associated with severe pain.

Diagnosis and Differential Diagnosis

Neuropathic disorders can be broadly divided into those that are acquired and those that are hereditary (Table 121-8). Acquired disorders are the more common and have many causes: metabolic or endocrine disorders (diabetes mellitus, renal failure, porphyria); immune-mediated disorders (GBS, CIDP, multifocal motor neuropathy, antimyelin-associated glycoprotein neuropathy); infectious causes (human immunodeficiency virus [HIV], Lyme disease, cytomegalovirus [CMV], syphilis, leprosy, diphtheria); medications (HIV drugs, chemotherapies); environmental toxins (heavy metals); or paraneoplastic processes. Diabetes

TABLE 121-8 HEREDITARY NEUROPATHIC DISORDERS

	INHERITANCE PATTERN	GENETIC DEFECT	CLINICAL FEATURES
Hereditary sensorimotor neuropathies	AR, AD, or X-linked	See E-Table 121-4	Pes cavus, distal atrophy and weakness, hammer toes
Familial amyloid polyneuropathy	AD	Transthyretin Gelsolin Apolipoprotein AI	Pain, autonomic dysfunction
Fabry disease	X-linked	α-Galactosidase	Cardiac ischemia, renal disease, stroke, cutaneous angiokeratomas
Tangier disease	AR	Apolipoprotein A	Low HDL levels, orange tonsils
Refsum disease	AR	Phytanic acid oxidase	Retinitis pigmentosa, cardiomyopathy, deafness, ichthyosis

AD, Autosomal dominant; AR, autosomal recessive; HDL, high-density lipoprotein.

mellitus and alcoholism are the most common causes of polyneuropathy in developed countries. As many as one third of acquired neuropathies are cryptogenic in which the etiology can never be identified. Causes of monneuritis multiplex include systemic vasculitis (rheumatoid arthritis, systemic lupus erythematosus, Wegener's granulomatosis, Churg-Strauss syndrome, polyarteritis nodosa) and primary peripheral system vasculitis (25% of cases).

Because of the many causes, it is important to approach the patient with neuropathy systematically, beginning with the patient's history and physical examination. It is essential to determine which nerves are involved (motor, sensory, or autonomic) and in what specific combination (Table 121-9). Small-fiber neuropathies often manifest with unpleasant or abnormal sensations such as a burning pain, electric shock-like sensations, cramping, tingling, pins and needles, or prickly feelings such as the limb "feeling asleep." Large-fiber neuropathies can manifest as numbness, tingling, or as gait ataxia. Symptoms suggesting motor nerve involvement include muscle weakness that typically involves the distal foot muscles. Autonomic nerve involvement is suggested by symptoms of orthostatic hypotension, impotence, cardiac arrhythmia, or bladder dysfunction.

The distribution of muscle weakness is important. In axonal neuropathies, the weakness predominantly involves the distal lower extremity muscles, and in demyelinating neuropathies the weakness can involve both proximal and distal muscles as well as facial muscles. Most neuropathies result in *symmetrical* weakness. If asymmetry is present, motor neuron disease, radiculopathy, plexopathy, compressive mononeuropathies, or mononeuritis multiplex should be considered. The intensity and distribution of painful dysesthesias can be informative. Although many axonal neuropathies are associated with a burning sensation in the feet, pain as the chief complaint suggests specific causes of neuropathy (Table 121-10). A neuropathy that manifests with acute, asymmetrical weakness, and severe pain suggests vasculitis.

In patients with severe, asymmetrical proprioceptive deficits, with sparing of motor function, the site of the lesion is usually the sensory neuron. This specific syndrome has a relatively limited differential diagnosis, including paraneoplastic process, Sjögren's syndrome, cisplatinum toxicity, vitamin B_6 toxicity, and HIV infection.

Most neuropathies are relatively insidious in onset, particularly those associated with metabolic or endocrine disorders. Acute neuropathies may be caused by a vasculitic process, toxin exposure, porphyria, or GBS. GBS is commonly preceded by

TABLE 121-9 DIFFERENTIAL DIAGNOSIS OF NEUROPATHIC DISORDERS BASED ON SYMPTOMS

MOTOR SYMPTOMS ONLY	SENSORY SYMPTOMS ONLY	AUTONOMIC SYMPTOMS
Porphyria	Cryptogenic sensory polyneuropathy	Amyloid neuropathy
Charcot-Marie-Tooth	Metabolic, drug-related, or toxic neuropathy	Diabetic neuropathy
Chronic inflammatory demyelinating polyneuropathy	Paraneoplastic sensory neuropathy	Fabry disease
Guillain-Barré syndrome		Guillain-Barré syndrome
Lead neuropathy		Hereditary sensory or autonomic neuropathy
Motor neuron disease		Porphyria

TABLE 121-10 NEUROPATHIES ASSOCIATED WITH PAIN

Alcoholic neuropathy	Heavy metal toxicity (arsenic, thallium)
Amyloidosis	Hereditary sensory or autonomic neuropathy
Cryptogenic sensorimotor neuropathy	HIV sensorimotor neuropathy
Diabetic neuropathy	Radiculopathy or plexopathy
Fabry disease	Vasculitis
Guillain-Barré syndrome	

HIV, Human immunodeficiency virus.

a viral illness, immunization, or a surgical procedure. The neurologic history must thoroughly explore potential toxic exposures such as prior medications and alcohol use (E-Table 121-3).

Because many neuropathies are hereditary, it is essential to obtain a detailed family history, specifically inquiring about a history of gait instability, use of adaptive equipment, or skeletal deformities of the feet. Hereditary neuropathies may be autosomal recessive, autosomal dominant, or X-linked. In some situations it may be helpful to actually examine family members because the severity of disease may vary considerably from one generation to the next. The most common hereditary neuropathy is CMT disease (see later discussion).

A complete neurologic examination should always be performed in a patient complaining of numbness. If the patient shows evidence of upper motor neuron involvement in addition to the sensory loss, vitamin B_{12} or copper deficiency should be considered, even in the absence of apparent anemia. An elevated methylmalonic acid or homocystine level can also help confirm this diagnosis in patients with borderline B_{12} levels. The presence of weakness and upper motor neuron signs without associated sensory loss suggests ALS.

If the neuropathy is associated with mental status abnormalities, then pyridoxine intoxication or deficiencies of thiamine, niacin ("dementia, diarrhea, dermatitis"), and vitamin B_{12} should be considered in the differential diagnosis. Lyme disease (see Chapter 90) may result in both peripheral nervous system symptoms (facial nerve palsies, paresthesias, weakness) and central nervous system symptoms (dementia, headache). Acquired immunodeficiency syndrome (AIDS) can also affect both the central and the peripheral nervous systems. GBS and CIDP usually occur at the time of HIV seroconversion, whereas sensory neuropathy, mononeuritis multiplex, and CMV polyradiculopathy generally occur in the context of low CD4 counts in the terminal stages of the disease.

Once a preliminary differential diagnosis is developed based on the history and neurologic examination findings, laboratory studies can confirm the diagnosis. Laboratory tests to identify potentially treatable causes of neuropathy are included in Table 121-11. Additional studies can be ordered based on the suspected diagnosis. An impaired glucose tolerance test is found in more than half of patients with cryptogenic sensory peripheral neuropathy and is more sensitive than tests of fasting glucose or hemoglobin A_{1c} (HbA_{1c}). In a patient with acute, asymmetrical weakness and sensory loss, screening for an inflammatory process (ESR, ANA, RA, SS-A, SS-B) is appropriate. In addition, genetic testing is now available for most patients with CMT disease. If a monoclonal protein is identified on serum protein electrophoresis, a skeletal survey, urine immunofixation electrophoresis, and bone marrow biopsy should be ordered to rule out an underlying lymphoproliferative disorder. If the patient has a monoclonal protein associated with autonomic dysfunction, congestive heart failure, or renal insufficiency, a biopsy (rectal, abdominal fat, or sural nerve) should be considered for diagnosis of amyloidosis. CIDP can be associated with a monoclonal gammopathy, and in this situation patients should be treated with immunosuppressive therapy. Monoclonal gammopathies observed in patients with an axonal peripheral neuropathy are frequently benign (monoclonal gammopathy of unknown significance) and do not necessarily warrant therapy.

A lumbar puncture is indicated only if an acquired demyelinating neuropathy such as GBS or CIDP is being considered. In these cases one expects to find "albuminocytologic dissociation" with an elevation in cerebrospinal fluid (CSF) protein and a relatively normal white blood cell (WBC) count. If the CSF WBC count is greater than $50/mm^3$, Lyme disease, HIV-associated disease, or a paraneoplastic process must be considered.

Electrodiagnostic studies consisting of nerve conduction testing and EMG can be a helpful extension of the physical examination. These studies are useful in defining whether the neuropathic process is caused by a primarily axonal or demyelinating process. In general, axonal degeneration decreases the amplitude of the compound muscle action potential out of proportion to the degree of reduction in peripheral nerve conduction velocity, whereas demyelination produces prominent reduction in conduction velocities. Nerve conduction testing can help determine, in the case of a demyelinating neuropathy, whether the process has an acquired or hereditary cause. A uniform slowing of nerve conduction usually suggests a hereditary cause. Electrodiagnostic studies can identify subclinical neuropathy (in patients receiving potentially neurotoxic medications) and can quantitate the extent of axon loss. Finally, these studies can localize the lesion in the case of radiculopathies, plexopathies, and multiple mononeuropathies.

Sensory nerve biopsies should be obtained for diagnosis of a vasculitic neuropathy because treatment involves potentially toxic medications. Performing a muscle biopsy in addition to the nerve biopsy may improve the diagnostic yield and should be considered because the inflammation is random and focal and easily missed. Nerve biopsies are not indicated in "cryptogenic" neuropathies, diabetic neuropathy, or motor neuron disease. If nerve conduction studies are normal, skin biopsies allow quantification of the number of epidermal nerve fibers. A length-dependent decrease in the number of these fibers can help confirm a small fiber neuropathy.

Treatment

Despite a very thorough history, examination, and laboratory studies, the cause of as many as one third of neourpathics remain unknown. In this situation, the focus of management is pain control. Patients with neuropathy frequently report a burning, searing, and aching sensation in their feet and hands that interferes with sleep. Neuropathic pain is difficult to treat but may respond to various medications having different mechanisms of action (Table 121-12). It is important to "start low and taper slow" and to treat for a minimum of 4 weeks before concluding that an agent is ineffective. In patients with a vasculitic neuropathy, therapy with corticosteroids in addition to a cytotoxic agent can stabilize and in some cases improve the neuropathy.

Prognosis

Peripheral neuropathies caused by axonal degeneration are generally progressive unless the underlying cause can be identified and treated. Recovery from axonal degeneration requires nerve regeneration, a process that often requires 2 to 3 years. Prognosis

TABLE 121-11 PERIPHERAL NEUROPATHY LABORATORY STUDIES

STANDARD TESTS	TESTS INDICATED IN SELECTED CASES
B_{12}	Anti-Hu antibody
Complete blood count	ESR, ANA, RF, SS-A, SS-B
Glucose tolerance test	Genetic studies for Charcot-Marie-Tooth
Rapid plasmin reagin	Human immunodeficiency virus
SMA20	Lyme antibody
Serum protein electrophoresis and immunofixation electrophoresis	Phytanic acid
Thyroid function tests	24-hr urine for heavy metals
Nerve conduction studies or electromyogram	Quantitative sensory testing
	Lumbar puncture
	Nerve biopsy
	Skin biopsy
	Tilt table testing

TABLE 121-12	SYMPTOMATIC TREATMENT FOR NEUROPATHIC PAIN
TRICYCLIC ANTIDEPRESSANTS	Topiramate 150-200 mg bid (Level U)
Amitriptyline 10-150 mg qhs (Level B)	Duloxetine 60-120 mg qd (Level B)
Nortriptyline 10-150 mg qhs (Level U)	Pregabalin 150-600 mg qd (Level A)
Imipramine 10-150 mg qhs (Level U)	Sodium valproate 250-500 mg BID (Level B)
Desipramine 10-150 mg qhs (Level U)	**ALTERNATIVE TREATMENTS**
Venlafaxine 75-225 mg qd (Level B)	Tramadol 50-100 mg qid (Level B)
ANTICONVULSANTS	Lidoderm patches (Level C)
Gabapentin 300-1200 mg tid (Level B)	Capsaicin cream (Level B)
Carbamazepine 100-200 mg tid (Level U)	Transcutaneous nerve stimulation Acupuncture

of demyelinating and vasculitic neuropathies is extremely variable, depending on the cause.

⬤ COMMON MONONEUROPATHIES

Common mononeuropathies are explored in Table 121-7.

Carpal Tunnel Syndrome

Carpal tunnel syndrome results from compression of the median nerve at the wrist as it passes beneath the flexor retinaculum. Precipitating factors include activities that require repetitive wrist movements, such as mechanical work, gardening, house painting, and typing. Predisposing causes include pregnancy, diabetes, acromegaly, rheumatoid arthritis, chronic renal failure, thyroid disorders, and primary amyloidosis.

Symptoms usually begin in the dominant hand but commonly involve both hands over time. Patients typically report numbness, tingling, and burning sensations in the palm and in the fingers supplied by the median nerve: the thumb, index finger, middle finger, and medial one half of the ring finger. Some patients report that all fingers become numb. Pain and paresthesias are most prominent at night and often interrupt sleep. The pain is prominent at the wrist but may radiate to the forearm and occasionally to the shoulder. Shaking the hand relieves both pain and paresthesias. Percussion of the median nerve at the wrist provokes paresthesias in a median nerve distribution in 60% of patients (Tinel sign), and flexion of the wrist for 30 to 60 seconds provokes pain or paresthesias in 75% of cases (Phalen sign).

The diagnosis is based on clinical symptoms and signs. Electrodiagnostic studies may demonstrate prolongation of the sensory or motor latencies across the wrist in up to 85% of patients. In more severe cases, EMG may demonstrate evidence of denervation in the abductor pollicis brevis.

Treatment initially includes avoidance of repetitive wrist activities and the use of a neutral wrist splint. If these conservative measures fail, injections of lidocaine and methylprednisolone can be given into the carpal tunnel or surgical treatment by section of the transverse carpal ligament can effectively decompress the nerve. Indicators that have been shown to predict failure with conservative management include age greater than 50 years, disease duration greater than 10 months, constant paresthesias, and a positive Phalen sign in less than 10 seconds.

Ulnar Palsy

The ulnar nerve may become entrapped at the elbow because of external compression in the condylar groove. Injury may also occur years after a malunited supracondylar fracture of the humerus with bony overgrowth. Contrary to the findings in carpal tunnel syndrome, muscle weakness and atrophy characteristically predominate over sensory symptoms and signs. Patients notice atrophy of the first dorsal interosseous muscle and difficulty performing fine manipulations of the fingers. Numbness of the little finger, the contiguous one half of the ring finger, and the ulnar border of the hand may be present. Ulnar nerve compression can be confirmed with electrodiagnostic studies demonstrating slowed motor conduction velocity across the elbow. Treatment includes the use of elbow pads to avoid compression or surgical procedures including transposition of the ulnar nerve or decompression of the cubital tunnel.

Peroneal Neuropathy

The peroneal nerve can become compressed as it wraps around the fibular head and passes into the fibular tunnel between the peroneus longus muscle and the fibula. Compression may occur as a result of habitual leg crossing, prolonged bedrest, knee casts, prolonged squatting, anesthesia, or profound weight loss. The nerve can also be compressed as a result of Baker cysts, fibular fractures, blunt trauma, tumors, or hematomas at the knee. Symptoms include "footdrop" with selective weakness of the ankle dorsiflexors and evertors as well as the toe extensors. Reflexes remain normal, and sensory loss generally involves the anterolateral leg and dorsum of the foot. Electrodiagnostic studies demonstrate slowing of the peroneal conduction velocity across the fibular head and may demonstrate denervation if axonal injury is present. Compressive injuries usually resolve spontaneously within weeks to months. Magnetic resonance imaging (MRI) and surgical exploration should be considered if symptoms are progressive.

⬤ SPECIFIC ACQUIRED POLYNEUROPATHIES

Guillain-Barré Syndrome: Acute Inflammatory Demyelinating Polyneuropathy

Since the advent of polio vaccination, Guillian-Barré (GBS) has become the most frequent cause of acute flaccid paralysis throughout the world. GBS is an immune-mediated disorder that follows an identifiable infectious disorder in approximately 60% of patients. The best-documented antecedents include infection with *Campylobacter jejuni*, infectious mononucleosis, CMV, herpesvirus, and mycoplasma. *C. jejuni* is often associated with more severe axonal cases.

The initial symptoms of GBS often consist of tingling and pins-and-needles sensations in the feet and may be associated with dull low back pain. By the time of presentation, which occurs hours to 1 to 2 days after the first symptoms, weakness has usually developed. The weakness is usually most prominent in the legs, but the arms or cranial musculature may be involved first. Muscle stretch reflexes are lost early, even in regions where strength is retained. Cutaneous sensory deficits (loss of pain and temperature) are relatively mild; however, large fiber function (vibration and proprioception) is more severely impaired. Other clinical features include pain (20%), paresthesias (50%), autonomic symptoms (20%), facial weakness (50%), ophthalmoparesis (9%), bulbar weakness, and respiratory failure (25%). Symptoms associated with GBS typically evolve over a 2- to 4-week period, with approximately 90% of patients showing no evidence of progression beyond 4 weeks. For this reason, patients who are seen within several weeks from onset continue to require hospitalization for close observation. Respiratory muscle strength should be monitored with bedside measurements of the forced vital capacity. Intubation should be initiated when the forced vital capacity falls below 15 mL/kg.

Treatment may include either intravenous gammaglobulin (0.4 g/kg/day for 5 days) or plasmapheresis (the exchange of the patient's plasma for albumin) (200 mL/kg over 7 to 10 days). Clinical studies have confirmed equal efficacy between these two therapies, with no additional benefit conferred with combination therapy. Corticosteroids are not effective in GBS. Indications for therapy include inability to ambulate independently, impaired respiratory function, or rapidly progressive weakness.

Clinical features predicting a poor prognosis or prolonged recovery time include rapidly progressive weakness, need for mechanical ventilation, and low-amplitude compound muscle action potentials. The mortality rate remains 5% to 10%, usually because of respiratory complications, cardiac arrhythmia, or pulmonary embolism. With appropriate supportive care and rehabilitation, 80% to 90% of patients recover with little or no disability.

Chronic Inflammatory Demyelinating Polyneuropathy

Chronic inflammatory demyelinating polyneuropathy (CIDP) has been considered the "chronic form" of GBS, because by definition the symptoms must progress for at least 8 weeks. The clinical features include proximal and distal weakness, areflexia, and distal sensory loss. Autonomic dysfunction, respiratory insufficiency, and cranial nerve involvement can occur but are much less common than in GBS. Treatment for CIDP includes the use of oral immunosuppressive agents such as prednisone, cyclosporine, mycophenolate mofetil, and azathioprine. Intravenous immune globulin and plasmapheresis are also indicated for severe or refractory cases.

Diabetic Neuropathy

Diabetes mellitus is the most frequent cause of peripheral neuropathy worldwide. The diabetic neuropathies take many clinical forms, including symmetrical polyneuropathies and a wide variety of individual plexus or nerve disorders.

Diabetes mellitus often causes a slowly progressive, distal, symmetrical sensorimotor polyneuropathy (DSPN). DSPN is uncommon at the time of diagnosis of diabetes, but its prevalence increases with duration of diabetes with a lifetime prevalence of 55% for type 1 and 45% for type 2. The precise pathogenesis is not defined, but, similar to the ocular and renal complications, diabetic neuropathy can be reduced in incidence and in severity by maintaining blood glucose levels close to normal.

Initial symptoms may consist of numbness, tingling, burning, or prickling sensations affecting the feet and toes. Mild distal weakness and gait instability may subsequently develop. The sensory symptoms can then slowly progress to involve a "stocking-glove pattern." The small-fiber dysfunction often produces spontaneous neuropathic pain in which unpleasant sensations can be evoked by normally innocuous stimuli, such as the bed sheets on the toes at night. Continuous burning or throbbing pain may occur, and prolonged walking is often distressing. In severe cases, patients may develop foot ulcers in insensitive areas that necessitate amputation. Autonomic dysfunction is also frequently associated with DSPN including impotence, nocturnal diarrhea, sweating abnormalities, orthostatic hypotension, and gastroparesis.

Other less common neuropathies associated with diabetes include cranial neuropathies (the sixth, third, and rarely fourth nerves), mononeuropathies, mononeuropathy multiplex, radiculopathies, and plexopathies. Diabetic amyotrophy (also known as *diabetic lumbosacral polyradiculopathy*) is a distinctive disorder characterized by severe thigh pain followed by proximal greater than distal lower extremity weakness that progresses over a period of months. The onset is invariably unilateral, but the condition may progress to involve both lower extremities. Physical therapy and effective pain management are essential; treatment with immune modulators is controversial.

Toxic-Induced Neuropathies

Toxic-induced neuropathies constitute a large number of disorders caused by alcohol, drugs, heavy metals, and environmental substances (E-Table 121-3). The majority of toxic neuropathies manifest as a distal sensorimotor axonal neuropathy that chronically progresses over time unless the offending agent is eliminated. Clinical evaluation should focus on the temporal relationship between exposure and the onset of sensory or motor symptoms as well as symptoms of systemic toxicity.

Critical Illness Polyneuropathy

Critical illness polyneuropathy (CIP) is a common cause of failure to wean from a ventilator in a patient with associated sepsis and multi-organ failure. Clinical features include generalized or distal flaccid paralysis, especially involving the lower extremities, depressed or absent reflexes, and distal sensory loss with relative sparing of cranial nerve function. The diagnosis can be confirmed with nerve conduction studies showing evidence of a severe, generalized axonal neuropathy. CSF protein should be normal and, in addition to conduction studies, distinguishes CIP from GBS.

⬤ SPECIFIC HEREDITARY POLYNEUROPATHIES

Charcot-Marie-Tooth Disease

The eponym Charcot-Marie-Tooth (CMT) identifies a group of heritable disorders of peripheral nerves that share clinical features but differ in their pathologic mechanisms and the specific genetic abnormalities (E-Table 121-4). CMT is the most common heritable neuromuscular disorder, with an incidence of 17 to 40 cases per 100,000.

CMT disease usually manifests during the first to second decades with symptoms related to insidious footdrop: frequent tripping and inability to jump well or run as fast as other children. Over time, distal upper extremity weakness develops, resulting in difficulty with buttoning, handling keys, and opening jars. Examination reveals distal weakness and wasting of the intrinsic muscles of the feet, the peroneal muscles, the anterior tibial muscles, and the calves (inverted champagne bottle legs). A variable degree of impaired large-fiber sensory function is reflected in reduced vibratory sensation at the toes. Muscle stretch reflexes are lost, first at the ankles. Typically, a foot deformity exists, with high arches (pes cavus) and hammer toes, reflecting long-standing muscle imbalance in the feet. Most patients with CMT disease have nearly normal occupational and daily activities, and they have a normal life span. Although no specific treatment has been developed, the foot drop can be treated by appropriate bracing of the ankle with ankle-foot orthoses. Genetic counseling and education of affected patients and their families are important, both for reassurance and to preclude unnecessary diagnostic evaluation of affected members in future generations.

Demyelinating forms of CMT are classified as CMT1 and axonal forms as CMT2. CMT is usually transmitted as an autosomal dominant trait; however, X-linked dominant transmission is responsible for approximately 10% of cases. Rare autosomal recessive forms are designated CMT4, and these patients tend to have an earlier onset and more severe phenotype. CMT1A is the most common form and accounts for 90% of CMT1 and 50% of all CMT cases. CMT1A is associated with the 17p11.2-p12 duplication in the *PMP22* gene expressed by Schwann cells. A deletion or a point mutation of the *PMP22* gene produces a different phenotype: HNPP, which is characterized by recurrent episodes of focal entrapment with attacks of weakness and numbness in the peroneal, ulnar, radial, and median nerves (in descending order of frequency) or in a brachial plexus distribution.

● FAMILIAL AMYLOID NEUROPATHIES

Amyloid neuropathy is an autosomal dominant disorder caused by extracellular deposition of the fibrillary protein amyloid in peripheral nerve and sensory and autonomic ganglia, as well as around blood vessels in nerves and other tissues. The age of onset varies from 18 to 83 years. In all forms of amyloidosis, the initial and major abnormalities affect the small sensory and autonomic fibers. Involvement of small fibers responsible for pain and temperature sensibilities leads to loss of the ability to perceive mechanical and thermal injuries and to an increased risk of tissue damage. As a result, painless injuries present a major hazard of this disorder; in advanced stages, they can lead to chronic infections or osteomyelitis of the feet or hands and the necessity for amputation. Amyloid deposition in the heart can lead to cardiomyopathy. Mutations in transthyretin, apolipoprotein A1, or gelsolin are responsible. Early recognition is essential, as liver transplantation has been shown to halt disease progression.

For a deeper discussion on this topic, please see Chapter 420, "Peripheral Neuropathies," in Goldman-Cecil Medicine, *25th Edition.*

SUGGESTED READINGS

Barohn RJ: Approach to peripheral neuropathy and neuronopathy, Sem Neurol 18:7–18, 1998.

Bril V, England J, Franklin GM, et al: Evidence-based guideline: Treatment of painful diabetic neuropathy–report of the American Association of Neuromuscular and Electrodiagnostic Medicine, the American Academy of Neurology, and the American Academy of Physical Medicine & Rehabilitation, Muscle Nerve 43:910–917, 2011.

Dyck PJ, Thomas PK, editors: Peripheral Neuropathy, ed 4, Philadelphia, 2005, WB Saunders.

Feldman EL: Amyotrophic lateral sclerosis and other motor neuron diseases. In Goldman L, Ausiello DA, editors: Cecil Textbook of Medicine, ed 23, Philadelphia, 2007, WB Saunders.

Jackson CE, Bryan WW: Amyotrophic lateral sclerosis, Sem Neurol 18:27–40, 1998.

Miller RG, Jackson CE, Kasarkis EJ, et al: Practice parameter update: The care of the patient with amyotrophic lateral sclerosis: drug, nutritional, and respiratory therapies (an evidence-based review):report of the Quality Standards Subcommittee of the American Academy of Neurology, Neurology 73(15):1218–1226, 2009.

Miller RG, Jackson CE, Kasarksi EJ, et al: Practice parameter update: The care of the patient with amyotrophic lateral sclerosis: multidisciplinary care, symptom management, and cognitive/behavioral impairment (an evidence-based review): report of the Quality Standards Subcommittee of the American Academy of Neurology, Neurology 73(15):1227–1233, 2009.

Shy M: Peripheral neuropathies. In Goldman L, Ausiello DA, editors: Cecil Textbook of Medicine, ed 23, Philadelphia, 2007, WB Saunders.

Wolfe GI, Baker NS, Amato AA, et al: Chronic cryptogenic sensory polyneuropathy: clinical and laboratory characteristics, Arch Neurol 56:540–547, 1999.

122

Muscle Diseases

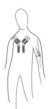

Jeffrey M. Statland and Robert C. Griggs

INTRODUCTION

Skeletal muscle fibers are the effector cells of the nervous system, turn thoughts into actions, and are the means by which we interact with our environment. Myopathies are primary diseases of the muscle and can be both inherited and acquired (Table 122-1). Myopathies can result in weakness and muscle wasting, myalgias, cramps, muscle breakdown, or contractures. Inherited disorders affect muscle proteins involved in transmission of signals from the neuromuscular junction, proteins involved in energy production or metabolism, or structural proteins that anchor and transmit force from the contractile apparatus to the extracellular matrix. Acquired myopathies are caused by external factors and can be due to metabolic derangements, toxic exposures or drugs, infections, or autoimmune dysfunction causing inflammation in the muscle. Acquired myopathies often improve with treatments geared towards eliminating or ameliorating the precipitating factors. To date, there have not been specific treatments for most inherited disorders of muscle, but as our understanding of the molecular pathological mechanisms of these disorders advances, new disease-directed therapies are entering clinical trials.

ORGANIZATION AND STRUCTURE OF MUSCLE

Each muscle is enclosed in a connective tissue sheath made up of collagen and extracellular matrix proteins called the epimyseum, which merges at either end to form the tendons, which attach muscle to bone. The epimyseum divides internally into the perimysium, which separates the muscle into individual bundles of muscle fibers called fascicles. The endomyseum surrounds and provides support for the individual fibers. Each muscle fiber is a single multi-nucleated syncytial cell and can be as long as 10 cm. On cross section, muscle fibers appear polygonal in shape and in adults range from 40 to 80 micrometers in diameter. Medium size arterioles and veins run in the perimysium, with capillaries between the individual muscle fibers. On hematoxylin and eosin stains, cytoplasm appears pink and the nuclei blue, with a thin rim of white, the epimyseum, between fibers (Fig. 122-1A). Each

individual muscle fiber has multiple nuclei, which are found beneath the sarcolemma membrane on the periphery of the cell. The amount of connective tissue between fibers, the position and number of myonuclei, and the amount and distribution of mitochondria can all be indicators of disease.

The plasma membrane around the muscle fiber is called the sarcolemma, and inside there are a large number of myofibrils made of thick (myosin) and thin (actin) filaments, which make up 70% to 80% of the volume of the cell, and when activated, create force. Electrochemical signals carry the signal from the nerve, through the neuromuscular junction, into the muscle fiber along the sarcolemma and t-tubule system. Muscle ion channels line this network and carry electrochemical signals. Mitochondria and enzymes involved in glycolysis and fatty acid metabolism provide energy for muscle. A network of proteins, the dystrophin-glycoprotein complex (DGC), anchors the myofibrils to the subsarcolema cytoskeleton and connects to the extracellular matrix (Fig. 122-2). Many inherited myopathies are due to mutations in these ion channels, metabolic enzymes, or structural anchoring proteins.

ASSESSMENT

The work-up of a patient with a suspected myopathy is a staged process and involves a history and physical examination, followed by laboratory studies, electrodiagnostic testing, muscle biopsy, and genetic testing (Table 122-2). The family history is important because muscle disease can run in the family and may not have been previously diagnosed. Questions about whether family members require assistive devices to walk or wheelchairs, and concerning common extra muscular manifestation of muscular dystrophies can be useful. The genetic myopathies can be inherited in an autosomal dominant or recessive fashion, be X-linked, show maternal inheritance, or be sporadic (Table 122-3).

The most common symptom of a patient with muscle disease is a loss of function caused by weakness (see Table 122-2). Other common symptoms, like fatigue or myalgias (muscle pain), are less specific than muscle weakness. Muscle cramping is most often benign, and can be secondary to neuropathic changes. Muscle contractures are sustained contractions that are distinguished from cramping on electrodiagnostic testing, where contractures are electrically silent. Tendon contractures, on the other hand, are a fixed shortening of the tendon, and associated with long-standing disuse.

EXAMINATION

The physical examination uses a standard modified Medical Research Council scale of motor strength to determine the

TABLE 122-1 OVERVIEW OF MYOPATHIES

HEREDITARY MYOPATHIES	ACQUIRED MYOPATHIES
Muscular dystrophies	Inflammatory myopathies
Congenital myopathies	Endocrine myopathies
Metabolic/Mitochondrial myopathies	Systemic illness/infectious myopathies
Channelopathies	Toxic/Drug-induced myopathies

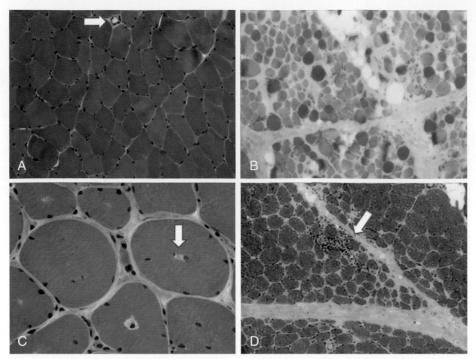

FIGURE 122-1 Muscle biopsies hematoxylin and eosin staining. **A,** Normal adult muscle medium power. Notice polygonal muscle fibers arranged in fascicles with blue staining nuclei on the periphery. A small arteriole is visible *(white arrow)*. **B,** Duchenne muscular dystrophy low power. Note the variability in fiber size with rounding of fibers, increase in connective tissue, and fatty deposition. **C,** Centronuclear congenital myopathy. Notice variability in fiber size, large rounded fibers, and characteristic central nuclei in most fibers *(white arrow)*. **D,** Dermatomyositis on low power. Notice the prominent perifascicular atrophy of fibers, with inflammatory infiltrates *(white arrow)*.

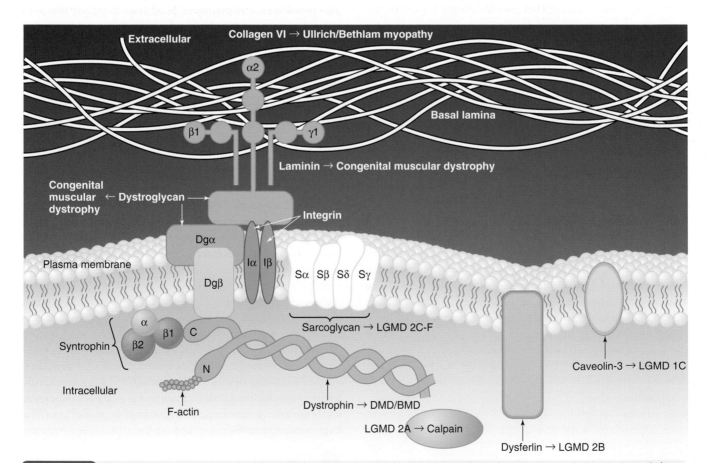

FIGURE 122-2 The dystrophin-glycoprotein complex. Muscle structural proteins connect the contractile apparatus to the internal cytoskeleton and the extracellular matrix. Mutations in proteins from the extracellular matrix to the anchoring proteins, which connect the extracellular matrix to the internal cytoskeleton to proteins, which attach the internal cytoskeleton to the contractile apparatus are all involved in the inherited muscular dystrophies and myopathies.

TABLE 122-2 WORK UP FOR A PATIENT WITH SUSPECTED MYOPATHY

FEATURE	DESCRIPTION
HISTORY	
Age of onset	Congenital, childhood, adult
Chronic, progressive, or episodic	Dystrophies are usually progressive; congenital static; metabolic/channelopathies episodic
Triggers	Exercise, foods, temperatures
FAMILY HISTORY	Dominant, recessive, or no family history
WEAKNESS ON EXAM	
Proximal	Difficulty lifting objects, climbing stairs, getting up from chair, scapular winging, waddling gait, Gower's sign
Distal	Difficulty making a tight fist, fastening buttons, opening jars, wrist drop, foot drop
Facial	Difficulty squeezing the eyes shut, transvers smile, inability to pucker or blow out cheeks, inability to whistle
Oculopharyngeal	Ptosis, restricted extra ocular movements, coughing after drinking, and difficulty swallowing
Cardiac	Cardiac conduction defects, cardiomyopathy
Respiratory	Using accessory muscles, difficulty lying flat
LABORATORY	
CK	Dystrophies/inflammatory myopathy increased >10x normal; congenital 3-5x normal; metabolic >10x normal during attacks
Thyroid / Parathyroid	High TSH, low T4, low PTH, Ca^{2+}
ELECTRODIAGNOSTIC STUDIES	Irritated muscle shows fibrillations and positive sharp waves; myopathic motor units are brief, low amplitude, and polyphasic; myotonia spontaneous waxing and waning motor unit amplitude and frequency
MUSCLE BIOPSY	Changes in muscle fiber shape and composition of fiber types, amount of connective tissue, presence of inflammatory cells, necrotic muscle fibers, regenerating fibers, number or morphology of mitochondria, or abnormal deposits of fat or glycogen
GENETIC TESTING	Confirmatory for inherited myopathies

TABLE 122-3 INHERITANCE PATTERN IN GENETIC MYOPATHIES

X-LINKED	Oculopharyngeal muscular dystrophy Channelopathies Central core myopathy
Duchenne/Becker muscular dystrophy Emory-Dreifuss muscular dystrophy	**AUTOSOMAL RECESSIVE**
AUTOSOMAL DOMINANT	Limb-girdle muscular dystrophy (2A-2S) Metabolic myopathies Recessive myotonia congenita
Myotonic dystrophy types 1 and 2 Facioscapulohumeral muscular dystrophy Limb-girdle muscular dystrophy (1A-1H)	**MATERNAL TRANSMISSION**
	Mitochondrial myopathies

TABLE 122-4 MODIFIED MEDICAL RESEARCH COUNCIL MOTOR STRENGTH TESTING SCALE

GRADE	DEGREE OF STRENGTH
5	Normal strength through entire range of motion and against resistance
5-	Equivocal, barely detectable weakness
4+	Able to move against gravity and resistance, but examiner can break
4	Able to move against gravity and some resistance
4-	Able to resist gravity but only minimal resistance
3+	Able to overcome gravity and transient resistance, but then quickly gives out
3	Able to overcome gravity but no resistance
3-	Able to resist gravity but not through full range of motion
2	Able to move through range of motion with gravity eliminated
1	Trace muscle contraction
0	No contraction

weakness occur in myopathies (Table 122-5). Most myopathies have the proximal, limb-girdle pattern. There are other, highly distinctive, patterns. Weakness that is asymmetric and includes the face, proximal arms and shoulders, and distal lower extremities is characteristic of facioscapulohumeral muscular dystrophy. Weakness that starts in the distal finger flexors (patients cannot curl fingers when making a fist) and proximal lower extremities (the quadriceps) is virtually pathognomonic for sporadic inclusion body myositis. A patient in middle age who presents with ptosis and difficulty swallowing is highly characteristic for oculopharyngeal muscular dystrophy. In all cases these patterns need to be distinguished from other diseases of the nervous system causing similar patterns of weakness (see Chapters 121 and 123.).

⬤ DIAGNOSTIC TESTING

The most useful initial laboratory study is the serum creatine kinase (CK), which is commonly elevated in both inherited and acquired myopathies. Despite the obvious localizing value of elevated muscle enzymes it is important to remember not all elevations in serum CK are due to myopathy (Table 122-6).

Electrodiagnostic testing can help distinguish between neurogenic and myopathic causes for weakness. In muscle disease nerve conduction studies are normal. Changes on electromyography characteristic for muscle disease include: chronic changes characterized by small, brief duration, polyphasic motor units; and more acute changes (irritable myopathic changes), which include fibrillations or positive sharp waves.

Muscle biopsies can be an important diagnostic test in patients whose family history and physical examination does not suggest a particular myopathic diagnosis. Characteristic morphological changes are hallmarks of the congenital myopathies (e.g., central core disease, or centronuclear myopathy), inflammatory myopathies (dermatomyositis and polymyositis), and metabolic myopathies (glycogen storage disorders), but most myopathies result in nonspecific muscle changes including rounding of muscle fibers, variation in fiber size, and increased number of internal nuclei.

In patients for whom the family history is suggestive of an inherited myopathy or in which the diagnosis is important to help guide surveillance or treatment, genetic testing is confirmatory.

pattern and degree of involvement of various muscles (Table 122-4). But just as important as isolated strength testing are functional motor tasks, particularly in children. Patients may have difficulty climbing stairs, rising from a low chair or toilet, getting up from the floor, trouble lifting objects over their heads and washing or brushing their hair, or difficulty opening jar tops and fastening buttons. Muscles should be inspected for atrophy or hypertrophy and range of motion around the joints for evidence of tendon contractures. Ten broad patterns of muscle

TABLE 122-5 CHARACTERISTIC PATTERNS OF MUSCLE WEAKNESS AND ASSOCIATED MYOPATHIES

PATTERN	WEAKNESS	DISEASES
Proximal limb-girdle	Symmetrical, pelvic and shoulder girdle muscles. Distal muscles to lesser extent. ± Neck flexor/extensor.	Nonspecific: Duchenne muscular dystrophy; limb-girdle muscular dystrophy; inflammatory myopathies; certain autoimmune neuropathies
Distal	Symmetrical, distal upper or lower extremity. Proximal muscles to lesser degree.	Nonspecific: Miyoshi myopathy (calves); Welander myopathy (wrist and finger extensors); Nonaka and Markesbery/Udd myopathy (tibialis anterior); rule out neuropathy
Proximal arm/distal leg	Scapuloperoneal distribution: periscapular muscles (proximal arm) and anterior compartment distal leg (tibialis anterior). Scapular winging. Can be asymmetrical.	When face involved highly suggestive of facioscapulohumeral muscular dystrophy; with elbow contractures Emory-Dreifuss dystrophy; scapuloperoneal dystrophies; certain limb-girdle dystrophies; congenital myopathies
Distal arm/proximal leg	Distal forearm muscles (distal finger flexors) and proximal leg (quadriceps). Other muscles variable. Often asymmetrical.	Highly suggestive of sporadic inclusion body myositis; also consider myotonic dystrophy
Ptosis ± ophthalmoparesis	Ocular weakness at presentation. Restriction of eye movements often without diplopia. Occasionally followed by pharyngeal weakness. Variable extremity weakness	Ocular and pharyngeal weakness highly suggestive of oculopharyngeal muscular dystrophy; ptosis and ophthalmoplegia without pharyngeal involvement mitochondrial myopathies
Neck extensor weakness	Neck extensors, "dropped head syndrome." Variable neck flexor. ± extremity weakness.	In isolation consider isolated neck extensor myopathy; rule out amyotrophic lateral sclerosis and myasthenia gravis
Bulbar weakness	Tongue and pharyngeal weakness	Certain myopathies (e.g., oculopharyngeal muscular dystrophy); significant overlap with neuromuscular junction and motor neuron disease
Episodic pain, weakness, and myoglobinuria	May be triggered by exercise or metabolic stress	Metabolic myopathies; may also occur in deconditioning
Episodic weakness delayed or unrelated to exercise	May be triggered by food, stress, rest after exercise	Characteristic of periodic paralyses
Stiffness and decreased ability to relax	May be episodic, triggered by cold	Characteristic of myotonic disorders; but may be seen in other myopathies; acquired conditions (e.g. stiff person syndrome)

Modified from Jackson CE, Barohn RJ: A pattern recognition approach to myopathy, Continuum (Minneap Minn) 19(6 Muscle Diseases):1674-1697, 2013.

TABLE 122-6 CAUSES FOR ELEVATED SERUM CK

MYOPATHIES	MEDICATIONS
Muscular dystrophies/carrier state	Statins
Congenital myopathies	Fibric acid derivatives
Metabolic myopathies	Chloroquin
Inflammatory myopathies	Colchicine
CHANNELOPATHIES	**ENDOCRINE ABNORMALITIES (THYROID/PARATHYROID)**
MOTOR NEURON DISEASE (ALS, SMA)	**SURGERY**
NEUROPATHIES (GBS, CIDP)	**TRAUMA**
VIRAL ILLNESS	**STRENUOUS EXERCISE**
	INCREASED MUSCLE MASS
	IDIOPATHIC

INHERITED MYOPATHIES

Muscular Dystrophies

The muscular dystrophies are inherited myopathies characterized by progressive weakness and mutations in genes coding for structural and other muscle proteins. Typically the muscular dystrophies are divided into the dystrophinopathies, the myotonic dystrophies, facioscapulohumeral muscular dystrophy, Emery-Dreifuss muscular dystrophy, and the limb-girdle dystrophies (Tables 122-7, 122-8, and E-Table 122-1). The limb-girdle muscular dystrophies (LGMD) are a diverse group of diseases due to mutations in more than 20 genes. The LBMDs are inherited in either autosomal dominant or recessive fashion, and present anywhere from childhood to later in life, having as the name implies, a limb-girdle pattern of weakness (E-Table 122-1). Another group of patients who have dystrophic changes in the muscle from birth, often with accompanying changes in the brain on

MRI, include congenital muscular dystrophies (see Table 122-8; not discussed in text). The traditional distinction between dystrophies and other inherited myopathies is becoming blurred as our genetic understanding advances because mutations for different diseases are often allelic.

Dystrophinopathies

Definition and Epidemiology

Dystrophinopathies are X-linked recessive disorders resulting from mutations of the large dystrophin gene located at Xp21. The incidence of Duchenne muscular dystrophy is 1 in 5300 male births; one third of the cases result from a new mutation. Becker muscular dystrophy is a milder form of dystrophinopathy and is less common than the Duchenne form, with an incidence of 5 per 100,000.

Pathology

Dystrophin is a large subsarcolemmal cytoskeletal protein that, along with the other components of the dystrophin-glycoprotein complex, provides support to the muscle membrane during contraction. Muscle biopsies are typically not required for diagnosis but show variability in fiber size; active and chronic changes, including necrotic and regenerating fibers; and, later in the disease, increased connective tissue and deposition of fat (Fig. 122-1B).

Clinical Presentation

Mutations in dystrophin result in a spectrum of disorders reflecting variations in the amount of functional dystrophin still expressed—from Duchenne muscular dystrophy and Becker's on the severe end, to isolated quadriceps weakness and isolated cardiomyopathy in the middle, and to cramps and myalgias with

TABLE 122-7 PREVALENT MUSCULAR DYSTROPHIES

DISEASE	INHERITANCE	MUTATIONS	AGE OF ONSET	PHENOTYPES	TREATMENT
Dystrophinopathies	X-linked recessive	Xp21; ~75% deletion or duplication; remaining sequence variant	Duchenne diagnosis by age 4; Becker variable	Limb-girdle pattern. Duchenne: severe progressive and life limiting. Becker progressive but not as severe, more variable. Calf pseudo-hypertrophy; isolated quadriceps weakness; isolated cardiomyopathy	Prednisone (or deflazacort) for Duchenne; ACE β-blocker for afterload reduction in cardiomyopathy; yearly to biannual surveillance for respiratory, cardiac and orthopedic problems
Myotonic dystrophy type 1	Autosomal dominant	19q13; CTG expansion > 50 repeats	Classic 20-30s; congenital at birth	Limb-girdle, can have distal weakness. Classic: myotonia and muscle wasting, temporal wasting, frontal balding; cataracts; cardiac conduction deficits; and diabetes. Congenital: severe and progressive, respiratory deficits, intellectual disability, and death ~45 years if survive neonatal period	Mexiletine for symptomatic myotonia; Yearly surveillance for cataracts, cardiac conduction deficits, and respiratory involvement.
Myotonic dystrophy type 2	Autosomal dominant	3q13; CCGT expansion > 75 repeats	30s	Limb-girdle pattern; multi-system involvement cataracts, cardiac conduction deficits; diabetes	Mexiletine for symptomatic myotonia; Yearly surveillance of ocular, cardiac, and respiratory involvement
Facioscapulohumeral muscular dystrophy	Autosomal dominant	4q35; ~95% between 1-10 D4Z4 repeats; ~5% decreased methylation <20% D4Z4 region	20s	Scapuloperoneal pattern with facial involvement; can have marked asymmetry; significant axial involvement	Supportive; screening dilated eye exam; hearing studies as indicated clinically; respiratory studies once wheelchair bound
Emery-Dreifuss muscular dystrophy	X-linked recessive; autosomal dominant or recessive	~70% Xq28 Emerin or FHL1 mutation; 1q21 lamin A/C, both dominant and recessive mutations reported	Joint contractures childhood; progressive weakness 20s-30s	Scapuloperoneal pattern; joint contractures, particularly at elbows, significant cardiac involvement	Yearly surveillance for cardiac and respiratory involvement; orthopedic evaluation for symptomatic contractures
Oculopharyngeal muscular dystrophy	Autosomal dominant and recessive	14q11 PABPN1 (Polyadenylate-binding protein) GCG repeats 7-13	40s (range 20s-60s)	Typically ptosis 2-3 years before dysphagia; limb-girdle pattern weakness	Swallow study; consider blepharoplasty for ptosis, consider cricopharyngeal myotomy for severe swallowing difficulty

TABLE 122-8 CONGENITAL MUSCULAR DYSTROPHIES

NAME / AKA	GENE	INHERITANCE	PHENOTYPE	CNS INVOLVEMENT
Merosin-deficient	6q22; laminin alpha-2	Autosomal recessive	Hypotonia; contractures; scoliosis or rigid spine; respiratory involvement; external ophthalmoplegia	MRI diffuse white matter changes; 20-30% seizures
Bethlam myopathy / Ullrich muscular dystrophy	21q22; 2q37; COL6 (collagen 6 spectrum disorders)	Autosomal dominant or recessive	Hypotonia; contractures; distal joint laxity; keloid; respiratory involvement	
Dystroglycanopathy	9q34 (POMT1); 14q24 (POMT2); 9q31 (fukutin); 19q13 (FKRP); 22q12 (LARGE); 1q32 (POMGnT1); 7p21 (ISPD)	Autosomal recessive	Spectrum of disorders but characteristic intellectual, eye, and brain involvement; motor early death, to acquiring ambulation	Walker Warburg Syndrome: severe eye involvement, cobblestone lissencephaly, hypoplastic cerebellum and brainstem. Muscle eye Brain Syndrome: common eye involvement, pachygyri/polymicrogyri, hypoplastic cerebellum and brainstem. Fukuyama: mild eye involvement, cortex mild changes, hypoplastic cerebellum but normal brainstem
SEPN1 related myopathy	1q36 (SEPN1)	Autosomal recessive	Cervicoaxial weakness, rigid spine syndrome, early nocturnal hypoventilation, medial thigh wasting	
LMNA related	1q22 (lamin A/C	Autosomal dominant and recessive	Cervicoaxial weakness, dropped head, rigid spine syndrome, respiratory and cardiac involvement	

elevated serum CK on the mild end. Duchenne muscular dystrophy manifests as early as age 2 to 3 years with delays in motor milestones and difficulty running. Patients can have marked pseudo-hypertrophy of the calf muscles. And when asked to get up from the floor, boys use a Gower's maneuver (use hands to push up). The average age of diagnosis is around 4 years of age. The proximal muscles are the most severely affected, and the course is relentlessly progressive. Patients begin to fall frequently by age 5 to 6, have difficulty climbing stairs by age 8 years, and are usually confined to a wheelchair in their early teens. The smooth muscle of the gastrointestinal tract is involved and may cause intestinal pseudo-obstruction. The average IQ of boys with Duchenne muscular dystrophy is low, reflecting central nervous system involvement.

Diagnosis and Differential Diganosis

Diagnosis is based on clinical history, physical examination, serum CK, and is confirmed by genetic testing. The majority of patients have deletions or duplications in the dystrophin gene. In the remaining patients, mutations can be small insertions or deletions, point mutations, or splicing errors. Other differential considerations are congenital myopathies and muscular dystrophies, and limb-girdle muscular dystrophies.

Treatment

Duchenne muscular dystrophy is a combination of surveillance for respiratory, orthopedic, and cardiac involvement, and the use of prednisone. Prednisone and deflazacort (a synthetic derivative of prednisolone available in other countries) improve strength and motor function in boys with Duchenne muscular dystrophy. Cardiac evaluation should begin at the time of diagnosis and, if cardiac involvement is found, afterload reduction is recommended (ACE inhibitor, β-blocker). Respiratory function should be monitored beginning prior to wheelchair use or when the forced vital capacity drops below 80%. Regular orthopedic screening for scoliosis and bone health is recommended. New investigational strategies for treatment include gene therapy, exon skipping strategies, and readthrough of premature stop mutations, all of which are designed to make the cell produce some form of dystrophin. There are no guidelines for the treatment of Becker muscular dystrophy and clinical presentation is highly variable, but monitoring for cardiac and respiratory involvement is warranted. Some female carriers of dystrophin mutations may become symptomatic later in life, and may have severe cardiomyopathy.

Prognosis

Patients with Duchenne muscular dystrophy die of respiratory complications in their 20s unless they are provided with respiratory support. Congestive heart failure and arrhythmias can occur late in the disease. The disease course for other dystrophinopathies is highly variable.

Myotonic Dystrophy
Definition and Epidemiology

Myotonic dystrophies are autosomal dominant diseases characterized by muscle wasting and myotonia. There are two types and both are due to expanded DNA repeats: type 1 (DM-1) due to CTG expansion on chromosome 19; and type 2 (DM-2) to CCGT expansion on chromosome 3. DM-1 is the most prevalent adult muscular dystrophy, with an incidence of 13.5 per 100,000 live births.

Pathology

In both myotonic dystrophy types 1 and 2, accumulation of aberrant RNA in the nucleus binds regulatory proteins and causes aberrant splicing of a variety of proteins. Both disorders are multisystem diseases, affecting skeletal, cardiac, smooth muscle, and other organs, including the eyes, the endocrine system, and the brain. Muscle biopsies are not required for diagnosis but characteristic findings include rows of internal nuclei (boxcar appearance), ring fibers, type 1 fiber predominance, and later, fibrosis and fatty infiltration.

Clinical Presentation

DM-1 can present at any age, with the usual onset of symptoms in the late second or third decade. However, some affected individuals may remain symptom-free their entire lives. A severe form of DM-1 with onset in infancy is known as congenital myotonic dystrophy. The severity of DM-1 generally worsens from one generation to the next (anticipation). Typical patients exhibit facial weakness with temporalis muscle wasting, frontal balding, ptosis, and neck flexor weakness. Extremity weakness usually begins distally and progresses slowly to affect the proximal limb-girdle muscles. Percussion myotonia can be elicited on examination in most patients, especially in thenar and wrist extensor muscles. DM-2 is typically milder but can present in an identical fashion to DM-1; however, some patients can only have a mild proximal limb-girdle pattern of weakness. Associated manifestations in the myotonic dystrophies include cataracts, testicular atrophy and impotence, intellectual impairment, and hypersomnia associated with both central and obstructive sleep apnea.

Diagnosis and Differential Diagnosis

The diagnosis is based on clinical examination, demonstration of myotonia on electromyography, and is confirmed by genetic testing. Myotonic dystrophy needs to be distinguished from other adult onset muscular dystrophies and non-dystrophic myotonic disorders.

Treatment

Yearly surveillance for cardiac and respiratory involvement is recommended. Mexiletine, a type IB anti-arrhythmic medication, can be used for symptomatic myotonia. There is currently no treatment to halt disease progression but many therapies targeting the interaction between RNA accumulations and regulatory proteins, or RNA accumulations themselves, are under investigation.

Prognosis

Respiratory muscle weakness may be severe, with impairment of ventilatory drive. Chronic hypoxia can lead to cor pulmonale. Cardiac conduction defects are common and can produce sudden death. Pacemakers may be necessary.

Facioscapulohumeral Muscular Dystrophy

Definition and Epidemiology

The majority of patients with facioscapulohumeral muscular dystrophy (FSHD) have disease inherited in an autosomal dominant fashion due to a deletion of a large repetitive element on chromosome 4 (FSHD-1). An additional 5% of patients (FSHD-2) will have disease with digenic inheritance, which occurs through a deletion-independent pathway. The prevalence of FSHD is 1 : 15,000.

Pathology

Both forms of FSHD lead to changes in methylation on chromosome 4 leading to the de-repression of the gene, *DUX4*, which is typically silenced in adult muscle; it is believed to cause disease in a toxic gain-of-function fashion. Muscle biopsy is typically not required for the diagnosis, but shows nonspecific myopathic changes. Up to 30% of biopsies can show inflammatory infiltrates.

Clinical Presentation

Patients typically present in their late teens or early twenties with weakness in a characteristic pattern, often with dramatic side-to-side asymmetry: typically first in the face, shoulders, and arms, later involving the trunk and distal lower extremities. Patients are unable to squeeze their eyes shut, have a transverse smile, scapular winging, loss of proximal muscle mass with often preserved forearm muscles, and a positive Beevor's sign (movement of the umbilicus up or down when asked to tense the abdominal muscles). Extramuscular manifestations of FSHD are rare: retinal vascular changes, which can occasionally lead to symptomatic retinal vasculopathy termed Coat's syndrome, high frequency hearing loss, and often asymptomatic atrial arrhythmias.

Diagnosis and Differential Diagnosis

Diagnosis is based on clinical examination, family history, and is confirmed by genetic testing. The differential diagnosis includes other myopathies or neuropathies with a scapuloperoneal pattern of weakness.

Treatment

There is no treatment for the weakness of FSHD. A dilated eye examination is indicated at the time of diagnosis, and surveillance for respiratory involvement for patients with pelvic girdle weakness or who are confined to wheelchair.

Prognosis

FSHD is not life limiting, but approximately 20% over the age of 50 will require a wheelchair.

⬤ CONGENITAL MYOPATHIES

Congenital myopathies are defined by their appearance on biopsy (see E-Table 122-2; Fig. 122-1C), and have a large number of genetic mutations associated with them. They are usually present at birth with hypotonia and subsequent delayed motor development. If the child survives the perinatal period, most congenital myopathies are relatively nonprogressive and may not be diagnosed until the second or third decade. Clinical findings

common in the congenital myopathies are reduced muscle bulk, slender body build, a long and narrow face, skeletal abnormalities (high-arched palate, pectus excavatum, kyphoscoliosis, dislocated hips, and pes cavus), and absent or reduced muscle stretch reflexes.

⬤ METABOLIC MYOPATHIES

Metabolic myopathies are muscle diseases due to mutations in enzymes responsible for energy production including glycogen, lipid, and mitochondrial metabolism (see E-Table 122-3). Classically, these disorders present in older children or adults with episodes of exercise intolerance, muscle cramping, or pain associated with myoglobinuria. Newborn and infants present with severe multisystem disorders that are often fatal.

Glucose and Glycogen Metabolism Disorders

Definition and Epidemiology

Glucose, and its storage form glycogen, is essential for the short-term, predominantly anaerobic energy requirements of muscle (see E-Table 122-3). Disorders of glucose and glycogen metabolism (called glycogenesis) have two distinct syndromes: static symptoms of fixed weakness without exercise intolerance or myoglobinuria, and dynamic symptoms of exercise intolerance, pain, cramps, and myoglobinuria. Acid maltase deficiency (Pompe disease) is an example of the first and is notable for enzyme replacement therapy, which is life extending for the childhood variant. McArdle's disease is an example of the second. These are rare disorders with incidence rates for the individual disorders of around 1 : 100,000. The incidence varies between region and ethnic group. For example, acid maltase deficiency has an incidence as high as 1 : 14,000 in African Americans. The prevalence of McArdle's disease is approximately 1 : 100,000.

Pathology

All are due to mutations in enzymes responsible for glucose or glycogen metabolism. Muscle biopsies usually show subsarcolemmal accumulation of glycogen.

Clinical Presentation

Acid maltase disease typically has a severe infantile form with respiratory and cardiac involvement and a slowly progressive adult myopathy, which can affect the diaphragm, so surveillance for respiratory involvement is important. However, McArdle's disease presents with severe episodes of muscle cramping and contractures associated with exercise and a fixed myopathy later in life. Many patients note a "second wind" phenomenon after a period of brief rest so that they can continue the exercise at the previous level of activity.

Diagnosis and Differential Diagnosis

Diagnosis is made by characteristic appearance on muscle biopsy with subsequent study of the enzyme activity or by searching for specific genetic mutations. The differential diagnosis includes other glycogen storage disorders, disorders of lipid metabolism, or mitochondrial disorders.

Treatment

The only glycogen storage disorder with a therapy approved by the U.S. Federal Drug Administration is enzyme replacement for infantile or adult-onset acid maltase deficiency. Treatment for the other glycogen storage disorders is supportive.

Prognosis

Severe infantile forms of most these disorders can often involve multiple organs and be fatal. A less severe adult myopathic phenotype is also common.

DISORDERS OF FATTY ACID METABOLISM

Disorders of lipid metabolism differ from glucose and glycogen disorders in that the metabolic derangement is in the enzymatic breakdown of fatty acids (see E-Table 122-3). Many present in childhood with episodes of encephalopathy precipitated by fasting with hypoketotic hypoglycemia. Serum fatty acid profiles often show reduced carnitine and increased longer chain fractions, depending on whether the mutation is in very long chain, long chain, or medium chain fatty acid metabolism. Adults typically show exercise intolerance and myoglobinuria and may developed a mild limb-girdle pattern myopathy. The most prevalent disorder of fatty acid metabolism is carnitine palmitoyltransferase II deficiency. This disease ranges from a lethal neonatal form to an adult form with muscle pain and recurrent myoglobinuria, often precipitated by intense exercise, febrile illness, or fasting. The diagnosis is usually made by detection of reduced carnitine palmitoyltransferase enzyme activity in skeletal muscle.

Mitochondrial Myopathies

Definition and Epidemiology

Mitochondrial myopathies can present at any age, with varying degrees of severity or weakness, affect multiple organ systems, and have any pattern of inheritance (see E-Table 122-3). Mutations affect enzymes necessary for normal mitochondrial function, and can be mitochondrial or nuclear. The overall prevalence for mitochondrial disorders is thought to be approximately 1:8500; however, the prevalence of individual mitochondrial syndromes is much lower and ranges from just a handful of cases, to 1to 6 per 100,000.

Pathology

Mutations can occur in both mitochondrial DNA (in which case inheritance is maternal) and nuclear DNA (autosomal dominant, recessive, or x-linked). Mitochondrial disorders produce biochemical defects proximal to the respiratory chain (involving substrate transport and usage) or within the respiratory chain. On muscle biopsy, muscle fibers contain abnormal mitochondria. Pathologically these fibers have a "ragged red" appearance on biopsy stains (trichrome) and may fail to react for cytochrome c oxidase.

Clinical Presentation

Despite the diversity, there are certain patterns that are characteristic for mitochondrial disorders, including slowly progressive myopathy and myalgias, which worsen with exertion or illness,

and ptosis and/or ophthalmoplegia. E-Table 122-3 lists common clinical mitochondrial syndromes.

Diagnosis and Differential Diagnosis

The diagnosis is based on clinical history, serum lactate levels, which are often elevated at rest, and characteristic findings on muscle biopsy. Diagnosis is confirmed by mitochondrial or nuclear genetic testing.

Treatment

Treatment is largely supportive, and includes identification of other multisystem involvement, including diabetes, cardiac and ophthalmological involvement, and hearing loss. Many agents have been tried in mitochondrial diseases, including coenzyme Q10, creatine, and carnitine; however, a meta-analysis showed no clear evidence for benefit for any treatment. Aerobic exercise may reduce fatigue and improve muscle function, although there are no large trials of efficacy.

Prognosis

The severity and prognosis depends partially on the load of abnormal mitochondrial DNA as well as the degree of multisystem involvement. Certain clinical syndromes with more predictable prognosis have been described (see E-Table 122-3).

MUSCLE CHANNELOPATHIES

The muscle channelopathies are a spectrum of disorders due to mutations in muscle ion channels commonly divided into the nondystrophic myotonias and periodic paralyses. Most are inherited in an autosomal dominant fashion, with episodic symptoms, often triggered by temperature or certain foods.

Nondystrophic Myotonias

Definition and Epidemiology

Nondystrophic myotonias are due to mutations in muscle chloride (CLCN1 on chromosome 7) or sodium (SCN4A on chromosome 17) channels resulting in hyperexcitable muscle and myotonia. The overall worldwide prevalence for nondystrophic myotonias is 1:100,000.

Pathology

Mutations in chloride channels cause a loss of function. Loss of hyperpolarizing chloride conductance cannot counteract a buildup of potassium in the t-tubule system during repetitive contractions, which results in a depolarized sarcolemma. Sodium mutations, on the other hand, cause anomalous depolarizing sodium currents due to alterations in fast or slow channel inactivation, or hyperpolarizing shifts in channel activation curves.

Clinical presentation

The nondystrophic myotonias have myotonia in common; on examination this can be seen as delayed muscle relaxation after contraction. Patients have trouble opening their eyes or fist when instructed to squeeze them shut. On percussion of the thenar eminence or wrist extensors there is a catch then delay in the relaxation phase. Electromyography shows a characteristic waxing and waning motor unit amplitude and frequency that when amplified sounds like a dive bomber or motorcycle revving. Symptoms usually start in the first decade, and patients can have a characteristic muscular build. Chloride channel mutations can be both dominantly and recessively inherited and have a characteristic warmup of myotonia with repetition. Sodium channel myotonias typically have more myotonia on eye closure and can demonstrate a paradoxical worsening of myotonia with activity (paramyotonia).

Diagnosis and Differential Diagnosis

Diagnosis is based on family history, myotonia on clinical examination, and electrodiagnostic testing. It is confirmed by genetic testing. The differential diagnosis includes myotonic dystrophy and secondary causes of myotonia (other myopathies and drugs associated with myotonia—e.g., statins, fibric acid derivatives, and colchicine).

Treatment

Treatment for nondystrophic myotonias consists of non-mutation–specific sodium channel blockade: mexiletine, a class IB antiarrhythmic, is the first line therapy but phenytoin, procainamide, and flecainide have also been used. Certain sodium channel myotonias respond to the carbonic anhydrase inhibitor acetazolamide.

Periodic Paralyses

Definition and Epidemiology

The periodic paralyses are disorders due to mutations in the calcium (CACN1AS on chromosome 1), sodium (SCN4A on chromosome 17), and potassium channels (KCNJ2 on chromosome 17) that result in depolarized but inexcitable sarcolemma and episodes of paralysis. Overall prevalence for the primary periodic paralyses is greater than $1:100,000$ and varies between conditions from $1:100,000$ to $1:1,000,000$.

Pathology

Hyperkalemic periodic paralysis is due to sodium mutations that lead to persistent inward sodium current causing both myotonia and paralysis depending on the relationship of depolarization to the sodium channel inactivation potential. Hypokalemic periodic paralysis is due to an anomalous gating pore current that, in low potassium conditions, produces a depolarizing current larger than hyperpolarizing potassium currents. Andersen Tawil syndrome is due to loss of function in a potassium inward rectifier.

Clinical Presentation

Common to all is attacks of flaccid tetraplegia, often brought on by rest after exercise, or in the mornings, and is associated with changes in extracellular potassium. Hyperkalemic periodic paralysis is due to mutations in sodium channels and is associated with either high or normal extracellular potassium. Triggers include potassium-rich foods. In hypokalemic periodic paralysis attacks are associated with low extracellular potassium, and are triggered by carbohydrates, stress, alcohol, or rest after exercise. Andersen-Tawil syndrome is due to mutations in a potassium inward rectifier and is characterized by the clinical triad of attacks of flaccid paralysis, dysmorphic features (wide-set eyes, narrow mandible,

low-set ears, bent fifth finger, and common origin for the second and third toes), and polymorphic ventricular tachyarrhythmias.

Diagnosis and Differential Diagnosis

Diagnosis is based in family history and clinical history, supported by electrodiagnostic testing and confirmed by genetic testing.

Treatment

In all of the periodic paralyses disorders mild exercise at onset of weakness can abort attacks of paralysis. Treatment for acute attacks consists of carbohydrates (hyperkalemic periodic paralysis) or potassium supplementation (hypokalemic periodic paralysis). Prophylactic treatment for all the periodic paralyses consists of carbonic anhydrase inhibitor acetazolamide.

⬤ ACQUIRED MYOPATHIES

Unlike the inherited myopathies, the acquired myopathies are typically secondary to another process: toxic, inflammatory, or infectious. Pathological changes can be distinctive and are not due to mutations in muscle-related proteins. Clinically, symptoms appear acutely or subacutely. Treatment often includes eliminating the precipitating factor.

Inflammatory Myopathies

The idiopathic inflammatory myopathies can be divided into dermatomyositis/polymyositis and sporadic inclusion body myositis (Table 122-9).

Dermatomyositis/Polymyositis

Definition and Epidemiology

Dermatomyositis/Polymyositis (DM/PM) are acquired idiopathic diseases of muscle characterized by inflammation and variable symmetrical proximal muscle weakness, associated with elevated serum creatine kinase and irritable features on electromyography. The overall annual incidence is approximately 1 in 100,000.

Pathology

Dermatomyositis shows a characteristic pattern on muscle biopsy of perifascicular atrophy with perivascular inflammatory infiltrates and positive pericapillary membrane attack complex staining (Fig. 122-1D). In contrast, polymyositis shows endomyseal inflammatory infiltrates with invasion of non-necrotic fibers, without other pathological changes.

Clinical Presentation

Dermatomyositis has a bimodal age of onset with peaks in childhood and adulthood, with an acute to insidiously progressive onset of painless symmetrical proximal muscle weakness with characteristic skin changes, which include heliotrope rash, shawl sign (maculopapular violaceous rash in v-shape around neck), Gottron's nodules (erythematous papular rash on the extensor surfaces of the hands or fingers), and mechanic's hands (dry, cracked skin on the dorsal or ventral hands). In contrast, Polymyositis is largely a diagnosis of exclusion, occurring in adults and not associated with skin changes. Myalgias are more common in polymyositis. In both DM/PM can be associated with respiratory

TABLE 122-9 IDIOPATHIC INFLAMMATORY MYOPATHIES

MYOPATHY	SEX	TYPICAL AGE AT ONSET	PATTERN OF WEAKNESS	CREATINE KINASE	MUSCLE BIOPSY	RESPONSE TO IMMUNOSUPPRESSIVE THERAPY
Dermatomyositis	Women > men	Childhood and adult	Proximal > distal	Increased (up to 50× normal)	Perifascicular atrophy, inflammation, complement deposition on capillaries	Yes
Polymyositis	Women > men	Adult	Proximal > distal	Increased (up to 50× normal)	Endomyseal inflammation; invasion of non-necrotic fibers	Yes
Sporadic Inclusion Body Myositis	Men > women	Elderly (>50 yr)	Proximal and distal; predilection for finger and wrist flexors, knee extensors	Increased (<10× normal)	Endomyseal inflammation, rimmed vacuoles; electron microscopy: 15- to 18-nm tubulofilaments	No

involvement, difficulty swallowing, or cardiomyopathy. Both DM/PM can be associated with underlying malignancy (dermatomyositis more frequently than polymyositis), so screening for malignancy is recommended especially in patients over age 40.

Diagnosis and Differential Diagnosis

Diagnosis is based on clinical history and examination findings in conjunction with irritable changes on electromyography (e.g., fibrillation potentials and positive sharp waves) and characteristic muscle biopsy. Both can be associated with autoantibodies (e.g., ANA). The most useful is the anti-Jo-1 antibody, which can be seen more frequently in patients with pulmonary involvement.

Treatment

For both DM/PM the first line of treatment is prednisone. Steroid-sparing immunosuppressive therapies (e.g., methotrexate, azathioprine) are often added for those patients requiring long-term therapy in order to reduce the required dose of prednisone or to replace prednisone completely. In patients who do not respond to conventional therapy, intravenous immunoglobulin or rituximab may be effective.

Prognosis

Most patients respond to immunosuppressive therapies.

Sporadic Inclusion Body Myositis

Definition and Epidemiology

Sporadic inclusion body myositis (s-IBM) is an idiopathic, slowly progressive muscle condition in older adults (occurring in more men than women), associated with inflammation and characteristic pathological changes on muscle biopsy. It is the most common inflammatory muscle disease in patients over 50, affecting 3.5 per 100,000.

Pathology

Muscle biopsies resemble polymyositis with endomyseal inflammatory infiltrates and invasion of non-necrotic fibers. Distinctive for IBM are vacuoles rimmed by mitochondria and electron microscopy, which shows 15 to 18 nm tubulofilamentous inclusions.

Clinical Presentation

S-IBM is a slowly progressive, often asymmetric weakness occurring usually after 50 years of age initially in a distinctive pattern, including distal forearm muscles (distal finger flexors) and quadriceps wasting and weakness. This can progress to involve almost any muscle and can affect swallowing in up to 70% of patients.

Diagnosis and Differential Diagnosis

Diagnosis is based on clinical history and examination and characteristic muscle pathology. The main differential diagnosis is other idiopathic inflammatory myopathies or late-onset inherited myopathies, including a hereditary form of IBM.

Treatment

Unlike the other inflammatory myopathies, IBM does not respond to immunosuppression. Treatment is supportive.

Prognosis

Most patients with s-IBM progress to need a wheelchair over 10 to 15 years. Swallowing difficulty can be life threatening.

Infectious Myositis

An acute viral myositis can occur in the setting of an influenza viral upper respiratory tract infection. In addition to typical influenza-associated myalgias, affected patients develop muscle pain, proximal weakness, and elevated CK levels. The disorder is self-limited, but when severe it is often associated with myoglobinuria and occasionally with renal failure. A similar syndrome can complicate infections with other viruses.

An inflammatory myopathy can occur in the setting of human immunodeficiency virus infection, either in early or in later acquired immunodeficiency syndrome. The clinical presentation resembles polymyositis. The patient's condition may improve with corticosteroid therapy. The disorder must be distinguished from the toxic myopathy caused by zidovudine, which responds to dose reduction. Although rarely seen, tuberculosis can present with muscle abscess (pyomyositis) either in the setting of pulmonary or disseminated disease or in isolation.

Myopathies Caused by Endocrine and Systemic Disorders

Thyroid studies should be obtained in any adult coming in with a new complaint of muscle weakness. Patients with hyperthyroidism often have some degree of proximal weakness but this is rarely the presenting manifestation of thyrotoxicosis. Hypothyroid myopathy is associated with proximal weakness and myalgias, muscle enlargement, slow relaxation of the reflexes, and marked (up to 100-fold) increase of the serum CK level.

Excess corticosteroids can result from endogenous Cushing's syndrome or can be caused by exogenous glucocorticoid administration. Iatrogenic corticosteroid myopathy (or atrophy) is the most common endocrine-related myopathy. However, muscle weakness is rarely the presenting manifestation of Cushing's syndrome and, in virtually all instances of corticosteroid myopathy, other factors contributing to weakness are also present. Therapy consists of reducing the corticosteroid dose to the lowest possible level. Exercise and adequate nutrition prevent and may improve weakness.

Toxic Myopathies

Many drugs have been associated with muscle damage, proximal weakness, elevated CK levels, myopathic EMG readings, and abnormalities on muscle biopsy. Symptoms generally improve after stopping the medication. Some drugs can produce acute, rapidly progressive muscle destruction and myoglobinuria, particularly the hypocholesterolemic drugs, including the statins and fibric acid derivatives. In some patients statin use has been associated with a subsequent autoimmune necrotizing myopathy associated with antibodies to HMG-CoA.

Critical illness myopathy (CIM), also termed, acute quadriplegic myopathy, develops in a patient in the intensive care setting and is often discovered when a patient is unable to be weaned off a ventilator. The cause of the diffuse weakness is the prolonged daily use of either high-dose intravenous glucocorticoids or nondepolarizing neuromuscular blocking agents, often both. Patients often have had sepsis and multi-organ failure. The diagnosis of critical illness myopathy can be confirmed by muscle biopsy, which shows the loss of myosin-thick filaments on electron microscopic examination. Treatment is supportive after discontinuation of the offending agents.

SUGGESTED READING

Amato AA, Griggs RC: Overview of the muscular dystrophies, Handb Clin Neurol 101:1–9, 2011.

Jackson CE, Barohn RJ: A pattern recognition approach to myopathy, Continuum (Minneap Minn) 19(6 Muscle Disease):1674–1697, 2013.

Lemmers RJ, Tawil R, Petek LM, et al: Digenic inheritance of an SMCHD1 mutation and an FSHD-permissive D4Z4 allele causes facioscapulohumeral muscular dystrophy type 2, Nat Genet 44(12):1370–1374, 2012.

Matthews E, Fialho D, Tan SV, et al: The non-dystrophic myotonias: molecular pathogenesis, diagnosis and treatment, Brain 133(Pt 1):9–22, 2010.

Pfeffer G, Majamaa K, Turnbull DM, et al: Treatment for mitochondrial disorders, Cochrane Database Syst Rev (4):CD004426, 2012.

Statland JM, Bundy BN, et al: Mexiletine for symptoms and signs of myotonia in nondystrophic myotonia: a randomized controlled trial, JAMA 308(13):1357–1365, 2012.

Statland JM, Tawil R: Facioscapulohumeral muscular dystrophy: molecular pathological advances and future directions, Curr Opin Neurol 24(5):423–428, 2011.

Wheeler TM, Leger AJ, Pander SK, et al: Targeting nuclear RNA for in vivo correction of myotonic dystrophy, Nature 488(7409):111–115, 2012.

Wu F, Mi W, Burns DK, et al: A sodium channel knockin mutant (NaV1.4-R669H) mouse model of hypokalemic periodic paralysis, J Clin Invest 121(10):4082–4094, 2011.

Wu F, Mi W, Hernández-Ochoa EO, et al: A calcium channel mutant mouse model of hypokalemic periodic paralysis, J Clin Invest 122(12):4580–4591, 2012.

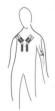

123

Neuromuscular Junction Disease

Emma Ciafaloni

Neuromuscular junction diseases are caused by abnormal neuromuscular transmission of the action potential from the nerve terminal to the muscle, and they can be autoimmune (myasthenia gravis, Lambert Eaton Syndrome), hereditary (congenital myasthenic syndromes), or toxic (botulism, organophosphate intoxication).

MYASTHENIA GRAVIS

Definition/Epidemiology/Pathology

Myasthenia gravis (MG) is a rare autoimmune disease caused by antibodies against the postsynaptic acetylcholine receptors (AChR Ab) in the neuromuscular junction. All ages are affected but incidence is higher in women younger than 40, and in men older than 50. Prevalence is approximately 20 in 100,000. Transient neonatal MG occurs in about 12% of newborns of myasthenic mothers and is caused by transplacental passive transfer of antibodies from the mother to the fetus. Thymoma is found in 10% of patients with MG and thymic hyperplasia is present in 65%.

Clinical Presentation

MG is characterized by fluctuating, fatigable weakness either isolated to the ocular muscles (ocular MG), or involving ocular as well as limb, bulbar, and respiratory muscles (generalized MG). The majority of patients present first with ocular symptoms (blurred vision, double vision, droopy eyelids), but about 15% of cases present with bulbar symptoms first (dysarthria, dysphagia, shortness of breath), or limb weakness. Ptosis is usually asymmetric. Myasthenia crisis is a true neurological emergency that occurs in 15% to 20% of patients and consists of severe dysphagia or respiratory failure requiring ventilator support and/or tube feeding in an ICU setting.

Diagnosis and Differential Diagnosis

The diagnosis of MG is based on a combination of clinical history, physical examination, and confirmatory tests. The ice pack test is a simple and relatively sensitive test to differentiate ptosis caused by MG from other causes of ptosis. In this test an ice pack is applied to the ptotic eye for 2 minutes and an improvement of 2 mm or more in ptosis supports MG.

Edrophonium chloride (Tensilon) is a short-acting acetylcholinesterase inhibitor administered IV to demonstrate symptom improvement in patients with MG. A positive Tensilon test is defined as an unequivocal improvement in strength in an affected muscle after 2 to 5 minutes from administration of 2 mg incremental doses up to 10 mg. Atropine should be available during a tensilon test because bradychardia and hypotension are possible side effects. Edrophonium testing can be positive in other disorders.

Electrodiagnostic testing with 3 Hz repetitive nerve stimulation (RNS) demonstrates a compound muscle action potential (CMAP) decrement more than 10% in about 50% to 75% of patients with generalized MG, but is abnormal in less than 50% of patients with purely ocular symptoms. Single fiber electromyography (SFEMG) is the most sensitive test in the diagnosis of MG and reveals increased jitter and blocking in 99% of patients with generalized MG, and in 97% of those with purely ocular MG when a weak muscle is tested. SFEMG is usually available only in specialized EMG laboratories.

Serum antibody testing for AchR Ab (binding antibody) is positive in about 80% of patients with generalized MG, and 50% of patients with purely ocular symptoms. Anti MuSK antibody is detected in a portion of seronegative patients, usually men.

Chest CT should be performed to rule out thymoma. Thyroid function should be evaluated because thyroid disease is commonly associated with MG. Electrodiagnostic and serum antibody testing help with differentiating MG from motor neuron disease, Lambert-Eaton myasthenic syndrome (LEMS), and Guillain-Barre syndrome (GBS).

Treatment

Pyridostigmine 30 to 60 mg every 4 hours improves symptoms in most patients with MG; it is used alone to treat purely ocular and generalized cases with only minimal or mild weakness, or in combination with immunosuppressant drugs in patients with more severe manifestations. Prednisone is effective in improving muscle weakness in a short period of time, but long-term use is associated with side effects. Azathioprine and mycophenolate mofetil are used for long-term treatment and as steroids-sparing agents. Plasmapheresis and IVIG are used for cases with severe bulbar or generalized weakness, respiratory crisis, and in refractory patients who do not respond to oral immunomodulating medications. Thymoma resection is indicated in all patients with MG and thymoma. Thymectomy is also recommended as an option in patients with nonthymomatous autoimmune MG to increase the probability of remission or improvement. Thymectomy is usually not recommended in patients over age 60. Some medications may exacerbate the symptoms of MG or precipitate the initial signs and symptoms of the disease (Table 123-1).

Prognosis

Most patients with MG who are optimally treated experience improvement or remission of their symptoms. About 10% of

TABLE 123-1 DRUGS TO BE AVOIDED OR USED WITH CAUTION IN MYASTHENIA GRAVIS

DRUGS TO BE AVOIDED

- D-penicillamine and α-interferon should not be used in myasthenic patients because they can cause Myasthenia Gravis (MG)
- Botulinum toxin treatment should be avoided as it blocks NMT

DRUGS TO USE ONLY WITH CAUTION AND MONITOR FOR EXACERBATION OF MG SYMPTOMS

- Selected antibiotics, particularly aminogylcosides, telithromycin (Ketek) and ciprofloxacin (many other antibiotics have been reported to increase weakness in occasional patients with MG)
- Magnesium, magnesium salts contained in some laxatives and antacids
- Neuromuscular blocking agents such as succinylcholine and vecuronium should only be used by an anesthesiologist familiar with MG
- Quinine, quinidine or procainamide
- Beta-blockers (propranolol; timolol maleate eyedrops)
- Calcium channel blockers
- Iodinated contrast agents

patients with MG experience refractory symptoms despite optimal treatment. Mortality is currently less than 5%.

LAMBERT-EATON MYASTHENIC SYNDROME (LEMS)

Definition/Epidemiology/Pathology

Lambert-Easton myasthenic syndrome (LEMS) is an acquired, presynaptic neuromuscular transmission disorder caused by antibodies against the P/Q type voltage-gated calcium channel (VGCC). P/Q VGCC antibodies cause reduced Ca^+ influx into the presynaptic nerve terminal resulting in decreased acetylcholine release and neuromuscular transmission failure. LEMS is associated with cancer, usually small cell lung carcinoma, in 60% of cases. LEMS may predate tumor detection by up to 3 years. LEMS is very rare and more common in men (3:1).

Clinical Presentation

LEMS should be suspected whenever the triad of muscle weakness, dry mouth, and decreased or absent reflexes is present. Patients have fluctuating weakness and fatigability of proximal limb and trunk muscles, with the lower limbs more severely affected than the upper ones. Difficulty walking is a common symptom. Dysphagia, dysarthria, and ocular symptoms (ptosis, blurred vision, and diplopia) are less common than in MG. Tendon reflexes are hypoactive or absent and may increase following short exercise of the muscle. Autonomic manifestations (dry mouth, impotence, decreased sweating, orthostatic hypotension, and slow pupillary reflexes) occur in 75% of patients.

Diagnosis and Differential Diagnosis

Serum antibodies against P/Q VGCCs are found in nearly all cases of paraneoplastic LEMS, and in about 90% of non-paraneoplastic cases. Electrodiagnostic testing can help confirm the diagnosis by demonstrating reduced CMAP amplitudes in distal hand muscles; CMAP facilitation of at least 100% after 10" maximal voluntary contraction or high frequency RNS (posttetanic facilitation); and CMAP decrement greater than 10% with low frequency RNS. Patients diagnosed with LEMS

should be screened and monitored with chest CT for lung cancer, especially if they are smokers and over age 50. LEMS and MG can be differentiated with electrodiagnostic and antibody testing.

Treatment

Symptomatic treatment with 3,4-DAP 5 to 10 mg every 3 to 4 hours and up to a maximum daily dose of 80 to 100 mg is most effective in improving muscle strength in patients with LEMS. Side effects at doses up to 60 mg per day are rare. Acral and perioral paresthesias occur within minutes from a dose and resolve in about 15 minutes. It is contraindicated in patients with seizures. 3,4-DAP is not currently FDA approved in the United States, but it can be obtained in specialized neuromuscular centers. Pyridostigmine 60 mg every 4 hours is also used to improve symptoms. In patients in whom symptoms are not adequately controlled with 3,4-DAP and pyridostigmine, immuno-modulation with prednisone, azathioprine, or mycophenolate mofetil is used. Severe weakness is treated with plasmapheresis or IVIG. The underlying cancer should be treated.

Prognosis

In paraneoplastic LEMS the prognosis is determined by the underlying cancer. The presence of LEMS in patients with small cell lung cancer (SCLC) is associated with longer survival from the malignancy. Non-paraneoplastic LEMS, when optimally treated, has an excellent prognosis and normal life expectancy, although patients may continue to experience various degrees of muscle weakness.

BOTULISM

Definition/Epidemiology/Pathology

Botulism is a rare, potentially lethal, paralytic illness caused by the neurotoxin produced by the anaerobic, spore-forming bacterium *Clostridium botulinum*. Botulinum toxin blocks voluntary and autonomic cholinergic neuromuscular junctions by binding irreversibly to the presynaptic nerve endings where it inhibits the release of acetylcholine. Human forms of the disease include foodborne botulism most commonly caused by home-canned food, wound botulism with most cases occurring among "black tar" heroin users, and infant botulism occurring usually in the second month of life due to intestinal colonization. Outbreaks of foodborne botulism occur in prison inmates due to ingestion of pruno, an alcoholic drink made illicitly in prison. About 145 botulism cases are reported each year in the United States; approximately 15% are foodborne, 65% are infant, and 20% are wound botulism.

Clinical Presentation

The disease is characterized by symmetric descending flaccid paralysis starting with blurred or double vision, ptosis, dysphagia, dry mouth, dysarthria, and muscle weakness. Symptoms usually start 18 to 36 hours after ingesting contaminated food.

Botulism should be suspected in any infant with poor feeding and sucking, constipation, dilated pupils, weak cry, poor tone, and respiratory distress. Sensory examination and mental status are normal.

Diagnosis and Differential Diagnosis

All suspected cases of botulism need to be reported to public health authorities immediately. Local health department and CDC laboratories can confirm the diagnosis by detecting the toxin in serum, stool, or gastric or wound aspirate specimens. Electrodiagnostic testing can also confirm the diagnosis by demonstrating persistent post-tetanic facilitation of CMAP of at least 20%, a decremental response greater than 10% with slow RNS, and increased jitter and blocking on SFEMG. Electrodiagnostic tests are also helpful in differentiating botulism from Guillain-Barré syndrome and myasthenia gravis.

Treatment

Prompt intensive care support with mechanical ventilation and parenteral feeding as needed are crucial in reducing mortality. Timely administration of equine antitoxin within the first 24 hours may arrest the progression of paralysis and decrease the duration of illness. The antitoxin is provided by the CDC through the local health departments. Children less than 12 months old should not be fed honey because it can contain *Clostridium botulinum*.

Prognosis

The proportion of patients with botulism who die has fallen from 50% to between 3% and 5% in the past 50 years. Recovery of muscle strength may take several months. Mortality in untreated botulism is 60%.

● ORGANOPHOSPHATE POISONING

Organophosphorus compounds (OPs) are used as pesticides and developed for chemical warfare. Exposure to even small amounts of an OP can be fatal and death is usually caused by respiratory failure. OPs cause inhibition of acetylcholinesterase (AChE) accumulation of acetylcholine at the cholinergic receptor sites, producing continuous stimulation of cholinergic fibers throughout the nervous system. A combination of an antimuscarinic agent (e.g., atropine), AChE reactivator, such as one of the pyridinium oximes (i.e., pralidoxime, trimedoxime, obidoxime, and HI-6), and diazepam are used for the treatment of OP poisoning in humans.

For a deeper discussion on this topic, please see Chapter 422, "Disorders of Neuromuscular Transmission," in Goldman-Cecil Medicine, *25th Edition.*

SUGGESTED READINGS

Gronseth GS, Barohn RJ: Practice parameter: Thymectomy for autoimmune myasthenia gravis (an evidence-based review), Neurology 55:7–15, 2000.

Palace J, Newsom-Davis J, Lecky B: A randomized double-blind trial of prednisolone alone or with azathioprine in myasthenia gravis, Neurology 50:1778–1783, 1998.

Passaro DJ, Werner SB, McGee J: Wound botulism associated with black tar heroin among injecting drug users, JAMA 279(11):859–863, 1998.

Pascuzzi RM, Coslett HB, Johns TR: Long-term corticosteroid treatment of myasthenia gravis: report of 116 patients, Ann Neurol 515:291–298, 1984.

Sobel J, Tucker N, Sulka A: Foodborne botulism in the United States, 1990-2000, Emerg Infect Dis 10:1606–1611, 2004.

Tim R, Massey J, Sanders D: Lambert-Eaton mysthenic syndrome: electrodiagnostic findings and response to treatment, Neurology 54:2176–2178, 2000.

Underwood K, Rubin S, Deakers T: Infant botulism: a 30 year experience spanning the introduction of botulism immune globulin intravenous in the intensive care unit at Children's Hospital Los Angeles, Pediatrics 120(6):1380–1385, 2007.

Vugia DJ, Mase SR, Cole B: Botulism from drinking pruno, Emerg Infect Dis 15:69–71, 2009.

Wirtz P, Lang B, Graus F: P/Q-type calcium channel antibodies, Lambert-Eaton myasthenic syndrome and survival in small cell lung cancer, J Neuroimmunol 164:161–165, 2005.

XVII

Geriatrics

124 The Aging Patient
Mitchell T. Heflin and Harvey Jay Cohen

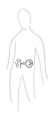

The Aging Patient

Mitchell T. Heflin and Harvey Jay Cohen

INTRODUCTION

Over the last century, the number of Americans over the age of 65 years increased from 3 million to nearly 45 million in 2013, accounting for 13% of the population. During the same period the population over age 85 grew rapidly, expanding from 100,000 in 1900 to nearly 6 million in 2013. By 2030, the number of adults over age 65 will likely reach 72 million, or just over 20% of the total population. Ten million of those people will be over age 85 (Fig. 124-1). A report from the National Institute on Aging and the U.S. State Department points out that this phenomenon is not isolated to the United States. Around the globe, the percentage of the population over 65 years of age will increase by 25% to 50% over the next 25 years and by 140% in developing nations.

The aging of the world's population compels virtually all health care providers to gain competency in geriatrics, the clinical science of assessment, prevention, and treatment of illness in older adults. A basic grasp of geriatrics requires understanding at epidemiologic, biologic, and clinical levels. The provider must appreciate the impact of aging on presentation of and predisposition to certain conditions, identification of goals of care, and selection of treatment strategies. Moreover, care of older adults demands a multifaceted approach, accounting for individual, family, and community resources for caregiving. Finally, the practice of geriatrics requires an appreciation for systems of care that include interprofessional teams working in a variety of settings ranging from home to hospital to long-term care. This chapter will provide an introduction to geriatrics and the essentials of caring for older adults.

EPIDEMIOLOGY OF AGING

Most experts believe that the rapid growth of the population of older adults reflects the many health care successes of the twentieth century. Fries, in his landmark paper, attributes the extension of the human lifespan to "the elimination of premature death, particularly neonatal mortality." Improvements in other aspects of public health, including adequate nutrition and housing, safe drinking water, immunizations, and antibiotics, have led to lower rates of mortality throughout childhood and early adulthood, affording an opportunity for more people to

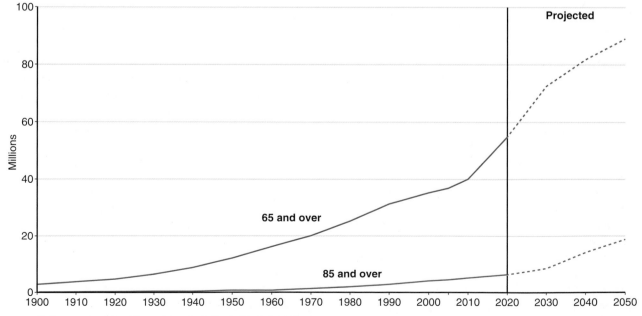

Population Age 65 and Over and Age 85 and Over, Selected Years 1900–2010 and Projected 2010–2050

Reference population: These data refer to the resident population.

FIGURE 124-1 Number of people aged 65 years and older, by age group, for selected years 1900 to 2010 and projected years 2010 to 2050. (From Federal Interagency Forum on Aging-Related Statistics: Older Americans 2012: key indicators of well-being. Federal Interagency Forum on Aging-Related Statistics, Washington, D.C., 2012, U.S. Government Printing Office.)

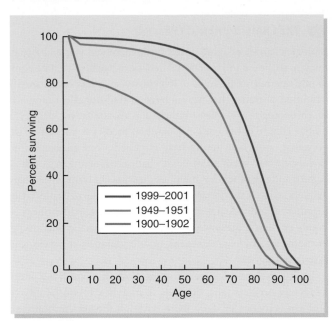

FIGURE 124-2 Percent surviving by age. Deaths tracked by state registries, 1900 to 1902, and by national registry, 1949 to 1951 and 1999 to 2001. (From Arias E, Curtin LR, Wei R, et al: U.S. decennial life tables for 1999-2001, United States life tables, Natl Vital Stat Rep 57:1–10, 2008.)

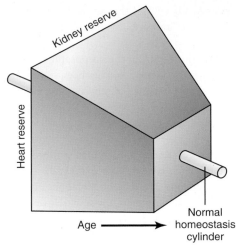

FIGURE 124-3 Classic schematic representation of decreased homeostatic reserve. (From Fries J, Crapo LM: Vitality and aging: implications of the rectangular curve, San Francisco, 1981, WH Freeman.)

survive to late life. Examination of survival curves across the twentieth century demonstrates a marked change in the shape of the overall graph from nearly linear in 1900 to rectangular in the 1990s, with much of the mortality compressed into late life (Fig. 124-2). Although the life expectancy at birth over the same period has risen dramatically from 47 years to nearly 77 years with up to 10% of the birth cohort surviving to age 95, the maximum lifespan defined as the age of the oldest surviving humans has remained remarkably stable.

THE BIOLOGY OF AGING

The relatively static nature of the maximum lifespan reflects the human body's limits at the cellular, tissue, and organ level in dealing with the stresses of aging. Across cell types and organ systems, certain consistent age-related alterations in function exist. Variability in tissue and organ function decreases, as evidenced by less fluctuation in heart rate or hormone secretion. Organ systems also exhibit predictable declines in function over time. These changes are most evident at times of stress, and ultimately these systems are slower to react and recover. The overall result is an impaired ability to deal with any demands beyond a narrow range outside the normal. This progressive restriction in the capacity to maintain homeostasis can be depicted as a steady tapering in the reserve available in multiple organ systems as time progresses (Fig. 124-3). In this situation an individual may function within the normal range in the absence of crisis, but stress such as acute illness may exceed his or her capacity to restore function and recover health. The result at best may be a decline in health and ability, and at worst, death.

THEORIES OF AGING

Scientific research provides a number of plausible theories of aging, which can be grouped into two major categories. *Error* or *damage theories* propose that aging occurs because of persistent threats from damaging agents and an ever-declining ability to respond to or repair this damage. *Program theories* postulate that genetic and developmental factors most significantly determine the biologic life course and the maximal age of the organism. In actuality, biologic aging may reflect a complex combination of many types of events.

The free radical theory of aging proposes that oxidative metabolism results in an excess of highly reactive byproducts, called *oxygen free radicals*, which damage proteins, DNA, and lipids. Molecular injury eventually leads to cell dysfunction and ultimately to tissue and organ disrepair. A second theory asserts that the accumulation of glucose-related molecules on proteins contributes to their dysfunction and degradation. These "glycosylated" molecules become more abundant over time and lead to impaired function at the tissue and organ level. Theory proponents point to the many chronic problems that routinely arise in patients with diabetes mellitus as proof of the significance of this phenomenon.

A different line of reasoning asserts that human lifespan and aging result from genetic-based timing mechanisms. Older theories suggest that evolutionary pressures are biased for traits that promote health and reproduction in early adulthood, possibly at the expense of health and function in late life. Furthermore, little selective pressure exists against negative traits that emerge in late life, leaving humans prone to the ill effects of aging. Geneticists have identified, among species of fruit flies and certain nematodes, specific genes that result in a significant prolongation in the organism's lifespan. Work is ongoing to discover similar genetic sequences among mammalian models.

Study of the enzyme telomerase has also generated much interest among theorists on aging. In a process called apoptosis, cells undergo programmed death to be replaced by younger cells. These divisions and replacements are limited by the number of generations intrinsic to a specific cell line (the Hayflick phenomenon). As telomeres located on the ends of chromosomes are depleted, cell aging and demise eventually occur. The enzyme telomerase prevents telomere shortening and may increase a cell's number of allotted replications and thereby extend the lifespan of the organism. Of course, this advantage must be weighed against the price of "immortality," namely the increased risk of malignancy.

Caloric restriction (CR), or the purposeful reduction of food intake, is the only intervention that has been shown to reproducibly extend maximal lifespan in certain laboratory animal models. In rats, lifespan increases an average of 20 months with a 40% reduction in calories. Rhesus monkeys enrolled in a trial of caloric restriction appear to have improvements in metabolic markers and a lower disease burden than controls after 15 years but have had no definitive extension in lifespan. The mechanism is not well understood but may be metabolically mediated. In observational studies in humans, those with lower average body temperature, lower insulin levels, and higher dehydroepiandrosterone sulfate (DHEAS) levels (all changes found in calorically restricted monkeys) appeared to survive longer. Current research is focused on reproducing this phenomenon in human subjects and discovering chemical agents that mimic or mediate these metabolic effects, including resveratrol and sirtuins.

To understand the changes in the individual's ability to cope with physiologic stress with age, one must also examine the changes at the level of the organ system. Table 124-1 provides an overview of these changes by system. As will be evident, although normal aging is not itself a diagnosis, it is, indeed, fertile ground for disease and disability.

TABLE 124-1	CHANGES IN PHYSIOLOGIC FUNCTION WITH AGE
ORGAN SYSTEM	**AGE-RELATED DECLINE IN FUNCTION**
Special senses	Presbyopia
	Lens opacification
	Decreased hearing
	Decreased taste, smell
Cardiovascular	Impaired intrinsic contractile function
	Increased ventricular stiffness and impaired filling
	Decreased conductivity
	Increased systolic blood pressure
	Impaired baroreceptor function
Respiratory	Decreased lung elasticity
	Decreased maximal breathing capacity
	Decreased mucus clearance
	Decreased arterial PO_2
Gastrointestinal	Decreased esophageal and colonic motility
Renal	Decreased glomerular filtration rate
Immune	Decreased cell-mediated immunity
	Decreased T-cell number
	Increased T-suppressor cells
	Decreased T-helper cells
	Loss of memory cells
	Decline in antibody titers to known antigens
	Increased autoimmunity
Endocrine	Decreased hormonal responses to stimulation
	Impaired glucose tolerance
	Decreased androgens and estrogens
	Impaired norepinephrine responses
Autonomic nervous	Impaired response to fluid deprivation
	Decline in baroreceptor reflex
	Increased susceptibility to hypothermia
Peripheral nervous	Decreased vibratory sense
	Decreased proprioception
Central nervous	Slowed speed of processing and reaction time
	Decreased verbal fluency
	Increased difficulty learning new information
Musculoskeletal	Decreased muscle mass

PO_2, Partial pressure of oxygen.

THE FRAILTY PHENOTYPE

Biologic changes of aging portend the increased vulnerability of humans to illness and functional decline in late life—a state commonly referred to as "frailty." Recent research has established a definition of frailty that moves beyond traditional components of chronologic age, comorbidity, and disability to identify a unique clinical entity with independent predictive capacity. Two prevailing models of frailty have emerged—one focused more exclusively on a set of physiologic changes occurring in a cyclical pattern and the other that includes measures of both physiologic markers as well as disease burden. The "cycle of frailty" ties together the individual system-specific changes and identifies key events or clinical presentations that create a specific phenotype, including weight loss, weakness, poor endurance, slowness, and inactivity (Fig. 124-4).

Frailty, defined as three or more of these conditions, independently predicts falls, declines in mobility, loss of ability to perform activities of daily living (ADLs), hospitalization, and death. This definition seems to provide a defined link between aging-related disease and disability and, perhaps, a target for interventions to prevent the onset of functional decline. Many believe, however, that this model remains difficult to recognize or measure in the clinical setting. The other definition conceives of frailty as a result of accumulation of problems (or deficits) that ultimately exceeds an individual's ability to maintain function and health. This count of deficits generates an index predictive of disability and death. To some degree both models capture different aspects of complex and heterogeneous phenomenon of vulnerability to declines in health and function with aging.

CLINICAL CARE OF OLDER ADULTS

Caring for older adults requires a strong foundation in the basics of internal medicine integrated with an appreciation for the complexity and heterogeneity of the impact of aging on health and well-being. The clinician must possess strong diagnostic skills, given that older adults may have atypical presentations or multiple comorbid conditions and functional decline. In addition, the clinician must monitor for a number of nonspecific conditions, such as problems with mobility, mood, or mentation that affect self-care capacity and safety. Treatment strategies present unique challenges as well, often requiring a balance of pharmacologic and nonpharmacologic interventions with careful consideration of the individual's goals for care. This section presents the core components of the comprehensive assessment of the older patient.

COMORBID CONDITIONS, FUNCTION, AND LIFE EXPECTANCY

With advancing age and declines in reserve, older adults experience high rates of chronic illness and related functional decline. Eighty percent of those over age 65 years have at least one chronic illness, and 50% have two or more comorbid conditions. Some of these conditions contribute directly to increased rates of mortality, including the leading causes of death among older adults—heart disease, cancer, stroke, lung disease, and Alzheimer's disease. Many common diseases, however, primarily threaten

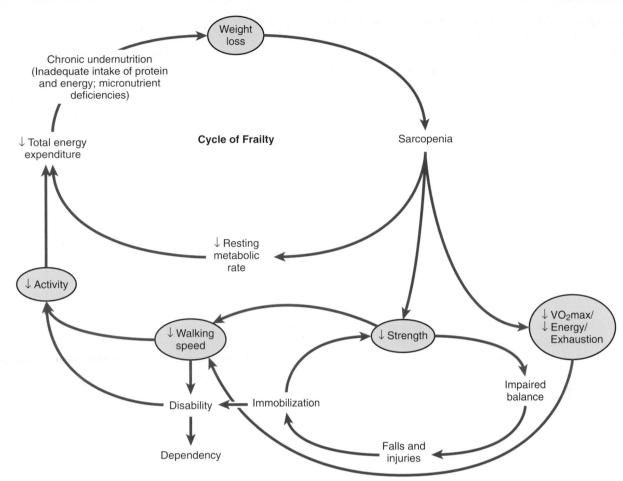

FIGURE 124-4 Cycle of frailty. (From Xue QL, Bendeen-Roche K, Varadhan R, et al: Initial manifestations of frailty criteria and the development of frailty phenotype in the Women's Health and Aging Study II, J Gerontol A Biol Sci Med Sci 63:984–990, 2008.)

function and result in disability and institutionalization. Arthritis, hearing loss, and vision impairment are all important problems in this respect. The presence of multiple comorbid conditions compounds the disabling effects of individual diseases and further complicates management. In the era of evidence and guidelines, a provider caring for a patient with several common chronic conditions, such as diabetes mellitus, coronary artery disease, and osteoporosis, may feel compelled to prescribe six or seven medications to remain in compliance with current recommendations. This practice can result in significant cost to the patient and with limited accounting for risks, benefits, and individual preferences. In addition to considering the discrete management of individual diseases, care of the older adult requires assessment of the overall impact of treatment on symptoms, function, and life expectancy. To address this common clinical challenge, the American Geriatrics Society has recently published guiding principles on care of older persons with multiple comorbid conditions that highlights the importance of accounting for complex interactions between conditions, risks and benefits of various treatment options, overall prognosis, and patient goals and preferences.

Function, defined formally by Reuben et al, is "a person's ability to perform tasks and fulfill social roles across a broad range of complexity"—more succinctly, self-care capacity. Assessing this ability provides the clinician with a means of understanding the impact of illness, assessing quality of life, identifying care needs, and estimating progress and prognosis. Comprehensive assessment of function should include questions about self-care capacity as well as objective measures of cognition and mobility (see later sections for details about the latter two). Self-care capacity is most often divided into basic, instrumental, and advanced ADLs. Basic ADLs include those actions that maintain personal health and hygiene, including transferring, bathing, toileting, dressing, and eating. Instrumental ADLs (IADLs) include activities necessary for living independently, specifically driving or using public transportation, cooking, shopping, managing medications and finances, using the telephone (or other communication device), and doing housework. Advanced ADLs include social or occupational functions associated with activities such as hobbies, employment, or caregiving. Approximately 30% of adults over age 65 and 78% of those over age 85 have difficulty with IADLs or one or more basic ADLs. Predictably, as the incidence of disability rises, so does the rate of dependence and nursing home residence. Long-term care in skilled facilities increases from 2% among those aged 65 to 74, to 14% among those older than 85 years. Impairment in ADLs is also associated with an increased risk of falls, depression, and death in the affected elder. Among older adults the assessment of self-care capacity provides key health status information independent of age and comorbid conditions.

For clinicians, navigating the myriad options for management of multiple chronic conditions requires individualized assessment of risks, benefits, and specific goals of various therapies. Estimates of life expectancy, integrating the impact of age, comorbid illness, and function, have been generated to assist in medical decision making. These estimates assist providers in predicting median survival and thus can help in estimating the potential life remaining in which one might benefit from a given procedure or therapy (Fig. 124-5). For example, the options offered to a frail 85-year-old man with less than 3 years left to live may be quite different from those presented to his healthy counterpart of the same age with a median life expectancy of 5 to 7 years. In addition, any decision should take into account the individual patient's goals and preferences. A variety of prognostic tools exist to assist clinicians with estimating survival in different populations and care circumstances. These tools can be accessed online in an interactive fashion for clinicians at http://eprognosis.ucsf.edu/.

PRESENTATION OF DISEASE IN THE OLDER ADULT

Competent care of the frail older adult starts with recognition of disease, even in the absence of typical signs and symptoms. Presentation of disease among older adults may differ dramatically from that expected in younger patients; manifestations of distress may be subtle or nonspecific, and improvement is less obvious and slower. These phenomena occur for a number of reasons. As noted previously, older adults experience high rates of comorbid illness, which may confound the clinician's ability to diagnose a problem accurately. For example, a patient with heart disease and chronic obstructive pulmonary disease who visits the office because of dyspnea may be experiencing a flare of his or her pulmonary disease or an atypical presentation of ischemic heart disease or both. Reporting of symptoms may also be affected by psychosocial factors, including limited access to the health care system, cognitive problems, or minimization of symptoms as "normal aging." Likewise, health care providers may minimize complaints by older adults with complex medical illness or frail health.

The alert clinician may anticipate "geriatric" presentations for certain conditions (Table 124-2). Hyperthyroidism can manifest with apathy, malaise, depression, and fatigue, while lacking classic symptoms of tremor, tachycardia, or sweating. It can also manifest with heart failure and is highly prevalent among older adults with new-onset atrial fibrillation. Likewise, older patients with hypothyroidism may atypically demonstrate

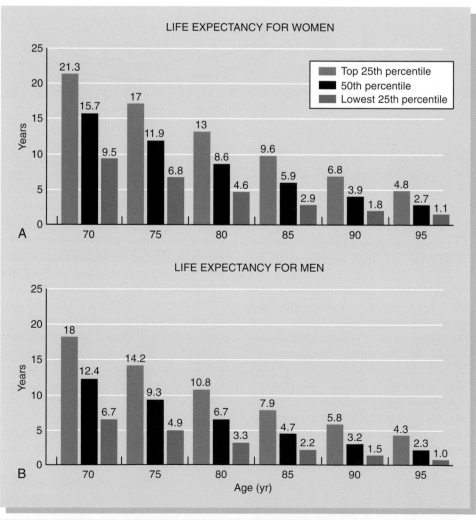

FIGURE 124-5 Upper, middle, and lower quartiles of life expectancy for women and men at selected ages. (From Walter LC, Covinsky KE: Cancer screening in elderly patients: a framework for individualized decision making, JAMA 285:2750–2756, 2001.)

TABLE 124-2	PRESENTATIONS OF DISEASE IN OLDER ADULTS*	
DIAGNOSIS	**POTENTIAL PRESENTING SYMPTOMS AND SIGNS**	
Myocardial infarction	Altered mental status	
	Fatigue	
	Fever	
	Functional decline	
Infection	Altered mental status	
	Functional decline	
	Hypothermia	
Hyperthyroidism	Altered mental status	
	Anorexia	
	Atrial fibrillation	
	Chest pain	
	Constipation	
	Fatigue	
	Weight gain	
Depression	Cognitive impairment	
	Failure to thrive	
	Functional decline	
Electrolyte disturbance	Altered mental status	
	Falls	
	Fatigue	
	Personality changes	
Malignancy	Altered mental status	
	Fever	
	Pathologic fracture	
Pulmonary embolus	Altered mental status	
	Fatigue	
	Fever	
	Syncope	
Vitamin deficiency	Altered mental status	
	Ataxia	
	Dementia	
	Fatigue	
Fecal impaction	Altered mental status	
	Chest pain	
	Diarrhea	
	Urinary incontinence	
Aortic stenosis	Altered mental status	
	Fatigue	

*This table represents only a limited list of select disease processes and presentations; it is not meant to serve as an exhaustive reference for use during patient care activities.

failure to thrive, weight loss, cognitive decline, or depression. In the presence of infection, older adults may not reliably mount fever or experience localized symptoms. Studies have demonstrated that lowering the threshold definition of fever can improve the diagnostic utility of body temperature as a sign of bacterial infection. Although chest pain remains the most common and important symptom of ischemic heart disease, dyspnea in the absence of chest pain is a commonly reported symptom, particularly in older adults and those with multiple comorbidities.

In truth, any medical illness may manifest nonspecifically among older adults, particularly those in frail health. Nonspecific symptoms related to an underlying illness include changes in mentation, difficulty with balance and falls, new urinary incontinence (UI), and a general change in functional ability. These presentations are often referred to as the "geriatric syndromes" and are detailed later. A lack of understanding of how disease presentation differs among older adults can lead to delays in diagnosis and treatment and result in worse outcomes. Research indicates that altered presentation predicts not only suboptimal care, but future functional decline and increased mortality.

MEDICATIONS

Medication-related problems are very common in older adults. In the United States, outpatients over age 65 take, on average, three to five medications. Although medications may be indicated for specific medical conditions, use of multiple medications increases the risk for drug-drug interactions and associated adverse drug events. Altered pharmacokinetics and pharmacodynamics contribute to adverse drug events, which are a common cause of hospitalization and morbidity in older persons. Common changes in pharmacokinetics include changes in body composition, with increased fat stores and decreased body water. Fat-soluble medications, such as benzodiazepines, have a prolonged duration of effect because of this phenomenon. Age-related declines in glomerular filtration rates result in decreased clearance of many medications, including such drugs as atenolol, digoxin, and lithium. Accurate calculations of creatinine clearance will inform drug choice and dosing and improve prescribing safety. Pharmacodynamic changes include decreased sensitivity to certain commonly prescribed drugs, such as β-blockers, and increased sensitivity to other agents, such as narcotics and warfarin.

Given the risks of medication use in older adults, health care providers and systems must employ strategies to improve both the effectiveness and safety of prescribing. Evidence-based recommendations include the following:

- Maintain an up-to-date medication list, including over-the-counter medications and herbal supplements.
- Comprehensively review medications at least once annually (if not at every visit) and, in particular, at the time of transitions between care settings (e.g., after hospitalization). A clear indication for each medication, and documentation of response to therapy (particularly for chronic conditions) should be included.
- Assess for duplication and drug-drug or drug-disease interactions. Using a drug information database will help with this process.
- Assess adherence and affordability and inquire about the patient's system for administering medications (e.g., a pillbox).
- Assess for specific classes of medications commonly associated with adverse events: warfarin, analgesics (particularly narcotics and nonsteroidal anti-inflammatory drugs [NSAIDs]), antihypertensives (particularly angiotensin-converting enzyme [ACE] inhibitors and diuretics), insulin and hypoglycemic agents, and psychotropics.
- Be suspicious that new symptoms arise from adverse effects of current drugs, not new disease.
- Minimize or avoid use of anticholinergic medications, which present specific risks.

In addition to following these general principles, prescribing providers also benefit from consulting lists of potentially inappropriate medications. The Beers List of Potentially Inappropriate Medications (PIMs) provides an evidence-based guide to drugs that should be avoided if possible or used with caution in older adults. A clear and rational approach to prescribing and ongoing management of medications that accounts for indication, interactions, and adherence may reduce the risk of common adverse events.

COGNITION

Dementia

The prevalence of dementia increases with age, with estimates ranging from 20% to 50% after age 85. The most common forms of dementia include Alzheimer's disease, Lewy body dementia, and vascular dementia. The latter is commonly present in combination with Alzheimer's disease in a condition termed *mixed etiology dementia*. Dementia is characterized by impairment in one or more cognitive domains severe enough to disrupt function or occupation. Mild cognitive impairment (MCI) is present when an individual has discernible cognitive limitations without apparent functional impact. Patients with MCI develop dementia at a rate of approximately 15% per year. Dementia is associated with a higher risk of falls, functional impairment, institutionalization, and death. Caregivers of demented individuals also face increased rates of stress and health problems. Clinicians diagnose dementia through symptom and functional history (often including the input of caregivers), cognitive assessment, and physical examination. A number of instruments, including the MOCA (see Chapter 108), clock-drawing test, and the Mini-Cog, are validated screening tools. The time-tested Mini Mental State Examination (MMSE) offers an assessment of multiple cognitive domains but does not provide adequate measure of executive function and is prone to lack of sensitivity in individuals with high premorbid intelligence and lack of specificity in those with low levels of education. Validated assessments of executive function include the clock-drawing test, verbal fluency test, and the Trail B test. Instruments also exist for collecting data regarding patient function from a relative or caregiver. In patients suspected of having dementia, personal safety with respect to firearms, driving, and the home environment should be assessed. A careful medication review and physical examination, including vital signs, complete neurologic assessment, including gait and balance, are, of course, essential in dementia to reveal findings that point to a specific cause (see Chapter 116).

Delirium

The differential diagnosis for cognitive problems other than dementia is broad, and includes delirium, mood disturbance, and drug effects. The differentiation of dementia and delirium may present the most significant challenge, particularly in hospitalized elders (Table 124-3). Delirium is characterized by its acuity and alteration in global cognitive function, whereas dementia is chronic and affects specific cognitive domains. Differentiation often hinges on history, which may be lacking at presentation. Delirium affects more than 2 million hospitalized persons each year. Its incidence is variably estimated at 25% to 60% among patients in acute care settings and results in extra hospital days and related expenditures. Delirium is also associated with prolonged hospital stay, increased costs, increased readmission rates to the hospital (12% to 65% at 6 months), higher in-hospital and 1-year mortality, and incident dementia. The Confusion Assessment Method (CAM) offers a validated tool to diagnose delirium. Per the CAM, delirium is likely present if the patient has both an acute onset of confusion with fluctuating course and inattention, and either disorganized thinking or altered level of consciousness. Key risk factors for delirium include older age,

TABLE 124-3	FEATURES OF DELIRIUM VERSUS DEMENTIA	
FEATURE	**DELIRIUM**	**DEMENTIA**
Onset	Acute	Insidious
Course	Fluctuating, lucid at times	Generally stable
Duration	Hours to weeks	Months to years
Alertness	Abnormally low or high	Usually normal
Perception	Illusions and hallucinations common	Usually normal
Memory	Immediate and recent impaired	Recent and remote impaired
Thought	Disorganized	Impoverished
Speech	Incoherent, slow, or rapid	Word-finding difficulty
Physical illness or medication causative	Frequently	Usually absent

cognitive impairment, comorbid illness, and impairments in vision and hearing. Precipitating factors related to acute illness include hypoxia, electrolyte abnormalities, dehydration, and malnutrition as well as medications and alcohol withdrawal. Although treatment of delirium is difficult and revolves around the underlying medical issues, controlled trials have demonstrated that a multi-modal intervention is effective in reducing rates of delirium in high-risk patients. There is evidence that the use of restraints in combative or confused older adults leads to increased morbidity and mortality. Nonpharmacologic management strategies include reorientation and preservation of sleep patterns, family or caregiver presence at the bedside, and early mobilization. The use of pharmacologic agents, specifically neuroleptics, should be reserved for patients in whom nonpharmacologic strategies do not help and the patient presents a risk of harm to self or others.

MOOD

Older adults commonly experience depressive symptoms, with prevalence estimates as high as 15% to 19% among those over age 75, although in community-dwelling elders, major depressive disorder is actually less common than in younger adults. The presence of comorbid illness and grief often confound the presentation of depression. As a result, it can remain undetected despite its significant adverse impact on quality of life, morbidity, and mortality. Suicide rates are almost twice as high among older persons when compared with the general population, with the rate highest for white men over 85 years of age. Among older adults, depression can manifest atypically with cognitive, functional, or sleep problems, as well as complaints of fatigue or low energy. Several instruments have been developed and validated for screening for depression in elders. Asking two simple questions about mood and anhedonia ("Over the past 2 weeks have you felt down, depressed, or hopeless?" and "Over the past 2 weeks have you felt little interest or pleasure in doing things?") may be as effective as using longer instruments. Longer screening questionnaires, such as the Geriatric Depression Screen (GDS) or Patient Health Questionnaire (PHQ-9), are also useful tools in the ambulatory setting. Any positive screening test result should trigger a full diagnostic interview. When screening for depression in elders, it is particularly important to have systems in place to provide feedback of screening results, a readily accessible means of making an accurate diagnosis, and a mechanism for providing treatment and careful follow-up. Recent trials indicate that the addition of counseling to pharmacologic therapy confers additional benefit for older, frail patients with depression. Anxiety is more common than depression among older adults and may similarly result in physical and cognitive symptoms, insomnia, agitation, psychosis, and isolation. Clinicians should consider a diagnosis of generalized anxiety, panic, or agoraphobia in older adult patients with any of these symptoms.

⬤ MOBILITY

Problems with mobility are common among older persons. Among those over age 65, 20% of men and 32% of women report difficulty with one or more of five specific physical activities (stooping or kneeling, reaching overhead, writing, lifting 10 pounds, or walking two to three blocks). Among these, respondents cite problems with walking most commonly. Difficulties with balance and gait present significant risks for older adults. Approximately 30% of community-dwelling elders fall each year. The annual incidence of falls approaches 50% in patients over 80 years of age. Five percent of falls in older adults result in fracture or hospitalization. Risk factors for falls include a history of falls, fear of falling, decreased vision, cognitive impairment, medications (particularly anticholinergic, psychotropic, and cardiovascular medications), diseases causing problems with strength and coordination, and environmental factors. Effective interventions for people with a history of falls or who are at risk for falling involve addressing multiple contributing factors. Providers should regularly inquire about recent falls or a fear of falling in older patients. For patients who report falling, the assessment should include review of circumstances of the fall(s), measure of orthostatic vital signs, visual acuity testing, cognitive evaluation, and gait and balance assessment. A brief physical examination maneuver called the "timed get up and go" has the patient arise from a sitting position, walk 10 feet, turn, and return to the chair to sit. A time of more than 12 seconds to complete the process, or observation of postural instability or gait impairment, suggests an increased risk of falling. Gait speed, an additional measure of mobility, predicts changes in ability and health status in older adults. Gait speed is measured over a 10-meter span with the patient walking at a comfortable pace. A speed of less than 1.0 m/sec is associated with increased mortality; 0.8 m/sec predicts difficulty navigating outside the home, and a speed of less than 0.6 m/sec predicts a high risk of falls and functional decline. For those found to be at risk for falls, providers should also review all medications for possible causative agents and inquire about home safety. High-risk patients should be evaluated for assistive devices and a supervised exercise program (Table 124-4).

⬤ VISION AND HEARING

Problems with vision and hearing are very common among older adults and frequently complicate the management of comorbid conditions and accelerate functional decline. Significant vision loss occurs in 16% to 18% of adults over age 65. Common causes include glaucoma, cataracts, age-related macular degeneration, and retinopathy from hypertension and diabetes. Decreased visual acuity increases fall risk and has been associated with all-cause mortality. Such problems may be detectable with regular testing via bedside tools such as the Snellen or Jaeger eye chart. Given the implications of vision loss for function and safety, a general ophthalmologic examination every 1 to 2 years is recommended for all older adults. Furthermore, ophthalmologic centers have recognized the multifaceted challenges faced by older adults with vision impairment and have developed specialized low vision clinics offering evaluation by optometrists, occupational therapists, and social workers with a focus on improving quality of life and maintaining independence.

Hearing loss is the third most common ailment in older adults (behind hypertension and arthritis), affecting an estimated 40% to 66% of those over age 75. It is associated with depression, social isolation, poor self-esteem, cognitive decline and functional disability. Pure tone audiometry is the reference standard for screening for hearing loss, but a simple whispered voice test is also highly sensitive and specific. Ideally all older adults would undergo annual hearing screen by questionnaire and handheld audiometry. Unfortunately, the lack of reimbursement for hearings aids under most insurance plans, including Medicare, presents a major barrier for many older adults.

⬤ CONTINENCE

UI affects up to 30% of community-dwelling older adults and at least half of those residing in skilled nursing facilities. It occurs more frequently in women, but this gender disparity narrows as the rate of UI in men increases after age 85. The impact of UI on health ranges from increased risk of skin irritation, pressure wounds, and falls, to social isolation, functional decline, and depression. For caregivers of older adults, UI complicates physical care and can contribute to decisions for placement in skilled nursing facilities. Common comorbid conditions include diabetes mellitus, heart failure, arthritis, and dementia.

A systematic approach to the investigation of UI can often reveal a cause and potential solution. It is important to first determine if the incontinence is acute or chronic in nature. Acute causes of incontinence are often attributable to specific medical problems, including infection, metabolic disturbance, or medication effects. The pneumonic DIAPERS recalls the various potential acute causes of UI (*D*, delirium; *I*, infection; *A*, atrophic vaginitis; *P*, pharmaceuticals; *E*, excess urine output from congestive heart failure [CHF] or hyperglycemia; *R*, restricted mobility; and *S*, stool impaction). If the UI is chronic, then further history can characterize the nature of the symptoms from among four types. Urge incontinence from detrusor overactivity is the most common type. Patients with this problem will complain of urinary frequency, nocturia, and a sudden onset of urge to void. Stress incontinence occurs with incompetence of pelvic musculature or urethral sphincter, and is characterized by small amounts of leakage with laughing, sneezing, coughing, or even standing. Overflow incontinence results from urinary retention, often related to prostatic hyperplasia in men or bladder atony in patients with diabetes or spinal cord injury. Patients often have constant dribbling or leakage without a true sense of needing to void. Finally, functional incontinence results from comorbid conditions that limit a patient's ability to act on or interpret the need to void, mobility problems such as arthritis, and weakness or cognitive problems. Table 124-5 describes the various types of incontinence and suggested approaches. Of course, older adults

TABLE 124-4 RECOMMENDED COMPONENTS OF CLINICAL ASSESSMENT AND MANAGEMENT FOR OLDER PERSONS LIVING IN THE COMMUNITY WHO ARE AT RISK FOR FALLING

ASSESSMENT AND RISK FACTOR	MANAGEMENT
Circumstances of previous falls* Medication use • High-risk medications (e.g., benzodiazepines, other sleep medications, neuroleptics, antidepressants, anticonvulsives, or Class IA antiarrhythmics—including Quinidien, Procainamide, and Disopyramide)*†† • Four or more medications†	Change in environment and activity to reduce the likelihood of recurrent falls Review and reduction of medications
Vision* • Acuity <20/60 • Decreased depth perception • Decreased contrast sensitivity • Cataracts	Ample lighting without glare; avoidance of multifocal glasses while walking; referral to an ophthalmologist
Postural blood pressure (after ≥5 min in a supine position, immediately after standing, and 2 min after standing)† • ≥20 mm Hg (or ≥20%) drop in systolic pressure, with or without symptoms, either immediately or after 2 min of standing	Diagnosis and treatment of underlying cause, if possible; review and reduction of medications; modification of salt restriction; adequate hydration; compensatory strategies (e.g., elevating head of bed, rising slowly, or performing dorsiflexion exercises); pressure stockings; pharmacologic therapy if the above strategies fail
Balance and gait†† • Patient's report or observation of unsteadiness • Impairment on brief assessment (e.g., the "get up and go" test or performance-oriented assessment of mobility)	Diagnosis and treatment of underlying cause, if possible; reduction of medications that impair balance; environmental interventions; referral to physical therapist for assistive devices and for gait, balance, and strength training
Targeted neurologic examinations • Impaired proprioception* • Impaired cognition* • Decreased muscle strength††	Diagnosis and treatment of underlying cause, if possible; increase in proprioceptive input (with an assistive device or appropriate footwear that encases the foot and has a low heel and thin sole); reduction of medications that impair cognition; awareness on the part of caregivers of cognitive deficits; reduction of environmental risk factors; referral to physical therapist for gait, balance, and strength training
Targeted musculoskeletal examinations of legs (joints and range of motion) and examination of feet*	Diagnosis and treatment of underlying cause, if possible; referral to physical therapist for strength, range-of-motion, and gait and balance training, and for assistive devices; use of appropriate footwear; referral to podiatrist
Targeted cardiovascular examination† • Syncope • Arrhythmia (if there is known cardiac disease, abnormal electrocardiogram, and syncope	Referral to cardiologist; carotid-sinus massage (in case of syncope)
Home-hazard evaluations after hospital discharge††	Removal of loose rugs and use of nightlights, nonslip bathmats, and stair rails; other interventions as necessary

From Tinetti ME: Clinical practice. Preventing falls in elderly persons, N Engl J Med 348(1):42–49, 2003.
*Recommendation of this assessment is based on observations that the finding is associated with an increased risk of falling.
†Recommendation of this assessment is based on one or more randomized controlled trials of a single intervention.
‡Recommendation of this assessment is based on one or more randomized controlled trials of a multifactorial intervention strategy that included this component.

TABLE 124-5 CAUSES, TYPES, AND TREATMENT OF URINARY INCONTINENCE

TYPE	DEFINITION	CAUSE	TREATMENT
Stress	Leakage associated with increased intra-abdominal pressure (coughing, sneezing)	Hypermobility of the bladder base, frequently caused by lax perineal muscles	Pelvic muscle exercise, timed voiding, α-adrenergic drugs, estrogens, surgery
Urge	Leakage associated with a precipitous urge to void	Detrusor hyperactivity (outflow obstruction, bladder tumor, detrusor instability), idiopathic (poor bladder), compliance (radiation cystitis), hypersensitive bladder	Bladder training, pelvic muscle exercise, bladder-relaxant drugs (anticholinergics, oxybutynin, tolterodine, imipramine)
Overflow	Leakage from a mechanically distended bladder	Outflow obstruction, enlarged prostate, stricture, prolapsed cystocele, acontractile bladder (idiopathic, neurologic [spinal cord injury, stroke, diabetes])	Surgical correction of obstruction, intermittent catheter drainage
Functional	Inability or unwillingness to void	Cognitive impairment, physical impairment, environmental barriers (physical restraints, inaccessible toilets), psychological problems (depression, anger, hostility)	Prompted voiding, garment and padding, external collection devices

with multiple comorbid conditions often have incontinence that results from a combination of chronic and/or acute causes.

Continence problems are frequently treatable but are often not raised by patients as a concern. A targeted history and physical examination can often identify the cause of UI and lead to appropriate intervention. Asking about and documenting the presence or absence of UI should be done biannually, as well as determining whether the UI, if present, is bothersome to the patient or caregiver. In addition to a history of acute and chronic causes, a targeted physical examination should include an assessment for fluid overload, genital and rectal examination, and neurologic evaluation. Urine and blood tests are indicated to evaluate for infection, metabolic causes, and renal dysfunction. In addition, for patients suspected of having urinary retention, catheterization or ultrasound can help define the postvoid residual and determine any need for catheter placement and further urologic evaluation. Many institutions now offer more specialized evaluation and care through incontinence clinics, which offer a multidisciplinary approach to management, addressing both pharmacologic and nonpharmacologic options. Effective non-pharmacologic options include scheduled toileting, bladder training, and biofeedback. Use of these strategies may avoid the use of medications with frequent adverse effects, such as anticholinergic medications for detrusor overactivity.

NUTRITION

Older adults experience high rates of malnutrition related to multiple causes, including medical illness, dental problems, or access issues related to limited mobility, cost, or cognitive problems. Approximately 15% of older outpatients and half of hospitalized elders are malnourished, and have associated increases in morbidity and mortality. The utility of general laboratory testing is limited, but a combination of serial weight measurements and inquiries about changing appetite can reveal nutritional problems in the older adults. Vulnerable elders with an involuntary weight loss of 10% or more in 1 year or less should undergo further evaluation for undernutrition, including assessment of medical or medication-related causes, dental status, problems with acquiring or preparing food, appetite and intake, swallowing ability, and previous directions for dietary restrictions.

SOCIAL AND LEGAL ISSUES

The social history for older persons includes assessment of resources for direct caregiving and financial support available. These issues become particularly important for frail older adults, given their physical and economic vulnerability.

Caregiving

The clinician should always inquire about who is providing care for the older patient, including both personal care with ADLs and help with IADLs, such as transportation, medications, food preparation, finances, and housekeeping. This list should include both formal caregivers, such as home health professionals or hired aides, and informal caregivers, such as family members, neighbors, or friends. The majority of elder care provided in the United States is delivered by informal caregivers. Over 34 million people in the United States provide informal care for older adults and, of these, 8.9 million are caring for persons suffering from dementia. The majority of informal caregivers are women and elderly themselves, with an average age of 63 years. The stress of providing daily care can have serious deleterious effects on the caregiver's health. Studies have demonstrated adverse effects on blood pressure and immune function, and increased rates of cardiovascular disease and death. In addition, caregivers have alarmingly high rates of psychological illness, with symptoms of depression reported in up to 50%. This problem is particularly prevalent in those providing care for patients with dementia. The presence of mental illness further raises the risk of verbal or physical abuse or neglect of the patient. The clinician must recognize caregiver problems early and consider referral to a social worker, patient resource manager, or, when available, a geriatric assessment team. Key risk factors for stress include a frail family caregiver; a patient with cognitive impairment, emotional disturbance, substance abuse, sleep disruption, or behavioral problems; low income or financial strain; and acute illness or hospitalization. Providers should recognize signs and symptoms of physical

or mental strain, and regularly inquire about caregiver burden with an offer to talk apart from the patient if need be.

A number of resources exist to support caregivers and provide strategies for problem solving and self-care. Community-based programs provide assistance with meals, transportation, and respite care options through volunteer organizations or subsidized programs. Counseling on both the physical and emotional aspects of care has been demonstrated to reduce health risks to the caregiver and delay institutionalization, including in-home or institutional respite stays to provide caregivers with precious time off. Studies consistently demonstrate that such services are underused by caregivers.

Mistreatment

Older adults are particularly vulnerable to mistreatment due to poor health, functional dependence, and social isolation. Mistreatment is defined as either elder abuse (harm caused by others) or self-neglect. Self-neglect is thought to be the most common form of mistreatment, but true rates are difficult to estimate. Risk factors include cognitive impairment and recent functional decline. Elder abuse has been reported in 3% to 8% of the older adult population in the United States, although this is likely an underestimate due to underreporting by patients and lack of recognition by health care providers. Abuse assumes many forms including psychological, financial, physical, sexual abuse, and neglect. Studies have demonstrated that neglect and abuse are associated with higher rates of nursing home placement and mortality among older adults. Signs of physical abuse include contusions, burns, bite marks, genital or rectal trauma, pressure ulcers, or unexplained weight loss. Other forms of abuse may be more difficult to discern on examination, but can be improved with direct questions such as "Has anybody hurt you?"; "Are you afraid of anybody?"; or "Is anyone taking or using your money without your permission?" Any suspicion of abuse or neglect should be reported to Adult Protective Services. Of note, 44 states and the District of Columbia have laws mandating reporting of suspected elder abuse.

Finances

The older adult population in the United States varies widely in measures of wealth. Although the overall rate of poverty among adults over age 65 has declined over the last 50 years, 10% of older adults still live at or below the poverty line, and the percentage is higher among African Americans (24%) and Hispanics (21%). Providers should screen for financial problems because these issues have direct implications for health status and well-being. Older adults with limited means are more prone likely to have problems affording medications, meals, and basic amenities. Referrals to community resource networks can help identify options for help with basic needs, including housing options and congregate meals. Information on agencies and services in specific locales can be identified at www.eldercare.org.

Advance Directives

Advance directives come in a number of different forms and serve a variety of purposes. Ideally these documents articulate a person's preferences for care in the event of serious illness or incapacitation. Often they will describe limits on care and circumstances in which life sustaining or restoring measures may be withheld or even withdrawn. Traditionally, advance directives have included a living will and health care power of attorney. The living will often addresses situations in which the patient has a terminal illness, persistent vegetative state, or progressive neurologic condition and can include explicit directions for care management including withdrawal or withholding of specific measures, including artificial nutrition and hydration. Living wills are ideally paired with a companion document, the health care power of attorney, which designates the person's preferred decision maker, or proxy, in the event of an incapacitating illness. For patients who have not created a health care power of attorney, typically the spouse or other first-degree relative is the default decision maker. If no proxy is designated and no next of kin is available, guardianship may be obtained. Guardianship is a legal proceeding whereby the court appoints a surrogate decision maker. The physician's responsibility includes determination of a person's capacity for independent decision making in the event of altered sensorium or progressive cognitive impairment. This involves an assessment of his or her ability to understand the situation, ask questions, weigh options and render an opinion and, in certain situations, may require a full geriatric or neuropsychological assessment. Traditional advance directives, particularly the living will, have been criticized as having limited utility in conveying specific preferences. Recently, more detailed forms have emerged to record very specific preferences and limits for measures such as hydration, nutrition, hospitalization, and resuscitation. Examples include the Medical Orders for Scope of Treatment (MOST) and Physician's Orders for Life Sustaining Treatment (POLST) forms. Of course, effective completion and application of any of these forms should include a goals of care conversation conducted with the primary care provider ideally involving family caregivers. In addition, as preferences change over time depending on health status, health care providers should encourage older adults to revisit and renew their advance directives on an annual basis.

HIGH-RISK CIRCUMSTANCES
The Hospitalized Patient

Millions of older adults are hospitalized in the United States each year for a variety of acute illnesses and elective procedures. Fortunately, in the United States, Medicare Part A covers much of the cost associated with acute care, including hospitalization and follow-up rehabilitation. While in the hospital, however, older adults are vulnerable to myriad complications related to both their compromised health state and problems inherent to the acute care environment itself. As noted previously, delirium afflicts hospitalized elders at a very high rate and increases risk of prolonged hospital stays, nursing home admission, and death. Hospitalized older adults also experience the effects of immobilization, with loss of muscle strength and deconditioning. Acutely, these factors increase the risk of falls and impair function and ability to provide self-care. In addition, poor oral intake may result in malnutrition, and illness-related fluid losses cause dehydration. As a result, hypotension and protein-calorie malnutrition are common problems. Immobility and malnutrition both predispose the acutely ill patient to the development of pressure

wounds, which can develop in under 2 hours. All these problems worsen in the presence of delirium or depressed mood. Environmental factors also contribute to problems, including tethers such as catheters and intravenous lines (which increase risk of falls), noisy wards, and frequent tests and procedures that further disrupt diurnal rhythms and sleep. Up to one third of hospitalized older adults experience a decline in their ability to perform ADLs in the course of their hospitalization. Patients who experience declines in function during hospitalization have higher rates of rehospitalization, prolonged institutionalization, and mortality after discharge, and many (41%) never return to their preadmission level of function. To combat these problems, some hospitals have created specialized inpatient geriatric care units, often termed *acute care for elders (ACE) units*. These units incorporate adaptations in the physical environment and specially trained staff to provide safe, patient-centered care designed to maximize restoration of function and prevent common complications of hospitalization. In randomized trials, ACE units and their consultative counterpart, the Mobile ACE (or MACE), have reduced lengths of stay, improved care transitions, and lowered readmissions. Likewise, geriatric evaluation and management (GEM) units (described later) offer specialized, team-based post-acute care with an emphasis on rehabilitation and return to prior level of function.

Care Transitions

As noted previously, older adults experience high rates of complications during acute illness and require prolonged periods of time to recover. For this reason, management in the post-acute period represents a critical and complex time in their care. Specifically, older adults with acute illness often find themselves transferred among different care settings and providers. Nearly one quarter of hospitalized older adults are discharged to skilled nursing facilities, and another 12% are discharged with home health care. Of those discharged to skilled facilities, about one fifth will return to the hospital within 30 days. Transitions in care represent high-risk episodes, and evidence shows that patients and caregivers frequently experience miscommunication, medication errors, and missed essential laboratory tests or appointments during this period. Recent trials have demonstrated a reduction in rehospitalization through a structured discharge and transition plan that includes medication reconciliation before and after discharge, careful planning for laboratory and appointment follow-up, communication with patients and caregivers about expectations and preferences, and specific coaching for patients and caregivers in symptom management and care. More information on care management in transitions is available at www.caretransitions.org.

SYSTEMS OF CARE
Ambulatory and Home Care

The majority of care for older adults occurs in the outpatient setting. Much of the cost of this care, including visit fees, laboratory tests, x-ray studies, and vaccinations, is covered under Medicare Part B, for which patients pay a monthly premium. Outpatient visits may occur with the physician, physician assistant, nurse practitioner, or clinical nurse specialists, depending on the nature of the problem and the structure of the setting. Other key members of the care team include social workers, pharmacists, psychologists, and physical and occupational therapists. Most assessments discussed in this chapter can be performed in outpatient settings, including functional assessments, cognitive and mood screening, gait and balance assessment, medication review, eye and ear examinations, and continence evaluations. Interview of a caregiver can augment the information collected. Care in this setting can be complicated, though, by problems with transportation and ineffective or inefficient communication among multiple providers, particularly for patients with multiple specialists.

Over the last several years, home care has reemerged as an effective means of providing health care for older adults. As with the outpatient setting, Medicare Part B will reimburse providers in part for services rendered in the home. In addition, if a rehabilitative or skilled service is needed, Medicare Part A provides coverage. Patients receiving services in the home must be "homebound," implying that they are significantly functionally impaired and travel with assistance out of the home infrequently and usually only for medical purposes. Services rendered in the home include a full range of evaluations by teams of providers from a variety of health professions depending on needs. Social workers often lead these visits and perform case management, assessing financial and other resource needs. Nurses, clinical nurse specialists, and/or nurse practitioners provide skilled services when necessary, including health education, symptom monitoring, or wound care. Physical and occupational therapy can assess mobility and home safety and greatly enhance function and independence. Furthermore, examination of a person's home environment can reveal much about his or her safety and nutrition, and can facilitate education or intervention in these areas. Physicians may serve as medical directors of such programs, but may also perform visits themselves to learn more about a given patient's health status. If significant concerns exist about a patient's safety, particularly in the setting of cognitive impairment, a home visit may provide information about the need for more urgent interventions, including referrals to Adult Protective Services. Research has demonstrated that coordinated home care programs can improve management of chronic disease, including dementia, diabetes mellitus, and congestive heart failure, as well as to reduce rehospitalization in patients with congestive heart failure.

Long-Term Care

The phrase *long-term care* describes the array of services available to provide care for patients with disability from chronic and acute conditions. This definition includes the services offered in the outpatient and home settings described previously. Most associate the term, however, with the system of nursing facilities providing personal and medical care for disabled adults of all ages. Skilled nursing facilities provide long-term care for those with permanent disabilities from chronic illness or short rehabilitative stays after acute illness (e.g., stroke) or procedures (e.g., joint replacement). The scope of services may also include end-of-life care in conjunction with a hospice care team. Facility staff includes licensed nurses who give 24-hour supervision, with much of the personal care provided by certified nursing assistants. Each facility also has a medical director overseeing various

aspects of medical care. An attending physician, who may or may not be the medical director, performs patient visits every 30 to 60 days. Most SNFs also employ physical, occupational, and speech therapists for rehabilitation care, dietitians, social workers, and recreational therapists. Patients with moderate or severe dementia constitute approximately 60% of patients living in skilled nursing facilities. Although Medicare Part A provides payment for rehabilitative stays of 100 days or less (with a copayment for days 21 to 100), it does not finance long-term stays. Such patients pay out of pocket, through long-term care insurance, or through Medicaid, a joint federal and state assistance program. Medicaid constitutes 47% of all payment sources for skilled nursing facilitie care.

For patients with less complex care needs, assisted living facilities or domiciliary care homes provide an alternative arrangement for long-term care. Although these facilities vary dramatically in their size and structure, most provide nonskilled care for patients who need some assistance with activities of daily living. Licensed nurses may be present during some specified periods of time, and other professions may visit the facility intermittently to provide services such as physical therapy. Facilities do not have medical directors, and patients normally continue to see a primary care provider in the outpatient setting. Unlicensed staff, including nursing aides, provides most of the personal care and assistance. Medicaid provides some reimbursement for this type of care, but the majority of residents pay out of pocket or through other assistance programs, such as Social Security. For those with adequate means, a living option has emerged that combines independent living, assisted living and skilled care in one location. Continuing care retirement communities allow residents to live within the same community while moving through or between levels of care. They offer residents convenient central resources, such as recreational and dining facilities, transportation, and onsite health care.

PACE

In the 1970s, a group providing care for older Chinese adults in San Francisco developed a model of long-term care centered in the community. Proponents of this model, entitled the Program of All-inclusive Care for the Elderly (PACE), believed that the community (rather than the institution) provided a better location to meet the chronic care needs of older adults. From its start as a community-based effort in California, the PACE model has grown with the support of private foundations and Medicare demonstration projects; now PACE is a benefit for elders who qualify for both Medicare and Medicaid. Reimbursement is at 95% of the cost of nursing home care in the area where the patient lives. Participants must be over 55 and certified by the state to be eligible for nursing home care. The PACE program then uses combined Medicare and Medicaid funds otherwise slated to pay for the individual's long-term care to provide care in the community; much of it coordinated through senior centers offering an array of resources and services, including the following*:

- Adult day care, offering nursing; physical, occupational, and recreational therapies; meals; nutritional counseling; social work; and personal care

*Information from the National PACE Association website at www.npaonline.org.

- Medical care provided by a PACE physician familiar with the history, needs, and preferences of each participant
- Home health care and personal care
- All necessary prescription drugs
- Social services
- Medical specialists such as audiology, dentistry, optometry, podiatry, and speech therapy
- Respite care

When necessary, PACE participants are admitted to the hospital or nursing home. These services are provided under the auspices of the PACE program as part of the care package, and the program bears full financial risk. The benefits of care for older adults, particularly those of limited means, appear to be substantial.

Geriatric Care

In caring for frail older adults with complex care needs, consultation with a geriatrician or geriatrics-focused team can often provide highly useful information. The geriatrician can assist in the assessment and management of the specific conditions or situations described earlier. He or she can help with difficult decisions regarding treatment options in the context of multiple comorbidities and limited life expectancy, and offer advice on appropriate level or setting of care for an older adult. Geriatricians complete a minimum of 1 year of fellowship after residency training in internal medicine or family practice. After training they are eligible for board certification and qualified to work in a number of different settings, including the hospital, long-term care, home care, and outpatient clinics. Comprehensive assessment by a geriatrician or geriatrics team includes components detailed previously, including evaluation of the patient's medical condition, function, and social support. Normally the consultant will work with an interdisciplinary team that may include a nurse case manager, physician's assistant, social worker, physical or occupation therapist, pharmacist, psychologist and others. The outcome of the geriatric assessment is a comprehensive plan for safely restoring the patient to optimal function with mutually agreeable and realistic goals of care.

In the setting of acute illness, geriatricians also provide important services. As described earlier, acute-care-for-elders units can improve patient care and prevent iatrogenic complications. Similarly, once patients are medically stable, transfer to a specialized geriatrics care unit, often termed a geriatric evaluation and management unit, may be possible, to provide a comprehensive medical assessment and plan for transition of care. Early consultation with a geriatrician and an interdisciplinary team in the acute care setting can help in the management of complex medical illness and with communication with patients and caregivers about post-hospitalization options. Subsequent to hospitalization, locating facilities or services that offer comprehensive care by a geriatrician and interdisciplinary team would be ideal, including a coordinated approach that uses specific strategies to manage transitions of care.

For a deeper discussion on this topic, please see Section IV, "Aging and Geriatric Medicine," in Goldman-Cecil Medicine, 25th Edition.

SUGGESTED READINGS

American Geriatrics Society 2012 Beers Criteria Update Expert Panel: American Geriatrics Society Updated Beers Criteria for Potentially Inappropriate Medication Use in Older Adults, J Amer Geriatr Soc 2012. http://www.americangeriatrics.org/files/documents/beers/2012BeersCriteria_JAGS.pdf.

American Geriatrics Society Expert Panel on the Care of Older Adults with Multimorbidity: Guiding Principles for the Care of Older Adults with Multimorbidity: An Approach for Clinicians, J Am Geriatr Soc 2012. http://americangeriatrics.org/files/documents/MCC.principles.pdf.

Boyd CM, Darer J, Boult C, et al: Clinical practice guidelines and quality of care for older patients with multiple comorbid diseases: Implications for pay for performance, JAMA 294:716–724, 2005.

Campisi J: Aging, Cellular Senescence, and Cancer, Annu Rev Physiol 75:685–705, 2013.

Covinsky KE, Pierluissi E, Johnston B: Hospitalization-Associated Disability: "She Was Probably Able to Ambulate, but I'm Not Sure," JAMA 306:93–2011, 1782.

Eckstrom E, Feeny DH, Walter LC, et al: Individualizing Cancer Screening in Older Adults: A Narrative Review and Framework for Future Research, J Gen Intern Med 28:292–298, 2012.

Federal Interagency Forum on Aging-Related Statistics: Older Americans 2012:Key Indicators of Well-Being. Federal Interagency Forum on Aging-Related Statistics, Washington, DC, June 2012, U.S. Government Printing Office. http://www.agingstats.gov/main_site/data/2012_documents/docs/entirechartbook.pdf.

Flood KL, Maclennan PA, McGrew D, et al: Effects of an Acute Care for Elders unit on costs and 30-day readmissions, JAMA Intern Med 173:981–987, 2013.

Fries JF: Aging, natural death, and the compression of morbidity, N Engl J Med 303:130–135, 1980.

Goode PS, Burgio KL, Richter HE, et al: Incontinence in Older Women, JAMA 303:2172–2181, 2010.

Hung WW, Ross JS, Farber J, et al: Evaluation of a Mobile Acute Care of the Elderly (MACE) service, JAMA Intern Med 173:990–996, 2013.

Kim CS, Flanders SA: In the Clinic: transitions of Care, Ann Intern Med 158:ITC3-1, 2013.

Li RM, Iadarola AC, Maisano CC, editors: Why Population Aging Matters: A Global Perspective. A booklet prepared in follow-up to the 2007 Summit on Global Aging hosted by the U.S. State Department and the National Institute on Aging, March 2007, National Institute on Aging and the National Institutes of Health.

Libert S, Guarente L: Metabolic and Neuropsychiatric Effects of Calorie Restriction and Sirtuins, Annual Rev Physiol 75:669–684, 2013.

Marcantonio ER: In the Clinic. Delirium, Ann Intern Med 154:ITC6-1, 2011.

Mosqueda L, Dong X: Elder Abuse and Self-neglect: "I Don't Care Anything About Going to the Doctor, to Be Honest…," JAMA 306:532–540, 2011.

Pacala JT, Yueh B: Hearing Deficits in the Older Patient: "I Didn't Notice Anything," JAMA 307:1185–1194, 2012.

Reuben DB: Medical Care for the Final Years of Life: "When You're 83, It's Not Going to Be 20 Years," JAMA 302:2686–2694, 2009.

Reuben DB, Wieland DL, Rubenstein LZ: Functional status assessment of older persons: concepts and implications, Facts Res Gerontol 7:232, 1993.

Steinman MA, Hanlon JT: Managing Medications in Clinically Complex Elders: "There's Got to Be a Happy Medium," JAMA 304:1592–1601, 2010.

Tinetti ME, Kumar C: The Patient Who Falls: "It's Always a Trade-off," JAMA 303:258–266, 2010.

Xue QL: The Frailty Syndrome: Definition and Natural History, Clin Geriatr Med 27:1–15, 2011.

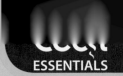

XVIII

 Palliative Care

125 Palliative Care
Robert G. Holloway and Timothy E. Quill

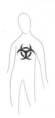

Palliative Care

Robert G. Holloway and Timothy E. Quill

INTRODUCTION

Palliative care is both a philosophy of care and an area of specialization within several medical fields. The primary goal of palliative care is to minimize suffering and to support the best possible quality of life for patients and their families. Patients with serious and debilitating illness need and deserve excellent symptom control, assistance with difficult medical decisions, effective communication and collaboration among their providers, addressing of psychosocial problems, and an empathetic presence that fosters hope and healing relationships. Palliative care affirms life by supporting the patient's goals for the future in light of a full understanding of their medical condition, potentially including their hopes for cure, life-prolongation, relief from suffering, as well as preparation for death when time is short. This process includes exploring what would be left undone if treatment does not go as hoped, who should make medical decisions for the patient if decision-making capacity is lost, and what, if any, limits might be set on aggressive therapy.

Palliative care provides an organized, highly structured system for delivering care by an interdisciplinary team, including physicians, nurses, social workers, chaplains, counselors, as well as other health care professionals. Palliative care should be integrated within various health care settings including the hospital, emergency department, nursing home, home care, assisted living facilities, and outpatient settings. Palliative care remains very unevenly available, so many patients and families needlessly suffer having either no, limited, or delayed access to appropriate palliative care. Basic palliative care should be part of the tool kit for all physicians who care for seriously ill patients, and specialty palliative care should be available for the more challenging symptom management and complex and often conflictual medical decision making.

The integration of palliative care into the experiences of patients and families is designed to meet several objectives. First, to ensure that pain and symptom control, psychosocial distress, spiritual issues, and practical needs are addressed throughout the continuum of care. Second, to make certain that patients and families obtain the information they need in an ongoing and comprehensible manner to understand their prognosis and treatment options. This process incorporates their values and preferences and is sensitive to changes in the patient's condition over time. Third, palliative care seeks to provide seamless care coordination across settings with high-quality communication among providers. Finally, for those patients who are not going to recover, palliative care prepares patients and families, to the extent possible, for the dying process and for death, including options for hospice care and opportunities for personal growth and bereavement support.

COMMON ILLNESS TRAJECTORIES AND PALLIATIVE CARE

There are four distinct trajectories of functional decline before dying (E-Fig. 125-1). These trajectories have major implications for palliative care and health care delivery. Patients and families likely have different physical, psychological, social, and spiritual needs depending on the trajectory of their illness before they die. Being aware of these trajectories can help providers deliver appropriate care that integrates both disease-directed and palliative treatments.

Trajectory 1: Short Period of Evident Decline before Death

Cancer typifies this trajectory. Function is preserved until rather late, followed by a predictable and precipitous decline over weeks to months. The onset of decline usually suggests metastatic tumor. A more predictable decline in function can assist in anticipating care needs, transitioning away from curative treatments toward a more exclusive emphasis on palliation, and eventually into hospice care. Not all malignancies follow this trajectory (e.g., prostate, breast) and some non-malignant conditions may follow this course.

Trajectory 2: Chronic Illness with Exacerbations and Sudden Dying

Congestive heart failure (CHF), chronic obstructive pulmonary disease (COPD), end-stage liver disease, and AIDS typify this trajectory. These organ system diseases represent chronic illnesses with occasional, acute exacerbations (e.g., physiological stress that overwhelms the body's reserves), often requiring hospital admission. Patients can have a return of function after an exacerbation, but often not to the level of their baseline. They also may die suddenly during an exacerbation, but it is difficult to predict in advance. Prognosticating is very challenging in this trajectory. When patients choose to forego or stop aggressive life support, planning for aggressive symptom relief during a future exacerbation is essential.

Trajectory 3: Prolonged Dwindling

Dementia and frailty typify this trajectory. These patients have a prolonged course of physical and cognitive decline and become increasingly frail. Additional diagnoses include other neurodegenerative conditions (e.g., Parkinson's disease, amyotrophic lateral sclerosis) and patients with multiple moderate to severe comorbidities (e.g., arthritis, visual impairment, past mild strokes, diabetes with neuropathy). Gradual decline in function, weight loss, fatigue, and low levels of activity are core features. Caregiver burden is usually immense. Prognosticating survival is difficult and complications, such a pneumonia and fractures, may be terminal events. The benefits and burdens of artificial nutrition and hydration must be balanced in the late stages.

Trajectory 4: Sudden, Severe Neurological Injury

Sudden impairment trajectories are those that stem from sudden neurological injury that can lead to profound cognitive and functional impairment. These include stroke, hypoxic ischemic encephalopathy, and traumatic brain injury. The vast majority of deaths occur either early after the event when treatments are withheld or withdrawn, or in the chronic stage in survivors who have accumulating debility (these events represent the leading cause of adult disability). At the extremes of impairment are persistent vegetative states, minimally conscious states, and locked-in syndrome. But there is a vast spectrum of severe impairments short of these extremes that raise questions about how to manage potentially severe debility with little or uncertain chances of improvement. This trajectory requires a health care system responsive to negotiating goals of treatment with patients and surrogates who may consider these future health states to be "worse than death."

⬤ COMMUNICATION SKILLS AND NEGOTIATING GOALS OF TREATMENT

Excellent communication skills are central to palliative care: communication with patients, family, other physicians, nurses, and other members of the health care team. The overarching aim is to assist the patient and family in establishing the goals of current and future treatment in a process of shared decision making. When negotiating goals of treatment in palliative care, the focus is often to assist with the following decisions: to help decide types and aggressiveness of disease-directed therapies; to ensure optimum palliation of symptoms; to assist in hospice determinations; to discuss initiating, withholding or withdrawing therapies; to facilitate advance care planning; and to initiate surrogate decision-making if the patient lacks capacity. These discussions occur at various time points in the course of advancing illness when new and important information is learned and needs to be communicated to the patient and family. The need to renegotiate goals should also be anticipated when triggers of advancing disease suggest limited life expectancy or excessive suffering. These discussions are almost always variants of "bad news" discussions.

The overall approach to communication and negotiating goals of care in each of these scenarios is similar (Table 125-1). This includes running an effective family meeting with or without the patient present. Initial elements include establishing the proper setting, identifying key stakeholders, and "doing your homework" (i.e., discussing potential plans with all relevant subspecialties who may have communicated with the patient and families). When the meeting begins, find out what the patient and family understand about the medical condition and ask about what added information they want. Keeping an open mind and trying

to hold back on a fixed agenda (e.g., to "get the DNR" or to "stop futile care") helps clinicians allow patients and families sufficient time to "tell their stories" and provides the context within which effective decision making can occur. In general, the more patients and families speak in the early parts of such meetings, the better.

The provider then needs to share prognostic information and discuss the benefits and burdens of the available treatment options. Alerting the patient or family of impending bad news (e.g., *"I am afraid I have some difficult news to share with you"*) is a useful initial communication strategy. The amount of information should be paced with frequent pauses to allow time for emotional responses. Comprehension should be frequently checked, and questions should be encouraged using an "ask-tell-ask" strategy. The skilled clinician can flexibly assess, probe, and pace the content and depth of the discussion in an emotionally responsive (acknowledge, explore, empathize, and legitimize) and culturally competent manner. This includes the ability to understand and respect diverse religious practices and differing preferences about degree of truth telling. When appropriate, the clinician should make recommendations based on scientific knowledge as well as awareness of a patient's values and preferences, and be prepared to help resolve conflicts among patient, family members, and providers. Finally, providers need to develop strategies to preserve and potentially reframe hope, including ways to *"hope for the best"* and simultaneously *"prepare for the worst."* Commitments to minimize suffering and to not abandon the patient and family are essential. At the end of the discussions, the provider should summarize key aspects of what was reviewed and establish a follow-up plan for future communications and treatments.

Estimating and Communicating Prognosis

A core component of information shared in the palliative care setting is prognosis. Understanding prognosis is central to making decisions (e.g., treatment, comfort measures, hospice). Prognosis is a prediction of possible future outcomes of a disease (e.g.,

TABLE 125-1	GENERAL STRATEGY FOR COMMUNICATING AND NEGOTIATING GOALS OF CARE IN COMMON PALLIATIVE CARE SETTINGS
Step 1	Prepare and establish setting Do not have a rigid preset agenda
Step 2	Ask patient and family what they know and understand Provide sufficient time for patients and families to "tell their story" Active listening skills
Step 3	Find out how much patient and family want to know Acknowledge and explore emotions
Step 4	Give information in small amounts, and frequently check understanding Discuss prognosis and benefits and burdens of treatment options Be mindful of overly optimistic and pessimistic predictions Be prepared to make recommendations
Step 5	Respond to emotions and empathetic response Convey honesty and reframe hope Use "I wish" statements
Step 6	Summarize, establish and implement plan, follow-up Possible time-limited trial

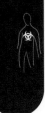

survival, symptoms, function, quality of life, family and financial impact) with or without treatment. Most patients and families want to know prognosis. Since there are some patients and families that may not want to know prognosis or want it communicated in a particular way, it is essential to begin by finding out what the patient and family knows and wants to know.

Inaccurate predictions may lead to poor decision making. Indeed, physicians tend to overestimate survival in patients with advanced cancer by about 30%, and the bias is more pronounced the longer the physician-patient relationship. Overly optimistic predictions can lead to overuse of ineffective or unwanted disease-directed treatment, delay in hospice referrals, false expectations, unnecessary tests and procedures, and poor symptom control. Therefore, accurately estimating and communicating prognosis is central to optimal decision making in advanced illness and at the end of life.

In advanced illnesses, common factors found to be predictive of short-term survival (i.e., less than 6 months) include performance status, anorexia-cachexia syndrome, delirium, and dyspnea. In addition to a physician's subjective predictions of survival, there exist models to assist with prognostic estimates, including generic models for particular populations (e.g., hospice enrollees) as well as disease-specific models (e.g., cancers, heart failure, liver disease, stroke, AIDS, spinal cord compression). Hospice eligibility criteria also differ for specific diseases. While not uniformly reliable, they can be useful in formulating estimates where prognosis might be 6 months or less if the disease is allowed to run its natural course (a prognostic criterion).

For an individual patient, however, prognostic uncertainty remains the rule. Therefore, it is important to integrate both evidence and experience-based medicine, and present the information in formats tailored to the particular patient (verbal descriptions, numeric, frequencies, or graphics). Prognostic estimates should be bounded with ranges to convey realistic uncertainty, being sure to allow for exceptions in both directions. For example, *"in my experience, patients with your condition live on average a few weeks to a few months. It could be longer, but it could also be shorter."* For survival-predominate prognoses (e.g., *"How long do I have?"*), be mindful of overly optimistic prognoses, remembering to think of and convey the lower bound (e.g., *"some may live longer, but others may, unfortunately, live shorter"*). For outcome-predominant prognoses (e.g., *"What will life be like?"*), be mindful of overly pessimistic predictions, remembering the power of adaptation and engendering hope by helping patients and families find new meaning.

● SUFFERING AND SYMPTOM MANAGEMENT

Palliative care aims to relieve suffering, which is defined as severe distress related to events that threaten the stability of personhood or interconnectedness of the physical, psychological, spiritual and social aspects of self. Beginning with simple, open-ended screening questions, such as *"In what ways are you suffering most?"* and following with more domain-related screening questions (e.g., physical, psychological, spiritual, social) may allow for more probing and multidimensional inquiries to better understand the various sources of and contributions to an individual's suffering.

One of the first steps in the care of any seriously ill patient is to control pain and other forms of physical suffering. There are

striking similarities between the burden of symptoms experienced in patients dying of cancer and non-cancer conditions. Although the profile of symptoms may differ, each disease carries with it troubling symptoms that can potentially be addressed and managed.

Physical Symptoms

Pain

Uncontrolled pain dominates all other experiences, and most pain can be relieved using basic pain management strategies. This includes a detailed history and physical examination, categorizing the likely type or types (i.e., somatic, visceral, neuropathic) and severity (rated on a 0-10 scale) of pain, knowledge about proper opioid dosing strategies, and judicious use of consultations and invasive interventions (e.g., nerve blocks, epidural analgesia). The overarching three-tiered approach is to use nonopioids (e.g., acetaminophen, nonsteroidal anti-inflammatory drugs) for mild pain, weak opioids (e.g., hydrocodone or codeine) for mild-to-moderate pain, and strong opioids (e.g., morphine, hydromorphine, fentanyl, methadone) for moderate to severe pain.

Risk factors for potential opioid abuse or misuse should be screened for even in the presence of clearly defined terminal illness, including any lifetime personal or family history of opioid, alcohol, or other substance abuse. If risk factors are present (about 20% of the population), special precautions should be taken to minimize the risk of abuse, including clearly defined and adhered to prescribing contracts and strict limits and expectations about renewals and dose alteration processes. One single prescriber should be responsible for all opioid prescriptions and renewals, and one pharmacy should be used. If clinicians are inexperienced with such prescribing, formal consultation with specialists in palliative care and/or addiction medicine should be considered.

Most seriously ill patients with chronic moderate to severe pain should be initially started on around-the-clock dosing using a short-acting opioid. Table 125-2 shows the equianalgesic dosing, usual starting doses, half-life, and duration for the commonly available opioid agents. Once the total daily dosing has been determined (sum of all scheduled and "as needed" doses), the patient may be switched to a long-acting opioid to cover the baseline requirements. As needed opioids for breakthrough pain should be approximately 10% of the total daily dose every 1 to 2 hours orally or every 30 to 60 minutes subcutaneously or intravenously. If a patient is requiring more than 4 to 6 breakthrough doses per day, he should be in contact with the prescribing clinician for re-evaluation of dosing. Continuous intravenous or subcutaneous infusions of opioids may be needed for rapid control of severe pain. Methadone is useful in palliative care because of its excellent oral bioavailability, lack of active metabolites in renal impairment, low cost, flexible route of administration (PO, IV, SC), and possible effect on both neuropathic and somatic pain. However, it does have a dose-dependent, progressively long half-life and arrhythmogenic potential.

Constipation occurs with all opioids, and it should be anticipated and treated. Other predictable but less common side effects include nausea, myoclonus, urinary retention, pruritis, and delirium. Some of these side effects are time-limited with

TABLE 125-2 EQUIANALGESIC TABLE FOR ADULTS

PAIN	MEDICATION	EQUIANALGESIC DOSE (for chronic dosing)		USUAL STARTING DOSES ADULT >50 KG; FOR OPIOID NAÏVE PATIENTS (♦ ½ dose for elderly, or severe renal or liver disease)		HALF-LIFE	DURATION	RELATIVE GENERIC COST
		IM/IV onset 15-30 min	PO onset 30-60 min	PARENTERAL	PO			
Moderate to Severe	Morphine	10 mg	30 mg	2.5-5 mg IV/SC q3-4h (♦1.25-2.5 mg)	5-15 mg q3-4h (IR or Oral Solution) (♦2.5-7.5 mg)	1.5-2 h (includes active metabolites)	3-7 h	$ (IR tablet) $$ (solution) $$ (ER generic) $$$$ (ER brand)
	Oxycodone	Not Available	20 mg	Not Available	5-10 mg q3-4h (♦2.5 mg)	3-4 h	4-6 h	$$ (comb. w/APAP) $$ (IR tablet) $$$ (solution) $$$ (ER brand)
	Hydromorphone	1.5 mg	7.5 mg	0.2-0.6 mg IV/SC q2-3h (♦0.2 mg)	1-2 mg q3-4h (♦0.5-1 mg)	2-3 h	4-5 h	$ (tablet) $$$ (solution) $$$$ (ER tablet)
	Methadone	Oral: IV 2:1	24 hr oral morphine dose — morphine:methadone ratio: <30 mg = 2:1; 31-99 mg = 4:1; 100-299 mg = 8:1; 300-499 mg = 12:1; 500-999 mg = 15:1; 1000-1200 mg = 20:1; >1200 mg = Consider consult	1.25-2.5 mg q8h (♦1.25 mg)	2.5-5 mg q8h (♦1.25-2.5 mg)	15-190 h (N.B. large variation)	6-12 h	$ (tablet) $ (solution)
	Fentanyl (Duragesic Patch)	100 µg (single dose) (T1/2 life and duration of parenteral doses variable)	24 hr oral morphine dose — Initial patch dose: 30-59 mg = 12.5 µg/hr; 60-134 mg = 25 µg/hr; 135-224 mg = 50 µg/hr; 225-314 mg = 75 µg/hr; 315-404 mg = 100 µg/hr	25-50 µg IV q1-3h (♦12.5-25 µg)	12.5 µg/hr q72h (transdermal) (♦Not recommended for opioid naive)	7 h (lozenge) 12-22 h (buccal) 13-22 h (transdermal)	60+ min (lozenge) 120+ min (buccal; not well studied) 48-72 h (transdermal)	$$$ (transdermal) $$$$ (buccal) $$$$ (buccal)
Mild to Moderate	Codeine	130 mg (IM only)	200 mg	15-30 mg IM/SC q4h (♦7.5-15 mg) IV Contraindicated	30-60 mg q3-4h (♦15-30 mg)	3 h	4-6 h	$$ (combination with APAP) $$$ (tablet)
	Hydrocodone	Not Available	30 mg	Not Available	5 mg q3-4h (♦2.5 mg)	3 h	4-6 h	$$ (comb. with ibuprofen) $ (combination with APAP)

initiation (e.g., nausea), while others can be managed by dose reduction or opioid rotation (e.g., myoclonus, delirium). Major respiratory depression is extremely rare if the opioid is dosed appropriately and proportionate to the severity of symptoms. In the absence of a prior personal or family history of drug and alcohol abuse, addiction is rare in the presence of serious illness, but physical dependence (i.e., withdrawal symptoms upon abrupt cessation) and tolerance (i.e., decrease in drug effect over time) should be expected. Naloxone should be rarely used unless a clear overdose is suspected, or if life-threatening complications occur. Special caution about opioid prescribing is needed in the elderly and debilitated patients, and recommended starting doses should be reduced by approximately 50%. There are additional opioid selection recommendations for patients with renal insufficiency (avoid morphine and codeine; use hydromorphone and oxycodone with caution; methadone and fentanyl (optimal) and hepatic insufficiency (cautiously use fentanyl, hydromorphone, oxycodone, or methadone; avoid or decrease dose of morphine).

Non-pain

There are numerous non-pain physical symptoms that can dominate and overwhelm the clinical picture in any given patient. These include dyspnea, nausea and vomiting, constipation, anorexia-cachexia, fatigue, bleeding, agitation, apathy, myoclonus, pruritis, and specific functional deficits. Each symptom requires a structured approach to the history and physical examination with a full exploration of the potential etiologies and treatment options; informed by the prognosis and preferences of the patient and family. (For practical information geared to basic palliative management of pain and other symptoms, see Quill TE, Holloway RG, Shah MS, et al: Primer of Palliative Care, ed 5, Illinois, 2010, American Academy of Hospice and Palliative Medicine.)

Psychological Distress

Depression, anxiety, and delirium are all common in the palliative care setting. They are frequently under-recognized and under-treated. Appropriate diagnosis and treatment can improve quality of life.

Nearly all patients in palliative care and their families experience sadness, preparatory grief, and transient anxiety as illness advances. Grief or normal sadness is often experienced in waves with retained capacity for pleasure. Depression is more enduring, persistent and intense, and may be associated with hopelessness, helplessness, worthlessness, and guilt. Two screening questions assessing depressed mood and anhedonia include: *"Are you depressed?"* and *"Do you have much interest and pleasure in doing things?"* One should be cautious about overusing somatic symptoms to diagnose depression (e.g., fatigue, anorexia, sleep disturbance) because they frequently overlap with physiological changes associated with advanced disease. For depression and anxiety, consider and rule out contributions from physical symptoms (e.g., uncontrolled pain), medical causes (e.g., hypothyroidism, hyperthyroidism), and medications. Effective pharmacological and non-pharmacological treatments exist for both depression and anxiety, though treatment selection depends on symptom intensity, patient prognosis, and treatment benefits

and burdens. Other members of the interdisciplinary team (social worker, chaplain, and psychologist) often play a critical role in assessment and ongoing management.

Delirium, an acquired and fluctuating disorder of consciousness and cognition, occurs commonly in the palliative care setting. The level of psychomotor activity can vary from hyperactive ("agitated" delirium) to hypoactive ("quiet" delirium). Nearly 80% of the delirium in the palliative care setting is the hypoactive variant. As a result, it is often under-diagnosed or misdiagnosed as depression and fatigue. The most common causes of delirium in palliative care include medications (e.g., opioids), metabolic disorders due to progressive organ failure, and infection. Meticulous attention to the history from collateral sources (e.g., nurses, caregiver) and a detailed medication history are essential for an accurate diagnosis. While delirium may reverse if an obvious cause is identified and removed, frequently it represents an important marker of progressive illness so cognitive improvements may be transient and incomplete. In addition to etiology-specific treatment (e.g., change or stop medications, treat infection, oxygen, hydration, biphosphonates), environmental interventions are recommended for all patients (e.g., quiet reassurance, gentle re-orientation, optimize sensory input, minimize night disruptions). Pharmacological management should be used sparingly and cautiously, and may include antipsychotic medications, benzodiazepines, and pyschostimulants (for the hypoactive variant).

Spiritual and Existential Pain

Spiritual and existential distress is prevalent in patients and families with serious illness, especially at the end of life. Spirituality is about one's relationship with and responses to transcendent questions that confront one as a human being (e.g., search for meaning and purpose in life). Religion is a set of texts, practices, and beliefs about the transcendence shared by a community. Spirituality is broader than religion. The spiritual issues of seriously ill and dying patients often center on questions of meaning, value, and relationships. Dying patients want to be assured of their value in the face of actual or perceived threats to their intactness as a human being (e.g., physical and cognitive declines, altered appearances). Spirituality can help people find hope in despair and help restore purpose.

One of the goals of palliative care is to relieve spiritual and existential distress. Patients and families often welcome such discussions. Examples of open-ended questions to facilitate this dialogue include: *"Are you at peace with all of this?"* and *"Is faith (religion, spirituality) important to you?"* Acknowledgement and empathetic listening are the most important responses for most clinicians, as opposed to trying to provide "correct answers."

Other strategies for fostering hope and meaning include developing caring relationships, setting attainable goals, involving the patient in the decision-making process, affirming the patient's worth, using lighthearted humor (when appropriate), and reminiscing with life review. It is important, however, to know one's professional boundaries and refer to chaplains or clergy from the patient's faith traditions if questions move beyond the realm of general exploration (e.g., *"It sounds like it would be good to explore this with someone with more experience than I have. Would it be okay for me to send our chaplain in to discuss this with you?"*).

The Role and Use Of Diagnostic Tests and Invasive Procedures

Several questions should be considered in determining the appropriateness of aggressive medical or palliative interventions near the end of life: What is the goal or expected outcome of the proposed intervention? What is the probable efficacy of the intervention? What is the patient's baseline level of function and life expectancy? What are the potential side effects and burdens of the intervention? What are the patient's and family's wishes, values, and preferences?

The range of medical and palliative options available is huge, so the challenge is to determine what makes sense to enhance the well-being of this patient at this particular stage of illness. Palliative interventions range from pure symptom management and support to invasive options, such as chemotherapy, radiotherapy, surgical/endoscopic interventions, stenting procedures, thoracentisis, paracentesis, pericardiocentesis, home inotropic therapy, non-invasive ventilation, antibiotics, or transfusions. The challenge is to individualize discussions, so that patients can take full advantage of treatments that will help them meet their goals without having their experience dominated by near futile invasive interventions.

The Role of Hospice

Hospice care is a specialized form of palliative care aimed at those patients and families in the terminal stages of illness. In 2011, 1.65 million patients were served by hospice programs in the United States. Median length of stay on hospice is less than 3 weeks. In order to qualify for the Medicare Hospice Benefit, two physicians must sign a statement certifying that the patient's prognosis for survival, if the disease runs its natural course, is likely to be 6 months or less. Hospice criteria exist to assist in making these determinations for common medical conditions. Hospice care can be delivered in hospitals, patient's homes, nursing homes, or dedicated "hospice houses." The Medicare Hospice Benefit covers most costs related to terminal care without a deductible, which includes palliative medications, nursing oversight, supplies, and bereavement care. Hospice also covers up to 4 hours of custodial caregiver services per day; however, family and/or friends must provide the remaining care if the patient is to stay at home. Hospice it does not cover custodial caregiver serives if the patient is admitted to a nursing facility.

Cancer continues to be the most common diagnosis for patients dying in hospice programs. However, the prevalence of non-cancer diagnoses is increasing and now represents more than 50% of all hospice admissions. Discussing hospice with patients and families can be challenging. First, it is often initially viewed as a "bad news" discussion given that patients and families need to confront the fact that disease-directed treatment is no longer effective and that prognosis is likely to be 6 months or less. Second, given the reimbursement restrictions, patients may also need to forgo particular types of treatment that are important to them (e.g., acute hospital or ICU-level care, dialysis, chemotherapy, milrinone for heart failure).

Request for Hastened Death and Last Resort Options

The prevalence of suicidal ideation and suicide attempts is higher in patients with advanced life-limiting illness compared to those without serious disease. In Oregon where physician-assisted suicide is legally permitted (subject to safeguards), the prevalence of a patient's wanting to explore a health care professional's willingness to help hasten death is about 1/50, whereas only about 1/500 die using physician-assisted suicide. The motivation behind such initial explorations may relate to relentless physical suffering, disfigurement, hopelessness, loss of dignity, fear of being a burden, or a "cry for help." Most enduring requests from patients with progressive medical illnesses, however, arise not from inadequate symptom control, but from a patient's belief about dignity, meaning, and control over the circumstances of death. Although some providers might be uncomfortable with exploring such requests, they need to be approached systematically with a diligent search to understand the root causes before responding.

A careful evaluation includes a precise clarification and exploration as to exactly what the patient is asking and why. Is the request based on transient thoughts about ending life (common) or a serious appeal for assistance (relatively rare)? Does the request occur in the context of intense physical suffering, psychological despair, an existential crisis, or a combination of factors? Does the patient have full decision-making capacity? Is the request proportionate to the level of suffering? Evaluating such requests can be emotionally fatiguing and conflicting, and clinicians need self-awareness in distinguishing their emotions from the patient's, including tending to one's own support by sharing the burden of such requests with trusted colleagues.

Responding to such a request should first include intensification of a search for potentially reversible contributions to suffering. This will often include treating physical and psychological symptoms, aggressive attempts to foster hope, consulting psychiatrists or spiritual counselors, and creative brainstorming with trusted colleagues and team members. Some requests for hastened death persist, despite optimal palliative care. In such circumstances, the clinician should seek out a second opinion and confront the possibilities. These possibilities include withdrawal of life-sustaining interventions, palliative sedation, voluntary cessation of oral intake, and assisted suicide (illegal in the United States except for the states of Oregon, Washington, Vermont, and Montana). While it is important to support the patient, the clinician must balance integrity and non-abandonment. This may include drawing specific boundaries of what the clinician can and cannot do, while still searching in earnest for a mutually acceptable solution.

COMMON ETHICAL CHALLENGES IN PALLIATIVE CARE

Inadequate Treatment of Pain and the Myth that Pain Medication Hastens Death

Evidence abounds that pain is under-treated in many medical settings, including those patients who are severely and even terminally ill (especially women, the elderly, minorities and those who are cognitively impaired). Some under-treatment stems from fears about addiction as well as concerns about the possibility of hastening death. When patients with prior addiction problems are excluded, the incidence of new addictive behavior when opioids are used to treat pain in those with a well-defined, serious illness is rare. Similarly, there is very little data to suggest that properly prescribed opioids hasten death. In fact, current evidence supports the idea that opioids may prolong life in these patients and enhance quality of life in those with advanced illness and major pain or dyspnea.

Addiction and diversion exist in medically ill populations. Alcoholism and substance abuse exist in medically ill populations as they do in all other parts of society. When patients with such risk factors develop painful, potentially life-limiting medical conditions, they deserve adequate pain treatment, but with extreme caution because of the risk of reactivating or aggravating abuse behavior, including diversion of prescription drugs for recreational purposes. Prescribing contracts that specify one single medical prescriber, set amounts around the clock and as needed limits, face-to-face encounters for all renewals, and dose adjustments only after direct conversation with the prescriber, are all essential parts of the plan. Consultations with experts in palliative care and/or substance abuse should be requested if there is any difficulty adhering to the contract.

When Patients and Families Want Near Futile Treatment

The patient autonomy movement in medicine has led to patients and families taking an active role in their own medical decision making. This is generally a positive development except in two circumstances: 1) when physicians stop taking an active role using their expertise to guide patients in their decision making, thereby abdicating their professional responsibility of advocating for the best possible treatment based on the patient's medical condition and personal values, and 2) when patients or their families want and even demand near futile treatment toward the end of their lives despite physician's advice that treatment has much more burden than benefit. Physicians might try to respond to patients who want "everything" by suggesting that they want to try everything that is "more likely to help than harm," but avoid any treatment that is most likely to "do more harm than good." However, some patients and families will accept no limits on treatment no matter what the burden and the improbability of success. Of course, truly futile treatment should not be offered or provided upon request, but absolute futility has been difficult to define in many cases.

Feeding Tube Questions When Patients Stop Eating and Drinking

Many patients gradually stop eating and drinking as a natural part of the dying process, but this can be very hard for patients and families to accept in light of fears about "starving to death" and in view of seemingly simple technologies that can potentially combat and even reverse the problem. In fact, with few exceptions, feeding tubes have not been show to prolong life in most advanced illnesses such as metastatic cancer or advanced Alzheimer disease. It is important to know about the exceptions (e.g. esophageal and oropharyngeal cancers, amyotrophic lateral

sclerosis, acute stroke), but also to have an open discussion about the naturalness of diminished eating and drinking as many illnesses progress. If there is uncertainty about whether a particular patient might benefit from a feeding tube, and patient and family are clear about wanting to give it a try, the clinician can frame the decision as a "time-limited trial" to see how the patient tolerates tube feeding psychologically as well as physiologically in a specified timeframe. A nasogastric tube has a built-in time limit of about a month before a PEG tube needs to be inserted as a potential framework for such a trial. Explaining to patients and families about the positive aspects of natural feeding, even in small amounts, of real food (smell, taste, and enjoyment) may help focus the decision on important quality of life issues (that may otherwise be ignored), rather than more technical, physiological issues.

● LAST HOURS AND DAYS OF LIVING

An integral aspect of palliative care is preparing and guiding the patient and caregivers through the dying process. When prognosis is measured in hours to days there are typical signs and symptoms that usually occur. Patients become weak and fatigued and gradually lose mobility. There is also a gradual and predictable decrease in food and fluid intake. Most patients do not experience hunger and thirst, and the associated mouth dryness that occurs is easily palliated with small sips or sponges of cold water. Caregivers will frequently ask about intravenous hydration. In rare instances, intravenous or subcutaneous fluids may temporarily improve mental status and energy in the final days of life. Most of the time, however, the benefits are difficult to discern and the excessive fluids may contribute to end-of-life physiologic conditions (edema, ascites, effusions, and pulmonary secretions) that do not improve longevity and may worsen comfort.

As patients become weaker, there is a predictable decrease in the level of consciousness with increasing periods of somnolence eventually giving way to a comatose state. Education about this process should include associated changes in respiratory patterns and to anticipate progressive periods of apnea, interspersed with episodes of hyperpnea and deep breathing (Cheyne-Stokes respirations). During this process caregivers often feel they are on "a roller-coaster ride" and gentle guidance on what to expect can allay concerns. As consciousness wanes, swallowing slows and the cough reflex weakens. As a result, saliva pools in the oropharynx and can result in noisy respiration ("death rattle"), which can usually be palliated to some degree with transdermal scopolamine, gylcopyrrolate (PO, IV, SC) or sublingual atropine ophthalmic drops. Families should be reminded that these symptoms are a natural part of the dying process, and that persistent shortness of breath is relatively uncommon, but can be treated with opiates and benzodiazepines, if needed.

As death approaches, reduced perfusion causes cooling and cyanosis of the extremities and a decrease and darkening of the urine. Most deaths are relatively peaceful, but a few can be preceded by periods of intense agitation and restlessness (hyperactive terminal delirium). Antipsychotic medications and conventional doses of benzodiazepines can usually treat terminal delirium. Prior to and when death occurs, families should be encouraged to carry out cultural or religious rituals that are important to them. Providers should express condolences, be available for questions and responsive to intense emotional reactions that sometimes occur. A short condolence card or letter is almost always appreciated. If possible, efforts should be made to follow-up with family members and caregivers deemed at risk for complicated bereavement and grief.

PROSPECTUS FOR THE FUTURE

Palliative care became an officially recognized subspecialty within the United States in 2006. Physicians from 10 specialties can be board certified in hospice and palliative medicine including: family medicine, internal medicine, emergency medicine, pediatrics, physical medicine and rehabilitation, anesthesiology, psychiatry, neurology, radiology, and surgery. As patients live longer with chronic illness, there will be an increasing need to fully integrate palliative care providers and programs within hospitals, nursing homes, and the outpatient setting; and to ensure that all primary care providers and non-palliative specialists develop the skill sets needed to provide basic palliative care.

There is a compelling need for research to better define the optimal timing, setting, and delivery of palliative care to improve the quality of life and lessen the suffering of patients and families with advanced illness.

SUGGESTED READINGS

Goldstein NE, Morrison RS, editors: Evidence-Based Practice of Palliative Medicine, Philadelphia, 2013, Elsevier.

Moryl N, Coyle N, Foley KM: Managing an acute pain crisis in a patient with advanced cancer: "This is as much of a crisis as a code", JAMA 299:1457–1467, 2008.

National Consensus Project for Quality Palliative Care: Clinical Practice Guidelines for Quality Palliative Care, ed 3, Pittsburgh, PA, 2013. http://www.nationalconsensusproject.org.

Quill TE, Abernethy AP: Generalist plus specialist palliative care–creating a more sustainable model, N Engl J Med 368:1173–1175, 2013.

Quill TE, Holloway RG, Shah MS, et al: Primer of Palliative Care, ed 5, Glenview, 2010, American Academy of Hospice and Palliative Medicine.

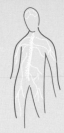

XIX

Alcohol and Substance Abuse

126 **Alcohol and Substance Abuse**
Richard A. Lange and L. David Hillis

Alcohol and Substance Abuse

Richard A. Lange and L. David Hillis

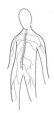

ALCOHOL ABUSE

Alcohol abuse is a major public health problem. In 2010, an estimated 2,735,511 deaths worldwide were attributable to alcohol use. About 58.3 million people in the United States (nearly one quarter of persons aged 12 years or older) participate in binge drinking, and almost 16 million (6.2% of the population aged 12 or older) report heavy drinking, defined as binge drinking on at least 5 days in the past month. Alcohol use is the third leading preventable cause of death in the United States (exceeded only by cigarette smoking and obesity) and claims over 80,000 lives annually. In 2011, an estimated 11% of persons aged 12 years or older drove under the influence of alcohol at least once. Alcohol use contributes to roughly 31% of all fatalities caused by motor vehicle accidents, or approximately 10,000 vehicular deaths annually, and is a major contributor to risky sexual behavior, domestic violence, homicide, and suicide. For the year 2006, the estimated economic cost of excessive drinking in the United States was $223.5 billion: 72% from lost productivity, 11% from healthcare costs, 9% from criminal justice costs, and 7.5% from other effects.

DEFINITION AND EPIDEMIOLOGY

The American Psychiatric Association has specific criteria for the diagnosis of *alcohol use disorder;* these 11 criteria are described in the *Diagnostic and Statistical Manual of Mental Disorders,* fifth edition, and are listed in Table 126-1. Alcohol use disorder is further characterized as mild, moderate, or severe, based on the number of criteria the individual meets; 2 to 3 criteria indicate a mild disorder, 4 to 5 criteria a moderate disorder, and 6 or more a severe disorder. The so-called *binge drinker* is defined as one who typically consumes five or more drinks on a single occasion.

Among individuals aged 12 or older, whites are more likely to report current alcohol use than other racial groups (Fig. 126-1), and men are more likely than women to be drinkers (57% versus 47%, respectively). The average age at first alcohol use is 17 years; 65% of college students currently use alcohol (Fig. 126-2); and more than half of all college students admit to heavy episodic drinking. Although the prevalence of ethanol use is highest in individuals younger than 30 years of age, survey data suggest that about two thirds of persons over age 30 consume it.

PHARMACOLOGIC AND METABOLIC FACTORS

After oral ingestion, alcohol is absorbed predominantly in the small intestine, and its rate of intestinal absorption is accelerated by the simultaneous ingestion of carbohydrates and carbonated beverages. Prolonged retention of alcohol in the stomach, as occurs when food is consumed before drinking, delays alcohol absorption because absorption in the stomach is considerably slower than in the duodenum. Once in the blood, alcohol equilibrates rapidly across all membranes, including the blood-brain barrier, thereby accounting for the prompt onset of its euphoric effects. Maximal blood alcohol concentrations are reached 45 to 75 minutes after alcohol is ingested.

The liver metabolizes approximately 90% of ethanol to acetaldehyde via the alcohol dehydrogenase pathway; subsequently, acetaldehyde is converted by aldehyde dehydrogenase to acetate, which enters the Krebs cycle. At low or moderate serum concentrations of ethanol, the alcohol dehydrogenase pathway functions almost exclusively in metabolizing ethanol. At high concentrations, the microsomal ethanol oxidizing system (CYP2E1) contributes to metabolism. Less than 10% of ethanol is excreted unchanged through the skin, kidneys, and lungs. Elimination of alcohol from the body is affected by obesity, food intake, previous exposure to alcohol, and variability among individuals in the efficiency of the alcohol and aldehyde dehydrogenase systems.

TABLE 126-1	CRITERIA FOR THE DIAGNOSIS OF ALCOHOL USE DISORDER

TWO OR MORE OF THE FOLLOWING IN THE PREVIOUS 12 MONTHS

Recurrent alcohol use resulting in a **failure to fulfill major** obligations at work, school, or home

Recurrent alcohol use in situations in which it is physically **hazardous**

Continued alcohol use despite having persistent or **recurrent social or interpersonal problems** caused or exacerbated by the effects of alcohol

Tolerance, as defined by:
- need for markedly increased amounts of alcohol to achieve intoxication or desired effect; and/or
- markedly diminished effect with continued use of the same amount of alcohol

Withdrawal, as manifested by:
- characteristic alcohol withdrawal syndrome; and/or
- alcohol is taken to relieve or avoid withdrawal symptoms

Alcohol is often taken in **larger amounts** or over a longer period than was intended

Persistent desire or **unsuccessful efforts to diminish** or to control alcohol use

A great deal of **time** is spent in activities necessary to obtain, use, or recover from the effects of alcohol

Important social, occupational, or recreational **activities are relinquished or reduced** because of alcohol use

Alcohol use is **continued despite knowledge** of having a persistent or recurrent physical or psychological problem that is likely to have been caused or exacerbated by alcohol use

Craving or a strong desire or urge to use a specific type of alcohol

Modified from the American Psychiatric Association: Diagnostic and statistical manual of mental disorders, ed 5, Washington, D.C., 2013, American Psychiatric Press.

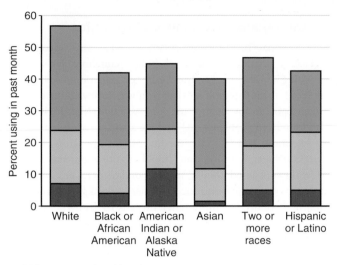

□ Current use (not binge)
□ Binge use (not heavy)
■ Heavy alcohol use

FIGURE 126-1 Current, binge, and heavy alcohol use among persons aged 12 or older, by race and ethnicity, according to the National Survey on Drug Use and Health (2011). Binge drinking is defined as having five or more drinks on a single occasion. Heavy alcohol use is defined as having had five or more drinks on the same occasion on each of five or more days in the previous 30 days. (From Substance Abuse and Mental Health Services Administration: Results from the 2011 National Survey on Drug Use and Health: Summary of National Findings, NSDUH Series H-44, HHS Publication No. [SMA] 12-4713, Rockville, Md., 2012, Substance Abuse and Mental Health Services Administration.)

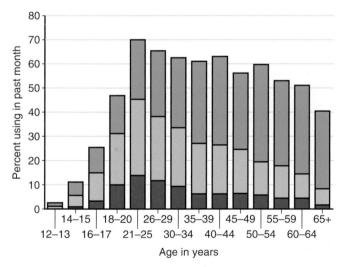

□ Current use (not binge)
□ Binge use (not heavy)
■ Heavy alcohol use

FIGURE 126-2 Current, binge, and heavy alcohol use among persons aged 12 or older, by age, according to the National Survey on Drug Use and Health (2007). Binge drinking is defined as having five or more drinks on a single occasion. Heavy alcohol use is defined as having had five or more drinks on the same occasion on each of five or more days in the previous 30 days. (From Substance Abuse and Mental Health Services Administration: Results from the 2011 National Survey on Drug Use and Health: Summary of National Findings, NSDUH Series H-44, HHS Publication No. [SMA] 12-4713, Rockville, Md., 2012, Substance Abuse and Mental Health Services Administration.)

These enzymatic variations also influence a person's risk of developing an alcohol use disorder. The mechanism is thought to involve elevated acetaldehyde levels resulting from a more rapid conversion of ethanol (in cases of alcohol dehydrogenase variants with higher enzymatic activity) or slower elimination of acetaldehyde oxidation (in cases of aldehyde dehydrogenase variants with reduced enzymatic activity). Acetaldehyde causes facial flushing, nausea, and tachycardia, which make individuals reduce their intake of alcohol.

● MECHANISMS OF ALCOHOL-INDUCED ORGAN DAMAGE

The major organs that are susceptible to damage by alcohol are the liver, pancreas, heart, brain, and bone (Table 126-2). Several alcohol-related medical disorders are caused by various nutritional deficiencies; ethanol is deficient in proteins, minerals, and vitamins. Therefore, the initial management of the alcoholic patient must attend to suggested dietary deficiencies (e.g., thiamine) and electrolyte deficiencies, including potassium, magnesium, calcium, and zinc.

Alcohol-related liver disease is the leading preventable cause of hepatic failure in the industrialized world. Genetic factors are thought to play a role in susceptibility to this disorder, since alcoholic liver disease is more prevalent in whites than in other ethnic groups (despite a similar magnitude of ethanol consumption). The histopathologic features of alcoholic liver disease

TABLE 126-2	MEDICAL COMPLICATIONS OF ALCOHOL ABUSE	
NEUROLOGIC		**ELECTROLYTE OR NUTRITIONAL**
Encephalopathy (Wernicke, with oculomotor dysfunction; gait ataxia)		Thiamine deficiency
		Niacin deficiency
		Folate deficiency
Marchifava-Bignami disease (demyelination of corpus callosum)		Vitamin B12 deficiency
		Vitamin D deficiency
		Zinc deficiency
Central pontine myelinosis		Hypokalemia
Cognitive dysfunction		Hypomagnesaemia
Amnesia (i.e., Korsakoff syndrome)		Hypocalcaemia
Dementia		Ketoacidosis
Cerebellar degeneration		Hypoglycemia
Peripheral neuropathy		Hypertriglyceridemia
Seizures		Malnutrition
HEMATOLOGIC		**ENDOCRINE**
Anemia (often with macrocytosis)		Diabetes mellitus
Leukopenia		Gynecomastia
Thrombocytopenia		**MUSCULOSKELETAL**
GASTROINTESTINAL		
Esophagitis		Myopathy
Esophageal varices		Osteoporosis
Gastritis		Testicular atrophy
Gastrointestinal bleeding		Amenorrhea
Pancreatitis		Infertility
Hepatitis		**MISCELLANEOUS**
Cirrhosis		
Splenomegaly		Spontaneous abortion
		Fetal alcohol syndrome
CARDIOVASCULAR		Increased risk of cancer (breast, oropharyngeal, esophageal, hepatocellular, colorectal)
Hypertension		Accidents, trauma, violence, suicide
Cardiomyopathy		
Stroke		
Arrhythmias (especially atrial fibrillation)		

include fatty infiltration, hepatitis, fibrosis, and end-stage cirrhosis.

● CLINICAL PRESENTATION
Acute Alcohol Intoxication

Mild ethanol intoxication produces slurred speech, ataxia, irregular eye movements, and poor coordination. Signs of CNS depression and associated cerebellar or vestibular dysfunction include dysarthria, ataxia, and nystagmus. Although blood alcohol concentrations are not precisely correlated with the degree of intoxication and the clinical effect of ethanol widely varies among individuals, stupor and coma usually develop at blood concentrations approaching 400 mg/dL. Blood levels of 500 mg/dL often are fatal; however, it is important to understand that death may occur even when the blood alcohol concentration is as low as 300 mg/dL.

Withdrawal Syndrome (Convulsions)

Alcohol withdrawal occurs in three stages. The signs of minor withdrawal usually appear 6 to 12 hours after the discontinuation of ethanol and are caused by central adrenergic hyperexcitability; they consist of anxiety, tremors, sweating, tachycardia, diarrhea, and insomnia. Additional evidence of autonomic nervous system hyperactivity often appears within 12 to 24 hours and includes increased startle response, nightmares, and visual hallucinations. Alcohol withdrawal seizures (so-called *rum fits*) are generalized clonic-tonic convulsions that occur 12 to 48 hours after the discontinuation of ethanol and are estimated to occur in 2% to 5% of alcoholics.

Delirium Tremens

Delirium tremens (DTs) is characterized by delirium (a confused state with varying levels of consciousness), hallucinations, disorientation, agitation, tremor (caused by marked autonomic nervous system over activity), tachycardia, hypertension, fever, and diaphoresis. It occurs in approximately 5% of alcoholics, most often in chronic heavy abusers with underlying neurologic damage. If unrecognized and untreated, the in-hospital mortality rate of DTs approaches 25%; with early recognition and treatment the mortality is only 5%.

● TREATMENT

Intervention strategies in alcohol abusers are designed to modify the individual's attitudes, knowledge, and skills to prevent alcohol misuse. In the outpatient setting, increased frequency of contact between the primary care physician and the patient increases the likelihood of detection, intervention, and prevention of heavy alcohol consumption. All scheduled office visits should include alcohol screening, assessment, and brief attempts at intervention (one or more discussions lasting 10 to 15 minutes), if indicated, as studies show that this approach decreases alcohol intake and its consequences. Behavioral or pharmacologic treatment should be considered because two thirds of treated patients have a reduction in the amount of consumption (by more than 50%) as well as the consequences of consumption (e.g., alcohol-related injury or job loss). A year after treatment, one third of patients are either abstinent or drink moderately without consequences.

Screening and Intervention Strategies

The National Institute on Alcohol Abuse and Alcoholism (NIAAA) provides several web-based guidelines for alcohol screening during the routine health examination (www.niaaa.nih.gov). A four-step plan exists with which physicians can (1) screen patients for alcohol use, (2) assess for the presence of alcohol-related problems, (3) provide advice concerning appropriate action, and (4) monitor the patient's progress. For the current drinker, the physician should inquire about the number of drinks consumed per day, number of days per week on which ethanol is consumed, and total number of drinks consumed per month. Alcohol consumption that exceeds 14 drinks per week or three drinks per day should trigger an in-depth assessment of alcohol-related problems. The physician should ascertain if the individual is at risk for alcohol-related problems, has an existing problem, or may be alcohol-dependent. Difficulties with work-related, interpersonal, or family relationships and/or evidence of high-risk behavior despite self-reported low-risk consumption indicate that the individual is at risk for alcohol use disorder.

The CAGE questionnaire (each of the letters in the acronym refers to one of the questions) (Table 126-3) is a useful screening tool for identifying alcohol-dependent individuals. A positive response to two or more of the four questions is indicative of a potential alcohol problem and should prompt questions regarding the quantity and frequency of consumption. The Alcohol Use Disorders Identification Test (AUDIT) (Table 126-4) is the most widely validated instrument for use in primary care settings. Utilizing 10 items and taking two to three minutes to complete, it is better suited to settings where visit times are longer or when it can be completed and scored before a clinician visit. On physical examination, evidence of alcoholic liver disease may be exhibited as jaundice, hepatomegaly, palmar erythema, male gynecomastia, spider angiomata, and ascites. The serum γ-glutamyltransferase concentration typically is elevated in individuals who drink excessively.

Low-Risk Drinking

A standard drink contains 12 g of alcohol, an amount similar to that found in one 12-oz bottle of beer or wine cooler, one 5-oz glass of wine, or 1.5 oz. of distilled (e.g., 80 proof) spirits. In men older than age 64 years and in women older than 21 years, the limit for moderate drinking is one drink per day. For younger men, moderate drinking is defined as no more than two drinks per day. For the same amount of ingested ethanol, women and older adult men achieve a higher blood concentration of ethanol than younger men owing to their smaller volume of body water. A reasonable blood alcohol level should not exceed 50 mg/dL.

A blood-alcohol level as low as 80 mg/dL may exceed the legal definition for driving under the influence (DUI) or driving while

TABLE 126-3	CAGE: AN ALCOHOLISM SCREENING TEST

1. Have you ever felt you should *cut down* on your drinking?
2. Have people *annoyed* you by criticizing your drinking?
3. Have you felt *guilty* about your drinking?
4. Have you ever had a drink first thing in the morning to steady your nerves or to get rid of a hangover (i.e., as an *eye-opener*)?

TABLE 126-4 COMMONLY ABUSED DRUGS

SUBSTANCE: CATEGORY AND NAME	EXAMPLES OF COMMERCIAL AND STREET NAMES	HOW ADMINISTERED*	INTOXICATION EFFECTS AND POTENTIAL HEALTH CONSEQUENCES
CANNABINOIDS			Euphoria, slowed thinking and reaction time, drowsiness, inattention, confusion, impaired balance and coordination, enhanced perception, cough, frequent respiratory infections, impaired memory and learning, increased heart rate, anxiety, panic attacks, tolerance, addiction
Hashish	Boom, gangster, hash, hash oil, hemp	Smoked, swallowed	
Marijuana	Blunt, dope, ganja, grass, herb, joint, bud, Mary Jane, pot, reefer, green trees, smoke, sinsemilla, skunk, weed	Smoked, swallowed	
K2/Synthetic Marijuana	Spice, K2, fake weed, Yucatan fire, skunk, moon rocks,	Smoked, swallowed	Vomiting, agitation, hallucinations, hypertension, myocardial infarction, death, withdrawal and addiction symptoms.
SEDATIVE-HYPNOTICS (CNS DEPRESSANTS)			Reduced pain and anxiety, feeling of well-being, lowered inhibitions, labile mood, impaired judgment, poor concentration, fatigue, confusion, impaired coordination and memory, respiratory depression and arrest, addiction
Benzodiazepines (Other Than Flunitrazepam)	Ativan, Halcion, Klonopin, Librium, ProSom, Restoril, Serax, Tranxene, Valium, Xanax, Doral; candy, downers, sleeping pills, tranks	Swallowed	Sedation, drowsiness, dizziness
Flunitrazepam[†]	Rohypnol; forget-me pill, Mexican Valium, R2, roach, Roche, roofies, roofinol, rope, rophies	Swallowed, snorted	Visual and gastrointestinal disturbances, urinary retention, amnesia while under drug's effects
Sleep Medications	Ambien (zolpidem), Sonata (zaleplon), Lunesta (eszopicline)	Swallowed	Sedation, drowsiness, dizziness
Barbiturates	Amytal, Nembutal, phenobarbital, Seconal; barbs, reds, red birds, phennies, tooies, yellows, yellow jackets	Injected, swallowed	Sedation, drowsiness, depression, unusual excitement, fever, irritability, poor judgment, slurred speech, dizziness
GHB[†]	γ-hydroxybutyrate; G, Georgia home boy, grievous bodily harm, liquid ecstasy, soap, scoop, goop, liquid X	Swallowed	Drowsiness, dizziness, nausea and vomiting, headache, loss of consciousness, hallucinations, peripheral vision loss, nystagmus, loss of reflexes, seizures, coma, death
DISSOCIATIVE DRUGS			Increased heart rate and blood pressure, impaired function, memory motor loss, numbness, nausea and vomiting
PCP and Analogues	Phencyclidine; angel dust, boat, hog, love boat, peace pill	Injected, smoked, swallowed	Possible decrease in blood pressure and heart rate, panic, aggression, violence, suicidal ideation; loss of appetite, depression
Ketamine*	Ketalar SV; cat Valiums, K, Special K, vitamin K	Injected, smoked, snorted	At high doses: delirium, depression, respiratory depression and arrest, amnesia while under drug's effects
Salvia Divinorum	Salvia, shepherdess's herb, maria pastora, magic mint, sally-d	Chewed, smoked swallowed	
Dextromethorphan (DXM)	Found in some cough and cold medications: Robo, Robotripping, Triple C	Swallowed	Euphoria, slurred speech, confusion, dizziness, distorted visual perceptions
HALLUCINOGENS			Altered states of perception and feeling, nausea, chronic mental disorders, persisting perception disorder (flashbacks)
LSD	Lysergic acid diethylamide; acid, blotter, cubes, microdot, yellow sunshines, blue heaven	Swallowed, absorbed through mouth tissues	LSD: flashbacks, hallucinogen persisting perception disorder LSD and mescaline: increased body temperature, heart rate, blood pressure, loss of appetite, sleeplessness, numbness, weakness, tremors, impulsive behavior, rapid shift in emotion
Mescaline	Buttons, cactus, mesc, peyote	Smoked, swallowed,	
Psilocybin	Magic mushrooms, purple passion, shrooms, little smoke	Swallowed	nervousness, paranoia, panic
OPIOIDS AND MORPHINE DERIVATIVES			Pain relief, euphoria, drowsiness, respiratory depression and arrest, pinpoint pupils, nausea, confusion, constipation, sedation, unconsciousness, seizures, coma, tolerance, addiction
Codeine	Empirin with Codeine, Fiorinal with Codeine, Robitussin A-C, Tylenol with Codeine, OxyContin, Roxicodone, Vicodin; Captain Cody, Cody, schoolboy (with glutethimide: doors and fours, loads, pancakes and syrup)	Injected, swallowed	Less analgesia, sedation, and respiratory depression than morphine

Continued

TABLE 126-4 COMMONLY ABUSED DRUGS—cont'd

SUBSTANCE: CATEGORY AND NAME	EXAMPLES OF COMMERCIAL AND STREET NAMES	HOW ADMINISTERED*	INTOXICATION EFFECTS AND POTENTIAL HEALTH CONSEQUENCES
Other Opioid Pain Relievers			
Oxycodone, hydrocodone bitartrate hydromorphone, oxymorphone, meperidine, propoxyphene	Tylox, Oxycontin, Percodan, Percocet; Oxy, O.C., oxycotton, oxycet, hillbilly, heroin, percs	Chewed, injected, snorted, suppositories, swallowed	For oxycodone—muscle relaxation/twice as potent an analgesic as morphine; high abuse potential
	Vicodin, Lortab, Lorcet; vike, Watson-387		
	Dilaudid; juice, smack, D, footballs, dillies		
	Opana, Numorphan, Numorphone; biscuits, blue heaven, blues, Mrs. O, octagons, stop signs, O bomb		
	Demerol, meperidine hydrochloride; demmies, pain killer		
	Darvon, Darvocet		
Fentanyl	Actiq, Duragesic, Sublimaze; apache, China girl, China white, dance fever, friend, goodfella, jackpot, murder 8, TNT, Tango and Cash	Injected, smoked, snorted	80-100 times more potent an analgesic than morphine
Heroin	Diacetylmorphine; brown sugar, dope, H, horse, junk, skag, skunk, smack, white horse, China white, cheese (with OTC cold medicine and antihistamine)	Injected, smoked, snorted	Staggering gait
Morphine	Roxanol, Duramorph, M, Miss Emma, monkey, white stuff	Injected, smoked, swallowed	
Opium	Laudanum, paregoric; big O, black stuff, block, gum, hop	Smoked, swallowed	
STIMULANTS			Increased heart rate, blood pressure, body temperature; feelings of exhilaration, increased energy and mental alertness, tremors, rapid or irregular heart beat; reduced appetite, irritability, anxiety, panic, paranoia, violent behavior, psychosis, weight loss, insomnia, heart failure, seizures, coma
Amphetamine	Adderall, Biphetamine, Dexedrine; bennies, black beauties, crosses, hearts, LA turnaround, speed, truck drivers, uppers	Injected, smoked, snorted, swallowed	Rapid breathing, hallucinations, loss of coordination, restlessness, delirium, panic, impulsive behavior, Parkinson's disease, tolerance, addiction
Methamphetamine	Desoxyn; chalk, crank, crystal, fire, glass, go fast, ice, meth, speed, yaba, fire, tina, tweak, uppers, trash, yellow barn, methlies quick, stove top, go fast	Injected, smoked, snorted, swallowed	Memory loss, cardiac and neurologic damage, impaired memory and learning, tolerance, addiction, severe dental problems
Methylphenidate	Ritalin, Concerta; JIF, MPH, R-ball, Skippy, the smart drug, vitamin R	Injected, snorted swallowed	Increase or decrease in blood pressure, psychotic episodes, digestive problems,
Cocaine	Cocaine hydrochloride; blow, bump, C, candy, Charlie, coke, crack, flake, rock, snow, toot	Injected, smoked, snorted	Chest pain, respiratory failure, nausea, abdominal pain, stroke, malnutrition, nasal damage from snorting
MDMA† (Methylenedioxymethamphetamine)	Adam, clarity, ecstasy, Eve, lover's speed, peace, uppers, Molly	Injected, snorted, swallowed	Mild hallucinogenic effects, increased tactile sensitivity, empathic feelings, chills, sweating, nystagmus, ataxia, teeth clenching, muscle cramping, impaired memory and learning, lowered inhibition
Synthetic Cathinone (Methylenedioxypyrovalerone (MDPV), Mephedrone ("Drone," "Meph," or "Meow Meow"), and Methylone)	Bath salts, drone, meph, meow meow, ivory wave, bloom, cloud nine, lunar wave, vanilla sky, white lightning, scarface	Injected, smoked, swallowed	Chest pain, paranoia, hallucinations, panic attacks, excited delirium, rhabdomyolysis, renal failure, high abuse and addiction potential
OTHER COMPOUNDS			
Inhalants	Solvents (paint thinners, gasoline), glues, gases (butane, propane, aerosol propellants, nitrous oxide), nitrites (isoamyl, isobutyl, cyclohexyl); laughing gas, poppers, snappers, whippets	Inhaled through nose or mouth	Stimulation, loss of inhibition, headache, nausea or vomiting, slurred speech, loss of motor coordination, wheezing, unconsciousness, cramps, weight loss, muscle weakness, depression, memory impairment, damage to cardiovascular and nervous systems, sudden death
Anabolic Steroids	Anadrol, Oxandrin, Durabolin, Depo-Testosterone, Equipoise; roids, juice, gym candy, pumpers	Injected, swallowed, topical	No intoxication effects. Hypertension, blood clotting and cholesterol changes, hostility and aggression, acne, prostate cancer, reduced sperm production, shrunken testicles, breast enlargement. In females: menstrual irregularities, beard development, and other masculine characteristics

CNS, Central nervous system.

*Taking drugs by injection can increase the risk of infection through needle contamination with staphylococci, human immunodeficiency virus, hepatitis, and other organisms.

†Associated with sexual assaults (e.g., date rapes).

intoxicated (DWI). In national surveys, the strategy of the *designated driver* appears to be effective at preventing unsafe driving by drinkers at risk for DWI. Complete abstinence is recommended for people with a history of alcohol use disorder, other serious medical conditions (e.g., liver disease), and pregnancy.

Nonpharmacologic Therapies

Pharmacologic agents are complementary and adjunctive to the traditional approaches of abstinence, group therapy, coping mechanisms, and behavior modification. The most widely employed behavioral approach is the 12-step program administered by Alcoholics Anonymous (AA), with which the recovering alcoholic moves through 12 specific steps aided by his or her attendance at regular meetings within a self-help peer group. Cognitive behavioral therapy is based on the principle that the alcoholic first must identify the internal and external cues to drinking so that he or she can develop effective countermeasures for drinking behavior. Motivation enhancement therapy is a four-session, brief contact intervention program that encourages self-awareness and behavioral changes in the alcoholic. These therapies provide similar efficacy.

Considerations for Drug Interventions

If desired, medications can be administered in conjunction with behavioral modification. Disulfiram, naltrexone, and acamprosate have been approved by the U.S. Food and Drug Administration (FDA) for adjunctive therapy.

Disulfiram (Antabuse) inhibits aldehyde dehydrogenase (i.e., the enzyme that converts acetaldehyde to acetate), resulting in a 5- to 10-fold increase in serum acetaldehyde concentrations when alcohol is consumed. This produces uncomfortable symptoms (e.g., facial flushing, tachycardia, nausea, vomiting, and headache), which act to deter alcohol consumption. Because of low medication compliance and limited efficacy, disulfiram is rarely prescribed.

Naltrexone is an opioid receptor antagonist. In clinical trials, a combination of naltrexone and psychosocial intervention reduced the number of drinking days, induced a longer period of abstinence from ethanol, and decreased the relapse rate in heavy drinkers when compared with psychosocial intervention alone. Naltrexone is administered orally in a dose of 50 mg daily for 12 weeks, although larger doses (i.e., 100 to 150 mg daily) and a longer duration of administration may improve its success in preventing relapse. In 2006, the FDA approved a once-a-month injectable form of naltrexone (380 mg) for the treatment of alcohol use disorders; this form appears to be more effective than the pill form at maintaining abstinence, since it eliminates the problem of medication compliance.

Naltrexone can be initiated while the individual is still drinking, thereby permitting treatment to be provided in a community-based setting without the need for enforced abstinence or detoxification. Some recovering alcoholics develop nausea when it is initiated. Because hepatic toxicity may occur at high doses (≥300 mg), periodic testing of liver function is recommended. Naltrexone is contraindicated in subjects receiving opioids, given that opiate withdrawal is an unintended adverse effect of the drug.

Acamprosate (Campral), a structural analog of γ-amino butyric acid (GABA), decreases excitatory glutamatergic neurotransmission during alcohol withdrawal. The recommended dosage is 666 to 1000 mg 3 times daily, and its most common side effects are diarrhea and intestinal cramping. In placebo-controlled trials involving almost 7000 alcoholic patients, acamprosate reduced relapse rates and increased abstinence from ethanol. In comparative trials, it did not appear to be as efficacious as naltrexone. Acamprosate should be used once abstinence is achieved; since it is not metabolized by the liver, it can be given safely to individuals with alcoholic liver disease.

The use of several other pharmacologic agents has been associated with a reduction in alcohol consumption, including ondansetron (a selective serotonin reuptake inhibitor), topiramate (an anticonvulsant), baclofen (a GABA agonist), nalmefene (an opioid antagonist), and varenicline (a nicotinic acetylcholine-receptor and dopamine partial agonist), but none of these agents has been approved by the FDA for treatment of alcohol dependence.

Fetal Alcohol Spectrum Disorders

Alcohol freely crosses the placenta and is teratogenic. It is a leading preventable cause of birth defects with mental deficiency, with up to 1 in 100 children in the United States being born with fetal alcohol spectrum disorders (FASDs). The scope of disabilities and malformations varies and depends on the amount of alcohol consumed, the frequency of exposure, the stage of fetal development when alcohol is present, maternal parity, nutrition, genetic susceptibility, and individual variation in maternal and fetal alcohol metabolism.

The term *fetal alcohol spectrum disorder* (FASD) is used to characterize the full range of prenatal alcohol damage, varying from mild to severe and encompassing a broad array of physical defects and cognitive, behavioral, and emotional deficits. It includes conditions such as fetal alcohol syndrome (FAS), alcohol-related neurodevelopmental disorder (ARND), and alcohol-related birth defects (ARBDs).

FAS, the most severe form of FASD, is characterized by (a) growth retardation (i.e., height or weight ≥10th percentile); (b) neurodevelopmental abnormalities (i.e., microcephaly, hyperactivity, irritability, altered motor skills, learning disabilities, seizure disorders, and mental retardation), and (c) dysmorphic facial features (i.e., short palpebral fissures, smooth philtrum, and a thin upper lip). Children with typical dysmorphic facial features who lack the other features have partial FAS. Children with ARBDs have typical facies associated with FAS as well as anomalies in other organs (i.e., cardiac, renal, skeletal, auditory) but no growth retardation or neurodevelopmental abnormalities. Children with ARND exhibit behavioral or cognitive abnormalities in the absence of dysmorphic facial features.

Although the damage from prenatal exposure to alcohol cannot be reversed, children with FASDs benefit from early diagnosis and aggressive intervention with physical, occupational, speech and language, and educational therapies. Early recognition can also benefit the impaired mother, resulting in access to alcohol treatment and a better social situation for the entire family.

Although the recognition of FASD is important, its prevention is essential. Given that no safely established level of alcohol consumption in pregnancy exists, recommendations suggest that pregnant women maintain abstinence. In addition, women who are considering pregnancy or are already pregnant must be counseled about the effects of alcohol on the fetus.

Medical Management of Alcohol Withdrawal and Delirium Tremens

For the patient with probable alcohol withdrawal, comorbid conditions that may coexist or mimic the symptoms of withdrawal (e.g., infection, trauma, hepatic encephalopathy, drug overdose, gastrointestinal bleeding, and metabolic derangements) should be excluded. Once this has been accomplished, the patient should be placed in a quiet and protective environment and should receive parenteral thiamine and multivitamins to decrease the risk of Wernicke encephalopathy or Korsakoff amnestic syndrome.

The Revised Clinical Institute for Withdrawal Assessment for Alcohol (CIWA-Ar) scale (available at https://umem.org/files/uploads/1104212257_CIWA-Ar.pdf), a measure of withdrawal severity, is useful in guiding symptom-triggered therapy in medically stable (i.e., non ICU or postoperative) patients. Benzodiazepines are the only medications proved to ameliorate symptoms and to decrease the risk of seizures and DTs in patients with alcohol withdrawal. Typically, diazepam (5 to 20 mg), chlordiazepoxide (50 to 100 mg), or lorazepam (1 to 2 mg) is administered intravenously every 5 to 10 minutes until symptoms subside, with the last of these medications preferred in patients with advanced cirrhosis, considering that the liver minimally metabolizes it. All benzodiazepines appear to be similarly efficacious in treating alcohol withdrawal, but long-acting agents may be more effective in preventing withdrawal seizures and are associated with fewer rebound symptoms. Conversely, short-acting agents may offer a lower risk of oversedation. For the patient who is resistant to benzodiazepines, intravenous phenobarbital (130 to 260 mg administered intravenously every 15 minutes until symptoms are controlled) may be given.

⬤ PRESCRIPTION DRUG ABUSE

According to the National Survey on Drug Use and Health, an estimated 6.1 million Americans aged 12 years or older used prescription-type psychotherapeutic drugs nonmedically in the past month (Fig. 126-3). This estimate represents 2.4% of the population aged 12 years or older. In 2011, the illicit drug category with the largest number of recent initiates was marijuana use (2.6 million), followed by nonmedical use of pain relievers (1.9 million) and nonmedical use of tranquilizers (1.2 million). More people in the United States now die of prescription drug overdose (i.e., the nonmedical use of prescription-type pain relievers, tranquilizers, stimulants, and sedatives) than accidental vehicular trauma.

Sedatives and Hypnotics

Benzodiazepines and barbiturates are the major sedative-hypnotic drugs among the commonly abused agents that are listed in Table 126-4. The patient with sedative-hypnotic intoxication may have slurred speech, incoordination, unsteady gait,

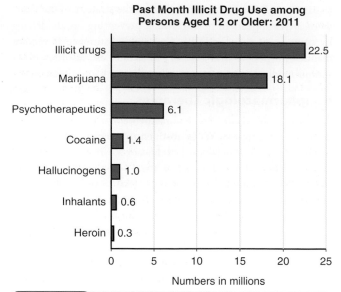

FIGURE 126-3 Past-month illicit drug use among persons aged 12 or older, according to the National Survey on Drug Use and Health (2011). (From Substance Abuse and Mental Health Services Administration: Results from the 2011 National Survey on Drug Use and Health: Summary of National Findings, NSDUH Series H-44, HHS Publication No. [SMA] 12-4713, Rockville, Md., 2012, Substance Abuse and Mental Health Services Administration.)

impaired attention or memory, stupor, and coma. The psychiatric manifestations of intoxication include inappropriate behavior, labile mood, and impaired judgment and social functioning. On physical examination, the person may have respiratory depression or even arrest, nystagmus, and hyper-reflexia. Although benzodiazepines rarely depress respiration to the extent that barbiturates do (and, as a result, have a much wider margin of safety), the effects of these drugs are additive with those of other CNS depressants, such as ethanol. Chronic use may produce physical and psychological dependence and a potentially dangerous withdrawal syndrome.

Benzodiazepines potentiate the effects of GABA, which inhibits neurotransmission. They are available as short-acting agents (temazepam [Restoril] and triazolam [Halcion]), intermediate-acting agents (alprazolam [Xanax], chlordiazepoxide [Librium], estazolam [ProSom], lorazepam [Ativan], and oxazepam [Serax]), and long-acting agents (clorazepate [Tranxene], clonazepam [Klonopin], diazepam [Valium], flurazepam [Dalmane], halazepam [Paxipam], Prazepam [Centrax], and quazepam [Doral]). Flunitrazepam (Rohypnol, also known as *roach, roofies, circles, Mexican valium,* or *rope*) is a popularly abused benzodiazepine that is not legally available in the United States but is often smuggled here from other countries. It has been implicated in cases of date rape and is known as a club drug because adolescents and young adults often use it at nightclubs and bars or during all-night dance parties called raves.

In persons with an acute benzodiazepine overdose, respiratory depression is the major danger. Flumazenil (Romazicon), a competitive antagonist of benzodiazepines, can be given intravenously for acute overdose. Although it reverses the sedative effects of benzodiazepines, flumazenil may not completely reverse respiratory depression, and it may cause seizures in patients with physical dependence or concurrent tricyclic antidepressant poisoning.

Benzodiazepine cessation may precipitate withdrawal symptoms, depending on the half-life of the specific agent, the duration of use, and the dose. Such withdrawal is characterized by intense anxiety, insomnia, irritability, perceptual changes, hypersensitivity to light and sound, psychosis, hallucinations, palpitations, hyperthermia, tachypnea, diarrhea, muscle spasms, tremors, and seizures. Withdrawal symptoms usually peak 2 to 4 days after the discontinuation of a short-acting agent and 5 to 6 days after discontinuation of a longer-acting one; however, panic attacks and nightmares may recur for months. In general, agents with shorter half-lives produce more intense withdrawal symptoms compared with agents with longer half-lives. Detoxification requires a change to a longer-acting benzodiazepine (e.g., clonazepam, diazepam) or phenobarbital and a tapering regimen of 7 to 10 days for short-acting agents or 10 to 14 days for longer-acting ones. For hemodynamically unstable patients who require very rapid medication titration to control withdrawal symptoms and for those with severe hepatic failure, short-acting medications are indicated in lieu of phenobarbital. Propranolol can be given to decrease tachycardia, hypertension, and anxiety.

Barbiturates may be short acting (pentobarbital and secobarbital), intermediate acting (amobarbital, aprobarbital, and butabarbital), or long acting (mephobarbital and phenobarbital). The symptoms of acute intoxication with the withdrawal from barbiturates are similar to those of benzodiazepines. For acute barbiturate overdose, oral charcoal and alkalinization of the urine (to a pH >7.5) with forced diuresis are effective in lowering the blood concentration. For patients with hemodynamic compromise refractory to aggressive supportive therapy, barbiturate elimination can be increased by hemodialysis or charcoal hemoperfusion. The effective treatment of withdrawal symptoms requires estimating the daily dose of the abused drug and substituting an equivalent phenobarbital dose to stabilize the patient, after which the dose of phenobarbital is tapered over 4 to 14 days, depending on the half-life of the abused drug. Benzodiazepines may also be used for detoxification, and propranolol and clonidine may help reduce symptoms.

Abuse of γ-hydroxybutyrate (GHB) has increased substantially over the last decade in the United States. This drug is abused for its sedative, euphoric, and bodybuilding effects. GHB is a metabolite of the neurotransmitter GABA, and it also influences the dopaminergic system. It potentiates the effects of endogenous or exogenous opiates. The ingestion of GHB results in immediate drowsiness and dizziness, with the feeling of a *high.* These effects can be potentiated by the concomitant use of alcohol or benzodiazepines. Similar to flunitrazepam and ketamine, GHB is a popular club drug, and it has been implicated in cases of date rape. Its street names include *G, liquid E, liquid X, fantasy, Georgia home boy, and grievous bodily harm.* Adverse effects that may occur within 15 to 60 minutes of its ingestion include headache, nausea, vomiting, hallucinations, loss of peripheral vision, nystagmus, hypoventilation, cardiac dysrhythmias, seizures, and coma. In rare instances, these adverse effects have led to death. The withdrawal from GHB becomes clinically apparent within 12 hours and may last up to 12 days.

Opioids

Opioids include the natural and semisynthetic alkaloid derivatives of opium as well as the purely synthetic drugs that mimic heroin. They bind to opioid receptors in the brain, spinal cord, and gastrointestinal tract; in addition, they act on several other CNS neurotransmitter systems, including dopamine, GABA, and glutamate, to produce analgesia, CNS depression, and euphoria. With continued opioid use, tolerance and physical dependence develop. As a result, the user must use larger amounts of the drug to obtain the desired effect, and withdrawal symptoms may occur if use is discontinued. The commonly abused opioids include heroin, morphine, codeine, oxycodone (OxyContin, OxyIR, Oxectya, Roxicodone, or combination products, such as Percocet, Percodan, Tylox, Combunox), meperidine (Demerol), propoxyphene (Darvon), hydrocodone (Vicodin, Lortab, Lorcet), hydromorphone (Dilaudid), buprenorphine (Temgesic) and fentanyl (Sublimaze). In 2000, retail pharmacies dispensed 174 million prescriptions for opioids; by 2009, 257 million prescriptions were dispensed, an increase of 48%. The 2011 National Survey on Drug Use and Health reported that over 70% of subjects who abused prescription pain relievers obtained them from friends or relatives, whereas approximately 5 percent procured them from a drug dealer or over the internet.

Acute opioid overdose produces pulmonary congestion, with resultant cyanosis and respiratory distress, and changes in mental status that may progress to coma. Other manifestations include fever, pinpoint pupils, and seizures. Unsterile intravenous practices can lead to skin abscesses, cellulitis, thrombophlebitis, wound botulism, meningitis, rhabdomyolysis, endocarditis, hepatitis, or human immunodeficiency virus (HIV) infection. Neurologic complications from intravenous heroin use include transverse myelitis, inflammatory polyneuropathy, and peripheral nerve lesions.

For acute opioid overdose, the patient's respiratory status must be assessed and supported. Naloxone should be administered intravenously and repeated at 2- to 3-minute intervals, often in escalating doses; the patient should respond within minutes with increases in pupil size, respiratory rate, and level of alertness. If no response occurs, opioid overdose is excluded, and other causes of somnolence and respiratory depression must be considered. Naloxone should be titrated carefully, since it may precipitate acute withdrawal symptoms in opioid-dependent patients.

Withdrawal symptoms may appear as early as 6 to 10 hours after the last injection of heroin. Initially the individual often has feelings of drug craving, anxiety, restlessness, irritability, rhinorrhea, lacrimation, diaphoresis, and yawning; these signs are followed by dilated pupils, piloerection, anorexia, nausea, vomiting, diarrhea, abdominal cramps, bone pain, myalgia, tremors, muscle spasms, and, in rare cases, seizures. These symptoms and signs peak at 36 to 48 hours and then subside over 5 to 10 days, if untreated. A protracted abstinence syndrome characterized by bradycardia, hypotension, mild anxiety, sleep disturbance, and decreased responsiveness may occur for up to 5 months.

Withdrawal from opioids can be managed with methadone, a long-acting synthetic agonist drug; withdrawal symptoms of methadone develop more slowly and are less severe than those caused by heroin. Methadone can be given twice daily and tapered over 7 to 10 days. Methadone use, in both therapeutic doses and overdoses, has been associated with QTc interval prolongation and torsade de pointes, which, in some cases, has been fatal. Alternatively, buprenorphine, a partial agonist, can be given; it is combined with naloxone in a formulation (Suboxone) developed to decrease the potential for abuse. Clonidine reduces autonomic hyperactivity and is particularly effective if combined with a benzodiazepine. Patients with repeated relapses can be maintained on methadone or buprenorphine.

Naltrexone, a long-acting opioid antagonist that blocks impulsive opioid use, is an option for maintenance treatment to prevent relapse. It can be given orally daily or via injectable depot and implantable formulations every 60 to 90 days. It should only be administered after the patient is thoroughly detoxified because it may precipitate withdrawal. Pharmacotherapy must be combined with psychotherapy and structured rehabilitation to achieve an optimal outcome.

Amphetamines

Amphetamines have been used therapeutically for weight reduction and treatment of attention-deficit disorder and narcolepsy. Similar to cocaine, they cause a release of monoamine neurotransmitters (dopamine, norepinephrine, and serotonin) from presynaptic neurons. In addition, however, they have neurotoxic effects on dopaminergic and serotonergic neurons. Their euphoric and reinforcing effects are mediated through dopamine and the mesolimbic system, whereas their cardiovascular effects are caused by the release of norepinephrine. Chronic use leads to neuronal degeneration in dopamine-rich areas of the brain, which may increase the risk for the eventual development of Parkinson's disease.

Amphetamines can be abused orally, intranasaly, intravenously, or by smoking. The most frequently used drugs are dextroamphetamine (Dexedrine), methamphetamine (Desoxyn), and methylphenidate (Ritalin). Methamphetamine is known on the street as *ice, crank, meth, crystal, tina, glass, and yaba*. Illicit use of amphetamines has increased substantially, in part because (a) it is easily and quickly synthesized from ephedrine or pseudoephedrine (Fig. 126-4), and (b) its psychotropic effects persist for up to 24 hours. The anorexiants, phenmetrazine and phentermine, which are structurally and pharmacologically similar to amphetamine, also have been used illicitly.

Tolerance to the stimulant effects of amphetamines develops rapidly, and toxic effects can occur with higher doses. Acute amphetamine toxicity is characterized by excessive sympathomimetic effects, including tachycardia, hypertension, hyperthermia, cardiac tachyarrhythmia, tremors, seizures, and coma. The patient may experience irritability, hypervigilance, paranoia, stereotyped compulsive behavior, and tactile, visual, or auditory hallucinations. The clinical picture may simulate an acute schizophrenic psychosis. The symptoms of withdrawal are similar to those seen with cocaine (see discussion of cocaine), but the acute psychosis and paranoia are often pronounced.

The treatment of amphetamine abuse centers on a quiet environment, benzodiazepines for anxiety, and sodium nitroprusside for severe hypertension. Antipsychotics, such as haloperidol, can reduce the agitation and psychosis by blocking the effect of

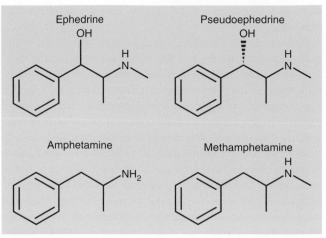

FIGURE 126-4 The chemical structures of amphetamine and methamphetamine, which can be easily manufactured from ephedrine or pseudoephedrine given that they are structurally similar and widely available.

dopamine on the CNS receptor. Urine acidification with ammonium chloride accelerates amphetamine excretion.

ILLICIT DRUG ABUSE
Cocaine

Among individuals 12 years old or older in 2011, 1.4 million had used cocaine within the previous month, and 670,000 had used it for the first time within the previous 12 months. Cocaine can be taken orally or intravenously; alternatively, because it is well absorbed through all mucous membranes, abusers may achieve a high blood concentration after intranasal, sublingual, vaginal, or rectal administration. Its freebase form (called *crack* because of the popping sound it makes when heated) is heat stable, and it can be smoked. Crack cocaine is considered to be the most potent and addictive form of the drug. Euphoria occurs within seconds after crack cocaine is smoked, and is short lived. Compared with smoking crack cocaine or intravenous injection of the drug, mucosal administration results in a slower onset of action, a later peak effect, and a longer duration of action. The blood half-life is approximately 1 hour. The drug's major metabolite is benzoylecgonine, which can be detected in the urine for 2 to 3 days after a single dose.

An intense, pleasurable reaction lasting 20 to 30 minutes occurs after cocaine use, after which rebound depression, agitation, insomnia, and anorexia occur, which are then followed by fatigue, hypersomnolence, and hyperphagia (the *crash*). This crash usually lasts 9 to 12 hours but occasionally may last up to 4 days. Users often ingest the drug repetitively at relatively short intervals to recapture the euphoric state and to avoid the crash. On occasion, sedatives or alcohol are ingested concomitantly to reduce the intensity of anxiety and irritability associated with the crash. The combination of cocaine and intravenously administered heroin (so-called *speedball, snowball, blanco, boy-girl, Bombita, Belushi,* or *dynamite*) is often used so that the abuser can experience the cocaine-induced euphoria and then *float* down on the opiate. Unfortunately, this combination has been reported to cause sudden death. People who use cocaine in temporal proximity to the ingestion of ethanol produce the metabolite cocaethylene, which has also been implicated in cocaine-related deaths.

Cocaine blocks the presynaptic reuptake of norepinephrine and dopamine, producing an excess of these neurotransmitters at the site of the postsynaptic receptor. Thus, cocaine acts as a powerful sympathomimetic agent, resulting in tachycardia, hypertension, tachypnea, hyperthermia, agitation, pupillary dilation, peripheral vasoconstriction, and seizures. Cocaine causes potent vasoconstriction of cerebral arteries and, therefore, may result in a stroke. It is associated with myocardial ischemia and arrhythmias and, in rare cases, with myocardial infarction in young persons with normal or only minimally diseased coronary arteries. The principal mechanisms of ischemia and infarction are coronary arterial vasoconstriction, thrombosis, platelet aggregation, tissue plasminogen activator inhibition, increased myocardial oxygen demand, and accelerated atherosclerosis (Fig. 126-5).

For patients with cocaine-induced hypertension or tachycardia, labetalol and benzodiazepines are usually effective in lowering systemic arterial pressure and heart rate. Patients with acute myocardial infarction should receive aspirin, heparin, nitroglycerin, and, if indicated, reperfusion therapy (with a thrombolytic agent or primary coronary intervention). The use of β-adrenergic blockers should be avoided, since ischemia may be worsened by unopposed α-adrenergically mediated coronary arterial vasocon-striction. Patients with a normal electrocardiogram or nonspecific changes can be managed safely with observation.

The immediate treatment of acute cocaine intoxication includes obtaining vascular and airway access, if needed, and careful electrocardiographic monitoring. Benzodiazepines can be given to control CNS agitation; haloperidol or risperidone can be used in the severely agitated patient. A supportive environment is needed, but detoxification is not required, given that few physical signs of true dependence are present.

Most chronic cocaine abusers have psychological dependence and an intense craving for cocaine. Personal and group therapies are important adjuncts to pharmacologic treatment, but relapse is common and is difficult to manage. Although no medication is FDA approved for treatment of cocaine addiction, disulfiram, modafinil, anticonvulsants (e.g., topiramate and tiagabine), serotonin reuptake inhibitors (e.g., citalopram), serotonin receptor antagonists (e.g., ondansetron), and GABA receptor agonists (e.g., baclofen) have shown some promise in promoting cocaine abstinence.

Cannabis

The cannabinoid drugs include marijuana (the dried flowering tops and stems of the hemp plant) and hashish (a resinous extract of the hemp plant). Marijuana is the most commonly used illicit drug in the United States. (It has been recently legalized for recreational use in Alaska, Colorado, Oregon, and Washington.) In

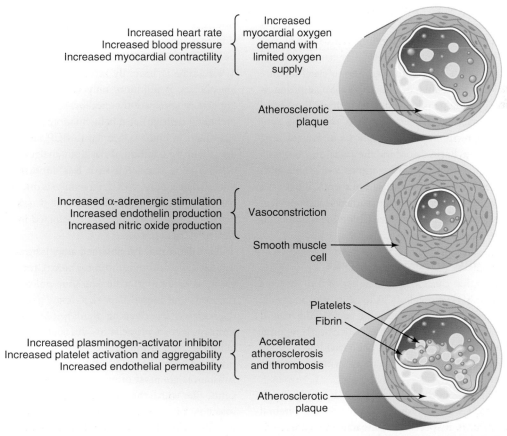

FIGURE 126-5 The mechanisms by which cocaine may induce myocardial ischemia or infarction. Cocaine may cause increases in the determinants of myocardial oxygen demand when oxygen supply is limited *(top)*, when intense vasoconstriction of the coronary arteries occurs *(middle)*, or when accelerated atherosclerosis and thrombosis are present *(bottom)*.

2011, an estimated 18.1 million Americans had used it in the past month. Between 2007 and 2011, the rate of use increased from 5.8 to 7.0%, and the number of users increased from 14.5 million to 18.1 million. Nearly 5.0 million persons used marijuana on a daily or almost daily basis over a 12-month period. Marijuana and hashish are among the drugs most commonly used by adolescents, with approximately one half of 12th graders admitting use at least once and 20% reporting that they are current users. Most of their pharmacologic effects come from metabolites of δ-9-tetrahydrocannabinol, which bind to specific cannabinoid receptors located in the CNS, spinal cord, and peripheral nervous system. The primary mode of use is smoking, with mood-altering and intoxicating effects noted within 3 minutes and peak effects in approximately 1 hour. The acute physiologic effects are dose-related and often include increased heart rate, conjunctival congestion, dry mouth, fine tremor, muscle weakness, and ataxia. Psychoactive effects include euphoria, enhanced perception of colors and sounds, drowsiness, inattentiveness, and inability to learn new facts. Tolerance and physical dependence occur, and chronic users may experience mild withdrawal symptoms of irritability, restlessness, anorexia, insomnia, or mild hyperthermia. Rarely, acute psychosis with panic reactions occurs. The treatment of withdrawal is supportive and includes reassurance; benzodiazepines may be used in severely agitated patients. Cannabinoids have been used as antiemetic agents in patients with cancer receiving chemotherapy, for weight stimulation (in patients with cancer or HIV infection), and in the treatment of glaucoma.

Synthetic marijuana is a psychoactive designer drug composed of a mixture of herbs, spices, or shredded plant material that is sprayed with synthetic chemicals that mimic the effects of cannabis when smoked or prepared as a tea. They have been sold widely in "head shops" as well as through the internet and are best known by the brand names K2 and Spice. Spice products are popular among young people; of the illicit drugs most used by high school seniors, they are second only to marijuana. Synthetic cannabis can precipitate acute psychosis or a worsening of previously stable psychotic disorders; they also may trigger a chronic (long-term) psychotic disorder among vulnerable individuals, such as those with a family history of mental illness. K2 ingestion has been associated with myocardial infarction and death. Regular users may experience withdrawal and addiction symptoms.

Hallucinogens and Dissociative Drugs

Hallucinogens (drugs that cause hallucinations) include lysergic acid diethylamide (LSD), mescaline, psilocybin, and ibogaine. *Dissociative drugs* distort perceptions of sight and sound and produce feelings of detachment (dissociation) without causing hallucinations. They include phencyclidine (PCP), ketamine, salvia, and dextromethorphan (a widely available cough suppressant).

LSD is the most potent of the hallucinogenic drugs. Although it is known to interact with serotonin receptors in the cerebral cortex and *locus ceruleus*, its precise psychoactive mechanism is unknown. Within 30 minutes of its oral ingestion, sympathomimetic effects appear, including mydriasis, hyperthermia, tachycardia, elevated blood pressure, diaphoresis, dry mouth, increased

alertness, tremors, and nausea. Within 2 hours, the psychoactive effects become apparent, with heightened perceptions (highly intensified colors, smells, sounds, and other sensations), body distortions, mood variations, and visual hallucinations. An acute panic reaction may occur, sometimes leading to self-injury or suicide. After approximately 12 hours, the syndrome begins to subside, but fatigue and tension may persist for another day. Flashbacks (brief recurrences of the hallucinations) may occur days or even weeks after the last dose but tend to disappear without treatment. Acute panic reactions are best treated in a supportive environment; benzodiazepines can be given to severely agitated patients.

PCP is a potent, addictive hallucinogen that produces a prompt stimulant effect similar to that of amphetamines, with feelings of euphoria, power, and invincibility. Patients may have hypertension, tachycardia, hyperthermia, bidirectional nystagmus, slurred speech, ataxia, hallucinations, extreme agitation, and rhabdomyolysis. With more severe reactions, patients may be brought to medical attention in a coma-like state, with open eyes and pupils that are partially dilated, a decreased pain response, brief periods of excitation, and muscle rigidity. On occasion, PCP users may have hypertensive urgency, seizures, and bizarre (often violent) behavior, which lead to suicide or extreme violence toward others. Tolerance and mild withdrawal symptoms have been seen in daily users, but the major problem is drug craving. Treatment entails a quiet environment, sedation with benzodiazepines, hydration, haloperidol for terrifying hallucinations, and suicide precautions. Continuous gastric suction and acidification of the urine with intravenous ammonium chloride or ascorbic acid may aid in the drug's excretion, but acidification may increase the risk of renal failure if rhabdomyolysis is present.

Ketamine is a rapidly acting general anesthetic; unlike most anesthetics, it produces only mild respiratory depression and appears to stimulate the cardiovascular system. Adverse effects, including delirium and hallucinations, limit its use as a general anesthetic in humans. Similar to PCP, ketamine is a dissociative anesthetic. In addition, it has both analgesic and amnestic properties and is associated with less confusion, irrationality, and violent behavior than PCP. Ketamine is one of the club drugs that have been implicated in date rape.

Inhalants

The inhalants may be classified as (1) *organic solvents,* including toluene (airplane glue and spray paint), paint thinners, kerosene, gasoline, carbon tetrachloride, shoe polish, acetone (nail polish removers and Liquid Paper), xylene (permanent markers), and degreasers (dry cleaning fluids); (2) *gases,* such as butane, propane, aerosol propellants, and anesthetics (ether, chloroform, halothane, and nitrous oxide); and (3) *nitrites,* such as cyclohexyl nitrite, amyl nitrite, and butyl nitrite (room deodorizer). These substances are most often inhaled by children or young adolescents, after which they produce dizziness and intoxication within minutes. Prolonged exposure or daily use may lead to hearing loss, bone marrow depression, cardiac arrhythmias, cerebral degeneration, peripheral neuropathies, and damage to the liver, kidneys, or lungs. A characteristic "glue sniffer's rash" around the nose and mouth is sometimes seen after prolonged use. In rare instances, death may occur, most likely from hypoxemia, cardiac arrhythmias, pneumonia, or aspiration of vomit while unconscious. Detoxification is rarely required for the patient who has abused these substances, but psychiatric treatment may be needed to prevent relapse.

Designer Drugs

The term *designer drug* refers to illicit synthetic drugs, many of which have increased potency in comparison with their parent compounds. The most common designer drugs include analogs of fentanyl, meperidine, piperazine, and methamphetamines. The best-known fentanyl derivatives are α-methyl fentanyl *(China white)*, parafluorofentanyl, and 3-methyl fentanyl. Because these drugs are approximately 1000 times as potent as heroin, it is not surprising that fatal overdoses from respiratory depression have been reported.

The major meperidine derivatives are 1-methyl-4-phenyl-4-propionoxypiperidene (MPPP) and 1-methyl-4-phenyl-1, 2, 3, 6-tetrahydropyridine (MPTP), each of which produces euphoria similar to that caused by heroin. In some users, MPTP causes neuronal degeneration in the substantia nigra, which produces an irreversible form of Parkinson's disease.

Piperazines, a new class of designer drugs of abuse, are commonly sold as party pills in the form of tablets, capsules, or powders on the drug black market and in so-called head shops or over the internet under the names of Frenzy, Bliss, Charge, Herbal ecstasy, A2, Legal X and Legal E. 1-Benzylpiperazine (BZP) is the most prevalent of these compounds. Aside from BZP and 1-(3,4-methylenedioxybenzyl) piperazine (MDBP), the phenylpiperazine derivatives 1-(3-trifluoromethylphenyl) piperazine (TFMPP), 1-(3-chloro phenyl) piperazine (mCPP), and 1-(4-methoxyphenyl) piperazine (MeOPP) are often abused. Because piperazines and amphetamines cause similar pharmacologic symptoms, piperazine poisoning can easily be wrongly diagnosed as amphetamine poisoning. Furthermore, piperazines are not detected by routinely used immunochemical screening procedures for drugs of abuse, but they require an appropriate toxicologic analysis (e.g., by gas chromatography-mass spectrometry). The methylenedioxy synthetic derivatives of amphetamine and methamphetamine are generally referred to as *ecstasy* and include 3, 4-methylenedioxy methamphetamine (MDMA, also known as *Adam*); 3, 4-methylenedioxy-ethylamphetamine (MDEA, also known as *Eve*); and N-methyl-1-(3, 4-methylenedioxyphenyl)-2-butanamine (MBDB, also known as *Methyl-J* or *Eden*). These drugs have CNS stimulant and hallucinogenic properties. They produce elevated mood and increased self-esteem and may cause acute panic, anxiety, paranoia, hallucinations, tachycardia, nystagmus, ataxia, and tremor. Deaths in some users have been attributed to cardiac arrhythmias, hyperthermia with seizures, and intracranial hemorrhage.

Prospectus for the Future

Recent research is focused on so-called vaccine strategies, whereby protein-conjugated analogues of cocaine would be administered to produce anti-cocaine antibodies that bind cocaine, thereby preventing its passage across the blood-brain barrier. A novel pharmacokinetic approach to the treatment of drug toxicity involves the development of compounds that can be administered safely to humans and that accelerate the metabolism of the drug to inactive components. For example, catalytic antibodies have been developed to accelerate cocaine metabolism and are administered parentally. In experimental animals, mutations of human butyrylcholinesterase (one of the enzymes responsible for the metabolism of cocaine) accelerate cocaine metabolism and antagonize cocaine's behavioral and toxic effects.

SUGGESTED READINGS

Amato L, Minozzi S, Davoli M: Efficacy and safety of pharmacological interventions for the treatment of the Alcohol Withdrawal Syndrome, Cochrane Database Syst Rev (6):CD008537, 2011.

Anton RF: Naltrexone for the management of alcohol dependence, N Engl J Med 359:715–721, 2008.

Arbo MD, Bastos ML, Carmo HF: Piperazine compounds as drugs of abuse, Drug Alcohol Dep 122:174–185, 2012.

Capriola M: Synthetic cathinone abuse, Clin Pharm Adv Appl 5:109–115, 2013.

Centers for Disease Control and Prevention: Alcohol Related Disease Impact (ARDI) application, 2012. Available at: http://apps.nccd.cdc.gov/DACH_ARDI/Default.aspx. Accessed November 2014.

Edenberg HJ: The genetics of alcohol metabolism: role of alcohol dehydrogenase and aldehyde dehydrogenase variants. Available at: http://pubs.niaaa.nih.gov/publications/arh301/5-13.htm. Accessed October 2014.

Ferri MMF, Amato L, Davoli M: Alcoholics Anonymous and other 12-step programs for alcohol dependence, Cochrane Database Syst Rev 4:1–26, 2008.

Jonas DE, Garbutt JC, Amick HR, et al: Behavioral counseling after screening for alcohol misuse in primary care: a systematic review and meta-analysis for the U.S. Preventive Services Task Force, Ann Intern Med 157:645–654, 2012.

Kao D, Bartelson BB, Khatir V, et al: Trends in reporting methadone-associated arrhythmia, 1997-2011, Ann Int Med 158:735–740, 2013.

Lim SS, Vos T, Flaxman AD: A comparative risk assessment of burden of disease and injury attributable to 67 risk factors and risk factor clusters in 21 regions, 1990–2010: a systematic analysis for the Global Burden of Disease Study 2010, Lancet 380:2224, 2012.

Pruett D, Waterman EH, Caughey AB: Fetal alcohol exposure; consequences, diagnosis, and treatment, Obstet Gynecol Surv 68:62–69, 2013.

Rosner R, Hackl-Herrwerth A, Leucht P, et al: Acamprosate for alcohol dependence, Cochrane Database Syst Rev (9):CD004332, 2010.

Schindler CW, Goldberg SR: Accelerating cocaine metabolism as an approach to the treatment of cocaine abuse and toxicity, Futuer Med Chem 4:163–175, 2012.

Substance Abuse and Mental Health Services Administration: Results from the 2011 National Survey on Drug Use and Health: Summary of National Findings, NSDUH Series H-44, HHS Publication No. (SMA) 12-4713, Rockville, Md., 2012, Substance Abuse and Mental Health Services Administration. Available at http://store.samhsa.gov/product/Results-from-the-2011-National-Survey-on-Drug-Use-and-Health-NSDUH-/SMA12-4713. Accessed November 2014.

Warner M, Chen LH, Makuc DM, et al: Drug poisoning deaths in the United States, 1980-2008, NCHS Data Brief 1–8, 2011.

Index

Page numbers followed by "f" indicate figures, "t"
indicate tables, and "b" indicate boxes.

1139

Pulmonary artery catheter/catheterization, 60
  intraoperative, in noncardiac surgery, 277
  in shock, 263
Pulmonary capillary wedge pressure, 48-49
  as measure of preload, 19
  in pulmonary arterial hypertension, 164
Pulmonary circulation, 192, 196
  physiology of, 21
Pulmonary disease, 183-184
  as cause of death, 183
  classification of, 184, 184f
  epidemiology of, 183-184
  future prospects for, 184
  Sjögren's syndrome and, 817
Pulmonary edema
  in acute respiratory distress syndrome, 262
  management of, 60
  noncardiogenic, 262
Pulmonary embolism, 165-167, 166f-167f, 243
  acute coronary syndrome and, 101
  dyspnea in, 25
  evaluation of, 243f
  obstructive shock secondary to, 263
  in older adults, 1107t
  pain in, 24
  in pregnancy, 572-573
  risk factors for
    acquired, 567-568
    inherited, 565-567, 566t
Pulmonary endothelial cells, 240.e1f
Pulmonary fibrosis
  idiopathic, computed tomography, 227f
  lung compliance in, 193-194, 194f
  in spondyloarthritis, 776
Pulmonary function testing, 188, 200, 200f-202f, 200.e1f
  in chronic obstructive pulmonary disease, 212
  indications for, 200, 200t
  patterns in, 184, 188, 200
Pulmonary hemorrhage, diffuse alveolar, 232-233
Pulmonary hypertension, 163-164
  arterial, 164
  atrial septal defects and, 67
  chest pain in, 186
  in chronic obstructive pulmonary disease, 213
  classification of, 164t
  in connective tissue disorders, 231
  definition of, 163-164
  in obesity, 252
  secondary, 241, 240.e1f
  sleep apnea with, 245
  in systemic sclerosis, 789, 792
Pulmonary infiltrates, in immunocompromised patients, 943-944
Pulmonary regurgitation, 85
  pulmonary valve stenosis and, 72
Pulmonary rehabilitation program, 214
Pulmonary-renal syndrome, 233
Pulmonary stenosis, 85
Pulmonary thromboembolism, 242-243
Pulmonary valve stenosis, 72
Pulmonary vascular diseases, 184, 184f, 240-244
Pulmonary vascular resistance, 192
Pulmonary vasculitides, 233-234
Pulmonary vasculitis, 232-234
Pulmonary veins, 192

Pulmonary venous congestion, chest x-ray in, 37-38
Pulmonary venous flow, in transposition of great arteries, 74
Pulse, arterial, 28-30, 29f
Pulse oximetry, 188, 202-203
Pulse pressure, aging and, 176, 176f
Pulsus bisferiens, 142
Pulsus paradoxus, 30, 137
  in asthma, 219
  in severe asthma, 187
Pulsus parvus, 76-77
Pulsus parvus et tardus, 29-30
Pupillary reactivity, in coma, 967
Pupils, examination of, 1002-1004, 1004f
Pure water loss, 301-302
Purified protein derivative (PPD) testing, in HIV-infected patient, 932
Purine metabolism, 799-800, 800f
Purkinje cells, 17
Purpura
  Henoch-Schönlein, 234, 547-548
  immune thrombocytopenic, 550-551
  palpable, 547-548
  post-transfusion, 552
  senile, 548
  steroid-induced, 548
  vascular, 547
Purpura fulminans, neonatal, 567
Pursuit eye movements, 1004
Pyloric sphincter, 402
Pyoderma gangrenosum, in inflammatory bowel disease, 420
Pyomyositis, 884-885
Pyramids, in kidneys, 282
Pyridostigmine
  for Lambert-Eaton myasthenic syndrome, 1099
  for myasthenia gravis, 1098
Pyroglutamic acidosis, 310
Pyropoikilocytosis, hereditary, 510

Q

Q fever, 838t, 841
  infective endocarditis and, 878-880
Q wave
  and myocardial infarction, 41, 44t
  with ventricular aneurysm, 41
QRS complex, 38
QT interval, 38
Quadrantanopias, 1002
QuantiFERON-TB Gold (QFT-G), 257
Quincke's pulse, in chronic severe regurgitation, 79
Quinidine
  for malaria, 953
  side effects of, 113, 115t
Quinsy, in pharyngitis, 869

R

R prime, 38
Rabeprazole, for peptic ulcer disease, 407-408
Rabies, encephalitis and, 861
Rachitic rosary, 754
Radiation, cancer risk and, 582
Radiation nephritis, 331

Radiation therapy, 586
  acute effects of, 586, 586t
  late effects of, 586, 586t
  in prostate cancer, 607
  for spinal cord compression, 619
Radiculopathy, cervical, 1000
Radiographic findings, on renal calculi, 337t
Radionuclide imaging
  in chronic kidney disease, 297
  of gallbladder, 395
  gastrointestinal, 395
Radionuclide scintigraphy, gastrointestinal, gastric-emptying scan, 415
Radionuclide stress testing, in angina pectoris, 91-92
Radionuclide ventriculography, 92-93
Radon, lung cancer and, 266, 592
Raloxifene, for osteoporosis prevention and treatment, 762t, 763
Ramelteon, for insomnia, 974
Ramsay Hunt syndrome, 887, 1000
Randomized Aldactone Evaluation Study (RALES), 63
Range of motion, assessment of, 810
Ranitidine, for peptic ulcer disease, 407
Ranolazine, for angina pectoris, 95
Rapamycin, 370
Rapid eye movement behavior disorder, 975
Rapid-onset dystonia, 1021
Rapid urease test, 407
Rapidly progressive glomerulonephritis (RPGN), 315, 315f
  glomerular diseases with, 320-323
  microscopic polyangiitis with, 233-234
Rash
  fever and, 837, 838t-839t, 842-843
  from syphilis, 923
  viral infections associated with, 843
Raynaud's disease, systemic sclerosis and, 790
Raynaud's phenomenon, 163, 781, 814
  in systemic sclerosis, 789, 791
Reactivation tuberculosis, 256-257
Reactive arthritis, 767t, 775, 777, 777f, 779
Reciprocating atrioventricular tachycardia, 121
Recombinant human PTH (1-34), 763
Recombinant tissue-type plasminogen activators (rt-PA), in acute STEMI, 105-106
Recombination, 8, 9f
Rectal cancer, in HIV-infected patients, 933
Rectal examination
  in abdominal pain, 373
  in prostate cancer, 721
Red blood cells
  carbonic anhydrase in, 197
  congenital, membrane abnormalities, 510t
  disorders of, 502-514
  metabolism of, 511f
  normal structure and function, 502
  prospectus for future, 513
5α-Reductase, lack of, 654
5α-Reductase inhibitors, for benign prostatic hyperplasia, 722
Reduviid bug, 955.e1f
Reentry, 111, 112f
Refeeding syndrome, with parenteral nutrition, 688